1 MONTH OF FREE READING

at
www.ForgottenBooks.com

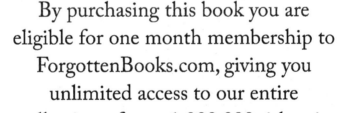

By purchasing this book you are eligible for one month membership to ForgottenBooks.com, giving you unlimited access to our entire collection of over 1,000,000 titles via our web site and mobile apps.

To claim your free month visit:
www.forgottenbooks.com/free895081

ISBN 978-0-265-82576-1
PIBN 10895081

Medical Times and Gazette.

Dec. 31st 1881.

19122

THE

Medical Times and Gazette.

A

JOURNAL OF MEDICAL SCIENCE,

LITERATURE, CRITICISM, AND NEWS.

VOLUME II. FOR 1881.

LONDON:

PUBLISHED BY J. & A. CHURCHILL, 11, NEW BURLINGTON STREET;

AND SOLD BY ALL BOOKSELLERS.

MDCCCLXXXI.

LONDON :
PARDON AND SONS, PRINTERS,
PATERNOSTER ROW.

ORIGINAL LECTURES.

CLINICAL LECTURES
ON DISEASES OF THE ABDOMEN.

By FREDERICK T. ROBERTS, M.D., B.Sc., F.R.C.P.,
Professor of Materia Medica and Therapeutics at University College,
Physician to University Hospital, and Professor of
Clinical Medicine, etc.

LECTURE II.
GENERAL ÆTIOLOGY AND PATHOLOGY OF ABDOMINAL DISEASES.

ÆTIOLOGICAL facts are often of considerable importance in relation to the diagnosis, prognosis, and treatment of abdominal affections, and, without entering into details, I purpose now to give a general summary of the causes of these affections, and of the conditions under which they occur. The consideration of particular causes, and of the special ætiological points relating to individual organs or diseases, will claim our attention on future occasions. In giving this summary, it will be practicable to indicate at the same time the nature of the principal diseases to which the abdominal structures are liable; and for convenience sake the causes may be arranged under certain groups and subdivisions.

GROUP I.—In many cases an abdominal disease is *primary, independent,* or *local,* that is, it is induced by causes acting more or less locally and directly, generally coming from without. Different organs or structures will be affected according to the precise nature of the cause, and the part it affects, while the effects produced will also necessarily vary. Under this group come the following subdivisions :—

1. All kinds of physical injury and mechanical causes originating from without, such as strains, contusions, or wounds, swallowing foreign bodies, and external pressure, especially that produced by tight stays or belts.

2. Excessive local heat or cold, either directly applied to the abdomen externally, or coming into contact with internal parts, as the result of swallowing hot or scalding liquids, or, on the other hand, very cold liquids or ice.

3. Chemical agents, including certain recognised poisons, medicines of various kinds, and some articles of food, or such as have undergone decomposition or other deleterious changes. These act mainly on the alimentary canal, and the poisons belong either to the corrosive or irritant class; but it must also be remembered that certain medicinal agents, especially when taken injudiciously—as is often the case with regard to purgatives—injuriously affect this canal. Moreover, some poisons and medicines are liable to produce a remarkable local effect upon the kidneys, when introduced into the system in any way, and may thus cause more or less functional derangement of, or even structural damage to, these organs, such as cantharidis, turpentine, and copaiba.

4. Various causes connected with food and drink. These are but too familiar as originating numerous abdominal disorders and organic diseases, and in many cases they act locally and directly in connexion with the alimentary canal and its appendages. Not only may · ticles of food and drink be hurtful in themselves, but there are various errors in relation to diet which are prolific causes of local affections, and which will need hereafter to be considered at some length. Liquids are often highly injurious in this way, as may be exemplified by the effects of drinking water in excess or bad water, abuse of tea, and, above all, intemperance in the use of alcoholic drinks, which act locally as well as generally.

As regards the nature of the affections produced by the causes belonging to this group, they include wounds and other forms of mechanical injury, burns or scalds, corrosion, active congestions, acute and chronic inflammations, spasmodic affections, functional disorders, and displacement of organs. The alimentary canal is, on the whole, far more liable than other structures to be affected by this class of causes.

GROUP II.—In a comparatively few instances abdominal complaints result from causes originating from without, which act upon the *general system,* but tend to affect particular organs or structures in the abdomen. The connexion of this group of causes with the complaints which they are

supposed to produce is not always so clear and definite as could be wished, but their reality cannot be doubted. Thus, exposure to cold and wet, or general chilling of the body, may originate abdominal affections. In exceptional instances acute peritonitis seems attributable to such causes. Unquestionably they may disorder the functions of the digestive apparatus; but their most obvious effects are noticed in connexion with the kidneys, where they may produce congestion, acute Bright's disease, or probably, by their long-continued action, even chronic organic changes. Excessive heat is another agent to be noticed here. When the body is exposed for a prolonged period to a high temperature, especially in connexion with residence in tropical climates, not only functional disorders, but also serious organic changes are very liable to be set up in the liver and other abdominal organs. Summer diarrhœa is another illustration of a condition which probably depends, in many instances, at any rate in part, upon the injurious effects of a high temperature upon the body. Overcrowding, bad hygienic conditions, offensive effluvia, and allied causes, frequently cause gastric and intestinal disorders, and assist in producing more serious complaints. Want of cleanliness of the skin deserves particular notice here, as probably not uncommonly materially disturbing the renal functions, and assisting in the development of organic renal disease. Lastly, causes arising from food and drink, and especially alcohol, must again be mentioned under this group, for although their primary effects are local, secondarily they affect the entire system, and their injurious effects are often observed in connexion with organs and structures altogether remote from those with which they come into direct contact.

GROUP III.—There is a group of abdominal affections which may be referred ætiologically to *derangement of some normal function or action,* in consequence of which certain organs are liable to become more or less damaged, either functionally or organically.

1. A function may be entirely neglected or imperfectly attended to by the patient, either habitually or on some particular occasion, and in this way mischief may be set up. For instance, neglect of mastication and of proper ensalivation is a potent cause of digestive disorders, and may ultimately originate organic changes in the stomach. A want of attention to habit and regularity with regard to meals, as influencing the gastric functions, may produce similar effects. The injurious consequences resulting from neglect of the act of defœcation are but too familiar; and not only do the intestines themselves suffer, but the other organs engaged in the process of digestion are also often implicated, while in some instances serious results ensue from accumulation of fœces in the bowels. Neglect of micturition is another cause of mischief to be mentioned here. I have recently seen a marked case in which temporary paralysis of the bladder resulted from the patient allowing his bladder to remain over-distended for a considerable time. Habitual carelessness in this respect may not improbably lead to permanent damage to the urinary apparatus.

2. Abdominal functions are not uncommonly disordered by remote causes, especially those connected with digestion, and in this manner certain complaints may be originated. These causes are often associated, and may be illustrated by the effects of deficient exercise, over-study, excessive smoking, and other injurious habits.

3. Disordered actions may give rise to serious conditions in the abdomen. Thus, severe vomiting or retching may lead to hæmorrhage or even rupture of the stomach under certain circumstances; straining at stool is often highly injurious; and even irregular and abnormal movements of the intestinal tube itself may cause its own displacement, or drive one part of it into another, thus originating intussusception.

GROUP IV.—This is a very important group, for it includes those cases in which an abdominal disease is a part or complication of, or a sequel to, some *general disease or condition,* and they are of very common occurrence. The local disease may be comparatively insignificant and unimportant, or it may be of great consequence. This group can be arranged in certain subdivisions, according to the following plan :—

1. Abdominal structures are frequently affected in connexion with acute febrile and allied diseases. In the first place, you must remember that mere fever or pyrexia always

tends more or less to disturb the functions of abdominal organs, as may be exemplified by the furred tongue, loss of appetite, and constipation, indicating disturbance of the alimentary canal. But, further, there are certain acute complaints which have a special connexion with the abdomen, and these may be illustrated by typhoid fever, cholera, dysentery, and yellow fever. Scarlatina tends specially to affect particular organs, namely, the kidneys, and often permanently damages them. Malarial fevers and malaria act mainly upon the spleen. Pyæmic and septicæmic conditions are often evidenced by lesions which have their seat in abdominal organs. Peritonitis is liable to occur not only in these conditions, but also in other acute diseases, such as small-pox, erysipelas, glanders, and possibly in rheumatic fever. Diphtheria sometimes implicates certain abdominal organs. From these examples it will be seen that a large number of acute febrile and allied diseases are in some way or other associated with organs in the abdomen.

2. The second subdivision includes certain abdominal disorders, or sometimes obvious diseases, which depend upon the general condition of the patient. Thus they are often associated with anæmia, debility, plethora, scurvy or purpura, hysteria or nervous exhaustion. In all these conditions, for instance, dyspeptic symptoms are common. In scurvy and purpura hæmorrhages may occur. Hysteria may cause various phenomena. In this connexion may also be noticed the effects of chronic lead-poisoning upon certain abdominal organs.

3. The third subdivision is an extremely important one, for it comprehends the so-called *constitutional diseases* or *diatheses*, which are often manifested by lesions connected with abdominal structures, several of which may be implicated in some of these disease. At present it will suffice to enumerate them thus:—(a) Malignant disease or cancer; (b) albuminoid disease; (c) tubercular or scrofulous disease; (d) syphilis; (e) gout, and perhaps rheumatism; (f) the fatty diathesis; (g) the condition giving rise to lymphadenosis or leucocythæmia. It is a question how far some local injury or irritation may help to bring out the manifestations of some of these diatheses in connexion with abdominal structures.

4. Another subdivision may be made to comprise those abdominal complaints which have been attributed to chronic skin diseases, to the rapid cure of these diseases, or to the suppression of chronic discharges. Burns and scalds of the body may also be referred to here, which, when extensive, have been found to give rise to a peculiar ulceration of the duodenum.

5. Lastly, in connexion with this general group, do not forget the effects of the natural decay incident to age, and the consequences of the degenerations which form such an important element in senile changes. These often account for symptoms referred to the abdomen.

GROUP V.—The next group to which I would call attention comprises those abdominal affections which are *secondary to some disease or disorder in other parts of the body.*

1. First and foremost must be mentioned those which follow, and are due to morbid conditions within the chest. And I would take this opportunity of impressing upon you very strongly the intimate pathological and clinical relations existing between the thorax and abdomen, diseases in either cavity very often giving rise to symptoms or even important organic changes associated with the other region. To illustrate the point at present under consideration, any condition within the chest which interferes with the general venous circulation, and especially certain cardiac and pulmonary diseases, will lead to mechanical congestion of all the abdominal viscera, and thus symptoms, and ultimately permanent organic lesions, are commonly originated. Thoracic diseases may also mechanically interfere with the structures contained within the abdomen, as may be exemplified by the effects of extreme emphysema, pleuritic effusion or pneumothorax, and intra-thoracic tumours. Phthisis is commonly attended with abdominal disorders, and may give rise to secondary organic lesions, by an infective process or in other ways. Again, morbid conditions, such as cancer, sometimes extend directly through the diaphragm from the chest to the abdomen. A rupture or perforation in exceptional instances takes place through the diaphragm, as of an empyema or a hydatid cyst in the lung, so that morbid products find their way into the abdominal cavity, up secondary mischief there.

2. The relation of the nervous system to the abdominal viscera is also worthy of consideration, and especially in setting up various functional disorders, but organic diseases may also have their origin in the nervous system. The effects of powerful emotions upon the digestive organs are well known; they influence secretions, disturb digestion, and may cause diarrhœa. Hysteria and general nervous exhaustion have already been alluded to as causes of abdominal disorders. Migraine or sick headache affords another illustration of a nervous complaint affecting abdominal viscera. Cerebral diseases have often a remarkable effect upon the alimentary canal, as evidenced by a thickly coated tongue, loss of appetite, and obstinate constipation. The urinary organs may also be disturbed. Spinal diseases frequently cause a sensation of pain around the abdomen, so that the patient will refer his ailment to this part; or, on the other hand, they destroy sensation here; while they are also liable to interfere seriously with the functions of the intestines and bladder. How far abdominal disorders may depend upon the sympathetic system cannot at present be determined, although their connexion must be recognised. Dentition may be mentioned here as a frequent cause of abdominal disorders in children, probably acting mainly by reflex irritation, and thus through the nervous system.

3. Embolism may be alluded to under this group as an occasional cause of lesions affecting certain of the abdominal organs. The embolus may come from various parts of the body.

GROUP VI.—This group includes those cases in which an abdominal disease is *secondary to some previous disease or disorder in the abdomen itself.*

1. In the first place, a disease, though it has ended in apparent recovery and cure, may leave behind it permanent organic changes, which may prove more or less serious. Thus peritonitis may terminate in recovery, but adhesions form, which may afterwards prove very troublesome, or even cause grave mischief, such as strangulation of the intestine. Cicatrisation of an ulcer may lead to contraction or complete closure of a canal or duct, such as the intestine, bile-duct, or ureter. In such cases, unless one knew the previous history, much difficulty might be experienced in explaining the cause of the patient's illness. It must also be remembered that repeated irritation is liable to bring about serious conditions, which may even terminate fatally. For instance, the passage of gall-stones may set up inflammation in the gall-duct.

2. A secondary disease may be originated in a structure or organ by some previous disease affecting it. Thus, tubercular and cancerous peritonitis imply peritonitis set up by the irritation of tubercle or cancer; ulceration of the stomach or intestine is likely to set up inflammation or catarrh of these organs respectively. Further, disordered secretions may irritate, and in this way set up secondary lesions. Some conditions are almost necessarily combined. For instance, an obstruction at any orifice or tube, such as the pylorus or intestine, is almost certain to be followed by more or less dilatation and hypertrophy, of the stomach in the one case, and of the bowel above the obstruction in the other. Of course an organ may be the seat of two or more diseases which are quite independent of each other.

3. A disease may extend directly from one organ to another within the abdomen, or from one structure to another. It is therefore very necessary to bear in mind the anatomical relations of the different parts to each other, as regards contiguity, as well as how certain structures are united by peritoneal folds, vessels, absorbents, communicating tubes, or in other ways; and thus you will be enabled to understand how morbid conditions are most likely to be transmitted from one organ to another. This may be exemplified by the extension of cancer of the pancreas to the duodenum, and by the spreading of inflammation from the intestine to the liver along the gall-duct, or from the kidney along the ureter to the bladder, or in the opposite direction.

4. Secondary deposits may form in organs within the abdomen, when other organs have been the primary seat of disease. This event frequently happens in cases of malignant disease, and it also occurs in pyæmia.

5. It must further be remembered that the anatomical connexions of organs, by means of vessels, tubes, etc., as well as their physiological relations, often account not only for a variety of symptoms referable to structures not obviously diseased, but also for certain pathological con-

ditions, or even permanent morbid changes. In some instances the secondary disturbance is direct, and its cause is obvious and easily explained; in others it is sympathetic or reflex in origin. As illustrations may be mentioned the effects produced as the result of portal obstruction from hepatic disease—ascites, gastric and intestinal disorders, enlargement of the spleen, etc.; the disturbances excited by abnormal secretions on parts with which they come into contact, such as the gastric juice, the bile, or the urine; and the numerous derangements of the abdominal viscera which are attributed to uterine and ovarian disorders.

6. Secondary mischief in the abdomen frequently results from the mechanical effects produced by many diseases in this region. They may cause irritation and inflammation; diffused or local pressure; obstruction of orifices, tubes, hollow viscera, or vessels; or actual injury to and destruction of tissues: and thus a variety of phenomena are often induced. This may be exemplified by the effects of enlarged organs, tumours of all kinds, accumulations in hollow organs, calculi, and ruptures or perforations.

7. Finally, disease of an abdominal organ may originate a condition of the blood which sets up some other disease in the abdomen. For instance, peritonitis may have its origin in the unhealthy state of the blood resulting from certain forms of renal disease.

GROUP VII.—It will suffice to mention this group, which includes those abdominal diseases due to *animal parasites* which have gained access into the body. They are an important class, as they include the affections associated with intestinal worms, and hydatid disease. Trichinosis also comes under this head; and there are other rare parasitic affections.

GROUP VIII.—A mere notice will suffice also for this group, which is that including morbid conditions that are either *congenital*, or originate from subsequent *anomalies as regards growth and development.* They belong mainly to the class of malformations and malpositions of organs.

GROUP IX.—A group may be formed of *doubtful or inexplicable diseases,* so far as their ætiology and pathology are concerned, which may be illustrated by acute atrophy of the liver, and certain non-malignant growths, the origin of which is often so extremely doubtful, that they cannot be attributed to any special causes.

GROUP X.—Lastly, a class of cases must be mentioned which are due to the long-continued working of *several causes in combination,* often both *local* and *general.* Thus, to take a common complaint—the so-called dyspepsia—this is often due, not to any special cause, but to a number of causes, each of which calls for recognition and attention in treatment.

Having thus given you this general summary of the ætiology and pathology of abdominal diseases, you will now understand why I warned you at the outset against looking upon these affections as a separate and independent class.

THE RECENT ACTION FOR MALPRAXIS IN NEW YORK. —The result of this case, and of several similar cases, is likely, the *New York Med. Record* observes, to give a check to the practice of bringing the preposterous actions that had become so common in the United States. Dr. Sayres, having to do with what was represented as a case of obstinate constipation, prescribed for a woman some pills containing each a grain of extract of nux vomica, directing her to take one of them and repeat it in four hours if required. The patient took four at once, and declared that one of her lower limbs became paralysed, which, however, was ascertained to be untrue. She was afterwards attended by a gynæcologist for an abrasion of the os uteri; and a twelvemonth after taking the pills brought an action, claiming $25,000 for the mischief they had done to her health! So ridiculous a suit would not have been persevered in had not a complaisant medical witness been ready to testify that the symptoms described were those of strychnia-poisoning. This was nonsense; but had it been true it would not have availed her case, as it was proved that she had taken four pills when ordered to take but one, while the symptoms she complained of were those of hysteria dependent upon uterine disease. The judge summed up strongly in favour of the defendant, and the jury at once found for him. A motion for appeal was refused, and an allowance of $1250 was made to the defendant.

LECTURES ON OPHTHALMOLOGY.
By J. R. WOLFE, M.D., F.R.C.S.E.,
Lecturer on Ophthalmic Medicine and Surgery in Anderson's College; Surgeon to the Glasgow Ophthalmic Institution.

LECTURE VII.
ON GLAUCOMA.

GENTLEMEN,—The disease called glaucoma (γλαυκος, green), from the peculiar sea-green appearance of the pupil, is one of the most dangerous and insidious affections of the eye. The study of it has of late years become particularly interesting from the fact that it has been removed from the category of incurable diseases, and in many cases rendered remediable by the timely operation of iridectomy; and for this practice we are indebted to the genius of von Graefe. The disease is characterised by hardness of the eyeball; excavation of the optic nerve, rendering it cup-shaped or pitcher-shaped; hyperæmia and inflammation of the deep structures; spontaneous arterial and venous pulsation of the optic nerve; and disturbance of vision, ranging from mere dimness to complete abolition of sight. The inflammatory symptoms may be entirely absent, and the other symptoms may exist only to a slight extent; but the characteristic symptom which is never absent, is hardness of the eyeball, and this is due to an abnormal increase of intra-ocular pressure. As this increase of pressure may exist without an inflammatory process, we must conclude that it cannot be the product of inflammation. The disease may be divided into—

I. Inflammatory glaucoma ("glaucoma c. ophthalmia" of Donders), comprising those cases in which an inflammatory process is present, which may be either (a) acute or (b) chronic.

II. Glaucoma simplex, comprising those cases in which there is only increased tension without apparent inflammation.

I. (a) ACUTE INFLAMMATORY GLAUCOMA forms the majority of cases. It sets in with ciliary neuralgia, in which there is pain in the eyeball, the brow, and the temple, and which sometimes extends to the entire half of the head, and is reflected to the stomach, producing vomiting. The patient complains of dimness of vision and of a halo surrounding any flames, the outer margin of the halo being red, the inner margin bluish-green, and between these the ordinary prismatic colours. He sees sparks of various colours before his eye, which may be owing to dilatation of the pupil, to change in the lens, or more particularly, to disturbance of the circulation. You may find, on inquiry, that he has been troubled for some time past with frequently recurring symptoms of neuralgic pain in the head on the affected side, and an occasional dimness of vision in trying to look at near objects; and as he is most likely of a gouty or rheumatic diathesis, the attention is apt to be diverted from the real nature of the disease, which is therefore regarded as a simple case of neuralgia.

Whenever such a case presents itself before you, examine the eye most carefully, and on putting your finger upon the eyeball and comparing it with the other eye (if that be still free from the disease) you will find the affected eye to be harder than the normal one—the pericorneal and episcleral regions hyperæmic, and the pupil slightly dilated and sluggish—which of itself is an untoward symptom, for in no other disease of the eye is the pupil in a condition of symptomatic mydriasis.

On ophthalmoscopic examination you will not discover any sign of disease in the choroid nor in the lens or vitreous, but the optic nerve will present an excavation —a peculiar cup-shaped appearance. The colour of the disc inclines at the beginning of the disease to blood-red on account of the venous congestion, and is encircled by a yellowish-white arch or ring, which is characteristic. On the outermost border of the optic nerve entrance the vessels are bent by a lateral displacement at the point of exit, and spontaneous pulsation is seen at first in the veins only, but, when tension increases, also in the arteries, showing the disturbance in the circulation of the eye. This condition, which is the expression of a sudden increase of the intra-ocular pressure, may intermit—the tissues accommodating themselves to the tension for a short time ; but the acute stage may progress, the ocular pressure continue, and when we next see the patient we may find the ciliary pain increased, the headache more excruciating, the eyeball harder, the arteries and veins of the pericorneal region highly distended, the episcleral tissues inflamed, the aqueous chamber narrower (the iris and lens being pressed forward as if the aqueous humour were exhausted), the iris immovable, and the pupil not effaced though widely dilated. The cloudiness of the dioptric media and the dilatation of the pupil produce the peculiar greenish colour of the fundus, formerly regarded as the pathognomonic symptom of the disease. The ciliary nerves in their passage to the anterior hemisphere of the globe being suddenly compressed, both sensation and conduction are interfered with, and the iris becomes more atrophied, and may be reduced to a small border, unless pre-existing iritis have caused adhesions of that membrane. The pressure upon the ciliary nerves causes some anæsthesia of the cornea, which becomes insensible to the touch ; and von Graefe has shown that the sensibility of the cornea returns after the aqueous humour is drawn off by a paracentesis. The motor fibres of the ciliary nerves become paralysed, and the range of accommodation is limited. There is, as you may expect, disturbance of vision from cloudiness of the cornea and from paralysis of the optic nerve fibres both in the retina and in the lamina cribrosa, due to pressure. In this form of the disease vision is affected from the commencement, and may be reduced to mere perception of light in a few days, or even hours ("glaucoma fulminans" of Graefe) ; but in the largest number of cases it commences with indistinctness of vision, which gradually increases until a thick fog lies over the visual field. The limitation of the visual field begins at the inner side, and gradually advances to the middle, then the upper and lower peripheries become contracted and gradually narrowed from all sides, the fog thickens and envelopes objects, the field becomes obscured, and absolute darkness covers the field.

(b.) Chronic Inflammatory Glaucoma.

An acute attack of glaucoma, although most distressing to the patient, is the least dangerous form of the disease, because it is most amenable to treatment. The form most to be dreaded is chronic inflammatory glaucoma, in which the intra-ocular pressure creeps on slowly and insidiously, with only occasional slight neuralgic attacks. The increase of pressure is not sudden, but gradual, causing excavation of the disc and mischief to the retina and optic nerve, and inducing complete blindness without warning to the patient. Unfortunately we generally see these cases after the whole process has been gone through, and the eye is as hard as marble, so that we have not even an opportunity of examining the interior of the eye, because the cornea is hazy, the aqueous and vitreous humours cloudy, and perhaps the nucleus of the lens opaque. In cases where we have a chance of making ophthalmoscopic examination, we find the excavation has progressed ; the disc, which was red, has become greyish or green, and, later on, the floor of the excavation is spotted with a dirty yellowish-grey colour, while arterial pulsation is more marked.

II. Glaucoma Simplex.

In this form of the affection the intra-ocular pressure comes on gradually, without any symptom of inflammation, which, indeed, is absent during the whole course of the disease. The increasing pressure creeps on imperceptibly, and the place of entrance of the optic nerve, being the weakest point, yields, so that at first the tension is not recognisable by the sense of touch, although excavation has already taken place. The peculiarity of this form is that the pressure is at the expense of the posterior hemisphere, whilst the cornea, aqueous chamber, and lens are not affected ; the iris is atrophied, and the pupil dilated, but not to such an extent as in the inflammatory form. There is no chromatopsia ; the disc is generally white, and is situated in a hollow, the walls of which are formed by the sclera, and the retinal vessels are forced against the walls of the excavation, sometimes to such an extent that the floor of the excavation is destitute of vessels. The depth of the excavation may be calculated from the optical differences of the correcting lenses required to enable us to see distinctly the erect image, first in the plain of the retina, and then in

the floor of the excavation. In the inverted image the difference in parallax produced by moving the convex lens is directly dependent upon the difference of level : the greater the parallax, the deeper the excavation. The margin of the excavation is often surrounded by a narrow, characteristic bright ring, due to atrophy of the choroid surrounding the optic disc ; and this atrophied choroidal ring may be staphylomatous. This state of things may last for years without apparent progress, the only marked symptom being the progressive hardness and the gradual contraction of the visual field. In connexion with the subject of excavation, we must, however, bear in mind that in some cases there exists a natural physiological cup or hollow of the disc without disease, and it is therefore of importance to compare the two eyes, for physiological excavation is symmetrical, and does not extend over the whole disc, and there is no displacement of the vessels.

Causes.—As the disease rarely occurs before the age of fifty, it is now believed to be a senile change in the tissues, although it was formerly thought to be connected with an atheromatous condition of the bloodvessels, and was regarded as an expression of rheumatism or gout. There is no doubt that there is an inherent tendency or predisposition to the affection. When such a tendency exists, the disease may be induced by a very slight injury, in which case it is called *secondary glaucoma*.

Von Graefe regarded glaucoma as a form of choroiditis, or irido-choroiditis, with effusion, by endosmosis, into the vitreous and aqueous humours.

In a paper(a) I maintained that there is no trace of iritis in glaucoma, neither is there choroiditis, but that the affection is owing to perturbation of the ciliary nerve. This view had been advanced by Tavignot in 1846 ; and I further maintained(b) that the whole range of glaucomatous symptoms may be accounted for, and the *modus operandi* of iridectomy in effecting its cure explained, on that hypothesis. I took the disease to be the result of hyperæsthesia of the sympathetic, the vaso-motor nerve which presides over the process of circulation, and can produce changes in the local circulation of the organ, by which the amount of blood, and consequently the temperature, may be increased or diminished. This will account for dilatation of the pupil, and also for engorgement of the humours, which gives rise to dragging of the filaments of the trigeminus ; and this in its turn produces anæsthesia of the cornea, and vitiated nutrition of the organ, the tension rendering the phenomena more complex, and the *tout ensemble* invariably tending to blindness. About the same time there appeared a reference in the *Annales d'Oculistique* to the opinion of Donders that "we must seek the proximate cause of glaucoma in hyperæsthesia of the fifth nerve, which regulates the secretion of the ocular fluid," for Donders found that after division of the fifth nerve the tension of the eyeball decreased and became soft.

Grenhaggen and Hippel also found that electric irritation of the root of the fifth nerve produced a remarkable increase in intra-ocular pressure. Dr. Brailey's recent observations on the dilatation of the ciliary arteries which he found in dissecting glaucomatous eyes only tend to corroborate the theory of paralysis of the sympathetic being the cause of the tension. But the main question which has still to be answered is, "What is the genesis of that disease?" We only know that grief, anxiety, protracted night-watching, in old nervous persons generally induces eye-tension. Sometimes it may be brought on by a very slight injury to the eyeball, but apparently there must be an inherent tendency to the affection.

Treatment.—The introduction of the operation of iridectomy for the cure of glaucoma opened a new era in ophthalmic surgery, and although the theory upon which the operation was founded was not reconcilable with the phenomena of the disease, yet the results, as proved on a large scale, were hailed as evidence of a great conquest over a previously incurable affection. I believe that its undoubted efficacy is due to neurotomy, for Nélaton obtained satisfactory results in tic douloureux by removing a part of the diseased nerve—an operation which was suggested by Allan Burns.(c)

In removing a part of the iris, we remove a portion of the diseased nerves ; and this, I think, has a modifying influence by cutting through the vicious circle which keeps up the

(a) Lancet, 1859.   (b) British Medical Journal, 1864.
            (c) "Surgical Anatomy of the Head and Neck."

disease. Mr. Hancock published some papers in the *Lancet* in 1860, on the cure of glaucoma by the section of the ciliary muscle, and both he and Mr. Power were practising this operation; and I have no doubt that the results must have been satisfactory, on the principle just indicated—viz., a section of the ciliary nerves, which are distributed in the muscle of accommodation. I have, however, never tried the operation myself, being averse to the surgery of that region, from anatomical considerations.

The suggestion which has been made, that the cystoid union of the scleral wound relieves the intra-ocular pressure, has been sufficiently answered by Hirschberg that he never saw any cystoid union; (d) and Schweigger very justly maintains that the cicatrix, instead of becoming more pliable, is, on the contrary, harder than the natural tissues. More recently the operation of sclerotomy has been introduced for the cure of this affection.

This operation is performed by introducing von Graefe's knife at the extreme periphery of the cornea at the sclerotic limbus, and pushing it in a horizontal direction to the opposite side, just as if it were intended to make a flap extraction; then by two or three sawing motions an opening is effected at the outer as well as the inner side of the scleral border, about a quarter of an inch in length. Fig. 13 shows the nature and extent of the section. You will see, therefore, from the very nature of the performance, that sclerotomy must be limited to those affections in which the pupil is contracted and rigid, and where there is no risk that the peripheric puncture will induce hernia iridis, as otherwise it is apt to complicate matters. De Wecker's opinion, that the operation is applicable to cases of *glaucoma simplex*, is a

FIG. 13.

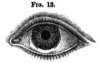

very safe one, for it may at least be said that if anyone should try it in a case of inflammatory glaucoma, he will be certain to produce traumatic cataract. His suggestion, however, that it must be aided by eserine and pilocarpine, somewhat retracts from its merits, for no operation can be worth much which requires the help of drugs. There is no doubt, however, that this operation yields good results in some cases, for it gives free exit to the aqueous humour, and relieves tension to a considerable extent. I have practised it with success in some cases of secondary glaucomatous affection, where glaucomatous symptoms supervened on disease of the cornea, recurrent cyclitis, or keratoglobus; and in a case of the latter I found it reduced the globe, while it was beneficial in every case where the cornea being opaque, an iridectomy might have had to be performed in the dark, as it were; but with regard to primary glaucoma, my confidence in iridectomy is too well founded to allow me to try any other treatment.

The operation of iridectomy is performed in the following manner:—Chloroform is administered only to nervous patients, and in cases where the eye is very painful. The patient being in a recumbent position, and the eyelids kept open by a speculum, the surgeon stands behind the patient; or if section is to be made downwards, he takes his position in front of the patient, who is ordered to look downwards; with the conjunctival forceps in the left hand, a part of the conjunctival and sub-conjunctival tissue is seized in order to steady the eye, and with a curved lance in the right hand, the anterior chamber is entered through the conjunctiva half a line from the corneo-scleral junction. The lance should then be held with its point looking to the cornea, for, owing to the shallowness of the aqueous chamber, the lens runs risk of being wounded. Then taking the curved iris forceps in the left hand, and the scissors in the right, the forceps are introduced, and the iris is seized at its pupillary margin and a segment of it withdrawn. Into this part a vertical incision is made from the pupillary margin to its ciliary attachment, a flap of iris thus remaining within the forceps, and, this being put upon the stretch, by means

(d) *Centralblatt.*

of two other cuts with the scissors, first in a horizontal and then in a vertical direction, the section is finished. Fig. 14 shows the appearance of the pupil after iridectomy performed downwards. By this method the exact portion of the iris can be measured, which it is proposed to remove. When there is some blood in the aqueous chamber, slight pressure of the probe on the scleral lip of the wound is sufficient to

FIG. 14.

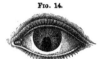

cause its expulsion. An assistant is required for this operation to hold the speculum a little forwards, in order to prevent the pain caused by its pressure on the orbit. The forceps is dispensed with in the second stage, and the operation is thus performed with a minimum of pain, most of which is caused by the pressure of the speculum and fixation forceps. The dressing consists of lint secured by a bandage.

Case 1.—Acute Glaucoma—Sudden Invasion of Symptoms caused by a Slight Injury and Fright—Double Iridectomy —Cure in one Eye.

Miss T., aged seventy-nine, of a highly nervous temperament, enjoyed good health till May, 1878, never having suffered from gout or rheumatism, and not being subject to any eye-affection, her sight being normal. About the time mentioned, the chimney of the room in which she was sitting caught fire, and in the midst of the confusion her hands and face were slightly singed. This accident frightened her exceedingly. The same night pain was experienced for some time in the top of the head, and this returned with greater severity on the succeeding night, depriving her of sleep. Two or three days later she appeared to herself to be enveloped in a cloud, as if the house were full of smoke, and this mist before her eyes gradually thickened until vision was almost abolished. She remained in this condition for five weeks, when I was called in to see her, and found both cornea hazy-looking. The conjunctive were hyperæmic; tension T + 3, and vision almost *nil*; while focal illumination revealed the commencement of cataract in both eyes; opaque striæ advancing from the periphery of the lenses.

I performed iridectomy in both eyes on July 1, 1878. The headache from which she had previously suffered was abated, the mist disappeared, and four days after the operation vision in the right eye was tolerably good, as she was subsequently able to walk about, and also to read ordinary type. The optic disc is represented in Fig. 15. In the left

FIG. 15.

eye, however, excavation had advanced too far, the disc being found white and cupped, the vessels displaced from the floor of the excavation, and luminous perception entirely abolished.

A London ophthalmic surgeon, a relative of the patient, saw her, and expressed the opinion that, if the iridectomy had been performed sooner, the sight of both eyes would have been saved; and of this there can be little doubt, for on January 6, 1881, notwithstanding the advance of the cataract, and consequent limitation of the visual field, as represented in Fig. 16, she was able to read with ease No. 3½ Snellen's test-type, with twelve inches convex glasses.

Case 2.—Glaucoma Fulminans—Iridectomy—Cure.

Mrs. K. (from Dundee), aged about fifty, consulted me on May 14, 1881. Sixteen years ago she began to suffer pain and dimness of vision in the left eye, and Mr. White Cooper pronounced it to be a case of glaucoma. Some years later an iridectomy had been performed upon it. She had never had any pain in it since, but the eye is cataractous and perception of light abolished. Some time ago she began to feel occasionally some uneasiness in the right eye, but on May 13 violent pain set in. She became "fog-bound," suffered excruciating pain on the right side of the head, attended with sickness during the night, and next morning vision was completely gone. In this condition she was brought to me. On examination I found the eyeball hard (T. 3), the cornea clear, the aqueous chamber shallow, iris forming a concavity forwards. Ophthalmoscopic examination showed the vitreous

Fig. 16.

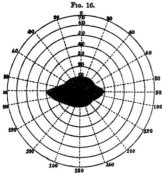

humour opaque, and the fundus invisible, as if masked by some dark body. As evening was approaching, I determined, for the sake of immediate relief, to perform a paracentesis, fearing lest by waiting another night every chance of saving vision would be lost. Immediately after, she could see distinctly; went to bed, saying that she "was in paradise," and slept well. Two days after she could tell the time to a minute on a watch. The same night, however, pain returned, and I again resorted to paracentesis on the 17th. She then had other two quiet days with good sight; after which the symptoms returned, although they were not so violent as before. I then performed an iridectomy on the 19th. Sight is now more distinct than it has been for years past. Reads No. 2 Jaeger fluently with suitable glasses. According to the last report, four weeks after the operation, "vision is brilliant, and the eye feels more comfortable than it has done for some years past." The encouraging and hopeful feature of this case is the healthy appearance of the eye and the depth of the aqueous chamber, showing that a new condition has been induced. It is quite conceivable that the fencing with the disease by paracentesis has contributed to the ultimate success of the iridectomy. I shall try it in similar cases.

THE MEDICAL WITNESS.—Dr. Legrand du Saulle, lecturing at the Salpêtrière, on the Mental Condition of the Hysterical (*Rev. Méd.*, June 11), thus cautions his hearers :—"When you are called as a physician before a court of justice, never step beyond the limits of science, and, above all, do not give yourself up to your imagination. Say what you know; describe, but never become either judge, accuser, or advocate, but remain the physician. He who quits the limits of his position to become accuser or judge, who seeks to become the public minister or the presiding officer, such a man is no longer the physician. 'That is my opinion,' you will simply state; 'it is based upon such and such facts and considerations; such is the condition of the accused; this or that may exist. Make what applications you choose, for I am not here to render justice.'"

ORIGINAL COMMUNICATIONS.

ACUTE PROSTATITIS.

By REGINALD HARRISON, F.R.C.S.(a)

OF all the complex structures from the kidneys downwards, which together constitute the genito-urinary tract, the prostate gland may be regarded as the least liable to attacks of acute inflammation, and in this respect it seems to serve a wise purpose in acting as a check against the extension of inflammation from the much exposed and susceptible urethra below it to the more vital organs above it.

Structural differences of this kind play a most important, though not, I believe, sufficiently appreciated, part in limiting the progress of a variety of pathological actions, which otherwise, by continuity, would spread almost unrestrained.

Under the term "acute prostatitis," I have been in the habit of recognising two varieties, presenting distinct pathological features, each disposed to pursue a tolerably definite course, and determined by different circumstances.

The one I shall speak of as acute follicular prostatitis, the other as acute general or parenchymatous prostatitis. I think that these terms will not only be found convenient in localising the effects of inflammation as observed in the gland, but also are free from anything like an artificial distinction.

A very brief reference to the structure of the prostate will suffice for my purpose. It is essentially glandular and muscular, the former consisting of numerous follicular pouches, opening into elongated canals, which join to form from twelve to twenty small excretory ducts. The glandular element is, so to speak, embedded in muscular fibres of the involuntary kind, the whole being enclosed in a thin, but firm, fibrous capsule distinct from the posterior layer of the deep perineal or triangular ligament.

I think it will be at once conceded that in the prostate we have two elementary structures—one, the glandular, which is not at all opposed to inflammatory attacks; and the other, the muscular, which only becomes inflamed when the provocation is extreme. Further, as being explanatory of some of the symptoms which are met with in the course of a prostatitis, we must not forget the unyielding nature of the covering with which the gland is invested.

Acute follicular prostatitis is not by any means a very uncommon event. It is most frequently seen in connexion with gonorrhœa. A person with this affection suddenly finds the discharge either diminished or altered in character, and this is immediately followed by a sensation of weight or uneasiness in the perineum. The prostate gland is found to be hot, tender, or swollen; micturition becomes frequent or impeded in accordance with the extent to which the bladder structurally sympathises, or the swollen prostate obstructs. In some cases there is complete retention.

In such instances as these, it will be found that the inflammation is almost entirely confined to the follicles of the gland. These may individually suppurate, or a limited abscess may form by the fusion of two or more of them which have thus become obstructed.

"There is never, then," as Bumstead remarks, "at the outset one abscess of considerable size. Such occurs only by the coalescence of a number of small ones seated in the follicles. Meanwhile, the muscular tissue, which constitutes so large a portion of the prostate gland, is unaffected, except that it is in a constant state of contraction, thereby inducing urethral and rectal tenesmus."

And what is true of the normal prostate, in regard to the insusceptibility of its muscular portion to inflammatory action, is still more apparently so when it is hypertrophied and the proportion of muscular and connective structure is increased. And if proof of this were required I would point to the tolerably hard usage the gland sometimes receives, when in the course of its growth it impedes micturition and becomes an obstacle to the introduction of the catheter.

Though nearly every museum furnishes instances where, either by accident or design, the outgrowth has become more or less riddled with perforations, or shows other signs of hard,

(a) Paper read at the Medical Society of London, April 11, 1881.

though possibly necessary, treatment, yet examples of suppuration or inflammation occurring under these circumstances are comparatively rare.

The impunity with which forced catheterism in enlarged prostate has sometimes been practised is, I believe, in a measure owing to its adoption being sanctioned by some writers, if not also by some practitioners of eminence.

The follicular, then, is the simplest form of acute prostatitis. Though painful and distressing whilst it lasts, the symptoms are not usually protracted, and the prognosis is favourable. Recovery most frequently follows by resolution, suppuration being the exception, and not the rule. And when suppuration does take place under these circumstances, it is to be inferred rather than demonstrated, for rigors are often absent, and most careful examination with the finger in the rectum fails to discover fluctuation, though an escape of matter by the urethra may almost immediately follow the introduction of the catheter, which has been found necessary either for the purpose of completing the examination or relieving the retention. And where there has been reason for believing that matter has so formed, I have never known any evil effect result.

The other form of prostatitis, acute parenchymatous or general, is a much more serious condition. It is as if the whole gland within the capsule were at one and the same time invaded with the inflammatory action. Suppuration usually rapidly supervenes, and unless treatment is prompt and decisive on the first appearance of fluctuation, as revealed by rectal examination, the most serious results, both to structure and life, are likely to follow.

This form of prostatitis is rare. I can find no specimen of the kind described in the *Transactions of the Pathological Society* since 1865, nor do I see any reference to it amongst the *Proceedings of the Clinical Society* from its commencement. I have looked through a considerable number of the volumes of hospital reports published by several metropolitan institutions, all of which show how seldom this affection is met with. Instances of it will, however, be found scattered throughout the medical journals; and the experience of those who have seen much of this class of disorders will include some examples. Here, owing to the violence of the inflammation, the structures outside the prostatic capsule become more or less infiltrated with serous effusion, or even pus—a condition which has been described as peri-prostatitis. This I have never seen to any appreciable extent, except as secondary to acute suppurative inflammation of the whole gland, and I believe that it has no other significance.

At the outset it is not easy to determine which of the two conditions I have referred to we have to deal with. The causes producing them are much the same, and we must look for other circumstances as determining whether the inflammation will be limited to the follicles or will involve *en masse* the entire gland. And we shall find that the very circumstances which lead to the latter are such as, if they happened to be present when any part other than the prostate was inflamed, would render the occurrence of suppuration, if not of gangrene, probable.

We have only to look at the kind of persons who suffer from acute parenchymatous prostatitis to learn the circumstances favouring it. Speaking generally, they may be indicated as individuals of either much deteriorated constitutional powers, or as possessing urinary organs more or less damaged by long-standing obstructive disease. Belonging to the former class, we see it occasionally happening in persons whom we are accustomed to speak of as highly tubercular, and who have been unfortunate enough to contract a gonorrhœa. I have seen it occur in such subjects, and have had reason to suspect (though I have never been able to prove it) that a previous state of tuberculosis of the gland had determined this particular consequence. Here it is not the follicles that alone suffer, but the whole gland, the capsule of which serves the purpose of a bag for the pus which is the result.

Again, it is seen in prostates that have been rendered unhealthy by old-standing strictures and cystitis. In these, on the occurrence of some fresh exciting cause, such as the gonorrhœal poison, or even, I believe, by disordered urine, the gland seems to have lost its power of resisting inflammation, and may speedily suppurate.

Under these circumstances the occurrence of suppuration must be carefully looked for, as the spontaneous escape of matter, in such directions as the rectum, bladder, and peri-

toneal cavity, is likely to be much more detrimental than the opening which the surgeon would afford.

Gangrene of the prostate as a result of inflammation is exceedingly rare, but I believe it occasionally happens. I have certainly seen it after lithotomy in a very unhealthy adult, and I thought that the softened and putrescent condition in which I once found the gland of a young man who died after symptoms of prostatitis, with other renal complications, was no other than an example of this termination of inflammation. With this brief reference to the circumstances under which we see acute prostatitis, let me refer to two conditions which simulate it, one of which, I believe, has led to the impression that this disease is far more common than it really is.

The first is inflammation and suppuration around the membranous portion of the urethra as a consequence of urethritis; and the second, inflammation and plugging of the veins constituting the prostatic plexus. I have seen many instances of the former where inflammation and suppuration around the membranous urethra have led practitioners into the belief that the case was one of metastasis of the gonorrhœal inflammation from the urethra to the prostate gland. And the points of resemblance are by no means isolated—there is, in fact, a remarkable likeness between the two conditions. In both there is a cessation or an alteration in the character of the urethral discharge: in both there is a feeling of weight and uneasiness about the perinæum; in both there is some difficulty in micturition, perhaps amounting to retention; and in both there is some tumefaction to be felt, and much distress is occasioned on introducing the finger into the rectum. So painful is the latter to the patient, that it often leads to an imperfect examination being made, and hence an error in diagnosis arises in exactly fixing the position of the tumefaction, which might have been avoided.

It must, on the other hand, be remembered that in inflammation and suppuration around the membranous urethra, though this part lies between the layers of the perineal fascia, there is more or less perineal tumefaction, and that matter so formed may make its way forward, and be discharged by means of the perineal opening.

In the cases of acute prostatitis I have seen, neither of these two indications have been present, whilst in urethritis I have usually observed them.

Considering the relations of the prostate and the denseness of the fascia immediately in front of it, I do not see how perineal tumefaction is to be expected as a consequence of prostatitis, any more than swelling in this locality is to be associated with the hypertrophy of the gland as it is seen in old age.

I should not have thought it necessary, even to this extent, to have referred to this particular source of error without knowing, of my own verified experience, of the necessity for it, and without feeling that even in some of our best literature there is ambiguity upon this point.

Though I would speak with the greatest possible deference of the writings of the late eminent surgeon Sir Benjamin Brodie, the description he gives in his opening remarks on inflammation of the prostate are, to my mind, much more applicable to the condition I have been referring to, rather than to the one it is intended to depict. And what Sir Benjamin wrote, many others have copied, and hence the obscurity to which I have referred. The other disordered condition which may simulate prostatitis is rare, and it is also curious. I have only seen two cases of it, and they both came under my notice recently, about the same time.

The primary lesion was rapid œdema of the prepuce, dependent upon plugging of the dorsal vein of the penis. This was quite obvious. In the course of a few days each complained of perineal weight, frequent rather than painful micturition, with great uneasiness referred to the neck of the bladder, which led to its being suggested that in each case the prostate was inflamed. Both patients were gouty; in one the œdema was attributed to gonorrhœa, in the other to a strong injection.

In each I was able to determine, by rectal examination, that the vesical pain and irritability were not due to any inflammation of the gland, but to the extension of the vein-blocking to the prostatic plexus. Each patient certainly had some ground for believing that prostatitis was imminent. And now I will say a few words about treatment.

I know of nothing which at the outset of an attack of

prostatitis gives greater relief than free leeching of the perineum, followed by hot applications. Some practitioners, I know, advise the use of ice by the rectum, but, as a rule, I have found heat preferable to cold. I am opposed to the employment of all purgatives in this affection. When we consider how closely related the levator ani muscle is to the prostate gland—how every movement of it necessarily aggravates the sufferings of the patient—I am at a loss to understand how such measures can be advised by anyone, who appreciates the good work of the late John Hilton in reference to the importance of rest in the treatment of an inflammation. I should just as soon think of advising a patient with an acutely inflamed knee-joint to walk a mile as I should of administering purgatives to one with a prostatitis. If a distended rectum requires relief, a copious enema of hot water will answer every purpose, and, in addition, will be found most soothing. Guthrie, in his admirable lectures, refers to the great benefit attending the use of hot enemata in these cases. In one instance of threatened suppuration of the prostate, under my observation, the patient experienced great relief from frequently injecting hot water into the bladder by means of a syringe, which I have found serviceable in certain affections of the urethra; and this experience corresponds with a remark of Guthrie's to the same purport. I believe such injections tend to prevent the accumulation of mucus within the prostatic urethra, and in this way avert the formation and collection of matter in the follicles. The use of opium in some form or other will be found essential in protecting the powers of the patient from being worn down by the irritation and pain which to some degree are always present. The occurrence of suppuration must be carefully looked for; and it appears to me, in reference to this point, that a conclusion may be formulated to the effect that any formation of matter in the gland which is not appreciable to the finger in the rectum may with safety be left to evacuate spontaneously, but that when fluctuation is detected by rectal examination, a perineal incision becomes imperative.

When the finger detects that suppuration has taken place there should be no hesitation in giving exit to the pus by an incision into the prostate with a long-bladed finger-knife, the finger of the opposite hand being retained within the bowel as a guide. Unless this is done the matter will most probably find its way into the rectum, and a permanent fistula may be the result, or it may burrow in other directions, all of them likely to be more disastrous to the patient than the course the surgeon would afford.

Rectal puncture, I know, has been advocated, but I am not in favour of it; a cut, in the treatment of an acute abscess, is, as a rule, far better than a puncture.

If there is one point upon which I would desire to lay particular stress as bearing upon diagnosis and treatment, it is the importance of a thorough examination by the rectum in all cases where there may be ground for suspecting that the prostate is inflamed or suppurating.

Pain and tension have often rendered this incomplete, and an error has been the result—an error which would possibly not have arisen had all source of obstacle been removed by the use of an anæsthetic.

It must not be forgotten that abscesses, sometimes of very considerable size, may form within the limits of the prostate without giving rise to such symptoms as are usually provoked. A case in point is recorded by Dr. Pitman at St. George's Hospital, where prostatitis supervened upon an attack of gonorrhœa, and terminated in suppuration and death of the patient, with entire absence of rigors and the ordinary symptoms of abscess.

In conclusion, let me say one word about an occasional consequence of follicular prostatitis. I refer to a more or less permanent state of dilatation of the follicles, and consequently a fruitful source of a chronic discharge—namely, prostatorrhœa—a condition which has been well described by the eminent American surgeon, Professor Gross. Whether these dilated follicles, as furnishing receptacles in which urine may become stagnant, have any connexion with the formation of calculi in the prostate, is a direction of inquiry which is hardly within the scope of this communication. In these few observations on prostatitis I have aimed at conciseness rather than at elaboration, knowing that I should the more certainly advance knowledge by eliciting your experience than by occupying your time to any great length.

DISTOMA RINGERI.(a)
By Dr. PATRICK MANSON, Amoy.

THE list of parasites inhabiting the human body is gradually becoming a long one; another addition—the latest, I believe—has recently been made by Dr. Ringer, of Tamsui, Formosa. The following notes embrace all that is yet known of the new parasite.

Some time ago, November 6 to December 18, 1878, I had in hospital here a Portuguese suffering from symptoms of thoracic tumour presumed to be an aneurism. He improved with rest and treatment, and returned to Tamsui, whence he had come and where he had resided for many years. He did not live long after his return, and died suddenly (June, 1879), from rupture of an aneurism of the ascending aorta into the pericardium. Dr. Ringer made the post-mortem examination, and, knowing I took an interest in the case, kindly wrote me the particulars of the examination. Besides describing the immediate cause of death, he told me he had found a parasite of some sort in making a section of the lung, and promised to send the animal to me for inspection. He wrote:—"After making a section I found the parasite lying on the lung tissue—it might have escaped from a bronchus. Whilst alive a number of young (microscopic) escaped from an opening in the body. There were some small deposits of tubercle, no cavities, and, if I remember aright, slight congestion of the lungs."

Last April a Chinaman consulted me about an eczematous eruption he had on his face and legs. The eruption had been out for some time, and had its origin, he believed, in an attack of scabies. Whilst he was speaking to me I observed that his voice was rough and loud, and that he frequently hawked up and expectorated small quantities of a reddish sputum. At that time I was making examinations of lung-blood in connexion with another subject, and as this man's sputum afforded a favourable opportunity for examination, I placed a specimen under the microscope. The sputa, which to the naked eye appeared to be made up of small pellets of rusty pneumonic-like spit, specks of bright red blood, and ordinary bronchial mucus, contained, besides ordinary blood and mucus corpuscles, large numbers of bodies evidently the ova of some parasite. These bodies were oval in form, one end of the oval being cut off or shut in by an operculum, granular on the surface, blood-stained, measuring on an average $\frac{1}{30} \times \frac{1}{60}$". Firm pressure on the covering glass caused them to rupture and their contents to escape, the shell being left empty, and fractured at the opercular end. Though empty, the shell had a pale brownish-red colour. No distinctly organised embryo could be made out in the uninjured ovum, but when the contents were expressed they resolved themselves into oil masses, and granular matter having very active molecular movements. A delicate double outline could be made out in most of the ova. They were so numerous that many fields of the microscope showed three or four of them at once.

Two days afterwards I again examined this man's sputum, and found it full of ova as on the previous occasion. I asked him to come again and to supply me from time to time with sputum, but he did not return, and has left the neighbourhood, I believe. I hoped to attempt successfully the hatching of the ova, as has already been done in the case of other distomata, but his disappearance and my failure to get another and similar case oblige me to postpone the experiment.

At his first visit I obtained the following particulars of his case:—Tso-tong, male, aged thirty-five, native of Foochow, a secretary in the Salt Office, resident in Amoy about one year. He was born in Foochow city, and lived there till he was twenty-one years of age; he then went to Tecktcham, a town in North Formosa, about two days' journey from Tamsui, and resided there for four years; then he returned to Foochow for a year and a half. He was again sent to Tecktcham for a second service of four years. He returned again to his native town for a year, and was then sent for six months to Henghwa. Afterwards he lived successively in Foochow, one year; Amoy, a year and a half; Foochow, four months; and again Amoy for one year, where he is at present stationed. A year after his arrival in Tecktcham, when he was twenty-two years of age, he first spat blood.

(a) From the *Medical Reports of the Imperial Maritime Customs of China.*

Every day for nineteen days he brought up from an ounce to half an ounce of blood; he emaciated slightly, but had very little cough. Hæmoptysis returned about six months later, smaller in quantity, but, as in the former attack, the blood at first was pure, unmixed with mucus, and of a bright red colour; this second attack lasted for a few days only. Since then he says he has spat blood for two or three days at a time, in small quantities, every second or third month. He has never had much cough, and he says the blood is always mixed with mucus after the first mouthful. Once during two years he had no blood-spitting. Though rather thin, he enjoys good health. I could discover no signs of lung-disease on auscultation. His father is dead, but never had a cough; his mother had a cough and died ten years ago. He has had two brothers and two sisters; they are all of them alive and in good health.

When I discovered the ova in this man's sputum I recollected Dr. Ringer's parasite, and that the Portuguese in whose lungs it was found had also lived for many years in North Formosa; and I came to the conclusion that this Chinaman's lungs probably contained a similar parasite, and that it was the cause of his blood-spitting. At my request Dr. Ringer sent me the solitary specimen he had found a year before. It was preserved in spirits of wine. I placed a little of the sediment in the spirit under the microscope, and found in it several ova of the same shape, colour, and dimensions as those I had some time before found in the Chinaman's sputum. Most of the ova were ruptured; a few, however, were still perfect. The parent parasite was of the shape, size, and outline represented. It was of a light brown colour, firm, leathery texture, and measured ⅛″ × ⅛″ × ¹⁄₁₆″. It was evidently a distoma; but, not feeling sure if it was a new species or not, I sent it to Dr. Cobbold, who has pronounced it to be new, and has named it *Distoma Ringeri* after the discoverer.

We are as yet not in a position to say much about the pathological significance of this parasite. I do not think it common in this locality, but when practising in South Formosa I recollect seeing many cases of chronic and oft-recurring blood-spitting without apparent heart or lung lesion, and it is just possible that the hæmoptysis in many of these cases was caused by distoma Ringeri. My patient told me that blood-spitting was a very common complaint in Tocktcham.

The intermediary host or hosts, the geographical distribution, and the mode of entrance of the parasite into the lungs, offer a very interesting field for future investigation.

DEATH FROM EMPLOYMENT OF A CARBOLIC ACID SOLUTION.—Dr. Bradford relates, in the *Boston Medical Journal* for April 7, the case of a boy, five years old, who had been under treatment for hip-joint disease during six months. A cold abscess having formed in the thigh, this was evacuated, and the cavity hyper-distended by a solution of carbolic acid (one to forty), which was then allowed to flow out, pressure being used to secure its full discharge. Vomiting supervened, and the boy, soon becoming enfeebled, died in collapse two days after.

IODOFORM IN THE TREATMENT OF WOUNDS.—Dr. Mikulicz, in a paper read to the Vienna Medical Society (*Wien. Med. Zeit.*, May 31), gave an account of the results he had obtained from the use of iodoform in old or recent wounds, ulcers, cavities of abscesses, fistulous passages, etc. The mode of employing it was very simple, consisting in sprinkling some of the powder on the surface, and covering up with wadding and a bandage; or it might be combined with gelatine, mucilage, or cacao-butter in the proportion of one to ten. For parenchymatous injection, also, a solution in ethereal oil, one to five, may be used. It has been tried in nearly two hundred cases of the most various description. It forms a complete substitute for the Listerian dressing, its application is simple, and healing takes place rapidly under its use. In military surgery so simple a mode of dressing will be found of great utility. Its antiseptic power is shown by its influence on phagedænic and cancerous wounds; and it exerts a powerful effect when it is brought into immediate contact with fungous growths and caries of tubercular origin. In the cases of two feeble children suffering from caries it did harm, exerting a toxical effect, which proved fatal. Its employment, therefore, on children has to be watched, especially when it has to be used for months.

REPORTS OF HOSPITAL PRACTICE

IN

MEDICINE AND SURGERY.

LONDON HOSPITAL.

CASE OF ACUTE BASILAR MENINGITIS (IDIOPATHIC).

(Under the care of Dr. ANDREW CLARK.)

[Reported by Dr. NORRIS WOLFENDEN.]

History.—Patient, a strong healthy seaman, aged twenty-four, was admitted on November 14, 1880, in a helpless and unconscious condition. A fortnight ago he came from Calcutta, and would be exposed to cold in coming up Channel. He also was upset on hearing of the death of a mate. On the Friday he was sick after a cup of tea; has not eaten anything since. On Saturday morning he crawled out of bed to the fireplace, grovelling in the ashes. Asked what he was doing, he muttered unintelligibly, and has not spoken one intelligible word from the beginning of the illness to the end. The following notes were taken soon after admission:—
" He is half unconscious; face dusky, eyes half open, breathing through the nose, teeth clenched; extremely restless. Temperature 104·8°; pulse 120; respirations 42. Right arm and leg retain perfect motor power; slight pricks with a pin produce excessive response (hyperæsthesia). The left arm and leg are paralysed, and exhibit marked anæsthesia. The fingers of the left hand are flexed; the limb is not rigid. There is some excess of tendon reflex in the left leg. The head is constantly directed towards the right side, not drawn back. There is very decided internal strabismus of the left eye, which has only appeared during the last day or two. Pupils are normal, and both respond well to light. Right cornea extremely sensitive to touch; left cornea not at all. The eyelids are half closed, but there is no real ptosis. The muscles of expression of the left side of face are paralysed. The sphincters are intact. Skin hot, burning, and dry."

Treatment.—A bath of 70°, lowered till absolutely cold, was given, and patient kept in fifteen minutes. The temperature fell to 102·5°, and the pulse to 102. Respirations were no longer stridulous, and he was no longer restless, otherwise the same.

November 15.—The strabismus of the left eye disappeared, and there is now internal strabismus of right eye. The right eyelid droops a little. There is much muscular tremor in the right arm, with twitching. The left arm is still useless and still anæsthetic. Pulse 140; temperature 104·2°; respirations 44, chiefly nasal. At 6 p.m. the temperature had risen to 109°; the pulse 150; respirations 48. Great beads of perspiration all over, and the skin burning hot. Internal strabismus of right eye, and ptosis. A cold bath was immediately given as before. At 6.40 the temperature was taken again, and found to be 102°; pulse 120; respirations 32. At 7.30, temperature 103·8°. Sponging with ice-cold water ordered. At 8, temperature 101°. At 10 p.m., temperature 104°. Again sponged. After sponging, temperature 100°.

16th.—Patient remains the same. Tongue dry, swollen, with dirty brown patches. Breathing 60, noisy, but not stertorous. Pulse 148, full and bounding. Skin burning. Temperature at 1 a.m. 104°, steadily rose to 107° at 10.20, and fell to 104° after sponging with ice-water. Shortly afterwards the patient died.

Post-mortem, made November 17.—On opening the skull the brain-surface looked sticky and yellowish. Over the outer surface of the right hemisphere, extending upwards over the anterior lobe, and over the parietal lobe to the base, was a thin layer of yellow thick pus. A small quantity also was found at the base of the left lobe. No disease of tympanum or bones could be found. The grey matter of the cortex was pink and sticky. There was no effusion in the ventricles. In the posterior fossa were some points of ecchymosis on the dura mater. There was a congested appearance of the base of the brain, but no trace of tubercles to be found anywhere. The heart and lungs were perfectly normal, except that the latter were engorged and œdematous. The spleen was large and very soft. The liver and kidneys healthy. No tubercle to be seen anywhere, and no pus about the medulla oblongata.

Remarks.—This case, though very rare, is clinically distinctive. Its rapid course, its acuteness, and its manner of onset are characteristic. The prodromal stage was marked by a certain wildness of manner, evidenced by the patient getting out of bed and grovelling in the ashes; by sickness; followed by unconsciousness, hemiplegia, and involvement of certain nerves about the base of the brain in an irregular manner; and throughout characterised by an intense fever and quick bounding pulse. The coma was not complete, since the patient could be got to say a word or two occasionally; but there was never any return to consciousness. It is impossible to divide these symptoms into the three stages described as tubercular meningitis. As to the causation of this disease, it is involved in obscurity. In this case it seems not improbably to have been emotional, joined to exposure to heat and cold possibly. There was not the slightest occasion to suspect syphilis, though this is accused of being a cause of meningitis (in children alone, I believe).

A CASE OF GLOSSO-LABIAL PALSY.
(Under the care of Dr. ANDREW CLARK.)
[Reported by Dr. NORRIS WOLFENDEN.]

J. B. was admitted into the London Hospital on July 31, 1880, and died on August 5. He is a printer's assistant, and works in a very hot room, and is obliged to have the windows open, which makes it very draughty. Three months ago, he states, he experienced pain in the back of the neck, and could not eat much; this was followed by "pain in the back and top of the head." The voice failed occasionally, but got well again, and was never so bad as it is at present. He now has no pain in his head. His friends state that he appeared almost quite well a month ago, and then he began to feel weak and to lose his appetite. It was only eight days ago that he could not swallow, and lost his voice permanently.

Present Condition.—He is emaciated and pale; very intelligent, and can readily write down answers to questions. It is impossible to understand what he says, for his speech is mumbling and inarticulate, and his voice very nasal in quality. The lips are not at all pendulous, and there is no accumulation of saliva or dribbling at the mouth. Attempts to swallow fluids are followed by ejection through the mouth, but not through the nares. He will not attempt to swallow anything solid. He is able to grin fairly well, but the left side of the mouth is a little more drawn than the right. He is able to blow out the cheeks well, and to whistle moderately well. The tongue when protruded is directed a little to the left side; he is unable to touch the roof of the mouth with the tip, and it is with great difficulty that he directs his tongue at all to the right side. His sense of taste is good, as far as acids and bitters are concerned; he recognises tartaric acid as "acid," and quinine as "bitter," but does not know what sugar is. The uvula is directed slightly towards the left. Both pillars of the fauces are perfectly immovable on the left side, but act normally on the right. Bougies (Nos. 13 and 15) readily passed into the stomach. For four days he was fed regularly with enemata of beef-tea and port wine, and the misturæ potass. iodidi given. There was nothing abnormal in the lungs and heart, and all the limbs and muscles were normal. The temperature was always from 97° or a little below to 98°, and never above; the skin always moist and cold, especially that of the feet. On August 5, while raising the patient in bed, he fell back, and died in a few seconds from syncope.

A post-mortem examination was forbidden by the friends.

Remarks.—The chief features of this case are its rapid course (the patient being quite well three months ago), the transient attacks of loss of voice, the progressive emaciation, and the supervention of permanently dangerous and symptomatic phenomena only a fortnight before death—viz., inability to swallow, and loss of voice, and paralysis of the muscles of the pharynx—and the sudden death by syncope. The nerves involved in this disease are generally stated to be the seventh, the ninth, and the eleventh. In this case, the seventh was only very slightly involved, as evidenced by the slight drawing of the right side of the face. The ninth nerve, evidently, was chiefly implicated, as evidenced by paralysis of the azygos uvulæ and the palato-pharyngeus and palato-glossus of the left side, and the paralysis of the posterior portion of the pharynx. Some amount of loss of taste appears to point to impairment of its gustatory fibres also. The vagus had, no doubt, a share in producing the paralysis of the pharynx, and possibly in slowing the circulation by its inhibitory fibres, and causing the final attack of syncope. It is curious to note how partial is the paralysis in this disease very often. I have seen a case which had apparently become quite well under iodide of potassium, and in which the only lesion left was paralysis of the uvula. When we remember, however, how many individual fibres go to make up a nerve—e.g., in the optic nerve probably some 100,000—the selection of these individual muscles becomes more intelligible. Glosso-labial palsy is somewhat rarer as an idiopathic disease than when occurring along with other well-marked nervous diseases. The causation is obscure, and in this case would appear to be from excessive heat and cold. These changes of heat and cold have a remarkable influence in inducing certain diseases of the nervous system—e.g., progressive muscular atrophy, which Charcot has asserted to be very common amongst stokers. No doubt, had a post-mortem been made, a sclerosis in the medulla would have been found, involving the nerve-roots (or their cells) of the seventh, ninth, tenth, and twelfth. The disease is not always easy to recognise, but in a well-marked case the features are distinctive enough. The above case, however, had been treated for "liver complaint" before being sent to the hospital.

TERMS OF SUBSCRIPTION.
(Free by post.)

			£	s.	d.
British Islands	. . . .	Twelve Months	1	8	0
,, ,,	. . . .	Six ,,	0	14	0
The Colonies and the United } States of America . . . }		Twelve ,,	1	10	0
,, ,, ,,	. . . .	Six ,,	0	15	0
India	. . . .	Twelve ,,	1	10	0
,, (viâ Brindisi)	. . . .	,, ,,	1	15	0
,, ,, ,,	. . . .	Six ,,	0	15	0
,, (viâ Brindisi)	. . . .	,, ,,	0	17	6

Foreign Subscribers are requested to inform the Publishers of any remittance made through the agency of the Post-office.

Single Copies of the Journal can be obtained of all Booksellers and Newsmen, price Sixpence.

Cheques or Post-office Orders should be made payable to Mr. JAMES LUCAS, 11, New Burlington-street, W.

TERMS FOR ADVERTISEMENTS.

			£	s.	d.
Seven lines (70 words)	. . . .		0	4	6
Each additional line (10 words)	. .		0	0	6
Half-column, or quarter-page	. .		1	5	0
Whole column, or half-page	. .		2	10	0
Whole page	. . . .		5	0	0

Births, Marriages, and Deaths are inserted Free of Charge.

THE MEDICAL TIMES AND GAZETTE is published on Friday morning: Advertisements must therefore reach the Publishing Office not later than One o'clock on Thursday.

Medical Times and Gazette.

SATURDAY, JULY 2, 1881.

DR. BARCLAY'S HARVEIAN ORATION.

IT is but a trite observation that he who receives the honour of being appointed to deliver the annual Harveian Oration at the Royal College of Physicians has a thorny crown presented to him. So many of these Orations have now been delivered that the whole subject has been worn threadbare, and it would only be by the merest good fortune that any new Orator could have anything new to say with regard to Harvey's life and career. In sheer despair, therefore, we take it, Dr. Barclay has broken away from the accustomed trammels, and sought new directions of thought. These he has embodied in an Oration distinguished by those scholarly tastes for which Dr. Barclay is well known, and which in certain passages rises to veritable eloquence.

Briefly, the Oration may be said to divide itself into three parts. The first we might describe as the logic of the

Infinite; the second as that of Darwinism (which, by the way, Dr. Barclay always speaks of as Darwinianism); and the third, that of Listerism. Passing over introductory matter, we come to the portion relating to the logic of Harvey; this, as Dr. Barclay points out, was essentially that of Bacon—not, however, as the Orator inclined to think, from any careful logical training, but from that intuitive sense which enables great minds to spring from point to point, overleaping many intermediate steps, but always coming to a safe conclusion. Undoubtedly this was so with Harvey, but we cannot commend the example. We are not all born Harveys or Bacons, or even like unto that now despised man, Aristotle.

It is not perfectly easy to follow Dr. Barclay in the paragraphs which succeed. They are, if anything, too closely reasoned, though assuredly there are flaws in the reasoning. Thus, when he says that when Harvey saw that the blood propelled from the heart must return to it he discovered a law of nature, we cannot see the sequence, for Harvey never traced the blood from one side of the heart to the other—he only inferred it. Moreover, there is no necessity about the matter, as those experience who are unfortunate enough to bleed to death. But Dr. Barclay's object would seem to have been to attain the domain of law only for the purpose of reaching that of the Lawgiver, and thence to obtain that old and exploded argument for the necessary existence of a Supreme Being. Law, as we take it, means simply uniformity of action, and if we were to draw such an argument from it we should be rather inclined to go to the exceptions than to the rule itself—the irregularities, for which we cannot account, rather than to that uniform action which has been known ever since the "time" we know of existed.

The philosophy of the Infinite is perhaps a strange subject to introduce into a Harveian Oration, but, putting that on one side, we may do well to quote the following section of the address on a cognate subject :—

"So, too, of eternity. I make bold to say in this place that the man who talks of the eternity of matter knows not of what he speaks. It is a question that human reason cannot grasp, that logic cannot reach. One thing, however, comes out very clearly in the argument, which might almost have been predicated of the dictum when evolved out of the finite human understanding. Every speculation tacitly assumes a beginning for this evolution of matter. Eternity counts no beginning in its history! History, indeed, it knows not; duration is not of it; it is ever the same; a thousand years and a thousandth part of a second are just alike in that calendar; the limits of time and space are unknown; the present, the finite, the tangible, can scarcely be regarded as fragments of that great unfathomable abyss."

Next follows a passage referring to that curious dispute between Tyndall and Bastian with regard to the origin of life. Dr. Barclay does not, however, though drawing some useful lessons from it, impress that one which, to our mind, has always been the most appropriate and most important—this, namely: that when a man accustomed to examine into uniformly acting laws, such as Dr. Barclay elsewhere alludes to, turns his attention to biological phenomena, he is more likely to be deceived than one who deals with phenomena apparently subject to no laws except those which are liable to vary from an infinite number of unknown causes.

Suddenly there comes a break in Dr. Barclay's Oration. He goes at once to Harvey and his relations to the College, and we cannot but commend the bold, clear, and outspoken language of the speaker when referring to the bygone days of the College, and the risks that are yet to be encountered. Harvey wanted, and eagerly laboured to accomplish his wish, to make the College of Physicians the centre of all medical knowledge in this country. What his aim came to we all know, but Dr. Barclay does well to speak a word in favour of the spirit which now animates the majority of the Fellows of the College. We quote again :—

"It must be confessed that until recently his hopeful anticipations have not been realised, for a narrow and exclusive jealousy grew up in place of the large-hearted sympathy which he had hoped would guide the steps of the Fellows of the College. It was not until the fatal Act of 1815 brought the certain Nemesis of overweening pride in the general lowering of the status of the profession, that anyone seemed to think that a nobler future might be in store for the College. It had become little better than a gossiping club for Oxford and Cambridge graduates in medicine, with the select few whom they admitted into the Fellowship.

"The origin of all this is not far to seek. The first failure lies at the door of the older universities of this kingdom. I will not venture to inquire how all the trusts placed in their hands have been discharged, but there can be no doubt that one of the most sacred—the encouragement of the study of medicine—has not had in times past the fostering care of either *Alma Mater*. Harvey himself left Cambridge to study in Italy, and from that day forward so little has that branch of science been regarded, that foundations set apart for its advancement have been awarded wholly on account of other distinctions, even to men who never opened a book on medicine and the allied sciences. It is true, indeed, that the English character has developed in her public schools and universities in a way that seemed to defy all antecedent probability—that the majority of those who have passed through the curriculum bear in after-life the hall-stamp of gentlemen, and that a few have distinguished themselves as critical scholars or as pioneers in the path of scientific research. For teaching purposes beyond the limits of classical and mathematical study, the English universities were for long ages practically without resource. Medicine seemed to a certain extent to be secured by the foundation of professorships, fellowships, and scholarships; but in the general lethargy it failed to awake any enthusiasm in England, and Edinburgh stands pre-eminent as the teacher that first drew away students from the foreign universities. The titular M.D. of Oxford and Cambridge necessarily sank in general estimation, while the graduates arrogated to themselves the rights and privileges conferred by the charter of the College.

"From such a state of languor and depression a reaction was unavoidable. Outside the College, a strong phalanx of medical practitioners arose; inside the College, many a keen-sighted observer foresaw the doom which awaits exclusive mediocrity. Measures to stop the advancing tide have been eagerly grasped. Much has of late been done to raise the status of the profession; but at the present moment no prophetic eye can clearly discern the issue. So long as scientific workers are content to labour in a field where the hire is so small and the fruit so slow in its growth, increase of knowledge must be gained; progress must be made. But whether practical medicine is to drift into a trade in which the breath of popularity alone raises a man above his fellows, or is to mount into that position in which the esteem of those competent to judge shall be the only portal to eminence, who can say? It is for the younger Fellows of this College to choose which path they will follow."

We have, however, said enough to indicate the line of the Orator's address. Space forbids us to enter into his discussion of Darwinism and Listerism, though both will well repay perusal. We have, however, said enough to indicate that the Harveian Oration of 1881 is inferior to none of its predecessors in its originality of thought and manner, and certainly not as regards conventionality.

ACUTE MILIARY TUBERCULOSIS.

THE various clinical phases, under which miliary tuberculosis presents itself, is no doubt the reason why its diagnosis cannot often be made with the same accuracy and certainty as that of many other diseases. For it is only in a certain number of cases that the diagnosis is possible; while, on the other hand, it is frequently mistaken for some other malady.

Dr. Heitler contributes an interesting and instructive article on this subject to our Vienna contemporary, the *Wiener Medizinische Wochenschrift*, No. 20. Guided by clinical symptoms, he divides the cases into five chief groups. The first, from the nature of the most prominent symptoms, he calls the typhoid form. The second, from the fact that the membranes of the brain and cord chiefly suffer, he calls the cerebro-spinal form. Very frequently the tuberculosis shows itself as a capillary bronchitis, the sufferers dying of asphyxia; this he calls the "asphyctic" form. In a certain number of other cases, the effects are due to the localisation of the disease on the serous membranes, and then the symptoms are those of inflammation of these membranes: this may therefore be called the tubercular form; while, in a given proportion of cases, the presence of the tubercles gives rise to so few symptoms that this variety merits the name of latent tuberculosis. The localisation of tubercle in the liver, the spleen, or the kidneys does not generally lead to any very well marked symptoms; sometimes a little albumen is present in the urine, sometimes there may be acute nephritis. Rigal last year published a case of miliary tuberculosis which presented all the symptoms of a parenchymatous nephritis, but the kidneys were found to be quite free from tubercles. The most common varieties are the typhoid, the "asphyctic," and the cerebro-spinal.

As regards the typhoid form, Dr. Heitler holds that cases of general tuberculosis occur, which present all the symptoms and run the course of typhoid fever. The temperature curves correspond, and may either be high throughout with very slight morning decrease, or even imitate those abnormalities for which typhoid is remarkable so as to be indistinguishable from it. There may be nothing unusual in the relation of the pulse to the temperature; and even a slight diffused catarrh of the lungs, with swelling of the spleen, tympanitic abdomen, diarrhœa, and roseolous rash, may still further complicate, instead of helping to clear up, the diagnosis. Moreover, the absence of roseola in many cases of typhoid is well known. The presence of slight apex dulness, under such circumstances, would not add much real information; for individuals with lung mischief at the apices are in no way exempt from typhoid fever. Under such conditions, the diagnosis is a matter of great difficulty, even when one can observe the case for two or three weeks, and it becomes one of almost impossibility when, as is usual, one's observation is limited to a shorter period.

The history of the case may, in many cases, raise a suspicion of tuberculosis; while the seemingly typical symptoms of typhoid, on the other hand, for a while incline one to the latter diagnosis. There are other cases in which the difficulty is soon cleared up by the appearance of certain symptoms which indicate the implication of special organs—the brain, for instance; or in yet other cases the lungs become implicated. Again, irregular symptoms in some cases almost exclude typhoid fever—such as abnormal temperature, early dyspnœa, either with or without cyanosis, and with or without appreciable lung changes, or, at all events, without any changes which would account for the dyspnœa. The early appearance of anæmia, such as is not common in typhoid, would speak in favour of tuberculosis. The history of wasting some time previous to the onset of the acute symptoms, would suggest tuberculosis rather than typhoid.

Continued irregularity of temperature, with an increasing frequency of pulse, with increasing dyspnœa and cyanosis, are all symptoms in favour of tuberculosis, and against typhoid.

The "asphyctic" variety of tuberculosis is, according to Dr. Heitler, one of the most common forms of the disease. In many cases the symptoms prevent any chance of mistaking the disease. Clinically they present themselves as those of a bronchitis extending into the minutest ramifications of the tubes, giving rise to severe constitutional disturbance, which points clearly to the seat, and probable source, of the malady. The outbreak of the acute disease is usually preceded by a prodromal stage, during which an indefinite feeling of illness, gastric disturbance, frequent and purposeless vomiting, rapid emaciation, cough, hoarseness, sometimes hæmoptysis, irregular fever, or regular intermittent fever, may be present. The early onset of dyspnœa would probably lead to a suspicion of tuberculosis in cases which otherwise much resembled typhoid, and the doubt would soon be set at rest by the occurrence of lung symptoms.

Further, if the history affords any reliable suggestions of tuberculosis, such as hereditary tendency, or if there is apical dulness, or if scrofulous scars are present, then the diagnosis is materially strengthened. On the other hand, it is well to remember that acute tuberculosis may attack those in whom none of the aforementioned points are to hand, and who appear to be in the most blooming health.

The onset of cerebro-spinal tuberculosis does not usually present the same or any difficulties. Sometimes the symptoms are not very apparent; on the other hand, in cases of general tuberculosis, with affection of the meninges, the symptoms often point solely to the brain. Tuberculosis of the spinal cord does not seem to occur as a separate disease, or else it occurs but very seldom, or perhaps its symptoms are not clearly recognised.

In the tuberculosis of the serous membranes (pleura and pericardium) we refer, of course, to the cases of primary acute disease, and not to those forms where there is a general scrofulous affection, and in which the tuberculosis follows on the resorption of a large quantity of exudation into their respective cavities. Such cases are undoubtedly very rare, and the opportunity of making differential studies is consequently wanting. As important points to remember, however, and as aids to diagnosis, may be mentioned a certain want of connexion between the local and the general conditions at the very commencement of the disease—intense dyspnœa and cyanosis, even before the exudation has attained any considerable height, a rapid increase in its quantity, with early collapse.

There is not much to say about what Dr. Heitler calls the latent form of the disease. The patients become greatly prostrated, and waste unaccountably, without there being any objective signs of disease. There may be a little occasional rise of temperature or not, with or without bronchial catarrh. Thus the diagnosis is very uncertain, and its rectitude cannot be verified during life.

Dr. Senator contributes to the *Berliner Klinische Wochenschrift*, No. 25, an article bearing on this subject, in which he relates a case of acute miliary tuberculosis that during life was supposed to be typhoid fever. The patient was a man aged forty-eight, who, three years before coming under observation, had gone through a severe attack of typhoid. During its third week a very stubborn and intractable hiccough came on, which lasted eight days. There had also been attacks of epistaxis, with hawking up of blood-stained mucus from the posterior nares; but he quite recovered. He subsequently broke his arm, and again recovered without further trouble. His last illness commenced, about five weeks before he came under Dr. Senator's care, with slight shiverings, malaise, depression, and dyspnœa, which obliged him to keep his bed for a few days. When taken into the hospital he was observed to be a fairly well-built man, well nourished, without cachexia, and with a good family history. There were no abnormalities in the circulatory or respiratory apparatus. After some days the spleen was felt to be enlarged, and several roseola spots showed themselves; then epistaxis came on, and some pulmonary catarrh also; and later, hiccough and slight deafness. About three weeks after admission some inflammation and suppuration occurred over and about the left parotid gland, sanious and fœtid pus being discharged. The temperature varied from 100° to 104° Fahr. The patient then died. In view of the enlargement of spleen, the fever, and the roseola, a diagnosis of typhoid was made. The man, it is true, had once before passed through an attack of typhoid, but authentic cases are recorded where an individual may have the disease twice. Moreover, the occurrence of epistaxis and hiccough (which were marked symptoms during the first attack) occurred during his last illness. Finally, the occurrence of a suppurative parotitis seemed to favour the typhoid view. But at the autopsy, not only were there no appearances of typhoid,—there were not even any traces of the previous attack. On the other hand, there was a general tuberculosis of both lungs, with enlargement of the bronchial glands. The spleen, the liver, and both kidneys were also tuberculous.

Dr. Heitler's paper is interesting in a negative way; while Dr. Senator's case is doubtless one of great rarity, though not entirely unique. But they show in a practical manner the difficulties which beset the practitioner in the recognition of a disease at once common, intractable, and fatal.

REPORT OF THE METROPOLITAN BOARD OF WORKS FOR THE YEAR 1880.

THE matters over which this Board exercises its jurisdiction are of the most varied description. On it devolve directly the drainage and sewerage of the whole metropolitan district, the prevention of floods and extinction of fires, the improvement of thoroughfares and of unhealthy areas, the care of the bridges and the preservation of open spaces; while it exerts a control over buildings in general, the means of locomotion, street-lighting and water-supply, offensive and dangerous trades, cowsheds and dairies, the contagious diseases of animals, and the protection of infant life, so far as attained by the registration of "baby farms."

With some of these we have no greater concern than other citizens, but several have so direct a bearing on the public health that it behoves us as sanitarians to watch closely the conduct of so powerful a body, and to point out any mistakes or shortcomings we may detect.

The general impression left after a perusal of this report is certainly a favourable one. We shall not attempt to criticise the financial aspects of such transactions as the freeing of the bridges, etc., believing that the members of the Board have in all such questions acted to the best of their judgments. It is only to their half-hearted acceptance of the 33rd Section of the Metropolitan Streets Improvement Bill of 1877 that we take grave exception. They complain bitterly of this clause, which requires that whenever such improvement involves the demolition of fifteen or more houses occupied by the labouring classes, a sufficient accommodation shall be provided in the vicinity for the persons about to be unhoused. They pray for a relaxation of this rule, which, they argue, paralyses their action in nearly every instance, since they can seldom begin the improvement without pulling down so many houses tenanted mainly by the poor, while the suspense in which the owners and occupiers are kept during the delay brings the Board into undeserved unpopularity. We cannot, however, help thinking that the difficulty is greatly exaggerated, and that the real explanation is to be found in their unwillingness to let ground already cleared on unremunerative terms. Indeed, they admit as much when, on page 32, they describe the letting of a certain plot on a building lease at 2½ per cent. as a loss of half the outlay. One of the schemes which they adduce as arrested by this condition is the much needed widening of Gray's-inn-road; but we cannot see why ample provision for the present inhabitants of Baldwin's-gardens and the neighbouring courts could not be provided in the now vacant ground along Theobald's-road, though it might be more profitably let for shops and warehouses. We would appeal to philanthropists of all kinds to support the Home Secretary in resisting this narrow-minded and £ s. d. complaint. Wide and handsome streets are greatly to be desired, but we must urge that they should not be obtained at the cost of increasing the overcrowding which is already a disgrace to our boasted wealth and civilisation, and a source of untold misery, disease, and crime. If valuable property be once erected on sites hitherto covered by dilapidated tenements, the golden opportunity of providing decent habitations for the London poor will have passed by, never to return.

The inadequacy of the present main drainage system to carry off the occasional heavy rainfalls, not only in the low-lying districts of East London and Westminster, but also in Kentish Town and Holloway, has determined the Board to supplement it by a number of new sewers and storm relief lines at an estimated cost of £708,000, and they are preparing to carry out the provisions of the Thames River Prevention of Floods Act of 1879, by causing the walls of wharves and river frontage to be sufficiently raised to prevent further overflow.

The charge brought against the Board by the Conservators of the Thames, of causing, by their main drainage outfalls, the formation of certain banks in the Barking and Halfway Reaches, has been rebutted by the inquiries of a joint commission, who have come to the conclusion that the said deposits are partly the alluvium incidental to any large river, partly the result of the dredging required to keep the channels of navigation open, and only in small part formed of sewage matters held in suspension in the tidal waters.

The Board congratulate the ratepayers of London on the failure of Sir R. Cross's Water Companies Bill, pointing out the extravagant compensation which would have been made to the companies proposed to be bought up, and express a hope that ere long a more satisfactory arrangement may be reached. They remark that five only of the existing companies have even partially provided a constant supply, no notice of such intention having been made by the Grand Junction, Chelsea, or Southwark and Vauxhall.

Under the head of cattle diseases they report 383 cases of pleuro-pneumonia, and 92 of swine typhoid, all of which were slaughtered or died; and 626 of foot-and-mouth disease, of which 1 died and 13 were killed, the rest having recovered or were progressing favourably. The increase in the number of cases of glanders and farcy during the last few years calls for special notice—in 1877-78-79-80, the cases reported having been 486, 571, 997, and 1806 respectively. Whether the prevalence of this grave disease, as dangerous to man as to the horse, has actually doubled since 1879, or whether greater vigilance only in its detection can explain these figures, demands careful inquiry.

The provisions of the Cowsheds Order of 1879 have been rigorously enforced. Already nearly three hundred of the worst sheds have been abolished, and many others improved. The number of private slaughter-houses has been gradually reduced from 1429 in 1874 to 903 in 1880, and during the last year no new ones have been sanctioned.

The number of houses registered under the Infant Life Protection Act has been reduced to twenty-three ; and the Board, in reply to a communication from the Home Secretary, have suggested several amendments, the most important of which are that the operation of the Act be extended to infants under five years instead of one, and to the keeping for hire of any number, i.e., of even one ; also that parents shall not be relieved of their responsibilities in respect of their infant children by the payment of sums of money to other persons for adopting them. The expediency of these amendments is only too obvious.

THE WEEK.

TOPICS OF THE DAY.

THE Whitechapel District Board of Works have recently had under discussion the large displacements of the population which have been caused by the improvements and clearances of the Metropolitan Board, and the railway and dock companies. In Whitechapel alone the Metropolitan Board of Works have condemned areas giving accommodation to 8000 persons, half of whom have already been evicted. The remainder cling to the dwellings which, thus marked for removal, are fast falling into decay, and are without the commonest provisions for the preservation of decency and health. On a report to this effect being submitted by the local sanitary inspector, the Survey Committee took steps to assure themselves of its correctness, and the reality proved far worse than the description given. In many of the places visited there was neither ventilation nor light, and health, decency, and modesty were impossibilities. The Committee of Survey found that paraffin lamps were necessarily kept burning at noon in the month of June in the rooms where the people not only lived, but worked, slept, and died. Spaces on the bare floors of some of these hovels were let for nightly accommodation, and both sexes, without discrimination, paid for the privilege of sleeping on the bare boards. Major Munro, representative of Whitechapel at the Metropolitan Board of Works, denied that the overcrowding had been increased by the clearances of the Metropolitan Board. Four thousand persons, he said, had been removed from the condemned Whitechapel areas, and the Census return showed that the population of the district had been correspondingly reduced. To a very large extent these people had sought accommodation in the suburbs, where rents were low, and to which access had been made easy by cheap trains. Ultimately the Board ordered the report of the sanitary officer to be forwarded to the Metropolitan Board of Works for their information.

At a recent meeting of the Select Committee of the House of Commons engaged in considering the working of the Artisans' and Labourers' Dwellings Improvement Act, Dr. Tidy, Medical Officer of Health for Islington, was examined, and, in reply to Sir Richard Cross, stated that he had made three representations to the Metropolitan Board of Works for improvement schemes in Angel-court, Little Pierrepont. road, and Essex-road. In the Angel-court representation there were seventy-eight houses affected, with a population of 504 people. The condition of the place had been exceedingly bad ; in fact, the premises were almost falling to pieces. There was no possibility of dealing with the houses unless under an improvement scheme. He might have done something under Mr. Torrens' Act, but he preferred to submit a scheme to the Board of Works. There was practically no valuable property mentioned in the representation, and as for the population, it consisted principally of Irish costermongers and a large number of people who sold

newspapers in the street. Epidemic diseases in these parts were especially virulent. There was no special reason why the people should live there. At present three out of the seven courts were empty, and in the others notices that the people were to clear out within a certain period had been put up. These might be dealt with in several ways, but it seemed to him desirable that they should be dealt with, if possible, by a scheme, and therefore he made them the subject of a representation. The Essex-road scheme was a larger one, the number of the population affected being 1052. Many of the houses in this case were in a very bad condition, and even before the scheme was proceeded with many of the houses were shut up by the magistrates. There were some model dwelling-houses in the district, in Peabody-square, and he had reason to believe that the death-rate in those houses was not much greater, or much less, than elsewhere in the neighbourhood. After Dr. Tidy's evidence was concluded, some other persons were examined.

Lord Dorchester recently presided at a meeting of the Council of the Society for the Prevention of Street Accidents and Dangerous Driving. An official document laid before the meeting showed that during the first complete year of the Society's operations there had been, for the first time, an actual diminution in the number of fatal street accidents resulting from vehicles. A communication was read from the Chief Commissioner of the Metropolitan Police on the subject of " crawling cabs," the Commissioner observing that he did not wonder at the number of these noted in the streets; but the police could not help it, as some of the magistrates declined to enforce the law. The Chairman expressed an opinion that the matter was one which ought to be at once brought under the notice of Parliament ; and it was ultimately decided that the representatives of the metropolitan constituencies should be asked to attend the next meeting of the Council.

The latest communication on the subject of the papers on the subject of the Islington Small-pox Camp Hospital may, we suppose, be regarded as official, or, at any rate, as " communicated." It refers to the " considerable amount of alarm " caused in Finchley, Edmonton, and the surrounding localities by the statement that the newly opened Islington camp hospital for small-pox patients is within four hundred yards of inhabited houses, and that there may be danger of infection from the sewage matter of the camp escaping into an open brook close by; and then asserts, " on the authority of the Superintendent of the Sanitary Department of the Islington Vestry," that the new camp hospital is three-quarters of a mile from Colney Hatch Asylum, and that there are a few houses, not in blocks, but built here and there, about a quarter of a mile from the camp. A long distance down the road at Fortis Green is the nearest block of inhabited houses. The Superintendent adds that " for all sanitary purposes the camp is, as it were, on a common. It is enclosed, in no place comes within a hundred feet of other people's land, and there are three acres of land between it and the road. For drainage of the sewage the Vestry are using seventeen acres of land, without reference to the brook referred to, which will not be in any way utilised, and the system of earth-closets is also adopted. Only a few patients have been as yet received, but there will be accommodation for 128 eventually. Seventeen tents or marquees have been pitched, and of these eight are hospital tents, each containing sixteen beds. A disinfecting chamber of the best kind has also been constructed."

We have received the forty-sixth annual report of the British Medical Benevolent Fund for the year 1880, and are glad to find that the Fund is progressing satisfactorily. The number of the annuitants was forty-seven, and the donation department was able, during the year under notice, to make 148 grants to urgent cases. One of the most pleasing features of this charity is its inexpensive working; there are no salaries, and no office expenses, so that donors and subscribers have the satisfaction of knowing that the whole of their contributions, less a perfectly insignificant sum for the most necessary items, such as printing and postage, go to the relief of the most deserving cases. Another distinguishing feature of the Fund is that applicants for aid are put to the least possible trouble and expense, and they are not required to make public their distress by canvassing. For these reasons alone it is deserving of the utmost recognition at the hands of the profession and the public, and we most willingly commend it to the attention of those of our readers who like to do good in an unostentatious and thoroughly effective manner. We may add that Dr. W. H. Broadbent, 34, Seymour-street, Portman-square, W., is the honorary treasurer.

Up to Wednesday evening last about £25,000 had been paid in at the Mansion House to the credit of the Hospital Sunday Fund. This is stated to be nearly £2000 in excess of the amount received during a corresponding number of days in 1880. We still doubt, however, judging by the experience of former years, whether the mysteriously settled limit of £30,000 will be much exceeded upon the present occasion. Amongst some of the larger contributions may be mentioned St. Peter's, Eaton-square, £479; St. Stephen's, Westbourne-park, £402; St. Paul's, Onslow-square, £331; St. Paul's, Wilton-place, £250; All Saints, Knightsbridge, £211; Holy Trinity, Paddington, £182, etc.

At a recent meeting of the Health Committee of the Liverpool City Council, it was stated that the medical officer had received the official statement of the population of the city from the Registrar-General. The total population had been ascertained to be 552,425. Of these 210,161 were in the parish of Liverpool, and 342,264 in the out-townships. In 1871 the population of Liverpool was 492,935; there has thus been an increase of 59,490 in the ten years.

THE TROUBLES OF THE METROPOLITAN ASYLUMS BOARD.

At the fortnightly meeting of the Metropolitan Asylums Board, held on Saturday last, a letter was read from the Thames Conservancy Board, sanctioning the mooring of the *Endymion* close to the *Atlas* at Deptford, but stating that both vessels must be removed as soon as the present epidemic of small-pox is over. Considerable discussion ensued on this subject, during which it was stated that the site was not selected by the Asylums Board, but by the Local Government Board. Sir E. Hay Currie observed that he had a very great objection to the small-pox hospital-ship being moored at Deptford, and thought it ought to be stationed lower down the river. The vessel would be ready for the reception of patients on the 7th inst. After some debate, and with the view of relieving themselves of the responsibility of the selection of the site, it was resolved to inform the Local Government Board that the Managers would proceed to have the vessels moored off Deptford Creek unless any objection the Local Government Board might have was immediately communicated. The Darenth Committee had experienced the greatest difficulty in getting any wharf or place suitable for the embarcation of patients, but premises on the north side of the Thames, nearly opposite Greenwich pier, had at last been obtained from the Thames and Channel Steamship Company. A communication was next read from the Guardians of the City of London, declining to sell the Holloway Workhouse for use as a small-pox hospital; and one of the Managers remarked that the Board encountered the same difficulties wherever

they went, and unless the Local Government Board acted with a high hand they would never get a place for a small-pox hospital. The City Guardians had resolved to sell the workhouse; but the moment it was known for what purpose it was to be used, they refused to part with it. It was stated that, during the fortnight ended June 24, 653 patients had been admitted to the asylums; the deaths had been 113, and 559 persons had been discharged; the numbers now under treatment were 1030, together with 538 convalescents, making a total of 1568, as compared with 1680 for the previous fortnight. Sir E. H. Currie then proposed—"That application be made to the Local Government Board to authorise the Managers to purchase two sites, in the north and south of the metropolis respectively, whereon to erect administrative blocks to form the nucleus of hospitals for the accommodation, in huts, tents, or otherwise, of convalescent patients in times of epidemic. That, upon the consent of the Local Government Board being obtained to this proposal, the General Purposes Committee be empowered to take such steps as may be necessary for giving effect thereto." This was going rather too fast for these active and much-maligned Managers; and, after some discussion, the matter was referred to the General Purposes Committee "for consideration and report."

ASSASSINATION OF A MEDICAL OFFICER OF A LUNATIC ASYLUM.

While Dr. Marchant, Director of the Lunatic Asylum near Toulouse, was paying his daily visit, one of the patients, a captain, going behind the doctor, discharged at him a revolver which he had managed to conceal on his person when admitted, about three weeks before, for the form of insanity known as *délire des persécutions*. Dr. Marchant expired in the course of the night.

THE RIGHT HON. W. H. SMITH, M.P., AT CHARING-CROSS HOSPITAL.

The Right Hon. W. H. Smith, M.P., recently presided at the distribution of prizes at the Charing-cross Hospital Medical School. After congratulating all who took an interest in the School, in the Hospital, and in the advance of science and education in London, the right hon. gentleman remarked that the cause of medical education was also very much the cause of charity. It seemed to him that the character of the medical profession was much influenced by the fact that the young men who entered it had, at a time of life when their impressions were the strongest and their characters most easily formed, to devote a large portion of their energies to the relief of the sick and suffering poor. They were responsible often for the lives, the health, and the happiness of large numbers of persons, and in the discharge of their duty they did not wait to weigh the risk to their own lives. Devotion to duty was a motive which must influence the conduct of every man or woman who would pass to the grave honoured and revered. But for the assistance of medical men, many persons doing good work in the world would have their careers of power and usefulness prematurely cut short. Just as that lawyer was said to be the best lawyer who kept his clients out of court, so, he conceived, that physician was the best who kept his patients from bringing upon themselves all the misfortunes and disasters which prevailing carelessness and recklessness would bring upon them. It was hardly possible to exaggerate the importance of medical men to the happiness of the family and of society. If he was a gentleman in feeling and instincts, and thoroughly realised his responsibility, he was sure to be honoured, in however humble a neighbourhood his residence might be fixed. No one exercised a greater influence on the progress of society. He did not even except the clergyman, great though the latter's influence for good was. He said this, because there seemed to be an impression abroad amongst medical men that their position was not properly recognised. It depended, of course, very much upon the man himself whether he should be regarded as the equal of the first gentleman in the land, or should be considered of little account. But a man who acted on the motives he had mentioned was sure to be an honour to his profession and to be properly appreciated by the world.

MEDICAL EDUCATION IN INDIA.

THE Lahore Medical School, to judge from the report of the year 1879-80, is rendering excellent service in training native youths of the North-Western Provinces and Punjaub for the medical profession. The *Indian Medical Gazette* notes that the English class numbered sixty-eight, of whom forty-eight remained at the close of the session. Eleven completed their five years of study, passed their final examination, and entered the service of Government as assistant-surgeons. The Hindustani class numbered 140, of whom ninety remained; twenty-one were passed out after having been examined and found qualified. Fifteen of the recently passed assistant-surgeons on the Punjaub establishment volunteered for special duty with the Kabul forces, and did good service in base-hospitals and on the several lines of communication. Four women who attended lectures on midwifery for three years, passed a final examination in that subject with credit.

THE WARNEFORD ASYLUM.

THE Warneford Asylum at Oxford is a charity which has for its special object to supply suitable accommodation to insane persons belonging to the middle and upper classes of society, who are not paupers, but may be too poor to bear unaided the necessary expenses of insanity. Recent extensive additions have been made to the buildings on the female side of the Asylum, but most of the accommodation thus provided is still vacant. "If the institution were more extensively known," say the visiting Commissioners in Lunacy, "we doubt not that applications for admission would be more numerous than could be met." As soon as the finances of the Asylum will permit, the male department of the Asylum is also to be enlarged. During the year 1880, seventy-seven patients were under care and treatment in the Asylum, and amongst forty-eight of these £1207 was distributed in charitable aid of maintenance, giving on the average £25 to each recipient of relief. But, of course, all patients treated in the Asylum participated to some extent in the benefits of the charity, being kept at a much cheaper rate than would have been possible but for the bequest out of which the buildings were erected, and the endowment fund, which yields upwards of £2000 of revenue, out of which many establishment charges are defrayed. Dr. Bywater Ward is in medical charge of the Warneford Asylum,

THE PARIS WEEKLY RETURN.

THE number of deaths for the twenty-fourth week, ending June 16, 1881, was 1047 (viz., 568 males and 479 females), and among these there were from typhoid fever 17, small-pox 16, measles 13, scarlatina 9, pertussis 13, diphtheria and croup 52, dysentery 1, erysipelas 13, puerperal infections 3, and acute tubercular meningitis 54. There were also 27 deaths from acute bronchitis, 61 from pneumonia, 90 from infantile athrepsia (36 of the infants having been wholly or partially suckled), and 34 violent deaths. The diminution in the number of deaths for the twenty-third week (1098)

is of importance, as bearing upon epidemic diseases, all of which have considerably diminished with the exception of diphtheria. As indicating a change in manners, it is noticeable that the civil funerals have been 16 per cent. of the entire number, varying from 1 in 10 to 3 in 10 in different arrondissements. The births for the week amounted to 1055, viz., 555 males (394 legitimate and 161 illegitimate) and 500 females (380 legitimate and 120 illegitimate); 78 children (45 males and 33 females) were born dead or died within twenty-four hours.

SCARLET FEVER CONVALESCENT HOMES.

ON Monday last an influential meeting was held at the Mansion House to promote the establishment of a Scarlet Fever Convalescent Home. We have before this drawn attention in our columns to the effort being made to provide a home for patients convalescent from scarlet fever, and we are glad to see the matter has now been so well and prominently placed before the public. Of the many homes open for the convalescent sick poor, none take in patients recovering from infectious disorders; and no sufferers are more in need of pure air, good food, and well-warmed and well-ventilated houses than are the convalescent from scarlet fever, both for their own sakes and for the sake of the public. A few people have formed themselves into a provisional committee, with the view of arousing public interest, and of promoting the establishment of at any rate one home for such convalescents. Sir Rutherford Alcock and the Earl of Aberdeen proposed—"That in view of the great mortality from scarlet fever in the metropolis, and the spread of infection from patients in various stages of convalescence, especially among the working-classes, where isolation from the healthy is impossible, the establishment of convalescent homes for such cases is of the greatest importance, as a means of checking the spread of infection, and as an aid to the more rapid recovery of the patients themselves; and the meeting pledges itself to promote the establishment of such homes"; and this was carried unanimously. Sir E. H. Currie and Dr. Andrew Clark moved the appointment of a committee, headed by the Lord Mayor, to carry out this object; and Dr. A. Clark observed that every medical man was painfully well acquainted with the need of such homes. A medical council was appointed to advise on all medical and sanitary matters; and Sir Risdon Bennett, Sir Joseph Fayrer, Dr. Brewer, and others, spoke in warm approval of the project. We trust it will meet with hearty and general support.

INTERNATIONAL MEDICAL AND SANITARY EXHIBITION.

THE Committee engaged in organising the Exhibition to be held at South Kensington on and after July 16, have agreed to set apart a considerable space for the purpose of illustrating the various appliances in ordinary use for the treatment of the sick at the chief London hospitals. Their request to exhibit a bed with its full equipment of ward furniture, along with splints or other apparatus in common use for fractured limbs at each hospital, has been readily acceded to by the governing committees of the twelve hospitals associated with medical schools, as well as by the Medical Departments of the Army and Navy and Local Government Board. It had been felt that although the surgical appliances referred to would be best shown on the living model, it would have been unwise to introduce such in a miscellaneous exhibition, and considerable difficulty has been experienced in providing efficient substitutes, since lay figures are expensive and unobtainable in sufficient number from commercial sources; while the papier maché figures in common use in shops are without joints, and are otherwise ill adapted for the purpose indicated. This difficulty has now been surmounted by the result of an appeal made to several members of the Royal Academy for the loan of their lay figures during the time the Exhibition is open. Sir F. Leighton, Messrs. Millais, Calderon, Leslie, Frith, Yeames, etc.—in fact, all the leading academicians—have responded so readily to the request made to them that the number of applicants for relief considerably exceeds the number of beds at the disposal of the Committee. It is proposed to have the hospital appliances arranged in saloons in the Albert Hall, contiguous to and in direct communication with the Exhibition buildings, and it may be confidently predicted that the department, which will possess a scientific and humanitarian interest apart from the character of the rest of the Exhibition, will prove especially attractive to foreign and country visitors, who will thus have an opportunity of seeing within small compass what is done at the best hospitals, without having to make a tour of the metropolis.

THE NEW ST. MARYLEBONE INFIRMARY.

On Wednesday, June 29, the Prince and Princess of Wales opened the new infirmary buildings at Notting-hill for pauper patients of the parish of St. Marylebone. This is the latest-built of the sick asylums erected under the provisions of the Gathorne Hardy Act of 1867; and, owing to the great difficulty and cost of obtaining a suitable site in the parish itself, has been erected at the western extremity of the Ladbroke-grove-road. The buildings are arranged on the pavilion plan in the form of blocks, communicating with each other by covered ways. Each ward contains twenty-eight beds, and has a cubic capacity of 24,192 feet, or 864 cubic feet per bed. All the arrangements seem to be excellent; all necessary appliances have been liberally supplied; and the water-supply is obtained from an artesian well sunk on the premises to a depth of 500 feet, of which 211 feet are in the chalk. A supply reckoned at 4600 gallons per hour of pure and excellent water will be thus obtained; and in this respect the sick poor of St. Marylebone will be better off than the ratepayers. The Infirmary will accommodate 700 persons. The medical staff consists of a resident superintendent, an assistant medical officer, and a dispenser; and the nursing is entrusted to a staff of nurses under the Nightingale system. The night-nursing is but scantily provided for, as there is to be only one head night-nurse for the whole building, with one night-nurse for each pavilion. An address was read to the Prince of Wales, who made a felicitous reply; and the Infirmary having been declared open, the Royal party made the tour of the buildings. One of the male wards was named "Alexandra" by the Princess of Wales, and one of the female wards "Albert Edward" by the Prince of Wales.

SOCIAL SCIENCE CONGRESS: DUBLIN MEETING, 1881.

The Committee for the Health Department met at the Mansion House, Dawson-street, Dublin, on Tuesday, June 28. The following were appointed Secretaries of the Department: —Charles A. Cameron, Esq., Ph.D., and Stewart Woodhouse, Esq., M.D. The following were nominated as Vice-Presidents of the Department, viz.:—The Hon. F. R. Falkiner, Recorder of Dublin; George Johnston, Esq., M.D., President of the King and Queen's College of Physicians in Ireland; Samuel Chaplin, Esq., President of the Royal College of Surgeons in Ireland; Thomas Wrigley Grimshaw, Esq., M.D., Registrar-General for Ireland; Charles Crokor King, Esq., M.D., Medical Commissioner of the Local Government Board for Ireland; and Edward Dillon Mapother, M.D., Consulting Medical Officer of Health for the City of Dublin. The following special questions were selected for discussion at the Congress, subject to the approval of the Standing Committee of the Department, namely:—1. "Is it desirable that there should be a system of Compulsory Notification of Infective Diseases? If so, what is the best method of carrying such a system into effect?" 2. "Is any further legislation desirable in order to more effectually prevent the Overcrowding of Dwelling-Houses?" 3. "Is it desirable that Hospitals should be placed under State Supervision?"

DEATH OF PROFESSOR HESCHL.

By the death of Richard L. Heschl, the successor of Rokitansky as Professor of Pathological Anatomy, the Vienna school has lost one of its ablest teachers. Born in 1824, and taking his degree in 1849, he became Rokitansky's assistant in 1850, continuing with him for four years. He was then appointed to professorships in succession at Olmütz, Cracow, and Graz, and finally became the successor of his celebrated master at Vienna in 1876. He attained great fame as a most successful teacher; but although a frequent contributor of articles on pathological anatomy to the leading medical journals, he produced no book since 1855, when his "Compendium of Pathological Anatomy" appeared.

THE SANITARY CONDITION OF THE ROMAN HOTELS.

The Italian Times Sanitary Commission is making steady progress with its inquiry into the sanitary condition of the hotels of Rome, though at one time it was threatened with serious opposition from a very unexpected quarter. A general meeting of the Italian Medical Society was summoned to discuss, among other subjects, "Measures to be taken in view of the arbitrary interference of certain foreign medical practitioners with the hygienic condition of the Roman hotels." This proposal appeared to be very absurd and uncalled for, for the hotel-keepers themselves welcomed this inquiry, and two of the most distinguished members of the Society, Drs. Manassei and Fiordespini, are members of the Sanitary Commission. However, in consequence apparently of a letter from Dr. Fiordespini, the proposed discussion was allowed to drop. But the Popolo Romano has published an article from an Italian physician, denying the right of foreign physicians to interfere with Roman sanitary questions, in which he tells a little story that shows how desirable it is that hotel-keepers in Rome should be supervised and educated in other matters besides questions of drainage, ventilation, and other structural defects. He says: "A short time since a Protestant clergyman attended a lady, one of his co-religionists, who died of typhoid fever in one of the principal hotels of Rome. The next day the same clergyman called on the Bishop of Gibraltar, who had just come to Rome, and had gone to lodge in the same hotel. To his great surprise, he found him occupying the very room in which the lady had died of typhoid fever the day before." The Italian Times remarks: "The Italian physician apparently sees nothing disquieting or improper in this." English visitors to Rome will take a very different view of it from that of the Italian physician, and it is to be hoped the Sanitary Commission will "make a note of it." It is very satisfactory, meanwhile, to learn that the Quirinale, Constanzi, Bristol, Europa, Molaro, Anglo-Americano, Parigi, Russie, and Victoria Hotels have already been inspected; and that the proprietors have in all cases expressed their willingness to carry out the reforms suggested. We are glad to learn, also, from the Italian Times of June 4, that the Municipal Council of Rome had just recently appointed a committee to examine and report upon the town drainage, especially with reference to the connexion between the hotel drains and the general system of sewers.

THE REGISTRAR-GENERAL OF SCOTLAND'S RETURN FOR THE FIRST QUARTER OF 1881.

DURING the quarter ended March 31, 1881, the number of births registered in Scotland was 30,860, which gives a birth-rate 0·166 per cent. less than the average of the corresponding quarter of the ten years immediately preceding, and equal to 3·33 per cent. of population. Of the eight principal towns, Paisley showed the highest, and Perth the lowest, proportion of births. For every ten thousand of estimated population the birth-rate was 394 in Paisley, 369 in Leith, 338 in Aberdeen, 318 in Greenock, 312 in Glasgow, 304 in Dundee, 298 in Edinburgh, and 280 in Perth. Of the 30,860 births, 2618, or 8·5 per cent., were illegitimate; the rate of illegitimacy showing highest in the mainland rural districts, and lowest in the large towns. During the whole quarter there were registered on an average 342·9 births per diem. The first three months of the present year proved fatal in Scotland to 21,284 persons, giving a death-rate which was 0·178 per cent. below the average of the ten preceding corresponding quarters, and constituting an annual proportion of 230 deaths to every ten thousand of estimated population. The lowest death-rate was recorded in Greenock, the highest in Paisley, so that the latter town was at the head for both increase and decrease of population. Zymotic diseases caused 1174 deaths in the three months under notice, or 13·9 per cent. of all deaths referred during the quarter to specified causes. Only 1 death from small-pox was recorded; it occurred in Dundee in January, in the case of a man aged thirty-seven, who is said to have been vaccinated, and who contracted the disease in London. The details respecting the weather during this quarter are somewhat singular. The unique characteristic of January, 1881, was the low mean temperature—lower than ever chronicled before for the same or for any other month. This remarkable cold was further accompanied by an equally remarkable and abnormal depth of snowfall, and that again characterised by terrific drifting and accumulation in special localities. Both cold and snow were the result of a terrestrial influence interfering with the direct rays of the sun, and have been more particularly traced up to an abnormal cyclone which entered Europe east of the North Cape, and came whirling down the Gulf of Bothnia, and thence across Sweden and Norway from a north-easterly path, so contrary to the south-west path of the regular West Indian and Atlantic cyclonic storms. February was distinguished by its coldness, its mean temperature being 4·1° lower than the average, and by a deficiency of westerly, and preponderance of easterly, winds, turning the rain, which was rather over-abundant as to quantity, into snow. The barometric pressure was less than the average. The cold of March was extreme, and was accompanied, or expressed, by heavy drifting snowstorms, for the wind was also in extra strength. The general direction of the wind was west.

ASYLUM CASUALTIES.

IN his thoughtful report, presented last January to the Committee of Visitors of the Hereford County Asylum, Dr. Chapman expresses his thankfulness that another year has passed without a death from homicidal or suicidal violence in the institution over which he presides. No instance of either has occurred in the Hereford County Asylum since its opening, and in this respect it probably stands alone amongst the county asylums of England. Good luck, no doubt, has had something to do, Dr. Chapman observes, with the immunity from serious misadventures which the Asylum has enjoyed, as no justifiable amount of precaution will secure absolute and permanent freedom from accidents in houses in which large numbers of lunatics of all classes are congregated together. Still, allowing for good luck, he thinks there is a considerable margin to be carried to the credit of the care and attention of the officers of the Asylum. It would not be fair also to leave out of account the cheerfulness of tone promoted by the frequency of the associated amusements in the Asylum—a cheerfulness of tone so difficult to obtain among a population, many of whom keenly feel the evils inseparable from their position, namely, loss of mental soundness, deprivation of liberty, and association with the insane.

MEDICAL PARLIAMENTARY AFFAIRS.

Poor-Law Medical Officers.—In the House of Commons, on Thursday, June 23, Mr. Dodson, in reply to Mr. Firth, said he could not lay on the table a copy of the correspondence between Mr. Hele, the district medical officer of Plomesgate Union, in respect of an accident to a boy whose leg had afterwards been amputated. The Board of Guardians had refused to pay the fee to which Mr. Hele was entitled under Article 177 of the General Consolidated Orders of 1847.

Dust-Carts.—Mr. Dodson, replying to Viscount Newport, said that he had no control over the vestries as regards the construction of their dust-carts, but he hoped the attention of the vestries would be directed to the complaint, and that they would be disposed to consider how far they could comply with the proposal to have covered dust-carts such as are used in some continental towns.

Militia Surgeons.—On Friday, June 24, Dr. Farquharson asked if the Government intended to grant compensation for loss of expectation of pensions to Militia surgeons who joined previous to the circular of 1854, and to other Militia surgeons for the loss of income incurred by recent changes, and especially by the withdrawal of fees for the examination of recruits.

The Opium Traffic.—On Monday, June 27, the Marquis of Hartington informed Sir W. Lawson that the principal recommendations of the Chief Commissioner of British Burmah with respect to the opium traffic had been carried out. The number of opium shops had been reduced from sixty-eight to twenty-seven, and the rates at which opium was supplied to the farmer, licensed vendor, and medical practitioner had been raised.

Small-pox.—Dr. Cameron said that after the notice of the Prime Minister in regard to the urgency of public business, he must either give up all opportunity of discharging a very urgent piece of public duty or move the adjournment of the House. He wished to call attention to the conduct of the Local Government Board in connexion with the small-pox epidemic. Since the beginning of the year there had been 1500 deaths from small-pox in London, and 9000 cases had occurred. On the appeal of Mr. T. Collins, Dr. Cameron said he would take his motion off the paper, and would postpone the motion for the adjournment of the House to some future day. He merely wished to get something done, as great loss of life had arisen from the refusal of the Local Government Board to exercise its powers.

Supply of Fish.—In reply to an inquiry, Sir J. McGarel Hogg said the Metropolitan Board of Works were fully sensible of the defects in the metropolitan fish-supply, and on Friday last they appointed a Committee to consider the subject and confer with the Home Secretary.

Coroners in Ireland.—The Coroners (Ireland) Bill, as amended, was considered, and read a third time.

Veterinary Surgeons.—In Committee of the House of Lords, on Tuesday, June 28, a new clause in the Veterinary Surgeons Bill was inserted, on the motion of the Earl of Camperdown, providing for examinations in Scotland. The Marquis of Salisbury proposed that the period of practice which should qualify for the profession of veterinary surgeons without examination should be reduced from five to three years. This was agreed to. A proposal of Lord Aberdare's to exempt veterinary surgeons from serving on juries was rejected. The remaining clauses were then agreed to.

Vaccination.—In the House of Commons, Mr. Dodson, in reply to Mr. P. H. Taylor, said that, so far from the child, F. M. Woodley, having died from exhaustion due to vaccination, the jury returned a verdict that the child died from natural causes. The medical man who gave evidence at the inquest stated that the vaccination had nothing whatever to do with the child's death.

SANITARY INSTITUTE OF GREAT BRITAIN.

At the ordinary meeting of the Sanitary Institute of Great Britain, held at 9, Conduit-street, on Tuesday, June 21, Dr. A. Carpenter in the chair, a paper was read by Professor W. H. Corfield, M.A., M.D., on "The Present State of the Sewage Question."

After some introductory remarks on the importance of removal of refuse matters, and the results of their non-removal as shown by the spread of black death, Oriental plague, cholera, and enteric fever, the entire depopulation of many ancient cities being doubtless due to such causes, and after pointing out that utilisation, though no doubt important, was a secondary matter, and indeed was what an athlete would call "a very bad second," the reader of the paper proceeded to consider the systems of sewage removal and treatment at present in use under the two heads of conservancy systems and water carriage.

In the former the refuse matters were either collected unmixed with anything else, or mixed with ashes, earth, etc. The first of these plans was now being adopted in several large towns, as Birmingham, Rochdale, etc., and it might be said to be the only successful one among the conservancy systems—it is certainly the only one from which a profit has been obtained. The manure in all the other plans is nearly valueless, and the results obtained by the Sewage Committee of the British Association show that the earth compost, after having been used in the closets six times, is only as rich as a good garden soil, and will not bear the cost of carriage.

After a summary of the results obtained by the conservancy systems, in which they were shown not to be solutions of the questions, especially as they leave the liquid sewage still to be treated, but in which it was admitted that under certain circumstances, as where it was necessary to reduce the bulk of the sewage, they might, with proper precautions, be adopted, the water carriage system was considered somewhat in detail; its advantages in the continuous removal of refuse from houses pointed out, its disadvantages shown not to be inherent in the system, but to be mistakes made in carrying it out, as, for instance, sewers pervious to water, or too large, or not ventilated, or without sufficient fall, or with a blocked outlet, or discharging into rivers, house draining not properly disconnected. The folly of turning surface waters, and, in many instances, even springs and streams, into sewers, and so increasing the difficulty of dealing with the sewage at the outfall, was insisted on. The various chemical processes for the treatment of sewage were passed in review, and all shown to be quite inadequate to cope with the difficulty, though some might be useful as preliminary aids to purification.

Filtration through soil and wide irrigation were next treated at some length, and the results obtained by them described. Certainly the sewage had been satisfactorily purified in many cases, the conditions for satisfactory purification in winter being that the sewage passes through the soil, and not merely over it. Crops of all kinds had been grown by means of it, and in soil that would otherwise bear nothing; and the British Association's Sewage Committee had shown that as great a percentage of the manurial constituents had been utilised as was, on an average, utilised of the best commercial manure. Although, for various reasons, it had seldom been found to be remunerative, the reader adhered to his opinion, formulated ten years ago, that sewage irrigation would ultimately be remunerative in many instances; and that opinion was shared by the committee appointed by the Local Government Board in 1876 to inquire into modes of treating town sewage. An irrigation farm should be supplemented by a filterbed, to receive and purify sewage when it is not wanted on the farm. The supposed dangers from the proximity of such farms, or from the spread of entozoic disease, were found to be purely imaginary; it was, on the whole, a better solution of the question for a large number of places than any other, and if, as was very likely, we had a series of dry years, its adoption would receive a great impulse. Where towns cannot make sewage utilisation pay, they must be content to be taxed to a slight extent to get rid of a most serious nuisance and to secure a low death-rate.

In the discussion which followed, Mr. W. C. Sillar, Mr. E. F. Bailey Denton, Mr. Douglas Onslow, Mr. R. W. P. Birch, Mr. G. B. Jerram, and Mr. Wilson Grindle took part.

The Chairman made a few remarks relative to the successful working of the Sewage Farm at Croydon; and Professor Corfield replied briefly to some of the points raised in the discussion.

NAVAL MEDICAL DEPARTMENT.

REGULATIONS FOR ENTRY OF CANDIDATES FOR COMMISSIONS IN THE MEDICAL DEPARTMENT OF THE ROYAL NAVY.

The following are the newly issued regulations as to entry into the Naval Medical Service:—

ADMIRALTY, June 20, 1881.

1. Every candidate for admission into the Medical Department of the Royal Navy must be not under twenty-one nor over twenty-eight years of age on the day that he presents himself for examination. He must produce a certificate from the District Registrar of the date of his birth; or, in default, a declaration made before a magistrate, from one of his parents or other near relative, stating the date of birth. He must also produce a certificate of moral character, signed by a clergyman or a magistrate, to whom he has been for some years personally known, or by the president or senior professor of the College at which he was educated.

2. He must be registered under the Medical Act in force at the time of his appointment, as possessing two diplomas or licences recognised by the General Council, one to practise medicine and the other surgery in Great Britain and Ireland.

The certificates of registration, character, and age must accompany this Schedule, which is to be filled up and returned as soon as possible, addressed as above.

3. He must be free from organic disease, and will be required to make a declaration that he labours under no mental or constitutional disease or weakness, or any other imperfection or disability that can interfere with the most efficient discharge of the duties of a medical officer in any climate.

His physical fitness will be determined by a board of medical officers, who are to certify that his vision comes up to the required standard, which will be ascertained by the use of Snellen's test-types.

He must also declare his readiness to engage for general service at home or abroad as required.

4. Candidates will be examined by the Examining Board in the following subjects:—Anatomy and Physiology; Surgery; Medicine, including therapeutics and the diseases of women and children; Chemistry and Pharmacy, and a practical knowledge of drugs. (The examination in medicine and surgery will be in part practical, and will include operations on the dead body, the application of surgical apparatus, and the examination of medical and surgical patients at the bedside.)

The eligibility of each candidate will be determined by the result of the examinations in these subjects only.

Candidates who desire it will be examined in Comparative Anatomy, Zoology, Natural Philosophy, Physical Geography, and Botany, with special reference to Materia Medica, also in French and German; and the number of marks gained in these subjects will be added to the total number of marks obtained in the obligatory part of the examination by candidates who shall have been found qualified for admission, and whose position on the list of successful competitors will thus be improved in proportion to their knowledge of natural science and modern languages.

5. Every candidate, immediately after passing this examination, will receive a commission as a Surgeon in the Royal Navy, and will undergo a course of practical instruction in naval hygiene, etc., at Haslar Hospital.

THE FRENCH CONSCRIPTION OF 1879.—Of 316,662 young men inscribed on the lists for drawing for the conscription, 24,857 have been exempted as unfit for any kind of service. With respect to education, the 316,662 conscripts are distributed as follows:—Unable to read or write, 46,686; knowing how to read only, 9931; knowing how to read and write, 64,409; having received primary instruction, 181,680; bachelors of letters, 3496. Thus there were nearly 47,000 young men of the class for 1879, or 14·50 per cent., who were completely illiterate.—*Lyon Méd.*, June 19.

REPORT OF THE MEDICAL OFFICER OF THE LOCAL GOVERNMENT BOARD FOR 1879.

THE supplement to the ninth annual Report of the Local Government Board, which contains the report of the Medical Officer for the year 1879, has recently been published. In the outset Dr. Buchanan pays a graceful tribute to the memory of his lamented predecessor, Dr. Seaton, who was compelled by ill-health to retire during the year under notice, and whose death took place shortly after his retirement. The usual statistics as to the work of the department in the supervision and the promotion of vaccination are contained in an appendix; and in the Report opportunity is taken to remind medical practitioners that the purpose of the National Vaccine Establishment " is not the provision of indefinite supplies of lymph for the vaccination of each person who may require it in a district, or a medical practice, but the supply of such an amount of lymph as shall suffice for the establishment of local ' stocks,' and for the replacement by lymph of a new stock, and of undoubted efficiency, of any local stocks that may be found to be giving unsatisfactory results "—a highly correct view, we dare say, but reeking of officialism of the straitest and narrowest kind. It is carefully stated, also, that it was more especially with this object, and in order to know whether any better lymph can be obtained than that furnished by the experienced public vaccinators of the establishment, that the Board caused examination to be made of the effects upon children of lymph which had been derived from the Animal Vaccine Institution of Brussels. The experiments in this direction were entrusted to Dr. Cory, of St. Thomas's Hospital, who undertook the investigation; and the Report states that the results which followed his employment of Dr. Warlomont's lymph may be summed up as follows :—" In some respects they differed from those which he habitually obtains with long-humanised lymph; that there was no reason for preferring the results of the calf-lymph; and that the humanised lymph had, in its arm-to-arm transmissions, the advantage over the calf-lymph of showing greater uniformity of action."

In commenting upon the intelligence and interest displayed by medical officers of health for urban and rural sanitary districts throughout the kingdom, in the annual reports submitted by them to the Board, Dr. Buchanan remarks that these returns bear testimony to the fact that throughout the country the promotion of health and the prevention of disease are each year receiving wider and more intelligent interest from local communities, and he is not slow to recognise what our frequent notices of these annual reports so often record—namely, that in too many cases the sanitary authorities select as officers of health gentlemen with no better qualification for the appointment than the tenure of some other medical office, or have taken no counsel with their officers of health, and for fear of incurring expense ignore these gentlemen's representations. This latter fact will principally answer Mr. Buchanan's complaint that as regards special occurrences of infectious diseases the reports required by the order of the Board have often not been sent, leaving the central authority without information of serious outbreaks of disease until it learned of them from private individuals, or from the Registrar-General's returns. During 1879 no less than thirty local inquiries into serious and exceptional outbreaks of this kind were conducted by the Board's medical inspectors—scarlatina, diphtheria, and enteric fever being the diseases mostly requiring to be traced to their origin in the affected locality. Three of these reports are specially mentioned as of more than usual interest. The first is by Mr. Power on the particulars of a remarkable outbreak of " fever " on board the reformatory school-ship Cornwall. It will be remembered that Mr. Power found, on post-mortem examination, evidence of a parasitic disease, " in certain essential particulars resembling that produced in the human subject by the presence of trichina," and that we pointed out some reasons for strongly objecting to this view. Dr. Buchanan now observes, " Some anatomical peculiarities of this Cornwall parasite (noted at the time by Mr. Power, but by him regarded as of no generic importance) tended, indeed, to throw doubt on its identity with Trichina,

and a further report on the subject by Dr. Bastian (given in the appendix) refers the parasite to the genus Pelodera, which has not heretofore been known to invade the human body. This view adds materially to the interest and importance of Mr. Power's observations of the disease on board the Cornwall."

The second report is one by Dr. Thorne, on an outbreak of enteric fever at Caterham and Redhill; and the last by Dr. Airy on a sudden outburst of scarlet fever at Fallowfield, near Manchester. It may be mentioned that full particulars of these three outbreaks have already appeared in our columns.

In recording, under the head of " Auxiliary Scientific Investigations," the work inaugurated by the Board during the year 1879, the Report enumerates the result of investigations by Dr. Klein " on the lymphatic system of the skin and mucous membranes," and results of experiments by the same gentleman " in the inoculation of bovine animals with small-pox." Dr. Thudichum also contributes a report " on the chemical constitution of the brain, and of the organoplastic substances." In the spring of 1877 the President directed that a portion of the Parliamentary grant which is made to the Board for purposes of scientific investigation should be appropriated to an inquiry, to be undertaken by the Pathological Society of London, into the nature, causes, and prevention of the infectious diseases known as pyæmia, septicæmia, and by other names. The report, already well known to our readers, of the committee of the Society charged with this study will be found in the second appendix issued with the present Report.

FROM ABROAD.

PROFESSOR PASTEUR'S DISCOVERIES.

AT the meeting of the Académie de Médecine on June 24, Prof. Bouley, who is the confident and authorised exponent of the views of this great experimenter, furnished an interesting account of the various steps taken by Prof. Pasteur in the investigation of the nature and the attenuation of viruses, which have already led to such important conclusions, to be followed, doubtless, by others of still wider application. The different treatment required by the microbes of chicken-cholera, and those of charbon, to secure their innocuity and their prophylactic influence, was described with an eloquent lucidity which completely carried the Academy with it. For an account of the communication, for which we have not space, we must refer to the Bulletin of the Academy of the above-named date.

TREATMENT OF PLEURISY IN CHILDREN.

A paper upon this subject was read at the Obstetrical Section of the New York Academy of Medicine by Dr. Lewis Smith (New York Medical Record, No. 15).

He observed that at the commencement of idiopathic pleurisy the abstraction of blood may be beneficial if judiciously employed, from one to three leeches being applied in a robust child from two to four years of age. As a rule, bleeding is injurious in all cases of secondary pleurisy (as after scarlatina, etc.), and when the quantity of effusion is large. Emollient and simply irritating poultices (as a mixture of one part of mustard to sixteen of linseed) are serviceable in the first stage. The poultice should be made very wet, spread thin, and applied over the chest in front and behind, covered with oiled silk, and changed twice in the twenty-four hours. For children under six or seven months, rubbing the chest with camphorated oil, and applying a poultice, may be sufficient. Blistering at this early stage should not be employed, as it increases the inflammation. The indications for internal remedies in the first stage are to diminish the frequency of the pulse, relieve the pain, and allay the cough. To a child three years of age the tincture of aconite may be given in doses of half a drop, and to one of six years one drop, every three hours for two or three days. In the first stage of primary pleurisy the cardiac sedatives may be used; but digitalis is a safer and better remedy in all other cases, and it may be used in the second stage. One drop of the tincture may be given every three hours to a child of two years, and two drops to a child of five. An opiate is ordinarily required, as from one to three grains of Dover's powder every three hours. Hyoscyamus may be used to relieve pain and cough; digitalis may be combined with an opiate, and morphia with aconitia. In secondary pleurisy digitalis is preferable to aconitia.

In the second stage, unless the effusion is small, measures for its removal are required; but the propriety of using blisters is very doubtful. A relaxed condition of the bowels favours absorption, but diaphoretics are not of much use; while pilocarpin produces depression, which renders it unsafe. Diuretics and tonics are useful, and digitalis with acetate of potash is very serviceable (infus. digital. ℥iv., pot. acet. ℨj.; teaspoonful every three hours for a child four or five months old). Bitter tonics are especially useful, and acetate of potash may be combined with dec. cinchonæ with good results. A full amount of nutriment should be taken, with but little fluid. When the appetite and general health are good, and there are no symptoms due to the presence of the fluid, but little medication is necessary. If there are such symptoms, and the fluid does not disappear, the question of surgical interference arises; and the indications for it are—1. Oppressed breathing. 2. The flat percussion-note over the whole affected side, with displacement of the heart (it is called for in this case, even when no dyspnœa is present, as this may occur suddenly). 3. Moderate effusion, without material decrease in quantity by absorption, after some weeks of treatment. There is here danger that catarrhal pneumonia, terminating in cheesy pneumonia and tuberculosis, may occur in portions of the compressed lung. Besides, the longer the lung is compressed, the slower will it return to normal expansion after the pressure has been removed. 4. A moderate quantity of fluid co-existing with disease of the opposite lung, or of the lung of the affected side. 5. Extension of the inflammation to the pericardium—a not infrequent occurrence. 6. The existence of valvular lesion of the heart. 7. The presence of pus, empyema. The operation of thoracentesis should be performed in the eighth intercostal space, on a line perpendicular with the angle of the scapula, the admission of air being carefully avoided. The thickness of the thoracic wall is about half an inch (less in emaciated children), so that introduction of the canula to the depth of one inch suffices to pass beyond the exudation, and allow the liquid to flow out through the canule. The sharp needle should not be used. Washing out the pleural cavity is injurious rather than beneficial, except in cases in which the pus is offensive. To empty the pleural cavity and approximate the pleural surfaces is the indication. Dr. Smith believes that there will be a reaction against the removal of a portion of the ribs in cases of empyema.

At the discussion of the paper, Dr. Caro observed that he disapproved of bleeding even in the first stage. He uses the bromide of potash in doses of two or three grains every one or two hours, for the purpose of reducing the capillary congestion. Aconitia may be used when there is much elevation of temperature. He especially favoured the use of acetate of potash in free doses in the second stage. Large doses of calomel also diminish capillary congestion and favour resolution of the inflammation. Externally, he recommended tincture of iodine or Lugol's solution, covered with oiled silk. He was in favour, also, of the internal use of jaborandi in infusion, and believed it to be preferable to hypodermic injections of pilocarpin. Take two drachms of the leaves to three or four ounces of water, and give the whole in two or three doses.

Births and Deaths in Berlin during 1880.

The following preliminary statement has been furnished by the Berlin Municipal Statistical Bureau, and is published in the supplement to No. 14 of the *Veröffentlichungen d. Deutschen Gesundheitsamtes* of the present year :—

The population amounted in the middle of the year to 1,107,000. During the year there were born 44,112 living children (viz., 22,380 male and 21,732 female), or 39·84 per 1000 of the entire population. Of this number, all but 5922 were born in wedlock. There were also 1749 (997 male and 752 female) born dead, or 1·58 per 1000. The number of deaths (exclusive of the born-dead) amounted to 32,823 (or 29·65 per 1000), viz., 17,358 males and 15,465 females. Of the deaths, 13,838 (or 42·16 per cent.) took place in infants under one year, 10,875 being legitimate and 2963 illegitimate.

Between one and five years there died 5694 (or 17·35), 5267 being legitimate and 427 illegitimate. Between five and ten there were 1211 deaths (3·69); between ten and fifteen, 324 (0·99); between fifteen and twenty, 482 (1·47); between twenty and thirty, 2024 (6·17); between thirty and forty, 2332 (7·10); between forty and sixty, 3552 (10·82); between sixty and eighty, 2870 (8·74); and above eighty, 496 (1·51). Among the *causes* of death are returned—measles 376 (1·15 per cent.), scarlatina 872 (2·66), small-pox 9 (0·03), erysipelas 81 (0·25), diphtheria 1198 (3·65), angina 224 (0·68), purulent infection 83 (0·25), puerperal fever 173 (0·53), typhoid fever 506 (1·54), typhus 21 (0·06), dysentery 129 (0·39), pertussis 354 (1·08), acute rheumatism 41 (0·12), apoplexy 773 (2·36), pulmonary phthisis 3830 (11·67), pneumonias 1864 (5·68), acute bronchitis 100 (0·30), laryngitis and tracheitis 811 (2·47), diseases of the stomach and intestinal canal and diarrhœa 2476 (7·54), cholera 3477 (10·59). The violent deaths constituted 1·95 per cent. of the whole number of deaths, 325 of the number being returned as accidental or incapable of verification, and 308 as suicidal.

This return shows an increase of the general mortality of 1·92 per 1000 over that of the preceding year; the mean annual mortality of Berlin from 1872 to 1875 amounted to 32·6 per 1000 ; it then slowly decreased, until 1879, when it had sunk to 27·7. In 1880 it has again risen to 29·65, being almost as high as in 1877, when it was 29·78. The maximum mortality took place in July, when there were 4184 deaths (1804 of these arising from diarrhœa and cholera), and the minimum fell in November, when there were 2163 deaths. The explanation of the remarkable increase of the rate of mortality in 1880 is not found in the increase of diarrhœa and cholera of children, since the total deaths from these causes were only 7·54 and 10·59 per cent., as compared with 6·87 and 10·57 of the preceding year. It is rather to be attributed to prolonged epidemics of measles, scarlatina, and diphtheria, and especially to a bad epidemic of typhoid fever occurring at the latter end of the year. The typhoid fever epidemic was, however, the chief cause of the excess of mortality. After the epidemic of 1879 a remission took place, the deaths falling to 290, or only 1 per cent. They have now risen again to 506, or 1·54 per cent. As in former years, the maximum occurred in autumn and winter, the greatest number of cases occurring in September, and of deaths in October ; the minimum was observed in April and May. From an official table which is given it is seen that in the months when the subsoil water was at its lowest there was a maximum of cases and deaths of typhoid ; while, when this was highest, the cases and deaths were fewest. Typhus only occurred sporadically, the entire number of deaths only amounting to 21, of which 12 occurred in July. Relapsing fever appeared as a prevalent epidemic at the early part of the year, but pursued a very moderate course, so that out of 620 cases only 32 (0·1 per cent.) deaths occurred. Small-pox only showed itself occasionally, causing but 9 deaths in the year.

Harveian Society of London.—The *conversazione* given at the South Kensington Museum on Wednesday evening last, by Mr. Henry Power, the President, and the Council of the Harveian Society, to celebrate its fiftieth anniversary, was an eminent success. The weather was delightful—a matter of importance for even indoor assemblings,—excellent music was performed by the band of the Grenadier Guards, and by Kalozdy's admirable Hungarian band, and there was equally excellent singing of glees and part-songs. The arrangements were perfect, and some two thousand guests spent a most enjoyable evening. One object of great interest in the rooms was Mr. Joy's statue of Harvey, shortly to be erected at Folkestone, which deservedly excited much admiration.

Ventnor as a Health-Resort for the Consumptive.—In an article in the *New-York Med. Journal* for May, Dr. Thornton Parker strongly recommends to his American countrymen Ventnor as the best existing resort for such consumptive patients as can be properly recommended to leave their homes. With its unrivalled climate, he says, it unites advantages—such as quietude, domestic comforts, pleasant intercourse, and beautiful scenery—most favourable to the amelioration of diseased conditions, and not to be met with, so combined, at any other resort either in the United States or on the continent of Europe.

REVIEWS.

Human and Animal Variola: A Study in Comparative Pathology. By GEORGE FLEMING, F.R.C.V.S., Army Veterinary Inspector. London: Baillière and Co. 1881.

THE appearance of this pamphlet at the present time is most opportune. The importance of the subject can scarcely be over-rated; and yet, judging by recent correspondence in the medical press, and the opinions expressed at the conference on vaccination, the greatest ignorance seems to prevail in the profession itself on the mutual relations of the variola incident to man and the lower animals. It seems to be commonly held among medical men in this country that cow-pox is not a disease natural to the bovine species, but merely small-pox conveyed to them from man by inoculation, and that in the operation of vaccination we avail ourselves of the modification which it has undergone in the body of the cow, precisely as Dr. Greenfield confers immunity from anthrax on cattle by inoculation with bacilli which have passed through the system of a rabbit.

In support of this view it is usual to adduce the supposed rarity of the cow-pox now that small-pox has become almost unknown in rural districts, the asserted exemption of the male sex among cattle, the successful inoculation of cattle with small-pox, with the production of what Thiele and Ceely believed to be cow-pox, and the vaccination of infants therefrom by the same observers.

Mr. Fleming has collected a vast amount of evidence from French, German, Scandinavian, and Italian sources, and has carefully scrutinised the scanty records of English experimenters. He gives irresistible evidence of the prevalence of cow-pox in countries where small-pox is almost unknown, of the equal susceptibility of bulls if exposed to the contagion with cows, and satisfactorily proves that the supposed vaccinations of Mr. Ceely were, in fact, nothing more or less than inoculation with small-pox unchanged by its transmission through the cow. Such inoculation of the cow is not often successful, but in several instances the real nature of the lymph thence taken and implanted in children has been manifested not only by the eruption following, but by the communication of unmistakable and fatal small-pox to other infants by ordinary infection—a caution to those who would attempt to reproduce a more active vaccine through such a procedure as mediate variolation.

The space at our disposal does not permit of our describing in detail the experiments conducted by the Academy of Sciences under Professor Chauveau, between 1863 and 1866, or by the Italian Commission under Professor Bassi, from 1871 to 1874, on a scale and with a scientific accuracy unattempted in this country. For these we must refer our readers to Mr. Fleming's work. We must content ourselves with stating the conclusions arrived at by them and the author of this essay. These are, that man, the horse, cow, sheep, goat, camel, swine, and dog, with perhaps some other animals, have each their own peculiar and independent variola or pox, agreeing with and differing from one another in various ways, *e.g,* the human, ovine, cameline, canine, and porcine variola are *infectious, i.e.,* communicable to other individuals of the same species by simple proximity or by fomites, though rarely so to any other species; that the bovine, *caprine,* and equine are only *contagious,* or communicable to other individuals by actual contact or inoculation. In the former group the fever is severe and fatal; in the latter there is little constitutional disturbance and no danger to life. The horse, cow, and small-pox are capable of indefinite or continuous cultivation by transmission in animals of each other species and in man, and are mutually protective against each other and against small-pox, and may therefore be indifferently employed for the purpose of "vaccination"; whereas small-pox, though communicated with great difficulty to the horse and cow, producing a trifling local result, if any, is in no way modified as a disease by such transmission, and though incapable of being continued in these animals, it recovers its original character on being reconveyed to man. Monkeys alone are as susceptible as mankind to small-pox, which is not only fatal to them in captivity, when they can impart it again to us by infection, but even in the wild state seems to affect them epidemically.

Cow-pox, it is said, could be continued indefinitely in man and horse. It is communicable to, but not continuous in,

the sheep, goat, and dog, losing its activity after the first or second transmission.

Sheep-pox in its visible features, its fatality and infectiousness, most resembles the human small-pox, and is communicable to man, etc., by inoculation, but it confers no protection against small-pox, cow-pox, horse-pox, etc., nor they against it.

The vesicles resulting from the use of lymph derived from the natural horse or cow-pox are larger, but slower in development, than those produced by humanised lymph; and vaccinations with humanised lymph are more certain of success than those with the lymph of the horse and cow. In retro-vaccination the same twofold change of lessened certainty with greater energy in the event of success is obtained, so that in default of the natural cow-pox, retro-vaccination, or the vaccination of the calf from the child, may be resorted to as a means of revivifying the stock of vaccine—if, indeed, such revivification be at all called for,—though it seems doubtful whether after several transmissions the humanised lymph retains any advantage from having been thus retro-vaccinised. Humanised lymph, too, as recent experience has amply proved, keeps better, or possesses what the Italians call far greater " tenacity of activity," than bovine—a fact of vast practical importance, especially in the presence of epidemics of small-pox.

On the all-important question of the elimination of any syphilitic taint from human lymph by this process the Italian Commission are very decided. They state that, though monkeys alone are capable of true and general syphilisation, the result of their experiments shows that a local syphilis can be produced by inoculation in the cow, and reconveyed to man, just as we have seen small-pox to be. It does not appear that they had the opportunity of using syphilised lymph, and the possibility of the syphilitic virus itself retaining its activity after such transmission, however remote the probability of such a contingency, upsets, unfortunately, one popular argument in favour of retro-vaccination.

Jenner was well aware of the non-identity of small-pox and cow-pox, but erroneously supposed the latter to have been derived from the horse-pox, which, as has been shown, is readily communicated to and continued in the bovine and human species. He, and after him Dr. Loy, spoke of this disease as the "grease." Much confusion and many contradictory statements have arisen from the fact that under this name, as also under its foreign equivalents, *le javart* and *der Mauke,* is also included a simple non-infectious and incommunicable catarrh of the sebaceous follicles, which, in the hands of experimenters who failed to distinguish the diseases, has, of course, proved incapable of producing vaccinia in the cow. Such blunders, and the disastrous results of mediate variolation instead of vaccination, in America and India show the value of a knowledge of the diseases of domestic animals. Comparative anatomy and physiology are already taught in all our medical schools. Why, asks Mr. Fleming, have we not chairs of comparative pathology ? —a subject of far greater practical importance to the medical man.

A System of Oral Surgery : being a Treatise on the Diseases and Surgery of the Mouth, Jaws, and Associate Parts. By JAMES E. GARRETSON, M.D. With numerous illustrations. Third Edition. Philadelphia: Lippincott and Co. 1881. Pp. 916.

THIS volume represents the "experience of thirty years, fifteen of which were spent as a dentist, and the last fifteen as a practitioner of general surgery." The author ought also to have added that it includes a vast amount of bibliographical research, for it would be difficult to name a textbook which has not been put to contribution either to supply cases, drawings, or references.

The book is a very complete *exposé* of the diseases of the face in the widest sense of the word, for it includes the teeth from a dentist's point of view, the gums, the salivary glands, the tonsils, the tongue, the trachea, cysts of the neck, palatine defects, the nose and its cavities, the antrum, the maxillæ, giving their various diseases, and the operations which are done for their relief; the subject of neuralgia is also discussed, and the book finishes with a long chapter on anæsthesia.

Such a work must have cost the author no small amount of labour, and those who are specially interested in the surgery of this region will here find an immense mass of information, compiled from the most varied sources, which cannot but prove of great value. When we add that there are 541 engravings, in addition to nine steel plates, our readers will be able to judge what the book is.

That we find a lack of individuality is, perhaps, our own fault, but it is one which we can overlook in the presence of such a mass of general information on "oral surgery" as is not to be found in any other work on the subject with which we are acquainted. The general "get-up" of the work is beyond praise.

Contributions to Military and State Medicine. By JOHN MARTIN, Surgeon A.M.D. Vol. I. London: J. and A. Churchill. 1881.

THE present volume contains two essays—the one which received the Howard Prize given by the Statistical Society, having for its subject, "The Effect of Health and Disease on Military and Naval Operations"; and the other, to which was awarded the Alexander Memorial Gold Medal and Prize of the Army Medical department, treating of " The Influence of Drinking-Water in Originating or Propagating Enteric Fever, Diarrhœa, Dysentery, and Cholera."

The former essay is the shorter, but by far the more satisfactory, since it deals with well-recognised facts, and advances no theories on disputable points. Naval operations are only referred to incidentally once or twice, but the experiences of every campaign, not only of our own but of foreign armies, in the present and past centuries are freely quoted. In the second chapter the author discusses the operations, whether preparatory to war, as mobilisation and transport of troops, or those of actual war, as strategy and tactics, as affected by the physical condition of the soldiery; in the next, the diseases, whether inseparable from life in camp, frequently coincident with, or independent of but occasionally appearing in the course of, a campaign; and in the last, the influence of disease in general on the numerical strength or the efficiency of troops. He concludes with some remarks on the effects of diseases of cattle on the operations of war.

The commemorative character of the essay requiring some allusion to the labours of Howard. Mr. Martin selects for this purpose the state of the military hospitals of Russia as seen by that good man in his last pilgrimage preceding his death—a frightful picture of indifference to human life.

He then shows by statistics the great improvement which has taken place, especially within the last ten or twenty years, in our own and other armies. One remarkable result of the greatly increased precision and range of modern rifles is an actual decrease in the proportion of men put *hors de combat*, although the wounds inflicted are more serious, the fact being that the terrible accuracy of our arms necessitates a change in, and gives a greater importance to, tactics in place of mere brute force, at the same time lessening the duration of campaigns. The increased facilities of locomotion afforded by railways also aid the removal of the wounded from the unfavourable surroundings of camps. On other matters there is little that has not been already well given by Dr. Parkes in his great work; and the writer does not notice the measures to be taken for averting disease and maintaining the efficiency of armies in the field, except so far as regards the duty of not exposing any but mature men to the hardships of actual warfare.

The second essay, though occupying the larger part of the book, and making higher pretensions to a scientific character, seems to us eminently unsatisfactory. A treatise on the origin and propagation of specific and communicable diseases which entirely ignores the researches of Chauveau and Pasteur, Sanderson, Greenfield, and Klein, Koch, Obermeier, Buchner, etc., is, to say the least, an anachronism, though the honoured names of Parkes, Aitken, Murchison, Radcliffe, Pettenkofer, etc., are freely quoted. Convinced as we are that the causation of all these diseases by various forms of bacilli has passed from the region of conjecture to that of ascertained facts, only awaiting further elucidation by experimental research on the lines already laid down, we must protest against any attempt to revive "pythogenic" theories, and to maintain the origination of zymotic diseases, not excluding small-pox! (page 208) from indifferent, various, and non-specific causes, as a sadly retrograde course.

With a great show of logic, and grave charges of erroneous reasoning against others, the author's own arguments are pervaded by—and, indeed, founded on—a fallacy. Assuming that a *specific* disease is "one which maintains a certain individuality," he includes under this description cancer, as well as enteric and other fevers, and argues that if the first do arise *de novo*, so may the latter, without the agency of bacterial or other specific causes. If his opponents reply that the former "are not specific in the same sense that enteric fever is specific, the specificity of the latter meaning that each case must spring from a foregoing one, after the manner of species in the animal kingdom," he charges them with reasoning in a circle, and asserts that such a statement is "absurd." The fact is that our knowledge has outstripped our language, and the term "specific" has become ambiguous and inadequate. We may admit the *individuality* of carcinomatous neoplasia, and also of small-pox, and yet maintain that every case of the latter disease is derived from a pre-existing one. It is Mr. Martin himself who falls into the fallacy of ambiguous middle scarcely less glaring than the example of the schools, that "feathers dispel darkness because they are light."

Many of his statements will startle those of our readers who have studied the etiology of these diseases—as, for example, that the possession by enteric fever of "a period of incubation, and a subsequent exhaustion of susceptibility, are only apparent," and that its propagation by drinking-water "is infrequent and of very limited extent," that in cholera water acts "only as an excitant" (!), that in certain cases of diarrhœa it acts "by being a carrier of a specific modification of vitality"—whatever that may be!—that infection is "something impalpable and intangible," and, lastly, the proposition in which he embodies the outcome of all his experience, that in diarrhœa, dysentery, enteric fever, and cholera alike, the "nature of the influence of drinking-water in originating or propagating" the disease may be referred to "(1) mechanical irritation, (2) chemico-physical irritation, and (3) probably other more obscure influences of the nature of which we are ignorant."

The Student's Guide to the Diseases of Women. By Dr. GALABIN. Illustrated. Second Edition. London: J. and A. Churchill. 1881. Pp. 395.

THE first edition of this little volume has been quickly disposed of, thus testifying to its popularity amongst those for whom it was written. In this edition the author has revised his work, made several additions, and added some new engravings. We so fully reviewed it on its first appearance that there is no need to do so on the present occasion; suffice it to say that it retains its original form and characteristics. Both the student and practitioner will find the mechanical treatment of displacements of the uterus carefully considered and copiously illustrated in this useful volume of "Churchill's Medical Class-Books."

On the Diseases of Children. For Practitioners and Students. By WILLIAM HENRY DAY, M.D. London: J. and A. Churchill. 1881. Pp. 752.

IT is some years since a general work on children's diseases has been published in London, although it has long seemed to us that such a work was wanted. Pathology nowadays makes rapid strides, and the examining boards are becoming so exacting that new works, or new editions, are constantly being called for. Under these circumstances, therefore, the work before us has ample *raison d'être.* The book conforms also in other respects to a requirement of the times—we refer to the multiplicity of sources from which the doctrines it contains have been culled. To say that a better selection of descriptions and opinions might possibly have been made, and that some additional personal experience ought to have been given, are perhaps matters on which there is room for difference of opinion. Our author, nevertheless, has managed to condense into a volume, which now forms one of Churchill's well-known "Manuals," a large amount of very useful information.

In the introductory remarks he says: "The diseases of children have a claim to be considered separately and specially. It is before mental training has worked its influence, and the body has undergone the wear and tear of adult life, that we are able to study disease in its most natural form. An opportunity is presented to us of seeing disease, as it were, unrestrained and free, running its course in a tender frame, keenly sensitive to exaltation and depression, without the complications and the thousand collateral circumstances which determine the form and character of the disease which is to assail it in subsequent life. All practitioners of medicine will admit that the diseases of children should be regarded in a distinct light from like diseases of adults, where too frequently disease acts upon shattered organs and worn-out tissues." We are much inclined to agree with our author in these remarks; but with us our belief is a result of practice rather than a profession; while with Dr. Day the opposite would seem to obtain, if the long list of prescription formulæ at the end of the book is any index to the amount of physic which he considers it necessary to advocate in the treatment of "unrestrained and free" disease.

The chapter on "Milk Diet and Hygiene" is good; that on "Acute and Chronic Disease" might well have been omitted—it is indefinite in scope, in detail, and in application. The chapter on "Debility" would be more practical if divided into sections, with the plans of treatment given under the respective headings of those diseases which had caused the debility. Surely it would be better to treat of the debility arising from loss of blood under its cause than under a general heading, for the treatment of this form of debility would be quite different from that which proceeds from starvation or "free purgation."

The subject of "Marasmus or Atrophy," "which is a common disease among infants and young children, as the out-patient practice of any London hospital amply testifies," is dismissed in a very short chapter. This is really a subject which is essentially "special," and ought, therefore, to be fully dealt with in such a work as this; but we get no new ideas from our author, no pathological inquiry into the causes of the condition spoken of. Atrophy is defined as "the decrease of size of a tissue or of the whole body, with consequent impairment of function." For our own part, we have always reversed this order of events, and regarded the wasting as the *result* of impaired function. As regards treatment, a remedy which sometimes acts like a charm—we mean mercurial ointment—is not even referred to.

On the other hand—probably by way of counterpoise—there is a long chapter on "Asthma." We are told that "neither West, Underwood, Meigs and Pepper, Steiner, Churchill, nor Niemeyer alludes to asthma in childhood," and that the author himself has "only seen a few cases." We believe the disease occurs so very infrequently that this chapter could with great advantage have given place to a more detailed account of marasmus, which is unfortunately so common, and often so intractable.

Speaking of laryngismus stridulus, our author, quoting Dr. Marshall Hall, says: "Spasm of the glottis is an excitation of the true spinal, or excito-motory system." Perhaps this sentence may convey information to some of our elderly readers, but to us who have lived since the days of Marshall Hall it is absolutely meaningless.

The chapter on "Chorea" concludes: "Finally, sea air, shower-baths, cold-water douches, gymnastic exercises, are useful in properly selected cases." Might it not have been as well, in a book intended for students, to have specified the particular form of the disease for which such powerful remedies as cold-water douches, for instance, are useful? Then the author says: "Galvanisation and faradisation are also to be recommended. A gentle constant current, applied for four or five minutes to the suffering portion of the brain (sic), generally arrests the choreic movements at once. In hemichorea the opposite side of the brain must be galvanised"! (The interjection is our own, and it is the only comment we shall make.)

One other criticism, and we have done. Alluding to the causes of infantile paralysis, Dr. Day says: "I have known the attacks follow cold and ulceration of the throat, diphtheria, and the eruptive fevers. Blows and falls upon the hip have produced this form of paralysis." This does not actually say the disease is caused in this way, although the above quotation is taken from the paragraph enumerating the "causes." We almost wonder to find such statements in this place, for it might mislead the student; especially as the author relates one or two typical cases, and mentions disease of the anterior horns of the cord as the most recently accepted pathology of the disorder.

We have ventured on the foregoing criticisms, because, in a work intended for students, information must be precise as well as practical. We well know the difficulties of compiling such a work, and doubt not that in its later editions the book will be much improved. In view of this, we would recommend a more careful study of the various diseases at the bedside or in the out-patient room; the author will thus greatly improve his book, add to his reputation, and will then find less difficulty in making suitable selections from our current literature of cases in support or otherwise of any theories which he may wish to advocate, either of symptoms, treatment, or pathology of the "Diseases of Children."

REPORTS OF SOCIETIES.

ODONTOLOGICAL SOCIETY OF GREAT BRITAIN.

MONDAY, JUNE 13.

Mr. T. ARNOLD ROGERS, President, in the Chair.

MR. HILDITCH HARDING showed an upper central incisor which he had extracted from the mouth of a boy at St. Thomas's Hospital, on account of abscess about the fang. Half of the crown had been broken off by a fall some time before. After extraction a splinter of wood was found projecting a quarter of an inch beyond the apical foramen. The boy said he had a habit of chewing wood occasionally, but had no idea how this piece got into the tooth.

Mr. COLEMAN showed an upper wisdom-tooth which he had extracted for caries. One of the fangs was missing, and, on probing the alveolus, a hard substance was felt which he at first took to be the missing root. It proved, however, to be a second wisdom-tooth, coming down above the first, and which had, by its pressure, caused absorption of the root of the tooth which he had extracted.

Mr. DAVID HEPBURN read a paper on "Chronic Suppuration connected with the Teeth." After briefly referring to the most common form, that of ordinary alveolar abscess, in which a fistulous opening existed on the surface of the gum, communicating by a short canal with the root of a tooth, Mr. Hepburn proceeded to describe those more complicated cases in which the pus had penetrated to a part remote from the original source of the mischief. Of this he related several instances which had come under his own observation, as where an impacted wisdom-tooth had given rise to a large abscess which opened in the neck. In most cases the extraction of the tooth which had been the original cause of the mischief would be followed by the closure of the sinuses; but it was not always easy to discover which tooth was the cause of the mischief, and sometimes, even when this had been extracted, little improvement would result. This was generally due to the presence of a small piece of necrosed bone, and this, again, was often most difficult to discover, and might remain for months keeping up irritation before it could be removed. Mr. Hepburn related several cases illustrating these points. In one the patient was under treatment for five months, and was then cured by the extraction of an upper lateral incisor. In another the patient had been suffering for seven months before he applied for advice for a profuse discharge of offensive pus coming from the socket of an extracted lateral. Active treatment was persisted in for eight months, with little result, when suspicion fell upon the central incisors. These were extracted, and at the bottom of the socket of the right central a piece of dead bone was found, and a canal which communicated in a circuitous manner with the sinuses that had been so long discharging. Immediate improvement followed. In the treatment of these cases, Mr. Hepburn spoke highly of the value of eucalyptus oil; it was a powerful antiseptic and a useful stimulant, whilst its taste and smell were not generally considered disagreeable; it was altogether far preferable to carbolic acid. Tincture of iodine was also useful; but the great point was to find out and remove the cause of the irritation as soon as possible.

An interesting discussion followed.

ROLLESTON MEMORIAL.—A general meeting of the friends and pupils of the late Professor Rolleston will be held at the house of Dr. Shepherd, 17, Great Cumberland-place, Hyde-park, W., on Wednesday, July 6, at 3 p.m.

NEW INVENTIONS AND IMPROVEMENTS.

MODIFIED FERGUSON'S SPECULUM (PATENT).

This modification was suggested, we are informed, by Dr. J. H. Aveling to Mr. Hicks, of Hatton-garden, and the following advantages are claimed for it:—In consequence of the frequency with which the ordinary speculum is rendered useless and dangerous by its bevelled edge becoming denuded of its protective covering of varnish. Friction, and the chemical action of solutions, are the causes of this peeling. When it has taken place, a sharp, rough edge presents itself. In this modification, instead of having the bevelled edge ground, it is fused, and being thus made smooth, no covering of varnish is required. The silvering and varnishing are stopped an eighth of an inch from the edge, leaving a bare polished rim of glass, which cannot be affected by any ordinary usage.

Cleanliness and economy are secured by this modification. It is more cleanly, because the slightest flaw in the varnished edge of the ordinary instrument offers a home for septic or specific discharges. It is more economical, because the speculum cannot be rendered useless by its bevelled edge becoming roughened and sharp.

[We have more than once objected to patented medical wares. Here it does not appear who the patentee is; we therefore give Dr. Aveling the benefit of the doubt, and so publish the notice.—Ed. Med. Times and Gas.]

DR. DUDGEON'S POCKET SPHYGMOGRAPH.

Some little time ago we had a sample of this little apparatus submitted to us. We were at once convinced of its neatness and the ingenuity of its contrivance; the question that remained to be settled was whether or no it would work well. Here we have to deal with a somewhat difficult subject, but it appears to us that it may be easily divided into three parts—the delicacy or coarseness of the instrument; the skilfulness or its reverse on the part of the operator; and the mental and bodily condition of the patient under examination. With regard to the delicacy of Dr. Dudgeon's appliance

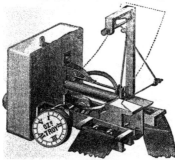

there can be no question; indeed, we doubt if it would not be better as regards the two descending levers if they were made heavier. The little pen is almost too light to do its work except on very carefully prepared paper (which, by the way, is best done by camphor-smoke). A piece of camphor can be set on fire anywhere, and in a few minutes any number of good slips can be prepared from it and these of the most delicate kind; if the first tracing is not satisfactory, it can be wiped off in a moment, and a new

layer of carbon applied. Even with paper thus prepared, the delicate pen is hardly heavy enough to do its duty. The instrument undoubtedly requires skill in its use, its great delicacy rendering this all the more important, and we have seen the slightest excitement give rise to all kinds of aberrations. Nevertheless, with due care, excellent tracings can be got from it—always, we are inclined to think, more delicate than those that are to be got by the ordinary apparatus in use, but consequently requiring more care in reading. Some tracings we have got are really extraordinary; we scarcely know how to read them. As compared with other sphygmographs it is a marvel of cheapness; and, we may add, it is manufactured by Mr. J. Ganter, 19, Crawford-street, W.

MEDICAL NEWS.

UNIVERSITY OF DURHAM.—At the final examinations for the degrees of Medicine, concluded on the 24th inst., the following candidates satisfied the Examiners:—

For the degree of Doctor in Medicine (for practitioners of fifteen years' standing)—

Deane, Andrew, L.R.C.S., etc.
Leach, John Comyns, B.Sc. Lond., M.R.C.S., L.S.A.
Orton, Charles, M.R.C.P. Edin., M.R.C.S., L.S.A.
Reed, Thomas Sleeman, M.R.C.S., L.S.A.

For the degree of Doctor in Medicine—

Bowman, Hugh Torrington, M.B., M.S., M.R.C.S.
Dodd, John Richard, M.B., M.R.C.S.
Morton, Shadforth, M.B., M.R.C.S.
Powell, Scudamore Rydley, M.B., M.R.C.S.
Tyson, William Joseph, M.B., F.R.C.S. Eng., L.R.C.P.
Woodman, William Edwin, M.B., M.R.C.S., L.S.A.

For the degree of Bachelor in Medicine—

Austen, Henry Hinds, M.R.C.S.
Baker, John Hopper.
Burton, Francis Henry Merceron, M.R.C.S.
Clowes, Herbert Alfred, M.R.C.S.
Cripps, Charles Couper, M.R.C.S.
East, Frederick William, L.S.A.
Kempster, William Henry.
Kennedy, William Adam, L.R.C.P., M.R.C.S.
Prowde, Edwin Longstaff, M.A. Cantab.
Robinson, William.
Smith, William Harvey, M.R.C.S.
Thomson, George James Crawford.
Walker, Basil Woodd, L.R.C.P., M.R.C.S.

For the degree of Master in Surgery—

Burton, Francis Henry Merceron, M.R.C.S.
Clowes, Herbert Alfred, M.R.C.S.
Cripps, Charles Couper, M.R.C.S.
Robinson, William.

UNIVERSITY OF DUBLIN: SCHOOL OF PHYSIC IN IRELAND.—At the Trinity Term examination for the degree of Bachelor in Surgery (B.Ch.), held on Monday and Tuesday, June 20 and 21, the successful candidates passed in order of merit as under:—

Jencken, Francis John.	Nangle, Edward C.
Irwin, James M.	MacCarthy, William Ft.
Young, Louis T.	Macquillan, John W.
Myles, Thomas.	O'Hara-Hamilton, Thomas W.
Donnelly, Thomas.	Robinson, James J.
Grant, Donald St. John.	Miller, Alfred.
Hall, Edward G.	Gloster, Charles.
Elliott, William S.	Moore, Reginald H.
Cochrane, Edward.	

ROYAL COLLEGE OF SURGEONS OF ENGLAND.—The following gentlemen, having undergone the necessary examinations, were admitted Licentiates in Dental Surgery of the College at a meeting of the Board of Examiners on the 27th inst., viz.:—

Amoore, John S., Balham.
Davis, Charles D., M.R.C.S., Kilburn, N.W.
Ewbank, Francis, M.R.C.S., Queen Anne-street, W.
Harris, U. A. C., M.R.C.S., Brighton.
Hern, William, St. Mary's-square, W.
Matthews, William, Hereford-road, W.
Oakley, Archibald H., Tunbridge Wells.
Pidgeon, William J., Finsbury-park, N.
Price, Ross, Blythe-road, W.
Rose, Frederick, North-crescent, W.C.
Stuck, Thomas J., Gower-street, W.C.
Tothill, Walter, North-crescent, W.C.
Treman, Charles E., M.R.C.S., Southwick-street, W.
White, Henry F., Hill-street, S.W.

Only two candidates failed to acquit themselves to the satisfaction of the Board. The following were the questions submitted to the above candidates at the written examination on the 24th inst., when they were required to answer at least one of the two questions, both on Anatomy and Physiology and on Surgery and Pathology, from two to four o'clock p.m., viz. :—Anatomy and Physiology : 1. Describe the course and distribution of the arteries and nerves which supply the teeth. 2. What are the changes which the food undergoes in the mouth and stomach ? Surgery and Pathology : 1. Describe the causes, symptoms, and appropriate treatment of ununited fracture of the lower jaw. 2. What is meant by "abscess of the antrum"? How does it differ from common abscess, such as occurs in the cellular tissue ? Give its symptoms, and the treatment which is generally adopted. The following were the questions on Dental Anatomy and Physiology and Dental Surgery and Pathology ; the candidates were required to answer at least two out of the three questions, both on Dental Anatomy and Physiology and on Dental Surgery and Pathology, from five to eight o'clock, viz. :—Dental Anatomy and Physiology : 1. Describe the crowns of the following permanent teeth, viz. :—Upper central incisors, lower bicuspids, first molars, upper and lower ; make special mention of those peculiarities of form which predispose to caries. 2. Give a general account of the dentition of snakes : explain the mechanism by which they are enabled to swallow large objects: describe the special contrivances found in the teeth of poisonous species. 3. Describe specimens 1 and 2 under the microscope ; and state the manner of formation of the structures under observation. Dental Surgery and Pathology : 1. What are contour fillings ? What is the *rationale* of their employment ? Describe the relation of two contiguous teeth to each other in a perfectly normal arch, pointing out the methods by which overcrowding of teeth tends to their destruction. 2. Explain the nature of dentigerous cysts ; give their symptoms, diagnosis, and treatment. 3. Describe the operation of pivoting a recently fractured tooth. Mention the difficulties and complications ordinarily encountered.

NAVAL, MILITARY, Etc., APPOINTMENTS.

ADMIRALTY.—Surgeon John Francis Enright, M.D., has been placed on the retired list of his rank from May 6, 1881.

BIRTHS.

BUTLER.—On June 18, at 168, Holland-road, Kensington, the wife of William John Butler, Surgeon H.M.'s Indian Medical Service, Madras (retired), of a son.
CAPON.—On June 21, at 159, Edgware-road, W., the wife of Herbert J. Capon, M.D., L.R.C.P., of a daughter.
FINZI.—On June 25, at 89, Sutherland-gardens, W., the wife of L. M. Finzi, L.R.C.P., M.R.C.S., of a son.
GUTHRIE.—On June 25, at Ashley Lodge, Esher, the wife of J. Guthrie, M.D., of twin daughters.
HALL.—On June 26, at 46, Queen Anne-street, Cavendish-square, the wife of F. de Havilland Hall, M.D., F.R.C.P., of a daughter.
PARISH.—On June 25, at 14, Steyne, Worthing, the wife of Frank Parish, M.R.C.S., L.R.C.P., of a daughter.
PHILLIPS.—On June 19, at Woodville, New Ferry Park, Cheshire, the wife of Edward J. M. Phillips, M.R.C.S., L.D.S., of a daughter.
PRINGLE.—On May 29, at Mussoorie, North-West Provinces, India, the wife of Surgeon-Major R. Pringle, M.D., of H.M.'s Indian Medical Service, of a daughter.

MARRIAGES.

BROWNING—TODD.—On June 23, at Camberwell, Percy, second son of Robert S. Browning, Esq., of St. Martin's, Leicester, to Charlotte Elizabeth, only daughter of G. M. Todd, M.D., of Old Kent-road.
COHEN—COHEN.—On June 28, at 11T, Gower-street, W.C., Algernon A. Cohen, M.B., to Priscilla, eldest daughter of A. Cohen, Esq., of Farringdon-street, E.C.
DIPLOCK—STANTUS.—On June 23, at Chiswick, the son of T. B. Diplock, M.D., of Arlington House, Gunnersbury, to Evelyn Geraldine, fourth daughter of General Stannus, C.B.
DURRANT—HOLLAND.—On June 9, at Petworth, Charles Aubrey Durrant, Esq., youngest son of C. M. Durrant, M.D., of Ipswich, to Catherine Louisa, second daughter of the Rev. C. Holland, Rector of Petworth.
EMERSON—AINSWORTH.—On June 22, at Rivington, Peter Henry Emerson, M.R.C.S., of Clare College, Cambridge, to Edith Amy, youngest daughter of the late J. Ainsworth, Esq., of The Thorns, Bolton-le-Moors.
HARDEN—TERRY.—On June 21, at Richmond, Surrey, Walter Harden, M.D., of Tonbridge, to Fanny, second daughter of the late Mr. Terry, of Richmond.
HART—LAZARUS.—On June 22, at Portland-place, W., Dr. Alfred Hart, of Maison Lacodée, Biarritz, to Lizzie, youngest daughter of the late Henry Lazarus Esq., of Pembroke-square, Dublin.
LOWE—COWPAR.—On June 24, at St. Andrew's, Fifeshire, John Lowe, M.B., C.M., of Coupar-Angus, to Annie Willis, daughter of the late James Cowpar, Esq., formerly Surgeon Madras Medical Service.
MACKINNON—MUNRO.—On June 18, at Kensington, Surgeon-Major Henry William Alexander Mackinnon, A.M.D., to Dora Jessie, second daughter of Surgeon-General W. Munro, C.B.

MATTHEWS—WATT.—On June 22, John Matthews, M.D., of Colebrooke-row, London, N., to Miss Isabel Watt, of Anstrey, Warwickshire.
NANKIVELL—POTTS.—On May 21, at Butterworth, South Africa, John Howard Nankivell, M.R.C.S., District Surgeon, of the Transkei, to Minnie, daughter of Rev. Henry J. Potts, of Llangarron, Herefordshire.

DEATHS.

ATKINS, ALFRED, L.R.C.P., of 91, New North-road, London, N., on June 26, in his 68th year.
DAVIES, WILLIAM, M.R.C.S., L.S.A., at Yorktown, Surrey, on June 27, aged 75.
FOLKARD, HENRY, M.R.C.P., M.R.C.S., L.S.A., A.K.C., at 18, Blenheim-crescent, Bayswater, on June 25, aged 53.
MORRIS, EDWIN BETHUNE, eldest son of Edwin Morris, M.D., F.R.C.S., of Spalding, Lincolnshire, at Mafeteng, Basutoland, South Africa, on April 4.
OSBORNE, JAMES, M.R.C.S., L.R.C.P., L.S.A., at Echuca, Victoria, Australia, on May 5, aged 24.
PEATSON, JOSEPH CHADWICK, M.D., M.R.C.S., L.F.P.S.G., at 28, St. John street, Manchester, on June 26, aged 52.
STEVENSON, WILLIAM, M.D., late of Kingston, Jamaica, at Oporto, on June 8, aged 52.

VACANCIES.

In the following list the nature of the office vacant, the qualifications required in the candidate, the person to whom application should be made and the day of election (as far as known) are stated in succession.

CHESTERFIELD FRIENDLY SOCIETIES' MEDICAL AID ASSOCIATION.—Physician and Surgeon. Candidates must be doubly qualified, and are requested to forward their applications, together with testimonials of recent date, to the Secretary, Durrant-road, Chesterfield, from whom further information can be obtained, on or before July 4.
DEWSBURY AND DISTRICT GENERAL INFIRMARY AND DISPENSARY.—House-Surgeon. Candidates must be doubly qualified and unmarried. Applications, with testimonials, to be sent to the Secretary, Charles J. Abbs, Dewsbury.
EAST LONDON HOSPITAL FOR CHILDREN AND DISPENSARY FOR WOMEN, SHADWELL, E.—Resident Medical Officer. (*For particulars see Advertisement.*)
HOSPITAL FOR CONSUMPTION AND DISEASES OF THE CHEST, BROMPTON.—Assistant-Physician. (*For particulars see Advertisement.*)
HOSPITAL FOR WOMEN, SOHO-SQUARE, W.—House-Physician. (*For particulars see Advertisement.*)
ST. BARTHOLOMEW'S HOSPITAL.—Two Casualty Physicians. Applications, with testimonials, must be left at the Clerk's office on or before July 8, where particulars of the duties and all necessary information may be obtained on personal application. Candidates must attend the meeting of the Committee which takes place at 11 a.m. on July 14.
STOCKTON-UPON-TEES HOSPITAL AND DISPENSARY.—House-Surgeon (non-resident). Candidates must be doubly qualified. Applications, stating age, with recent testimonials, to be sent to the Secretary, John Settle, not later than August 9.

UNION AND PAROCHIAL MEDICAL SERVICE.

‡ The area of each district is stated in acres. The population is computed according to the census of 1871.

RESIGNATIONS.

Penistone Union.—Dr. William Gruggen has resigned the Silkstone District : area 9330 ; population 5213 ; salary £96 per annum.
Upton-upon-Severn Union.—Mr. Edward Watkins has resigned the Fifth District : area 9968 ; population 9867 ; salary £35 per annum.
West Derby Union.—Mr. Patrick O'Connor, Assistant Medical Officer at the Walton Workhouse, has resigned, as from October 1 next : salary £120 per annum.

APPOINTMENTS.

Hackney Union.—George Birch, M.R.C.S. Eng., L.S.A., to the First District.
Norwich Union.—Charles Firth, M.B. Lond. and F.R.C.S. Eng., to the Eighth District. Robert James Mills, M.B. and C.M. Aber., M.R.C.S. Eng., and L.S.A. Lond., to the Second District.

THE annual exhibition of additions about to be made to the Museum of the Royal College of Surgeons will be on view in the Council Room of the College, from the 5th until the 13th inst. inclusive, with the exception of the 7th, when the institution will be closed to all except Fellows attending the annual election into the Council.

MR. CADGE.—The Fellows of the Royal College of Surgeons will regret to hear that, owing to a severe domestic loss, this gentleman will be unable to take the chair as the annual festival on the 7th inst. Mr. T. Crosse, of Norwich, having been invited, has consented to take his place on that occasion.

SEA-WATER BATHS IN LONDON.—Brill's Sea-water Baths at Brighton have long enjoyed a high reputation, and now a company, entitled "Brill's Sea-water Baths, London, and Savoy Mansions Company," has been formed to supply for London "tepid sea-water swimming baths" for gentlemen and for ladies, "hot sea-water baths," and "douche, vapour, and shower baths." A site has been obtained for the establishment, on the Thames-embankment, on the western side of Waterloo-bridge ; and the sea-water is to be brought to the very doors of the baths by steam-vessels especially constructed for the purpose.

Deodorisation of Iodoform.—Dr. Burn observed at the Vienna Medical Society (*Wien. Med. Zeit.*, June 14) that the deodorising of iodoform is a matter of great importance in private practice, and that the different means of effecting this hitherto proposed, such as tincture of musk, bergamot oil, balsam of Peru, oil of mint, etc., either insufficiently conceal the odour or produce one that is as unpleasant as that of the iodoform itself, while they prevent the iodoform being sprinkled as a powder. The addition of a split tonquin-bean, so well known to snuff-takers, will suffice to deodorise effectually from 150 to 200 grammes of iodoform; or if a small quantity of iodoform has to be rapidly deodorised, this may be done by a drop of an alcoholic or ether solution of the bean. The specific smell of the iodoform is lost in a few minutes, and is replaced by a scarcely perceptible bitter-almond odour. Prof. Dittel observed that most of these means act well enough in bottles, but when applied to a wound the smell of the iodoform still prevails. He mixes gypsum-tar with the iodoform in this proportion: beech-tar one part, sulphate of lime four to five parts, and iodoform one hundred parts. This entirely conceals the smell, but cannot be used for union by the first intention. Gypsum-tar is a very useful means also in gangrenous wounds.

How to make a Doctor.—A French journal gives the following account of an examination for a medical degree. We might locate the incident in this city, if it were not for the Latin:—Q. Quid est creare?—A. E nihilo facere. Q. Bene; te doctorem creavimus.—*New York Med. Record*, June 4.

APPOINTMENTS FOR THE WEEK.

July 2. Saturday (this day).

Operations at St. Bartholomew's, 1½ p.m.; King's College, 1½ p.m.; Royal Free, 2 p.m.; Royal London Ophthalmic, 11 a.m.; Royal Westminster Ophthalmic, 1½ p.m.; St. Thomas's, 1½ p.m.; London, 2 p.m.

4. *Monday.*

Operations at the Metropolitan Free, 2 p.m.; St. Mark's Hospital for Diseases of the Rectum, 2 p.m.; Royal London Ophthalmic, 11 a.m.; Royal Westminster Ophthalmic, 1½ p.m.

Royal Institution, 5 p.m. General Monthly Meeting.

5. *Tuesday.*

Operations at Guy's, 1½ p.m.; Westminster, 2 p.m.; Royal London Ophthalmic, 11 a.m.; Royal Westminster Ophthalmic, 1½ p.m.; West London, 3 p.m.

6. *Wednesday.*

Operations at University College, 2 p.m.; St. Mary's, 1¼ p.m.; Middlesex, 1 p.m.; London, 2 p.m.; St. Bartholomew's, 1½ p.m.; Great Northern, 2 p.m.; Samaritan, 2½ p.m.; King's College (by Mr. Lister), 2 p.m.; Royal London Ophthalmic, 11 a.m.; Royal Westminster Ophthalmic, 1½ p.m.; St. Thomas's, 1½ p.m.; St. Peter's Hospital for Stone, 2 p.m.; National Orthopædic, Great Portland-street, 10 a.m.

Obstetrical Society, 8 p.m. Specimens will be shown by Mr. Heath, Dr. Godson, and others. The following Papers will be read:—Dr. James Braithwaite, "On Non-capsulated Fibroids resembling Retained Placenta." Dr. Galabin, "On a Case of Labour with Cancer of Cervix followed by Septicæmia, with Symptoms simulating Diphtheria." Dr. Godson, "On Four Cases of Spasmodic Dysmenorrhœa, with Sterility, successfully treated by Dilatation."

Ophthalmological Society, 8½ p.m. Annual General Meeting for Electing Officers and Council and receiving Treasurer's Report. Mr. J. E. Adams, "On Endocarditis with Embolic Panophthalmitis." Drs. Brailey and Edmunds, "On Certain Ocular Changes in Bright's Disease, and similar Changes from Local Causes." Mr. Snell, "On Hemeralopia, with Patches on Conjunctiva." Mr. Spencer Watson, "On Intraocular Tumour ending Fatally six years after Excision of Eye." Mr. Nettleship and Dr. Edmunds, "On Central Amblyopia in Diabetes; Microscopical Examination." Mr. Nettleship and Dr. Fox, "Sequel to a Case of Multiple Growths on Irides." Dr. Knaggs (by Mr. Swanzy), "On a Case of Vaccinal Ophthalmia." Living specimens and card specimens at 8 o'clock. Mr. Brudenell Carter, "On the Result of Optic Neuritis from Injury to Head." Mr. McHardy, "On a Case of Persistent Hyaloid Artery." Mr. Miles—(1) Specimens of Disease of Vitreous; (2) New Instruments.

7. *Thursday.*

Operations at St. George's, 1 p.m.; Central London Ophthalmic, 1 p.m.; Royal Orthopædic, 2 p.m.; University College, 2 p.m.; Royal London Ophthalmic, 11 a.m.; Royal Westminster Ophthalmic, 1½ p.m.; Hospital for Diseases of the Throat, 2 p.m.; Hospital for Women, 2 p.m.; Charing-cross, 2 p.m.; London, 2 p.m.; North-West London, 2½ p.m.

8. *Friday.*

Operations at Central London Ophthalmic, 2 p.m.; Royal London Ophthalmic, 11 a.m.; South London Ophthalmic, 2 p.m.; Royal Westminster Ophthalmic, 1½ p.m.; St. George's (ophthalmic operations), 1¼ p.m.; Guy's, 1½ p.m.; St. Thomas's (ophthalmic operations), 2 p.m.

Quekett Microscopical Club (University College), 7 p.m. Conversation and Exhibition of Objects.

VITAL STATISTICS OF LONDON.

Week ending Saturday, June 25, 1881.

BIRTHS.

Births of Boys, 1264; Girls, 1240; Total, 2504.
Corrected weekly average in the 10 years 1871-80, 2480·4.

DEATHS.

	Males.	Females.	Total.
Deaths during the week	742	657	1399
Weekly average of the ten years 1871-80, corrected to increased population ...	742·8	663·6	1406·4
Deaths of people aged 80 and upwards ...	...	...	41

DEATHS IN SUB-DISTRICTS FROM EPIDEMICS.

	Enumerated Population, 1881 (unrevised).	Small-pox.	Measles.	Scarlet Fever.	Diphtheria.	Whooping-cough.	Typhus.	Enteric (or Typhoid) Fever.	Simple continued Fever.	Diarrhœa.
West	668993	15	7	2	1	4	...	...	...	4
North ...	905677	27	22	9	5	7	...	2	...	11
Central ...	281793	2	6	2	...	5	...	1	1	4
East	692530	3	24	3	3	6	...	3	...	16
South... ...	1265578	41	12	8	5	11	2	1	...	9
Total	3814571	88	71	24	14	33	2	7	1	44

METEOROLOGY.

From Observations at the Greenwich Observatory.

Mean height of barometer	29·788 in.
Mean temperature	60·6°
Highest point of thermometer	77·2°
Lowest point of thermometer	47·5°
Mean dew-point temperature	52·3°
General direction of wind	S.W.
Whole amount of rain in the week	0·19 in.

BIRTHS and DEATHS Registered and METEOROLOGY during the Week ending Saturday, June 25, in the following large Towns:—

Cities and boroughs (Municipal boundaries except for London.)	Estimated Population to middle of the year 1881.*	Persons to an Acre. (1881.)	Births Registered during the week ending June 25.	Deaths Registered during the week ending June 25.	Temperature of Air (Fahr.) Highest during the Week.	Lowest during the Week.	Weekly Mean of Daily Mean Values.	Temp. of Air (Cent.) Weekly Mean of Daily Mean Values.	Rain Fall. In Inches.	In Centimetres.
London	3829751	50·8	2504	1399	77·2	47·5	60·6	15·90	0·19	0·48
Brighton	107934	45·9	58	30	74·4	50·4	59·0	15·00	0·14	0·36
Portsmouth ...	128335	28·6	91	42	...	...	...	...	...	...
Norwich	88038	11·8	43	38	75·0	52·0	59·5	15·28	0·04	0·10
Plymouth	75262	54·0	61	14	65·8	45·0	56·7	13·72	1·06	2·69
Bristol	207140	46·5	12[illegible]	69	67·5	43·8	56·3	13·50	0·97	2·46
Wolverhampton ...	75934	22·4	56	17	70·8	43·3	55·6	13·12	0·89	2·26
Birmingham ...	402296	47·9	291	139	70·4	45·7	58·2	14·55	·44	1·12
Leicester	123120	38·5	105	40	73·2	48·8	58·5	14·72	0·49	1·24
Nottingham ...	188035	18·9	122	49	...	...	...	...	...	...
Liverpool	553988	106·3	383	244	...	...	...	...	...	...
Manchester ...	341269	79·5	300	121	...	...	...	...	...	...
Salford	177760	34·4	120	52	...	...	...	...	...	...
Oldham	112176	24·0	92	34	...	...	...	...	...	...
Bradford	184037	25·5	127	73	69·6	45·1	57·7	14·28	0·47	1·19
Leeds	310490	14·4	226	107	71·0	43·0	58·2	14·55	0·50	1·27
Sheffield	285621	14·5	2[illegible]6	113	71·0	45·5	57·8	14·34	0·74	1·88
Hull	155161	42·7	103	44	...	...	...	...	...	...
Sunderland ...	116753	42·2	116	82	...	...	...	...	...	...
Newcastle-on-Tyne	145675	27·1	120	45	...	...	...	...	...	...
Total of 20 large English Towns ...	7608775	38·0	5252	2700	77·2	43·0	58·0	14·44	0·54	1·37

* These figures are the numbers enumerated (but subject to revision) in April last, raised to the middle of 1881 by the addition of a quarter of a year's increase, calculated at the rate that prevailed between 1871 and 1881.

At the Royal Observatory, Greenwich, the mean reading of the barometer last week was 29·78 in. The lowest reading was 29·41 in. on Tuesday morning, and the highest 30·07 in. on Friday morning.

NOTES, QUERIES, AND REPLIES.

Be that questionath much shall learn much.—Bacon.

Fairplay.—You cannot prevent his practising. But it is illegal for either of them to sign an ordinary certificate of cause of death for a case which they have never seen.

Septimus.—Yes; in Prince Edward's Island the sale of spirituous liquors on Sundays has been prohibited for more than the last hundred years. But the conditions of existence in the colonies are obviously different from those which prevail at home. We believe in some parts of the United States a woman having a drunken husband has a right to go to the keeper of a public-house and give him notice not to sell liquor to her husband. If the publican does sell liquor to the husband he becomes responsible for what may be termed "consequential damages." As to these damages, if the husband should, after the notice given, be supplied with liquor, and commits an assault or any act which brings him within the law, the publican has to pay damages.

Lex.—Gideon de Lawne was one of the first Assistants of the Apothecaries' Company after their separation from the "Grocers" in 1617. A bust and portrait of him are preserved at Apothecaries' Hall.

Impartial: No Enthusiast.—We imagine the treatise to which you refer is Mr. Charles Loring Brace's, entitled, "The Dangerous Classes of New York, and Twenty Years' Work among them." He writes with judgment and impartiality, and lays great stress upon workmen's clubs, the provision of better public amusements, the introduction of lighter alcoholic beverages, and of drinking-gardens in lieu of public-houses. The treatise may be obtained from Trübner and Co., London.

Liquor "Treating."—The American society which some time ago started a crusade against "treating in liquor," boasts of having secured upwards of 190,000 subscribers to its anti-treating pledge.

Antiquary.—Drinking-fountains, now becoming general in London and other large towns, were provided by benevolent persons nearly two centuries ago. Sir Samuel Morland, who resided in Hammersmith in 1684, observing the scarcity of good drinking-water in the neighbourhood, and knowing how seriously the poor would suffer from the want of such a necessary of life, had a well sunk near his own house, and constructed over it a pump (a rare convenience in those days), and conveyed it gratuitously for the use of the public. A tablet fixed in the wall of his own house recorded this benefaction. The pump has been removed, but the stone bearing the inscription was preserved in the garden of the house, afterwards known by the name of Walbrough House.

G. G., Sussex.—The Local Government Board has no power, under the Public Health Act, to prescribe any particular qualification, or mode of appointment, or salary, or tenure of office, of a medical officer of health or inspector of nuisances. Upon these matters the local authorities, so far as they are not controlled by Act of Parliament, are uncontrolled. The central authority, however, offers half the salaries of these officers on condition that it is allowed to have a paramount voice in appointing them and setting out their duties. The regulations, which are published, constitute the terms of this subsidy.

J. F. F., Borough.—Buchan's "Domestic Medicine" first appeared in 1769. It was written in Sheffield; it went through nineteen editions in the author's lifetime.

The Homœopathic Medical Officer Agitation at Hastings.—Public meetings were held last week, in reference to the recent appointment of the Medical Officer of Health, under the auspices respectively of the Conservative and Liberal Associations of the borough. The former manimously passed resolutions condemning the appointment, and the refusal of the Mayor to call a meeting, and supporting freedom of speech, etc. The latter adopted resolutions in favour of the appointment, and condemned the agitation of the Conservative party as detrimental to the borough.

Sea-Water in London.—1, 1877. 2. The threatened opposition in the House of Lords to the London Sea-Water Supply Bill has been withdrawn, and the success of the measure may almost be regarded as assured.

A Publican "a Life-long Testotaler."—The Preston Board of Guardians have recently had under discussion a proposal to petition Parliament in favour of closing public-houses on Sunday. Mr. Ashcroft, a publican, but a Sunday-closer, and a "life-long teetotaler," in opposition to the motion, stated that he did not agree with compulsory total closing on Sunday. In his young days public-houses were opened till half-past ten on Sunday morning; and since the hours had been altered, twice as much beer was sold in bottles on Saturday night. The motion was rejected by twelve votes to eleven.

The Society for Improving the Condition of the Labouring Classes.—From the thirty-seventh annual report of this Society it appears that the houses of the Society had been largely used by the class of persons for whom they were intended. The death-rate throughout the property was only twenty per thousand, and there had not been a single case of small-pox in any of the dwellings.

Revaccination in the Navy.—The Admiralty, in consequence of the prevalence of small-pox, has directed a general examination of the officers and men of Her Majesty's ships at the home ports, for the purpose of ascertaining the extent to which revaccination may be necessary. The medical officers of the ships are to perform the operation.

Quis.—It was Mr. John Bright, M.P., when at the Board of Trade, who somewhat startled a deputation by stating that adulteration was only a form of competition.

Increased Mortality in the Male Population.—A noteworthy fact in the Annual Report of the Registrar-General is, that the mortality of males, as compared with the mortality of females, has been undergoing increase for many years past. From the commencement of civil registration until 1851-55, the mortality of males diminished in comparison with that of females. The change began at that period, and, after a short cessation, has continued in the new direction ever since. The proportion in 1879 was 113 to 100.

Seats for Shop Employés.—It is announced that the Legislature of the State of New York has unanimously passed a Bill making it compulsory for shopkeepers to provide seats for their employés. This is a grievance in our own country in regard to which much has lately been said, but it would appear the cruel system is likely to prevail till it is abrogated by a similar legislative enactment.

"A Winter in Madeira."—Lord Henry Lennox, M.P., has, under this title, re-published in a pamphlet form (Hamilton, Adams, and Co., London) a lecture delivered by him before the Chichester Working-Men's Institute. Lord Henry went to Madeira last autumn, being in a precarious state of health, and has returned "from that beautiful spot in renewed health and strength." He has given a detailed and graphic account of the island, but the pamphlet is not one of indiscriminate praise. It points out the several drawbacks to a *rendezvous* of invalids, and contains valuable recent information on Madeira interesting to intending visitors.

Sanitary Wards: Llanelly.—A public meeting has been held at Llanelly to consider a proposal to divide the urban sanitary district into wards. After considerable desultory discussion, a motion to petition the Local Government Board on the subject was lost by a bare majority.

An Epitaph "On a Quack."

"I was a quack, and there are men who say
 That in my time I physick'd lives away;
 And that at length I by myself was slain
 With my own drugs, ta'en to relieve my pain.
 The truth is, being troubled with a cough,
 I, like a fool, consulted Dr. Gough,
 Who physick'd me to death at his own will,
 Because he's licensed by the State to kill:
 Had I but wisely ta'en my own physic,
 I never should have died of cold and 'tisick.
 So all be warned, and when you catch a cold,
 Go to my son by whom my medicine's sold."

COMMUNICATIONS have been received from—

Dr. Norris Wolfenden, London; Dr. James Anderson, London; Dr. Langmore, London; The Secretary of the Local Government Board, London; Dr. J. Russell, Birmingham; The Director-General of the Naval Medical Department, London; Dr. Crighton Browne, London; Dr. Robert Saundby, Birmingham; Dr. Fraser, Plymouth; The Secretary of the Ophthalmological Society, London; The Registrar of the Durham University; Miss Yates, London; Mr. W. W. Oberyn, London; The Secretary of the Obstetrical Society, London; Dr. Anderson, London; Mr. Patrick Chalmers, London; Mr. J.J. Steele, London; The Honorary Secretary of the Rolleston Memorial, London; Dr. A. Sangster, London; Mr. J. Crafto, London; Mr. T. M. Stone, London.

BOOKS, ETC., RECEIVED—

Chemical Vade-Mecum, by George Jones, F.C.S.—Charitable and Parochial Establishments, by E. Saxon Snell—The Sanitary Chronicles of the Parish of St. Marylebone during May, 1881—Reports on "Sanitas"—Medical Societies, by J. Collins Warren, M.D.—The Patent Rottan Transport Splint of C. De Mooy—Annual Report of the British Medical Benevolent Fund for the Year 1880—A Dictionary of Chemistry, by Henry Watts, B.A., F.R.S., F.C.S.—Furton 8pa—Annual Report of the Board of State Viticultural Commissioners—Borough of Newcastle-upon-Tyne: Notice on the Prevention of Infectious Diseases—The Principles of Myodynamics, by J. S. Wight, M.D.—The Laryngoscope, by Gordon Holmes, L.R.C.P.—On Cancer, by F. Albert Purcell, M.D., M.R.C.S.—Report of the Health of Liverpool for 1880—On Vaccination, by J. W. Miller, M.D.—How to make the Best of Life, by F. M. Granville, M.D.

PERIODICALS AND NEWSPAPERS RECEIVED—

Lancet—British Medical Journal—Medical Press and Circular—Berliner Klinische Wochenschrift—Centralblatt für Chirurgie—Gazette des Hôpitaux—Gazette Médicale—Le Progrès Médical—Bulletin de l'Académie de Médecine—Pharmaceutical Journal—Wiener Medizinische Wochenschrift—Centralblatt für die Medizinischen Wissenschaften—Revue Médicale—Gazette Hebdomadaire—National Board of Health Bulletin, Washington—Nature—Occasional Notes—Deutsche Medicinal-Zeitung—Boston Medical and Surgical Journal—Louisville Medical News—Japan Weekly Mail—Gazeta Científica—Chicago Medical Review—Queensland Government Gazette—Archives of Medicine—Indian Medical Gazette—Weekblad—Our Times—The Pilot—Bicycle Annual—Sunday at Home—Boy's Own Paper—Leisure Hour—Friendly Greeting—Girl's Own Paper—National Anti-Compulsory Vaccination Reporter—The American—Dublin Journal of Medical Science.

ORIGINAL LECTURES.

CLINICAL LECTURE ON FOUR CASES OF PNEUMONIA.

By C. HANDFIELD JONES, M.B. Cantab., F.R.S.,
Physician to St. Mary's Hospital.

Case 1.—Bacteria in Urine, Kidney and Spleen probably—Albuminuria—Pneumonia—Autopsy.

E. D., female, aged twenty-three, admitted December 6, 1880. An emaciated woman, of slight make, with anxious countenance. Left hospital in tolerable case about middle of last November. She had disease of aortic valves and albuminuria. On December 3, after a visit to hospital, she was seized with retching and diarrhœa. She got worse, and was admitted. Her breath was then very short; she had to be propped up in bed. Face pale, with circumscribed malar flush. Temperature 104·2°; pulse 120; respirations 32. Double aortic murmur heard at mid-sternum, none at apex. Resonance impaired in both lower bases; entry of air is weak, and crepitation is heard. Urine acid, smoky; specific gravity 1025; contains much albumen and some blood. No œdema. Mist. ammon. citrat. efferv. ℥j., ammon. carb. gr. iij., quater die.

December 7.—Temperature 104°; pulse 140. Skin burning hot and dry. Complains of pain about umbilicus, and tenderness in splenic region. Dulness and tubular breathing in upper right back; harsh breathing and crepitation elsewhere. In evening an ice-bag was applied to both backs, and was borne well. Liq. opii sed. ♏v. was added to each dose. Brandy four ounces. At 11.30 p.m., temperature 104·2°, pulse 120, respirations 40.

8th.—Passed a better night, but dyspnœa troublesome. Bowels open once. Face pallid, ashy. Extremities rather cold. Temperature 108·4°; pulse 150 to 160; respirations 36. 9th.—She steadily got worse, and died at 6 a.m.

Post-mortem (on 10th).—Bright flush on cheek; lineæ albicantes on abdomen; breasts show signs of lactation; brain arteries at base healthy, no signs of embolism. Left lung healthy; right upper lobe is consolidated, passing from red to grey hepatisation; there is some red hepatisation at the posterior borders of middle and lower lobes. Bronchi of right lung congested and contain some blood-stained frothy mucus. Heart: Right cavities are dilated and full of clot; left cavities nearly empty. Wall of left ventricle of firm healthy consistence, three-quarters of an inch thick. Mitral valve shows chronic fibroid thickening, and is slightly incompetent. Aortic valves intensely ulcerated, and utterly incompetent, beset with large vegetations, partly soft and partly calcareous. Aorta: Acute ulceration of the elastic coat has given rise to an aneurism of the size of an ordinary nut, the sac being formed entirely of the adventitia or outer coat. The aneurism exactly corresponds with the position of the calcified mass on the left posterior flap of the aortic valve when thrown back. The ulcer seems to have been produced by the impact of the mass. Liver very coarsely granular, especially on its under surface; its consistence much denser than usual. Spleen very large, pale, and firm; it contained a recent infarctus involving one-fourth of its substance. Kidneys: Capsules not adherent, or but slightly; surface smooth; cortex of normal depth and appearance. Microscope showed nothing remarkable in the splenic infarct, except vast numbers of granules much resembling micrococci, and some rods like short vibrios; none were seen moving. The examination was made on December 11. The kidneys appeared quite normal to the eye, but microscope showed in very many tubes a very narrow epithelial lining and a very wide lumen, sometimes equalling two-thirds or three-fourths of the whole diameter. In thin sections the wide lumens of the tubes at certain spots looked much like round vacuoles; in one spot the tubes seemed quite full of some refracting material or quite empty of epithelium. In many detached fragments of epithelium of the cortical tubes that were lying about the observation was made, and confirmed by another observer, that the wall appeared to consist of a coarse

granular matter, the granules very much resembling micrococci. The convoluted tubes and straight tubes were in some parts quite opaque and infarcted with granular matter. The Malpighian tufts were pretty normal, but greyish and unduly refractive.

This post-mortem record derives additional value from the record made November 15, and which I had quite forgotten, that the urine of that date was light-coloured, notably albuminous, and deposited a notable flocculent sediment. In this sediment were found very many red blood corpuscles; casts tolerably wide, granular, pigmented, and corpuscular, and some renal epithelium. The epithelial scales and casts, and leucocyte-like corpuscles, often contain much opaque granular matter, the granules much resembling micrococci. The tracing on October 30, when she appeared in fair health, but had albuminuria, double aortic murmur, and marked pulsation and thrill at the sternal notch, presented a moderate rather low rise, a very flat top, and a notchless fall. The pulse felt cordy.

As regards the pneumonia, there is nothing of any special moment in this case, except it be that the application of cold to the chest was well borne and seemed beneficial. It is possible that the hepatisation of the left lung might have been much more extensive had not the process been checked by the local application. The fatal issue was due quite as much to the general unsoundness of the system, seriously damaged in two most important organs—the heart and the kidneys—as to the acute lung disease. The production of the aneurism in a most manifestly mechanical method, viz., by the rapidly repeated impact and pressure of a calcareous mass against the wall of the aorta, is very noteworthy as showing the effects of rapidly recurring "usure" on a tissue, which, as being feebly vascularised, has probably but slender power of repair. Of course the impossibility of rest to the part was also most unfavourable.

The probable presence of micrococci in the splenic infarct, in the urine—near a month before the fatal disease—and in the kidney, seems to me of great interest. I say the probable presence, for my experience of micrococci is not large, and I am not positively certain that the objects I saw were micrococci. Moreover, I did not have recourse to the tests for bacteria proposed by von Recklinghausen, or to the methods of staining and illumination employed by Koch. Still, as I have long been familiar with the appearances presented by the urine and kidneys in states of disease, I can hardly doubt that there was something peculiar in both in the case of E. D., or that my interpretation of the phenomena was correct. There is no novelty in the detection of micrococci in the kidneys; they have been found there by von Recklinghausen, Orth, and Heiberg, in typhus, pyæmia, and puerperal fever. E. D.'s case may be regarded as in some measure allied to these, seeing that her cardiac valves were severely ulcerated, and that her spleen presented the lesion commonly attendant on arterial pyæmia. Still, it is to be noted that her urine presumably contained bacteria, as it certainly did albumen, long before she had any fever or any appearance of general disease. In two other cases bacteria have been present for a longer or shorter period in the urine, quite independent of any putrefactive change. One of these was a male aged twenty-three, who had an attack of nephritis two years previously, and a second shortly before he came under my care. His urine persistently contained albumen, often also hæmatin, was alkaline, and deposited phosphates. The other was of a male, aged fifty-eight, suffering under what some would term renal dropsy, but which I prefer to regard as arterio-capillary fibrosis. His urine was constantly cloudy throughout with bacteria, though none of the other patients' urines were in a like state. In these two cases the presence of bacteria in the urine cannot be referred to cardiac valve lesions. The one thing common to them and to Case 1 is persistent albuminuria. This may have been caused by the bacteric growth in the kidney. If so, we have here a new form of chronic renal disease not necessarily associated with any general infective disorder.

Case 2.—Pneumonia of Right Lung, chiefly affecting Apex—Delirium—Recovery.

A. B., aged twenty-four, a groom, admitted February 18, 1881. Dark hair and eyes. Ill seven days. Was first taken with shivering and giddiness. Lost his voice about same time, and became rather deaf; is so still. Never ill before. Very restless the night after admission, and is so still

(4 p.m. of 19th). In left lung breathing is full and good, and resonance also. Right front dull at upper part, and back more or less dull also, especially at upper third. Breathing in upper right lung, both in front and behind, markedly tubular, and voice bronchophonic; breathing in middle and lower right back defective, weak, harsh, semi-tubular, attended with some half-moist râle. Has a bad cough; expectorates about two ounces of muco-purulent, thickish brown sputa. Heart-sounds normal. Tongue brown and dry. Pulse 96; respirations 54. Last night was bad; he had bad dreams, got out of bed twice, had delusions. Ammon. carb. gr. iv., tinct. cinch. ʒj., dec. cinch. ʒj., ter die; opii gr. j., ter die; brandy four ounces. Spoon diet—milk, beef-tea.

February 21.—Tongue clean and moist. Pulse 114, jerky, soft, very compressible. Physical signs same, except that in lower half or so of right back the breathing is very weak, and very little is heard except peculiarly small, almost fine, crepitation. In left back there is some slightly marked bronchial breathing in supra-spinous fossa, with small moist râle in all the rest of back, especially at the base. Aspect of face is much improved. Omit opium.

22nd.—Rather delirious and wandering in night. Pulse 114; respirations 36; expectoration rusty, one ounce.

24th.—At right supra-spinous fossa there is exquisite bronchial breathing and bronchophony; lower down the breathing gradually loses its tubular character, and the voice becomes less bronchial, whilst vesicular breathing mingled with small crepitations becomes well-marked. Good, full breathing in all left back, but rather harsh, and expiration rather long. Sputa tinged; but little chloride in urine—two or three days ago there was a mere trace. Has broth diet, two eggs, milk Oij., rice-pudding, beef-tea. Takes opii gr. ? p. r. n., liq. ferri pernitratis ℥xv., quin. disulph. gr. ij., aq. piment. ʒj. t. d.

On 28th the urine contained an abundance of chloride. Pulse 84; respirations 24. The consolidation signs were gradually disappearing. Sputa about two ounces. A little sweating at night.

March 14.—Percussion-note under right clavicle woody, under left good. Good, pure breathing in upper left front, in right almost equally good throughout the whole front, but rather "divided" at the mid-region. Breathing in right supra-spinous fossa fairly good, but somewhat wanting in purity and fulness. Good full breathing without râle all through right back. Perfectly good breathing in all left front and left back. No sputa. Feels weak.

Went to Walton on 16th.

TEMPERATURE TABLE.

Date.	Morning.	Evening.
Feb. 18 ...	...	—	108° (8 p.m.) ; 102·8°
„ 19 ...	...	108°	108·8
„ 20 ...	...	102·6	101·8
„ 21 ...	...	100·2	98·6 (8 p.m.) ; 99
„ 22 ...	...	100·2	100·6
„ 23 ...	...	99·6	99·4
„ 24 ...	...	98·8	100·6
„ 25 ...	...	99·4	100·6
„ 26 ...	...	99·4	99·2
„ 27 ...	...	98·4	98·6
„ 28 ...	...	98·6	99·6
After this	...	Normal.	

In this instance the nervous system was severely affected, the patient had delusions, and was delirious and wandering as late as the eleventh day of his illness. Opium, given pretty freely for two days, was decidedly beneficial, and subsequently a small occasional dose was found useful. The pneumonic process chiefly affected the right lung, but extended also to the left about the ninth or tenth day. Defervescence ensued late (not till about eleventh day), and was much more gradual than is often the case.

Case 3.—Pneumonia—Albuminuria—Delirium—Recovery.

A. L., aged seventeen, baker, admitted March 14, 1881.

March 15.—He never had any serious illness before. On March 1 he felt out of sorts; he had had a toothache for some time before. He got pain at right side of chest, felt chilly, and shivered, had cough, was sick at times, breathed with difficulty, felt dyspnœa on the slightest exertion. He had thirst, loss of appetite. At present is very restless, hot and flushed. Pulse 114, irregular. Expectoration rusty,

two ounces and a half; not much cough. Herpetic eruption on lips. Urine thick, acid, albuminous. Temperature 104·2°. Tongue red at tip, brown at dorsum. Well marked dulness in right front down to third rib. In all right front entry of air is weak; in quiet respiration no crepitation or bronchial breathing is heard, but in deeper breathing the bronchial quality becomes evident, with moist sounds extending as far down as fourth rib. In lower three-fourths of right back air enters pretty well and breathing is good; in supra-spinous fossa it is harsh, with unduly prolonged expiration. Good resonance and breathing in all left chest. Ammon. carb. gr. iij., tinct. cinchon. ʒj., dec. cinch. ʒj., ter die; opii gr. ss., h. n.; brandy three ounces. Diet—broth, milk, beef-tea.

16th.—Rather delirious during night, did not sleep well. Takes nourishment well. Tongue coated. Bowels not open three days. Pulse 84, weak. Sputa in less quantity, not tinged, but streaked with blood. Is drowsy. Pil. hydr. c. coloc. gr. v. statim.

19th.—Complains of pain in abdomen. Slept fairly. Breathing much easier. Sputa chiefly mucus, slightly streaked with blood. First right space dull; second gives woody tympanitic resonance; third is pretty normal. Air enters more freely in upper right front; air enters well in all right back, but expiration is prolonged in supra-spinous fossa. No râles heard. Good breathing in left back.

21st.—Slight quasi-bronchial breathing in upper and middle right front; air enters more freely. Expectoration scanty, tinged with blood, dark-coloured. Takes food well. Liq. ferri pernitratis ℥xv., liq. strychniæ ℥iv., æth. chlor. ℥xv., aq. ʒj., t. d. Chop, rice pudding; omit brandy for beer.

24th.—Perfectly good resonance and breathing in both upper fronts; condition of right equal to that of left. He seems quite well. Went out on 31st.

TEMPERATURE TABLE.

Date.	Morning.	Evening.
March 14 ...	...	—	104·2°
„ 15 ...	...	108·6°	108
„ 16 ...	...	102	101·4 (3 p.m.) ; 108·4° (6 p.m.)
„ 17 ...	...	102	102 (6 p.m.) ; 97·8° (11.30 p.m.)
„ 18 ...	...	98·4	98 (6 p.m.)
„ 19 ...	...	98	100·2
„ 20 ...	...	96	98·8
Subsequently normal.		

If the patient's account is correct, the pneumonia in this case was unusually prolonged. Defervescence occurred on the evening of 17th, the initial symptoms having appeared on the 1st, as stated. This gives a duration of sixteen days—five days longer than in Case 2, and eleven days longer than in Case 4. Possibly the longer duration of the illness may be in connexion with the longer delay before the patient came under hospital care. This view accords with the short duration of Case 4. The absence of breath-sounds in quiet respiration over the inflamed lung was not due to over-distension of the air-cells by exudation preventing the entry of more air, nor yet to obstruction of the tubes, as shown by the result of a more forcible inspiration. The part of lung affected was not large, and the air-hunger not great.

Case 4.—Previous Rheumatic Pains for five days—Sudden Invasion of Pneumonia while in Hospital—Severe Cough.—Agitation—Opium used pretty freely—Recovery.

A. B., aged eighteen, barmaid, admitted December 20, 1880.

December 21.—Has been ill in bed a week with aching in all her limbs; knees and right wrist have been swollen, are not tender now. She had shivering several times for two to four minutes during the day before the pains came on. Attributes her illness to sleeping in a damp bed. Catamenia regular now, but had amenorrhœa with pains in head and fainting fits and nausea for three months a year ago. Pulse 92, regular and weakish. Bowels constipated. Mist. sodæ salicylicat. ʒj. o.h. ad vices 6.

23rd.—Murmurs at apex presystolic and systolic, the former temporary. Lungs normal. Salicylicate not repeated. Temperature was 100·8° on 20th in evening; 99·6° on 21st p.m., then for the next three days at same time 99°, and on 25th p.m. 98·6°. She was apparently quite well at midnight of 25th, and until an early hour of 26th. Then she had short shiverings, and on sitting up she felt very giddy. Her breathing has been getting bad since, and she has felt pain in respiration chiefly along the sternum, pains also in both legs. Six leeches were applied to left side this morning, with relief to pain, which was acute there, but it continues very bad in the middle of chest. Temperature at 9.30 a.m. of 26th, 105°. In evening she had six doses of salicylicate, one o.h. ; they did not affect the temperature much.

27th.—Respirations 52 ; pulse 120, weak. She is very deaf. Expectoration scanty, watery, and rusty. In the afternoon she was in a state of great agitation, coughing almost continuously, and retching now and then. In lower left back quasi-tubular breathing was heard, and now and then crepitation. This part was very tender to pressure. The lower right back was dull, and the breathing weak, but not decidedly tubular. Opii gr. ss. 2dis horis ; mist. ammon. citrat. efferv. ℥j. 4tis horis. Poultices to left side.

28th.—Patient has had a fairly good night ; was sick once. She has a good deal of bronchial irritation ; coughs up muco-watery fluid, sometimes vomits a little. She complains much of headache. Can sit up well. Pulse 140. No normal breathing in either back—in right, tubular breathing is heard very extensively ; in left, there is tubular breathing about middle, and almost silence below. More or less dulness in both lower backs. Quin. disulph. gr. v., acid. sulph. dil. ℳvj., aq. ℥j., 4tis horis.

29th.—Slept fairly ; cough is troublesome, provokes sickness. She has brought up about twelve ounces of greenish watery fluid. Perspires a good deal. Expectoration rather rusty, about one ounce and a half since last night. Bowels not open since 25th. Tongue quite moist. Much pain in left side. Pulse 110, regular, soft ; respirations 36. Opium taken 2dis vel 3tiis hor.

30th.—Bowels well opened by enema ; has great thirst. Pulse 112, quite distinct and regular. Left side where pain is felt expands well and air enters well. Subcut. morphia gr.¼.

31st.—Good night ; pain in left side quite gone ; coughing and retching almost ceased.

January 1, 1881.—Restless in night ; did not sleep, though she had a morphia injection. Some vomiting. At 3 p.m. pulse 80, good. First sound at apex prolonged, with some tendency to reduplicate ; second sound clear at apex. No murmur except at left third space near sternum.

4th.—Doing well ;=taking food with appetite. Pulse 78, weak ; respirations 33, very shallow. Breathing quite good throughout both backs. Taking quinine ter die since the 3rd ; port wine four ounces.

10th.—Omit brandy.

12th.—Doing well. Good breathing in both backs, except at right base posteriorly, where air enters weakly, and there is some obscure crepitation. Ferri et quinæ citrat. gr. viij., tinct. nucis vom. ℳx., aq. ℥j. ter die.

26th.—Is very well ; walking about. Her heart's sounds appear quite normal, except that the first sound is mainly valvular—a sharp flap. (A sister of nearly the same age has a well-marked, long, presystolic murmur, abruptly terminated.) Went out soon after.

TEMPERATURE TABLE.

Date.	Morning.	Evening.	Date.	Morning.	Evening.
Dec. 20	...	100 8°	Dec. 24	...	98·6°	99°
„ 21	... 99°	99·6	„ 25	... —	98·6
„ 22	... 99	99	„ 26	... 105	104·4
„ 23	... 99·2	99			

Hourly Observations.

Dec. 26, 12 p.m.	... 103·4°	Dec. 28, 7.30 a.m.	... 102·2°
Dec. 27, 1 a.m.	... 103	„ 10	... 103·8
„ 2	... 104	„ 12	... 104·2
„ 3	... 103·8	„ 2 p.m.	... 105
„ 4	... 104	„ 6	... 104·8
„ 5	... 105	„ 9	... 105
„ 6	... 102·5	„ 11	... 103·6
„ 10	... 102·5	Dec. 29, 1 a.m.	... 102·6
„ 12	... 103·6	„ 3	... 101·4
„ 2 p.m.	... 106·6	„ 5	... 101·2
„ 6	... 105	„ 7	... 102·5
„ 9	... 104·2	„ 9	... 104
„ 11.30	... 103	„ 11.30	... 104
Dec. 28, 1.30 a.m.	... 101	„ 1.30 p.m.	... 103·4
„ 3.30	... 101·8	„ 3.30	... 102·4
„ 5	... 101	„ 5.30	... 103·6

Dec. 29, 7.30 p.m.	... 104·6°	Jan. 1, 4 a.m.	... 104°
„ 9.30	... 101·6	„ 5	... 103·2
„ 11.30	... 100·8	„ 7	... 101·2
Dec. 30, 1.30 a.m.	... 100	„ 8	... 100·8
„ 3.30	... 100	„ 10	... 100·6
„ 5.30	... 103·6	„ 12	... 99
„ 7 a.m.	... 103·2	„ 2 p.m.	... 99
„ 9	... 103	„ 4	... 99·2
„ 11.30	... 104·4	„ 6	... 99
„ 1.30 p.m.	... 104	„ 12	... 99·6
„ 3.30	... 103·6	Jan. 2, 2 a.m.	... 99·2
„ 6.30	... 103	„ 4	... 99·6
„ 10	... 101·6	„ 8	... 98
„ 12	... 100·6	„ 10	... 100
Dec. 31, 2 a.m.	... 99·6	„ 1 p.m.	... 98·6
„ 5	... 98·6	„ 5	... 98·6
„ 8	... 99	„ 12	... 98·6
„ 9.30	... 99	Jan. 3, 5 a.m.	... 98·6
„ 2 p.m.	... 99·2	„ 10	... 99
„ 6	... 99·8	„ 2 p.m.	... 99
„ 12	... 101	„ 6	... 99·2
Jan. 1, 2 a.m.	... 101·4		

The interest of this case lies chiefly in the circumstance that the pneumonia commenced some days after the patient's admission for slight rheumatism, while she was therefore directly under observation. The invasion was quite sudden ; the temperature was certainly normal on the previous evening. It rose rapidly, and attained its maximum height in about three hours from the setting in of the rigor. Considerable irritation of the bronchial and gastric nerves, and great general agitation, occurred early and called for the free use of opium. The pyrexia was decidedly of remittent type, the culmens occurring chiefly at a late evening or night hour, and the bases at the morning hours, but not without notable exceptions, as the subjoined table shows :—

	Culmens on		Bases.
First day	at 9.30 a.m.	6 a.m. and 10 a.m.
Second	„ 6 p.m.	10 a.m.
Third	„ 2 p.m. and 9 p.m.	1.30 a.m. and 5 a.m.
Fourth	„ 7.30 p.m.	11.30 p.m.
Fifth	„ 11.30 a.m.	1.30 a.m. and 3.30 a.m.
Sixth	„ 12 p.m.	5 a.m.
Seventh	„ 4 a.m.	8 a.m.

This variability is unfortunate, as it interferes with the use of preventive measures intended to anticipate abnormal elevations of temperature.

The daily averages are shown in the accompanying table, and it is evident that on the whole the temperature declined pretty constantly from the commencement to the close, the only exception being the seventh day, when the average was ·9° above that of the previous day. It is to be observed, however, that only seven readings are recorded for the sixth day against eleven on the fifth day and eleven on the seventh, so that it is possible the low figure on the sixth day was owing to omission of some higher elevations. Also it appears that the culmens of the seventh, which occurred at 4 and 5 a.m., may have properly belonged to the sixth day, but were postponed, as we know to occur in ague paroxysms when the malady is on the wane. The gradual lowering of the temperature harmonises with the view that the body-heat is controlled by the nervous system, and that fever is, in fact, a paralysis of a regulating centre. If fever proceeded from combustion of protoplasm solely, irrespective of loss of nerve control, how could we explain its subsidence as long as any protoplasm remained to burn ?

Daily Averages.

First day	... ... 104·7°	Fifth day	... ... 102·4°
Second „	... ... 103·7	Sixth „	... ... 99·4
Third „	... ... 103·2	Seventh „	... ... 100·3
Fourth „	... ... 102·7	Eighth „	... ... 98·9

Complete defervescence ensued on the seventh day, a small rise followed on the eighth, its culmen at 4 a.m. with a speedy fall. Thenceforward the temperature remained normal or very nearly so. The quinine may have favoured the subsidence of the pyrexia, as it certainly lessened from the time this medication was commenced. The opium certainly appeared to do good. The disease, though it affected both lungs, was not of long duration, and the convalescence was speedy. The treatment in all the cases was mainly directed to sustain the general power, and especially the action of the heart, which were to some extent imperilled by the morbific influence. This aim is quite consistent with measures intended to mitigate the local inflammation of lung or pleura, as the ice-bag or leeches. In acute disease of all kinds the object of rational treatment seems to be to control the morbid process, lessen its dangers, mitigate its sufferings, and conduct it to a favourable issue, but not to arrest the malady. In this sense we may very beneficially treat pneumonia, but attempts at cutting short its course are, I fear, unwise. The disease is self-limiting, and, once started, will have its way like a fever, which, in fact, it is. How it came to pass that the exudation did not caseate in the three cases which recovered I should be glad to be informed by those who think that phthisis is essentially an inflammatory disorder. The situation of the pneumonia in two cases was specially favourable to phthisis, and inflammation was present. Why was this result awanting?

ON THE CAUSES AND SIGNIFICANCE OF REDUPLICATION OF THE SOUNDS OF THE HEART.

By ARTHUR ERNEST SANSOM, M.D. Lond., F.R.C.P.,
Physician to the London Hospital; Physician to the
North-Eastern Hospital for Children, etc.

THERE are few questions in cardiac pathology more difficult than that of the causation of reduplication of the heart-sounds. This can scarcely be surprising when it is considered that observers are by no means agreed as to the causes of the normal uncomplicated sounds of the heart. As regards reduplication of the first sound, the theory which long seemed with greatest probability to be correct ascribed it to non-synchronous contraction of the two ventricles—a right ventricular systole being followed by a left ventricular systole, or vice versâ. Many observers have, however, found it difficult to accept this theory on account of the structural unity of the ventricles and the observed consentaneousness of their action. That such derangement of synchronism is possible, however, some physiologists consider to be well proved by physiological research. Dr. Barr has pointed out that each side of the heart has to a certain extent its own nerve-supply, and can accomplish its own peristaltic action, and, though both sides are set to the same time and have a complex interlacement of fibres, "it is an experimental fact that one side can begin or end contraction before the other."(a) It has been considered, too, that in some rare cases this want of synchronism on the part of the ventricles can be clinically demonstrated.

Dr. Barr has related to me a case in which the impulse of the left ventricle could be first felt, and then that of the right ventricle, and this succeeded by a weak impulse of the left. In this case the two periods between the three impulses were of about equal duration, while the pause that intervened between the last impulse and the first was quite equal to, or rather longer than, the other two intervals combined. On auscultation there were heard three distinct sounds over the ventricles, the first being loudest around the apex, the second over the right ventricle, and the third at the apex. The second sound was not audible over the ventricles, very feeble at the base, and double at the aortic cartilage. The pulse at the wrist was weak and infrequent, and exhibited the following rhythm with great regularity, viz.: a comparatively strong beat, followed by a weak and scarcely perceptible beat, and then, after a considerable pause, a strong beat again.

At a late period in the history of the case the second systole of the left ventricle was abolished, but the same asynchronous contraction of the two ventricles was plain to the eye when little levers were attached over the sites of visible pulsation, and was easily and distinctly felt on palpation. At this time the first sound at the apex was accompanied by a short systolic murmur, and this was followed by a sharp, clear sound, which was especially loud and ringing over the right ventricle. Following these two first sounds,

a duplex second sound was heard over the whole præcordium and at the aortic and pulmonic cartilages—the first element being loudest over the left ventricle and at the aortic cartilage, the second over the right ventricle and pulmonic cartilage.

The proximate cause of reduplication, then, as advanced by those who first adopted the theory of asynchronous systole of the ventricles, was the retarded closure of the tricuspid valve owing to the excess of blood-pressure in the right cavities. Dr. Barr, however, whose investigation of the subject is a very careful one, whilst adopting the theory of asynchronism of the ventricles, gives an opposite explanation of the proximate cause. He considers that excess of blood-pressure in the right heart (such as occurs in the normal heart during deep expiration when physiological reduplication of the first sound is heard) stimulates the right ventricle to commence contraction before the left; so the tense closure of the tricuspid valves occurs before that of the mitral. One of the chief objections urged against the theory of ventricular asynchronism has been that the disturbance in systole ought in the nature of things to be accompanied by disturbance in diastole; that the non-simultaneous impletion of the aorta and pulmonary artery respectively should be followed by non-simultaneous closure, by reflex of the aortic and the pulmonary semilunar valves; that,'therefore, doubling of the first sound should be invariably accompanied by doubling of the second—which is not the case. Dr. Barr meets this difficulty by advancing the view that though the right ventricle commences its systole before the left, it is longer in emptying itself, owing to its overloading and to the increased obstruction in the pulmonary circuit: hence, "although it had the start of the left, it has not completed its contraction before it, so there is no reduplication of the second sound under these circumstances."

Of other theories which have been advanced to explain reduplication of the first sound may be mentioned that of Guttmann, which ascribes it to non-synchronous tension of the individual segments of the auriculo-ventricular valves owing to absence of perfect uniformity in the contraction of the papillary muscles. This hypothesis appears to me in the highest degree improbable; it would seem much more likely that such irregularities on the part of the papillary muscles would produce not reduplication, but murmurs.

Dr. Hayden's view is that the doubling is equivalent to the resolution of the first sound into its two constituent elements, viz., the ventricular impulse and the click of valvular tension. According to this the click of valve-tension should occur at the very latest period of systole, the "thud" of muscular impulse always preceding it. This cannot, however, be sustained, for cardiographic evidence abundantly shows that the closure of the auriculo-ventricular valves occurs early in the systole, and that the first sound is prolonged subsequently to their closure. The "click," therefore, ought always to precede the "thud," whereas Dr. Hayden says that, in his experience, without exception, the first element of the double sound has been dull and muffled, and the second sharp and clear.(b)

Dr. George Johnson has advanced a theory totally distinct from the others. He considers that the so-called reduplication of the first sound consists in the rapidly following sounds of first an auricular, and then a ventricular systole. The contraction of a dilated, and especially of a hypertrophied, auricle becomes audible, and the first division of the double first sound is the result of the auricular systole.(c) It appears to me very difficult of belief that sound can be the direct effect of the muscular contraction of the auricle. It is a familiar fact that auscultation over the auricle demonstrates the existence of no sound during the period which we know to be occupied by the muscular contraction. In all conditions of its hypertrophy or dilatation the result is the same. I have had abundant opportunities of auscultating the auricle when through pulmonary disease it was wholly uncovered by lung, and the result has been always the same—the contraction of its muscle is soundless.

Whether sound may not be the indirect effect of the auricular systole is quite a different question. "During the period of rest," says Guttmann, "the auriculo-ventricular valves hang loosely down into the ventricular cavities, but are floated upwards when the latter are filled with blood, and belly out in the direction of the auricles, shutting off

---

(a) Vide a paper "On Reduplication of the Heart-Sounds," Medical Times and Gazette, 1877.

(b) "Diseases of the Heart and Aorta," 1875, page 112.
(c) Cf. British Medical Journal, December 23, 1876, and Lumleian Lectures, loc. cit., April 26, 1877.

he' lower from the upper chambers of the heart ; the short auricular systole, which precedes by an instant that of the ventricles, renders them somewhat tense, but to such a slight degree as to give rise to no audible sound."(d) Such is the case in the state of health, but it is quite conceivable that sound may be produced by the sudden tension given to the valve-curtains by the auricle when the systole of the latter is exaggerated, or when the valve-curtains are so altered by disease as to be more readily put upon the stretch. Potain has described a form of reduplicated first sound which he met with in cases of hypertrophy of the heart associated with chronic Bright's disease. Here occurred what he termed the "*bruit de galop*,"—" besides the two normal sounds, a third was heard, coming immediately before the first sound, and separated from it by a short pause ; this additional sound was therefore presystolic." I have already said that Guttmann adduces as an explanation of reduplication of the first sound a theory which I find it impossible to accept, viz., "non-synchronous tension of the individual segments of the semilunar valves." Nevertheless, Guttmann says that he has heard in a number of instances of cardiac hypertrophy a presystolic sound which might be referred to the systole of a hypertrophied auricle. He adds, "The auriculo-ventricular valves are to a certain extent rendered tense, even at the end of the diastole—that is, in the presystole,—but this tension is normally so feeble that no sound results ; but if the walls of one of the auricles undergo hypertrophy as the consequence of some valvular lesion, the corresponding auriculo-ventricular valve is put more sharply and thoroughly on the stretch by the contraction of the auricle, and in this way the conditions necessary to the production of a presystolic sound are realised."(e)

It appears to me that in the present state of our knowledge as regards the phenomenon known as doubling of the first sound, we are face to face with two theories—(a) that the reduplication is *real*, and is due to non-simultaneous tension of the curtains of the valves of the right and the left sides of the heart respectively ; (b) that the reduplication is *simulated* by a sudden tension of the mitral curtains, caused, under abnormal conditions, by the systole of the auricle closely followed by the production of tension again by the closure of the mitral orifice by the valve-curtains, due to the systole of the ventricle. It is possible that either of these theories, or both, may be right.

As regards the first, if we agree with Dr. Barr that the systole of the two ventricles may occur independently and non-simultaneously, we must acknowledge that the instances in which this can be proved are very rare. Yet it would seem probable that if such disturbance of rhythm were due to the variations of pressure or variations in the balance of pressure in the right and left ventricles it would be likely that the manifold perturbations induced by disease would afford us more numerous examples. It is acknowledged that reduplication of the first sound of the heart is, apart from the physiological reduplication at the end of expiration or beginning of inspiration, of by no means common occurrence. Dr. Hayden objects to Dr. Richardson's assertion that reduplication of heart-sounds is rare, but he mentions only twelve cases of reduplicated first sound as having occurred in his wide experience. Of these, "four were examples of hypertrophy with dilatation of the left ventricle, and two of fatty heart. The condition of heart, however, with which, *par excellence*, reduplicated first sound is associated, is that of nervous instability, as exhibited in proneness to palpitation. Of this no less than six of my cases are examples, but of these one was also gouty, and one exhibited contraction of the mitral orifice and reduplication of both sounds."(f)

(*To be continued.*)

POISONING BY MISADVENTURE.—Last April, the Correctional Tribunal of Bordeaux condemned to a fine of 200 fr. and 1000 fr. damages a *pharmacien* of St. André-de-Cubzac, who had caused the deaths of two children from having dispensed strychnine in place of santonine. Dissatisfied with the punishment, the family appealed, and the fine has been increased by the Court to 500 fr. and the damages to 3000 fr.—*Union Méd.*, June 30.

(d) "Handbook of Physical Diagnosis," New Sydenham Society's translation, page 282.
(e) *Ibid.*, page 277.   (f) *Loc. cit.*, page 165.

ORIGINAL COMMUNICATIONS.

THE MEDICINAL AND DIETETIC USES OF CITRATE OF CAFFEINE.

By LEWIS SHAPTER, M.D.,
Physician to the Devon and Exeter Hospital and to the West of England Institution for the Deaf and Dumb.

MEDICINALLY, caffeine or theine in the form of a soluble citrate has gained a certain degree of favour in a variety of complaints which may at first sight appear of more or less distinctive pathological causation. In doses of a grain, it has been used in tic douloureux, hemicrania, and varied forms of neuralgia. Coffee, in the form of strong decoction, has further been recognised as an astringent in certain forms of diarrhoea, as a febrifuge in fevers, and as a tonic and stimulant in cases of adynamy. In all probability, the therapeutic action is similar, if not identical, in all these different classes of cases. The forms of diarrhoea in which it has proved useful are those which are termed atonic, colliquative, sympathetic, or vaso-paralytic as in extreme cachexia ; and its action is, therefore, not probably dependent upon the presence of tannic acid, but upon that of theine, which is tonic to the vaso-motor nerves, and consequently relieves atony and hyperæmia of the intestinal mucous membrane. So, also, theine is febrifuge because through the vaso-motor nerves it induces a slight increase in perspiratory functions ; and it is stimulant only in so far as it braces the nerves which govern the calibre of vessels, and so sustains the circulation. These hypotheses receive support from the recognised value of citrate of caffeine in the group of neuralgias. In cases of migraine or sick headache, which, according to M. Hervey, is an arterial neurosis taking origin in the great sympathetic nerves, and having its seat in the nervous filaments accompanying the arteries, citrate of caffeine may be looked to to remove vascular relaxation, allay pain, and induce sleep. In protracted attacks of spasmodic asthma, where the nervous system is fatigued and exhausted by the continuance of spasm, caffeine in sufficient doses will prove of signal service. In melancholia, in the brain of overworkers, in the sleeplessness and depression of spirits of drunkards, and in asthenic mania, a similar indication is to be met, and the citrate in doses of from three to five grains will prove calmant and restorative. The most interesting therapeutic property, however, of the citrate of caffeine, in doses of not less than three grains, is its diuretic action in cases of advanced cardiac dropsy, where muscular embarrassment and neurosal inco-ordinate cardiac action are amongst the striking indicators of progressive cardiac mural decay. Through the agency of the sympathetic system, and specially of the intrinsic cardiac ganglia, we can, with the aid of citrate of caffeine, promote co-ordinate cardiac power, without of necessity increasing cardiac action ; and through the agency of the vaso-motor nerves we can excite contraction of the arteries and increase arterial blood-pressure and power of the pulse. It probably also acts like belladonna in overcoming the controlling effect of the splanchnic nerve, and through this medium that of the abdominal vascular system generally ; and although this may be induced indirectly as a reflex act commencing in the sensory nerve (depressor nerve of Ludwig and Cyon) of the heart itself, the effect is practically the same, for increased power of cardiac contraction and diuresis are promoted by the increase in vascular pressure.

All these points bearing upon the therapeutic properties of citrate of caffeine I have ventured to discuss at length, and in detail, elsewhere (*Brain and Practitioner*, 1879) ; but the practical outcome of these observations is suggestive to another point, for citrate of caffeine is shown therapeutically to be anything but a stimulant to the central and peripheral vascular system ; it is a tonic or restorative agent to the nervous system which governs and co-ordinates the circulation, and may therefore be given to relieve a palpitating adynamic heart with no fear of increasing turbulent action either of heart or vessels. Dietetically, therefore, if infusions of tea and coffee are judged by the presence of their active principle—theine, which is their sole restorative[agent,—these substances are not stimulants as alcohol is a stimulant, but in sustaining the circulation through the nervous system they perform the true physiological need for which alcohol is erroneously taken, and might effectually be looked to to take the place of alcohol, if only they were rid of their injurious adjuncts, and the theine alone were producible as a beverage in a palatable form.

Theine, as is well known, is the active principle not only of tea and coffee, but also of Paraguay tea and *Paulinia sorbilis* (guarana), and probably also of cocoa. The essential oil of tea, from which the dried leaves derive their flavour, is opposed to the action of theine; it excites the nervous system, and is the substance to which must be ascribed disquieting disorders of the nervous system which result undoubtedly from tea-drinking, such, *e.g.*, as palpitation of the heart, excitability, and wakefulness. The tannic acid, again, which is present to a considerable extent in the ordinary form of infusion, is a powerful astringent, and is the cause very often of indigestion and constipation which result from constant tea-drinking. Theine, on the other hand, is the only restorative or tonic agent in these substances; and the mere fact that the dietetic use of infusions of tea and coffee has alone led to the acceptation of the active principle as a medicine of value is of itself sufficient to give some stable position to theine as a tried and recognised article of dietary. Dr. Lankester has ascribed to theine an action similar to that of quinine as a nervine tonic; and Dr. Mapother has compared it with kreatine, one of the principles of meat, asserting that both seem to have *invigorating power* irrespective of their *nutritive value*. Professor Liebig has shown that theine, with the addition of oxygen and the elements of water, can yield taurine, the nitrogenised compound peculiar to bile; a little more than two grains of theine giving to an ounce of bile the nitrogen it contains in the form of taurine. Or, in other words, one-tenth of a grain of theine—the probable amount in an ordinary cup of tea—constitutes an important aid to the requirements of the system for the maintenance of health. Too much stress must, of course, not be placed, in the present day, upon this observation of Professor Liebig's: it is, perhaps, doubtful how far it could be maintained as the basis of any physiological teaching; but reference to it is important, because it shows, in conjunction with the other observations referred to, that theine is a substance that has long been recognised of undoubted value as a dietetic agent, although it has hitherto not been popularly or generally utilised as such. In the present day, however, when the excessive and immoderate use of alcohol has become a national question, and a question affecting public health, it is a step in the great work of preventive medicine to acknowledge the value of some dietetic substance which can hopefully be looked to as the required physiological substitute for alcohol.

From the medical point of view, alcohol is a useful medicine, and there is, perhaps, no other medicine which, under certain conditions, can effectually take its place. Thus, in protracted fevers, it is a food and prevents tissue-waste; it preserves life, because, in many instances, it is the only substance that can be assimilated to prolong vital power and energy over the critical time. It may also be a preserver and preventer of disease, for, judiciously given, it may be made to aid and promote digestion and to act as a refrigerant; as a heat-giving food also it may be useful to check overfeeding or the excessive use of nitrogenous food; and as a wine it may not only be a nutrient tonic *when pure*, but perhaps derivative and slightly diuretic. The danger of the use of alcohol really arises in cases of exhausted or deficient nerve-power when this occurs as a condition of itself, and not as the result especially of disease; for here alcohol is used erroneously as a remedy, and it is partly on this account used to excess.

Exhausted nerve-power may arise from a variety of causes—such, for example, as the exigencies of society, unhealthy employment, intemperance, and excessive mental labour. The difficulty, indeed, which has to be practically contended with in the present day is the tendency of the age to work the brain rather than the body, to overstrain the mental faculties and to overtax mental capacity. "Cram" at high pressure is the dictum of scholastic life; the competitive examination or a feat of memory is the high road to successful life; and the ever increasing literature of the day must be made the food of everyday life. Add to all this the fact that the resources of machinery are continually replacing the need for manual labour, and that the education of all classes to some higher level is the prevailing passion of the age, and have we not cumulative evidence of the strain on mental vigour, with its result—a desire or need for temporary support or restoration when that power becomes exhausted?

Now, a brief reference to physiological teaching will at once tell us that alcohol as an agent for restoring exhausted nerve-power is unreliable, and our worst and most dangerous and delusive friend. It offers truly enough a means of temporarily rousing a failing vascular system to renewed energy, and thereby affording an increased supply of nutrient material to the nervous system for a time; but what then? There is no means of continuing this nutrient supply: it is like expecting a steam-engine to work by putting more fuel into the furnace when there is no more water put into the boiler: the overworked vascular system, stimulated for a time, must itself become all the more exhausted; and the nervous system, temporarily invigorated, will again fail for want of nourishment. All this is seen in its full development in the intemperate inebriate as a person distinct from the simple drunkard. There is confirmatory evidence in the case of the inebriate of deficient nerve-power, it may be in a tendency to mental depression or irritability, in an absolute incapacity for mental exertion of any kind whether even of reading or writing, in a consequent inclination to pursuits of the field as least irksome, in an insensibility to moral delicacy and position, or in dreaming, recklessness, and insomnia; but, in the main, the effect is the same—he is an intemperate man in every sense of the term, and even if at one time the desire to overcome what is recognised as a failing is strong within him during what may with some degree of propriety be termed a "lucid interval," yet the favourable promise of reform to the unobservant is but short-lived. There is still a predominant symptom which has only to be awakened by a passing word or thought, and the power of the weakened will is no longer able to adjust the balance: it is the feeling of nervous exhaustion or prostration; and it is a part and parcel of the man himself, for his disease is defective nerve-power or defective nerve-nutrition.

Now, alcohol in small quantity is found practically to relieve this main symptom which is the manifestation of a disorder, and it enables the man for a time to exert himself to labour or employment. What wonder, then, if that which has once proved a relief should grow powerlessly into an infatuation! The alcohol which has relieved exhaustion through an indirect channel will undoubtedly produce exhaustion, and the so-called remedy will become the growing cause of still greater disorder, even to the production of organic disease or morbid growth, the result of arterial relaxation, malnutrition, and vaso-motor paresis. A similar train of results dependent upon what is probably a poisoning or paresis of vaso-motor nerves controlling arterial calibre, and manifestly affecting nutrition, is often to be observed in cases of plethora and obesity and gout, where there is a retention of waste materials in the system, and too large and inappropriate supplies are unguardedly given to cope with legitimate demand. A prominent symptom in these cases is weakness, sinking, and exhaustion; and the medical adviser can scarcely induce the conviction that this feeling of weakness is a morbid and a false one, and that a lowering and a diluent dietary, rather than a feeding and a stimulating one, are the reliable measures to remove the indications of abnormal brain and nerve nutrition, which may be evidenced in general anasarca or localised œdema, giddiness, occasional epileptiform attacks, drowsiness, or even temporary unconsciousness. In many cases of dyspepsia also a prominent symptom is often observed, which is very justly attributed to nervous atony. This is a feeling of sinking at the pit of the stomach, and gives rise to a craving, insatiable feeling or appetite, often to be relieved by stimulants, but probably only to be met medicinally by nervine tonics. This same teaching holds true with all the greater force in minor states of nervous exhaustion—in, for example, the occasional weariness or exhaustion resulting from a daily occupation or a little extraordinary mental work.

It is not always wise to take extra food to rebuild the nervous system, because to constantly tax the digestive functions is proportionately to weaken them; but what is required is a readily assimilated tonic and restorative, which will from the physiological point of view support the nervous system, and neither stimulate like alcohol, nor overload and overfeed the system like iron and phosphorus. Physiology even tells us that, in speaking of the normal circulation of the blood, the nervous system must be regarded as a most important factor in both central and peripheral circulation. The nervous system may very properly be considered as the controller, regulator, and co-ordinator of the entire vascular system, and, as such, too hasty conclusions must not be drawn of defective vascular power, when possibly defective nerve-force is the primary cause of disorder. At any rate, alcohol is a remedial agent to be used cautiously and advisedly, and, as a dietetic agent, no more dangerous weapon can perhaps be placed in the hands of the general public. The only restoratives, on the other hand, which have stood the test of practical acceptation and experience are infusions of tea and coffee and similar beverages. It needs no medical knowledge to speak of the increased sense of respiratory power and muscular vigour, the promotion of general warmth and comfort, the cooling of the body the result of the slight increase of perspiratory function, and the general feeling of reaction when the body is overcome with fatigue, which is the generally accepted result of the use of tea and coffee. These substances, as has been already shown, have but one active and restorative principle—theine; and if ill results are to be attributed to the uses of the infusions of the leaf and berry, these are dependent upon the presence of the essential oil, which is excitant and stimulant, and the tannic acid, which is astringent. That the action of theine is tonic and restorative to the nervous system, and specially the sympathetic system, is almost self-evident even by the reasoning of exclusion; and, as such, it may therefore be looked to to relieve nervous depression and want of vigour, and not indirectly the results of that depression.

Theine is agreeably used in the form of an aërated distilled water, and, as such, it may be regarded as an efficient substitute for alcohol. I have now used the aquathëin (made at my suggestion by Mr. Ham, of 29, North-street, Exeter) in a variety of cases where it has been advisable to omit the use of stimulants; in all cases the requirement has been completely fulfilled. To inebriates it seems to take the place of alcohol, and to quench the desire for it; to the plethoric and obese it is a sufficient beverage; and in many cases of heart disease, where ordinary infusions of tea and coffee are avoided from fear of exciting palpitation, aquathëin is readily taken, and appears to be calmative and tonic to the nervous system. Dietetically, also, to those in health aquathëin has proved its position in a number of instances as supplanting the necessity for alcoholic stimulants of any kind. If further experience can confirm these facts we have a remedy for the excessive misuses of alcohol which can with safety and propriety be placed in the hands of the public as a physiological substitute.

CLINICAL HISTORY OF

HYDATID DISEASE AFFECTING THE RESPIRATORY ORGANS.

By J. DAVIES THOMAS, M.D. Lond., F.R.C.S. Eng.,
Lately Senior House-Surgeon of the Adelaide Hospital;
formerly Resident Medical Officer of University College Hospital.

(Continued from page 700 of last volume.)

Symptoms of Hydatid of the Lungs.—In nearly all respects the symptoms of cysts of the lungs, pleura, and mediastina are identical, but reference will hereafter be made to some characters by which it is alleged that cysts of the pleura may in some cases be distinguished during life from true pulmonary cysts. The symptoms of cysts in these various localities may vary from such slight and indefinite phenomena as to completely escape the observation of the patient and physician, up to a condition the gravity of which cannot fail to claim the attention of both. If the cyst be small there will be absolutely no symptoms. Thus Andral relates the case of a woman who died of uterine cancer; her right lung contained a cyst of the size of a large nut, and in her case "respiration was easy and there was no cough."

The severity of the symptoms will vary with the size and, to some extent, with the situation of the cyst, with its condition as regards integrity or rupture, and with the condition of the surrounding lung-tissue.

The study of the symptoms of this, as of all other diseased states, resolves itself into the consideration of (a) subjective, or those appreciable by the patient alone—the chief symptoms of this class being pain in the chest of varying seat and severity and a sense of shortness of breath; (b) objective signs, i.e., those capable also of being observed by the physician. These require detailed notice.

The morbific influence of the unruptured hydatid cyst is confined to the direct results of the local lesion occasioned by its presence, and it neither causes nor is accompanied by any constitutional state primarily due to the presence of the parasite.

After the cyst has burst, there may either be only very slight constitutional disturbance (as in Case No. 2),(a) or a state may be induced similar to that present in cases of phthisical vomicæ, but exhibiting a far greater tendency towards cure (s.g., Case No. 4).

In general terms, then, it may be stated that the subjective symptoms and the physical signs may be divided into two great classes:—1. Those dependent upon the presence of the unbroken cyst. 2. Those caused by the ruptured cyst.

1. *Cyst unbroken.*—Cough, dyspnœa, hæmoptysis, and pain may be present.

Cough.—There is usually some cough, and this very frequently possesses a paroxysmal character. While the cyst is but small, and causes no local congestion or inflammation, it is unaccompanied by any expectoration. The cough, however, by no means always possesses a paroxysmal character, for it may be "short" and dry like that of early phthisis. Cough having these characters may persist for months or even years, especially in the case of cysts occupying the pleural cavity. Although the cyst usually causes scarcely any local irritation, yet it may at times set up a localised bronchitis or pneumonia, and more rarely even gangrene. The case will then present the characters of cough and expectoration proper to these conditions.

Hæmoptysis.—Scarcely any, perhaps no single, case of hydatid cyst of the lung runs its entire course without some expectoration of blood.

Hearn observes that there was scarcely one-fifth of the recorded cases in which the presence of hæmoptysis had not been noted; and in many, even of the latter group, it was stated that the patient had a phthisical aspect, and hence very probably hæmoptysis had been present, although it was not recorded. More or less hæmoptysis is the rule in cysts of the lung, the rare exception in those of the pleura (Hearn).

Copious hæmoptysis is rare in the early history of cysts —when it is usually, as in early phthisis, small in amount and not of long continuance. It is rarely more than a mere streak accompanying the mucous or muco-purulent sputa often present at this period. Sometimes rusty sputa are present, indicative of a local pneumonic process.

Hæmoptysis is usually repeated at intervals of perhaps months or years. The blood may be florid and frothy, or dark and less aërated.

Bird remarks that hæmoptyses connected with pulmonary cysts ought to be divided into two classes—first, those preceding the rupture; second, those accompanying or following this event.

The hæmorrhages of the first class are not abundant, and often consist only of a mere streak of blood in the expectoration; while the hæmoptyses of the second period are far more profuse, and are accompanied with suffocative dyspnœa, and they may prove fatal at once, either from suffocation or by occasioning fatal anæmia, or death may take place within a few days from the uncontrollable loss of blood, as in Case No. 5.

Lebert quotes a case where death occurred during an hæmoptysis. The patient had previously suffered from numerous hæmoptyses, and had brought up large quantities of hydatids. At the autopsy there were found a large cavity in the inferior lobe of the right lung, and a long erosion of a branch of the pulmonary artery. Haberahon relates the case of a youth aged seventeen years, the subject of an hydatid cyst, in whom death suddenly resulted from the rupture of a dilated pulmonary vein into the interior of the cyst-cavity.

_____

(a) "Cases of Hydatid Disease," etc., reported at pages 64 and 235 of last volume.

These cases show a strong resemblance to the frequent cases of fatal hæmoptysis of the third stage of phthisis, where the hæmorrhage is due to the rupture or erosion of a large vessel; and just as in the case of phthisical vomica, bloodvessels may be seen on the walls of the exocyst of an hydatid, denuded and, as it were, dissected out (see Cases Nos. 15 and 16, Hearn, page 122). It is highly probable that, under these circumstances, aneurismal dilatations of the vessels similar to those so common in phthisis may occur.

In a case recorded by Pillon, and cited by Davaine(b) and by Hearn,(c) a large quantity of blood was found at the post-mortem examination contained in a cyst of the lung, and yet none was expectorated for some time before death.

Hæmoptysis is not uncommonly the earliest symptom of hydatid of the lung as it is of phthisis, and it may occur two, or even three, years before the patient consults a medical man.

Pain in the chest may be slight, severe, or absent. In most cases where the cyst is unbroken, severe pain is very rare. Far more commonly there is a sense of discomfort or weight, which in some instances may even amount to the actual sense of the presence of a foreign body in the chest. Very severe pain, however, follows the rupture of a cyst into the pleura. But this is fortunately an uncommon event; far more frequently a local pleurisy is set up in the immediate vicinity of the cyst. Pain is said to be more pronounced in cysts of the pleura than in those of the lungs.

Dyspnœa may range from mere shortness of breath up to the mortal agony of intense orthopnœa. More or less shortness of breath is always present if the cyst attain any material size, but owing to the gradual growth and comparatively unirritating character of the unbroken cyst, urgent dyspnœa is rare. However, cases have been recorded of severe dyspnœa resulting in death from the mere bulk of the unruptured cyst invading and compressing the lung-tissue until the respiratory area was too limited to sustain life (see Cases Nos. 4 and 7, Hearn.(d) Exertion always materially increases the shortness of breath.

Nothing in the whole pathology of chest disease is more remarkable than to observe how large an amount of lung area may be slowly and imperceptibly invaded by an hydatid cyst, and yet only slight shortness of breath result. Thus, in Case No. 1, a large part of the left lung was disabled by the large cyst, and yet the man scarcely suffered from shortness of breath. In some cases recorded the dyspnœa had a paroxysmal character, but this is not common. The presence of some intercurrent local disease, such as bronchitis, pneumonia, or gangrene, adds greatly to the difficulty of breathing. The presence of the cyst, especially of the ruptured cyst, may determine and possibly even actually cause the development of phthisis, and this will of course cause increased impairment of respiratory power. Intense orthopnœa may be present under the following circumstances :—1. From rupture of the cyst into the pleural cavity, with the production of very severe pleurisy. 2. From rupture into a bronchial tube. At the moment of rupture a large quantity of fluid is suddenly poured out into the bronchial tubes, the trachea and larynx being forcibly ejected by the joint influence of violent cough and the natural elasticity of the endocyst. By the next inspiration a large quantity of the fluid in the air-passages is sucked into the entire bronchial tract of both lungs, and for the time the whole of both lungs is disabled. Under these circumstances sudden death may occur; while in other cases the patient may live on for forty-eight hours in urgent dyspnœa, and then die.(e)

Another cause of urgent dyspnœa ending in death is the detachment and impaction in the larynx or air-tubes of a large piece of cyst-wall, and this peril exists throughout the whole period of the spontaneous cure of pulmonary cysts.

In some cases, such as No. 2, the endocyst may be rapidly and completely separated, but far more frequently months or years elapse before the whole of the endocyst is detached and cure results. More or less cyst-wall may be detached and expelled from the lung at the moment of rupture; or, as frequently happens, weeks or months may intervene between the moment of rupture and the expulsion of the first portion of cyst-wall. Rupture may occur simultaneously into the pleura and into the bronchial tract, and pneumothorax result, with intense pain and difficulty of breathing. In Budd's case of hydatids in the branches of the pulmonary

vein there was intense dyspnœa. As already mentioned, severe dyspnœa may occur from the mere amount of lung-area invaded by the acephalocyst.

The State of General Health bears a strong resemblance to the condition of a phthisical patient. Thus, there are progressive debility and loss of flesh, cough, expectoration, pain in the chest, night-sweats, and pyrexia. The two last named occur especially after the rupture of the cyst. Pyrexia, however, may arise antecedently to the rupture of the cyst, in consequence of local pneumonia, gangrene, or pleurisy. Again, the pyrexia is usually most marked immediately after the rupture of the cyst, and is then due to inflammation set up in the neighbourhood of the cyst. Later on pyrexia diminishes, and may often be wanting. Records of temperature in cases of hydatid disease are wanting in sufficient number to permit many general statements upon this point yet. There is a very important relation between the damage to general health and the evidences of local lesion in hydatid cysts of the lungs. Thus, in phthisis there is a certain proportion between the amount and degree of local lung lesion and the impairment of general health; and although this relation is one not yet capable of being described by any definite formula, yet individual experience enables us to form a fair estimate of the probable amount of lung affection, from the observation of the general state of the patient, the amount of pyrexia, loss of flesh, etc. Now, in hydatid disease this ratio is often entirely altered, and a patient may exhibit a fair amount of muscularity, and even of plumpness, and yet, upon physical examination, he may be found to have a large cavity in one of his lungs. This characteristic, although common, is not universal.

The Physical Signs of the Unbroken Cyst. — We are indebted to Dr. Bird, of Melbourne, for much of our knowledge of the diagnosis of the presence of the unbroken cyst in the lungs. The diagnosis will depend much upon the size and situation of the cyst. Thus, at the apex, the physical signs will simulate those of the first stage of phthisis; at the base, those of pleural effusion. If the cyst be very small, there may be absolutely no physical signs to be found. It is impossible to assert what the minimum size of cyst capable of being discovered during life is, but "from eight to sixteen ounces of fluid is about the average capacity when they should be diagnosed with certainty."—Bird.(f)

The following is a sketch of the physical signs of the unbroken cyst when of moderate dimensions : — "Expansion more or less deficient on the affected side measurement but little affected; absolute dulness on percussion, with absence of respiratory sounds over a space of the chest-wall not smaller than the palm of the hand, generally in the lateral or infra-clavicular regions, with absence of vocal fremitus in most cases. This dull space always presents a rounded outline; is limited by a line of demarcation so exact that it can be mapped out with pen and ink, and is unaltered by position, i.e., posture of patient. Beyond the boundary line percussion is clear and normal. The respiratory sounds, though inaudible over the dull surface, commence immediately beyond the pen line, and, though probably rather harsh and puerile in character, are indicative of healthy lung-tissue.

. . . . A localised pleuritic effusion confined by adhesions would fulfil the above physical signs, but such a state of things is very rare, and would probably be preceded by a history of pain and febrile symptoms. In fact, one is reduced to the conclusion that there is a sac containing fluid within the chest-wall, slowly enlarging, causing little or no pain or local irritation—not the result of any inflammatory effusion, but foreign to, though growing in, the thoracic viscera. A hydatid cyst alone combines all these characters, so that the diagnosis may be reduced almost to a certainty."—Bird.(g)

This summary of the physical signs is so complete that but little remains to be added.

Difficulties in Diagnosis vary according to the seat of the cyst; thus, when seated at the apex, it may be mistaken for the consolidation of phthisis; if at the base, for hydrothorax, pleuritic effusion and empyema, etc. Reference has been already made to various diagnostic points, and others may be added as follows.

Cyst at apex from phthisical consolidation :—1st. If phthisis be sufficiently advanced to cause dulness over a considerable part of one apex there will generally be some damage inflicted also upon the opposite lung. 2nd. The unbroken cyst causes absolute loss of all respiratory sound

(b) Op. cit., page 433.   (c) Op. cit., page 184, Case 22.
(d) Op. cit., pages 114 and 116.
(e) Case by Simon, cited by Davaine and Hearn.

(f) Op. cit., page 12.   (g) Op. cit., pages 14, 17.

over a certain area. Around this part there may be, and usually is, perfectly healthy respiration, but there may be signs of irritation or consolidation of the adjacent tissue—*e.g.*, local bronchitis or pneumonia. In phthisis, on the other hand, respiration-sound would not be lost, but altered to divided respiration, bronchial breathing, etc. 3rd. Probably pyrexia would be the rare exception in unruptured hydatid, the rule in phthisis. 4th. A marked amount of dulness from phthisis would necessarily be accompanied by material damage to the general health, while a moderate-sized cyst would cause far less impairment of health in most cases. 5th. In a doubtful case in any situation, an exploratory puncture with No. 1 aspirator needle would clear up the diagnosis and aid cure in hydatid. Hydatid fluid cannot be mistaken for any other (see Case No. 1).

Diagnosis from Cancer of the Lung.—Centripetal pressure signs are very rare in hydatid cysts, common in cancer because of the frequent association of tumour with carcinoma. Infiltrated cancer is characterised as follows :(h)—

(a.) *Retraction or depression* of the affected side, with more or less deepening of intercostal spaces. Hydatid cysts unbroken (and sometimes even when ruptured) are characterised by bulging or local fulness rather than by retraction (see Cases No. 1 and No. 3).

(b.) *Vocal fremitus* varies in cancer according to varied local states of amount of infiltration, etc.; almost universally lost over a certain area in cysts.

(c.) *Percussion-note* in infiltrated cancer is most commonly of "raised pitch, and hard wooden or tubular quality; but true simple dulness may be the prominent character." —Walshe.(i) In the unbroken cyst, toneless dulness like that of pleural effusion, and often there is the same character in the ruptured cyst (see Cases 1, 3, and 4).

(d.) *Auscultation.*—"Strongly marked, diffused, blowing respiration" is most usual in infiltrated carcinoma. In the unbroken cyst, an area of silence. *After softening in cancer*, cavernous respiration, with bubbling or metallic râles. In the ruptured cyst, may have all these, but the constitutional state is far less cachectic, as a rule.

(e.) *Progress* of hydatid slow, of cancer fast.

(f.) Infiltrated cancer lessens the size of the lung, hydatid increases it.

If *cancer, mainly tuberous.* Very liable to get tumour; signs and evidences of centripetal pressure. Hydatid cysts are centrifugal. In tuberous carcinoma, tubular or blowing respiration is most common; in the unbroken cyst, silence; in the ruptured one, cavernous or amphoric breathing.

In very rare cases, cysts other than hydatid ones exist in the lungs. Thus, Dr. Sedgwick, of Boroughbridge,(k) has recorded the case of a man, aged forty years, who for some years had been subject to attacks of hæmoptysis, but one day he was seized "with his usual symptoms, but along with the blood he expectorated a considerable quantity of mortary-looking matter, mixed with numerous hairs, some short and fine, others long and well grown. The solid stuff under the microscope showed indications of cells, but was mainly composed of granular matter, soluble in ether." The physical signs pointed to the upper part of the left lung as the seat of the mischief.

Diagnosis of the Unbroken Cyst from Aneurism.—In thoracic aneurism there is evidence of "the existence in some part of the thorax of a pulsating tumour other than the heart, which beats isochronously with it, and at least as forcibly, and which at each pulsation expands in every direction."—Balfour.(l) Add to this the extreme frequency with which aneurism attacks the arch of the aorta, the almost universal occurrence of centripetal, and often also of centrifugal, pressure-signs, the frequent presence of one or more murmurs and of hypertrophy of the heart, and the risk of confusion is not very great.

Cysts seated towards the base may be readily confused with aneurisms of the descending aorta. If either be of small size, the diagnosis may be impossible; but when a hydatid becomes sufficiently large to cause evident physical signs, it could only be confused with an aneurism of considerable magnitude, and in that case signs of centripetal pressure —*e.g.*, pain from erosion of vertebræ and pressure on nerves, a pulsatile and expansile tumour, one or more murmurs, etc.—would probably, one or more of them, be present.

(h) See Walshe, "Diseases of Lungs," fourth edition, 1871.
(i) *Op. cit.*   (k) *Lancet*, vol. i. 1860, page 612.
(l) "Diseases of the Heart," page 340.

In the *Lancet*, vol. ii. 1859, page 617, there is recorded a very interesting case where an aneurism of the size of a small cocoanut communicated directly with a bilocular cavity in the base of the right lung. There were present—dysphagia and a loud mitral murmur, also "a firm, resisting, but movable, swelling above the umbilicus, pulsating synchronously with the heart, and a muffled whirring sound was heard below the ensiform cartilage."

The concurrence of such signs of disease in the vascular system with centripetal pressure effects would prevent any difficulty in the diagnosis between such a case as the above and a hydatid cyst.

Perhaps the most common difficulty in diagnosis is between fluid in the pleura and a cyst, especially when the fluid is circumscribed by adhesions.

Hydrothorax is generally bilateral; hydatid disease very rarely so. Again, there is always some disease present to account for the hydrothorax—*e.g.*, cardiac or Bright's disease, etc.

From Pleuritic Effusion.—There is generally pyrexia or a history of pyrexia, pain, friction-sound, and fremitus, etc., in pleurisy. The pleurisy would be very unlikely to cause some peculiar displacements not uncommon in cysts—*e.g.*, to push the heart bodily forwards (see Case No. 1). Again, it often happens in hydatid disease that there is resonance on percussion somewhere where it ought not to be in pleurisy with effusion. Finally, aspiration, which is a valuable therapeutic measure in either case, will definitely clear up the diagnosis, and it should always be promptly undertaken.

The Pressure Effects of Hydatid Cysts.—Hydatid cysts have the characteristic of growth in the direction of least resistance; consequently their effects are centrifugal rather than centripetal. Hence bulging of the chest-wall, fulness or bulging of the interspaces, dislocation of the mediastinum, heart, and liver, are very common; but pressure on bloodvessels, nerves, or large bronchial or air tubes is rare. So that local dropsies, severe pain, and dyspnœa from compression of large tubes are very uncommon. This characteristic will very often permit a diagnosis to be made between hydatid cysts and other intrathoracic tumours.

The direction and amount of displacement of organs will vary with the situation and size of the cyst.

The lungs may be compressed towards the root, just as in pleural effusions; but, unlike the latter condition, a hydatid cyst may press the lung forwards. Thus Geoffroy and Dupuytren relate a case where there were large cysts in both pleuræ which exerted pressure effects, so that "the heart was pushed towards the epigastrium; the lungs compressed, flattened out, and pressed towards the anterior part of the chest."

Again, in unilateral pleural effusion the heart is merely pushed over to the opposite side (*i.e.*, if it be free to move at all), but in hydatid cases it might be pressed in any direction according to the situation of the cyst. Thus in Case 1 the heart was not much, if at all, pushed to the right, but it was pressed bodily forwards to the front of the chest (*e.g.*, Case 1). Although centripetal pressure is rare, yet it does sometimes occur. Thus, Leraux describes a case where there was œdema of the upper extremities (and not of the lower ones); the right side of the chest was filled with a large cyst containing multiple acephalocysts in great numbers. Other similar cases are on record. In rare cases even cartilages and bones are eroded by hydatid cysts. Thus, in the *Gazette Hebdomadaire* (July 23, 1875), there is a case where "the intervertebral cartilage between the ninth and tenth vertebræ was destroyed, and the bodies of these two vertebræ were hollowed out into cavities, in which hydatid vesicles were seen." In this case probably the cysts commenced in the substance of the vertebræ.

Diagnosis of the Ruptured Cyst.—The physical signs are those of a cavity (see Cases 1, 3, 4), but there often are certain additional characters. Thus, in Case 1, for some time there was a curious interrupted character of the respiration sounds, especially pronounced during inspiration. This I attributed at the time to the presence at the orifice into the bronchus of a valve-like piece of cyst-wall; at any rate, it disappeared after the expectoration of a piece of endocyst. Then, again, any signs of dislocation of organs present before rupture often continue after. Thus, in the little boy H. R. (Case 4), the apex-beat was displaced to the left, although there were certain evidences of a large cavity. Now, a lung containing a phthisical vomica is contracted, not enlarged. In this little boy, again, it would have been extraordinary, firstly, to get signs of so large a cavity at such an age, and secondly, to find such very extensive disease on one side while the opposite remained healthy.

The history, too, will at times give some assistance. For example, a patient who for some time—possibly for months or years—has been suffering, slightly or severely, from cough, hæmoptysis, loss of flesh, shortness of breath, etc., suddenly experiences a sense of something giving way in his chest, brings up a large quantity of watery fluid mixed with or followed by blood, and perhaps " bits of skins," suffers for a time from intense dyspnœa, and is laid up for a longer or shorter time with " inflammation of the lungs," from which he does not completely recover, and is now believed to be " consumptive." Such was the history in Cases 3 and 4. However, the patient's history per se is usually of very small value.

The expectoration of laminated membrane, hooklets, or echinococci of course sets all doubt at rest, but months may elapse between the first examination of a case of ruptured cyst and the moment when the patient can produce a piece of endocyst for examination. As a rule, echinococci and hooklets soon disappear from the sputa after the rupture of the cyst. In none of the cases of ruptured cyst that I have yet examined could I find lung-tissue in the sputa ; and it seems probable that the absence, after repeated examinations (by Dr. Fenwick's method), of any elastic tissue from sputa apparently derived from a vomica would be a negative sign of some value in a case doubtfully hydatid. The presence of local gangrene would, of course, vitiate this test. Offensive sputa are more common in cases of hydatid than in phthisical cavities.

The frequent alteration of ratio between general and local damage in hydatid cases as compared with phthisical ones has already been referred to.

In many cases the differential diagnosis between hydatid and phthisis is very difficult, in some probably impossible, but in the majority of cases careful physical examination will usually show the presence of some sign or signs not readily to be accounted for by the supposed existence of the more common forms of chest-disease.

Treatment.—In the case of the unbroken cyst there is no doubt that the evacuation of the contents of the cyst by the aspirator or a fine trocar is the mode of treatment. In the case of a large recently ruptured cyst, the patient's chances of recovery are greatly increased by the establishment of a free opening into the cyst through an intercostal space. The orifice should be made at the point where the cyst presents most distinctly to the chest-wall. A most interesting series of cases are recorded by Dr. Bird (m) where this bold and judicious measure proved successful. At present further data are required as to the best mode of performing this operation, and as to the circumstances connected with the cyst which render it judicious. However, there is but little doubt that operative interference offers a better prospect of speedy recovery in cases of large old cysts than the long and perilous process of natural elimination through the bronchial tubes does.

THE International Medical and Sanitary Exhibition, to be held at South Kensington from July 16 to August 13, 1881, will be opened on Saturday, the 16th. The President, the Right Hon. Earl Spencer, K.G., will take the chair, in the Royal Albert Hall, at 4·30 p.m., and will be supported by the Right Hon. Earl Granville, K.G. ; the Right Hon. John G. Dodson, M.P. ; Sir James Paget, Bart., D.C.L., LL.D., F.R.S. ; John Eric Erichsen, Esq., F.R.S.

CHLORHYDRATE OF MORPHIA IN INSANITY.— Dr. Voisin, of the Salpêtrière, has published twenty-seven additional cases (Bulletin de Thérapeutique, May 15 and 30) showing the great value of the hypodermic injection of the chlorhydrate of morphia in certain forms of insanity. Fifteen of the cases were treated at home, twelve being examples of melancholia and hallucination, and three of maniacal hysteria. Twelve were treated in the hospital, viz., eight cases of melancholia and hallucination, and four of religious insanity—the form admitted as the most difficult to cure. The maximum doses generally employed were from five to eight centigrammes per diem.

(m) Op. cit., page 83 et s

REPORTS OF HOSPITAL PRACTICE
IN
MEDICINE AND SURGERY.

LONDON HOSPITAL.

ABSCESS IN ILIAC REGION ATTENDED WITH INSIGNIFICANT RISE OF TEMPERATURE.
(Under the care of Mr. HUTCHINSON.)
[Reported by Mr. J. HUTCHINSON, jun.]

HARRIET W., aged forty, was healthy until January, 1881, when she was laid up with " gastric fever " for six weeks, and if this was true typhoid it is very probable that the subsequent abscess was dependent in some way upon it. About this time the right groin felt painful and heavy, but no swelling was noticed about the hip until the end of April. Very soon after this she was admitted into the medical ward, and subsequently transferred to the surgical one. From admission her temperature was regularly taken. On the first evening it was 100·4° (as is common with many hospital patients), but it fell to 99° next day, and continued to be normal until May 24.

On examination, there was a reddened swelling between the right iliac crest and the trochanter major, with doubtful fluctuation and enlarged superficial veins over it. It was tender and painful. There was a harder swelling above the ilium.

On the 16th there was no doubt about the presence of pus.

On the 23rd she had a rigor and headache with nausea ; and next evening her temperature stood at 101° ; on the 25th, 100° and 103° ; on the 26th, 99° and 101°. On this date the abscess was opened, and no further rise of temperature occurred. A large quantity of fluid pus was let out, having a distinctly fæcal smell, so that Lister's antiseptics were not used. She recovered speedily and completely.

Remarks.—This was not a case of chronic abscess, for the whole time during which it lasted was little more than three weeks ; it was very painful, and occurred in a woman. Under these circumstances the absence of fever was remarkable, and caused some uncertainty in the diagnosis. Although she was not aware of having passed any matter with her motions, yet it seems possible that a communication with the intestine prevented any tension in the abscess-cavity, as well as accounted for the fæcal odour of the pus discharged from it.

CHARING-CROSS HOSPITAL.

CASE OF POISONING BY BITTER ALMONDS.
(Under the care of Dr. GREEN.)
[Reported by Mr. J. B. BAKER, Resident Medical Officer ; partly from notes by Mr. LYSTER, Assistant Medical Officer.]

A MAN, aged thirty-eight, was brought here on Wednesday, June 1, at 9.30 p.m., insensible. He was said to have fallen down in a fit, and was brought to this hospital at once. When seen he was quite insensible and collapsed, with gasping and laboured breathing ; he was cyanotic ; the pulse hardly perceptible, rapid, and flickering ; some dark mucus about his mouth ; his jaws were fixed, teeth firmly closed ; pupils contracted, and perfectly insensible to touch and light.

On examination, his apex-beat was weak and rapid ; abdomen somewhat distended, and he had passed his fæces unconsciously ; and he had some mucous râles over his chest.

The stomach-pump was at once used, and about a pint of thick brown fluid containing a quantity of small white particles smelling strongly of hydrocyanic acid was removed. His stomach was then washed out with warm water. After this the patient became more collapsed, and his radial pulse almost ceased. The battery was used for ten minutes, one pole over the apex of the heart, the other on the neck over the course of the pneumogastric nerve. Respiration now slightly improved, so the patient was put to bed, and hot fomentations placed on his chest and abdomen, with hot water to his feet. At 10 p.m., liquor ammon. fort. was inhaled every ten minutes, and twenty-five cells of a Leclanché's battery were applied as before, contact being made and broken with inspiration. His breathing became deeper and more regular. Pulse 120 to 140. Twelve (midnight): Patient remained in about the same condition. The battery and inhalations of liquor ammon. were continued alternately every half-hour until 2 a.m. Pulse 130, stronger. At 2 a.m., turpentine stupes were applied over the chest, and one-twenty-fourth of a grain of sulphate of atropia was injected hypodermically. Soon after this he perspired freely, and had a slight convulsion, his breathing improved, and his jaws were no longer fixed. From 2 to 5 a.m. he had several slight convulsions, his breathing gradually became easier, his pupils more sensitive; and at 3 a.m. he was able to swallow, although still very cyanotic and insensible. At 5 a.m. he opened his eyes for the first time, and his pupils became sensitive; his pulse, stronger and regular, 140; breathing 30. The mucous râles had ceased, and he was given brandy ʒss. in beef-tea every hour. He was now undressed and cleaned. 10 a.m.: Patient had slept for two hours, and was conscious, but still dull, and very cyanotic; respirations 20, easy; pulse 120; perspiring freely. The brandy continued every hour with beef-tea or milk until 6 p.m., when he was sleeping quietly; breathing 18; pulse 80, good.

June 3.—Patient passed a good night, and was discharged this afternoon at his own request, well, though weak. Patient said he had eaten nothing during the day, but in the evening had had two handfuls of bitter almonds and a pint of beer; had then returned to work, and felt quite well until he fell down, after which he remembered nothing. The contents of the stomach were tested at once, and gave reactions for hydrocyanic acid. Throughout the night his pulse varied from 120 to 140; his respirations were very rapid, and his breath smelt strongly of prussic acid.

TERMS OF SUBSCRIPTION.
(Free by post.)

British Islands	. . . .	Twelve Months	.	£1 8	0
"	"	Six	"	. 0 14	0
The Colonies and the United } States of America . . . }		Twelve	"	. 1 10	0
"	"	Six	"	. 0 15	0
India	"	Twelve	"	. 1 10	0
" (vid Brindisi)	"	"	"	. 1 15	0
"	"	Six	"	. 0 15	0
" (vid Brindisi)	"	"	"	. 0 17	6

Foreign Subscribers are requested to inform the Publishers of any remittance made through the agency of the Post-office.

Single Copies of the Journal can be obtained of all Booksellers and Newsmen, price Sixpence.

Cheques or Post-office Orders should be made payable to Mr JAMES LUCAS, 11, New Burlington-street, W.

TERMS FOR ADVERTISEMENTS.

Seven lines (70 words)	.	.	.£0	4	6
Each additional line (10 words)	.	.	. 0	0	6
Half-column, or quarter-page	.	.	. 1	5	0
Whole column, or half-page	.	.	. 2	10	0
Whole page	.	.	. 5	0	0

Births, Marriages, and Deaths are inserted Free of Charge.

THE MEDICAL TIMES AND GAZETTE is published on Friday morning: Advertisements must therefore reach the Publishing Office not later than One o'clock on Thursday.

Medical Times and Gazette.

SATURDAY, JULY 9, 1881.

THE COUNCIL OF THE ROYAL COLLEGE OF SURGEONS.

THE annual election of Fellows to fill vacancies in the Council of the Royal College of Surgeons of England, which always excites much interest at this time of the year, will have been decided shortly before we go to press; consequently, we hope to be able to place the result before our readers this week. It is not our custom to lecture the Fellows of the College as to the choice that they ought to make of the candidates who contend for the honour of a seat in the Council. Did we care to do so on this occasion, it would now be too late. Nevertheless, the contest is this year unusually exciting and interesting, and it may therefore be well that we notice once more the claims which the respective candidates have on the support of the Fellows. There are three vacancies to be filled up, owing to the retirement, in the prescribed order, of Sir James Paget, Mr. Haynes Walton, and Mr. C. G. Wheelhouse. Sir James Paget and Mr. Haynes Walton present themselves for re-election; but Mr. Wheelhouse, the well-known Senior Surgeon of the Leeds Infirmary, declines to seek that honour. Four candidates, however, besides the above-mentioned gentlemen are before the electors, so that there are altogether six candidates for the three vacancies.

On reviewing the respective merits of these candidates, it must be acknowledged that the electing Fellows cannot well help choosing three good men and true. Sir James Paget's re-election may, we suppose, be regarded as certain. He became a Member of the College in 1836, was elected a Fellow in 1843, and has served it, in various capacities, for nearly thirty-five years. He is author of the Pathological Catalogue of the Museum of the College, and for two or three years past has been working at a new edition of it. In 1847 he was appointed Arris and Gale Professor of Human Anatomy and Surgery, and in that capacity delivered his valuable and well-known Lectures on Surgical Pathology. In 1863 he became a member of the Council, was re-elected in 1873, and in 1875 was President. From 1876 until a month or two ago he represented the College in the General Medical Council; and in 1877 he delivered his eloquent Hunterian Oration. Who can doubt his re-election into the Council on the present occasion? Mr. Haynes Walton was elected a member of Council in 1873, and has filled the office for eight years. The Fellows ought, therefore, to be well able to judge of the value of his services. Mr. John Whitaker Hulke, F.R.S., the senior candidate among those who have not yet been on the Council, obtained, in 1859, the Jacksonian Prize for his essay "On the Morbid Changes of the Retina, as seen in the Eye of a Living Person and after Removal from the Body"; in 1868 he was appointed Arris and Gale Lecturer; for four years he was a member of the Board of Examiners in Anatomy and Physiology, and in 1880 he was elected on the Court of Examiners. He is well known to the profession as an eminent surgeon and teacher, and he has taken an active interest in the welfare of the College for very many years. He deserves to be, and doubtless will be, strongly supported. Mr. Croft, known as Surgeon to, and Lecturer on Practical Surgery at, St. Thomas's Hospital, has not yet held any office in the College of Surgeons; but he has been Examiner in Surgery at the sister College of Physicians. This is the first time, we think, that he has come forward as a candidate for election into the Council of the College of Surgeons. Mr. Christopher Heath, the next in seniority, Surgeon to University College Hospital, and Holme Professor of Clinical Surgery in University College, also gained the Jacksonian Prize, in 1867, for his essay on "Diseases and Injuries of the Jaws," in 1875 was elected a member of the Board of Examiners in Anatomy and Physiology, and was for a time chairman of the Board. He has also served as an Examiner for Medical and Surgical Degrees of the Universities of Cambridge and of Durham, and as Examiner in Surgery at the Royal College of Physicians, London. Mr. Reginald Harrison, the junior candidate, is brought forward as a provincial candidate, and as such specially appeals to the provincial Fellows for support; but he has deservedly gained great repute as a surgeon and a teacher, and is a man of much energy and working capacity.

Here is undoubtedly a great plenty of excellent candidates; and it is not often that the Fellows have such men to select from. But when professional and collegiate services and distinctions have been considered, personal, school, and hospital predilections will no doubt come into play, and may perhaps considerably affect the voting. We venture, however, to say that we much doubt whether Mr. Harrison is well advised in standing a contest this time. We have more than once objected to the drawing of any invidious contrast between provincial and metropolitan candidates as such. Men should be elected into the Council on the strength of the services they have rendered and are likely to render to the profession and the College, not as representatives of metropolitan or of provincial hospitals or schools; and further, we are inclined to think that the Fellows should remember just now that a very large part of the real business of the College is done by committees, and by committees that must meet at short intervals and often; and that though there can be no doubt that Mr. Harrison has in him all the qualities to make a valuable member of Council, yet it is a far cry to Liverpool. Anyhow, we feel confident that three good men will be chosen from among the candidates for the distinction of Councillor; and it must be owned that, though we have not ourselves ventured to advise the Fellows in the matter, plenty of advice, often of a very questionable kind, has not been wanting from some of our contemporaries.

There is one other subject of great importance connected with the College of Surgeons upon which we may say a few words. The Council have on this occasion to elect the President of the College; and one of our medical contemporaries has thought fit to warn them against following the usual course of electing to that high office the Senior Vice-President, on the ground that he is not truly a representative of English surgery. But Mr. Erasmus Wilson was a surgeon before he was a dermatologist. He has, indeed, done good and great work as a student and teacher of the characters and treatment of diseases of the skin, having been one of the earliest, the ablest, and the most energetic of the physicians and surgeons who have, during the last fifty years, made dermatology a recognised department of scientific medicine. But it need not generally be forgotten—surgeons certainly will not forget it—that Mr. Wilson made his name known far and wide, and won the blue ribbon of the learned societies, the F.R.S., as an anatomist. His "Anatomists' Vade-Mecum" was a wonder and a joy to demonstrators and dissectors when it first appeared—we know not exactly how many years ago,—we think in 1841, but in 1847 it had reached a fourth edition,—and it is still one of the best books of its kind; and not many years ago, Quain and Wilson's great anatomical plates were well known and were much valued by all who could gain opportunities of using them. It appears to us extremely improbable that the Council of the College of Surgeons forget this, or that they will overlook the services the College has accepted from Mr. Wilson, so as to withhold from him, even for a time, the honour of the Presidency. There is no danger or possibility that British Surgery and the Royal College of Surgeons of England will not be fully and fittingly represented at the International Medical Congress. Is not Sir James Paget to be President of the Congress itself, and Mr. Erichsen President of the Surgical Section?

THE ASPIRATOR IN HYDATID DISEASE OF THE LIVER.

WHEN the aspirator came into common use in medicine and surgery the expectations regarding its utility were perhaps somewhat over-sanguine. We now know that the evacuation of an abscess or an empyema with the aspirator frequently fails to cure where the free evacuation of the pus and subsequent drainage under antiseptic precautions succeeds, and that speedily. Of this fact we noticed lately a most striking example reported in a German medical paper —a case of purulent pericarditis in a boy with serous effusion into the left pleural cavity. Two successive aspirations of the pericardium and pleura produced only very temporary relief, and ultimately, first the pericardium, and soon after the pleura, were incised antiseptically— the double operation being followed by a cure within six weeks. A similar treatment of hepatic abscess is now freely recommended and practised by the most experienced authorities on the subject. While, however, the use of the aspirator as a means of treating collections of serous or purulent fluid may not have produced results so brilliant as were expected of it, as a means of diagnosis it holds the first rank, and in this respect alone has been a most valuable addition to our armamentarium. In hydatid disease of the liver its use as a means both of diagnosis and of treatment has been most satisfactory, and Dr. Mortimer Balding(a) has done a good work in collecting and tabulating with their results all cases of hydatid disease reported since 1866—both those in which the aspirator has been used, and those in which it has not.

To be convinced of the necessity of establishing a diagnosis in hydatid disease, and of proceeding to some decided form of treatment, we have only to look at Dr. Balding's Table VII., which includes 35 cases where the disease was either not diagnosed or was treated with drugs only. Of these 35 cases, 7 recovered, 28 died, and in 5 the result is not stated—giving a mortality very much higher than any other method of treatment. Is there any danger, however, in establishing the diagnosis by the introduction into the tumour of a fine trocar or an aspirator-needle? That the liver is an organ marvellously tolerant of surgical interference we know from the results of post-mortem examinations. In a case of hepatic abscess lately exhibited at the Pathological Society, where the liver, ten days or a fortnight previous to death, had been freely punctured in various directions, there was very considerable difficulty in finding the traces of the operation. But, at the same time, there undoubtedly is a certain amount of danger in introducing a trocar into the liver. This is proved by several cases recorded by Dr. Balding, the most rapidly fatal of these being one in which a branch of the portal vein had been punctured, causing death in five minutes. In these two or three fatal cases, however, Dr. Balding notes that the instrument used was a fine trocar, not a fine needle, such as is generally used with the aspirator, and which here, in consequence of the thinness of the fluid, has not the same disadvantage as in cases of thick curdy pus. Where such a needle has been used no accident of the above nature has been recorded.

In Table VI., Dr. Balding records nine cases treated with electrolysis or simple acupuncture, and all with good results. It is to be noted, however, that the tumours were all in young persons, and of small size. Also, in several of the cases, fluid evidently escaped into the peritoneum, which, in the case of purulent contents, would in all probability be fatal. Table V. records thirty cases in which, by means of caustics or incisions, a considerable opening was maintained from the first. The results are not favourable, prolonged suppuration having generally followed, with a fatal result in ten cases. The first four tables record those cases in which the cyst was punctured with a small trocar. Out of 155 cases the fluid on the first puncture was clear in 106, thick or purulent in 49. Among the 49 cases we have 26

(a) "Hydatid Disease of the Liver: its Diagnosis and Treatment." By Mortimer Balding, B.A., M.D. Cantab. London: Harrison and Sons.

cures, 20 deaths, and 3 results not stated; while among the 106 we have 86 cures, 17 deaths, and 3 results not stated—the class in which the contents were clear thus showing 81 per cent. of cures, as against 53 per cent. where the contents were purulent. Again, of the 106 cases in which the fluid was clear at the first puncture, in 35 cases the contents subsequently became purulent, while in 71 there was no evidence that suppuration ever took place. Of these 71 cases last mentioned, there were 58 cures, 11 deaths, and 2 results not given.

The conclusions to which Dr. Balding comes, and which are fully justified by the cases and the statistics he adduces, are as follows:—1. So soon as the tumour is actually felt, establish the diagnosis by the introduction of a fine aspirator-needle. 2. Should the fluid be clear, withdraw the greater part or the whole of it, and close the wound. 3. Should the fluid be purulent, introduce a large trocar, leave the canula in situ, and wash out the cavity once or twice daily, maintaining a free opening and keeping the abdomen well bandaged. Several cases recorded by Harley belonging to this last class did not do well till a free opening was made.

THE WEEK.

TOPICS OF THE DAY.

AT the recently held annual meeting of the Victoria-street Society for the Protection of Animals from Vivisection it was stated that the Society's Bill for the Total Abolition of Vivisection is down for second reading in the House of Commons on the 13th inst. This Bill is in the charge of Sir E. Wilmot, M.P., and prohibits the vivisection of animals with or without anæsthetics. By a strange coincidence a House of Commons return, issued about the time that this meeting was being held, shows the number of experiments performed on living animals during the year 1880 by medical men and others licensed under the Act. The experiments were in most cases performed at laboratories connected with the universities in England and Scotland, or at hospitals or veterinary institutions. The experiments numbered 311, of which only 114 can have been the cause of any pain, and of these all but seventeen were of a kind involving no more pain than is experienced by ordinary vaccination. The painful part of the proceeding in the seventeen cases involving pain was made under anæsthesia, and no appreciable suffering can be said to have been inflicted beyond confinement until the wounds healed, or until the animals were killed. The most important results have been acquired in the elucidation of an obscure and fatal disease (anthrax) which attacks sheep and cattle, and also persons engaged in wool-sorting. Of this series of experiments, twenty-nine were undertaken at the instance of the Royal Agricultural Society, and forty at that of the Medical Department of the Local Government Board.

The Sanitary Committee of the City Commission of Sewers, at the last meeting of that body, brought up a report on a circular communication from the Metropolitan Poor-law Guardians' Association relative to the isolation and treatment of small-pox and fever cases. They at first suggested that they should join the Association in urging on the Government the need of an Act to define and, if requisite, enlarge the powers of the Metropolitan Asylums Board and the several local authorities, in order to prevent the serious consequences which might, in the present uncertain state of the law, result from an epidemic of small-pox or fever, and to include provision for the compulsory notification of infectious diseases, for the compulsory removal to hospitals of persons suffering from such diseases

obtained, and for the non-pauperisation of recipients of that form of relief. The suggestion was referred back to them upon a previous occasion for reconsideration, and the Committee then made a fresh report, stating that, having fully gone into the matter, they were not now prepared to recommend the carrying out of their previous advice. This latter decision the Court now confirmed. Dr. Sedgwick Saunders, the Medical Officer of Health, reported that four cases of small-pox had happened in one house in Ropemaker-street, the patients being a girl of seven and her three elder brothers. The girl took the disease first, and was treated by a private practitioner for some weeks, but he had not informed the authorities of the outbreak, and the result had been that the three brothers had also taken the disease. They were now well enough to be conveyed, with the necessary precautions, to the hospital-ship Rhin, off Gravesend, where they would be properly attended to.

We are rather sorry to hear of the imminent collapse of the Society for the Prevention of Street Accidents. Of course, imperial and parochial legislation is directed, as far as possible, to preserve the lives of the people; but there are many minor details of traffic regulation and street rule, such, for instance, as the erection of street refuges, which can be more promptly carried out by a society such as the one now called upon to perform its happy despatch. At a recent special general meeting the chairman, the Rev. W. Rogers, M.A., with some tinge of bitterness, reproached the public for not properly supporting the Society. He remarked that, judging by results, the public did not want them or their help, and, therefore, the sooner they wound up, the better. It was folly to endeavour to save people if they were determined not to be saved. The Society's best friends had left them, and there was no use in carrying on, although they had done their utmost, had met time after time, and even had called an indignation meeting at the Mansion House; still the people did not seem to take an interest in their proceedings. The public, it appeared, liked to be run over; they wished for a little excitement in that way. The meeting then adopted a resolution directing that a report up to date be sent out to the subscribers, and that a final meeting be called for the purpose of winding up the Society.

The Almoner and Sub-Almoner of the Order of St. John of Jerusalem in England have addressed a communication to the Press which runs as follows:—"We venture to ask your indulgence to enable us to bring to the notice of the public a movement second only in importance, we believe, to the support of hospitals themselves—the system of supplying nourishing diets to discharged convalescent patients at their own homes. It is now fourteen years since a scheme was set on foot by the English branch of the Order of St. John of Jerusalem, for the supply of such diets as are medically ordered by the hospital surgeons, and so to continue the work of the recovery of the patients after leaving the hospitals as to enable them to return, at the earliest possible time, to the business of life and the support of their families. The object of the Order in this, as in all its works, is purely unsectarian. All communications should be addressed to the Sub-Almoner, at St. John's-gate, Clerkenwell, E.C., who will be glad to supply all information that may be desired."

We have to record the first general meeting, in the Hall of the Institute of Civil Engineers, Great George-street, of the new "Society of Chemical Industry." Though only inaugurated as recently as April 4 last at the rooms of the Chemical Society, Burlington House, it already numbers more than three hundred members, and its chief aim is to bring more closely together the scientific chemist and the acquisition and practice of that species of knowledge which constitutes the profession of a chemical engineer." Professor Roscoe, F.R.S., the President of the Chemical Society, and also of the new Society, acted as chairman, and after his address three papers were read—" On Recent Legislation on Noxious Gases," by Mr. E. K. Muspratt; " The Brewing of Lager-Beer," by Professor C. Graham; and " Mechanical Furnaces," by Mr. James Mactear.

At the last meeting of the Metropolitan Board of Works, two deputations were received from the Vestry of Bermondsey, respectively presenting memorials on the subject of widening Tooley-street and Bermondsey-street, and the formation of a thoroughfare to the Kent-road. The Chairman explained that the operations of the Board in this direction were greatly restricted by Section 33 of the Metropolis Improvement Act, which had the effect of delaying many valuable improvements. The Works and General Purposes Committee recommended that the Board should contribute one-half of the cost (estimated at £1700) of the improvement and laying-out by the Vestry of Bermondsey of the parish churchyard, upon condition that the same be maintained in perpetuity as an open space for the use and benefit of the public, such contribution not to exceed the sum of £850. This was ultimately agreed to.

Dr. Andrew Clark, the Senior Physician of the London Hospital, delivered, on Thursday last week, before an audience consisting chiefly of ladies—of subscribers to the institution, —together with many of the nurses of the Hospital, the inaugural lecture of a popular course on nursing. He defined nursing as simply a ministration to the necessities and comforts of the sick. He reminded his hearers that it called for qualities not always nor often united—some knowledge of the nature of disease, of the bodily functions, of the wants of the sick, and of how they were to be met. It was, he said, the medical man who possessed most of the knowledge requisite for successful nursing; he must guide, and the nurse must be the skilled hand to carry out his instructions along with clinical assistants and dispensers. Nursing was thus a secondary and ministerial, although not necessarily an inferior, function. To suppose the nurse degraded by her work was against the true view of the dignity of the labour. The nurse would minister not only to the alleviation and cure of the disease, but even to the advancement of knowledge. The lecturer then dwelt on the physical, intellectual, and moral qualifications of nurses, which, however, would not suffice without long, patient, and assiduous practice, for which the eight hundred beds of the London Hospital afforded ample scope. Dr. Clark concluded by inculcating on nurses the necessity of self-sacrifice and humility if they wished their sacred office to become, like charity, twice blest.

The Medical Acts Commission met at Victoria-street, Westminster, on the 24th, 25th, and 27th of last month. The evidence of Dr. A. H. Jacob, Dr. Glover, and Dr. R. Scott-Orr was taken. There were present—The Earl of Camperdown, Chairman; the Bishop of Peterborough; the Right Hon. W. H. F. Cogan, the Master of the Rolls; the Right Hon. G. Sclater-Booth, M.P., Sir William Jenner, Bart., K.C.B., Mr. Simon, C.B., Professor Huxley, Dr. McDonnell, Professor Turner, Mr. Bryce, M.P., and the Secretary.

In consequence of the increasingly numerous cases of myopia developed in French schools through bad arrangement of seats and distribution of light, the Minister of Public Instruction has nominated a commission, named " De l'Hygiène de la Vue dans les Écoles," whose object will be to study the influence of the material conditions of school arrangement on the progress of myopia, and to discover the means of counteracting the evil.

The latest returns from the Mansion House show that over £27,000 has been paid in to the credit of the Hospital Sunday Fund, and it is now considered certain, in some quarters, that last year's amount will be far exceeded.

THE COLLEGE OF SURGEONS' ANNUAL ELECTION.

THE numbers of votes given to the several candidates for the vacant seats in the Council of the Royal College of Surgeons were as follow :—Sir James Paget, 228 votes, including 1 plumper; Mr. John Whitaker Hulke, 187 votes, 8 plumpers; Mr. Christopher Heath, 133 votes, 5 plumpers; Mr. John Croft, 113 votes, 18 plumpers; Mr. Reginald Harrison (Liverpool), 87 votes, 12 plumpers; Mr. Haynes Walton, 72 votes, 5 plumpers. The choice of the Fellows has thus fallen on Sir James Paget, Messrs. Hulke and Heath.

INTERNATIONAL MEDICAL CONGRESS.

THE arrangements for the coming meeting in London during the early part of August are now all but completed. The Executive have, unfortunately, received news of the sudden death (from angina pectoris) of Professor Maurice Raynaud, who was to have given one of the four chief addresses. His subject was " Le Scepticisme en Médecine, au Temps Pass et au Temps Présent." We believe that a substitute has not yet been chosen; and it will be by no means easy to find anyone willing and able to attempt, at so short a notice, to fill the place of such a physician and orator as M. Raynaud. It is whispered that Dr. G. de Mussy will be asked to read the address of his former friend, which, fortunately, the author had completed just before his death. Under any circumstances, we believe that a Frenchman will be invited, in order to make this series of the addresses as representative as possible. Professor Virchow has quite lately decided to be present at the Congress; he will also give an address, the subject of which will probably be " Pathological Experiment in Medicine." The attendance of Professor Volkmann, of Halle, is rather uncertain; his health has been indifferent for some time past, and he has been obliged, in consequence, to rest during the past session and spend his winter in Italy. The opening of the Congress takes place on August 2, at the College of Physicians, on which occasion Sir William Jenner will preside.

KING AND QUEEN'S COLLEGE OF PHYSICIANS IN IRELAND.

AT a special business meeting of the College, recently convened to consider the minutes of evidence to be submitted by the Registrar on behalf of the College to the Royal Commission on the Medical Acts, the following resolution was adopted, namely :—" That it be an instruction to the Registrar to state to the Royal Commission that this College is prepared to accept legislation based upon the following lines :—1. That no person shall be allowed to hold a public appointment until he shall have passed a public examination conducted under the authority of the Government. 2. That no candidate shall be admitted to such public examination without the production of diplomas in medicine, surgery, and midwifery from bodies authorised to confer the same."

THE VICTORIA CROSS.

THE London Gazette of June 28 announced that the Queen has been graciously pleased to signify her intention to confer the decoration of the Victoria Cross upon Surgeon John Frederick M'Crea, of the 1st Regiment Cape Mounted Yeomanry, whose claim has been submitted for Her Majesty's approval, for his conspicuous bravery in South Africa, as recorded against his name. The act of courage for which Mr. M'Crea was recommended is thus described :—" For his ment with the Basutos on January 14, 1881, at Tweefontein, near Thaba Tsen, when, after the enemy had charged the Burghers in the most determined manner, forcing them to retire with a loss of sixteen killed and twenty-one wounded, Surgeon M'Crea went out for some distance, under a heavy fire, and, with the assistance of Captain Buxton, of the Mafeteng Contingent, conveyed a wounded Burgher named Aircamp to the shelter of a large ant-heap, and having placed him in a position of safety, returned to the ambulance for a stretcher. While on his way thither Surgeon M'Crea was severely wounded in the right breast by a bullet, notwithstanding which, he continued to perform his duties at the ambulance, and again assisted to bring in several wounded men, continuing afterwards to attend the wounded during the remainder of the day, and scarcely taking time to dress his own wound, which he was obliged to do himself, there being no other medical officer on the field. Had it not been for this gallantry and devotion to his duty on the part of Surgeon M'Crea, the sufferings of the wounded would undoubtedly have been much aggravated, and greater loss of life might very probably have ensued."

THE MASSACHUSETTS MEDICAL SOCIETY.

THE oldest surviving medical society in America, the Massachusetts Medical Society, has lately celebrated its centennial anniversary. "A medical society in Boston" seems to have been established in 1735 or 1736, but it did not live many years, and on November 1, 1781, the Massachusetts Society, embracing the broad limits of the State, was incorporated, its charter being signed by Samuel Adams, President of the Senate, and John Hancock, Governor of the Commonwealth—names strongly suggestive of revolutionary days and of patriotism. In honour of this centennial celebration, our ably and energetically conducted contemporary, the *Boston Medical and Surgical Journal*, devoted the whole of its issue of June 8 to illustrate and commemorate the event. The number contains portions of the centennial address delivered before the Society by Dr. Samuel Green; numerous documents relating to the foundation of the Society; a memoir of the venerable Dr E. A. Holyoke, the founder of the Society, who died in 1829, with a silhouette portrait of him, and a fac-simile of the toast offered by him at a dinner given on his one-hundredth birthday, August 13, 1828. And it contains also many summaries, articles, fac-simile letters, and other documents of interest of the Society relating to the history and the times of the Society: among others, a fac-simile of two pages from Dr. Holyoke's day-books, 1750-1828, with explanations; a fac-simile of a certificate of fumigation after small-pox, 1776; and "the diary of Mr. W. Pyncheon, relating his personal experiences during inoculation against small-pox, 1776." The whole number is very interesting and curious, and does great credit to the patriotism and enterprise of our contemporary.

SCHOOL OF PHYSIC IN IRELAND.

AT the usual monthly business meeting of the King and Queen's College of Physicians in Ireland, held on Friday, July 1, Dr. Aquilla Smith tendered his resignation as King's Professor of Materia Medica and Practical Pharmacy in the School of Physic in Ireland. The appointment to the vacant chair is vested by Act of Parliament in the President and Fellows of the King and Queen's College of Physicians. It will probably be made on next St. Luke's Day, October 18. As the King's Professor also holds the office of Clinical Physician to Sir Patrick Dun's Hospital, that post is also now vacant. Dr. Henry Kennedy has been appointed *locum*

THE PARIS WEEKLY RETURNS.

THE number of deaths for the twenty-fifth week, ending June 23, 1881, was 944 (viz., 471 males and 473 females), and among these there were from typhoid fever 11, smallpox 24, measles 24, scarlatina 10, pertussis 11, diphtheria and croup 43, erysipelas 7, puerperal infections 5, and acute tubercular meningitis 46. There were also 22 deaths from acute bronchitis, 54 from pneumonia, 72 from infantile athrepsia (26 of the infants having been wholly or partially suckled), and 25 violent deaths. The mortality continues to diminish, and especially with respect to the chief epidemical diseases. Still, deaths from small-pox have increased from 16 to 24. Diphtheria, too, although diminished from 52 to 43, is still in excess of the mean for the week (34 to 40) of former years. The births for the week amounted to 1154, viz., 580 males (426 legitimate and 154 illegitimate) and 574 females (432 legitimate and 132 illegitimate); 84 children (48 males and 36 females) were born dead or died within twenty-four hours.

THE REPORT ON THE METROPOLITAN WATER-SUPPLY FOR MAY LAST.

THE report on the examination made of the water supplied by the metropolitan water companies during the month of May last states that the condition of the water in the Thames at Hampton, Molesey, and Sunbury (where the intakes of the West Middlesex, Grand Junction, Southwark and Vauxhall, Lambeth, Chelsea, and East London Companies are situated) was good in quality during the whole of the month, with the exception of the last two days, when it was slightly turbid. The water in the river Lea was also very good during the whole of the month. The foregoing remarks refer to the condition of the water previous to filtration. The Examiner again calls attention to the fact that, in the absence of a duly authorised and official "standard of filtration" regulating the quantity of water to be passed through a given area in a given time, it has been found during the past nine years that when the rate of filtration does not exceed 540 gallons per square yard of filter-bed each twenty-four hours, the filtration is effectual, and this has been generally recognised as a tentative standard rate of filtration. Dr. Frankland reports that the Thames water supplied by the Chelsea, West Middlesex, Southwark, Grand Junction, and Lambeth Companies, which was unusually free from organic matter in April, exhibited a further improvement during May, being of better average quality than at any time during this or the preceding year. The water was also uniformly well filtered before delivery. Of the water derived from the Lea, Dr. Frankland found that that sent out by the New River Company was but slightly inferior in chemical quality to the best of the deepwell waters, whilst the East London Company's supply resembled average Thames water. Both these waters were distributed in an efficiently filtered condition.

DURHAM UNIVERSITY MEDICAL GRADUATES' ASSOCIATION.

THE first annual meeting of the above Association was held in the Divinity Lecture-room of the University of Durham, on the 28th ult., when a code of by-laws was framed and other business transacted. The members afterwards dined together (by the kind permission of the Reverend the Master of University College) at the High Table in the Hall of University College. The next annual meeting will be held in London. The following are the officers for the ensuing year 1881-82:—*President:* G. H. Philipson, M.A., M.D., F.R.C.P. *Vice-Presidents:* Luke Armstrong, M.D.; W. Travers, M.D., F.R.C.S. Eng. *Council:* W. C. Arnison.

F.R.C.S. Eng.; Bedford Fenwick, M.D.; Shadforth Morton M.D.; W. S. Porter, M.B.; D. Drummond, M.A., M.D.; W. Robinson, M.B.; R. H. Wilson, M.D.; J. R. Dodd, M.D.; S. Fielden, M.D.; G. P. Goldsmith, M.D. *Hon. Secretary for the North and Treasurer*: W. P. Mears, M.B. *Hon. Secretary for the South*: R. H. Wilson, M.D.

NEW EXAMINERS AT THE ROYAL COLLEGE OF SURGEONS.

THE following candidates have applied to be elected to the offices of Examiners in Medicine and in Midwifery at the Royal College of Surgeons for the ensuing year, viz., for Medicine—Dr. W. H. Allchin, Dr. H. C. Bastian, Dr. A. J. Pollock, Dr. F. T. Roberts, and Dr. I. B. Yeo; and for Midwifery—Dr. J. B. Potter. Doubtless other candidates (who must be Fellows of the Royal College of Physicians of London) will be nominated at the meeting this day (Friday.)

THE NEW OUT-PATIENT CONSULTATIONS AT THE SALPÊTRIÈRE.

THE *Gazette des Hopitaux* of June 28 gives the following account of this new arrangement:—" These external consultations are to take place every day at half-past nine, on patients suffering from nervous and mental diseases. Medicines are to be supplied, and a little later, baths and douches. The public is received on Mondays by M. Moreau (de Tours), on Tuesdays by M. Charcot, on Wednesdays by M. Luys, on Fridays by M. Auguste Voisin, and on Saturdays by M. Legrand du Saulle. On Thursdays there is to be a surgical consultation by M. Terrier. A special building has been raised at the entrance of the Salpêtrière on purpose for this consultation, which evidently will have a very great success. The possibility for the district-physicians and for families to be able to obtain immediately and gratuitously a certificate of insanity in urgent and very difficult cases will, in fact, give rise to the disappearance of a crowd of embarrassments or perils. The responsibility which often presses so heavily upon district-physicians (*médecins de quartier*) would be entirely covered by the authorised signature of one of the physicians of the hospital. On the other hand, the formalities necessary for the entrance of patients into the special services will be somewhat simplified. The delivery of medicines to all the consultants appears also a very great benefit to the hysterical, epileptic, apoplectic, ataxic, choreic, and insane patients, who have already been submitted to the examination of the medical *personnel* of Salpêtrière.

THE REGISTRAR-GENERAL OF IRELAND'S RETURN FOR THE FIRST QUARTER OF 1881.

THE return of the Registrar-General in Ireland for the first quarter of the present year shows that there were registered during that period 31,527 births (a number equal to an annual birth-rate of 23·8 in every 1000 of the estimated population), and 28,786 deaths, representing an annual rate of 21·7 per 1000. The English returns for the corresponding quarter give a birth-rate of 35·5 and a death-rate of 21·8 per 1000. The birth-rate in Ireland for this first quarter of 1881 is under the average of the rate for the corresponding quarter of the previous five years to the extent of 3·2 per 1000, and 2·5 per 1000 under the death-rate for the corresponding quarter of the year 1880. The death-rate for this quarter is also below the average of the corresponding quarter of the five years 1876-80, to the extent of 0·2 per 1000, being also 1·2 below the first quarter of the preceding year. In the report of the Registrar-General now under notice, two improvements are noticeable; the first of these consists of a separate table, constructed so as to give the rate of mortality in each of the fifty-six urban sanitary districts of Ireland,

of death as have hitherto been published for the various territorial divisions used for registration purposes. This arrangement affords a means for comparing the causes and rates of mortality in towns, with the country at large and with one another. Secondly, three new headings have been introduced into those portions of the tables relating to zymotic diseases; instead of the simple heading "fever," we find now a separate column for typhus, typhoid, and simple fevers. This change has been made with the view of affording a more accurate indication of the unhealthy conditions which promote fever, inasmuch as it is now conclusively ascertained that the promoting causes of the various forms of fever differ in kind and degree. The death-rate in Leinster for the first quarter of the present year was 26·0 per 1000, in Munster it was 21·5, in Ulster 21·2, and in Connaught 16·7 only. The county death-rates range from 15·4 per 1000 in Roscommon and Sligo to 35·0 in Dublin; between these rates the lowest five are— Kerry, 16·1; Mayo, 16·4; Longford, 16·8; Leitrim, 16·9; and Donegal, 17·8; and the highest five are—Antrim, 22·9; Louth, 23·8; Wexford, 24·6; Limerick, 26·4; and Waterford, 27·8. The returns for this quarter present a favourable aspect with regard to the principal zymotic diseases, the deaths from which show a substantial diminution as compared with the corresponding quarters of 1880 and 1879, and with each of the four quarters of the preceding year. Small-pox caused 10 deaths, against 17 in the preceding quarter, and compared with 94 in the corresponding quarter of 1880; all the deaths took place in the Dublin Registration District. The Registrar's notes appended to the Return, as usual, contain much information regarding the prevalence of disease, and the sanitary conditions under which the inhabitants of their several districts are placed. There were 787 inquests reported to the Registrars during the quarter, this number being equal to 1 in every 37 of the total deaths registered.

MEDICAL SOCIETY OF LONDON.

IT is intended to elect the following gentlemen as Honorary Fellows:—Professor Bamberger, Dr. J. H. Billings, Dr. Bigelow, Professor Billroth, Professor Charcot, Professor Da Costa, Dr. Emmett, Professor Haller, Professor von Nussbaum, Professor Tarnier, Professor Verneuil, Professor Volkmann. Professor Raynaud, of Paris, whose death we have elsewhere recorded, would also have been proposed for a similar honour.

ST. PETERSBURG REGISTRATION RETURNS.

FOR the week ending May 30 the number of deaths in St. Petersburg (exclusive of dead-born children, 29 in number) was 805, or 62·50 per 1000 (507 males and 298 females). Among these there were 132 deaths below one year, 95 between one and ten years, 51 between ten and twenty, 247 between twenty and forty, 177 between forty and sixty, and 86 above sixty. Of the deaths, 71 arose from typhus fever, 50 from typhoid fever, 60 from relapsing fever, 22 from unspecified forms of typhus, 7 from small-pox, 4 from measles, 13 from scarlatina, and 10 from diphtheria and croup. Accidental deaths were 13 in number, and suicides 4. During the week ending June 7, on account of the want of room, 544 patients were refused admission to civil hospitals. The pressing necessity for more room is to be met by devoting 400 additional beds in the Nikolai Military Hospital to civilian patients. For the week ending June 7 there were admitted to the civil hospitals 6521 (4394 male and 2127 female) patients; into the children's hospitals 280 (137 male and 143 female) patients; and into the military hospitals 1039 (1021 male and 18 female) patients. Among the female), 1673 (1102 male and 571 female) were cases of typhoid and typhus fever, 29 (13 male and 16 female) scarlatina, 20 (12 male and 8 female) small-pox, and 1083 (626 male and 457 female) venereal diseases. The out-patients of the children's hospitals numbered 2124.

REPORTS ON OUTBREAKS OF TYPHOID FEVER, BY DR. FRANKLIN PARSONS.

In November, 1880, Dr. Parsons was despatched by the Local Government Board to examine and report upon the general sanitary condition of the Totnes Urban and Rural Sanitary Districts. This inspection was ordered in consequence of typhoid fever having been unduly prevalent in 1879-80 in the borough of Totnes, and for several years past in different parts of the rural district. Dr. Parsons instituted inquiries at Harberton, Galmpton, South Brent, Ugborough, and Buckfastleigh, and he found that, although there had been some scattered cases (mostly of doubtful nature) in isolated places, the great majority of fatal cases had occurred in distinct groups, and in certain particular localities. The grouped cases may be considered, he thinks, without much risk of error, to have been all cases of enteric fever, although in some of them the cause of death was certified as typhus. In reviewing the sanitary arrangements of the districts, Dr. Parsons expresses an opinion that in the generality of cases the infection has probably been received through the medium of sewage-poisoned air. In many of the houses in which cases occurred, there have been opportunities for the entry of sewer air, such as indoor water-closets with unventilated soil-pipes, defective drains running under the house, or untrapped or inefficiently trapped sinks in or near it. In other cases the effluvia from foul privies on neighbouring premises was complained of. In the low-lying streets called Warland, there are, or were, old stagnant sewers, and the tide occasionally backs up the drains and floods the houses. In other cases the infection may have been conveyed, the report goes on to say, by polluted well-water; but there are no facts to show that the quality of the public water-supply had any share in propagating the disease, though the insufficiency of the supply as regards quantity has, in all probability, tended largely to the result. The persons attacked had obtained milk from various sources, and no special incidence of the fever upon the customers of any particular dairy was observed. The recommendations appended by Dr. Parson's to this report are principally calculated to secure an improved system of sewerage, and he remarks that as most of the places in the rural district have abundance of irrigable land in their vicinity, the diversion of sewage from the streams would be a comparatively easy matter.

Dr. Parsons has also furnished a report to the Local Government Board on the prevalence of typhoid fever in the borough of Haverfordwest, Pembrokeshire, and the general sanitary condition of that place. In the beginning of August, 1880, several cases of typhoid fever commenced nearly simultaneously in different parts of the town, and it soon attained a widespread prevalence. Of the origin of the outbreak Dr. Parsons admits he can give no explanation; the earliest of the cases, so far as dates could be obtained, lived in widely separated localities, in some instances unconnected with the town sewers or water service, and no direct communication between them, or common cause, could be discovered. Sanitary defects certainly existed at the houses in which they occurred, but similar defects were to be found at only too many of the houses in Haverfordwest. To account satisfactorily for the occurrence of the earlier cases it should be shown how these particular patients came about the same time to be exposed to the specific poison of the disease; and this Dr. Parsons is un-

able to do. The number of cases which had come to the knowledge of the Medical Officer of Health up to the middle of December, when this inspection was made, was eighty-eight, and it is a noteworthy feature that twenty of these sufferers were domestic servants. Female servants, from the nature of their duties, are, of course, especially exposed to exhalations from sinks and water-closets, and the Medical Officer of Health considers that at Haverfordwest they are mostly in the habit of using water as a beverage. Without being able to affirm it, Dr. Parsons remarks that it seems likely that the origin of the epidemic was in some way connected with the condition of the water service of the borough, but what the nature of the connexion may have been, he is unable to say. He has no doubt, however, that the various unsanitary conditions existing in the town have conduced to the spreading of the disease, but how much of the result may be attributable to each of those conditions there are no means of ascertaining. At the request of the Town Clerk, and with the sanction of the Local Government Board, Dr. Parsons attended a meeting of the Haverfordwest Town Council, when he had an opportunity of pointing out to them the state of matters conducing to the spread of fever which he had discovered to be existing, together with such recommendations as occurred to him to be necessary.

DEATH OF DR. MAURICE RAYNAUD.

Another sudden death (it is said, from angina pectoris) has to be added to the great number of such occurrences that have told so disastrously of late on the profession in France, in the persons of Lorain, Chauffard, Broca, Delpech, and Peisse. Although of late suffering much at times from overwork, Dr. Raynaud furnished no indication of approaching danger, and had recently been more than usually cheerful, in consequence of his having been selected to deliver the French address at the approaching Medical Congress. Indeed, he was playing with his children three hours before his death. Scarcely fifty years of age, he commenced his medical career by the production of a thesis, "Les Médecins du Temps de Molière," which attained great popularity. He was an indefatigable worker, both at his profession and in literature, and at the time of his death last week was Physician at La Charité, Agrégé of the Faculty of Medicine, member of the Section of Medical Pathology of the Academy of Medicine, and Officer of the Legion of Honour. Possessed of great oratorical power, much was anticipated from the address he was commissioned to deliver.

UNIVERSITY OF DUBLIN : SUMMER COMMENCEMENTS.

The Summer Commencements for the conferring of degrees were held on Thursday, June 30, in the Examination Hall of Trinity College. More than usual interest was attached to the proceedings owing to the fact that the Chancellor (Lord Cairns) was to preside for the first time since his appointment to that high office fourteen years ago. There was a large attendance of the members of the University and of the students; while the occasion was graced, as usual, with the presence of a considerable number of ladies. The Chancellor having taken the chair, with the Rev. John H. Jellett, D.D., Provost, to his right, and the Rev. J. W. Barlow, Senior Master non-regent, to his left, thus constituting the *Caput*, the Public Orator (Dr. Webb) addressed him as follows (we take this from print copy) : —"Ad Cancellarium—Gratus hic nobis affulsit dies, qui nunc aspicit in hac aulâ Senatum omnibus numeris absolutum. Cancellarium salvere jubemus. Hactenus inter Academiæ Cancellarios adnumerantur Reges, Principes, Pontifices, Primores Civitatis, sed omnes adventitii ; nunc primum nostratem, nostrum, nostræ Academiæ alumnum, jactamus. Te, vir summe, salutamus Cancellarium vere nostrum. Neque hæc sola gloriandi causa. Academiæ Cancellarius, Cancellarius idem Angliæ, sanctissimum illud tribunal, haud impar, ascendisti ne tot et tanta ingenia orbi terrarum jus dixerunt. Nec juris tantam peritia enituisti. Rempublicam summa prudentia, summa auctoritate tractasti. Miraculum illud ingeni quod optimatum partibus nuper lumen affudit, eheu citius occidit. Te spem alteram intuetur Patria. In te oculi intenduntur omnium Imperi majestatis et libertatis antiquæ propugnatorem. Cressa ne careat nota hic dies. Te iterum iterumque salvere jubemus." The Chancellor, who on rising was greeted with cheers, in reply, said : " Libentissime, hanc Universitatem, almam meam matrem, post longam, sed non sine causa, absentiam, rursus adspicio; atque ex officio meo, Universitatis Cancellarius, hæc comitia ad gradus conferendos habeo." The number of degrees in medicine, surgery, and midwifery which were conferred was unusually large. In addition the " Gradus honoris causâ" was conferred :—Doctores in Utroque Jure : Præhonorabilis Edvardus Sullivan, Mag. Rot. in Hibernia; Præhonorabilis Edvardus Gibson, M.P.; Jacobus Carolus Mathew, Eques Auratus, Justiciarius Summæ Curiæ apud West; Evelyn Philippus Shirley; Doctor Weiss; Rev. Archibaldus H. Sayce; Johannes Mulholland, M.P.; Bindon Blood Stoney. Doctor in Medicinâ : Achmuty Irwin. The gentlemen were introduced collectively by Dr. Webb in the following words : —" Præsto, sunt viri, variis artibus egregii, quos honoris causâ Universitas, Cancellari, purpurâ suâ decorandos elegit." Dr. Achmuty Irwin, C.B., Surgeon of the Royal Navy, on coming forward to receive the degree of Doctor of Medicine, was received with very loud cheering. Of him Dr. Webb said : " Præsento Machaonem nostrum Achmuty Irwin. Hujus artis, pietates, virtutis testis Sinope, testis Odessa, testis Alma; testis et Seres et Afri. Numismatis ecce cintillat. Hunc insignibus suis honoris causâ quatuor ornavere Reges; hunc honoris causâ, nostro insigni ornamus."

THE MUSEUM OF THE ROYAL COLLEGE OF SURGEONS.

FROM the annual report of the Conservator of the Museum of the Royal College of Surgeons, it appears that the additions to the Pathological department about to be made to the Museum are unusually numerous; and especially interesting as including a series of preparations presented by Mr. S. G. Shattock, showing the repair of wounds, cicatrisation after the fall of the petiole, the union of grafts, and other processes of vegetable pathology. M. Parrot, Drs. Barlow and Herman, and Messrs. Parker and Shattock, have contributed a number of specimens illustrating the pathology of rickets, infantile syphilis, and combined or allied forms of these diseases in fœtal life and in childhood, which have been the subjects of papers published in the *Proceedings of the Pathological Society* and in the medical journals. Sir Joseph Fayrer has contributed several valuable specimens of dysenteric intestines and abscess of the liver. The staff of the Samaritan Hospital have presented some interesting examples of diseases of the female organs, including a series demonstrating the twisting of ovarian pedicles, and the pathological effects of that lesion.

Numerous specimens have been added to the series of Normal Anatomy and Physiology—some of great interest. The additions in Human Anatomy comprise a preparation showing the muscles of the abdominal wall, evidently requiring great skill and care in dissection. In Comparative

Anatomy are several preparations made by Mr. William Pearson with great care of the manatee which had lived for seventeen months in the Brighton Aquarium, the directors of which company presented the body to the Museum. The larger number of other specimens of this series have been presented by the Zoological Society, of which Mr. Flower is the President.

Mr. S. G. Shattock has continued his valuable aid in preparing a series of human bones, on which the attachments of the various muscles are neatly delineated; the additions he has made during the past year of the sternum, the foot, and the pelvis nearly complete the series.

In the Osteological department, the "Barnard Davis" collection, of which we have already published a full account, has been thoroughly cleaned, and the varnish and dust with which nearly all the skulls were covered carefully removed; the lower jaws, which in many cases had become transposed, have been adjusted to their respective crania, and the skeletons have all been partially re-articulated and placed upon stands. The thorough examination of the collection has satisfactorily shown that its value was never over-estimated, and that its acquisition and preservation in the College Museum is a solid and permanent increase to the scientific wealth of the country; for even if the methods of investigation now used are superseded by others, and the present descriptive catalogues come to be looked upon as obsolete, the specimens will always remain as materials for building up the history of the human race. As the interest in the subject increases, many of these evidences of the physical structure of people passed or passing away will come to be objects of priceless value.

Attention is directed to a very fine specimen of a sea lion (*Otaria jubata*), obtained for the Museum by Mr. F. Coleman, Secretary of the Falkland Islands Company; it has been well mounted and articulated by Mr. John Marle. A remarkably fine skull of the great elephant seal (*Macrorhinus leoninus*), considerably larger than any existing in the other museums in Europe, has been presented by Mr. H. Mansel.

To the series of Human Osteology, Mr. W. R. Kynsey, Principal Civil Medical Officer and Inspector-General of Hospitals in Ceylon, has contributed a valuable collection of skulls and skeletons of the Veddahs, or aboriginal inhabitants of that island, and promises to send corresponding specimens of the Cingalese. Dr. Shortt, Deputy Surgeon-General, has continued his donations of crania of the inhabitants of Central and Southern India, and Surgeon-Major Mackenzie has presented two complete skeletons and four others are now on their way from the same source; and Captain Burton, H.M. Consul at Trieste, has sent a large collection of Egyptian skulls, about one hundred in number.

In his report of 1871, Mr. Flower alluded to the necessity for a change in the Museum staff, and recognising the supreme importance to the Museum that its pathological collections should be kept up in the best manner, and that every specimen sent to it should be examined and described according to the most recent phases of knowledge of the subject, it was determined, for the first time in the history of the Museum, to appoint permanently upon the staff a gentleman devoting himself especially to surgical pathology, whose hours of attendance could be so arranged as not to interfere with hospital studies carried on simultaneously, or with some cultivation of the more practical part of the profession. This arrangement has been highly successful, and the additions made to this department during the time the Pathological Assistantship was held, for six years by Dr. Goodhart, and for four years by Mr. Doran, have been numerous and valuable, while the condition of the whole collection has been greatly improved. As our readers already know, a further step is to be taken in the same direction by the appointment of a "Pathological Curator."

The new catalogue by Sir J. Paget, Dr. Goodhart, and Mr. Doran is steadily progressing, and it is expected will be ready for press before the end of the year.

In concluding his report, Mr. Flower states the interesting fact that art students, both male and female, avail themselves of the Museum in constantly increasing numbers, as in the numerous articulated skeletons and dissected preparations of muscles they find facilities for their studies which they can obtain nowhere else in London.

THE HARVEY TERCENTENARY MEMORIAL.

A MEETING of the subscribers to this fund was held, by permission of the President of the Royal College of Physicians, at the College, on Wednesday, June 29. There were present —Sir George Burrows, in the chair; Dr. Owen Rees, Dr. Sieveking, Dr. Fincham, Dr. R. Barnes, Dr. Begley, Mr. John Simon, Mr. Prescott Hewett, Mr. John Gay, Mr. Edwin Saunders, Mr. J. B. Tolputt (Mayor of Folkestone), and other gentlemen, with Mr. George Eastes and Mr. W. G. S. Harrison, the Honorary Secretaries.

Mr. Eastes read a statement respecting the arrangements sanctioned and carried out by the Executive Committee appointed in June, 1878. It is generally known, however, that the statue of Harvey, by Mr. A. B. Joy, will be unveiled at Folkestone on Saturday, August 6, during the meeting in London of the International Medical Congress. Sir E. Watkin, Bart., M.P., has kindly promised a special train for conveying from London to Folkestone and back the guests invited from London to take part in the ceremony; and Lord Radnor had granted a site for the statue on the Leas, Folkestone, which had been selected by Mr. Joy, and approved by the Folkestone Committee. This meeting was summoned to make the final arrangements for presenting the statue to the future care and custody of the Mayor and Corporation of Folkestone; to designate some eminent person to unveil the statue and make the presentation in question; and to settle any other matters having reference to the Memorial Fund. As regarded funds, there was then a sum of £358 in hand, whilst the amount still to be paid to the sculptor and for other purposes was about £530. There was thus a deficit of about £172 which would require to be collected before the receipts and expenditure quite balanced, and before the fund could be closed. But thirty-three promised subscriptions, probably good for about £80, were still unpaid, and the remaining sum of about £90 or £100 it was thought would be collected within the next few weeks.

The report was received and adopted. The meeting then resolved—"That the statue of Harvey be presented to the Mayor and Corporation of the borough of Folkestone, as the elected representatives of that borough, to be preserved by them in honour of the memory of William Harvey, the discoverer of the circulation of the blood."

The Mayor of Folkestone (Mr. J. B. Tolputt) returned thanks on behalf of his fellow-townspeople for the honour done them by this committal to their custody of the statue of Harvey, and said that it would always be highly valued and well cared for by them.

It was proposed by Mr. John Simon, C.B., seconded by Dr. Owen Rees, and resolved—"That Professor Owen, C.B., be invited to unveil the statue at Folkestone, and to make such presentation on behalf of the subscribers to the Harvey Tercentenary Memorial Fund." Mr. Simon, in introducing Professor Owen's name, said he was the patriarch of British physiologists, a master of much learning and eloquence; and that he (Mr. Simon) was sure it would be agreed upon all hands that Professor Owen was most eminently qualified in all respects to undertake the duties connected with the unveiling of the statue. The proposition was carried unanimously with much applause.

It was proposed by Mr. Edwin Saunders, seconded by Dr. Robert Barnes, and unanimously resolved—"That the Executive Committee, consisting of Sir George Burrows, Mr. Prescott Hewett, Dr. Quain, Dr. Owen Rees, Mr. John Simon, Mr. E. H. Lushington, Mr. J. J. Lonsdale, the Mayor of Folkestone, Mr. W. Bateman, Mr. W. G. S. Harrison, and Mr. George Eastes, have full power to act in the future, on behalf of the subscribers, in all matters connected with the fund, and with the settlement of the accounts, and in the final closing of the fund."

Some formal business was transacted, and finally the meeting, on the motion of Dr. Sieveking and Mr. Prescott Hewett, resolved by acclamation—"That a cordial vote of thanks be, and is hereby, given to Mr. George Eastes for his energy and ability in all matters connected with the Harvey Tercentenary Memorial Fund, and the deep obligation of the subscribers is due to him for originating the fund, and perseveringly bringing it to a successful issue."

THE CLIMATE OF THE ORANGE RIVER FREE STATE.

WE have received from Dr. Symes Thompson the following graphic account of the experience of an invalid who went to Bloemfontein in search of health:—

"You will remember seeing me in the spring of 1880; that I belong to a consumptive family, and have for two years been subject to recurrent hæmorrhage. I have tried Hyères, Mentone, Algiers, and Madeira. The sirocco in the eastern bay of Mentone set up hæmorrhage. Algiers was more beneficial than the Riviera, especially in the early spring.

"Last summer I had a bronchial attack, with further mischief at the base of the unsound lung. I was shipped off to Madeira, and thence went on to South Africa, expecting to find a dry air, with freedom from rain, at Bloemfontein, the capital of the Free State. I was disappointed to find that between January 28 (when I began to keep a register) and March 31 (sixty-three days) there were thirty-one wet and thirty-two fine days. On the wet days torrents of rain generally fell day and night. On eleven or twelve of these rainy days there was a thick fog, and the difference between the wet and dry bulbs of the thermometer was only one or two degrees. The fine days were sometimes windy. One could sit out in comfort on about two-thirds of the fine days—i.e., on about twenty days during the three months; on these days the difference between the wet and dry bulbs was about ten degrees (from 82° to 72°).

"During this, the rainy season, reports were arriving from all sides of coaches stuck in the mud and at the sides of rivers for some days and nights. The coaches are leaky, and very bad in every way. A few days ago a Boer's house was cruelly shut in the faces of some passengers, who were obliged, supperless, to spend the night on the 'veldt.'

"Official records have only been kept at the Meteorological Office here from April, 1878. The rainfall during the wet season (between January and March) was twenty inches, whereas in this last exceptionally wet season it has been thirty-five inches.

"The rainfall at Bloemfontein greatly exceeds—is, in fact, nearly double—that of the plateau of Cradock and Beaufort West. Here the rainfall occurs about the winter season, and it is usually dry on the Karroo about Cradock when wet at Bloemfontein.

"Travelling during the rainy season is full of risk for invalids. Those who come out to avoid the English winter should delay at Cradock or near Beaufort until March; and for those who are weakly the hardships of the long journey to the capital of the Free State are too great—for such it is best to remain near Beaufort (2500 ft. ?)

"Bloemfontein has lately increased greatly in population; the cesspits and cattle kraals have increased. The dirt common to Dutch and Africander towns is terrible; there is no drainage, and the filth is often four or five feet thick in the cattle places. Piggeries are abundant, and the air is at times redolent with odours from the outskirts, where the town refuse is deposited. The town is situated in a hollow, is close, confined, and relaxing.

"There are many sent out as a last resource, who have gained health in the neighbouring country, but only just keep their health in the town.

"The town has changed much for the worse since the great increase of population.

"Soon after my arrival I lost appetite, and fell away much. After great difficulty I secured a place fit to live in at Hartbeesthoek, twelve miles off, and, notwithstanding the violence of the rain, I am now doing well. The wet season is now (April 8, 1881) over, and to-day at 2 p.m. we had 83° dry and 63° wet bulb, and the favourable conditions of climate are reasserting themselves.

"The proposed sanatorium cannot flourish unless established outside the town. Heaven knows a sanatorium is badly needed! The hotels are awfully dirty in sitting-room and bedroom, with bad cooking and worse food. All except one are unbearable.

"I hope to go 'trekking' for six months in September, getting down to the Karroo when the wet season commences here. No doubt I shall in the end confirm the general view of the climate. It is clear that one is liable here, as in other places, to very bad seasons.

"Those who get on best are young men who have had to work at home, and have not been spoilt by luxury: the annoyances of sleeping two or three in a room, and the rough food, are sooner acquiesced in, especially if the health improves; but for those who have lived in English comfort, the place is simply killing. The hardships and jolting of the post-carts make travelling quite unfit for ladies.

"I keep a pair of horses, and have had six coachmen in two months—thieves, drunkards, fools, fellows who did not know a horse's head from his tail; and so it is everywhere—worry, worry, with these dreadful niggers."

FROM ABROAD.

A FRATRICIDAL MEDICAL TRIAL.

THE May number of the *Canada Med. and Surg. Journal* contains an account of a medical action, which, whether we consider the provocation which gave rise to it, or the delay which so long frustrated justice being done, must surely be unprecedented.

The action of Levi v. Reed took place between two medical men. Plaintiff is a graduate of M'Gill University, of 1876, and alleged that soon after he commenced practice in the locality inhabited by the defendant, a practitioner of more than twenty-seven years' standing, he became the object of his enmity and slanderous misrepresentation. The immediate cause of the action arose from Dr. Levi having been called in to a case of obstinate vomiting in a woman then pregnant about six months. After trying the usual remedies without success, he asked for a consultation with Dr. Reed, the senior practitioner of the place. At this, having expressed his fears for the patient's safety, he proposed discussing the propriety of resorting to the induction of premature labour. To this Dr. Reed objected, and eventually the woman did well, and went on to her full time. It appears that, on the strength of this occurrence, the defendant mentioned to several persons that the plaintiff had suggested to him an operation which would have been death to both mother and child, and did not hesitate to apply to him the words "abortionist" and "murderer." To Roman Catholics he gave the information that the Church condemns the operation, and that anyone guilty of the same is damned.

Dr. Levi treated these slanders with contempt for some six months, in the hope that the defendant would cease employing his libellous language; but on his remonstrating with him at their continuance, the defendant declared that Levi had asked him to assist him in committing a crime. Dr. Levi therefore brought this action for $10,000 damages in October, 1877; and after the case had dragged on two years (during which there were eight *enquêtes*, and fifty-four witnesses were examined), the Supreme Court gave judgment for the plaintiff, the defendant being adjudged to pay $1000 damages and the costs. Reed then took the case into the Court of Review, but, failing to appear, it was dismissed; and he then brought it before the Court of Appeal at Quebec. There, two of the five judges agreed with the judgment of the first court, but the other three, while declaring the conduct of Reed wholly unjustifiable, reduced the damages to $500, and ordered Levi to pay the costs of the Court of Appeal, which amounted to $784—leaving him with a judgment in his favour and $300 out of pocket. The three judges also considered that the summoning of some eminent men at great expense by Levi, to prove that Reed's slanders were scientifically erroneous, was illegal. The case was now carried by Dr. Levi into the Supreme Court at Ottawa, which on February 11, 1881, unanimously reversed the judgment of the Court of Appeal, and restored to Levi the judgment of the first court, with all costs; also declaring that the medical expert evidence which he produced was legal and necessary.

Commenting upon this remarkable case, the editor of the Journal whence we have quoted it observes:—"It is, indeed, lamentable to think how utterly lost to all self-respect—how utterly wanting in the generous instincts of professional courtesy—how completely unmindful of the Hippocratic act of every medical graduate—must that man be, who, appealed to by a junior *confrère*, receives his confidential communications, goes through the farce of a so-called consultation, and then immediately proceeds so to distort and misrepresent what passed between them as to carry the most horrid ideas to the minds of the whole community. Such a use to be made of secrets learned from a confiding colleague at a professional consultation is calculated to excite the anger and contempt of every right-thinking medical man, and we congratulate Dr. Levi on having thoroughly vindicated his professional name and private character. And, more than this, he deserves the thanks of the profession of this country for the stand he has taken and the perseverance he has exhibited in carrying his case even up to the Supreme Court. For the result of this trial shows that the law of the land will punish the slanderous innuendoes of a jealous rival, if he cannot be prevented from indulging therein by a proper respect for medical ethics. The tardiness and the expense of legal proceedings have been fairly exemplified here. It took the plaintiff three years and three months, during which he had expended $1500, before the final judgment was obtained."

TREATMENT OF SPRAINS BY COLLODION.

In a paper read at the Suffolk District Medical Society, and published in No. 13 of the *Boston Med. Journal*, Dr. Blodgett draws attention to the value of "Collodion in the Treatment of Strains and Sprains." After describing the conditions attendant upon sprains, the tediousness in recovery from them, and the usual inefficacy of the treatment adopted in regard to them, he goes on to give an account of the means which he successfully adopted in treating a sprain of the ankle which occurred in his own person, and which he has since put into force in seven other cases. After, in his own case, trying the usual remedies with very little benefit, he was induced to employ collodion so prepared that it would contract on drying. For some minutes no appreciable result followed the application, but after several coatings had been put on, a contraction of the whole layer of collodion in all directions at once took place, to a much greater degree and in a much more efficient manner than could have been brought about by any bandage. So great was the contractile power of the collodion that it seemed as if it would divide the skin at the border of the film; and some of the hairs around the ankle which were accidentally included were so violently pulled upon that they were drawn out from the skin. The discomfort produced ceased in a short time, and gave way to a feeling of coolness around the ankle and relief from the pain. The skin was drawn into wrinkles in all possible directions, with a positive and marked diminution in the measurements of the ankle. After some hours, the collodion film cracked in many directions, becoming divided into small scales, which could be picked off. The skin was not in the least irritated. Another coating, consisting of several layers of collodion, was at once applied before putting the foot to the ground; and the same powerful contraction, with a similar diminution of the swelling, resulted. In three days the ankle was restored to its usual size, and there was a total absence of pain and tenderness, even on walking, except when the foot came in contact with an inequality of the ground. "In a week I found myself quite well, and have never had a relapse, which I consider the more remarkable as I am not particularly careful, and am upon my feet a great deal."

In all the cases in which he has tried this means Dr. Blodgett has met with the same satisfactory results, and has found it unattended with any inconveniences. Thus, although the contraction around the ankle is very powerful, it does not interfere with the circulation, no swelling or puffiness about the toes or any part beyond the ankle being produced. It would be scarcely possible to apply a bandage exerting a similar amount of compression upon the parts beneath without occasioning swelling of the parts beyond the bandage. A very desirable feature in the collodion also is the protection which it gives to any wounded surface which may happen to accompany the sprain. Its adaptability to cases requiring the cooling or evaporation ordinarily obtained by lotions is also of great advantage. Its refrigerant power is applied exactly where it is wanted, and reduces the temperature of the part without actually *touching* the skin, so that a *dry cold* is produced instead of a wet and chilling one. The skin does not become macerated and soggy, and the sensation is much more agreeable to the patient than that produced by the *contact* of a refrigerating application. Through the thin transparent film, spread evenly over the surface, the injured part can be inspected, and every shade of colour in the skin be clearly discerned. After some hours this film becomes cracked in the lines of its wrinkles, when it may be easily peeled off and another film immediately applied to the same spot, by which all the benefit of a renewed compression is at once obtained. Before applying the collodion the greasy or oily matters should be gently washed off the part by means of soap-and-water, drying rather by pressing the towel against the part than by rubbing. The collodion should then be at once applied, and each additional coat strengthens the layers already applied, and adds to the compressing power.

" The degree of contraction depends much upon the quality of the collodion employed. There is a *flexible* collodion which contains castor oil that does not contract at all, or only very slightly, and will not do the work. The so-called ' *contractile* ' collodion must be employed. It yields uniform and satisfactory results, and is quite durable. It is very volatile and should be kept stoppered, and when being used the finger should be tightly applied to the mouth of the bottle. It is also liable to explode, from the ether it contains, if brought too near a flame; but it is fully as safe as ether, and we all use this agent by day or by night without accidents. To obtain the contractile effect of collodion it is necessary to apply several coats successively one upon another. I think that I have never applied less than six layers, which is easily accomplished, as the collodion dries very quickly, and a second coat can be applied almost as soon as the first is finished. If, for any reason, it should become desirable to remove that which has been applied, this can readily be done by means of a small quantity of ether, which dissolves the collodion with great readiness."

REVIEWS.

The Diagnosis of Diseases of the Spinal Cord. An Address delivered to the Medical Society of Wolverhampton, October, 1879. By W. R. GOWERS, M.D., F.R.C.P., Assistant-Professor of Clinical Medicine in University College; Senior Assistant-Physician to University College Hospital; Physician to the National Hospital for the Paralysed and Epileptic. Second Edition. London : J. and A. Churchill. 1881. Pp. 86.

WE are very glad to see that a second edition of this admirable address has already been called for. It was first placed before the profession generally in our pages, at the end of 1879, and was soon after published in a separate form, with additions and illustrations. Now it has again been carefully revised by Dr. Gowers, and numerous additions been made in order to render it more complete as an outline of the subject dealt with. The address sets forth, concisely but very clearly, what is known at present about the symptoms and diagnosis of diseases of the spinal cord, a subject to which Dr. Gowers has, as is well known, paid much attention, and upon which he has earned the right to speak as an authority. At the outset he remarks that — " A tendency is sometimes observable among many members of the profession to underconvalue diagnosis." It matters little, they say, whether your diagnosis of a diseased condition is minutely exact, if you are able to cure it. This, Dr. Gowers observes, is true ; " but a very superficial study of practical medicine will show that much diagnosis, which is of no direct avail for treatment, is essential for the diagnosis which enables us to treat successfully." For some diseases of organs much can be done ; for others, but little ; and without accurate diagnosis, we cannot apply our skill where it will be effective. Further, he remarks, very truly, " in systematic treatises, types of disease are described. But the mutual relations of all parts of the nervous system are very complex, and its morbid states are equally complex. Typical cases are rare, and the untypical cases are often puzzling, and can only be understood by a clear conception of the general principles of diagnosis."

The first section of the work deals with "The Medical Anatomy of the Spinal Cord." The relations of the cord to the spinal column are described, and illustrated with great exactness by a new and most useful diagram, prepared by Dr. Gowers himself, which shows " the average relations of the spines to the bodies of the vertebræ, and of both to the origins of the spinal nerves." The general structure of the cord is next clearly described, and illustrated by diagrams ; and the secondary degenerations are spoken of. Section II. treats of the physiology of the cord in relation to the symptoms of its disease ; and here the superficial and the deep forms of reflex actions are considered, and the subject of " tendon-reflex " is most carefully and thoroughly gone into. The best modes of exciting these deep reflexes are separately described and illustrated, and the value and meaning of each set forth. Dr. Gowers objects, with great force, to the term " tendon-reflex," on the sufficient ground that the phenomena are dependent on a " muscle-reflex " irritability, which has nothing to do with the tendons. He argues that if they are to be described by a general term, it will be best to employ one which does not involve any special theory of their nature. " They may be termed," he says, " ' tendon-muscular phenomena,' but the intervention of tendons is not necessary for their production ; the one condition which all have in common is that passive tension is essential for their occurrence, and they may more accurately be termed *myotatic* contractions (*τείνως*, extended). The irritability on which they depend is due to, and demonstrative of, a muscle-reflex action which depends on the spinal cord." All the rest of the section, dealing with co-ordination of movement, controlling functions, nutrition of muscles, the use of electricity in diagnosis, etc., is clearly and simply written, and very interesting and instructive. Section III. treats of "Indications of Position of Disease: Anatomical Diagnosis"; and Section IV. of "Indications of Nature of Disease: Pathological Diagnosis"; and these parts are as valuable and clear as the parts of the work previously noticed. To aid the due comprehension of anatomical diagnosis, Dr. Gowers gives a diagram and table showing the approximate relation to the spinal nerves of the various motor, sensory, and reflex functions of the spinal cord. In Section IV. he divides the lesions into six classes, according to their onset, and gives a table showing the common relation of the lesions to the modes of onset :—

Sudden (few minutes)
Acute (few hours or days) } Vascular Lesions.

Pressure }
or } Subacute (one to six weeks) } Inflammation
Growths } Chronic (six weeks to six months) } (Myelitis).

Very chronic (six months and upwards) { Degeneration (Sclerosis).

When speaking of syphilis as a cause of disease of the cord, Dr. Gowers agrees with Fournier, Vulpian, Erb, and others in thinking that " the majority of cases (about 70 per cent.) of locomotor ataxy, primary posterior sclerosis, occur in individuals who have had syphilis many years before." He says, however, " it is not suggested that syphilis is the cause in this proportion ; in some the coincidence of the two diseases may be incidental. The facts seem to justify the assertion that half the patients would not suffer from ataxy had they not previously suffered from syphilis."

Dr. Gowers does not devote any portion of his address to the consideration of "anæmia" or of "hyperæmia" of the cord, but observes: " I cannot help thinking that a vigorous scientific imagination has contributed much more than observation has supplied " in current descriptions of these conditions.

In concluding this section, Dr. Gowers speaks briefly, but very pertinently, on the subject of the nomenclature of diseases of the cord. He observes : " If we wish to obtain clear ideas, it is essential to use terms, when we can, which shall be pathological, and which shall be at once simple and descriptive. To obtain these, we must avoid the error, too common, of striving after extreme brevity " ; we should endeavour to substitute the idea of morbid processes for that of definite diseases. We have only to combine the terms indicating the place and the lesion to have a system of terminology already partly in use, and which will altogether suffice for our present needs. " Thus we may have a columnal or a cornual myelitis, hæmorrhage, sclerosis, degeneration, or growth. We may have, for instance, an 'anterior cornual myelitis '; or, for shortness (since we cannot yet diagnose posterior cornual diseases), a 'cornual myelitis'; or we may have a 'cornual degeneration.'" Anterior cornual myelitis has been termed "tephromyelitis" by Charcot, and "anterior polio-myelitis" by Kussmaul. The last-named term is very widely employed, but the meaning of it is certainly much less obvious than that of the term proposed by Dr. Gowers, viz., "anterior cornual myelitis."

The fifth and last section of the book contains the histories of six instructive cases, as illustrations of the methods of diagnosis; and the work closes with a very well executed coloured plate representing some of the more important lesions of the spinal cord.

The whole of Dr. Gowers' little work is excellent. It bears in all parts the stamp of having been written by one who is not only a master of his subject, but also a master of clearness with conciseness of description. It cannot be read by any practitioner without pleasure and profit, and it may be especially recommended as a valuable guide and help to senior students, and practitioners away from the teaching centres and the societies.

REPORTS OF SOCIETIES.

THE OBSTETRICAL SOCIETY OF LONDON.
WEDNESDAY, JUNE 1.

Dr. MATTHEWS DUNCAN, President, in the Chair.

DR. GODSON presented a cast of the child's head, showing a depression after delivery by forceps, which he had shown at a previous meeting of the Society.

Dr. GALABIN showed microscopic sections from two cases, illustrating the histology of cancer of the internal surface of the body of the uterus. They showed a transition from cylinder epithelioma to carcinoma. The tissue was removed by curette. In the first case, in which the uterus was movable and but slightly enlarged, there was proliferation of glands with upgrowth of processes from their walls filling up the lumen. In the second case, in which the uterus was fixed and nodular, there was, in addition, infection of the stroma with epithelial masses. He had found cancer of the body of the uterus relatively not uncommon in virgins, but had hardly ever met with the ordinary cancer of the cervix where there was proof of virginity.

Dr. WILTSHIRE related a case in which, after thorough removal of the malignant growth, and the use of perchloride of iron, the patient, a lady sixty years of age, lived three years all but one month. When cancer of the body of the uterus was diagnosed, removal was desirable where practicable.

Dr. CLEVELAND hoped that the time would come when such an exact diagnosis of the disease in its early stage might be established as to warrant recourse to more radical measures than had been carried out by Dr. Wiltshire, namely, entire removal of the uterus.

Dr. HEYWOOD SMITH added his testimony to Dr. Galabin's as to the relative frequency of cancer of the body of the uterus in virgins, and cited a case of a lady aged fifty. He considered that when such cases could be diagnosed early enough, the uterus should be removed, leaving the cervix as a stump.

Mr. DORAN urged the importance of the fact mentioned by Dr. Galabin that cancer of the cervix was almost peculiar to impregnated women, since it was among such that the numerous forms of erosion were so frequently found. The cure of such a form of erosion as preceded cancer might absolutely avert malignant disease.

The PRESIDENT considered that total extirpation of the uterus was at present too dangerous an operation. He had known a case of cancer of the cervix in a virgin.

Dr. WILTSHIRE showed the uterus, foetus, and placenta from a case of utero-vaginal rupture. The placenta, which was praevia, was found in the vagina, and the head, which was low down, was delivered by the obstetric house-surgeon. The patient rapidly sank. The uterus was large and thick, containing many small fibroids.

Mr. ALBAN DORAN showed for Dr. Bantock a large thick-walled single cyst of the great omentum, removed by operation. The symptoms had resembled those of ovarian cyst. Once the cyst had ruptured and filled again, and several times it had been tapped. At the operation there was great difficulty in separating the cyst from its connexions.

A fold of mesentery separated the cyst from the pelvic organs, which were absolutely normal. The patient was doing well four days after operation.

Dr. GODSON showed "Marshall's Patent Sectional Feeding Bottle," which had a movable front, enabling the fingers to be introduced to clean the interior.

A CASE OF PLACENTA PRAEVIA COMPLICATED BY A LARGE MYOMA.

Dr. HICKINBOTHAM related this case. The patient was a delicate primipara, of small stature, at full term. She had previously aborted. She had been in labour six hours, and had lost much blood. The os was dilatable, large enough to admit two fingers. The placenta presented completely; no edge could be felt, and through its centre, which seemed to be the thinnest part, a rounded mass was felt, and supposed to be the foetal head. The author decided to break through the centre of the placenta with the view of turning. Having torn through it, he discovered that the round mass was a large tumour upon which the placenta was attached. The delivery of the placenta was therefore completed, after which the haemorrhage greatly abated. Version was performed, the after-coming head perforated, and extraction effected with the aid of the crotchet. A terrible attack of septicaemia followed, and for a fortnight the patient's life was almost despaired of. The tumour sloughed, and became protruded through the os. On the tenth day a softened and foetid portion was extracted, and the remainder painted with pure carbolic acid. In three months the uterus was freely movable and its cavity of normal length, but the patient had not again menstruated after eleven months. If the placenta had not been praevia, the author would have preferred Cæsarian section.

Dr. BARNES said that no general rule could be laid down for labour complicated by fibroid tumours. Sometimes necrosis occurred when the tumour did not obstruct delivery, and the cases might do well. Sometimes the tumour might be pushed out of the way, and delivery effected by craniotomy or turning, or enucleation might be available. In extreme cases Cæsarian section might be necessary; and in such cases it should be considered whether Porro's method of removing uterus and ovaries would not be best.

Dr. HICKINBOTHAM said that the size and wide base of the tumour precluded enucleation. He did not agree with Dr. Barnes as to the advisability of removing the uterus, considering that the results of the operation had been very unsatisfactory, and he thought it would be sufficient to remove the ovaries and Fallopian tubes in performing Cæsarian section.

CASE OF MYXOEDEMA.

Dr. C. W. MANSELL-MOULLIN read a paper on a case of myxoedema. The patient was aged thirty-eight; mother of four children; at the commencement of her last pregnancy she had been troubled with swelling about the eyes, which continued for a month or two. Shortly after delivery the swelling about the eyes reappeared, and from this period she dated her present symptoms, which were those characteristic of myxoedema, as recently described, the urine being free from albumen.

Dr. GERVIS had had three cases of myxoedema referred to him to examine the pelvic organs, but found nothing abnormal. Two had passed the climacteric, but one had not.

Dr. WILTSHIRE suggested that the patient should be shown. The affection was, he believed, degenerative, and often occurred about the approach of the climacteric.

The PRESIDENT had two examples of the disease now under his care; one was a married lady, under forty, who had borne children, but came to him on account of amenorrhoea. In the other patient, aged forty, the periods were regular and copious, but the disease was described as beginning with exophthalmos and amenorrhoea for a year.

ON THE (SO-CALLED) LITHOPAEDION.

Dr. BARNES read a note on the (so-called) lithopaedion, being a supplement to his paper on so-called "Missed Labour." The author had examined the specimen in the Hunterian Museum from Dr. Cheston's historical case, which was undoubtedly one of extra-uterine foetation, and it had been minutely examined by Mr. Doran. The abdominal viscera and thoracic organs were quite soft, but impregnated with lime-salts. The skin and subcutaneous tissue of the front of the thorax and abdomen were thick and infiltrated with lime-salts, so as to feel gritty and friable. The same structures in the posterior part of the body were very thin and converted into calcareous plates. Another specimen in the Hunterian Museum, without a history, but apparently a fœtus of not more than seven months' development, had also been examined by Mr. Doran. It showed a more advanced calcification of the shrunken soft parts. The surface was brittle and not remarkably hard. The lungs were powdery, and effervesced with hydrochloric acid. In a specimen in St. Thomas's museum, the cyst-wall was calcified, and there were calcareous plates in the skin. The viscera and muscles were soft.

The PRESIDENT said that the paper impressed him with the necessity for greater care than he and other authors had used in applying the word "lithopædion." The observations confirmed the remarks which he made on the reading of Dr. Barnes' paper, that there was never a stone-child really, but only petrifaction of the membranes and adjacent fœtal parts.

OBITUARY.

HOFRATH PROFESSOR JOSEPH SKODA.

WITH the death of this distinguished man, the last of the founders of the new Vienna medical school has disappeared; and if in some of his qualities and acquirements he was surpassed by Rokitansky, Schuh, Oppolzer, Hebra, and others, he excelled them all in that justness of judgment and acuteness of the logical faculty that enabled him to utilise at the bedside the acquisitions which his labours with Rokitansky in the dead-house had furnished him. Born of poor parents at Pilsen, in Bohemia, in 1805, he had to face a hard struggle while studying for his doctor's degree at Vienna, which he obtained in 1831. After having obtained an appointment as Cholera-Physician in Bohemia during the epidemic which prevailed there, when this had terminated he returned to Vienna; and in 1833 he succeeded in obtaining a subordinate post to the Vienna General Hospital. Here he attached himself to the small band who were then zealously cultivating pathological anatomy—Draut, Kolletschka, and Rokitansky,—and continued working with these industriously during two years; but having acquired a thorough knowledge of this subject, he felt the necessity of utilising his knowledge at the bedside, clearly perceiving that without such practical application morbid anatomy is a mere dead letter. This was no easy task, for it was evident that by the means hitherto pursued the end would never be attained. He it was who first employed the inductive method in medicine in Germany. He drew all his conclusions from what he had observed in the anatomical theatre or at the bedside; and he was enabled in the most complicated cases, by reason of his great penetrative power, and working with the then new mode of exclusion, to arrive at a diagnosis of remarkable precision. With his reforming tendencies, he met with the most vigorous opposition, so that while his friend Rokitansky was enabled to pursue his labours in quietude, Skoda was met with all kinds of obstacles, some of which were of so serious a character that his career would probably have been cut short had not a far-seeing member of the Ministry, Baron Türkheim, had the sagacity to appreciate his merits, and afford him the necessary protection. He especially devoted himself to the development of the work begun by Avenbrugger and Laennec, which, although well known, was little utilised at that time. After delivering private courses of lectures on the subject, which were attended by great numbers both from at home and abroad, he brought out in 1838 his solitary but "epoch-marking" book on Auscultation and Percussion. By the intervention of Baron Türkheim he obtained in the Vienna Hospital two wards devoted to diseases of the chest. Before this, numbers of young physicians continued to arrive at Vienna from all countries, and this was now more than ever the case, and the Vienna Hospital became the scene of the most active work carried on in all directions. Skoda and Rokitansky were now regarded throughout the civilised world as the founders of the Vienna school. Indeed, Skoda's work had then obtained much more renown and influence abroad than at home. After having received promotion at the Hospital, he was appointed in 1846 Professor of Clinical Medicine; but this post was only obtained after a hard struggle, for the upholders of the old school were still numerous and powerful. He held pos-

session of it until 1871, when his increased sufferings from gout obliged him to give it up. To this disease he had long been a victim in an aggravated degree, so that he on more than one occasion was brought to the brink of the grave. His equanimity under these sufferings was most remarkable, for, after terrible paroxysms and sleepless nights, he recovered all his strength and serenity of mind; and it was a marvel to his friends to listen to his dissertations on scientific and social topics, stated with all the conciseness, logical acumen, and appropriateness characteristic of the great thinker. During his last illness he suffered also from terrible paroxysms of dyspnœa, which were thought to be explained by the existence of an aneurism of the ascending aorta. This, however, proved erroneous, for at the autopsy no aneurism was found, although there were stenosis and insufficiency of the aortic valves and general hypertrophy of the heart.

Skoda was much beloved and venerated by the students, not only by reason of the excellence of his teaching, but because they regarded him as a paternal and influential guardian of their interests. Within the small circle of friends in which of late years he lived, his relations seem to have been of the most affectionate and almost enthusiastic character; and certainly the appreciation of his qualities by some of them since his death do not err on the side of lukewarmness. To those coming less intimately in contact with him he seemed somewhat cold and hard, owing to his reserved manner, but although a severe critic of his own life and acquisitions, he was mild in his judgment of others, and sympathetically responded to all that was noble and good.

In estimating the position of Skoda, it would seem that his friends exhibit some exaggeration in regarding him as the leading clinical teacher of Europe; or, at all events, that will remain a mere tradition, as he has not left works behind him justifying that position. It may be that he was not the mere "lung and heart" doctor which the public at large believed him to be and abundantly consulted him as such; but, although so acute and able a mind would doubtless feel equally at home in any case brought before him, yet he has left no evidence that such was the case. In the province of the diagnosis of diseases of the heart and chest he was unrivalled; and, indeed, Professor Bamberger would seem to believe that the labours of Laennec and the French school were of comparatively little import, and sometimes carried on in an erroneous direction, until taken in hand, recreated, and reformed by Skoda. Skoda has been charged with nihilistic therapeutical views, but while utterly discarding the farragos which so long have continued to overload German pharmacopœias, there were many remedies which he had ample faith in, and frequently employed to relieve his own severe suffering.

A CASE OF REMARKABLY LOW TEMPERATURE.—Dr. Mendelson, House-Physician of the New York Hospital (New York Medical Record, June 4) relates the case of a German aged forty-six, who was brought into hospital in a state of semi-starvation, not having had food for several days. He was very much emaciated, and his voice and the sounds of his heart were almost inaudible. The pulse was 45, and the temperature, taken in the rectum three or four times with two different thermometers, was only 90·6° Fahr. Heat was applied, and warm milk administered at intervals. In twelve hours his temperature had risen to 91·6° in the axilla. After the first day the temperature remained nearly normal, sinking to 97·5° early in the morning, but always reaching 98·8° or a little more in the afternoon. There was no febrile reaction, 99·6° being the highest temperature reached. The digestion was undisturbed, for on the third day the patient was eating heartily. His appetite became enormous, and he gained flesh rapidly. At the end of about two weeks a mild form of dementia was developed, but whether he had exhibited this prior to admission could not be ascertained. In the above abstract it is omitted to be stated that a drachm of a mixture of equal parts of brandy and ether was administered hypodermically at the commencement of treatment, and Dr. Mendelson thinks highly of the combination where promptness of action is desirable. The annoyance of the barrel of the syringe becoming filled with the vapour of ether, and the expansion of this forcing out the liquid portion prematurely, when ether is used alone, is entirely done away with.

NEW INVENTIONS AND IMPROVEMENTS.

DR. WARD COUSINS' PATENT BED-CLOTHES ELEVATOR, WITH FRACTURE SWING, EXTENSION APPARATUS, ETC.

WE have received the following account of certain important inventions made by Dr. Ward Cousins, of Portsmouth:—The whole contrivance is very simple and convenient. It can be used with great facility for a great number of medical and surgical purposes by making slight alterations in the component parts. Its special feature is the application of lever action over the bed, without weight or contact with the bed itself. By a mechanical contrivance of great simplicity the lever is sustained immovably in any position, and by this means all the ordinary surgical instruments, including the fracture swing, the bed cradle, the extension pulley, the bath, the splint elevator, and bed-rest, are reduced to the form of one efficient, durable, portable, and economical apparatus. Messrs. Arnold and Sons, of West Smithfield, are the sole manufacturers. The following is a short description of some of the principal applications:—

The bed-clothes elevator is suitable in every case in which part or all of the bed-clothes must be raised from the body of the patient. It can be instantly applied and adjusted to any part of the bed, and it will be found both in hospital and private practice far more convenient than the old-fashioned bed-frame. The elevator never comes in contact with the patient, and never rests on the bed. It can be fixed to any bedstead, and at the same time it can be applied

FIG. 1.

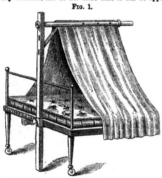

either at the ends or the sides of the bed. It can be adjusted inside or outside the bed-clothes, and it can be also regulated so as to raise them any convenient height from the patient. It will support all the bed-clothes at once, or it can be fixed to elevate only a part of them in any required position; and thus it becomes a complete substitute for any size of the ordinary bed-cradle. The elevator serves also many other useful purposes. It will suspend a weight or icebag in any position over the body, or it can be converted into a very convenient stand for a vessel, as in the application of an evaporating lotion. The annexed engraving shows the instrument in position. The upright can be fixed to any part of the lower edge of the sides or ends of the bedstead; a spike holds it to the floor, and a clamp secures it to the angle iron of the bedstead. The part of the bed-clothes to be elevated is then pushed with one of the short rods through the clamp or lever, and this is closed firmly with a metal ring. The degree of elevation can then be regulated, and the lever fixed in the upright by a bracket and screw.

PATENT BED-CLOTHES ELEVATOR AND EXTENSION APPARATUS.

Extension by weight is now universally employed in many forms of injury and joint-disease, and this kind of treatment is regarded by all surgeons as extremely simple and efficient. Up to the present time, however, extemporary, and often very imperfect, means have been employed for this important purpose; but with convenient apparatus the surgeon is provided with every requisite so that this method can be very readily and efficiently carried out, both in hospital and private practice. This new apparatus consists of a

FIG. 2.

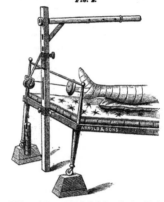

special form of the patent bed-clothes elevator fitted with a pulley, which is suspended by means of a sliding bracket from the back of the instrument, and is thus capable of adjustment at any convenient height. A sliding collar with a clamp working on a hinge is also supplied for the purpose of fixing securely the upright to the bedstead in those cases in which counter-extension is obtained by raising the foot of the bed. The whole contrivance is extremely easy of application, and can be applied to any bedstead, fulfilling at once the double purpose of elevating the bed-clothes from the body of the patient, and supplying a ready and convenient method of extension in any case in which such treatment is essential. The apparatus is fitted with two counter-extension blocks, each giving three elevations, movable weights, and in fact everything necessary for the immediate use of surgeons practising in the country, or of medical officers going abroad.

NEW FRACTURE SWING.

This is another novel and efficient application of this very convertible apparatus, adapted for the treatment of simple

FIG. 3.

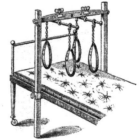

and compound fractures, and other diseases of the joints and bones. It consists of a very simple form of swing in combination with the patent bed-clothes elevator, and will be found a very valuable contrivance for hospital and private practice. The swing is supported by two uprights which are secured firmly to the sides of the bedstead, and a cross-bar carrying a beam in which the slings are attached by sliding hooks. It can be used with any kind of ordinary splint, and it supports the limb at any required height; at the same time it can be made to swing both legs without any addition to the apparatus. It is a far more handy instrument than the ordinary fracture cradle; it does not rest on the bed, and does not interfere with the comfort of patient. Moreover, it occupies no space in the bed, permits a free circulation of air under the bed-clothes, and does not required to be removed in dressing the limb.

The apparatus is convertible by a very simple arrangement with wooden rods into an elevator of the bed-clothes, which

Fig. 4.

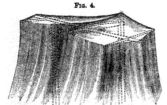

will be found of great service in the application of hot air and vapour baths, and also in the treatment of injuries and diseases of the chest, abdomen, and pelvis. The cross-bar can also be placed on the bed for a rest in cases of lung and heart disease, in which the patient is unable to lie down. It will be found a simple and efficient support during the attacks of dyspnœa, and a wooden stand can be adjusted to it to hold an inhaler or other vessel.

THE SPLINT ELEVATOR AND REST.

The elevator can be used as a splint rest, and it will be found invaluable in those cases in which the limb requires

Fig. 5.

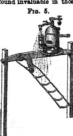

elevation. Special arm wire splints, fitted with shifting bars, and movable hand and foot pieces, are supplied with the apparatus, and by means of a sliding metal rest they can be adjusted on the cross-bar at any convenient height. This application of the apparatus will be found very convenient in practice, and is especially adapted for the treatment of injuries and fractures, wounds of the hands and feet, amputation cases, and many other affections in which absolute rest and elevation of the limb are essential. It occupies no space in the bed, permits free circulation of air, cannot get out of position, and during the dressing of a stump or wound the steam spray can be conveniently placed on the stand.

PREVENTION OF PITTING IN SMALL-POX.—Dr. Karrik, discussing this subject at the St. Petersburg Medical Society, stated that the application recommended by Dr. Smart, of Edinburgh, in 1863, has proved in his hands far more efficacious than any other. A four-ounce phial is half-filled with chloroform, and small pieces of the finest caoutchouc are added until the bottle is three parts full. The bottle is then shaken until complete solution is effected. With this solution the eruption is painted by means of a fine pencil from three to five times a day, forming a thin layer of a blackish colour, which excludes air and light and exercises a gentle elastic pressure.—St. Petersb. Med. Woch., June 13.

MEDICAL NEWS.

UNIVERSITY OF DURHAM. — EASTER TERM. — At a Convocation of the University, held in Bishop Cosin's Library on June 28, the following medical and surgical degrees were conferred :—

Doctor of Medicine (for practitioners of fifteen years' standing)—
    Deane, Andrew.
    Leach, John Comyns, B.Sc. Lond.
    Orton, Charles.
    Reed, Thomas Sleeman.

Doctor of Medicine—
    Bowman, Hugh Torrington, M.S., M.B. Durh.
    Morton, Shadforth, M.B. Durh.
    Powell, Soudamore Rydley, M.B. Durh.
    Tyson, William Joseph, M.B. Durh., F.R.C.S. Eng.
    Woodman, William Edwin, M.B. Durh.

Bachelor of Medicine—
    Austen, Henry Hinds, M.R.C.S.
    Baker, John Hopper.
    Burton, Francis Henry Merceron, M.R.C.S.
    Clowes, Herbert Alfred, M.R.C.S.
    Cripps, Charles Couper, M.R.C.S.
    East, Frederick William.
    Kempster, William Henry.
    Kennedy, William Adam, M.R.C.S.
    Prowde, Edwin Longstaff, M.A. Cantab.
    Robinson, William.
    Smith, William Harvey, M.R.C.S.
    Thomson, George J. Crawford.
    Walker, Basil Woodd, M.R.C.S.

Master in Surgery (M.S.)—
    Burton, Francis Henry Merceron, M.R.C.S.
    Clowes, Herbert Alfred, M.R.C.S.
    Cripps, Charles Couper, M.R.C.S.
    Robinson, William.

Examiners for the above degrees :—G. Y. Heath, M.D., C. J. Gibb, M.D., J. C. Nesham, M.D., Professor G. H. Philipson, M.D., F.R.C.P., H. E. Armstrong, F. Page, M.D., J. Barron, M.B., O. Sturges, M.D., F.R.C.P., H. G. Howse, M.S. Lond., F.R.C.S. For the M.S. degree :—Dr. Heath, Mr. Howse, M.S.

At 3 p.m., the first annual meeting of the Medical Graduates' Association was held in the Divinity Lecture-room of the University, Professor Philipson in the chair. At 6 p.m., the members of the Association dined together in the Great Hall of University College, the Reverend the Master of University College in the chair.

UNIVERSITY OF DUBLIN.—At the Second Summer Commencements held in the Examination Hall of Trinity College, on Thursday, June 30, the following degrees and licences in Medicine, Surgery, and Midwifery were conferred by the University Caput—viz., the Right Hon. Earl Cairns, Chancellor of the University; the Rev. John H. Jellett, D.D., Provost of Trinity College; and the Rev. James W. Barlow, M.A., Senior Master non-regent :—

Baccalaurei in Chirurgiâ.—Edvardus Cochrane, Thomas Donnelly, Gulielmus Solomon Elliott, Donald Grant, Carolus Gloster, Thomas W. O'Hora Hamilton, Edvardus Gordon Hull, Jacobus Murray Irwin, Franciscus Johannes Jencken, Gulielmus Ffennell MacCarthy, Johannes Macquillan, Alfredus Miller, Thomas Myles, and Jacobus Johnston Robinson.

Baccalaurei in Medicinâ.—Thomas Arthur Baldwin, Edvardus Cochrane, Thomas Donnelly, Thomas Jacobus Dowse, Gulielmus Solomon Elliott, Carolus Gloster, Donald Grant, Thomas W. O'Hora Hamilton, Dawson Henry, Edvardus Gordon Hull, Achmuty Irwin, Jacobus Murray Irwin, Franciscus Johannes Jencken, Thomas White Lewis, Gulielmus C. Lucas, Gulielmus Ffennell MacCarthy, Alfred Miller, Johannes W. Macquillan, Reginald Lawson Moseley, Thomas Myles, Augustus Nickson, Henricus R. Pope, J. Allsann Powell, Thomas Stanton, Jonas C. Stawell, and Augustus W. Woodroffe.

Magistri in Arte Obstetriciâ.—Thomas Dennelly and Jacobus Murray Irwin.

Doctores in Medicinâ. —Achmuty Irwin (honoris causâ), Gulielmus Hume Hart, Johannes Carolus Hogan, Johannes Franciscus Houghton, and Alfredus Hubertus Kelly.

Licentiati in Medicinâ.—Reginald Moore, Edvardus Cuthbert Nangle, and Ludovicus Tarleton Young.

Licentiati in Chirurgiâ.—Reginald Moore, Edvardus Cuthbert Nangle, and Ludovicus Tarleton Young.

ROYAL COLLEGE OF SURGEONS OF ENGLAND.—The following gentlemen passed their primary examinations in Anatomy and Physiology at a meeting of the Board of Examiners on the 4th inst., and, when eligible, will be admitted to the pass examination, viz. :—

Anderson, Fitzgerald U., student of the Edinburgh School.
Brooke, H. St. John, of the Dublin School.
Dawson, Rankine, of McGill College.
Dupuis, Thomas R., of Kingston, Canada.
Graham, George R. M., of the Dublin School.
Jameson, Granville, of the Edinburgh School.
Karanjia, Merwanji D., of the Bombay School.
Lyon, Thomas G., of St. Thomas's Hospital.
Sutcliffe, Victor E., of the Leeds School.
Weir, Richard R., of the Aberdeen School.
Whyte, Herbert, of Guy's Hospital.

Seventeen candidates were rejected. The following gentlemen passed on the 5th inst., viz.:—

Annacher, Ernest, student of the Manchester School.
Buxton, William M., of the Newcastle School.
Carmichael, William, of the Manchester School.
Clarke, J. McFarlane, of the Manchester School.
Dutton, William H., of the Edinburgh School.
Fisher, Alfred, of the Liverpool School.
Garman, Edwin C., of the Birmingham School.
Hanson, Alfred, of University College Hospital.
Hare, Arthur W., of the Edinburgh School.
Matthews, H. E. Hamerton, of the Manchester School.
Mercer, Frederic, of the Liverpool School.
Palmer, Septimus, of the Manchester School.
Perry, Allan, of the London Hospital.
Quennell, Robert W., of St. Bartholomew's Hospital.
Smith, Albert, of St. Thomas's Hospital.
Tilley, William J., of University College Hospital.
Walton, George A. T., of St. Bartholomew's Hospital.

Twelve candidates were rejected. The following gentlemen
passed on the 6th inst., viz.:—

Beattie, Robt., student of the Belfast and Galway Schools.
Dearden, William F., of the Manchester School.
Hartley, Horace, of St. Thomas's Hospital.
Hillstead, Herbert J., of Guy's Hospital.
Howitt, George H., of the Newcastle School.
Huret, Walter, of the Manchester School.
Jenkins, John, of the Bristol School.
Parsons, John J., of the Newcastle School.
Rainbird, Alfred F., of Guy's Hospital.
Smailes, Robert, of the Leeds School.
Stericker, George F., of the Leeds School.
Whittendale, James J. G., of the Birmingham School.
Wilde, Robert P., of the Liverpool School.

Twelve candidates were rejected.

Primary Examinations.—The following were the questions
on Anatomy and on Physiology submitted to the 202 candidates now undergoing their primary examination for the
diploma of Member of the Royal College of Surgeons, viz.:—
Anatomy (four, and not more than that number, of the
questions were required to be answered between one and
three o'clock): 1. Describe the ilium. 2. Describe the
articulations of the dorsal vertebræ one with another, and
also their articulations with the ribs. 3. Describe the course
and relations of the ulnar artery, and its branches. 4. Describe the right auricle of the heart. 5. Give the dissection
by which you would expose the whole of the anterior surface
of the adductor magnus muscle. 6. Describe the lumbar
plexus of nerves, and its branches, so far as they lie within
the abdomen. The following were the questions on Physiology (four out of the six were required to be answered from
four till six o'clock), viz.:—1. Describe the distribution of
the bloodvessels in the kidney. Under what physiological
conditions does the blood-pressure in the renal arteries vary?
What effect have such variations on the secretion of urine?
2. How is the act of mastication performed? What nerves
and nerve-centres are engaged in its performance? 3. Give
an account of the innervation of the heart. 4. What is the
composition of the blood? How are the corpuscles renewed?
5. Describe the structure and uses of the pleura. How are
the visceral and parietal layers kept in apposition? 6. Explain what is meant by sound-vibrations, and describe the
manner in which they are transmitted to the auditory nerve.

APOTHECARIES' HALL, LONDON.—The following gentlemen passed their examination in the Science and Practice of
Medicine, and received certificates to practise, on June 23
and 30:—

Clark, William, Wotton, Gloucester.
Inger, John William, Nottingham.
Kilham, Charles Speight, Millhouse, near Sheffield.
Pike, Charles James, Hobart, Tasmania.

At the recent examination for the Prizes in Botany given
annually by the Society to medical students, the Gold Medal
has been awarded to James Kecheid Forrest, of St. Bartholomew's Hospital, and the Silver Medal to William Ayton
Gostling, of University College, London.

NAVAL, MILITARY, ETC., APPOINTMENTS.

BENGAL MEDICAL ESTABLISHMENT.—To be Surgeons-Major:—Surgeons
Christopher William Calthrop, Richard Careless Bandars, Edwin Sanders,

Benjamin Franklin, Frederick Pooly Edis, Robert Temple Wright, M.D.,
George McBride ,Davis, M.D., Kali Pada Gupta, and Henry James
Linton.

BOMBAY MEDICAL ESTABLISHMENT.—To be Surgeons-Major:—Surgeons
John Alexander Howell, Charles Thomas Peters, Edwar Colson, and
Colin William MacRury.

MADRAS MEDICAL ESTABLISHMENT.—To be Surgeons-Major:—Surgeons
William Price, M.D., Samuel Matthias Tyrrell, William Hope Boalth,
and Joseph Backhouse.

BIRTHS.

BATTERSBURY.—On June 28, at Wimborne Minster, the wife of George
Henry Battersbury, M.B., of a son.

CABLE.—On July 1, at Royal Hill, Greenwich, the wife of G. H. Cable,
M.R.C.S.E., of a son.

CASEMENT.—On July 4, at Magherintemple, Ballycastle, co. Antrim, the
wife of Brabazon N. Casement, M.B., of Ballymena, of a daughter.

HARTLEY.—On June 28, at Great Dunmow, Essex, the wife of Charles
Hartley, M.R.C.S., of a son.

MAYBURY.—On June 18, at 362, Mile-end-terrace, Portsmouth, the wife of
Aurelius Victor Maybury, M.D., of a son.

PAGE.—On June 30, at Netherfield, Kendal, the wife of David Page, M.D.,
of a daughter.

RENNER.—On June 29, at 80, Portsdown-road, the wife of Charles Renner,
M.D., of a son.

WALLACE.—On June 19, at Cardiff, the wife of Thomas Wallace, M.D., of
a daughter.

MARRIAGES.

CHALMERS—MARTIN.—On June 25, at St. Mary's, Paddington, the Rev.
R. S. Chalmers, eldest son of the late Matthew Chalmers, M.D., of
Kingston-upon-Hull, to Adela Gertrude, elder daughter of the late
Robert Edward Martin, of Holbrook, Suffolk.

COLT—NICHOLSON.—On June 27, at Southsea, Thomas Archer Colt,
L.R.C.P., M.R.C.S., to Mabel Aileen, second daughter of the Rev.
Horatio Langrishe Nicholson, D.J., Vicar of St. Paul's, Southsea.

CRUICKSHANK—McIVER.—On July 1, at 5, Ravelston-terrace, Edinburgh,
Brodie Cruickshank, M.D., of Nairn, son of the Rev. J. A. Cruickshank,
of Mortlach, to Johanna, fifth daughter of the late Norman McIver,
banker, of Stornoway.

HAY—TUCKER.—On June 28, at the parish church, Bridport, William
Henry Hay, M.D., of Bridport, to Grace Elizabeth, youngest daughter of
W. D. Tucker, of Askerswell.

LOCKE—GARLAND.—On June 29, at St. John's Church, Yeovil, the Rev.
Cecil F. H. Locke, Rector of Lufton and Curate of St. John's, Yeovil,
to Ethel Mary, only daughter of E. C. Garland, L.R.C.P., of Yeovil.

MARSHALL-ALLEN—McCOMBIE.—On June 30, at St. Mary's, Paddington,
Robert Marshall-Allen, Esq., F.R.C.S.E., of Welbourn Hall, Grantham,
Deputy Inspector-General of Hospitals (Army Medical Department),
to Mary, elder daughter of the late Hon. Thomas McCombie, M.S.A.
and M.E.C., of Melbourne, Australia.

ROSS—SCRATCHLEY.—On June 27, at St. Andrew's, Well-street, Henry
Cooper, eldest son of Henry Cooper Ross, M.D., of Hampstead, to
Constance Evelyn, daughter of Arthur Scratchley, Esq., of the Inner
Temple, barrister-at-law.

WATHEN—EDWARDS.—On June 30, at Stoke Bishop Church, near Bristol,
by the Rev. D. Claxton, John Hanocoks Wathen, L.R.C.P.E., of Coburg
Villa, Clifton, eldest son of William Dean Wathen, Esq., M.R.C.S., of
Fishguard, Pembrokeshire, to Edith Mary, eldest daughter of Alderman
George William Edwards, of Sea Walls, Stoke Bishop, near Bristol.

DEATHS.

ALFORD, STEPHEN S., F.R.C.S., from injuries received in a railway accident near Willesden, a few days ago.

BIDDLE, HENRY COOPER, M.R.C.S., at Addison House, 'Edmonton, on
July 2, aged 46.

BRITTAN, ELIZA, wife of Frederick Brittan, M.D., at 16, Victoria-square,
Clifton, Bristol, on June 25.

SKAPE, JOSEPH, M.R.C.S. Eng., L.R.C.P. Edin., at Southport, on June 27,
aged 41.

TWEDDELL, AUGUSTA, younger daughter of the late H. M. Tweddell,
Esq., Deputy Inspector-General of Hospitals, Bengal Army, on July 1.

WHITSED, JOHN, M.B., at Twickenham, Middlesex, after a week's illness,
on June 25, aged 26.

WILSON, SURGEON, M.D., of the Army Medical Department, at Prahsu,
from fever.

VACANCIES.

In the following list the nature of the office vacant, the qualifications required in the candidate, the person to whom application should be made
and the day of election (as far as known) are stated in succession.

EAST LONDON HOSPITAL FOR CHILDREN AND DISPENSARY FOR WOMEN,
SHADWELL, E.—Resident Medical Officer. (*For particulars see Advertisement.*)

HOSPITAL FOR WOMEN, SOHO-SQUARE, W.—House-Physician. (*For particulars see Advertisement.*)

NEWTON ABBOT UNION.—Medical Officer and Public Vaccinator. Applications to be sent to the Clerk's office, Newton Abbot, on or before Monday,
July 11. Election will take place on July 18.

NORTH STAFFORDSHIRE INFIRMARY.—Two Resident Medical Officers. (*For
particulars see Advertisement.*)

ST. BARTHOLOMEW'S HOSPITAL.—Two Casualty Physicians. Applications,
with testimonials, must be left at the Clerk's office on or before July 8,
where particulars of the duties and all necessary information may be
obtained on personal application. Candidates must attend the meeting
of the Committee which takes place at 11 a.m. on July 14.

SOMERSET AND BATH LUNATIC ASYLUM, WELLS.—Medical Superintendent Candidates to send testimonials to the visitors (under cover), addressed to Mr. B. T. Duke, their clerk, at the said Asylum, not later than July 20, endorsed, "Superintendent Candidate." Candidates must not exceed the age of thirty-five, and are required to be graduates of medicine of any university in the United Kingdom—L.R.C.P. Lond., M.R.C.S. Lond., Edin., or Dub. Testimonials must state past medical career, and their experience in the treatment of insanity.

STOCKTON-UPON-TEES HOSPITAL AND DISPENSARY.—House-Surgeon (non-resident). Candidates must be doubly qualified. Applications, stating age, with recent testimonials, to be sent to the Secretary, John Settle, not later than August 9.

UNION AND PAROCHIAL MEDICAL SERVICE.

⁂ The area of each district is stated in acres. The population is computed according to the census of 1871.

RESIGNATIONS.

Chertsey Union.—Mr. Charles Mott has resigned the Walton District: area 6859; population 5381; salary £75 per annum.

Dover Union.—Dr. W. J. Simpson has resigned the St. Mary's District: salary £70 per annum.

Pembroke Union.—The First District is vacant: area 24,293; population 5908; salary £80 per annum.

Tynemouth Union.—The North Shields District is vacant by the death of Mr. Thomas Stephens: area 5641; population 21,314; salary £80 per annum.

West Derby Union.—Mr. J. W. H. Watling has resigned the Childwall and Wavertree Districts. Childwall District: area 890; population 177; salary £3 3s. per annum. Wavertree District: area 1390; population 7880; salary £35 per annum.

APPOINTMENTS.

Cardiff Union.—John Llewellyn Treharne, M.R.C.S. Eng., L.S.A., to the Splottlands District. Daniel Thomas Edwards, M.R.C.S. Eng., L.S.A., to the Pentyrch District. Richard Frederick Nell, M.R.C.S., L.S.A., to the Penarth District.

Kensington Parish.—Alfred Godrich, M.R.C.S. Eng., L.R.C.P Lond., L.S.A., to the South District.

St. Marylebone Parish.—John R. Lunn, L.R.C.P. Lond., M.R.C.S. Eng., L.S.A., to the New Infirmary.

Toxteth Park Township.—Alfred Meeson, L.R.C.S. Edin., L.S.A. Lond., as Assistant Medical Officer at the Workhouse.

Wantage Union.—Ashwin C. Newman, M.R.C.S. Eng., L.S.A., to the Harwell District.

THE RULING PASSION STRONG IN DEATH.—The bright, mirthful soul of Senator Carpenter was not overawed even in the shadow of death. The evening before he died he suffered excruciating pain, and in his agony asked for an explanation of its cause. "The pain is caused, Senator," replied a physician, "by a stoppage of the colon." "Stoppage of the colon, eh?"—and again the sense of humour overcame pain itself—"Well, then, of course, *it isn't a full stop!*"—*N. Y. Med. Record.*

APPOINTMENTS FOR THE WEEK.

July 9. Saturday (this day).

Operations at St. Bartholomew's, 1½ p.m.; King's College, 1½ p.m.; Royal Free, 2 p.m.; Royal London Ophthalmic, 11 a.m.; Royal Westminster Ophthalmic, 1½ p.m.; St. Thomas's, 1½ p.m.; London, 2 p.m.

11. *Monday.*

Operations at the Metropolitan Free, 2 p.m.; St. Mark's Hospital for Diseases of the Rectum, 2 p.m.; Royal London Ophthalmic, 11 a.m.; Royal Westminster Ophthalmic, 1½ p.m.

12. *Tuesday.*

Operations at Guy's, 1½ p.m.; Westminster, 2 p.m.; Royal London Ophthalmic, 11 a.m.; Royal Westminster Ophthalmic, 1½ p.m.; West London, 3 p.m.

13. *Wednesday.*

Operations at University College, 2 p.m.; St. Mary's, 1¼ p.m.; Middlesex, 1 p.m.; London, 2 p.m.; St. Bartholomew's, 1½ p.m.; Great Northern, 2 p.m.; Samaritan, 2½ p.m.; King's College (by Mr. Lister), 2 p.m.; Royal London Ophthalmic, 11 a.m.; Royal Westminster Ophthalmic, 1½ p.m.; St. Thomas's, 1½ p.m.; St. Peter's Hospital for Stone, 2 p.m.; National Orthopædic, Great Portland-street, 10 a.m.

14. *Thursday.*

Operations at St. George's, 1 p.m.; Central London Ophthalmic, 1 p.m.; Royal Orthopædic, 2 p.m.; University College, 2 p.m.; Royal London Ophthalmic, 11 a.m.; Royal Westminster Ophthalmic, 1½ p.m.; Hospital for Diseases of the Throat, 2 p.m.; Hospital for Women, 2 p.m.; Charing-cross, 2 p.m.; London, 2 p.m.; North-West London, 2½ p.m.

SANITARY INSTITUTE OF GREAT BRITAIN (9, Conduit-street), 8 p.m. Prof. F. S. B. F. De Chaumont, "On Modern Sanitary Science." The medals and certificates awarded to the successful exhibitors at the Exhibition at Exeter, in 1880, will be presented.

15. *Friday.*

Operations at Central London Ophthalmic, 2 p.m.; Royal London Ophthalmic, 11 a.m.; South London Ophthalmic, 2 p.m.; Royal Westminster Ophthalmic, 1½ p.m.; St. George's (ophthalmic operations), 1¼ p.m.; Guy's, 1½ p.m.; St. Thomas's (ophthalmic operations), 2 p.m.

VITAL STATISTICS OF LONDON.

Week ending Saturday, July 2, 1881.

BIRTHS.

Births of Boys, 1254; Girls, 1232; Total, 2486.
Corrected weekly average in the 10 years 1871-80, 2467·8.

DEATHS.

	Males.	Females.	Total.
Deaths during the week	767	678	1440
Weekly average of the ten years 1871-80, corrected to increased population ...	730·5	667·9	1398·4
Deaths of people aged 80 and upwards ...	...	...	45

DEATHS IN SUB-DISTRICTS FROM EPIDEMICS.

	Enumerated Population, 1881 (unrevised).	Small-pox.	Measles.	Scarlet Fever.	Diphtheria.	Whooping-cough.	Typhus.	Enteric (or Typhoid) Fever.	Simple continued Fever.	Diarrhœa.
West	668993	7	10	1	1	5	...	...	...	14
North ...	905677	18	19	11	4	11	1	4	...	16
Central ...	281793	...	11	4	2	5	...	...	...	8
East	692530	5	15	4	3	9	...	1	1	20
South	1265578	22	9	15	8	13	1	3	1	14
Total	3814571	52	64	35	18	43	2	8	2	72

METEOROLOGY.

From Observations at the Greenwich Observatory.

Mean height of barometer	29·941 in.
Mean temperature	61·9°
Highest point of thermometer	82·6°
Lowest point of thermometer	47·2°
Mean dew-point temperature	51·1°
General direction of wind	S.W. & N.W.
Whole amount of rain in the week	0·01 in.

BIRTHS and DEATHS Registered and METEOROLOGY during the Week ending Saturday, July 2, in the following large Towns:—

Cities and boroughs (Municipal boundaries except for London.)	Estimated Population to middle of the year 1881.*	Persons to an Acre. (1881.)	Births Registered during the week ending July 2.	Deaths Registered during the week ending July 2.	Temperature of Air (Fahr.): Highest during the Week.	Temperature of Air (Fahr.): Lowest during the Week.	Temperature of Air (Fahr.): Weekly Mean of Daily Mean Values	Temp. of Air (Cent.): Weekly Mean of Daily Mean Values.	Rain Fall: In Inches.	Rain Fall: In Centimetres.
London	3829751	50·8	2486	1440	82·6	47·2	61·9	16·61	0·01	0·03
Brighton	107934	45·9	57	39	76·8	49·9	59·4	15·22	0·09	0·23
Portsmouth ...	128335	28·6	76	49	...	...	...	...	...	...
Norwich	88038	11·8	57	31	80·0	50·0	60·4	15·78	0·26	0·66
Plymouth	75262	54·0	53	19	68·2	46·8	57·2	14·00	0·34	0·86
Bristol	207140	46·5	142	75	70·0	46·0	56·2	13·44	0·15	0·38
Wolverhampton ...	75934	22·4	56	27	69·6	42·4	54·6	12·56	0·25	0·63
Birmingham ...	402296	47·9	268	132	72·2	45·0	58·2	14·55	0·14	0·36
Leicester	123120	38·5	101	52	71·5	46·0	57·5	14·17	0·08	0·20
Nottingham ...	188035	18·9	132	59	76·7	44·4	58·7	14·83	0·37	0·94
Liverpool	553988	106·3	388	267	65·3	50·9	55·8	13·23	0·00	0·00
Manchester ...	341269	79·5	247	122	...	...	...	...	...	...
Salford	177760	34·4	132	47	...	...	...	...	...	...
Oldham	112176	24·0	77	52	...	...	...	...	...	...
Bradford	184037	25·5	112	80	64·3	48·6	55·6	13·12	0·08	0·20
Leeds	310490	14·4	213	126	66·0	48·0	56·1	13·39	0·20	0·51
Sheffield	285621	14·5	220	90	72·0	47·0	56·2	13·44	0·11	0·28
Hull	155161	42·7	150	44	...	...	...	...	...	...
Sunderland ...	116753	42·2	72	41	77·0	48·0	58·1	14·50	0·25	0·63
Newcastle-on-Tyne	145675	27·1	87	57	...	...	...	...	...	...
Total of 20 large English Towns ...	7608775	38·0	5126	2849	82·6	42·4	57·8	14·23	0·17	0·43

* These figures are the numbers enumerated (but subject to revision) in April last, raised to the middle of 1881 by the addition of a quarter of a year's increase, calculated at the rate that prevailed between 1871 and 1881.

At the Royal Observatory, Greenwich, the mean reading of the barometer last week was 29·94 in. The lowest reading was 29·74 in. on Monday afternoon, and the highest 30·14 in. on Thursday morning.

NOTES, QUERIES, AND REPLIES.

Is that questioneth much shall learn much.—Bacon.

Health of Cowes.—Dr. W. Hoffmeister, the Medical Officer of Health, in his recent report states that he never knew West Cowes healthier than at the present time, and he is not aware of the existence of any case of infectious or contagious diseases. During the first five months of the year, out of the forty-one deaths, there had not been a single one from enteric or other fever, small-pox, scarlatina, measles, whooping-cough, or diphtheria.

Alms.—The system of supplying such diets as are medically ordered by the hospital surgeons to discharged convalescent patients at their own homes was set on foot fourteen years since by the English branch of the Order of St. John of Jerusalem. The work has been limited to the Charing-cross and King's College Hospitals; the only funds at the disposal of the Order having been supplied exclusively by its own members.

Diseased Cattle from America.—We learn from Philadelphia that the Treasury Department has now control of a fund for the inspection of cattle shipped to Europe. Special inspectors are to be immediately appointed for each port; bills of health being given of the cattle cargoes on the inspector's recommendation.

Sea-Water Supply to London.—We understand that already boards of works and local authorities are making arrangements to secure the advantages the Sea-Water Company will be enabled to offer them—the Company having obtained the Act of Parliament. Clauses were, at the special request of some of these bodies, inserted in the Bill to enable them to use the water for sanitary and other purposes.

Impure State of the Regent's Canal.—The Bethnal-green Guardians have directed their Clerk to draw the attention of the directors of the Regent's Canal Company to the foul and unwholesome condition of the water, and to the fact that numerous houses along its banks use it as a common sewer. Some time ago the foul state of the Canal was the subject of public complaint. But the secretary of the Company then represented that the canal had lately been "satisfactorily" cleansed—a statement which was disputed, and the recurrence of the noxious impurities was early anticipated.

Fruit in Tins.—In reference to the increasing consumption of American tinned apples, a correspondent of the *Daily Telegraph* writes that there is great danger in eating fruit so packed, the acid of the fruit acting upon the tin and solder, and leaving a deposit of acetate of lead which mixes with the fruit. A case has come under his notice of a whole family exhibiting grave symptoms of poisoning through eating these apples.

Medical Charlatans.—Sir Henry Holland, in his "Recollections," gives the following useful hint how to deal with charlatans:—"I have witnessed in my professional career many charlatanries coming rapidly in succession to one another, and each drawing largely on public credulity. Argument is seldom of much avail with those thus imposed upon, and the time and temper of the physician are both grievously wasted if submitted to controversies utterly useless, where ignorant asseveration takes the place of that evidence which alone can establish a medical truth. In such cases I have myself generally found the refusal of discussion a more effectual answer than any train of reasoning. One of the sharpest weapons in argument is silence."

London Churchyards.—The Honorary Secretary of the City Church and Churchyards Protection Society has just issued a report on the condition of City churchyards, the principal object of which is to call attention to such of these burial-grounds as yet await improvement so as to adapt them to recreation purposes. Some of them are terribly neglected—even in a disgraceful state. We hope this interesting report will largely serve towards the promotion of its praiseworthy object—the reclaiming these open spaces for public use.

The Surrey Coroners.—The Surrey magistrates have increased the respective salaries of the coroners of the county as follows:—Mr. Carter, Eastern District, from £990 to £1204; Mr. Hall, Western District, from £655 to £797; Mr. Payne, Southwark and Duchy of Lancaster, from £153 to £167 per annum.

Unqualified Medical Practitioners.—Mr. D. R. Flinn, District Medical Officer of the Lichfield Union, in a recently published pamphlet, draws attention to the singularly large increase in the number of unqualified medical practitioners. In his own district, he believes he is under the mark in saying that over one-fourth of the deaths returned to him by the registrars are attended by these unqualified persons, who are, as a class, men whose preliminary education and training have been of the lowest order. The matter may well (and it is stated, will) be brought before the Royal Commission now sitting on the working of the Medical Acts.

The Death-rate, Keswick.—Dr. Robertson, the Medical Officer of Health, reported to the Cockermouth Rural Sanitary Authority, at their last fortnightly meeting, that the death-rate in the Keswick Rural Sanitary District had been *nil*.

"Better Late than Never."—Dr. W. S. Simpson, Dover, was last week appointed by the Aberdeen Town Council, Medical Officer of Health for the city. The office is an entirely new one, and the duties combine those of the officer of public health, of police surgeon, examiner of quality of gas, and inspector under the Milkshops Acts. The salary is £300 per annum.

An Unsatisfactory Verdict: Subsequent Unofficial Post-mortem Examination.—A rule *nisi* for a *certiorari* has been granted by the Queen's Bench Division to set aside an inquisition held by the Coroner for Somersetshire in the matter of a man—the Quartermaster-Sergeant in the 1st Somerset Militia—who was taken ill suddenly, suffered from sickness, and of which illness he died. In April the coroner's jury sat on the body. There was an absence of direct evidence as to the cause of death, but the jury returned a verdict that the deceased had "died suddenly by the visitation of death." On a post-mortem examination being subsequently made at the request of the relatives, a large quantity of arsenic was discovered in the body, and in consequence the finding of the jury was not considered satisfactory; moreover, the coroner had written a letter, verified by affidavit, that in his opinion there ought to be further inquiry. The inquest will be quashed, and another coroner's inquiry held.

Iona.—1. The Committee of the Liverpool Hospital Sunday Fund have decided to distribute £9600 amongst the medical charities. The allotment will be on the same scale as last year. 2. Yes; the Eye and Ear Dispensary at Birkenhead is to be conducted in future as a public institution.

Llandudno.—A cottage hospital, which has been erected chiefly through the liberality of a lady (Mrs. Nichol), has just been opened in this town.

Holograph Wills.—A layman making his own will is a sight to delight the lawyers. A probate suit was heard last week in the Probate Division, in which the Society for Improving the Condition of the Working Classes were the plaintiffs; and Miss Saffery, the administratrix under the will of the late Dr. Edward Lambert, of Bath, was the defendant. By the will the Society received £2000. The only question involved in the suit, which was a friendly one, arose from the fact that in the testator's will, which was a holograph, the word "two" before the thousand was somewhat indistinct, owing to its having been written over some letters which had apparently been made by the testator; and the jury had to decide whether this alteration had been before or after the execution of the will. The evidence was dependent on that of two experts, which was somewhat conflicting. The jury returned a verdict in favour of the plaintiffs, and the judge gave directions for the insertion of the word "two" before the thousand.

Inquirer.—The total numbers of medical students in the last and present Sessions of Owens College, Manchester, were—1879-80, 222; 1880-81, 237.

COMMUNICATIONS have been received from—

Dr. Ward Cousins, Portsmouth; Dr. Kassowitz, Vienna; The Registrar of Durham; Dr. A. E. Sansom, London; The Secretary of the Sanitary Institution, London; The Registrar-General, Edinburgh; Dr. Mears, Newcastle-on-Tyne; The Secretary of the Royal Institution, London; Dr. M. Mackenzie, London; Dr. G. W. Moore, Dublin; Mr. J. Chatto, London; Messrs. Fletcher, Fletcher, and Stevenson, London; Mr. Mark H. Judge, London; Dr. Barnardo, Stepney; Mr. T. M. Stone, London.

BOOKS, ETC., RECEIVED:—

A Treatise on Comparative Embryology, vol. II., by Francis M. Balfour, LL.D., F.R.S.—Contribution à l'Etude des Traumatismes de la Vessie, par le Docteur P. Maltrait—Advantages of Wheat and Whole-meal Breads—The Micrognaphic Dictionary, by J. W. Griffith, M.D., and Arthur Henfrey, F.R.S., F.R.S.—Report of the Sanitary Condition of the Whitechapel District for the Quarter ended April 2, 1881—Rheumatism, its Nature, its Pathology, and its Successful Treatment, by T. J. Maclagan, M.D.—Transactions of the American Dermatological Association—An Interesting Case of Malformation of the Female Sexual Organs, by Edward Swasey, M.D., New York—Metropolitan Asylums Board Tenth Annual Report—Diseases of the Nervous System, by Prof. Charcot—Colles' Works, by Robert McDonnell, M.D., F.R.S.—That Free Trade in "Drink" is the only Cure for National Drunkenness, by Claud Warren—Die Normale Ossification und die Extraanhängen des Kirchenwesens bei Rachitis und Hereditäre Syphilis, von Dr. M. Kassowitz—Metropolitan Asylum District Annual Reports for 1880 of the Stockwell Fever and Small-pox Hospitals.

PERIODICALS AND NEWSPAPERS RECEIVED:—

Lancet—British Medical Journal—Medical Press and Circular—Berliner Klinische Wochenschrift—Centralblatt für Chirurgie—Gazette des Hopitaux—Gazette Médicale—Le Progrès Médical—Bulletin de l'Académie de Médecine—Pharmaceutical Journal—Wiener Medizinische Wochenschrift—Centralblatt für die Medizinischen Wissenschaften—Revue Médicale—Gazette Hebdomadaire—National Board of Health Bulletin, Washington—Nature—Occasional Notes—Deutsche Medicinal-Zeitung—Louisville Medical News—Chicago Medical Review—The American Medical Temperance Journal—Night and Day—Homœopathic Review—Edinburgh Medical Journal—Specialist—Veterinarian, July—Glasgow Medical Journal, July—Revista de Medicina—L'Imparzialità Médicale—Archives Générales de Médecine—Manchester City News—Analyst—Students' Journal—Ophthalmic Hospital Reports, vol. x. part 3—Therapeutic Gazette—Australian Medical Journal—Italian Times—Church of England Pulpit and Ecclesiastical Review—Progress Medical Roman—Modern Review, July—Il Popolo Romano—Philadelphia Medical Times—Braithwaite's Retrospect, January to June, 1881.

ORIGINAL LECTURES.

ON THE

CAUSES AND SIGNIFICANCE
OF REDUPLICATION OF THE SOUNDS OF
THE HEART.

By ARTHUR ERNEST SANSOM, M.D. Lond., F.R.C.P.,

Physician to the London Hospital ; Physician to the
North-Eastern Hospital for Children, etc.

(*Concluded from page 23.*)

I WILL now call your attention to the evidence upon the question afforded by cases under my own care. I have met with twelve examples of reduplication, real or apparent, of the first sound. Of these seven were males and five females. They could, in my opinion, be classed under three categories—1. Cases of disease of the mitral valve. Six cases, viz., four of mitral stenosis, and two of mitral regurgitation. 2. Cases in which there was hypertrophy of the left ventricle. Four cases: in one a murmur existed, attributable to aortic obstruction ; in another there were the murmurs of combined aortic obstruction and regurgitation. 3. Cases in which the prominent feature was dyspnœa with engorgement or dilatation of the right chambers of the heart. Two cases.

I will first call attention to cases in which the mitral valve was diseased. In two of these the phenomenon which closely resembled a reduplication of the first sound I had, after sufficient observation, no hesitation in ascribing to the auricular systole rendered audible just before the ventricular. In one of these the sound immediately preceding that of the ventricular systole was on many occasions a brief roll drum-beat (*Trommelschlag*). In another the cardiographic tracing gave a remarkable delineation of the powerful systole of the left auricle. In these cases, therefore, though there was the closest resemblance to reduplication of the first sound, there could be little doubt of the correctness of the theory which ascribes the first element of the reduplication to the contraction of a hypertrophied auricle in conjunction with disease of the mitral valve.

The first case requires a little more detail. A female, aged thirty, was admitted, under my care, at the London Hospital for Epilepsy. She had suffered occasionally from subacute rheumatism from the age of six. She was pregnant. The physical signs in regard to the heart showed, briefly, the apex in normal condition, the first sound subdued but accompanied by murmur conveyed towards axilla, at the base of the heart the second sound pronounced but uncomplicated. On the day following admission I found that the first sound was reduplicate, the reduplication being heard in a line leading from the fourth interspace to the anterior border of the axilla. Two days afterwards the patient aborted. The reduplication persisted, but changed in certain characters. At the end of a fortnight it was heard from the third interspace to the apex. A little internal to the apex, reduplication was distinct and uncomplicated by murmur. On nearing the apex, a soft systolic murmur was observed to tail off from the *second* element of the reduplication ; and at the apex, reduplication was lost, a first-sound murmur only being heard. Sphygmographic tracings gave evidence of tension above the normal, with irregularities in time and occasional disturbances of rhythm (double pulse). Cardiographic tracings indicated hypertrophy of the left ventricle ; in the diastolic portion it is seen that the eminence due to the auricular systole has a broad base and is decidedly marked. There can be no doubt that in this case the second element of the reduplication was the voice of the left ventricle ; this is attested by the fact that a mitral systolic murmur tailed off from it. To what, then, was the first element due ? It seems scarcely probable that it could be the tension of the tricuspid valve effected by the muscular effort of the right ventricle, for the reduplication was at one time not even audible over the right apex, though distinct in the fourth interspace. The progress of the case seems to offer a clue for the interpretation. I lost sight of the patient for eight months ; at the end of that

period I found that there was no reduplication of the first sound, but a *presystolic murmur typical and distinct*. It would seem to me most probable, therefore, that the reduplication of the first sound which we formerly heard was an *apparent* reduplication, due, as in the cases I have previously mentioned, to the auricular systole rendering tense the mitral valves, which were already thickened, and permitting regurgitation. Subsequently the orifice became more and more contracted, and the force of the auricular contraction was expended in urging the blood into the ventricle until the moment of ventricular systole.

Another very marked case of reduplication of the first sound has lately been under my care in the London Hospital. Ellen L., aged sixteen, admitted August 30, 1880, in her third attack of rheumatic fever. The following were the cardiac signs :—Heart's action irregular both in time and volume ; apex in normal position ; palpation occasionally demonstrated a *double impulse ;* pulmonary second sound accentuated ; first sound reduplicated—reduplication best heard at fifth left costal cartilage, and thence downwards towards the apex ; from the second element of the reduplication tailed off a systolic murmur. The sphygmograph in this case demonstrated very low tension, with irregularities in time. The cardiograph gave evidence of a very marked auricular systole. This case seems to present considerable analogy with the preceding, but there is one point which may seem to differentiate it—the existence of double impulse. It may be thought by some that this sign is conclusive of non-synchronous contraction of the two ventricles. It has been thus interpreted by Skoda, Bamberger, Leyden, and others. But it is worth while to inquire whether this double impulse may not be due to auricular preceding ventricular systole. It is clear that no evidence of this double ventricular systole is in this instance afforded by the cardiograph, as we might reasonably expect ; and it seems to me not improbable that an auricular impulse which so tilts the apex as to cause it to lift the cardiographic needle to the extent of one-fifth or more of the altitude effected by the systole of the ventricle may be distinctly appreciated by the finger.

So far, therefore, as regards the cases of reduplicated first sound occurring in cases of mitral disease, I am inclined to think the balance of evidence is in favour of the auriculoventricular causation of the phenomenon in the manner I have described. In the other classes of cases the evidence is by no means strong of any participation of the auricle in the mechanism, and certainly does not point to the auricular systole as a *universal* cause of the phenomenon. In the class of cases attended with prolonged systole of the left ventricle, it is quite probable that the theory so ably argued by Dr. Barr may be correct, and the tension of the tricuspid curtains may occur at an earlier period than those of the mitral, for it is well proved that the contraction of hypertrophied muscle is comparatively slow. Dr. Galabin has shown that in aortic disease the time which the ventricles take to become fully hardened may be increased to double the normal.(a)

One of my cases presented doubling of the first sound on the nineteenth and twentieth days of an attack of typhoid fever, doubling of *both* sounds having been manifest on the seventeenth. In this instance it is most probable that there was an *immediate* disturbance of the rhythm of the ventricles by the myocarditis (in scattered areas) which is known to occur in typhoid.

As regards the reduplication of first sound in the cases in which engorgement of the right cavities of the heart was the prominent feature, it seems quite probable that they may be explained by the theory which accounts for *physiological* reduplication of the first sound thus enunciated by Dr. Barr : —"At the end of expiration the great veins of the chest have become engorged, while the surplus in the lungs has been disposed of, so the right ventricle becomes over-distended, and is stimulated to initiate contraction, thus giving rise to reduplicate first sound ; but the same overloading and the increased obstruction in front prolong the right ventricular systole : hence there is no doubling of the second sound." Whilst quite admitting that this is highly probable, however, I think the auricular theory here also affords a possible explanation. For it must be admitted that the engorgement of the right ventricle leads directly to engorgement of

(a) *Vide Med.-Chir. Trans.*, vol. lix., page 268.

the left auricle, and that the systole of the latter may be exaggerated owing to such engorgement.

So far as the extant evidence justifies conclusions, they are, therefore, I consider, these :—

That reduplication of the first sound may be apparent or real.

That an apparent reduplication is the indirect effect of the auricular systole.

That real reduplication of the first sound is a phenomenon of rare occurrence, and is due to want of synchronism in the systolic tension of the tricuspid and the mitral curtains respectively.

I now ask your attention to the phenomenon of reduplication of the second sound.

It is undoubted that by far the most common condition in which double second sound is heard is mitral stenosis. Next in point of frequency, according to Dr. Hayden, is aortic insufficiency. With considerable unanimity the phenomenon has been ascribed to a *want of synchronism in the closure of the valves of the aorta and of the pulmonary artery respectively*. The sequence of closure may vary. In cases of aortic insufficiency Dr. Hayden is satisfied that the second element is aortic because the murmur of aortic regurgitation accompanies it. He believes that in such cases the left ventricle is dilated, and so it is slower to become emptied in systole; consequently the aortic reflux is postponed. On the other hand, in mitral stenosis the derangement is chiefly in the pulmonary artery, "the entire pulmonary system and the right chambers being engorged by obstruction at the mitral orifice. In the effort to overcome this obstruction systole of the right ventricle is protracted, and the reaction of the pulmonary artery proportionately postponed. The reaction of the aorta is, on the other hand, in mitral stenosis most probably anticipated, where the left ventricle is reduced in capacity, as always is the case where mitral or aortic reflux does not co-exist. Hence it is likely that in simple mitral stenosis two causes of doubling of the second sound are in operation, namely, diminished capacity of the left, and dilatation of the right, ventricle."(b)

It seems a truism to assert that conditions of blood-pressure in the two great vessels respectively cannot be the *vera causa* of such reduplication, for until the occurrence of diastole there can be no reflux, and consequently no second sound. The causation of reduplication, as of the first so of the second sound, under the theory we are now discussing must revert to the ventricles. When their systole is simultaneous, the second sound, produced by reflux against the semilunar valves of the two great vessels at the moment of their relaxation, must be simultaneous also. When their systole is not simultaneous, or does not last through equal periods, the diastolic reflux cannot be simultaneous; if the discrepancy be such as can be appreciated by the ear, the second sound is doubled.

The following is Dr. Barr's view:—"As I have ascribed reduplication of the first sound to asynchronism in the initial stage of ventricular contraction, so I believe reduplication of the second sound to be due to asynchronism at the end of contraction, and in the consecutive reaction of the aorta and pulmonary artery with the tension of their respective valves."

The comparative rarity of cases of reduplication of the first sound is explained by the much greater length of time occupied by the first than by the second sound, whence is required a correspondingly greater want of synchronism between the closure of the tricuspid and mitral valves than between the closure of the pulmonic and aortic to produce a reduplication.

Physiological reduplication at the end of inspiration is accounted for by the fact that the capacity of the pulmonic system being increased, the obstructive burden upon the right ventricle is lessened—consequently the systole of the latter is shortened. The lessening of the duration of the systole of the right ventricle implies anticipation of the diastolic closure of the pulmonary semilunar valves; so there is a reduplicate second sound, the primary element being pulmonic. In pathological reduplication the origin may be in either the right or the left ventricle. If from any cause the systole of one of the ventricles be protracted, the diastolic closure of the valves of its great vessel of exit will be delayed also, and so the second sound will be double.

Guttmann supports the view of non-simultaneous closure of the aortic and pulmonary valves, without giving reasons for the proximate cause. He says, however, that it is not unreasonable to explain it by a change in a single set of the semilunar valves causing their tension to take place in two distinct movements. This hypothesis appears to me impossible to accept: such change would surely be likely to produce murmur rather than reduplication. But Guttmann says that reduplication of the second sound in mitral stenosis is difficult to account for satisfactorily, and in this I quite agree with him. He adds, "The broken diastolic sound is (so far as I have observed) certainly not loudest over the large vessels, but at the lower part of the sternum and near the apex of the heart, and is further absent in the more marked cases of mitral contraction, precisely in the cases in which the conditions most favourable to the postponement of the closure of the pulmonary valve are present in their highest degree." Reduplication, however, does not occur in mitral regurgitation where the conditions of relative blood-pressure are profoundly altered. Guttmann considers it probable that the reduplication may arise at the narrowed mitral orifice itself, that it may be a component part of a presystolic (or, as he terms it, diastolic) murmur, and adds that it has been conjectured that the first element of the reduplication is the diastolic pulmonary sound, and the second is produced, towards the end of diastole, by the contraction of the hypertrophied left auricle.(c) In fact, the hypothesis reverts to the last I have mentioned as probably explaining some cases of reduplication of the first sound.

I consider, then, that there is a theory of auricular causation of reduplication of the second sound which is well worth considering, and that we have before us as plausible explanations of the phenomenon—

a. That it is due to non-simultaneous closure of the semilunar valves in the aorta and the pulmonary artery respectively.

b. That it is the effect of a sudden tension of the mitral curtains after the normal second sound.

I now proceed to discuss the evidence on this question that my own cases have afforded me. The total number of such cases was 22; of these 11 occurred in mitral stenosis. Of 27 instances of such reduplication noted by Dr. Hayden, no less than 26 were cases of mitral constriction.(d) The phenomenon occurred in 26 out of 68 cases of mitral stenosis in Dr. Hayden's experience. Guttmann gives the proportion of doubled second sound in all cases of mitral stenosis as 1 in 3; and my own cases give a proportion of 11 in 37. These proportions agree pretty closely. It is obvious, therefore, that mitral stenosis is a condition which especially disposes to reduplication of the second sound, and it is *à priori* probable that in this form of valve-lesion there should be some special reason for its manifestation.

I will consider then (1) cases of reduplication of the second sound met with in conjunction with mitral stenosis.

The following is an illustration :—A lady, aged fifty, had been frequently under my care for symptoms of dyspepsia. There was no history of rheumatism, nor development at any time of articular phenomena. I had frequent opportunities of physical examination of the heart, but I found no evidence of lesion. After the lapse of a few months, however, during which interval no special symptoms had manifested themselves, the patient complained of "fluttering of the heart." I then discovered a rough presystolic murmur just internal to the apex, with a short systolic murmur at and outside the apex. There was *distinct reduplication of the second sound* heard at the aortic cartilage and down the left border of the sternum, but ceasing at the point internal to the apex, where the presystolic murmur became audible. At the next examination the reduplication was heard as far as the apex. A subsequent note states, "Reduplication very marked, but no presystolic murmur heard." Afterwards, "No reduplication heard at any part of the base ; commences well below the region of the pulmonary valves, and is certainly loudest at, or even a little outside, the apex." A subsequent note, "Reduplication still very pronounced; not heard at left third interspace nor anywhere left of the sternum until the level of the fourth costal cartilage; it is well heard at the apex and marked in the axilla." Afterwards the reduplication was plainly heard at the back near the angle of the left scapula.

(b) "Diseases of the Heart and Aorta," page 126.

(c) "Physical Diagnosis," page 279.   (d) *Loc. cit.*, page 165.

Let us ask whether the phenomena in this case can be explained by the theory which postulates a want of synchronism between the aortic and pulmonary second sounds. Supposing this theory to be correct, it would be the aortic that would be the first element of the reduplication, because as the aortic region was receded from, the second element of the reduplication undoubtedly became more and more pronounced. But to accept this theory, even under the conditions first noted, we must agree that the aortic second sound was audible not only over its normal area, but as far as the apex. We had in this case, however, abundant reason for knowing that the aortic tension, instead of being above, was far below the normal. A reference to the record of one of Dr. Hayden's cases points to the same difficulty. Here "the second sound was double and heard all over the præcordium." Under the accepted theory, therefore, the sound of reflux against the aortic valves, its first element, must of course have been audible all over the præcordium; that is, over a wider area than we might expect the normal aortic second sound to be heard. But the case was fully observed, and diagnosis confirmed by post-mortem examination; and Dr. Hayden adds: "The quantity of blood which, in this case, passed into the aorta at each systole of the left ventricle must have been very small, owing to the twofold lesion of mitral obstruction and incompetency." Moreover, the aortic orifice was reduced to the diameter of the point of the little finger, and its valves thick, and therefore less disposed to give the "click" of closure.

The difficulty of accepting the asynchronism theory is further greatly increased by consideration of the subsequent areas of audibility in my case, for the reduplication was not even *audible in the area of the aortic valves*. Here only a single second sound was heard. On the other hand, the reduplication, with increasing intensification of both its elements, approached nearer the apex, and afterwards the maximum pronunciation of both elements was in the axilla. Such being the case, I consider that in this instance the aortic second sound could have had no share in producing the phenomena of reduplication. In two cases the only point at which reduplication was audible was at, or just internal to, the apex; in four cases it was audible down the sternum approaching near the apex, where the presystolic murmur became manifest.

It appears to me most probable that the reduplication of the second sound which occurs in mitral stenosis is apparent, not real, and that it is caused (as in apparent reduplication of the first sound) by sudden tension of the mitral curtains. In reduplication of the first sound (so-called) this tension is effected by the auricle just before the ventricular systole, and the mechanism for its production postulates a hypertrophied auricle with an inconsiderable degree of stenosis of the mitral aperture. In reduplication (so-called) of the second sound the tension of the mitral curtains is effected early in diastole. The moment the ventricle becomes relaxed after its systole, the blood retained in a state of tension (the pressure in the pulmonary circuit being heightened) in the left auricle enters with force into the ventricular cavity, and, finding its way on the parietal side of the curtains of the mitral valve, causes these to bulge towards the centre of the ventricle, and in so doing occasions the click of valve-tension, which click, coming so soon after the second sound, closely resembles a reduplication of the latter. The extrusion of the blood being continued, and the force causing such extrusion being reinforced by the auricle, the presystolic *murmur* is produced.

I think it may be considered fully proved that the murmur of mitral stenosis may be diastolic as well as presystolic—that is, as Dr. Wilks long ago considered probable, it may be due to the flow through the mitral orifice from the distended auricle previously to the period at which such flow is quickened by the auricular systole. I have narrated a case in which such view is confirmed. The truth of it is also further shown by cardiograms which I have obtained in cases of mitral stenosis, wherein, although there was a prolonged (so-called) presystolic murmur and thrill, the eminence due to the auricular systole is shown to occupy its normal position just before the ventricular systolic upstroke.

It can also be considered proved, in my opinion, that the blood-pressure in the auricle in diastole is often a *variable* blood-pressure, enhanced at various times out of its normal rhythm by the auricle, the contractions of which may be multiple. This was shown long ago by Dr. Galabin, whose cardiograms demonstrated that occasionally (sometimes when mitral stenosis was not proved) repeated eminences due to auricular systoles were seen in the diastolic portion of the tracing. This observation I have many times confirmed.

It is obvious that, if my view be correct, a distinct interval (just such as our experience shows to occur) should separate the second sound caused at the moment that the ventricles have become relaxed from the little flap of the mitral curtains, which could only be effected when sufficient blood had entered the ventricular cavity to lift them. I have obtained some cardiograms in cases in which there was typical reduplication of the second sound, in which there is (1) a highly pronounced notch in the downstroke, indicating abrupt closure of the semilunar valves; (2) in the horizontal (diastolic) portion of the tracing an eminence indicating a rise of blood-pressure which might reasonably indicate the period at which the so-called reduplication might become audible.

Whilst offering this as the probable explanation of the phenomenon known as reduplication of the second sound when it is met with in conditions of mitral stenosis, I would by no means urge that it is the universal explanation of reduplication of the second sound met with under other circumstances.

I have observed reduplication of second sound in eleven instances in which I had no proof that there was any constriction at the mitral orifice. Of these, the most frequent examples were in conditions of respiratory distress, especially where the right chambers of the heart were in a marked degree dilated. It is noteworthy that in these cases *the area of audibility of the reduplication was strikingly different from that noted in the cases of mitral stenosis.* It was always over the pulmonic valves or the right ventricle, where, supposing the theory which ascribes the phenomenon to asynchronism of pulmonary and aortic second sounds to be correct, it most probably would occur. In these cases it is most probable that the reduplication is *real*, and is explicable on the theory of Dr. Barr and others.

In the cases of hypertrophy of the left ventricle it is also quite probable that the theory of asynchronism may be correct, though the difficulties are greater, in my opinion, than in the class of cases just considered.

The following case illustrates these difficulties:—A female, aged fifty, was admitted under my care at the London Hospital, suffering from chronic renal disease, with thickened arteries, albuminuric retinitis, hypertrophy of left ventricle with mitral regurgitation. Whiffing systolic murmur with marked reduplication of second sound *heard at apex*; at next examination, reduplication heard at base as well as at apex. Of the two elements of reduplication, the *first* the loudest; over area of pulmonary valves this first element is louder than over aortic valves. Below this area, and near apex, the two elements are about equally loud. The *microphone* demonstrated the reduplication in the *neighbourhood of the apex.*

At the next examination, patient then being extremely ill, reduplication heard only at base, and best at aortic cartilage. The conditions as demonstrated by post-mortem examination were great hypertrophy and dilatation of the ventricles and auricles. Left auriculo-ventricular orifice much thickened, but no stenosis. In this case, too, it would appear to me more probable that the first element of the reduplication was the second sound, accentuated in the aortic region by the greatly heightened tension in the aorta, and in the pulmonary region by that in the pulmonary artery. Careful examination in the two regions could not convince me otherwise than that the two second sounds, though not of equal intensity, were simultaneous.

It is difficult to understand why, if the phenomenon were due to asynchronism of the second sound, the reduplication should be heard only *at the apex*. On the other hand, it seemed quite probable that, as in mitral stenosis, there might have been diastolic tension of the thickened mitral curtains.

SEATS FOR SHOP-GIRLS.—A Bill to provide seats for shop-girls has passed the State Legislature. It provides that employers shall allow the girls a reasonable length of time in which to rest during the day. We fear, however, that shopkeepers cannot be legislated into humanity.—*New York Med. Record,* June 11.

ORIGINAL COMMUNICATIONS.

ON THE USE OF THE ŒSOPHAGOSCOPE IN DISEASE OF THE GULLET.

By MORELL MACKENZIE, M.D.,

Senior Physician to the Hospital for Diseases of the Throat; late Physician to the London Hospital.

NOTWITHSTANDING the facility with which instruments can be passed down the gullet, the examination of that organ by means of tubes is always likely to be attended with considerable difficulty; for, unlike the larynx and trachea, which are nearly always open to inspection, the orifice of the gullet is closed, and lower down the walls of the canal are usually more or less in apposition. Further difficulty arises from the spasmodic contraction of the muscular tunic of the œsophagus, which is so easily set up, and also from the pharyngeal irritation which almost unavoidably occurs.

The older surgeons do not appear to have endeavoured to overcome these difficulties, and the first attempt to examine the gullet during life would seem to have been made by Semeleder and Stoerk in 1866.(a) This experiment, however, yielded only negative results. The instrument employed appears to have consisted of a forceps with spoon-shaped blades. The idea of the instrument originated with Semeleder, who offered himself to Stoerk for experiment. After the introduction of the instrument the laryngeal mirror was placed in the ordinary position, but it was at once found that the view was obstructed by a kind of figure-of-eight projection of the mucous membrane between each blade of the forceps.(b)

Two years afterwards, the late Dr. Waldenburg(c) invented an œsophagoscope. This instrument was made of gum-elastic and was eight centimetres in length. It was slightly conical in shape, the diameter above being one centimetre and a half, and below one centimetre. It was connected to the extremity of a two-pronged fork fourteen centimetres in length, in such a way that considerable movement was permitted. After the introduction of the instrument it was held with the left hand, and the tongue being slightly pressed down, the laryngeal mirror was put into the mouth. In the case in which Dr. Waldenburg used the instrument, there was a pouch at the upper part of the gullet on the left side, and he was able to keep the instrument in situ for ten or fifteen seconds, and to see that the mucous membrane of the œsophagus was not ulcerated or in any way diseased. On introducing the speculum into the diverticulum itself, that cavity was seen to contain a small quantity of broth. Subsequently, Waldenburg had an instrument made of metal instead of gum-elastic, consisting of two tubes arranged telescopically, each tube being six centimetres in length, the one playing on the other by means of a slot. Waldenburg's instrument was exhibited and used on a patient by Professor Stoerk before the Society of Physicians of Vienna.(d)

Subsequently, Stoerk employed an instrument resembling Waldenburg's, but consisting of three tubes. In February of the present year, Professor Stoerk described a new œsophagoscope which consists of a lobster-jointed tube covered

with india-rubber, with a small mirror attached its upper extremity, and with a handle, consisting of a two-pronged fork like that of Waldenburg's. This tube is provided with a pilot or director, consisting of a piece of elastic tubing terminating in a small bag which projects beyond the end of the œsophagoscope, the diameter of the bag being a little larger than that of the tube. The ball being inflated, the instrument is passed into the gullet, when the air is allowed to escape and the pilot withdrawn.

My own attempts to examine the gullet with an œsophagoscope commenced in February, 1880. From the following description it will be seen that the instrument which I have introduced(e) is altogether different from those hitherto employed. It consists of two parts—a stem and a skeleton tube. The stem is made up of a handle and a shank, between which there is a hinge. The skeleton tube is only formed when the instrument has been introduced into the gullet; before that, it consists of two flattened wires placed anteriorly and posteriorly, connected above and below, and at certain intervals between these points, by rings. When the rings lie in the vertical position, the wires are separated from each other only by the thickness of the rings, but when the latter are thrown into the horizontal position the two wires become separated, and, with the rings, constitute a kind of skeleton speculum.(f) At the top of the back wire there is a slot, into which the stem of a laryngeal mirror is fitted. In the upper figure of the annexed cut it will be seen that the handle and shank are almost in a line—a position which greatly facilitates the introduction of the instrument. When the "body" has been passed down the œsophagus, the operator, holding the handle in his hand, but leaving the index-finger free, presses with the latter on the upper part of the shank near the handle.

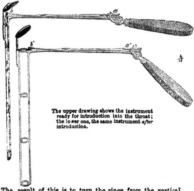

The upper drawing shows the instrument ready for introduction into the throat; the lower one, the same instrument after introduction.

The result of this is to turn the rings from the vertical to the horizontal position, and thus to open the speculum and expand the gullet. With a view of causing as little irritation as possible, before withdrawing the instrument the operator should close the speculum by pressing the under part of the shank (near the handle) with his thumb. Tubes varying in length from three to five inches can be bolted so securely to the end of the shank that they are as safe as if the whole instrument were made in one piece.(g)

For the sake of convenience, I prefer to have several instruments of different lengths. In November, 1880, I had attempted to use the instrument on fifty patients, and I had succeeded thirty-seven times. Subsequently I have used it from time to time, whenever a suitable case presented itself. In the three following cases I have been able to carry out

(a) Private letter from Professor Stoerk, November 13, 1880. Dr. Stoerk has since published a description of this experiment in the same paper, in which he gives an account of his more recent invention (Wien. klin. Wochenschrift, No. 8, February, 1881).

(b) In 1866, Bevan (Lancet, vol. i., April, 1866) published a description of various instruments for examining the pharynx, larynx, and posterior nares, fitted to a lamp, on the principle of the endoscope. In this paper there is no detailed description of the œsophagoscope, but merely a few lines describing the figure which illustrates it. As far as I can make out from this drawing, the œsophagoscope appears to be a straight tube, four inches long, by three-quarters of an inch in diameter, which has attached to its upper extremity, by means of a wire on each side, a ring slightly larger in diameter and about one inch in length. This ring is placed at an angle of about forty-five degrees to the tube, and to it the pharyngoscopic tube of the endoscope was, to use the words of the inventor, "very easily applied." It is not stated that any mirror was used, but as a reflector is seen in the drawing of the pharyngoscope it was probably employed for inspecting the gullet. A perusal of Bevan's paper will convince any reader that the experiments were the results of work in the laboratory rather than in the wards of a hospital; and, in fact, the instrument was of no practical value.

(c) Berlin. klin. Wochenschrift, No. 48, November 29, 1870.

(d) Letter before quoted. The Professor does not recollect the exact date of the exhibition of the patient, but, no doubt, an account of it would be found in the Transactions of the Imperial-Royal Society of Physicians of Vienna soon after 1871.

(e) The instrument was made for me by Messrs. Mayer and Meltzer, Great Portland-street.

(f) In the earlier instrument which I employed there were a great number of rings, and the speculum was opened and closed by means of a movable slide on the upper part of the shank.

(g) A skeleton speculum has, I believe, been used for the vagina.

treatment which could not have been accomplished without the use of the œsophagoscope.

Case 1.—Mrs. B., aged sixty-two, was sent to me by Mr. Yate, of Godalming, on June 28, 1880, on account of difficulty of swallowing, which had commenced two years previously. She was able to take liquids easily, but could not swallow solids. The dysphagia gradually increased, and at the beginning of August, Mrs. B. could only take liquids with the greatest difficulty. At last, liquids could not be swallowed. With the œsophagoscope a ragged projecting growth was seen about three inches below the lower border of the cricoid cartilage. On August 18, in the presence of Mr. Yate, Mr. Hovell, and Mr. Bayley (who administered chloroform), I succeeded in removing with the œsophageal forceps a piece of growth about the size of a cherry. The effect of the operation was most satisfactory. The patient felt some pain for two or three days, but a week after the operation she was able to swallow semi-solids with ease. Microscopic examination showed that the tumour was an epithelioma. The patient lived rather more than six months after the operation, which may fairly be considered to have prolonged life for four or five months.

Case 2.—Miss P., aged twenty-seven, consulted me in August, 1880, on account of difficulty of swallowing, which had been coming on for six or seven years. Examination with the œsophagoscope revealed an oval, semi-transparent polypus, situated on the right of the gullet, one inch below the cricoid cartilage. On August 28, in the presence of Mr. C. L. Taylor, I removed a growth about the size of a white currant. The patient felt some slight pain for twenty-four hours after the operation ; but at the end of a week she was able to swallow perfectly, and has never since had any recurrence of the symptoms. The following is the report of Dr. Stephen Mackenzie on the specimen :—" The surface of the growth is covered with squamous epithelium, beneath which is a very lax œdematous and highly vascular mass with numerous lymphoid cells (leucocytes) infiltrated into the tissue. It appears, in fact, to be a polypus arising from chronic inflammation of the œsophageal mucous membrane."

Case 3.—The third case was that of Mrs. B., aged fifty-one, sent to me by Dr. Spitta, of Clapham, in February, 1881. She complained of great difficulty of swallowing and a feeling of something sticking in her throat. The symptoms commenced suddenly whilst she was taking a meal, a fortnight previously. At the first examination with the œsophagoscope, the interior of the gullet was seen to be highly inflamed, but no foreign body could be seen. At a second sitting, a few days later, a flat lamella of bone, about four millimetres square, was seen about two inches below the cricoid cartilage on the anterior wall of the œsophagus. This was easily removed by the aid of forceps, together with a small piece of decayed meat which was found adherent to the bone after its removal. This patient felt some slight inconvenience for three or four weeks after the removal of the foreign body, but when last seen was able to swallow without any difficulty.

CLINICAL ILLUSTRATIONS OF

EMOTIONAL EXCITEMENT AS A CAUSE OF CHOREA.

By JAMES RUSSELL, M.D., F.R.C.P.

Among the causes usually assigned in explanation of an attack of chorea, fright or some other powerful emotion frequently occupies a place. Probably few of the so-called causes of disease are more open to the fallacy of the *post hoc ergo propter hoc* than strong emotion ; and accordingly, in analysing any group of cases in which this influence figures as an alleged cause, it will be apparent that the evidence on which the allegation is founded possesses very different degrees of force in different instances. Without entering into the question as to the sufficiency of strong emotion of itself to account for the phenomena of chorea, there will nevertheless be found a certain proportion of cases of this malady which are so closely related to states of mental excitement, that a distinct connexion must be admitted between the emotion and the disease ; whilst, in comparing the particular cases with one another, it will be

further observed that the emotion holds many different relations both as regards the force of the particular development and the directness of the influence it seems to have exerted over the patient.

I have taken the first hundred cases of chorea from my hospital case-books, and I find that in twenty-three an emotional influence has been asserted, more or less directly, to have had a share in producing the symptoms. I subjoin a brief abstract of the histories given in these cases, for the purpose of illustrating the different characters of the ground on which the allegation of the cause is based.

There is, however, another reason which gives interest to a comparison of cases in the production of which mental excitement appears to have taken a part. Nothing need be said in order to establish the truth that the condition of the emotional element has a large share in determining the state of physical well-being. By no one has the intimate relation which subsists between mental and bodily health been more strikingly illustrated, because illustrated on a large scale, than by our naval and military surgeons, and some of the best demonstrations may be obtained from the papers and essays which were produced by the many eminent medical men who adorned our Army and Navy during the protracted warfare with which the present century so unhappily opened. " It is related," writes Sir Gilbert Blane (" Select Dissertations," 1822, page 79), " that when the fleet under Admiral Matthews in the year 1744 was off Toulon, in the daily expectation of engaging the combined fleets of France and Spain, there was a general suspension of the progress of sickness, particularly of scurvy, from the influence of that generous flow of spirits with which the prospect of battle inspires the British seaman. . . . This is the place, therefore, to remark of what importance it is, in point of health, to support the spirits of the men ; depression of mind not only damping the courage, but being favourable to the invasion of disease in every form." I may also quote a very striking case given by the late Dr. Stokes (" Diseases of the Heart and Aorta," 1854, page 22, note), in which recovery from a severe case of pericarditis was seriously delayed by a state of melancholy in the patient, due to religious doubts. Dr. Stokes asked a clergyman, distinguished for his talent and eloquence, to visit his patient. " The interview was followed by the best results. Next day the rubbing sounds had become softer. The visit was repeated ; and on the third day all morbid signs had disappeared." " The bowl that rolls easiest along the green," writes Sir Walter Scott, " goes farthest and has least clay sticking to it. I have often noticed that a kindly, placid good-humour is the companion of longevity, and I suspect frequently the leading cause of it."

In virtue of this direct influence over the nutritive processes, morbid emotional states become powerful agents, under favouring circumstances, in the production of disease. " I could give," writes Esquirol, " the history of our revolution, from the taking of the Bastile to the last advent of Buonaparte, by that of certain insane, whose delusions associated themselves with the events which have marked that long period of our history." A curious account in the *Daily News* (October 3, 1874) of the effect produced on the animals in the Zoological Gardens by the alarm excited in consequence of the explosion of gunpowder on the Regent's-park Canal, shows that consequences of intense emotion even dangerous to life are not restricted to the highly developed brain of man.

Dr. Hughlings-Jackson has very ably employed the different phenomena presented by an epileptic fit to support and illustrate his doctrine of the general representation in the brain of most of the functions of the body. The pathological phenomena of vascular changes which take place in different parts of the body from injury or disease of the brain, described by Vulpian (" L'Appareil Vaso-moteur "), and especially those changes of which he speaks under the title " Congestions Émotives" (vol. ii., page 509), afford material corroboration of Dr. Jackson's descriptions, and connect together, in the same category, both injury to the physical tissues of the brain, and excess in its functional activity. There is a very striking remark by Andral (" Clinique," 1840, vol. v., page 128) in anticipation of the later pathology, which deserves quoting in the present connexion :—" I suspect that a certain number of inflammations are preceded by a simple nervous perturbation, in which, at the outset, consists all the malady ; at that time narcotics dissipate the symptoms marvellously. But suffer this condition to remain, and it will soon have changed its nature : those functional derangements which hitherto were the expression of an isolated disorder of innervation, will be henceforth produced and maintained by inflammatory action ; then narcotics become injurious—other measures must replace them." This passage, I may add, embodies the discussion respecting "irritation" as opposed to "inflammation," which was connected with the publication of Dr. Marshall Hall's essay "On the Effect of Loss of Blood."

The part which is played by the emotional element in producing the phenomena of health or disease is a complex problem ; in part, no doubt, it is regulated by the amount of emotional force implanted in each individual ; but in comparing different individuals with reference to the emotional development they severally display under the ordinary circumstances of life, a second highly important element will force itself upon our notice—namely, the amount of control which each habitually exercises, consciously or unconsciously, over the action of his nervous centres. It is this restraining power, this " control over the passions," which largely determines the nature of each man's character, according as it keeps the more movable part of the brain under its command, limiting its activity within bounds suitable to the occasion, and maintaining it in a state of quiescence when action is out of place, or according as its restraint is unstable, irregular in its operation, and easily disturbed. Now, this fact, which is embodied in the most ordinary conception of the formation of character, embodies a highly important doctrine in relation to the pathology of the nervous system. This doctrine, especially developed by Dr. Ringer, with particular reference to forms of nervous disease (e.g., tetanus) supposed to be the consequence of abnormal increase in the activity of nerve-cells, lays greater stress upon variations in the strength of the controlling or inhibiting power in accounting for the phenomenon than upon any supposed production of nervous energy. Referring to the pent-up force normally contained in nerve-cells, which, as Dr. Gowers justly observes, " may be infinitely greater than any manifestation which we perceive could possibly suggest," Dr. Ringer would explain the unstable equilibrium of nerve-tissue rather by instability of resistance than by added production of nervous energy.

Of the action in which this power of inhibiting action operates we are very ignorant, but there can be no doubt that a healthy state of nutrition in the physical structure of the central organs is one of the most important conditions. It is from the application of this doctrine that those forms of disease which are attributable in any degree to emotional causes, derive considerable interest by rendering broader the ground on which their causation may be discussed. So long as the emotional excitement is regarded in the light of a supply of active energy to the excited tissue, we shall be met by the difficulty created by the disproportion between the supposed cause and the presumed effect, whilst at the same time a certain obvious connexion between the two forbids our ignoring altogether this operation of the emotion in causing the disorder. But if, on the other hand, we can apply to the cases the analogy of the electric spark, which, embodying in itself but a small amount of energy, has yet the ability to release an enormous amount of force in a mine of explosive material, our attention is fixed on the prior condition of the nerve-cells, and the question to be answered will then be, whether there is reason for believing that the inhibiting force by which these cells are habitually controlled has been altered or diminished. It is this inquiry which must be satisfied before the full share of the emotional disturbance in producing the immediate phenomena can be satisfactorily adjusted.

A curious illustration of what has just been said was afforded in a paper read some years ago by M. Charbonneau before the French Academy on the case of Louise Lateau. M. Charbonneau regards it as a necessary condition for a man to reach the "mystic stage" that he " should submit himself to a debilitating regimen, which, while diminishing the activity of his physical functions, suppresses the superior faculties of the soul, to the advantage of the imagination." In other words, the aspirant must adopt the treatment best calculated for removing from the most excitable part of the brain the inhibitory influence which a healthy state of nutrition would exert upon it. With respect to chorea, the disease with which I am immediately concerned, the truth of this doctrine has been acknowledged by the different controversies which have been conducted respecting the nature of its fundamental cause.

It is worth while to mention, in passing, one circumstance which may often be noticed in cases of disease wherein reference is made to emotion as a cause—viz., that the effect produced is by no means necessarily immediate. It is the most serious part of the evil which results from the operation of morbid excitement upon a susceptible subject, that its results cannot be judged by the immediate consequences ; the change which is determined may be gradual in its operation, and the more enduring on that account. It frequently happens that during the interval sufficient attestation to the operation may be noticed in the behaviour of the patient before the final explosion takes place. I may quote a curious illustration which occurred to myself. A married woman informed me that when nine years of age she went one day upstairs to bring a coat from a room where a dead body had lain a short time before. A man who followed her, doubtless observing that she was unnerved, in a thoughtless jest, said to her, " The devil is behind you !" She made no reply, but retired with so much precipitation as to fall downstairs ; nor did she make any reference to what had happened. But during the following week she was less alert than usual, disliked to move about after dark, and positively refused to go into the cellar ; nor would she go to bed unless one of her sisters stood by her whilst she undressed. On the evening of the seventh day, without anything having occurred afresh, whilst getting into bed, she suddenly turned to her sister. " Mr. Jones says the the devil is behind me !" and instantly fell into a state of violent and destructive mania, which lasted in a modified form for four months. It was significant that even at so great a distance of time this woman shrank from recalling the original cause of her illness. This tendency in a susceptible mind to retain deep impressions made upon it, constitutes an important fact to be dealt with in considering the influence of strong emotion. I recall a case mentioned by Dr. George Johnson, in which a man had unfortunately run over a child and killed it : the painful recollection of the occurrence was testified by the continual recurrence of frightful dreams, in most of which the child figured, for seven years, and probably also by epileptic fits to which he became subject two years after the accident. In my own case, just narrated, it would seem that the excitement, first produced and then repressed, had been gathering force day by day, until it burst forth with accumulated violence.

I should like to prefix to my histories of chorea the following details of a case of intense mental disorder, of a temporary character, which occurred under my own observation. The symptoms concerned the mental function alone, but I quote the case in order to show how nearly mental and motor derangement approximate in the nature of their development when affected by violent disturbance. The case occurred in a middle-aged lady of strumous constitution, and of excitable temperament, liable to nervous derangements ; and of a very neurotic family. She was exposed for a period of twenty-four hours to a state of peculiar and intense anxiety. She sat up all night and took little food. On the following evening the cause of anxiety was completely and satisfactorily removed, but the night was passed without sleep, and in the morning, obeying a hasty summons, I found the room darkened, the patient intolerant of the faintest light or slightest noise, scarce venturing to speak, and complaining of intense headache. In the evening she became violently delirious. She did not know me, declared that she heard noises and saw people about her bed ; and she referred to the late occurrence as if giving me information respecting it. The delirium which occurred then and subsequently was of a curious, half-rational character ; the subjects referred to were accurate in their nature and in their reference ; but the error consisted in the unrestrained and violent manner in which they were adduced, and in the want of co-ordination in associating them with one another.

The night was again sleepless, but by the evening of the following day she was quiet and almost rational, when it was necessary to mention the arrival of a sister, who was associated in my patient's mind with the original occurrence. In an instant the whole scene was changed. She started up, indignantly denied being ill, again asserted the presence of people, and almost in a shriek repeated what they said ; then she recurred to the preceding events, and repeated her account of them. She did not recognise her sister, but, referring to my having said that she was come to nurse her, she told me that a tall, rude nurse had been in the room and had shaken her.

On the day after, the patient had come to herself, but still could not bear light nor noise, nor take food on account of the irritability of her stomach. She entered into conversation about affairs, which it was necessary to permit her to do, but at the close of a perfectly coherent conversation a chance remark, having the remotest connexion with the original provocation, was dropped by one of us, and instantly the former scene, with every detail wonderfully alike, was renewed; but in a short time she regained composure, and, having been reminded by something of what she had before been saying, she returned to her family affairs, and repeated her directions with perfect precision. Sixteen days later, when recovery was progressing, delirium and excitement occurring unexpectedly, revealed the presence of uneasiness and suspicion, over which she had been brooding. The death of this lady, some few years after, affords a striking comment on the foregoing details: it was occasioned by anæmia apparently due entirely to the removal by death of the one relative to whom every thought of her life had for a long succession of years been entirely given up.

My first three cases of chorea are examples of intense excitement from fright, which had made a profound and lasting impression upon the patient. A marked alteration in their nervous and physical health dated from the occurrence of the original excitement, and remained through a considerable length of time. The attack of chorea which resulted was but one element in a generally altered state of the nervous functions; it was but one of the consequences of the violent excitement to which the patient had been exposed. It did not show itself at any fixed period after the receipt of the shock, nor did it observe any close relation with intensity of the apparent cause.

Case 1.—A very emotional girl, aged twenty-one, was greatly alarmed by a dog flying at her; and fell into a succession of hysterical fits. She remained "sickly and low" afterwards. Six weeks after, in going to work, she saw a little boy nearly knocked down by a horse. On arriving at her shop she was asked what was the matter with her; her appearance was said to be changed; she was told that she was not like the same person. She cried a good deal, and on setting to work found that she could not hold things in her right hand; when going home she staggered as if tipsy. She was very feverish during the night, and had violent headache the next day, when chorea (right unilateral) set in with some severity, much increased by agitation and sleeplessness. Heart healthy (one examination). Patient was not rheumatic.

Case 2.—A girl, aged fourteen, stated to have been of even temper, and favourably circumstanced. She was sitting by her father when he fell dead; she was greatly excited, and had been quite changed ever since. The same day, or the following, she was attacked with rheumatic fever, for which she was in bed for three weeks. Six months later, after some return of rheumatic symptoms, she was taken quite suddenly with chorea. She was "seized as though she were going to 'have a fit,'" and in one night the movements extended over the entire body. Sleep entirely deserted her, and the movements continued without intermission, night and day. The chorea rapidly assumed its most violent form; articulation and then deglutition became impracticable, and she died on the tenth day of the chorea. It is to be noted that in her agitation during the night she often called for her father, whose sudden death seemed to have constituted the original disturbing cause. A post-mortem was refused. The condition of her heart could not be satisfactorily ascertained.

Case 3.—A girl, aged seventeen, badly fed and over-worked, not rheumatic, was upset in a boat whilst menstruating, and was in much danger. She was greatly altered by the accident: menstruation was at once arrested; she became nervous and frightened, afraid of going to bed in the dark (she was never nervous before); she had disturbed nights and frightful dreams; became violently passionate; wasted considerably; her aunt, to whom she came after her illness began, noticed a great change in the girl's temper and general nutrition. The choreic movements began very gradually directly after the accident, and were hardly noticed at the time; but she was compelled to leave work at the end of the first week from inability to thread her needle.

The movements have been confined to the left side, and have never exceeded a medium degree of severity; but the emotional excitement was very prominent throughout. The girl was thin and ill-nourished, and menstruation had been suspended for four months. She presented a mitral bruit, possibly due to scarlet fever.

(*To be continued.*)

OVARIOTOMY AT LIVERPOOL WORKHOUSE.

By WILLIAM ALEXANDER, M.D., F.R.C.S.,
Visiting Surgeon to the Workhouse.

TEN ovariotomies is a small number to write about in these days, when such cases are usually published in series of fifty each. But this larger experience has only fallen to the lot of three or four special ovariotomists. Ten cases is a comparatively large number from a workhouse hospital and from a general surgeon, and may prove as interesting to general readers as a larger number would from specialists.

Besides, several of these cases presented peculiarities in symptoms, operative details, or in subsequent treatment, and in Case 6 the complications, treatment, and result are almost, if not quite, unparalleled in the annals of ovariotomy.

To secure a paper of reasonable length, the cases will be divested of all unnecessary details, and the uncomplicated successes will be dismissed in a very few words.

Case 1.—The first ovariotomy ever performed in this hospital was on a woman sixty years of age, a hawker of vegetables. Her family and personal history were favourable to the operation: her state of health, though much reduced, did not contraindicate it; whilst her indomitable spirit encouraged the hope that she would survive. Eighteen months before operation the tumour was noticed in the left iliac region, and ascribed to a bruise produced by carrying heavy loads in her apron. The tumour gradually increased until, in six months, she thought it necessary to seek medical relief. The result was that paracentesis was performed, and thirty-one pints of fluid removed. Five months after this, thirty-three pints were removed. In seven months more she became alive to the necessity for a more radical operation, and was admitted to hospital. Dr. Graham, *locum tenens* for my predecessor, Mr. Barnes, operated on July 10, 1872, and removed a multilocular cyst which weighed five pounds and a half. A few adhesions required to be cauterised, and the pedicle was secured by the clamp. Half an hour after the commencement of the operation the patient was comfortably in bed. No spray was used, but a large ward had been disinfected, in which the operation and subsequent treatment were carried out. Brandy and beef-tea were administered frequently by enemata during the first few days. Sickness and vomiting were troublesome symptoms during the 12th, 13th, and 14th, but were relieved by oxalate of cerium. Diarrhœa nearly carried the patient off on the 18th and 19th; it was checked by laudanum injections. The clamp was removed on the 20th. From this date the patient progressed rapidly. This case is an example of a success in a very old woman. I saw her some time ago; she was becoming very feeble, and a fistula was discharging at the seat of the operation-wound.

Case 2.—Margaret W., aged fifty-five, married, the mother of one child, was admitted under my care on January 21, 1879, suffering from a right ovarian tumour of seven months' duration. She had been tapped on several occasions, and after each tapping had suffered from abdominal pains and feverishness for some days. I performed the operation on January 29, and removed a multilocular cyst that weighed 18 lbs. 6 ozs. The peritoneum was covered with lymph, both on its visceral and parietal layers, and large masses of inspissated pus were removed from dependent spots in the abdominal cavity. The operation was performed under the spray, the pedicle was clamped, and the wound was dressed with carbolic oil. Owing to the large size of the tumour and its gelatinous contents, the wound reached from the umbilicus to the pubes. Small quantities of iced water and beef-tea were allowed during the first forty-eight hours. On the third day, the temperature, which had previously ranged from 102° to 104·2°, fell to 99° to 101·4°. Thirst and a short cough that had troubled her very much the day before began to abate, and in the evening she went to sleep without the morphia injections which had been required since the operation. Next morning I got an urgent message to visit her, and found her semi-conscious, with rapid, noisy breathing, and feeble, intermittent pulse. She had passed a good night, and felt comfortable until an hour before I was sent for, when her breathing began to trouble her. Her temperature was 104·2°. Death took place two hours afterwards.

On post-mortem examination the lungs were found to be very much congested; the left one being much smaller than usual, and collapsed. The heart was thin and flabby, but without distinct valvular disease. The peritoneum was in exactly the same state as at the time of operation, except that some more pus was found. The abdominal wall was healthy, its edges adherent. A small quantity of pus was found on the pedicle beneath the clamp. The other organs were fairly healthy.

Remarks.—I am inclined to think this patient was underfed after the operation, and a more liberal diet has been prescribed to my cases since. Had her strength been kept up a little more, the effusion into the lungs might not have taken place, and a little extra movement of the bowels could hardly have aggravated the serious peritonitis that existed. Although a certain amount of peritonitis was suspected before the operation, neither the temperature, the state of the patient, nor the abdominal tenderness seemed at all proportionate to the amount of mischief that was then found.

Case 3.—Margaret M., aged twenty-four, who has a brother afflicted with Pott's curvature, was admitted on May 5, 1879, suffering from an ovarian tumour of eighteen months' duration. Ovariotomy was performed on May 21, and a monocystic growth was removed, which contained twenty-four pints of straw-coloured fluid. A few adhesions were broken down easily by the finger, and did not require cauterisation. The temperature only reached 102° on the second day. Except flatulence and a little cough, no bad symptoms occurred. When dressing the wound on the second day I inserted a small piece of oiled lint beneath the clamp and round the pedicle, with the object of keeping the parts free from suppuration. On the fourth day I removed the clamp altogether—a practice which I have since followed to the comfort and advantage of the patients. The after-treatment in this and the subsequent cases consisted in giving the patient a morphia and atropine injection as soon as she recovered from the effects of the anæsthetic (ether). When she again awoke she had Liebig's extract and iced water in small and frequent doses for several days, until she complained of being hungry; then small quantities of tea and dry toast were allowed. No morphia was ever used unless the patient complained of pain or became restless, when an injection was at once administered. Charcoal lozenges were of great benefit in relieving flatulence. The patient went to town on July 14, quite well.

Case 4.—Mary M., aged fifty-four, a general servant, the mother of one child, was admitted to hospital on May 20, 1880. Had intermittent fever twenty years ago. Had no other illness till last last year, when she began to suffer from exoruciating pains in her stomach, accompanied by frequent vomiting. By poulticing and some medicine obtained at the Stanley Hospital she was completely relieved. On April 14 the pains returned, and have continued more or less up to the time of her admission. Menstruation ceased six years ago. On examination at the time of admission a moderate-sized movable tumour was felt, and diagnosed as ovarian. The abdomen was rather tender, but there was no evidence of peritonitis. Ovariotomy was performed on June 23, when a unilocular, semi-solid cyst, one pound in weight, was removed. The interior of the cyst was partially decomposed, dark-coloured, and smelt badly. The future progress of the case gave no cause for anxiety, except that on July 5 the temperature ran up from 99° to 103·6°, on account of a small abscess that had formed in the seat of a catgut ligature. The patient was quite well by July 10. The decomposed state of this tumour serves as an introduction to the more serious state of matters found in the next case.

Case 5.—Ellen R., aged thirty-one, married, three children; admitted June 23, 1880. Her parents are still alive, and her grandfather died at the age of 104. She has had no serious illness, and her confinements have been favourable. The last confinement occurred fifteen months ago. Three months ago she began to complain of cramps in the abdomen,

"dry retching," and dysuria, accompanied by a menstrual flow—the first since her last child was born. She has been "regular" since, but the above symptoms have troubled her constantly. A unilocular, freely movable ovarian cyst was diagnosed, and as the patient was a strong, clean-limbed, well-developed, and courageous woman, an operation was contemplated with satisfaction by both surgeon and patient. A fortnight was to have elapsed before operation.

On June 30 the patient complained of great pain in the abdomen and down the left thigh, vomiting, and dysuria. She was very thirsty, and her temperature 108°. The tumour could not be felt in the abdomen, but had fallen into the pelvis. Under ether it was partially returned to its original place. Next day it was again in the pelvis, whence it could not be dislodged. Peritonitis had now commenced, and means directed to check this and to relieve pain were employed. On the morning of July 6 the patient was much reduced and in great distress, praying that something might be done for her. I opened the abdomen in the usual way. The normal-sized uterus presented, pressed upwards and forwards by a tumour lying behind. Above the uterus the tumour was covered by an adherent coil of dark inflamed intestine. In all my ovariotomies it has been a custom to keep the abdominal wall well pressed against the tumour, so that no blood, air, or spray can get into the abdominal cavity, and it was well that this was being done now. On attempting to turn aside the before-mentioned coil of intestine, the ovarian cyst burst, and about two quarts of abominably foul-smelling material ran away over the patient's legs and outside of the abdomen. The cyst was then completely emptied by sponges; and a large quantity of material like dirty wet tow, similar to the contents of the cyst in Case 4, but more offensive, was thus removed. As the cyst was adherent over a very large area of the posterior wall of the abdomen as well as to the intestines it could not be safely removed. The lower wall of the cyst was closely contiguous to the posterior wall of the vagina close to the uterine neck. Through the most contiguous parts a half-inch drainage-tube was passed per vaginam, and the cyst was thoroughly washed out with Condy's fluid, the tube left in, and the abdominal walls closed. Carbolic oil dressings were applied, surmounted by an ice-bag. The vaginal tube projected over the edge of the bed into a basin of carbolic acid solution. Five minims of morphia and atropine were injected. Midnight: Temperature 106·2°; respirations 24; pulse 96. Has taken some ice and four ounces of Liebig's extract. Six ounces of urine drawn per catheter.

July 7.—4 a.m.: Temperature 105°; pulse 96; respirations 31. Slept two hours. 8 a.m.: Temperature 100·8°; pulse 81; respirations 31. Much pain in abdomen; three ounces of urine drawn off; wound dressed; cyst syringed from below with Condy's fluid. 12 p.m.: Temperature 99°; respirations 20; pulse 86; restless. Wound dressed; the fresh lint gives her ease.

8th.—8 a.m.: Temperature 99·6°; respirations 20; pulse 98. 12 p.m.: Temperature has not risen all day—now 93·2°; perspiring.

9th.—8 a.m.: Temperature 100·8°. At 11 a.m. much pulmonary oppression; abdomen tense; wound bulging. Three stitches taken out, and a pint of fœtid pus removed from abdomen by syringing with Condy's fluid. Vaginal tube ceased to act and was withdrawn. (For a week afterwards the vagina was syringed at each dressing, although scarcely any matter came from it.) The ovarian cyst had collapsed, and the discharge came through the abdominal wound from a large cavity in the right iliac fossa. Until July 14, morning and evening washings were persevered with, the temperature during that time fluctuating between 99° and 101°, and the patient taking a fair quantity of food.

14th.—Bowels much distended. At 8 a.m. a starch enema administered to induce a mild action of the bowels, which have not been moved since the operation. At 9 p.m., temperature 102·4°; pulse 86; respirations 20. Distension so great that breathing very distressing. A purified aspirator-needle passed into colon. Gas came away for about a minute with a noise as loud as that produced by opening the safety-valve of a primed steam-spray. The relief was immediate and intense.

15th.—8 a.m.: The distension is increasing; temperature 102°; respirations 22; pulse 101. Vomiting; bowels not opened. Long tube of stomach-pump passed up to sigmoid flexure, and a small turpentine enema given. Some flatus came down through tube. Some flatus during the day Vomited twice.

16th.—8 a.m.: Temperature 100°; respirations 22; pulse 96. Has had a restless night. Long tube again passed, and enema given. Patient slightly delirious. 4 p.m.: Bowels rumbling.

17th.—Bowels opened this morning. Patient much relieved.

18th.—8 a.m.: A bedsore forming over right trochanter; abdominal cavity granulating; cystitis and increase of temperature (102·4°). Bladder washed out with carbolic acid.

21st.—Cystitis has subsided. Ceased to wash out bladder. Abdomen strapped, and patient laid on side.

August 9.—Wound almost closed. Patient has got a strong abdominal belt, which gives her much relief. Is getting stout. To sit up daily.

September 4.—Walked about for the first time; feels fairly strong.

October 4.—Discharged strong and well, with uterus in position, abdominal wall closed, and wearing an abdominal belt, which she was warned always to use.

Case 6.—Mary G., aged thirty-seven, single, was admitted to the medical wards in the beginning of June, 1880, suffering from rheumatism of the legs. An ovarian tumour of about six months' standing was found, and about the size of the adult human head. It was freely movable, monocystic, and apparently free from adhesions. On September 1 the abdomen was opened. A thick, fleshy pedicle came into view, running from the right side of the uterus over the front of the tumour, where it was attached to its upper and anterior part. The pedicle was detached, clamped, and held out of the way. The tumour, though freely movable, was found to lie behind the peritoneum, the peritoneum being so stretched as to allow considerable movement. Enucleation was impossible, and to remove both tumour and peritoneum would have stripped the greater part of the pelvis of that membrane. The cyst was cleared of fluid. Its interior was clean and pearly in hue. Half the cyst was removed, ligatures being applied to any vessels, and the pelvic cavity was then sponged out. All went on well till next evening. The temperature was then only 99°; but vomiting began. No remedies had the slightest effect upon the vomiting, and the patient died exhausted at 4 a.m. on September 3. The temperature remained at 99° till six hours before death, when it rose to 105°.

A post-mortem showed a healthy wound, a clean pelvis, and congested intestines covered with a clammy fibro-sanguineous effusion.

This case might be excluded from our list as an *incomplete* ovariotomy.

Case 7.—Mary Ann H., aged twenty-four, single, unfortunate; three children. She suffered from dropsy four months ago, when she was tapped, and seventeen quarts of water taken away. The abdomen enlarged again, and she was admitted May 25, 1880, with a large ovarian tumour. The operation took place on June 5. Twenty pints of dark-coloured fluid were removed from the cyst, and the cyst itself weighed 2 lbs. 6 oz. She was treated as the others, and made an excellent recovery.

Case 8.—Alice R., aged eighteen, single, hawker. Has been much exposed to cold and wet. Twelve months ago she suffered from abdominal pains and subsequent abdominal swelling. She was admitted June 30, 1880, with an enormous quantity of fluid in abdomen, and with the rest of the body much emaciated. On July 7, paracentesis abdominis was performed, and twenty-one pints of sero-purulent fluid were removed. A large movable tumour was then felt, and diagnosed as ovarian. The patient was impatient to have an operation performed, and, though the case was admittedly a forlorn hope, her age and eagerness induced me to perform ovariotomy next day. Great masses of pus were found in the abdomen, and everything therein was covered by a layer of lymph. A large multilocular cyst weighing seven pounds was removed, and the pedicle (four inches broad and one inch and a quarter thick) was partly ligatured and partly clamped. The abdomen was carefully and gently cleaned out, the wound closed, and the patient laid between warm blankets. After the first morphia-induced sleep a slight cough troubled her; but this was not greater than in several other cases, and was a small complication in view of a thoroughly unreasoning and cross-grained obstinacy that characterised

her until an hour before her death. She was not delirious, but got out of bed, struck the nurses, tore off her bandages, called for potatoes, refused medicines—in a word, was perfectly unmanageable. The congestion of the lungs increased, and the patient died on the fourth day after operation, to the intense relief of all concerned.

After her death I heard that her unmanageable temperament was habitual. In subsequent cases I have looked more to the temperament as an important factor in the chances of recovery.

On post-mortem examination both lungs were collapsed and saturated. The abdomen was in almost the same condition as at the time of the operation.

Case 9.—Ellen M., aged forty, a charwoman; married, no children. Admitted December 1, 1880. A "lump" came in abdomen fifteen years ago, and has been slowly increasing till the present time. She suffered no inconvenience from it till lately, when it began to pain her. Ovariotomy was performed on December 16, and a multilocular, semi-solid, gelatinous tumour removed, weighing 3 lbs. 2½ ozs. Pedicle clamped, and spray-gauze treatment used. The temperature rose during the first few days to 100°, but there were no accompanying symptoms, and in a month the patient was quite well.

Case 10.—Mary C., aged thirty-nine; married, no children. Was admitted in May, 1880, suffering from a large multilocular cyst of two years' duration. It was removed a fortnight after. The notes of this case have been lost, but she made an uncomplicated recovery.

Remarks.—Such are all the ovariotomies that have ever been *attempted* in the Liverpool Workhouse, and although the shortest readable sketch has been given, the paper is already too long to permit further remarks. Besides, my experience is too limited for generalisation. I would only say that the employment of the clamp did not seem to influence the mortality, and that the more Listerian the anti-septicity the better the result.

CASE OF MICROCEPHALUS.—In the *New York Medical Record* for June 11, Dr. Mary Putnam Jacobi publishes a paper which she read at the Neurological Society, giving a detailed account of a case of microcephalus which recently came under her notice.

DURING a residence of eighteen months in Ningpo, I have been very much struck by the absence from amongst the members of the community of the habitual deposit of urates in the urine—the condition termed lithuria,—whereas during a long residence in Chefoo I found it frequently existing amongst the foreigners. This pathological difference between the two localities led me to make inquiry of an individual who had removed from Chefoo to Shanghai, and who had formerly been very much subject to the deposit. As to his present state, he told me that after the change of locality he became entirely free from it, even after moderate excesses in diet. In Chefoo he had, like others similarly affected, to exercise the greatest caution in regard to diet, as any strain upon his liver was at once followed by the deposit. In those subject to lithuria, as a rule, the deposit immediately appeared after the consumption of an immoderate amount of any article of diet, solid or liquid, with the exception of two, in which excess would be difficult, viz., bread and water. From another individual who had resided in Chefoo I got a like experience. Previous to his taking up his abode in Chefoo he had not been troubled with the affection. After residing there for some time he lost weight considerably. This he was able to regain in part when in full exercise, but it was lost again when the exercise was relaxed. Now, with change of residence to the south, he has recovered his original weight. A third individual, with a strong tendency to lithuria, was compelled periodically to seek temporary refuge in a moister climate, and invariably returned in a state of vigour, which he could not otherwise have attained. A fourth was so affected with lithæmia that his medical adviser ordered him to leave Chefoo, and the change was followed by the happiest results. The explanation of the presence of the deposit in the one locality and its absence in the other seems to be found in the difference between the two climates—the northern being dry, and the southern moist.—*Dr. W. A. Henderson, in the "Medical Reports of the Imperial Maritime Customs of China."*

REPORTS OF HOSPITAL PRACTICE
IN
MEDICINE AND SURGERY.

ST. THOMAS'S HOSPITAL.

A SERIES OF CASES OF MAMMARY CANCER, WITH REMARKS ON TREATMENT AFTER OPERATION.(a)

(Under the care of Mr. JOHN CROFT.)

Case 1 (Dresser, Mr. Davies).—A. H., aged fifty-four, married; mother of twelve children, eight of which died during infancy, remaining four healthy. Her father died at the age of eighty-six, her mother at seventy; her brothers all healthy; had no sisters. Her husband is healthy; two of his sisters died of cancer of the breast.

Tumour had been noticed ten months; it is about as large as a walnut; there is some sharp pricking pain in it. It appears to be increasing slightly in size. It occupies left breast; skin is not adherent, and it is freely movable over the pectoral muscle. The nipple is retracted. There is one small gland, high up in the axilla, doubtfully enlarged.

She was admitted March 31, 1873, and on April 2 the breast was removed. The tumour measured two inches and a half transversely, and was about three-quarters of an inch thick. It was intensely hard. On section, a quantity of fluid escaped from what proved to be dilated tubes and acini. It was surrounded by a large quantity of fat, and had no adhesions to the pectoral fascia. The wound was closed with silk sutures, and covered with a compress of lint soaked in carbolic oil (one to twenty). A drainage-tube was put in.

April 3.—Temperature 100° Fahr.

4th.—Temperature 99° Fahr.

9th.—The wound looked well, "but there was not much union"; the discharge slight.

12th.—Had a sharp attack of hemorrhage; wound had to be opened up, and the vessel ligatured.

15th.—"Wound granulating; free discharge of pus."

April 22.—To get up. Wound healed, except just in centre; scar rather puckered; no tenderness. Discharged.

Case 2 (Dresser, Mr. Armstrong).—E. W., aged thirty-nine, married; mother of three children, all of whom were suckled, and are healthy. There was no history of tumours in the family. Catamenia commenced at the age of twelve; have been very irregular during the past few months. The tumour occupies the right breast; it has been coming for twelve months, during which time there has been a slight but constant discharge from the nipple, which is now retracted. The tumour is hard and nodular, adherent to the skin; there is constant pain of a pricking, shooting character, running down the arm.

Admission, April 17, 1874. Amputation of breast, May 6. After removal, the tumour was found to be a typical scirrhus. The wound was dressed in the same manner as the preceding case.

May 17.—Erysipelas supervened, and patient was removed to isolation ward. She recovered, and was discharged on June 19.

Case 3 (Dresser, Mr. Boys).—H. B., aged forty-nine, unmarried. She had first noticed a discharge from the nipple of the left breast twelve months ago; two months later (that is, ten months before admission), she found a lump near the nipple, which was retracted. The tumour gradually increased in size until lately, when the increase had been much more rapid. There was a stabbing pain in the breast, which extended down the back. There were no enlarged glands in the axilla. The skin over the breast was not involved, and the tumour moved freely on the subjacent structures. Two of her sisters had died of "tumours—one with stoppage of bowels, and another with tumour over the stomach."

Admitted October 28, 1874. Operation, October 30. The entire breast was removed under chloroform. There was

some considerable hæmorrhage. A drainage-tube was inserted, and the wound covered with a compress of lint soaked in carbolic oil (one to twenty).

November 5.—The sutures were removed; the sternal end of the wound was healed, but from the other extremity there was an offensive discharge. A drainage-tube was put in. Temperature since operation has varied from 97·9° to 102·8° Fahr.

10th.—Patient was removed to a separate ward on account of difficulty in breathing.

November 14.—She died. During this day the temperature rose to 103·4° Fahr.; pulse 140; and respirations 50. There was no *post-mortem* examination, but the symptoms indicated pretty clearly that death resulted from broncho-pneumonia. She had suffered from bronchitis for some time previous to the operation.

Case 4. (Dresser, Mr. Moullin).—E. D., aged forty; married, no children. There is no family history of tumours of any kind. First noticed eighteen months ago, when it was the size of a nut. Has grown much during last two months. There is pain of a stabbing character in it. Nipple is not retracted. The tumour is now as large as a hen's egg, and very hard; freely movable. There is no œdema of arm, no axillary glandular swelling; and the skin is not visibly involved, but is adherent to the tumour.

Admitted, March 11, 1875. Operation, March 27. The whole breast was removed. All the bleeding vessels were twisted. A small hardened gland was felt in, and removed from, the axilla. Flaps were closed by silver sutures, and were rather tense. Drainage-tube was put in, and the wound covered with a compress of lint soaked in carbolic oil.

March 29.—Wound dressed; looked well; was washed with carbolic lotion, strapped, and a pad of oiled lint applied; over this a quantity of cotton-wool.

April 1.—Sloughing at edges of wound where the tension was greatest. A poultice was ordered for a day or two, after which the carbolic oil and lint were resumed.

May 13.—Was discharged. The wound was not quite healed.

Case 5 (Dresser, Mr. Green).—F. F., aged fifty-six, widow. Has had several children, the last fifteen years ago; catamenia ceased at the age of fifty-one. She first noticed a tumour in her (right) breast sixteen months ago; it was then as large as a good-sized walnut, situate at the upper and outer part of the breast, close to the nipple, which was retracted. The skin over the tumour was adherent to it and puckered; it was not very circumscribed, but diffused itself gradually into the surrounding tissue, especially towards the axilla. She knew of no cause to account for it; there was no family history of tumours. Two sisters and one brother had died of consumption. The tumour moved freely on the pectoral muscle. On examining the axilla an enlarged and indurated gland could be distinctly felt; this had been known of four months. On pressing the nipple a brown watery fluid was expelled.

Admitted into the Hospital, December 7, 1874. Operation, December 19. The whole breast was removed under chloroform, and the affected glands from the axilla were dissected out, exposing the vessels and nerves. The skin at the bottom of the wound was pierced for a drainage-tube. The flaps were brought together and secured by silver-wire sutures. A compress of lint soaked in carbolic oil was applied.

December 27.—The last of the sutures was removed to-day. Edges of the wound were found united. There was no gaping anywhere. Patient is feeling quite well, and wants to get up.

January 15, 1875.—She was discharged.

(To be continued.)

IMPRISONMENT FOR NOT REPORTING INFECTIOUS DISEASES.—Dr. Alphonso Oulman, of Brooklyn, having refused to pay a fine of $50 imposed on him for failing to report a case of small-pox, has been sent to gaol. The law which compels physicians to report cases of infectious disease, whether they will or not, and without any compensation for the trouble, is arbitrary and without any foundation in equity. Since the law exists, however, physicians must abide by it, unless they wish to break it for the purpose of testing its legality.—*New York Med. Record*, June 11.

(a) The series of tumours at our disposal embraces forty cases, and represents what may be called the time before antiseptics were generally used, and the present period of strict Listerian precautions. Typical cases will be selected from each, and then some remarks will be made on the series.

TERMS OF SUBSCRIPTION.

(*Free by post.*)

British Islands	*Twelve Months*	.	£1	8	0
„	*Six*	„	.	0 14	0
The Colonies and the United }	*Twelve*	„	.	1 10	0
States of America . . . }					
„ „ „	*Six*	„	.	0 15	0
India	*Twelve*	„	.	1 10	0
„ (*viâ Brindisi*) . . .	„	„	.	1 15	0
„ „ „	*Six*	„	.	0 15	0
„ (*viâ Brindisi*)	„	„	.	0 17	6

*Foreign Subscribers are requested to inform the Publishers of
any remittance made through the agency of the Post-office.*

*Single Copies of the Journal can be obtained of all Booksellers
and Newsmen, price Sixpence.*

Cheques or Post-office Orders should be made payable to Mr.
JAMES LUCAS, 11, *New Burlington-street, W.*

TERMS FOR ADVERTISEMENTS.

Seven lines (70 words) . . .	.£0	4	6
Each additional line (10 words) .	. 0	0	6
Half-column, or quarter-page .	. 1	5	0
Whole column, or half-page . .	. 2	10	0
Whole page	. 5	0	0

Births, Marriages, and Deaths are inserted Free of Charge.

THE MEDICAL TIMES AND GAZETTE *is published on Friday
morning: Advertisements must therefore reach the Publishing Office not later than One o'clock on Thursday.*

Medical Times and Gazette.

SATURDAY, JULY 16, 1881.

THE SANITARY CONDITION OF THE ROMAN HOTELS.

THE *Italian Times* of the 2nd of this month contains a report of its Sanitary Commission, giving the general results
of the inspection of the hotels of Rome. The Commissioners
inspected the Hotels Quirinale, Constanzi, Bristol, Molaro,
Anglo-Americano, Inghilterra, Europa, Russie, Vittoria,
Parigi, Pace, Roma, Della Città, Aliberti, Londra, Minerva,
and Louvre; and the Pensions Tullenbach and Smith; and
they found that in all of them the appliances adopted for the
exclusion of sewer-gas were inadequate. The water-closets,
built usually one above the other, open, as a rule, freely into
the air, but into courts so narrow that real ventilation is impossible; and as the doors of the closets generally open directly
on to corridors, passages, or staircases, any gases from the
closets would escape into the hotel at least as easily as into
the air. The Commissioners made "such recommendations for
better ventilation of the closets as their construction and position rendered practicable." The closets in all the hotels, with
but one exception, were provided with pan-basins; but in
many the water was quite insufficient in quantity, though in
some of the hotels the supply for the closets was very fair.
The pans, themselves untrapped, discharged into soil-pipes,
which were trapped at their entrance with the house-drains
in one or two instances only. The soil-pipes were generally
carried up to open above the roofs or under the cornices;
but frequently the rain-water pipes were used as their ventilators. The pipes were usually made of glazed earthenware,
and were almost always built into the walls so as to be
hidden from the sight, but the walls so used were rarely the
walls of bedrooms. House-drains were always built of
brick or tufa; were almost universally square in shape; and
were never specially ventilated, nor had any flushing arrangements, save in one hotel. The man-holes into these
drains were, as a rule, untrapped, and the coverings often
perforated or not hermetically sealed. The openings of sink,
lavatory, and bath waste and overflow pipes were usually
untrapped. Urinals existed in only a few hotels. They
had always a constant water-supply, but were untrapped.
These are the chief defects and imperfections noticed by
the Commission, and they are just what might have
been expected to be found. The Commissioners say they
"think it right to state their belief that the same faults
of construction and want of sanitary appliances found by
them in Rome, would probably be found in every hotel in
Italy, and in almost all the hotels on the Continent"; and
we will add that we more than suspect they may be found to
exist, in varying degree, in very many hotels in England.
The Commissioners made various recommendations in the
way of syphons, bell-traps, and ventilation pipes; and all
the landlords and proprietors have promised that these recommendations shall be carried out, and have invited the
Commissioners to revisit their hotels in October, to ascertain in what manner the improvements have been effected.
We fear that, considering the description given of some
of the most marked defects, as the construction of the
water-closets, it will be almost impossible to effect any
very great improvement in them in the existing hotels;
but no doubt the inspection and the recommendations
made will result in really considerable benefits; and
it must be allowed that great credit is due to the
proprietors of the *Italian Times*, and to the physicians who
gave so much time and unpaid labour to the work of the
Commission, for the public spirit displayed by them all.
We only further observe that the Commissioners' report
that the drinking-water in every hotel was found good.
The closets had often a quite distinct supply from that
used for drinking. No pozzo (or well) water was used in any
of the hotels; and in only one hotel, supplied with Trevi
water, was the water-pipe led into an underground pit, and
thence pumped into the cistern; and attention was called to
the risk attending the use of the pit. The Commissioners
report that the water-supply, which is so abundant and so
good in Rome, cannot be a source of danger in any of the
hotels inspected.

The Italian Medical Association, to whose hostility to the
Commission we have before referred, have not been able
to resist casting some pebbles at the proceedings of the
Commission and at the *Italian Times*. The Roman Committee of the Association held extraordinary general meetings to consider the whole matter in May and June, and
on July 1 agreed to several resolutions regarding the Commission, the condition of the hotels, the health of Rome, and
the action of the *Italian Times*. They consider, among other
things, that the "criticisms of the said journal are offensive
to the dignity of the medical community and the interests
of the city of Rome"; and that the hotels to which strangers
resort are found in regular hygienic condition as regards the
construction of water-closets; they "deplore the action of
the *Italian Times*"; and they pray that the municipal
authority may always show more and more interest for
the hygiene of the city, and may publish the operations
of the Special Commission it has already nominated for
the purpose." The last resolution really justifies the action
of the *Italian Times* Commission, though of course that
was not by any means the intention of the Committee.
Certainly neither the journal concerned nor the Commission
need care for these proceedings. Such resolutions as were
agreed to cannot hurt them, and they amuse the Italian
Medical Association.

DIPHTHERIA IN GLASGOW AT THE BEGINNING OF THE NINETEENTH CENTURY.

THE current number (for July) of our contemporary the *Glasgow Medical Journal* contains some interesting contributions to the subject of diphtheria, its history and relations to croup. Dr. James Finlayson, of the Glasgow Western Infirmary, when commenting, a short time ago, to his clinical class on a case where a membranous exudation was found in the trachea only, stated that one of the most serious difficulties felt by many in accepting the identity of croup and diphtheria "might be termed the historical difficulty." By way of lessening this difficulty he has contributed a "Historical Note on the occurrence of Laryngeal and Tracheal Diphtheria in Glasgow at the Beginning of the Nineteenth Century"; and further has induced the editor (Dr. Joseph Coats) to print, for the first time, an admirable essay by Dr. Thomas Brown, Lecturer on Botany in the University of Glasgow, which was read before the Glasgow Medical Society in 1820, and which has been preserved in the manuscript volumes of their *Essays*.

Dr. Finlayson says:—"While it is generally admitted now that undoubted diphtheria, occurring, it may be, in the midst of ordinary cases of this disease, may begin and also end with an affection of the larynx or trachea only, it is also admitted that such an exclusive limitation is certainly rare in proportion to any given number of cases of diphtheria as the disease is met with at the present time." If cases of "cynanche trachealis," or "croup," were frequently recognised in this country at the end of the eighteenth or beginning of the nineteenth century by the physicians of the day, how can we account for the silence of such acute observers with regard to diphtheria affecting the fauces—supposing this disease were really prevalent at that time, and that the laryngeal cases formed only a fraction of the total number?

In reply to this it may be pointed out, and it has been pointed out frequently, that the silence alleged did not exist, although, of course, the word "diphtheria" was not employed.

Dr. Finlayson then refers to Home's original essay on croup, and points out that the first two fatal cases narrated (by Home) occurred in the same family, apparently within ten days of each other, and in the second of these there is some question of the tonsils being involved. Cheyne, also, in his treatise on Croup (1809) admits that he had repeatedly supposed he had to do with cases of croup in the second stage until he examined the fauces and found them seriously affected, and he was of opinion that all such cases, although closely resembling croup, ought to be classed separately.

As early as 1816, Dr. Robert Perry read a paper on Croup before the Glasgow Medical Society, in which he laments the want of success which attended the treatment of this affection, and he says that he lost two cases in the same family within eight days. We almost regret that this paper, the manuscript of which is preserved in one of the volumes of the Society's *Essays* in the Library of the Faculty of Physicians and Surgeons of Glasgow, has not been reprinted along with the others on the same subject to which we are now referring, for the above-mentioned fact alone would suffice to suggest that Dr. Perry had to do with an infectious disease, such as real croup (at that time) was not allowed to be.

In 1819, Dr. Finlayson tells us, an actual epidemic of typical diphtheria seems to have occurred in Glasgow. The cases are described in an admirable essay by Dr. Thomas Brown (to which we shall presently refer), which was read before the Glasgow Medical Society in 1820, and which is likewise preserved in manuscript in one of the volumes of the Society's *Essays*. The title of this paper—"Cases of Ulcerated Sore Throat, terminating in Croup"—is almost conclusive. It will be seen that most of the cases were complicated with croup; but others ran their course without this complication. Dr. Brown, in his introductory remarks, says that this disease "was remarkable for its intractable nature and for its almost uniform fatality, in spite of the most active and varied practice." The first case recorded is that of "Joan M'Gregor, aged two, September 2, 1819. After having been slightly indisposed or feverish for a day or two, she seemed to have some difficulty in swallowing, and on examining the throat, it was ascertained that the tonsils were covered with white-coloured aphthous crusts surrounded with some degree of inflammation. This complaint occasioned little alarm, and she continued without any marked fever or uneasiness for three days, when, without any obvious cause, she became affected with constant and alarming dyspnœa, arising from obstruction at the larynx, and attended with all the usual symptoms of croup. After suffering severely for two days, she died of suffocation."

"In this case, emetics, purgatives, and the warm bath were employed. Blood was taken from the arm till fainting came on. The throat was leeched and blistered. Calomel was most liberally exhibited. The tonsils were deeply scari[?]. and on the second day of the croupy symptoms a consultation was assembled to deliberate on the propriety of performing bronchotomy, but from the age of the child and from other considerations, it was thought unadvisable. No opportunity was obtained of inspecting the throat after death."

This child's sister, aged six, became affected with a similar kind of sore-throat about the same time. "These covered sores continued unabated for eight or nine days, when they gradually disappeared." In consequence of the striking similarity of this condition to that observed in the previously recorded fatal case, great alarm and anxiety were felt both by the physician and the patient's friends, and active measures were carried out. The larynx, however, never became affected, and at length health was restored. These children resided in the country, about a mile from the town, in an airy situation, and in a well-ventilated house.

Dr. Brown next relates some cases all occurring in the same family. He was called in to see a boy, aged nine, and was then informed that a child had just died of "croup, following ulcerated sore-throat." The patient, he says, "had all the symptoms which attend an extreme case of croup, joined to aphthous ulceration of the throat, if such an expression can be employed with propriety. The throat was studded with superficial excavations, and these were covered with crusts resembling curdled milk, though not so opaquely white. The surrounding inflammation was but trifling." The child coughed up large fragments of membrane with variable relief. The disease ran a typical course, and proved fatal from exhaustion on the eleventh day. "The usual practice of bleeding, blistering, vomiting, and purging was adopted." A little girl, aged five, "at the same time was confined to an adjoining room with an ulcerated sore-throat, which, however, differed materially from that of her brother. The ulcerations of the tonsils were quite distinct, and were not covered with aphthous crusts. There was also more inflammation around them. Along with this there was a considerable degree of fever, but there was no eruption on the surface of the body. In short, this case resembled exactly what is named 'cynanche maligna.' After nine days the ulcers of the throat were sensibly worse: they had become more deep and sloughy; and they had extended so far towards the larynx that the clear voice was quite lost, and there was some degree of croupiness in the cough, though the breathing was scarcely, if at all, affected. The skin was rather cold. The throat, which had been blistered eight days before, and which had been scarcely attended to, began to inflame, and the inflammation to extend over the breast. By the next day the blistered part was gangrenous, and she died soon after."

"In this same family there were four other children. Two of them, when the alarm was taken, were sent to Stirling, and these two, in a few days after the rest, took the aphthous sore-throat, but they recovered well without having any croup or any eruption."

"The two others remained in Glasgow, and of these a boy, aged four, also took the aphthous form of sore throat, but without much fever or any croup. He recovered in a short time under the use of laxatives, followed by bark and wine. The other child, an infant under a year old, did not take the disease. In this ill-fated family, therefore, of seven children, six took the disease, and of these three died."

We need hardly abstract the remaining cases contained in Dr. Brown's interesting paper. We, however, will mention one other—that of a child "affected with croup, which had followed a sore throat of the appearance formerly described"; for in this case the autopsy was made by the well-known ophthalmic surgeon, Dr. W. Mackenzie. He says: "We found the larynx inflamed, and covered with a firm membranous exudation, so thick as nearly to have obstructed the passage of the air. The same inflamed appearance and membrane, though less firm in its texture as you receded from the larynx, extended far into the lungs, and could even be traced to many of the minute ramifications of the trachea."

This author recapitulates in a few sentences the leading symptoms of the disease. "After a slight fever of one or two days' duration without vomiting, and indeed without much marked derangement, the throat was complained of, and when examined, the tonsils and velum palati were observed to be studded with aphthous crusts or specks of an opaque whitish appearance. These were surrounded with more or less inflammation. In the majority of instances these aphthæ were stationary, and after remaining for eight or ten days, they, as well as the attendant feverishness, were gradually removed, and health was restored. But in other cases this aphthous inflammation appeared to have a disposition to extend downwards to the larynx, creeping from one mucous membrane to the other, but without leaving the parts originally affected."

"In consequence of the mechanical obstruction to the passage of the air through the rima glottidis, both from the swelling occasioned by the inflammation and from the inflammatory exudation, the symptoms of croup were induced, which appeared to be of a very intractable nature and soon proved fatal."

In some "remarks" which follow this paper, Dr. Brown asks "Is this complaint a new disease?" He briefly alludes to various accounts of the "morbus strangulatorius," and its modes of onset at different times, and then says: "I have, therefore, now no doubt that this complaint has been often observed and described, and that it is merely a variety of cynanche maligna, in which, from some peculiarity in the causes acting on the constitution, there is an increased disposition to an affection of the windpipe. It is a fact well known in the history of different epidemics, that in particular seasons almost invariably every case shall be disposed to assume a character different from what is observed in the same disease at a different period. We are to regard this peculiar modification of cynanche maligna as produced by causes of whose nature we are ignorant. It is not heat, or cold, or moisture or its opposite, that disposed to this form of disease, for it prevailed from the month of August till December, in spite of every variety of weather."

Our author refers to its infectious nature; and in discussing its identity or relations with scarlet fever, he says in all these cases "the disease differed materially in its symptoms from those of scarlatina, and in none of the families was there any case of scarlet eruption."

He then comes to the question, *Are the ulceration of the throat in this disease, and that affection of the larynx which produces croup, of the same nature?* After posing this question, Dr. Brown says: "I am inclined to believe that there is a great similarity between these two affections, although at first sight they seem to differ from each other. On the tonsils and neighbouring parts we have inflammation attended with the effusion of detached portions of lymph, forming what is named aphtha, and in the larynx we have also an inflammatory exudation, which, however, appears to be effused with greater uniformity, and not in detached spots as on the fauces; and perhaps in this respect alone does one disease differ from the other. In short, I consider the croupy exudation as merely an extension of the aphthous crust from the tonsils and velum to the larynx and trachea, in the same manner as erysipelas diffuses itself, creeping from one surface to a neighbouring one, or as other inflammations extend to structures similar to those they have originally attacked."

This essay concludes as follows:—" . . . . This aphthous sore-throat, which in most instances has lately been so mild and trifling in its appearance as scarcely to attract attention, is in all probability highly infectious, and is nothing less than a mild variety of cynanche maligna or putrid sore-throat, a complaint which occasionally has been most fatal, even though confined to the fauces, and which in a different form, viz., that of croup, has been sufficiently alarming in this district."

There is also the reprint (from the *Edinburgh Medical and Surgical Journal*, April, 1825) of an article "On the Symptoms and Cure of Croup," by Dr. William Mackenzie (whose name we have already referred to), from which, as bearing on the identity of croup and diphtheria, we may quote the following passage:—"There is one fact, however, in the history of this disease which has not as yet been noticed by authors on this subject. . . . The fact to which I refer is that the exudation of fibrin very frequently commences on the surface of the tonsils, thence spreads along the arches of the palate, coats the posterior surface of the velum palati, sometimes surrounds and encloses the uvula; and at last descending, covers the internal surface of the pharynx and œsophagus, the larynx and trachea. That this is the frequent progress of the fibrinous exudation, I am convinced, from the careful and repeated observation of the phenomena during life and upon dissection."

Want of space alone prevents our commenting on these exceedingly interesting papers. Enough has been quoted to show that Dr. Brown gave a most accurate clinical as well as pathological description of what Bretonneau, a year later, described as diphtheria, and that Dr. William Mackenzie anticipated him (Bretonneau) in the opinion that "croup" was identical with membranous disease of the fauces, and that, although it might occur in the larynx alone, it (the membrane) not infrequently spread from the fauces to the larynx, when it at once became "croup."

Dr. Finlayson is to be congratulated for having unearthed these valuable essays, and Dr. Coats for having made them public. We must express a hope that, if the manuscript volumes of the Glasgow Medical Society contain any other such memoirs on this obscure subject, they too may in due course appear.

PLAGUE AND QUARANTINE.(a)

ALL who are interested in the advancement of epidemiological science—and the list should embrace the whole of the medical officers of the Army, Navy, and East Indian Service, as well as our professional brethren resident in the colonies or elsewhere abroad—will find much instructive matter in the new official Report on the late progress of the Levantine Plague, and on Quarantine.

The two elaborate documents prepared by Mr. Netten Radcliffe—(1) "On the Progress of Levantine Plague in 1878-79, including the Reappearance of the Disease in Europe," and (2) "On Quarantine in the Red Sea, and on the Sanitary Regulation of the Pilgrimage to Mecca," contain numerous trustworthy details and diverse information on various points that are little known to the public generally, and which yet promise to be of no small moment alike to the legislator and to the enlightened physician in the future elucidation of State medicine.

As our limited space precludes our doing more in regard of these subjects than to express our admiration of the industry of the author's researches, and the ability with which the whole narrative of his labours is drawn up and put forth in his pages, we shall at present merely extract two or three passages from the prefatory letter of Dr. Buchanan to the President of the Local Government Board, which will give the reader some idea of the important and varied value of Mr. Radcliffe's papers.

"In continuation of the memoranda concerning plague then (March, 1880) submitted to Parliament, Mr. Radcliffe now records the results of his study of the disease in its still more recent movements. By the help of a variety of documents, among which were the reports of the English, French, German, and Roumanian Commissioners on the Volga, he has brought the history of plague down to the end of 1879. Accordingly his present Report gives a detailed account of the Russian outbreak in the previous winter, and records the progress of the disease in the Assyr district of Western Arabia. Further, it gives detailed information as to the existence of plague during recent years in Western China, particularly in the province of Yunnan. Chief interest attaches to the history of the outbreak on the Lower Volga, where, after its many years of absence, plague reappeared in Europe." . . . .

"The outbreak on the Volga has been variously ascribed to importation of contagion from Resht, in Persia, in the course of trade along the Caspian, and to conveyance from infected places in Asia Minor by Cossacks returning from the seat of the Russo-Turkish War of 1877-78. But it would seem to be of little avail to demonstrate, if it were possible, one definite place of origin for this particular outbreak. Its analogies appear to be with occurrences of the disease in Mesopotamia, in Benghazi (North Africa), in the Assyr country, where, during the years 1874 and 1875, plague made its appearance in circumscribed epidemics of limited duration, coming and going under unknown or unexplained conditions, more after the fashion of a disease that requires for its prevalence some fresh development in customary unhealthy circumstances, than like a disease that depends altogether for its appearance upon the importation of a specific contagion from elsewhere. Mr. Radcliffe's Memorandum contains reasons for regarding in this light the outbreak on the Volga, as his former papers had led him to a like view of plague in other districts. There are, indeed, in the series of reports a good many indications of plague resembling typhus fever

(a) "Report and Papers on the Recent Progress of Levantine Plague, and on Quarantine in the Red Sea, submitted by the Medical Officer of the Local Government Board, in supplement to his Report for the year 1879." 8vo. Pp. 246. 1881.

(if not, as some have contended, in its nature) in its behaviour among populations living under conditions of privation, of squalor, and of overcrowding; and, just as it may be affirmed, from our knowledge of the condition of typhus, that European populations need no longer suffer from this scourge, so it may be expected that, as civilisation carries with it a knowledge of the elementary conditions for health, plague may, at least as an epidemic, be driven behind a more and more remote Asiatic and African frontier."

The maps accompanying the descriptions of the progress of plague in late years vividly illustrate what an amount of additional benefit to our correct knowledge of the natural history of epidemic diseases may be derived from accurate geographical and chronological details.

Besides the information respecting this form of pestilence, Mr. Radcliffe gives a highly interesting account of the past history of quarantine in respect of epidemic cholera during the last thirty or thirty-five years in this and other countries of Europe, and the present condition of this much debated question as to the real or the fancied utility of the restrictive measures included under that term.

"Mr. Radcliffe's Memorandum finds much matter for criticism in the administration of quarantine in the Red Sea, and, indeed, contains not a little in confirmation of views that have been often expressed to the Board by its medical officers, respecting the small assurance to public health that is afforded by quarantine imposed under such conditions as the necessities of modern existence ordain. But in the course of consideration of the whole subject, given in the Memorandum, there has arisen occasion for suggesting many ways in which progress can be made towards due regulation of the pilgrimage and efficient control over communicable diseases that may show themselves in the Red Sea. Under the present circumstances of the pilgrimage and of traffic through the Red Sea, it is seen, indeed, that there are difficulties to be overcome and international agreements to be arrived at, before the risk of cholera travelling towards Europe by way of the Red Sea can be reduced to its earlier proportions; but the object is of real importance, and is well worthy of pains for its attainment."

THE WEEK.

TOPICS OF THE DAY.

As the time for the assembling of the International Medical Congress approaches, the arrangements are gradually developing. His Royal Highness the Prince of Wales, whose intention to attend the opening ceremony was recently announced, has accepted an invitation to lunch with Sir James Paget after the meeting, and to dine in the evening with Sir William Gull, who has asked the Vice-Presidents and Council of the Medical Section, the Presidents of the other Sections, and several distinguished foreign visitors to meet His Royal Highness. The Prince has also intimated his intention of being present at the reception at the South Kensington Museum the same evening, when it is expected the Princess of Wales will accompany him. It has further been decided that the Corporation of the City of London shall give their entertainment to the members of the Congress on Friday, August 5, which will necessitate the postponement of the reception by the College of Surgeons until Monday, August 8. The Reception Committee of the Congress have had placed at their disposal 2000 cards of invitation for the Corporation soirée. Up to the present time nearly two thousand members of the profession have signified their intention of attending the Congress.

The Select Committee appointed to inquire into the subject of Artisans' and Labourers' Dwellings, requested the attendance of the Medical Officer of the Parish of St. George's-in-the-East, to give evidence. This gentleman stated that he made a representation to the Metropolitan Board, in 1875, under the Act of that year. In one district between the London Docks and the Thames, with an area of three acres and a quarter, there were 207 houses, and the population was 1593, or about 7·6 per house. One or two of the alleys were inhabited by the lowest class of labourers, and others by watermen and lightermen. There were a great number of Irish among the former, but not among the latter. The houses were generally unhealthy—in one, containing two rooms, there were as many as twelve people living. In others there were six persons living in two rooms of about 750 cubic feet each. The death-rate in the worst part of the district was 31 per 1000, and the rate all over the district was 25 per 1000. The No. 1 District only contained 27 or 30 houses, with a population of 200 or 250, and his representation was rejected because the place was too small. In the No. 2 District there were 55 houses, and the population was 254. His scheme in this case also had been rejected, and it was impossible to make use of the Torrens Act. It was in one of these courts that Charles Dickens' opium-smokers lived. The Medical Officer of Health from St. George's, Southwark, was also examined, and gave similar evidence. With the view of prosecuting their inquiries in every direction, the Select Committee recently paid a visit to East London for the purpose of viewing some of the sites taken for the erection of blocks of buildings under the Act, and to inspect some of the houses already finished. The districts visited were Upper East Smithfield, Lower Well-alley, Whitechapel, Salter's-alley, Flower-and-Dean-street, Spitalfields, and Limehouse, at some of which places the Peabody trustees are erecting large blocks of commodious dwellings, intended to supersede the horrible dens and rookeries with which these places now abound.

Our contemporary *Iron* draws attention to the fact that the New York Legislature have passed an Act which has caused great excitement among the plumbers of Brooklyn. It is now required, on sanitary grounds, that all new plumbing work shall be officially inspected before being covered, and the inspector, of course, has to be satisfied that there are no defects which are likely to endanger health. We agree with our contemporary in wishing that law-makers would pass a like common-sense and valuable law. On this side of the Atlantic we give lectures on plumbing, and tender advice wholesale and gratis, but we could not think of interfering with a class of artisans at whose mercy householders have been only too long. It is true we have made considerable progress in the matter of sanitary regulations, but we have not ventured yet even to talk of going to the length that our republican cousins in America have, in this and other instances, in interfering with that greatly worshipped idol, the liberty of the subject.

We are glad to aid in giving publicity to the fact that the Board of Trade has officially declared the exhibition of smoke-consuming apparatus, fuel, etc., to be held at South Kensington in October and November next, to be "calculated to promote British industry, and prove beneficial to the industrial classes." By this step protection is conferred on all inventions exhibited during the time of exhibition and for six months afterwards (in virtue of the Protection of Inventions Act, 1870). The Secretary of the Admiralty has also forwarded a communication, promising that the Admiralty will favourably consider applications for trials of apparatus at one or other of the dockyards, in case the size and character of the appliances shown in particular cases should exceed the capabilities of the testing places already

provided. These communications were announced at a special meeting of the Smoke Abatement Society, and it was also mentioned that, in addition to premiums conferred by the committee, a series of extra prizes would be arranged, including a "ladies' prize" for the best smoke-consuming domestic grate.

At the instance of the Registrar-General, William Hollingworth, keeper of a people's dispensary, was recently fined £5 at the Manchester County Police-court, for issuing a false certificate regarding the death of a child named Page. The defendant had signed the document in the name of a medical man who had not seen the child. At the same time a surgeon was committed for trial for perjury. He had certified, in a similar case, that he had seen and prescribed for a child, which was stated to be untrue.

At the usual fortnightly meeting of the Managers of the Metropolitan Asylums District, held on Saturday last, Dr. Brewer presiding, a letter was read from the Local Government Board, acknowledging the receipt of a communication of the Board of the 28th ult., and stating that they approved of the proposal of the Managers to discontinue the arrangement under which small-pox patients had been received into the Fever Hospital at Homerton, and to again appropriate that Hospital to the reception of fever cases. An important report was also brought up from the Stockwell Committee with regard to vaccination. This, after giving the number of the cases admitted, said :—" As evidencing the negligence displayed by the authorities, upon whom the responsibility of enforcing the laws relating to primary vaccination rests, your Committee have ascertained from the Medical Superintendent of the Small-pox Hospital that, of the 704 patients admitted to that establishment during the past seven months, no fewer than 191 were children under twelve years of age. Of these, 83 were imperfectly vaccinated, 13 'doubtful' if vaccinated, and 95 absolutely unvaccinated. Of the vaccinated cases, 2 died (death in neither case, however, being attributable to small-pox). Among the 'doubtful' if vaccinated, 9 deaths were recorded, whilst among the unvaccinated 42 succumbed." After the meeting the President and some of the officials of the Local Government Board paid a visit of inspection to the two ships which have been lent by the Admiralty to the Managers for the reception of small-pox patients. The vessels are fitted-up to accommodate upwards of 200 patients, and Sir E. H. Currie explained that the entire cost had been about £11,000, whereas, if the Managers had had to erect a building to accommodate the same number of patients it would have cost about £60,000. The President of the Local Government Board complimented the Managers on the prompt manner in which they had acted with a view of checking the further progress of the epidemic of small-pox. A report of the *Atlas* will be found elsewhere in our columns.

A meeting was recently held at the residence of Dr. Andrew Clark, to discuss the feasibility of devising some scheme which shall provide the same kind of advantages for those who are discharged as certified sane patients from lunatic asylums as are conferred on convalescents from bodily illness confined in convalescent homes. Lord Shaftesbury presided, and amongst those present were Dr. Bucknill, Dr. Lockhart-Robertson, and Mr. E. H. Lushington. The Rev. Henry Hawkins, Chaplain of the Colney Hatch Asylum, who has devoted some years and much work to this project of "after-care," read an account of what had been done so far, and after some explanations it was resolved, on the motion of Mr. Lushington, to appoint a sub-committee to co-operate with the Convalescent Committee of the Charity Organisation Society. It was pointed out by Dr. Andrew Clark that the new society was not a begging one, as a wise provision of the Lunacy Act enables the visiting magistrates of lunatic asylums to defray the cost of pauper lunatics for such time after they leave the asylums as they think necessary. But the difficulty being to find private houses where they will be received, the Society's great want is publicity, in order that by having correspondents in many parts of the country it may have a better chance of learning of suitable accommodation. All persons desirous of forwarding this work are requested to apply to the Rev. Henry Hawkins, at Colney Hatch Asylum.

The Conservators of the Thames recently preferred a charge against a brewer, of Goring, on the Oxfordshire side of the river, about nine miles below Reading, of polluting the stream. It appeared that in the sample of water taken by Mr. Wigner, the analyst to the Conservators, there were germs of the yeast-plant in full-growth, which remained alive in the stream, and within twenty-four hours would get to the source of the London water-supply. If imbibed, they would be highly injurious. The amount of dissolved matter in the water was 130 grains to the gallon, eighty being of organic matter. The defence was, that the nuisance complained of did not arise from the brewery, but from some cottages. The magistrates before whom the inquiry was held, however, decided that the refuse was from the brewery, and inflicted a fine of £5 and costs. Notice of appeal was given.

The Municipal Council of Paris has recently made a great improvement in the arrangements of the Morgue by adopting the refrigerating apparatus of MM. Mignon and Rouart, at a cost of 53,000 fr. The bodies on view will thus be enabled to be preserved for any length of time within reason, and the sanitary conditions of the Morgue will be greatly altered for the better, while the longer period of exposure will frequently further the ends of justice, and give greater opportunities for identification.

ROYAL COLLEGE OF SURGEONS.

At a meeting of the Council yesterday, the 14th inst., Mr. Erasmus Wilson, F.R.S., was elected President of the College, and Mr. T. Spencer Wells, of Grosvenor-street, and Mr. John Marshall, F.R.S., of Savile-row, Vice-Presidents for the ensuing year. Mr. Wilson, who, as the senior Vice-President, succeeds to the chair vacated by Mr. Erichsen, is well known to the medical profession, of which he is such a distinguished member, by his numerous and valuable contributions to science; and as late Professor of Dermatology, the chair of which in the College of Surgeons he endowed with £6000. To the Medical Benevolent College he has been equally generous; and at Margate he is enriching and completing the Sea-bathing Infirmary, structurally, at a cost of upwards of £30,000. To the nation he is known as the eminent and patriotic surgeon who, at his own cost, brought Cleopatra's Needle to London, and placed it in its present position on the Thames Embankment. At this meeting the recently elected Councillors, Messrs. Hulke and Heath, were sworn in and took their seats.

THE MEDICAL ARRANGEMENTS AT THE WINDSOR REVIEW.

Although the weather at Windsor on Saturday last was hot, and during the early part of the day very bright, it is satisfactory to be able to record that the Review passed off with few really serious casualties, and without loss of life. The whole of the medical regulations were suggested by Surgeon-Major Shelton, the head of the medical branch of the Army Medical Department; and Surgeon-Major Gasteen, A.M.D., was on the field in command of the Volunteer Ambulance Corps. Two field-hospitals were established in the Great Park, each composed of about seven tents, with the necessary medical and surgical equipment, field stretchers, water-carts, etc., and in addition to other medical comforts, each was provided with an ample store of ice. The corps was composed of the Volunteer Bearer Company and a detachment of the Army Hospital Corps, its strength, in addition to the medical officers, being ninety-four non-commissioned officers and men. From first to last the total number of cases receiving treatment was about 150, twenty-five of which were at the first of a serious character. Ten of these were from sunstroke, the remaining fifteen being cases of faintness caused by exposure to the extreme heat, and the fatigue which had been endured in the long railway journey undertaken by many of the Volunteers. All but eight of the sufferers were able to rejoin their corps or leave for home in the course of the evening, the worst case—one of sunstroke—being eventually removed to the Guards' Hospital at Windsor. The arrangements of the Army Medical Department on Saturday not only comprised the scene of action itself, but, with much forethought, a medical officer of the Department, with orderlies and a small equipment of medicines and comforts, was stationed at the Paddington, Waterloo, Ascot, Slough, Datchet, Virginia Water, and Windsor Stations, to be in readiness to afford medical assistance to any case requiring it en route. With so much willing and able tuition, it will not be long, we should think, before the Volunteer Medical Department will be able to rely upon itself on similar occasions.

THE FELLOWS' FESTIVAL.

The annual festival of the Fellows of the Royal College of Surgeons took place on the evening of the elections into the Council, when Mr. T. W. Crosse, of Norwich, took the chair, in place of Mr. Cadge, who was unhappily prevented from attending by a severe domestic affliction. About seventy sat down to dinner. In proposing the Medical Schools, Professor John Wood, F.R.S., said that to the Fellows of the Royal College of Surgeons no toast could possibly possess more interest and importance than the toast which had been entrusted to his care, and none could be more pleasant to him to propose. It was the health and prosperity of the medical schools, which furnished the elementary atoms composing the body corporate of the College—which maintain the changes and supply the reliefs to recompose and reanimate that living and growing institution. We cannot pretend to give our readers the benefit of nearly all Mr. Wood said; but among other things he remarked: as the medical schools grow and increase, and preserve an emulative and critical spirit of observation, the examining bodies are kept up to the mark, and the standard and fairness of the examinations are maintained. If they languish, so do the examinations, for without competition there is no emulation. To wish for the health and prosperity of the medical schools was therefore, he thought, a mark of wisdom, and well became the occasion on which the Fellows were assembled, that recorded the yearly changes in the Council of the Royal College of Surgeons. Unmitigated commendation, he further observed, was said to be necessarily dull to the hearer, and by way of critical variety he would point out a fault. This was the tendency, already observable, to a neglect, by the students sent up from all the schools, of close practical attention to anatomical details—a neglect which had recently produced failure to the students and disappointment to the examiners in the primary examinations. An increased familiarity with physiological methods of investigation would, in his opinion, be dearly purchased by a want in the surgeons of the future of acquaintance with surgical anatomy. But there was no reason whatever why both should not be equally and proportionately developed. They need not fall on the other side of their ambition.

He coupled with the toast the name of Mr. Reginald Harrison, whose recent American experiences would, he suggested, be of much interest. Mr. Harrison, however, while appreciating highly, he said, the kind personal reference made to himself, declined, on the ground of want of time, speaking of the medical schools of America, several of which he had visited, and had found in a condition of great vigour and activity. He said that wherever he went, either in the States or in Canada, he had met with the greatest hospitality, and he had heard universally the kindest expressions of cordiality towards the profession in the Old Country. He strongly advised his professional brethren, "in search of an interesting and invigorating holiday, to pay a visit to the American continent, where they would find every variety of intellectual and physical relaxation." Mr. F. Woodhouse Braine, F.R.C.S., of Maddox-street, has succeeded Mr. B. Thompson Lowne as Hon. Secretary to the Festival.

INTERNATIONAL MEDICAL CONGRESS.

WE are asked to state that it is urgently desirable that intending members of the International Medical Congress should at once make known their intention to the Secretary-General, Mr. W. Mac Cormac, as a knowledge of the probable number of persons likely to attend the Congress is essential to the completion of the needful arrangements.

THE LATE DR. MAURICE RAYNAUD.

IN the oration pronounced at Raynaud's grave, Prof. Peter indicated the cause of his premature death in these words: —"A bitter grief gnawed at his heart and poisoned his existence. This chagrin arose from his not having obtained the chair at the Faculty which his great acquirements, numerous aptitudes, and incontestable talent entitled him to." And, in fact, everybody was surprised at the time that he did not obtain the chair of the History of Medicine when it fell vacant, for which he was so well adapted. But that this disappointment had anything to do with generating the terrible disease which has also so recently carried off Delpech, Chauffard, and Broca, is quite disbelieved by those who knew him best. "This," says his friend, Dr. Amédée Latour, "is very contestable for all who knew the profound convictions and energetic faith of this austere Christian, who accepted with submission all that it pleased his Master to impose upon him. 'They will not have me at the Faculty because I go to mass,' said he to me one day; 'but I must avow I like this pretext better than that of ignorance and incapacity,' accompanying this with a smile which at once betrayed the resignation of the believer, and the ruffled self-esteem of the savant."

THE BOARD OF WORKS AND THE FISH-SUPPLY OF THE METROPOLIS.

THE promptitude with which the Works and General Purposes Committee of the Metropolitan Board of Works has reported on the subject of the fish-supply of the metropolis has certainly taken everybody by surprise, more especially as the Corporation of the City of London Committee engaged on the same work seems scarcely to have opened the question. The report now presented, which was put in the form of a motion at the last meeting of the Board, and carried almost unanimously, states that the present market at Billingsgate is utterly inadequate to the needs of the metropolis, and that the deficiency of market accommodation has a prejudicial effect in limiting the supply and increasing the price of an important article of food. The Board will be perfectly willing to undertake to remedy the existing state of affairs, but as the City holds a charter, granted by Edward III., to construct and manage all markets within a radius of seven miles, it would be essential to obtain an Act of Parliament to confer the necessary authority upon them. It has long been clear, to everyone not directly interested in the monopoly of Billingsgate, that the one fish market for the metropolis is utterly and ludicrously inadequate; and it is not so much a question as to what authority shall deal with its enlargement, and the formation of others, as how soon some remedy can be provided to do away with the present unsatisfactory state of affairs. If the Board of Works would only act as promptly as they have reported on the matter, there would appear to be no reason why the City Corporation should not be deprived of a charter which is decidedly opposed to the interests and convenience of the community, since they do not "construct or create" new markets themselves, while they prevent them being constructed by others. Moreover, such a charter as the one referred to is an anachronism; "the City," which a century or two ago was London, is but a very small portion of the metropolitan province of houses now known as London.

MATER MISERICORDIÆ HOSPITAL, DUBLIN.

IN accordance with the will of the late Mark Leonard, Esq., the annual interest of the Leonard bequest of £1000 was on Thursday, July 7, awarded by the Senior Physician of the Hospital, Dr. J. Hughes, in equal proportions to Messrs. J. J. O'Hagan, John M'Donagh, and Thomas Donnelly, for the best reports of cases occurring in the Hospital during the clinical session just terminated.

THE BOYLSTON MEDICAL PRIZE.

THE Boylston Medical Committee, appointed by the President and Fellows of Harvard University, U.S., have announced that at the annual meeting, held June 1, this year, the prize of $300 was awarded to Herbert W. Page, F.R.C.S., Assistant-Surgeon of St. Mary's Hospital, London, for his essay on "Injuries to the Back, without apparent mechanical lesion, in their surgical and medico-legal aspects." It will be remembered that last year the Boylston Prize was carried off by Mr. W. Watson Cheyne, of King's College Hospital. The following are the questions proposed for 1882:—1. "Sewer Gas, so-called (the gas found in sewers): what are its physiological and pathological effects on animals and plants? An experimental inquiry." The author of a dissertation considered worthy of a prize will be entitled to $300. 2. "The Therapeutic Value of Food, administered against or beyond the patient's appetite and inclination." The best dissertation, if worthy of a prize, will be awarded $200. Dissertations must be sent to Dr. D. H. Storer, 182, Boylston-street, Boston, Massachusetts, on or before the first Wednesday in April, 1882. The following are the questions proposed for 1883:—1. "Measles; German Measles; and their Counterfeits." 2. "The Differential Diagnosis of Abdominal Tumours; especially those connected with the genito-urinary organs." The author of a dissertation considered worthy of a prize on either of the subjects for 1883 will be entitled to a premium of $300. Preference will be given to dissertations which exhibit original work.

THE REGISTRATION, ETC., OF MEDICAL STUDENTS.

A CONFERENCE of delegates appointed by the various licensing bodies in Ireland was held on June 15 and 16, 1881, in the Hall of the King and Queen's College of Physicians, Kildare-street, Dublin. The conference was convened, at the instance of the College of Physicians, for the purpose of considering the advisability of introducing a uniform system of registration of the entries in, and the certificates granted by, the various medical schools and clinical hospitals in Ireland. Propositions embodying the main points for consideration, which had been drawn up by a joint committee of the Colleges of Physicians and Surgeons in February, 1881, were submitted to and discussed by the conference, which was composed of the following representatives, nominated by the licensing bodies, viz.:— *The University of Dublin:* Rev. Dr. Samuel Haughton, M.D., S.F.T.C.D., Representative of the University on the General Medical Council; Alexander Macalister, Esq., M.D., University Professor of Anatomy and Surgery. *The Queen's University in Ireland:* J. T. Banks, Esq., M.D. F.C.P., Physician to the Queen, Representative of the University on the General Medical Council; Peter Redfern, Esq., M.D., Member of the Senate of the University, and Professor of Anatomy, Queen's College, Belfast. *The King and Queen's College of Physicians in Ireland:* Thomas Hayden, Esq., F.C.P., Professor of Anatomy, Catholic University; Reuben J. Harvey, Esq., M.D., F.C.P., Lecturer on Physiology in Carmichael College. *The Royal College of Surgeons in Ireland:* J. K. Barton, Esq., M.D., Vice-President and Member of Council, Royal College of Surgeons, and Lecturer on Surgery, Carmichael College; A. H. Jacob, Esq., M.D., Fellow and Member of Council, Royal College of Surgeons. *Apothecaries' Hall, Ireland:* Thomas Collins, M.R.C.S.E., Director, Apothecaries' Hall; C. F. Moore, M.D. Glasg., Director, Apothecaries' Hall. Dr. J. Magee Finny, F.C.P., was requested to act as honorary secretary to the conference. The following resolutions were adopted, and the honorary secretary was requested to forward the same to the medical authorities, as the unanimous recommendations of the delegates:—"1. That it is advisable that the last day of entry for students in schools and hospitals shall be the *fifteenth* day of the winter and the *tenth* day of the summer sessions. 2. That it is desirable that a return should be made to the Branch Medical Council for Ireland of the names of all students entered at any school or hospital, together with the courses for which they are severally entered, within three days after the days specified above. 3. That it is desirable that within *fifteen* days after the close of each session each school and hospital should furnish a return to the Branch Medical Council for Ireland of the several attendances of each student; and that the Branch Council be requested to print, and forward to each licensing body in Ireland, a copy of the foregoing returns. 4. That it is desirable that the undermentioned qualifying bodies pledge themselves not to admit to examination any student whose attendance has not been duly returned as sufficient to the Branch Medical Council—viz., the University of Dublin; the Queen's University in Ireland; the King and Queen's College of Physicians, Ireland; the Royal College of Surgeons, Ireland; and the Apothecaries' Hall, —and that no attendance on medical lectures or clinical instruction be deemed sufficient which does not at least include *two-thirds* of the course."

ST. ANDREWS GRADUATES' ASSOCIATION.

THE thirteenth anniversary session of the Association was held at the house of the Medical Society of London on Wednesday, the 6th inst. The following gentlemen were elected officers and Council for the year ending June 30, 1882:—*President of Council:* Dr. B. W. Richardson, F.R.S. *Treasurer:* Dr. Paul. *Secretary:* Dr. Leonard Sedgwick. *Council:* Dr. Holman, Mr. Menzies, Professor Pettigrew, Drs. Seaton, Bransby Roberts, Christie, Cleveland, Dudfield, MacIntyre, Royston, Wiltshire, Cooper Rose, Falls, Mott, Gramshaw, Semple, Samuel Hill, Dale, Kershaw, Archibald, Cholmeley, Davey, C. A. Gordon, C.B., Stedman, Crosby, W. H. Day, Griffith, Wynn Williams, Alderson, Cassells, Corner, Lush, Rhys Williams, Gillespie, Wilkinson, Henty, and Longhurst.

THE COLLEGIATE ELECTION.

AT the recent election of Fellows into the Council of the Royal College of Surgeons, 303 gentlemen recorded their votes, viz.:—Metropolitan Fellows, 189; provincial, 93; with no address, 18; of the Royal Navy, 2; and 1 of the Indian Army. In the list of stewards of the annual festival there were, out of the seventy-seven so acting, twenty-two provincials.

THE HOSPITAL-SHIP "ATLAS."

ON Saturday last, July 11, we had an opportunity of inspecting the *Atlas,* which is about to be used as a hospital-ship for small-pox patients. The *Atlas* was formerly a 100-gun line-of-battle ship, of the good old type, which has now almost completely disappeared from our navy. Her former officers would hardly recognise her in her new capacity as a hospital-ship. There are three decks, the lowest of which has been made available by cutting thirty-four new ports, of about three feet square each. This must have been an immense labour, for the wood is untouched oak, and nearly a yard thick. It is from this deck, too, that the patients gain access to the ship through an entrance port level with a dummy which has been moored to the ship, and on which the patients are landed. Adjoining this entrance is a lift, which communicates with the upper decks (wards) and with the weather deck, where convalescents can air themselves. Speaking-tubes are fitted all over the ship, so that there is easy and rapid communication with all parts, and without any expenditure either of time or labour. The lower hatchways have been uncovered, and are now enclosed with louvre boarding, open to the weather deck, where a skylight provides ample ventilation, and at the same time keeps out the rain. To each ward is attached a nurse's room, scullery, and bath-room in the after part of the vessel; and at this end, also, the screw aperture has been utilised for the formation of a staircase to lead from the entrance port to the various decks without passing through the wards. At the fore end of each deck, water-closets and slop-sinks 'have been placed in such a position as to secure the greatest amount of ventilation possible under the circumstances. We did not quite gather what is to become of the soil from these water-closets, but presume it will find its way direct into the river; if this is the case we much doubt the expediency of the arrangement, for the fæces of those attacked with the specific fevers may, for all we know to the contrary, be a mode of propagating the disease. The wards are necessarily very low indeed—barely eight feet high, we should guess; each one contains about sixty beds. We could not help thinking that the beds were packed very much too closely. On the upper (weather) deck are special wards, male and female, as well as wards for doubtful cases; there is also a mortuary. The administrative department is in the *Endymion,* a forty-gun frigate, connected with the *Atlas* by a bridge. The *Endymion* is not yet ready, but the work of adaptation is being pushed on with great spirit. The arrangements for the reception of patients is very complete. The Managers have secured a wharf for embarkation of patients, known as "Potter's Ferry," situate on the north side of the Thames, almost immediately opposite Greenwich Pier. Here a barge is moored, on to which patients can be shipped from the ambulances at any state of the tide. Running between the *Atlas* and this wharf is a specially constructed barge (not unlike what boating-men will know as a "house-boat")· towed by a small steam-launch, which has been either hired or purchased for this work. There is an ambulance-station at George-street, London Fields, a position central to the several parishes allocated to the ship. Here will be retained, ready for immediate use, horses and ambulances, with the necessary staff of drivers and nurses. All the *employés* will be boarded on the premises, thus preventing contact with the public. This ambulance-station will be in telephonic communication with the chief offices of the Metropolitan Asylums Board in Norfolk-street, Strand. On discovery of a small-pox patient in any of the allocated parishes, a telegram is despatched by the parochial officer to the Norfolk-street office, whence immediate directions for the prompt removal of the case will be telephoned to the ambulance-station. The ambulance, specially constructed by Messrs. Holmes, of Derby, accompanied by one of the nurses, will proceed to the address of the patient, who will be conveyed to the wharf, where the steam-launch will be in waiting ready to carry the patient to the hospital-ship. The cost of fitting up the ships will be about £11,000.

HONOURS TO FRENCH SCIENTIFIC MEN.

PROF. PASTEUR, of the Institut, has been made Grand-Croix of the Légion d'Honneur, and his assistants in his investigations of contagious diseases, Drs. Chamberland and Roux, have been made Chevaliers. Dr. Brouardel, Professor of Legal Medicine at the Faculty of Medicine, has been made Officier. Dr. Wurtz, Professor of Chemistry at the Faculty, was elected a Senator for life by 146 of the 157 votes given.

MEDICAL DEFENCE ASSOCIATION.

THE Medical Defence Association having been invited to give evidence before the Royal Commission on the Medical Acts, the Council of that body is making arrangements to hold a representative meeting of the medical profession at Exeter Hall before the end of the present month, to discuss the question of medical reform, and to pass resolutions thereon.

THE PARIS WEEKLY RETURNS.

THE number of deaths for the twenty-sixth week, ending June 30, 1881, was 1025 (viz., 527 males and 498 females), and among these there were from typhoid fever 38, small-pox 23, measles 22, scarlatina 11, pertussis 8, diphtheria and croup 46, erysipelas 9, puerperal infections 6, and acute tubercular meningitis 44. There were also 29 deaths from acute bronchitis, 47 from pneumonia, 99 from infantile athrepsia (31 of the infants having been partially or wholly suckled), and 40 violent deaths. There was an increase of 81 deaths upon the preceding week, of which 27 arose from typhoid fever and 23 from athrepsia among infants brought up by hand. The births for the week amounted to 1150, viz., 600 males (416 legitimate and 184 illegitimate) and 550 females (393 legitimate and 157 illegitimate); 95 children (51 males and 44 females) were born dead or died within twenty-four hours.

DEATH OF DR. LOUIS MANDL.

THE Gazette Hebdomadaire notices the death of Dr. Mandl, who, by his relations with the artistic world and his much-frequented weekly receptions, has obtained great notoriety. Mandl, however, before making a speciality of the larynx, especially with singers, had been one of the earliest and most zealous of the employers of the microscope in anatomico-pathological investigations, and besides many communications to the medical journals, he published a large work in two folio volumes, with ninety-two plates, "Anatomie Microscopique" (1838-57), which is still consulted. Besides several smaller publications relating to the voice, he also issued in 1872 his "Traité Pratique des Maladies du Larynx et du Pharynx." He was born at Pesth in 1812, and, having taken his medical degree there in 1836, he repaired to Paris to complete his studies, and obtained the doctorate there in 1842. He was also naturalised in 1849.

UNIVERSITY OF DUBLIN.

THE following honours have recently been awarded in the School of Physic in Ireland:—Medical Travelling Prize: Louis Tarleton Young. Medical Scholarships: In Anatomy and Institutes of Medicine—Alfred Middleton, Sidney Gerald Turpin, and Thomas Wilfred Haughton; in Chemistry, Physics, Botany, and Materia Medica—Frederic Conway Dwyer. The following resolution was adopted by the Council of the University at the meetings of June 1 and July 6, 1881:—"That instead of a course of lectures on Materia Medica and Pharmacy now required from candidates for the degree of Bachelor of Medicine, a course of lectures on Pharmacology and Therapeutics be required."

AT the quarterly meeting of the Directors of the Naval Medical Supplemental Fund, held on the 12th instant, H. J. Domville, Esq., C.B., M.D., Inspector-General of Hospitals, in the chair, the sum of £95 was distributed among the several applicants.

ENTERIC AND OTHER FEVERS IN AFGHANISTAN.

IN the Indian Medical Gazette of May 2, 1881, there is an interesting and valuable paper by Dr. J. Pedlow, of the Army Medical Department. Considering the mooted and disputed points in regard to the etiology of enteric fever the author thinks it would be of advantage to review the facts connected with an outbreak of this fever in Afghanistan, during which he had the opportunity of observing a considerable number of cases, "especially as it occurred under circumstances hardly reconcilable" with the usually accepted conditions of origin. Along with these cases of enteric or typhoid fever, Dr. Pedlow says, there were at the same time and place "cases of fever returned as remittent or simple continued."

The fevers described in the article in question were prevalent at a place called Peshbolak, on the Khyber line. It was a temporary station, and during its occupation was garrisoned by one British regiment and a battery of field artillery, in addition to a large native force. The writer thus describes the place:—"The site chosen for the camps was on the slopes which rise by a gradual ascent from the Cabul River and the Jellalabad Valley to the Sufraid Koh range of mountains, and about midway between them. The European camp was pitched on a sandy, sterile tract of virgin soil, almost devoid of vegetation. Beneath the upper layer was a bed of 'kankar' irregularly disposed. For a depth of six or seven feet there was scarcely sufficient moisture in the soil to give even a sensation of dampness to the hand. The Native camp was pitched on ground which, some thirty years before, had been fields cultivated by irrigation. It was, however, at the time of its occupation, as arid and free from moisture as the European site. The water-supply was very abundant, and in proximity to both camps. It was obtained from the 'karezes' characteristic of the country. These were simply tunnels with branches which tapped subterranean springs, and conducted the water to a point of exit. The length of these tunnels depended on the slope of the ground and the depth at which the spring was tapped. As a rule, this was from twelve to eighteen feet from the surface of the ground. From these 'karezes' an abundant stream of pure water was poured into reservoirs temporarily constructed by us. It will thus be seen that the water was non-surface, and probably derived from the snows and ice of the Sufraid Koh range, which, melting and percolating into the deeper layers of the soil, was finding its way by gravitation to the low-lying spring in the Jellalabad Valley. The question of its contamination by animal matter as well as stagnation may, I think, be dismissed as very improbable. Local pollution by surface-water was impossible, as during the whole period of the occupation of the camp, about four months, there was only five hours' rain." Dr. Pedlow, accordingly, dismisses water as a factor in the causation of his cases of typhoid. He also excludes putrid emanations, in the absence of moisture to favour decomposition. In regard to importation, he brings forth some positive evidence, which, taken into consideration with his via exclusionis reasoning, is, we are inclined to think, of moment. We are told that cases of typhoid fever had occurred at Lundi Kotal in men of the same regiment afterwards quartered at Peshbolak. Thirty-five days after the regiment left Lundi Kotal the first case occurred after arrival at Peshbolak; this case, we learn, was followed by "a run of others." Dr. Pedlow says, guardedly —"It is hardly likely that it would remain latent during that period; besides, a number of patients attacked belonged to the Artillery who had been quartered in the station for nearly two months." "Its existence previous to this in a mild form, without being recognised, is possible, but very improbable considering the fatality of the disease at the commencement of the outbreak." He then proceeds to discuss the question of the introduction of typhoid into Peshbolak. Admitting this to be possible, he thinks the propagation of the disease has to be accounted for. Excreta, he says, would in a very few hours be dried to powder in the hot sun, and the dry wind and sand-storms —which are peculiar to the country—might possibly have carried the disease-germs to drinking-water, food, etc. Dr. Pedlow tells us that the sanitary arrangements were good. "As far as I can recollect," says our author, "there was only one case in the native camp considered typhoid." The exclusion, therefore, of bazaars, etc., as foci of origin considerably limits the inquiry into causation, yet every effort to trace the fever to definite causes failed. It appeared at a time when the heat was intense, running up daily in the occupied tents to 108° and 110°, often to 116°, and when the debilitating effects of high temperature were felt by every European." (The italics are ours.)

Dr. Pedlow records ten cases of which he took notes, and out of these eight proved fatal. As to their ages, we learn that four were under twenty-seven years, four under thirty, and two were in their thirty-first year. He made a post-mortem examination in all these eight cases. With the exception of one, he found "extensive typhoid lesions" in all; and in that one there was "considerable enlargement of one of Peyer's patches," and "congestion of solitary glands." In the seven cases the spleen was enlarged and congested; "its pulp broke down on slight pressure between the fingers into a semi-fluid jelly."

It is interesting to find that "in five out of eight cases in which the temperature was observed and noted, it failed to indicate anything characteristic." Some of the thermometric observations are given in the paper.

The report teems with suggestive remarks and indications for future research, but pressure on our space precludes our noticing it farther. We, nevertheless, commend Dr. Pedlow's paper to the notice of our readers in general, and to the Epidemiological Society in particular, especially with reference to the papers read last year by Sir Joseph Fayrer, Surgeon-Major Don, Surgeon-General Gordon, Dr. Ewart, and others.

FROM ABROAD.

COPYRIGHT IN LECTURES.

A CASE has been before the American Law Courts for some time, which has led to the authoritative statement—or rather re-statement, for it has been often laid down before—as to the right of lecturers to prevent the publication of the addresses they deliver. This right, as laid down by Lord Eldon in the case of Abernethy v. the Lancet, more than half a century ago, has since been repeatedly affirmed in America, and has just been made the subject of a decision in the Supreme Court of the State of New York, in the case of the firm of Putnam and Sons v. Leo Meyer and others. Messrs. Putnam are the publishers of Profs. Darling and Ranney's "Essentials of Anatomy," being lectures delivered by Prof. Darling, and they brought this action against Meyer for publishing these lectures under the title of "A Guide to the Study of Anatomy," as an infringement of the copyright of the former work. A complication in the present case arose from Prof. Darling having granted Meyer permission to print the reports of his lectures for the use of the students attending the class, afterwards entering into a contract with Messrs. Putnam for their publication—the case, therefore, turning on the legal difference between the terms "to print" and "to publish." The Court held that lectures delivered to a class were the property of that class for their own use only, and that no member of the class could publish them without permission of the lecturer. It seems that Darling's previous permission given to Meyer to print the lectures allowed the latter to sell the report to students in actual attendance. There is, however, no right to print a report, even for this limited circulation, unless the lecturer's permission has been obtained. Although no respectable journal would think of publishing a lecture without the author's permission, or against his wish, there would seem to be several of another description in America which would not hesitate to do so. "In congratulating the Messrs. Putnam upon the termination of their suit," the New York Medical Journal for June observes, "we may express the hope that the decisions bearing upon the points at issue may be turned to account by medical lecturers for their own protection. There can be no doubt that many a clinical lecture has been published against the wish of the lecturer, and to the detriment of his reputation. From an ethical point of view, there has never seemed to us to be the slightest doubt that anything uttered in the way of a medical lecture, or read as a paper at a society meeting, or spoken in debate at such meeting, should not be published, even in abstract, without an opportunity being afforded the author to revise it or to object to its publication at all. Now that the law of the matter has been shown to be at one with its ethics, we trust that lecturers and speakers at society meetings will muster the courage to enforce their rights. By so doing they will also guard the profession against being misled by inaccurate reports. From time to time we receive communications, generally on postal cards, from persons wholly unknown to us, asking how much we will give for a report of a clinical lecture by this, that, or the other professor. We invariably decline such offers, but we cannot avoid the conclusion that much of this matter finds its way into print—such drivel do we find attributed to men whose scholarly attainments are well known, and who never talk without saying something."

CONSUMPTION OF QUININE IN THE UNITED STATES.

The New York Med. Record (June 18) directs attention to the enormous consumption of the cinchona alkaloids in America, in order to advert to some points of importance. First, are not quinine and its allied alkaloids being used in an excessive, if not dangerous, amount? It is said that the total annual consumption throughout the world amounts to 220,000 lbs., and that a fourth of this is used in the United States alone. Nearly half a million of ounces of quinine were imported in 1880, besides over 32,000 bales of cinchona bark—these figures not including the other alkaloids, which, however, exist in the bark, on an average, in two or three times the amount of quinine. Of the four chief alkaloids—quinine, quinidia, cinchonia, and cinchonidia—none are wasted by the manufacturer. The prescribing quinine has become excessively frequent in New York, and the inevitable diagnosis of "malaria" is a matter of ridicule with the laity; and yet, for every doctor's prescription of quinine, the druggist receives ten or twelve calls for the drug by persons who are treating themselves, and who resort to it for every possible ailment, real or supposed. "Quinine has become thus a mainstay of the physician, and the panacea of an enormous circle of self-medicating citizens. There is no question that a great deal of this dosing is ill-advised and useless, and it can hardly fail to be in some cases positively injurious. The people in this matter are a little stupid. A certain share of them have the idea that medicine can always counteract sanitary indiscretions. It is considered easier to take quinine or a cathartic than to take good care of oneself. There is undoubtedly a great deal of malarial poison in this city, and physicians are very often justified in their diagnosis and treatment. But, often also, hepatic derangements, indigestions, simple continued fevers, fevers from filthy exhalations, fevers from nervous or gastro-intestinal disturbance, or inflammatory changes, are incorrectly diagnosed as due to malaria. We repeat that there is a great deal of carelessness in the prescribing and consumption of quinine."

Secondly, it is stated that nine persons out of ten who go to a drug-store get quinidia, cinchonidia, or even cinchonia, in its place. Most druggists, perhaps, give quinine when written for in a prescription; but it is said that the number is very small who do so when it is asked for by ordinary customers. The druggists, indeed, justify the practice, stating that these other alkaloids are nearly as powerful, while the public would not purchase them if sold under their own names. In the South and West, and in the country generally, these allied salts are enormously sold. As to their relative value, no absolute statement can be made, although it is probable that their rank as follows:—Cinchonidia, quinidia, cinchonia. Cinchonidia is largely used in hospitals and dispensaries, and among country practitioners; and the results of the trials it has been submitted to are very satisfactory. It is claimed to be almost, if not quite, equal to quinine; and in some cases it seems to produce less gastric or cerebral disturbance. Quinidia is nearly equal to cinchonidia, but is more irritating to the stomach. Cinchonia is the weakest of the four alkaloids. There are good reports of some allied preparations, as dextro-quinine; while of others, as quinquinia, less can be said. On the whole, it seems that quinine, though still the best and surest alkaloid, is not to be considered so pre-eminent as formerly.

PROFESSOR VOLKMANN'S MODE OF DRESSING.

Dr. Allen, after giving some account of Prof. Volkmann's beautiful new Surgical Clinic at Halle (*New York Med. Record*, June 18), proceeds to speak of his mode of dressing. "In operating, Prof. Volkmann does not use a spray. Before beginning to operate, the part is most thoroughly scrubbed with soap-suds and a nail-brush, until no dirt can possibly remain, and it is then shaved, without regard to what part it is. The sponges used in the amphitheatre are kept in seven earthen pails (containing a 10 per cent. carbolic acid solution), marked for each day of the week; so that no sponge is used in operating unless it has been soaked for at least a week. Before operating, the sponges are placed in a 3 per cent. solution, as are the instruments. From time to time the wound is flooded with a 3 per cent. solution from a small ordinary watering-pot without the sprinkler; and the pot is held high above the wound, so that the stream may fall upon it with considerable force. The catgut and silk used for sutures and ligatures are kept on spools which lie continually in carbolic oil, and the ligatures are cut off and handed to the operator only when required. At the completion of the operation, after the wound has been thoroughly flooded and closed, a hand-spray is used during the application of the dressing. The wound is dressed first with a piece of prepared oil-silk protective, only large enough to cover the wound. Above this is placed a wad of very soft carbolised gauze, the first folded, but is shaken apart, and made into a soft mass. An abundance of this is used, and then it is covered by an ample piece of gutta-percha protective, reaching far beyond the limits of the wound, and sufficient to render difficult the communication of any discharge with the air. This is held in place with a carbolised gauze bandage. All the interstices are carefully closed with wads of salicylic cotton, the elasticity of which tends to render the dressing more secure; and when complete, the dressing, though seemingly sometimes redundant, fully realises the object for which it was applied—the occlusion of the wound. When the wounds are opened and dressed, a simple hand-spray is used, and the wound is thoroughly rinsed. For this purpose a can filled with a 3 per cent. solution is used, having an opening in its side just at its lower border, to which a rubber tube is attached. This tube has a small nozzle which can be inserted if necessary into sinuses. The can is held above the head by an assistant, and the water thus runs into the wound with considerable force, or by lowering it, with as little force as may be desired. Sponges are used only in the primary operations, and never in dressing wounds; but pledgets of absorbent cotton, which after being used are thrown away. The free use of carbolic acid in the amphitheatre often floods the floor (constructed of tesselated marble), but an opening in the centre serves to carry most of it away; still the feet of the operator and assistants are often wet. Although so much carbolic acid comes in contact with the wound, I was told that cases of carbolic acid poisoning are very rare, being less frequent when the pure acid is used instead of the impure, as frequently is the case. Bandages which are very little soiled are washed, disinfected, and used again in the polyclinic, but not in the operating theatre. Other dressings are burned. . . . Very few patients are received into this hospital who are not able to pay something, unless their cases are very urgent or very interesting. Very poor patients must pay 20 cents daily, and others 37 cents, and they must pay extra for Lister dressings. If tramps are admitted, the city from which they come is charged for their support. Fortunately, there does not seem to be the large class, such as we have, who pay nothing for hospital treatment; but most of the patients belong to some mutual society that assists them during sickness."

DR. E. P. McFARLANE'S REPORT ON THE HEALTH OF ICHANG.(a)

THE town of Ichang, situated in latitude 30° 14′ 25″ N. and longitude 111° 18′ 34′ E., lies on the north bank of the Yangtse, about 1000 miles from the sea. The foreign population of the town is seventeen, and this includes five ladies and two children. The general health of the community since my arrival in Ichang, nearly two years ago, has been, upon the whole, very good. This is more especially to be noted as all the foreigners are living in native houses, and the majority of them inside the city wall, in localities where it is hardly possible for them to escape the effluvia caused by the inefficiency of sanitary arrangements.

The sanitary conditions of Ichang are most deplorably neglected, notwithstanding the comparatively good health enjoyed by foreigners in it. Efficient drainage is utterly uncared for by the Chinese in this town, and no precautions whatever are taken to prevent obnoxious smells or to clear away from the entrance of the drains the rubbish which collects there. The whole town is drained after some method, but no sooner does a heavy shower of rain fall than the streets are flooded with water, and passengers may be seen walking up to their knees in it. Privies are very numerous, and as they are emptied, as a rule, only once a week, their contents have ample time to undergo putrefaction. The farmers, who buy the soil for manure, come at all hours of the day and carry off their purchase through the streets of the city. As the latrines are never thoroughly emptied or washed out, the consequence is that the nuisance caused is never absent. People of the poorer class live, as a rule, in the open air all day, but notwithstanding their absence, their sleeping apartments remain laden with abominable odours, against which no precautions are taken by means of ventilation.

The piece of ground marked out as the English Concession is perhaps the best spot that could be chosen about the city for foreigners to reside on. It is situated on the north bank of the river, about three hundred yards from the south gate of the city. The distance will prove sufficient to enable residents to escape the obnoxious smells consequent on the bad sanitary arrangements of the town. The space is quite open and commands a magnificent view on all sides, the only native houses near being those on both sides of the street leading up to the city, and a few huts on the south side. The Concession is bounded by the river in front, and immediately to the back is a large piece of land where the Chinese in former days buried their dead. So far as I know, no interment is now made there. Here the river flows in a south by south-east direction, and is about a quarter of a mile broad in summer, and somewhat less than that in winter. The city side, although not hilly, rises to a considerable extent at a distance of about half a mile from the banks of the river. The country on the opposite side (south) is rather hilly, and a few miles inland it becomes quite mountainous. Another great advantage, and perhaps the most enjoyable for a foreigner in the summer, is that the wind, as a rule, is from the south and blows up river. It is therefore hardly possible that it should bring anything deleterious to health, as it passes over a long stretch of mountainous country, with very little, if any, decomposed

(a) From the *Medical Reports of the Imperial Maritime Customs of China.*

vegetable matter, and afterwards blows up river a distance of about ten miles. This breeze, which invariably blows in the afternoon, is very fresh and invigorating in the summer. Any decomposed vegetable matter about the rice-fields, which lie at a considerable distance to the back of the Concession, is blown in a northerly direction. The plot of ground has also all the sanitary advantages that could be desired, as it slopes towards the river.

The disadvantage in this piece of ground lies mainly in its liability to be inundated should the river rise several feet above its usual height in the summer. I am inclined to believe myself that, should the water rise high enough to inundate the Concession, the whole city would likewise be flooded. Such catastrophes are expected every ten years, and great anxiety prevailed this summer, as it is now ten years since the last flood. Foreigners as well as natives were, however, happily disappointed. In the case of merchants or others building houses on the Concession, precautions should be taken to raise the foundations at least six feet high as a safeguard against the more serious inconveniences to which a householder is put when such a disaster as a flood occurs. I am decidedly of opinion that Ichang is healthy. I infer this from the facts already mentioned regarding the Concession ground, and from the general good health of the foreigners at present residing in and about the town. On the hills and in the valleys on the opposite side of the river pleasant walks can be got, although the roads are bad. The air is bracing and enlivening in all the surrounding country, and only about three miles up river is the commencement of the renowned gorges of the Yangtze, where a complete change is experienced by the visitor.

INTERNATIONAL MEDICAL CONGRESS, 1881.

We have received from the Honorary Secretary-General the following revised programme of arrangements for the forthcoming Congress :—

GENERAL ARRANGEMENTS.

An Informal Reception will take place at the Royal College of Physicians, Pall-mall East, on Tuesday afternoon, August 2, from 3 p.m. to 6 p.m., at which the Executive and Reception Committees will meet the members of the Congress.

The Opening Meeting of the Congress will be held in St. James's Great Hall, on Wednesday, August 3, at 11 a.m. Entrances in Regent-street and Piccadilly.

The other General Meetings will be held in the Theatre of the University of London. Entrance in Burlington Gardens. The Sections will meet in the places assigned to them.

The offices of the Reception Committee are in the College of Physicians, Pall-mall East, at the north-west corner of Trafalgar-square.

The Reception Committee will meet daily during the week at 3 p.m. in the Censor's Room of the College of Physicians.

The office of the Reception Committee at the College of Physicians will be open for the registration of members on and after Monday, July 18. Members are requested to call as soon as possible, after their arrival in London, to enter their names and addresses in the register, when they will be supplied with programmes of business and tickets for membership, excursions, and entertainments. Every possible information will be given as to the prices and situation of convenient hotels and lodgings.

By the kindness of the Directors of the United Telephone Company, the Medical Congress has been placed in direct communication with the exchange system of that Company. It will therefore be competent for anyone attending the Congress to hold conversation by means of the telephone with any of the subscribers to the above Company.

The United Telephone Company has also erected for the use of the Congress a private line, which connects the College of Surgeons, in Pall-mall East, with Burlington House, and thus affords facilities for verbal communication between those two points.

Members wishing to take part in any of the excursions, or to visit any of the private and public places of interest open on the occasion, must enter their names in the proper book, at the College of Physicians, at the earliest opportunity, in order that the necessary arrangements may be made.

The office of the Editors of the Daily Programme is on the first floor in the College of Physicians, where MSS. of all business to be transacted in the Sections on the next day must be handed in before 4 p.m.

The Hon. Secretary-General's room is at the College of Physicians, on the ground floor, at the right hand side of the staircase.

A reading and writing room is provided at the College of Physicians, where members can see the journals and write letters. Letters of members may be addressed here during the meeting of the Congress.

A postal and telegraph office is situated on the left-hand side of the entrance to the courtyard of Burlington House, Piccadilly.

Facilities will be afforded every day during the session of the Congress, between the hours of 2 p.m. and 3.30 p.m., to members desirous of visiting the London hospitals and medical schools and their museums. Special arrangements have been made for afternoon hospital visits on Thursday, August 4, and Friday, August 5, when the members of the staff of each hospital and school, so far as is practicable, will attend. The officers of the Sections will afford information respecting visits which members may desire to make to special hospitals other than those mentioned in the Programme, or institutions of interest to members of the Section.

Members of the Congress are admitted free, on presentation of their tickets of membership, to view the International Medical and Sanitary Exhibition at South Kensington, at which will be exhibited the various materials and apparatus employed in the prevention, detection, cure, and alleviation of disease.

SECTIONS.

The Sections will meet in the following places from 10 a.m. to 1 p.m. and from 2 p.m. to 3.30 p.m :—

1. Anatomy—Linnean Society's Council Room, Burlington House.
2. Physiology—Royal Institution, Albemarle-street.
3. Pathology—Chemical Society's Meeting Room, Burlington House.
4. Medicine—The Theatre, University of London, Burlington-gardens.
5. Diseases of the Throat (Sub-section)—Astronomical Society's Meeting Room, Burlington House.
6. Surgery—The Library, University of London, Burlington-gardens.
7. Obstetric Medicine and Surgery—South-East Examination Hall, University of London.
8. Diseases of Children—Antiquaries' Society's Meeting Room, Burlington House.
9. Mental Diseases—The Asiatic Society's Meeting Rooms, Albemarle-street.
10. Ophthalmology—Royal Society's Meeting Rooms, Burlington House.
11. Diseases of the Ear—The Assembly Room, Royal Academy of Arts, Burlington House.
12. Diseases of the Skin—Linnean Society's Secretary's Room, Burlington House.
13. Diseases of the Teeth—Linnean Society's Meeting Room, Burlington House.
14. State Medicine—Royal School of Mines, Jermyn-street.
15. Military Surgery and Medicine—The Graduates' Meeting Room, University of London.
16. Materia Medica and Pharmacology—Geological Society's Meeting Room, Burlington House.

Museum—Geological Society's Museum, Burlington House.

DAILY PROGRAMME.

Tuesday, August 2.—10 a.m. to 6 p.m. : Registration of members and issue of tickets at the office of the Reception Committee in the Royal College of Physicians, Pall-mall East. 3 to 6 p.m. : Reception of the members of the Congress by the Committees at the Royal College of Physicians.

Wednesday, August 3.—9 a.m. to 6 p.m. : Registration of members and issue of tickets at the Royal College of Physicians. 11 a.m. : First General Meeting, St. James's Great Hall. The chair will be taken by the President of the Royal College of Physicians, Chairman, ex officio, of the General Committee, in the presence of H.R.H. the Prince of Wales. Presentation of the report of the Executive Committee by the Honorary Secretary-General. The constitution of the Congress and the election of officers will be proposed by the Chairman of the Executive Committee, and seconded by the President of the Congress of 1879. 2 p.m. : Meeting of the Sections. Constitution of the Sections, and other business. 4.30 p.m. : Second General Meeting. Address by Professor Virchow, of Berlin, on "The Value of Pathological Experiment." 5 to 6.30 p.m. : Musical Promenade at the Royal Botanic Society's Gardens, Regent's-park. 8.30 p.m. : Conversazione at South Kensington Museum (entrance Exhibition-road), given by the English members of the Congress to the foreign members. Every member of the Congress may on this occasion be accompanied by one lady.

Thursday, August 4.—10 a.m. to 1 p.m. : Sectional Meetings. 1.30 to 3.30 p.m. : Visits to hospitals (Guy's Hospital, London Hospital, St. George's Hospital, St. Mary's Hospital, St. Thomas's Hospital, Westminster Hospital). The medical officers and lecturers will be prepared to receive such members of the Congress as may desire to visit these hospitals and to inspect their schools and museums. 3 to 3.30 p.m. : Additional meeting time for the Sections. 4 to 5.30 p.m. : Third General Meeting, St. James's Great Hall. The address by the late Professor Maurice Raynaud, Paris. "Le Scepticisme en Médecine, au temps passé et au temps présent," will be read by Dr. Féréol. 6.30 p.m. : Banquet given to a certain number of the members of the Congress by the Lord Mayor of London, at the Mansion House.

Friday, August 5.—10 a.m. to 1 p.m. : Sectional Meetings. 1.30 to 3.30 p.m. : Visit to Hospitals (Bethlem Hospital, Charing-cross Hospital, King's College Hospital, Middlesex Hospital, St. Bartholomew's Hospital, University College Hospital). The medical officers and lecturers will be prepared to receive such members of the Congress as may desire to visit these hospitals and to inspect their schools and museums. 2 to 3.30 p.m. : Additional meeting time for the Sections. 4 to 5 31 p.m. : Fourth General Meeting, St. James's Great Hall. Address by Dr. Billings, Washington, U.S., on "Our Medical Literature." Visit to Messrs. Penn's Works. 8 to 11 p.m. : Conversazione at the Guildhall, given to members of the Congress by the Lord Mayor and Corporation of the City of London.

Saturday, August 6.—10 a.m. to 1 p.m. : Sectional Meetings. 12.15 p.m. : Excursion to Croydon Sewage Farm. 1.45 p.m. : Excursion to Folkestone. 2 p.m. : Excursion to Hampton Court. 4 to 7 p.m. : Reception of a certain number of the members at Kew Gardens, by Sir J. D. Hooker. 4 to 7 p.m. : Garden Party will be given by Mr. and Mrs. Spencer Wells, at Golder's-hill, Hampstead. 4 to 7 p.m. : A Garden Party will be given by Mr. and Mrs. Saunders, at Fairlawn, Wimbledon. 6.30 p.m. : The United Hospitals' Club will entertain a party of the members of the Congress at Dinner at the "Star and Garter," Richmond-hill.

Sunday, August 7.—10 a.m. : A Full Choral Service will be held in Westminster Abbey; sermon by the Very Rev. Dean Stanley, D.D., F.R.S. 3.15 p.m. : A Full Choral Service will be held in St. Paul's Cathedral; sermon by the Rev. Canon Liddon, D.D., D.C.L. 1.30 p.m. : Excursion to Boxhill. Visit to Sir Trevor Lawrence. 2 p.m. : The Royal Botanic Society's Gardens, and the Gardens of the Zoological Society in the Regent's-park, will be open free to members on this, and on every day of the week, on presentation of their tickets. The Royal Gardens at Kew may be visited on Sunday, from 9 a.m. till sunset, and Hampton Court Palace and Gardens from 2 p.m. till sunset.

Monday, August 8.—10 a.m. to 1 p.m. : Sectional Meetings. 2 to 3.30 p.m. : Additional meeting time for Sections. 4 to 5.30 p.m. : Fifth General Meeting, St. James's Great Hall. Address by Professor Volkmann, Halle, "Ueber Moderne Chirurgie." Visit to the Docks. 6.30 p.m. : Dinner given to a certain number of the foreign members of the Congress by the Worshipful Master and Wardens of the Society of Apothecaries in their Hall in Blackfriars, 9.30 p.m.; Conversazione given by the Royal College of Surgeons to the members of the Congress.

Tuesday, August 9.—10 a.m. to 1 p.m.: Sectional Meetings. 2 to 3 p.m.: Sixth General Meeting, St. James's Great Hall. Address by Professor Huxley, F.R.S., D.C.L. London, "The Connexion of the Biological Sciences with Medicine." 5 p.m.: Concluding Meeting of the Congress.

INFORMAL DINNER AT THE CRYSTAL PALACE.

After the concluding meeting, the members, accompanied by their friends, including ladies, will proceed to Victoria Station, for High Level Station (London, Chatham, and Dover Railway), where special trains will be in waiting at four o'clock to convey them to the Crystal Palace. After a visit to the Palace and grounds, an Informal Dinner will take place in the Concert-room, about seven o'clock. At dusk, the fountains will play during a display of fireworks, which may be viewed by members of the Congress from the Queen's Corridor.

PLACES OF INTEREST.

The following places of interest may be visited by members of the Congress on conditions which can be ascertained at the office of the Reception Committee:—The Hunterian Museum of the Royal College of Surgeons, Lincoln's-inn-fields, 8 a.m. to 6 p.m.; the Library of the Royal College of Surgeons, 10 a.m. to 8 p.m.; the Library of the Royal Medical and Chirurgical Society, 53, Berners-street, W., 1.30 to 6 p.m.; the Tower of London, 10 a.m. to 4 p.m.; the Royal Mint, Tower-hill; the Bank of England; the Royal Botanic Society's Gardens, Regent's-park, 9 a.m. till sunset; the Gardens of the Zoological Society, Regent's-park, 9 a.m. till sunset; the Royal Gardens at Kew, 1 p.m. till sunset; Hampton Court Palace and Gardens, 10 a.m. till sunset; the Inner and Middle Temple Halls and Temple Church; Her Majesty's Prison, Holloway, N.; the General Post Office, St. Martin's-le-Grand; the British Museum, Great Russell-street, Bloomsbury, W.C., Monday, Wednesday, and Friday, 10 a.m. to 6 p.m., Saturday, 12 noon to 8 p.m.; the National Gallery, Trafalgar-square, W.C., 10 a.m. to 6 p.m.; the Soane Museum, Lincoln's-inn-fields, W.C., daily, 11 a.m. to 6 p.m.; the Dulwich Gallery, Dulwich, S.E., daily, 10 a.m. to 5 p.m.; the Natural History Museum, Cromwell-road, South Kensington, S.W., daily, 10 a.m. to 6 p.m.; the South Kensington Museum, S.W., Monday, Tuesday, and Saturday, 10 a.m. to 10 p.m., Wednesday, Thursday, and Friday, 10 a.m. to 6 p.m.; the National Portrait Gallery, South Kensington, daily, 10 a.m. to 6 p.m.; the Indian Museum, South Kensington, daily, 10 a.m. to 6 p.m.; Stafford House (the residence of the Duke of Sutherland), St. James's, S.W.; Apsley House (the residence of the Duke of Wellington), Hyde-park-corner, W.; Bridgwater House (the residence of the Earl of Ellesmere); Hertford House (the residence of Sir Richard Wallace), Manchester-square, W.; Dudley House (the residence of the Earl of Dudley), Park-lane, W.; Dorchester House (the residence of R. S. Holford, Esq.), Park-lane, W.; Messrs. Barclay and Perkins' Brewery, Southwark, S.E.; Messrs. Mandslay's Works, Westminster-bridge-road, S.E., daily, 2 to 3 p.m., except Saturday; Messrs. Penn's Engine Factory, Greenwich, S.E.; Messrs. Siemens' Telegraph Construction Works, Woolwich; the Royal Arsenal, Woolwich; the Docks; Buckingham Palace; Windsor Castle; the Houses of Parliament.

Clubs.—The following clubs are, by the courtesy of the committees, open to such foreign members as shall inscribe their names in the book lying for the purpose at the office of these Committees, at the the Oriental College of Physicians:—The East India United Service Club, 14, St. James'-square, S.W.; German Athenaeum, 93, Mortimer-street, W.; Hanover-square Club, 4, Hanover-square, W.; Société Nationale Française, 20, Bedford-street, W.C.; The Science Club, 4, Savile-row, W. The Army and Navy Club, 36, Pall-mall, W., will be open to foreign medical officers, either naval or military.

EXCURSIONS.

Friday, August 5.—12.45 p.m.; Mr. John Penn will receive a certain number of the members of the Congress on board a special steamer at Charing-cross Pier, in order to proceed down the river to Greenwich, and after luncheon there with Mr. Penn, to visit the engine works of the Messrs. Penn, returning either by water or rail to Charing-cross.

Saturday, August 6.—1.45 p.m.: Excursion to Folkestone. A certain number of members will leave Charing-cross Station by special train, provided free of cost by the South-Eastern Railway Company, to witness the unveiling of the Harvey Memorial Statue. After the ceremony the Mayor and Corporation of Folkestone will entertain the visitors at a Banquet in the Town Hall. 5 p.m.: Excursion to Hampton Court. Under the guidance of Dr. Langdon Down, a party will visit Hampton Court Palace and Gardens, proceeding thence by river to Hampton Wick, where they will be entertained by Dr. Down at a garden party at his residence, Normansfield. The members can reach Hampton Court either by the road, the river, or the rail. A special train will leave Waterloo Station (South-Western Railway) at two o'clock. 12.10: Excursion to Croydon Sewage Farm and Beddington Female Orphan Asylum. A limited number of members, under the guidance of Dr. Alfred Carpenter, will inspect the Farm and the Asylum. A luncheon, consisting mainly of the produce of the farm, will be provided by Dr. Carpenter in the Old Hall at Beddington—a place of favourite resort by Queen Elizabeth in the time of the Carews. Trains leave Victoria at 12.10, London-bridge at 12.15, for Beddington, where vehicles will be waiting for the party. Trains return from Croydon about five o'clock.

Sunday, August 7.—1.30 p.m.: Excursion to Boxhill. A special train will leave Victoria Station (Brighton and South Coast Railway) for Boxhill, situated in a beautiful part of the county of Surrey. At Burford Lodge, close to the station, Sir Trevor Lawrence, Bart., M.P., will receive a party of the members of the Congress at luncheon. The train will return from Boxhill to London about 6 p.m.

Monday, August 8.—11 a.m.: Visit to the Docks, under the guidance and hospitality of Sir George Chambers, Chairman of the London, St. Katharine, and Victoria Dock Company. A limited number of members will proceed to the St. Katharine Dock House on Tower-hill at 11 a.m., where the indigo and tobacco floors will be inspected, and, in the adjoining London Dock, the ivory, drug, spice, and wool floors, and also the largest wine vault. From the Shadwell Basin a steamboat will then take the party, for whom Sir George Chambers will provide luncheon on board, down the river to the Victoria Docks. Having passed through the Royal Victoria and Royal Albert Docks, the party will return by the river to Charing-cross Pier.

REVIEWS.

A Treatise on Diphtheria. By A. JACOBI, M.D. New York: William Wood and Co. 1880. Pp. 252.

THE book before us is to be considered as an augmented edition of a monograph which appeared in Gerhardt's *Handbuch der Kinderkrankheiten*, 1877.

Dr. Jacobi seems to have enjoyed large opportunities for studying diphtheria, as he tells us that his experience is based on several thousand cases.

As regards the identity or non-identity of "croup" and diphtheria, and of the bacteric causation or character of the diphtheritic poison, the author thinks "that the safest verdict of the sober critic is still 'not proven.'" Fortunately, non-acceptance of the bacteria doctrine "does not at all interfere with the success of the rational practitioner."

The book is divided into nine chapters; each chapter closes with a "summary" of its contents, which is a great help to the reader. We shall not attempt any critical review, for, to do the author justice, it would be necessary to transcribe his summaries just as they stand. We may say that the practitioner will find both instruction and interest in the perusal of the chapters, while a would-be critic is disarmed by the "non-proven" expression of opinion just quoted. We may select a few sentences from the summaries as samples of the remainder. Thus, in speaking of the mode of infection, our author says, "There are cases in which the origin of the disease is decidedly local." "There are others in which the poisoning of the blood through inhalation is the first step in the development of the disease"; while "in many cases, both a sore integument and the lungs are the inlets of the poison simultaneously."

Dr. Jacobi says, "Diphtheria is very contagious. Both the patient and his surroundings, dwelling, furniture, towels, etc., convey the disease. In dwellings it rises to the upper storeys with the current of warm air. The poison clings mostly to mucous membranes. Mild cases may communicate serious ones, and *vice versâ*. The period of incubation lasts two days or more; it may last a fortnight." He divides diphtheria in the fauces into the "croupous," the "diphtheritic," and the "necrotic." The symptoms must be carefully studied, and therefore we make no attempt to transcribe them in this place.

In the last chapter, that on Treatment, we are told that "Every case should be treated on general principles; thus it is not possible to lay down a routine treatment for every individual case. High fever should be reduced by sponging and baths, quinine and sodium salicylate; collapse speedily treated, and severe reflex symptoms, as vomiting, etc., checked at once. Whether to employ for this purpose ether, wine, cognac, champagne, or coffee, must be decided by the physician in individual cases. The administration of the remedy, whether by mouth, by injection into the bowels, or subcutaneously, as I have employed cognac, ether, alcohol, and camphor dissolved in ether or alcohol, in some cases with decided and rapid success, must depend on the condition of the organs and on the urgency of the case. At all events, it may be stated that all the above remedies are frequently of no service, because they have been administered too late and in too small doses; and hence we may infer that to obtain the proper results both from external and internal treatment the remedy must be employed early and often and in sufficient quantity. If I have ever had cause to feel contented with the results of treatment in diphtheria, it is owing to the fact that I did not lose time. Moreover, the nourishment of the patient is a matter of very great importance, and should not be neglected, and no medicines resorted to which are apt to derange the digestion of the patient. It is true that caution must be exercised in the food administered to febrile patients, but we must bear in mind that when the lymphatic vessels are kept empty, and no new and proper material is introduced into them, the absorption of locally existing poisonous substances is proportionally increased." After these general remarks, the author discusses the value, mode of action, and methods of employing all the long string of medicaments which have been suggested by various authors, beginning with chlorate of potassium. This drug has enjoyed a large reputation, and those who would wish for a *resumé* of what has been said in its praise cannot do better than read what Dr. Jacobi (who does not believe in its cure-all properties) has written. He says—"The practical point I wish to make is this, that chlorate of potassium is by no means an indifferent remedy; that it can prove, and has proved, dangerous and fatal in a number of instances, producing one of the most dangerous diseases—acute nephritis." The use of disinfectants is also advocated—"In times of an epidemic every public place, theatre, ball-room, dining-hall, tavern, ought to be treated like a hospital. Where there is a large conflux of people, there are certainly many who carry the disease with them. Disinfection must be enforced by the authorities at regular intervals."

This will show what broad views the author holds, and assist the curious in guessing that he inclines to the doctrine of identity rather than of non-identity of all membranous inflammations of mucous surfaces.

GENERAL CORRESPONDENCE.

OMISSION OF NAMES FROM THE MEDICAL REGISTER.
LETTER FROM MR. J. W. BARNES.

[To the Editor of the Medical Times and Gazette.]

SIR,—Finding, quite by accident, that my name had been omitted from the Medical Register I went directly to the Registrar for explanation, and was informed that it was now the rule to strike off the names of all who did not reply to their circular, whether the address had been changed or not. Feeling that others might be ignorant of this (to my mind) summary regulation, makes me think it of sufficient importance to trouble you with this communication.

I am, &c., J. WICKHAM BARNES.
3, Bolt-court, Fleet-street, July 13.

OBITUARY.

MICHAEL FRANCIS WARD, M.D.

WE regret to record that tidings have been received in London of the death of Dr. Michael Francis Ward, M.P. for Galway in the last Parliament. Dr. Ward was the second son of the late Mr. Timothy Ward, merchant, of Galway, by his marriage with Catherine, daughter of Mr. John Lynch, of that city. He was born in 1845, and was educated at the College of St. Ignatius, and at Queen's College, Galway, where he matriculated in 1861; he afterwards studied medicine at Steevens's Hospital, Dublin, and became a licentiate of the College of Surgeons, Ireland, in 1868. Dr. Ward was for some time Curator of the Anatomical Museum of the Catholic University of Ireland, and he was also Surgeon to the Infirmary for Children in Buckingham-street, Dublin. He was elected in the Liberal or "Home Rule" interest as member for the borough of Galway in June, 1874, in the place of Mr. O'Donnell, who had been unseated on petition. Dr. Ward went out about a twelvemonth since to Demerara, where he was employed in the Government Medical Service, and where his death occurred.

JOSEPH A. BOND, L.S.A.

THIS estimable gentleman expired, at the age of sixty-eight, at his residence in Polesworth, where he had practised upwards of forty-seven years, having succeeded his father, who there began the career of the profession in 1798.

Mr. Bond possessed a conscientiousness, benevolence, and humour which made him of sterling value to his friends and patients, and a genial companion to all who enjoyed his society. Possessed of rare natural abilities, his quiet country life enabled him to cultivate those habits of keen observation, and that quick grasp of the nature of disease, for which his opinion was so highly valued and which rarely betrayed him. Fond of rural life with its associated sports, in which he excelled, he was thus enabled to qualify the monotony of a large general practice, in which he commanded the confidence and respect of all. During the last twelvemonth of an unusually active life his health began to fail, and after bronchitis he suffered from asthma, complicated with anasarca. His loss will be felt far beyond the limits of the old village in which he spent his life.

NEW INVENTIONS AND IMPROVEMENTS.

FLETCHER'S CONCENTRATED LIQUORS.

FROM Messrs. Fletcher and Fletcher, North London Chemical Works, Holloway-road, we have lately received samples of their concentrated liquors for chemical syrups. There is no disputing the great convenience of these preparations for dispensing purposes, as, when any one of the syrups is required, the dispenser has only to add the proper proportion of Fletcher's concentrated liquor to a certain volume of simple syrup in order to obtain the required combination; or, if desired, the concentrated liquor may be added to pure water, and thus the medicine, as to be taken, may be prepared at once. Of these liquors, the most useful are, probably, those of. the hypophosphate and lactophosphate of lime, of the bromide and the hypophosphate of iron, of the iodide of iron, and of the compound phosphates of iron, quinine, and strychnine. Messrs. Fletcher also prepare a liquor ferri phosphatis compositus, with which a "chemical food" may readily be prepared, and syrups of the hydrobromates. All these preparations are very elegant, and, so far as our observation of them goes, they are stable and trustworthy.

HEWLETT'S MISTURA PEPSINÆ CO.

THIS elegant preparation, brought out by Messrs. C. J. Hewlett and Sons, manufacturing chemists, of Cree Church-lane, Leadenhall-street, E.C., is a compound of pepsine, liquor bismuthi, purified solution of opium, hydrocyanic acid, and tincture of nux vomica, in such wise that each fluid drachm contains two minims of hydrocyanic acid (P.B.) and three minims and a half of solution of opium. It will no doubt be found a handy and convenient form for use whenever such a combination of drugs is required. It is of a pretty colour, is bright and clear, and, of course, is miscible in water, and the dose would be from half a drachm to a drachm, diluted.

McKESSON AND ROBBINS' CAPSULED PILLS.

AMERICAN chemists are wonderfully ingenious in inventing new, especially convenient and handy, and even enticing, forms of medicines; and the latest examples we have seen of this praiseworthy ingenuity are the "McKesson and Robbins' Capsuled Pills." The drug or drugs to be taken are enclosed in a thin but perfect envelope of pure transparent gelatine, which is applied while the pill-mass is soft; and while the contents of the capsule are thus preserved from damp and atmospheric influence, the envelope is perfectly and quickly soluble. The pills are really beautifully made, and are unusually elegant preparations. They are ovoid in shape, and it is claimed that this makes them much more easy to swallow than are round pills. We rather doubt this, but will admit this much—that confidence is an immense aid in the swallowing of pills; to hesitate about it is to be lost : and consequently we have no doubt that people who believe that an ovoid can be more easily swallowed than a round one, will be able to prove in themselves the soundness of their faith. Anyhow, these pills are very pretty, and very convenient—qualities that deserve to be widely recognised. We will add a special word of recommendation for the capsule pills of the bisulphate of quinine. This salt is much more soluble than the ordinary sulphate is, and these little pills of it will be found very convenient for travellers as well as for practitioners. Burroughs, Wellcome, and Co., Snow-hill, London, are the agents for the "McKesson and Robbins" pills.

THE SO-CALLED RUPTURE OF THE INTERNAL LATERAL LIGAMENT OF THE KNEE-JOINT.—After describing two cases under the above designation, and some experimental attempts to produce the injury, Dr. Jersey formulates, in the New York Med. Jour. for June, the following conclusions:—1. Many cases of the so-called rupture are in reality cases of fracture of the internal tuberosity of the condyle. 2. Many of the more severe sprains are fractures of the tuberosity. 3. The absence of a bony crepitus is no certain sign of the non-existence of fracture at this part. 4. The diagnosis rests upon the extreme lateral motion, the severity of the pain on manipulation, the localised pain always found at a certain point, and the length of time required for complete recovery.

MEDICAL NEWS.

KING AND QUEEN'S COLLEGE OF PHYSICIANS IN IRELAND.—At the usual monthly examinations for the Licences of the College, held on Monday, Tuesday, Wednesday, and Thursday, July 4, 5, 6, and 7, the following candidates were successful :—

For the First Professional Examination—

M'George, Mary, London.
Morice, Margaret, London.

For the Licence to practise Medicine—

Acheson, Howard William, New Ross, co. Wexford.
Anderson, Louis Edward, Rathmines, Dublin.
Atkinson, James Law, Ballyshannon.
Birmingham, Herbert Joseph, Ballinrobe, co. Mayo.
Brownrigg, Herbert Watson, Camolin, co. Wexford.
Chance, Arthur Gerald, Dublin.
Colgan, Francis Philip, Kilcock, co. Kildare.
De la Cherois, Annie, Belfast.
De Lisle, Samuel Ernest, Dublin.
Gallagher, Thomas Mark, Killala.
Hayes, Alfred Adolphus, Dublin.
Jones, William Percy, Dublin.
Lane, John Lilly, Cabinteely, co. Dublin.
Lynch, Francis John, Armagh.
Macmullen, James Carnegie, Dublin.
MacSwiney, Claude Henry, Dublin.
Mahon, Henry Greenwood, Sandycove, co. Dublin.
Mitchell, Adam, Parsonstown, King's Co.
Murphy, Edmond, Dublin.
Murray, Arthur Hill, Edenderry, King's Co.
Nelis, George, Blackrock, co. Dublin.
O'Brien, Francis Randolph, Ennis, co. Clare.
Power, Robert Ignatius, Carrick-on-Suir.
Robinson, Frederick, Dublin.
Waterhouse, William Dakin, Kingstown, co. Dublin.

For the Licence to practise Midwifery—

Acheson, Howard William.
Anderson, Louis Edward.
Atkinson, James Law.
Birmingham, Herbert Joseph.
Brownrigg, Herbert Watson.
Chance, Arthur Gerald.
Colgan, Francis Philip.
De la Cherois, Annie.
De Lisle, Samuel Ernest.
Dempsey, Patrick Joseph, Dublin.
Gallagher, Thomas Mark.
Jencken, Francis John, Kingstown, co. Dublin.
Jones, William Percy.
Lane, John Lilly.
Lynch, Francis John.
Macmullen, James Carnegie.
Mahon, Henry Greenwood.
Mitchell, Adam.
Murphy, Edmond.
Murray, Arthur Hill.
Nelis, George.
Nickson, Augustus, Ardee, co. Louth.
O'Brien, Francis Randolph.
Power, Robert Ignatius.
Robinson, Frederick.
Waterhouse, William Dakin.

The following Licentiates in Medicine, having complied with the by-laws relating to membership, have been duly elected Members of the College :—

Graham, William, 1868, Fleet-Surgeon Royal Navy.
Clune, Michael Joseph, 1878, Sydney, New South Wales.
Harrison, Damer, 1876, Liverpool.

ROYAL COLLEGE OF SURGEONS OF ENGLAND.—The following gentlemen passed their primary examinations in Anatomy and Physiology at a meeting of the Board of Examiners on the 8th inst., and, when eligible, will be admitted to the pass examination, viz. :—

Bate, John F., student of University College Hospital.
Bird, Henry, of University College Hospital.
Ellis, Charles C., of St. George's Hospital.
Hall, Fred, of the Manchester School.
Harper, John M., of the London Hospital.
Hitchcock, Alfred J., of the London Hospital.
Hodge, William T., of Guy's Hospital.
Hugill, George F., of Guy's Hospital.
Kidd, Leonard J., of Guy's Hospital.
Manders, Neville, of St. Mary's Hospital.
Rowe, Arthur W., of St. Mary's Hospital.
Saville, Henry W. B., of the Manchester School.
Sidebottom, Richard B., of the Manchester School.
Williams, George H., of the Manchester School.
Woods, Everard, of St. Bartholomew's Hospital.

Nine candidates were rejected. The following gentlemen passed on the 11th inst., viz. :—

Adams, Gofton G., student of St. George's Hospital.
Bean, Charles M., of Guy's Hospital.
Des Voeux, Harold A., of St. George's Hospital.
Edgelow, Herbert, of St. George's Hospital.
Gilkes, Norton G., of the London Hospital.
Hale, George M., of St. Mary's Hospital.
Jones, Harry J., of Guy's Hospital.
Kirkhouse, George, of St. Bartholomew's Hospital.
Ruck, John R., of St. Bartholomew's Hospital.
Sharpley, Edward, of Guy's Hospital.
Starr, William H., of St. Bartholomew's Hospital.
Taylor, Charles H., of King's College Hospital.
Watson, James, of the Charing-cross Hospital.
Whitworth, William, of St. Bartholomew's Hospital.

Ten candidates were rejected. The following gentlemen passed on the 12th inst., viz. :—

Brickwell, Henry T., student of the London Hospital.
Buck, Lewis A., of King's College Hospital.
Carroll, Edward R. W., of the Westminster Hospital.
Cook, Robert J., of Guy's Hospital.
Edwards, William L., of the London Hospital.
Harvey, James, of Guy's Hospital.
Haydon, Hildyard W., of King's College Hospital.
Howard, Edmund G., of the London Hospital.
Jones, Hugh E., of Guy's Hospital.
Law, Charles W., of St. Bartholomew's Hospital.
Rogers, William F. C., of St. George's Hospital.
Warren, William J., of Guy's Hospital.

Thirteen candidates were rejected. The following gentlemen passed on the 13th inst., viz. :—

Anderson, W. Dunlop, B.A. Cantab., of St. George's Hospital.
Clarkson, Edward, University College Hospital.
Duke, Robert E., of University College Hospital.
Hewer, Henry J., of St. Bartholomew's Hospital.
Howard, Herbert, of Guy's Hospital.
Koele, J. Rushworth, of St. Thomas's Hospital.
Kindle, F. Wellesley, of King's College Hospital.
Linnell, Edward, of Guy's Hospital.
Lockwood, Harry, of King's College Hospital.
Parry, Herbert L., of the London Hospital.
Penfold, Frederick W. H., of Guy's Hospital.
Reeks, John, of St. Bartholomew's Hospital.
Roe, Montagu W., of St. George's Hospital.
Sumpter, Walter J. E., of University College Hospital.
Thomas, Samuel R., of Guy's Hospital.
Winn, T. Cromwell, of the London Hospital.

Eight candidates were rejected.

APOTHECARIES' HALL, LONDON.—The following gentlemen passed their examination in the Science and Practice of Medicine, and received certificates to practise, on Thursday, July 7 :—

Alexander, Alexander Charles Archibald, Ardrossan, Ayrshire, N.B.
Brewitt, James Bunning Brewitt, Melton Mowbray.
Johnson, James Bovell, 364, Kingsland-road.

APPOINTMENTS.

⁎ The Editor will thank gentlemen to forward to the Publishing-office, as early as possible, information as to all new Appointments that take place.

BENNETT, STOKES, L.R.C.P. Lond., M.R.C.S. Eng., L.D.S. Eng.—Assistant Dental Surgeon to the Middlesex Hospital.
LAYCOCK, G. LOCKWOOD, M.B.—Physician to the North-West London Free Dispensary for Sick Children.
PAYNE, HENRY, M.R.C.S. Eng., L.R.C.P. Edin.—House-Surgeon to the Infirmary at Ashton-under-Lyne.

BIRTHS.

BROWNRIGG.—On July 5, at Hill House, Gravesend, the wife of J. Annesley Brownrigg, M.A., M.D., of a daughter.
LYLE.—On June 5, at 19, Westbourne-terrace, the wife of W. V. Lyle, M.D., of a son.
MEREDITH.—On July 6, at 84, Week-street, Maidstone, the wife of John E. Meredith, M.D., of a daughter.
NOLAN.—On June 8, at Colaba Point, Bombay, the wife of Surgeon-Major W. Nolan, M.D., Superintendent Colaba Asylum, of a son.
STROVER.—On July 3, at Mill Hill, Hendon, the wife of Walter Strover, M.R.C.S., of a daughter.

MARRIAGES.

CAMPBELL—TWEEDIE.—On July 6, at the British Consulate, Geneva, Surgeon-Major Alexander Dugald Campbell, Bengal Medical Service, third surviving son of the late Rear-Admiral Donald Campbell, of Barbreck, Argyleshire, to Isabella Leslie, elder daughter of the late Alexander George Tweedie, Madras Civil Service, and grand-daughter of Alexander Tweedie, M.D., F.R.S., of Bute Lodge, Twickenham.
MACBRAYNE—WOODBURN.—On July 7, at Camlarg, Dolmellington, N.B., David Robert MacBrayne, of Glasgow, to Jean, third daughter of David Woodburn, M.D., late H.E.I.C.S.
SQUIRE—BURRIDGE.—On July 6, at the Church of St. Martin on-the-Hill, Scarborough, William Wilkinson Squire, C.E., eldest son of William Squire, M.D., of Orchard-street, Portman-square, to Beatrice Elizabeth, second daughter of the Rev. John Burridge, Vicar of Emanuel Church, Everton, Liverpool.
TULK—YOXHALL.—On March 9, at the residence of the bride's parents, Arthur Tulk, son of Alfred Tulk, M.R.C.S., of London, to Mary Adelaide, fourth daughter of John Yoxall, of Beechworth, Victoria.
TURNER—LINGEN.—On July 5, at St. Paul's, Tupsley, near Hereford, Thomas Turner, of Hereford, to Ellen Mary, eldest surviving daughter of the late Charles Lingen, M.D.
TURNER—TIZARD.—On July 5, at the parish church, Weybridge, George Sydney Turner, solicitor, of Southampton, to Ethel, second daughter of Henry Tizard, M.D., of Baycliffe, Weymouth.
WILSON—MILLAR.—On July 6, at 28, East Claremont-street, Edinburgh, Thomas Jackson Wilson, solicitor before the Supreme Courts, Edinburgh, to Jessie Guthrie Millar, eldest daughter of Robert Mungle, Staff-Surgeon R.N.

DEATHS.

BEALES, GEORGIANA, wife of Robert Beales, M.D., J.P., at Chapel House, Congleton, on July 8, aged 88.

GOLDIE-SCOTT, HELEN MARY DOROTHY, eldest daughter of the late Thomas Goldie-Scott, of Craigmuir, M.D., Deputy-Inspector of Hospitals, at Craigmuir, Kirkcudbrightshire, on July 9, in her 13th year.

HENDERSON, HAROLD BRUCE, infant son of J. B. Henderson, M.D., at Essex House, Waltham Abbey, on July 6.

POLLOCK, MARGARET, wife of T. Pollock, M.D., late of Hatton-garden, at Rose Hill Cottage, Hornsey, on July 5, aged 77.

PURNELL, THOMAS, M.D., J.P., late of Wells, Somerset, at 1, Weymouth-villas, Gunnersbury, aged 64.

VACANCIES.

In the following list the nature of the office vacant, the qualifications required in the candidate, the person to whom application should be made and the day of election (as far as known) are stated in succession.

ARASAIG DISTRICT OF ARDNAMURCHAN PARISH.—Medical Officer. (*For particulars see Advertisement.*)

CHARING-CROSS HOSPITAL MEDICAL SCHOOL.—Chair of Comparative Anatomy. (*For particulars see Advertisement.*)

HOSPITAL FOR WOMEN, SOHO-SQUARE, W.—House-Physician. (*For particulars see Advertisement.*)

NORTH STAFFORDSHIRE INFIRMARY.—Two Resident Medical Officers. (*For particulars see Advertisement.*)

SOMERSET AND BATH LUNATIC ASYLUM, WELLS.—Medical Superintendent. Candidates to send testimonials to the visitors (under cover), addressed to Mr. B. T. Duke, their Clerk, at the said Asylum, not later than July 20, endorsed, "Superintendent Candidate." Candidates must not exceed the age of thirty-five, and are required to be graduates of medicine of any university in the United Kingdom—L.R.C.P. Lond., M.R.C.S. Lond., Edin., or Dub. Testimonials must state past medical career, and experience in the treatment of insanity.

STAFFORDSHIRE GENERAL INFIRMARY, STAFFORD.—Honorary Physician. Applications, with testimonials, to be sent under cover to the Secretary, F. Marsh, at the Infirmary, on or before July 20. Further particulars can be obtained on application to the Secretary.

STOCKTON-UPON-TEES HOSPITAL AND DISPENSARY.—House-Surgeon (non-resident). Candidates must be doubly qualified. Applications, stating age, with recent testimonials, to be sent to the Secretary, John Settle, not later than August 9.

UNION AND PAROCHIAL MEDICAL SERVICE.

⁎ The area of each district is stated in acres. The population is computed according to the census of 1871.

RESIGNATIONS.

Crediton Union.—Mr. Richard Bartlett has resigned the Morchard Bishop District: area 13,200; population 2608; salary £52 10s.

APPOINTMENTS.

Alderbury Union.—James Kelland, L.R.C.P. and L.R.C.S., to the Fifth District.

Cockermouth Union.—Robinson James Hutchinson, M.D. and M.C. Edin., to the Second Cockermouth District.

Leeds Union.—Richard Tippetts Richardson, M.R.C.S. Eng. and L.S.A. Lond., to be Assistant Medical Officer at the Workhouse.

Peterborough Union.—Lawrence Clapham, M.R.C.S. Eng. and L.S.A. Lond., to the Thorney District.

St. Columb Major Union.—John Cawful Mackay, L.R.C.P. and L.R.C.S. Edin., to the Workhouse.

Sheffield Union.—Louis Gibson Hunt, M.D., L.R.C.P., and L.F.P.& S. Glasg., to the Workhouse. William Francis Blyth, L.R.C.P. and M.R.C.S. Edin., to be Resident Assistant Medical Officer at the Workhouse.

Wharfedale Union.—Walter H. Cheetham, M.B. Durh., M.R.C.S. Eng., to the First District.

Whitchurch Union (Hants).—William Fleming Phillips, L.R.C.P. and M.R.C.S. Edin., to the St. Mary Bourne District.

MR. BISHOP'S "THOUGHT-READING."—After quoting the account of the so-called thought-reading which has been going the round of our newspapers, the *New York Med. Record* (June 18) observes:—"American readers will recognise all these performances as having been made familiar to audiences in this country not long ago by Brown and others. It was then quite well settled that the explanation lay in the fact that the persons experimented on made unconscious muscular movements which gave the clue to the former. It is really a case of muscle-reading, and not of mind-reading. We are not aware who first suggested this physiological explanation of the phenomena. It is one that probably would occur to any person scientifically trained, who had studied the matter. In the *Popular Science Monthly* for 1877 there appeared a very full account of the whole subject, with a full explanation of it, by Dr. George M. Beard, who investigated it thoroughly at that time. A comparison of that article with what has been done and said across the Atlantic recently, shows that the eminent scientific gentlemen there are only repeating what has been seen and fully studied here. We believe that Mr. Bishop, though a very clever young man, and in no sense a charlatan, does not accept the unconscious muscular action theory himself. He thinks that he possesses some occult power, but what it is he does not profess to understand."

THUMB-SUCKING.—In a paper read at the American Medical Association, Dr. Goodwillie, of New York, concluded—1. Thumb-sucking is more disastrous to the health of the child than the sucking of the other fingers, for, once in the mouth, it more readily remains there during sleep. 2. It interferes with the child's proper rest, which should be continuous and undisturbed, and so becomes a source of nervous irritation and exhaustion. 3. It interferes with the natural respiration through the nose, and sets up abnormal conditions. 4. It malforms the anterior part of the mouth, and affects proper mastication. The treatment consists in breaking off the habit by applying a leather pad to the elbow, preventing the hand from coming to the mouth.—*Boston Med. Jour.*, May 19.

MEDICAL ACTS COMMISSION.—This Commission met at 2, Victoria-street, Westminster, on the 8th, 9th, and 11th inst. The evidence of Mr. John Marshall, Dr. D. R. Haldane, Dr. T. S. Byass, and Dr. Edward Waters was taken. Present—The Earl of Camperdown (chairman), the Bishop of Peterborough, the Right Hon. W. H. F. Cogan, the Master of the Rolls, Sir William Jenner, Bart., K.C.B., Mr. Simon, C.B., Professor Huxley, Professor Turner, Mr. Bryce, M.P., and Mr. John White (Secretary).

PILOCARPIN IN DIPHTHERIA.—Dr. Jacobi, discussing the treatment of diphtheria at the meeting of the American Medical Association (*Boston Med. Jour.*, May 19), adverted to the statements published by Dr. Guttmann that he had been invariably and rapidly successful in all the eighty-one cases he had treated by pilocarpin. Assertions like these differ in nowise from those made concerning their remedies by the most reckless quacks. The action of pilocarpin in increasing the secretion from the skin or mucous membrane is well known. Diphtheritic membranes are of two kinds—they are either deposited on the surface, or they are imbedded in the mucous membrane and submucous tissue; and although a mucous membrane may throw off a diphtheritic membrane only deposited upon it, it is not easy to see how it can cast off one embedded in its tissue. Cases in which membrane is only deposited on the surface will recover under the influence of any treatment, and even without any treatment at all. But severe cases, in which the mucous membrane and the submucous tissue are the seat of a necrotic process, are of a very different character. They are generally of a septic character, and do not heal by simple removal of the deposit. Dr. Jacobi has tried this pilocarpin in severe cases, which are the only ones proper for testing a new remedy, and in not a single case was it of the least utility, while in some it seemed to hasten the fatal termination.

APPOINTMENTS FOR THE WEEK.

July 16. *Saturday (this day).*

Operations at St. Bartholomew's, 1½ p.m.; King's College, 1½ p.m.; Royal Free, 2 p.m.; Royal London Ophthalmic, 11 a.m.; Royal Westminster Ophthalmic, 1½ p.m.; St. Thomas's, 1½ p.m.; London, 2 p.m.

18. *Monday.*

Operations at the Metropolitan Free, 2 p.m.; St. Mark's Hospital for Diseases of the Rectum, 2 p.m.; Royal London Ophthalmic, 11 a.m.; Royal Westminster Ophthalmic, 1½ p.m.

19. *Tuesday.*

Operations at Guy's, 1½ p.m.; Westminster, 2 p.m.; Royal London Ophthalmic, 11 a.m.; Royal Westminster Ophthalmic, 1½ p.m.; West London, 3 p.m.

20. *Wednesday.*

Operations at University College, 2 p.m.; St. Mary's, 1¼ p.m.; Middlesex, 1 p.m.; London, 2 p.m.; St. Bartholomew's, 1½ p.m.; Great Northern, 2 p.m.; Samaritan, 2½ p.m.; King's College (by Mr. Lister), 2 p.m.; Royal London Ophthalmic, 11 a.m.; Royal Westminster Ophthalmic, 1½ p.m.; St. Thomas's, 1½ p.m.; St. Peter's Hospital for Stone, 2 p.m.; National Orthopædic, Great Portland-street, 10 a.m.

21. *Thursday.*

Operations at St. George's, 1 p.m.; Central London Ophthalmic, 1 p.m.; Royal Orthopædic, 2 p.m.; University College, 2 p.m.; Royal London Ophthalmic, 11 a.m.; Royal Westminster Ophthalmic, 1½ p.m.; Hospital for Diseases of the Throat, 2 p.m.; Hospital for Women, 2 p.m.; Charing-cross, 2 p.m.; London, 2 p.m.; North-West London, 2½ p.m.

22. *Friday.*

Operations at Central London Ophthalmic, 2 p.m.; Royal London Ophthalmic, 11 a.m.; South London Ophthalmic, 2 p.m.; Royal Westminster Ophthalmic, 1½ p.m.; St. George's (ophthalmic operations), 1¼ p.m.; Guy's, 1½ p.m.; St. Thomas's (ophthalmic operations), 2 p.m.

QUEKETT MICROSCOPICAL CLUB (University College), 8 p.m. Annual General Meeting; Election of Officers, etc.

VITAL STATISTICS OF LONDON.

Week ending Saturday, July 9, 1881.

BIRTHS.

Births of Boys, 1216; Girls, 1192; Total, 2408.
Corrected weekly average in the 10 years 1871-80, 2470·1.

DEATHS.

	Males.	Females.	Total.
Deaths during the week	809	776	1585
Weekly average of the ten years 1871-80, corrected to increased population ...	737·0	677·8	1414·8
Deaths of people aged 90 and upwards ...	...	...	48

DEATHS IN SUB-DISTRICTS FROM EPIDEMICS.

	Enumerated Population, 1881 (unrevised)	Small-pox.	Measles.	Scarlet Fever.	Diphtheria.	Whooping-cough.	Typhus.	Enteric (or Typhoid) Fever.	Simple continued Fever.	Diarrhœa.
West ...	668906	11	9	3	2	2	...	2	...	26
North ...	905677	25	16	16	1	14	...	...	...	26
Central ...	261798	...	11	9	1	5	...	...	...	12
East ...	692580	1	14	5	...	11	1	1	2	30
South ...	1265576	36	20	8	4	5	1	7	...	39
Total ...	3814571	73	70	41	8	37	2	10	2	135

METEOROLOGY.

From Observations at the Greenwich Observatory.

Mean height of barometer	29·966 in.
Mean temperature	65·1°
Highest point of thermometer	92·5°
Lowest point of thermometer	47·6°
Mean dew-point temperature	55·0°
General direction of wind	W.S.W.
Whole amount of rain in the week	1·00 in.

BIRTHS and DEATHS Registered and METEOROLOGY during the Week ending Saturday, July 9, in the following large Towns :—

Cities and boroughs. (Municipal boundaries except for London.)	Estimated Population to middle of the year 1881.*	Persons to an Acre.	Births Registered during the week ending July 9.	Deaths Registered during the week ending July 9.	Temperature of Air (Fahr.) Highest during the Week.	Temperature of Air (Fahr.) Lowest during the Week.	Temperature of Air (Fahr.) Weekly Mean of the Week.	Temp. of Air (Cent.) Weekly Mean of Daily Mean Values.	Rain Fall. In Inches.	Rain Fall. In Centimetres.
London ...	3629751	50·8	2406	1585	92·8	47·6	65·1	18·39	1·00	2·54
Brighton ...	107934	45·9	51	35	82·0	49·5	61·3	16·28	0·37	0·94
Portsmouth ...	128355	28·6	82	28	...	...	...	...	...	...
Norwich ...	88038	11·6	42	26	85·0	50·0	64·7	18·17	0·43	1·09
Plymouth ...	75262	54·0	51	28	79·0	49·4	60·1	15·62	0·35	0·89
Bristol ...	207140	46·5	125	62	86·0	48·0	59·4	15·22	0·77	1·96
Wolverhampton ...	75934	22·4	47	31	87·7	46·6	61·4	16·33	0·87	2·21
Birmingham ...	402296	47·9	277	162	...	...	...	...	...	...
Leicester ...	123120	38·5	78	48	85·5	46·8	61·2	16·22	0·60	1·52
Nottingham ...	188255	18·9	114	75	91·6	46·1	63·8	17·67	0·59	1·50
Liverpool ...	552998	106·3	389	255	84·2	49·7	59·6	15·34	0·77	1·96
Manchester ...	341289	79·5	252	143	...	...	...	...	...	...
Salford ...	177760	34·4	130	63	...	...	...	...	...	...
Oldham ...	112176	24·0	81	42	...	...	...	...	...	...
Bradford ...	184037	25·5	106	44	83·3	48·3	61·0	16·11	1·80	4·57
Leeds ...	310490	14·4	211	114	87·0	50·0	62·5	16·95	0·50	1·27
Sheffield ...	295621	14·5	178	107	85·0	48·0	62·5	16·95	0·75	1·90
Hull ...	155161	42·7	89	65	85·0	47·0	61·2	16·22	1·25	3·17
Sunderland ...	116753	42·2	52	41	80·0	48·0	60·8	16·31	1·00	2·54
Newcastle-on-Tyne ...	145675	27·1	114	62	...	...	...	...	...	...
Total of 20 large English Towns ...	7505775	36·0	4918	3022	92·8	46·1	61·8	16·56	0·79	2·01

* These figures are the numbers enumerated (but subject to revision) in April last, raised to the middle of 1881 by the addition of a quarter of a year's increase, calculated at the rate that prevailed between 1871 and 1881.

At the Royal Observatory, Greenwich, the mean reading of the barometer last week was 29·87 in. The highest reading was 30·06 in. at noon on Monday, and the lowest 29·52 in. on Wednesday morning.

NOTES, QUERIES, AND REPLIES.

He that questioneth much shall learn much.—Bacon.

M.D., Obstetrician.—The following gentlemen were nominated for the Examinership in Midwifery of the Royal College of Surgeons, viz., Drs. G. E. Herman, W. M. Grally Hewitt, Alfred Meadows, J. B. Potter, and John Williams.

Anæsthesia.—The lines of Middleton, the old dramatist, are—
"I'll imitate the pities of old surgeons
To this lost limb—who, ere they show their art,
Cast one asleep, then cut the diseased part."

M. O. E.—1. Yes. 2. The Act of Parliament passed in the session of 1871, fusing the Poor-law Board, the Home Office, and the Privy Council, so far as their sanitary functions were concerned, into one new department—the Local Government Board,—had the special advantage of creating a Minister specially charged with the duty of preparing sanitary Bills. 3. Centralisation means a superseding of the local authorities by a central authority for correcting inefficient local government.

AN APPEAL.

TO THE EDITOR OF THE MEDICAL TIMES AND GAZETTE.

Sir,—I trust you will allow me to make an appeal in your paper to the profession on behalf of Dr. Stainthorpe, of Wareham, who has lately been subjected to a vexatious prosecution.

The following are the facts as given in evidence, and copied from a local paper:—

The case was tried in the County Court held at Wimborne, before Mr. Serjeant Tindal Atkinson, the County Court Judge, and two assessors, Mr. C. H. Watts Parkinson and Mr. W. Wyke-Smith, surgeons, of Wimborne, appointed by the Judge, with the consent of the two legal gentlemen engaged in the case, Mr. Howard, of Weymouth, for the prosecution, and Mr. G. Symonds, of Dorchester, for the defence. The plaintiff, Jesse Still, journeyman miller, of Wareham, claimed £200 damages against the defendant (Dr. Stainthorpe) for the unskilful setting of his broken thigh on June 18, 1880.

The trial commenced on March 24 in the present year, and was concluded on the 31st, the judgment being delivered on April 29. After the plaintiff had given his evidence, in which he stated he could walk a mile or two, and in his cross-examination said he did not tell the Rev. Mr. Stokes (of Wareham) that he was in the hands of his solicitor and the doctors—at least, he did not think he did, he could not be positive,—

Dr. R. F. Philpots, of Poole, was called, and stated that the fractured limb was two or the two and a half inches shorter than the other. The fracture was an oblique one. He would not say the splints used were improper, but he had not seen such splints used before for an oblique fracture. It was more than probable that if extension had been used the shortening would not have taken place.

Mr. Nunn, surgeon, of Bournemouth, deposed that he found the limb which had been fractured two inches shorter than the other. To his mind nothing had been stated to show that extension had been used. In his cross-examination he said, "Shortening of limbs after fracture was the exception, and not the rule, so far as his experience of fifteen years taught him. It should be the exception, and was so. He had set a great many thighs, and had never had a case of shortening of the limb. If skilfully treated it would be impossible for a limb to shorten through a simple fracture like the one in the present case."

Mr. Tudor, surgeon, of Dorchester, said he agreed with the last two witnesses as to the splints not being properly adapted for counter-extension. He considered that in the present case the obliquity of the fracture rendered extension specially necessary.

Dr. Aldridge, of Dorchester, stated that the case in question was one in which he should most certainly have used the principles of extension.

For the defendant, Professor Longmore, of Netley Hospital, stated that the fractured limb was shortened over two inches and under two inches and a quarter, which was above the average. With the exception of the shortening, the limb was in its normal position, and there was nothing to show any unskilful treatment. He did not believe that, whatever the mode of treatment was, there would be a uniting of the bone without more or less shortening, but he had seen cases of greater shortening than the present. He would say that the man had an excellent limb. Mr. Enson, of Dorchester, and Surgeon to the County Hospital, said the plaintiff walked remarkably well, and he did not think there had been any unskilful treatment.

Dr. Leach, of Sturminster Newton, said the plaintiff walked in an easy and quick manner, and he could see nothing to complain of in the treatment the man had received. Mr. Lys, surgeon, of Bere Regis, was surprised to see the plaintiff walk so well after what he heard, and he did not consider there had been any unskilful treatment.

The Judge, on delivering his decision, read the report of the assessors at length, in which they exonerated the defendant from the charge of negligence and unskilful treatment. He stated that he found no reason to differ from them in the conclusions they arrived at, and that the evidence failed to satisfy him that the treatment had been negligently performed. The verdict was therefore for the defendant with costs.

I may be allowed to mention that I am not acquainted with Dr. Stainthorpe in the slightest degree, and that I make this appeal on his behalf purely out of sympathy for him. I have reason to know that in consequence of the plaintiff being a poor man, the trial has been the cause of considerable loss and anxiety as well as expense to the defendant.

I venture to hope that the profession will come forward and help Dr. Stainthorpe with pecuniary support, which will carry with it the moral sympathy which is so precious and gratifying to us all when in trouble and anxiety. Subscriptions will be thankfully received by me, and acknowledged in the medical papers. I am, &c.,

S. Leonards, Blandford, July 9. G. W. DANIELL.

The defendant, in his evidence, said that, finding there was no shortening, he put on a long splint on the outside and a short one on the inside. The fact of his not using the long Liston's splint with the perineal bandage appears to be the cause of the action being brought against him.

OUR YOUNG SOLDIERS.

TO THE EDITOR OF THE MEDICAL TIMES AND GAZETTE.

SIR,—I don't know whether you have read the report of the inquest on the men who died of sunstroke at Aldershot! The jury considered the troops should not have been subjected to the fatigue of a field day on that Monday, owing to the excessive heat, and that during the hot weather field days should be held in the early morning. So far as I am concerned, I have no objection to make to this, though perhaps it would be still better to have field days in the *middle of the night!* Officials might then publicly proclaim in Parliament that they *saw* nothing to complain of in the *physique* of the men. But I must say the jury overlooked one part of the evidence sadly. The soldiers had no water in their water-bottles! Now, anyone who knows anything of Tommy Atkins must be aware that if he is directed to take a water-bottle with him he will strictly obey, but it is sheer folly to suppose that he would *put water (inside the bottle)* without a specific order. We hear from the War Minister that the present recruits are infinitely superior in intelligence to the old class under long service, but as to their ever mastering the idea that water should be put into bottles, the Commander-in-Chief and the Secretary for War know, that the British nowhere-else-to-go-to, nothing-else-to-do, workhouse-or-glory volunteer is incapable of it. Decidedly the military authorities were to blame in some measure for the effects of the sun on the parched and thirsty troops. But the jury should also have added a rider to their recommendation. The moral was pointed out to them by the senior medical officer, when he stated that "when coffee-taverns were properly established throughout the army, there would be less sunstroke, for a good deal of it was due to the men drinking." What were the jury thinking of, not to snap at this bright idea! They should have recommended perambulating coffee-stalls to accompany each regiment, and portable furnaces to keep the pot a-boiling! Of course it would have been necessary to give *explicit orders* as to the coffee being put into the pots, and water to be put on the coffee, and fire to be put *under* the water, and so on; but still the gain would be enormous, for sunstroke would be erased from the list of possible diseases! My aunt, to whom I have read this, says, "Why not tea!" My uncle suggests "Date-coffee!" My grandmother says, "Pap!" However, these are matters of detail, and we must be guided by the opinion of the medical officer, who may possibly have based his theory on the fact that the Commander-in-Chief felt no ill effects whatever from the heat, and had probably taken coffee for *his* breakfast!   Yours as ever,

Temperance Hall.   THE ROVING CORRESPONDENT.

A Member.—Messrs. Thomas Cook and Son have organised excursions for members of the International Medical Congress and of the British Medical Association.

P. C. S.—The alleged right of the Corporation of London as to the election of presidents of the four great City hospitals was decided by the St. Thomas's Hospital case, in the Court of Queen's Bench, in November, 1866. Judgment was given for the Hospital. The result of the decision is, that the governors of the great hospitals have free choice in the election of their presidents.

Vigilans.—Mr. Bryce's City (London) Parochial Charities Bill includes the providing and maintaining of open spaces and recreation grounds. The income of these charities has been steadily increasing, and now amounts to upwards of £100,000 a year. Some of the ancient churchyards in the City and other parts of the metropolis are closed, even to the parishioners to whom they belong. Why should the public be excluded from the moat of the Tower, and be admitted only by special favour? Formerly, this ground was open to the public; but in 1845, for some unexplained reason, it was enclosed. The Government have granted free admission to the Tower itself; to throw open the moat for the enjoyment of the people would be a boon sure to meet with high appreciation.

A Laudable "Requisition."—The Board of Guardians of Preston are about to erect a new infectious hospital at a cost of £10,220. The erection of this hospital has been required by the central authority.

The Metropolitan Drinking Fountain and Cattle Trough Association.—From the recently issued annual report of this Association it appears that during the past year 81 new fountains and 44 new troughs have been erected. There are now in use 462 fountains for human beings, and 450 troughs for animals. The statistics show that more than five hundred thousand men, women, and children drink every day at these fountains. A size has been granted in Smithfield, by the City Corporation, for a large trough, with two fountains attached, to be erected, the gift of Mrs. Philip Twells, widow of the late Mr. P. Twells, M.P.

M.D. Oxon.—Mr. Barraud has just published an admirable photograph of the late Professor Rolleston. In his studio, 96, Gloucester-place, Portman-square, we saw several excellent photographs of distinguished members of our profession, especially one of Mr. Spencer Wells, just taken.

Enquirer, Lambeth.—Jenner's discovery was recognised by the Legislature in 1802, and sums were annually voted by Parliament to the National Vaccine Establishment, founded in 1808, to maintain the supply of lymph. An Act passed in July, 1840, made lawful the contracts of guardians with the Poor-law medical officers and other practitioners for the vaccination of all persons resident in unions or parishes, but the Act prohibited inoculation with variolous matter, under penalties, and an Act passed in 1841 declared that vaccination at the public expense was not to be considered parochial relief. In 1853, vaccination was made compulsory by a measure introduced by Lord Lyttleton, who was not a member of the Government.

J.—Dean Swift founded the St. Patrick's Hospital, Dublin. The funds which finally devolved upon the Hospital amounted to about £12,000, which was the sum of Swift's savings.

A Pension.—A Greenwich Hospital pension of £50 a year has been awarded to Fleet-Surgeon Gerald Yeo.

"The Old Story."—The cases of thirty-two persons prosecuted for having neglected or refused to comply with the Vaccination Act were heard before the magistrates at Brighton on the 8th inst. Most of the defendants pleaded conscientious objections. One woman alleged that one of her children was suffering, and two had died, from vaccination. The magistrate ordered vaccination to be performed, and fines were inflicted in cases where previous orders had been discharged.

Erasmus.—The charge of the Liverpool Water Company for supplying the Haydock Local Board District with water from Rivington is 6d. per 1000 gallons.

An Excellent Example: Dorking.—Dr. E. L. Jacob, Medical Officer of Health, at the meeting of the Local Board of Health last week, reported cases of typhoid and scarlet fevers and small-pox, and requested the Board to offer a fee to medical practitioners for giving him prompt notice of fresh cases—a request which the Board granted.

Extensive Illegal Sale of Liquors.—A shopkeeper living near Trentham has been fined £50 by the stipendiary magistrate at Fenton for selling spirits and beer without a licence. The defendant has a cottage near to his shop, where he has been carrying on a very extensive illegal business for some years, and where, a few days ago, a heavy stock of all kinds of drinks was seized by the police.

" Unimpeachable."—We extract the following from an official report by Messrs. W. Crookes, William Odling, and C. M. Tidy, just published. " Judged by our daily examinations, the water supplied to London is, in our opinion, whether considered as to its proper aëration, or as to its purity and wholesomeness, unimpeachable. The result of our six months' work, and the examination during this period of 1197 samples, enable us to state that as an excellent drinking supply it leaves nothing to be desired."

Homoeopathy on the Continent.—It is reported that at Leipsic a medical paper has been fined 100 marks, and costs, at the suit of seventy-five homoeopathic doctors, for publishing a lecture, delivered to a Berlin medical society, in which homoeopathy was denounced as quackery and swindling.

W. K. C.—It is said that the first Christian asylum designed expressly for lunatics was founded at Valencia in 1409, though the Knights of Malta had previously admitted them into their hospitals, and there seem to have been regular asylums for Mohammedan countries at a certain date. It was not till the eighteenth century that any general and systematic effort was made throughout Europe for the relief of this malady.

Medical Responsibility.—Dr. J. Addington Symonds' "Miscellanies." He writes:—" In debating these questions of responsibility, we are taken somewhat beyond our strictly medical functions. Sometimes we willingly, almost officiously, pass out of our province; but oftener we are dragged out of it. I do not think that it is our business to say what is moral, much less legal, irresponsibility. It might be well for us to resolve and agree to say no more than what we know as medical practitioners. Let us declare the man to be, in our judgment, sane or insane; just as, in examining for an insurance office, we pronounce the candidate to be sound or unsound in body. Having declared him to be unsound in mind, let moralists and legal judges settle the question whether he was responsible for his actions. We have burthens enough on our minds—enough of difficult problems to solve,—and it is hard to have forced on us those which do not belong to our calling."

COMMUNICATIONS have been received from—
Dr. LUCAS, Bombay; Dr. DOWN, London; Mr. A. A. KNIGHT, London; THE REGISTRAR OF APOTHECARIES' HALL, London; Mr. DANIELL, Blandford; Mr. NEWBER NIXON, London; Dr. M. MACKENZIE, London; Dr. LEONARD SEDGWICK, London; THE CLERK OF THE LOCAL GOVERNMENT BOARD; Dr. B. NICHOLSON, London; THE CLERK OF THE LOCAL BOARD OF HEALTH, Ventnor; Mr. WHITE WALLIS, London; Mr. GEORGE BROWN, London; Mr. FLETCHER, Warrington; THE REGISTRAR-GENERAL, Edinburgh; THE SECRETARY OF THE STATISTICAL SOCIETY, London; THE HONORARY SECRETARY OF THE QUEKETT MICROSCOPIC CLUB, London; Messrs. BURROUGHS, WELLCOME, and Co., London; Dr. J. W. MOORE, Dublin; Mr. J. WICKHAM BARNES, London; Mr. H. C. HOWARD, London; Mr. W. F. JESS, London; THE REGISTRAR OF THE UNIVERSITY OF DUBLIN; Dr. HOWARD MURPHY, Twickenham; Mr. W. MACCORMAC, London; THE ACCOUNTANT-GENERAL OF THE NAVY, Admiralty; Messrs. STREET BROS., London; Mr. J. CHATTO, London; THE COMMITTEE OF MANAGEMENT OF THE CATERHAM ASYLUM.

PERIODICALS AND NEWSPAPERS RECEIVED:—
Lancet—British Medical Journal—Medical Press and Circular—Berliner Klinische Wochenschrift—Centralblatt für Chirurgie—Gazette des Hopitaux—Gazette Médicale—Le Progrès Médical—Bulletin de l'Académie de Médecine—Pharmaceutical Journal—Wiener Medizinische Wochenschrift—Centralblatt für die Medizinischen Wissenschaften—Revue Médicale—Gazette Hebdomadaire—National Board of Health Bulletin, Washington—Nature—Deutsche Medicinal-Zeitung—Revista de Medicina—Italian Times—Louisville Medical News—Boston Medical and Surgical Journal—Occasional Notes—Brain, July—Centralblatt für Gynäkologie—Birmingham Medical Review, July—Welcome, July—Westminster Review, July—Weekblad van Het Nederlandsch Tijdschrift voor Geneeskunde—Edinburgh Daily Review—Newcastle-on-Tyne Borough Lunatic Asylum Sixteenth Annual Report, 1880—Journal of Anatomy and Physiology, July—Indiana Medical Reporter—New York Medical Record—The Colonies and India—Boston Journal of Chemistry—Liverpool Daily Courier—Wells Journal—Canadian Journal of Medical Science.

ORIGINAL LECTURES.

CLINICAL LECTURE
ON A
CASE OF TREPHINING FOR ANOMALOUS CONVULSIVE ATTACKS,
SUPERVENING SEVERAL MONTHS AFTER INJURY TO THE HEAD.

By J. W. HULKE, F.R.C.S., F.R.S.,
Surgeon to, and Lecturer on Surgery at, the Middlesex Hospital.

GENTLEMEN,—The subject of my last clinical lecture was a little child who had undergone secondary trephining for abscess following a punctured wound of the vault of the skull, with lodgment of splinters of bone and hair in the brain. The case to which I invite your attention to-day is that of a young man in Bentinck ward who has recently been trephined for fits following an injury in the right temple.

The following is the record abridged from my dresser's (Mr. Thane) notes:—

A ticket-clerk, aged twenty-one years, who as a youth was considered delicate and to have phthisical tendencies, was admitted into the hospital on January 23, 1879.

Six months previously, at 5 a.m., he slipped off a railway-platform, which was greasy with wet, and falling upon the line, about four feet lower than the platform, struck his right temple, it was supposed against the parapet of a dwarf wall. He was stunned by the blow, which was severe, for although the distance through which he fell was not great, he was running quickly at the moment, which increased the impetus. How long he continued unconscious is not known—probably not longer than a few minutes. On recovering consciousness he found himself upon the ground. He managed to rise, get upon the platform, and reach the next station, about three-quarters of a mile distant, where he reported his accident to the station-master. A bruise and a bump of about the size of the last joint of the thumb, were seen on his right temple by his father, a guard, and by others. His head ached greatly, and it felt very confused, but he managed to perform his duty until midday, by which time the headache and confusion of mind had become so great that he was compelled to leave work, and he then went to a friend's lodgings near the station, where he sat down in a chair. About 4 p.m. he first thought he had fallen asleep; he had, however, become deeply unconscious, and could not be roused. He was therefore put to bed, where he remained unconscious of what was happening during twenty-four hours, when he awoke, and was startled to find himself undressed, in his friend's bed, with two doctors examining him.

During about one month he continued deeply soporose, sleeping heavily during several hours, then waking and taking food. He did not, however, feed himself, appearing to be unable to hold the cup or to manage a spoon. He had complete control over his bladder, but it was necessary to place the vessel, for he seemed unable to arrange it or hold it himself. He had also control of the bowels, and he always intimated his wants to those in attendance upon him. Throughout this month he did not leave his bed; he seemed to have become too weak to stand.

In the condition just described he was next taken to his parents' home in a seaport seventy miles distant. He did not appear to be much exhausted by the journey. The quiet, the surroundings of home, and the fresh sea-breezes appeared to benefit him, and he slowly and gradually recovered, becoming able, at the end of a few weeks, to creep about in the garden. At the end of two months (three months after the accident) he had improved so much that he made an attempt to resume work, which this aggravated the headache, which had never left him, and he could not bear even slight mental strain without becoming confused; so that, after a fortnight, he was obliged to return into the country to his parents, with whom he remained until his admission into this hospital. During all this time he was never free from headache, and latterly he occasionally had what were called slight seizures, twitchings, and very transient unconsciousness.

Five days before being brought to the hospital he was violently convulsed—in twenty-four hours he had fourteen

very severe fits; the convulsions were so strong that three men could not restrain him. During the fits and for some time after he seemed to be quite unconscious. In the course of the next day and night he had ten similar fits, and on the third night he was convulsed with little intermission from 10 p.m. till 2 p.m. on the fourth day. He did not bite his tongue nor foam.

When I saw him on the fifth day after his journey of 100 miles, he looked like a convalescent from a severe illness. His face was pale, his pulse weak (100 per minute). The surface of his body was mottled, and it felt cold to the hand. The thermometer in the axilla, however, marked 99° Fahr.

His mind appeared to be unclouded; his memory was good; he gave a coherent account of the accident and his subsequent illness; and when questioned, his answers were always pertinent. His statements (corroborated by his father) were remarkably clear and consistent.

He complained of constant headache and dizziness, of a tightness as if a cord were tied round his forehead, and of a hammering in the back of the head. His visual acuteness was unimpaired, but he said that on reading his sight soon failed. No indications of inflammatory or congestive disorder of optic nerves was discernible. Just behind the right temporal ridge, about one inch above its origin, in the spot where the bump was noticed on the day the accident occurred, was a very limited area, pressure on which caused, he said, a darting sensation through his head. This spot was marked with an ink-dot, and diverting his attention by questions referring to other matters, the smooth end of a pencil was repeatedly made to cross it in different directions, with the result that he always winced and exclaimed, "It darts through my head." No scar was discernible here; the soft coverings seemed to be quite natural, and no unevenness of the underlying bone could be felt.

At 7.30 p.m. he made a curious noise, so like a snarl or bark that the patients in the neighbouring beds thought a dog had got into the ward. His hands were then noticed to be clenched, and he became violently convulsed. The House-Surgeon, who saw him within a very few minutes of this attack, found him then quiet and apparently quite insensible; his eyes were strongly rolled upwards—the left appeared more elevated than the right. After about five minutes, the masseter muscles were observed to stand in tense relief, and the upper lip was raised, showing the teeth and gums. The teeth were tightly clenched. Then his fingers became flexed, and the arms rigidly stiff through violent contraction of their muscles. The muscles in the nape of the neck were soft, and not contracted. Seven such fits occurred at intervals of about five minutes, ushered in by the strange barking noise. There was then a calm interval of half an hour, followed by another fit, after which consciousness returned. He then asked for a chamber-pot, and micturated. At 11 p.m. he had two more fits. He passed the rest of the night quietly, appearing to sleep.

January 24th.—9 a.m., temperature 98·4°, pulse 84. Calm and sensible. Headache continued. At 3 p.m., two fits.

25th.—9 a.m.: Temperature 97·4°; pulse 86. Slept from eleven o'clock last night till seven this morning. Headache and dizziness unchanged. 9 p.m.: Temperature 98·4°. At 10 p.m., whilst apparently sleeping, began to mutter, then made a barking noise, and was convulsed six times in half an hour—after which he became conscious. In these fits there was extreme opisthotonos.

26th.—9 a.m.: Temperature 98°; pulse 78. More headache. At 7 p.m. a convulsion lasting five minutes; after which he continued unconscious during half an hour.

27th.—In the course of the morning, five fits; and in the evening, four fits. Temperature 98·4°; pulse 84.

28th.—During forenoon, three fits. Temperature 98·6°; pulse 96. Up to this time he had been taking large doses of potassium bromide. At midday he was placed under the influence of chloroform, and trephined at the spot in the right temple, where, as already mentioned, pressure always caused a darting pain through the head. In the soft coverings, and in the disc of bone removed, no trace of injury or structural change was discernible. The dura mater also appeared normal. An aspirator-needle was therefore pushed through this to the depth of rather more than an inch, upon which, as nothing escaped through it, the needle was withdrawn. For a few moments, cerebro-spinal fluid spurted in a slender stream through the prick in the dura mater to the distance of nearly a foot. The middle of the scalp-wound was purposely left open. Throughout the operation, and subsequently, strict antiseptic measures were observed.

During the next forty-eight hours no fits occurred. The temperature ranged between 98·4° and 99°, and the pulse averaged 80. He was cheerful but calm, and took fluid nourishment freely. His headache was, he said, much less. Movements of the lower jaw caused much pain, obviously referable to the division of the temporal muscle in the operation.

In the afternoon of the 30th he was allowed to see his father, which appeared to excite him. Later, at 5.30 o'clock, he seemed to become unconscious, and at 6.15 he was slightly convulsed.

February 1.—At 1.15 a.m., a slight fit; at 11.45, a slight fit, preceded by unconsciousness of about twenty minutes' duration; and at 9.30 p.m., unconsciousness, which lasted twenty-five minutes, when he came-to without convulsion. Temperature ranged from 98° to 99°.

2nd.—One slight convulsion. Temperature 98·2°; pulse 84. Potassic iodide gr. x. t. d. now ordered.

3rd.—At 12.15 p.m., a strong fit.

4th.—Had a calm day, followed at 8.40 p.m. by several violent fits.

5th.—Between 7 and 9 a.m., six fits.

7th.—Temperature 98°; pulse 56, in afternoon intermittent. The dose of iodide of potassium was diminished by half—to gr. v. t.d. 8.30 p.m.: Unconscious during five minutes, after which a severe fit of convulsions, lasting half an hour; followed by four more fits between 3.30 and 4 a.m.

On the 12th he began to take valerianate of zinc in doses of gr. iss. t. d. On the 15th this was increased to gr. ij. 4ta quaque hora; then to gr. iij., gr. iv., and finally (on the 24th) to gr. vj. 4ta q. h.

After this date he had no fits until March 6, when he was unconscious during several hours, and was violently convulsed several times.

7th.—Allowed to leave his bed and sit in an easy chair. The valerianate of zinc pills were now taken only four times in twenty-four hours. From this time he appeared to improve.

On the 15th he declared himself quite free from headache, and he had not had any fit for eight days.

On the 16th he returned home. At this time he could walk a little; had a good appetite, and was free from headache.

The early symptoms in this most remarkable case are those which are generally thought to indicate severe concussion of the brain. When death has occurred soon after an injury to the head, followed by such symptoms, not infrequently bruisings, slight lacerations, and small hæmorrhages in the cortex of the brain have been demonstrated. The severity of the early symptoms, the tardy and imperfect recovery, warranted the belief that such surface-damage of brain had occurred here. The unconsciousness which supervened later on the day of the accident raised the suspicion that a coarse hæmorrhage had happened; but the interval—twelve hours—between the accident and this unconsciousness was exceptionally great for it to have been due to pressure through hæmorrhage, and the subsequent progress was also inconsistent with such a supposition.

What were the fits which came on six months after the time of the injury?

In those which occurred on the day he was taken into the hospital, the House-Surgeon noticed very marked trismus; the masseters became like rigid bars, and the lower jaw was tightly clenched.

In subsequent fits extreme opisthotonus occurred. The occiput and rump nearly touched.

Trismus and opisthotonus are, as you know, characteristic features in tetanus. Our patient, however, certainly had not tetanus, for during the cramp of the masseters the muscles of the nape were soft and uncontracted, those of the hands and forearms were as violently convulsed as those of the trunk, and in the intervals between these terrible fits none of the muscles were unnaturally rigid; whilst in tetanus, rigidity of the muscles of the nape is early associated with trismus, and it precedes the implication of the muscles of the trunk, the muscles of the hands and forearms usually escape, and between the convulsive paroxysms all the implicated muscles continue stiff through inordinate tonic contraction. It was evident, then, that these convulsive fits were not tetanic: were they epileptic?

The earliest seizures noticed at home, a few days before the first convulsions, were not unlike those of the least severe form of epilepsy—transient unconsciousness ("he seemed to lose himself for a moment") and slight twitchings. That epilepsy sometimes has a traumatic origin cannot be doubted. Its sequence upon injuries of the head affecting the brain has been observed too frequently to allow this to be regarded as a casual coincidence. We have had in the surgical wards within the last two years two instances of this. In the present case the increase of headache in the right temple, which often, he said, shortly preceded a fit, and the darting pain through the head on touching the site of the bruise at this part, favoured the supposition of a causal relation between the injury and the fits; and this supposition was strengthened by the continuance of headache and dizziness during the intermediate time between the injury and the occurrence of the fits—symptoms suggestive of the existence of some chronic irritative process at the injured spot.

Against the idea that the fits were epileptic was the manner in which they often began: the patient, who, a few moments previously had been talking rationally and coherently, appeared to lose the thread of the sentence; he muttered disconnected words, repeating the same word again and again—mostly a word occurring in the last coherent sentence he had himself spoken, or in the last sentence addressed to him. He did not become unconscious instantly, but gradually, and a period varying from a few minutes to half an hour often preceded the convulsions. Occasionally the first convulsions had the aspect of purposive movement. He, on two occasions when I was myself present and saw it, distinctly made a snap at a dresser who happened to be at his bedside, and tried to seize him with his teeth. His tongue was never bitten.

As, however, the fits seemed to differ least from epilepsy, bromide of potassium, so useful in this disorder, was tried in large and frequent doses. It had not any controlling influence; the fits continued with great violence. It was now that recourse was had to trephining. As you have already heard, nothing abnormal was discovered. The high intracranial pressure, sufficient to project a spurt of cerebrospinal fluid to the distance of nearly one foot, is worth notice. The fluid continued to leak during several hours afterwards in quantity enough to wet the boric charpie with which the wound was covered, and the pressure will have been for some time lowered. Had this lessened tension any causal connexion with the absence of fits during the next sixty hours or so? On their return, iodide of potassium was next tried in doses of ten grains, diminished one-half when, after a few days, the pulse began to be very weak and to intermit. It was, however, soon apparent that this drug also was without influence over the malady. The similarity of the fits in respect of the occasional purposive character of the initial convulsions, and also in respect of the opisthotonus which sometimes occurs in violent hysterical convulsions, next led to a trial of valerianate of zinc, which was begun to be taken in doses of one grain and a half, and finally in six-grain doses at short intervals. Under this treatment the fits subsided, which favours the idea of their hysterical nature. In some recently published cases of violent hysterical convulsions in young women, it was related that pressure in the inguinal regions, directed so that it might be supposed to reach the ovaries, quickly arrested the convulsions. As an experiment, compression of the homologous organs, the testes, was tried here during some fits, but without any effect upon them.

Upon the whole the conclusion which has the largest support in the facts of this case is that the fits were hysterical, induced by the shock of the accident in a person whose nervous system was not particularly stable, and that they were not immediately dependent upon a local irritative process set up by the blow on the temple; trephining, therefore, whilst it did not appear to have done any harm, was useless. In the case which I very recently brought before you, you will remember that the symptoms of cerebral disorder were one-sided: this gave them a very different signification to that of the convulsions in the present case, which were not restricted to one side, but implicated both sides equally.

Note.—After the patient's return home, he fell into what was called a "galloping consumption," and died on July 14 following. An examination of the head showed that the trephine-hole in the skull, which had measured eleven millimetres across, had been completely closed by new bone—a result probably referable to the small size of the trephine and the preservation of the pericranium, which was in a normal condition at the time of operation. No trace of the puncture with the aspirating-needle was discernible in the dura mater or brain.

The brain weighed forty-eight ounces; it was well formed and symmetrical. The pia mater, especially that covering the posterior lobes, was congested. No trace of injury could be detected by most careful examination—no scar or depression or mark of former contusion or laceration ; the surface of the brain appeared quite normal. The white and grey matter of the hemispheres were firm ; the puncta vasculosa rather more conspicuous than usual. Each hemisphere was carefully sliced for traces of previous injury ; none whatever were found. The only pathological conditions were four small yellowish nodules. One of these, about the size of a large pin's head, was in the grey matter of the anterior part of the corpus striatum, close to its upper surface ; a second, slightly larger, was in the grey matter of one of the convolutions of the left frontal lobe ; the two others were one in each cerebellar hemisphere—also in the grey matter, that in the right side being the larger, and about the size of a horse-bean.

ORIGINAL COMMUNICATIONS.

CLINICAL ILLUSTRATIONS OF
EMOTIONAL EXCITEMENT AS A CAUSE OF CHOREA.

By JAMES RUSSELL, M.D., F.R.C.P.

(Continued from page 63.)

I TAKE next three cases which place in a clear light the varied position held by the emotion to the disease which followed it. In all the patients the attack of chorea was of the most severe description—in one, was fatal,—yet in each instance the fright was, by comparison, of a trivial description, and, but that it appeared closely connected with the occurrence of the chorea, and certainly impressed the patient, would have been ignored by the clinical inquirer. Supposing, however, the nerve-cells in the patients to have been already in an explosive condition, the immediate excitement would be sufficient to afford the force which removed the restraining influence.

Case 4.—A finely-developed, high-spirited, and passionate, but healthy girl, aged sixteen, was much frightened by a slight cut on her finger, from which much blood flowed ; at the time, too, she was in a violent passion with her mother. On the same evening choreic movements came on " in the arm on the same side." In a week the leg became involved, and in a day or two the face and tongue. In the course of fourteen days the choreic movements became greatly exaggerated, and continued to augment in violence, causing general excoriation from constant friction, but without emotional development, for nine days, when she died. Her heart was found healthy, as were all the other organs.

Case 5.—This case related to a girl aged sixteen, in good health, and living under favourable conditions, passionate, but not hysterical nor in any way nervous ; the sounds of her heart pure. She was very much frightened by a fall on her left side, doubling her wrist under her. She soon recovered from the fright, and thought no more about it. Choreic movements commenced on the following day, and became very severe in four days. The disease presented its most violent form for three days, and then gradually subsided.

Case 6.—A chlorotic-looking girl, an orphan, aged nineteen, overworked and underfed, not rheumatic, was preparing to emigrate to America, her passage having been paid, when she " spent silly " some money sent over to her to defray her expenses. She was much troubled thereby, and the present illness began, and put an end to her intention of leaving the country. The movement came on gradually, increasing in severity, and at the end of a fortnight or three weeks attained great violence, which for ten days seriously threatened the patient's life, and only subsided tardily.

I may adduce in this connexion two other illustrations of

a large amount of energy having been released through the application of a comparatively low degree of force, when, as in chorea, the explosive material lies ready to hand, and the restraining influence by which it is normally controlled has been lowered. The incidents did not occur as a primary cause of the chorea, but produced severe aggravation of the disease. In one case a girl, aged twenty-one, had been suffering from choreic movements of a mild character for two days, when her attention was directed to her condition : she immediately burst into tears, and from that time the movement became greatly aggravated, and speedily developed into a very severe form of the disease, with much emotional development. The second instance occurred in an emotional girl who entered the hospital with mild chorea of a month's duration. Ten days afterwards she was much excited by hearing a band of music ; she jumped out of bed, and was worse directly ; the movements became so violent that she was placed in a private ward, and it was a month before any permanent amendment was effected. The late Dr. Hughes, in his paper on Chorea in *Guy's Reports*, narrates a case of chorea of a mild character for five days, when the girl was derided; she immediately fell into a fit, the movements became universal, and the patient died in four days. A second case mentioned by the same writer seemed to have been converted from a mild form of the malady into fatal violence by a slight fright in the ward.

The next case presents us with a state of severe emotional excitement in a young susceptible subject, which had evidently produced a profound impression of a very persistent character. The effects which resulted were of a very marked description, but among them the motor disorder, which alone seemed to have attracted special attention, was the least important. Both intellectual and physical health were permanently and seriously lowered, and it was doubtless to this latter circumstance that the long persistence of this mild form of motor derangement was mainly due.

Case 7.—A thin, small-made boy, aged seven, but healthy, with pure cardiac sounds and no rheumatism, was taken to see his dead mother. He did not seem to be particularly affected at the time, but a day or two after, the servant in whose charge he was, desiring to take a holiday surreptitiously, shut the boy up in a room with the shutters closed. He was there for eight hours, when, his cries and screams having aroused the neighbourhood, he was taken out through the window by help of a ladder. The day after he was observed to be ill, " shaking in every joint," and unable to hold anything. The occurrence just mentioned took place ten months before admission, but the chorea (right unilateral) had continued throughout the period in a mild form. After the fright his sleep became disturbed, his spirits were depressed, and he was afraid to go to bed in the dark. He seemed to lose his recollection. He lost his appetite and wasted, so that when admitted he was much emaciated. Since the setting-in of the chorea his mental vigour had materially declined ; from having been a very quick child he had declined in intelligence, and had become unable to learn. He mended slowly, but improved greatly in nutrition.

The following group of six cases do not require to be specialised. They illustrate in a minor degree one or other of the phenomena connected with the influence of emotion on choreic patients, to which attention has been more fully directed in the preceding instances. The degree of excitement encountered by some of the patients was of a less severe character, and the connexion between the apparent cause and the chorea, in one or two of the cases, is open to much question.

Case 8.—An excitable, impressible, and very timid child, not rheumatic, and with a healthy heart, was brought to the hospital with right unilateral chorea. It was the second attack, the earlier one having happened three years previously. The relapse was occasioned by a fright. She was going along the street after dark, carrying a bundle, when she was pursued by some lads with the intention of robbing her. She came home much frightened. The movements did not show themselves for a fortnight, but during that period her nights were disturbed, as, indeed, had been the case before the occurrence in question.

Case 9.—A boy, aged seven, with rheumatic tendency, but with pure sounds of his heart, intelligent and good-tempered, had suffered from chorea of some severity for a

month, and during that time had had three epileptic fits.
For two months preceding the attack of chorea he had been
much disturbed by frights in his sleep, and had lost flesh;
and the day before the movements appeared he had been
frightened by having upset a board of meat in the shop; he
went away and hid himself for some time. Some hours
before the movements were observed he had been sitting as
in a melancholy state. With the chorea occurred a renewal
of rheumatic pain in some of the joints. The attack was
protracted. Four years afterwards he returned to the
hospital with a return of the movements. He had been
employed in carrying out meat, and was often subjected to
fatigue. Immediately before the return of the movements
he had followed a procession of Foresters to Aston Park,
and at the fête which followed the "Female Blondin" was
killed. The boy was greatly excited by the procession and
by the subsequent accident, though he did not witness the
latter. The relapse occurred "directly afterwards." He had,
however, been observed to be dull for some days previously.

Case 10.—A married woman, aged twenty-three, said to
have been very nervous for two months, and three months
advanced in pregnancy (her third), on coming downstairs
one evening at dusk, after having put her child to bed, saw
"a black face with red lips" pressed against the window.
It proved to be the face of an intoxicated sweep. She was
much alarmed and "shook for two hours"; she could not get
the better of it. A series of short paroxysms of hysterical
aphonia followed, and three weeks after she had an
attack of hysteric hemiplegia on the right side, and the
paresis was followed by choreic movements of some severity,
also limited to the right side. She had a return of the hemiparesis afterwards, but she soon ceased her attendance.
Her former pregnancies had been free from any similar
phenomena.

Case 11.—A boy, aged nine years, not rheumatic, reported
to have quite good health, and having good appetite, had
the misfortune to have a severe mother. She had often
"beaten him well" for playing truant, and he was much
afraid of her. On one occasion she took him to two police-
men on account of his truancy; this occurred four months
before the chorea. He lost some money with which he had
been entrusted, and came back "all of a tremble." The
trembling was most marked in his right arm, but extended
to the leg and impaired his speech. Occasionally it has
extended all over him. Since this occurrence he has been
gloomy and disinclined for play. His mother insists that
his health was perfect before this incident. The chorea was
not severe, but very persistent. His heart-sounds were
pure.

Case 12.—S. A. B., aged seven years, was described as
irritable, impressible, liable to have things dwell on her
mind, and apt to dream. When seven years old, a neighbour
alarmed her by reading of a murder, and then blowing out
the candle, leaving the child in the dark. She appeared
very sad and trembled, and was much frightened through
the night. She remained dull afterwards, but the movements did not show themselves for two months. The movements seem never to have left entirely for five years, and at
times were rather severe. This period ended in a considerable aggravation of the movements through nine weeks, after
which they entirely cleared away, though the child remained
dull and careless to play. She was brought to the hospital
with a renewed attack, after six months' immunity, produced immediately by a severe scolding from a neighbour
during the absence of her mother. She came to her mother
frightened and trembling, was dull the next day, and in a
few days twitching showed itself in the left hand, and
gradually extended over all the limbs. She made a brief
attendance only.

Case 13.—A girl, aged eleven years, morbidly nervous and
timid, irritable, and of low intelligence, fell down the cellar
steps. She was not hurt, but was much frightened. Two or
three days afterwards, her mother observed that her limbs
shook a good deal, and she could not articulate distinctly.
She had been living badly for two years, not having meat
for weeks together. She had chorea for five weeks, and was
an in-patient of the Queen's Hospital. One night, two years
afterwards, a fellow-workwoman alarmed her by throwing a
sheet over her; in two days the shaking returned, and proved
the opening of more severe chorea than on the preceding
occasion, of three months' duration. A third followed, four
years after the one just mentioned.

The concluding cases exhibit a further decline in the value
of the incidents assigned as causes of the chorea; and if
admitted in that capacity at all, must have operated on a
foundation already well prepared to receive their action.
They, however, require to be mentioned in any report purporting to take complete notice of the influence which
emotion is asserted to have exerted in the disease in question. Many of them illustrate the fallacy of the *post hoc
ergo propter hoc*, to which an incident of a striking character preceding a personal change in any individual is
peculiarly exposed.

Case 14.—A girl aged sixteen, who had not had enough
to eat, was very much "put about" by the return of her
brother from abroad, who had enlisted two years before. At
the same time her agitation was increased by the falling off
of work, and by lessened means of subsistence. It was just
at this time that the movements began, and they increased
through six weeks, when she entered the hospital with chorea
of moderate severity, from which she speedily recovered.

Case 15.—A married woman, aged twenty, with good
health, but acknowledging "a nasty temper," a fortnight
after her first confinement had an aching in her right
shoulder. This continued, and a month after, when in a
passion with her husband, she noticed a shaking in the
shoulder, which lasted a quarter of an hour, but returned
the same evening, then affecting also her right thigh and
right side of her face and tongue, so that she could not
speak. The movements recurred in frequent paroxysms.
She became timid, and lost flesh considerably. A week
before admission, pain came on in the right knee, and she
entered the hospital with quite characteristic chorea (right
unilateral), and decided rheumatic swelling in the right
wrist and hand. She had not suffered from rheumatism
before. Her heart was healthy. The rheumatism did not
extend, and the chorea did not prove intractable.

Case 16.—A girl aged twelve, irritable, but well-fed, with
an imperfect history, ascribed a moderate attack of chorea
to some one speaking sharply to her. Her mother so far
confirmed the allegation as to say that the child was much
frightened, and fell downstairs in consequence. She had
a restless night, and the chorea showed itself on the following
morning.

Case 17.—A girl aged eight years, apparently ill-managed,
and stated by her mother to be "passionate and peevish,"
was greatly frightened by a thunder-storm "some time ago."
She screamed frightfully, and her mother had to hold her.
The chorea, of a mild character, affecting the left side, was
ascribed immediately to a fall, which severely bruised her left
temple, causing subcutaneous effusion. The mother, on returning home from a day's washing, found her child very nervous
and crying. A week or ten days after, she was clumsy in
using her left arm, and the chorea then appeared. Her
sleep became impaired, and the girl lost flesh. She had
enjoyed good health.

Case 18.—The chorea (left unilateral) in an emotional
girl aged fourteen, was confidently referred to an alarm she
encountered from having been left in a new house and
believing she heard some one trying to force an entrance.
She had not had rheumatism. Whilst in the hospital she
evinced a tendency to emotional development. In the attack
the paralytic element was prominent.

Case 19.—A boy, aged fourteen, free from rheumatism,
had had choreic movements of slight character, "on and off,"
for two years, but increased in severity for three months.
He referred the origin of his complaint to being kept in a
state of alarm by the workman who was "set over him"
and was constantly "frightening him very much." His
mother also stated that he was nervous in using a hammer
which he was required to employ in his business. The left
arm gradually moved irregularly; then the left side of his
face and the left leg. The right side does not seem to have
been entirely spared. The condition of his heart was doubtful. His health has been very good, but since he became
subject to his present complaint he has been much disposed
to cry, and apt to "sit down and seem full of grief."

Finally.—A girl aged eleven, and her mother, both concurred in explaining the first attack of chorea (left unilateral)
one year ago, by a fright which the child had undergone
on getting up early in a morning, from the cat, in a dark
room, throwing over a glass of gold-fish. She ran upstairs
"as white as a sheet." The movements began in a week or
two, and lasted two or three months. They returned about

nine months after with greater severity. Between the fright and the commencement of the movement the child was markedly timid and refused to go upstairs in the dark. She was quite strong and well up to the day of the fright. She was free from rheumatism; her heart was healthy.——The mother of a girl aged ten, who had suffered from right hemi-chorea for five weeks, confidently explained the attack by her brother having beaten her, sent her to school, and then fol-lowed her for some distance. The "dance" came on in a fortnight. Her nervous and bodily health were good. She never had rheumatism, and the sounds of her heart were pure.——A girl, aged ten, free from rheumatism, who had lived chiefly on bread-and-butter, cheese, and tea, when crossing the road was frightened by a carriage, which nearly went over her foot. She seemed very nervous and frightened on reaching home, and cried severely. She was at the time in her usual health. A fortnight after, right hemichorea developed. Her heart was healthy.——A delicate, emotional child, subject to convulsive seizures, aged ten, referred a return of her chorea to a smart caning at school, by which she was frightened. The sounds of her heart were pure.

It is worth while to complete my subject by noticing in conclusion the patients belonging to the same group of one hundred, in whom, though no mental excitement was credited with having been the cause of the attack, more or less of emotional disturbance was distinctly observed in connexion with the chorea. The chief value of the observation is from the evidence it affords of an abnormal condition of the nerve-cells antecedent to the application of any cause tending further to release these cells from their natural control. The emotional excitement displayed in these cases is paralleled by Dr. Gowers' observation " that in most, though not in all, cases " of chorea which he had examined " a distinct increase in the irritability of both nerve and muscle on the affected side" existed, "extending to both faradisation and the voltaic current " (British Medical Journal, March 30, 1878).

1. The chorea in a female, aged seventeen, coexisted with a dangerous maniacal attack, after amputation. The illness was a very grave one. 2. A girl, aged twenty-three, after slight twitching for a day or two, had a frightful dream, from which she woke up in great excitement, rousing the dormitory. Next night she refused to undress, and became quite wild, but not delirious, threatening to go out by the window if the door were locked on her. She ran about the school in great excitement all night. She was admitted in this condition with violent choreic movements, which were quieted when the mental condition improved under Indian hemp. 3. A girl, aged nineteen, manifested great emotional development with disturbed sleep; twice she became almost maniacal, and required a special nurse. 4. A girl, aged fourteen, presented absence of sleep, outbreaks of crying and shrieking, and maniacal tendency. 5. A girl, aged ten, whilst being examined, burst into a fit of crying and then laughed as readily; burst into tears at her mother's visit, and again at the medical visit; she had become very irritable. 6. A girl, aged fourteen, since the chorea had shown decline in intelligence, and had become subject to fits of laughing and crying impossible to restrain, with great tendency to emotional development; she had never been so before. 7. A girl, aged fifteen, had two brief attacks of epileptic delirium (apparently) ten days after the chorea set in. 8. A child, aged four years and a half, seemed going silly before the chorea—had a foolish expression and an unmeaning laugh, and lost her memory. 9. A girl, aged sixteen, since the chorea had become bad-tempered, passionate, was frightened and screamed in the night. 10. A girl, aged fifteen, had fallen into a low way; sat before the fire and cared for no play; afterwards was very movable, excitable, and foolish. 11. A female, aged eleven; since the chorea her nights had become very restless; she was stupid, talked foolishly, and got laughed at. Previously had been acute, and was trusted with considerable sums of money. She quite altered in the hospital.

The remaining patients are characterised more briefly. 12. A female, aged sixteen; emotional; sleep had become disturbed; she was depressed; dreamt and talked in her sleep. 13. A boy, aged thirteen, had become very irrit-able with the chorea, and cried at the least thing. 14. A woman, aged twenty-one, had become excitable and liable to frightful dreams; never was so before. 15. A boy, aged eleven, had become much more irritable. 16. A girl, aged

eleven, had become very passionate. 17. A girl, aged fifteen, had become excitable since chorea, and subject to frightful dreams; never was so before. 18. A girl, aged thirteen, at each of two choreic attacks had very bad sleep; was disturbed by frightful dreams. 19. A girl, aged seventeen, had her fears easily excited since the chorea. 20. A girl, aged ten, is described as sitting without speaking for a considerable time. 21. A boy, aged thirteen, has been very stupid since the chorea. 22. A girl, aged eleven, has been duller since the chorea; previously was very sharp and quick; sleep has been very much disturbed. 23. A girl, aged seventeen, had been at times dull and incapable of being understood since the chorea; at times she had been clear. 24. A girl, aged thirteen, burst into a violent fit of sobbing on being looked at. Three other patients made marked complaints of bad sleep since the chorea; and one patient was epileptic.

ANEURISM OF THE AORTA
SIMULATING ANEURISM OF THE PULMONARY ARTERY.

By THOMAS OLIVER, M.D.,
Physician to the Infirmary, Newcastle-upon-Tyne.

THE difficulties which surround the diagnosis of intra-thoracic aneurism are many; and even when a diagnosis has been made, the attempt to localise the seat of the dila-tation on the vessel is not always a matter of ease. It is true that when we are able to map off the area of dulness and pulsation much of the difficulty disappears, especially if there be added to this a careful interpretation of the symptoms and physical signs dependent upon the pressure exercised by the bulging vessel. As showing what pecu-liarities may be met with in cases of thoracic aneurism the following notes may prove of some interest :—

J. W., aged forty-three years, a goods guard on the rail-way, was admitted into the Newcastle Infirmary on June 10, 1880, complaining of cough and shortness of breath. Patient, who is a strongly built man, and upwards of six feet in height, states that he enjoyed good health until about seven weeks before his admission, when he began to complain of cough and of epigastric pain. For the last twenty years he has been in the service of the railway company, but states that although he has been frequently exposed to wet and cold, he has never had to lift heavy weights. He has been temperate and regular in his habits, and has never had hæmoptysis.

At the time of his admission it is noted that there is a good deal of dyspnœa, but so long as the semi-recumbent posture is maintained his breathing is easy, and there is little cough. Both legs are swollen, and there is scrotal dropsy. The urine, which is passed in fair quantity, has a specific gravity of 1022, is acid and free of albumen.

Chest.—There is enlargement of the area of the apex-beat. The apex is felt beating outside the line of the left nipple. Area of cardiac dulness is enlarged, measuring transversely six inches and a half. There is also well-marked epigastric pulsation. Over the mitral area a very soft but roughened systolic bruit is heard, followed by a well-developed clicking second sound. A similar murmur, but louder, coarser, and of longer duration, is heard over the right ventricle, and it is noticed that the murmur increases in intensity as the stethoscope is carried upwards along the left side of the sternum to the third left costal cartilage, whence it is con-ducted to the left along a line which takes the form of an arc. The arc which corresponds to the line of conduction of the murmur just surmounts the left base of the heart. A very faint systolic murmur is detected over the aortic area, but it is not conducted into the vessels of the neck. Although faint it is followed by a well-developed clicking second sound. The pulse is very rapid, 120 in the minute, fairly full and strong.

On June 25, after having rested in bed and having had small doses of digitalis, it is noted in the journal that he is better; that he is eating and sleeping well, that his cough has nearly all gone, but that shortness of breath is still experienced, especially when he awakens in the morning. The systolic murmur is well marked over the base of the heart; it follows the curved line which surmounts the left base of the heart, the ends of the arched line being respectively the second left intercostal space and the left nipple. A faint systolic bruit is again described as having been detected over the aortic area—a murmur, however, which diminishes in intensity as the right side of the manubrium is approached, in contradistinction to what is observed on auscultating leftwards. Bronchial râles are heard over the right lung anteriorly. Coarse crepitation is heard over the base of the left lung.

The lividity of the lips had diminished by June 30. On this date it is stated that his breathing is better, that he is passing a larger quantity of urine, and that the dropsy is considerably diminished. Two areas of pulsation are noticed in the cardiac area—one over the apex, the other over the second and third left intercostal spaces about an inch and a half from the sternum. The conduction of the systolic murmur remains unaltered. Along the whole length of the left border of the sternum there is heard an accentuated clicking second sound. The murmur described on former occasions as having been detected over the aortic area is to-day inaudible.

Repeated examination from this date onwards showed that the murmur was always loudest over the left base of the heart, and that its line of conduction was to the left, the point of maximum intensity corresponding to the centre of the arched line already mentioned. On August 2 he expressed a wish to go home to his father, who lived in the country, feeling, as he remarked, " very well."

On August 23, patient came in from the country and consulted me at my own house; he stated that he had been keeping very much better, and that he intended beginning work on the following day at one of the railway sidings near town, where he said the work was comparatively light. At this time there was marked lividity of the lips and slight dyspnœa, which was increased on exertion. The dyspnœa was somewhat nocturnal in character; it came on, as a rule, soon after he got into bed, and was generally relieved when he lay upon his face. He could now sleep with a low head. The area of cardiac dulness remained unaltered; it measured still six inches and a half. The systolic murmur had a peculiar creaking, vibrating, and musical character; it obeyed the line of conduction already mentioned, becoming extremely musical at the centre of the arched line. Its localisation seemed to be over the pulmonary area.

His wife came to me on September 19, and asked me to see him at his own house, as he was confined to bed. The dyspnœa had by this time increased in severity—he could now only get his breath by occupying the semi-upright position in bed, and the lips were very blue. The area of cardiac dulness had increased in both directions, being continuous with an area of dull percussion which existed over the lower third of each lung. The pulsation formerly noticed over the left base of the heart had disappeared, and the systolic murmur over the base of the heart was only faintly audible. Bronchial râles were general.

During the early part of the following morning patient died suddenly, and, with the assistance of my resident clinical clerk, Mr. Milburn, I made a post-mortem about sixteen hours after death.

The diagnosis was aneurism and mitral disease—*aneurism presumably of the pulmonary artery*—from the fact of an area of dull percussion locating itself over the second and third left intercostal spaces; the conduction of the murmur leftwards and downwards, more frequently absent than present in the aortic area; a murmur accompanied by well-marked lividity of the features, without the attendant circumstances of small weak pulse and the condensation of lung of mitral disease and its sequela.

Autopsy.—Both pleura contain about two pints of clear serum. The lungs are emphysematous at their margins in front, and towards the base are in a state of congestive œdema. With this exception the lungs are healthy. Heart: The pericardium contains about a pint of serum. On slitting open the pericardium, it is noticed that there is adhesion between it and a roughened bulging which is lying anteriorly to and upon the pulmonary artery just at its commencement. It was thought, at first, that the bulging was an offshoot of the pulmonary artery, and it was not until the heart and its great vessels were removed from the body that the true condition of matters was realised. It then became apparent that the pulmonary artery was displaced and encircled by an aneurism which had compressed it. The ·urism itself, however, which is about the size of a small

tennis-ball, arises from the inner—and somewhat, too, from the anterior—part of the very commencement of the ascending portion of the arch of the aorta. It arises a little to the left of the right coronary artery, so that in its development it may be said to have coursed outwards to the right, then to the left in front of the pulmonary artery, and, having entirely encircled it, formed adhesions with the left auricle. The aorta presents numerous patches of atheromatous deposit. The aortic valves are also atheromatous, and are fringed with vegetations. Numerous fibrinous bands stretch from the margin of the valves to the border of the aneurism. The left ventricle is dilated, and its walls are thickened. Patches of endocardial thickening run from the lower border of the aortic valves downwards amongst the columnæ carneæ. The tips of the mitral valve are firm and hard to the touch, and its orifice is dilated. The valves of the pulmonary artery have undergone extreme thinning—they are almost diaphanous; they look as if the internal structure of the valve had been worn away—that is to say, the sustaining fibres which radiate from the corpora aurantii alone remain; and there stretch from the margin of the valve to the wall of the artery tendinous cords similar to what have already been described as existing in the aorta. The portion of the left auricle which is attached to the wall of the aneurism is undergoing softening. The walls of the right auricle are thinned, and its cavity is dilated; the tricuspid orifice admits five fingers.

Remarks.—The diagnosis of aneurism was easy enough; it was when we tried to localise it that we experienced the difficulty. I leaned towards the suspicion of aneurism of the pulmonary artery—a rare condition of matters, no doubt, but one which the symptoms and physical signs suggested to me, viz., an accentuated second sound heard over the pulmonary artery; an area of dulness and pulsation over this region; extreme lividity of countenance; and, above all, a peculiar conduction of the murmur leftwards. And for all practical purposes the interpretation of the physical signs was correct, for it cannot be proved that a great part of the systolic bruit was not really generated in the pulmonary artery. That vessel was constricted and pressed upon by the aneurism, which surrounded it and naturally offered great resistance to the onward flow of blood—the very conditions which caused the murmur to be conducted along the line already mentioned. And, in addition, the musical element in the murmur must have depended upon vibration of the fibrinous cords which stretched across the pulmonary artery, and not upon those in the aortic orifice, otherwise the murmur would have been conveyed into the vessels of the neck. This case shows us that a bruit may be carried along a certain vessel; and yet, while it is a physical fact announcing disease, it cannot be taken as an indication of disease of that vessel, but of one juxtaposed to it. This remark applies forcibly, I think, to cases of abdominal aneurism, where—say in aneurism arising near the origin of the cœliac axis or the superior mesenteric artery— the murmur may be carried along one or other of these vessels, the aneurism the while being in the aorta, and surrounding or pressing upon the mouth of these vessels just mentioned. The simple conduction of a murmur, therefore, proves nothing when vessels are near each other, and may mislead if attention is too exclusively devoted to it. It is true that greater stress might have been laid upon the fact of the relief to the breathing which patient experienced when he lay on his face, but that symptom seemed to me to apply to aneurism of the anterior part of the pulmonary artery as much as to aneurism of the aorta. Again, the accentuated second sound was so distinctly of pulmonic origin—occurring, too, in a case of mitral disease—that it could not be considered a sign of aortic aneurism. This record shows us the advisability of not excluding the probability of aneurism of the aorta—even of the ascending portion of the arch—in cases where the physical signs and symptoms distinctly point to disease at the left base of the heart.

PRESERVATION OF VACCINE VIRUS.—Dr. Benoit, a vaccination medical officer, states (*Lyon Méd.*, June 5) that during the last three years he has found a very simple plan succeed in preserving vaccine virus in an active condition for a very long period. After filling completely two or three vaccine-tubes and sealing them, he places them in a test-tube filled with lard so as entirely to cover them with this. They are then placed in a cellar until wanted.

REPORTS OF HOSPITAL PRACTICE
IN
MEDICINE AND SURGERY.

ST. THOMAS'S HOSPITAL.

A SERIES OF CASES OF MAMMARY CANCER, WITH REMARKS ON TREATMENT AFTER OPERATION.

(Under the care of Mr. JOHN CROFT.)

(Continued from page 66.)

Case 6 (Dresser, Mr. Robinson).—Constance H., aged forty-five; no brothers or sisters. Her father died of heart-disease at the age of fifty-two; her mother, "of tumour of the stomach," at the age of forty-two. She is married twenty-seven years, and has eight children—five alive and healthy; three have died. She has had two miscarriages. She never suffered from her breasts during lactation.

Three or four months ago she felt a pain in the left breast, which has continued up to the present time. A week or two ago she found a lump in the lower part of the breast, about as large as a walnut. At the time of admission there was a hard, ill-defined swelling, deeply seated in the substance of the mamma, as large as a small orange. Skin over it was dimpled and adherent to the growth. The nipple was more retracted on the diseased than on the other side. There was no implication of axillary glands. [*] The pain is rather severe, and is referred to the back and shoulders.

She was admitted on March 15, 1876, and operated on March 26. The tumour was removed by elliptical incisions; the whole breast was not removed, only the affected portion. The vessels were twisted; there was but little hæmorrhage. The edges of the wound were brought together with cat-gut sutures, and dressed with Lister's antiseptic gauze. "The whole operation was done under a carbolic acid hand-spray."

March 27.—Patient quite comfortable. Temperature 99·6° Fahr. No oozing through the gauze.

28th.—Dressed under the carbolic spray. Slight sanguineous discharge on the dressings; wound looking healthy. Temperature 99·6° Fahr. Wound syringed with carbolic acid lotion.

30th.—Dressed. Copious sanguineo-purulent discharge; somewhat offensive. Union in middle of wound; none at side. Temperature 99·7° Fahr.

31st.—Dressed. Sanguineo-purulent discharge. No offensive smell. Temperature 98·5° Fahr.

April 1.—No blood in discharge to-day; less in quantity. No offensive smell. Edges of wound gaping a good deal; brought together by strips of strapping, dipped in hot carbolic acid solution. Temperature 97·4° Fahr.

2nd.—Discharge of healthy pus from wound.

4th.—Skin above and below wound much excoriated, apparently from the rubbing of the antiseptic gauze upon it. Gauze left off to-day in consequence.

5th.—Dressings changed to-day—not quite sweet. Discharge copious. Lower and outer part of wound uniting, but no signs of union in the upper and inner parts. Pad of lint and isinglass plaster applied.

10th.—The spray has not been used since the 6th. Pad of lint again applied, with chlorinate of soda lotion.

20th.—Discharged. The wound granulating slowly up; discharge slight in quantity and perfectly healthy in character.

Re-admitted into hospital, January 15, 1877, on account of local recurrence. The scar appeared healthy, but there were several small nodules around the nipple, which was much more retracted than before. Axillary glands not enlarged.

January 17.—The remainder of the breast was removed under chloroform. No vessels tied. A drainage-tube was put in, catgut sutures were used, and the wound was dressed with a compress of lint soaked in carbolic oil, and then covered with salicylic wool.

Case 7 (Dresser, Mr. Gover).—Julia C., aged thirty-four, married; has no children. Appears a strong, robust woman. She first noticed a slight watery discharge two years and a half ago from nipple of right breast; then, twelve months ago, a lump appeared; at first this was not painful and grew very slowly, but six months ago it became painful, and then began to grow rather rapidly. The pain was of a shooting character. On admission the tumour was found to involve the whole mammary gland; not tender; hard and inelastic. It is movable on the deep structures, but adherent to the skin over its outer half, which is here infiltrated and puckered. Bands can be felt radiating from it into the surrounding structures. The nipple is retracted. The axillary glands do not appear to be involved.

Admitted January 25, 1878. Operated February 2. The entire breast was removed under ether. While dissecting out the tumour, a cyst was opened, which contained about one ounce of clear, yellow, glairy fluid. There was free hæmorrhage. The operation was performed under the carbolic spray. Two drainage-tubes were inserted, and gauze dressing applied.

February 3.—Dressed. Temperature 100° Fahr. There has been no sickness. She has had a fair night, dozing at intervals, with two and a half hours' sound sleep.

11th.—The wound has been dressed antiseptically daily. There was slight bagging of the discharge, for which a carbolised lint was applied.

21st.—Is now dressed every other day. One-half of the incision has united; the other is granulating.

March 10.—Has gradually healed up from the bottom. Still dressed antiseptically. Patient gets up every day.

19th.—Healed. Was discharged this day. The highest recorded temperature has been 101° Fahr. in the evening; for the most part, however, it has not exceeded 99° Fahr.

Case 8 (Dresser, Mr. Smith).—M. H., aged forty-eight, married, no children. Her mother is alive, aged eighty-six; her father died of congestion of brain; brothers and sisters all alive and healthy; an aunt died of internal cancer, aged fifty-five. The patient still menstruates. The right breast is occupied by a tumour of the size of a fist, most obvious on the right side of the breast; nipple is retracted. About an inch above and outside the nipple there is "a boss of elevated skin" as large as a shilling, adherent to the tumour beneath, and of a livid colour. There are some enlarged veins over the tumour, and some shotty glands in the axilla. The tumour was first noticed fifteen months ago. It was painful at times; the pain was of a stabbing character, sometimes absent for three or four days. The pain was aggravated by using the right arm. She has not lost flesh, nor has her appetite failed.

Admitted into hospital, September 16, 1878. Operated on, September 23. The breast was removed by elliptical lateral incisions, including the nipple. Structure of the tumour very dense, undergoing degeneration in the centre. Antiseptic spray and dressings were used.

29th.—Was dressed under the spray. Temperature 99·6° F.

October 7.—All the sutures were removed.

21st.—No bagging; wound almost healed; no discharge from the deep parts.

29th.—Patient was discharged from the hospital. Her temperature since the operation has never exceeded 99 6° F.; for the most part it has been about normal.

Case 9 (Dresser, Mr. Gover).—Amelia L., aged fifty-six, married; no children; a short, robust, healthy-looking woman. One month ago she first noticed a small lump in the left breast, which has grown steadily and slowly since. It has not been painful, but there is a sense of fulness. Her mother died of cancer of the breast; her father and a brother of phthisis.

On admission, a small, hard, nodulated lump as big as a pigeon's egg is felt in the outer and lower part of the breast. The skin is not adherent to it, nipple is but little retracted, and there are no enlarged glands in the axilla. The tumour is freely movable on deeper structures.

Admitted February 23, 1878; operation, March 2. It was removed under chloroform, a small cyst being incised, which contained a bloody fluid. There was not much hæmorrhage. The operation was performed under the antiseptic spray; drainage-tubes were inserted; silver-wire sutures were put in.

March 5.—Wound has been dressed antiseptically every day since last date. The sutures were removed, and a pad of carbolised oil lint was applied (to keep the edges of wound in position).

9th.—A pad of salicylic wool was put on the wound, the

lower angle of which was packed with strips of lint dipped in carbolic oil.

11th.—Wound gaping a little at its lower part.

14th.—There was some redness about the wound (? from the carbolic dressings, which were now left off).

25th.—Wound much improved since warm-water dressings have been used. The upper three-fourths of the wound have firmly united.

The temperature was 101° Fahr. on one occasion ; it has ranged from normal in the morning to 99·8° in the evening, occasionally reaching 100° Fahr.

April 4.—Was discharged cured.

(To be concluded.)

TERMS OF SUBSCRIPTION.
(Free by post.)

British Islands	. . . .	Twelve Months	. £1 8	0
,, ,,	. . . .	Six ,,	. 0 14	0
The Colonies and the United } States of America . . . }		Twelve ,,	. 1 10	0
,, ,, ,,		Six ,,	. 0 15	0
India		Twelve ,,	. 1 10	0
,, (viâ Brindisi) . . .		,,	. 1 15	0
,, ,, . . .		Six ,,	. 0 15	0
,, (viâ Brindisi) . . .		,,	. 0 17	6

Foreign Subscribers are requested to inform the Publishers of any remittance made through the agency of the Post-office.

Single Copies of the Journal can be obtained of all Booksellers and Newsmen, price Sixpence.

Cheques or Post-office Orders should be made payable to Mr. JAMES LUCAS, 11, New Burlington-street, W.

TERMS FOR ADVERTISEMENTS.

Seven lines (70 words)	. . .	.£0 4	6
Each additional line (10 words)	. .	. 0 0	6
Half-column, or quarter-page	. .	. 1 5	0
Whole column, or half-page	. .	. 2 10	0
Whole page	. . .	. 5 0	0

Births, Marriages, and Deaths are inserted Free of Charge.

THE MEDICAL TIMES AND GAZETTE *is published on Friday morning: Advertisements must therefore reach the Publishing Office not later than One o'clock on Thursday.*

Medical Times and Gazette.

SATURDAY, JULY 23, 1881.

THE MORALITY OF THE MEDICAL PROFESSION.

THERE must surely be some inscrutable reason why the Medical Profession should so often be attacked from without, as compared with those of Divinity and Law. We often hear jokes about the readiness with which a clergyman finds it his duty to exchange a worse for a better living, and equally bad jests as to lawyers' bills of costs; but it is seldom that we hear such downright abuse of these as is from time to time showered on the medical profession. The latest example of this is contained in the April number of the *Modern Review*, which for scurrility and malignancy we do not remember ever to have seen equalled, certainly never surpassed. Such is its character, that we should never have thought of answering or attempting to reply to it had not this task been taken in hand by Dr. William Carpenter in the current number of the *Review*. Dr. Carpenter's paper has been reprinted in pamphlet form, and circulated somewhat widely, so that the existence of the offensive article may thus be made known where otherwise people would have remained ignorant of its very existence.

It is a well-known saying that we never hate so well as when we hate those who have done us a good turn; and if this be true, the benefits which the writer of the first-named article has received must indeed have been

many and great. The first thing to be noted with regard to this article is that it is the only one in the number which is unsigned, though the editor speaks of the author as "an esteemed contributor." He also speaks of the writer as "him," but from internal evidence it would be hard to arrive at any other conclusion than that it ought to be "her." It is easy, therefore, to estimate the moral courage of this wholesale libeller, who seeks to hide his or her identity by anonymity and the additional mask (if we are not mistaken) of change of sex. It is not to be supposed that this is the work of a raw novice in the art of writing, for the style is vigorous and clear. Evidently the article is from one well trained to wield the pen ; but vile abuse takes the place of argument, and in many places falsehood that of truth. We hardly know whether the writer is altogether to be blamed for this last ; for it is plain that, whilst possessed of a certain smattering of knowledge with regard to our profession, he or she has totally failed to master its details.

Turning, however, to the substance of this extraordinary production, we find the writer first of all oppressed with a terrible sense of the growing power of the medical profession, which is destined, apparently, to override everything, even Parliament, in whatever relates to health. But next comes the pertinent inquiry, Who are these who are thus to rule over us? Why, vulgar upstarts! In America, and several countries of Europe, medical practitioners, we learn, often spring from the "upper ten," and in France even nobles become doctors nowadays, but in England they come from among the secondary professional class, or from tradesmen, or even from among intelligent artisans. This is a fearful denunciation truly, and one which the profession is not likely soon to get over.

With magnificent carelessness of logic, we are told that the higher ranks of society do not habitually send their sons to our hospitals in preference to Eton or Christ Church. Our humble notion was that men began to study medicine when they had got some smattering of letters, that gentlemen are even vain enough to take a degree in Arts before entering on special studies, but we did not suppose there was anyone mad enough to entertain the idea of substituting the one course or kind of training for the other.

With characteristic malignancy which will see nothing that is good about us, the writer next proceeds to assume that the chief motive which induces a man to take to medicine is what it will bring in the shape of money. For is not, says the writer, the average income of the medical practitioner £50 a year more than that of a clergyman? and then look at the enormous prizes in medicine and surgery! Alas, alas! were there no blinding by evil feeling here, the story would be very different. Next we are treated to a fancy sketch of the medical student of the present day, and of his sudden transformation into the full-blown practitioner, "to flit evermore softly through shaded boudoirs, murmuring soothing suggestions to ladies suffering from headaches, and recommending mild syrups to teething infants"! It is not easy to say whether "this is wrote sarcastical," but the *animus* is there, and well betokens the spleen and venom with which the writer was bursting.

Then immediately follows a full dose of innuendo of the most filthy kind, as to the crimes of doctors "committed on narcotised victims," for do they not possess facilities which fall to no other lot? And then the reader is invited to fall back on memory for illustrations of this, as well as cases where men who have thus guilty have been screened by their professional brethren. Nay, more; it is asserted to be doubtful whether a medical coroner would not hesitate to commit a brother practitioner in a case of poisoning brought home to him.

Next comes a string of accusations, all insulting, if not untruthful. Here is the first:—"Honour is justly due to the physician who studies science in order to cure his patients; but is it equally honourable to study patients in order to acquire science?" This happy mortal knows nothing of clinical work and its necessities. A tirade on the feelings of a woman surrounded by a crowd of students gives the keynote as to what is meant. Not less worthy of notice is the assertion that surgeons operate needlessly to keep their hands "well in." Then follows a reiteration of the old charge, that gold, gold, gold, is the sole moving spring in our profession, with a broad accusation that medical men deliberately make patients ill for the sake of continuing their services. So too in consultation, we are told, the consultant invariably backs up what has been said or done before his visit, whether that be good or ill for the patient. So that it comes about that " in the sight of God he has told a shameful and cruel lie, and has taken money from the very victim of his falsehood. He has betrayed the trust of loving and simple hearts, and left them to break, when with a word he might have done what in him lay to save their earthly treasure." Do any of our readers recognise the faintest inkling of truth in this picture? We confess we cannot.

Then we have the unfailing topics of vivisection and of vaccination, which, we are assured, doctors back up simply for the money it brings, together with that darkest charge, the Contagious Diseases Acts. Space forbids us to say more now on certain other topics, but we shall end with a quotation to show what manner of fanatic is here disclosed. The author writes thus: respecting "the horrible proposal to compel parents, children, husbands, and wives to submit to be separated from their beloved ones in cases of infectious disease, and to send them to be treated at the discretion of a medical man. The day when this atrocious scheme is legalised, either in Switzerland (where it has made some progress through the Legislature), or here in England, will be ' the beginning of the end ' of all family happiness. Cowardice is always cruel, but the cruelty of this proposal to tear asunder the holiest ties in the hour when they ought to be closest drawn, is a surprising revelation of the poltroonery to which we are advancing in our abject terror of disease. Better would it be that pestilence should rage through the land, and we should die of 'the visitation of God,' than that we should seek safety by the abandonment of our nearest and dearest in the hour of mortal trial, and leave them to the tender mercies of the men who could call on us for such a sacrifice of affection and duty."

It is useless to argue with such people. Theirs is certainly ignorance which is invincible; but still more apparent is the spite and malignancy which lie at the bottom of all such productions. Their utter untruthfulness is perhaps their least demerit.

"MODERN SANITARY SCIENCE."

IT is many years since Mr. Chadwick, C.B., first began to agitate for public sanitary reform; but his advice and suggestions for a long time fell on comparatively barren soil, and brought forth but little fruit. To-day, however, sanitary science has gained for itself an amount of public recognition more worthy the object it has in view, and in more fitting proportion with the importance which wholesome sanitation exercises, not on individuals alone, but on the nation at large.

The past week will be remembered as a notable and, we will hope, an epochal period by promoters of this science, as then a first great International Medical and Sanitary Exhibition was opened at South Kensington. The Exhibition has been organised by the Executive Committee of the Parkes Museum of Hygiene, itself founded to perpetuate the memory of a great and successful sanitarian, and the present time was selected on account of the meeting of the International Medical Congress, which is to be held in London during the early days of August. A very large concourse of medical men from all parts of the world will take place, and it is to be hoped that they will carry away with them much practical information concerning the art and science of preventive medicine and the promotion of public health.

During the week, also, the Sanitary Institute of Great Britain held its annual meeting, at which Professor de Chaumont delivered an interesting and important address, in which he demonstrated the value and bearing of sanitation on our life-prospects. He contrasted the present sanitary condition of England with earlier periods, and showed that, had the death-rate between 1871 and 1881 continued the same as during the period from 1861 to 1871, some 300,000 persons in England and Wales alone, who are now living, would have been dead—a convincing proof, we think, " that modern sanitary legislation had produced useful and important effects."

Few can doubt that public hygiene is one of the great questions of the day. When we look around us, especially when we go into some of the poorer districts of London and come face to face with the masses of population inhabiting these districts, we must admit that we have to do with a very large and a very complicated problem. Next to thrift —by which we mean making the most of what one has— there is hardly a subject of which the poorer classes are more ignorant than of the value of hygiene. It is true, they live in surroundings where it is very difficult to carry out even such notions of hygiene as they may possess; and, until very lately, this unsanitary condition has not attracted much attention, while even now it is neglected in one of its most important and fundamental principles—that of house-building. The vast mass of dwellings for the poor are small cottages, which were probably intended for single families when they were first planned; but which, as the population has grown, have now come to be occupied by several families. They were probably never very perfect in their arrangements; indeed, in many of these houses—as we can testify from personal inspection—sanitary regulations are prominently conspicuous by their absence. Nor is this absence of sanitary forethought alone confined to the dwellings of the poor. Our readers need only call to mind the condition in which, on careful inspection, Marlborough House was found a year or two ago, for confirmation of the statement we have just made. But the rich are able to look after themselves in this respect. When sickness, or its early symptoms, threaten, a change of air or of residence at once suggests itself, and is carried out, often before the ill effects of bad drainage have had time to do much damage. A vigorous health, as the result of a better food-supply, renders the system better able to withstand the effects of unsanitary conditions, and hence for awhile their effects fail to produce much tangible mischief. But with the poorer classes the question of healthy homes is one of paramount importance; for circumstances oblige them—year in, year out—to live in the same house, it may be in the same room, and to subsist on a diet which is hardly in accordance with what physiologists would regard as scientifically sufficient, even if partaken of under more favourable conditions both of light and of air.

We have already had an opportunity of just looking over the Sanitary Exhibition, though we have not made any attempt to examine any of the many interesting objects which are there to be seen. This will be done later, and a full report will appear in our columns in due course. An amount of skill and forethought is, however, obvious, which will surprise many who come to see this kind of work for the first time. An amount, too, of luxury will be observed, which will make young householders almost shudder, while those who have yet to establish themselves will certainly hesitate before encountering the vast expenses which modern notions of sanitation, house decoration, and house furnishing almost necessarily lead to.

In the midst of all this, we would urge on the public officials the necessity of extending the benefits of "modern sanitary science" to the poor, and to the classes who cannot do much in this direction for themselves.

First and foremost, we believe that there should be an official inspection of the plans of all houses not built for the personal occupation of the builder, and that an official supervision should be exercised during the actual building. In this manner, without interfering with the rights of private property or of private individuals, the authorities could see that the water-supply and drainage connexions were of the best description. Such supervision would doubtless be little acceptable to speculative builders and to such as run up houses at the cheapest rate to sell in the dearest market. The growth of our London suburbs might possibly be somewhat slower, but we question whether this can be regarded as any serious drawback. As things stand at present, houses are run up in a few weeks which look very pretty from the outside, but the occupiers, after a year or two, soon begin to find out, to their cost, that "all is not gold which glitters."

In the East of London—among other districts—where house-room is much wanted, there are miles of streets, bordered by small, ill-built, two-storey four-roomed houses. When we think of this, and hear so much about the value of land, the expense of living far away from one's occupation, we wonder why these small houses do not give place to others more convenient, and better adapted for the occupation of small families—such houses, for instance, as those known as Peabody-buildings. These houses have long since outlived the prejudice which existed in the minds of a few. The idea of having a house to oneself is doubtless a pleasant one; but eight-tenths of the houses to which we have just referred, if inspected, would prove to contain two or three, and some even four, families.

"Modern sanitary science" is establishing itself on a secure basis. It has been taken up by those who can demonstrate—with almost mathematical precision, what can be accomplished by it. It is, however, a costly luxury as those can testify who have had to call in the assistance of a sanitary surveyor to inspect and set in order their houses. Let us not forget this; but while enjoying all the advantages which it secures for us, let us not cease to advocate adequate supervision of the homes of those who are too poor to look after themselves.

THE CONTAGIOUS DISEASES ACTS.

SOME of the evidence lately given before the Select Committee on the Contagious Diseases Acts is especially worthy of notice, as being the testimony of men who have had special opportunities of minutely and carefully observing the working of them, who might have been expected to have strong prejudices and feelings against the Acts, and yet who were convinced by experience and observation that they have had a most beneficial effect.

Early in June the Rev. Thomas Tuffield was called before the Committee. He is a "Congregational" minister living in Woolwich, and is a member of the Board of Guardians and of some other local bodies. He said that he had had

ample opportunity of observing the operation of the Acts in the Woolwich district; that he had been familiar with the district before the Acts came into force; and that it was impossible not to be struck with the much more orderly condition of the streets, the diminution in the number of common women, and the more decent and cleanly appearance of the few now seen—a result he was unable to attribute to any other agency than the Acts, as all other police regulations remained precisely the same.

As to the frequently repeated statement, that it was unsafe for respectable women to walk about the street for fear of interference by the official appointed to carry the Acts out, he declared that, on the contrary, the order and decorum now established rendered it possible for respectable women to go out with perfect security, where formerly it was impossible. And he further stated that it was well known that he was willing to aid those who had any grievances, particularly as the champion of the poor; nevertheless, during all these years, he had never once had any complaint made to him of an attempt to subject a virtuous woman to the operation of the Acts. He was strongly of opinion that the working of the Acts was a most valuable means of getting at women with a view to their reformation; and with regard to juvenile prostitution, he thought it had decidedly diminished. The fear of the Acts, he considered, acted as a most wholesome deterrent to many young minds. Clandestine prostitution had also decidedly decreased; and the class known as "officers' girls," if they still existed, were at all events no longer seen flaunting on the parade-ground. He was decidedly of opinion that voluntary hospitals would not work; women could not be got to enter them, still less kept in them. His own experience in the matter had convinced him that the women would not listen to advice now, any more than they had in former days, till it was too late.

Mr. Tuffield thought that many Nonconformists opposed the Acts on religious grounds. They considered the Act a human attempt to oppose a God-made punishment for sin, and this idea prevailed extensively among the fervently religious; but there was a sort of religious fervour that did not always lead to the best practical results. In supporting the Acts he was taking, he said, a view opposed to that held by many other Congregational ministers, and he had suffered no little loss of popularity in consequence. But he had been unable to resist the strong conviction that had forced itself upon him, as to the beneficial effects of the Acts; and he was sure that if other ministers had had his opportunities, and had seen what he had seen, they would be of his opinion.

Mr. Tuffield was examined by Mr. Osborne Morgan, and cross-examined by Dr. Cameron, Mr. Hopwood, and Mr. Stansfeld, but his evidence was clear and unshaken. He declared that, without exception, all the points he had dealt with had been matters of his own personal observation, owing to his official position in Woolwich.

A few days later, the Rev. E. P. Grant, who has for fifteen years been the Vicar of Portsmouth, was before the Committee, and was examined by Mr. Osborne Morgan, by Messrs. Stansfeld and Hopwood, and some other members of the Committee. Mr. Grant had made it his business to inquire carefully into the working of the Acts, and the conclusion he had arrived at was that they have been of the greatest service in diminishing the number of prostitutes and of brothels, in checking disease, and in providing greatly increased facilities for the reclamation of fallen women. As Chairman of the Hospital Committee he was able to describe with full knowledge and authority the management of it, and the various influences for good brought to bear on the women; and as a member of the Council of he Penitentiary at Basingstoke, it was within his knowledge that during the last three years sixty-eight girls had been received into the Portsmouth Refuge on leaving the Lock wards. As, with two exceptions, all those had since done well, he thought a great success had been achieved, and that this was entirely due to the working of the Acts. He corroborated the evidence given by Inspector Anniss and other witnesses as to the facilities afforded by the operation of the Acts for rescuing girls who were on the borderland between levity and immorality, or who had been induced to actually take the first step towards prostitution; and he spoke also of the decided reduction in the number of juvenile prostitutes, and the great decrease of public solicitation in the streets. With regard to voluntary hospitals, he, like Mr. Tuffield, thought that girls would not be got to enter them, and consequently the opportunity of bringing good influences to bear on them would be lost. When questioned as to whether it did not seem to him a gross deed that men should fetch in and examine women compulsorily for the benefit of men, he admitted that it did seem so to a certain extent; but observed that, on the other hand, it must be remembered that it was still more for the benefit of women, and especially for the benefit of posterity; and that though the individual liberty of the women was interfered with to a certain limit or extent, still the remedy was always in the women's own hands—they had only to give up the life they were leading. Considering the machinery of the Acts, and that an information had to be laid before a justice of the peace, who would not make an order for a woman to attend for examination unless he was satisfied as to the truth of the charges brought against her, he thought it impossible for an innocent woman to be brought under police control. During the thirteen years he had lived in Portsmouth, he had not heard of a single authenticated case of abuse by the police of the special powers entrusted to them; and he believed that, had there been such, he could not have failed to hear of it.

The Rev. Prebendary Wilkinson, D.D., for eleven years vicar of St. Andrew's, Plymouth, who also was before the Committee, gave evidence to the same effect. He likewise had been led to actively support the Acts by the benefit he had observed to result from them. And this witness said that he did not think that immorality was in any degree fostered among men by a feeling of security given by the knowledge that the Acts were in operation. He did not believe that men entered into any cold calculations in the matter, and held, moreover, that, supposing any such feeling prevailed in a very slight degree, the absence of solicitation in the streets was an advantage that quite counterbalanced it.

We place this summary of the evidence of these three gentlemen before our readers, in the belief that it will be useful to such of them as may be called upon to justify the extension or the continuance of the operation of the Contagious Diseases Acts, to have a knowledge of the witness borne to their value by men who have had prolonged opportunities of observing the effects of them closely and minutely, and who cannot be accused of the prejudices in their favour that some of the opponents of them so kindly attribute to the medical profession.

THE WEEK.

TOPICS OF THE DAY.

THE report of Dr. Collingridge, the Medical Officer for the Port of London, for the month of June last, shows that during that period 1859 vessels of all classes were inspected, 886 in the river and 973 in the docks. The small-pox epidemic in London, though from time to time exhibiting a diminished severity, still continued. The number of deaths during June was 311, as against 352 in May. Due publicity was given to the offer of free vaccination of sailors and others in the port of London, and during the month under notice 106 persons had been vaccinated or revaccinated at a cost for lymph of under £2. Out of every hundred cases of revaccination, it has been shown that 88 per cent. have been successful. Understanding that the Metropolitan Asylums Board proposed to place their small-pox hospital-ships off Deptford, and knowing that to be a most unsuitable place, for many reasons, Dr. Collingridge wrote to the Board, calling their attention to the state of the river at that spot, and showing that excellent positions were available a little distance below. To that, however, he received a reply that the Local Government Board had decided to accept all the responsibility in the matter, and he was requested to advise as to the best locality for embarking patients. Dr. Collingridge enumerates the various cases of small-pox found on board vessels, and he states that all the cases were distinctly traceable to the epidemic in London, and were in no way imported. The number of emigrants passing through London to New York was very much smaller than during the previous month—viz., from Hamburg, 749; Antwerp, 136; and Havre, 5—and among these no cases of disease were discovered.

The ceremony of laying the foundation-stone of the Vyrnwy Embankment of the new waterworks at Llanwyddyn, intended to supply the city of Liverpool with water, was performed last week by Earl Powis, in the presence of nearly 200 guests invited by the Mayor and Corporation of Liverpool, and a vast concourse of spectators. The district in question (though not the immediate site of the Liverpool Works) has long been known to engineers as one affording peculiar facilities for the construction of waterworks, and was mentioned by Mr. Bateman in his evidence before the Royal Commission in 1867 as being suitable for the supply of London. Our readers will remember that some time ago we regularly, from time to time, recorded the steps taken by the Liverpool authorities to obtain Parliamentary sanction to their scheme; and after protracted operations, and in the face of much opposition, they at length, in August of last year, obtained the Royal assent to their Bill. The works just commenced, alike by reason of their magnitude and the novelty of some of their features, are among the most important which have been undertaken in modern times—their only rival, in point of magnitude, being the Thirlmere project of Manchester, which has not yet been thoroughly developed. The length of the reservoir, or lake, to be formed at Llanwyddyn is four miles and three-quarters, the area 1115 acres, and it will afford a daily supply of 52,000,000 gallons of water to Liverpool. The river Vyrnwy is the chief upper tributary of the Severn, and the waters of this stream, together with those of two other affluents, will be impounded at Llanwyddyn by a dam or embankment of masonry built across the valley, which will be 140 feet high, and 1255 feet long. The water will be conveyed to Liverpool—a distance of nearly seventy miles—in a triple set of pipes, each of a diameter of from four feet to five feet. In this long distance three tunnels have to be got through, one about two miles and a quarter in length, and two others under a mile each. Oswestry and other towns on the route will take water from these pipes. The works now commenced are expected to occupy from eight to ten years in their completion, but when finished it is claimed for this gigantic scheme that by its adoption Liverpool will be provided with a water-supply sufficient for all time, and for all increase of population. The development of these works, so recently inaugurated, will be watched with some curiosity and much interest by those amongst us who are of opinion that the time will come when a similar colossal scheme will have to be undertaken to place the metropolis itself in a satisfactory position as regards its water-supply.

It is an unfortunate circumstance that the London magistrates are not entirely unanimous in supporting the efforts of those who are bound, as far as possible, to protect the public from the risk of infection. Recently, at the Wandsworth Police-court, a man was summoned, at the instance of the Wandsworth Board of Guardians, for exposing himself without taking proper precaution while suffering from small-pox. Dr. Nicholas, the Medical Officer of Health for Wandsworth, deposed that on May 17 last the defendant walked into his surgery suffering from small-pox, stating that he was barman and potman at the "French Horn" Tavern, Lambeth-walk, and that his master sent him in a cab to his sister in Bendon Valley for the purpose of applying to the medical officer of the district for an order to admit him to a small-pox hospital. The defendant walked from Garrett-lane to witness's surgery. Mr. Sheil, the magistrate, wanted to know how it was possible for the defendant to obtain the advice of a doctor without going to him; perhaps he could not afford to pay a doctor to visit him. The Clerk to the Board of Guardians explained that the defendant should have applied for an order in Lambeth, and not come to Wandsworth. Mr. Sheil, however, considered it would be harsh to punish in such a case, and dismissed the summons. The defendant may, possibly, have obtained some knowledge of Mr. Sheil's peculiar views, which prompted him to avoid Lambeth, since about the same time a Mrs. James Williams was summoned to the police-court of the latter district for having, without proper precaution, wilfully caused her maidservant to expose herself in the public street while suffering from small-pox. In this case Mr. Ellison, the Lambeth magistrate, ordered her to pay a fine of £5 and costs.

The preliminary report of the City Day Census, taken three weeks after the Imperial Census of this year, has just been published. From this it appears that the total residents, occupiers, and persons employed was—males, 195,287; females, 44,095; children, 21,288; total, 260,670. The Imperial Census gives for the resident night population alone, on Sunday night, April 4, 1881 – males, 25,085; females, 25,441; total, 50,526. The mercantile and commercial population in 1881 is 210,144; in 1866 it was 170,133—being an increase of 40,011. The decrease in the night residents and caretakers, since the Imperial Census of 1871, is 24,371. The number of persons resorting to the City on foot and in vehicles has greatly increased. In 1881, in a day of twelve hours, 5 a.m. to 5 p.m., 589,468; in 1866, in a day of twelve hours, 5 a.m. to 6 p.m., 549,613—an increase of 39,855. In 1881, in a day of sixteen hours, 5 a.m. to 9 p.m., 739,640; in 1866, in a day of sixteen hours, 5 a.m. to 9 p.m., 679,744—an increase of 59,896.

On Saturday last a meeting was held at Grosvenor House to promote the movement for extending to the working-classes of London the benefits of provident dispensaries. In the absence of the Duke of Westminster, Mr. Stansfeld, M.P., presided, and in the course of his address remarked that rich people had no difficulty in providing medical attendance for their families, but it was unreasonable to expect working-men to be able to pay the ordinary fees of even moderate-charging doctors in the event of illness. The common method of insuring against sickness was by resorting to a sick club, but that was a somewhat primitive institution, and was not always successful financially. Moreover, it took the man only into account, ignoring the wife and children. The same defect characterised the majority of the friendly societies of England. The great hospitals of London were the marvel of the

civilised world, but they had diverged from their true work by encouraging a system of gratuitous out-relief, which exercised a pauperising and demoralising influence on the people. With a view of remedying such a state of things partially, if it could not be done wholly, the Metropolitan Provident Medical Association had been founded, its aim being to give the working-classes in every part of London and its environs —on terms within their means, and consistent with their independence and self-respect—the advantage of medical treatment on the same satisfactory footing as was enjoyed by the upper classes, including skilled and tender nursing. The dispensary would occupy the place of the family doctor to the working-man. The work which they had undertaken was, in fact, a great and practical one, and with energy and patience he felt certain it would succeed. After speeches by Sir C. Trevelyan, Mr. Timothy Holmes, Dr. A. Carpenter, and others, resolutions were passed approving the plan of the Association.

One, if not the most universal, topic of the day during the past week has been the exceptional heat-wave which has visited the whole of Europe and America. In this country, though of late years we have scarcely experienced our full share of the sun's rays, the casualties from sunstroke (as far as at present reported) have been insignificant, but from France several cases are recorded. It is, however, from America, as usual, that the gravest results are received. According to official returns, 500 deaths have occurred from heat in Cincinnati in six days. It seems almost impossible to suppose that this enormous mortality is due to sunstroke only; probably in the majority of cases the heat has simply accelerated death. To make the return complete the number of deaths from all causes ought to be reported, and it should also be stated how much the mortality is in excess of the average.

The agitation to secure a park for Paddington still continues, and unless the promoters persevere, there is a great chance of this most desirable project entirely falling through. Since we last mentioned the subject, another meeting has been held, presided over by Mr. J. R. Holland, M.P. In the course of the proceedings Lord Brabazon pointed out that the Census just taken showed a growing depopulation of some of the more central parishes, like Marylebone, with a corresponding overflow to the districts of Paddington and Kilburn, where the proposed park was badly needed. Other speakers urged the importance of securing the site selected for the proposed park, and it was eventually decided to form a local committee to aid in collecting the fund of £100,000, which it is proposed to raise by voluntary contributions. It was announced that the amount already received or promised exceeded £21,000.

THE ROYAL COLLEGE OF SURGEONS OF ENGLAND.

At the quarterly meeting of the Council of the Royal College of Surgeons, held on Thursday, July 14, the minutes of the ordinary meeting of June 9 were read and confirmed. Sir James Paget, whose re-election by the Fellows we have already reported, was readmitted a member of Council, and Mr. J. W. Hulke and Mr. Christopher Heath were also admitted as members of the Council for the first time. Reports were received from the Board of Examiners and the Court of Examiners on the candidates passed and rejected at the several primary and pass examinations held during the collegiate year 1880-81; and from the several annual committees and the Nomination Committee. The professors, lecturers, and other officials were re-elected for the ensuing year. Mr. Erasmus Wilson, F.R.S., the Senior Vice-President, was elected President by a large majority, and Mr. Spencer Wells and Professor John Marshall, F.R.S., were elected

Senior and Junior Vice-Presidents respectively. The annual committees and the Nomination Committee were appointed. Mr. J. Hutchinson was re-elected Hunterian Professor of Surgery and Pathology; Mr. W. H. Flower and Mr. W. K. Parker were re-elected Hunterian Professors of Comparative Anatomy and Physiology; and Mr. Gerald Yeo was re-elected Arris and Gale Lecturer on Anatomy and Physiology. Dr. Bristowe and Dr. Dickinson were re-elected Examiners, and Professor F. T. Roberts and Dr. S. Gee were elected additional Examiners in Medicine; and Dr. G. E. Herman, F.R.C.S., and John Williams, F.R.C.P., were elected Examiners in Midwifery for the ensuing year. Mr. Frederick S. Eve, F.R.C.S., was appointed to the newly-made office of Pathological Curator of the Museum of the College. A letter from the Royal Commission on the Medical Acts was read, and was referred to a committee consisting of the President and Vice-Presidents and seven other members of the Council—viz., Sir James Paget, Dr. Humphry, Mr. Erichsen, Mr. Savory, Mr. Holmes, Mr. Lund, and Mr. Lister—for consideration and report.

THE HEALTH OF KENSINGTON FOR THE MONTH OF MARCH LAST.

DR. T. ORME DUDFIELD, in his report on the health, etc., of Kensington for the four weeks, February 27 to March 26 last, remarks that the health of the district, as gauged by the Registrar-General's weekly returns, continues favourable. The death-rate in the parish was only 17·2, or 3·4 per 1000 below the decennial average, and 4·6 below the metropolitan rate—this, too, being 2·7 per 1000 below the decennial average. The deaths from diseases of the chest have diminished considerably, viz., from 61 and 60 in the two previous months, to 46; the deaths from phthisis, however, were numerous (33), a considerable proportion of these having occurred in the Brompton sub-district. The deaths from the principal diseases of the zymotic class were only 14, or less than one-half the corrected average (29). The cases of scarlet fever recorded during the four weeks under notice were 18, as against 24 and 31 in the two previous months. Eleven of these cases occurred in the district north of Uxbridge-road, and 7 in the remainder of the parish south of that road. All the cases in the north had been concealed, and consequently not one was removed. Thirty-six cases of small-pox (one less than in the previous month) have been recorded since March 2 last; thirty-two of the sufferers were removed to hospital; in three of the remaining four cases such removal was unnecessary. Speaking generally, Dr. Dudfield adds, there is too often a longer interval between the beginning of the illness and the removal of the case than there should be, probably due to failure to recognise the nature of the disease at the outset. Only one death, however, from small-pox was registered in the parish during the month, viz., of a woman shortly after her confinement.

SOCIETY FOR RELIEF OF WIDOWS AND ORPHANS.

THE Quarterly Court of Directors was held at 53, Berners-street, on Wednesday last, at 5 p.m.; the President, Sir George Burrows, B.A., in the chair. A sum of £1302 was voted for the sixty-one widows and twelve orphans now on the list of recipients of grants. The expenses of the quarter were £41 14s. One fresh application was made by a widow for a grant, and her claim was admitted. Two orphans ceased to be eligible through age for any further assistance. One new member was elected, and the deaths of three were reported. It was resolved at the meeting to send a circular to all the medical men residing in the area comprised between the old and new limits of the Society, now extended to all places within twenty miles of Charing-cross.

THE PARIS WEEKLY RETURN.

THE number of deaths for the twenty-seventh week, ending July 7, 1881, was 1125 (viz., 576 males and 549 females), and among these there were from typhoid fever 38, small-pox 27, measles 26, scarlatina 21, pertussis 11, diphtheria and croup 38, dysentery 1, erysipelas 6, puerperal infections 4, and acute tubercular meningitis 59. There were also 36 deaths from acute bronchitis, 56 from pneumonia, 134 from infantile athrepsia (44 of the infants having been partially or wholly suckled), and 39 from violent deaths. The mortality has increased by 100 over that of the preceding week, which in so hot a season might be expected. Several of the epidemic diseases have somewhat increased, especially scarlatina (from 11 to 21); and the diseases liable to aggravation during great heat have much augmented in mortality. Thus there were 134 deaths from athrepsia instead of 93, 59 from meningitis instead of 44, and from other cerebro-spinal diseases 111 instead of 87. The proportion of civil to religious interments for the month of May was more than 16 per cent., or 1 civil interment to 5 religious interments. The births for the week amounted to 1225, viz., 644 males (473 legitimate and 171 illegitimate) and 581 females (426 legitimate and 155 illegitimate); 95 children (49 males and 46 females) were born dead or died within twenty-four hours after birth.

SANITARY INSTITUTE OF GREAT BRITAIN.

AT the anniversary meeting of the Sanitary Institute of Great Britain, held at the Royal Institution, Albemarle-street, on Thursday, July 14, Right Hon. Earl Fortescue in the chair, an address was delivered by Professor F. S. B. F. de Chaumont, M.D., F.R.S., Chairman of the Council, entitled "Modern Sanitary Science," and the medals and certificates were awarded to the successful exhibitors at the Exhibition held at Exeter in October, 1880. At the close of the address, which will be found elsewhere in our columns, the Chairman called upon Dr. A. Carpenter to propose a vote of thanks to Professor F. S. B. F. de Chaumont, M.D., F.R.S., which was seconded by G. J. Symons, F.R.S. Earl Fortescue, in putting the motion, spoke of the pleasure with which he had listened to the address, and fully endorsed the wisdom of the paper, and spoke of the interest he had formerly taken in the sanitary condition of the Army. A vote of thanks to Earl Fortescue was moved by Mr. W. H. Michael, Q.C., and seconded by E. Chadwick, Esq., C.B.

VACATION LECTURES FOR GENERAL PRACTITIONERS.

WE learn from the Berliner Klinische Wochenschrift that the next course of vacation lectures for general practitioners in Berlin will commence on September 21, and terminate towards the close of October. The course will embrace:— 1. Normal and Pathological Anatomy; 2. Physiology and its Relation to Medicine; 3. Materia Medica and Toxicology; 4. Medicine and Methods of Physical Examination 5. Psychology and Brain Disease; 6. Nervous Disease and Electrotherapeutics; 7. Surgery; 8. Diseases of the Eye; 9. Disease of the Ear; 10. Gynæcology; 11. Skin Diseases and Syphilis; 12. Legal Medicine and Hygiene. Such lectures are sure to be appreciated by general practitioners. Modern improvements, as they are somewhat complacently called, are going on so fast, that without study, practitioners in the country are apt to "get rusty," and lose their facility in the use of ophthalmoscope, laryngoscope, etc. The Germans are decidedly ahead of us in having successfully set such a movement as this on foot, and in having provided special facilities like the above for country practitioners. Although a similar plan has been tried in this country, it has always conspicuously failed. Not only will it keep up a good feeling of *esprit de corps*, but it will serve to keep fresh that theoretical knowledge of professional work which is the more valuable when combined with a sound knowledge of how to apply it practically.

MEDICAL EDUCATION: WHAT NEXT?

THE *Glasgow Medical Journal* for July thinks that those in charge of medical education ought to afford students some practical instruction in cookery! "The universities and licensing boards still insist on a certain experience in preparing and dispensing medicines, although the graduate is not expected to be a druggist, and surely some similar elementary knowledge as to the preparation of food is no less important, and no less desirable. Arrangements might be made with the schools of cookery to provide such instruction with regard to the cooking of ordinary food, as well as the preparation of special articles for the sick-room."

HEALTH CHRONICLES OF ST. MARYLEBONE, MAY, 1881.

THE Sanitary Chronicles of the Parish of St. Marylebone for the month of May last contain a statement by Mr. A. W. Blyth of the steps taken by the authorities to obtain a site for an infectious hospital. The Vestry having failed to get any suitable land in the parish, has acquired, on what must be considered favourable terms, the right of using a large piece of land, thirteen acres in extent, in the parish of Finchley, for the purpose of erecting a temporary hospital for infectious diseases should occasion require. For the present there is no necessity to provide any accommodation, as the epidemic, so far as Marylebone is concerned, is distinctly on the decline; the successive numbers of cases reported at the Court House during the four weeks of May were 7, 24, 11, and 7. It will, however, Mr. Blyth thinks, be wise to prepare the site by the provision of suitable drainage, etc. Unnecessary anxiety and apprehension is, he believes, felt in certain quarters as to the erection of an infectious hospital on the site thus acquired by the Vestry, but he explains that should such a building become a necessity, it will be established on a small, easily manageable scale, and every precaution will be taken that it shall in no way be injurious to the vicinity. In commenting on the results of the late Census, Mr. Blyth states that in five out of the six registration divisions of the parish of St. Marylebone there is a smaller number of inhabitants than there was ten years ago.

DEATH OF DEAN STANLEY.

UNFORTUNATELY the untimely death of Dr. Maurice Raynaud has not proved the only loss sustained in anticipation by the International Medical Congress. Now we have to record, what we feel more keenly here in England, the lamented death of Dean Stanley, who had undertaken to conduct a special service for members of the Congress in Westminster Abbey on the Sunday which occurs during Congress week.

IT will be observed from our advertising columns that a meeting of the profession, to discuss the question of Medical Reform, will be held in St. James's Hall (not Exeter Hall, as previously announced) on Friday next, at 4 p.m. The meeting is being held under the auspices of the Medical Defence Association.

WE hear that the King of Bavaria has recently conferred on Mr. Mac Cormac the Knight's Cross of the Military Order for Merit. The services for which this cross has been conferred were rendered to the Bavarian wounded during the Franco-German war. It is to be regretted that, through an oversight, this unusual delay has occurred in acknowledging them.

ROLLESTON MEMORIAL.

IN pursuance of a resolution passed at a preliminary meeting held at the house of Dr. A. B. Shepherd, a General Committee is being formed for the purpose of founding a Prize or Scholarship in memory of the late Professor Rolleston. The following gentlemen, among others, have already allowed their names to appear in support of the proposed memorial. A complete list will be published later, as well as a list of subscribers to the fund.

Preliminary List.

The Most Honourable the Marquis of Salisbury, K.G., D.C.L., Chancellor of the University.

Right Hon. J. G. Mowbray, M.P., D.C.L.
John G. Talbot, Esq., M.P., D.C.L.
The Rev. the Vice-Chancellor.
The Very Rev. the Dean of Christ Church.
The Rector of Lincoln.
The Master of Balliol.
The Principal of Brasenose.
The Warden of Merton.
The Provost of Queen's.
The President of the Royal Society.
The President of the Royal College of Physicians.
Charles Darwin, Esq.
Prof. Virchow.
Prof. Pettenkofer.
Prof. Charcot.
George Busk, Esq.
Prof. Acland.
The Bishop of Exeter.
The Bishop of Gibraltar.
Canon Pusey.
Canon Liddon.
Canon Bright.
Canon Rawlinson.
Canon Greenwell.
Canon Duckworth.
The Head Master of Eton.
Rev. W. W. Jackson, Sub-Rector of Exeter.
Rev. E. T. Turner, Registrar of the University.
Sir Thomas Watson, Bart.
Sir George Burrows, Bart.
Sir W. W. Gull, Bart.
Sir James Paget, Bart.
Sir J. Risdon Bennett.
Sir Joseph Fayrer.
John Evans, Esq.
Dr. King Chambers.
Dr. Monro.
Prof. Turner.
Prof. Humphry.
Prof. Burdon Sanderson.
Dr. Clifford Allbutt.
T. Pridgin Teale, Esq.
A. W. Franks, Esq.
E. B. Tylor, Esq.
Prof. Sayce.
Prof. Fowler.
Prof. Boyd Dawkins.
Prof. Henry Smith.
Prof. Clifton.
Prof. Westwood.
Prof. Bonamy Price.
Prof. Huxley.
Prof. Flower.
Prof. Fawcett, M.P.

Prof. Michael Foster.
Henry Power, Esq.
Prof. Bartholomew Price.
Capt. Douglas Galton.
Joseph Lister, Esq.
G. Herbert Morrell, Esq.
Prof. Allman.
Warren de la Rue, Esq.
Prof. Gamgee.
Prof. Samuel Haughton.
G. J. Romanes, Esq.
Dr. J. W. Ogle.
Dr. Andrew.
Dr. W. H. Broadbent.
Prof. Prestwich.
Prof. Bryce.
Dr. G. W. Child.
Prof. Lionel Beale.
John Simon, Esq.
W. J. C. Miller, Esq.
General Pitt Rivers.
Sir John Lubbock, M.P.
Prof. Stubbs.
Prof. Allen Thomson.
Prof. Corfield.
Dr. Church.
W. S. Savory, Esq.
Prof. Reinold.
Prof. Rücker.
C. S. Tomes, Esq.
A. G. Vernon Harcourt, Esq.
Prof. Max Müller.
E. W. Willett, Esq.
H. N. Moseley, Esq.
Prof. Story Maskelyne, M.P.
C. H. Roberts, Esq.
Prof. St. George Mivart.
Prof. Odling.
Sir T. D. Acland, Bart., M.P.
Matthew Arnold, Esq.
Dr. J. F. Payne.
Prof. Earle.
Charles Robertson, Esq.
A. Neubauer, Esq.
W. H. A. Jacobson, Esq.
Dr. Pye-Smith.
Prof. Ray Lankester.
R. F. Freeborn, Esq.
Dr. C. Creighton.
Dr. Gray.
Dr. Tuckwell.
Dr. G. Buchanan.
Rev. Brooke Lambert.
Ingram Bywater, Esq.
Dr. Pavy.
R. W. Raper, Esq.
P. L. Sclater, Esq.
Rev. J. W. Horseley.
Rev. Hayward Joyce.
W. W. Fisher, Esq.
J. H. Morgan, Esq.

Gentlemen desirous of adding their names to the above Committee are requested to communicate with the Secretaries.

Subscriptions will be received by the Honorary Secretaries, C. W. Mansell-Moullin, M.D., Theodore D. Acland, M.B., E. B. Poulton, M.A., and A. P. Thomas, M.A., at 17, Great Cumberland-place, W.; or by the Treasurer, Edward Chapman, Esq., Frewen Hall, Oxford.

INTERNATIONAL MEDICAL AND SANITARY EXHIBITION, 1881.

THIS Exhibition was formally opened on Saturday last by the Earl Spencer, Lord President of the Council, in the presence of a large concourse of people who had assembled to witness the ceremony. The formal opening took place in the Royal Albert Hall. Earl Spencer was supported by Earl Granville, Sir James Paget, Bart., Mr. Erichsen, Professor de Chaumont, and other gentlemen interested in the work of public hygiene.

Earl Spencer regretted the absence of H.R.H. the Duke of Edinburgh, in whose stead he was really officiating that day. The improvements which had been made in all matters concerning the public health during the few preceding years were manifest even to outside observers. Marshes, formerly the beds of malarial poisons, had been drained, and made not only habitable but healthy; while improved drainage, improved water-supply, improved dwellings, were so many public measures, each of which had been of great benefit to the world at large, and testified to the activity which had been going on in this direction during the past few years. The recent census returns showed that in consequence of a lessened death-rate during the last decennial period, as compared with that immediately preceding, some 300,000 lives had been saved, which would otherwise have been sacrificed.

Dr. G. V. Poore next read the Report of the Executive Committee of the Parkes Museum of Hygiene; after which Mr. Mark Judge read the statement of the Exhibition Committee. Both reports were commendably short and to the point.

Earl Granville congratulated the Committee on the large attendance, as clearly showing the interest taken by the public in the Exhibition. He thought everyone, at some time or other, talked or thought something about health. Indeed, if one by chance mentioned any slight indisposition to which one was liable, one was immediately besieged by a host of prescriptions as to medicine, diet, or *régime*. He himself had some years ago while staying in Rome an attack of gout, and on its becoming known, he was inundated with prescriptions in English, Italian, French, German, and even Russian. The Cardinal Secretary of State gave him some kindly advice based on personal experience; while a Foreign Minister from the North tendered him exactly the opposite. On another occasion he had been advised by one unknown friend to try whisky, and by another to avoid it; another suggested claret; while yet a third advised strict abstinence. One old gentleman had strongly recommended him to get a complete set of artificial back teeth. The moral of it all was that neither experience nor study alone sufficed. It must be by a combination that good results could be obtained. He begged to state that the present Government were fully alive to the great importance of sanitation, and, although he regretted that the present session had not been very fertile in work of this kind, yet one great measure—the Flooding of Rivers Bill—was so far advanced that they had a hope of being able shortly to pass it into law.

Sir James Paget, Bart., next spoke. He said that we had very much to show for the results of the teaching of sanitary science in this country during the last few years, thanks to the intelligence and industry of a comparatively small band of sanitary reformers. Such exhibitions as the one which they were assembled to open must do much to promote a knowledge of sanitation. In his opinion, "health" and "wealth" were synonymous terms. Amongst the exhibitors themselves a wholesome rivalry in the attainment of what was as near perfection as possible was set up. Mutual criticism of each other's appliances was likely to bring out the weak and the strong points in such things, and perhaps exhibitors looked at each other's goods with keener eyes for defects or improvements than were possessed by the eminent judges of the awards. A spirit of emulation was set up, and the public in the long run were the gainers. He next pointed out in what various ways the Exhibition might serve as a means of educating the public in matters of sanitation, and concluded by saying that he had one other reason for wishing it success, and it was that he reverenced the memory of Edmund Parkes. He therefore hoped that the success of the Exhibition would be such as to help in placing the Parkes Museum of Hygiene on a more permanent footing, seeing that that institution sought to perpetuate the work to which Parkes devoted the best years of his life.

The proceedings terminated with a vote of thanks to the Earl Spencer for presiding, proposed by Mr. Godwin, seconded by Mr. Erichsen.

In addition to the general purposes in view of which this Exhibition is held, the Executive Committee of the Parkes Museum of Hygiene hope to be able to establish a permanent exhibition for the use of the public. When Dr. Parkes' lamented death occurred in the spring of 1876, it was strongly felt by his professional and personal friends, as well as by those who had known him officially, that some steps should be taken to perpetuate the memory of a man whose life had been of almost unparalleled utility to others. With this object a public meeting was held at University College, London, on June 18, 1876, under the presidency of Sir William Jenner, Bart., when it was unanimously resolved to establish a museum of hygiene, to be called by his name.

This idea met with considerable favour, and an Executive Committee having been appointed, the subscriptions, headed by a donation of £50 from Her Majesty the Queen, soon exceeded £1000. This money enabled the Executive Committee of the Museum to proceed with their work, but little could have been done had it not been for the liberality of the Council of University College, who, on February 7, 1877, placed a large room at the disposal of the Committee in which to temporarily arrange the collection. The Museum was formally opened to the public on June 28, 1879, by Sir R. A. Cross, G.C.B., then Secretary of State for the Home Department, and from that date it has been open gratuitously to the public on every Tuesday, Thursday, and Saturday.

From that time the Museum has grown rapidly, and at present it contains, in addition to a library of some 500 volumes having reference to sanitary science, a large collection of articles illustrated of (a) engineering and local hygiene; (b) architecture; (c) furnishing; (d) clothing; (e) food; (f) preservation and relief. The work of the Executive Committee has been entirely gratuitous. No charge has been made to visitors at any time, neither has any charge been made for space, suitability being the only conditions for the acceptance of any article.

The moderate amount of funds at the disposal of the Committee has not deterred them from making the greatest possible use of the museum. A number of demonstrations and lectures have been given, and these have been very well attended. The first series in the winter of 1879-80 was given for the benefit of the Working Men's Club and Institute Union, and comprised the subjects of house-drainage, ventilation, lighting and warming, food, and the management of the sick-room. The second series was given to members of the Institution of Builders' Foremen and Clerks of Works, and comprised the subjects of ventilation and house-drainage. During the past winter, 1880-81, in response to a suggestion made to the Executive Committee by the "Nineteenth Century Building Society," a course of five lectures was delivered to members of metropolitan building societies. These, which comprised the same subjects as the lectures of the previous year, were attended by numbers so large that the museum was found barely adequate for their accommodation.

The Committee regard this as proof that the museum has supplied an existing want, and they therefore no longer hesitate to ask the public for funds to enable them to continue and extend a work so important to the future well-being of the country. They desire to see the work carried on in a building specially erected for the purpose in some central situation, and they therefore appeal to all classes of the community for subscriptions for this purpose.

We may attempt to give a general idea of its scope and extent by saying that the various objects exhibited have been divided into the following seventeen classes :—1. Surgical Instruments and Apparatus; 2. Obstetrical Instruments, etc.; 3. Ophthalmic Instruments, etc.; 4. Dental Instruments, etc.; 5. Aural Instruments, etc.; 6. Appliances for the Ward and Sick-room; 7. Drugs, Disinfectants, Dietetic Articles, and Mineral Waters; 8. Electrical Instruments and Appliances; 9. Microscopes and Optical Apparatus; 10. Appliances used in teaching Medicine, and other Medical Apparatus; 11. Physiological Instruments; 12. Street Ambulances and other Appliances used for the Treatment of Sick and Wounded; 13. Domestic Hospital Architecture, Planning, Construction, Decorative Materials; 14. Ventilation, Lighting, and Warming; 15. Waterclosets, Sinks, Baths, etc., Sewerage and Drainage; Water-supply and Filtration; 17. School Furniture, Window Blinds, Clothing, Books, etc.

Some idea of the extent of the Exhibition will be got from this index of subjects. We shall draw attention to the most interesting and novel points in each of the sections, and endeavour to assist our readers to a right estimation of their merits.

The Exhibition will remain open until the middle of August. The members of the International Medical Congress will be admitted without payment, on showing their membership card.

FRENCH REGISTRATION RETURNS FOR 1879.—There were during the year 282,976 marriages, 936,529 births, and 839,882 deaths, or only an excess of 96,647 of births over deaths. In 1872, the first year after the national disasters, the marriages were 325,754, the births 966,000, and the deaths 793,064, or an excess of 172,936 of births. The proportion of dead-born to living-born has not varied of late years, being 4·65 per cent. for 1879 ; and the proportion of natural births to the total of births is about the usual mean, 7·15 per cent.—*Lyon Méd.*, July 3.

INNOCUITY OF CEMETERIES IN CITIES.—M. Robinet terminates an able article in the *Revue Scientifique* (June 18) with the following statement :—" We are able to affirm that up to our own times not a single positive example of injury can be laid to the charge of the cemeteries of Paris. We may thus with a good conscience assure the public in this respect, and deplore with the illustrious Fourcroy the abuses which some persons have made of discoveries in physics and modern chemistry to increase and multiply the complaints against the air of cemeteries and against its effects on the neighbouring houses. Let those say so who have not the courage to bear it, that the spectacle of mortality should be removed from our sight, and that in our present life of feverish industrialism we have no time to spend over the dead, and let the speculator banish from Paris the fields of sepulture. But, at all events, let them cease to invoke science and hygiene, and to declare that cemeteries are really centres of infection, and that they are able to develope the germs of the most serious diseases. Let them cease frightening the ignorant public by mere phrases and sonorous words. It is very easy to declare and repeat everywhere that cemeteries are the source of dangerous emanations, but assertions are not proofs."

SYMPATHETIC PAIN OF THE FEET.—In a paper read at the Boston Society of Medical Improvement (*Boston Jour.*, No. 14), Dr. Curtis enumerated the various affections in which *pododynia* or *podalgia*, or painful affection of the feet, may exist independently of all signs of disease of the part itself. These are—1. *Urethral stricture*, as observed by Luxmoor, Brodie, and many others. 2. *Vesical calculus*: Pitha relates a remarkable case of a patient who was enabled by the diminution of a sense of burning of the sole of the foot to indicate precisely the progress of the diminution of the calculus by means of lithotrity. 3. *Cysto-prostatitis*, or inflammation of the neck of the bladder : In a case met with by Dr. Curtis, the pain in the neck of the bladder was constantly accompanied in corresponding degree with pain in the feet of a similar character. 4. *Cystalgia*, or neuralgia of the neck of the bladder. Pitha is himself a well-marked example of the co-existence of the two affections. 5. *Gout*: Under this head the observations of Paget, Duckworth, and Weir Mitchell are referred to. 6. *Renal calculus* occasionally gives rise to pain irradiated to the heel. 7. Fournier and others describe this pain as occasionally met with in *syphilis* and gonorrhœa. 8. In *locomotor ataxy* the heel may be the first or, for a while, the principal seat of the lancinating or boring pains characteristic of the first stages. 9. Prof. Gross describes an obscure form of pain in the feet, under the name *pododynia*, which is met with in certain sedentary classes of artisans, especially tailors.

INTERNATIONAL MEDICAL AND SANITARY EXHIBITION, 1881.

ELSEWHERE we have alluded to the opening of this Exhibition, the results of which may be of the greatest possible benefit to medical and sanitary science, but which may likewise, if due care be not taken, give rise to some degree of ill-feeling on the part of exhibitors. To-day we begin certain reports which we are desirous of making as full and as perfect as possible, and to that end would earnestly bespeak the help of those most deeply interested.

SECTIONS I. TO VI.
SURGICAL INSTRUMENTS AND APPLIANCES.

[*First Notice.*]

The exhibits in these sections, though none of them are very large, contain many novelties in the way of surgical instruments. If their practical utility is at all commensurate with the general excellence of their finish and ingenuity in their construction, they may be regarded as almost perfect. It is needless to say that the antiseptic apparatus is everywhere prominent ; sprays of all kinds and sizes are on every stall—testifying, doubtless, to the great demand which exists for them. The dental instruments, too, are multiplying in number at an extraordinary rate ; some of them are beautifully made, in spite of their smallness. There is, too, a number of dental engines, worked, for the most part, with a treadle, which are marvels of ingenuity. It is difficult to know where to begin first; we must therefore trust to chance, hoping to notice all that is noteworthy before the Exhibition closes. We shall also publish details, with woodcuts of some of the more novel and useful of these instruments, in future numbers, in our column of " New Inventions."

Messrs. J. WEISS and SON, Strand, W.—showed us some very complete cases of ophthalmic instruments. The firm are well known for the excellence of all their goods, and we need hardly say, therefore, that these cases were perfect in all their details. To attempt anything like an enumeration of their contents would be impossible, but we have little doubt that the surgeon who is provided with one of them might safely venture into the country, and feel quite prepared for all emergencies.

Their carbolic spray-producers in copper and brass are very beautiful instruments; those we saw are provided with a five-flame lamp, by means of which steam can be got up in a very short space of time. The fluid to be sprayed is contained in a metal stand, thus doing away with the necessity of a side bottle, such as is found on most of the spray instruments. Our only objection to this arrangement would be the fear lest this stand should not contain a sufficient supply for a long operation. The sprays are provided either with single or double steam-jets and have a water-gauge.

We saw a portable amputation case which will prove very serviceable. The blade of its long knife closes into the handle in an ingenious way, and the handle of the saw also shuts up. In this way the case is very small; it will be found convenient for country use.

Messrs. EVANS and WORMULL, Stamford-street, S.E.—exhibit, among other novelties, Mr. Spanton's corkscrew-like instruments for the radical cure of hernia. They are arranged in a neat little case, and consist of four sizes. A continuous-suture needle is also to be seen. It also resembles a corkscrew, except that the blade is flat and is provided with an orifice to carry a thread. Its mode of action is obvious ; it only remains to be seen whether it works as well in practice as in theory.

Here are to be seen some inexpensive dressing-basins of various shapes and sizes, designed by Surgeon-Major Fitzgerald, made of tin ; they are either triangular or square-shaped, and their sides curve inwards—thus they adapt themselves to any part of the body. Circular pans only touch the surface of the limb at one point and to a very limited extent, so that fluids run down into the bed and make all wet and uncomfortable. We can recommend these trays to the attention of all hospital managers.

Mr. P. BOURJEAURD, 49, Davies-street, Berkeley-square, V.—exhibits a variety of elastic spiral appliances, made on an especial plan of his own. Instead of a single piece of elastic webbing, of the same strength or thickness throughout, these appliances are made of narrow elastic bands sewn together at the edges in a spiral manner. Among the advantages claimed may be mentioned that elastic bands of different thicknesses are used, so that, although the whole limb, for instance, is covered with a uniform-looking stocking, the amount of support afforded varies considerably. The thickest and strongest elastic is inserted where the greatest amount of pressure is required. We cannot doubt that the method of making elastic apparatus which can localise pressure will prove very useful. They show also a novel truss, with regulating spring. First of all, a plaster-of-Paris cast is made, from which a mould is taken; the truss is then made to fit this mould very accurately. The advantages of such a mode of measuring and fitting trusses will be obvious, quite independently of any advantages which the truss itself confers.

They have invented a neat little respirator. It is made of tortleshell, fits inside the lips (and is therefore invisible), and it can be carried in the waistcoat pocket. For those whose occupation obliges them to run in and out of a hot room into the cold air, and this "Bijou Respirator" may prove useful.

Their riding belts also deserve attention.

Messrs. JAMES ALLEN and SONS, Marylebone-lane, W.—show their steam spray-producers. They are large, and well adapted for theatre use, and are, comparatively speaking, inexpensive. Made either of block tin or of copper, they are both sightly and strong, are provided with safety-valves, and will work for two or three hours without replenishing. Messrs. Allen have devised a stand, which rises to any required height, and rotates; this will be found very convenient for ward or theatre use. We also saw a small steam-spray for the throat; it will work for half or three-quarters of an hour, and might even be used for a short antiseptic dressing. For applying lotion to the eyes, in the form of a spray, it will be found useful.

Their appliances for the ward and sick-room are already well known to the public. Bronchitis-kettles, vapour-baths, invalids' and nursery baths, are to be seen. Their combination of hot-air or vapour or mercurial bath will be found very convenient. The ventilating croup-kettle is also worthy of notice. It is chiefly intended for diphtheria cases; it supplies air as well as steam into an enclosed bed, and if desired the steam can further be medicated. We consider this far superior to the ordinary bronchitis-kettles; for while steam alone makes the air heavy and depressing, moistened and warmed air proves highly beneficial in many forms of lung disease.

Messrs. BAILEY and SON, 16, Oxford-street, W.—show a collection of trusses, which deserve especial attention, both on account of their external finish and their practical utility. They are light, and yet strong enough for all purposes. When fitted, they are applied on the opposite side of the body to the hernia, and the pads cross over. In this way the pressure of the truss meets, so to speak, that of the hernia. They are reversible, and hence can be worn for either side. The pads are not fixed, and thus they accommodate themselves to the varying movements of the body. Their price is very moderate. The patent abdominal belts maintain their excellence. We have already expressed a favourable opinion of them, in which we are now even more confirmed. We saw some elastic stockings of a very fine material, which support the limb without producing that sense of heat so commonly complained of by wearers of elastic stockings.

Messrs. MAYER and MELTZER, Great Portland-street, W.—exhibit a variety of instruments, including some very fine and delicate forceps of different kinds, for removal of foreign bodies from the auditory meatus, nostrils, urethra, etc. The stem is bent at an angle, more convenient for use, and allowing the operator to see what he is about. The forceps itself has a crocodile mouth, is self-closing, and it is worked by means of a lever handle. They are neat little instruments, well adapted for the delicate work they have to perform.

We saw a self-feeding steam-spray apparatus—an arrangement which allows of steam being rapidly got up, and of being kept up indefinitely without any interruption. The instrument is of medium size, and is supposed to be more convenient for carrying than the larger-sized ones. If preferred, a simple arrangement converts it into an ordinary spray. It can, on the other hand, be as easily furnished with two steam nozzles as with one. Its price is moderate.

Mr. Mayer has been working at a new clinical thermometer; it is made of metal, and is about as large as a lady's watch, with a dial and hand as in a watch. It appeared very sensitive to changes of temperature, but we have not, of course, had any opportunity of testing it. The index can be fixed at any point by merely turning a handle, which, of course, ought to be done before the thermometer is removed from the axilla, etc. Its shape and size allow of its easy insertion in cavities, while, from its being made of metal, it cannot be broken by any accidental fall.

Their metal trusses, with a celluloid covered spring pad, struck us as excellent.

Messrs. DAVID MARR, Little Queen-street, W.C.—shows a small but select display of instruments, prominent among which we observed the especial instruments, sprays, surgical dressings, which are patronised—not to say invented—by the great master of "antiseptics," Professor Lister. The steam sprays struck us as solid, well-made instruments, without any needless refinements, either nickeled or bronzed, to suit the taste of the surgeon. Their prices are still too heavy, we think, considering the time such have been in use, and the numbers which have been made. All kinds of gauze, and catgut ligatures, carbolised silk, drainage-tubing, absolute phenol, lead buttons, and all the most recent additions to the antiseptic paraphernalia, will here be found, and may certainly be relied on as first-rate.

Messrs. J. F. MACFARLAN and Co., Edinburgh and London —The antiseptic appliances exhibited by this firm, and to which they have devoted great attention, include the well-known antiseptic gauze, carbolised jute, lint, tow, and wool, also catgut ligatures and silk sutures—in all of which carbolic acid is the active agent. Among other exhibits in this class are oiled silk protective, and pink jaconet, boric lint and wool, salicylic jute and wool, thymol gauze (which for some time has been used in antiseptic treatment), and also gauze (more recently introduced) prepared with eucalyptus oil.

Messrs. LLOYD, of Harborne, Birmingham—exhibit some useful appliances for the sick-room or nursery. Their combined bronchitis-kettle, food-warmer, and vapour-bath is a neat and well made apparatus; it fully answers the purposes for which it is intended. The lamp and the kettle are so adjusted as to their contents that the lamp will burn from three to five hours, during which time it will evaporate nearly the whole contents of the kettle. It requires very little attention.

SECTION XIII.

DOMESTIC AND HOSPITAL ARCHITECTURE.

PLANNING, CONSTRUCTION, DECORATIVE MATERIALS.

[First Notice.]

With a permanent Exhibition at the Parkes Museum, and an annual one at the Agricultural Hall, it could scarcely be expected that this at South Kensington should present many really new features. The stalls, too, being for the most part ranged along the walls of narrow corridors, are cramped for space, and do not permit of the same variety and disposition in the display of exhibits as was enjoyed at Islington. The total number of exhibitors is perhaps greater, but the ground covered is not quite coincident. Architectural design, water-supply, disinfecting apparatus, and other matters nearly absent from the Building Exhibition, are here fairly represented; but we miss the goodly show of bricks and tiles—hard, impervious, and artistic—on which we commented so favourably on that occasion.

The arrangement of the catalogue is open to criticism. While the stalls are numbered as a rule consecutively, and with some rough attempt at a division into sections—this division is carried out rigidly in the catalogue, the exhibitors' names being arranged alphabetically in each section. The probable place in such a classification of each exhibit has to be determined, and the name of the exhibitor, not the inventor or patentee, to be known, before it can be found in the catalogue. For instance, the name of Professor Barff will be looked for in vain; iron goods prepared by his process are exhibited by Mr. Maguire. But though shown in the same stall, pipes and corrugated sheet-iron are referred to different sections in the catalogue. Again, Dr. Scott's disinfecting chamber will be found in the Section XV., headed "Water-closets, Sinks, Baths, Sewage, and Drainage," and under the name of the exhibitor, Mr. Maguire.

Such errors will occur in any exhibition opened for the first time, but their existence must be our excuse if the order followed in our notice is not so methodical as might be desired.

Among the exhibits in Section XIII. of most practical interest are those intended for the covering and decoration of the interior walls of dwellings. We do hope that the time is fast coming when people generally will recognise that such should be washable, non-absorbent, and free from noxious pigments, as well as, if possible, durable and artistic.

Papers, distempers, and lead paints are alike objectionable, but in the Albissima, the Sanitary, and the Silicate paints, Duresco and Lincrusta, we have a complete solution of the problem, in materials suited to every description of dwelling, from the palace to the cottage. Between the merits of the three great rival paints, time alone can decide, but so far as we have been able to judge, we are certainly inclined to give the preference to the Silicates, which seem to possess a fuller body and covering power than the others; all, however, are free from the sickening and unwholesome odour of fresh lead paints, and dry with great rapidity. They are at least as cheap as common lead paints, if not cheaper, and the whites are entirely unaffected by the sulphur compounds given off from coals, drains, etc., and which so soon turn white lead paint to a dingy brown—especially in London. They are manufactured in all varieties of colour, but free from mercurial, arsenical, and other poisonous pigments, though fully rivalling vermilion, orpiment, etc., in brilliancy, and are sold in the dry, pasty, or fluid state, with the pigments separate or combined.

The ALBISSIMA (34, Lime-street, E.C.), consists, we believe, mainly of oxide of zinc.

The SANITARY PAINT COMPANY, of Liverpool, and 34, Leadenhall-street, E.C., use a sulphide of zinc and barium, gaining, as they believe, weight and body thereby. To this compound they give the name of Griffith's white; but their right so to do will soon be decided by the courts of law.

The SILICATE PAINT COMPANY, of Charlton, Kent, and 107, Cannon-street, E.C., employ an improvement on the original Griffith's white—the Charlton or Orr's white, consisting of a sulphide of zinc obtained by precipitation by an alkaline sulphide from solutions of sulphate, chloride, or nitrate of zinc. The alkaline sulphide used may be that of barium, but they now prefer strontium. After sundry processes of grinding, washing, and drying, it is combined with a soluble silicate, which gives it a cohesion and hardness above any other paint.

The Duresco is essentially the same, but mixed with a special thinning. It is admirably adapted for the walls of hospitals, churches, halls, staircases, and bedrooms—the silicate permeating the plaster, and converting it into a hard, non-absorbent surface. Some flock papers saturated with colourless Duresco acquire the appearance of a tinted plaster, from which the pattern stands out in bold relief. Duresco of a neutral ground may be beautifully stencilled or otherwise decorated when desired, as may be seen on the wall behind the stall occupied by the Company.

The distempers in ordinary use are, on sanitary grounds, delusive. They, like common plaster, absorb organic emanations from the breath, and, though repeated application of fresh coats may give an appearance of cleanliness, they do not remove or destroy what is already absorbed; besides, every drop of water leaves an unsightly stain.

Recent revelations have, as is well known, shown that arsenic is by no means confined to green papers. Arsenite of copper (Scheele's green) and emerald green are not the only pigments of this class—yellows, browns, and dull or neutral shades are frequently as highly arsenical,—but if we must have wall-papers there is no need to have them containing anything injurious to health. Messrs. W. WOOLLAMS and Co. exhibit a large variety of wall-papers of the richest hues

and most artistic designs, all of which are guaranteed to be free from any poisonous colouring.

Lincrusta is a production entirely *sui generis*, the conception of Mr. Fred. Walton, the inventor of linoleum, and composed, like it, of oxidised linseed oil and wood powder spread on canvas. Flexible, tough, and elastic, almost indestructible, a non-conductor of heat and impervious to moisture, uninjured by soap-and-water or weak acids, it is the perfection of a wall covering. Richly embossed with highly artistic designs, of delicate neutral tints or capable of being painted by block or hand, or of gilding, it is adapted alike for wide areas of walling, or for panels, dadoes, cornices, friezes, etc., in which various patterns may be combined, or it may be coloured so as to closely simulate wood-carving. Its prime cost must restrict its use to houses of the better class, but compared with the decorations which in such cases it will supersede, it is really inexpensive. Already it is extensively adopted at home and abroad, and certainly it has a magnificent future in prospect.

The exhibits in bricks are not so numerous as they were in the Building Exhibition held last April at the Agricultural Hall, to which we called attention at the time, but LANCHESTER's facing bricks deserve a passing notice. Messrs. STIFF and SONS exhibit a goodly collection of art stoneware and faience, as do also Messrs. DOULTON, FINCH, and others.

The EUREKA CONCRETE Co. show the method of laying pavements or floors with their speciality, which seems to be the best of its kind. It is simply mixed like Roman cement with water, when it speedily sets into a mass of extreme hardness, smooth and white. Pavements at 8d. per square foot are capable of withstanding the heaviest traffic, and floors at 6d. are fire and water proof. Sills, cornices, etc., sinks, chimney-pieces, and a variety of appliances usually made of stone, are also moulded of this material; and large drains, egg-shaped, such as are commonly built of brick, are exhibited in Eureka, each length being made of a few segments fitted with flanged joints longitudinally and transversely, which may be put together with a great saving of time and labour, forming a sewer perfectly water-tight, and presenting the smoothest possible surface.

Messrs. MAGUIRE exhibit corrugated iron roofing and iron pipes prepared by Professor Barff's process, which renders the iron incapable of oxidation, thereby superseding the use of paint. For water-mains these pipes seem admirably adapted, and they might be jointed with Spence's metal, like them, unaffected by water or moist air. This is a higher sulphide of iron obtained by fusing the ordinary sulphide with an excess of sulphur, forming a fusible metal melting at a temperature little above that of boiling water, and adhering alike to iron or stone. It is already adopted by the South Metropolitan Gas Company, and has the special merit in this case of requiring no caulking, as lead joints do. It may be used for fixing rails into stone, and for repairing lead or zinc roofs and gutters when corroded.

We regret to find so few visitors at the Exhibition, and are not surprised to hear of a good deal of discontent among the exhibitors in consequence. Whether it is the weather, or the charge for admission, or the want of activity on the part of the executive in not making the Exhibition more known, we cannot say; but the fact remains, the Exhibition is almost deserted. We hope, for the sake of the exhibitors, who, at considerable expense, have made great efforts to please as well as instruct expected visitors, that something will be done with a view to make the undertaking as successful from a commercial aspect as it will doubtless prove to the Committee of the Parkes Museum from their own point of view.

HYDROPHOBIA IN PRUSSIA.—In Berlin a tax on dogs has existed since 1829, and a law for compulsory muzzling since 1853. There were 318 dogs which died mad between 1846 and 1853, and 466 between 1853 and 1880 inclusive. Of deaths from hydrophobia there were 6 between 1846 and 1853, and 13 between 1853 and 1880 inclusive. In 1878 there were 19,487 dogs taxed in Berlin, 25,897 in 1875, and 37,000 in 1880. In the Prussian States there died 21 persons (18 males and 3 females) of hydrophobia in 1876; 13 (9 males and 4 females) in 1877; and 15 (13 males and 2 females) in 1878.—*Berlin. Klin. Woch.*, June 20.

ROYAL COLLEGE OF SURGEONS OF ENGLAND.

The following is the report from the Board and the Court of Examiners of the number of candidates who have presented themselves for the Primary and Pass Examinations for the diploma of Member of the College during the collegiate year 1880-81, showing the numbers of those who have passed and of those who have been rejected from each medical school during that period:—

Primary Examinations.

Medical School.	Totals.	Number passed.	Number rejected.
St. Bartholomew's .	135	80·50	54·50
University College .	101·6	52·83	48·83
Guy's . . .	97	67	30
King's College .	68	43·50	24·50
St. Thomas's . .	58·50	40	18·50
London . . .	46	37	9
Middlesex . .	35·50	21	14·50
Charing-cross .	34	24	10
St. George's . .	27	18	9
St. Mary's . .	23·3	10·83	12·50
Westminster . .	17·50	13	4·50
Manchester . .	54	25·50	28·50
Leeds . . .	29·83	14·50	15·3
Cambridge . .	22·83	17·50	5·3
Liverpool . .	22·50	16·50	6
Newcastle-on-Tyne.	21·50	10·50	11
Bristol . . .	17	14	3
Birmingham . .	16	12	4
Sheffield . . .	7	3	4
Dublin . . .	9	5	4
Belfast . . .	3·50	—	3·50
Edinburgh . .	52·83	34·83	18
Glasgow . . .	11·50	4·50	7
Aberdeen . .	7	6	1
Toronto . . .	4·50	2·50	2
McGill Col., Montreal	3	2	1
Halifax . . .	·50	·50	—
New York . .	2	1	1
Yale . . .	·50	—	·50
Harvard . . .	·3	·3	—
Bengal . . .	2	1·50	·50
Calcutta . . .	1	·50	·50
Bombay . . .	1	1	—
Melbourne . .	2·50	2·50	—
Leipzig . . .	1·50	1·50	—
Heidelberg . .	1	—	1
Berlin . . .	·3	·3	—
Paris . . .	1·50	1·50	—
Seville . . .	1	—	1
Vienna . . .	·3	·3	—
Bâle . . .	1	1	—
Totals . .	**942**	**588**	**354**

Pass Examinations.

Medical School.	Totals.	Number passed.	Number rejected.
St. Bartholomew's .	106·16	75·83	30·3
Guy's . . .	85	47·50	37·50
University College .	73·16	52	21·16
St. George's . .	41·50	26·50	15
London . . .	39·6	20	19·6
St. Thomas's . .	38·50	26	12·50
King's College .	30	13·50	16·50
St. Mary's . .	27·50	19·50	8
Middlesex . .	27·50	16·50	11
Charing-cross .	18·6	12	6·6
Westminster . .	17·50	9·50	8
Manchester . .	24·6	13·50	11·16
Birmingham . .	19	11	8
Leeds . . .	15	6	9
Cambridge . .	11	8	3
Liverpool . .	9·6	7·83	1·83
Newcastle-on-Tyne	8·3	4	4·3
Bristol . . .	5·50	3·50	2
Sheffield . . .	3·3	1·83	1·50
Dublin . . .	5	2	3
Galway . . .	1·50	1·50	—
Cork . . .	·50	·50	—
Edinburgh . .	17	12·50	4·50
Glasgow . . .	4·3	1·3	3
Aberdeen . .	1	1	—
Madras . . .	1	·50	·50
Toronto . . .	2·50	2·50	—
McGill Col., Montreal	2	1	1
New York . .	1·50	1·50	—
Ohio . . .	·50	·50	—
Harvard . . .	·3	·3	—
Colombia . .	·3	·3	—
Melbourne . .	3	1·50	1·50
Adelaide . . .	·50	·50	—
Hobart Town . .	·3	—	·3
Leipzig . . .	1	1	—
Berlin . . .	·83	·83	—
Vienna . . .	·3	·3	—
Bâle . . .	1	1	—
Paris . . .	1·83	·83	1
Malta . . .	1	—	1
Totals . .	**649**	**406**	**243**

Note.—In the above list, candidates who are indicated by a fraction have received their education at more than one school of medicine.

PROFESSOR DE CHAUMONT ON MODERN SANITARY APPLIANCES.

The anniversary meeting of the Sanitary Institute of Great Britain was held on July 14, when Professor De Chaumont, M.D., F.R.S., delivered an address on "Modern Sanitary Appliances," of which the following is a short summary.

Dr. De Chaumont said that we should be prepared to take up the subject on as strict a scientific footing as existing circumstances would allow, and to treat it in the same way as we treat astronomy and physics.

At present in sanitary matters we are working to a great extent, not perhaps actually in the dark, but by the light of somewhat indifferent illumination, resembling, in some instances, that darkness visible which gives weird outlines to objects that would be simple and ordinary enough in the broad light of day—outlines that impress the visual faculties of different observers so variously, that each is apt to draw his own conclusion, and treat with contumely that of his neighbour.

Every step that we can take in the direction of mathematical precision, by reducing to weights and measures all phenomena capable of such resolution, is a step in the true direction of scientific accuracy, and will lead to the advancement of the less certain sciences to a higher status.

It may now be legitimately asked what modern sanitary science really is, and how far it justifies the demand that we should regard it with favour. We may consider this question with reference to the following points:—

1. What are the objects of sanitary science? These are simple and obvious. It desires to preserve the lives and health of the community. It seeks to diminish the inordinate waste of life which is continually going on. Even now, one-half of the population, dying in childhood, is throughout its existence absolutely unproductive. The average age at death throughout the United Kingdom is only thirty-nine, of which barely one-half has been productive. Sanitary science further proposes that lives shall not only be preserved, but that they shall be preserved under the best possible circumstances, with health and strength to enable them not only to find means of supporting themselves and those dependent upon them, but also of adding to the wealth and productiveness of the community and nation at large.

2. How are those objects to be carried out, and how are those principles to be applied? Bearing in mind the principle of the redistribution of matter, we may say that this may be best carried out by seeing that the appropriate place be found for all kinds of matter, and that matter (particularly organic matter) be allowed to remain nowhere

where it is likely to expend its energy in the propagation of such low forms of life as are believed to be inimical to human economy. We must further try and scatter our town population more, by attempting to provide better dwellings, and by providing more open spaces so as to form lungs for the towns. The advantages of this last principle are very considerable, and have been dwelt upon by many writers. Another great work of sanitation is the improvement of the food of the people. To insure also that the food shall be good and wholesome, in a sound condition itself, and free from dangerous or deteriorating adulteration, is another branch of the subject of the utmost importance.

3. What has been achieved up to the present time? It has sometimes been said, that with all our boasted efforts sanitation has not done much to diminish the death-rate of the community. Is this true? Hardly, I think. The returns of the last Census have just shown two points—first, that the birth-rate is larger than was expected, and secondly, that the death-rate was smaller than was expected, during the last ten years.

4. What are our prospects for the future? I think we may say that they are, on the whole, encouraging. The great hold that sanitary matters have got upon the public attention is evinced in many ways—by the number of writings and discussions on the question; by the great impetus given to the production of sanitary apparatus and requirements, as shown by the success of sanitary exhibitions in various places, notably those in connexion with this Institute, and the great Exhibition about to open this week. There is one point on which we ought to insist, and that is, more extended means of instruction for all classes, and the exaction of certificates of competency from all who are officially charged with sanitary duties—medical officers of health, borough and district surveyors, and inspectors of nuisances.

FROM ABROAD.

OBSTETRICAL AUSCULTATION.

In a clinical lecture (reported in the *Revue Médicale*, No. 7) Prof. Depaul, after adverting to the history and progress of obstetrical auscultation, to which no one has contributed more than himself, proceeded to explain to his class how best to perform it. The woman should be laid on a bed on her back—for although she can be auscultated while standing, this is very inconvenient, and may give rise to serious mistakes. The abdomen should be exposed free from all garments, especially among common women, whose coarse clothing might give rise to difficulty in the perception of sounds. In private practice it may be possible to make an examination over a chemise of fine linen. The physician must place himself on her left and right side, so as to make the examination of both sides, alternately, the most complete silence being observed. The auscultation must be made by means of the stethoscope; and after having tried the various forms of this instrument, Prof. Depaul has finally adopted one of medium length, having its auricular surface slightly excavated and the edges of the opposite aperture sufficiently thick to prevent disagreeable or painful sensations being caused. The wall of the abdomen and that of the uterus must be somewhat depressed, but only moderately so, as any strong pressure would modify the sounds to be perceived, and especially the *souffle*. Some women refuse to allow of auscultation, but a little persuasion and explanation of the objects in view usually overcome their objections. There are others, again, who have the abdominal surface in a state of hyperæsthesia, the slightest touch, according to their account, causing pain. Moreover, in morbid conditions of the respiratory organs, the various pathological sounds produced may render the uterine auscultation difficult.

It is towards the third month and a half or the fourth month that auscultation is of service: and the sounds produced are of two kinds, those proceeding from the pregnancy itself, and those which are independent of it. Of the first, there are the uterine *bruit de souffle* and the double sound resulting from the contractions of the fœtal heart, the fœtal *souffle* dependent upon the circulation of the fœtus, and the uterine *souffle* dependent upon the maternal circulation. Finally,

there are sounds due to the active movements of the fœtus, as the *bruits de choc*, which may be both perceived by the hand and heard by the ear. We may also perceive by palpation, as well as by the ear, a friction sound (*bruit de frottement*). As to the sounds independent of pregnancy which are heard in women with child, it is of importance not to confound them. They may arise from the constriction of the muscles of the abdomen, or from the vesicular expansion of the lungs, which in some women extend from above downwards. So also the sounds produced by the beating of the heart of the mother may be transmitted to the cavity of the abdomen, and these are to be distinguished from those of the fœtus by their isochronism with the pulse. Finally, there are the pulsations of the aorta and the sounds due to the presence of gas in the digestive canal, especially in nervous and impressionable women.

The maternal *souffle* has been designated by various names, but Prof. Depaul prefers that of "uterine *souffle*," given it by Paul Dubois; and although it is not the most important of the sounds inherent to pregnancy, it is very desirable that it should be known. It is a *souffle* without pulsations isochronous with the maternal pulse. It is more or less strong and intermittent in the great majority of cases, having a certain interval between two successive *souffles*. It is sometimes musical or sibilant, analogous to the sound produced by a large bass string—at least, these are the typical sounds, of which, however, numerous shades exist, and which may be modified at intervals of a few instants in the same subject. There is no part of the uterus at which this may not be heard, but still there are generally three points of predilection—at the right and the left (sometimes both sides in the same woman), and at the fundus. This uterine maternal *souffle* may sometimes be absent on the first examination, for it is capricious, and not like the beatings of the heart, being constant, it may disappear and reappear occasionally. It is heard from the fourth or fifth month until the end of pregnancy. Nearly everybody is agreed in admitting that this sound is produced within the interior of the walls of the uterus, and that its mobility is due to the movements of the child, which compress this or that artery according to the position it occupies at the moment.

PHYSIOLOGY OF CLIMATE.

Dr. Rattray, of San Francisco, terminates as follows a series of papers on "The Physiology of Climate, Season, and Ordinary Weather-Changes" (*Phil. Med. Times*, No. 349):—

"To conclude, the following may be given as a summary of the most important of the preceding facts and inferences resulting from change of climate, season, or ordinary weather fluctuations, when the thermometric rise is from 42° to 83° F., or the reverse:—1. An increased spirometric capacity of the lungs to an average of 19¼ per cent., or 31 cubic inches, equivalent to a reduced vascularity by 17·88 fluid ounces. 2. A diminished respiratory function, as shown by a slower respiration to the extent of 8·9 per cent. These combined phenomena diminish the amount of air consumed daily by 36·85 cubic feet, or 18·43 per cent. of carbon excreted daily by the same percentage, or 1·843 oz., and of watery vapour excreted by the same percentage, or 4 fluid ounces nearly. 3. A diminished pulse by 2¼ beats per minute, and perhaps a reduction in its force also. 4. An increased body-temperature by from 1° to 2° F. 5. A diminished urinary secretion by 17½ per cent. 6. An increased perspiratory secretion to the extent of 22·38 per cent., and perhaps a correspondingly increased elimination of carbonic acid by the skin. 7. A diminished hepatic secretion to the extent of 0·15 per cent. 8. A diminished weight of the body in the majority, and a like impairment of the physique, often to the extent of 14 per cent., and average of 5 lbs. 9. Retarded growth in the majority of youths. 10. A correspondingly increased supply of blood or vascularity of some of the involved organs, and a similarly diminished turgescence of others, according as their function is increased or diminished. 11. Phenomena of an exactly reverse kind, and to a like extent, on making a change of temperature from hot to cold. 12. A corresponding fluctuation, both in vascularity and functions of corresponding organs, after each successive change of temperature. 13. The occurrence of similar phenomena as a result of change of *season*, and also of ordinary weather fluctuations. 14. The occurrence of like results, and from a like cause, from change of *altitude*.

15. The dependence of one and all of these phenomena on a definite cause, which may be termed the *climatic law* of the circulation, by which internal organs are congested at the expense of external ones under the influence of cold, and external ones congested at the expense of internal ones under heat. 16. The greater extent of these phenomena in adults and persons of large frame, and that for an obvious reason—the greater bulk of the blood. 17. The existence of a certain range in this redistribution of the blood and the resulting functional and morphological changes, which varies according to size, age, sex, and individual peculiarities, and beyond which they become pathological. 18. This physiological rise and fall, especially when great, as during zonal migrations, tends to increase both the ordinary and the vicarious action of the different involved organs. 19. The climatic law and its results affect the white and the black race, and therefore, presumably, every other race and variety of mankind, though each, doubtless, has its physiological differences. 20. They likewise manifest themselves in all latitudes and climates, in every change of season, and even during local variations in the weather. 21. In all cases, whether from climate, season, or weather-change, the primary and essential cause of these physiological phenomena is change of temperature. 22. As the aërial temperature is everywhere, and at all times, varying, so these physiological phenomena are not only of universal occurrence, but also in more or less constant progress in every individual over the entire face of the globe. 23. Temperature being their exciting cause, they necessarily vary with this in extent, and therefore may alter as greatly and much more speedily within the twenty-four hours than they do during a more slowly accomplished change of season or zone. 24. Their ultimate object in health is hygienic. 25. Seeing that they are as evident in morbid as in healthy states of the frame, they may thus act, according to circumstances, as therapeutic agents or the reverse."

RUPTURE OF THE BLADDER.

In a paper read at the German Medical Society of St. Petersburg (*St. Petersburg. Med. Woch.*, June 11), Dr. Assmuth stated that he had brought forward two cases of rupture of the bladder from muscular exertion in consequence of the rarity of the accident; for, although these two cases were admitted into the Obuchow Hospital in two successive years (1879 and 1880), yet Bartels, in his monograph on the subject, states that among 10,867 surgical cases, treated at the Bethanien in Berlin (1869-76), only three cases of rupture of the bladder occurred, and in 16,711 surgical cases at St. Bartholomew's only two cases occurred. Of the 169 cases collected by Bartels, not one arose from mere muscular exertion.

The subject of the *first* case was a man, thirty-two years old, who, while removing a heavy sack of flour from a railway platform to a cart, was seized with a violent pain in the hypogastrium. Trying some time after to make water, he only passed a few drops of blood. He came to the hospital on foot two days afterwards. His pulse was then 88, and his temperature 37·7° C. There was great tenderness in the hypogastrium, and a catheter only withdrew a few drops of blood. His general condition, and the apparent absence of any cause for it, prevented the diagnosis of a ruptured bladder, which the local symptoms would have justified. He soon, however, became much worse, and died on the sixth day after the accident, without having passed a drop of urine. The autopsy exhibited recent general peritonitis, and a rupture, two centimetres and one-third in length, at the upper part of the posterior wall of the bladder, a little to the right of its apex. The *second* case occurred in the person of a man forty years of age, who, two days prior to admission, had been seized with a violent pain in the hypogastrium while endeavouring to raise a very heavy burthen. He died on the sixth day after the accident. Peritonitis with purulent exudation was found, together with a rupture, three centimetres in length, at the right side of the posterior wall of the bladder, about two centimetres from the apex. The mucous membrane of the bladder was quite normal in appearance, and no trace of coagulum was found within the organ or in its vicinity. Of the urine, which during life had in both cases collected in the right hypogastrium, there was but little found after death, it having evidently become diffused by the intestinal movements. The local tenderness in that region became less concentrated in that spot; and after death a diffused peritonitis was found to be present.

In both these cases the muscular exertion required to raise a heavy burthen was obviously the cause of the rupture, and although hitherto no example of such an occurrence has been published, yet an analogous action in the production of fractures and dislocation is not rare. Although both patients denied that the urine had been long held in the bladder, there can be little doubt that considerable distension must have existed. In practice we frequently meet with very erroneous statements as to the fulness of the bladder, and that not only from defective self-observation, but also from impaired elasticity of the walls of the bladder, preventing a right judgment being formed as to its distension. In both cases the localisation of the rupture of the bladder was the same; and Dr. Assmuth deduces from Hyrtl's description of the anatomy of the bladder that this was at the feeblest part of the organ.

A CASE OF SEPTICÆMIA.

THE following interesting extract is from the pen of Dr. Alexander Jamieson, Shanghai(a):—

With Dr. Pichon's permission, I take his account of it from his recently issued Report on the Medical Branch of the French Municipal Service for the year 1880:—

"Mr. Charrier was called on January 3, 1880, to visit a cow standing in a shed on the French Concession, and which had reached the last stage of typhus. While he was examining its mouth the animal coughed violently, spattering his face with a fœtid discharge. A portion of this matter entered his mouth, and the stench which it emitted provoked during some ten minutes uncontrollable attempts at vomiting. Returning home, Mr. Charrier washed his mouth with brandy, hoping thus to escape danger. But it was too late—the poison had already entered his system. Next day sharp pain attacked his mouth and head, which soon became so severe that, attributing it to dental neuralgia, he had the two posterior upper molars on the right side extracted. Instead of obtaining relief from this operation, he found all the symptoms gaining in intensity, and at length on the 17th he sought my advice.

"By this time, fourteen days after inoculation, the disease had made considerable progress. The right cheek was much swollen, the saliva was thick and stringy, and the breath fœtid. As these symptoms are common to all forms of stomatitis, I might have attributed them to mere dental disturbance, were it not that the interior of the mouth revealed a condition of things of far from usual gravity. On the right side, the anterior pillar, the gums, and the outer border of the tongue where it came into contact with the teeth, were covered with scattered ulcers in various stages of development. Some presented a bright red border with a greyish-white centre. Over others a white exudation had spread, which entirely concealed them. Others, again, were completely gangrenous. In spite of all this, the glands were but little affected, and there were no general symptoms.

"I proceeded to cauterise the parts with a mixture of fuming hydrochloric acid and honey; but the application was only partial, as the swelling hardly permitted the patient to separate his jaws. I ordered chlorate of potash in large doses, and for local use 'coal-tar saponiné' with carbolised washes. In some days there was evident improvement: the spots reached by the acid became clean, and lost their greyish hue, and I was hoping that the lesions had been arrested in their progress, when they manifested themselves afresh, especially on the left side, and with greater intensity, as though they were the result of a new infection. Every symptom became aggravated, while the breath remained indescribably fœtid. Salivation was so abundant that the patient could not lie down, but was forced to remain in a sitting posture all night, lest the saliva should suffocate him. He complained of severe pain, which seemed to have its seat in the interior of the maxilla. The true gangrenous stage now set in. The greyish patches sloughed, and the sloughs separated very slowly, leaving behind stationary ulcers, which, instead of healing, developed a white false membrane so closely

(a) From the *Medical Reports of the Imperial Maritime Customs of China.*

adherent by its attached surface that it seemed to occupy the entire thickness of the mucous membrane. When destroyed by hydrochloric acid, it reappeared next day. In two months the disease advanced by successive outbursts, penetrating each time more deeply into the tissues. The areolar membrane of the walls of the mouth was next attacked. An indurated nodule would form in the substance of the cheek, would invade the mucous membrane, and, becoming attached to it, would impart a scirrhous hardness to it. For about three weeks no active pathological change would occur in these indurated regions, but then mortification seized the patches, and, advancing from within outwards, cast off day by day sphacelated pieces, producing a cadaveric odour and a putrid and bloody discharge. Under these infective conditions, fever soon lighted up, and those general symptoms were manifested which betray profound blood-change. The pulse was small, frequent, and irregular; the skin was dry, but the temperature was not excessive. From time to time there were attacks of profuse and fœtid diarrhœa. The patient's exhaustion was increased by nightly recurring attacks of facial neuralgia, which deprived him of sleep. So painful had become the muscular movements needed for speech that writing took the place of speaking, and the act of swallowing caused so much suffering that nourishment could only be administered in very small quantities.

"To combat this profoundly adynamic condition, I ordered wine and quinine under every imaginable form, while I gave carbolic acid internally, with a view to neutralise the evil effects of the decomposing fluids which reached the stomach.

"At length the advance of the mortification was arrested, and the ulcers healed; but the extensive loss of substance now produced grave trouble. The teeth were left bare, the periosteum was exposed at various points of the alveolar borders, while superficial necroses gave rise to suppuration, which maintained the mouth in an extremely fœtid condition. The folds of mucous membrane corresponding to the angles of the jaw were replaced by scar tissue, which fixed the lower jaw almost immovably, and every attempt to separate the jaws produced unbearable agony. Mr. Charrier left hospital early in April. The mouth-affection was cured, but his extreme weakness, and the smallness and frequency of his pulse, testified to the poisonous action exerted on his entire system by the absorption of putrid substances. For some weeks there was obvious improvement in the general condition: strength increased notwithstanding the difficulties which, in consequence of the anchylosis of the jaw, lay in the way of suitable nourishment. But the patient, who was not very obedient, soon deviated from his instructions, and anæmia reappeared, with all the train of symptoms indicative of hectic fever. He lived miserably for two months longer, and died on July 18.

"The following conclusions flow from the history just related:—

"The salivary secretion of a cow suffering from contagious typhus produced, by its direct action on the buccal mucous membrane of a human subject, a specific disease marked by a specially gangrenous tendency.

"This secretion therefore contained a virus endowed with the power of originating the pathological process described.

"The affection did not declare itself by ataxo-adynamic symptoms following quickly on the development of the local lesion—thus contrasting with malignant pustule.

"The patient was not killed by the malignancy of the local lesion, but by septic poisoning due to long-continued ingestion of hurtful substances.

"Were I to seek a place for this disease in the common classification of inflammatory affections of the mouth, I should couple it with diphtheritic stomatitis. With this it has a greater number of characters in common than with any other; but it is separated from it by its greater malignancy, inasmuch as it invades not only the entire thickness of the mucous membrane, but also the areolar tissue of the mouth-walls."

Dr. Pichon relates this case in connexion with an account of the epizootic among horned cattle, which, appearing in November, 1879, prevailed for several months in the settlements:—"In the reports submitted by Mr. Charrier, in his capacity of Inspector of Markets, the commencement of the epizootic was traced back to November 7, 1879. The first case that he had under observation was a heifer imported from France. The scourge spread ra idly through the sheds on the French Concession, whence it invaded the English

Settlement, proving disastrous at the 'farm,' where 122 head of cattle were lost within a few weeks."

I take the opportunity of enforcing the recommendations with regard to the boiling of milk which have often been offered in these Reports, by quoting the remarks with which Dr. Pichon closes his account of the epizootic of 1879.80:— "Most authors are silent as to the quality of the milk yielded by cattle during the prevalence of epizootics. It is possible that experience has not as yet supplied sufficient ground for its condemnation, and it is true that while a diminution of milk secretion is usually an early symptom in almost all diseases of the cow, complete suppression of that secretion accompanies any aggravation or prolongation of disease. The source of danger is thus removed by the operation of natural causes, and the discussion is narrowed to the question whether milk secreted at the very onset may not have acquired hurtful properties. In this state of uncertainty, which has not been cleared up by any authority on hygiene, the precaution of boiling the milk should be adopted. Boiling destroys any infective germs that it may contain."

REVIEWS.

A Manual and Atlas of Medical Ophthalmoscopy. By W. R. GOWERS, M.D., F.R.C.P., Assistant-Professor of Clinical Medicine in University College; Assistant-Physician to University College Hospital, and to the National Hospital for the Paralysed and Epileptic. J. and A. Churchill. 1879. Pp. 352.

WE owe an apology to Dr. Gowers and to our readers for not having noticed this valuable work much sooner.

As indicated in the title, the subject of the work has reference rather to the medical employment of ophthalmoscopy than to its special uses. The introduction consists of descriptions of methods to be used for ophthalmoscopic examination. The author reminds his readers that morbid appearances may be strictly ocular, or may be dependent on disease in other organs. He points out the necessity of distinguishing these, and gives a few descriptions of purely optical changes.

The body of the work itself is divided into two parts. In the first the author treats of "changes in the retinal vessels and optic nerve, of general medical significance." That is to say, he describes the various morbid appearances which are of importance, from a general medical point of view, giving full and clear descriptions of the ophthalmic appearances they present. He traces their history, gives their general causes, and enters very fully into their pathological phenomena. In fact, the morbid appearances to which this work has reference are in this part considered apart from their connexions with special disease.

The retinal vessels are first considered. These are very carefully described, and the reader is reminded of their insignificant size as compared with their apparent magnitude, when seen in direct ophthalmoscopic examination. Another point, the importance of which certainly would not strike a beginner, is here placed before us—it is that the red lines, which are commonly spoken of as the retinal arteries and veins, are in reality only the columns of blood in those vessels, and not the vessels themselves. As a rule, in the normal state the vessels are actually invisible.

It is in speaking of the increased size of the retinal veins due to distension that we first find a hint of a departure on the part of the author from the generally accepted doctrine as to the cause of this condition.

Von Graefe in 1866 attached great importance to constriction at the sclerotic ring as a cause of such distension. Clifford Allbutt, following him, attributed the condition he called "ischæmia of the disc," or "choked disc," to the same cause. Dr. Gowers, however, considers this condition of constriction at the sclerotic ring as unproven. He admits its *à priori* possibility, but asserts that he has never been able to discover evidence of such pressure, microscopically. The distended condition of the veins, in certain circumstances, he considers more probably due to their constriction in the papilla by the products of inflammatory action.

This explanation of the mechanism which gives rise to the appearances under discussion repeatedly recurs throughout this first part. Thus, under "Anæmia of the Retinal Vessels" (page 20), we find mention made of the undue narrowing of the arteries and distension of the veins; and we read, " This condition is constantly seen during the contraction of the inflammatory tissue in the papilla." Again, when treating of neuritis under the heading " Pathological Anatomy " (page 51), we find the following description of microscopical appearances in the papilla :—" The vessels do not usually present any evidence of compression at the sclerotic ring, but commonly appear to be narrowed, often considerably, in the thickest part of the swelling, and the veins are again enlarged as they pass down on the outer sides." When the relation of optic neuritis to encephalic disease is considered (page 63), we find the question still more fully discussed. The views of Von Graefe and Allbutt are given, and those of the authors who have opposed them, and there seems to be no doubt that the theory of constriction at the sclerotic ring will not hold as accounting for the condition of the vessels ; and it may be said, we think, that Dr. Gowers' view of the cause of this venous distension and other congestive signs has rightly been accepted.

We next come to the morbid conditions of the optic nerve, with descriptions of the symptoms which are shown to be indicative of their presence.

The author's views of the causes and the pathology of all of these conditions differ somewhat from those propounded by previous writers. For example, simple congestion is described as a morbid condition existing *per se*, and is compared to the condition described by Dr. Allbutt as chronic neuritis. It is supposed not to have any connexion with the inflammatory process, even when followed by atrophy of the nerve ; it is not to be regarded even as " the first stage of an actual neuritis."

As regards optic neuritis itself, the first variety is described as one of congestion with œdema ; he second and the third are distinctly inflammatory, and are termed " moderate " and " intense " papillitis.

In speaking of the relation of this complaint to encephalic mischief, the author says (page 67)—" The first point to be borne in mind is that optic neuritis, limited to, or at least most intense in, the optic papilla may occur without any obvious cranial or cerebral disease." This view is rather gaining ground, we think ; but it appears to us that the case given in illustration of this view does not quite bear it out. Reference to the case (29, page 289) will show that there was headache, intense and persistent ; strabismus ; and nearly constant sickness.

Dr. Gowers objects to the use of the old term " optic neuritis," and would adopt in its place the term " papillitis," as being pathologically accurate, while not assuming a knowledge which he thinks is not yet clear and definite. We can well sympathise with him in this ; but we confess that our experience leads us to doubt—except, possibly, when caused, as is suggested by the author, by hypermetropia or some other intraocular mischief—the possibility of the existence of this disease without intracranial causal accompaniments. Even in cases of renal disease the brain cannot be described as normal, as there would certainly be changes in the cerebral vessels.

With regard to the treatment of optic neuritis, Dr. Gowers very truly observes that this consists in the treatment of " the intracranial mischief, or general disease." Leeches and the like are of little or no use. It may be asked, Would this be the case if papillitis ever existed as a disease *per se ?* especially when we bear in mind the connexion between the orbital and frontal veins mentioned on pages 64 and 65.

The atrophic changes in the nerve are, as is usual with Dr. Gowers, most carefully and accurately described, and the first part of the work concludes with descriptions of the changes in the retina and choroid.

In the second part of this work the ophthalmoscopic appearances of general medical interest are viewed in the connexion with special diseases—that is to say, the various appearances belonging to the different complaints which present ophthalmic changes are here described, and not only so, but many diseases are mentioned in which the author has failed to find any ophthalmic changes, and thus valuable evidence of a negative character is adduced. To enumerate these diseases and their ophthalmic symptoms in a notice like the present would be impossible ; but a few extracts taken hap-hazard will show the accuracy and completeness with which this portion also of the work has been written.

Under " Lead-Poisoning " it is pointed out that " The eye is occasionally affected, apart from the effects of induced kidney-disease. The eye may be affected in three ways. There may be, first, amblyopia, usually transient, without ophthalmoscopic changes ; second, atrophy of the optic nerve ; third, " optic neuritis." Each of these conditions is fully described and explained, the causes and ophthalmic symptoms being carefully pointed out.

Under the heading of functional diseases of the nervous system, we find the ophthalmic appearances in nine distinct forms of disease. The appearances observable in " epilepsy " are very fully discussed, and are divided into those observed before and during the paroxysm. Throughout this part of the work, constant reference is made to the cases which are given in full further on, also to the plates. The concluding chapter relates to the ophthalmoscopic signs of death, and almost in the concluding words the author adduces powerful evidence in support of the assertion which we noticed at the commencement of the first part, viz., that the red lines which are observed on the fundus of the eye are in reality not the vessel themselves, but the columns of blood by them contained. In this concluding chapter we read as follows :—" After death . . . . the arteries quickly cease to be recognisable on the disc, appearing to commence at its edge. . . . The indistinctness of the arteries, which is due to their contraction emptying them of blood, quickly extends towards the periphery, and in the course of half an hour, sometimes in ten minutes, they are unrecognisable."

In the appendices we have some valuable hints on the use of the various ophthalmic instruments and other methods of diagnosis, and some eighty pages of cases bearing on the points treated of in the text. These are followed by the plates illustrative of the cases—some of which are chromolithographs, some autotypes, and some lithographs. The execution of these is excellent, and undoubtedly as true as is possible.

On the whole, the book is invaluable to all who really care to go into their cases thoroughly. It supplies very completely a long-felt want ; and we cannot too strongly recommend it to students and practitioners. It teaches how skill in the use of the ophthalmoscope is to be acquired, and shows what a grievous mistake men make who regard the employment of the ophthalmoscope as an aid to diagnosis as being of value to ophthalmologists only.

GENERAL CORRESPONDENCE.

HOW TO RENOVATE A SPECULUM.

LETTER FROM DR. R. NEALE.

[To the Editor of the Medical Times and Gazette.]

SIR,—In your journal, at page 25, you publish a plate and description of a speculum bearing Dr. Aveling's name. Any speculum that has become useless, owing to the varnish being worn away from the bevelled edge, may be converted into a useful instrument by cutting away the varnish for an inch from this edge, and running round a stream of collodion half an inch broad, one quarter of an inch being on the bared glass, and one quarter of an inch being on the remaining varnish. A damaged speculum so repaired has stood good service for more than a year, and accurately represents the form of instrument devised by Dr. Aveling.　　I am, &c.,　RICHARD NEALE, M.D. Lond.
60, Boundary-road, South Hampstead, N.W., July 20.

THE Library of the Obstetrical Society will be closed during the month of August.

COVERING NAUSEOUS MEDICINES.—Dr. Stillwell, after protesting (*Phil. Med. Times*, May 21) against the prevalent practice of prescribing very nauseous medicines in unnecessary bulk, supplies a formula for an elixir that he keeps prepared, half an ounce of which, added to a four-ounce mixture containing disagreeably tasting medicines (as bromide and iodide of potassium, bichloride of potassium or sodium, sulphate of quinine, etc.), covers a multitude of imperfections in a prescription as regards colour, taste, etc. —℞. Cort. aurant. rec. ℥j., sem. anisi contus. ℈j., sem. cardam. contus. ℥j., sem. fœniculi ℨij., cocci. cacti ℥j., saccharalb. ℥xxxvj., sp. vini rec. ℥iv., aquæ Oiss. ; macerate in the alcohol and water for four days, filter and dissolve the sugar by the aid of a gentle heat, and strain while warm.

MEDICAL NEWS.

ROYAL COLLEGE OF SURGEONS OF ENGLAND.—The following gentlemen having undergone the necessary examinations for the diploma, were admitted Members of the College at a meeting of the Court of Examiners on the 19th inst., viz. :—

Allan, Robert J., Scarborough.
Birt, Cecil, Stourbridge.
Blore, Isaac, Manchester.
Bush, James P., Clifton.
Dupuis, Thomas R., Kingston, Canada.
Hodgson, Robert H., Clapham.
Holdsworth, Arthur T., Birmingham.
Kirkpatrick, Roger, M.B. Edin., Edinburgh.
Meyers, Herbert R., L.R.C.P. Edin., East Dulwich.
Odling, Alfred E., L.S.A., Wendover.
Phillips, Henry W., M.B. Edin., Atherstone.
Robinson, Frederick G., Manchester.
Ward, Edward, B.A. Cantab., Horbury, York.

Thirteen candidates were rejected. The following gentlemen were admitted on the 21st inst., viz. :—

Austin, Henry H., Lee, S.E.
Bird, Ashley, Clifton, Bristol.
Brown, James W. H., Leeds.
Chappell, Walter T., Toronto.
Cook, Philip J., Brixton.
Crookshank, Edgar M., Belsize-park-terrace.
Deeble, William B. C., Southampton.
Ellison, John C., Brisbane, Queensland.
Gilbert, Harry P., Southwater, Sussex.
Kilham, Charles S., Sheffield.
Laimbur, Frederick J., Liverpool.
Orr, William Y., Elgin, N.B.
Robinson, William, Stanhope, Durham.
Rogerson, John T., Manchester.
Sewart, John H., Burton.
Stacey, Herbert G., Leeds.
Wallers, William, Manchester.

Ten candidates were rejected.

The following gentlemen passed their primary examination in Anatomy and Physiology at a meeting of the Board of Examiners on the 14th inst., and, when eligible, will be admitted to the pass examination, viz. :—

Auwyl, James N., student of St. Bartholomew's Hospital.
Bell, John, of University College Hospital.
David, Evan T., of the London Hospital.
Dodson, Arthur E., of the Charing Cross Hospital.
Ellis, William, of St. George's Hospital.
Finch, Richard T., B.A. Cantab., of St. George's Hospital.
Hawkins, G. Cæsar, of St. George's Hospital.
Lewis, David T., of Guy's Hospital.
Maling, W. Haygarth, of King's College Hospital.
Parker, Herbert, of St. Bartholomew's Hospital.
Spong, C. Stuart, of Guy's Hospital.
Tetley, Charles, of Guy's Hospital.
Tuckett, Walter R., of the London Hospital.
Turner, Frederic S., of University College Hospital.
Webb, Hugh, of St. George's Hospital.
Westbrook, R. Talbot, of Guy's Hospital.
Whish, Martin S., of University College Hospital.
Woodson, Arthur A., of University College Hospital.

Six candidates were rejected.

Collegiate Examinations.—It is stated that at the last primary examination for the diploma of membership of the Royal College of Surgeons, when 200 candidates presented themselves, no less than eighty-five out of that number, having failed to acquit themselves to the satisfaction of the Board of Examiners, were referred to their anatomical and physiological studies for three months, including fourteen who had an additional three months. At the corresponding period last year there were 157 candidates, of which number fifty-four were referred for three months, and eight for six months.

Collegiate Finances.—The following is an abstract of the receipts and expenditure at the Royal College of Surgeons in the year from Midsummer-day, 1880, to Midsummer-day, 1881, viz. :—The receipts amounted to £16,848 17s. 6d., derived principally from fees paid on examinations for the diplomas of the College, which amounted to £13,872 8s.; the receipts from investments in house property and dividends on stock amounted to £2553 9s. 5d.; the fees paid by Fellows of the College on admission to the Council and Court of Examiners, and of Members to the Fellowship, produced £158 10s.; trust funds yielded £246 14s. The expenditure for the same period amounted to £16,380 13s. The principal item under this head appears to be £6761 13s. in fees paid to Courts and Board of Examiners and members of the Council; followed by salaries and wages paid to the large staff of officers and servants of the College, amounting to £4076 1s. 2d.; taxes, rates, and diploma-stamps are re-

presented by £1395 14s. 2d. In the "extraordinary expenditure" there is £112 15s. 2d. for the Hunterian Festival and Oration, in addition to receipts from that fund. There appears the respectable balance at the bankers of £852 19s. 1d. Altogether, the report may be considered very satisfactory.

NAVAL, MILITARY, ETC., APPOINTMENTS.

ADMIRALTY.—Staff-Surgeon Martin Magill, M.D., has been promoted to the rank of Fleet-Surgeon in Her Majesty's Fleet, with seniority of June 23, 1881.

BIRTHS.

DAVIS.—On July 13, at Hythe, Kent, the wife of Arthur Randall Davis, M.R.C.S., of a son.
HILL.—On July 14, at 55, Wimpole-street, W., the wife of Berkeley Hill, F.R.C.S., of a daughter.
MILSOME.—On July 19, at Addlestone, Surrey, the wife of J. R. Milsome, M.D., of a son, stillborn.
MORISON.—On July 11, at La Motte House, Jersey, the wife of John Morison, M.D., of a son.
MYERS.—On July 17, at Instow, North Devon, the wife of Arthur B. R. Myers, Surgeon Coldstream Guards, of a daughter.
RAPER.—On July 12, at Great Wakering, Essex, the wife of W. A. Raper, M.D., of a son.
RENDALL.—On July 14, at Maiden Newton, Dorsetshire, the wife of William Rendall, M.R.C.S., of a son.
RIORDAN.—On July 8, at Ivy Bank Villa, Gravesend, the wife of Surgeon Major W. E. Riordan, A.M.D., of a son.

MARRIAGES.

BAKER—PUDDICOMBE.—On July 13, at Silverton, Devon, Walter Baker, Esq., youngest son of the late Emanuel Baker, M.D., of York-place, Portman-square, to Eugenia Morgan, only daughter of Edward M. Puddicombe, M.R.C.S., of Silverton.
GRIMWOOD—APPLEBY.—On July 13, at Rusholme, Manchester, Harry Charles Grimwood, M.R.C.S., of Pontefract, Yorkshire, to Harrietta, eldest daughter of Frederick Appleby, Esq., C.E., of Rusholme, Manchester.
HALL—SHEKLETON.—On July 14, at Stoke Bishop, Bristol, Edwin, youngest son of Robert Hall, Esq., J.P., of Linsdale, co. Cork, to Ada Georgina, eldest daughter of J. F. Shekleton, M.D., Deputy Surgeon-General, of Chelsfield, Stoke Bishop.
POLLOCK—LENY.—On July 12, at Hanover-square, the Rev. Edward Downing Pollock, curate of Stoke-on-Trent, son of James E. Pollock, M.D., of 54, Upper Brook-street, Grosvenor-square, to Patricia Charlotte Macalpine, youngest daughter of the late James Macalpine Leny, Esq., of Dalswinton, Dumfries.
RAMSBOTHAM—CHADWICK.—On July 14, at Broadwater, Tunbridge Wells, Edward Geoffrey Ramsbotham, Esq., to Octavia Lucy Newbould, daughter of Charles Chadwick, M.D., of Tunbridge Wells.
WESTALL—CAMERON.—On July 14, at St. Marylebone, London, Alfred Charles Westall, Esq., of Shanghai, to Alice, only daughter of G. F. Cameron, M.D., of 39, Devonshire-place, London.

DEATHS.

ASH, A. A., wife of John Ash, M.D., of Victoria, Vancouver's Island, at Great Malvern, Adelaide, on July 13, in her 44th year.
FLEMING, J. N., M.D., at South Lodge, Champion-hill, S.E., on July 13, aged 53.
RICHARDSON, F. H., M.D., formerly of Cheltenham, at Dunedin, Otago, N.E., on July 16, aged 74.

VACANCIES.

In the following list the nature of the office vacant, the qualifications required in the candidate, the person to whom application should be made and the day of election (as far as known) are stated in succession.

LAMBETH PARISH.—Medical Officer of Health. (*For particulars see Advertisement.*)
LEEK DISPENSARY.—Assistant Medical Officer and Dispenser. Candidates must be registered, and not over thirty-five years of age. Preference will be given to a L.A.C. Lond. Applications to be sent to Mr. W. Ball.
NATIONAL DENTAL HOSPITAL, 149, Great Portland-street, W.—Dental Surgeon and Lecturer on Dental Surgery and Pathology. Candidates must possess the L.D.S.R.C.S. Eng., and are requested to send in their applications, with testimonials, to Arthur G. Klugh, Secretary, on or before August 10.
NORTH STAFFORDSHIRE INFIRMARY.—Two Resident Medical Officers. (*For particulars see Advertisement.*)
QUEEN CHARLOTTE HOSPITAL, MARYLEBONE-ROAD, W.—Resident Medical Officer. (*For particulars see Advertisement.*)
QUEEN'S HOSPITAL, BIRMINGHAM.—Resident Surgeon. Applications and testimonials, with certificates of registration, to be sent under cover to the Secretary, at the Hospital, from whom all further information may be obtained, on or before August 2.
ROYAL HOSPITAL FOR DISEASES OF THE CHEST, CITY-ROAD.—House-Physician. Candidates must be registered under the Medical Act, and must not engage in private practice. The post is tenable for six months. Particulars as to the duties of the office may be had of C. Lowther Kemp, Secretary to the Council, to whom applications and copies of testimonials should be sent by July 28.
ST. MARYLEBONE GENERAL DISPENSARY, 77, WELBECK-STREET, CAVENDISH-SQUARE.—Dental Surgeon. Applications and testimonials must be forwarded, not later than August 1, to Frank Stokes, Secretary, and candidates must attend the Medical Committee at the Dispensary on August 3, at 4.30 p.m. precisely.

STOCKTON-UPON-TEES HOSPITAL AND DISPENSARY.—House-Surgeon (non-resident). Candidates must be doubly qualified. Applications, stating age, with recent testimonials, to be sent to the Secretary, John Settle, not later than August 9.

TRINITY COLLEGE, GLENALMOND.—Resident Medical Officer. For particulars apply to the Rev. the Warden.

UNION AND PAROCHIAL MEDICAL SERVICE.

. The area of each district is stated in acres. The population is computed according to the census of 1871.

RESIGNATIONS.

Berwick-on-Tweed Union.—Mr. Robert Carr Fluker has resigned the Berwick District: area 5790; population 9155; salary £45 per annum.

Boston Union.—The office of Medical Officer for the Sutterton District is vacant: area 11,310 acres; population 2688; salary £50.

Chipping Sodbury Union.—Mr. Edwin Day has resigned the Second District: area 8594 acres; population 4723; salary £54 per annum.

APPOINTMENTS.

Hemstead Union.—Robert James Mills, M.B. and M.C. Aber., M.R.C.S. Eng., and L.S.A. Lond., to the Second District.

Lewisham Union.—John Edward Buckland Burroughs, M.R.C.S. Eng. and L.S.A. Lond., to the Lee District.

Oswestry Union.—John Thomas Jones, L.R.C.P. and M.R.C.S. Edin., to the Llansilin District.

Stratford-on-Avon Union.—John Gairdner, M.R.C.S. Eng. and L.S.A., to the Welford and Alveston Districts and the Workhouse.

York Union.—William Preston, M.B. and M.C. Edin., to the First District.

ANALYST.

Huntingdon.—Mr. James West Knights, reappointed as Analyst for the County for one year. Remuneration by fees.

LEGAL LIABILITIES OF HOSPITALS.—The Rhode Island Hospital was sued by a paying patient to recover damages for a dangerous hemorrhage which he attributed to unskilful treatment by a surgical *interne*, who assumed to treat a wound beyond his skill, instead of sending for the attending surgeon as he should have done. The results were gangrene and amputation. The suit gave rise to a statement of the legal rules governing the responsibility of an incorporated hospital for its medical attendants. These two are declared:—1. A hospital is not exempt from liability for unskilfulness or neglect, but is responsible for the exercise of reasonable care by the governing authorities in selecting physicians, surgeons, and *internes*, and, if incompetent persons are appointed, is responsible for the results of their neglect or want of skill. 2. If the rules of the hospital require that in specified cases an *interne* shall summon an attending surgeon, and the *interne* fails to do so, the corporation may be liable for the consequences of his neglect.—*New York Med. Journal*, June.

DANGER OF COD-LIVER OIL FOR YOUNG INFANTS.—At a recent meeting of the Académie de Médecine, the Préfet de Police addressed to it a question whether it would deem it desirable to add to the elementary advice which it had issued for mothers in relation to their infants a note to the same effect as a conclusion of the Conseil d'Hygiène du Département de la Seine:—"The ingestion by young infants of different substances, and especially of cod-liver oil, may induce dangerous diarrhœa." In support of this proposal, Dr. Ricklin calls attention (*Gas. Méd.*, June 11) to the aid that may be derived from physiology in explaining many of the deaths of young infants, and in this case by showing the impropriety of administering any fatty substances at this early age. That rickets may be induced by animal diet is seen by the numerous experiments performed on puppies; and although milk contains casein which is perfectly absorbed, this exists in a diluted and assimilable form—existing almost as a peptonised albumen in the cells of the mammary gland. Fatty matters have, however, been added to milk under the erroneous idea of increasing its nutritive quality; but the juices required to emulsify this scarcely exist in the economy of the infant. The liver, which is large in the new-born infant, secretes very little bile; and at birth the pancreas is in a state of functional inertia, the pancreatic juice possessing at this age little or no emulsifying power. The aptitude for digesting fatty matters is then very feeble, and the non-emulsioned fat may give rise to great irritation and arrest the process of digestion.

As will be seen by our advertising columns, a Company has been formed for carrying out certain patents for purifying and proving yeast. Undoubtedly, if this become successful, it will be a great boon to the public. Brewers' yeast is not at all times pleasant in the rough state, and the dried (so-called German) yeast, though excellent, is terribly dear, and does not keep well.

VITAL STATISTICS OF LONDON.

Week ending Saturday, July 16, 1881.

BIRTHS.

Births of Boys, 1262; Girls, 1271; Total, 2533.
Corrected weekly average in the 10 years 1871-80, 2491·7.

DEATHS.

	Males.	Females.	Total.
Deaths during the week	979	837	1816
Weekly average of the ten years 1871-80, corrected to increased population ...	790·7	721·7	1512·4
Deaths of people aged 80 and upwards ...			42

DEATHS IN SUB-DISTRICTS FROM EPIDEMICS.

	Enumerated Population, 1881 (unrevised).	Small-pox.	Measles.	Scarlet Fever.	Diphtheria.	Whooping-cough.	Typhus.	Enteric (or Typhoid) Fever.	Simple continued Fever.	Diarrhœa.
West	669998	11	13	2	1	4	1	...	...	45
North	905677	20	22	24	1	11	...	5	1	53
Central ...	281758	...	9	1	3	5	...	...	...	25
East	692530	3	18	9	1	11	...	1	...	80
South	1285578	15	11	17	3	13	1	2	1	84
Total ...	3814571	49	73	53	7	44	2	8	2	292

METEOROLOGY.

From Observations at the Greenwich Observatory.

Mean height of barometer	29·977 in.
Mean temperature	70·1°
Highest point of thermometer	97·1°
Lowest point of thermometer	53·9°
Mean dew-point temperature	58·9°
General direction of wind	S.W.
Whole amount of rain in the week	0·04 in.

BIRTHS and DEATHS Registered and METEOROLOGY during the Week ending Saturday, July 16, in the following large Towns:—

Cities and boroughs (Municipal boundaries except for London.)	Estimated Population to middle of the year 1881.[*]	Persons to an Acre.	Births Registered during the week ending July 16.	Deaths Registered during the week ending July 16.	Temperature of Air (Fahr.) Highest during the Week.	Temperature of Air (Fahr.) Lowest during the Week.	Temperature of Air (Fahr.) Weekly Mean of Daily Values.	Temp. of Air (Cent.) Weekly Mean of Daily Mean Values.	Rain Fall. In Inches.	Rain Fall. In Centimetres.
London	3829751	50·8	2533	1816	97·1	52·9	70·1	21·17	0·04	0·10
Brighton	107984	45·9	48	35	81·0	53·7	64·5	18·06	0·00	0·00
Portsmouth ...	128335	28·6	83	52	...	...	...	...	...	...
Norwich	88038	11·5	48	31	92·2	58·0	65·6	20·34	0·04	0·10
Plymouth	75392	54·0	44	28	82·0	53·4	61·8	16·56	0·01	0·03
Bristol	207140	46·5	143	72	79·0	52·3	61·9	16·61	0·05	0·13
Wolverhampton ...	75934	22·4	48	24	82·3	50·7	63·0	17·22	0·00	0·00
Birmingham ...	402296	47·9	286	156	88·2	53·3	63·5	18·61	0·00	0·00
Leicester	123120	39·5	77	51	...	...	...	...	...	...
Nottingham ...	188035	18·9	146	73	89·7	51·9	64·6	18·12	0·08	0·08
Liverpool	553998	106·3	417	298	75·3	53·3	61·1	16·17	0·00	0·00
Manchester ...	341289	79·5	265	144	...	...	...	...	...	...
Salford	177760	34·4	140	59	...	...	...	...	...	...
Oldham	112176	24·0	79	45	...	...	...	...	...	...
Bradford	184037	25·5	126	52	81·0	54·0	63·5	17·50	0·01	0·03
Leeds	310490	14·4	215	150	84·0	55·0	65·7	18·72	0·10	0·25
Sheffield	285621	14·5	194	102	83·0	54·0	64·2	17·89	0·00	0·00
Hull	155161	42·7	111	63	84·0	52·0	64·3	17·95	0·00	0·00
Sunderland ...	116753	42·2	68	41	91·0	54·0	65·8	20·45	0·04	0·10
Newcastle-on-Tyne	145675	27·1	98	84	...	...	...	...	...	...
Total of 20 large English Towns ...	7608775	38·0	5149	3361	97·1	50·7	64·8	18·23	0·02	0·05

* These figures are the numbers enumerated (but subject to revision) in April last, raised to the middle of 1881 by the addition of a quarter of a year's increase, calculated at the rate that prevailed between 1871 and 1881.

At the Royal Observatory, Greenwich, the mean reading of the barometer last week was 29·98 in. The lowest reading was 29·84 in. at the beginning of the week and on Friday afternoon, and the highest 30·16 in. on Thursday morning.

NOTES, QUERIES, AND REPLIES.

He that questioneth much shall learn much.—*Bacon.*

Mr. J. Cornish.—If it is not a story, it is very like one.

J. T. Y.—During the time that the Contagious Diseases Acts have been in operation, their efficiency has been supported and impugned; but every trustworthy account of their operation has shown that they have markedly diminished the ravages of a cruel disease, and that, from a moral point of view, they have produced, undoubtedly, satisfactory results.

J. More N.—In the days of Henry VI., before even a College of Physicians existed, it was the duty of the Privy Council, when the princes were ill, to "make choice of some one to attend, out of the many pretenders to the science of physick" (Rot. 32., Hen. VI.: De Ministrando Medicinas).

A Member.—We understand that only those Fellows and Members of the Royal College of Surgeons who are members of the International Medical Congress will be admitted to the *conversazione* to be held on Monday, the 8th proximo.

Disused Burial-Grounds.—The St. Pancras Vestry has agreed to undertake the management of the present disused burial-grounds belonging to the parish of St. George, Bloomsbury, and St. George the Martyr, at the rear of the Foundling Hospital, so soon as the same are laid out as a public garden to the satisfaction of the Vestry, which the Kyrle Society, upon this undertaking, has consented to do.

Goats' Milk.—A show of goats was last week held at the Alexandra Palace, Muswell Hill, under the auspices of the British Goat Society. The goats were arranged in several classes, with a distinct reference to their value as milk-producing animals, and various prizes were distributed. The object of the Society in this exhibition is to encourage the keeping of milch-goats, the characteristics of a good milch-goat being, *mutatis mutandis*, the same as those of a good milch-cow.

Evading the Friendly Societies Act.—Several convictions have lately been obtained in London against friendly and sick benefit societies for default in returning valuations to the Registrar of Friendly Societies, as required by law. The valuation of a friendly society is taking stock of its engagements and of the means it has for meeting them. An important fact, often not sufficiently considered, is, that, taking any number of men or women together, it is beyond all doubt or question that the rate of sickness becomes greater with age, and death more frequent.

Syrus.—London, as included in the Census, is, we believe, a district extending along the Thames from Hammersmith to Woolwich, and across it from Hampstead to Norwood.

"Tidy Homes."—Any scheme which tends to promote a greater regard for domestic cleanliness and neatness in the homes of the poorer classes is worthy of public attention and support. At the Jews' Infant School-room, in the Commercial-road, Whitechapel, a few days since, Lady Goldsmid presented the prizes annually distributed in connexion with the "Tidy Homes Society." The Society awards premiums periodically to such of the parents of the children attending the school as have merited the reward by paying proper attention to the sanitation and general tidiness of the houses in which they dwell. The Society has been in existence for some eight years, and home associations have been largely promoted by its influence in the district of its exertions. The giving of these prizes has answered so well that it has become an annual ceremony. It is a system almost, we believe, confined to this school.

Pig-Fever: a Precaution.—In consequence of the prevalence of pig-fever in the neighbourhood of Bridgwater, the local authority has ordered the issue of a notice prohibiting the exposure and sale of pigs within the division until the 31st instant.

A Student.—Competitive examination was originally advocated on the assumption that it was equivalent to appointment by merit instead of by personal interest. A man who comes out at the head of an examination list shows that he possesses certain qualities of intellect; whereas a man appointed merely by interest or jobbery may be an idiot.

"Nips."—The American bar system has unfortunately, with all its various pernicious enticements, taken at length a somewhat firm hold in London. The habit of indulging in irregular "nips," "pick-me-ups," etc., is rapidly extending itself in our midst. The custom of drinking liquors of this kind at odd times as a mere "nip" is said to be greatly on the increase amongst our business men. It is most injurious to health, the forerunner of insobriety, and a habit to be deprecated from every point of view.

COMMUNICATIONS have been received from—

The Secretary of the Hospital for Sick Children, Brighton; Dr. Pearse, Plymouth; Mr. W. W. Cheyne, London; The Secretary of the British National Veterinary Congress, London; Mr. J. Chatto, London; The Secretary of the Sanitary Institute, London; The Secretary of the Dalrymple Home for Inebriates, London; Dr. E. F. Willoughby, London; Mr. J. B. Blackett, London; Mr. Cornish, Plymouth; Dr. Mansell-Moullin, London; The Sub-Librarian of the Obstetrical Society, London; Mr. George Brown, London; Messrs. Lloyd, London; Mr. T. Bird, London; Messrs. Low, Marston, and Co., London; The Registrar of the Royal College of Surgeons, London; Lieut.-Col. F. Bolton, Local Government Board, London; Mr. Bordian, Brussels; The Secretary of the Society for the Abolition of Compulsory Vaccination, London; The Correspondent of the "Liverpool Journal of Commerce," Paris; The Secretary of the International Medical and Sanitary Exhibition, London; Dr. Richard Neale, South Hampstead; The Secretary of the International Pharmaceutical Congress, London.

BOOKS, ETC., RECEIVED—

Homœopathic Remedies do not act Homœopathically—Importance of a Knowledge of the Diseases of the Ear, by Thomas Barr, M.D.—Report on the Health of Bolton, by Edward Sergeant—Justus von Liebig, by Prof. Dr. F. W. Beneke—The Morality of the Medical Profession, a Reply by W. B. Carpenter, C.B., M.D., F.R.S.—Belper Union Rural Sanitary Authority, Eighth Annual Report—The Classics for the Million, by Henry Grey—Report of Surgeon-General forwarding Returns for Half-year ended December 31, 1880—Ether Death, by John B. Roberts, M.D.—Beiträge zur Gerichtlichen Medicin, von Prof. Dr. Hermann Friedburg in Breslau—Die Augen der Medicin, Studirenden von Prof. Dr. Hermann Cohn in Breslau—Trade Marks—Gangrena Scroto-Peniena, da Eresipela Oscheoplastia, memoria del Dottor Mariano Menzalora—Materia Medica and Therapeutics of the Skin, by Henry G. Piffard, A.M., M.D.—Diseases of the Nervous System, by M. Rosenthal, vols. i., ii.—On Therapeutics, by A. Trousseau and H. Pidoux, vols. i., ii., iii.—Venereal Diseases, by E. L. Keyes, A.M., M.D.—Foreign Bodies in Surgical Practice, by Alfred Poulet, M.D., vols. i., ii.—Minor Surgical Gynecology, by Paul F. Mundé, M.D.—Diagnosis and Treatment of Ear Diseases, by Albert H. Buck, M.D.—The Harrogate Waters, by George Oliver, M.D.

PERIODICALS AND NEWSPAPERS RECEIVED—

Lancet—British Medical Journal—Medical Press and Circular—Berliner Klinische Wochenschrift—Centralblatt für Chirurgie—Gazette des Hopitaux—Gazette Médicale—Le Progrès Médical—Bulletin de l'Académie de Médecine—Pharmaceutical Journal—Wiener Medizinische Wochenschrift—Centralblatt für die Medizinischen Wissenschaften—Revue Médicale—Gazette Hebdomadaire—National Board of Health Bulletin, Washington—Nature—Deutsche Medicinal-Zeitung—Boston Medical and Surgical Journal—Practitioner—American Journal of Medical Sciences—Journal of the British Dental Association—Revue des Sciences Médicales—Revue de Chirurgie—Philadelphia Medical Times—Students' Journal and Hospital Gazette—The American—Canada Lancet—North Carolina Medical Journal—Revue d'Hygiène—St. Louis Courier of Medicine—Mornington Mirror—New York Medical Journal and Obstetrical Review—Uniao Medica—Occasional Notes—Charity Record—Louisville Medical News.

APPOINTMENTS FOR THE WEEK.

July 23. *Saturday (this day).*

Operations at St. Bartholomew's, 1½ p.m.; King's College, 1½ p.m.; Royal Free, 2 p.m.; Royal London Ophthalmic, 11 a.m.; Royal Westminster Ophthalmic, 1½ p.m.; St. Thomas's, 1½ p.m.; London, 2 p.m.

25. *Monday.*

Operations at the Metropolitan Free, 2 p.m.; St. Mark's Hospital for Diseases of the Rectum, 2 p.m.; Royal London Ophthalmic, 11 a.m.; Royal Westminster Ophthalmic, 1½ p.m.

26. *Tuesday.*

Operations at Guy's, 1½ p.m.; Westminster, 2 p.m.; Royal London Ophthalmic, 11 a.m.; Royal Westminster Ophthalmic, 1½ p.m.; West London, 3 p.m.

27. *Wednesday.*

Operations at University College, 2 p.m.; St. Mary's, 1¼ p.m.; Middlesex, 1 p.m.; London, 2 p.m.; St. Bartholomew's, 1½ p.m.; Great Northern, 2 p.m.; Samaritan, 2½ p.m.; King's College (by Mr. Lister), 2 p.m.; Royal London Ophthalmic, 11 a.m.; Royal Westminster Ophthalmic, 1½ p.m.; St. Thomas's, 1½ p.m.; St. Peter's Hospital for Stone, 2 p.m.; National Orthopædic, Great Portland-street, 10 a.m.

28. *Thursday.*

Operations at St. George's, 1 p.m.; Central London Ophthalmic, 1 p.m.; Royal Orthopædic, 2 p.m.; University College, 2 p.m.; Royal London Ophthalmic, 11 a.m.; Royal Westminster Ophthalmic, 1½ p.m.; Hospital for Diseases of the Throat, 2 p.m.; Hospital for Women, 2 p.m.; Charing-cross, 2 p.m.; London, 2 p.m.; North-West London, 2½ p.m.

29. *Friday.*

Operations at Central London Ophthalmic, 2 p.m.; Royal London Ophthalmic, 11 a.m.; South London Ophthalmic, 2 p.m.; Royal Westminster Ophthalmic, 1½ p.m.; St. George's (ophthalmic operations), 1¼ p.m.; Guy's, 1½ p.m.; St. Thomas's (ophthalmic operations), 2 p.m.

Dalrymple Home for Inebriates.—Dr. Norman Kerr has been appointed Hon. Secretary to the Committee of Management of the proposed Dalrymple Home for Inebriates in succession to the late Mr. S. S. Alford. A strong effort is being made to raise the necessary funds for the acquisition and equipment of a suitable house and grounds. It is hoped that many will testify their appreciation of the late Mr. Alford's devotion by liberally contributing to this undertaking, for which £5000 is needed. Donations may be sent to the Chairman, Dr. Alfred Carpenter, J.P., Duppas House, Croydon, Surrey; or to the Hon. Secretary, Dr. Norman Kerr, 42, Grove-road, Regent's-park, London, N.W.

ORIGINAL LECTURES.

———

ON SOME OF THE EFFECTS OF
THE CHRONIC IMPACTION OF GALL-STONES
IN THE BILE-PASSAGES,

AND ON THE "FIÈVRE INTERMITTENTE HÉPATIQUE"
OF CHARCOT.(a)

By WILLIAM OSLER, M.D., M.R.C.P. Lond.,

Professor of the Institutes of Medicine, McGill University, Montreal.

GENTLEMEN,—I propose to call your attention this morning to some of the effects of the impaction of gall-stones in the biliary passages. The specimen before you, obtained from an old woman who died this week of septicæmia (Case 5) after a fracture, illustrates the distension of the gall-bladder and ducts which follows the lodgment of calculi, and it has served to remind me of other cases which have come under my observation. I shall therefore occupy the hour with this subject, and shall, moreover, depart somewhat from my usual custom in this course, and speak of certain clinical features in these cases which have not received much notice at the hands of English writers.

I will first speak of the effects of impaction of a gall-stone in the cystic duct. This tube is narrower than the common duct, and its mucous membrane is not uniformly smooth, but presents numerous transverse and oblique folds, so that it is almost impossible to pass a probe up or down its course. These valvular folds (valvula Heisteri) often form definite pockets, and the entire arrangement is certainly not the most favourable for the easy passage of a calculus.

The following effects may result from the plugging of this duct:—1. Dilatation of the gall-bladder. 2. Inflammation of its coats—catarrhal, diphtheritic, suppurative, or phlegmonous. 3. Obliteration. 4. The formation of fistulæ with contiguous organs.

The dilatation may attain a very high grade, and the organ contain several pints of fluid. The following instance is remarkable, as the distended gall-bladder reached to the pelvis, and was diagnosed as an ovarian tumour:—

Case 1.—On March 23, 1877, I performed an autopsy on a patient of the late Dr. Bell, a woman aged fifty-eight. In August, 1876, she consulted Dr. Bell for pains in the back and loins. He made a vaginal examination, and determined the presence of a tumour, apparently connected with the right side of the uterus. She became jaundiced on December 25, and gradually began to get emaciated. The tumour was evident anteriorly, but it could not be traced to the costal border, a zone of resonance intervening. On March 3, when it was being examined in the lower part, it was suddenly felt to give way, as if something had ruptured. At the post-mortem the gall-bladder was found enormously distended, reaching to within two inches of the pubes. On the surface of the right broad ligament was a round space covered with fibrin and deeply hæmorrhagic. On the apex of the gall-bladder was an irregular surface corresponding in size to that on the broad ligament; it looked as if the tumour had been attached at this point, and had been dislodged at the examination on March 3. There was no uterine or ovarian disease. The gall-bladder contained a quantity of a turbid and bloody fluid, and a large, recent-looking clot of blood. On the posterior wall there was a large ulceration, the base of which was hæmorrhagic. Nine or ten gall-stones were found, one being lodged in the duct. An irregular mass of cancer occupied the neck of the gall-bladder, and several nodular masses were found scattered throughout the substance of the liver.

More commonly, the dilatation which results from the impaction of a gall-stone in the cystic duct is of very moderate dimensions, and may produce no symptoms during life, as in the following examples:—

(a) Delivered in the Demonstration Course on Morbid Anatomy, January 15, 1881.

Case 2.—M. G., aged thirty-five. Death from abscess in broad ligament. Liver fatty. Gall-bladder of average size, contained about twenty concretions, the size of small cherries, and an ounce of a turbid, viscid fluid. A gall-stone the size of a large pea was lodged in the upper part of the cystic duct. So far as could be ascertained, this woman had not suffered from any symptoms referable to biliary derangement.

Case 3.—J. B., aged thirty-eight, died of heart-disease twenty-two hours after admission to the hospital. Liver congested; nutmeg. Gall-bladder moderately distended; contained a clear, slightly viscid fluid, with thirty concretions of various sizes, one of which, as large as a cherry, plugged the mouth of the cystic duct.

Case 4.—J. S., woman, aged sixty-five, died of emphysema. No history of any biliary disorder. Liver small and soft. Gall-bladder projected two inches below the edge of the organ, and contained about two ounces and a half of a clear, slightly viscid fluid, with two gall-stones; one, the size of a walnut, lay free in the sac, the other, as big as a marble, was firmly wedged in the first part of the cystic duct. The mucous membrane of the bladder looked normal.

Case 5.—Mary G., aged seventy-five, died from septicæmia after a fracture. Was not jaundiced. No history of biliary colic. Liver not enlarged; soft and fatty. Common bile-duct dilated to the size of the little finger, and the enlargement extended to the branches in the liver. They contained bile. Mucous membrane looked normal. A small calculus was situated in the terminal portion of the duct, about 8 mm. from the papilla. The gall-bladder was moderately dilated, and contained an opalescent, viscid fluid and fifteen calculi, chiefly of small size. Two, the size of peas, were lodged in the fossæ of the cystic duct and completely obstructed its lumen.

A fortunate termination in a case of distended gall-bladder, which produced symptoms during life, is illustrated by the following, in which obliteration of the sac took place:—

Case 6.—E. B., aged forty, a large, powerfully-built man; patient of Dr. Finnie's. Death from pneumonia. Eight years before his final illness he had suffered with an abdominal tumour, situated in the right hypochondriac region, which caused uneasiness and pain, but no serious trouble. He was seen by a great many medical men, and very diverse opinions appear to have been given as to the nature of the tumour. It lasted for many months, and then gradually disappeared. He left instructions that his body should be examined, in order to find out the cause of the tumour which had given him so much anxiety. Liver of large size, but healthy. Common duct pervious. Cystic duct dilated at its distal end, occluded in its upper part. Gall-bladder was small and shrunken, and its coats tightly embraced two gall-stones, the size of large cherries. A membranous septum separated the stones, and the walls of the bladder were so closely adherent that it was difficult to strip them off from the rough surface of the calculi.

I have seen another instance in which this condition of the gall-bladder occurred, but I have no notes of the case.

Inflammation of the gall-bladder (cholecystitis) not infrequently follows obstruction of the duct. More or less catarrh is probably a constant sequence, but the severer affections are rare. Diphtheritic inflammation is met with, leading to ulceration and even perforation. Gangrene is mentioned as occasionally occurring in and about the ulcers. A remarkable instance of primary inflammation passing on to gangrene happened recently in the practice of Dr. Howard, and I had an opportunity of inspecting the body:—

Case 7.—J. C., aged forty-eight, an old soldier, temperate and healthy. Taken ill on Tuesday, October 12. Chief symptoms—vomiting, pain in abdomen (particularly on right side). On account of the obesity a satisfactory examination of the abdomen could not be made. Many of the symptoms were those of obstruction of the bowels. No previous history of gall-stones. At the autopsy, localised purulent peritonitis about anterior border of liver, and between it and the transverse colon. Gall-bladder moderately distended; walls tense, and of a dark livid aspect; when slit open, a dirty, brownish-red, ill-smelling fluid escaped, and six or eight light coloured gall-stones. A calculus was found in the orifice of the cystic duct. The mucous membrane was not ulcerated, but was dark, and the coats looked sphacelated, particularly towards the fundus. The common and hepatic ducts were free, and there were no other special morbid features.

Between a dilated and inflamed gall-bladder and contiguous parts adhesions may form and fistulous communications be established by ulceration. Thus it may happen that the dilated sac adheres to the abdominal wall, ulceration at the fundus occurs, and by suppuration the skin is perforated and an external fistula established. Murchison has noted over eighty-seven cases of this kind. It is not uncommon for a fistula to form with the duodenum, more rarely with the colon or stomach. The following cases illustrate these latter varieties:—

Case 8.—S. J., a man aged forty-six; death from a low pneumonia after a severe fracture. No history of biliary colic. Liver not enlarged; common and hepatic ducts normal. Gall-bladder was of small size; but the pylorus and first part of the duodenum were adherent to it. When opened, a small quantity of purulent fluid escaped, and two large calculi, the size of filberts, occupied the cavity. Two wide fistulæ led into the duodenum and stomach; that to the latter did not perforate the mucous membrane directly, but formed a small abscess beneath it, the orifice being about 2 cm. within the ring. The one to the duodenum was shorter, and would have permitted the passage of a pea.

Case 9.—E. S., aged forty-eight, a stout, well-nourished person; patient of Dr. Rodger, of Point St. Charles. Fifteen years before her fatal illness she had an attack of what was called inflammation of the liver; there was no jaundice. but ever since she had been troubled with dyspepsia, and more or less feeling of discomfort in the region of the stomach. Her last illness extended over about three months, and the chief symptoms were jaundice, epistaxis, and occasional melæna. Death took place by hæmorrhage from the stomach and bowels. Stomach, duodenum, and transverse colon were closely adherent to the under-surface of the liver near the gall-bladder. Immediately outside the pyloric ring, in the upper and back part of the duodenum, was a large orifice 3·5 × 1·5 cm. partially blocked with clots, and communicating with the gall-bladder and an irregular cavity at the hilus of the organ. The source of the hæmorrhage was found to be an ulceration of the right branch of the hepatic artery. The gall-bladder was much ulcerated and communicated freely with the duodenum and with the irregular cavity at the hilus. At its fundus there was a fistulous opening into the colon, 7 mm. in diameter. Whether this represented the perforation of a duodenal ulcer into the gall-bladder, or the orifice caused by the passage of a large gall-stone into the duodenum, it is impossible to say. The extensive ulceration of the gall-bladder and the fistulous communication with the colon rather favour the latter view.

The very large calculi, which are sometimes passed per rectum, and which may induce symptoms of obstruction, most probably ulcerate into the bowel, and do not pass the common duct.

We will turn now, gentlemen, to the consideration of some of the effects of impaction of gall-stones in the common duct. The usual site for the lodgment of the calculus is in the terminal portion of the duct, the pars intestinalis, as here the calibre is considerably narrower than elsewhere. You see in this specimen taken from Case 5, above mentioned, how small a stone may find difficulty in getting through. It is impossible to say exactly how large a concretion may pass. Von Schweppal(b) places the limit at about 1 cm. in diameter. It is important for you to bear in mind that a gall-stone may remain permanently lodged in the pars intestinalis, and yet not be impacted. In such instances it may still permit the passage of bile past it, or it may act as a ball-valve and only permit of the flow when the distension behind has reached a certain point. Dilatation of the bile passages is the constant effect of permanent obstruction. At first they contain bile, but subsequently, if the channel is not re-established, this may be absorbed, and a clear mucoid fluid take its place. In obstruction from the pressure of tumours, etc., the enlargement of the ducts and gall-bladder may be excessive, and even the finer branches in the substance of the organ become dilated into tortuous canals which can also be seen beneath the capsule.

Inflammation of the bile-ducts (cholangitis) not infrequently succeeds dilatation, and may go on to suppuration, as in the following instance:—

(b) "Ziemssen's Encyclopædia," art. "Bile Passages."

Case 10.—*Calculus at Orifice of Common Duct—Dilatation and Suppuration of Bile Passages and Gall-Bladder.*

Unfortunately I have no history of the case, but it occurred in an old man who had been ill for nearly a year with symptoms pointing to hepatic disorder.

When the duodenum was laid open a dark spot was noticed at the papilla biliaria, which proved to be a gall-stone as large as a marble, lodged just within the orifice. It was freely movable, and could readily be pushed away. Behind it the common duct was much dilated, measuring 4·5 cm. in circumference at the orifice of the cystic duct, and 5·5 cm. at the hilus. The contents were purulent and tinged with bile. The ducts throughout the liver were dilated, and several as large as goose-quills coursed beneath the capsule of the right lobe. They all contained pus, and the walls were thickened. The gall-bladder was greatly dilated, and had formed close adhesions with the anterior abdominal wall, the duodenum, and the colon. When slit open, nearly a pint of pus escaped, and two small calculi. The walls were extensively ulcerated, and the contiguous part of the liver was rough and suppurating.

I wish more particularly to direct your attention to some remarkable symptoms, which occur in patients the subject of chronic obstruction of the common duct, and which are described at length by Charcot in his "Leçons sur les Maladies du Foie et des Reins." Under the name "fièvre intermittente hépatique" he has given an account of attacks, resembling closely paroxysms of ague, characterised by severe rigors, fever, and sweating. He states that these must not be confounded with the rigors and fever which sometimes accompany an attack of hepatic colic.

The following cases, which have been lately under my care, illustrate this symptom in a most admirable manner:—

Case 11.—*Obstruction of the Common Bile-Duct by a Large Calculus for over Nine Months—Repeated Ague-like Paroxysms—Jaundice—Passage of Gall-Stone—Recovery.*

N. K., aged thirty, a dark-complexioned, slightly-built woman, was admitted to hospital, under Dr. Wright, on November 17, 1879. She had been subject to attacks of indigestion, but otherwise appears to have been healthy. About four years ago she had several attacks of severe cramp-like pains in the abdomen, but she had no more for over two years, until the middle of September, 1879, when they came on again after a wetting. She had vomiting at this time, and such severe pains that morphia had to be administered hypodermically. Two days after she became deeply jaundiced. The attacks of pain recurred, and the vomiting was very troublesome, but in about two weeks she was able to go to her home, where she remained until her admission to hospital. The jaundice had persisted, and the "painful spells," as she called them, came on at intervals. When admitted she was suffering with jaundice, dyspepsia, and general debility. She remained in hospital during the winter, and I found her in Ward 23 when I took charge in April; and many of you had an opportunity of seeing her during the early part of the summer session. During a residence of five months and a half in hospital the chief symptoms were (1) jaundice, varying greatly in intensity, sometimes almost disappearing, but only to recur again in a few days; (2) ague-like paroxysms, chills, fever, and sweating, accompanied with severe abdominal pain, coming on at intervals of from three to ten days; (3) great impairment of appetite, dyspepsia, and frequent vomiting, especially during and about the time of the paroxysms; (4) great tenderness, particularly at times, in the epigastrium, most marked near the right costal border.

The way in which these paroxysms came on was usually as follows:—After an interval of a week or ten days, during which time the jaundice would diminish, the bile almost or entirely disappear from the urine, the fæces become slightly bile-tinged, the appetite improve, and the patient sit up, she would have a chill, sometimes only a transitory feeling of cold, at others a severe rigor in which she would shake as in an ague-fit. This stage lasted a variable time, from fifteen minutes to four hours, depending on the severity of the attack, and was followed by heat of skin and general feeling of warmth, after which sweating came on. The entire paroxysm, when well marked, lasted several hours. The temperature, which was normal, or even subnormal, rose during the attacks, reaching from 102° to 104°, and subsided quickly, sometimes sinking to 97°. The fever rarely lasted for twenty-four hours.

On the evening of March 28 a severe paroxysm came on, and the temperature rose to 103°. She had a very bad night, and the thermometer indicated 104° at nine o'clock in the morning of the 29th. At 7 p.m. it was 97°, and she was feeling comparatively comfortable.

Among the concomitant symptoms of these attacks, vomiting and severe gastric pain were the most common. The pain usually gave indication of the onset, and resembled that of hepatic colic, being epigastric, radiating, and often complained of beneath the right shoulder-blade. It was scarcely the agonising pain of genuine biliary colic, but was often severe enough to require morphia. Before and after the attack the epigastrium was very tender, so much so that she even complained of the weight of the bed-clothes.

Vomiting was a marked feature throughout the course of the disease, usually accompanying the paroxysms, and also frequent enough in the intervals, particularly after taking food. Bowels were moved each day, sometimes two or three motions. Colour depended on the intensity of the jaundice. For a long time the motions were filtered in the hopes of finding gall-stones. Invariably, after an attack the jaundice deepened, and we could generally tell the next day by her appearance alone whether she had had a paroxysm. The urine became bile-tinged, often deeply, and the stools clay-coloured. This would last for a day or so, and then the urine would get clearer, the bile-pigments disappear, and the stools get a little colour. In the intervals the pain subsided, the nausea and vomiting were less troublesome, but the appetite was very poor; for days she could not take anything but a little biscuit and milk. She usually remained in bed, but during a longer interval than usual would sometimes get up. Itching of the skin was occasionally a prominent symptom.

On April 8 I examined her carefully, and the following condition was noted :—" Is jaundiced and moderately wasted. Nothing special to be noted on inspection of abdomen. On palpation, decided tenderness in epigastric region, most marked towards the right costal border ; no special fulness or sense of increased resistance in this part. Hepatic dulness in nipple line extends from upper border of sixth rib to within half an inch of the costal margin. To the left the dulness can be traced well into the hypochondriac region. Splenic dulness of two inches and a half. Nothing abnormal on examination of heart and lungs. Urine is bile-tinged, gives a play of colours with nitric acid ; specific gravity 1020. Numerous darkly granular bile-stained casts, some containing epithelial cells. Fæces clay-coloured, soft, a little offensive. Tongue is clean. Pulse 85 ; temperature normal.

About the end of April she left the hospital, and went to her home in St. John's, where she was attended by Dr. Robert Howard, who diagnosed gall-stones, and gave bicarbonate of potash. She had several paroxysms, and continued jaundiced. On June 3 she passed a large round gall-stone weighing sixty grains and measuring over 1 cm. in diameter. She improved very rapidly after this ; the jaundice disappeared, and she has recovered her usual health and strength.

Case 12.—Obstruction of the Common Duct lasting over Eighteen Months—Jaundice of Varying Intensity—Numerous Ague-like Paroxysms.

On November 9, 1880, I was asked to see Mrs. S., aged fifty-five, a well-nourished woman, wife of a florist, and accustomed to work in the greenhouse. I found her deeply jaundiced, and suffering with intolerable itching. She had always been a healthy woman, and had borne five children. Present illness began in July, 1879, and I am indebted to Dr. Simpson for the following particulars of the onset and development of the disease :—" On July 8 and 12, 1879, Mrs. S. consulted me at my house for a mild attack of jaundice, which she ascribed to having lately seen a disgusting object, emitting a most offensive odour, which had caused her to feel sick. When a young girl she had a similar attack from fright. On August 4 I was sent for to visit her. In the interval the jaundice had become less intense. I found her deeply jaundiced, and complaining of nausea, dull pains in the region of the liver, and general discomfort. She remained in this state until the morning of the 6th, when she was seized with an alarming chill and intense pain below the ribs on the right side, extending to the epigastrium and to the right shoulder. It was increased by pressure and

motion. The breathing was oppressed, and the anxiety of the patient most distressing. The chill in a couple of hours gave place to a high fever, which was followed by a copious sweating, that stained the sheets of a deep yellow colour. The liver was found to be slightly enlarged. The intense pain gradually abated, but the tenderness persisted for several days. All of the essential phenomena of jaundice were present. She remained under my care until January, and during this period she suffered every two or three weeks from a paroxysm, varying somewhat in intensity and duration, such as I have described, except that the acute pain became less and less on each occasion, until at last there was scarcely any ; but the chill, fever, and perspiration were invariably present, constituting, with an increase of the jaundice, the entire paroxysm. Itching of the skin was a most distressing symptom throughout, often preventing sleep and rendering life almost unendurable. The stools were repeatedly strained for days together, but no gall-stones were found. The slight enlargement of the liver disappeared."

I ascertained from her that during the early part of last year the attacks continued, but during the summer (under homœopathic treatment) the jaundice almost disappeared, and she had not a paroxysm for several weeks. Latterly they have recurred every week or ten days. On the occasion of my first visit, she was intensely jaundiced, and suffering from the most terrible itching of the skin which I have ever witnessed, and for this she specially sought relief. Finding that most of the usual remedies had been tried, I ordered a warm alkaline bath, which had a very beneficial effect. During the night she became quite incoherent, and greatly alarmed her friends, who of course blamed the bath. In the morning the itching had almost disappeared and she was rational, but complained of a deep throbbing pain in the heart. I examined her carefully, and made the following notes :—Body well nourished ; thick layer of panniculus on abdomen. She says, however, that she has lost flesh in the past year. Skin of a deep greenish-yellow tint. In examining the abdomen, the edge of the liver cannot be felt ; no tumour is evident below right costal border. She winces on firm pressure midway between navel and ensiform cartilage. Area of liver-dulness somewhat diminished ; no tenderness over it. Splenic dulness a little increased ; seven inches in vertical diameter. Heart and lungs normal. Tongue red, and indented with the teeth. Bowels regular ; stools clay-coloured and offensive. Urine very dark-coloured, and contains much bile-pigment. Pulse 80 ; temperature 98·4°. Appetite is poor and she can only take soft food. During the next three days she improved, and the itching disappeared, except from the palms of the hands and soles of the feet. These she stated had been most troublesome throughout the attack, and the pads of the palms, at the bases of the fingers, were swollen and tender. By the 15th she was feeling much better, and the jaundice had begun to disappear. About noon on the 16th she had a severe paroxysm, the chill lasting nearly two hours, and at 5 p.m. I found her sweating profusely and much prostrated. During the cold stage she had constant relays of hot flannels wrapped round her, and hot bottles applied to the feet. The shaking was sometimes violent enough to move the bed and cause the room to vibrate. There was no vomiting with the attack, nor any special abdominal pain. On examination of the hepatic region no change was noticed. The following day the jaundice had become intensified and the urine much darker. From this time until Christmas-day she had seven attacks of varying intensity, five of which followed each other on the Fridays, coming on at noon. The temperature in one of the paroxysms reached 104°. The itching had come on again, but for some time starch powder gave relief ; then it failed, and she returned to the use of cloths wrung out of hot brine, which had been found very serviceable. The "shake," on Friday, December 10, was very slight, and there was but little fever after it. The jaundice, which had been fading since the 3rd, did not become intensified, and on the 13th and 13th was less marked than at any time during my attendance. The urine was clear, and the fæces were of a brownish colour. On the 15th and 17th there were paroxysms, and on the 18th she was again deeply jaundiced. From this date she improved very much, and has not had a definite paroxysm since. The jaundice has almost gone, and she has been able to be up and to get about the house. The appetite, also, has improved, and she has gained strength. On two occasions she has had severe headache, accompanied with great bodily depression, lasting for an entire afternoon, and followed by copious sweating. The itching has been much less, but the palms of the hands have at times been very sore. A troublesome symptom has been profuse sweating about the waist, sufficient to saturate the clothes and necessitating the wearing and constant renewal of cloths. The urine has been clear, free from bile-pigments, and the fæces have been dark-coloured. I have examined the liver on several occasions, but have not found any alteration; the spot of tenderness in the right of the epigastrium persists.

The temperature throughout the illness has been from 96° to 98·2°, rising in the paroxysms as high as 104°.

The pulse has ranged from 60 to 90 per minute.

During last summer there was an interval of nearly six weeks during which she had no paroxysm and the jaundice disappeared.

The daily amount of urea was estimated for me by Dr. Henderson during a period of three weeks, but there did not appear to be any special diminution during the paroxysms. Acting on the suggestion of Dr. Kennedy, of Bath, Ontario, I gave her large doses of oil, in the hopes of inducing the passage of the calculus. She took three Florence flasks of it without any effect. Latterly she has been taking potassium bicarbonate and Bethesda water.

The similarity of the clinical histories of these two cases is very striking; the chronic jaundice, varying in intensity, and the febrile paroxysms are, with trifling deviations, the exact counterparts, and let us hope that the parallelism will be still further carried out by the passages of a gall-stone in the second case.

Considering how rich is the literature of gall-stones, I have been surprised to find very few references to this symptom. Occasionally in the reports of cases of chronic obstruction by English writers, shivering fits are mentioned. Thus, Budd,(c) in the history of a case of impaction of a large gall-stone in the common duct, which lasted many months, says: "Has lately had many fits of shivering, and sweats much at night. Never had ague, and the spleen is not enlarged." In the second edition of his work on the Liver, Dr. Murchison speaks briefly of periodic paroxysms of intermittent fever occurring in connexion with the lodgment of gall-stones in the ducts. The only full account which I know of is in Charcot's work. He has been able to collect twenty cases for analysis, and his conclusions, briefly put, are as follows:— 1. The paroxysm begins suddenly with a chill, often severe enough to shake the bed; the temperature rises to 102° or 105·8°, and profuse sweating succeeds. 2. The periods of apyrexia are clearly defined. The fever comes on with the regularity of a quotidian, tertian, or quartan ague; but to this rule there are many exceptions. 3. In one instance Reynaud determined that the amount of urea was diminished during the paroxysm, whereas in true intermittent fever it is increased. 4. The paroxysms usually come on in the evening, while in genuine ague they most frequently occur in the morning. 5. The hepatic fever is chronic, and may last two or three months, with intervals of eight, ten, or fifteen days between the paroxysms. As many as thirty-nine attacks have been known to occur. 6. A favourable termination is possible, as shown by a case of Henoch's; but a fatal issue is the rule. Death may take place suddenly, with symptoms like a pernicious malarial fever, or as a remittent fever with typhoid characters.

Dr. Charcot states that the condition of the bile passages which accompanies this fever is dilatation with inflammation of the mucous membrane, and the presence of pus or muco-pus. He suggest, in explanation, that a septic principle or pyrogenic material is developed by changes in the bile, and getting into the blood induces the chills and fever.

Though the cases which I have detailed to you conform in all essentials with Charcot's description, there are a few additional points of interest.

In both the course of the disease seems to have been, compared with other cases, greatly prolonged; nine months in the one, eighteen in the other.

The recurrence of the pyrexial attacks did not fellow any definite order like true ague, but came on irregularly at

(c) "On Diseases of the Liver," second American edition, page 219.

intervals of from two to sixteen days. In Case 2, the "shakes" recurred on Friday, at noon, for five weeks.

One very remarkable feature in these cases I do not see mentioned, and that is the deepening of the jaundice after the attacks. No symptom was more constant, as some of you doubtless remember, in Case 1. It was rarely necessary to ask whether there had been a paroxysm, the colour of the face was a sufficient index. In the case of Mrs. S. the jaundice intensified very rapidly, often within eight or ten hours after the onset of the chill.

The cause of these repeated paroxysms must be confessed to be very obscure. Charcot supposes, as I told you, that a septic principle is developed in the dilated bile passages. Murchison suggests that "they are due to the simple irritation of the stone, and are analogous to the febrile paroxysms resulting from the passage of a catheter along the urethra." Certainly, in Case 12, the deepening of the jaundice and the absence of bile in the stools after the paroxysm favour the idea that a calculus, permanently lodged in the common duct, had shifted its position and had become for a time more closely wedged.

ORIGINAL COMMUNICATIONS.

CASE OF PNEUMONIA.
By E. SYMES THOMPSON, M.D., F.R.C.P., Physician to Hospital for Consumption, etc., Brompton.

FRANK J. F., alias General Mite, aged sixteen, born in New York, of healthy, well-grown parents. At birth, October, 1864, he weighed two pounds. Began to walk at fifteen months, and to talk at two years. His height is twenty-six inches; weight nine pounds. His general health is good, but he has been subject to asthmatic attacks for some years. In America, two years ago, he had a dangerous attack of double pneumonia, and was closely watched by Drs. Willard Parker, Stempson, and Wyld. Eventually he rallied and recovered completely. Since his arrival in England his health has been good. He has been much confined to the house.

On June 6 and 8 it was noticed that he ailed somewhat, and his nights were disturbed by asthmatic attacks.

On Sunday, June 12, he went for a drive, had a long walk (more than a quarter of a mile) in the park, and was chilled when perspiring while driving home. He slept badly, and on the following day was weary and depressed.

The day after (14th), he was in the Hall as usual. In the night asthma recurred, necessitating an emetic (syrup of ipecacuanha, twenty drops).

June 15.—He was restless, thirsty, and complained of pain in the right side of the chest. I found him sitting up in bed, fully dressed in frock coat, etc., tongue white and dry, unduly red at tip and edges. His face was pinched and pale. Chest barrel-shaped, shoulders high. Expansion fair. Percussion-note hyper-resonant on the left, but dull on the right, the dulness being absolute posteriorly below the spine of the scapula. Here the breathing was bronchial, voice bronchophonic, and a thrill was communicated to the hand. No vesicular murmur was audible. The heart-sounds were loudly conducted. No crepitation could be detected. Cough hard and frequent; saffron-coloured tenacious expectoration was got rid of with some difficulty. The pulse was 156; temperature 101·2°; skin dry and pungent. There was no appetite, but considerable thirst; urine high-coloured, otherwise normal—ten ounces daily; bowels regular. I ordered liq. amm. acet. ℥xv., spt. chloroformis ℥v., spt. amm. aromatici ℥x., secundâ quâque horâ; and linseed poultices to be applied constantly to the right side. During the night there was not any recurrence of asthma, and he slept fairly.

16th.—I found him at 9.30 a.m. less oppressed in the breathing and more cheerful. Pulse 142; respirations 34; temperature 100 4°. Physical signs unaltered. At 6.30 p.m.: Pulse 134; temperature 99·8°. On coughing, a slight, fine, crackling crepitus was heard at the base, but the bronchial breathing and bronchophony and dulness were unaltered.

17th.—After a good night, the pulse fell to 128; temperature 99·2°; respiration quiet. Expectoration free, frothy, and less tenacious and rusty. Bronchial breathing at the base less marked. Crackling sounds ("crepitatio redux") everywhere, and some vesicular murmur audible even to the base. Dulness very marked, but less absolute and extensive. Appetite returning. Eats porridge and bread-and-milk.

18th.—Aspect more natural. Pulse 118; temperature 99·4°; respirations 22. Tongue clean. On percussion, dulness at extreme base only. Elsewhere percussion-note on both sides equal. No bronchial breathing or bronchophony. A few scattered crackles, with sibilant sounds, audible on coughing. Expansion on both sides equal. To return to natural diet and take four drops of dialysed iron solution twice daily.

19th.—Running about in full dress as light and airy as ever. Pulse 128; temperature 93·6°. No dulness, and only slight crepitant and sibilant sounds audible at right base.

He is now (July 13) as well as usual. His nights are occasionally interrupted by asthmatic attacks, and sibilant sounds are audible posteriorly. He is still pale, and the temperature in the afternoon usually rises to 99°. He is quite well in all other respects.

Remarks.—The rapidity and completeness with which the pneumonia was resolved in General Mite's case seems worthy of notice. The consolidation of the lower lobe was absolute on the third day; but before the end of the fourth day, signs of resolution set in, and, with the exception of a few loose crepitant râles, all signs of the attack had passed from the lung within seven days of the onset. It seemed natural to anticipate that, in so fragile and diminutive a subject, an attack of pneumonia would prove more serious and alarming than in a boy of normal dimensions; but the contrary appears to be the case, and notwithstanding the long-existing emphysema with tendency to asthmatic complication, the removal of the pneumonic products was unusually rapid and complete.

OPERATING WITH NITROUS OXIDE UNDER HIGH PRESSURE.

By MR. TOM BIRD,

Instructor in the Use of Anæsthetics at Guy's Hospital.

MANY months ago there appeared in the *Times* a short but very faulty account of the results obtained by M. Paul Bert, of Paris, from some experiments conducted by him with a mixture of nitrous oxide gas and air on animals, under increased atmospheric pressure. The British *Medical Record* afterwards briefly noticed the subject. This week Mr. Allinson, in the "correspondence" of a contemporary, writes of an "operating travelling-car"; and as I am given to understand a stationary theatre on a like principle is to be built in Paris for the express purpose of not only holding the patient, operators, and assistants, but also the students to the number of 200, a short outline of the principle and practice may be of interest to your readers, the more especially as the public are often better informed about nitrous oxide and its use in practice than the majority of the profession.

The warm blood of an animal dissolves its equal volume of pure nitrous oxide gas under the ordinary variable pressure of the atmosphere in which we live.

To completely anæsthetise with nitrous oxide gas, it should be given perfectly pure, without admixture of air.(a) When the patient is anæsthetised with pure gas, it is possible, as my experience extending over four or five years tends to show, by introducing a small percentage of air, well mixed, to maintain the anæsthesia even through such an operation as ovariotomy.

It occurred to M. Paul Bert, that if the necessary amount of gas could be introduced into the blood, mixed with oxygen sufficient to preserve the normal conditions of respiration, anæsthesia could be safely maintained for a longer time than usual. This he first tried by increasing the pressure of the surrounding atmosphere as much again, so that, for example, he would have "a mixture of 50 for 100 of nitrous oxide, and 50 for 100 of air in the blood." The theory was completely justified by experiment: animals subjected to a

pressure of a fifth atmosphere, and made to respire a mixture of five-sixths of nitrous oxide and one-sixth of oxygen, fell into a profound anæsthesia, which was maintained for some time without any of the symptoms of asphyxia; on being withdrawn, their sensibility was immediately restored, without any unpleasant after-effects. M. Peau has demonstrated most unmistakably the feasibility, both in public and private hospitals, of this form of anæsthesia.

At the aëropathic establishment of Dr. Fontaine, assisted by M. Paul Bert, MM. Séquard, Lutaud, Brochin, Barraux, Nitot, and Boucheron, a carcinoma of the mammary gland was operated on. Under a pressure of 17 to 19 centimetres, the patient breathed from a bag containing 200 litres of a mixture of "gas" 85·2, oxygen 14·8, prepared by M. Limousin. The operation lasted fourteen minutes, and the patient breathed 150 litres.

Any adequate description of the theatres in which the operations have been conducted would take too much of your space; besides, they are being improved in detail from time to time.(b)

M. Paul Bert has noticed that the pulse and breathing both increase in frequency at the commencement of the inhalation. This occurs always on inhaling pure gas, to nearly all patients about to undergo an operation, and certainly to all persons on their first introduction to an extra pressure of atmosphere.

Practically, it has been noticed that should the mixture fail to keep the patient at rest, this object is almost immediately brought about by increasing the atmospheric pressure; the mixture being continued in the same way.

To sum up, the advantages claimed are—1. The absence of any period of excitement on commencing the inhalation. 2. The confidence given to the surgeon in the maintenance of the same degree of anæsthesia throughout. 3. The rapid return of consciousness. 4. The absence of vomiting. 5. Its complete harmlessness. With regard to these, the first and second are of no relative importance; the third is not always required; the fourth is a good and substantial reason—the case of ovariotomy which I had, had not an abnormal symptom, no depression, no sickness, no acute sensibility after the operation; the fifth is too sanguine at this period of its history.

38, Brook-street, W.

MIDLAND MEDICAL SOCIETY.—The inaugural address for the session 1881-82 of the Midland Medical Society will be delivered by Dr. Clifford Allbutt.

I HAVE now had frequent opportunities of observing that foreign residents in localities where so-called malarious influences exist may ward off their deleterious effects for a considerable period, even for years, but may suddenly, although living apparently under precisely similar circumstances, be seized with an attack of ague or remittent fever, and with no further cause that one can discover than perhaps a slight chill or a very brief exposure to the sun, such as would usually be passed by without a thought; and in some cases absolutely nothing out of the ordinary routine of daily life can be called to mind by the patient to account for the attack. My experience has further shown me that when once a patient has suffered severely from remittent or intermittent fever, it requires, as a rule, but a slight cause, such as getting wet or being exposed to the sun for but a short period, to start the blood poison fermenting, if I may so express it, and produce another attack. One or two instances of continued fever lasting for two or three weeks, with a high temperature, sometimes up to 103° or 104° Fahr., with no skin eruption, and apparently unaffected by medication, certainly not improved by quinine, have been under treatment. In these cases long exposure to the heat of the day seems to have an exciting cause. All such cases as the foregoing are generally put down to the influence of malaria, from which it seems to me that our knowledge of the pathology of malarious disorders is at present somewhat imperfect; and much good work might, I think, be done in this direction by careful records of all such cases in different localities; with notes of habits of life and age of patients, condition of dwellings, influence of treatment, etc.—*Dr. B. S. Ringer, in the "Medical Reports of the Imperial Maritime Customs of China."*

(a) I have just heard from Dr. Sternfeld, of Munich, that Professor Nüssbaum, of Munich, has had two deaths from nitrous oxide in 260 cases, and that he does not intend to use it again: but the alleged reason of the fatality ought not to occur in England, where we can get the gas as pure as we like.

(b) *Union Médicale,* September 18, 1879.

REPORTS OF HOSPITAL PRACTICE
IN
MEDICINE AND SURGERY.

ST. THOMAS'S HOSPITAL.

A SERIES OF CASES OF MAMMARY CANCER, WITH REMARKS ON TREATMENT AFTER OPERATION.

(Under the care of Mr. JOHN CROFT.)

(Concluded from page 92.)

Case 10 (Dresser, Mr. Butler).—Elizabeth O., aged sixty-five, married. There is no family history of tumours. A small lump began to form, apparently in the skin, three years ago, which has grown gradually, and has been painful during the past three months. The pain is of a shooting character.

On admission, the position of the left nipple is indicated by a deep depression, the skin being drawn upwards and inwards towards a hard lump in the breast. Two inches from the nipple inwards there is a hard circular discoloured patch. The tumour occupies the upper and inner part of the gland, and is very hard superficially, and apparently adherent by bands below. It has limited movement with the breast, with which it is continuous. The axillary glands are not enlarged. The right breast is larger than the left (diseased) one; the nipple is very flat, but there is apparently no disease.

Admitted January 12; operated January 24, 1881. The breast was removed under ether. The tumour was a typical scirrhus. Full Listerian precautions and dressings were adopted.

January 26.—Dressed; doing well. No rise of temperature. The wound rapidly healed, without any pus. Three dressings only were required.

February 14, 1881.—Discharged.

Case 11 (Dresser, Mr. Alpin).—Sarah M. F., aged sixty-one, married. Her mother was delicate, and died in childbirth. She had three sisters, two of whom died of phthisis. No member of her family has ever suffered from any breast affection. She first noticed this tumour about one month ago, retraction of the nipple having drawn her attention to it. It has grown very slowly. Some months ago she received a blow on the breast. The tumour is now as large as an orange, hard and circumscribed; it moves freely with the general mass of the breast. The skin over it is adherent, and the nipple is retracted. The axillary glands are not enlarged.

March 17.—The breast was removed under ether and chloroform. The carbolic spray and Lister's dressings were used. The new growth was not collected into one mass, but was scattered amongst the breast-tissue, chiefly between the nipple and axilla. All the arteries were twisted.

18th.—Dressed. There was a good deal of oozing.

19th.—Dressed again.

24th.—Dressed. The discharge is quite sweet; wound healthy, no irritation about the edges. Some of the sutures were removed, and the drainage-tube was shortened.

April 2.—All the dressings were discontinued. The temperature was normal throughout.

9th.—Discharged, well.

Case 12 (Dresser, Mr. Butler).—Caroline H., aged fifty, married twenty-three years. Has had six children, one of which has died. After one of her confinements she suffered from acute abscesses in each breast. The tumour was only noticed fourteen days ago.

On admission, a circumscribed tumour, hard and lobulated, two inches by three inches, was felt in the right breast. Skin over it slightly adherent; no tenderness except after handling. Axillary glands rather hard and enlarged; the nipple was retracted. Admitted into hospital, March 21; operated, March 28, 1881, under ether. The axillary glands were removed, together with the breast, under full Listerian precautions.

March 30.—Doing well. Temperature 98·6°; pulse 96.

April 2.—One-half of the drainage-tube was removed. Temperature normal.

8th.—Tube removed, as also the sutures. Healing complete.

16th.—Discharged from the hospital.

Remarks.—The cases which we have recorded in this and the two preceding numbers have been selected from among a series of forty, as showing pretty accurately what has been accomplished within the last few years by the gradual introduction of "antiseptic surgery," and the perfecting of the details of its application in actual practice. In the early cases there were an almost constant rise in the temperature, more or less suppuration, and a prolonged stay in the hospital; while during the early Listerian period suppuration was less frequent, yet primary union could not be absolutely relied on. The three last cases, however, representing typical "Listerism," all healed by primary union, without fever, rise of temperature, or suppuration. Three or four dressings only were required. The patients were up about the tenth day, and were able to be discharged from the hospital within a further few days. Experience alone can teach us whether this rapid closing of the wound without any suppuration is desirable in the interest of the patient. For it can hardly be doubted that suppuration, from its very nature, must have removed a considerable amount of the tissue which immediately surrounded the tumour; and it may therefore have removed any possible epithelial infiltration (from which recurrence takes place) from the nearest lymphatic structures, which, under the new method of healing, will necessarily be inclosed and shut up in the wound.

TERMS OF SUBSCRIPTION.
(Free by post.)

British Islands		*Twelve Months*	£1	8	0
,,		*Six* ,,	0	14	0
The Colonies and the United States of America	}	*Twelve* ,,	1	10	0
,, ,, ,,		*Six* ,,	0	15	0
India		*Twelve* ,,	1	10	0
,, (*viâ Brindisi*)		,,	1	15	0
,,		*Six* ,,	0	15	0
,, (*viâ Brindisi*)		,,	0	17	6

Foreign Subscribers are requested to inform the Publishers of any remittance made through the agency of the Post-office.

Single Copies of the Journal can be obtained of all Booksellers and Newsmen, price Sixpence.

Cheques or Post-office Orders should be made payable to Mr JAMES LUCAS, 11, *New Burlington-street, W.*

TERMS FOR ADVERTISEMENTS.

Seven lines (70 words)	£0	4	6
Each additional line (10 words)	0	0	6
Half-column, or quarter-page	1	5	0
Whole column, or half-page	2	10	0
Whole page	5	0	0

Births, Marriages, and Deaths are inserted Free of Charge.

THE MEDICAL TIMES AND GAZETTE *is published on Friday morning: Advertisements must therefore reach the Publishing Office not later than One o'clock on Thursday.*

Medical Times and Gazette.

SATURDAY, JULY 30, 1881.

THE SANITARY CONDITION OF THE ISLE OF WIGHT.

AT the commencement of the present year, a Report, by Dr. Ballard, one of the Medical Inspectors of the Local Government Board, on the Sanitary Condition of the Isle of Wight, was published, and excited no little stir and consternation among the medical officers and the inhabitants of the Island; and, indeed, not a little alarmed the general public. But we are happy to say that the Report has already produced very good results in at least one of the most popular of the Isle of Wight health-resorts, viz., in Ventnor; and it may be expected that still wider spread benefit will follow in the improvement of the sanitary condition of that favoured island in general. We are glad to learn from the Report of the Sanitary Committee of the Ventnor Local Board, the sanitary condition of which town appeared in a far from favourable light, even when compared with some other towns and districts in the Island, that the Board has taken active means to remove the very unfavourable impression left after the perusal of Dr. Ballard's Report. The Board had the advantage of a long conference with Dr. Ballard, and the result has been that sanitary work has since been carried out with increased vigilance and understanding; and many marked improvements have been made. In the Report it was most clearly shown how very insufficiently the sewers were ventilated; and the Local Board has carefully carried out Dr. Ballard's instructions on this important subject. The public may now feel certain that there is ample ventilation to prevent any undue pressure of sewage-gas on the traps of the house-drains, as the full number of ventilators recommended have been placed along the roadways, on the plan especially commended by the medical inspector, in addition to those which were already in existence. The main supply of water to the town is typically pure, and more than adequate to the demand. The greater part of it is derived from the chalk hill above the town, and is received into a reservoir near the railway-station, from which a portion is pumped to a smaller reservoir on the downs for the accommodation of the houses at the highest elevations. A second source of water is the Grove-road reservoir, supplied by neighbouring springs; and only a few houses are wholly dependent on well-water. Dr. Ballard found, on examination, that all the water supplied to the town from the two former sources had been for many years open to the possibility of contamination by sewer-gas, in consequence of a free communication having existed between the town sewers and the reservoirs by means of the waste or overflow pipes. In one of these pipes the trap was shown to be imperfect; while the overflow pipe from the lower reservoir, although it was supposed to be perfect in its arrangements, proved on inquiry to be entirely innocent of any attempt at trapping. As soon as the serious consequences likely to result from such a condition were pointed out to the Company, immediate steps were taken to disconnect the overflow from the sewers, and now all superabundant supply from the Grove-road reservoir is directed in an open stream down Grove-road. As we before mentioned, a small proportion of houses are dependent for their water-supply on wells. Specimens of water from these sources have been submitted to Mr. Hebner, the Public Analyst for the Island, and all wells polluted or tainted in even the slightest degree have been closed. A thorough house-to-house sanitary inspection has been made, and we shall no longer hear of the waste-pipes of cisterns from which drinking-water is obtained being connected with the pans of water-closets. The Local Board of Ventnor is also to be congratulated on having obtained a suitable site for a mortuary. We shall be glad to hear before long that the plans which are now being prepared by the Surveyor to the Board are being carried into effect. By issuing sanitary certificates to approved houses, the authorities have given the general public a most valuable plan of self-protection. We trust that visitors will be careful in asking to see the certificates before engaging houses, and that the plan will be appreciated—as indeed it deserves to be; for although we are well aware that the inhabitants for the most part are desirous of carrying out the improvements which have been suggested, yet there are always to be found a few who, from ignorance or other causes are not quite so zealous for sanitary reforms as their neighbours. We think that Ventnor, owing to the great improvements carried out there during the last

eighteen months, may now be considered as a fairly safe watering-place for invalids to be sent to, and we hope that the popularity so long enjoyed by the town as a health-resort may not be materially lessened. At any rate, it is improbable that it will be the fault of the local authorities if there is any falling-off of its old reputation. In his report of the district of Shanklin, Dr. Ballard dwelt at some length on the state of the drainage, and there also the all-important subject of ventilation for the sewers was found to have been very much neglected. The inspector calculated that only one small ventilator was provided for 390 yards of pipe-sewer. We are informed that the number of ventilators has been very much increased of late, and that their condition is now made a subject of proper care. A perfect scheme for augmenting the quantity of the water has also been devised, and before long, the need of water, which has always been such a drawback in Shanklin, will be a thing of the past. We are told that the disagreeable odour which issues from the ventilators in Ryde is considerably less than formerly. In other respects the town remains in much the same condition as at the time of the inspection. Although no part of the Island received a more favourable notice from Dr. Ballard than the urban sanitary district of St. Helen's, yet there are many improvements which might easily be brought about. In the Report mention is made of the fact that in the greater part of this district the domestic refuse is obliged, by by-law, to be removed at the expense of the inhabitants. The consequence of this law is, that much annoyance is given to the visitors and better class of residents, by animal and vegetable matter, often in a state of incipient decomposition, being thrown over the sea-wall to undergo further decay among the rocks, or to wait for a high tide to carry it away. We wish to remind the local authorities of the existence of a group of cottages on the outskirts of Seaview, situated not many yards from the main drain, and which are at present only accommodated with cesspools. It seems to us incomprehensible that, although it was in this block of cottages that a severe epidemic of typhoid fever broke out in 1876, nothing has as yet been done to connect them with the main drain. On the whole, St. Helen's is a very healthy district, but much of the illness which does occur among the visitors might easily be obviated by improved drainage, as a large proportion of the cases met with in practice can often be clearly traced to the inhalation of noxious gases. In consequence of the reclamation of Brading Harbour, all the sewage from the village of St. Helen's now passes into the Channel above the embankment thrown up by the Company. Although the refuse matter passes through a sewage farm, two cases of typhoid fever were reported during last month both of which occurred in night-labourers employed near the farm. We trust, therefore, that the Company will take the hint which they have received, and will see that everything is done to protect the interests of the men in their employ and of the inhabitants of the village.

ASCITES DURING CHILDHOOD.

Dr. Seiler recently read, before a Dresden Medical Society, a paper on Ascites during Childhood. He first related two cases which had been under his own care, and then discussed the subject in the light of as many recorded cases as he was able to find scattered in our medical literature. His first case may be summarised as follows:—Emily T., aged thirteen years. Her parents were healthy, as also her brothers and sisters. When two years old she had measles and "nerve fever"; when six years old, inflammation of the brain, about which no clear history could be obtained. Two years previously she had suffered from an inflammation of the lungs. There was no history of ulcers of any kind, nor of keratitis; but she not infrequently complained of general debility, without having anything very manifest to account for it. Four months before her admission she began to swell in the abdomen, and applied at the hospital on account of this. When admitted, she was noted as a slender-made girl, with light hair and pale mucous membranes. The abdomen was greatly distended with free fluid. No anasarca, and no other signs of disease. The liver could not be felt. On puncturing, nine pints of fluid were withdrawn; the fluid was amber-coloured, and contained a slight amount of albumen. After the tapping, the liver could be felt to be enlarged, and extending for some distance below the ribs. Mercurial ointment was ordered to be rubbed in, and iodide of potash prescribed for internal use. The fluid never re-accumulated; while the liver rapidly shrank under this treatment. She was examined eighteen months later, and found in good health.

A second case was that of Ida W., aged four years, taken into hospital with considerable ascites. There was, however, no constitutional disturbance nor pain. About six pints of an opal, serous fluid were withdrawn, after which the liver could be felt as an enormous tumour reaching down to the right anterior superior spine of the ilium. The same treatment (as in last case) was ordered. A second tapping became necessary some six weeks after the first; but only a moderate amount of fluid was drawn off. The above treatment was continued for two months, and then a tonic treatment was substituted. The general health was excellent, but the liver still reached as low as the line of the umbilicus. This patient was again seen when aged thirteen years, and was found to be in good health, with the liver normal. The author also mentions two other similar cases —one aged seven, the other aged fifteen years.

In proceeding to analyse these cases, our author of course excludes abnormalities—such as a case of chylous ascites (recorded by Winckel), fatty degeneration of the peritoneum (recorded by Klebs), and cases of ascites when combined with general hydrops. Ascites proper may be divided, he says, into two chief classes. The one includes local disease of the peritoneum; the other depends on disturbances in the portal circulation. To the first may be reckoned cases of tubercular peritonitis, as found either in children or adults; it is a rare complication, if we include only those cases in which the disease is very chronic and confined to the peritoneum, and in which the fluid is found free in the peritoneal cavity. These cases—in children, at all events—are generally accompanied by remissions and irregular temperatures; and, as other organs of the body may be free from tuberculosis, the diagnosis may remain uncertain for a long time.

In this class must also be reckoned cases of primary carcinoma of the peritoneum, which run a very chronic course, in some cases even without at first disturbing the general health. The exudation in these latter cases, says Dr. Seiler, is always blood-stained, while in the tubercular cases it is always serous. The form of cancer is usually colloid, as neither cylindrical nor endothelioma ever occur during childhood. A third variety of local disease of peritoneum, which might come into question, is the so-called "primary peritoneal exudation." This is the analogue of the pleuritic exudation due to inflammation, either with fever or without, or it may be the residuum of a past disease, remaining behind in the abdominal cavity. doubtless rare and obscure as to causation. Thus, Bauer (in Ziemssen's "Cyclopædia") says —"Chronic idiopathic peritonitis is a very rare form of disease, the existence of which is even doubted by many pathologists." The female sex, he says, during youth are especially disposed to it. Prognosis is favourable, the most

so during childhood. Iodine applications are recommended. Henoch, too, uses iodine; he inclines to regard the exudation as possibly dependent on traumatic causes.

To the second class of cases, due to circulatory disturbances in the portal system, belong malignant disease of the liver, pressing on the portal vein. Primary cancer of this organ is not so rare, Dr. Seiler thinks, as is generally believed, but whether it occurs in children he is not prepared to say. Pressure on the portal vein may also be brought about by syphilitic gummata, or by cicatricial contraction after gummata have healed, should they occur near the hilus; cases of the kind have often been recorded.

But the most important of the liver-diseases which are accompanied by ascites is cirrhosis. In his own country, he says, where malarious diseases, so often the cause of ascites, are quite exceptional, the practitioner will not go far astray in regarding cirrhosis as the cause of the ascites in any given case where cancer can be excluded. The patients are mostly men, and generally over forty years of age. There are, however, exceptions. Dr. Seiler thinks that spirit-drinking is not the most common cause in Dresden. The livers of drinkers, he says, are fatty. Both the hypertrophic and the atrophic stages may lead to ascites, but the latter is the more frequent. Neoplastic connective tissue in the interior of the organ causes ascites, either by collecting around the acini, or by shrinking and so pressing on the interlobular veins. The occurrence of this genuine cirrhosis of the liver in children is very doubtful, according to the most recent authors (Birsch-Hirschfeld, Gerhardt's "Handbook"). Probably the cases described as such are syphilitic.

Apart from the history and course of the disease, it is almost impossible microscopically to distinguish diffuse syphilitic hepatitis from cirrhosis during the hypertrophic stage. Dr. Seiler quotes recorded cases in support of the syphilitic theory, and his address finishes with the following conclusions :—1. Simple ascites during childhood, provided tuberculosis be excluded, always depends on syphilitic hepatitis, circumscribed or diffuse, even in cases where no syphilitic history can be obtained. The cases hitherto recorded depend on a late development of congenital syphilis. 2. It is always curable either by mercurial inunction, the internal use of iodide of potassium, or the two combined. The only other possibility during childhood is the occurrence of a simple hypertrophic cirrhosis of the liver (which is curable).

THE WEEK.

TOPICS OF THE DAY.

THE Prince and Princess of Wales visited Brighton last week for the purpose of opening the new building of the Hospital for Sick Children. Their Royal Highnesses were received by Dr. Taaffe, one of the vice-presidents, who presented the Prince with a golden key commemorative of the occasion. The Hospital was opened for out-patients in the year 1868; and in December of the same year a private house was hired for a limited number of in-patients in the Western-road. So liberally, however, were the Committee supported, that in 1871 they determined to purchase a private house standing in its own grounds, and this was fitted up for the reception of forty patients. About two years since, the funds being available, it was determined to erect a new building, and this, fitted up with all the modern appliances, was only finished in time for the opening ceremony. After the usual formalities, the Prince of Wales declared the Hospital open, and before leaving the building, the Princess granted Dr. Taaffe permission to name the institution the "Royal Alexandra Hospital for Sick Children."

The Urban Sanitary Authority of Wallingford were recently summoned to the Berkshire Petty Sessions, held at that town, at the instance of the Thames Conservancy, for failing to comply with a notice served upon them under the Thames Conservancy Act of 1866, requiring them to discontinue the flow of sewage or other offensive matter into the Thames from their district. It appeared that for many years past the sewage of the town of Wallingford had been allowed to flow into the Thames. As far back as the year 1867 notice to discontinue the nuisance was served upon the Board. In 1869 a further and final notice was again served; but from that date until the present time no steps had been taken by the local authorities to abate the nuisance. Under these circumstances the Thames Conservancy determined to put in force the Act in question, and the present summons was granted. Ultimately the magistrates convicted the Sanitary Authority, and fined them in the mitigated penalty of £10, together with a further fine of 10s. a day so long as they shall allow the nuisance to continue.

In the face of a determined opposition on the part of the residents of the locality, and of the parochial boards of Hackney, the arrangements made by the Metropolitan Asylums Board for the erection of a small-pox ambulance station in George-street, London-fields, are nearly completed. The buildings erected are intended for the accommodation of the parishes of Hackney, Bethnal-green, Shoreditch, Poplar, Bow, and Islington. Upon the discovery of a case of small-pox in any of these localities, a telegram will be despatched by a parochial officer to the office of the Asylums Board, Norfolk-street, Strand, and immediate directions for the prompt removal of the patient will be conveyed by telegram to the ambulance-station. An ambulance, accompanied by nurses, will then proceed to the address of the patient, who will be conveyed to Potter's Ferry, where a steam-launch will be in readiness, and the patient, still accompanied by nurses, will be conveyed to the *Atlas*, moored off Deptford. At the East-end station it is intended to keep ten ambulances, and the nurses, drivers, and stablemen will reside on the premises, to prevent any loss of time. At a recent meeting of the Hackney Board of Guardians, Dr. G. C. Millar stated, as the result of two visits to the proposed station, that he was decided as to the unsuitableness of the site chosen. It was close to two church buildings and to the militia barracks, and was surrounded by a number of densely populated courts, which gave the poorer class of inhabitants but little cubic space. His inspection of the ambulances led him to consider them highly unsuitable, as the furniture and matting would retain small-pox matter, and could not very well be freed therefrom. It was also stated that close to the locality there were schools, which had an aggregate attendance of 4000 children. The Guardians, by eighteen votes to one, decided that the action taken was a "huge blunder," and proffered co-operation with the committee of residents to protest against it. It is also stated that the Sanitary Committee of Hackney have decided to apply for an injunction against the Metropolitan Asylums Board to restrain them from the further use of the building for any such purpose.

The third annual meeting of the Home Hospitals Association for Paying Patients has just been held, and we are glad to find that so far the movement has been successful. In the unavoidable absence of the President, the Duke of Northumberland, Earl Percy, M.P., took the chair. The Secretary read the report, which gave a most favourable account of Fitzroy House, No. 16, Fitzroy-square, the Association's first hospital, established to test the soundness of their principles, and recommended the purchase of the next house (that in which the meeting was held), which might then be set aside for lady patients, reserving Fitzroy House for gentlemen. The report was adopted on the motion of the Chairman, seconded by Sir Rutherford Alcock, K.C.B. Dr. Quain proposed—"That it is desirable to raise £5000, with the object of purchasing the freehold of No. 17, Fitzroy-square, and for finding funds for the necessary fittings and furniture, for providing additional accommodation of a similar kind to that already afforded at Fitzroy House." This was seconded and carried unanimously.

The annual visit of the members of the Metropolitan Asylums Board to the Caterham Asylum was recently paid. It will be remembered that this is one of the four imbecile asylums erected by the Board under the Act of 1867. It contains nearly 2000 patients of the adult imbecile class, chargeable to the London rates; and altogether the Board has under its care nearly 5000 persons of this class, who were formerly in the wards of the London workhouses. At Caterham, as at Leavesden and Darenth, under the influence of good air and proper treatment, many patients formerly classed as "chronic imbeciles" have wholly recovered; while many others have so far improved as to be employed in useful work on the farm or in the workshops of the establishment, whereby the cost of their maintenance is considerably reduced. The establishment is, as far as possible, self-maintained, growing a great deal of its food, drawing its own water, making all the gas consumed, and utilising the sewage. After the inspection, the managers congratulated Mr. George Ward, of the Committee, upon the satisfactory condition of the Asylum, and Dr. Eliot, the medical superintendent, upon the manner in which he discharged the very onerous duties of his post.

A feeling of much dissatisfaction has been created in some parts of the West of England by the growing custom of coroners relying on their own subordinates, or other unqualified persons, to give evidence as to the cause of death, also of allowing juries to return verdicts without previously hearing medical testimony. A case of this description has been submitted to the Home Secretary, with a view of eliciting his opinion on the subject, and it is satisfactory to learn that he has addressed a letter to the coroner complained of, expressing a strong opinion "that in the case mentioned a medical man should have been required to attend, and, moreover, a post-mortem examination should have been ordered."

The latest information respecting the International Medical Congress is to the effect that, up to the present, the number of foreign medical men announced to attend is about 800, and the aggregate attendance of members of the profession is expected nearly to reach 2000. The general meetings are to be held in St. James's Hall, and although the inaugural address will not be delivered by Sir James Paget until Wednesday, August 3, in St. James's Hall, the Council of the Congress will practically be commenced the previous day, when there will be an informal reception at the College of Physicians, and a *conversazione* by the President of the Odontological Society. There will be a clinical morning for rare cases of skin diseases in the Skin Section of the Congress on Saturday, August 6, commencing at ten o'clock. Members of the profession are invited to communicate personally to Dr. Thin, 22, Queen Anne-street, W., as soon as possible, their intention to demonstrate rare cases of skin disease. Earl Granville has intimated to the Committee his intention to hold a reception of the foreign members of the Congress on Saturday, August 6. The New York Academy of Medicine is to be represented at the Congress by its President, Dr. Fordyce Baker, and Drs. J. G. Adams and R. P. Farnham, the secretary and treasurer of the Academy.

At a recent meeting of the Bristol Sanitary Authority, the Medical Officer reported an outbreak of small-pox in Clifton

College, the leading educational establishment in the West of England. A pupil belonging to a family "afflicted with a superstitious belief in the imaginary evil effects of vaccination" was allowed to visit his home in a neighbouring city, and on his return to college he exhibited all the symptoms of small-pox and was isolated. Two pupils who broke through the quarantine were also compulsorily isolated. There had been only this one case in the College, the authorities of which have since required every pupil to be revaccinated who had not been successfully vaccinated during the past seven years. Every person who has not been revaccinated, the Medical Officer added, is a danger to the whole community, and ought not to be admitted into any public institution such as Clifton College. The report incidentally stated that the two sisters of the pupil who contracted the disease, both unvaccinated, last year took small-pox, and one died.

By the latest accounts the total amount received at the Mansion House for the Hospital Sunday Fund collection of June last exceeds £31,000, and is the largest yet recorded. It is also stated that some churches have yet to account for their collections;—and one is tempted to ask why this is so. A certain amount is subscribed on a given day, and when its total has been ascertained the same has to be paid in at the Mansion House. Surely this does not require five weeks to carry out! Meanwhile the Distribution Committee cannot begin their duties, the long vacation is close at hand, and everything is delayed through the dilatoriness of a few unbusinesslike people.

An application was made to the Judge of the Consistorial Court (Dr. Tristram, Q.C.), on Monday last, in the case of St. Mary, Stoke Newington, in which a faculty has been ordered to erect a mortuary chapel, to set aside the proceedings on the part of a lady named Jephson, whose property would be depreciated by such erection. It was suggested that there were other eligible sites. The Chancellor said that he would give the applicant leave to appear, and another site could be proposed. However, the fact that property would be depreciated was no reason for preventing the erection of public mortuaries.

THE THREATENED WATER-FAMINE.

VERY recently we recorded the commencement of a masterly scheme by which Liverpool is to be provided with a water-supply that will be practically inexhaustible; and in doing so we mentioned that, many years ago, the very same source was proposed to be utilised for the benefit of the metropolis. That the time has come when some second source of supply for London should be provided, can hardly be doubted, since a few weeks of dry, warm weather has sufficed to put such a strain upon the capacities of the metropolitan water companies that grave inconvenience has been felt in more than one quarter. If the affairs of Ireland are ever sufficiently settled to permit the Government to turn its attention to our own country, the long-delayed legislation on this point will have to be faced at once, and seriously. The authorities of Liverpool, Manchester, Sheffield, and some other large provincial towns, have set us an example which in the due course of affairs we should have afforded to them, and it is not unlikely that we may find, when fairly roused to the immediate importance of the question, that they have monopolised sources of supply which should have been made available for the capital. Nor can it be said that this matter has come upon us by surprise. Many years ago it was authentically stated that, by an agreement between two great brewery proprietors, on either bank of the Thames, where it flows through London, their pumping operations only took place on alternate days, and our position is suffi-

ciently alarming if the bursting of one or more mains in our midst is to necessitate a warning as to how we empty our cisterns. We do not pretend to point out any scheme for the acceptance of the Government, but we warn them that, looking at the matter from only a sanitary point of view, the position of affairs is sufficiently grave to justify their immediate action when more than one magistrate is appealed to for advice by householders who find themselves deprived of one of the first necessities of our existence. The London water companies enjoy a monopoly so huge as to be almost an anachronism in the present day; and in return for their vast privileges they should, at least, be compelled to insure a supply, unaffected by any periods of drought known to England. The individual inconveniences experienced at the present time will not have been endured in vain, if the cry of alarm now raised has been sufficient to call the attention of Parliament to the actual importance which exists for dealing with the subject at once. Every month's delay is of consequence,—even the magnificent scheme provided for Liverpool is not expected to be in full working order under a period of from eight to ten years,—and were we in London at this present time in possession of a plan equally comprehensive and promising, it would not be reassuring to have to look forward to a probable recurrence, every summer for the next ten years, of the last few weeks' discomfort. Meanwhile, every class of society should agitate to call attention to the subject, and it is satisfactory to find that the Bishop of London has promised to present to the House of Lords a petition from the National Health Society, asking whether any measures have been taken, or are in preparation by Her Majesty's Government, for improving the water-supply of the metropolis.

AMERICAN APPRECIATION OF ENGLISH SURGERY.

AMERICAN appreciation of English surgery has always been cordial, and has been as warmly reciprocated by us. A pleasant example of this friendly feeling has lately reached us in the shape of resolutions by the New York Academy of Medicine, and the Medical Society of the County of New York, forwarded to Mr. Spencer Wells, congratulating him on the completion of one thousand cases of ovariotomy. The Academy forwarded a resolution of congratulation to their foreign associate for his "remarkable and unprecedented achievement," and the Society "recognises the great service rendered by Mr. Wells in bring this operation to its present perfection, by which a large proportion of formerly hopeless cases may be rescued from death, and by which lustre is shed on the healing art." These resolutions must necessarily be very gratifying to the recipient, as well as to every one interested in the credit of English surgery.

THE CITY COMMISSIONERS OF SEWERS.

AT a meeting of the City Commissioners of Sewers, held on Tuesday last, Dr. Sedgwick Saunders, the Medical Officer of Health, reported that during the past week 280 houses in the City had been inspected, 19 of which required sanitary improvement in various particulars. At the markets and slaughter-houses, 31 tons 11 cwt. of meat had been seized and destroyed as unfit for human food. No fresh case of small-pox had occurred in the City during the week; but, he said, there seemed to be a threatening of another zymotic wave in the shape of scarlet fever, several cases, including one death, having been reported. He recommended that all the courts and alleys of the City should be thoroughly flushed and disinfected, some daily and others twice a week. Thirty-one articles had been disinfected at the mortuary, and five bodies received. A report was received from the Finance and Improvements Committee on the steps to be taken under the City of London Artisans' Dwellings Act, recommending that the whole of the money authorised by the Act, amounting to £500,000, should be raised as a 3 per cent. loan, at one operation, 97 per cent. being the minimum price; the loan to be for thirty years, and one-thirtieth part to be paid off yearly by drawings at par. The Report was adopted. The Court sanctioned an arrangement to effect improvements in Ave Maria-lane, Amen-corner, and Stationers' Hall-court, at an expense of £2500.

THE METROPOLITAN ASYLUMS DISTRICT BOARD.

AT the last meeting of the Metropolitan Asylums Board a letter was read from the Local Government Board relating to the report of Dr. Bridges respecting the hospital-ships *Atlas* and *Endymion*, and recommending that not more than forty patients be placed on each of the three lower decks, the upper deck being reserved for exceptional cases. Sir E. H. Currie said all the decks were not of the same size, but he supposed a considerably larger number would eventually be accommodated. A letter was also read from a firm of shipbuilders, complaining of the position chosen for mooring these vessels. As usual, a discussion ensued as to who was really responsible for the position selected, and eventually both these letters were referred to the Ship Committee. A deputation from the inhabitants of Hackney and Shoreditch waited upon the Board in order to protest against the establishment of the ambulance station at George-street, London-fields, and presented a memorial embodying all the objections to the scheme. On the motion of Sir E. H. Currie, this memorial was referred to the Works and General Purposes Committee. The comparative return of the number of small-pox patients in the several hospitals of the Board showed that during the past fortnight 334 persons had been admitted, 65 had died, 416 were discharged, and 779 still remained under treatment. Including 263 convalescents remaining at Darenth camp, the total of those under treatment is 1032, showing a decrease of 242 as compared with the previous fortnight. Speaking upon a motion instructing a committee to seek out sites for the erection of convalescent homes, Sir E. H. Currie said that unless immediate steps were taken for this purpose, they would probably return from their vacation to find themselves in the midst of an epidemic of scarlet fever, without means of coping with it. Much opposition was shown to the motion, many Managers being opposed to taking any action without further statutory powers, and on a division it was rejected; and it was decided to defer the question until the judgment of the House of Lords in the Hampstead Hospital appeal case has been given.

INTERNATIONAL MEDICAL CONGRESS.

THE eventful week is now close at hand; and, thanks to an immense activity on the part of Mr. Mac Cormac and his assistants, the arrangements are not only completed, but they appear to be very nearly perfect. A final meeting of the secretaries of the various sections on Wednesday last was held at the College of Physicians, when some formal business was transacted. The volume of abstracts of all the papers to be read during the Congress will be ready for members on Monday, August 1, and can be had on application at the College of Physicians. A daily programme will be published; and members will do well to secure one each morning, for in it any slight variation in the business of the day will be duly recorded, although efforts will be made to abide as nearly as possible by existing arrangements. On Tuesday, August 2, the chief business will be that of greeting one's friends at the College of Physicians, where, from three to six, the Executive will assemble to welcome members. On Wednesday the amount of business is very large. The first general meeting will take place in St. James's Great Hall, at which H.R.H. the Prince of Wales will be present. On this occasion Sir William Jenner will preside, and the report of the Executive Committee will be read by Mr. Mac Cormac. The formal constitution of the Congress will be proposed by Sir Risdon Bennett, after which the Prince of Wales will declare it open. Sir James Paget, the President, will then deliver the Inaugural Address. After luncheon, the sections will be constituted, a short address will be delivered by each of the Presidents, and then the ordinary work will be commenced. During the afternoon a second general meeting will be held, at which Professor Virchow will deliver an oration on "The Value of Pathological Experiment." A *conversazione* at South Kensington, which is to be graced by the presence of ladies, will bring this day's work to a close. We need hardly say that we wish the members of the Congress a very happy and successful meeting. If the success of the undertaking is at all commensurate with the immense labour which has been so unstintingly bestowed on it, we have nothing to fear on this score.

THE PARIS WEEKLY RETURN.

THE number of deaths for the twenty-eighth week, ending July 15, 1881, was 858 (viz., 464 males and 394 females), and among these there were from typhoid fever 28, small-pox 17, measles 19, scarlatina 15, pertussis 8, diphtheria and croup 37, dysentery 1, erysipelas 6, puerperal infections 5, and acute tubercular meningitis 42. There were also 14 deaths from acute bronchitis, 49 from pneumonia, 115 from infantile athrepsia (41 of the infants having been partially or wholly suckled), and 52 violent deaths. The births for the week amounted to 994, viz., 502 males (366 legitimate and 136 illegitimate) and 492 females (371 legitimate and 121 illegitimate); 75 children (37 males and 38 females) were born dead or died within twenty-four hours. (The returns for this week are imperfect, owing to those of the last day not having been made up in consequence of the national *fête* of July 14.)

PRESENTATION TO PROFESSOR SPENCE.

A VERY interesting ceremony took place in Edinburgh on the 18th inst., in the presentation to Professor Spence of his portrait, painted by Mr. James Irvine. The portrait is the gift of members of the profession in Great Britain and Ireland and the colonies, as an expression of their esteem and regard for Professor Spence as a surgeon and a friend. The scene of the ceremony was the Hall of the Royal College of Surgeons, Mr. Imlach, the President of the College, being in the chair; and the presentation was made by Dr. Haldane, the President of the Royal College of Physicians. A replica is to be placed in the Hall of the College of Surgeons, and subscribers will receive an etching of the portrait by Durand, of Paris.

THE REPORT OF THE HEALTH OFFICER OF THE PORT OF LONDON.

THE half-yearly report of the Medical Officer of Health for the Port of London, to December 31 last, has been printed and published. In the outset Dr. Collingridge records a very satisfactory sign of the good influence which such an authority must exercise, namely, that although the number of vessels inspected during the period was unusually large, the proportion requiring cleansing and whitewashing again showed a marked decrease. In 1873 the number of uncleanly vessels was 17 per cent. of the total number inspected, whereas during the six months referred to in the present report, it was only 3 per cent. The health of the port of London during the latter half of 1880 was extremely good; but little sickness of an infectious nature was prevalent, with the exception of some outbreaks on board the different training-ships, and a few scattered cases of small-pox. Seventy sick seamen were referred to hospital during the period for various diseases, but it was only found necessary to disinfect clothing in the case of six patients suffering from small-pox, and six suffering from fever. It is not reassuring to find that Dr. Collingridge, whose experience should be considerable from the nature of his duties, comments strongly on the insanitary condition of the river Thames : the water, he says, is at all times in a very unsatisfactory condition, and must remain so while such enormous quantities of sewage are thrown into it. During July last it became very much worse than usual ; its colour, at all times bad, had become decidedly darker, and it gave a most intolerable smell. Though generally of a dark colour, it had still darker slate-coloured patches, over which the odour was more intense ; samples taken from these slate-coloured patches proved them to consist simply of sewage more or less sewage diluted. The quality of the drinking-water carried by vessels has been the subject of special attention : in the larger and better equipped vessels it is, as a rule, of good quality; in smaller vessels, especially barges, however, much improvement is still needed. Owing to the ignorant carelessness of crews, water is often taken from impure sources, and, even where a good supply is obtained, it is frequently spoiled by improper storage, dirty casks, etc. In one sample analysed, evidence was found of an appreciable amount of urine, and other equally bad specimens have been obtained. In such case the inspectors invariably see that the foul water is at once thrown away, and a fresh supply procured. On July 27 last, the *Orient*, belonging to the Orient Steam Navigation Company, entered the Royal Albert Dock with a clean bill of health. On the 30th of the same month, however, two cases of typhoid fever were discovered on board. These were at once removed, and proper disinfection carried out. A close investigation failed to give any clue as to the origin of the disease. On September 5, a case of small-pox was reported on the same vessel ; the patient was a carpenter engaged on board, and there seemed to be no doubt that the infection was derived from the neighbouring district. These two diseases on board the same vessel are referred to in the report to show the necessity that exists for a daily visit of inspection to all vessels lying in docks. The Port Sanitary Committee have, indeed, recognised the importance of these inspections, and, on the representations of Dr. Collingridge, an additional inspector has been added to the staff to render it more efficient. Before closing this notice it may be mentioned that the hospital-ship *Rhin*, moored off Gravesend, has been found extremely useful as a means of isolation in outbreaks of any epidemic, but the report adds, being an old vessel, and the timbers in many places spongy, it would hardly be a wise course to use her for cases of acute infectious disease, since it would be nearly impossible to thoroughly disinfect her afterwards.

ROYAL COLLEGE OF PHYSICIANS OF LONDON.

THE first Bradshaw Lecture will be delivered by Dr. G. Vivian Poore at the College of Physicians on Thursday, August 18, at five o'clock. The subject will be " Nervous Affections of the Hand."

MEDICAL PARLIAMENTARY AFFAIRS.

Cottage Dwellings in Ireland and Scotland.—In the House of Lords, on Friday, July 22, Lord Waveney presented a Bill framed for the purpose of providing sanitary supervision and sufficient accommodation in the dwellings of the cottiers

of Ireland and the islands and Highlands of Scotland, together with an adequate amount of ground to be cultivated as allotments. The opinion of the Government was that the Land Bill should not be overweighted by the introduction of any extraneous matter, though latterly special clauses had been introduced on the subject of labourers' dwellings. The Artisans and Labourers' Dwellings Act only applied to England, and in every English union frequent visits were paid to the cottages of the poor by the sanitary officials. The same evils of insanitary dwellings were at work in Scotland as in Ireland. The Bill was read a first time.

Alkali Works.—In the House of Commons, the report of amendment to the Alkali Works Regulation Bill was brought up and agreed to.

Wool Sorters' Disease.—On Monday, July 25, Mr. Mundella, in reply to Mr. Egerton, said that the report of Mr. Spears upon the danger of " anthrax " being communicated to sheep and cattle from the use of foreign hair and wool as manure, said that the report had been referred to the Veterinary Department. Anthrax, however, is a comparatively rare disease in animals in England, and does not appear to have increased during the past forty years.

London Water-Supply.—Mr. Dodson, in reply to Mr. Rogers, said that Colonel Bolton had made inquiry respecting the capabilities of supply by the Vauxhall and Southwark Water Company, and he states that the Company pump 25,000,000 gallons of water daily into their district—equal to thirty-five gallons and a half per head of population. There need be no apprehension that the district is, as alleged, within an hour's risk of a water-famine.

Small-pox among Hop-pickers.—On Tuesday, July 26, Mr. Dodson, in reply to Mr. Talbot, said that instructions had been given for a circular to be sent to the guardians and rural sanitary authorities in the hop-growing districts of Kent and neighbouring counties, cautioning them of the danger likely to arise from the immigration during the hop-picking season of persons from the metropolis who had been exposed to the contagion of small-pox. Suggestions would be given for the proper isolation of any case that might arise, and for protecting the inhabitants of the district. The guardians are recommended to notify by handbills or otherwise the penalties which would be incurred by the exposure of infected persons and articles of clothing and bedding.

THE PAINS OF LOCOMOTOR ATAXY.—For the relief of these, Prof. Vulpian recommends that compresses of many folds, after having been immersed in water and wrung out, should be moistened with a teaspoonful of chloroform and then applied to the painful parts and covered with oiled silk. They produce both a revulsive and anæsthetic effect which relieves the pain. We may employ them also, or have recourse to chloroform ointment, in the case of neuralgia of nerves situated superficially, and in muscular rheumatism. If the cold of evaporation is sought to be obtained for local anæsthesia, ether should be substituted for chloroform.— *Union Méd.*, July 21.

AROMATISED GLYCERINE.—The following is Professor Jaccoud's formula :—Glycerine, 40 grammes ; rum or cognac, 10 grammes ; and essence of mint, 1 drop. This mixture, which is of an agreeable taste, is well tolerated by the stomach, so that after several months of its uninterrupted employment it gives rise neither to satiety nor disgust. The addition of the alcohol has simply in view the modification of the insipid taste of this drug, and to aid in its digestion. Its dose would be quite insufficient as an alcoholic medication. The quantity of glycerine mentioned in the formula is the minimum daily dose, and it may be increased to fifty or sixty grammes. This last quantity, however, should not be given except to persons who present no sign of abnormal excitement of the nervous system or of the action of the heart. Moreover, whenever there is any agitation or unusual loquacity, obstinate sleeplessness, or a persistent elevation of temperature (in the absence of any pyretogenic incident) of 0·5° C. in relation to the mean temperature of the period prior to taking the glycerine, it will be an indication that the serviceable dose has been exceeded. Glycerine should be employed for the purpose of stimulating the digestive functions, and saving the waste of tissue during the non-febrile period of phthisis, when cod-liver oil has ceased to be tolerated. The dose of aromatised glycerine should be divided into two or three takings.—*Progrès Méd.*, July 16.

INTERNATIONAL MEDICAL AND SANITARY EXHIBITION, 1881.

Section VII.

DRUGS, DISINFECTANTS, DIETETIC ARTICLES AND MINERAL WATERS.

It may be just as well to premise with regard to this section, as has already been said of it—a statement which we beg leave to reiterate—that, after a considerable experience of exhibitions, this is the very worst arranged, and the catalogue the most confusing of any we have ever encountered. The feeble attempts which have been made at grouping have only served to make confusion worse confounded. Two important exhibits are separated from their neighbours, and are to be found among surgical instruments; two others are in the sanitary department; yet the space which they might well have occupied is either vacant or filled with surgical mechanisms.

Turning from this irritating theme, however, we find on our right and left hand on entering this department from Exhibition-road, two stalls typical in their way. We all know that nothing succeeds like success, and in the world of natural and artificial beverages there have been of recent days two notable examples, namely, Apollinaris water and "Zoedone." The latter does not make its appearance here, but it has a host of imitators, some of which we vastly prefer to the original. The newspapers are crowded with advertisements of all kinds sounding the praises of these, and were all that is said of them true, the ills of life would soon be gone. But, joking apart, there are here some very nice and palatable non-intoxicating drinks, and we do not think that there is any better than that first encountered—the so-called "Vin Santé" exhibited by Evans, Lescher, and Webb, especially with the addition of a few drops of raspberry cordial (and, for our own part, we should say, half a bottle of seltzer). This we can strongly recommend. Next to it is another of the same class, but with a totally different flavour. All, in point of fact, have differences in this respect; but all are good, and, to those who relish such drinks, will all be welcome. The one we now especially refer to is the "Hedozone" of Messrs. Packham and Co., of Croydon; very pleasant and refreshing. The exhibit of Messrs. Samuel Gulliver and Co., of Aylesbury, is almost entirely confined to these artificial beverages: chief among these they would seem to place what they call their "Sparkling Vinta"; and one which deserves special notice is their "Quinine Tonic." This aërated water, though comparatively little known in this country, is used in immense quantities in the East—seldom, however, we suspect, without a dash of something in it; but we are persuaded that it would be a boon to many in this country (not necessarily with the "dash"), especially to those—and there are some such—to whom the taste of quinine is pleasant. Messrs. J. Moorhouse and Co., of Manchester, send some very pleasant specimens of these artificial drinks—one, which they call "Sparkling Rozo," and said to contain glycero-phosphoric acid, is particularly worth notice. Curiously enough, the North of Ireland has been rising in repute of recent years for the production of artificial mineral waters, which are now largely introduced into London. They are excellent, and sold at a very cheap rate. We have one example here from the Newry Mineral Water Company, who also show a very good "Ginger Champagne." The only other samples of this kind of drink we noticed were sent by the Andover Aërated Water Company. But shall we go thus far afield, and overlook those at our own doors. Who that is athirst, and wants a good bottle of homely soda-water, would pass by the well-known portals in Piccadilly of Blake, Sandford, and Blake?—whilst most of us have at some time or other been thankful to Hooper and Co. for a draught of their well-known "Brighton Seltzer."

We scarcely know if we ought to speak of the great variety of specimens of lime-juice preparations here shown, which, however, really belong to this class. At all events, we cannot do wrong in specially directing attention to Felton and Son's "Lime-juice Cordial," which, mixed with water, and in warm weather just tempered with a little pounded ice, constitutes an admirable beverage.

Turning next to the class of beverages which personally we prefer—namely, of the natural sort—we are brought face to face with a great group of those table-waters, headed by the two chief German and French waters, "Apollinaris" and "St. Galmier." Both of these are excellent in their way, but patriotism has much to do with the great success of the latter. Apollinaris may, however, easily give many points to St. Galmier, or to any of the others here shown, and we can readily tell how this is to be settled. We know of no more terrible ordeal than that of going through a long series of such drinkables as those of which we have spoken, and trying to do one's duty faithfully by tasting each in turn. It is worse than tasting a long series of wines, by a long way. But supposing you end off, for the sake of cleansing your palate, with the crisp, sparkling mineral waters, and try them all, you will find when you come to the Apollinaris, even when taken last, that there is still room left for its distinct appreciation, its keen yet pleasant savour giving it a decided character, distinguishing it from all others. Esperto crede. Next to these giants of fame we should place a very pleasant water of comparatively recent introduction, namely, the "Gerolstein." This keeps well, constitutes by itself a pleasant drink, and mixes well with wine or spirits. It is, perhaps, a pity that in their prospectus the company claim so much for it as a medicinal agent. People seldom like to make physic an habitual beverage. Only two other specimens of mineral waters belonging to this class are exhibited, and we are heartily glad to be able to speak well of both. The "Harzer" is from a new district as regards table-waters. As its name implies, it is a product of the Hartz Mountains. The other, the "Bellthal," is from that volcanic region on the west of the Rhine now so freely tapped, and possesses characters similar in most respects to the others of this group. We saw only a single bottle of our old friend "Gieshübler." Quite a new water from the district near Audenach, called the "Genoveva," and to which a somewhat romantic legend is attached, here presents itself for the first time.

There is still another group of natural mineral waters to which the term medicinal rather than dietetic might best apply. These comprehend what the Germans call the natural bitter waters, whilst in this country they are commonly designated as purgative. Only four kinds are shown, and of these only two are well known. But, seniores priores, let us first speak of our old, faithful, but well-nigh forgotten friend, "Püllna," exhibited by the proprietor, Anton Ulbrich, in his squat stone bottles. For many years this was almost the only purgative mineral water available in this country, except one paid a visit to Cheltenham or some such watering-place. That it was safe and active there is no questioning, but the taste was most unpleasant. Nevertheless we are glad to see our old friend raising his head again. "Friederichshall" (which has not, however, made its appearance at this Exhibition) came soon after, and for a long time the two had it all their own way, but still the taste was disagreeable, and it often made one sick. But by-and-by came a greater than they, in the shape of "Hunyadi János," a Hungarian water from the neighbourhood of Pesth, the only absurd thing about it being its name. The literal meaning of the term is simply John Hunyadi, a great Hungarian hero of the days when the Turk was overrunning the country, after whom the spring was named. It is the curious Hungarian custom to put the Christian name always after the surname. As an example, we might give the instance of one of the largest Transylvanian wine-growers, who by some curious accident bears the well-known and, in our profession, honoured name of Paget, and is there universally known as Paget János. But, putting that on one side, we had in the Hunyadi for the first time a bitter water sure in its effects, easily regulated in its force, and comparatively tasteless. These characteristic properties easily account for the success it has met with. This water is exhibited by the Apollinaris Company.

Three other waters of the same kind are likewise shown. They are comparatively new to us, so that we have the less to say of them, for you cannot taste these one after the other as you would sparkling table-waters. Two at least are from the same district as Hunyadi, and probably do not differ greatly in their properties. They are the "Victoria," and another called by the somewhat ridiculous title of "Æsculap." The former of these, the "Victoria," is without doubt an exceedingly powerful bitter water, containing a very high percentage both of sulphate of magnesia and sulphate of soda, the latter of which we, for our own part, look upon as by far the more important ingredient of the two, owing to its great and specific effect on the liver. The "Bákoczy," likewise a Hungarian bitter water of a high potency, is exhibited by E. GALLAIS and Co., who are the importers of St. Galmier, and of many other pleasant things besides, especially in the shape of wines, to which, however, we cannot here refer.

There are still two varieties of mineral water to be mentioned—the one is that of the Purton Spa, which is a decided addition to our somewhat scanty list of easily available sulphuretted waters. In this case the sulphur is accompanied by both bromine and iodine, which should render the water specially valuable in certain forms of skin disease. This is exhibited by the proprietors, T. T. HIRST and Co. There can be no mistake about the quantity of sulphur, as well as of iodine, contained in it, after twenty-four hours' standing. The only other water to be noted is one recently discovered near Ampthill, in Bedfordshire; it is highly ferruginous, the iron being chiefly in the form of carbonate or oxide, but it likewise contains a considerable proportion of sulphates of soda and magnesia, which we always look upon as a most important addition to chalybeate waters. It is exhibited by the proprietor, Mr. H. K. STEVENS, but may be obtained direct from the spring at Flitwick, Ampthill, Beds.

DIETETIC ARTICLES.

Turning next to the allied subject of Dietetic Articles, we cannot do better than begin with the now well-known preparations of BRAND and Co. Many a doctor and many a patient has had good cause to bless them, for of all meat products they are those which are best taken when the strength is lowest. They are most easy of digestion, and the patient seldom tires of them. If he does, the selection is large enough to secure ample variety. We remember pulling through one of the most desperate cases we have ever seen on essence of chicken and what some would think the somewhat incongruous addition of tinned asparagus. It cannot be too clearly understood that these preparations are essences, not extracts. Hence they are more palatable and more nutritious. A recent introduction by this firm will be welcomed. It is what is called Albuminous Extract of Beef. This is intended to be used when the patient is strong enough to discontinue the use of the essence, and contains certain elements or ingredients wanting in the former, but which add to its flavour and nutritious properties. Next to these we may mention two other sets of dietetic remedies—if we may use the term—those shown by VAN ABBOTT and BONTHRON, consisting of various kinds of food for diabetics. Here we must limit ourselves to the subject of bread, with regard to which Van Abbott may be said to constitute himself the champion of the French gluten bread, whilst Bonthron exhibits only his own manufacture. With this, from a somewhat extended experience, we may pronounce ourselves well satisfied, more especially as regards the rusks and biscuits, though the bread is also very good, especially when toasted to crispness.

What the AYLESBURY DAIRY COMPANY have done for the public with regard to an improved milk-supply, they have outdone as regards the invalid. It is not long since the only resource possible for the delicate child or the still more delicate invalid was plain cow's milk—good, bad, and indifferent,—taken with the risk of getting some zymotic super-added. The height of ingenuity could go no further than to secure the milk of one particular cow for the use of one particular person, or, by having two or more stopcocks to the milk-can, drawing off the richer or upper portion—by far the most indigestible, as containing most oil or butter—and calling this babies' milk. But cow's milk is to many people and in many conditions of stomach-ailment—as we know full well from practical experience—highly indigestible. It has a strong tendency, when coagulated, to run into solid knots or masses, which are difficult to keep down, and still harder to bring up. Now, the whole of this would be easily obviated by milk deprived of its casein—that is, whey; but where to get whey in London? Again, to many the excess of fat in cow's milk is more or less poisonous; but where to get milk with the fat removed (that is, butter-milk) in London? The Aylesbury Dairy Company have deliberately set themselves to work to remedy this state of things, and they deserve our hearty thanks for so doing. For now not only whey and butter-milk, but also milk treated by digestive ferments (peptonised milk); milk reduced with care to as nearly as possible the characters of human milk; as well as the so-called "Koumiss" (or fermented milk)—are to be obtained from this Company. And we have no reason to think that their exertions will stop here. To the last named preparation—koumiss—we would earnestly ask attention. The taste is somewhat peculiar—something like butter-milk; but it is in a highly digestible condition, almost invariably agrees with the stomach, and contains quite enough nutrient matter to support life. Being highly carbonated, it needs no dilution with effervescent waters, the gas from which, when swallowed with milk, from which it does not readily escape, often gives rise to most unpleasant flatulent distension. Though not exhibited here, it is possible to procure from this Company small bottles of fine Danish rennet, which should be found in every family where there are children, and can be freely consumed.

It is likewise to be noted that rennet may also be obtained from Mr. JAMES DAVIDSON, of Dundee, who exhibits it here, and sells it in small bottles, price 6d. per bottle. In using rennet to make curds-and-whey it must be remembered that the temperature of the milk should be that of the fluid as it comes from the cow, or what is commonly known as blood-heat. If the temperature exceeds this the coagulation of the caseine is prevented; and cold milk will not coagulate. Whilst speaking of this gentleman's exhibit, we may at once say that he shows some very admirable specimens of cod-liver oil emulsion, nearly solid, even as the weather goes.

One of the most interesting exhibits is that of KOPF, of Erbswurst fame, now converted into a limited liability company. We would especially notice his consolidated soups, of which the well-known pea-soup, so largely employed in the Franco-German War, may be taken as the type. His extract of beef (solid) is also very good, and he has a great variety of biscuits, mixed with nutritious substances of different kinds. He likewise shows some specimens of the Maté (leaves of the *Ilex Paraguayensis*), so universally used in South America, not as a substitute for, but really superseding the use of, tea. A curious preparation shown by this Company is a kind of liquid extract of Maté, together with certain other ingredients, which, whether or not it retains the fragrance, will certainly retain the properties, of the dried leaf.

An artificial food, very highly spoken of, and very well liked, termed "LLOYD'S Universal Food," is here shown. It differs from many in being highly palatable and equally suited for adults and infants. It is composed of ordinary cereal flour together with some leguminous products mixed with malt-meal, the whole well cooked and dried, so that it may be ready for use in a minute, requiring only to be mixed with boiling water or milk to make it immediately available.

And now we approach—in a certain sense, with fear and trembling—a department where food and medicine are closely allied, in the shape of Malt Extracts, many of which so closely resemble each other that it would be hard to distinguish them, and they are so numerous that they are hard to be enumerated. One thing is comforting—we are able to speak well of them all, and whichever the patient selects, he is sure to get a good article, even though they differ among themselves as to strength and flavour. To begin with that longest known in this country, we at once encounter difficulty, for here there are two HOFFS, each of whom says he is the real original Hoff—just such another story as that as regards the veritable Johann Maria Farina at Cologne. We are in no position to settle the dispute, only, as far as we remember, it was Johann Hoff who first brought his wares to this country; and we can certify that the Hamburg Hoffs exhibit a very nice malt jelly.

We further find two malt extracts from Scandinavians—namely, BJÖRKBORN'S and ECKELL'S. From Germany we find samples prepared by LOEFLUND, of Stuttgart, already favourably noticed in these columns. Samples of malt extract and Liebig's soluble food also come from PAUL LIEBE, of Dresden; whilst from America we have two which are well worth special notice—namely, the "Kepler" malt extract, which we venture to say is by far the best we have seen; it is exhibited by BURROUGHS, WELLCOME, and Co. for the Kepler Company. The other is the now well known "Maltine," shown by the MALTINE COMPANY, which is peculiar as containing more than barley-malt alone, and which is both pleasant and nutritious.

The only specimen of extract of meat we feel called upon to notice specially is that of the DELACRE COMPANY, prepared near Buenos Ayres. It is a most admirable preparation, highly to be recommended, mixing nicely with water, having no burnt taste or smell, and equally available as food or medicine. It is very well worthy of a trial, and may be procured from Messrs. Savory and Moore, New Bond-street. Last, though by no means least, we notice a meat preparation for which Messrs. CORBYN are agents. This is called " Valentine's Meat Juice." It is dark-coloured, almost like free bromine, and perfectly fluid. Taken by itself it is too strong to be pleasant; but mixed with a little cold water (very hot water destroys it), it is highly palatable and highly nutritious. It is the best food stimulant we have seen, and might well take the place of alcoholic liquors where it is desirable to discontinue the use of the latter.

DISINFECTANTS.

Of the Disinfectants here shown, little need be said. Standing face to face, are to be seen the old rivals, " Condy " and carbolic acid; but the relative merits of each are now too well known to need more than mention. Each has a very distinct function to fulfil, and each does its duty well, but neither can take the place of the other. By the way, we wonder that the manufacturers of the carbolic compounds do not send it out—at all events, they do not show it—in that beautiful form where it is mixed with glycerine. It can be made tremendously strong, and will readily mix with water. Here, too, is our old friend " Sanitas "; though we never liked the name, its perfume is so pleasant, its oxidising activity is so great, that it amply deserves its reputation as one of the best domestic disinfectants.

Among the exhibitors is the well-known house of EUGÈNE RIMMEL, and with regard to their articles a word need be said. Many strongly object to the use of perfumes at all, as likely to conceal rather than to reveal foul smells and putrefying material. Were this objection of any valid weight it would apply equally, if not more so, to carbolic acid, for it by no means follows that because a place smells strongly of carbolic acid every hole and corner in it has been thoroughly disinfected. No one can object to the use of such substances as the "Aromatic Ozoniser" in a room, and we can readily point to still more important uses to which even stronger perfumes may be put. All medical men know that very troublesome odours are often associated with the sick-room, where ventilation is, from the condition of the patient, impossible; still more is this the case where the frequent use of the night-stool is necessary. In such and such-like cases, we say that products similar to those of M. Rimmel, especially his fumigating ribbons and papers, are of inestimable value.

In a new product called " Glacialine " we have at last, it is said, that long-sought-for substance which shall be at once preservative, tasteless, and harmless. The manufacturers, the ANTITROPIC COMPANY, invite a trial; and as this may be made by anyone at the small cost of fourpence, it may well suit our readers to make it for themselves.

Another new material which yet needs more protracted experiment is what is called " JEYES' Perfect Purifier"; its basis is naphthaline and creasote, and it seems to act very powerfully. It is to be had fluid, in powder, and in soap.

DRUGS.

The display of drugs is not, perhaps, so large as might have been expected, but that there is taken rank as of a very high quality. Nothing, in point of fact, is more striking in the whole of this Exhibition than the enormous improvements which it represents in modern pharmacy. When we look back twenty or thirty years, and compare the pharmaceutical products of that day with those of our own, we cannot fail to be impressed with the great change for the better both in the form and substance of the various medicaments sent out. The drugs are better, and, we trust, purer; the preparations neater and more certain; and certainly there can be no comparison, as regards the elegance in the modes of putting up, of the past and present time.

Probably it will be best, in this division, to adopt the purely alphabetical arrangement, and to indicate only some of the most striking preparations shown by each exhibitor.

First comes the old and well-known firm of ALLEN and HANBURYS, of Plough-court. We shall only mention their very fine cod-liver oil—the so-called " Perfected " oil—and a very fine specimen of fluid extract of Tonga, so highly recommended by some as a remedy for neuralgia. They also show a vaporiser for Cresoline, a new specific for whooping-cough. This vaporiser may likewise be used instead of a spray-producer for the dissemination of perfumes and other volatile substances.

Next come BATTLEY and WATTS, famous for their Liquors. Well do we remember the time when their liquor opii was the only watery preparation of opium to be had. Not less well known or less useful are their liquor secalis and their liquor cinchonæ.

BRAVAIS has long been famous for his dialysed iron and an equally useful preparation of quinine. In connexion with the former, we would notice one of the neatest little inventions we remember to have seen. The arrangement for " dropping " by means of a little india-rubber cap attached to a small bit of glass tubing has long been known: here the glass tube was introduced into the fluid, the india-rubber cup compressed, so that when it was allowed to recoil the fluid was drawn in exactly as in a now familiar form of enema-bag or syringe; when again compressed the fluid could be expressed drop by drop. But on this plan the iron or other fluid came in contact with the india-rubber and corroded it. In the present apparatus the old mechanism is retained, but its action is reversed, and a long fine quill or glass tube drawn to a rough point is also inserted through the cork of the bottle so as to reach the fluid. When now the small india-rubber capsule is compressed, the air from it forces down the surface of the fluid, which is thus made to ascend the fine tube, whence it may be easily dropped.

BURGOYNE, BURBIDGES, and Co. show some curious products of vanilla, and some beautiful specimens of capsules prepared by Pohl, near Dantzig.

BURK, of Stuttgart's, specialty is medicated wines. We find here wines of pepsine, iron, cocoa, and bark; whilst Messrs. BUSH and Co., of London, have a choice collection of their own manufacture of essential oils and fruit essences, the finest and most useful we have seen.

One of the largest and most interesting stalls is that of Messrs. BURROUGHS, WELLCOME, and Co., of Snow-hill, who not only exhibit for themselves, but in this respect act as agents for many others. The two chief products of their own are a beef and iron wine, an excellent and most palatable tonic, if we can call it so, for anæmic individuals; and a new preparation called "Hazeline," got from the American " witch hazel," and which is credited with all sorts of useful properties, especially in bruises, sprains, chaps, and insect stings, being of special value as regards irritated piles and other surfaces covered with irritated mucous membrane. They also exhibit Wyeth's preparations, of which his dialysed iron and his compressed tablets of various substances are the most important. We would especially refer to the chlorate of potash tablets, for to do good, say in sore tongue, throat, etc., we hold that chlorate of potash should be applied as directly as possible. We have been accustomed to use the solid crystals, but the tablets are better. Something after the same kind are compressed tablets of powerful alkaloids for hypodermic injection, where the chief ingredient is combined with sulphate of soda (each small tablet containing one dose and being readily soluble) in three or four drops of water. The same gentlemen exhibit for Messrs. McKesson and Robbins a great selection of beautifully made pills, coated with a readily soluble material, which, however, completely covers them in swallowing. These are ovoid in form, on which the manufacturers lay great stress. We should rather incline to point to the excellence of their make and materials as their most praiseworthy feature. We can only allude to two other preparations—one a citrate of caffeine, prepared by a London firm, and highly useful in some forms of headache; and a very nice perfume called " Florida water," which has, however, no very distant resemblance to our own lavender-water.

The many and various uses of " Vaseline" are now so well known that no further reference to it is here needed than to mention that a great variety of substances, of which it is the basis, are here shown by the CHESEBOROUGH COMPANY, its manufacturers.

We have already alluded to the valuable meat products

shown by Messrs. CORBYN, STACEY, and Co. We would only further refer to a very excellent form of vegetable food—one of the best of its kind—which they prepare, and to which they have given the name of "Lactrose." Another highly useful invention is that of sending out nitrite of amyl in exact doses of three minims, each in a little glass capsule, which may be broken and the fluid inhaled from a hand-kerchief. Nitrite of amyl is such a dangerous substance that it is well to have it thus safely dosed, rather than to trust to dropping or measuring, especially in the hands of an uninstructed person.

There are two most magnificent exhibits of the various alkaloids and principles obtainable from opium—the one set shown by J. F. MACFARLAN and Co., the other by T. H. SMITH and Co. The latter house has long held a very high reputation in this department of pharmacy, but Messrs. Macfarlan's exhibit indicates that they must look well to their laurels. Both specimens of codeia are splendid, and both are well worthy of the notice of the visitor.

MACKEY, MACKEY, and Co. show a cinchona preparation—Quinquina—which we would invite our medical brethren to notice as a substitute for quinine. It is worth their notice.

One of the most interesting exhibits is that of Mr. MARTINDALE. It contains a vast number of new substances and new preparations, together with some rare alkaloids; visitors will do well to give it a few minutes' attention. The "Poison Bag," as it is called, is something of a specialty; it was fitted up at the suggestion of Dr. Murrell, and contains all the requisites for dealing with any ordinary case of poisoning.

Messrs. MOTTERSHEAD and Co., of Manchester, show the peptic and pancreatic ferments so highly lauded by Dr. W. Roberts.

Messrs. NEWBERY and SONS show (for Messrs. Warner, if we are not mistaken) a great variety of sugar-coated pills. The great point claimed for them is that this coating is so readily soluble as to disappear in a few moments after swallowing. Certainly, in this respect, they are a great improvement on certain forms of coated pills largely used in this country.

Mr. HENRY J. PRATT shows a very good preparation of cod-liver oil—namely, cod-liver oil jelly; whilst Mr. J. M. RICHARDS exhibits his now well-known and highly useful lactopeptine in various forms and combinations.

Messrs. RICHARDSON and Co., of Leicester, have made a kind of specialty of thymol. They show what to many is new—a preparation intended for lubrication in midwifery, and rendered antiseptic by thymol; this is called thymol jelly. They are likewise strong in pearl-coated pills.

ROBBERTS and Co., of New Bond-street, are the sole re-presentatives of French pharmacy, they having a branch house in Paris. Their exhibit is worth notice, were it on this account alone.

SAVORY and MOORE are larger exhibitors, the most inte-resting feature of their stall is the great variety of medicine chests they show. In this respect they are unique, and to ordinary visitors the display is most instructive. Nor will many of our brethren fail to learn a good deal of the essentials of field medicine by an inspection of the various army chests, from the huge waggon pharmacy down to that carried by the orderly on the march or on the field of battle. We confess we were both interested and instructed. A highly useful little invention shown is that of lamels in great divided sheets, each little square containing the exact dose of the remedy required. To travellers afar off from medical aid these must be highly useful. So too, nearer home, will be the gelatine lamels containing doses of remedies for subcutaneous medication. Visitors should also take a look at the exceedingly complete chemical chest devised by Dr. Parkes, and containing every-thing necessary for the analysis of air and water just as it is supplied to expeditionary corps.

The specialty of Messrs. SCHUFFLIN and Co. is coated pills. All we need say of them, therefore, is that this coating seems excellent, even, uniform, and perfect.

Messrs. SOUTHALL BROTHERS and BARCLAY, of Birming-ham, have particularly turned their attention to absorbent disinfecting materials, which they here exhibit in various forms, of which "Tenax" is best known, and which has now been fairly proved to be most effectual. Their cod-liver oil is also excellent.

We have left ourselves but scanty space to do justice to what is probably the most magnificent of all the exhibits to be here seen. It is that of A. and M. ZIMMERMANN, who act as agents for many German houses. No one passing can fail to be struck with the splendid preparations sent by Schering, Berlin, the equally valuable products of Finzel-berg, of Rhodius, and of the Brunswick Quinine Factory. Those who visit the Exhibition cannot fail to see these, and those who see them once will look at them a second time.

SECTIONS I. TO VI.

SURGICAL INSTRUMENTS AND APPLIANCES.

[Second Notice.]

Messrs. KROHNE and SESEMANN, Duke-street, Manchester-square, W.—exhibit a good selection of new instruments and new modifications of old ones. We would draw attention to the laryngo-phantom. The apparatus was devised by Dr. Isenschmid, of Munich, to familiarise medical students and practitioners with as many of the details connected with the use of the laryngoscope as it is possible to learn before the application of the instrument to the living subject. The "phantom" consists of three parts. First, there is a mouth of thin metal, with tongue and uvula made of red velvet. This is fixed on a laryngeal tube of metal, which has a slit into which any of the thirty painted images of different views of the larynx can be introduced. The anatomical dimensions are taken from nature.

They show a full-sized model, on which are fitted Leiter's temperature regulators. They are made of pliable metal tubing, of any and every shape and size, and are capable of being bent so as to fit any part of the body. Either hot or cold water is kept continuously circulating, by means of which either artificial cold or warmth can be applied to a diseased part.

Dr. Renner's instruments used in vaccination were also to be seen. Dr. Renner, it seems, never uses the same lancet twice, so as to avoid all possibility of conveying infection from one patient to another. They have made a Thomas's splint in aluminium, which combines great strength with extreme lightness. Their midwifery instruments are many and varied, and all of excellent finish. Their eye instru-ments are worthy of special mention, as also their artifi-cial eyes, which are light, durable, and inexpensive. They are makers of a good pocket-case, particularly suitable for private nurses or ward sisters, containing caustic-case, dressing and artery forceps, probe and director, scissors, and a gum-lancet and abscess-knife combined. The case is provided with a ring for attaching to a belt. They have a neat tracheotomy case, with all the needful instruments; it is provided with the angular tubes which have recently been advocated as corresponding with the direction of the trachea better than quarter-circle tubes.

They are the agents for Martin's pure rubber bandage, many samples of which were shown us, and which appeared to be of a superior quality. Martin's adhesive plaster is worthy of its name, for it adheres almost too much. Another feature is Martin's ivory vaccine points. It is perhaps not so well known in this country that Dr. Martin has a large animal vaccine establishment, and is a strong advocate of this form of vaccination.

THE INTERNATIONAL SOCIETY FOR WOUND-DRESSING MATERIALS, Schaffhausen, Switzerland (Krohne and Sese-mann London agents).—This firm has among its directors von Bruns, von Nussbaum, Esmarch, and Volkmann. Could we wish for higher guarantees as to the excellence of the antiseptic hospital materials which it supplies? Among its specialities we may mention ol. juniperi catgut (Kocher's), carbolised silk (Czerny's), and iodoform gauze (Mikulics's). All kinds of gauze, catgut, protective, absorbent wool, etc., can be obtained at moderate prices.

Mr. MARTINDALE, New Cavendish-street, W.—exhibits among other things, "The Antidote Bag." It contains stomach-pump, male catheter, hypodermic case, and a series of chemicals and physiological antidotes for all the poisons usually met with. The labels give the doses and general directions. The practitioner, summoned in a hurry to a case of poisoning, will find such a bag of incalculable service. We also saw some cheap and effective inhalers; also an ingenious throat insufflator, which, by the way, would answer many other purposes. His eucalyptus gauze is worthy attention, as being hardly less effective than carbolic gauze, but without any of the irritating effects which the latter unfortunately possesses for some skins.

MILLIKIN and DOWN, St. Thomas-street, Borough, show a variety of instruments, mostly the inventions or suggestions of the Guy's staff. We saw a flexible tracheotomy tube, which may be useful in some cases, but which we should think is inferior to that proposed by Mr. Baker. There is a neat and useful dilating tracheotome, which will prove useful to beginners. They exhibit a skeleton with artificial ligaments, for demonstrating dislocations, etc., which strikes us as a valuable addition to a course of lectures on practical surgery. Their nippers for removing Sayre's jackets are well deserving attention. The "General Practitioner's Midwifery Bag" is a neat and useful arrangement, and well suited as a little present. Their carbolic sprays are elaborate and well made.

Messrs. ASH and SONS, Broad-street, Golden-square, W.—exhibit a great variety of dental instruments, artificial teeth, materials for stopping, etc. Their dental engine is very effective, and struck us as exceedingly ingenious : the handle into which forceps, burrs, excavators, engine-drills, and mallets fit, is worked with a treadle, and is capable of any and every movement. The stand is firm, and is yet so light as to be easily moved about the room. They show chairs of different kinds, which seem capable of almost any adaptation ; mineral teeth of feldspar and silex ; rubbers of Paris rubber ; and stoppings, either of amalgam or oxychloride of zinc. Apparatus for nitrous oxide gas is also shown ; as also vulcanisers.

Messrs. POCOCK BROTHERS, Southwark-bridge-road, S.E.—show their "Universal" invalid tubular water and air bed, which consists of a series of separate and distinct cylinders, any diameter and suitable length, made of waterproof material, either for water or air, fitting into a case which keeps them side by side, but slightly apart. Its advantages over ordinary water or air beds are as follows :—1. In cost it is less expensive. 2. It is quickly filled and easily adjusted. 3. It is warm and light, and well adapted for a camp or field-bed, being waterproof. 4. It admits of ventilation in the space between the tubes. 5. It can be regulated so as to relieve pressure from any part required. 6. By the addition of tubes it will raise one part of the body higher than the rest. 7. By the temporary removal of one or two tubes it affords room for the introduction of a bed-pan. 8. It can be inclined to any angle (even when filled with water) to suit the condition of the patient. 9. It is free from noise and surging, so disagreeable to the invalid on changing his position on a water-bed. 10. In case of injury to a tube it can be withdrawn, and a fresh one substituted at a trifling cost, and without loss of time ; whereas the ordinary water-bed if injured in any part (from being in one compartment) is rendered useless. 11. In the treatment of invalids, especially the insane, who are paralysed and have no control over their evacuations, they cannot lie in a pool of wet, the fluid passing away between the tubes.

This firm are making a very efficient padded room, a model of which is to be seen in the Exhibition. Safety, cleanliness, ventilation, and even comfort, are all thoughtfully cared for. All kinds of indestructible articles used by lunatics and other persons not able to control themselves can be seen at this stall.

Messrs. CHORLTON and DUGDALE, Blackfriars-street, Manchester—have on view chairs, couches, and beds, all of which are provided with their patent "Excelsior" spring. The spring appeared to us certainly to insure all the advantages which the makers claim for it. They say :—"The patented method of construction insures the most uniform elasticity, and provides for the separate and independent action of each part and section of the bed, allowing of complete adaptation to the form of the body, and affording a position of comfort and ease which induces sound, refreshing sleep, effectually preventing the weariness and discomfort incidental to great pressure on prominent parts of the body, which so often produces bed-sores. The principle of arrangement permits the free movement of one sleeper without inconvenience to the other, admits of complete isolation of each, and effectually prevents depression in the centre. Only a thin hair mattress being necessary, feather beds, cumbrous straw and flock palliasses are dispensed with ; cost of bedding is much reduced, and bed-making

becomes far less laborious ; sweetness and purity—conditions so essential to health—result from the change." The beds and couches are made in different qualities to suit different customers ; but the essential part—the spring—is of course identical in each, the higher priced goods being of greater external finish. Their patent spring chairs, either with or without the leg-rests, are most comfortable, and for invalids with heart or breathing troubles will prove of immense service. The construction of the spring will effectually prevent their getting out of order. They also show a "pillow divider." "Whenever two people occupy the same bed, it is essential for their health's sake alone, irrespective of additional comfort, that a pillow divider should be used, for by this means the unwholesomeness of two persons inhaling, at times, each other's breath is completely avoided." They also show an "Excelsior" spring ship's berth, as supplied to the Union Company's South African line of steamers, the comfort of which we can vouch for.

Mr. W. HAMILTON, Ship-street, Brighton—showed us his "Grasshopper" couch—an inexpensive, comfortable couch, which possesses various movements, either to raise the head or the knees, according to the requirements of the occupier. If raised a little higher, it would prove useful for the professional man, either for examining patients or for operations in the consulting-room. The movements can either be by rackwork or by a screw—the former are the quicker and handier, the latter the more quiet and slow, and such as invalids would prefer. These couches can be had covered in cretonne, satin, damask, or silk and wool tapestry, so that, besides being very useful in any household, they may be made to look ornamental as well.

Mr. SEELEY, Broadway, New York, and Philadelphia—exhibits a new form of truss. They are made of hard rubber in every desirable pattern, fitting perfectly to the form of the body ; light, cool, cleanly, and free from all sour smell, padding, or strapping. They may be used in bathing, and seem always reliable.

Mr. JOHN CARTER, 6A, New Cavendish-street, W.—The inventions and specialties of this maker have long been known to the profession. One of his newest patents is an invalid couch or bed, with descending cushion for commode arrangement. Its novel features are—by turning a handle the centre part of the cushion under the seat descends or rises automatically, without any disturbance of the patient or disarrangement of the bed-clothes. When it is down, a trapped earthenware pan is inserted under the orifice, through a slide in the side. By this plan the offensiveness and inconvenience attendant on the use of the bed-pan are avoided, the greatest possible comfort and cleanliness secured for the patient, and bed-sores prevented, as the centre cushion can be raised or lowered so as to vary the pressure due to the weight of the body. The back, knees, and feet frames are adjustable to any inclination. The mechanism is simple, and can be easily managed by a servant. The reading-easels are very convenient—so much so, as to encourage the healthy to grow lazy ; for invalids, however, invaluable. His carrying-chairs, light, yet strong, are admirably adapted for private houses. Bath chairs, spinal carriages, are also shown, and deserve attention.

Messrs. MONK and Co., Great Russell-street, W.C., manufacturers of invalid chairs—show different patterns of spinal carriages, adjustable couches, bed-rests, and folding chairs. They are all deserving of attention, and will doubtless recommend themselves to the notice of those who are unfortunately in want of such furniture.

Mr. STIDOLPH, High-street, Dartford—exhibits his " Improved Institution Bedstead.' Among its special features may be mentioned—the frame is made of wrought iron, light and neat in effect, free from projections, is perfectly rigid, and cannot break ; as the canvas bottom requires no lacing, there is neither hole nor hem, and being double and endless, its place on the bearings (which are frictionless) and the portion lain upon may be constantly shifted, making it thereby almost indestructible ; the tension can be always kept extreme—any slackness resulting from use may be instantly rectified, and cannot go back. From the principle of construction and arrangement of sacking the greatest strength with the most agreeable buoyancy are combined, affording comfort with one light mattress equivalent to that obtained by the use of three times the quantity of bedding on an ordinary bedstead, promoting thereby health, cleanliness, and economy. The bedstead may be had in various qualities and prices. The maker has quite recently improved on the castors upon which these beds move. Made much larger than usual, and provided with a vulcanite tire, they move easily and noiselessly, and there is less wear and tear of the carpet. We consider this castor a great improvement on the older form.

Messrs. MATHEWS BROTHERS, Carey-street, W.C.—One of the special features of this exhibit is a very clever steam spray, with influx pump, the object being to economise time in getting up steam; it is provided with a safety valve, by which all fear of accident seems to be avoided. We saw a hæmorrhoidal clamp which ought certainly to be very effective. There is a truss worthy of notice, designed, we believe, by Mr. Wood.

Messrs. MAW, SON, and THOMPSON, Aldersgate-street, E.C. —have a large and varied collection of instruments, including the regulation operation and amputation cases. One of the features of this firm is the variety and excellence of the much-used aspirator. The best with which we are acquainted (Potain's, of Paris) seems to have been improved on by this firm, for the syringe has been so arranged that it answers equally well either for exhausting or injecting. Their bladder instruments seem to include all the latest improvements. They also show quite a number of electric batteries of various patterns and prices; they are too complicated to allow of any detailed description in such a notice as this one. India-rubber bandages, which are still largely used, are shown of different sizes; also the pure Para rubber from which they are manufactured. We need hardly say that a goodly number of spray-producers are on view.

Messrs. FERGUSSON, Smithfield, E.C.—show pocket cases and midwifery instruments, also aspirators of different forms and lithotomy apparatus. We noticed Dr. Steavenson's splint for fractured patella. It consists of india-rubber bands passing crosswise above and below the fractured halves of the patella, and so tending to bring them into apposition.

Messrs. W. and J. JAMIESON, Broad-street, W.—show a variety of dental instruments and appliances. Among their specialties must be mentioned the crystal gold cylinders, blocks, and polygon pellets for fittings. The qualities which they claim for their gold are—its being unequalled for softness and adhesiveness under manipulation, its density when finished, and the facility with which it can be adapted to irregularities of the walls of cavities. Also, they have on view pluggers of different kinds, burrs, excavators, scalers, chisels, etc. We saw an ingenious atmospheric suction-valve. They have prepared a new and improved impression plastic compound, which, after being placed in hot water, becomes so soft as to be readily moulded and compressed without the use of much force, whereby all fear of causing pain is obviated, as well as the danger of disturbing the relative position and form of the surfaces to be moulded.

Mr. T. McILROY, 115, Charlotte-street, Fitzroy-square, W. —exhibits several very ingenious contrivances, in the way of beds, chairs, and head-rests; also an operating-table and a post-mortem table, which can be raised to and will revolve at any height. It is provided with a flow-pipe, which carries off fluids and exerts a downward ventilation intended to draw off noxious smells. It also gives the weight of the body by means of a balance, the lever of which, as we saw for ourselves, is turned even by a shilling. All these appliances display great mechanical skill, and the large number of awards and prizes obtained by the inventor bespeak a large amount of public approval. An invalid carrying-chair is a marvel of ingenuity; it can be opened and shut up again in a few seconds, and is so light withal as to be easily carried about.

Mr. McIlroy is agent for the Chartaline Blanket Company, who exhibit samples of their Chartaline blankets, and the disinfectant hospital blanket of the same material.

The well-known properties of paper in preventing the too rapid radiation of heat have been utilised in the manufacture of these articles. They are composed of a layer of wadding between two outer sheets of prepared paper, perforated for ventilation; they are light, warm, cleanly, and very cheap. One is declared by competent authorities to be equal in warmth to two pairs of ordinary woollen blankets. The disinfectant hospital blanket is similar, with the addition of a disinfectant. It retains all the warmth of a

Chartaline blanket, and has the additional merit of disinfecting the bed-clothing, thus reducing the risk of infection almost to a minimum.

For the poor such blankets must prove very serviceable. Charitable people would do well to supply these in preference to the common things (which afford but little warmth) so frequently given. The hospital blanket may prove useful in checking bad smells, whether in hospitals or private houses.

Mr. THOMAS ALLEN, Bristol—shows his improved patent tubular bedsteads, invalid bed-rest, and children's cots. The bedsteads are formed entirely of metal tubes, and elastic wood laths or canvas bottom, and combine every advantage as regards solidity, cleanliness, comfort, and durability. They require only one mattress, and can be taken apart or put together in a few minutes; are specially adapted for hospitals and lunatic asylums, as well as for general use. The children's cots struck us especially as well made and very convenient; their sides let down by means of a simple contrivance not likely to get out of order. They are provided with trays, which move up and down on noiseless rollers. Their peculiar construction gives lightness with strength. They are used in many public institutions.

The LONDON HOSPITALS exhibit beds and ward appliances. Lay figures have been secured, instead of patients, but otherwise one might almost fancy oneself in a hospital ward. The beds are placed in a somewhat out-of-the-way position, and there are scarcely sufficient indications to direct visitors to them.

The London Hospital shows the methods in use there of treating fracture of the thigh and of the leg, the former by a long outside splint of peculiar construction, and a weight running over a pulley at the foot of the bed; the leg splint consists of a back piece and side splints. We noticed the method of recording what diet a patient is taking—a wire rack hangs at the head of the bed, and each article of diet (as recorded on a card) occupies a little niche provided for it. Thus we see "full," "two eggs," "wine," etc. This must be very convenient for the surgeon.

Guy's Hospital (which has monopolised nearly half the space, and sends eight beds out of the thirty-two exhibited) is about the only one which is at all adequately represented. This is a model of a nurse in uniform, full size; the lockers are fully equipped, while the very pots and pans used in the wards are duly represented by specimen delegates. There is also a model of a tracheotomy tent. We hope for the sake of the patients that the prototype of this model has long since ceased to exist. There is a very neat cot enclosed with curtains, very much better adapted for the purpose and more in accordance with modern notions, which teach that the patients who need enclosed beds shall not on that account be entirely shut off from fresh air.

The Hospital for Sick Children is represented by two beds and a cot; while name and diet cards, a half-used bottle of medicine, nursing chair, dolls, etc., serve to complete the show. The method of treating osteotomy and disease of the hip is represented on the dummies occupying the beds.

Charing-Cross Hospital has three beds, in one of which the method of after-treatment of excision of the hip is indicated; in another, that of excision of the knee joint; while the ordinary way of applying extension is indicated on a third case. A modified "anterior" splint is also shown.

King's College Hospital is chiefly represented by a very unsatisfactory croup tent. The child's cot is placed beneath a large tent made of thick red blanket—material which we should think would effectually shut out both light and fresh air. The method of applying extension is also shown, and Professor Lister's dressing may be seen too.

St. Thomas's Hospital is represented by one bed; the lay figure is completely swathed in well-applied bandages, whereby the limbs are so hidden from sight that gangrene might threaten and set in before the surgeon was aware of it. The Bavarian plaster splints for the arm can be well studied in this bed.

St. Bartholomew's Hospital has three beds and one child's cot. The arrangement for slinging the arm will commend itself; as also a splint for fractured leg. The long outside splint (apparently) for fracture of the femur has a joint at the pelvis, which may or may not be an advantage, though it is certainly a convenience to the patient.

The Middlesex Hospital is chiefly noteworthy on account of an ugly, but effectual, contrivance for lifting a patient into and out of a bath. The method of putting up a fractured leg in a box splint and slinging in a Salter's cradle is very neat and comfortable. De Morgan's splint for excision or disease of hip is good.

St. George's Hospital sends two beds, in which the dummy is splinted up in a good old style. The crockery articles stand on a framework above the head of the bed; whether this is the arrangement actually in use or not we cannot say, but it did not strike us as "quite up to mark."

From Netley is represented a figure with *estempore* dressings in the field. The rifle has been applied as a long outside splint, and is fastened on with what look like pockethandkerchiefs. The bayonet has been applied to the arm in a similar manner. On another leg are to be seen some cane splints.

A series of dhoolies of different kinds and ages is likewise exhibited.

Models of the windows in different hospitals are shown.

Many of the above hospitals send specimens of their croup beds. They mostly seem founded on the plan originated at Great Ormond-street, which consists essentially of an ordinary cot, to which an iron or wooden framework has been attached, and over which either a special tent or a couple of ordinary sheets have been thrown. The old blanket has long since been discarded, and, instead of an apparatus which simply supplies steam, the so-called ventilating croup-kettle (made by James Allen and Son) may most advantageously be adopted. By the latter arrangement, fresh, moistened, and warm air is conducted into these enclosed beds.

These hospital fittings and arrangements are doubtless of interest, if only to show how similar ends may be attained by different methods. It is hardly to be expected that one hospital will alter its usual mode, and adopt that of another one, without good reason. We should like to know whether the plans of treatment as shown represent hospitals or their surgeons—whether they are universally used by all the surgeons; for, if not, the purpose of this exhibition will have been but very partially carried out, except in the case of Guy's Hospital. We think, too, it would have been well to have supplemented the exhibits with details of the principle and with specimens of the various splints—for when a splint is put on, it cannot be examined, especially when, as in some cases, every part of it is bandaged over.

But it would certainly be of interest if the Parkes Museum Committee could get a series of small models from the different hospitals, from different surgeons, for permanent exhibition in their future building, each one absolutely correct, and all done to a common scale. In generations to come such a collection would no doubt prove amusing, if not actually very instructive.

Mr. S. R. J. WINTER, of Goodge-street—shows a variety of bandages. We have had an opportunity of examining and trying these bandages, and believe them to be good in quality and reasonable in price. The absorbent bandages are particularly good and worthy of trial. He supplies cottonwools of various qualities.

Messrs. SOUTHALL BROTHERS and BARCLAY, Birmingham—exhibit their now well-known sanitary towels, absorbent and antiseptic pads and sheets. Likewise prepared millboard splints and arm-pieces, which we should like to try when the opportunity serves.

Messrs. ROBINSON and SONS, Wheatbridge Mills, Chesterfield—exhibit cotton-wools, bandages, and lints of various qualities: some of the ordinary kind, some of an absorbent nature. The bandages appeared very soft, but we were unable to handle them, and therefore cannot express a decided opinion.

We were rather surprised to see so few exhibits of bandage materials; for there is at present considerable room for improvement in this article. Especially objectionable is the "dressing" or "facing" powder, with which so many of the bandage materials are charged: for besides lending to them a quality which they do not require—namely, harshness—it makes them sources of danger. This "facing powder," on being wetted, tends to decomposition, the prevention of which is the great end of all our present "antiseptic" precautions. Bandages of a soft yet strong material, which allows of easy and rapid absorption, are the great desiderata at present.

The SANITAS COMPANY'S preparations, though belonging to Section VII., may be mentioned in connexion with surgical dressings. Carbolic acid is doubtless a most important antiseptic, but it has the misfortune to cause considerable irritation of the skin in many persons, especially in children. In such cases, we believe, Sanitas will be found an efficient substitute. It is supplied as oil, a very powerful deodoriser, disinfectant, and antiseptic; as fluid; in the form of soap of different qualities; as a powder, and for toilet purposes. Over carbolic acid it has the advantage of being agreeable and aromatic; it does not stain or injure clothes; while we think it is almost equally effective.

SECTION IX.

Mr. MEDLAND, 12, Borough, London-bridge—exhibits a practical physiology cabinet and microscope companion. This cabinet has been arranged in as small and compact a manner as possible, so as to have all the necessary apparatus used in the practical physiology class, etc., ready for immediate use, and avoiding the inconvenience and delay occasioned by having loose a number of small articles, many of which are very liable to injury or breakage. The contents, which may be slightly varied, according to the requirements of the various hospitals, are as follows:—Scalpel, forceps (straight or curved), scissors, spatula or section-lifter, needles in handles, razor, spirit lamp, pipette, bottles with droppers, bottles with brushes, evaporating dishes, 3" by 1" glass slips, thin glass covers, watch-glasses, camel-hair brushes, glass rod, gummed labels, pencil, palettes for cleaning covers, note-book, together with trays for microscopic specimens. The cabinet seems to us to be well made. Every student would do well to be provided with such a useful companion.

SECTION X.

In this section we noticed Mr. WILLIAM COWAN'S Vaccination Shield, made of wire and cotton. It is intended to protect the vaccine pustule from friction during sleep and at other times. In times of epidemic such as the present it seems to us a very useful and effective little appliance, and one whose price places it within reach of everyone. It can be had of all chemists.

SECTION XII.

STREET AMBULANCES, ETC.

Messrs. EVANS and WORMULL, Stamford-street, S.E.—exhibit a well-arranged "Ambulance" bag, containing all the requirements for the first dressing of wounds in the field.

The ORDER of ST. JOHN of JERUSALEM—show an ambulance wheeled litter, from which the stretcher can be detached without disturbing the patient; it is made of wood, metal, and canvas.

The ST. JOHN'S AMBULANCE ASSOCIATION—show a folding stretcher, weighing about twenty-three pounds; also a portable hamper, containing articles required in rendering first aid to the injured, and other articles of a kindred nature.

The "Ashford" litter, built under the superintendence of, and exhibited by, Mr. J. FURLEY. This consists of a folding stretcher with automatic pillow and a waterproof cover placed upon a light two-wheeled carriage. One of the principal merits of this conveyance is that the stretcher requires no complicated additions to fix it, and the bearers can pass between the wheels over a crank axle without the necessity of lifting it over the wheels as is usually done. This litter only weighs 111 lbs., and costs £10 10s.

SECTION XVII.

SCHOOL FURNITURE, CLOTHING, BOOKS, ETC.

Messrs. COLEMAN and GLENDINNING, Wigmore-street, W., and Norwich—show a selection of their school furniture. The great importance of properly shaped seats and properly distanced desks has been referred to more than once in our columns, and is a matter of great importance to weakly children especially, who are nowadays obliged to sit long hours in schools. We examined various desks and seats, and would especially draw the attention of schoolmasters and others interested in the matter to this exhibit. They show also an "automaton" seat for drapers' assistants, the low price of which ought to recommend it.

There are two or three forms of window-sashes capable of

being reversed for cleaning, thus avoiding the danger to life incident to ordinary sash windows which can only be cleaned from outside; and a wonderfully cheap and clever little clamp, the "Toby," for fixing the cords of the heaviest venetian blind, or indeed for supporting any weight.

Mr. ALBERT FRADELLE, 246, Regent-street—shows a collection of medical photographic portraits. Whether they be regarded as likenesses, or as samples of the photographic art, they leave but little to be desired. We could wish to see a complete collection of all the expected visitors to the Congress next month; it would be a pleasing souvenir of what is sure to be an almost unique gathering of the medical profession.

Messrs. WILLIAM BENGER and SONS, Stuttgart, Germany (Messrs. Newberger, Wood-street, Cheapside, E.C., sole English agents)—showed us some "stocking net" hosiery of admirable texture and make—under-vests and drawers, single or combined, for both men and women, which they have patented. They are made of the finest and purest wool and are highly elastic. The chest and shoulders are of double thickness, thus protecting the parts which most require it. For travellers, officers of the army, navy, or mercantile service, we should have no doubt that they will prove most useful articles of underclothing. Their prices are such as to place them within the reach of all.

Messrs. CHURCHILL, New Burlington-street, the only firm who limit themselves to medical books, show a selection of their publications on medicine and its collateral branches. As would be expected, it embraces most of the best known text-books in all branches of medical science, besides some of the oldest series of periodical literature which the profession possesses. Their illustrated works of themselves form a very handsome library; among them may be mentioned:— Lancereaux's "Atlas of Pathological Anatomy," translated by W. S. Greenfield, M.D.; Godlee's "Atlas of Human Anatomy"; Braune's "Atlas of Topographical Anatomy, after Plane Sections of Frozen Bodies," translated by E. Bellamy, F.R.C.S.; Maclise's "Surgical Anatomy: a Series of Dissections illustrating the Principal Regions of the Human Body"; Sibson's "Medical Anatomy," 21 imp. folio coloured plates and text; Heath's "Course of Operative Surgery," with 20 plates drawn from nature by Léveillé; Hutchinson's "Illustrations of Clinical Surgery"; Maclise's "Dislocations and Fractures"; G. H. Fox's "Photographic Illustrations of Cutaneous Syphilis"; also Tilbury Fox's "Atlas of Skin Diseases," with 72 coloured plates.

Mr. DAVID BOGUE, 3, St. Martin's-place, W.C.—shows a collection of works on social and sanitary science, and on general literature. We observed his Twining's "Science made Easy"—a connected and progressive course of lectures, and accompanying diagrams, which appear excellent.

Messrs. SAMPSON LOW, MARSTON, and Co., Crown-buildings, Fleet-street, are also represented among other books by Ziemssen's huge Encyclopædia, the translation of which from the German was initiated and largely carried out by our American cousins over the water.

Messrs. TRÜBNER and Co., Ludgate-hill, E.C.—are represented by a selection of works on veterinary, chemical, dental, and sanitary science, largely of American origin. They are agents for an American patent revolving book-case of novel design and very convenient. Full particulars and drawings can be obtained at their stall.

Messrs. SMITH, ELDER, and Co., 15, Waterloo-place, Pallmall—exhibit books and diagrams both on medical and hygienic subjects.

SECTION XIV.
VENTILATION, LIGHTING, AND WARMING.

In America the superiority of the hard coals over the soft for all purposes, save that of making gas, has long been recognised; here, however, the use of ANTHRACITE (which must not be confounded with steam coal) has, until the last few years, been confined to the drying of malt and hops. Pure anthracite—stone-coal, as it is called in Wales—is found in a limited area only, and is the extreme term of the hard series, as Boghead cannel is of the soft. It contains 92 to 94 per cent. of carbon, 0·6 of sulphur, and 1 to 1·6 of ash; whereas the best of the time-honoured Newcastle coals give about 82 of carbon, 1·7 of sulphur, and 7 or 8 of ash. Anthracite is hard, clean, and almost free from smoke, ash,

and sulphurous fumes; it is, however, often hard to light, especially in old-fashioned stoves, but burns well in the "slow combustion," and, in fact, in all new and improved stoves and ranges. Some beautiful samples of anthracite are exhibited here by the company into which the owners of the true anthracite beds have formed themselves, with offices at 19, Spring-street, Paddington.

Mr. EDWARDS, jun., of Great Marlborough-street, well-known as a writer on warming and ventilation, shows his new smoke-consuming and slow combustion stove, founded on the original idea of Dr. Arnott. Like his, it is filled with coals sufficient for the whole day or night, and lighted from above, but instead of raising a coal-basket, Mr. Edwards lowers a blind in front, balanced by chains and weights like a window-sash, as the fuel burns down. The register in the chimney is opened or closed by means of a chain and button in the front, above the opening of the stove, thus avoiding soiling of the hands. Small coal or cinders falling from the grate are received in a wire basket concealed from view, the fine ash falling through into a pan below. It requires no coal-scuttle except at lighting, makes no smoke after it is fairly kindled, and burns for twelve or more hours without attention. The only fire-iron is a small trident, and the chimney will not need sweeping oftener than once in ten years. A neater, better grate for small rooms or bedrooms cannot well be conceived, though it may be had in sizes fitted for waiting-rooms at railways, halls, etc.

The Tortoise stoves, of iron, lined with fire-clay, and closed, exhibited by C. PORTWAY and SON, are also constructed to burn anthracite. One form is furnished with a boiler with pipes and coils, and will be found greatly preferable to the ordinary furnaces seen in greenhouses generally.

HUNT'S Crown Jewel stove for warming halls and waiting-rooms with anthracite is a handsome object; and Mr. SAXON SNELL'S noble-looking Thermohydric Stove, which ventilates, warms, and regulates the moisture of the air, is too well known to need description. So are George's Calorigens, exhibited by FARWIG and Co.

The closed chimney above a kitchen range has many advantages over the older open one, but it prevents the ascent of the smells arising from cooking. Messrs. STEVEN BROS. and Co. meet this objection by inserting two or more ventilators, each consisting of two cones, the lower truncated, the upper and larger one overlapping it and separated from it by a space of about an inch; free exit is thus afforded to the vapours, while the fall of soot is excluded.

The "Wonderful Grate" (Russell's Patent), exhibited by ARCHIBALD SMITH and STEVENS, and constructed to burn anthracite with a quick or a slow draught, is an ingenious but rather complex and costly contrivance. It admits warm fresh air, and, swinging on an axis with a counterpoise, can be enlarged or reduced at pleasure. It forms a kind of hopper at the end of a pipe charged with the day's supply of coal and serving as a feeder. By means of damper in the front compartment of a double chimney the products of combustion are directed down through the fire to be consumed with an increased draught. If the damper be opened it works as an ordinary slow combustion grate. It may be seen in operation, and is highly commended by the Engineer.

A clever idea of Mr. RENTON GIBBS, the patentee of many hot-water apparatus, etc., is an open grate, the bars of which form part of a hot-water coil by which an adjoining or other room may be warmed at the same time; if this be not desired the connexion can be cut off. Its application seems, however, limited.

RITCHIE'S Lux Calor is an elegant, inexpensive, and most ingenious contrivance for heating and lighting and ventilating at the same time. There is no flue required, no dust, smoke, or smell, and the products of combustion are entirely condensed and intercepted in water. It burns gas or, where that is not available, petroleum, but there is no naked flame. It consists of three columns; in the middle one there is an argand, the side columns are double cylinders, the burnt air with its aqueous vapour and gases pass into a box over the burner, and thence by branches right and left into the outer cylinders, warming the pure air admitted by the inner one, and are condensed in a receiver at the base.

The best possible testimony to its efficiency is that of Messrs. Veitch, the eminent florists, who tried it in a lean-to house, facing the north, 50 ft. × 12 ft., when there were 10° of frost outside, and found it absolutely innocuous to the most delicate foliage and flowers, even at six inches from the stove, while the whole space was satisfactorily warmed. Such a test was indeed a crucial one.

BOYLE's and BUCHAN's Ventilators have long established their reputation. We need here only remark that, being fixed, they cannot, like revolving ones, get out of order, while their exhausting power with the gentlest wind exceeds that of any others. They are really ornamental, which is more than can be said of many. Mr. Buchan has an ingenious ventilator for railway carriages, the so-called ventilators in which are worse than useless. In this he employs the motion of the carriage as a powerful abstractor, the fresh air entering by other inlets.

Dr. NEALE, of South Hampstead, exhibits diagrams and working models of his recently patented "Chemical Lung" for the removal from the air of tunnels, mines, and heated and crowded places of assembly, of noxious gases, especially carbonic acid and sulphur compounds, by causing the air to pass over or through caustic alkalies, lime and other chemicals. Applied to rooms and buildings it assumes the form of a punkah, combining mechanical ventilation with chemical purification; in shafts of mines the air is driven by a centrifugal fan or other mechanism through tanks of the reagent, and for special use in the underground railway he proposes to attach to each train a waggon carrying a number of screens charged with the requisite chemicals against which the air will impinge obliquely in the progress of the train. We believe that he had first proposed to conduct the smoke from the funnel of the engine through a tank containing the alkaline solution, but that this plan was abandoned as impracticable. The idea of the chemical lung is ingenious, and in some of its applications original, but we are not aware of its having been as yet tried on a large scale. The air of the Metropolitan Railway, of the law courts and theatres, to say nothing of mines, presents a wide field for some such scheme of purification.

Drs. DRYSDALE and HAYWARD, of Liverpool, exhibit a model of a house illustrating the system of combined warming and ventilation, devised by themselves and described in their work " Health and Comfort in House-building." Fresh air admitted in the basement and warmed by a special heating apparatus enters the house by openings in the rises of the stairs, and from the passages gains access to the rooms by apertures behind the architraves of the doors, etc. The foul air from each room rises through cornice ventilators to a chamber in the roof, whence it descends by a shaft, and ascends again by another encircling the kitchen chimney, its ascent being aided by the heat of that fire, or by a gas-jet in its absence, and by an exhausting cowl at the summit. It is not easily introduced into existing houses, but in those specially constructed for it, its success is complete. Entire freedom from draughts, a uniform pleasant temperature in passages and rooms, with constant purity of air in even the smallest apartments, are practically achieved.

Messrs. BENHAM and SONS show a common parlour grate altered into one of Dr. Siemens', which, burning both gas and coke, or anthracite, combines the convenience of a gas-stove with the economy and cheerful appearance of a coal fire. By discarding as useless the copper back and gills of his earlier form, he has greatly reduced the prime cost. The gas, unmixed with air, is kindled along a perforated iron pipe running parallel with the lowest bars, while the products of its combustion are completely burned by passing through the mass of incandescent anthracite above, the gaseous and solid fuel mutually aiding each other's combustion, and giving out the maximum of heat.

Of simple anthracite grates, that of Crane, exhibited by Messrs. DRANE and Co., seems to possess the greatest warming power.

Other exhibits in this section deserving of special notice are an ingenious screen for washing the air entering a room from dust and blacks, in the form of a double or V-shaped louvre of glass, the air impinging on the surface of the water in the troughs, shown by Mr. RENTON GIBB; architrave and other ventilators on Currull's plan, designed by Mr. MARK JUDGE; the ventilating tubes and brackets of Messrs. VERITY and of the SANITARY ENGINEERING COMPANY; the apparatus of the SUN AUTOPNEUMATIC LIGHTING

AND HEATING COMPANY, for making a pure gas in private houses, by the saturation of air with hydrocarbon vapour—the patentees having apparently overcome the difficulties hitherto found to arise from the condensation of the vapours by employing a larger surface and a lower temperature than others; E. W. WINFIELD's ventilating gas-lamps, shut off from the air of the room, and another by BENHAM and SONS.

The number and variety of stoves and heating apparatus are too great to permit of particular notice, and too many of them present no new features whatever.

W. J. FRASER and Co., 98, Commercial-road, E., exhibit three forms of disinfecting apparatus, in each of which the bedding, etc., are exposed to a current of air at a temperature of 250° to 300° Fahr., impregnated, if desired, with sulphurous or other vapours, the outgoing air being passed through the fire. One is adapted for use in hospitals, etc.; in another, intended for sanitary authorities, the articles are introduced in an iron truck, in which they are conveyed to and from the houses of the owners, closely shut during transit; the third, which obtained the prize medal at the Exhibition of the Sanitary Institute at Croydon in 1879, is designed for country and camp use, being in the form of a one-horse van, which can be taken to the infected house or village.

A self-regulating disinfecting chamber, designed by Dr. Scott, is exhibited by Messrs. MAGUIRE. In this the heat, which is, of course, dry, is obtained from gas-burners within the chamber. The specialty seems to consist in the adoption of Dr. Ransome's idea of taking advantage of the low melting-point of certain alloys. Whenever the temperature exceeds 300° Fahr., a button of fusible metal (Dr. Ransome used a link of a chain) softens, and giving way, causes the gas to be cut off.

But we must specially commend one conceived by Mr. WASHINGTON LYON, of Cowper's-court, Cornhill, consisting of an air-tight receptacle into which superheated and saturated, but not wet, aqueous vapour is driven under pressure regulated by a steam-gauge. Thus not only are the injurious actions of dry heat and of boiling water on horsehair, feathers, silks, etc., avoided, but the penetration of the heat to the centres of mattresses, feather beds, bundles of letters, etc., is insured, as experiments have proved, by the displacement of the air contained in their interstices by the compressed and heated vapour. The most delicate fabrics come out uninjured, but the presence of vapour in the air renders it far more fatal to living organisms, such as we believe disease germs to be, than even a higher temperature if dry. Like Fraser's, it too may be fixed or portable. We have no hesitation in pronouncing it in every way the best apparatus of its kind.

Messrs. BENHAM also show a disinfecting chamber on the same principle as Mr. Lyon's.

SECTION XV.

WATER-CLOSETS, SINKS, BATHS, ETC.; SEWERAGE AND DRAINAGE.

The earth column of Mr. BARNARD is an ingenious attempt to intercept and mix with earth not only the solid, but the liquid excreta, for subsequent application to the land. The soil-pipe of the w.c. passes into a cylinder of iron containing fresh earth; the liquids are then conducted through a series of earthenware chambers, also containing earth, until a well filtered and, as the inventor believes, purified fluid only enters the sewer. The gases are conducted up a ventilating shaft charged with charcoal. The first, or iron, receptacle is to be removed weekly, and immediately replaced by an empty one, the earthenware boxes at longer intervals. It seems to us open to all the objections that can be urged against the dry-earth system, but in a greatly enhanced degree. The wet earth, even if it do not become water-logged, cannot possibly retain the antiseptic properties that dry earth alone possesses; putrefaction must proceed, and gases escape from the earthenware boxes, which make no pretensions to impermeability; and should a case of enteric fever occur, the consequences might be disastrous. There is good evidence that even dry earth does not destroy disease germs, but this wet-earth system, whatever the manurial value of the products may be, seems to us the worst mode of "conservancy" yet proposed from a sanitary point of view. We must confess that the samples of the effluent water which are stated to have received forty and sixty discharges respectively, are free from all perceptible colour or smell, but this is entirely a different question.

THE ANTISEPTIC APPARATUS MANUFACTURING COMPANY exhibit their contrivance for destroying foul gases in water-closets by injecting into the pan a small quantity of Condy's or other fluid at the moment of flushing, or during use, at the will of the user.

There is an ample display of water-closets of the most approved patterns by all the principal makers—Jennings, Tylor, Underhay, etc.—which are already well known to our readers. BUCHAN'S patent "Carmichael" wash-down accessible appears to be as good as any. Bostel's, highly spoken of by competent judges, though most effectually excluding the escape of gases, seems to us to present to steep an ascent to the exit of the excreta—a defect from which Buchan's is especially free. His "Cascade" ventilating drain trap is the best of its kind.

A real novelty in drain-pipes are the ribbed pipes just brought out by EDWARD BROOKE AND SONS. Four short longitudinal ribs greatly increase the resistance of the pipe to the weight of the superincumbent earth, while the lowest one supports it in the space between the joints standing out flush with the flanges.

W. INGHAM exhibits another novelty in Stanford's joint —a band of composition at either end, accurately turned so as to present two conical surfaces in close apposition, but capable of a slight ball-and-socket movement. There is no need for luting, the joint being so correct that even without any grease or cement it is practically water-tight.

Messrs. STEVEN BROS. and Co. show an improved trough closet for schools, barracks, etc., made in lengths for any number of persons up to ten, which (or that of Messrs. Wilcocks), we heartily recommend to school architects as more cleanly than any we have seen.

There are many forms of flushing tanks on the syphon plan more or less resembling that of Mr. Roger Field, and one in the shape of an unequally balanced tip-up basin; but the chief novelty in this line is that of Messrs. MAGUIRE, in which the overflow is conducted into a bucket suspended to one arm of a balance, the other carrying the plug of the tank by a chain. When the bucket is full, the plug rises, and the tank is speedily emptied; the bucket, having a small aperture in its bottom (being, in fact, leaky), has time to discharge itself wholly or in part before receiving a fresh overflow. Its contents must be carried away by a small gulley or other conduit. The simplicity of the contrivance is almost amusing.

Among the numerous water-waste preventers, BRAITH-WAITE'S patent syphon stands pre-eminent for simplicity and efficiency, there being no valves or holes in the bottom of the cistern. This is divided into two compartments communicating with one another by a small opening : in one the ball-valve works, in the other the waste-preventer. The service-pipe of the closet passes over the brim in the form of a syphon, the shorter or inner leg of which is a cylinder in its lower half, and in this there works a piston that, being raised, forces the water over into the other leg, setting the syphon in action, when a loose plate in the bottom of the piston rises, and allows the water to flow until the compartment is emptied.

The sanitary pipes of Messrs. MATHESON and GARDNER (Haines' patent ?), made of block tin cased in lead, not of lead washed with tin, ought in all cases to take the place of the odious lead pipes for house service, as BARFF'S "Anti-corrodo" iron should for the ordinary mains. Sections of these pipes twisted like corkscrews are shown to demonstrate the intimate cohesion of the two metals, and the resistance of the tin core to the effects of torsion.

JOHN REYNARD PICKARD exhibits a carbonising oven and a furnace for the reduction of town refuse on the plan which we recently described in a notice of Fryer's cremation and carbonising processes, adopted in several of the great towns of the Northern counties. There is a large number of earth, ash, and charcoal dry closets, all good in their way.

It would be impossible to describe even a tithe of the water-closets, baths, and traps of every conceivable shape exhibited in this section, but POTTS' patent Edinburgh air-chambered trap, though rather cumbrous, is effective and accessible, but inferior to Buchan's on the score of size and cost.

SECTION XVI.
WATER-SUPPLY AND FILTRATION.

Among the many exhibitors of filters we miss the well-known name of Mr. Lipscombe, but besides the silicated carbon and manganous carbon (Dr. Bernays' patent) there are three which merit a separate mention—Major CREASE's, adopted in our Army, and found very efficient where rapid filtration is required; MAIGNEN's "Filtre Rapide"; and BISCHOF's Spongy Iron. Maignen's Filtre Rapide differs in its entire principle from those usually employed. It consists of a filter case, a conical perforated filter frame, covered with asbestos cloth, on the outside of which a layer of the filtering medium (called by the inventor carbo-calcis), consisting of the best animal charcoal boiled in lime-water, is automatically deposited by the current of the first water passed through the filter, and an earthenware diaphragm resting on the apex of the filter frame. An air-pipe, which may be plugged with cotton-wool, enters the apex of the cone to aërate the water in its transit. Depending on the relatively large filtering surface, and the lessened pressure resulting from lateral percolation in place of vertical filtration, the inventor claims to be able to filter large quantities of water with great rapidity and without the risk of forcing suspended particles through the strainer. In some forms there is an outer case or storage chamber, but in most it is considered needless. Brilliant success is claimed for it by the patentee, and testified to by many who have tried it, but we should like to have seen the result of careful analyses. We satisfied ourselves by the ammonium oxalate test of its power of removing lime from a hard water, and found a strongly ferruginous water to be absolutely tasteless after passing through it. It is already widely adopted in the wine trade, a special form for which is made, in which filtering-paper reduced to a pulp is substituted for the carbo-calcis, and canvas for the asbestos. Though we are primâ facie suspicious of rapid filtration, we must admit that M. Maignen's filter seems to be a success, and will prove especially useful in military operations and in the trades where a soft and fairly pure water is required. If rapid filtration is less imperative, the chamber may be filled with granular charcoal.

For our own part, we should prefer, for domestic use, to trust to Mr. Bischof's spongy iron filter, the superiority of which is borne out by the reports of the Rivers Pollution Commissioners, the Army Medical Department, and the Prussian Army—all of which concur in pronouncing it to be the only filter which not merely arrests suspended particles, oxidises organic matter, and absorbs gases, but removes many soluble salts and lead, reduces the hardness, and, *above all, destroys the living organisms which are found to thrive in charcoal, especially of the animal kind.* It is also remarkable for not fouling, or, at least, for not imparting, as others do, the organic matter it has arrested to the effluent water for an indefinite time. We must candidly admit that is not easy to explain these various actions, which are chemical rather than mechanical; but that a filter should render such a fair water as that of the Grand Junction, organically as well as inorganically purer than that of the Kent Company, reducing the total solids, the hardness, the total nitrogen, and the nitrates and nitrites each by 50 per cent., and the organic nitrogen and carbon by 90 per cent., is amply enough to establish its reputation without a rival. It is easily taken to pieces, and the media renewed or revivified. Several patterns, as well as samples of the filtering materials, spongy iron and pyrolusite—the latter used to fix the iron, which would otherwise be dissolved to some extent in the water—are to be seen in this Exhibition.

J. TYLOR and SONS exhibit their patent grooved joints for lead pipes, which require no solder, and several water meters, one made of glass to show its workings. They depend on the rotation of a fan wheel. In one of the building exhibitions we remember seeing an actual metre which measured the supply by the alternate discharge of two buckets on a balance. Such meters may be of use under certain circumstances; but we should decidedly object to any inducement being held out to stint the use of water in households on account of the cost.

Mr. TONKS shows a ball-valve (Meakin's patent), remarkable for its simplicity; there is no hinge or pivot to get out of order, and the copper ball, so prone to corrosion, is replaced by one of glass. The lever of galvanised iron raises by a central pin a valve formed by a circular horizontal plate of brass, with which the lever is in simple contact. Should the lever become displaced, the pressure of the water closes the mouth of the pipe, and there is no risk of overflow.

Referred in the catalogue to Section XIII., but displayed on the walls of another room, are numerous architectural drawings, illustrating the construction of actual or proposed hospitals, workhouses, baths, and industrial dwellings. The former are nearly all on the pavilion system, which seems likely to be the system of the future. Such are the Herbert Hospital at Woolwich, by Captain GALTON; the infirmaries of St. Marylebone, St. George's, Fulham, St. Olave's, and many others, by Mr. SAXON SNELL; and the scheme for the reconstruction of University College Hospital on its present site, by Dr. POORE and Mr. ALFRED WATERHOUSE. In this the whole area of the basement would be utilised for out-patient and administrative purposes, the inner rooms being lighted from the roof. On this base arise three pavilions with stair-cases and open corridors (all fire-proof) between them; the topmost storey being set apart for operating theatres, post-mortem room, laboratories, etc.

Mr. F. E. JONES shows a rival plan on the circular ward system, proposed by Professor Marshall, F.R.S., and capable of accommodating, without any reduction of cubic space, nearly one hundred more beds than Dr. Poore's. The extent of outer wall and the freedom of ventilation between the several blocks seem also to be greater in Mr. Marshall's; while its massive and imposing appearance harmonises with that of the adjoining college.

Another plan for a circular ward infirmary for 800 beds is shown by Mr. SAXON SNELL.

The Camden Turkish Baths, by Mr. BRIDGMAN, and the Roman Baths at Vienna, by Dr. VON HEINRICH, deserve inspection.

The most remarkable, however, of the many hospitals, the plans of which are here exhibited, is one in the course of erection by the Guardians of the Salford Union, from the designs of Mr. LAWRENCE BOOTH, containing 880 beds at a cost of £68 per bed! each bed having an allowance of eighty square feet of floor space and 1000 cubic feet of air. Though the whole cost will be but little over £50,000, the constructional and sanitary arrangements seem perfect, and the hospital will be replete with every resource of science and art which can conduce to the efficiency of the administration and the comfort and convenience of the inmates and staff.

Among the plans for the erection of houses suited to the requirements and within the means of the lower middle, working, and labouring classes, we notice with deep interest those of the Shaftesbury-park Estate, at rentals ranging from 6s. 6d. to 13s. per week, and five to seven rooms; the Artisans', Labourers', and General Dwellings Company, at the Queen's-park Estate, Harrow-road; the Freehold Cottage Dwellings Company, the specifications of which, from a sanitary and constructional point of view, would put to shame not merely speculative builders, but the architects of our most pretentious houses; the Workmen's Dwellings at Salford, and the three-roomed dwellings, on two or three floors or flats, independent of one another, and only 2s. 6d. per week, designed by Mr. Mark Judge. These are certain to be more popular with the poor than the huge barrack-like edifices of the Peabody Trustees and other companies, with their five or six flights of stairs, and may be erected at trifling cost on any vacant sites. It would be impossible here to do more than call the attention of our readers to these designs, but we hope at a future time to reopen the whole question of the housing of the poor, with due regard to morals, health, comfort, and means, which seems to have been at length solved by these companies together and severally.

THE FISH-SUPPLY.—It is officially stated that the average quantity of fish sent to Billingsgate in the course of a month is 17,000 tons. Of this, the quantity condemned as unfit for consumption has been during the last six months 240 tons. But it seems much of this wasted food becomes tainted before it reaches the market.

FROM ABROAD.

EPIDEMIC DROPSY IN CALCUTTA.

THE May number of the *Indian Med. Gazette* contains an interesting report on "Epidemic Dropsy in Calcutta," by Surgeon-Major Macleod, Health Officer of Calcutta. After referring to former outbreaks of the affection, he states that the present epidemic made itself known about the end of 1879; and that according to the police returns there have been 266 cases with 51 deaths in the "town sections" of Calcutta, and 376 with 163 deaths in the "suburban sections." The facts regarding the outbreak are as follows:—
1. It attacks houses in a village in a promiscuous way, these not necessarily being contiguous. 2. Several or all the members of a household were attacked, single cases being exceptional. 3. The seizures took place almost simultaneously, as if from a common cause. 4. The disease seems to have broken out all over the infected area about the same time. 5. Recent cases are rare, the disease seeming to be dying out.

The symptoms of the disease are very definite:—1. Swelling of the limbs—the lower always, sometimes the upper, and occasionally the body. 2. Fever, sometimes before and sometimes after the swelling, and in some cases altogether absent. 3. Bowel complaints in many cases—diarrhœa most commonly; dysentery in a few. 4. Burning and pain in the affected limbs at the commencement. 5. Shortness of breathing and cough, and palpitation in all cases. 6. Great emaciation, exhaustion, and anæmia in severe cases; slighter, but well marked, in all. 7. The duration of the disease appears to be about two months in cases of average severity, and it leaves its victim greatly enfeebled. 8. In fatal cases great disturbance of respiration and circulation have been described, and death has generally been sudden.

"As regards the nature of the disease, it is impossible to write as yet very definitely. The prevailing opinion is that it is the same disease as has been described by observers in Madras and Ceylon under the term 'beri-beri.' As regards causation, I am not able to pronounce a positive opinion. (a.) Though it is most prevalent among the poorer classes of Mahometans and Hindus, it is by no means confined to these—Eurasians, Armenians, and natives in good circumstances have also suffered. (b.) I cannot attribute it to poverty of living, high prices, or any dietetic condition or consequent constitutional taint—well-fed Mahometan butchers, accustomed to generous living, and in excellent bodily condition, have been seized; and although I have observed indications of anæmia and scurvy in some cases, I am inclined to consider them secondary conditions due to the disease, and not the cause of it. (c.) The sanitary conditions of the households and villages in which the disease has broken out are certainly no worse than those of hundreds of others in towns and suburbs where no disease has prevailed. In short, I have been unable to fix upon any one condition or assembly of conditions, personal or otherwise, peculiar to the affected places. (d.) As regards infectiousness, the evidence is very conflicting. Dr. O'Brien considers the disease to be very infectious, and gives good reasons for his belief. Facts have come to my knowledge which favour the impression that the disease is communicable, while others have opposed that view. If it is infectious (and I am not prepared to deny this), it is so under conditions, seasonal and otherwise, which strongly modify its manner of transfer from man to man. The gradual spread northward, the pronounced localisation, and the seizure of whole families, are the most remarkable circumstances in the natural history of the malady considered from an epidemiological point of view."

PROFESSOR PASTEUR'S "ANTHRACOID VACCINATION."

A new series of experiments has been recently tried at a farm near Chartres, under the direction of a special committee nominated by the Préfet. Nineteen sheep which had been previously inoculated by Prof. Pasteur's "attenuated virus," and sixteen sheep taken at random from a flock, were all inoculated on July 16 with the virus taken from a sheep that had died of *charbon* at a farm near Chartres.

Three days afterwards (July 19), fifteen out of the sixteen sheep that had not undergone the preliminary inoculation of diluted virus were dead, while the nineteen sheep which had been previously treated by Prof. Pasteur were all perfectly well, and did not exhibit any morbid symptom whatever. In this series of experiments special precautions were taken in making the injections. The blood taken from the veins of the limbs of the dead sheep was employed, as also were clots from the heart and the pulp of the spleen. A Pravaz's syringe was filled with the fluid to be used, and when half of this had been injected into an unprepared sheep, the remaining half was injected into a sheep that had undergone the preventive inoculation, so that the two experiments were absolutely comparable. A great number of the Beauce farmers, the *Progrès Medical* states, were present on the occasion, and on the results being made known, several of them requested that their flocks might at once be protected.

ELECTROLYSIS IN HIRSUTIES.

In a paper read at the Boston Medical Society for Medical Improvement (*Boston Med. Jour.*, May 5), Dr. White describes the procedure adopted with so much success by Dr. Michel, of the Missouri Medical College, for the destruction of hairs which appear in unsuitable localities, especially on the face in women. It is the only means yet devised that has proved more than a palliative for this annoying deformity, and operates by the complete destruction of the hair-papilla at the bottom of the hair-follicle. After employing the means successfully in trichiasis, Dr. Michel extended it to hirsuties in general, and his practice has since been successfully followed by others. A galvanic battery of ten or fifteen cells, supplying a current strong enough to decompose water, is required as well as a small sponge electrode, some of the slender steel needles used by dentists for extracting the nerves, a proper electrode needle-holder, and two cord conductors a yard in length. The needle, properly secured in its holder, is connected with the negative, and the sponge electrode with the positive pole. The needle is carefully introduced into the hair-follicle as far as the papilla, while the moistened sponge electrode is applied to the skin in the immediate vicinity of the part. A frothy matter oozes from the mouth of the follicle around the needle, which is held in its place for a few seconds, according to the size of the hair, after which the sponge electrode is to be removed, and the needle withdrawn. The hair should be then removed with a forceps, and the ease with which it comes away indicates the completeness of the operation. If force is required for its removal, the process should be repeated within the empty follicle. A considerable amount of pain is produced during the passage of the current, which ceases on the removal of the sponge. Ordinarily, the after-effects are very trivial unless a small area be acted upon at short intervals; and the parts finally return to their natural condition, leaving in some instances a small pit or depression. If the operation is successful the hair does not reappear. The degree of success depends largely on the skill of the operator. Dr. Michel claims that 90 per cent. of the longer hairs are at once permanently destroyed, but others are satisfied if 50 per cent. are dealt with successfully at the first attempt. The operation needs repeating only upon those hairs which reappear, until all are finally destroyed. When the hair is very coarse, so that the mouth of the follicle remains well defined after its extraction, it may be removed before the electrolysis; but when the hairs are fine and blond, their presence is necessary as a guide to the needle. It is usually easy to make the fine points of the needle enter the follicle, even when the hair remains; and, at all events, the tissues close to the papilla can be penetrated and the necessary electrolysis effected. The patient should be placed in the strongest light; and even under the most favourable conditions the eyes of the operator will tire after a sitting of an hour or less. Perhaps forty or fifty hairs are all that can be advantageously attempted at one sitting—although the patient generally bears the pain without flinching after the first few sittings. When an extensive hirsuties has to be treated, a long time is required for the successful primary removal of the hairs, and some of the follicles will, without fail, require a repetition of the operation. For the fine, downy hairs occurring alone or interspersed with a stronger growth nothing had better be done until they attain a more conspicuous development.

THE PHYSIOLOGICAL IMMUNITIES OF THE JEWS.

An interesting article bearing the above title, by an anonymous writer, in the *Revue Scientifique* (April 23 and May 14), commences as follows:—

"The history of the Jews is one of the most curious episodes in the annals of mankind. Their obstinate, and finally victorious, struggle against implacable persecutions, stimulated both by religious hatred and the desire to appropriate their immense personal wealth; a peculiar power of expansion, of *irradiation*, which induced them to emigrate, from the most ancient period, into every part of the known world; the concentration in their hands, at the most remote epochs, of a great part of international commerce, and that first by reason of an admirable special aptitude, and then because of their sound notions on the power of credits, at a time when hoarding and unproductive concealment constituted the sole means of saving, and finally, through the laws of the countries which consented to receive them prohibiting them all other branches of active humanity; the preservation of their religious faith; the preservation, no less persevering in the land of exile, of the manners, customs, and traditions of their primary country; their persistent refusal to commingle with the races which surrounded them; and finally, an energetic vitality superior to that of these races, manifesting itself especially by a smaller mortality, and by an incomparable facility of acclimatisation. Such are the principal features under which are revealed to the observer, the historian, and the philosopher this strange people so admirably organised for the struggle—dreaming without ceasing, in spite of their interminable trials, of their mysterious and elevated destinies, which should justify their pretension of having been, and still being, the people of God.

"We can study here but one of the problems raised by this continuous increase of the Jewish race, especially in Europe—a problem modest enough in appearance, but which is nevertheless one of the greatest interest that ethnic studies present. It is precisely this vitality, this congenital power, this *vis durans* (as Tacitus termed it, speaking of the Germans), which seems to endow the race with true physiological privileges, probably by preserving it from the dangerous influences of climate, soil, and the bad hygienic, moral, and economical conditions of the countries in which they resided."

Our want of space forbids our pursuing the interesting demonstration which ensues, and we must content ourselves with the following *resumé*:—

"We believe that we have been able to show that nearly everywhere the Jews enjoy the following physiological immunities, when compared with the inhabitants of the countries in which they are established:—1. Their general fecundity (the relation of births to population) is less. 2. According to locality, their marriages are more or less fertile, but everywhere they preserve a larger number of their children. 3. They have much fewer illegitimate births and infants born dead. 4 The proportion of male births is sensibly higher. 5. Their mortality is less, and their mean life is longer. 6. Their increase by the preponderance of births over deaths is more rapid. 7. If they do not completely escape contagious diseases, they are less severely affected by them. 8. They are protected from certain diseases, such as pulmonary phthisis and scrofula. 9. They become acclimatised and reproductive under every latitude. These immunities resist the generally miserable condition which all observers attribute to them, as they do the frequency of their consanguineous marriages and their sojourn in cities, remote from the salutary influences of rural life enjoyed by the majority of the other inhabitants. What can be the causes of these privileges? Must we regard them, with a large number of authors, as the result of a superior vitality inherent to the race, which has been preserved intact through ages, and in spite of the differences of climates, in consequence of an almost complete absence of crossing? Must we seek these only in the persevering observation of the laws of hygiene laid down in Deuteronomy? But these rules were only applicable to the climate under which the ancient Israelites lived, whether in Judæa, or in Egypt during the captivity. Or should we attribute them, first, to the salutary influence of marriage, which Jews contract at a less advanced age than Christians, and also to their following the less fatiguing occupations, and which are but little exposed to accidents? Can we admit, also, that they profit by the beneficial hygienic effects of the spirit of order and economy, of regularity in habits and moderation in tastes, in the relative severity of their manners and the completely private and family life which many observers attribute to them? Finally, are we to admit with others that their state of misery is only in appearance, and that, in reality, their well-being is generally superior to that of the populations amidst which they live? All these hypotheses are admissible."

ILL EFFECTS OF MOUTH-BREATHING.

The *Boston Journal* (May 5) contains a short account of a paper read by Dr. Clinton Wagner before the Medical Society of the County of New York, in which he called attention to the evils resulting from habitual mouth-breathing. Catlin had found, in his multiplied intercourse with the Indian tribes, an entire absence of deafness and disease of the air-passages, and he arrived at the conclusion that this was attributable to the fact that nasal breathing was universally practised by them; and Dr. Wagner, during his intercourse as an army surgeon with the inhabitants of a large Indian village, who were living in a bad sanitary state, observed that there was an entire exemption from ear, nose, and throat disease, which he also attributed solely to the total absence of mouth-breathing among them. The causes of this unfortunate habit in civilised communities must be attributed to defective conditions of the nose, mouth, or throat, now so readily detected by the modern improvements in exploration. Thus, in the nose we may have occlusion from more or less deviation of the septum, polypi, various morbid growths and false membranes resulting from syphilitic or strumous ulceration; in some there may be a general imperforation of the nares; and in others there may be a general thickening and hypertrophy of the mucous membrane; and in any of these pathological changes even a slight cold of the head renders nasal breathing very difficult, and by recurrence might lead to the establishment of mouth-breathing. In the mouth, chronic enlargement of the tonsils is the most common cause of this; and elongation of the uvula, by the irritation it causes, leads to frequent mouth-breathing. Among the characteristics of a person so breathing are retracted lips, protruding teeth, an open mouth with the peculiar wrinkles surrounding it, and a silly, almost idiotic, expression of countenance. The sense of smell is diminished or lost, while the whole contour of the nose is changed. Hearing also is more or less affected, the relaxation of the muscles controlling the eustachian tube leaving this continually open. The constant action of cold air, loaded with impurities, upon the pharynx leads to follicular or dry pharyngitis, one of the most distressing of all throat affections. The patient is for ever making efforts to dislodge the hard, dry, tenacious mucus; and the constant hawking which results is a nuisance in all large assemblages of persons. Chronic catarrhal laryngitis is also a common result of mouth-breathing; and where a strumous diathesis is present, tubercular laryngitis is very likely to follow. Snoring, also, is due to this habit, being unknown among those who breathe through the nose. The effects of mouth-breathing on the general constitution are also serious, for in young subjects it may result in the malformation of the thorax known as "pigeon-breast," and in the imperfect oxygenation of the blood and faulty nutrition. In regard to treatment, after referring to the operative procedures that may be required, Dr. Wagner dwelt upon the benefit he had derived from the employment of dilatation by metallic sounds in stenosis of the meati from hypertrophy of the mucous membrane. At first their passage was painful, but the hyperæsthesia soon passed off. The dilators varied in size from that of an ordinary probe to that of a No. 6 or 8 urethral sound; weeks, and sometimes months, being required for their employment. For the first week they should be used daily, but afterwards less often—patients being instructed in introducing them for themselves when necessary. The following application should also be employed: ℞ Iodini gr. ij., pot. iod. gr. iv., zinc. iod. gr. x., aqua ʒj. The chloride of zinc (gr. v. ad ʒj.) may sometimes be substituted for the iodide. Where the tissue is excessively hypertrophied the galvano-cautery may be used. When enlarged tonsils are the cause of mouth-breathing they should be excised, topical applications being useless. When infants and young children breathe through the mouth an examina-

tion for the cause of this should be made. Mothers and nurses, however otherwise careful as to cleanliness, almost always neglect the nose. It should in these subjects be cleansed by means of a small syringe and tepid water or a camel's-hair pencil. A little vaseline applied at night would prevent the hardening of the nasal secretions until the child was old enough to learn to snuff up water by the nostrils from the hand. When the mouth is found open during sleep the lips should be gently pressed together; and all children should be taught at an early age the vital importance of always breathing through the nose instead of the mouth.

GUNSHOT WOUND OF THE TRACHEA.

The following extract is from the pen of Dr. Alexander Jamieson, Shanghai(a):—

For the following interesting case I am indebted to Dr. L. Vincent, of the French Navy, Médecin-Major of the *Champlain*. Although the facts reported occurred during the winter half-year, they may fitly find a place here:—

Gunshot Wound of the Trachea: Cure.—On November 10, 1880, a detachment of sailors from the corvette *Champlain* was engaged in rifle practice at the range on the Hongkew Settlement at Shanghai, when the certificated marksman P., one of the markers posted in the mantlets, was struck by a ball, and immediately fell. His companion having signalled the accident, firing was stopped, and the officer in command, along with Dr. Ganivet, assistant-surgeon in charge of the party, hastened to the spot. They found P. lying in a state of unconsciousness, with a wound, measuring about one centimetre in extent, situated in the middle line of the neck in front. Dr. Ganivet, before making a careful examination of the wound, endeavoured to restore the patient's consciousness, in which he was quickly successful. P. showed by signs that he experienced great difficulty in breathing, and while doing so he was seised with a violent paroxysm of cough, during which he expelled a flattened piece of a chassepôt bullet, accompanied by a considerable quantity of blood. The fragment, which was of irregular shape, measured about one centimetre in length by three or four millimetres in thickness, and had reached the marker by rebound from the target.

Having rapidly cleansed the wound, through which air was freely passing, the assistant-surgeon applied a temporary dressing, placed the patient in a carriage, and removed him to his ship with every possible precaution, and without accident. A minute examination was now made under favourable circumstances, and it was found that the lesion was situated transversely almost immediately below the cricoid cartilage. The edges were almost as clean-cut as though the wound had been made with a sharp instrument, but they were smeared with earth and sand which had clung to the projectile. A probe passed easily through the wound into the trachea, and by this exploration I assured myself that no foreign body was present, and that the posterior wall of the trachea was uninjured. The tube had been opened on its anterior aspect, and in the interval between the first and second rings, but only to the extent of the skin wound. At each expiration a hissing sound, audible at a considerable distance, was produced by air escaping through the wound, and for a certain extent all round the latter the subcutaneous areolar tissue was emphysematous. Voice was preserved, but it was much subdued and markedly changed in quality.

In the fear of increasing the emphysema, it was resolved not to stitch the wound, but merely to draw its edges together with the greatest care by means of strips of adhesive plaster. These were covered with a thick layer of cotton-wool, intended to exert slight pressure and to limit the extension of the emphysema. The entire dressing was maintained in position by a bandage. During the examination and dressing the patient coughed up a certain quantity of pure blood. There was, however, no bleeding from the wound, as none of the vessels of the neck had been injured by the ball. Breathing was distinct over the entire chest, but the respiratory murmur was somewhat feeble at the bases, where also there was slight dulness on percussion. Dyspnœa was intense, respirations 36 per minute; the pulse

(a) From the *Medical Reports of the Imperial Maritime Customs of China.*

was small, compressible, and beating 60 per minute. The patient was ordered cold broth, acidulated lemonade, and twenty drops of solution of perchloride of iron (Baumé, 30°). He was kept lying on his back with his head raised, and he was directed to keep absolute silence and to avoid all movement. The poor fellow had always been extremely quiet and obedient, and this contributed materially to his rapid recovery.

He passed a good night, continuing, however, to spit blood. The pulse, without rising in frequency, increased in volume. Next day (November 11), on examining the dressing without disturbing the strapping, the emphysema was found stationary; dyspnœa had decreased, but deglutition was difficult and painful. Expectoration still blood-stained, but no longer consisting of pure blood. Pulse 64; respirations 20; temperature 37·2° (99° Fahr.). Cotton and bandage were reapplied. Medicine and nourishment as before. Thirty-five grammes of castor oil. By November 14 the expectoration had lost all trace of blood, and consisted of mucus. Dyspnœa had greatly diminished, and auscultation revealed only a few sibilant râles on the right side. Cough had been troublesome during the night, and some difficulty in swallowing remained. The emphysema had completely disappeared. The edges of the wound were not inflamed, and union was already in part accomplished. Air, however, still passed through the diminished opening. The dressing was reapplied, and tapioca with wine and water and a mucilaginous syrup ordered. On November 19, cough and expectoration had ceased, the general condition was excellent, and though there was still some difficulty in swallowing, this symptom had much diminished, so that certain articles of food passed without serious difficulty. The wound was nearly closed, and was air-tight. A few exuberant granulations were cauterised.

Cicatrisation was complete on November 22, thirteen days after the accident. The patient's voice had then recovered all its volume, and was changed neither in strength nor in quality. A very slight difficulty in swallowing remained, but this had disappeared a week later, when P. resumed duty, perfectly cured.

REVIEWS.

A Practical Treatise on the Diseases of Women. By T. GAILLARD THOMAS, M.D., Professor of Diseases of Women in the College of Physicians and Surgeons of New York, President of the American Gynæcological Society for 1879, Honorary Fellow of the Obstetrical Society of London, etc. Fifth Edition, enlarged and thoroughly revised. London: Henry Kimpton. 1880. Pp. 808.

THE words which follow "fifth edition" are in this case no mere formal announcement. The alterations and additions which have been made are both numerous and important. Still, they are not such as to affect the general character of the work; they merely embody those changes in opinion and extensions of knowledge which increased experience and close attention to the current literature of the subject have led the author to adopt.

The attraction and the permanent value of this book lie in the clearness and truth of the clinical descriptions of disease; the fertility of the author in therapeutic resources, and the fulness with which the details of treatment are described; the definite character of the teaching; and last, but not least, the evident candour which pervades it, the reader feeling throughout that Dr. Thomas is not in the least anxious to conceal his own mistakes and failures, or to affect certainty where his experience is limited. We would also particularise the fulness with which the history of the subject is gone into, and which makes the book additionally interesting, and gives it a value as a work of reference.

Having said this, we may be allowed to point out what we take to be its defects. First, as to pathology. Dr. Thomas is fond of large vague terms, which may mean anything or nothing; e.g., we repeatedly find such as the following given as causes of disease:—"Natural feebleness of constitution," "a depreciation of the vital forces from any cause," "prolonged nervous depression," "a torpid condition of the intestines and liver," and we might quote more of the like. Considered in their colloquial meaning, there is no disease to which the human body is subject, of which they may not be reckoned as predisposing causes. But what we understand by scientific knowledge and scientific writing, is exact knowledge and precision in the use of language; and terms like these, which denote nothing definite, seem to us out of place in a scientific treatise.

In the lists of causes which are given under the heading of each disease we find set down things, the causal effect of which is entirely matter of speculation. Thus, at page 347 we are told that laceration of the cervix and uterine displacements are among the causes of uterine fungosities; and at page 523 nulliparity is put as a predisposing cause of uterine fibroids.

The lists of symptoms also involve statements which many would be inclined to flatly contradict, or which are only true in the most indirect way. In illustration of these remarks, we may quote from page 411 the following list of the symptoms "very generally" produced by anteflexion: "pain over hypogastrium and in groins and back; irritable bladder; leucorrhœa; dysmenorrhœa; sterility; nervous disturbance and despondency; pain on locomotion; menorrhagia; tendency to abortion; pain on sexual intercourse; pelvic neuralgia; sense of depression at the epigastrium." Whether true or not, the connexion of anteflexion with these symptoms has never yet been proved, and many would altogether deny it. Again, page 524, we are told of fibroid tumours, that "they in some way interfere with hæmatosis and the functions of the ganglionic nervous system"—a statement in support of which not a particle of evidence is adduced, nor, so far as we are aware, does any exist, and that "they disorder the mind by creation of depression of spirits, from the fact that the patient recurs with gloomy apprehension to their existence almost constantly." This is more or less true of every disease to which the human body is subject; uterine fibroids have no specialty or pre-eminence in this direction; and the intensity of such fears depends far more on the patient's mental idiosyncrasy than on the kind of the illness which is causing anxiety.

It will perhaps be thought that in particularising faults of this kind in a book which has so many merits we are hypercritical. But the loose way of writing, the omission to critically examine the evidence upon which alleged facts rest, before stating them as such, which passages like those we have quoted show, become, when extended into the subject of treatment, likely to lead to evil consequences. The number of pessaries figured and recommended would seem, except to one with unbounded faith in the mechanical system of uterine pathology, deplorable. Still, these (except the intra-uterine stems) would seldom do more harm than disappoint doctor and patient. But we find, for instance, Dr. Marion Sims's operation for anteflexion recommended—a proceeding in favour of which no evidence has ever been brought forward. Its inventor himself has never published his cases. All we know is that it is dangerous, and many say entirely useless, even when recovery from it has been complete. Dr. Thomas refers to no cases, but accepts without question everything said in its favour. If he would state how many times he has done it, and how many of the patients were any the better for it, he would make his recommendation of it more valuable. Again, the exaggerated statements as to the consequences of laceration of the cervix, which are just now so prevalent in America, Dr. Thomas accepts, with the practical teaching which follows, as to the urgent necessity of repairing such lacerations. He still seems to think that Dr. Marion Sims's vaginismus operation is worth performing, although he admits that grave cases can be cured without it. It does not seem to have occurred to him that the cases he has cured by this operation might have been cured better without it. The worst cases of all, in which all treatment (including Sims's operation) is useless, Dr. Thomas puts separately, under the title of hyperæsthesia of the vulva.

The book gives good clinical pictures of disease. But he who follows out all its suggestions as to treatment will subject his patients to much unnecessary suffering, and himself, as well as them, to sore disappointment. If Dr. Thomas would ruthlessly expunge from his book every statement of which he has not himself examined the evidence, every recommendation as to treatment which he has not himself tested and verified, and would insert, instead of general commendatory expressions, a summary of his experience with regard to doubtful modes of practice, he would make his work a safer guide.

The Relations of the Abdominal and Pelvic Organs in the Female. Illustrated by a full-sized chromo-lithograph of the Section of a Cadaver frozen in the Genu-Pectoral Position, and by a series of woodcuts. By Professor ALEXANDER RUSSELL SIMPSON and Dr. DAVID BERRY HART. Edinburgh and London: W. and A. K. Johnston. 1881. Pp. 11.

THE objection we have to make to this is to the title. The cadaver is not in the genu-pectoral position, for this is a posture which it is impossible for an adult human being with limbs and spine of no more than ordinary flexibility to assume. This body seems to be supported by its knees and nose: the part of the chest which is nearest to the horizontal plane on which the knees rest is four inches and a quarter removed from it. The knee-elbow position is, we presume, what the authors mean.

Having stated this preliminary criticism, we desire to express our hearty thanks to the authors for their trouble in making this most instructive section, their ability in interpreting the lessons to be drawn from it, and their enterprise in publishing the costly and beautiful drawing before us. They cannot have anticipated a largely remunerative sale for the publication, it being of no direct use in practice, and only of very limited utility to the average student, and their public spirit in producing such a work is the more to be admired.

The contents of the work are sufficiently indicated by the title. It deserves the careful study and consideration of all who are working at gynæcology.

Treatise on Diseases of Joints. By RICHARD BARWELL, F.R.C.S., Senior Surgeon and Lecturer on Surgery, Charing-cross Hospital. Second Edition. London: Macmillan and Co. 1881. Pp. 690.

MUCH labour has evidently been bestowed upon the compilation of this volume, but we are of opinion that its practical utility would have been materially increased by compression within narrower limits. It suffers, especially in the earlier chapters, from want of careful revision. The style is at times laboured and confusing, and the author's meaning difficult of interpretation.

The book commences with a chapter devoted to the physiology of joints, and the author, by criticism of the experiments of E. Weber, of Bonn, and description of his own, refutes the vacuum theory of joints. The attempt to explain, by a possible electric change in the surface texture, the fact that in some cases of synovitis the thermometer applied to the joint will only mark a fractional rise, while the sense to the hand is that of very considerable heat, cannot be considered as satisfactory. In Chapter IV. a summary of the germ theory in its application to pyæmic joint-disease is given, though, the author adds, "We must not hastily conclude that all and every part of the mystery is already solved by these recent discoveries." In this chapter the author is very confused, and it is often quite impossible to catch his meaning. Objection is taken to the use of the term gonorrhœal rheumatism, and cases (of which Case 14 is most instructive) are cited to show that gonorrhœa will occasionally produce pyæmia, and expression is given to belief in the pyæmic nature of gonorrhœal rheumatism. We cannot agree with the author that "it is wiser to have no theory of the rheumatic poison." The antiseptic treatment of pyæmic joint-disease by carbolic infiltration and other methods is fully discussed. The correlation between lead-poisoning and gout—a well-established fact—is announced, to our surprise, somewhat in the light of a new revelation. The treatment of hydrarthrosis by free incisions and the removal of pendulous hinges is gone into, and illustrative cases are supplied. We fail to see that the substitution of the terms per-acute, acute, and chronic, for acute, subacute, and chronic articular ostitis, is a happy one.

In the chapter dedicated to movable bodies in joints, Mr. Rainey's excellent description of their formation by hypertrophy and metamorphosis of one or more of the synovial hinges is quoted, and the other modes of formation are dealt with.

The histology of chronic ostitis is treated at great length, and the author's disbelief in the view, that throughout the process of inflammation osseous tissue is merely passive and incapable of inflammatory action—held by Billroth, whom he considers to be misled by his view of the constitution of bone, and by his method of investigation—asserted. The

author's theory to account for the coincidence of hip-joint disease and congenital phimosis in males, by the frequent and long-continued priapism in such cases producing irritability or irritation of the lumbar spinal cord, with consequent trophic changes in the nerves of the pelvis and lower limbs, is at least ingenious, if far-fetched. He adds, however, "I have not overlooked the fact that hip-disease also occurs in female children."

The chapter devoted to hysteric pseudo-disease of joints appears to us unsatisfactory from the indefinite expression of the author's own opinion on this difficult subject. The last three chapters are given up to the treatment of the restoration of crippled joints, some deformities of the knee, and excision of joints, and contain matter of much practical value.

In conclusion, let us add that the value of the work is increased by the interpolation of numerous illustrative cases. We regret, however, that we cannot praise the woodcuts as triumphs of artistic skill, and we fear that the work cannot be looked on as one materially advancing, or even popularising, our present knowledge of joint-disease.

GENERAL CORRESPONDENCE.

LONDON SMELLS.

LETTER FROM DR. W. D. STONE.

[To the Editor of the Medical Times and Gazette.]

SIR,—In a letter recently published in one of your daily contemporaries I drew attention to the abominable smells in our London streets, and I ventured to suggest the free use of a solution of chloride of lead as the most powerful and economical agent for eliminating sulphide of hydrogen from the atmosphere, as well as from all organic matter in a state of decomposition or putridity—a disinfectant strongly recommended by the late Dr. Goolden. Exception has been taken to this by Mr. H. S. Carpenter, chemist, of Holborn Viaduct, who, judging from the editorial remarks in which he is spoken of as "this eminent man of science," has evidently been mistaken for Dr. W. B. Carpenter, C.B., F.R.S.

Mr. Carpenter states that "chloride of lead cannot be regarded as a disinfectant"; he then goes on to say that "the only way in which it could act, etc." Such reasoning (?) I cannot understand. To speak of a chemical fact as "could be" or "might be" is simply incomprehensible; and the idea of the correspondent in question crossing lances with a man of the late Dr. Goolden's reputation is, to my mind, very like a minnow attacking a triton! I am, &c.,

W. DOMETT STONE, M.D.

Oxford-terrace, Hyde-park, W.

STRANGULATED HERNIA AND PULMONARY CONGESTION.—Prof. Verneuil related two cases at the Société de Chirurgie (*Gaz. Hebd.*, July 22), with the object of showing that the cause of death in these cases may be due to rigidity and to congestion of the lungs, the appearances in the abdomen being by no means such as to explain death. This state of things adds very much to the unfavourableness of the prognosis, but still in all cases in which the operation is indicated it should be performed, and an endeavour also made to relieve the pulmonary congestion. In these cases fæcal vomiting occurs at an early period of the strangulation, and sometimes it comes on when there is no strangulation. The nature of this vomiting is, in fact, but little understood.

THE PARIS NIGHT SERVICE.—Dr. Passant reports that for the quarter ending June 30 there were 1412 night summonses, or 15¼ per night, and that of these, men constituted 36 per cent., women 50, and children 14. In 44 instances the patients were dead before the doctors could arrive. Of the others, 149 were cases of laryngitis, croup, and pertussis; 210 affections of the heart and lungs; 226 gastro-intestinal affections, strangulated hernia, and retention of urine; 225 labours, uterine hæmorrhages, abortions, etc.; 274 cerebral and nervous affections, alcoholism, tetanus (1), and hydrophobia (1); 139 rheumatism, eruptive and other fevers, and hæmorrhoids; and 145 wounds and injuries, poisonings (10), asphyxia from charcoal (6), and suicides (4)—total, 1412.

MEDICAL NEWS.

ROYAL COLLEGE OF SURGEONS OF ENGLAND.—The following gentlemen having undergone the necessary examinations for the diploma, were admitted Members of the College at a meeting of the Court of Examiners on the 21st inst., viz. :—

Atkinson, Thomas R., L.S.A., Fleet-street.
Collins, John S., M.D.G.U. Ire., Belfast.
Harris, Thomas, Fallowfield, Cheshire.
Haycock, Henry E., Shrewsbury.
Humphreys, William C., L.S.A., Bromsgrove.
Jones, J. H., L.K.&Q.C.P.I. Talsarn, Carnarvonshire.
Joseph, John B. E., Trinidad, W. I.
Lane, James O., B.A. Cantab., Hereford.
Ray, William B., Newtown, Montgomery.
Robertson, C. A. J., Manchester.
Robinson, G. W., L.S.A., North Shields.
Schacht, Franc F., B.A. Cantab., Clifton, Bristol.
Tait, Henry B., Highbury-park.
Teevan, Henry, L.S.A., Nottingham-place.
Whelan, George, Ticehurst-street.
Wilson, Henry, Sale, Cheshire.

Ten candidates were rejected. The following gentlemen passed on the 22nd inst. :—

Bagshaw, Thomas W., Birkenhead.
Boobbyer, Philip, Hendon.
Bray, Ernest E., Bognor.
Gale, Arthur K., Chilworth, Oxon.
Gaskin, Thomas L., Barbadoes.
Herringham, Wilmot P., Bedford-square.
Hardwicke, Richard E., Tonbridge.
Gross, Asher, Leeds.
King, William H. T., L.S.A., Plymouth.
Pittard, Marmaduke, Guernsey.
Pounds, Thomas H., Chatham.
Pratt, James J., Newtown, Montgomeryshire.
Rimell, Alfred T., Eardley-crescent, S.W.
Roberts, Richard P., Bangor.
Vincent, Philip, Hadham Cross, Herts.
Wickham, Walter, L.S.A., Chew Stoke, Somerset.
Woolley, George T., Upper Bedford-place.

Five candidates were rejected. The following gentlemen passed on the 25th inst., viz. :—

Alderton, Herbert, Shotley, Suffolk.
Brown, Clarence W. H., Godalming.
Coates, William, Worksop.
Davies, Evan N., L.S.A., Cymmer, Glamorganshire.
Draper, James W., Barnsbury-road.
Grindon, Francis J., L.S.A., Olney, Bucks.
Hern, John, M.B. Edin., Ashburton, Devon.
O'Reilly, Archibald T., Sydney, New South Wales.
Robinson, Hugh S., Sydenham-hill.
Walker, Charles E., Eckington, Derby.
Webber, Edward B., Abergavenny.

Nine candidates were rejected. The following gentlemen passed on the 26th inst., viz. :—

Bickle, Leonard W., St. Leonards-on-Sea.
Cork, Augustus H., Hampstead.
Dowson, John, St. John's-wood.
Edwards, Arthur R., Malmesbury.
Fitch, Richard A., Kidderminster.
Lyster, Cecil R. C., Lessness Heath, Kent.
Perks, Robert H., Cardiff.
Prothero, Richard, Liverpool.
Rice, Bernard, Stratford-on-Avon.
Rudd, Charles F., L.S.A., Wymondham.
Russell, John E., L.S.A., Waltham Cross.
Bygate, David J., L.S.A., Cannon-street-road.
Sergeant, George, Callington, Cornwall.
Steer, William, L.S.A., Salcombe, South Devon.
Tuke, Charles M., Chiswick.

Eight candidates were rejected. The following gentlemen passed on the 27th inst., viz. :—

Atterbury, Walter, L.S.A., Oppidans-road, N.W.
Burrows, Charles W. G., L.S.A., Eckington, Derbyshire.
Cahill, John, Albert-gate.
Clifton, Frederick W., Derby.
Cornish, Charles N., Taunton.
Duff, Charles E., Gray's-inn-road.
Groom, William, B.A. Cantab., Wisbeach.
Fell, Walter, Vincent-square, S.W.
Hill, William J., Croydon.
Robins, George N., Buxton, Derbyshire.

Ten candidates were rejected.

APOTHECARIES' HALL, LONDON.—The following gentlemen passed their examination in the Science and Practice of Medicine, and received certificates to practise, on Thursday, July 21 :—

Allwork, Frank, Wateringbay, Kent
Boyd, James Dunlop, Beith, Ayrshire, N.B.
Coffin, Arthur Bonari, Eastbourne-terrace, Hyde-park.
Fletcher, Howard Burnett, Hanover-square, Sheffield.
Hoff, George Framingham, Burdwar, Bengal.
Manby, Herbert Lynsey, Brewood, Stafford.

Morse, Thomas Bickett, Eton House, Cheltenham.
Roberts, Richard Fletcher, Bangor, North Wales.
Teevan, Henry, 7, Nottingham-place, W.

The following gentlemen passed their primary professional examination on the 14th inst. :—

Bott, Joseph, London Hospital.
Gostling, Thomas Preston, University College Hospital.
Squire, Edward Herbert, London Hospital.
Treasure, William B. C., Charing-cross Hospital.

And on the 21st inst. :—

Faunce, Charles Edward, Middlesex Hospital.
Fink, George Herbert, University College Hospital.
McMillan, John F., Middlesex Hospital.
Scott, Bernard, Guy's Hospital.
Tate, Alan Edmonson, Middlesex Hospital.
White, Ernest Alfred, St. Bartholomew's Hospital.

NAVAL, MILITARY, ETC., APPOINTMENTS.

ADMIRALTY.—Deputy Inspector-General of Hospitals and Fleets Alexander Watson, M.D., has been placed on the retired list from the 20th inst., with permission to assume the rank of retired Inspector-General of Hospitals and Fleets.

BIRTHS.

ARCHIBALD.—On July 20, at Lynton House, Brixton Rise, S.W., the wife of John Archibald, M.B., C.M., F.R.C.S., of a son.
HOLDEN.—On July 19, at Sudbury, Suffolk, the wife of J. Sinclair Holden, M.D., of a son.
HUDSON.—On July 21, at Redruth, Cornwall, the wife of R. S. Hudson, M.D., of twin daughters.
LESSON.—On July 19, at 10, Denmark-villas, Brighton, the wife of Dr. Oliver Leeson, of Ripon House, Russell-square, of a son.
PRICKETT.—On July 24, the wife of Marmaduke Prickett, M.D., of a son.
RAHILLY.—On July 20, at The Court, Hutton, Somersetshire, the wife of Surgeon-Major J. Roche Rahilly, A.M.D., 21st Royal Scots Fusiliers, of a daughter.
SANDERS.—On July 18, at Sharrow, near Ripon, the wife of Surgeon-Major R. C. Sanders, Indian Medical Department, of a daughter.
SAUNDERS.—On June 15, at Petermaritzburg, Natal, South Africa, the wife of Surgeon W. Egerton Saunders, A.M.D., of a son.
SMITH.—On July 21, at 15, Imperial-square, Cheltenham, the wife of William Robert Smith, M.D., F.R.S. Edin., of a daughter.
STEVENS.—On July 22, at Norton, Bury St. Edmunds, Suffolk, the wife of Dr. George Stevens, F.F.P.S. Glasg., L.M., L.S.A., of a son.
STRUGNELL.—On July 25, at 45, Highgate-road, the wife of F. W. Strugnell, L.R.C.P., M.R.C.S., of a daughter, stillborn.
TIPPETTS.—On July 24, at Fulford, York, the wife of Brigade-Surgeon A. M. Tippetts, A.M.D., of a daughter.

MARRIAGES.

HARRIS—BLATCHLEY.—On July 19, at Hornsey, Spencer Clabon, son of Frederick Hills Harris, M.R.C.S., of Mildenhall, Suffolk, to Annie Charlotte Fanny, eldest daughter of Edwin Blatchley, Esq., of Herne House, Hornsey.
LAING—THOMSON.—On July 19, at Edinburgh, John T. Laing, Esq., manufacturer, of Harwich, to Annie Drummond, eldest daughter of George William Thomson, M.D.
BINNON—STOCKWELL.—On July 20, at Bath, Edward Gardner Robinson, Esq., to Clary Constance, third daughter of T. G. Stockwell, F.R.C.S.
SAVORY—PAVY.—On July 19, at Hanover-square, the Rev. Barradaile Savory, only son of N. S. Savory, F.R.S., of Brook-street, to Florence Julia, only surviving daughter of F. W. Pavy, M.D., F.R.S., of Grosvenor-street.
STRONG—WOOD.—On July 19, at Northfleet, R. G. Strong, L.R.C.P., of Horndean, Hants, to Fanny, daughter of J. Wood, Esq., of Westfield, Northfleet, Kent.
WATERHOUSE—STERN.—On July 16, at the British Embassy Chapel, Vienna, Charles H. Waterhouse, M.D., B.A., to Cecille, eldest daughter of Ferdinand Stern, Esq., of Vienna.
WOOD—HOLBERTON.—On July 20, at Teddington, Edward J. Wood, M.B., of Yalding, Kent, to Ethel Vaughan, eldest daughter of Vaughan Holberton, Esq., of Hampton, Middlesex.

DEATHS.

BARROW, MARION CHARLOTTE, daughter of T. W. Barrow, Inspector-General of Hospitals, at Woolwich, on July 14, aged 18.
DICKSON, HANNAH, eldest son of Edward Dalziel Dickson, M.D., Physician of H.M. Embassy at Constantinople, in London, on July 21, aged 29.
HOLT, ROSA BEATRICE, daughter of William Holt, M.R.C.S., L.S.A., of 1, Norton Folgate, Bishopsgate-street, on July 21, aged 12.
MYERS, HONOR FRANCES, daughter of Arthur B. R. Myers, Surgeon Coldstream Guards, at Instow, North Devon, on July 21.
TAYLOR, ARTHUR, M.B., M.R.C.S., late of Wanganui, New Zealand, eldest son of David Taylor, M.R.C.S., at 150, Kennington-park-road, S.E., on July 14, aged 27.

VACANCIES.

In the following list the nature of the office vacant, the qualifications required in the candidate, the person to whom application should be made and the day of election (as far as known) are stated in succession.

CARNARVONSHIRE AND ANGLESEY INFIRMARY —House-Surgeon. Candidates must be registered to practise in medicine and surgery, and acquainted with the Welsh language. Applications, with testimonials, to be sent to the Secretary on or before August 11.

GENERAL INFIRMARY, LEEDS.—House-Surgeon. (*For particulars see Advertisement.*)

GLAMORGAN COUNTY ASYLUM, BRIDGEND.—Assistant Medical Officer. Candidates must be single, and not over thirty years of age. Applications, accompanied with recent testimonials, to be sent to the Medical Superintendent not later than August 2.

HAMPSTEAD PROVIDENT DISPENSARY, NEW-END.—Medical Officer. Candidates must be legally entitled to practise both medicine and surgery under the Medical Acts, and be resident in Hampstead. Applications, with evidence of qualifications, to be sent to the Secretary, J. W. Fenn, 28, High-street, Hampstead, not later than August 6.

NATIONAL DENTAL HOSPITAL, 149, GREAT PORTLAND-STREET, W.—Dental Surgeon and Lecturer on Dental Surgery and Pathology. Candidates must possess the L.D.S.R.C.S. Eng., and are requested to send in their applications, with testimonials, to Arthur G. Klugh, Secretary, on or before August 10.

NORTH STAFFORDSHIRE INFIRMARY, HARTSHILL, STOKE-ON-TRENT.—Resident House-Surgeon and Resident House-Physician. Candidates must be duly registered, and possess a diploma or degree in surgery from the College of Surgeons of London, Edinburgh, or Dublin, or from one of the universities, and a diploma, degree, or licence in medicine from a university or duly recognised licensing body of Great Britain or Ireland. Applications, with testimonials, to be sent to the Secretary on or before August 17.

QUEEN'S HOSPITAL, BIRMINGHAM.—Resident Surgeon. Applications and testimonials, with certificates of registration, to be sent under cover to the Secretary, at the Hospital, from whom all further information may be obtained, on or before August 2.

ST. MARYLEBONE GENERAL DISPENSARY, 77, WELBECK-STREET, CAVENDISH-SQUARE.—Dental Surgeon. Applications and testimonials must be forwarded, not later than August 1, to Frank Stokes, Secretary, and candidates must attend the Medical Committee at the Dispensary on August 3, at 4.30 p.m. precisely.

STOCKTON-UPON-TEES HOSPITAL AND DISPENSARY.—House-Surgeon (non-resident). Candidates must be doubly qualified. Applications, stating age, with recent testimonials, to be sent to the Secretary, John Settle, not later than August 9.

UNION AND PAROCHIAL MEDICAL SERVICE.

*** The area of each district is stated in acres. The population is computed according to the census of 1871.

RESIGNATIONS.

Cannock Union.—The Brewood District is vacant by the death of Mr. Samuel Walsh: area 20,721; population 5556; salary £50 per annum.

APPOINTMENTS.

Berkhampstead Union.—Richard L. Batterbury, B.M. Lond., M.R.C.S. Eng., L.S.A., to the Berkhampstead District and the Workhouse.

Croydon Union.—Mark Jackson, M.R.C.S. Eng. and L.S.A., to the Second District.

Dunmow Union.—Charles Hartley, M.R.C.S. Eng., L.S.A., to the High Easter District.

Skipton Union.—John Anthony, L.R.C.P. Edin., L.F.P.& S. Glasg., to the Kettlewell District.

OBSTETRICAL SOCIETY'S LIBRARY.—In consequence of the Medical Congress, the Library of the Obstetrical Society will remain open until August 10, when it will be closed until September 12.

APPOINTMENTS FOR THE WEEK.

July 30. *Saturday (this day).*

Operations at St. Bartholomew's, 1½ p.m.; King's College, 1½ p.m.; Royal Free, 2 p.m.; Royal London Ophthalmic, 11 a.m.; Royal Westminster Ophthalmic, 1½ p.m.; St. Thomas's, 1½ p.m.; London, 2 p.m.

August 1. *Monday.*

Operations at the Metropolitan Free, 2 p.m.; St. Mark's Hospital for Diseases of the Rectum, 2 p.m.; Royal London Ophthalmic, 11 a.m.; Royal Westminster Ophthalmic, 1½ p.m.

2. *Tuesday.*

Operations at Guy's, 1½ p.m.; Westminster, 2 p.m.; Royal London Ophthalmic, 11 a.m.; Royal Westminster Ophthalmic, 1½ p.m.; West London, 3 p.m.

3. *Wednesday.*

Operations at University College, 2 p.m.; St. Mary's, 1¼ p.m.; Middlesex, 1 p.m.; London, 2 p.m.; St. Bartholomew's, 1½ p.m.; Great Northern, 2 p.m.; Samaritan, 2½ p.m.; King's College (by Mr. Lister), 2 p.m.; Royal London Ophthalmic, 11 a.m.; Royal Westminster Ophthalmic, 1½ p.m.; St. Thomas's, 1½ p.m.; St. Peter's Hospital for Stone, 2 p.m.; National Orthopædic, Great Portland-street, 10 a.m.

4. *Thursday.*

Operations at St. George's, 1 p.m.; Central London Ophthalmic, 1 p.m.; Royal Orthopædic, 2 p.m.; University College, 2 p.m.; Royal London Ophthalmic, 11 a.m.; Royal Westminster Ophthalmic, 1½ p.m.; Hospital for Diseases of the Throat, 2 p.m.; Hospital for Women, 2 p.m.; Charing-cross, 2 p.m.; London, 2 p.m.; North-West London, 2½ p.m.

5. *Friday.*

Operations at Central London Ophthalmic, 2 p.m.; Royal London Ophthalmic, 11 a.m.; South London Ophthalmic, 2 p.m.; Royal Westminster Ophthalmic, 1½ p.m.; St. George's (ophthalmic operations), 1¼ p.m.; Guy's, 1½ p.m.; St. Thomas's (ophthalmic operations), 2 p.m.

VITAL STATISTICS OF LONDON.

Week ending Saturday, July 23, 1881.

BIRTHS.

Births of Boys, 1223; Girls, 1228; Total, 2451.
Corrected weekly average in the 10 years 1871-80, 2530·4.

DEATHS.

	Males.	Females.	Total.
Deaths during the week	1014	929	1943
Weekly average of the ten years 1871-80, corrected to increased population ...	862·9	774 0	1636·9
Deaths of people aged 80 and upwards ...	...	...	49

DEATHS IN SUB-DISTRICTS FROM EPIDEMICS.

	Enumerated Population, 1881 (unrevised).	Small-pox.	Measles.	Scarlet Fever.	Diphtheria.	Whooping-cough.	Typhus.	Enteric (or Typhoid) Fever.	Simple continued Fever.	Diarrhœa.
West	668993	4	14	5	...	5	1	...	...	74
North ...	905677	13	20	6	2	4	...	4	...	88
Central ...	281793	1	6	4	3	5	...	1	2	36
East	692530	6	8	6	1	14	1	2	...	115
South	1265578	19	19	14	3	17	1	4	1	136
Total	3814571	43	67	35	9	45	3	11	3	449

METEOROLOGY.

From Observations at the Greenwich Observatory.

Mean height of barometer ...	29·790 in.
Mean temperature ...	66·4°
Highest point of thermometer ...	90·2°
Lowest point of thermometer ...	51·6°
Mean dew-point temperature ...	54·8°
General direction of wind ...	Variable.
Whole amount of rain in the week ...	0·11 in.

BIRTHS and DEATHS Registered and METEOROLOGY during the Week ending Saturday, July 23, in the following large Towns:—

Cities and boroughs (Municipal boundaries except for London.)	Estimated Population to middle of the year 1881.*	Persons to an Acre. (1881.)	Births Registered during the week ending July 23.	Deaths Registered during the week ending July 23.	Temperature of Air (Fahr.): Highest during the Week.	Temperature of Air (Fahr.): Lowest during the Week.	Temperature of Air (Fahr.): Weekly Mean of Daily Mean Values	Temp. of Air (Cent.): Weekly Mean of Daily Mean Values.	Rain Fall: In Inches.	Rain Fall: In Centimetres.
London	3829751	50·8	2451	1943	90·2	51·6	66·4	19·11	0·11	0·28
Brighton	107934	45·9	58	35	80·2	51·0	62·6	17·01	0·12	0·30
Portsmouth ...	128335	28·6	92	47	...	...	...	...	...	...
Norwich	88038	11·8	49	29	88·2	51·0	64·8	18·23	0·43	1·09
Plymouth	75262	54·0	51	26	78·5	50·5	61·4	16·33	0·05	0·13
Bristol	207140	46·5	123	68	75·4	47·0	60·0	15·56	0·17	0·43
Wolverhampton ...	75934	22·4	55	27	79·9	45·5	59·5	15 29	0·09	0·23
Birmingham ...	402296	47·9	267	142	...	...	...	...	...	...
Leicester	123120	38·5	96	60	...	...	...	...	...	...
Nottingham ...	188035	18·9	122	105	91·6	43·3	63·4	17·44	0·11	0·28
Liverpool	553988	106·3	369	249	...	...	...	...	...	...
Manchester ...	341269	79·5	256	144	...	...	...	...	...	...
Salford	177760	34·4	135	59	...	...	...	...	...	...
Oldham	112176	24·9	65	33	...	...	...	...	...	...
Bradford	184037	25·5	115	52	...	...	...	...	...	...
Leeds	310490	14·4	227	154	75·0	46·0	60·3	15·73	0·03	0·08
Sheffield	285621	14·5	186	104	80·0	46·0	59·6	15·34	0·12	0·30
Hull	155161	42·7	108	66	80·0	45·0	60·6	15·90	0·15	0·38
Sunderland ...	116753	42·2	82	51	75·0	46·0	59·7	15·39	0·27	0·69
Newcastle-on-Tyne	145675	27·1	96	71	...	...	...	...	...	...
Total of 20 large English Towns ...	7608775	38·0	5003	3465	91·6	43·3	61·7	16·50	0·15	0·38

* These figures are the numbers enumerated (but subject to revision) in April last, raised to the middle of 1881 by the addition of a quarter of a year's increase, calculated at the rate that prevailed between 1871 and 1881.

At the Royal Observatory, Greenwich, the mean reading of the barometer last week was 29·79 in. The highest reading was 29·94 in. on Sunday morning, and the lowest 29·65 in. on Tuesday evening.

NOTES, QUERIES, AND REPLIES.

Je that questioneth much shall learn much.—Bacon.

L.R.C.S.I.—Apply direct to the Colonial Office. All the examination papers for the A.M.D. have been duly published in our columns.

N., Edgware.—The freehold of a common belongs to the lord of the manor, and, speaking generally, the only persons who have any right over it are the lord and the commoners of the manor.

Medical Certificates.—At Glasgow, in a case just decided in regard to an industrial life assurance, a medical certificate appears to have been given under circumstances which are to be regretted. A woman, whose age was at first given as sixty-one, but who afterwards turned out to be nearly seventy, was insured by an unscrupulous agent for £21, and the agent obtained a medical certificate from the medical officer on his own assurances, the medical officer never having seen the woman at all. The acceptance of a medical engagement with a provident society implies a moral obligation to protect it as far as possible against imposition.

How to create Disease.—Correspondents are multiplying in condemnation of the cartage of offal and all kinds of offensive refuse through our crowded thoroughfares in the open day, when the sun has greatest power, thus polluting the London atmosphere by these plague carts, to the peril of the health of the population.

Assaulting a Workhouse Physician.—A pauper inmate of Cork Workhouse has been sentenced to five years' penal servitude for a murderous assault with a poker on Dr. Wall, visiting physician. The prisoner frequently complained that his mutton-chops were too fat, and Dr. Wall having refused to interfere in the matter, the assault was the result.

Water-Supply, Paris.—The Paris Municipality has voted a sum of 3,300,000 francs for the improvement of the waterworks.

Factory Act Prosecution.—A firm of soap manufacturers in Brewhouse-lane, Wapping, has been fined £3 16s. for unlawfully employing four young women after the hour of seven o'clock in the evening. The magistrate considered the firm had not exercised due vigilance to enforce the carrying out of the provisions of the Act. The loose manner in which measures are taken by employers to comply with the law is, in the majority of these prosecutions, apparently their chief characteristic —a laxity, albeit, which rightly subjects them to legal penalties.

Open Spaces.—In the Chancery Division, last week, an action was heard to restrain the Corporation of Wallingford from doing anything which might destroy an old Roman camp near that town, which was now used as a recreation ground. The place was described as being an interesting relic of olden times, and worthy of preservation. The Corporation appeared on the motion, and submitted at once to a perpetual injunction being made upon the terms which had been arranged.——A new recreation ground near the Cemetery, at Cardiff, was opened on the 18th inst. Its area comprises eleven acres and a half.

The Profession.—"The world of medicine is a world of controversies—controversies the more difficult to decide from the variety and complexity of the phenomena of life and disease. A new case may be a weapon to fling at an opponent, or a conclusive demonstration of the truth of that opponent's system. But it always has, as it were, its scientific little pigeon-hole to fit into."

A Bad Case.—A shopkeeper at Hounslow has been summoned before the Brentford magistrates, in two cases, for adulterating butter. In one case the adulteration consisted of 7 per cent. of water, 2·40 per cent. of salt, and 90 per cent. of fat; in the other, 95 per cent. of insoluble fatty acids; and in neither was there a particle of butter. The Bench deemed these the worst cases they ever had brought before them, and fined the defendant £5 and costs.

Population and Temperature.—In the Census returns of the United States is one showing the distribution of the population as regards temperature. Arranged in groups, varying 5° of mean annual temperature, it is shown that 96 per cent. of the entire population live between lines marked by 40° and 70° Fahr. Dividing the population between two classes—that which has a high maximum temperature, and that which has a low minimum—it is found that 39 per cent. live where there is a maximum of between 95° and 105°, while 95 per cent. live where there is a minimum of 35° below and 10° above zero for extreme cold. It will be seen that nine-tenths of the population of the United States live where there are great ranges between the extremes of heat and cold, and where an "equable climate" is unknown.

Involuntary Criminals.—An Austrian physician of some distinction has recently published a book in which he endeavours to prove that habitual criminals are so because they are incapable of helping it. He appears to have examined the brains of a number of persistent criminals, and has invariably found that the superior frontal convolution is not continuous, but is divided into four sub-convolutions analogous to the parts found in predatory carnivorous animals, and he thinks that the mental characteristics of criminals are due to this peculiar formation of brain.

Lunacy.—It is as long ago as 1815 that a Committee of the House of Commons inquired into the barbarities which had up to that time been employed in the treatment of lunatics.

A Reconsidered Decision.—It is satisfactory to learn, in reference to the case of Mr. Hele, the District Medical Officer of Plomesgate Union, who by the overseer's order attended a boy for an injury and amputated his leg, but who had been refused payment of his fee by the Board of Guardians, that since Mr. Firth asked the President of the Local Government Board whether his attention had been called to the case, the Board of Guardians had reconsidered their decision, and that Mr. Hele is no longer required to perform the operation of amputation gratuitously.

A Seasonable Gift.—Last week a large quantity of fresh strawberries, placed at the disposal of the Hospital Saturday Fund by the growers at Halstead and Knockholt, in Kent, were distributed amongst the various London hospitals by the Honorary Secretary of the South London Local Committee.

Jealous of his Privileges.—Mr. W. T. Payne, the Coroner for the City of London, has, under the following circumstances, called the attention of the Court of Aldermen to the fact that, by the Act under which the City Prison at Holloway was built, the interior was considered and taken as part of the Court of London, and the City Coroner had sole jurisdiction to hold the inquests there. In June, 1878, the Prison was transferred to the Government, but the Aldermen were still the only visiting justices. He (Mr. Payne) had continued to hold the inquests there down to the present time; but the new Coroner for Central Middlesex (Dr. Thomas) now claimed to hold them. Being disinclined to give up any of the privileges of the Corporation, he had laid the matter before the Court. The question was referred to the Gaol Committee.

COMMUNICATIONS have been received from—
The Chairman of the Smoke Abatement Committee, London; Mr. T. M. Stone, London; Dr. Wolfenden, London; Dr. J. W. Moore, Dublin; The Registrar of Apothecaries' Hall, London; Mr. J. Chatto, London; Mr. Rickman J. Godlee, London; The Manager of the Sanitary Engineering and Ventilating Company, London; Dr. F. Hogg, Netley; Mr. George Brown, London; The Sub-Librarian of the Obstetrical Society, London; Dr. James Anderson, London; Mr. Spottiswoode Cameron, Huddersfield; Dr. Henry Harris, Redruth; The Secretary of the Zenana Medical Mission for Ladies; Dr. Dorety Stone, London; Mr. Bailey Walker, Didsbury; Dr. Roberts, London; Dr. Herman, London; Dr. W. H. Day, London; Professor W. H. Flower, London; The Honorary Secretary of the Midland Medical Society; The Lord Mayor of London; The Honorary Secretary-General of the International Medical Congress, London.

BOOKS, ETC., RECEIVED—
Anæsthetics, by Edward T. Reichert, M.D.—Annual Report of the Darenth Schools and Asylum for Imbeciles to December 31, 1880—Post-Paralytic Chorea, etc., by E. C. Seguin, M.D.—Hip Injuries, etc., by De F. Willard, M.D.—Hip-Joint Disease, by De Forest Willard, M.D.—Châtel-Guyon, by Dr. G. H. Brandt—American Nervousness, by G. M. Beard, A.M., M.D.—Annual Report of the Royal Albert Asylum—Ueber den Einfluss des Rückenmarks auf die Harnsecretion, von Burney Sachs aus New York—In Memory of Edouard Seguin, M.D.—Fashion in Deformity, by Wm. Henry Flower, LL.D., F.R.S., F.R.C.S., etc.—Sessional Proceedings of the National Association for the Promotion of Social Science.

PERIODICALS AND NEWSPAPERS RECEIVED—
Lancet—British Medical Journal—Medical Press and Circular—Berliner Klinische Wochenschrift—Centralblatt für Chirurgie—Gazette des Hopitaux—Gazette Médicale—Le Progrès Médical—Bulletin de l'Académie de Médecine—Pharmaceutical Journal—Wiener Medizinische Wochenschrift—Centralblatt für die Medizinischen Wissenschaften—Revue Médicale—Gazette Hebdomadaire—National Board of Health Bulletin, Washington—Nature—Deutsche Medicinal-Zeitung—Boston Medical and Surgical Journal—Centralblatt für Gynäkologie—Western Weekly News, July 23—The American—Louisville Medical News—Church of England Pulpit, etc.—Japan Weekly Mail—Liverpool Medico-Chirurgical Journal—Revista de Medicina—Nordiskt Medicinskt Arkiv —Archives de Neurologie—Monthly Index—Oil and Drug News.

A NEW LEECH FROM TUNIS.—At the Société de Biologie, Dr. Megnin exhibited several leeches of a kind unknown in France, and which arrived at Vincennes in a healthy state, having made the journey from Tunis in a singular manner. They were found, in fact, adhering to the mucous membrane of the mouths of horses which belonged to a battery that had just returned from Tunis. All the brooks in the north of Africa, it seems, abound with this species of leech, known by the name of *hæmopis sanguisuga*. Its jaws being too feeble to seize hold of the skin, it fixes on the mucous membrane of the mouths of the horses as they come to drink. They therefore have remained in the mouth for a fortnight or three weeks, causing very serious hæmorrhage. Indeed, asphyxia has been caused by the penetration of the animal into the larynx.—*Gaz. des Hop.*, July 19.

INTERNATIONAL MEDICAL CONGRESS, 1881.

INAUGURAL ADDRESS

BY

Sir JAMES PAGET, Bart., F.R.S., etc.,

President.

It is not necessary to defend the meeting of an International Congress. Such meetings have become one of the general customs of our time, and have thus given evidence that they are generally approved. Let me rather suggest to you some thoughts as to the work which, being in Congress, we have to do, and the spirit in which it may best be done, so that the good effects of our meeting may last long after our parting.

In the largest view of our design, it may seem to be that of bringing together a multitude of various minds for the promotion and diffusion of knowledge in the whole science and art of medicine, in their widest range, in all their narrowest divisions, in all their manifold utilities. And this design, I cannot doubt, will be fulfilled; for although the programme tells of selected subjects for discussion, and defines the order of our work, yet knowledge will be promoted in a much wider range in the meetings without order, which will be held every day and everywhere—meetings of men with all kinds of mental power and all forms of knowledge and of skill; every one ready alike to impart and to acquire knowledge.

It is safe to say that in the casual conversations of this coming week there will be a larger interchange and diffusion of information than in any equal time and space in the whole past history of medicine. And with this interchange will be a larger increase, for in the mart of knowledge he that receives gains, and he that gives retains, and none suffer loss.

The increase will be the greater because of the great variety of minds which will meet. As I look round this hall, my admiration is moved not only by the number and total power of the minds which are here, but by their diversity—a diversity in which, I believe, they fairly represent the whole of those who are engaged in the cultivation of our science. For here are minds representing the distinctive characters of all the most gifted and most educated nations—characters still distinctly national, in spite of the constantly increasing intercourse of the nations. And from many of these nations we have both elder and younger men; thoughtful men, and practical; men of fact, and men of imagination; some confident, some sceptic; various also in education, in purpose and mode of study, in disposition, and in power. And scarcely less various are the places and all the circumstances in which those who are here have collected and have been using their knowledge. For I think that our calling is pre-eminent in its range of opportunities for scientific study. It is not only that the pure science of human life may match with the largest of the natural sciences in the complexity of its subject-matter; not only that the living human body is, in both its material and its indwelling forces, the most complex thing yet known; but that in our practical duties this most complex thing is presented to us in an almost infinite multiformity. For in practice we are occupied, not with a type and pattern of the human nature, but with all its varieties in all classes of men, of every age and every occupation, in all climates and all social states; we have to study men singly and in multitudes, in poverty and in wealth, in wise and unwise living, in health and in all the varieties of disease; and we have to learn, or at least to try to learn, the results of all these conditions of life, while, in successive generations and

in the mingling of families, they are heaped together, confused, and always changing. In every one of these conditions, man, in mind and body, must be studied by us; and every one of them offers some different problems for inquiry and solution. Wherever our duty, or our scientific curiosity—or, in happy combination, both—may lead us, there are the materials and there the opportunities for separate original research.

Now, from these various opportunities of study, men are here in Congress. Surely, whatever a multitude and diversity of minds can, in a few days, do for the promotion of knowledge, may be done here. Every one has something he may teach, much more that he may learn; and, in the midst of an apparent utter confusion, knowledge will increase and multiply. It has been said, indeed, that truth is more likely to emerge from error than from confusion, and, in some instances, this is true; but much of what we call confusion is only the order of nature not yet discerned; and so it may be here. Certainly, it is from what seems like the confusion of successive meetings such as this that that kind of truth emerges which is among the best moving and directing forces in the scientific as well as in the social life—the truth which is told in the steady growth of general opinion.

But it is not proposed to leave the work of the Congress to what would seem like chances and disorder, good as the result might be; nor yet to the personal influences by which we may all be made fitter for work, though these may be very potent. In the stir and controversy of meetings such as we shall have, there cannot fail to be useful emulation; by the examples that will appear of success in research, many will be moved to more enthusiasm, many to more keen study of the truth; our range of work will be made wider, and we shall gain that greater interest in each other's views and that clearer apprehension of them which are always attained by personal acquaintance and by memories of association in pleasure as well as in work. But as it will not be left to chance, so neither will sentiment have to fulfil the chief duties of the Congress.

Following the good example of our predecessors, certain subjects have been selected, which will be chiefly, though not exclusively, discussed, and the discussions are to be in the sections into which we shall soon divide.

Of these subjects it would not be for me to speak, even if I were competent to do so; unless I may say that they are so numerous and complete that, together with the opening addresses of the Presidents of Sections, they leave me nothing but such generalities as may seem commonplace. They have been selected, after the custom of former meetings, from the most stirring and practical questions of the day; they are those which must occupy men's minds, and on which there is at this time most reason to expect progress, or even a just decision, from very wide discussion. They will be discussed by those most learned in them, and in many instances by those who have spent months or years in studying them, and who now offer their work for criticism and judgment.

I will only observe that the subjects selected in every section involve questions in the solution of which all the varieties of mind and knowledge of which I have spoken may find their use. For there are questions, not only on many subjects, but in all stages of progress towards settlement. In some the chief need seems to be the collection of facts well observed by many persons. I say by many, not only because many facts are wanted, but because in all difficult research it is well that each apparent fact should be observed by many, for things are not what they appear to each one mind. In that which each man believes that he observes, there is something of himself; and for certainty, even on matters of fact, we often need the agreement of many minds, that the personal element of each may be counteracted. And much more is this necessary in the consideration of the many questions which are to be decided by discussing the several values of admitted facts and of probabilities, and of the conclusions drawn from them. For, on questions such as these, minds of all kinds may be well employed. Here there will be occasion even for those which are not unconditionally praiseworthy, such as those that habitually doubt, and those to whom the invention of arguments is more pleasing than the mere search for truth. Nay, we may be able to observe the utility even of error. We may not, indeed, wish for a prevalence of errors; they are not more desirable than are the crime and misery which evoke charity. And yet in a Congress we may palliate them, for we may see how, as we may often read in history, errors, like doubts and contrary pleadings, serve to bring out the truth, to make it express itself in clearest terms and show its whole strength and value. Adversity is an excellent school for truth as well as for virtue.

But that which I would chiefly note, in relation to the great variety of minds which are here, is that it is characteristic of that mental pliancy and readiness for variation which is essential to all scientific progress, and which a great International Congress may illustrate and promote. In all the subjects for discussion we look for the attainment of some novelty and change in knowledge or belief; and after every such change there must ensue a change in some of the conditions of thinking and of working. Now, for all these changes, minds need to be pliant and quick to adjust themselves. For all progressive science there must be minds that are young, whatever may be their age.

Just as the discovery of auscultation brought to us the necessity for a refined cultivation of the sense of hearing, which was before of only the same use in medicine as in the common business of life; or, as the employment of the numerical method in estimating the value of facts required that minds should be able to record and think in ways previously unused; or, as the acceptance of the doctrine of evolution has changed the course of thinking in whole departments of science; so is it, in less measure, in every less advance of knowledge. All such advances change the circumstances of the mental life, and minds that cannot or will not adjust themselves become less useful, or must, at least, modify their manner of utility. They may continue to be the best defenders of what is true; they may strengthen and expand the truth, and may apply it in practice with all the advantages of experience; they may thus secure the possessions of science and use them well, but they will not increase them.

It is with minds as with living bodies. One of their chief powers is in their self-adjustment to the varying conditions in which they have to live. Generally, those species are the strongest and most abiding that can thrive in the widest range of climate and of food. And, of all the races of men, they are the mightiest and most noble who are, or by self-adjustment can become, most fit for all the new conditions of existence in which by various changes they may be placed. These are they who prosper in great changes of their social state; who, in successive generations, grow stronger by the production of a population so various that some are fitted to each of all the conditions of material and mode of life which they can discover or invent. These are most prosperous in the highest civilisation; these whom mature adapts to the products of their own arts.

Or, among other groups, the mightiest are those who are strong alike on land and sea; who can explore and colonise, and in every climate can replenish the earth and subdue it; and this not by tenacity or mere robustness, but rather by pliancy and the production of varieties fit to abide and increase in all the various conditions of the world around.

Now, it is by no distant analogy that we trace the likeness between these in their successful contests with the material conditions of life and those who are to succeed in the intellectual strife with the difficulties of science and of art. There must be minds which in variety may match with all the varieties of the subject-matters, and minds which, at once or in swift succession, can be adjusted to all the increasing and changing modes of thought and work.

Such are the minds we need; or rather, such are the minds we have; and these in great meetings prove and augment their worth. Happily, the natural increase in the variety of minds in all cultivated races is—whether as cause or as consequence—nearly proportionate to the increasing variety of knowledge. And it has become proverbial, and is nearly true in science and art, as it is in commerce and in national life, that, whatever work is to be done, men are found or soon produced who are exactly fit to do it.

But it need not be denied that, in the possession of this first and chiefest power for the increase of knowledge, there is a source of weakness. In works done by dissimilar and independent minds, dispersed in different fields of study, or only gathered into self-assorted groups, there is apt to be discord and great waste of power. There is, therefore, need that the workers should from time to time be brought to

some consent and unity of purpose; that they should have opportunity for conference and mutual criticism, for mutual help, and the tests of free discussion. This it is which, on the largest scale and most effectually, our Congress may achieve; not, indeed, by striving after a useless and happily impossible uniformity of mind or method, but by diminishing the lesser evil of waste and discord which is attached to the far greater good of diversity and independence. Now, as in numbers and variety the Congress may represent the whole multitude of workers everywhere dispersed, so in its gathering and concord it may represent a common consent that, though we may be far apart and different, yet our work is and shall be essentially one—in all its parts mutually dependent, mutually helpful; in no part complete or self-sufficient. We may thus declare that as we who are many are met to be members of one body, so our work for science shall be one, though manifold; that as we, who are of many nations, will for a time forget our nationalities, and will even repress our patriotism, unless for the promotion of a friendly rivalry, so will we in our work, whether here and now, or everywhere and always, have one end and one design —the promotion of the whole science and whole art of healing.

It may seem to be a denial of this declaration of unity that, after this general meeting, we shall separate into sections more numerous than in any former Congress. Let me speak of these sections to defend them; for some maintain that, even in such a division of studies as these may encourage, there is a mischievous dispersion of forces. The science of medicine, which used to be praised as one and indivisible, is broken up, they say, among specialists, who work in conflict rather than in concert, and with mutual distrust more than mutual help.

But let it be observed that the sections which we have instituted are only some of those which are already recognised, in many countries, in separate societies, each of which has its own place and rules of self-government and its own literature. And the division has taken place naturally in the course of events which could not be hindered. For the partial separation of medicine, first from the other natural sciences, and now into sections of its own, has been due to the increase of knowledge being far greater than the increase of individual mental power.

I do not doubt that the average mental power constantly increases in the successive generations of all well-trained peoples; but it does not increase so fast as knowledge does, and thus, in every science, as well as in our own, a small portion of the whole sum of knowledge has become as much as even a large mind can hold and duly cultivate. Many of us must, for practical life, have a fair acquaintance with many parts of our science, but none can hold it all; and for complete knowledge, or for research, or for safely thinking out beyond what is known, no one can hope for success unless by limiting himself within the few divisions of the science for which, by nature or by education, he is best fitted. Thus, our division into sections is only an instance of that division of labour which, in every prosperous nation, we see in every field of active life, and which is always justified by more work better done.

Moreover, it cannot be said that in any of our sections there is not enough for a full strong mind to do. If anyone will doubt this, let him try his own strength in the discussions of several of them.

In truth, the fault of specialism is not in narrowness, but in the shallowness and the belief in self-sufficiency with which it is apt to be associated. If the field of any specialty in science be narrow, it can be dug deeply. In science, as in mining, a very narrow shaft, if only it be carried deep enough, may reach the richest stores of wealth, and find use for all the appliances of scientific art. Not in medicine alone, but in every department of knowledge, some of the grandest results of research and of learning, broad and deep, are to be found in monographs on subjects that, to the common mind, seemed small and trivial.

And study in a Congress such as this may be a useful remedy for self-sufficiency. Here every group may find a rare occasion, not only for an opportune assertion of the supreme excellence of its own range and mode of study, but for the observation of the work of every other. Each section may show that its own facts must be deemed sure, and that by them every suggestion from without must be tested; but each may learn to doubt every inference of its own which is not consistent with the facts or reasonable beliefs of others; each may observe how much there is in the knowledge of others which should be mingled with its own; and the sum of all may be the wholesome conviction of all, that we cannot justly estimate the value of a doctrine in one part of our science till it has been tried in many or in all.

We were taught this in our schools; and many of us have taught that all the parts of medical science are necessary to the education of the complete practitioner. In the independence of later life, some of us seem too ready to believe that the parts we severally choose may be self-sufficient, and that what others are learning cannot much concern us. A fair study of the whole work of the Congress may convince us of the fallacy of this belief. We may see that the test of truth in every part must be in the patient and impartial trial of its adjustment with what is true in every other. All perfect organisations bear this test; all parts of the whole body of scientific truth should be tried by it.

Moreover, I would not, from a scientific point of view, admit any estimate of the comparative importance of the several divisions of our science, however widely they may differ in their present utilities. And this I would think right, not only because my office as President binds me to a strict impartiality and to the claim of freedom of research for all, but because we are very imperfect judges of the whole value of any knowledge, or even of single facts. For every fact in science, wherever gathered, has not only a present value, which we may be able to estimate, but a living and germinal power of which none can guess the issue.

It would be difficult to think of anything that seemed less likely to acquire practical utility than those researches of the few naturalists who, from Leeuwenhoeck to Ehrenberg, studied the most minute of living things, the *Vibrionida.* Men boasting themselves as practical might ask, "What good can come of it?" Time and scientific industry have answered, "This good: those researches have given a more true form to one of the most important practical doctrines of organic chemistry; they have introduced a great beneficial change in the most practical part of surgery; they are leading to one as great in the practice of medicine; they concern the highest interests of agriculture; and their power is not yet exhausted."

And as practical men were, in this instance, incompetent judges of the value of scientific facts, so were men of science at fault when they missed the discovery of anæsthetics. Year after year the influences of laughing-gas and of ether were shown: the one fell to the level of the wonders displayed by itinerant lecturers; students made fun with the other. They were the merest practical men—men looking for nothing but what might be straightway useful—who made the great discovery which has borne fruit not only in the mitigation of suffering, but in a wide range of physiological science.

The history of science has many similar facts, and they may teach that any man will be both wise and dutiful if he will patiently and thoughtfully do the best he can in the field of work in which, whether by choice or chance, his lot is cast. There let him, at least, search for truth, reflect on it, and record it accurately; let him imitate that accuracy and completeness of which I think we may boast that we have, in the descriptions of the human body, the highest instance yet attained in any branch of knowledge. Truth so recorded cannot remain barren.

In thus speaking of the value of careful observation and records of facts, I seem to be in agreement with the officers of all the sections; for, without any intended consent, they have all proposed such subjects for discussion as can be decided only by well-collected facts, and fair direct inductions from them. There are no questions on theories or mere doctrine. This, I am sure, may be ascribed not to any disregard of the value of good reasoning or of reasonable hypotheses, but partly to the just belief that such things are ill suited for discussion in large meetings, and partly to the fact that we have no great opponent schools, no great parties named after leaders or leading doctrines about which we are in the habit of disputing. In every section the discussions are to be on definite questions, which, even if they be associated with theory or general doctrines, may yet be soon brought to the test of fact; there is to be no use of doctrinal touchstones.

I am speaking of no science but our own. I do not doubt that in others there is advantage in dogma, or in the guidance of a central organising power, or in divisions and conflicting parties. But in the medical sciences I believe that the existence of parties founded on dominant theories has always been injurious; a sign of satisfaction with plausible errors, or with knowledge which was even for the time imperfect. Such parties used to exist, and the personal histories of their leaders are some of the most attractive parts of the history of medicine: but, although in some instances an enthusiasm for the master-mind may have stirred a few men to unusual industry, yet very soon the disciples seemed to have been fascinated by the distinctive doctrine, content to bear its name, and to cease from active scientific work. The dominance of doctrine has promoted the habit of inference, and repressed that of careful observation and induction. It has encouraged that fallacy to which we are all too prone, that we have at length reached an elevated sure position on which we may rest, and only think and guide. In this way specialism in doctrine or in method of study has hindered the progress of science more than the specialism which has attached itself to the study of one organ or of one method of practice. This kind of specialism may enslave inferior minds: the specialism of doctrine can enchant into mere dreaming those that should be strong and alert in the work of free research.

I speak the more earnestly of this because it may be said, if our Congress be representative, as it surely is, may we not legislate? May we not declare some general doctrines which may be used as tests and as guides for future study? We had better not.

The best work of our International Congress is in the clearing and strengthening of the knowledge of realities; in bringing, year after year, all its force of numbers and varieties of minds to press forward the demonstration and diffusion of truth as nearly to completion as may from year to year be possible. Thus, chiefly, our Congress may maintain and invigorate the life of our science. And the progress of science must be as that of life. It sounds well to speak of the temple of science, and of building and crowning the edifice. But the body of science is not as any dead thing of human work, however beautiful; it is as something living, capable of development and a better growth in every part. For as in all life the attainment of the highest condition is only possible through the timely passing-by of the less good, that it may be replaced by the better, so is it in science. As time passes, that which seemed true and was very good becomes relatively imperfect truth, and the truth more nearly perfect takes its place.

We may read the history of the progress of truth in science as a palæontology. Many things which, as we look far back, appear, like errors, monstrous and uncouth creatures, were, in their time, good and useful, as good as possible. They were the lower and less perfect forms of truth which, amid the floods and stifling atmospheres of error, still survived; and just as each successive condition of the organic world was necessary to the evolution of the next following higher state, so from these were slowly evolved the better forms of truth which we now hold.

This thought of the likeness between the progress of scientific truth and the history of organic life may give us all the better courage in a work which we cannot hope to complete, and in which we see continual and sometimes disheartening change. It is, at least, full of comfort to those of us who are growing old. We that can read in memory the history of half a century might look back with shame and deep regret at the imperfections of our early knowledge if we might not be sure that we held, and sometimes helped onward, the best things that were in their time possible, and that they were necessary steps to the better present, even as the present is to the still better future. Yes, to the far better future; for there is no course of nature more certain than is the upward progress of science. We may seem to move in circles, but they are the circles of a constantly ascending spiral; we may seem to sway from side to side, but it is only as on a steep ascent which must be climbed in zig-zag.

What may be the knowledge of the future none can guess. If we could conceive a limit to the total sum of mental power which will be possessed by future multitudes of well-instructed men, yet could we not conceive a limit to the discovery of the properties of materials which they will bend to their service. We may find the limit of the power of our unaided limbs and senses; but we cannot guess at a limit to the means by which they may be assisted, or to the invention of instruments which will become only a little more separate from our mental selves than are the outer sense-organs with which we are constructed.

In the certainty of this progress, the great question for us is, What shall we contribute to it? It will not be easy to match the recent past. The advance of medical knowledge within one's memory is amazing, whether reckoned in the wonders of the science not yet applied, or in practical results in the general lengthening of life, or, which is still better, in the prevention and decrease of pain and misery, and in the increase of working power. I cannot count or recount all that in this time has been done; and I suppose there are very few, if any, who can justly tell whether the progress of medicine has been equal to that of any other great branch of knowledge during the same time. I believe it has been; I know that the same rate of progress cannot be maintained without the constant and wise work of thousands of good intellects; and the mere maintenance of the same rate is not enough, for the rate of the progress of science should constantly increase. That in the last fifty years was at least twice as great as that in the previous fifty. What will it be in the next, or, for a more useful question, what shall we contribute to it?

I have no right to prescribe for more than this week. In this let us do heartily the proper work of the Congress, teaching, learning, discussing, looking for new lines for research, planning for mutual help, forming new friendships. It will be hard work if we will do it well; but we have not met for mere amusement or for recreation, though for that I hope you will find fair provision, and enjoy it the better for the work preceding it.

And when we part let us bear away with us, not only much more knowledge than we came with, but some of the lessons for our conduct in the future which we may learn in reflecting the work of our Congress.

In the number and intensity of the questions brought before us, we may see something of our responsibility. If we could gather into thought the amounts of misery or happiness, of helplessness or of power for work, which may depend on the answers to all the questions that will come before us, this might be a measure of our responsibility. But we cannot count it; let us imagine it; we cannot even in imagination exaggerate it. Let us bear it always in our mind, and remind ourselves that our responsibility will constantly increase. For, as men become in the best sense better educated, and the influence of scientific knowledge on their moral and social state increases, so, among all sciences, there is none of which the influence, and therefore the responsibility, will increase more than ours; because none more intimately concerns man's happiness and working powers.

But, more clearly in the recollections of the Congress, we may be reminded that in our science there may be, or, rather, there really is, a complete community of interest among men of all nations. On all the questions before us we can differ, discuss, dispute, and stand in earnest rivalry; but all consistently with friendship, and with readiness to wait patiently till more knowledge shall decide which is in the right. Let us resolutely hold to this when we are apart; let our international be a clear abiding sentiment, to be, as now, declared and celebrated at appointed times, but never to be forgotten. We may, perhaps, help to gain a new honour for science, if we thus suggest that in many more things, if they were as deeply and dispassionately studied, there might be found the same complete identity of international interests as in ours.

And then, let us always remind ourselves of the nobility of our calling. I dare to claim for it, that among all the sciences, ours, in the pursuit and use of truth, offers the most complete and constant union of those three qualities which have the greatest charm for pure and active minds—novelty, utility, and charity. These three are sometimes in so lamentable disunion, as in the attractions of novelty without either utility or charity, are in our researches so combined that, unless by force or wilful wrong, they hardly can be put asunder. And each of them is admirable in its kind. For in every search for truth we can not only exercise curiosity, and have the delight—the really elemental happiness—of watching the unveiling of a mystery, ---- on the way to truth, if we look well around us, we shall

see that we are passing among wonders more than the eye or mind can fully apprehend. And as one of the perfections of Nature is that, in all her works, wonder is harmonised with utility, so is it with our science. In every truth attained there is utility either at hand or among the certainties of the future. And this utility is not selfish: it is not in any degree correlative with money-making; it may generally be estimated in the welfare of others better than in our own. Some of us may, indeed, make money and grow rich; but many of those that minister even to the follies and vices of mankind can make much more money than we. In all things costly and vainglorious they would far surpass us if we would compete with them. We had better not compete where wealth is the highest evidence of success; we can compete with the world in the nobler ambition of being counted among the learned and the good who strive to make the future better and happier than the past. And to this we shall attain if we will remind ourselves that, as in every pursuit of knowledge there is the charm of novelty, and in every attainment of truth utility, so in every use of it there may be charity. I do not mean only the charity which is in hospitals or in the service of the poor, great as is the privilege of our calling, in that we may be its chief ministers; but that wider charity which is practised in a constant sympathy and gentleness, in patience and self-devotion. And it is surely fair to hold that, as in every search for knowledge we may strengthen our intellectual power, so in every practical employment of it we may, if we will, improve our moral nature; we may obey the whole law of Christian love, we may illustrate the highest induction of scientific philanthropy.

Let us, then, resolve to devote ourselves to the promotion of the whole science, art, and charity of medicine. Let this resolve be to us as a vow of brotherhood; and may God help us in our work.

AN ADDRESS ON THE

VALUE OF PATHOLOGICAL EXPERIMENTS.

Delivered at the Second General Meeting of the International Medical Congress, August 3, 1881.

By RUDOLPH VIRCHOW.

GENTLEMEN,—At the last International Medical Congress, holden in Amsterdam, when reporting on the subject of medical education, I discussed the question as to how far the experimental method of teaching was necessary; and I arrived at the conclusion that it must be applied in its widest sense, and in particular that vivisection was an indispensable means to that end. In a still higher degree, however, I admit the importance of this subject in research, and in opposition to those who, with ever-increasing vehemence, attack experimenting investigators on account of the nature of their investigations and of the means they employ. I was able, with the fullest concurrence of a numerous meeting, without one single dissentient voice, to say: "All those who attack vivisection as a means of science do not possess the least idea of the importance of science, and they are still more ignorant of the importance of this aid to its attainment."

In the two years which have since gone by, the agitation of the opponents (of vivisection) has grown in extent, as well as in its object. One country after the other has been drawn into their net, and international communications have been opened in order to secure greater results by means of united efforts. They are no longer satisfied with the results which legislation in England in 1876 gave them. Now, the demands have increased: a petition of the new Leipzig Animals Protection Society of March 8th last, demands from the German Parliament the passing of a law by means of which "the torturing of animals under the plea of scientific research shall be punishable with imprisonment of not less than four weeks to two years, together with deprivation of civil rights." True, all do not go so far as this. Some ask not for complete suppression all at once, but for more or less limitation of vivisection. They do not, however, make any secret that this is provisional, and they demand that even the official laboratories of the universities shall be placed under the control of a member of the Animals Protection Society so far as to secure for their members free access to all parts at all times.

It would be simple deception if we were to attempt to believe that this movement is unimportant, and, on account of its obvious exaggerations, free from danger. On the contrary, there are unmistakable evidences that it has numerous and powerful allies, and that in some countries the danger is nearer; that, indeed, State institutions set apart for experimental research have already been somewhat narrowed in the scientific freedom of their methods of research. Thus it would appear the more important for the representatives of medical science to defend their position, and that they too should establish international means of protection. *The most powerful means of protection, however, is the truth, and, before all, truth founded on special knowledge of the subject.* If we cannot demonstrate the rightness of our cause before the world, and on the ground of this right come to a mutual understanding among ourselves, then the cause may at once be considered as lost.

The attacks which are levelled against us, when carefully considered, may be divided into two chief classes. On the one hand it is believed that experimental medicine—indeed, medicine generally—is essentially materialistic, not to say nihilistic, in its ultimate objects: it offends against sentiment, against morality, against religion. On the other hand, it is denied that experimentation on animals can have any real value, that the cause of medicine has been really promoted thereby, and, more especially, that the healing of disease has since made any appreciable advance. Even those who allow some slight progress, urge that similar progress might have been obtained as easily by anatomical means as by experiments on living animals.

For those who know the history of medicine, such arguments are not novel. During centuries, similar, not to say identical, reasons interfered with the dissection of human bodies, and anatomists had to fall back on the dissection of animals, even if they were not—as was Paracelsus, the contemporary of Vesalius—taunted with the derisive question as to whether anatomy was any good at all! Against the dissection of the human body the populace long struggled, and it was only at the commencement of the fourteenth century that permission to dissect dead bodies was given by the Church, under restrictions even more severe than those under which the majority of anti-vivisectors would permit vivisection. It was no accident that the time of the Reformation first secured for the great Vesalius a free field to test the truth of the dogmas of Galen by personal observations on the human body, and to establish a true human anatomy in the place of that of animals, which alone had served for thousands of years as the basis of all medical ideas as to the internal structure of the human body. And as regards pathological anatomy, what opposition has not been met with here, even at a much later period! Few things are more instructive in this regard than the accounts which Wepfer, the distinguished discoverer of the hæmorrhagic nature of ordinary apoplexy, gives of the insults with which he was followed after the Mayor of the town of Schaffhausen had given him permission to open the bodies of those who had died in hospitals and infirmaries—it was towards the middle of the seventeenth century. To those who said it was disgraceful and disgusting to soil the hands with blood and filthiness, he simply replied that the hands would easily be cleaned with a little water: far more disgraceful and disgusting was ignorance of anatomical details, as it saddled inexperienced physicians and surgeons with a disgrace which not even the Rhine, nor the ocean itself, could wash away. Thus, therefore, the study of anatomy was to be praised rather, and supported, by those who were placed by the State in positions of trust.

And indeed, since that time, one government after the other has recognised the immense importance of anatomical science. As far as medical education reaches, dissection is nowadays practised. Even the laity understand that without the most accurate knowledge of the structure of the human body, and of the changes which disease and the healing process bring about, no true scientific treatment by the physician is possible. Can anyone escape such a conclusion? Whoever knows anything of the history of general science must be aware that the two great epochs of the regeneration and revival of medicine date back to the union of these two chief branches of human anatomy, and are largely due to it. It was in the sixteenth century that physiological anatomy brought about the great victory of empiricism over dogmatism, of science over tradition; it was in the eighteenth century that pathological anatomy replaced mysticism by realism, speculation by autopsy, obscure belief and supposition by well-regulated thought. Truly the opponents mentioned also materialism. But with truth Harvey(a) has said, "Sicut ænorum et boni habitus corporum dissectio plurimum ad *philosophiam*, et rectam physiologiam facit, ita corporum morbosorum et cachecticorum inspectio potissimum ad pathologiam philosophicam."

(*To be continued.*)

SECTION OF PATHOLOGY.

INTRODUCTORY REMARKS BY SAMUEL WILKS, M.D., F.R.S.,

President of the Section.

I WELCOME all of you here to-day. But are we not already of one brotherhood? Has not a common bond long ago united us in one family? Although we may not have shaken hands, we have been joined in spirit, or perhaps some of us have even been in more direct communication by means of winged words. Amongst all the ties which link man and man together, some of the closest are those forged by science. A special scientific inquiry will find two minds closely akin, although separated by thousands of miles, nationalities, or tongues. In our own department of pathology it creates a thrill of satisfaction to feel that the study of some morbid process may have led some of us to the discovery that another investigator, of whose existence we had been hitherto ignorant, has his thoughts and occupation in perfect unison with our own, and that, although oceans and continents may separate us, our minds are both attuned to the same string. It is not surprising that the vast subject which more immediately occupies us can never cease to interest man in all its details, whilst he has a resting-place on this globe.

I would fain have inaugurated this Section with a general address, but have refrained from doing so, daring not to sacrifice to platitude our too precious time when so much practical work has to be accomplished.

I cannot, however, but occupy you a few moments in order to take a glance at the immensity of the subject before us, embracing questions as it does in which humanity will be for ever interested, viz., those referring to disease, decay, and death.

Our subject, in a word, is Pathology. Pathology has received various definitions, the most common being that which contrasts it with physiology; for as the latter is regarded as the science of healthy organic life, so the former has been held to be the science of the unhealthy or of the abnormal course of life contrasted with the normal. This division of vital action into normal and abnormal is true in a superficial sense, and might be made theoretically to stand as a definition, but it is by no means applicable to our practical science of pathology, nor can it be made of any value as an expression of diagnostic knowledge in treating the thousand ills to which flesh is heir.

In the first place, it must be admitted that the changes which occur in every organic structure, as years roll on, are to be regarded as normal, unless we take an imaginary or ideal standard of a being living in some former golden age, where nought was known but perpetual youth, and regard every departure from this as morbid. Although we do not frame such a picture to ourselves, but know that the various changes in the bones, the cartilages, the lungs, the brain, and other parts, which take place in age, are in harmony with the dictates of nature, yet how often are we called upon to treat these changes as forms of disease! They are, however, no more unnatural or pathological than the sere and yellow leaf which falls from the oak in autumn.

If, however, these senile changes occur prematurely, they will then be abnormal, and may be strictly regarded as morbid. Herein is one form of a pathological condition with which we have to deal—a premature decay arising from the various causes which bring the organism to an end, either from their operating with unusual force or from some

(a) Guil. Harveji, "Exercit. Anat.," II. : "De Motu Cordis et Sanguinis Circulatione," page 174. Roterod, 1671.

inherent weakness in the body, which is unable to moderate their action. Now, if all these potent influences, instead of driving the mechanism too quickly, and so bringing it prematurely to an end, concentrate their forces upon one organ only, that organ would become, in ordinary parlance, diseased; but the process there set up may be of exactly the same nature as time would otherwise have produced. In comparatively young persons, for instance, we meet with fibroid and fatty-changes in the heart and vessels, distension of the air-cells, alterations in the structure of bones and joints, which resemble in every respect those which age would have ordinarily induced. Therefore many of the conditions which we call disease seem nothing more than the result of the concentration on a particular organ of all those agencies which, under ordinary circumstances, bring about senile changes. These changes, therefore, although senile in character, are abnormal, and hence may be rightly regarded as pathological.

The pathologist, therefore, cannot but regard the body in the first place in its physiological relations with its surroundings, and mark the alterations which time produces. The physiologist is aware that the production of force must be accompanied by loss elsewhere, seeing that gain and loss are equal, and therefore, in observing organic life, he must regard the destructive processes as well as the formative. Life seems to depend upon changes continually going on in relation with the atmosphere in which all living bodies are steeped. The burning of the fuel in oxygen supplies the forces necessary for living processes; we, therefore, although alive, are constantly being consumed. During so many years the body is undergoing combustion, or we might say, slow destruction, and this process occurs much more rapidly in some persons and in some animals than in others. Why one creature should live longer or burn out sooner than another is not clear: why, for example, should a dog be worn out in ten or twelve years, its limbs be stiff, its sight and hearing impaired, its intellect obtuse, and senile changes be discoverable in its brain and elsewhere, when a parrot may take a century for the production of the same destructive changes? Why tissues of the same composition should wear out in one animal after ten revolutions of the earth when it takes a hundred revolutions to destroy similar ones in another, is by no means apparent. In man, if the destructive and reproductive changes are normally counter-balanced, the ordinary duration of life is reached. If the balance be not kept, the destructive agencies may be in the ascendency, and life be shortened. If any of the ordinary surroundings which are always exerting their influences upon us, as various kinds of air, food, moral and mental moods, be in any way noxious, they may in time tend to premature death; and if they should act in such a manner as to cause localised organic changes, we should style these changes disease. There can be little doubt that a large number of maladies in England—as gout, Bright's disease, etc.—are induced by mere excesses or inequalities in a mode of life which is considered ordinarily correct. It ought to be one of our studies to consider the relations of the human race to the soil, and observe all the circumstances which centuries have induced to bring about this normal or healthy relation between them. We might then observe the effects of the concentration of some of the more untoward of the influences which ordinarily environ it, as well as inquire into the effects of transplantation into another country. It seems that all the usual surroundings of life in civilised society, acting in undue proportion or in a more determined manner, induce a very large number of the diseases which we are called upon to treat.

In considering all these agencies working for what we call evil, and leading to destruction, we must not overlook an opposing law—that of reparation. Not only do we observe a production of living force in necessary association with a dissolution of material, but an ever-existing tendency towards the remaking of the injured tissues. We can scarcely think of a morbid change in the body which is not attended by another which has an opposite tendency. Every phthisical lung showing destruction of the tissue exhibits at the same time the attempt to limit the process and to save life by shutting off the escape of air from the lung or sealing the ulcerated bloodvessels.

Then, in considering the definition of disease, after having observed how large a number of maladies are produced by the influences of all our ordinary surroundings, we have to recognise those external causes of an extraordinary or specific character which prey upon the human frame, and often bring its machinery to an end. Now, if these causes are obviously parasitic, we are not witnessing so much the case of disease as the spectacle of one animal preying upon another. As regards the parasite, it is pursuing its normal life-history; and as regards the patient or the host, he is simply being destroyed: the difference in his mode of death from that which would result from the onslaught of a wild animal would consist merely in time. If a man fall a victim to the bite of a cobra he is not said to die of disease; but the term is applicable if he die of glanders. There is this difference, however, in the latter case—the poison is not a natural one even in the infecting animal. If, however, in these infectious diseases the morbific cause be an animal or vegetable organism, although microscopic, then we really have to deal with the operation of one living being acting upon another, and the so-called specific malady exhibits nothing more than the natural course of life of certain specific organisms. The term "disease," according to the definition, is here again scarcely applicable.

All these abnormalities of the human organism, under whatever conditions they may arise, suggest that as every branch of biological science is being studied in relation to the lower organisations, and according to the law of evolution, so must pathology become the subject of a large field of inquiry, and be made to embrace the diseases of all animal and vegetable life. The comparison of disease in man and animals may throw much light upon its nature, and it is remarkable that so few persons have been stimulated to the work by considering the long controversy which has taken place as to the relation between vaccinia and variola, or hydrophobia and rabies. A true human pathology should have its basis in comparative pathology. Here lies a mine of wealth, but little worked. As at the present time every structure and function of the human body is being studied in reference to its antecedents in the lower animals, so there can be no doubt that the various morbid changes to which it is liable may be also profitably discussed in reference to similar actions in more simple forms of life. The truth of this has been clearly seen by philosophers who have had no special acquaintance with our department of science. Thus Buckle, in his "History of Civilisation in England," says: "The best Physiologists distinctly recognise that the basis of their science must include not only the animals below man, but also the entire vegetable kingdom, and that without this commanding survey of the whole realm of organic nature we cannot possibly understand even human physiology, still less general physiology. The Pathologists, on the other hand, are so much in arrear, that the diseases of the lower animals rarely form parts of their plan, while the diseases of plants are almost entirely neglected, although it is certain that until all these have been studied, and some steps taken to generalise them, every pathological condition will be eminently empirical on account of the narrowness of the field from which it is collected." This is almost as true now as when written several years ago; but we are pleased to think that our countryman, Sir James Paget, has already removed this slur upon our scientific procedure by his lecture on "Elemental Pathology," in which he shows the importance of observing the resemblances between the changes in the various tissues of man and the vegetable world, and also the deductions to be drawn therefrom.

Again, if the specific diseases be due to organisms, and the hypothetical contagium vivum be a reality, it must be subject to the same laws as other organic matter; and if the doctrine of evolution be true, it must have numerous relations with families of its own kind, and perhaps with others which are now obsolete. This idea has occupied the minds of several medical men in this country, and it will no doubt further fructify in their hands.(a)

A highly contagious disease prevailing in a particular locality may be exhibiting the differentiation of some more simple, less virulent and widely-spread disorder. For example, a slightly contagious epidemic sore-throat might in course of time develope into a more virulent one until it culminated in diphtheria; and if this disease be due to an organism, the latter might have found a more genial soil for its development, or be altered by propagation and time, so that new properties might at last have

(a) Dr. Airy, Dr. Thorne, etc.

been added to it. There may be a progressive development of infectiveness. Then, again, the doctrine of natural selection might obtain in the fact of some specific diseases remaining amongst us, while others have become obsolete. The same law, too, if allowed its full operation, might tend still more than it does to the subjugation of many hereditary diseases; for as these appear in youth, and often cause death, they would fade away by a process of self-destruction. As regards the specific diseases, we see again how the most susceptible persons would be struck out by the poison, and the least susceptible remain, so that the poison would be modified in its virulence. We witness this fact in the more moderate characters of the exanthemata in all civilised nations, in comparison with the more profound effects produced by them in nations where the diseases had been hitherto unknown—as, for example, the fatality in the Pacific Islands of our comparatively mild British measles.

Besides the maladies which are induced by the evil influences of our ordinary surroundings and those due to specific causes just named, there is a class of diseases styled new growths, which take a very large share in adding to man's mortality. The advance made in our knowledge of these structures is very considerable, and is still rapidly progressing towards a determination of their origin and the discovery of their relation to the normal tissues. These investigations are assisting us in discarding some of our older notions regarding their constitutional and malignant nature, and proving that many are accidental in their origin, and therefore may possibly be averted.

In these brief remarks, we see how the simple definition of Pathology as a deviation from the healthy standard fails in its application, and how wide is the range of subjects included in its domain. What these are, you, gentlemen, are about to illustrate in the different subjects which you will bring before the Section.

Section of Medicine.

OPENING ADDRESS BY SIR WM. GULL, BART., M.D., F.R.S.,

President of the Section.

The President opened this section on Wednesday afternoon by an address in which he reviewed the present position of "Medicine." We cannot give our readers the whole address, but the following is a fair abstract of it. "Solidism," Sir William Gull said, is widely reasserting itself in the science of living things—not as an *à priori* system, but through the progress of knowledge. The proximate conditions of pyrexia are no longer vaguely referred to nerve, but to definite nerve-centres; hyperæmia and inflammatory changes to sympathetic lesions; abnormal chemistry to the great respiratory centres; the strange conditions of Addison's disease, with its characteristic pigment, to the supra-renal bodies, themselves probably but nerve-centres, and related, at least by structure, to the system of the pituitary gland; epilepsy, supposed in Hippocratic times to be due to extraneous maleficent spiritual influences, is traceable to apparently trifling changes in a few grey nerve-cells. The specific fever-processes notoriously owe much of their character and intensity to the nervous system. Their relation to time, their occurrence only in warm-blooded animals, the great mortality they cause through nerve-exhaustion, and the immunity they leave behind them, indicate that, whatever may be the nature or mode of operation of their several poisons, it is by implication of nerve-elements that fever obtains its chief clinical characteristics. Further, in the advance of "solidism," what can interest us more than the recent investigations on contagia? Perhaps no more important step has been made in practical pathology than the proof that at least of these contagia are organised solids. This discovery, which it has tried the patience, experimental skill, and scientific criticism of the best observers to establish, has brought us at length within view of that which has hitherto been so mysterious. To have been able to separate, though imperfectly, the contagious particles; to have come to the conclusion that no fever-poisons are soluble—is a hopeful preliminary towards forcing them to yield up the secret of their nature. If "solidism," as a theory of organic processes, wanted confirmation, we could point to nothing more striking

than the present established views on putrefactive changes; and to the amazing fact that the normal textures and fluids of the body resist decomposition unless invaded by microscopic organisms. May we not hereafter find that all organic chemistry is the resultant of mechanical changes in organic solids?

Section of Surgery.

INTRODUCTORY ADDRESS BY JOHN ERIC ERICHSEN, F.R.S., etc.,

President of the Section.

Gentlemen,—Surgery is never stationary. To be stationary while all around is in movement would be practically to retrograde. But movement does not necessarily mean advance. The general direction of the movement may undoubtedly be forwards, but the factors of that movement do not all equally tend to progress. When the history of surgery comes to be written—and this has never yet been done—it will be found that the surgery of the nineteenth century has not been uniform in its progress in all departments; that its advance has not been continuously in one line, but that its progress has been materially affected by the prevailing bias of the professional mind of the day. Anatomical at one time, physiological at another, the tendency of the surgery of the present day is influenced in one direction by the mechanical spirit of the age, and in another by the advanced pathology which is one of its chief medical characteristics. Yet the continuous advance of our art is undoubted. The gain that thus results has been definitively secured to surgery and to mankind. It can never be lost. Every conquest that has been made has been permanent. Year after year some new position has been won, often, it is true, after a hot conflict of opinion; but, once occupied, it has never been abandoned. Thus our standpoint has ever been pushed on in advance. For knowledge in science is cumulative, and skill in art is a tradition that is hereditarily transmitted from master to pupil—if not by the individual, yet by the profession to which he belongs, from which he has acquired and to whom he bequeaths it, augmented and perfected by his own labours. With the knowledge of our predecessors we are familiar; to its stores each generation has added. What they have done has been transmitted to us, and we can readily accomplish. In what we can do, we may be sure, our successors will not fail.

It is well that from time to time this advance should be measured, this gain weighed. The business of this Section is not only to measure the extent of the advance, but to determine the value of the gain, and to do this not so much by the novelty of the advance, nor by the brilliancy of its exposition, as by an estimate of its intrinsic merit, as shown by its proved utility. Our business here has to do with practical considerations, having reference to the recent advances in, or the future lines to be followed by, modern surgery.

The Executive of this Section has proposed eight subjects for the consideration of its members. It is hoped that these will be found to include the more important surgical questions that are at present most prominently before the profession. The short time at our disposal, which will scarcely enable us to do full justice even to these subjects, has prevented the possibility of our bringing forward other and perhaps equally interesting questions: but some of these will be found to have received consideration in the papers, which will be read either *in extenso* or in abstract, as time may allow.

I will now briefly refer to the more important subjects that have been set down for our consideration.

I. In no department of surgery has a more marked or a more brilliant advance been made of late years than in that which concerns the operative treatment of intra-peritoneal tumours. The establishment of Ovariotomy as a recognised surgical operation has now long been matter of history; but the perfection of safety to which it has of late years been carried, by the improvement of its details, has led the way to a vast and rapid extension of operative surgery for the cure or relief of various diseased abdominal organs. The uterus and the spleen, the stomach, the pylorus and the colon, have each and all been subjected to the scalpel of the surgeon—with what success has yet to be determined; and it is for you to decide whether some, at least, of these operations constitute real and solid advances in our art, or whether they are rather to be regarded as bold and skilful experiments on the endurance and reparative power of the human frame—whether, in fact, they are surgical triumphs or operative audacities. There must, indeed, be a limit to the progress of operative surgery in this direction. Are we at present in a position to define it? There cannot always be new fields for conquests by the knife; there must be portions of the human frame that will ever remain sacred from its intrusion, at least, in the hands of the surgeon. May there not be some reason to fear lest the very perfection to which ovariotomy has been carried may lead to an over-sanguine expectation of the value and the safety of the abdominal section and exploration when applied to the diagnosis or cure of diseases of other and very dissimilar organs, in which but little of ultimate advantage, and certainly much of immediate peril, may be expected from operative interference?

II. In the discussion of the next great question, I would submit that we may, with advantage, direct our attention less to the mere mechanical—the simple operative part of the business, the details of which are now well understood—than to the consideration of those higher questions as to the diagnosis and nature of the various forms of renal disease in which Nephrotomy and Nephrectomy may be respectively used, with a reasonable hope of relief or cure. And in considering the prospects afforded by these operations in the improvement of the health and the mitigation of the sufferings of the patient, it is surely not the least interesting point for us to study the after-physiological effects produced on the system by the extirpation of so important an eliminatory organ as the kidney.

III. We naturally pass from the consideration of operations on the kidney to that of those which implicate the bladder; and in doing so we have specially to direct our attention to the question as to what advances have of late been made in Lithotomy and Lithotrity.

In lithotomy we see much of change, possibly something of novelty, but not so certainly anything of real progress. Have we, indeed, advanced one single step either in the perfection or in the results of that operation since the days of Cheselden, of Martineau, or of Crosse—not to mention the names of more recent but equally illustrious surgeons and successful operators? The revived median, the combination of it with lithotrity, the supra-pubic (whether done antiseptically or not), have certainly not been very encouraging in their results, and can scarcely claim to be considered in the light of an advance on the old lateral operation in skilful hands. But yet we must admit that these methods of lithotomy may deserve this consideration—that possibly, in some forms of calculus and in certain conditions of the urinary organs, a wise eclecticism may be exercised in the choice of one or other of them.

In lithotrity, however, it is probable that a great and real advance has been made, and certainly it is undoubted that a complete revolution has been effected by the enterprise and skill of one of our American brethren; for it cannot be questioned that " Bigelow's operation " has completely changed the aspect of lithotrity, and there is every reason to believe that it constitutes one of those real advances in a method which marks an epoch not only in the history of the operation itself, but in the treatment of the disease to which it is applicable.

But here a fertile field opens up for our deliberation. We have to consider not only in what cases as regards the mere size of calculus " Bigelow's operation " may safely be used, but also, and far more important than this, the ultimate result both upon the bladder and the kidney of prolonged intra-vesical instrumentation. The mere question as to the comparative advantages of removal of stone by one or by several sittings is dwarfed by the more important one of determining the state of the bladder that results—not, perhaps, so much as concerns the life as the future comfort of the patient. It is here that information is much needed, and it is here that, unfortunately, but for very obvious reasons, the lithotritist himself may in many cases be unable to furnish it.

IV. Pre-historic man was doubtless a victim of injury before he became the sufferer from disease, and the treatment of wounds constituted probably the first effort of the healing art. From the earliest dawn of human intelligence the attempt to cure a wound must have suggested itself to man, and yet at the close of the nineteenth century we are still discussing the best methods of doing this, and the causes of their failure. There is still difference of opinion and of practice amongst surgeons, not only as to the comparative advantages of the " open air " method, and that in which all atmospheric contact is carefully guarded against; of the " dry " and of the " moist " system of dressing; as to whether the " antiseptic method " in a modified form suffices, or whether the more elaborate system of local treatment before, during, and after an operation, which has been devised by the skill, and worked out by the unwearied labour of Lister, be essential in all cases of operation wound. Not, of course, for its primary union—for this may be obtained by any and every of the methods mentioned. If it be contended that this system is necessary for the safety of the patient, and the due healing of the wound in some cases, has it been proved to be equally essential in traumatic lesions of all tissues, of all organs, and of all regions? These are questions that may well deserve the consideration of this Section. But there are others of a yet wider character that must also engage our attention in any discussion on the best methods of securing primary union in wounds, for it is impossible to fail to recognise in the general constitutional state of the patient a most important factor in this direction; and we should be taking a narrow view of this many-sided question if we did not give due weight to the influence of those hygienic conditions which, if faulty, are inimical, or even destructive, to the due performance of those actions which are necessary for the maintenance of the organism in a healthy state, and for the proper nutrition and consequent repair of the tissues of the body. Is there no fear that in some of the modern systems of treating wounds we are in danger of expending all our precautions in the prevention of the local and of ignoring the risk of a constitutional infection?

V. The treatment of Aneurism is one of those great questions which from an early period in the history of modern surgery has occupied the attention of practitioners, and has undergone no little fluctuation. A few years ago the battle between the ligature and compression appeared to have been decided in favour of the latter; but the invention of improved ligatures, made of various kinds of animal tissue, and applied with antiseptic precautions, has once more inclined the balance of professional opinion towards the Hunterian operation. But now again the practice of compression has received renewed strength from the employment of Esmarch's elastic bandage in the cure of certain forms of external aneurism, and it is for you to determine in what cases it can be used with advantage, and in what way a cure is effected by its means. For in the treatment of aneurisms, as in that of so many other surgical diseases, the wiser and more scientific course is to follow a judicious system of selection in the method to be employed in each particular case, rather than to subject all to one unbending line of practice.

VI. The treatment by Resection of some forms of chronic and otherwise incurable joint-diseases has, in certain articulations, and at suitable ages, met with the universal approbation of surgeons, and the wide extension of the principles of " conservative surgery " is one of the most striking evidences of advance in our art in modern times. Resection has, however, of late years come to be extensively applied to the treatment of cases of articular disease which formerly were subjected to procedures of a less heroic character; and it will be for the members of this Section to weigh carefully the wisdom of such a measure, and to contrast its results, both as regards life of patient and after-utility of limb, with those which may be obtained from the employment of milder means, such as absolute immobility with extension, and possibly, in some cases, simple incision of the articulation.

VII. In considering the relations between adenoma, sarcoma, and carcinoma in the mammary gland of the female, I would venture to submit that this subject has to be discussed here from its clinical rather than from its pathological side. We have here less to do with the ultimate structure of the tumours, with their histological affinities, with the parts that are played by epiblasts and mesoblasts, with what epithelium or connective-tissue cells can or cannot do, than with their clinical history, their differential diagnosis in their earlier stages, the best time for their removal by operation, the liability to recurrence after operation, and the possibility in recurrence of the substitution of one form of disease for another. With these, and such questions as these, we, as clinical surgeons, may advantageously occupy ourselves.

VIII. The last subject set down for discussion is one that has practical bearings of an importance that cannot be over-estimated. There are few questions of the present day of deeper surgical or social interest than the far-reaching, the apparently illimitable, and most pernicious extension of a syphilitic contamination of organs and of tissues; of the modifications impressed by it on other diseases that are the local developments of diatheses, whether strumous, tuber-cular, rheumatic, or gouty. Does the diathesis exercise any influence upon the form assumed by the syphilitic disease, and to what extent does it modify the characters presented by it in its primary and its secondary affections, more especially when the latter manifest themselves upon the skin or in the bones? How far are gummata and caries, psoriasis, and rupia the consequences of a constitutional impress, influencing the direction of the syphilitic poison? To what extent may rickets and grey granulations be the ultimate products of the syphilitic taint? These and various other questions will probably occupy the attention of those who enter on the discussion of this wide-spreading subject.

We hope to be able to take the discussion of two questions on each day, so as to work through the eight in the time allotted to us. In addition to these there are various detached papers on subjects which are of much interest, but which scarcely admit of being classified under one or other of the above heads of discussion. These we shall take up as time and opportunity admit, but their number is so great that it is to be feared that full justice can scarcely be done to all, and that it will be unavoidable, on account of the limited time at our disposal, that a large number be read in abstract.

SECTION OF OBSTETRIC MEDICINE AND SURGERY.

OPENING ADDRESS BY ALFRED H. McCLINTOCK, M.D., LL.D.,

President of the Section.

IN opening the Obstetric Section of this seventh International Medical Congress, the first and most gratifying duty that devolves upon your President is to offer an earnest and hearty welcome to those obstetric members who have come from other nationalities, and from distant British colonies, to take part in this—the largest convention of medical men that has ever, perhaps, assembled together at any one time or place.

I present this cordial salutation, not only on the part of the officers and council of the particular Section over which I have the honour to preside, but also on the part of the obstetricians and gynæcologists of England, Scotland, and Ireland.

We are proud and happy to meet here, on British ground, so many of our brethren from various parts of the civilised world, but especially from Germany, France, and America, and to accord them a friendly greeting, not only out of respect to their individual merits and high reputation, but as representing those great obstetric schools over which the names of Mauriceau, Levret, Bandilocque, and Dubois, of Roederer, Siebold, Nägelé, Kiwisch, and Scanzoni, and of Bard, Dewees, Meigs, and Hodge, have severally shed such imperishable lustre.

Not the least of the important objects contemplated in this Congress is the interchange of friendly feelings among its members. I am fully persuaded that our reunions will be attended, not alone with benefit to us all by the attrition of mind with mind,—but that new friendships will be formed, and old friendships confirmed, and that sentiments of mutual respect and regard will be developed, so as to strengthen the bond of brotherhood which should unite us as fellow-workers in the same department of medicine.

Allow me before going further to express my deep sense of the unexpected, unmerited dignity which the Congress has conferred by putting me into the position of President of this important Section; I feel it to be the highest and most flattering honour of my long professional life. Such a compliment more than repays one for forty years of labour and devotion; for it sets the seal of approval by contemporaries on my past life, and leaves nothing further or higher to aspire to in the way of professional distinction. At the same time, gentlemen, this feeling of just pride and exaltation is mingled with a very poignant sense of incapacity, and I might well shrink from the responsibility of the post, but that in the discharge of its duties I shall have the aid and co-operation of such accomplished men as those who constitute the vice-presidents and Council of the Section; they, in truth, are the giants on whose shoulders I am raised to the exalted position it is my good fortune to occupy in this Congress.

Inasmuch as this is the first occasion of the International Medical Congress meeting in London, it may not be inappropriate if I pass in review some of the more prominent among the many eminent obstetricians who lived and practised in this city, who by their writings, teaching, and discoveries have contributed in no small measure to the development of midwifery and gynæcology, as well as to the medico-chirurgical fame of London.

I must, however, study brevity, being desirous, if possible, to keep within the fifteen minutes allowed for the reading of communications, so as to set an example of obedience to the rules of the Congress.

In this retrospective glance, I find only one name standing out in the sixteenth century—Thomas Raynald, the translator of Eucarius Rhodion's celebrated treatise "De partu Hominis." The original English edition, by Raynald, appeared about 1540, and was the first distinct treatise on midwifery in the English language, and for over one hundred years was the sole guide and text-book of obstetric practitioners, male and female.

In the early part of the seventeenth century, the immortal William Harvey (*tanto nomini nullum par eulogium*) stands forth conspicuous, the splendour of his fame increasing as years roll on. He spent most of his time here, being physician to the King; and he delivered courses of lectures at the Royal College of Physicians on anatomy and surgery. As a practitioner we know from the testimony of his contemporaries that Harvey excelled in midwifery, and in the treatment of female diseases.

Before the publication of his celebrated exercitations on generation, parturition, conception, etc., there were, according to Dr. Aveling, "but three works on midwifery in our language; these were translations from Rhodion, Rueff, and Guillemeau. His was the first book on midwifery written by an Englishman, printed in our own language, and the influence which it had upon the practice of the time would with difficulty now be estimated. His claim, therefore, to eminence in our department of medicine is beyond question." With this conviction in our minds, we shall the more heartily yield our applause when his magnificent memorial statue is unveiled at Folkestone, the place of his nativity, on Saturday next—a ceremony, I may remark, which has with good taste and judgment been purposely so arranged that this great Medical Congress may take a part in showing honour and respect to the memory of one of the greatest discoverers in the science of medicine, and, consequently, one of the greatest benefactors to the human race.

Contemporary with Harvey was another remarkable man—Peter Chamberlen—the inventor of the midwifery forceps, indisputably the most valuable instrument of the whole *armamentarium chirurgicum.* Unfortunately for him, however, the brilliancy of his reputation is obscured by the unworthy selfish conduct which caused him to keep the instrument a secret for the aggrandisement of himself and family. He was father of Dr. Hugh Chamberlen, the translator into English of Mauriceau's works. There is a handsome monument to the memory of this Dr. Hugh Chamberlen in Westminster Abbey, erected by his patron and friend the Duke of Buckingham. No less than five generations of the Chamberlen family were eminent in the medical profession here; and Dr. Peter, who attained a great age, had been physician to five English sovereigns.

Towards the close of this (seventeenth) century, Richard Wiseman, "Serjeant-Chirurgeon" to Charles I., published his treatise on Surgery, in which he gives an excellent description of pelvic abscesses consequent on parturition. He thus anticipated Puzos' essay on the same disease, and put forward much more rational and correct views as to its pathology.

The eighteenth century was destined to see a marvellous development of midwifery, as well as of many other arts and sciences. As might therefore be expected, London can boast of several eminent obstetricians at this period.

In chronological order, the first to be mentioned is Dr. John Arbuthnot, F.R.S. and F.R.C.P., Physician to Queen Anne. Although he has left no enduring evidence of obstetric superiority, yet he was an eminent accoucheur in his day, and reflected infinite credit on our order by his rare literary talents, his deep scholarship, and his exalted social position. He was skilled in everything that related to science, and held a prominent place among the ablest writers and wits of that Augustan age: one of whom (Swift or Pope) alludes in his poetry to

"Arbuthnot's soft obstetric hand."

A man who was considered a friend and an equal by Parnell, Gay, Bolingbroke, Swift, and Pope, could not fail to adorn any pursuit to which he devoted his vast intellectual powers. Speaking of him, Swift said, "He has more wit than we all, and his humanity is equal to his wit." A higher tribute could not have been paid him.

The next to be mentioned is Dr. John Maubray, not on account of any peculiar merit in either of his works—"The Female Physitian," and "Midwifery brought to Perfection," —but because he is reputed to have been the first public teacher of midwifery in this country. He lectured, Dr. Denman tells us, at his house in Bond-street, so far back as the year 1724.

Nearly contemporary with Maubray was Dr. Edmund Chapman. He was the second public teacher of midwifery in this city, and is entitled to our lasting gratitude for having been the first to publish to the world a description of that "noble instrument" (to use his own phrase), the obstetric forceps, the secret of which the Chamberlens kept to themselves for over fifty years. This he did in the *Edinburgh Medical Essays*, and subsequently in his treatise "On the Improvement of Midwifery, chiefly with regard to the Operation,"—the "operation" meaning the application of the forceps. The first edition of this book came out in 1733.

About this same period also lived Sir Richard Manningham, F.R.S., a man of considerable learning and of great reputation as a successful midwifery practitioner. He was author of some obstetric works of temporary consequence, and his claim to remembrance arises from the circumstance that in the year 1739 he opened a ward in the Parochial Infirmary of St. James', Westminster, exclusively for the reception of parturient women, which was the first thing of the kind in Great Britain. Shortly afterwards the idea was taken up and enlarged upon elsewhere, and the great Lying-in Hospital of Dublin was founded by Dr. Bartholomew Mosse, being the first hospital of the kind in the British dominions.

The very same year that Sir Richard Manningham opened his obstetric ward in St. James' Infirmary, as we have just seen, a surgeon from a small country town in Scotland established himself here in London as an accoucheur, who ultimately effected the greatest reformation that had yet taken place in the principles and practice of obstetrics. This man was William Smellie, a name always to be respected wherever midwifery is cultivated as a science. For twenty years Smellie practised and taught here; and published the first volume of his celebrated treatise in 1751, and his splendid anatomical plates in 1754. Amongst his pupils who later on became eminent in the same branch of medicine, were William Hunter, Denman, David McBride (of Dublin), John George Roederer (subsequently Professor of Midwifery at Göttingen), Dr. James Lloyd, of Boston, U.S., and Dr. William Shippen, afterwards Professor of Midwifery in the Pennsylvanian University: these last being, according to Professor Parvin, "the two first American obstetric practitioners." Most gladly would I linger over the life and works of this great man, but I must content myself with a few sentences.

Smellie possessed a wonderful capacity for work, and a clear judgment; but beyond and above this, he was endowed with a singularly accurate perception of facts, which made him a correct as well as a close observer of nature. Herein lay the secret of his unrivalled success as a reformer and improver of midwifery. He himself felt this to be so, for in reviewing his practice he says, "I diligently attended to the course and operations of nature which occurred in my practice, regulating and improving what by that infallible standard" (Case 186, Sydenham Society edition). Truly, he was, in the words of Dr. Hugh Miller, a "noble character and an example of earnest living."

A couple of years after Smellie settled in London, there came to live with him a young man from the Scottish county (Lanarkshire) of which Smellie himself was a native. This young man was no less a person than William Hunter—a name familiar to you all—whose plates and descriptions of the human gravid uterus have gained their author a foremost rank among obstetric writers. By his great reputation as a lecturer and as an anatomist, aided no doubt by his prepossessing appearance, polished manners, and cultivated mind, Hunter proved a successful competitor of Smellie's in practice. Like him, he also gave special courses of lectures on midwifery; MS. notes of which are to be found in many libraries. Dr. Matthews Duncan tells us the College of Physicians possesses two pretty complete volumes of such notes.

In 1748, Hunter was appointed surgeon and man-midwife to Middlesex Hospital, and soon afterwards to the British Lying-in Hospital; for though the physicians claim him as belonging to themselves, yet it cannot be disputed that Hunter was a surgeon and member of the Corporation of Surgeons of this city.

Besides being a rival he was in some respects a contrast to Smellie. The school of obstetrics founded by the latter was not inaptly described by the late Tyler Smith as the mechanical school, from the importance it attached to the resources of art in aiding parturition. Hunter, on the other hand, placed extraordinary reliance on the powers of nature, and trusted too much to tincture of time. Hence his followers have been designated the physiological school; and, through the influence of his commanding authority, they formed a large section of the profession, and could boast some great names.

Although we may regard Hunter as one of ourselves, and appropriate much of the glory with which his name is invested, "yet it is necessary (as Dr. Duncan observes), with a view to justice, to point out that his obstetrical fame is chiefly anatomical, and that his greatest claim on our admiration and gratitude arises from his anatomical work and influence" (Harveian Address, 1876).

It is a just boast of the English school of midwifery that what, in the truest and strictest sense, is "the most conservative of all the resources of our art," was first formally admitted a place among obstetric operations in this city and about the year 1756. The recognition by the profession of the artificial induction of premature labour was the outcome of a medical conference held at the time and place just mentioned. Who was the first or most strenuous advocate of the operation at that conference does not appear; but we do know that the first to put it in practice was Dr. Macaulay, a midwifery practitioner of this city. It is natural and just, therefore, to identify his name with this most beneficent measure, and to accord him a prominent place among the many distinguished accoucheurs who lived and practised here.

One of the greatest ornaments of that physiological school of accoucheurs—founded, we may say, by William Hunter—was Thomas Denman, a man of remarkably sound judgment, great prudence, and of the highest moral integrity. Throughout half a century he lectured and practised in this city. His work, entitled "An Introduction to the Practice of Midwifery," is well known to most of you; it has many peculiar excellences, but to my mind the chief is his classification of labour, which is at once comprehensive, pathological, and practical, and thereby serves the highest purposes of any system of classification.

Did time permit, I could multiply these brief sketches so as to include many other London obstetricians who lived since the commencement of the present century, of whom, it is true, but yet men who stood far above mediocrity, and who, by their writings, their teaching, and their practice, materially aided the advancement of midwifery and gynæcology. I must content myself, however, with a mere recital of their honoured names, viz.:—John Clarke, Osborne, Leake, Bland, Merriman, Charles Clarke, Gooch, David Davis, Blundel, John Ramsbotham, Marshall Hall, Robert Lee, Robert Ferguson, Rigby, jun., Francis Ramsbotham, Granville, Ashwell, Lever, Locock, Waller, Murphy, Tyler Smith, Oldham.

These men all lived so near our own times (at least, those of us who, like myself, have reached the grand climacteric), that the bare mention of their names at once recalls the titles and the nature of their respective contributions to the funded capital of our professional knowledge.

Of the living obstetric celebrities who make this city the scene of their work and their influence, I purposely refrain from speaking.

> " My thoughts are with the dead ; with them
>   I live in long past years,
> Their virtues love, their faults condemn,
>   Partake their hopes and fears ;
> And from their lessons seek and find
> Instruction with an humble mind."—*Southey.*

But to a more worthy occupant of this chair at some future meeting of the Congress, after we have played our little parts in life's drama, I bequeath the grateful, pleasing task of supplementing the above list with the names of those eminent London obstetricians and gynæcologists, whom to meet and to know is assuredly the most gratifying of the many privileges connected with this great international gathering.

SECTION OF DISEASES OF CHILDREN.

OPENING ADDRESS BY SAMUEL WEST, M.A., M.B.,
President of the Section.

GENTLEMEN,—My first duty on taking this chair is a most pleasant one. It is to express my deep sense of the honour done me by my countrymen when they selected me as not unworthy to represent that department of medicine in England which we all assembled here more especially cultivate. The honour, too, was enhanced by the fact that at the time when it was conferred I was on the point of leaving London in search of what I am thankful to say I found—perfect health in a land of constant sunshine.

That I have found there, too, a second home, I owe it to the kindness of you, my French friends, who received me so cordially and treated me so graciously. You did not regard me as a stranger, but as a fellow-member of that great "Société Internationale" which has for its object, not the upsetting of thrones, nor the changing of governments in quest of some grand social regeneration, to be accomplished in a few days by violence and bloodshed, but the improvement of mankind by gentle means. The one, like the thunderstorm and the torrent, does but lay waste ; the other is like the silent dew, which falls unseen and fertilises the land.

But while I thank you most heartily for all your goodness to me in what I may now call my adopted country, you will, I am sure, find it but natural that I rejoice in returning once more to my native land, in seeing again the old familiar faces, and in revisiting the spots where I studied as a youth, or where I laboured as a grown man.

> " Cœlum, non animam, mutant,
>   Qui trans mare currunt."

And my French sympathies are not one jot lessened because I still feel myself altogether an Englishman.

With these words, gentlemen, I should have wished to stop, and to have invited you to pass at once to the business for which we are met.

Some three weeks ago, however, I learned to my dismay that the Executive Committee desired that the President of each Section should open its meetings by a short address bearing on its special objects.

Far away from my books, moving each day from place to place, I felt my utter inability to do anything worthy of the occasion.

Moreover, there came to my recollection an anecdote which did not help to cheer me.

Dr. Johnson and his friend Boswell dined one day with a gentleman, by special invitation. The next day Dr. Johnson complained to his friend of the meagreness of the entertainment. "Well, sir," said Boswell, "but it was a good dinner." "Yes," replied Johnson, "a good enough dinner, but it was not a dinner to ask a man to."

And so, how scanty and commonplace soever what I say is, pray remember, gentlemen, the entertainment is not one which, had I been left to myself, I should have thought good enough to ask you to.

One accusation which I have heard brought against a meeting like the present is, that it is apt to resolve itself into a mutual admiration society, each member praising what the other has done, all joining to extol what their own generation has accomplished ; and that the gratification of personal vanities, not the promotion of science, is the chief outcome of the whole.

But just as travellers on a long journey halt from time to time, and, looking back on the road they have traversed, take courage to go further, so may we, with no feeling of undue self-gratulation, rejoice over what has been accomplished, even in our own day, as an earnest and a pledge of further progress, an inducement to more unwearied effort.

Thirty years ago, throughout the whole of England and America, there was not a single hospital set apart for children. It was but rarely that one saw these little waifs and strays in the wards of our general hospitals, for the maxim, " De minimis non curat lex," held good in medicine as in law. Germany, too, was in but little better case, and one was forced to go to Paris to study on a large scale those diseases which men like Guersant, and Blache, and Baron, and Trousseau and Roger, investigated with untiring zeal, and, in spite of hospital arrangements most painfully defective, strove to cure. We all know how this is altered now. In London there are six separate children's hospitals, each, I believe, with its convalescent branch, and children's wards are to be found in every one of the large London hospitals. There are special children's hospitals in every large town in England ; America and Germany have followed the same example ; and everywhere throughout Europe the opportunities for the study of children's diseases are almost as numerous as for those of the adult.

Nor has this wide field been without abundant husbandmen to till it, and we may count with satisfaction the fruit of their labours.

The vague phraseology which served for years to conceal our ignorance, even from ourselves, has been to a great degree done away with. We talk no longer of worm fever, remittent fever, gastric fever, and so on, for under these various names we recognise the one disease, typhoid fever, varying in severity, but marked always by its own characteristic symptoms. Half a page in a handbook was all that was to be found thirty years ago concerning heart-disease in childhood, while at the present time the frequency of heart-disease has been fully recognised, and it has been studied with as much care in the child as in the adult. The various inflammations of the respiratory organs are no longer looked on as a whole, but each is referred to its proper class, and we distinguish lobar and lobular pneumonia, bronchitis and capillary bronchitis, and assign to each its proper place and its characteristic symptoms. Nor have our therapeutics lagged behind. I remember the hesitation with which, some forty years ago, my dear friend and master, the late Dr. Latham, decided on tapping the chest of a boy eight years of age, who was received into St. Bartholomew's Hospital on account of a pleurisy which had terminated in empyema ; and the delight—the wonderment almost—with which we regarded the successful issue of the operation in a child so young. A few months ago I communicated to the Medical Society of Nice the particulars of fifty cases in my own practice, where paracentesis of the chest had been performed at my desire, and several of you gentlemen could relate as many cases or more. That once almost unrecognised disease, diphtheria, has been studied with the greatest care ; its relation to membranous croup has been investigated ; the close connexion of the two has been demonstrated. I for my part should not hesitate to say their absolute identity has been established. Much light has been thrown on various diseases of the nervous system. That once enigmatical affection, the so-called essential paralysis of infancy and childhood, has been shown (in the first instance by the researches of my friend M. Roger, and his able coadjutor M. Damaschino) to be due to an acute inflammatory softening of the grey matter of the anterior columns of the spinal cord ; and twenty-five recorded observations since that time attest the truth of their discovery. Though, strictly speaking, perhaps not a disease of the nervous system, the pseudo-hypertrophic muscular paralysis of Duchenne claims mention here as a new and important addition to our knowledge of the pathology of early life.

I fear to weary you by further enumeration, else it would not be difficult to increase largely the instances of new and most important knowledge added to our stores since my student-days.

In estimating the value of these gains, too, it must not be forgotten that each truth established means an error exploded; so much base metal, so much counterfeit coin withdrawn from circulation; or, to put it differently, so much sterling gold substituted for inconvertible paper money.

In this process surgery has, as everywhere, borne a large part. The treatment of hip-disease, the excision of scrofulous joints, the new modes of treatment of spinal curvature—some, indeed, still on their trial,—the operation for the cure of genu valgum, which one cannot mention without a fresh tribute of thanks to Joseph Lister, who in this instance has rendered a proceeding safe and salutary, from which, but a few years since, the common sense of the surgeon would have recoiled, are so many fresh instances of progress made during a period of little more than the half of my professional life.

I take it, however, that the great use of meetings such as the present, is to take stock far less of what we know, than of what we do not know, or know at best but imperfectly. A few of these problems have been submitted to you in the list of subjects for discussion. To some it is probable that the combined experience of so many, and such distinguished men as are here present, may furnish definite and conclusive answers. Other questions are introduced in the hope of gaining fresh information on points concerning which our knowledge is fragmentary; while there are many other problems still unsolved, on which it is hoped that fresh light will be thrown during the time of our meeting here.

And now, with your permission, I will conclude with an old apologue, which tells how, when the fabled Arabian bird renewed each hundred years its vigour and eternal youth, the birds of the air all helped to build its nest. The eagle and the wren contributed alike to this labour of love and duty; each brought what he could, nor ceased till the task was done. And surely science and art, especially our science and art, are old and new, renewing day by day, and burning by a voluntary self-cremation old theories, half facts, hasty conclusions, and substituting more accurate observations, truer inferences, more solid judgments. To this great end we may all do something; but, labour as we may, our task will never be finished, for not once in a hundred years, as the fable runs, but every day and all day long the process goes on—a daily death, a daily renewal, as in our bodies' growth, a death of error, a development of truth.

SUB-SECTION OF DISEASES OF THE THROAT.

INTRODUCTORY ADDRESS BY GEORGE JOHNSON, M.D., F.R.C.P., F.R.S.,

President of the Sub-section.

GENTLEMEN,—The first duty that I have to perform is to express my high appreciation of the honour conferred upon me in the appointment to preside over this important sub-section of medicine. I have next the pleasure to offer a hearty British welcome to the many very eminent laryngologists, who, from various parts of the continents of Europe and America, have done us the favour and the honour to join this Congress, and to make, as they are about to do, numerous important and highly instructive communications to this department of medicine. The history of the laryngoscope has been often written, and is well known to this learned assembly. I am sure, however, that I shall have your sympathy and your approval in giving a brief expression of our indebtedness to Signor Garcia—whom we have the pleasure to welcome amongst us here to-day—for the pre-eminent share which he has had in the invention of that instrument. While all previous attempts to inspect the living larynx had been incomplete, and barren of further results, Signor Garcia, who has the unquestionable distinction of having been the first man whose thoughtful ingenuity enabled him to see his own larynx, published the results of his utoscopic observations in the *Proceedings of the Royal Society* (vol. vii., 1855), and this publication led on, through the appreciative mind of Professor Türck, and the indefatigable zeal and exertions of the late lamented Professor Czermak, to the creation and the rapid development of the art of laryngoscopy.

It is scarcely possible to over-estimate the practical importance of this simple invention. I have been long enough in practice as a physician to have had ample experience of the enormous difficulties which often attended the diagnosis, and therefore the treatment, of diseases of the throat in the dark pre-laryngoscopic age. And now, by contrast, the result of the new light thrown upon this region by the throat-mirror has been that within the last twenty years our knowledge of laryngeal diseases, including accuracy of diagnosis, with certain and successful treatment, has made greater progress than that of any other department of medicine or surgery during the same period of time. In making this statement I am not unmindful of the immense advance which has been made in the diagnosis and treatment of eye-diseases since the genius of Helmholtz conferred upon mankind the inestimable gift of the ophthalmoscope.

It is not without interest to compare the practical gains with regard to both diagnosis and treatment, which have been derived respectively from the two analogous instruments—the ophthalmoscope and the laryngoscope. In regard to facility and accuracy of diagnosis, the ophthalmic surgeon and the laryngologist may be considered to have been about equally benefited by the use of their respective instruments. If we take into account the numerous remote diseases, more especially those of the nervous system, upon which the ophthalmoscope has thrown a new light, that instrument may, perhaps, be considered, in the matter of mere diagnosis, to take precedence of the laryngoscope. With regard, however, to improved methods of treatment, and in particular to the introduction of entirely new and previously impossible mechanical operations, there can, I think, be no question that the laryngoscope has done more than can fairly be claimed for the ophthalmoscope. Without doubt the exact diagnosis of eye-diseases has led to improved and more successful treatment, but the ophthalmoscope has afforded no direct aid to treatment comparable, for example, with the safe and easy removal of morbid growths and foreign bodies which the laryngoscope has made an everyday proceeding.

Amongst the most interesting and important of the scientific and practical gains which have resulted from the use of these two instruments—and which may be claimed alike, if not equally, for both—is the fact that, by the inspection respectively of the interior of the eye and of the larynx, valuable light is often thrown upon the diseases of remote but physiologically correlated organs. If, for example, the ophthalmoscopist sees in the eye a retinitis significant of renal disease, a neuritis indicating cerebral tumour, or an embolism the result of valvular disease of the heart, so in like manner the laryngologist is often led by the observation of the paralytic or spasmodic condition of one or more laryngeal muscles, to the diagnosis of a general neurotic condition to which the term hysteria is often applied, or of a special local disease in the nervous centre, or, it may be, of a tumour cervical or intra-thoracic pressing on the pneumogastric nerve or its branches.

It is obvious that all clinical facts of this kind, indicating, as they do, the interdependence and the close physiological relationship between various tissues and organs, are of great scientific and practical importance. There is reason for the belief that the more thorough and profound is the investigation of any disease or class of diseases, the more numerous and intimate will be found to be the relationship with other morbid states. The study of renal diseases affords abundant and most instructive illustrations of this proposition.

The more special therefore is any department of practice, the greater is the need to recur often to general principles, and to bear in mind that so close is the *solidarity* of the animal organism, that there is a literal and physiological truth in the apostolic statement—"If one member suffer, all the members suffer with it." The ill-informed portion of the public are apt to look upon a man who has a reputation for skill in the treatment of a particular class of diseases, as of necessity unacquainted with all other diseases. We, on the other hand, maintain that of the specialist it should be said with truth that he is one, not who knows less of disease in general, but who knows more of the particular class of diseases to which he has devoted most time and especial attention and study.

The Hippocratic maxim, "Life is short, and art is long," is as true now as it was two thousand years ago. Bearing this in mind, and knowing, as I do, how many valuable communications are in store for us, I will occupy no more of your time, but will at once call upon the gentleman whose name stands first on the list to read his promised paper.

SECTION OF MILITARY SURGERY AND MEDICINE.

ADDRESS BY PROF. T. LONGMORE, C.B., F.R.C.S.,
President of the Section.

COLLEAGUES of the Naval and Military Services of our own and foreign countries, and all friends who are good enough to assist in the work of this, the Section of Military Medicine and Surgery,—Allow me, in the first place, to say how sensible I am of the honourable and responsible nature of the position in which I have been placed as President of this Section, and to express my thanks for the trust you have reposed in me. I accepted the office with very great diffidence in obedience to expressed wishes which I felt I could not do otherwise than comply with. I only entertained the hope that I might be able to discharge its duties satisfactorily, with the help of the eminent vice-presidents, Council, and other officers of the Section, on whose support and assistance I felt assured I might confidently rely.

In the second place, I wish, in the name of my British colleagues, to say a word of welcome to our foreign friends who have not hesitated to come, in many instances from places at remote distances, to join in the labours of this Section. We feel honoured that men so distinguished in the science and practice of naval and military surgery should have come among us, many of whom bear names that are not only household words in their own respective countries, but familiar in every part of the world where the progress of military medical science is watched and improvements in its practice are studied. It is a peculiar pleasure to me to welcome those of our foreign *confrères* who have been able to attend the Congress: for among them are many who have been friendly colleagues at previous meetings in various parts of Europe for purposes closely akin to the objects of our present gathering—the advancement of surgical knowledge, and the improvement of the means of alleviating the sufferings inseparable from a state of warfare. We hope that our foreign friends may find themselves well repaid for their journey to London on the present occasion; and that, on returning to their respective countries, they may not only feel that the part of the time which has been devoted to the discussions at the sectional meetings, and to observation of the scientific collections which have been specially formed for the occasion, has been passed profitably, but that also the time spent in our social gatherings has afforded an opportunity of renewing old friendships and forming fresh associations which will remain sources of very many pleasant reminiscences in the future.

Although this is the seventh meeting of the International Medical Congress, it is the first, I am informed, at which there has been a special section for the consideration of subjects connected with military medical and surgical practice; and yet there seems to be a wide field of work for such a section in a professional congress of the kind. Although the true principles of medicine and surgery must be true everywhere, in military or in civil practice, yet everyone practically acquainted with the conditions inseparable from service in the field knows that the application of those principles has perforce to be so modified that the modes of application themselves become a distinct branch of study. In saying this I do not confine myself to the mere physical or manual application of these principles—to the performance of a surgical proceeding in this way or that way,—I refer to matters of far more general influence. Consider how the whole range of what is generally spoken of as "conservative surgery" has to be modified in field practice from the mere influence of the circumstances by which our patients are surrounded in campaigning. How many injuries are there that would be appropriately treated in civil hospitals by an expectant method of treatment, by methods calculated to preserve the injured parts, and with good grounds for hoping to secure restoration of their function, which on numerous occasions the military surgeon would not dare to undertake from his acquaintance with the dangers to life that such a practice would entail on his patients under the exposures, repeated changes from place to place, and other sources of disturbance to which they would have to be subjected in field practice! Remember also the special considerations which arise out of the characters and complications of the great bulk of the injuries themselves which have to be dealt with in military practice, those caused by gunshot.

How great, again, the organisation, the internal administration, the methods of actions of armies, affect everything bearing on surgical practice in them; the quantities and descriptions of surgical and medical materials that the military surgeon can have at his disposal; the amount of protection, care, and attention he can obtain for his patients; the means at his command for transporting them from place to place without aggravation of their injuries! How much patient thought, what prolonged examination and trials; what experience have already been brought to bear on these subjects; and how much still remains to be done in order to attain results which may harmonise with military necessities, and, at the same time, conduce to the welfare of the patients who are placed under our charge! I may allude, further, to the many subjects for deliberation which the crowding together of bodies of troops and animals in the close quarters in which they often have to be placed, give rise to the means of warding off the diseases which such conditions are apt to engender; the means of combating and extinguishing them when they have sprung into existence. In naval professional practice, too, in ships of war, the need of special attention being given to many subjects of medical and surgical interest seems to be obvious. Although the officers and men have the advantage of being in their ordinary house and home on board ship, with its usual furniture, and many things may be carried with them that are not available to soldiers in the field; still, in modern ships of war, with their artificial light below the water-mark, artificial supply of air, large amount of complicated machinery, and limited space for movement, what a necessity there must be for special consideration regarding the means of preserving health, and of the arrangements to be made and the means to be adopted for dealing successfully with injuries which may happen on board, especially when they occur in large numbers, as in case of an action with the enemy! I need not dwell further on the importance of a section in such an International Congress as the present being specially devoted to subjects bearing on the pursuit of medicine and surgery in fleets and armies. A large proportion of those who are present probably have some personal experience of military practice, and, if so, already know how much advantage may be anticipated from meetings at annual intervals for the purpose of discussing special professional topics which are still involved in doubt or obscurity; for making mutually known and sifting the experience gained under varied military circumstances and conditions; for trying to arrive at definite rules of practice; and, in short, for acquiring any knowledge which may particularly conduce to the benefit of the officers and men who depend, often without power of appeal, on our judgment and skill for restoration to health in sickness, and for safety and repair when subjected to wounds and injuries. Although belonging to all nations, we have the advantage of being able to meet together without national jealousy, and with no other rivalry than that of vieing with each other in endeavours to discover what may most benefit the sick and wounded. It is not with our province of thought and action, as it is in some measure with those other parts of military science and practice, on which national safety or superiority in power may depend. A certain amount of reticence in regard to them is justified by national self-interest. We can speak quite openly of all our professional plans and arrangements. If they contain any features better than those belonging to our neighbours of other countries we have no fear of imparting them. We hope, indeed, if they are really better, that they may be adopted and turned to account; for, if practically applied, our own people may possibly be among those who will be benefited by their adoption. And if we lack anything in our military hospital system which our neighbours have better than ourselves, we have no reason to suppose they will object to imparting information on the subject to us; they, in turn, may be benefited by our improvements. Neither surgeons nor patients on either side can be harmed by mutual confidence in matters appertaining to technical knowledge or departmental arrangements. Even in time of war there are no enemies within our sphere of action.

The subjects on which observations are to be read at the present meeting of this Section, and on which discussions are expected, are all subjects having an important bearing on naval and military surgery. I need not enumerate them, as they are already before you in the printed programme.

I will only observe that the most urgent of the questions named for debate at this meeting appears to be the manner in which the antiseptic treatment of wounds can be carried out in times of war. This question, more or less, covers and influences many of the other subjects put down for consideration, such as the advance of conservative surgery in field practice, the treatment of injuries of bloodvessels in the field, improvements in field-hospital equipment, and several others. As you well know, the experience that has hitherto been gained in the strict application of antiseptic principles to the treatment of wounds in the field has been obtained only under exceptional circumstances, and is, comparatively speaking, still exceedingly limited; but, such as it has been, the published results have been so largely superior, both as regards saving life and also as regards the restoration of the usefulness of wounded parts, and the published results of any other methods of treatment in the field, that, so long as this difference holds its ground, we are morally bound to try and extend the practice. All military surgeons, however, can readily perceive the practical difficulties that lie in the way of applying the antiseptic precautions and details of treatment inculcated by Lister, owing to the peculiar conditions incidental to military arrangements in time of war. It appears to me that one of the chief points to be settled, looking at the question from the point of view of military practice, is whether the action on the air by the antiseptic spray is an essential part of the treatment; whether some of the other forms of antiseptic treatment advocated by eminent surgeons are, or are not, capable of producing equally favourable results? If the action on the air by atomised antiseptics be an essential part of the proceeding, then the hope of applying it under the ordinary circumstances of warfare seems almost desperate—so free, not to mention other obstacles, is the access of air—and frequently so strong is its movement, in the field, at the dressing station, and in all tent hospitals. On the other hand, if this part of the process can be dispensed with, then the question will be greatly simplified, and attention will only have to be directed to the description of antiseptic applications and dressings which will best answer the intended purpose, and to the manner in which these dressings can be rendered available, consistently with other military requirements, when and where they may be needed, and in adequate quantities for meeting the wants of each particular occasion. Experience is not wanting of antiseptic treatment being carried out by eminent surgeons in some civil hospitals without the use of the spray at the operation-table, and in other instances without its use during any part of the course of treatment; and, it has been alleged, with no less beneficial results than when the spray has been employed. It remains to be proved how far these observations are thoroughly correct; and satisfactory proof on the point can be only arrived at when sufficient experience has been collected on the subject.

I have been asked to give at this meeting an explanation of the system by which help is arranged to be afforded to the wounded among troops on active service according to the existing regulations of the British Service. It has been suggested that to those who have not had occasion to study the subject this description would not only possess some features of novelty and interest in itself, but would also furnish indications of the extent to which particular modes of treatment of wounds and injuries might be capable of application under the arrangements described. In accordance with this suggestion I have brought the two diagrams which you see before you as a ready means of furnishing the explanation required.

The surgeons who are now entering the British Military Medical Service can scarcely realise the greatness of the changes which have occurred in their branch of the profession during the last twenty-five years. When I commenced my military service the British Army was scattered in comparatively small detachments over the kingdom and in every colony. It was for the most part engaged as a safeguard for peace and good order in our own possessions, and occupied in performing duties that are now discharged by police, rather than in preparing itself for the sterner necessities of a time of war. Still more marked was this aspect of matters with respect to the Army Medical Service. It was entirely a peace establishment; and its duties were conducted as if there were no liability to the state of peace being interrupted. Nothing was prepared for a condition of war, whether as regards places of administration for field service, organisation of field-hospital establishments, means of transporting sick and wounded during a campaign, or the descriptions of field-hospital equipment to be employed. The results of the practical experience in these matters which had been gained during the Peninsular campaigns had gradually disappeared. In conducting the duties of the Medical Service, the attention had come to be largely devoted to economical details in small matters, which, in the aggregate, produced but comparatively trifling results; while the general system on which the hospitalisation of the sick was conducted was cumbrous, wasteful, and needlessly costly. This condition of things received a rude shock when the Crimean war occurred, and when, as the Director-General of the Army Medical Department at the time testified, without any records or patterns to guide him, everything for active service in the field, both as regards the field-hospital establishments, kinds of supplies, and forms of ambulance vehicles, had to be improvised for the occasion. The breakdown from want of systematic preparation which then occurred (not a breakdown so far as the surgical staff were individually concerned, but a breakdown in respect to the establishments with which they were connected) led to prolonged investigations, which not only demonstrated the need for a thorough reform of departmental arrangements and regulations, but also showed the directions in which the changes were required to be made. The experience of successive wars on the continent of Europe and in the United States since that period has step by step led to further developments in military medical organisation for field service, no less than it has done in the purely combatant parts of the army.

The principal problem which the Medical Department has had to solve has been to devise a scheme by which help and protection should be afforded speedily and effectively to the wounded over the large area which modern battles in Europe now usually occupy, and to provide for their subsequent treatment so long as circumstances render their stay in the theatre of war a matter of necessity; one, at the same time, which should be capable of being modified and adapted to all the varying conditions of warfare—that is, variations as to features of country, difference of climate, seasons, numbers of troops engaged, opportunities of shelter, and other such matters; that should not only not impede, but, on the contrary, should work in harmony with all the other military arrangements; that should be economical in regard to the number of officers and men employed; that should include an equipment which, while adequate to the needs of the hospital service, should not exceed the means of transporting it; and lastly and particularly, a scheme that, as regards the *personnel* necessary for the field-hospital and ambulance duties, should be little more than a redistribution of the *personnel* ordinarily employed in the stationary hospitals at home; so that, acting as a peace establishment as long as peace might last, the *personnel* should, at very short notice, be capable of being organised and arranged into the different parts composing the war establishment.

The plan adopted for accomplishing these various objects may be conveniently divided into two parts, viz.—(1) that for the medical service from the base of operations to the area of active operations of the army in the field, and (2) that for the medical service with the army itself. The hospital establishments belonging to these two divisions of the medical service are shown separately in the two diagrams. They are mutually in a great measure independent of each other, although connected and working in concert; and they differ in their qualities, administration, and in many articles of their equipment, although the officers and men of the Army Medical Department serving in them are interchangeable. The establishments at the base of military operations and along the lines of communication with the army have more or less of a stationary character, while the others are organised for being as movable as the troops which they accompany.

In making a survey of these establishments it must necessarily be a rapid and rather superficial one. It will be convenient, perhaps, to start from the base and to follow them to the front, so far as the establishments along the lines of communication with an army in the field are concerned.

The insular position of our country leads to complications in the medical preparations for war from which continental nations are for the most part free. The officers and men of the medical service must at first be conveyed in detached bodies on board ship, as well as the hospital stores and equipment. The vehicles which are to convey the stores, as well as the carriages for the wounded, must be made capable of being folded up into convenient packages for being carried by sea to the place where the army is to be formed before commencing its operations. Continental armies can generally move in their accustomed ways and concentrate their forces in a convenient place on their own frontiers. Wherever a British army may be despatched for hostile purposes, whether it be on part of a coast belonging to a friendly ally, or whether it be a position secured by force from a hostile power, the establishment of a new hospital in the place is one of the first necessities experienced. It is at once required to receive the sick and hurt who have accumulated in the transports during the voyage from England, and will be wanted to receive the casualties that are sure to happen while the force is being collected and formed prior to starting for the special purpose of the expedition. It is required for the reception of all the medical and surgical stores that have been brought from England for use during the campaign. If the position is retained as the base of operations, the hospital thus established will continually grow in importance as long as the campaign lasts. When once the military operations are in progress, a large proportion of the patients that result from them will find their way ultimately to this hospital, and here they will be disposed of, whether they are sent back to activity in the field or are invalided to England. Again, as the military operations approach their termination, and other hospitals that have been formed successively in advance are broken up, their occupants will fall back upon this base hospital, so that it will be the last medical establishment to be closed, as well as the first to be opened in a campaign. The base hospital is consequently required to have a more permanent character than other hospitals in the field. Some available buildings are usually secured for its occupation, which may be supplemented by subsidiary buildings or encampments, according to circumstances. The administrative as well as the executive staff are large in number, especially the executive staff, not only on account of the extent and variety of the duties to be performed, but also because it is the principal position where reserves of medical officers can be conveniently retained for replacing casualties in the field, and for supplying the demands which the military movements occasion.

As soon as the army quits the place of rendezvous and commences its march, casualties will occur of various kinds, and often in larger numbers than might be anticipated by those who have not studied the experience of such occasions. While comparatively near to the base, those that become disabled can be sent back to the general hospital established there, but after the troops have advanced to some distance, this would be inconvenient, and fresh hospital establishments have to be opened at suitable positions along the roads which the troops are following. These then become the stationary field-hospitals along the lines of communication, or, as they were formerly called, the reserve or intermediate field-hospitals. They are placed in situations which are not only suitable as regards sanitary considerations and hospital needs, but also as regards safety; in positions which the military authorities believe to be safe from incursions of an enemy, and from which the communication with the front in one direction and with the base in the other direction, may be expected to remain secure. They may be established in buildings in villages or towns, or in camps near them, or near railway-stations. The equipment allotted to each of these hospitals is very similar to that of a field-hospital, only differing in having an increased quantity of hospital clothing, and in not being supplied with special transport vehicles.

In front of the stationary field-hospitals, between them and the movable field establishments, is the "advanced depôt." At this station a supply of medical and surgical supplies and appliances is stored, ready for issue to meet wants in the bearer companies and movable field-hospitals. This is the station, too, to which the sick and wounded are brought from the field by the bearer company's ambulance waggons, and from which they are forwarded by vehicles obtained from the commissariat department to the stationary hospitals along the lines of communication with the base.

These comprehend the establishments between the area of active military operations in the field and the base. The duties to be performed, so that the patients in the stationary field-hospitals may have their wants properly attended to, so that there may be no interruption of the movements of men and material between the field and the base, to and fro, are so onerous and important that they are placed in the separate charge of a particular surgeon-general named for the purpose, as the military duties are in that of a general officer distinct from the general commanding the troops in the field. A surgeon-general acting under the orders of a general officer commanding the lines of communication, has the special direction of all the medical duties along the lines and at the base. He is responsible to the surgeon general-in-chief of the army for their regular fulfilment. The hospitals and the movements of sick along each road of communication are supervised by a deputy surgeon-general, acting under the directions of the commandant of the road. The charge of the advanced depôt is placed in the hands of a surgeon-major. At the base are three deputy surgeons-general, whose respective duties are indicated on the plan before you. It is at the base hospitals and in the stationary field-hospitals along the lines of communication with the army, that the regulations direct all civilian surgeons and other persons affording voluntary aid to the sick and wounded to be employed.

The establishments with the army actually operating in the field must now be glanced at. They are of three kinds: —1. The regimental establishment; 2. The bearer company; 3. The field-hospital. It will be more convenient to trace these from the front to the rear, from the fighting line to the line of the field-hospitals, this being the direction in which help has to be afforded by them on the occurrence of an action with the enemy.

The first surgical establishment belongs to the battalions and other bodies of troops composing the brigades and divisions of the army, and is of a very spare character. It is only organised for giving temporary help during halts of the troops on the march or in case of action, affording such primary aid to the wounded as may be necessary before the second establishment, the bearer company, can reach the spot. Each corps has a surgeon with it, and two men of each company are trained as stretcher-bearers. These form the corps field surgical staff. The ordinary equipment consists of two "medical field companions," cases containing surgical materials and medicines, carried by straps over the shoulder, two water-bottles per company, and a stretcher per company carried in the company cart. In case of a corps being detached on outpost or other duties, larger cases, field panniers, carried on the backs of pack animals, and other equipment, according to circumstances, are supplied.

The second establishment, the bearer company, is the most important source of aid in case of the occurrence of an action, and is very fully and carefully equipped for its duties. It comprises the means of performing all surgical operations of urgent necessity, applying surgical dressings, and giving preliminary aid to all wounded whenever they may be met with before their removal to the field-hospitals in the rear. It is specially organised for giving this aid in a systematic manner at certain important stations—in the immediate rear of the fighting line, at places to which the badly wounded are first carried, and where they can be transferred to wheeled conveyances—but principally at the dressing stations. It is by the bearer company that the wounded are removed from help-station to help-station, on stretchers from the place of fighting to the transfer or collecting station, by ambulance waggons from the transfer to the dressing station, and again from the dressing station to the field-hospitals, and from them again subsequently to the advanced depôt. To accomplish all these purposes, each bearer company in the field has a considerable personnel, over two hundred in number, allotted to it; medical officers, officers of orderlies, transport officer, men of the army hospital corps, stretcher bearers, drivers, and artificers. The details of these establishments may be found in the Code of Army Medical Regulations. The equipment is also large, and includes all the supplies for forming the dressing stations, performing the necessary surgical duties, supplying medical comforts, the ambulance conveyances, and a variety of articles, the lists of which are also laid down in the Medical Regulations. Each bearer company is divisible into two "half bearer companies," with personnel and equipment complete for its duties. The whole company is under the command of a surgeon-major. Four such companies constitute a bearer company, the complement for an army corps; and one of these companies has its transport and equipment adapted for work in a mountainous country, where wheeled transport could not be employed. The command of a bearer company is a very responsible one; the movements of the company, whether in marching with troops, in camping, or in discharge of its special functions on the occasion of an action, have to be conducted with the same military discipline and precision as the movements of all other parts of the army; the bearers must be drilled and exercised in the proper modes of carrying the wounded, and both they and the men of the army hospital corps must be taught and practised in the modes of rendering first assistance in the absence of surgical aid. All this constitutes part of the work which is now systematically done in the Army Hospital Corps Training Depôt at Aldershot. I may here mention that arrangements have been kindly made by the principal medical officer and the medical staff at Aldershot, to receive a certain number of visitors who may wish to attend the bearer company exercises at that station on the 5th instant. It is all the more important that the duties of the bearer company should be performed with thorough efficiency, especially as regards the preliminary dressing and treatment of the wounded, as, owing to the great range of modern projectiles, the field-hospitals, as shown by modern experience in European warfare, are often established so far away from the place of conflict that many hours may elapse before the wounded in the transport vehicles will be able to reach them and get fresh surgical help. This is especially liable to happen when an action only ceases as daylight is declining, and the roads between the battle-ground and the places where the field-hospitals have been established become encumbered by military vehicles of all sorts, as well as by the movements of troops.

The field-hospitals remain to be noticed. A great deal of thought has been given to the proper constitution of the establishments so as to combine qualities of portability and readiness at any time for use with the requisite efficiency. A field-hospital must be so arranged as to be always within reach of the troops; ready for reception of the wounded from the bearer company, shortly after the occurrence of an action, with all requisite means for their protection, care, and treatment for at least several days, if necessary; and it must be capable, as soon as the patients have been removed from it to the advanced depôt, to be quickly packed up again and ready for further movement forward, so as to be available for the reception of a relay of patients in case of another action with the enemy. The field-hospital, as now arranged in the British service, is fitted for the reception of 200 patients. The requisite number of tents, each calculated for four patients, is carried for accommodating the whole number, but if a farmhouse with outbuildings be available, or suitable houses in a village can be obtained, the tents would probably not be employed. Each field-hospital has its *personnel*, equipment, and transport so arranged as to be capable of division into two half-field-hospitals complete for 100 patients. Twelve field hospitals form part of each army corps, two being allotted to each division of the army corps, the remaining six being reserved for disposal wherever they may be specially needed. In addition to four store waggons for the ward, and cooking material and medical stores, four for tentage and equipment, and two water-carts, each movable field-hospital has two pharmacy waggons, containing a complete equipment of instruments, surgical appliances, medicines, and means of dispensing them, with a stock of medical comforts. The contents of the waggons, and modes of packing them, the order to be observed on the line of march, and the plan of encamping a field-hospital, with other details regarding such establishments, may also be found in the Army Medical Regulations.

It will be seen from the account I have just given that the regulated plan of medical and surgical assistance for troops on active service is a very complete one, and that it anticipates all the wants that are likely to occur during a campaign. It is obvious that to carry out the arrangements when the strain of a general action occurs, and help is demanded for a large number of wounded, previous training, intelligence, and active exertion on the part of all concerned will be necessary for success. An adequate staff is provided by the Regulations for the purpose. In addition to the special surgical and subordinate staff of the field-hospitals and of the bearer companies the surgeon-general-in-chief with the army corps has a deputy as a field-inspector, whose duty it is to see that the circulation of the system of help is properly maintained, two orderly medical officers, and other officers to assist him in his charge. Each division of the army has a deputy surgeon-general at its headquarters, and each battalion and separate corps its surgeons. In all these arrangements the calamity of a state of warfare in Europe has been particularly had in view. But even in other parts of the world, even in half-civilised countries, the general principles of the system can be maintained; the manner in which they are carried out has alone to vary, according to the nature of the military operations, the condition of country, and other local circumstances.

The sketch I have laid before you of the existing arrangements for ensuring systematic help and skilled attention to the wounded in case of this country unhappily becoming involved in war has been unavoidably a superficial and imperfect one, and I must apologise for its incompleteness. The description, short and partial as it has been, may, however, not be without some advantage if it has succeeded in conveying a general idea of the arrangements under which any particular system of treatment, whether the strictly antiseptic treatment of wounds or any modification of it, will have to be applied among troops when on field service.

SECTION OF STATE MEDICINE.

OPENING ADDRESS BY JOHN SIMON, C.B., F.R.S.,
President of the Section.

THIS Section was opened in the presence of some seventy members by the President, Mr. John Simon, C.B., F.R.S., with an inaugural address marked by even more than his usual clearness and earnestness. Referring to the greater interest taken by the laity in the subject of this than of the other sections, he said that he considered his words as addressed as much to the outside public as to the members of the Section or Congress.

The name of State Medicine, which had been selected, implied that under certain circumstances the body politic may be called on to interpose between man and man for the better carrying out of the purposes they had in view, viz., the prevention of disease; but before it could be justified in so doing it must be assured that the science of preventive medicine was sufficiently exact, and either all must be in possession of such knowledge, or the public must look to the State to provide experts in whose judgments they might place implicit confidence. He would not now discuss the legislative or executive aspects of preventive medicine, but consider it simply as a branch of science.

In it, as in other sciences, discoveries had on rare occasions been made, as it were, by chance, but for the most part diseases could be prevented only by an exact knowledge of their causes; and though Hippocrates, twenty-three centuries ago, incurred the charge of impiety by asserting, with almost prophetic insight, that the causes of most diseases were to be sought in air, food, and habits, thus enunciating the first principles of preventive medicine, it was not until within the last quarter of a century that any real progress had been made, and even the most advanced nations are only beginning to apply its lessons. In physical and biological sciences we recognise but one source of knowledge, viz., experiment; and in the case of preventive medicine we have experiments of two sorts—(1) experiments, few in number, but carefully pre-arranged, performed mostly in the pathological laboratory, on the lower animals; and (2) those performed by man on fellow-men in the social state on a vast scale, but with many elements of uncertainty. In the former we proceed from cause to effect, in the latter from effect to cause, but in each case we recognise the power of experiment alone. Perhaps the best example of the two methods is to be found in the case of cholera and its propagation by means of drinking-water. On the one hand, we have the classical experiments of Thiersch on mice—few indeed, but absolutely conclusive; and on the other, those performed by two commercial companies on half a million inhabitants of South

London, which led to the same conclusions, though not without a certain amount of ambiguity.

Again, with regard to consumption, one of the most fatal of diseases, the experiments of Villemin, sixteen years ago, opened a new era by proving the inoculability of tubercle, followed up as they have been by others, showing its transmissibility by sputa diffused as spray in the air breathed; by tuberculous matter into the stomach with the food; and lastly, as Gerlach has demonstrated, by the milk of diseased animals. There is good reason to believe that these experiments are now being extensively performed on our children by dairymen, but without any means being taken for verifying the results, and in this respect all popular experiment performed by men on their fellow-men are inferior in value to those undertaken by men of science in the laboratory.

Mr. Simon declined to draw any distinction between the relative value of human life and that of the so-called lower animals, which might be deemed invidious by persons outside, but, assuming a perfect equality between men and brutes, he thought that we were bound to take by preference those which were commercially the less costly. Popular experiments on the effect of sewage water and gases involved the loss of thousands of pounds and hundreds of lives; scientific experiments, far more exact, sacrificed a few dozen mice. Experiments with milk on the popular method, performed on millions of human beings, led to no certain results; Creighton's, conducted with scientific accuracy, were conclusive from half a dozen examples.

In fact, within the last twenty or thirty years the whole aspect of practical medicine has been changed by laboratory experiments; and with regard to preventive medicine, the present age is fuller of promise than any which has gone before.

Pasteur's experiments, beginning with the study of fermentation, led on to that of infection. Chauveau opened up a new world of knowledge when he proved that the most fatal of diseases were due to the invasion of the living body by a lower form of life. Such being the case, it behoves us to study the natural history of these organisms by cultivation in test-tubes, and then to proceed to the more important question, to be answered only by experiments on the living animal, whether we can so modify the properties of the disease-germs as to render them innocuous, or can confer on the higher animal an immunity against them in the future.

Never has such a glorious field for discovery been presented to us, and rapid progress is being made on all sides. Lister has applied the results of Pasteur's investigations to surgical practice, reducing the danger of the most serious operations to a minimum, and greatly facilitating recovery in all. Toussaint and Greenfield have so mitigated the virulence of anthrax as, by the induction of a trifling ailment, to confer a perfect protection against that disease, achieving for our herds what Jenner did for man in the case of small-pox; and Pasteur has done the same for the so-called cholera of fowls.

Semmach, of Dorpat, finds that he can so modify septicæmia as to produce a harmless but protective form of the disease; and Schüller, of Greifswald, in a series of experiments originally undertaken with reference to certain diseases of dogs, has thrown light on the whole class of tubercular and scrofulous affections, confirming their microphytic nature first advanced by Klebs, and promising good results from a preventive point of view.

In conclusion, he referred to the Vivisection Acts, which, nominally permitting of experiments under certain restrictions, are so vexatious as to be practically prohibitive. For the present a stop has been put to such research in this country; but, believing that ere long a change must be effected in the law, he would make a public confession of faith.

To the question whether medical men may make use of the lower animals for painful experiments, appeal may be made to two tribunals—first, what says the voice of conscience in the experimenter himself? and secondly, what is the standard of popular conduct in analogous cases?

He does not consider the infliction of pain on the lowest thing that breathes a matter of indifference—in itself the very thought is repugnant to him,—but when he sees his way to the discovery by which the general mass of suffering in animals or man may be alleviated, his conscience tells him he is justified in causing pain to a few. Just as in

the case of surgical operations before the introduction of chloroform, but with this important difference: that in those instances the benefit was confined to the individual—here it extends to the whole race.

Next, it is a fact, that men by universal consent are in the habit of subordinating the lives and feelings of the lower animals to their own, whenever they may reap advantage by so doing. The most conspicuous example is to be found in the mutilation without licence or anæsthetics of nearly all the males and many of the females of all our cattle—a point he urged on the Royal Commission; and another illustration is afforded by the most legitimate forms of sport and the chase.

He demands some principle of conduct, and has no patience with those who would

"Compound for sins they are inclined to,
By damning those they have no mind to."

Sentiment and emotion cannot take the place of principle and moral right or wrong. This cloud hangs heaviest over preventive medicine, but no branch of our art has such triumphs before it. Successive generations of scientific workers pass away, but science itself advances; the masses at the same time are rising in education, and will ere long demand that they shall be heard and regarded; then we may hope that the science and the profession which more than any other cares for man as man, which takes for its aim as no other does "the greatest possible happiness of the greatest possible number," will be better understood and appreciated at its proper value.

FISH MARKETS.—At the last meeting of the Metropolitan Board of Works a letter was read from the Home Office in reply to a communication from the Board, stating that the Home Secretary had learned with satisfaction that the Board had interested themselves with the subject of the deficiency in market accommodation for the supply of fish to the metropolis, and hoping that the Board might be able to bring forward some satisfactory scheme for remedying an evil which had been so long felt, and which operated so injuriously on the population of London. On the motion of Mr. Dalton, the letter was referred to the Works and General Purposes Committee. Sir James Hogg (the Chairman) and several members of the Board recently visited the St. Katharine Dock, with the object of ascertaining its capabilities as a site for a general market. The goods stations of several railways meet almost on the spot, and might facilitate the discharging of fish there, without transference to vans, whilst the completion of the Inner Circle Railway, with a station at Tower-hill, would also afford facilities for persons attending the market.

SMOKE ABATEMENT.—A meeting was recently held at Grosvenor House, by permission of the Duke of Westminster, to receive and consider a report submitted by the Smoke Abatement Committee of the National Health and Kyrle Societies on the subject of an exhibition and trial of improved heating and smoke-preventing appliances, to be opened at South Kensington in October next. The Duke of Northumberland, who had promised to take the chair, was unavoidably prevented, and in his absence Mr. Ernest Hart presided. Her Royal Highness the Princess Louise and several other influential persons were present. The report of the Committee with reference to the arrangement of the coming exhibition having been read, Dr. Siemens moved a resolution declaring that the present smoky condition of the atmosphere of London had an injurious effect upon the health and happiness of the community, besides destroying public buildings, deteriorating perishable fabrics, and entailing unnecessary expenditure. Dr. Siemens adduced many arguments in favour of his proposition, and Sir H. Thompson, Dr. Quain, and Mr. Romanes supported the resolution. Another resolution, moved by Mr. Barton and seconded by Sir A. Brady, approved of the action taken by the Smoke Abatement Committee for carrying out the proposed exhibition. Lord Brabazon also asked the assent of the meeting to a resolution declaring the readiness of the meeting to support the efforts being made to reduce the evil arising from coal-smoke, and to assist in raising the funds necessary for completely carrying out, on a practical scale, the competitive testing of various appliances to be shown at South Kensington, and for providing suitable prizes.

TERMS OF SUBSCRIPTION.
(Free by post.)

British Islands	. . . .	Twelve Months	.	£1 8 0
,, ,,	. . . .	Six	,,	0 14 0
The Colonies and the United }		Twelve	,,	1 10 0
States of America . . . }				
,, ,, ,,	. . .	Six	,,	0 15 0
India	.	Twelve	,,	1 10 0
,, (viâ Brindisi)	. . .	,,	,,	1 15 0
,, ,,	. . .	Six	,,	0 15 0
,, (viâ Brindisi)	. . .	,,	,,	0 17 6

Foreign Subscribers are requested to inform the Publishers of any remittance made through the agency of the Post-office.

Single Copies of the Journal can be obtained of all Booksellers and Newsmen, price Sixpence.

Cheques or Post-office Orders should be made payable to Mr. JAMES LUCAS, 11, New Burlington-street, W.

TERMS FOR ADVERTISEMENTS.

Seven lines (70 words)	. . .	.£0 4 6
Each additional line (10 words)	. .	0 0 6
Half-column, or quarter-page	. .	1 5 0
Whole column, or half-page	. .	2 10 0
Whole page	. . . . .	5 0 0

Births, Marriages, and Deaths are inserted Free of Charge.

THE MEDICAL TIMES AND GAZETTE *is published on Friday morning: Advertisements must therefore reach the Publishing Office not later than One o'clock on Thursday.*

Medical Times and Gazette.

SATURDAY, AUGUST 6, 1881.

THE ADDRESS BY THE PRESIDENT OF THE CONGRESS.

THE highly philosophical and eloquent opening address delivered by Sir James Paget, the President of the Congress, will have been listened to with such eager interest and attention, that any lengthy notice of it here would be superfluous, the more so as we publish it in full for the benefit of all who could not hear it. He dwelt on the value and importance of such meetings in "the bringing together a multitude of various minds for the promotion and diffusion of knowledge in the whole science and art of medicine, in their widest range, in all their narrowest divisions, in all their manifold utilities," and on the benefits that may be confidently expected to result from the "meetings of men with all kinds of mental power and all forms of knowledge and of skill; every one ready alike to impart and to acquire knowledge." And with his customary felicity of expression he spoke of the pre-eminence of our calling in its range of opportunities for scientific study. "It is not only," he said, "that the pure science of human life may match with the largest of the natural sciences in the complexity of its subject-matter; not only that the living human body is, in both its material and its indwelling forces, the most complex thing yet known, but that, in our practical duties, this most complex thing is presented to us in an almost infinite multiformity. For in practice we are occupied, not with a type and pattern of the human nature, but with all its varieties in all classes of men, of every age and every occupation, in all climates and all social states; we have to study men singly and in multitudes, in poverty and in wealth, in wise and unwise living, in health and all the varieties of disease: and we have to learn, or at least to try to learn, the results of all these conditions of life, while, in successive generations and in the mingling of families, they are heaped together, confused, and always changing. In every one of all these conditions, man, in mind and body, must be studied

by us; and every one of them offers some different problems for inquiry and solution. Wherever our duty or our scientific curiosity—or, in happy combination, both—may lead us, there are the materials and there the opportunities for separate original research." · We have been tempted to quote this passage at length, because it well sets out one of the chief reasons why the study and practice of medicine attract men so strongly—the infinite variety of subjects necessarily presented for observation and study. Neither the scientific student nor the man born with the longing to be a healer can ever be satisfied or satiated, for there is no end to the varieties of disease as affected by the sufferer, or of the sufferer as affected by disease. We will not be tempted to follow the President through the many subjects he dealt with. We can only note here and there the conclusions, so to speak, at which, from time to time, he arrives in the course of his oration. Thus, in enlarging on the ways in which a Congress can and should be specially useful, he points out how and why there is need, for the full progress of our science and art, of "minds which in variety may match with all the varieties of the subject-matters, and minds which, at once, or in swift succession, can be adjusted to all the increasing and changing modes of thought and work"; and meetings such as the Congress show that we have, as a profession, these minds, and prove and augment their worth; and further provide dissimilar and independent minds with opportunity for conference and mutual criticism, for mutual help, and the tests of free discussion. Sir James Paget defends the division of the work of the Congress into so many sections as being only a natural further carrying out of what had been already recognised as a necessity, due to the increase of knowledge being far greater than the increase of individual mental power. He believes, with the poet, that "the thoughts of men are widened with the process of the suns," though he clothes his creed in different words, saying, "I do not doubt that the average mental power constantly increases in the successive generations of all well-trained peoples," but knowledge increases more rapidly. Knowledge comes, but the increase of mental power to assimilate it lingers; and "our division into sections is only an instance of that division of labour which, in every prosperous nation, we see in every field of active life, and which is always justified by more work better done." The President does not, of course, deny that there are dangers in specialism; but, he says, "the fault of specialism is not in narrowness, but in the shallowness and the belief in self-sufficiency with which it is apt to be associated." If the field be narrow, dig deep, and precious ore may be brought to the surface. Study, in such a gathering of minds as the Congress, may, moreover, be a useful remedy for self-sufficiency. We are warned next against thinking any facts in science small: "for every fact in science, wherever gathered, has not only a present value, which we may be able to estimate, but a living and germinal power of which none can guess the issue." A little farther on in the address we meet with a most ingeniously pictured idea of a likeness between the progress of scientific truth and the history of organic life. "We may read the history of the progress of truth in science as a palæontology. Many things which, as we look far back, appear, like errors, monstrous and uncouth creatures, were in their time good and useful, as good as possible. They were the lower and less perfect forms of truth which, among the floods and stifling atmospheres of error, still survived; and just as each successive condition of the organic world was necessary to the evolution of the next following higher state, so from these were slowly evolved the better forms of truth which we now hold." This thought, Sir James Paget thinks, may comfort us when despondent about our progress in true knowledge, and give us fresh and better courage in a work we cannot hope to complete, and in which we see continual and sometimes disheartening change. "We may seem to move in circles, but they are the circles of a constantly ascending spiral; we may seem to sway from side to side, but it is only as on a steep ascent which must be climbed in zig-zag."

We have been drawn on and on to quote from this address till our space is exhausted, and we must be content to close our notice of it with a quotation from the President's conclusion. Bidding us always to remind ourselves of the nobility of our calling, he claimed for it, that among all the sciences, this, "in the pursuit and use of truth, offers the most complete and constant union of those three qualities which have the greatest charm for pure and active minds—novelty, utility, and charity"; and after enlarging somewhat on this, he concluded thus: "We had better not compete where wealth is the highest evidence of success: we can compete with the world in the noble ambition of being counted among the learned and the good, who strive to make the future better and happier than the past; and to this we shall attain if we remind ourselves that, as in every pursuit there is the charm of novelty, and in every attainment of truth utility, so in every use of it there may be charity. I do not mean only the charity which is in hospitals or in the service of the poor, great as is the privilege of such employment of it in that we may be its chief ministers; but that wider charity which is practised in a constant sympathy and gentleness, in patience and self-devotion. And it is surely fair to hold that, as in every search for knowledge we may strengthen our intellectual power, so in every practical exercise of it we may, if we will, improve our moral nature; we may obey the whole law of Christian love, we may illustrate the highest indication of scientific philanthropy."

"Let us, then, resolve to devote ourselves to the promotion of the whole science, art, and charity of medicine. Let this resolve be to us as a vow of brotherhood; and may God help us in our work."

We now leave the address as a valuable possession of the profession. It is high-toned throughout, and in every way admirable; fully worthy alike of the speaker and of the occasion.

SECTIONAL ADDRESSES.

Dr. Wilks, the President of the Section on Pathology, in welcoming the members of the Congress, alluded to the brotherhood of science. Amongst all the ties that link man and man together, some of the closest, he observed, are those forged by science. "In our own department of pathology it creates a thrill of satisfaction to feel that the study of some morbid process may have led some of us to the discovery that another investigator, of whose existence we had been hitherto ignorant, has his thoughts and occupations in perfect unison with our own, and that though oceans and continents may separate us, our minds are both attuned to the same string." This is very good philosophy, happily expressed, and most appropriate to the occasion. Dr. Wilks spoke of the immensity of the subject before the Section—a subject embracing questions of such universal interest to humanity, as those referring to disease, decay, and death; and then, remarking that pathology had been defined to be the science of the unhealthy, or the abnormal course of life as contrasted with the normal, he pointed out that the division of vital action into normal and abnormal may be permitted theoretically, but is not applicable to the practical science of pathology. For, in the first place, the changes that occur in every organic structure in man as years roll on are no more unnatural or pathological "than the sere and yellow leaf which falls from

the oak in autumn." They are normal senile changes; but when they occur prematurely, they are then abnormal, and may be strictly regarded as morbid. Hence one form of a pathological condition—a premature decay, arising from the various causes which bring the organism to an end, either from their operating with unusual force or from some inherent weakness in the body, which is unable to moderate their action. Or should these potent influences concentrate their forces upon one organ only, that organ would become, as we say, diseased; though the process thus set up may be of exactly the same nature as time would otherwise have produced. Changes of this kind, although senile in character, are abnormal, and therefore may be rightly regarded as pathological. The physiologist must therefore "regard the body in the first place in its physiological relations with its surroundings, and mark the alterations which time produces." Life seems to depend upon changes continually going on in relation with the atmosphere in which all living beings are steeped; and in man, if the destructive and reproductive changes are normally counterbalanced, the ordinary duration of life is reached. But if the balance be not kept, the destructive agencies may gain the ascendency, and life be shortened. There is little doubt that very many maladies in England—as Bright's disease, gout, etc.—are induced by mere excess or irregularities in a mode of life which is ordinarily considered correct. We ought also to study the relations of the human race to the soil, and observe the effects of all the surroundings of civilised life.

While considering all these evil-causing agencies, we have to consider also the law of reparation; for an ever-existing tendency towards the remaking of the injured tissues works in association with the dissolution of them. Dr. Wilks also spoke of the peculiarities of parasitic maladies—those not caused by disease in the ordinary meaning of the word, but by one animal preying upon another; of the importance and value of a study of the diseases of all animal and vegetable life; of the questions whether the specific diseases be due to organisms, and whether the hypothetical *contagium vivum* be a reality; and of the question of the evolution and differentiation and progressive development of contagious diseases. His address is highly suggestive, and will, no doubt, have excited great interest.

The President of the Surgical Section, Mr. Erichsen, commenced his address with a few remarks on the advance of surgery during the nineteenth century. This, he observed, has not been continuously in one line, but "has been materially affected by the prevailing bias of the professional mind of the day. Anatomical at one time, physiological at another, the tendency of the surgery of the present day is influenced in one direction by the mechanical spirit of the age, and in another by the advanced pathology which is one of its chief medical characteristics. Yet the continuous advance of our art is undoubted. The gain that thus results has been definitively secured to surgery and to mankind. It can never be lost. . . . . Knowledge in science is cumulative, and skill in art is a tradition that is hereditarily transmitted from master to pupil, if not by the individual, yet by the profession to which he belongs, from which he has acquired, and to which he bequeaths it, augmented or perfected by his own labours. With the knowledge of our predecessors we are familiar; to its stores each generation has added." In the main, this is no doubt true; but may not some exception be taken to the statement as being rather too highly coloured? Does it not happen that modes of surgical treatment of disease are now and then, and not very rarely, brought forward as new, which, after they have been widely employed for a time, are discovered to be old methods, tried and found wanting long before? Or that, in some instances, a method of treatment or a remedy of price that had been long forgotten is disentombed from the too little studied writings of our predecessors? As a broad truth, however, surgical knowledge, like all other knowledge, does continuously advance and increase, and it is well that "from time to time this advance should be measured, this gain weighed." And this, Mr. Erichsen said, is to be the work of the Surgical Section of the Congress. Its business is "not only to measure the extent of the advance, but to determine the value of the gain, and to do this not so much by the novelty of the practice, or by the brilliancy of its exposition, as by an estimate of its intrinsic merit, as shown by its proved utility. Our business here has to do with practical considerations having reference to the recent advances in, or the future lines to be followed by, modern surgery. He then briefly noticed the more important subjects set down for the consideration of the section. Eight subjects are proposed for discussion. I. The recent advances in the surgical treatment of intra-peritoneal tumours; and as regards this the President observed that the perfection of safety to which the practice of ovariotomy has of late years been carried, has led the way to a vast and rapid extension of operative surgery for the cure or relief of various diseased abdominal organs. The uterus, the spleen, the stomach, the pylorus, and the colon have each and all been the subject of operative surgery. And the Surgical Section should endeavour to decide "whether some, at least, of these operations constitute real and solid advances in our art, or whether they are rather to be regarded as bold and skilful experiments on the endurance and reparative power of the human frame—whether, in fact, they are surgical triumphs or operative audacities." II. It is proposed to discuss the diagnosis of certain diseased conditions of the kidney admitting of surgical treatment, and the operations that may be practised for their cure; and as to this subject the President suggested that information is needed concerning the diagnosis and nature of the various forms of renal disease in which nephrotomy and nephrectomy may respectively be employed with reasonable expectation of benefit, more than concerning the operative details; and he referred to the interest and importance of exact study of the after-physiological effects produced by the removal of such an eliminatory organ as the kidney. III. deals with recent advances in the methods of extracting stone from the bladder of the male; on this Mr. Erichsen observed that it is doubtful whether any real progress has been made as regards lithotomy, though there has been some change, and he allowed that it may deserve consideration whether in some forms of calculus, and in certain conditions of the urinary organs, a wise eclecticism may not be exercised in the choice of one or other of the methods of operating. No one will dispute this; the question is whether the Congress can give an authoritative opinion to guide the choice. As to lithotrity, Mr. Erichsen acknowledged fully and heartily the value and importance of "Bigelow's operation," but cautiously pointed out that we have yet to learn what may be the ultimate result upon the bladder and upon the kidney of prolonged intra-vesical instrumentation. When speaking of subject IV.—the consideration of the methods best calculated to secure primary union in operation-wounds, etc.—the President of the Section expressed himself very cautiously as to the question whether the "elaborate system of local treatment before, during, and after an operation, which has been devised by the skill and worked out by the unwearied labour of Lister," be essential in all cases of operation wound; and called attention to the question, "is there no fear that in some of the modern systems of treating wounds we are in danger of expending all our precautions in the prevention of the local and of ignoring the risk of a constitutional, infection?"

In a similar and brief way, he pointed to the need of exact information and guidance in the treatment of aneurisms, the treatment of diseases of joints by resection; the relations between adenoma, sarcoma, and carcinoma—referring here to the greater importance of clinical history than of histological affinities, and to the great importance of the proposed discussion on syphilis, and its influence on the local manifestations of rheumatism, gout, and tubercle.

In his brief introductory address in the Sub-section of Diseases of the Throat, the President, Dr. George Johnson, whose skill in the employment of the laryngoscope is well known, paid a graceful compliment to Signor Garcia, Professor Türck, and the late Professor Czermak, as the inventors of the art of laryngoscopy; spoke of the great importance of the invention; and then occupied himself with drawing a comparison between the practical gains with regard to diagnosis and treatment that have been derived respectively from the ophthalmoscope and the laryngoscope. He thinks that if the numerous remote diseases, especially of the nervous system, upon which the ophthalmoscope has thrown new light, be taken into account, it must be admitted that, "in the matter of mere diagnosis," the ophthalmoscope takes precedence of the laryngoscope; but that with regard to improved methods of treatment, "and in particular to the introduction of entirely new and previously impossible mechanical operations," the laryngoscope has unquestionably done more than can fairly be claimed for the ophthalmoscope. No one will dispute this, probably, as nature has provided a way of direct access to the interior of the larynx, but not to that of the eyeball. But we have no doubt that Dr. Hughlings-Jackson could make out a very good argument in proof of the generally superior value of the ophthalmoscope. Dr. Johnson well and usefully insisted on the vast importance to the specialist of a thoroughly good knowledge of the science and art of medicine in general. "We maintain that of the specialist it should be said with truth that he is one, not who knows less of disease in general, but who knows more of the particular class of diseases to which he has devoted most time or especial attention and study."

Dr. McClintock, the President of the Section on Obstetric Medicine and Surgery, after gracefully welcoming all his fellow-labourers, and recognising the eminence and value of French, German, and American workers in his department of medicine, employed the fifteen minutes that he allowed himself for his address in giving brief notices of the "more prominent among the many eminent obstetricians who lived and practised in London," and by their writings, teaching, and discoveries contributed in no small degree to the development of midwifery and gynæcology. In this interesting retrospective glance, Dr. McClintock gave, we more than suspect, new information to many English obstetricians, as well as to their foreign brethren. For instance, how many—or rather, how few—among us knew that the first distinct treatise on midwifery in the English language was the translation of Eucarius Rhodion's treatise, "De partu Hominis," by Thomas Raynald, which appeared about 1540, and was "for over one hundred years the sole guide and text-book of obstetric practitioners, male and female"? Next after him, Dr. McClintock named Harvey, his exercitations on generation, parturition, etc., being "the first book on midwifery written by an Englishman, printed in our own language, and having exercised an influence upon the practice of the time which it would be difficult now to estimate." Contemporary with him was the celebrated Peter Chamberlen, the inventor of the midwifery forceps; but, as Dr. McClintock remarked, "The brilliancy of his reputation is obscured by the unworthy, selfish conduct which caused him to keep the instrument secret for the aggrandisement of himself and family." Then come Arbuthnot; Dr. John Maubray, the first public teacher of midwifery in England, in 1724; and Dr. Edward Chapman, the second public teacher of that art, and the revealer of the obstetric forceps. Sir Richard Manningham, in 1739, was the first to open a ward, in the Parochial Infirmary of St. James', Westminster, for parturient women; but the first obstetric hospital in the British dominions was the great Lying-in Hospital of Dublin, founded by Dr. Mosse. Then William Smellie (the first volume of whose celebrated treatise was published in 1751) is noticed, and some of his most eminent pupils are mentioned. Next come William Hunter and Thomas Denman; and a long list of later obstetricians, down to Locock, Murphy, Tyler Smith, and Oldham, are merely mentioned.

In opening the Section on Diseases of Children, the President, Dr. West, gracefully acknowledged the welcome he had received from his countrymen on his return to England, and the kindness and courtesy that had been shown him by his French friends in his second home in Nice. Then he spoke of the great change effected in the last few years in the establishment of children's hospitals. "Thirty years ago," he observed, "throughout the whole of England and America there was not a single hospital set apart for children. It was but rarely that one saw these little waifs and strays in the wards of our general hospitals." Germany also was not much better off, and one had to go to Paris to study on a large scale diseases which men like Guersant, Trousseau, Roger, and others investigated with untiring zeal. Now, London has six separate children's hospitals, and children's wards are to be found in all the large London hospitals. There are special children's hospitals in all our large towns; America and Germany have followed suit; and throughout Europe the opportunities for the study of the diseases of children are nearly as numerous as they are for those of adults. Dr. West must have felt no little satisfaction and pride in speaking of this, for the improvement is very largely due to his own efforts and labours. As the founder and persistent promoter of the first children's hospital in London, the now beautiful hospital in Ormond-street, he has been the father of the movement that has led to the happy change which he described. As a result of all this change, the vague phraseology which for years served, he said, to conceal our ignorance, has been to a great degree done away with. We no longer speak of worm fever, remittent fever, and the other terms we used for typhoid fever in children. Heart-disease in them has been studied as closely and carefully as in adults; and inflammatory lung-diseases in them have been minutely differentiated and studied. Nor have therapeutics lagged behind. He then spoke briefly of the labour before the Section over which he presided: its work being to take stock of our knowledge; to furnish definite and conclusive answers, if possible, to questions submitted to it; to give us fresh information on points concerning which our knowledge is still fragmentary; and to endeavour to solve such problems as may be brought forward.

THE INTERNATIONAL PHARMACEUTICAL CONGRESS.

It is much to be regretted that a most interesting meeting of Pharmacists from all parts of the world during the earlier part of this week has been so completely overshadowed by its gigantic congener the International Medical Congress. The Pharmaceutical Congress met on Monday, when Dr. Redwood was duly elected as President of the meeting which orthwith proceeded to business. The main work of the three days during which the Congress lasted was one with

which we most heartily sympathise, being neither more nor less than the compilation of a Universal Pharmacopœia—one, that is, which shall contain all the more important drugs, reduced as nearly as possible to the same strength. Of course, such a codex need not contain every substance used in medicine, but only the more important, leaving to each nation to add on to it those recipients, diluents, or what not, which they most delight to use. Again, it is plain that only one language is adapted for this purpose. Latin is not so widely or so deeply known among us as it used to be, but a little of it is known everywhere, and it would be easy for each country to have a translation of the authoritative volume bound up with the Latin, and to this might be added those secondary or tertiary groups of substances which we have already referred to. Already several foreign governments have agreed to adopt any such codex as may be compiled by the various national delegates, and some steps have been taken by a section of French pharmacists towards realising the project. The same question will come up in the Materia Medica Section of the Medical Congress, when a paper by Eulenburg of Greifswald will be read on the subject, and a discussion will probably follow. The French are eagerly desirous that their own codex should be taken as the basis of the new one, and in a certain sense it must be, for it is plain that any such universal work must be founded on the metric system. To us this will not be at first convenient, but almost every nation has now adopted the metric system, and at the worst it cannot be more troublesome than the old apothecaries' weight to prescribers or dispensers. Before the separation of the Congress the following resolutions were unanimously adopted:—

" The fifth International Pharmaceutical Congress, held in London, confirms the resolution passed at previous Congresses as to the utility of a Universal Pharmacopœia; but is of opinion that it is necessary at once to appoint a commission, consisting of two delegates from each of the countries represented at the Congress, which shall prepare within the shortest possible time a compilation in which the strength of all potent drugs and their preparation is equalised." "The Executive Committee of this Congress is requested to take the necessary steps so that the resolutions be speedily carried out." "The work, when ready, shall be handed over by the delegates to their respective governments or their Pharmacopœia Committee." "It is desirable that the Committee suggest a uniform systematic Latin nomenclature for the pharmacopœias of all countries." "It is desirable that the Committee take immediate measures that an official Latin translation be made of the pharmacopœias of different countries which are not now published in that language." "It is desirable that the Committee be put in possession of all manuscripts, including the documents relating to the Universal Pharmacopœia compiled by the labours of the Society of Pharmacy of Paris, and presented at the fourth meeting of the International Congress at St. Petersburg by the Society of Pharmacy of Paris," and "that the Pharmaceutical Societies of the respective countries be requested to nominate those members of the commission not appointed by this Congress, and to fill up any vacancies that may arise from time to time."

Brussels was decided upon as the place for the next meeting of the International Congress in 1884. The President then delivered the concluding address, and the proceedings closed.

We should not overlook one of the pleasantest episodes connected with the meeting. On Tuesday evening the members of the Pharmaceutical Society of Great Britain entertained their foreign guests at dinner at Willis's Rooms, the President, Mr. Greenish, in the chair. The dinner was excellent; the toasts limited; and the music of the Hungarian Band of the finest. These contained all the elements of a most successful and agreeable evening, and we have every reason to believe that the guests enjoyed themselves most heartily.

THE WEEK.

THE ROYAL COLLEGE OF PHYSICIANS OF LONDON.

AT an ordinary meeting of the Royal College of Physicians, held on July 20, Sir William Jenner, Bart., President, in the chair, members were admitted, licences granted, and reports received from the Examiners, the Council, the Library Committee, and the Curators of the Museum. A communication was read from the Secretary of the Medical Acts Commission, requesting an expression of opinion from the College on the following questions :—1. Is any alteration of the present licensing system desirable; and, if so, what changes therein would be most likely to prove beneficial to the public and the profession? 2. Are the present constitution, powers, and functions of the General Medical Council satisfactory; and if not, what changes therein would be most likely to prove advantageous, either by enlarging the usefulness of the Council, or increasing the confidence in it of the profession or the public? An answer drafted by Dr. Pitman, the Registrar, was submitted to the College, and after some discussion was adopted with a slight alteration. It stated, with regard to the first question, that in the opinion of the College an alteration in the present licensing system is desirable; and that the change which would be beneficial would, in effect, consist in the adoption of the well-known Conjoint Scheme. As to the second question, the draft reply stated that the Council has no opinion to offer on the subject. More than one amendment to this was proposed; and finally it was resolved, on the motion of Dr. Quain and Dr. Priestley, to substitute for the words "has no opinion to offer," the words "does not desire to offer an opinion." Some doubt was expressed, we believe, as to whether it was wise to adhere to the Conjoint Scheme; but it is said Sir William Jenner pointed out that a one-portal system would be recommended by the Commission, and the only alternative to the Conjoint Scheme would be a State Board independent of the corporations. Drs. E. H. Sieveking, E. H. Greenhow, Andrew Clark, and Lionel Smith Beale were elected Censors; Dr. F. J. Farre, Treasurer; Dr. Pitman, Registrar; and Dr. Munk, Treasurer; and the various Examiners, and Curators of the Museum, nominated by the President and Council, were appointed.

THE DEFICIENCY OF THE METROPOLITAN WATER-SUPPLY.

AT the Marlborough-street Police-court, last week, before Mr. Newton, one of several summonses was heard against the Grand Junction Waterworks Company for neglecting to supply water to persons entitled to receive it, and an important legal argument on the liabilities of water companies arose. The complainant was a poulterer, of Swallow-place, Oxford-circus, and Mr. Abrahams stated his case, whilst Mr. Poland defended the Company. The latter gentleman said the Company were exceedingly sorry that any of their customers had been put to inconvenience in not having a proper supply of water, but the complainant having thought fit to take proceedings for a penalty, and the Company having done all in their power to meet the wants of the consumers, he (Mr. Poland) thought it right to take the objection that the summons entirely failed, on the ground that the complainant had not, on July 16, paid for the water. A long discussion between the magistrate and counsel ensued, in which it was shown that, if such a defence were admitted,

the Company could get out of all their liabilities by the expedient of delaying for a little time the collection of their rates. Eventually, Mr. Newton said he would reserve judgment on the question, and some other complainants having withdrawn their summonses on the ground that their purpose had been answered by this investigation, the hearing of the remainder was adjourned until the 10th inst., when judgment in this representative case will be given. At the close of the hearing the magistrate remarked that the inhabitants in the district of his Court had undoubtedly suffered great inconvenience by the breakdown in the Company's water-supply; in some cases—and not a few—where there were boilers attached to the kitchen grates, it had been found to be absolutely necessary to discontinue the lighting of the kitchen fire. Every case of this description goes further to confirm the opinion we recently expressed, that a second source of water-supply for the metropolis has become an absolute necessity; and it is a matter of vital importance that a general and unceasing pressure should be brought to bear upon the Government until this most important object has been attained.

THE INTERNATIONAL MEDICAL AND SANITARY EXHIBITION.

THE preparation of a design for the diploma to be awarded by the Parkes Museum, in connexion with the Hygienic Exhibition now open at South Kensington, was entrusted to Mr. Cave Thomas, who has produced a very simple, effective, and original composition, in the centre of which a female figure, representing sanitary science, stands at the prow of a boat, in the act of casting her "life-buoy" (hygiene) into the seething ocean of human ills. The design is so plastic in its arrangement that it might be successfully worked out in sculpture. On Monday next, Mr. Eric Erichsen and the Exhibition Committee will be present at the Exhibition during the afternoon to receive the members of the International Medical Congress. The Exhibition will finally close on August 13.

MR. JOHN MARSHALL, F.R.S.

METROPOLITAN and provincial teachers and pupils will regret to hear that at the last meeting of the Court of Examiners of the Royal College of Surgeons, this highly popular gentleman resigned his appointment as an examiner, to which he was elected by the Council in 1873. Mr. Marshall, who is a Vice-President of the College, and Surgeon to University College Hospital, will, it is expected, be succeeded by a colleague of that Hospital, Mr. Christopher Heath, late Chairman of the Board of Examiners, and a recently elected member of the Council.

THE PARIS WEEKLY RETURN.

THE number of deaths for the twenty-ninth week, ending July 21, 1881, was 1480, and among these there were from typhoid fever 32, small-pox 29, measles 44, scarlatina 36, pertussis 17, diphtheria and croup 49, erysipelas 10, puerperal infections 4, and acute tubercular meningitis 69. There were also 27 deaths from acute bronchitis, 57 from pneumonia, 314 from infantile athrepsia (108 of the infants having been partially or wholly suckled), and 57 violent deaths. The present week's returns are, in reality, one-eighth less than reported above, one day's mortality from the last week being added on account of the National Fête having prevented their earlier record. Some of the deaths, too, have not been recorded in time. Taking the two weeks together, their mean has been at least 1160 deaths, in place of the normal mean of 900 to 1000. The great heat has been principally the cause of the increase. Thus, the deaths from infantile athrepsia have been quadrupled or quintupled. The deaths have really increased from about 1065 for the twenty-eighth week to (with the corrections) 1330 in the twenty-ninth, and will probably go on increasing for the next week, as the effects of this high temperature are not exhibited at first in their full force. During the twenty-ninth week, scarlatina and measles have been especially remarkable for the number of deaths which they have caused.

ARMY MEDICAL SCHOOL.

THE summer session of the Army Medical School at Netley was brought to a close on Monday last. The Earl of Morley, Parliamentary Under-Secretary of State in the War Office, came from London to deliver the prizes gained by the probationers.

Army Medical Department.

The following is a list of Surgeons on probation in the Medical Department of the British Army who were successful at both the London and Netley examinations (August, 1881). The final positions of these gentlemen are not affected by the marks gained at Netley:—

	Marks.		Marks.
1. A. M. Davies . .	2330	21. G. H. Younge . .	1675
2. H. W. Hubbard .	2290	22. W. G. Clements .	1670
3. P. C. C. Fitzsimon	2090	23. W. Babtie . . .	1625
4. T. E. Noding . .	2065	24. E. F. O'Brien .	1620
5. J. R. Yourdi . .	1992	25. C. W. Thiele . .	1610
6. J. C. Culling . .	1960	26. F. P. Nichols . .	1590
7. R. I. D. Hackett .	1955	27. T. Cox	1570
8. R. T. M'Geagh .	1950	28. J. M'Laughlin .	1570
9. G. T. Trewman .	1910	29. R. Fowler . . .	1560
10. H. H. Johnston .	1900	30. S. H. Creagh .	1510
11. E. M. Wilson . .	1900	31. F. J. Lambkin .	1500
12. E. J. E. Risk . .	1895	32. W. L. Reade . .	1490
13. J. D. Davies . .	1880	33. H. J. Peard . .	1475
14. W. G. Birrell . .	1850	34. G. S. O'Grady .	1455
15. M. Dundon . . .	1840	35. S. J. Rennie . .	1425
16. T. R. Lingard . .	1830	36. J. Carmichael .	1405
17. C. W. S. Magrath	1830	37. E. D. Farmar .	1390
18. A. V. Lane . . .	1780	38. G. W. B. Creagh	1370
19. J. W. Beatty . .	1740	39. F. T. Wilkinson	1370
20. G. E. Weston . .	1695	40. J. Semple . . .	1345

The first-named gentleman gained the prize in Military Surgery presented by Sir Joseph Fayrer, K.C.S.I., and the Martin Memorial Silver Medal.

Indian Medical Service.

Appended is a list of candidates for commissions as Surgeons in Her Majesty's Indian Medical Service who were successful at both the London and Netley examinations (August, 1881). The final positions of these gentlemen are determined by the marks gained in London added to those gained at Netley, and the combined numbers are accordingly shown in the list here given:—

	Marks.		Marks.
1. H. T. Griffiths . .	5210	12. R. G. Cooper . .	3885
2. A. Milne	4710	13. M. B. Braganza .	3875
3. F. D. Cæsar Hawkins	4485	14. A. T. L. Patch .	3835
4. J. A. Cunningham	4465	15. J. F. Maclaren .	3715
5. A. G. E. Newland	4456	16. S. T. Avetoom .	3705
6. H. C. Hudson . .	4290	17. H. W. Stevenson.	3680
7. R. J. Baker . . .	4290	18. R. Ross	3630
8. A. Silcock . . .	4071	19. C. Adams . . .	3483
9. P. Mullane . . .	3925	20. E. R. Da Costa .	3265
10. J. W. Rodgers . .	3920	21. J. K. Kanga . .	3205
11. W. A. Corkery . .	3900	22. A. J. O'Hara . .	2990

The first-named gentleman gained the Herbert Prize and the Martin Memorial Gold Medal; the second gained the Parkes Memorial Bronze Medal.

DEATH OF M. HENRI CLOZEL DE BOYER.

THIS distinguished and rising member of the new Paris school has just been carried off, like so many others, after a three days' illness from diphtheria, which he contracted at the Hôpital des Enfants while officiating under Prof. Parrot. One of the most active collaborateurs of the Progrès Médical, and the author of a thesis which has already acquired a high reputation ("Etudes Cliniques sur les Lésions Corticales des Hémisphéres Cérébraux"), when just about to reap the reward bestowed by a successful concours, he has been carried off almost at the commencement of what promised to be a most successful scientific career.

INTERNATIONAL MEDICAL CONGRESS.

THE Hunterian Museum of the Royal College of Surgeons will be open to the members of the Congress on Sunday next from two o'clock until six, when Professor Flower has kindly consented to be in attendance to go round with the distinguished foreign visitors invited to meet him. This is a great concession on the part of the authorities, and one which will no doubt be much appreciated by many.

THE MEDICAL ACTS COMMISSION.—The Medical Acts Commission met at Victoria-street, Westminster, on the 22nd, 23rd, and 25th ult. The evidence of Mr. J. S. Gamgee, Professor Spence, Dr. R. S. Semple, Dr. H. A. Pitman, and Mr. Christopher Heath was taken. There were present— the Earl of Camperdown (chairman); the Bishop of Peterborough; the Right Hon. W. H. F. Cogan, the Master of the Rolls; Sir William Jenner, Bart., K.C.B.; Mr. Simon, C.B.; Professor Huxley, Professor Turner, Mr. Bryce, M.P., and the Secretary. The Council of the Medical Defence Association have been invited to state the views of the Association on the subject of medical reform, and at a meeting held at St. James's Hall, the question was discussed and certain resolutions arrived at.

SPREADING SMALL-POX.—The Hampstead Vestry recently summoned a laundress for having unlawfully transmitted, without previous disinfection, certain clothing, or linen, which had been exposed to infection from small-pox, whereby she was liable to a penalty not exceeding £5. It appeared that on June 10 last the sanitary inspector received information from Dr. Gwynn, the Medical Officer of Health for the parish, that there was a case of small-pox in the defendant's house. He visited the premises the same day, and found that a lad, aged eighteen, was the patient; he and his mother occupied the second and third floor rooms, she also being a laundress. The inspector cautioned both of them against taking in any linen, or sending any away. Subsequently, however, it was found that the defendant had not obeyed these instructions, and on being questioned on the matter she admitted this to be the case. The magistrate inflicted a fine of 20s., including costs.

WATER-SUPPLY.—Now that the subject of the water-supply of the metropolis is so prominent a topic, it will be instructive and interesting to notice what is being done in this important matter in some provincial places. The Plynlimon scheme for supplying Aberystwith with water has been almost completed; the sixteen miles of pipes have been laid, and the lake on the mountain has been tapped fourteen feet below the surface. The lake is upwards of eleven acres in extent, and the water is among the purest in the United Kingdom. The total cost of the works will be only about £16,000, and they have been carried out for the amount absolutely estimated for. This scheme puts an end to an agitation that has disturbed Aberystwith for upwards of a quarter of a century, since the supply of water from the source selected is practically unlimited. A system of water-supply for Clacton-on-Sea was recently inaugurated by the Mayor of Colchester. Like most of the Essex watering-places, the town has hitherto depended for fresh water upon surface-wells. A very pure and plentiful source has now been found by tapping the chalk at a depth of 400 feet, although a corresponding bore a few yards distant yielded only salt water. A serious stoppage in the supply of water to the city of Oxford recently took place. About four o'clock in the morning the beam of the large engine at the pumping station cracked in the middle. The two smaller engines were being repaired, and by a singular coincidence the reservoir was being cleaned out. The city was thus without water from the works for the greater part of one whole day.

THE INTERNATIONAL MEDICAL CONGRESS.

THE seventh meeting of the International Medical Congress was formally opened on Wednesday morning, in St. James's Hall, by His Royal Highness the Prince of Wales. The great hall was crowded in every part, and it is believed that nearly 3000 members of Congress were present.

The Prince of Wales, on his arrival, was received by Sir William Jenner, Sir James Paget, Sir William Gull, the Hon. Secretary-General Mr. W. Mac Cormac, and other members of the Committee.

Sir William Jenner, K.C.B., President of the Royal College of Physicians, who was very warmly received, took the chair as chairman *ex officio* of the General Committee until the President-elect of the Congress had been formally installed. In opening the proceedings, he said : When the Queen, whose sympathy with all suffering is well known, consented to be the patron, and permitted her likeness to be imprinted on the medal struck in commemoration of the meeting, the success of the Congress as an International Congress was secured ; and when the Prince of Wales had announced his willingness to open the Congress, a guarantee was given to the world that our meeting would be conducted with gravity and dignity, and that the discussions would be on matters of a nature and importance calculated to support the dignity and honour of our profession. It would be contrary to my sense of propriety and of duty to you were I to detain you from the proper business of the Congress by any lengthened remarks, but it would be scarcely courteous to you, or congenial to my own feelings, were I not to express very briefly, though with very faltering tongue and with very imperfect language, my idea of the sentiments which animate the objects and aims of those who have collected here from all parts of Her Majesty's dominions—and not only from all parts of Her Majesty's dominions, but from all the great schools in the world where the science of medicine is cultivated and advanced, and from which, by means of their pupils, the science of practical medicine, and the practical arts it bears, are diffused throughout all the world. Sir William Jenner proceeded to contrast the effects of commerce and science in binding men and nations together, and to contrast gold and knowledge, from the point of view that a glut of the former would reduce its value ; while every addition to the latter only enhanced the worth of the previously accumulated stock. He claimed for the searchers after new truths in medical science a disinterestedness that no other discoverers could claim, and cited Dr. Parkes as the beau-ideal of a scientific worker. Their reward was the knowledge that the result of their labours was saving life, alleviating suffering, and preventing disease. He concluded by hailing the Congress as a means of knitting more closely the bonds of professional brotherhood.

The Hon. Secretary read the report of the Executive Committee, and, though we are unwilling to even hint at a fault where success has been so well deserved and gained, we venture to think this report had better have been taken as read.

Sir J. Risdon Bennett moved a resolution appointing Sir James Paget President, and Mr. William Mac Cormac General Secretary, and the several gentlemen whose names were mentioned in the report as Vice-Presidents of the Congress, and Vice-Presidents of the various Sections, and all the other officers. He referred to the very complete literature of the Congress which had been prepared. While he was welcoming, in very good French, the foreign delegates, the Crown Prince of Prussia arrived, and was greeted with great heartiness and cordiality by the immense assembly.

Professor Donders, of Utrecht, seconded the resolution, paying a compliment to British skill and talent in organisation, as evinced by the arrangements of the Congress, and prophesied from its sittings valuable additions to medical science.

The resolution was carried by acclamation ; and then

The Prince of Wales rose and said : Your Imperial Highness and Gentlemen,—I gladly complied with the request that I should be patron of the International Medical Congress of 1881, and among many reasons for so doing, was my conviction that few things can tend more to the welfare of mankind than that educated men of all nations should from time to time meet together for the promotion of the branches of knowledge to which they devote themselves. The intercourse and the mutual esteem of nations have often been advanced by great international exhibitions, and I look back with pleasure to those with which I have been connected ; but when conferences are held among those who in all parts of the world apply themselves to the study of science, even greater international benefits may, I think, be confidently anticipated, more especially in the study of medicine and surgery, for in these the effects of climate and of national habits must give to the practitioners of each nation opportunities, not only of acquiring knowledge, but of imparting knowledge to those of their *confrères* whom they meet in Congress. I venture to think, gentlemen, that the Executive Committee have acted wisely in instituting sections for the discussion of a very wide range of subjects, including not only the sciences on which medical knowledge is founded, but many of its most practical applications, and I am very happy to see that so great scope will be granted for the discussion of important questions relating to the public health, to the cure of the sick in hospitals and in the houses of the poor, and to the welfare of the Army and Navy. The devotion with which many members of the medical profession readily share the dangers of climate and the fatigues and dangers of war, and the many risks which must be encountered in the study of means, not only for the remedy, but for the prevention of disease, deserves the warmest acknowledgment from the public. I have great satisfaction in believing, in seeing this crowded hall, that I may already regard the Congress as successful in having attracted a number never hitherto equalled of medical men from all parts of this kingdom, as well as from every country in Europe, from the United States, and from other parts of the world. The list of officers of the Congress, including as it does the names of those distinguished in every branch of medical science, shows how heartily the proposal to hold the meeting in London has been received. I think it speaks well for the good feeling of the profession that there should have been so warm a response to the invitations. How cordially the proposal has been received may be seen not only in the large number of visitors, but in the fact that they include a large proportion of those who enjoy a high reputation, not only in their own countries, but throughout the world. I sincerely congratulate the Reception Committee on this good promise of complete success, and I trust that at the close of the Congress they will feel rewarded for the labour they have bestowed upon it. The report which the Secretary-General, Mr. Mac Cormac, has read will have explained how great have been his labours. He will hereafter be well repaid, and I am sure Mr. Mac Cormac is sensible that he will be recompensed even for his great exertions by the assurance that the progress of the important science of medicine has been materially promoted, for any addition to the knowledge of medicine must always be followed by an increase in the happiness of mankind.

The President, Sir James Paget, having now taken the chair, proceeded to deliver his Inaugural Address, which we elsewhere print.

After Sir James Paget's speech, the first general meeting of the Congress was dissolved ; and from and after 3 p.m. the various sections were constituted and began work.

At 4.30 in the afternoon of the same day, the second general meeting was held in St. James's Hall, under the presidency of Sir James Paget, when Professor Virchow, of Berlin, delivered in German, to a large and most appreciative audience, an address on the "Value of Pathological Experiment." Neither space nor time will permit of our giving more than a very small part of the address from this master in pathology this week, but we hope to publish it next week. Elsewhere in our columns will be found reports of the proceedings in the sections. They were all largely attended.

The number of names inscribed on the roll of the Congress is now very little, if at all, short of 3000. The following have come commissioned by their several Governments to attend the Congress and report its proceedings:—For the Argentine Government, Professor William Rawson, of Buenos Ayres; for the Austrian Government, Professor Schnitzler, and for the Minister of Public Instruction, Dr. Hans Ritter von Hebra; for the Hungarian Government, Dr. L. Gross de Csatar, and for the Minister of Public Instruction, Dr. A. Rozsahegyi; for the Belgian Government, Dr. Warlomont, Dr. Gille, and Dr. Spaack, and for the Minister of Public Works, Dr. Libbrécht of Ghent; for the Brazilian Government, the Baron de Theresopolis; for Egypt, Dr. Osman Bey; for the French Government, Professor Pasteur, and for the Minister of War, Professor Gaujot and Dr. Poncet of Paris, and for the Minister of Public Instruction, Dr. Worms; for Her Imperial Majesty the German Empress, Professor Küster, Berlin; for the Bavarian Government, Professor Ranke and Oberstabsarzt Dr. Port of Munich; for the Prussian Minister of War, Generalarzt Dr. Coler of Berlin; for the Saxon War Department, Generalartz Dr. W. Roth of Dresden, and Oberstabsarzt Dr. Starke of Colberg, for the Saxon Minister of Internal Affairs, Geheimrath Dr. Günther; for Italy, Professor Commendatore Semmola of Naples, Professor Chevalière Murri of Bologna, and Professor Mazzoni; for His Majesty the King of the Netherlands, Professor H. Snellen of Utrecht, and Dr. Guye of Amsterdam; for the Grand Duchy of Luxemburg, Dr. Paul Koch; for Roumania, Dr. Marcovitch; for the Russian Ministry of the Imperial Household, Dr. Higginbotam of St. Petersburg; for the Imperial University of Kazan, Professor Dr. Leon Levachin; for His Majesty the King of Spain, Inspector-General Don Nicasio di Landa y Alvares and Inspector-General Dr. Ferradas y Rodriguez; for the Spanish Minister of Marine, Dr. Juan Acosta, Inspector of Medicine in the Navy; for the Swedish Government, Professor Carl J. Rossander of Stockholm; for the Norwegian Army Medical Department, Dr. Charles Smith of Bergen, and Dr. L. Dahl; for the Swiss Confederation, Dr. Joël of Lausanne; for the United States of America, Surgeon J. S. Billings, Washington, D.C., for the War Department, and Surgeon Brown for the Navy Department. Some gentlemen also have come from our Colonies, as Dr. Grant, who, with some others, represents, we understand, the chief medical societies of Canada.

SECTIONAL WORK.

In many of the sections no regular work was done on Wednesday beyond constituting the section and hearing the president's address, and in some even the address was postponed till Thursday morning. For instance, this was the case both in Anatomy and Physiology, though it had been understood that, in the case of Anatomy, Professor Flower would postpone his to even a later date. In Physiology, Dr. Michael Foster devoted himself to a most interesting account of English physiology and physiologists from the time of Harvey downwards to as near our own time as a wise man would venture to go. Among these he enumerated and briefly referred to the works of Glisson, Thomas Willis, Lower Mayo, to Boyle and Priestley, to Hales, Hunter, Hewson, Young, and many more, concluding with Sir Charles Bell, Marshall Hall, and others, finally referring to the great personal influence of Sharpey. The address was admirable, and was listened to with the greatest attention. Contrary to the plan adopted in the other sections, the proceedings in this are to take the form of discussion only. Various interesting topics will be brought forward by someone well qualified to do so, when it is expected that some interesting and instructive remarks may be elicited. That selected for Thursday was Localisation as regards the Brain Functions. This was introduced by a speech of portentous length by Goltz, of Strasburg, which being delivered in German, and at a rapid rate, was intelligible but to few, though probably the physiologists represent a greater number of German scholars than does any other branch in our profession.

In Medicine there has been some attempt at grouping the various subjects—the first section treating of Nervous Diseases. Immediately, therefore, after Sir William Gull's excellent and highly characteristic address, a paper was read by Professor Langenbuch on Nerve-Stretching in Loco-motor Ataxy, the discussion on which lasted for some time, and was again resumed on Thursday morning. Langenbuch's views we have already laid before our readers, to whom they will be familiar. The discussion was interesting, Brown-Séquard and Benedikt, of Vienna, taking part in it. On Thursday morning, Brown-Séquard read a paper, which might well have been relegated to the Physiological Section, dealing as it did with Brain Localisation; and this was followed by a highly interesting paper by Hughlings Jackson on Convulsions.

In the Section of Obstetric Medicine and Surgery, on Wednesday, the President, Dr. McClintock, delivered his address, which we report elsewhere. Dr. Fordyce Barker proposed a vote of thanks to him, which was supported by Professor Winckel, of Dresden, and Professor Tarnier, of Paris.

On Thursday, Professor Tarnier explained the peculiarities of his new forceps, and the mode in which he was led to their construction, and he also demonstrated their mode of action. Professor Lazarewitch, of Kharkoff, Russia, followed with a paper on the Curves of the Forceps, in which he gave reasons for thinking the generally adopted pelvic curve unnecessary. Drs. Matthews Duncan, Budin of Paris, Robert Barnes (who spoke in French), Stephenson, and Atthill, expressed their views, which differed widely.

Dr. Braxton Hicks's paper was then read by one of the secretaries. Professor Simpson, of Edinburgh, advocated the adoption of a common nomenclature in obstetric subjects, and proposed that a committee should be appointed to draw up such a nomenclature—a motion which was carried unanimously. An able anatomical paper by Dr. Budin concluded the morning's work.

The work in the Section of Diseases of Children was inaugurated on Wednesday afternoon by the address of the President, Dr. West, which will be found reported at length elsewhere in our columns. After which, a discussion on the treatment of spinal curvature, with special reference to Sayre's method, was commenced. The following papers or abstracts were read on the subject:—By Dr. Da Cunha Bellem, of Lisbon, on "Spine Deformity and Sayre's Method"; by Mr. Golding-Bird, F.R.C.S., of London, on "The Treatment of Spinal Curvature, with special reference to Sayre's Method"; by Mr. Walter Pye, F.R.C.S., on "Some of the Abuses of the Jacket Treatment of Spinal Disease"; and by Mr. Henry Baker, on "The Treatment of Spinal Curvature, with special reference to Sayre's Method." The discussion was continued till after the suggested official hour for closing the sections, and then adjourned until Thursday afternoon at 2 p.m.

At the meeting on Thursday morning, papers were read by Dr. Cheadle, Dr. Squire, Dr. Kassowitz, Dr. Lewis Smith, and Dr. Shuttleworth, and a long and interesting discussion took place on the real position of the so-called rubeola, röthelm or German measles, and its relation to scarlatina and measles. The general feeling was in favour of its being quite distinct from both measles and scarlet fever.

A paper by Mr. Howard Marsh, "On the Nature of the so-called Surgical Scarlet Fever," was also read and discussed; it was evidently held that patients with open wounds are very liable to be attacked.

In the Section of Ophthalmology, the first meeting was opened by a short introductory address by the President (Mr. Bowman), who, after alluding to similar previous Ophthalmological Congresses, and to the scientific spirit which made such congresses possible, proceeded to give an outline of the work which would be undertaken by the section during the week. Several special and all important subjects had been selected by the organisers of the section, and to deal with these in the most exhaustive manner, the co-operation of those who had made these particular subjects their special study had been secured. On Thursday, Professor Horner would introduce a subject of the greatest importance—the use of the Antiseptic Method in Ocular Surgery—in a paper, which would be supplemented by others on the same to ic. On Friday, a discussion on the deeply interesting but still obscure subject of Sympathetic Ophthalmia would be initiated by Dr. Snellen. On Saturday, Professor Leber would introduce the subject of the relation of Optic Neuritis to Diseases of the Brain. Monday and Tuesday would be devoted to the consideration of glaucoma in two aspects: on Monday, its nature and etiology would be discussed by Professor Weber and others; whilst on Tuesday the problem of its curative treatment would be critically examined in a paper by Dr. de Wecker. Before concluding, the President urged strongly the necessity of establishing some uniform system of periodical examinations and tests, especially of the colour-sense, of all those whose occupations necessitate close and accurate observance of signals, as in railway servants, but more especially in the maritime service; and for this purpose suggested that an international committee should be appointed to consider this question, and report at the termination of the Congress.

At the conclusion of the address the constitution of the Section was completed by adding the names of the following foreign members to the Council:—Drs. Meyer, Galezowski, Javal, Landolt, De Wecker, Dor, Weber, Leber, Tehender, Horner, Ole Bull, Roessander, Warlomont, Holmgren, Doyer, Reymond, Ozio, Agnew, Knapp, Thompson, Loring, and Basinelli.

To give effect to the suggestion by the President of the International Committee on Colour-Blindness, the following resolution was read by Mr. Critchett:—"That a committee be appointed by the Section to deliberate concerning the tests of vision and colour-sense most applicable to persons employed in working or observing signals by land or sea, where the lives of others are involved, and to report thereon to the Section."

The President proposed that the following members of the Section form a committee representing their respective countries:—Professor Donders (chairman), Drs. Javal (France), Warlomont (Belgium), Reymond (Italy), W. Thompson (America), Magnostakis (Greece), Leber (Germany), Ozio (Spain), Ole Bull (Sweden and Norway), Brailey (England), Lobo (Brazil), Dufour (Switzerland), Knaggs and Rudall (Australia).

The Section of Diseases of the Skin was formally constituted by the President, Mr. Erasmus Wilson, when, in addition to the members of Council already published, the following gentlemen were announced as honorary members: —Dr. Boeck, of Christiania; Dr. Bulkley, of New York; Dr. Hardy, of Paris; Dr. Kaposi, of Vienna; Dr. Lewin, of Berlin; Dr. Schwimmer, of Buda-Pesth; Dr. Rasori, of Roma. Several interesting cases of leprosy, etc., were shown in the Museum in the morning by Mr. Hutchinson, Mr. Startin, and Dr. Radcliffe Crocker, which will be noticed next week.

In the Section of Materia Medica and Pharmacology, the two classes into which the therapeutists of to-day may be divided are both well represented. On the one hand, we have the advanced or "experimental" pharmacologists, hailing chiefly from abroad—thanks to our Vivisection Act. Rossbach (of Würzburg), Binz (of Bonn), Dujardin-Beaumetz (of Paris), Boehm (of Marburg), Eulenburg (of Greifswald), and Fokker (of Gröningen), worthily represent the continental schools, although we miss Nothnagel and Schmiedeberg. Professor Wood, of Philadelphia, the best known of American therapeutists, is prominent as an author of papers and as a debater. Our own country is chiefly represented on the executive of the Section, which includes most of the names associated with the teaching of materia medica in the three kingdoms. The second class of therapeutists to which we have referred is constituted by the sanguine practitioner who clings to the faith in remedies which he inherited from a generation fast passing away, and who is manfully upholding the value of drugs by the citation of cases in point. May the day speedily come when these two classes of pharmacologists may find their results scientifically consonant with each other.

The attendance in this section, whilst considerable, cannot be expected to rival the attendance in more attractive departmenta, but it is expected that when the question of an international pharmacopœia comes to be discussed, on a very early day, there will be a reinforcement from the Pharmaceutical Congress.

The principal subjects down for general discussion are—this question of an International Pharmacopœia; the action of Apyretics (introduced by Professor Binz); the nature and limits of Physiological Antagonism (introduced by Professor Wood); Remedies used to promote Absorption (introduced by Professor Dujardin-Beaumetz); and the action of remedies on the Circulation (introduced by Professor Boehm).

The regular work of the Section commenced on Wednesday, August 3, at 3 p.m., when the chair was taken by the President, Professor Fraser, F.R.S., of Edinburgh, who, after the necessary business, delivered an interesting and instructive address. Dr. William Squire, of London, proposed, and Professor Wood, of Philadelphia, seconded, the vote of thanks to Professor Fraser.

The reading and discussion of the various papers immediately began. Dr. William Squire, of London, ever an indefatigable observer in the field of practical medicine, opened with a paper on "Bromide of Ethyl," which he discussed in its various applications, as a local anæsthetic, a general anæsthetic, and a stimulant or sedative. We have ourselves had occasion to notice in these columns the introduction of the new anæsthetic, and the unfortunate results in certain cases which have checked the promising use of it as a substitute for chloroform or ether. Dr. Squire's account of bromide of ethyl was highly laudatory, whether used for relieving pain, or for freezing the skin; whether as a general anæsthetic, which is "safe, and does not depress the heart" (like all new anæsthetics!); or whether as an anti-spasmodic in certain cases of cough, neuralgia, etc. The paper was abundantly illustrated by cases in practice.

The discussion which followed showed, as was to be expected, the want of favour for bromide of ethyl amongst the most advanced therapeutists. Professors Wood and Ringer both dwelt upon the depressing effect of the drug on the circulation, whilst they confessed that in this respect it is "safer" than chloroform.

In the next discussion, the question of the value of Strychnia as an Expectorant was again threshed out. Our readers are familiar with this recent application of the action of strychnia on the nervous centre of respiration in the medulla to the treatment of certain bronchitic conditions in which expectoration is feeble. The effect of the alkaloid on the heart further increases its value in emphysema and chronic bronchitis in the advanced stage. Professors Charteris (of Glasgow), Wood (of Philadelphia), and Lauder Brunton (of London) confirmed Dr. Fothergill's experience.

On Thursday morning the discussion on Antipyretics was opened by Professor Binz, who gave a careful résumé of our knowledge of the subject as it stands at present. Professor Binz divided remedies employed in fevers into the two great classes of—(1) Refrigerants, or those which increase the discharge of pyrexial heat; and (2) Antipyretics proper, which check its production. Devoting his attention to the second class, he dwelt almost entirely upon the enormous influence which has to be attributed to the action of substances belonging to it, of which quinine is the type, upon the life of substances akin to ferments, to which fever commonly owes its origin. In this section, therefore, as in several others, we recognise what may be called the leading feature of the present Congress, namely, the general recognition of the paramount importance of molecular processes (and in some instances the presence of organisms) in the healthy life, in many of the principal morbid processes, and in the treatment of disease.

The Section of Diseases of the Teeth was opened by an address from the President, Mr. Edwin Saunders, after which Professor Owen, F.R.S., read a paper on "The Scientific Status of Medicine." There was a full attendance of very nearly one hundred members, including the leading members of the dental profession in this country, and the following representatives from abroad:—Dr. Brasseur, Dr. Andrieu, M. Gaillard, and Dr. Colignon, from Paris; Dr. Iszlai and Dr. Arkövy, from Buda-Pesth; Dr. Kölliker, of Zurich; Professor Wedl, of Vienna; Dr. Floske, of Bremen; Dr. Sternfeld, of Munich; Dr. Taft, of Cincinnati; Dr. Shepard, of Boston; Dr. McKellops, of St. Louis; Dr. C. D. Cook, of Brooklyn; Dr. Butler, of Cleveland; Mr. Dean, of Chicago; Dr. Bonwell, of Philadelphia; and Drs. Atkinson and Bogue, of New York.

The President, in the course of his address, said that congresses served a great social purpose apart from their intellectual and scientific aims. They afforded, indeed, a valuable stimulus to intellectual effort, but in these days of an everteeming Press such result was subordinate to the living interchange of thought which they facilitated. The modern congress owed its existence to an intense intellectual activity, combined with a wide eclecticism. It was more than a fortuitous assembly; it was the deliberate coming together of distinguished men and experts for a set purpose. Mr. Saunders then went on to refer to matters more especially connected with odontology, a branch of science which now for the first time had secured a distinct and prominent place in a medical congress; and concluded by a brief allusion to the services which had been rendered by Mr. J. Tomes and Mr. J. S. Turner in the passing of the Dentists Act.

Professor Owen commenced his paper, "On the Scientific Status of Medicine," by saying that it should be the aim of every student of medicine to raise the healing art to the status of a science—i.e., to endow its followers with the power of more or less accurate prediction. He then, by way of exemplifying the passage of medicine from the stage of an art to that of a science, gave a brief description of the discovery of the trichina spiralis, and of the various morbid changes which its presence excited in the human subject. In so far as this discovery had enabled us to demonstrate an efficient cause for a series of symptoms previously unexplained, it had helped to raise medicine to the dignity of a science, the pre-trichinal age exemplifying a stage in which medicine had not risen above an art. In the same way, there was a pre-scientific age in the history of chemistry and of astronomy, when the pursuits of alchemy and of astrology respectively held their own against those studies; and there was a strict analogy between the alchemist and astrologist, and those unrecognised practitioners who traded on the ignorance and obtained the countenance and support of peers, prime ministers, and others in high places. In like manner the amount of success obtained by uncertified dentists was exactly proportionate to the stage which inductive medicine had reached in its progress to an established science.

A vote of thanks to Professor Owen for his paper was proposed by Dr. Taft, of Cincinnati, and seconded by Mr. Thomas Warner, of Cirencester, the latter of whom, in the course of his remarks, claimed the honour of having been a fellow-student of Professor Owen's under the late Mr. Abernethy. The vote was carried unanimously, and the Section adjourned.

On Thursday, the 4th, the subject for discussion was "The Transplantation and Replantation of Teeth," papers being read by Dr. Magitot, of Paris, and Dr. Finlay Thompson, of London. In connexion with this subject, cases were shown in the Museum Section by Mr. Macnamara, illustrating the transplantation of bone, and the reunion of bone with periosteum.

In the Section on Military Medicine and Surgery, Surgeon-General Longmore prefaced his inaugural address by wishing a hearty welcome to his numerous and distinguished audience, composed, as it was, largely of members of the naval and military services of the various continental powers and of the United States.

Amongst those present we noticed Surgeon-General Maclean, C.B., Professor of Military Medicine at Netley; Professor Esmarch, of Kiel; Surgeon-General Coler, of the Prussian War Department; Surgeon-General Tommer, of Berlin; Surgeon-General Roth, of the Saxon Army; Dr. C. Smith, of Christiania; Professor Yandell; Dr. Carl Reyher, of St. Petersburg; Oberstabsarzt Dr. Starke; Dr. Sommerbrock; Dr. Da Cunha Bellem and Dr. Gunes, of Lisbon; Medical Director Browne, of the U.S. Navy; Surgeon-General Bostock, C.B.; the representatives of the Italian Army and Navy; Dr. Woods, Staff-Surgeon R.N., Royal yacht Osborne; and many others.

The President, in the course of his address, congratulated his hearers upon the fact that this was the first Congress in which Military Medicine had had assigned to it a distinct section. The true principles of medicine and surgery were necessary in military as well as in civil life, but required great modification in actual warfare. The Professor dwelt upon the importance of such a section, which should meet from time to time for the discussion and clearing up of most points of military medical practice. There could be no grander or happier rivalry of nations than the vieing with one another for the common relief of suffering humanity, than the struggle for the lead in practical philanthropy. He laid stress upon the importance and urgency of the discussion of the feasibility of extending the antiseptic method to the treatment of wounded in war, as to whether it would not require to be considerably modified in actual warfare. He referred to the published results—notably those of Professor Reyher with the Army of the Caucasus—as showing the incompar-

able advantages when it could be strictly carried out, not only in the increased saving of life and limb, but in the vastly improved usefulness of the preserved parts. Still there were practical difficulties in the way—whether the spray was essential, whether it would be possible to thoroughly antisepticise currents of air on the field, whether it could not be modified to suit the exigencies of actual service—these were the burning questions of the hour. A modified antiseptic treatment in civil hospitals was advocated and practised by many eminent surgeons, and had given undoubtedly good results. Professor Longmore then referred to the magnitude of the changes in the Army Medical Department during the last twenty-five years—changes which had their foundation in the utter collapse of the department in the Crimean War, though this was not due to failure on the part of individuals. The lessons and experience of recent wars had contributed much to produce the present high state of efficiency. Professor Longmore gave a detailed description, illustrated by diagrams, of the organisation, personnel, equipment, and transport of the medical service—first, in rear of the armies, comprising (1) the base hospital, (2) stationary field-hospitals along the lines of communication, and (3) the advanced depôt; and secondly, of that of the medical service in the field, comprising—(1) the regimental establishment; (2) the bearer company; (3) the movable field-hospitals.

Professor Longmore concluded his able and eloquent address by an invitation to the members interested in this Section to visit Aldershot and see the operations and practical working of the bearer company. Two days were mentioned, Saturday and Wednesday. Surgeon-General Roth, of the Saxon Army, moved that Wednesday be the day selected, Saturday being already full of engagements, and in view of the very interesting and important character of the work to be seen at Aldershot, he was of opinion that longer time should be given than could possibly be the case on Saturday. Dr. Christin Smith, a delegate from Sweden, seconded. A show of hands being called for, Wednesday was carried by a large majority. The members visiting Aldershot will be entertained at luncheon at the mess of the Army Medical Department.

THE CONGRESS MUSEUM.

VALUABLE as the Museum is as a companion to the work to be done in Congress, and as an illustration of contemporary research, yet, to many, not the least interesting of its contents are the historical specimens, the memorials of past labours and of great men gone from us. Such are Sir C. Bell's bold water-colour sketches of Waterloo victims; the original drawings for E. W. Smith's splendid monograph on neuromata, and those illustrating Mr. Ceeley's researches on vaccination; whilst amongst single specimens may be noted a skull which Sir Stephen Hammick trephined, and a calculus which Civiale perforated but failed to extract.

Later come Dr. Adams's specimens of rheumatic gout, Dr. Greenhow's of diseased lungs from stonemasons and the like, Professor Charcot's of ataxic joint-disease, specimens of mercurial and syphilitic teeth, and Dr. Clark's series of drawings of fibroid phthisis.

A most interesting object in the Museum is a life-like model in wax, shown by Charcot. There lies the patient, on her hard bed, with distorted or dislocated knees, hips, and shoulders; and were it not that her skeleton is shown close by, one might readily believe her to be a "living specimen." Though Englishmen have long admired French skill in modelling, they have never been amazed by such a triumph of art as this before.

The models, drawings, and specimens of aural disease shown by Professor Politzer form a fine collection, and are well worthy of close study. But with these exceptions the foreign exhibition is disappointing.

Those who are interested in rarities will find ample material in the number of drawings and photographs collected to illustrate Addison's disease, ainhum, leprosy, and encephalocele; whilst the specimens numbered 8 and 535 will satisfy the most exacting curiosity-hunter.

In the large room, a remarkable series of tree-outgrowths or tumours is shown, which well illustrates Sir James Paget's remarks of last year, and his wide range of pathological research.

To the anatomist we commend Dr. Laura's sections of the

spinal cord and brain, and some of Professor Struthers' and Professor Curnow's specimens.

We pass briefly over, for the more original exhibits, several series which have been transferred from other more or less public museums, noting that those most worthy of attention are from Guy's, St. Bartholomew's, St. Thomas's, and especially from the Irish College of Surgeons. The last contains many good specimens of fractures, including several of that rarely illustrated one—Colles' fracture of the radius.

The visitor should on no account omit to see the specimens showing the results of ligature of arteries with catgut, etc., shown by Mr. Bryant, Mr. Treves, and others; nor the specimens of coincident eczema of the nipple and cancer of the breast; nor the calculi removed by Bigelow's method, shown by Mr. Teevan; nor the specimens from successful and unsuccessful cases of nephrectomy, shown by Mr. Couper, Dr. Patterson, and Mr. Lucas—Nos. 642, 776, and 777.

The Museum is perhaps as rich in works of art (for such most of the drawings are) as in specimens. Besides those already mentioned, we would call particular attention to the microscopical drawings—to those from the Richmond Hospital, and to those illustrating diseases of the eye. Mr. Treves's beautiful drawings of scrofulous glands are only surpassed by Mr. Cripps's of adenoid rectal cancer in so far that pen-and-ink demands greater precision and greater clearness than pencil, and hence is the best, if the most difficult, means of portraying microscopical appearances. Mr. Cripps's drawings have rarely, if ever, been surpassed in their kind. Dr. Bornhaupt, of St. Petersburg, shows a series illustrating tuberculosis of the testicle, and Mr. Galton and Dr. Mahomed a number of ingenious and novel photographs of consumptive patients. An average of twenty faces is obtained by exposing a plate, which requires twenty seconds, to each patient for one second.

In conclusion, we would point out that a great many exhibits arrived too late to be mentioned in the catalogue, and for this no one is to blame but the senders; but we feel compelled to notice several grave defects which a little more judgment and energy might have avoided. There are very many bad errors in the catalogue, and, what is worse, several things should have been excluded from it—notably an advertisement of a cancer-doctor, and a tedious description of a "new ophthalmoscope." Besides this, some specimens are shown which are destitute either of novelty or of interest. Nevertheless, the Committee deserve credit for a very successful Museum.

MEMORIAL TO OFFICERS OF THE ARMY MEDICAL DEPARTMENT.—At the annual dinner of the Army Medical Department, on July 4, the Director-General expressed a hope that the officers would unite in erecting a memorial to their comrades who lost their lives in the late campaigns in Afghanistan and South Africa. A committee, composed of the following officers, has undertaken to give effect to this proposal:—Surgeon-General Thomas Longmore, C.B., Surgeon-General G. A. F. Shelton, Surgeon-General S. H. Fasson; Surgeon-Major Alfred Clarke, 6, Whitehall-yard, will act as honorary secretary. The subscriptions are to range from 5s. to £2. Medical officers desirous of contributing will be good enough to send their names and amount of contribution to the honorary secretary with as little delay as possible, as, until the amount raised is known, the form which the memorial shall take cannot be decided on.

MEDICO-PSYCHOLOGICAL ASSOCIATION.—The thirty-sixth annual general meeting of this Association was held on Tuesday, August 2, at University College, Gower-street, under the presidency of Dr. Hack Tuke. At the morning sitting the proceedings included a vote of thanks to Mr. G. W. Mould, the retiring President, and the resignation by Dr. Clouston of his post as an editor of the *Journal of Mental Science*. At the afternoon meeting the President read an address in which he reviewed the history of lunacy legislation and treatment during the past forty years. At its conclusion the Earl of Shaftesbury, who was present, moved a vote of thanks to Dr. Hack Tuke, adding from his own experience several detailed particulars in corroboration of the statements contained in the address. Dr. Bucknill seconded the vote, and it was carried with acclamation. The members of the Association dined together in the evening at the Freemasons' Tavern, where they were joined by several distinguished guests, including Mr. Justice Fry, Dr. Tamburini, Dr. Benedikt, Dr. Foville, and Professor Motet.

VITAL STATISTICS OF LONDON.

Week ending Saturday, July 30, 1881.

BIRTHS.

Births of Boys, 1443; Girls, 1312; Total, 2755.
Corrected weekly average in the 10 years 1871-80, 2530·6.

DEATHS.

	Males.	Females.	Total.
Deaths during the week	1052	948	2000
Weekly average of the ten years 1871-80, corrected to increased population ...	907·1	825·6	1732·7
Deaths of people aged 80 and upwards	...	...	36

DEATHS IN SUB-DISTRICTS FROM EPIDEMICS.

	Enumerated Population, 1881 (unrevised).	Small-pox.	Measles.	Scarlet Fever.	Diphtheria.	Whooping-cough.	Typhus.	Enteric (or Typhoid) Fever.	Simple continued Fever.	Diarrhœa.
West ...	666908	6	10	...	3	7	...	1	...	82
North ...	905677	10	17	16	6	9	...	2	...	128
Central ...	361798	...	4	6	2	3	...	1	...	33
East ...	692530	4	7	6	1	11	...	3	1	109
South ...	1365578	19	15	18	3	12	...	3	1	143
Total ...	3814571	39	63	46	13	41	...	10	2	495

METEOROLOGY.

From Observations at the Greenwich Observatory.

Mean height of barometer	29·718 in.
Mean temperature	60·2°
Highest point of thermometer	75·9°
Lowest point of thermometer	43·7°
Mean dew-point temperature	58·0°
General direction of wind	S.W.
Whole amount of rain in the week	0·54 in.

BIRTHS and DEATHS Registered and METEOROLOGY during the Week ending Saturday, July 30, in the following large Towns:—

Cities and boroughs (Municipal boundaries except for London.)	Estimated Population to middle of the year 1881.*	Persons to an Acre, (1881.)	Births Registered during the week ending July 30.	Deaths Registered during the week ending July 30.	Temperature of Air (Fahr.)				Temp. of Air (Cent.)	Rain Fall.	
					Highest during the Week.	Lowest during the Week.	Weekly Mean of Daily Mean Values.	Weekly Mean of Daily Mean Values.		In Inches.	In Centimetres.
London ...	3329751	50·8	2755	2000	75·9	43·8	60·5	15·84		0·54	1·37
Brighton ...	107994	45·9	76	49	70·3	47·0	59·0	15·00		1·08	2·74
Portsmouth ...	128335	28·6	78	39	...	...	...	...		...	...
Norwich ...	88038	11·8	49	30	72·5	46·8	58·3	14·61		0·36	0·91
Plymouth ...	75282	54·0	40	20	71·8	45·0	58·3	14·61		0·93	2·36
Bristol ...	207140	46·5	126	69	68·5	42·9	56·8	13·67		0·57	1·45
Wolverhampton	75934	22·4	43	18	66·7	42·5	55·2	12·89		0·53	1·35
Birmingham ...	402296	47·9	294	184	...	...	...	...		...	...
Leicester ...	123120	38·5	92	87	...	...	...	...		...	...
Nottingham ...	188635	18·9	123	106	75·4	41·0	57·3	14·08		0·73	1·85
Liverpool ...	553968	106·3	414	308	67·4	50·1	56·0	13·33		0·74	1·88
Manchester ...	341269	79·5	197	147	...	...	...	...		...	...
Salford ...	177760	34·4	108	63	...	...	...	...		...	...
Oldham ...	112176	24·0	77	37	...	...	...	...		...	...
Bradford ...	184037	25·5	113	64	66·4	49·0	55·9	13·28		0·90	2·29
Leeds ...	310490	14·4	185	147	69·0	49·0	58·7	13·72		0·78	1·98
Sheffield ...	285621	14·5	191	97	70·0	47·0	58·8	13·78		0·53	1·35
Hull ...	155161	42·7	109	86	73·0	45·0	57·7	14·28		0·37	0·94
Sunderland ...	116758	42·2	83	54	72·0	48·0	57·7	14·28		0·65	1·65
Newcastle-on-Tyne	145675	27·1	126	61	...	...	...	...		...	...
Total of 20 large English Towns ...	7608775	38·0	5274	3673	75·9	41·0	57·4	14·11		0·67	1·70

* These figures are the numbers enumerated (but subject to revision) in April last, raised to the middle of 1881 by the addition of a quarter of a year's increase, calculated at the rate that prevailed between 1871 and 1881.

At the Royal Observatory, Greenwich, the mean reading of the barometer last week was 29·72 in. The lowest reading was 29·39 in. on Tuesday morning, and the highest 30·06 in. on Thursday morning.

MEDICAL NEWS.

ROYAL COLLEGE OF PHYSICIANS OF LONDON.—The following gentleman was admitted Fellow on July 28 :—

Siordet, James Lewis, M.B. London, Mentone.

The following gentlemen were admitted Members on the same day :—

Anderson, James, M.D. Aberdeen, 37, Keppel-street, W.C.
Fenwick, Bedford, M.D. Durham, 5, West-street, B.C.
Gulliver, George, M.B. Oxford, St. Thomas's Hospital, S.E.
Hadden, Walter Baugh, M.D. London, 7, Coventry-street, W.
Marriott, Peter William, M.D. St. Andrews, Mentone.
Thursfield, Thomas William, M.D. Aberdeen, Leamington.
Tooth, Howard Henry, M.B. Cambridge, 25, Bernard-street, W.C.
Uthoff, John Caldwell, M.D. London, Sussex County Hospital, Brighton.

The following gentlemen were admitted Licentiates on the same day :—

Barratt, Herbert James, West London Hospital, Hammersmith, W.
Barton, William Edwin, Etchingham, Hawkhurst.
Bradshaw, Oswald George Dix, 88, Warwick-street, S.W.
Butler, Thomas Edward, 3, Sydney-villas, New Malden.
Clark, William, Wotton, Glo'ster.
Clegg, Walter Thomas, 76, Edge-lane, Liverpool.
Copley, William Henry, 156, Stanhope-street, N.W.
Corlett, William Thomas, M.D. Wooster, London Hospital, E.
Crook, John Siddon, Northfleet, Gravesend.
Hitch, Frederick, Poplar Sick Asylum, Bromley, E.
Inger, John William, Nottingham.
Jones, Robert Dennett, Bron'r Eryr, Conway.
Laimbeer, Frederick James, 75, Roscommon-street, Liverpool.
Lewis, William Henry Phillips, 42, Halsey-street, S.W.
Marsh, Frank, Infirmary, Stafford.
Neatby, Edwin Awdas, London Hospital, E.
Starling, Edwin Alfred, Widmerpoole, Sutton, Surrey.
Sutherland, William Ross, M.D. McGill, 3, Belsize-square, N.W.
Sykes, Matthew Carrington, 3, Greenville-street, W.C.
Tidswell, Herbert Henry, 63, Chepstow-place, W.
Wells, Alfred Ernest, St. Thomas's Hospital, S.E.

ROYAL COLLEGE OF SURGEONS OF ENGLAND.—The following gentlemen having undergone the necessary examinations for the diploma, were admitted Members of the College at a meeting of the Court of Examiners on the 28th ult., viz. :—

Alpin, William G. F., Calcutta.
Blatherwick, Henry, Rochester.
Draper, John B., Manchester.
Fletcher, George A. C., Hereford.
Hodge, Arthur, L.S.A., Liskeard.
Hunt, Howard W. Hunt, Bampton, Oxon.
Kenny, Alexander S., Guilford-street.
Marras, Ernest A., Halsey-street, S.W.
Marsden, Thomas, M.B. and C.M. Aber., Preston, Lancashire.
Milligan, Robert A., Kimbolton.
Rhodes, Thomas, Huddersfield.
Shaw, John A., L.S.A., Deal.
Unicume, Thomas, Headcorn, Kent.

Eight candidates were rejected. The following gentlemen passed on the 29th ult., viz. :—

Brewitt, James P., L.S.A., Melton Mowbray.
Colman, George M. H., L.S.A., Holland-road, Kensington.
Clough, Morley E., Worksop, Notts.
Daniell, Charles H., L.S.A., Derby.
Dashwood, Edmund S., L.S.A., Billingford, East Dereham.
Davis, Edward, L.S.A., Euston-square.
East, Frederick W., L.S.A., Lower Clapton.
Eminson, Thomas B. F., L.S.A., Scotter, North Lincolnshire.
Loveridge, Arthur W., L.S.A., Merthyr Tydfil.
Norvill, Frederick H., L.S.A., Chester-terrace, S.W.
Prentice, Zachariah, L.S.A., Canterbury.
Roberts, Richard F., L.S.A., Bangor.
Smith, Herbert, Weston-super-Mare.
Sumner, Joseph H. S., L.S.A., Chelsea.

Five candidates were rejected, making a total of seventy-six out of the 215 examined. With this meeting the examinations for the present session were brought to a close.

APOTHECARIES' HALL, LONDON.—The following gentlemen passed their examination in the Science and Practice of Medicine, and received certificates to practise, on Thursday, July 28 :—

Allnutt, John, Kidderminster.
Colman, George Maurice Holbyn, Holland-road, Kensington.
Cook, Philip Inkerman, Brixton.
Drysdale, Alfred, Stamford-road.
Gee, Thomas Ernest, 364, Kingsland-road.
Paine, George Ruben Robins, Goring, Sussex.

The following gentlemen also on the same day passed their primary professional examination :—

Bostock, John, London Hospital.
Cortis, Herbert Liddell, Guy's Hospital.
Rugg, George Lewis, King's College Hospital.

NAVAL, MILITARY, ETC., APPOINTMENTS.

ADMIRALTY.—Surgeon Philip Somerville Warren has been placed on the retired list of his rank from the 18th inst.

BIRTHS.

BAINBRIDGE.—On July 28, at 8, Selkirk-parade, Cheltenham, the wife of Surgeon-Major G. Bainbridge, Bombay Army, of a son.
GALTON.—On July 30, at Woodside, Anerley-road, S.E., the wife of John H. Galton, M.D., of a daughter.
HARRISSON.—On July 22, at 28, Gambier-terrace, Liverpool, the wife of James Harrisson, M.R.C.S., M.K.Q.C.P., of a son.
MILWARD.—On July 24, at Edinburgh, the wife of W. Clement Milward, Surgeon A.M.D., of a son.
NAISMITH.—On July 28, at Ayr, N.B., the wife of W. J. Naismith, M.D., of a daughter.
WALDO.—On July 22, at Bradstowe Lodge, Pembroke-road, Clifton, Bristol, the wife of Henry Waldo, M.D., of a son.
WHITE.—On July 31, at Fletcher House, Tottenham, the wife of Octavius M. White, M.R.C.S., of a son.

MARRIAGES.

HOBDAY—COOMBS.—On July 30, at Bedford, John Edward Hobday, Esq., to Helen, younger daughter of James Coombs, M.D., J.P., of Bedford.
HOWEY—WILSON.—On July 27, at Tunbridge Wells, Richard Taylor Nelson, second son of Edwards Werge Howey, M.R.C.S., of Clifton, York, to Violet, only daughter of John Atkinson Wilson, Esq., formerly of Alnwick, Northumberland.
LUPTON—OATES.—On July 28, at Warwick-square, S.W., Frederick Lupton, Esq., of Statham, Norfolk, to Emily, daughter of Parkinson Oates, M.D., of Cambridge-street, Eccleston-square, S.W.
ST. CLAIR—RICE.—On July 30, at Jubbulpore, Central Provinces, India, the Hon. Lockhart Matthew St. Clare, to Ellen Mary Margaret, daughter of Surgeon-Major W. E. Rice, M.D.
SHAW—LOMER.—On July 27, at Woolston, Surgeon-Major John Alexander Shaw, A.M.D., of Chatham, to Jessie, second daughter of Alderman W. A. Lomer, J.P., of Woolston House, near Southampton.
STEWART—JACKSON.—On July 28, at Wakefield, William Stewart, M.B., of Bacup, Lancashire, to Lucy Ellen, daughter of John Jackson, Esq., of Heathfield Lodge, near Wakefield.
WHITTLE—DE VITRÉ.—On July 28, at Brighton, Edward George Whittle, M.B., F.R.C.S., to Elizabeth, eldest daughter of the late Major John Denis de Vitré, Bombay Fusiliers.

DEATHS.

BURTON, THOMAS BEARD, M.R.C.S., at 46, Rich-terrace, Richmond-road, West Brompton, on August 1, aged 83.
FORSYTH, WILLIAM, L.R.C.P., L.R.C.S., of 118, St. Martin's-lane, Charing-cross, London, on July 25, aged 69.
HATCHELL, EBENEZER JOHN, M.D., Staff Assistant Surgeon h.-p. A.M.D., at Villa d'Este, Lago di Como, on June 30, aged 46.
HATMAN, PHILIP CHARLES, M.R.C.S., formerly of Axminster, Devon, at Ramsgate, on July 26.
HENDERSON, EMILY, wife of Andrew Henderson, M.R.C.S., of Great Malvern, at Cranfield, Great Malvern, on July 29.
RIORDAN.—The infant son of W. E. Riordan, Surgeon-Major A.M.D., at Ivy Bank Villa, Gravesend, Kent, on July 18.
TIDY, VIOLET FORDHAM, wife of C. Meymott Tidy, M.B., at 3, Mandeville-place, Manchester-square, on July 29, aged 27.
TURNBULL, ALEXANDER, M.D., late of Russell- and Berkeley-squares, London, at Neckeregat, Belgium, on July 24, aged 86.

VACANCIES.

In the following list the nature of the office vacant, the qualifications required in the candidate, the person to whom application should be made and the day of election (as far as known) are stated in succession.

CAERNARVONSHIRE AND ANGLESEY INFIRMARY.—House-Surgeon. Candidates must be registered to practise in medicine and surgery, and acquainted with the Welsh language. Applications, with testimonials, to be sent to the Secretary on or before August 11.
HAMPSTEAD PROVIDENT DISPENSARY, NEW-END.—Medical Officer. Candidates must be legally entitled to practise both medicine and surgery under the Medical Acts, and be resident in Hampstead. Applications, with evidence of qualifications, to be sent to the Secretary, J. W. Fenn, 23, High-street, Hampstead, not later than August 6.
LEEDS GENERAL INFIRMARY.—House-Surgeon. (For particulars see Advertisement.)
NATIONAL DENTAL HOSPITAL, 149, GREAT PORTLAND-STREET, W.—Dental Surgeon and Lecturer on Dental Surgery and Pathology. Candidates must possess the L.D.S.R.C.S. Eng., and are requested to send in their applications, with testimonials, to Arthur G. Klugh, Secretary, on or before August 10.
NORTH STAFFORDSHIRE INFIRMARY, HARTSHILL, STOKE-ON-TRENT.—Resident House-Surgeon and Resident House-Physician. Candidates must be duly registered, and possess a diploma or degree in surgery from the College of Surgeons of London, Edinburgh, or Dublin, or from one of the universities, and a diploma, degree, or licence in medicine from a university or duly recognised licensing body of Great Britain or Ireland. Applications, with testimonials, to be sent to the Secretary on or before August 17.
PRESTON AND COUNTY OF LANCASTER ROYAL INFIRMARY.—Senior House-Surgeon. Candidates must be duly qualified and unmarried. Applications, stating age, with testimonials, to be addressed to Mr. R. P. Basterby, Secretary, 54, Fishergate, Preston, on or before August 16.
STOCKTON-UPON-TEES HOSPITAL AND DISPENSARY.—House-Surgeon (non-resident). Candidates must be doubly qualified. Applications, stating age, with recent testimonials, to be sent to the Secretary, John Settle, not later than August 9.
SUSSEX COUNTY HOSPITAL, BRIGHTON.—House-Surgeon. (For particulars see Advertisement.)

UNION AND PAROCHIAL MEDICAL SERVICE.

⁂ The area of each district is stated in acres. The population is computed according to the census of 1871.

RESIGNATIONS.

Keynsham Union.—The office of Medical Officer for the Bitton District is vacant: area 5060; population 2969; salary £40 per annum.

Reigate Union.—Mr. E. E. Hooper has resigned the Fourth District: area 7162; population 2117; salary £40 per annum.

Towcester Union.—The Blakesley District is vacant: area 11,025; population 2266; salary £60 per annum.

APPOINTMENTS.

Isle of Wight Union.—Henry M. Barker, B.M. Aber., M.R.C.S. Eng., L.R.C.P. Edin., to the Brading District.

Luton Union.—David Thomson, M.D., M.C., to the Barton District.

Ormskirk Union.—George A. Coombe, M.R.C.S. Eng., L.S.A., to the Second District.

MR. P. TAYLOR AND VACCINATION.—In order to be in good time, Mr. P. A. Taylor has already given notice of his intention, early next session, to call attention to the undoubted failure of vaccination to prevent epidemics of small-pox, and to move that it is unjust and impolitic to enforce vaccination, under penalties, upon those who regard it as unadvisable or dangerous.

HYPERTROPHY OF THE SPLEEN IN CHILDREN.—Dr. Bouchut, in a clinical lecture at the Hopital des Enfants Malades, on hypertrophy of the spleen, due to palustral influences, and not amenable to ordinary treatment, referred to three cases—one of four years of age, another of two, and a third of ten—which presented enormous spleens, forming tumours, and inducing aneurism, leucocythæmia, and the cachectic condition, so difficult of removal. Quinine, arsenic, cold douches over the region of the spleen, had all been employed without success. Splenotomy had not been performed on any of them, but, in Dr. Bouchut's opinion, this operation is the only resource when ordinary therapeutic agents are without avail, and the patients would otherwise rapidly arrive at the fatal end.—*Rev. Méd.*, July 16.

INTERNATIONAL MEDICAL CONGRESS.—We are requested by the Honorary Secretary-General to state that a register is open at the College of Physicians of members of the Congress proposing to entertain visitors at dinner during the Congress, and willing to receive a certain number of guests recommended by the Reception Committee. Anyone who wishes to put such invitations at the disposal of the Committee is requested to be so good as to communicate to the General Secretary, at the College of Physicians, the details of the day and hour of the proposed entertainment, and the number of vacant places; and also to forward, at once, a corresponding number of blank invitation cards.

APPOINTMENTS FOR THE WEEK.

August 6. *Saturday (this day).*

Operations at St. Bartholomew's, 1½ p.m.; King's College, 1½ p.m.; Royal Free, 2 p.m.; Royal London Ophthalmic, 11 a.m.; Royal Westminster Ophthalmic, 1½ p.m.; St. Thomas's, 1½ p.m.; London, 2 p.m.

8. *Monday.*

Operations at the Metropolitan Free, 2 p.m.; St. Mark's Hospital for Diseases of the Rectum, 2 p.m.; Royal London Ophthalmic, 11 a.m.; Royal Westminster Ophthalmic, 1½ p.m.

9. *Tuesday.*

Operations at Guy's, 1½ p.m.; Westminster, 2 p.m.; Royal London Ophthalmic, 11 a.m.; Royal Westminster Ophthalmic, 1½ p.m.; West London, 3 p.m.

10. *Wednesday.*

Operations at University College, 2 p.m.; St. Mary's, 1¼ p.m.; Middlesex, 1 p.m.; London, 2 p.m.; St. Bartholomew's, 1½ p.m.; Great Northern, 2 p.m.; Samaritan, 2½ p.m.; King's College (by Mr. Lister), 2 p.m.; Royal London Ophthalmic, 11 a.m.; Royal Westminster Ophthalmic, 1½ p.m.; St. Thomas's, 1½ p.m.; St. Peter's Hospital for Stone, 2 p.m.; National Orthopædic, Great Portland-street, 10 a.m.

11. *Thursday.*

Operations at St. George's, 1 p.m.; Central London Ophthalmic, 1 p.m.; Royal Orthopædic, 2 p.m.; University College, 2 p.m.; Royal London Ophthalmic, 11 a.m.; Royal Westminster Ophthalmic, 1½ p.m.; Hospital for Diseases of the Throat, 2 p.m.; Hospital for Women, 2 p.m.; Charing-cross, 2 p.m.; London, 2 p.m.; North-West London, 2½ p.m.

12. *Friday.*

Operations at Central London Ophthalmic, 2 p.m.; Royal London Ophthalmic, 11 a.m.; South London Ophthalmic, 2 p.m.; Royal Westminster Ophthalmic, 1½ p.m.; St. George's (ophthalmic operations), 1¼ p.m.; Guy's, 1½ p.m.; St. Thomas's (ophthalmic operations), 2 p.m.

NOTES, QUERIES, AND REPLIES.

He that questioneth much shall learn much.—*Bacon.*

Homœopathy.—Hear O. Wendell Holmes:—

"Munchausen's fellow-countryman unlocks
His new Pandora's globule-holding box,
And as King George inquired, with puzzled grin,
How—how the devil got the apple in!
So we ask how—with wonder-opening eyes—
Such pigmy pills can hold such giant lies!"

Alleged Insanitary State of Margate.—Dr. E. A. White, Medical Officer of Health, in a letter recently addressed to the Town Council, refutes the false rumours, and states that there is not a single case of small-pox in the town, and that it is all but free from epidemic disease.

A Vexed Question.—A communication from the Local Government Board was read to a fully-attended meeting of the newly elected Board of Guardians of St. Pancras last week, again refusing to permit a reconstruction of the Workhouse on its present site, and adhering to the previous determination that the Guardians shall build a new and additional workhouse. After some discussion it was resolved that the whole Board of Guardians, with the county and borough members, should form a deputation to the Local Government Board on the subject.

The Salubrity of Beaumaris.—It was reported to the Town Council, last week, that but one death had occurred in the borough during the past quarter, and that in the corresponding period last year there was no death whatever.

Cabby.—From the annual report of the Cabdrivers' Benevolent Association, we are glad to learn that the institution continues to prosper financially, and otherwise. It numbers 1000 members; its funded capital, on March 31 last, was £5200; and, during the financial year, an investment of £500 had been made, raising the capital to about £5700.

Infringing the Factories Act.—The Wheelock Iron and Salt Company has been summoned at the Petty Sessions, Sandbach, by the Inspector of Factories, on five charges for breaches of the Factories Acts. Several boys had been employed for weeks without a medical certificate as to their fitness to work having been obtained. The offence was admitted, and the Company was fined £10 and costs.

Women-Doctors.—The Court of the Clothworkers' Company has sent another donation of twenty guineas to the London School of Medicine for Women, Henrietta-street, making in all £63 that they have granted to the institution.

Aiding the Frustration of the Law.—Lord Clifton paid the amount of the fine (£25) imposed at the Brighton Quarter Sessions on John E. Goble for an assault on Dr. J. H. Ross, on the occasion of an anti-vaccination demonstration. The Brighton Local Branch of the National Anti-compulsory Vaccination League has publicly acknowledged this gift and his Lordship's support to the League.

COMMUNICATIONS have been received from—

Mr. CLAUDET, London; REGISTRAR OF THE COLLEGE OF PHYSICIANS, London; Messrs. FLETCHER AND STEVENSON, London; Surgeon-Major A. CLARKE, London; Dr. A. CARPENTER, Croydon; THE VICE-DEAN OF THE UNIVERSITY OF GLASGOW; THE ALBISSIMA PAINT CO., London; Messrs. COXETER AND SONS, London; THE SECRETARY OF THE OBSTETRICAL SOCIETY, London; THE REGISTRAR OF APOTHECARIES' HALL, London; Messrs. CALVERT AND Co., Manchester; Mr. GEORGE BARNARD, London; THE SECRETARY OF THE CONSUMPTION HOSPITAL, London; Mr. J. CHATTO, London; Dr. LUCAS, Bombay; Mr. BOWMAN, London; Dr. GEORGE JOHNSON, London; THE SECRETARY OF THE MEDICAL FACULTY OF THE UNIVERSITY OF ABERDEEN; Mr. JUDGE, London; Mr. F. C. JARVIS, London; Mr. BALMANNO SQUIRE, London; Dr. R. CROCKER, London; Dr. R. RAYNER, Hanwell; THE SECRETARY OF THE ARMY MEDICAL SCHOOL, Netley; THE SECRETARY OF THE MEDICAL AID SOCIETY, London; Messrs. LONGDEN AND Co., Sheffield; THE ÆSCULAP BITTER-WATER COMPANY, London; SOCIÉTÉ d'HYGIÈNE PRATIQUE, London; Mr. T. M. STONE, London.

BOOKS, ETC., RECEIVED—

The Action of Alcohol upon Health, by Andrew Clark, M.D.—Throat Diseases and the Use of the Laryngoscope, by W. Douglas Hemming, F.R.S.—The Ocean as a Health-Resort, by William S. Wilson, L.R.C.P., M.R.C.S.—Dangers to Health, by T. Pridgin Teale, M.A.—Tropical Dysentery and Chronic Diarrhœa, by Sir Joseph Fayrer, K.C.S.I., M.D.

PERIODICALS AND NEWSPAPERS RECEIVED—

Lancet—British Medical Journal—Medical Press and Circular—Berliner Klinische Wochenschrift—Centralblatt für Chirurgie—Gazette des Hopitaux—Gazette Médicale—Le Progrès Médical—Bulletin de l'Académie de Médecine—Pharmaceutical Journal—Wiener Medizinische Wochenschrift—Centralblatt für die Medizinischen Wissenschaften—Revue Médicale—Gazette Hebdomadaire—National Board of Health Bulletin, Washington—Nature—Deutsche Medicinal-Zeitung—Boston Medical and Surgical Journal—Oil and Drug News—Maryland Medical Journal—Specialist—Veterinarian—El Observador Medico—Chemists' Journal—Enciclopedia Médico-Farmacéutica—Journal of the British Dental Association—Archives Générales de Médecine—Detroit Lancet—Philadelphia Medical Times—El Medico y Cirujano—Evening News, August 1—Glasgow Medical Journal—Indiana Medical Reporter—Monthly Homœopathic Review—Indian Medical Gazette—Sunday at Home—Friendly Greetings—Leisure Hour—Girl's Own Paper—Boy's Own Paper—Students' Journal and Hospital Gazette—The Analyst—Zoophilist—Edinburgh Medical Journal—Charity Record.

INTERNATIONAL
MEDICAL CONGRESS, 1881.

OUR MEDICAL LITERATURE.

ADDRESS BY JOHN S. BILLINGS, M.D.,
Surgeon U.S. Army.

WHEN I was surprised by the honour of an invitation to address this Congress, my first thought was that it must be declined; for the simple, but sufficient, reason that I had nothing to say that would be worth occupying the time of such an assemblage as it was evident this would be. But while thinking over the matter, and looking absent-mindedly at a shelf of catalogues and a pile of new books and journals awaiting examination, it occurred to me that perhaps some facts connected with our medical literature, past and present, from the point of view of the reader, librarian, and bibliographer, rather than from that of the writer or practitioner, might be of sufficient interest to you to warrant an attempt to present them; and, the wish being probably father to the thought, I decided to make the trial.

When I say "Our Medical Literature," it is not with reference to that of any particular country or nation, but to that which is the common property of the educated physicians of the world as represented here to-day—the literature which forms the intra- and inter-national bond of the medical profession of all civilised countries; and by virtue of which we, who have come hither from the far West and the farther East, do not now meet, for the first time, as strangers, but as friends, having common interests, and though of many nations, a common language, and whose thoughts are perhaps better known to each other than to some of our nearest neighbours.

It is usual to estimate that about one-thirtieth part of the whole mass of the world's literature belongs to medicine and its allied sciences. This corresponds very well to the results obtained from an examination of bibliographies and catalogues of the principal medical libraries. It appears from this that our medical literature now forms a little over 120,000 volumes properly so called, and about twice that number of pamphlets, and that this accumulation is now increasing at the rate of 1500 volumes and 2500 pamphlets yearly.

Let us consider the character of this annual growth, somewhat in detail, first giving some figures as the number of those who are producing it.

" There are at the present time scattered over the earth about 180,000 medical men, who, by a liberal construction of the phrase, may be said to be educated; that is, who have some kind of a diploma, and for whose edification this current medical literature is produced. Of this number about 11,600 are producers of, or contributors to, this literature, being divided as follows :—United States, 2900; France and her colonies, 2600; the German Empire and Austro-Hungary, 2300; Great Britain and her colonies, 2000; Italy, 600; Spain, 300; all others, 1000. These figures should be considered in connexion with the number of physicians in each country; but this I can only give approximately, as follows :—United States, 65,000; Great Britain and her colonies, 35,000; Germany and Austro-Hungary, 32,000; France and her colonies, 26,000; Italy, 10,000; Spain, 5000; all others, 17,000.

It will be seen from these figures that the number of physicians who are writers is proportionately greatest in France, and least in the United States. As regards France, this is largely due to the requirement of a printed thesis for graduation, which of itself adds between six and seven hundred annually to the number of writers.

Excluding popular medicine, pathies, pharmacy, and dentistry, all of which were included in the figures for the

annual product just given, we find that the contributions to medicine, properly so called, form a little over 1000 volumes and 1600 pamphlets yearly.

For 1879, "Rupprecht's Bibliotheca" gives as the total number of new medical books, excluding pamphlets, periodicals, and transactions, 419; divided as follows, viz : France, 187; Germany, 110; England, 43; Italy, 32; United States, 21; all others, 26. These figures are, however, too small, and especially so as regards Great Britain and the United States. The "Index Medicus" for the same year shows by analysis that the total number of medical books and pamphlets, excluding periodicals and transactions, was 1643; divided as follows : France, 541; Germany, 364; United States, 310; Great Britain, 182; all others, 246. This does not include the inaugural theses, of which 693 were published in France alone.

The special characteristics of the literature of the present day are largely due to journals and transactions, and this is particularly true in medicine. Our periodicals contain the most recent observations, the most original matter, and are the truest representations of the living thought of the day and of the tastes and wants of the great mass of the medical profession, a large part of whom, in fact, read very little else. They form about one-half of the current medical literature, and in the year 1879 amounted to 655 volumes, of which the United States produced 156; Germany, 129; France, 122; Great Britain, 54; Italy, 65; and Spain, 24. This is exclusive of journals of pharmacy, dentistry, etc., and of journals devoted to medical sects and isms. These are given in an appended table, from which it appears that the total number of volumes of medical journals and transactions of all kinds was for the year 1879, 850; and for 1880, 864. The figures for 1880 are too small, but the real increase is slight. During the year 1879, the total number of original articles in medical journals and transactions which were thought worth noting for the "Index Medicus" was a little over 20,000. Of these there appeared in American periodicals 4781; in French, 4608; in German, 4027; in English, 3592; in Italian, 1210; in Spanish, 708; in all others, 1243. The figures for 1880 are about the same. It will be seen that at present more of this class of literature appears in the English language than in any other, and that the number of journal contributions is greatest in the United States. The actual bulk of periodical literature is, however, greatest in Germany, owing to the greater average length of the articles. With regard to the mode of publication, I will only say that in all countries except Spain the greater number of medical periodicals are monthly, while in Spain they are semi-monthly. It is this periodical literature which, more than anything else, makes medicine cosmopolitan; and although, as regards new discoveries or methods of treatment, it is still somewhat farther from London or Berlin or Paris to New York, than it is from New York to either of these places, the discrepancy is gradually becoming less.

Many of the medical journals are very short-lived, but the total number is increasing. In 1879, twenty-three such journals ceased, but sixty new ones appeared, and in 1880 there were twenty-four deaths and seventy-eight births in this department of literature. Over one-third of this fluctuation occurs in the United States alone, France being next in the scale, Spain third, and Italy fourth, while Great Britain is the most stable of all.

This merely quantitative classification gives, of course, no idea as to the character, and very little as to the value, of the product. Let us now consider it by subjects. During 1879 there were published 167 books and pamphlets, and 1543 articles relating to anatomy, physiology, and pathology—that is, to the biological or scientific side of medicine. Dividing this again by nations, we find that Germany produced a majority of the whole, France being second. The proportionate production by nations of this class of literature is perhaps better shown by an analysis of the bibliography of physiological literature for the year 1879, as published by the *Journal of Physiology*. This shows 59 treatises and 500 articles in German, 17 treatises and 227 articles in French, 5 treatises and 77 articles from Great Britain, 8 treatises and 41 articles from Italy, and 2 treatises and 24 articles from the United States. The number of authors for this product was—German, 393; French, 119; English, 59; Italian, 39; United States, 19; all others, 41. For the year 1880 the same journal reports 62 treatises and 452 articles from Germany, 23 treatises and 216 articles from France, treatises and 76 articles from Great Britain, 4 treatises and 51 articles from Italy, 6 treatises and 25 articles from the United States, and 10 treatises and 31 articles from all other countries.(a)

When we turn to the literature of the art, or practical side of the profession, the figures are decidedly different. We find over 1200 treatises and 18,000 journal articles which come under this head, and the order of precedence of countries as to quantity is—France, United States, Germany, Great Britain, Italy, and Spain. The appended tables give still further subdivisions, showing by nations the number of works and journal articles upon the practice of medicine, surgery, obstetrics, hygiene, etc., for the years 1879 and 1880, and some of the figures will be found interesting. A marked increase has occurred in the literature of hygiene during the last two years, and this especially in England, France, Germany, and the United States. The literature of diseases of the nervous system, of ophthalmology, otology, dermatology, and gynaecology, is also increasing more rapidly than that of the more general branches.

It would of course be extremely unscientific to use these figures as if they represented positively ascertained and comparable facts, the accuracy of which, as well as of the classification, could be verified. They represent merely the opinions of an individual—first as to whether each treatise or pamphlet included in these statistics was worth noting, and second as to how it should be classed. Had everything been indexed, the figures, for journal articles at least, might have been nearly doubled; while if the selection had been made by a more severe critic they might have been reduced one-half.

If I had to do the work again I should not obtain the same results. The prevailing error is that, as regards journal articles, the figures are too large, for some of those included are of so little value or interest that they are, I fear, never read by more than two persons.

Be that as it may, I think we can take them as indicating certain differences in the direction of work of the medical authors of the great civilised nations of the earth; but they must be considered as approximations only; and the statistical axiom must be remembered that the results obtained from a large number of facts are applicable to an aggregate of similar facts, but not to single cases. There will be a certain number of medical books and papers printed next year, just as there will be a certain number of children born; and as we can within certain limits predict the number of these births and the proportion of the sexes, or even of monsters,—so we can within certain limits predict the amount and character of the literature that is yet to come, the ideas that are yet unborn. The differences are due to race, political organisation, and density of population. As Dr. Chadwick has pointed out, in speaking of the statistics of obstetric literature, one of the chief causes of the multiplication of medical societies is geographical. "In England it is possible for those who are specially interested in gynaecology and obstetrics to attend the meetings of the Obstetrical Society of London, whereas in America the distances are so great that this is impossible." Speaking broadly, we may say that at present Germany leads in scientific medicine, both in quantity and quality of product, and that the rising generation of physicians are learning German physiology. But the seed has gone abroad, and scientific work is receiving more and more appreciation everywhere.

Seven years ago Professor Huxley declared that if a student in his own branch showed power and originality he dared not advise him to adopt a scientific career, for he could not give him the assurance that any amount of proficiency in the biological sciences would be convertible into the most modest bread and cheese. To-day I think he might be bolder, for such a fear would hardly be justifiable; at all events, in America, where such a man as is referred to could almost certainly find a place, bearing in mind the Professor's remark that it is no impediment to an original investigator to have to devote a moderate portion of his time to giving instruction either in the laboratory or in the lecture-room. Within the last ten years the literature of France, Ger-

much with regard to medical education and the means for its improvement. In all these countries there is more or less dissatisfaction with the existing condition of things, although there is no general agreement as to the remedy. Solomon's question, " Wherefore is there a price in the hand of a fool to get wisdom, seeing he hath no heart to it ?" is now easily answered, for even a fool knows that he must have the semblance of wisdom, and a diploma to imply it, if he is to succeed in the practice of medicine; but to insure the value of a diploma as a proof of education is the difficulty.

This evidence of discontent and tendency to change is a good sign. In these matters stillness means sleep or death —and the fact that the stream is continually changing its bed shows that its course lies through fertile alluvium, and not through sterile lava or granite.

I have said that as regards scientific medicine we are at present going to school to Germany. This, however, is not the case with regard to therapeutics, either external or internal —in regard to which I presume that the physicians of each nation are satisfied as to their own pre-eminence. At all events, it is true that, for the treatment of the common diseases, a physician can obtain his most valuable instruction in his own country; among those whom he is to treat. Just as each individual is in some respects peculiar and unique, so that even the arrangement of the minute ridges and furrows at the end of his forefinger differs from that of all other forefingers, and is sufficient to identify him; and as the members of certain families require special care, to guard against hemorrhage, or insanity, or phthisis; so it is with nations and races. The experienced military surgeon knows this well, and in the United States, which is now the great mixing ground, illustrations of race-peculiarities are familiar to every practitioner.

Neither the tendency nor the true value of this current medical literature can be properly estimated by attending to it alone. It is a part of the thought of the age—of that wonderful kaleidoscopic pattern which is unrolling before us,—and must be judged in connexion with it. From several sources of high authority there have come of late years warnings and laments that science is becoming too utilitarian. For example, Professor Du Bois-Reymond, in his address upon civilisation and science, says that that side of science which is connected with the useful arts is steadily becoming more prominent, each generation being more and more bent on material interests. "Amid the unrest which possesses the civilised world, men's minds live, as it were, from hand to mouth. . . . And if industry receives its impulse from science, it also has a tendency to destroy science. In short, idealism is succumbing in the struggle with realism, and the kingdom of material interests is coming." Having laid down this rather pessimistic platform, he goes on to state that this is especially the case in America, which is the principal home of utilitarianism, and that it has become the custom to characterise as "Americanisation" the dreaded permeation of European civilisation by realism. If this characterisation be correct, it would seem that Europe is pretty thoroughly Americanised as regards attention to material interests and appreciation of practical results. But the truth of the picture seems to me doubtful. Science is becoming popular, even fashionable; and some of its would-be votaries rival the devotees of modern Æstheticism in their dislike and fear of the sunlight of comprehensibility and common sense. The languid scientific swell, who thinks it bad style to be practical, who takes no interest in anything but pure science, and makes it a point to refrain from any investigations which might lead to useful results, lest he might be confounded with mere "practical men" or "inventors," exists, and has his admirers. We have such in medicine, and their number will increase.

The separation of biological study from practical medicine, which has of late years become quite marked in the literature of the subject, has its advantages and disadvantages. Thus far the former have far outweighed the latter, and both the science and the art of medicine have been promoted thereby. But are not the physiologists, or as I believe they prefer to be called, the biologists, separating themselves too completely from medicine for the best interests of their own science, in that they are neglecting human pathology ? In our hospital wards and among our patients, nature is continually performing experiments which the most dexterous operator cannot copy in the laboratory—she is, as Professor Foster says, "a relentless and untraumelled vivisector, and there is no secret of the living frame which she has not, or will not, at some time or place, lay bare in misery and pain."

Now, while it is true that Professor Foster, in his address before the British Medical Association last year (which address is the clearest exposition of the aims of the physiology of the present day that I have seen), insists upon the fact that all distinctions between physiology and pathology are fictitious, and declares that attempts to divide them are like attempts to divide meteorology into a science of good and a science of bad weather, his conclusion that the pathologist should be trained in methods of physiological investigation seems to me to be only a part of the truth. The tacit assumption is that all, or at least the most important, phenomena of human disease may be reproduced in the physiological laboratory. If this were only true, what a tremendous stride would have been taken towards making medicine a science! Unfortunately, it is not so. Many of the most interesting of these phenomena—the most interesting because as yet the most unexplainable—can only be observed in the sick man himself. Nor have the physiologists as yet made much use of that field which ought to be specially inviting to them, namely, comparative pathology; although the literature of the present time already indicates that a change has begun in this respect.

While it is true that to the graduate of thirty ago much of the physiological literature of the present day is in an unknown tongue, it is also true that the physiologist of the present, who confines himself to laboratory work, will find himself distanced by the man who keeps his clinical and pathological studies and his experimental work well abreast.

The increase in both the amount and value of the literature of the several specialties in medicine is readily seen by a comparison of recent catalogues and bibliographies with those of twenty or thirty years ago, and this increase still continues at a greater rate than prevails in the more general branches. There are great differences of opinion as to the relative value of this increase and as to its future effect upon the profession, but there can be no doubt as to the fact. There must be specialties and specialists in medicine, and the results will be both good and evil; but the evils fall largely upon those specialists who have an insufficient general education—who attempt to construct their pyramid of knowledge with the small end as a foundation. It has been said by Dr. Hodgen that "in medicine a specialist should be a skilled physician and something more, but that he is often something else,—and something less." There is truth in this; truth which the young man will do well to consider with care before he begins to specialise his studies; but on the other hand it is also true that the great majority of men must limit their field of work very much and very clearly if they hope to achieve success. The tool must have an edge if it is to cut. It is by the labour of specialists that many of the new channels for thought and research have been opened, and if the flood has sometimes seemed to spread too far, and to lose itself in shallow and sandy places, it has nevertheless tended to fertilise them in the end.

The specialists are not only making the principal advances in science, but they are furnishing both strong incentives and valuable assistance towards the collection and preservation of medical literature and the formation of large public libraries.

Burton declares that a great library cannot be improvised, not even if one had the national debt to do it with; thinks that 20,000 volumes is about the limit of what a miscellaneous collection can bring together, and refers especially to the difficulty in creating large public libraries in America. My experience would show that these statements do not apply to medical books. Of these the folios and quartos of three and four hundred years ago seem to have had great capacity for resistance to ordinary destructive forces. Perhaps much of this is due to the fact that they are not usually injured by too much handling or perusal. True, they are gradually becoming rarer, but at the same time by means of properly organised libraries they are becoming more accessible to all who wish to really use them, and not merely to collect and hide them away. They drift about like the sea-weed, but the survivors are gradually finding secure and permanent resting-places in the score of great collections of such literature which the world now possesses. At present the currents

of trade are carrying them in relatively large numbers to the United States, where medical collectors and specialists are among the best customers of the antiquarian booksellers of Europe. I could name a dozen American physicians who have given to European agents almost unlimited orders for books relating to their several specialties, and upon their shelves may be found books of the fifteenth and sixteenth centuries, which may be properly marked as "rarissime."

Not that the rarest books are by any means the oldest. The collector who seeks to ornament his shelves with the "Rose of John of Gaddesden," or the "Lily of Bernard de Gordon," the first folios of Avicenna or Celsus, or almost any of the eight hundred medical *incunabula* described by Hain, will probably succeed in his quest quite as soon as the one who has set his heart on the first editions of Harvey or Jenner, the American tracts on inoculation for small-pox, or complete sets of many of the journals and transactions of the present century.

Whatever may be the chosen line of the book collector, he is the special helper of the public library, and this whether he intend it or not. In most cases his treasures pass through the auction room, and sooner or later the librarian, who can afford to wait, will secure them from further travel. Thanks to the labours of such collectors, I think it is safe to say—what certainly would not have been true twenty years ago —that if the entire medical literature of the world with the exception of that which is collected in the United States, were to be now destroyed, nearly all of it that is valuable could be reproduced without difficulty.

What is to be the result of this steadily increasing production of books? What will the libraries and catalogues and bibliographies of a thousand, or even of a hundred years hence, be like if we are thus to go on in the ratio of geometric progression which has governed the press for the last few decades? The mathematical formula which would express this, based on the data of the past century, gives a result so absurd and impossible conclusion, for it shows that if we go on as we have been going there is coming a time when our libraries will become large cities, and when it will require the services of every one in the world, not engaged in writing, to catalogue and care for the annual product. The truth is, however, that the ratio has changed, and that the rate of increase is becoming smaller. In Western Europe, which is now the great centre of literary production, it does not seem probable that the number of writers or readers will materially increase in the future; and it is in America, Russia, and Southern Asia that the greatest difference will be found between the present amount of annual literary product and that of a century hence.

The analogies between the mental and physical development of an individual, and of a nation or society, have been often set forth and commented on, but there is one point where the analogy fails as regards the products of mental activity—and that is, that as yet we have devised no process for getting rid of the exuviæ. Growth and development in the physical world imply the changes of death as well as of life—that with the increase of the living tissues there shall also be the excretion and destruction of dead, outgrown, and useless matters which have had their day and served their purpose. But—*litera scripta manet*. There is a vast amount of this effete and worthless material in the literature of medicine, and it is increasing rapidly. Our literature is in fact something like the inheritance of the Golden Dust-man, but with this important difference, viz., that when the children raked a few shells or bits of bone from the dustman's heap, and, after stringing them together and playing with them a little while, threw them back, they did not thereby add to the bulk of the pile; whereas our preparers of compilations and compendiums, big and little, acknowledged or not, are continually increasing the collection, and for the most part with material which has been characterised as "superlatively middling, the quintessential extract of mediocrity." A large medical library is in itself discouraging to many inquirers, and I have become quite familiar with the peculiar expression of mingled surprise, awe, and despair which is apt to steal over the face of one not accustomed to such work when he first finds himself fairly in the presence of the mass of material which he wishes to examine for the purpose of completing his ideal bibliography of—let us say epilepsy, or excisions, or the functions of the liver.

Let such inquirers, as well as those who regret that they

have no access to large libraries, and must therefore rely on the common text-books and current periodicals for bibliography, console themselves with the reflection that much the larger part of all our literature which has any practical value belongs to the present century, and, indeed, will be found in the publications of the last twenty years.

There are a few books written prior to 1800 which every well-educated medical man should—I will not say read, but—dip into, such as some of the works of Hippocrates and Galen, of Harvey and Hunter, of Morgagni and Sydenham; but this is to be done to learn their methods and style rather than their facts or theories, and by the great majority of physicians it can be done with much more profit in modern translations than in the originals. The really valuable part of the observations of these old masters has long ago become a part of the common stock, and the results are to be found in every text-book.

If, perchance, among the dusty folios there are stray golden grains yet ungleaned, remember that just in front are whole fields waiting the reaper. There is not, and has not been, any lack of men who have the taste and time to search the records of the past; and the man who has opportunities to make experiments or observations for himself, wastes his time, to a certain extent, if he tries to do bibliographical work so long as he can get it done for him. He wishes to know whether this problem has been attacked before, and with what result—whether there are accounts of any other cases like the one he has in hand. In ninety-nine instances out of a hundred, if the answer to these questions is not given in the current text-books or monographs, it is not worth prolonged search by the original investigator. Yet he should know how to make this search, if only to enable him to direct others, and it is for this reason that a little acquaintance with bibliographical methods of work ought to be obtained by the student.

When a physician has observed (or thinks he has observed) a fact, or has evolved from his inner consciousness a theory which he wishes to examine by the light of medical literature, he is often very much at a loss to know how to begin, even when he has a large library accessible for the purpose.

The information he desires may be in the volume next his hand, but how is he to know that? And even when the usual subject-catalogue is placed before him, he finds it very difficult to use it, especially when, as is often the case, he has by no means a well-defined idea as to what it is he wishes to look for. Upon the title-page of the "Washington City Directory" is printed the following aphorism:—"To find a name you must know how to spell it." This has a very extensive application in medical bibliography. To find accounts of cases similar to your own rare case you must know what your own case is.

To return to the subject-catalogue. If it is a classed catalogue—a catalogue raisonné—it will often seem to be a very blind guide to one who is not familiar with the classification and nomenclature adopted by the compiler. And certainly some of these classifications are very curious, reminding one of Heine's division of ideas into reasonable ideas, unreasonable ideas, and ideas covered with green leather. But if the inquirer has mastered the arrangement of the catalogue, it is two to one that it will not help him. It is a catalogue of the titles of books, but very often the title of a book gives very little information as to its contents, if, indeed, it is not actually misleading. Now, suppose the particular case he has in hand is one of a new-born infant having one leg much larger and longer than the other. He will find no book title relating to this. There may be a book in the library on diseases of the lymphatics which contains just what he wants; but unless he knows that his case is one affecting the lymphatics he will hardly get the clue. There may also be in the library twenty papers, in as many different volumes of journals and transactions, the titles of which show that they probably relate to similar cases, but the titles of such papers do not appear in the catalogue.

It should also be observed that subject-catalogues may easily be put to improper uses, or thought to give more information than they really do. They are not bibliographies, but mechanical aids in bibliographical work.

You will perhaps pardon me for taking as an illustration the index catalogue of the library of the Surgeon-General's Office, in Washington, as being one with which I am familiar, and which I can venture to comment on without risk of its

being thought that I wish to depreciate its value. Taking any given subject in medicine, it is possible for a fairly educated physician to obtain from this catalogue a large proportion of all the references which have any special value, and by so doing to save a vast amount of time and labour. On the other hand; he will find, when he comes to examine the books and articles referred to, that at least one-half of them are of no value so long as the other half are accessible, seeing that they are dilutions and dilatations, rehashes and summaries of the really original papers. If the seeker is in the library itself, this does not cause a great waste of time, as he can rapidly examine and lay aside those that do not serve his purpose. But if he is using this catalogue in another library—say, here in London—the case is different. It is highly improbable that he will find in any other collection all the books referred to; and then comes the annoyance of the doubt as to whether he may not be missing some very valuable paper. 'How is he to know whether or not Smith, in his pamphlet on the functions of the pneumogastric, has anticipated his own theory of its relations to enlarged tonsils? And in all such cases, *omne ignotum est pro magnifico*. In a bibliography of the subject, prepared from the same material as the catalogue, he would either find no mention of Smith's paper, or, better still, a note that his paper is merely an abstract or compilation. The fact that he does not find Smith's book in the London library, nor any allusion to it in the best works on the subject, ought to induce him to ignore it altogether.

In proportion to the energy of the young writer, and his determination to not only note everything that has been written about his subject, but to carry out the golden rule of verifying all his references, he is apt to be led off from his direct research into the many attractive by-paths of quaint and curious speculation which he will find branching off on every side; and this danger must be guarded against, or he will find that he is wasting his time and energy in turning over chaff which has long ago been pretty thoroughly threshed and winnowed.

It is, however, no part of my present purpose to set forth the methods and principles of bibliography—it is sufficient to point out their importance, and to call attention to the point that a knowledge of how and where to find the record of a fact is often of more practical use than a knowledge of the fact itself: just as we value an encyclopædia for occasional reference, and not for the purpose of reading through from cover to cover.

Instruction in the history and literature of medicine forms no part of the course of medical education in English and American schools, nor should I be disposed to recommend its introduction into the curriculum if it were to be based on French and German models, but it does seem possible to take a step in this direction which would be of great value, not only as a means of general culture, as teaching students how to think, but from a purely practical point of view, in teaching them how to use the implements of their profession to the best advantage—for books are properly compared to tools of which the index is the handle. Such instruction should be given in a library, just as chemistry should be taught in a laboratory. The way to learn history and bibliography is to make them; the best work of the instructor is to show his students how to make them.

In the absence of some instruction of this kind the student is liable to waste much time in bibliographical research. There has been much more done in this direction than many writers seem to suppose, and there are not many subjects in medicine which have not been treated from this point of view. Of course all is not bibliography which pretends to be such. Very many of the exhaustive and exhausting list of references which are now so common in medical journal articles have been taken largely at second hand, and thereby originate or perpetuate errors. It is well to avoid false pride in this matter. To overlook a reference is by no means discreditable; but a wrong reference, or an unwitting reference to the same thing twice, gives a strong presumption of carelessness and second-hand work. Journal articles, however, and especially reports of cases, undergo strange transmogrifications sometimes, and I have watched this with interest in the case of a French or German paper, translated and condensed in the *London Record*, then appearing in abstract under the name of the translator in a leading journal, then translated again, with a few new circumstances, in a continental periodical, and finally, perhaps, reversed and appearing as an original contribution in the pages of the *Little Peddlington Medical Universe*.

In this connexion it is well to remember that a mere accumulation of observations, no matter how great the number, does not constitute science, especially if these observations have been recorded under the influence of the same theories and in essentially similar conditions.

Science seeks the law which governs or explains the phenomena, and when this is found, the records of isolated instances of its action usually become of small importance so far as that law is concerned. We care little now for the records of the chemical experiments of a century ago, and the many detailed accounts of the earlier cases of the use of ether or chloroform are of so little interest at the present time that it is not worth while to refer to them in a bibliography of the subject. And although much has been done towards classifying and indexing our medical records (more, in fact, than most physicians suppose), still, as Helmholtz points out, such knowledge as this hardly deserves the name of science, since it neither enables us to see the complete connexion nor to predict the result under new conditions yet untried.

Do I seem to depreciate the value of the thoughts which our masters have left us, and which have furnished the foundations on which we build?—or to undervalue the importance of the great medical libraries in which are stored these thoughts?—or to speak slightly of the utility of the catalogues, and indexes, and bibliographies, without which such libraries are trackless and howling wildernesses? If so, I have said what I did not mean to say. The subject has been considered from the point of view of what used to be called the division of labour, but which now I suppose should be called evolution and differentiation; and this has been done because life is short and the art is long—with fair prospect of becoming longer. It is surely unnecessary for me to enter upon any panegyric of books or libraries. As Dr. Holmes says: "It is not necessary to maintain the direct practical utility of all kinds of learning. Our shelves contain many books which only a certain class of medical scholars will be likely to consult. There is a dead medical literature, and there is a live one. The dead is not all ancient, the live is not all modern. There is none, modern or ancient, which, if it has no living value for the student, will not teach him something by its autopsy. But it is with the live literature of his profession that the medical practitioner is first of all concerned."

In medicine, as in social science, we must depend for many facts upon the observation of conditions which occur very rarely, and which cannot be repeated at pleasure. I have already alluded to the importance of Nature's vivisections to the physiologist, and a record of a case written a century ago may be just the link that is needed to correlate the results of his experiments of yesterday with existing theories. The case which at first seems unique and inexplicable both receives and furnishes light when compared with ancient records.

A science of medicine, like other sciences, must depend upon the classification of facts, upon the comparison of cases alike in many respects, but differing somewhat, either in their phenomena or in the environment. The great obstacle to the development of a science of medicine is the difficulty in ascertaining what cases are sufficiently similar to be comparable; which difficulty is in its turn largely due to insufficient and erroneous records of the phenomena observed. This defect in the records is largely due—first, to ignorance on the part of observers; second, to the want of proper means for precisely recording the phenomena; and third, to the confused and faulty condition of our nomenclature and nosological classifications.

Let us consider each of these points briefly. Very, very few are the men who can, by and for themselves, see and describe the things that are before them. Just as it took thousands of years to produce a man who could see, what now anyone can see when shown him, that the star Alpha in Capricorn is really two separate stars, so we had to wait long before the man who could see the difference between measles and scarlatina, and still longer for the one who could distinguish between typhus and typhoid. Said Plato, "He shall be as a god to me, who can rightly divide and define." Men who have this faculty, the *Blick* of the Germans, we cannot produce directly by any system of education; they come we know not when or why, "forming

a small band, a mere understanding of whose thoughts and works is a test of our highest powers. A single English dramatist and a single English mathematician have probably equalled in scope and excellence of original work in their several fields all the like labours of their countrymen put together."(b)

But cannot we do something to increase the number of observers by telling them what to observe? It is probably that much may be accomplished in this direction, provided that care be taken to limit the field. Manuals of "what to observe at the bedside and in the post-mortem room" are very well in their way, but can never be made to reach the great majority of the profession, nor would they be of much use if they did. If a few, a very few, distinct specific questions are brought to the attention of the general practitioner, he will often be on the alert for their answer. And it should be remembered that chance may present to the most obscure practitioner an opportunity for observation which the greatest master may never meet.

The great difficulty is to get such questions prepared. They must relate to matters that are just in the nebulous region between the known and unknown—to points not yet clear, but of which we know enough to make it probable that by observing in a definite direction they can be made clear; and to prepare them requires not only knowledge, but a certain reaching out beyond knowledge. It usually happens that the man who has this faculty strives to answer his questions himself, and no doubt he can usually do it better than another. But much can be done towards defining and marking out what we do not know, and this has been a powerful aid to the progress of physiology in recent years.

I have had occasion to refer to this in speaking of Professor Foster's work on physiology, in each section of which an attempt is made to separate that which may be considered as proved from that which is merely probable; and thus almost every page becomes suggestive of work to be done.

Another example of what I mean will be found in a paper on the collection of data at autopsies by Professor H. I. Bowditch, of Boston (*Trans. Mass. Med. Legal Soc.*, i., 1880, page 189). Taking the results of an investigation into the absolute and relative size of organs at different periods of life, and in connexion with different morbid tendencies recently published by Professor Beneke, of Warburg,—Dr. Bowditch urges the securing as large a number as possible of such data, and selects certain of Professor Beneke's results for special inquiry; as, for instance, that "the cancerous diathesis is associated with a large and powerful heart, capacious arteries, but a relatively small pulmonary artery, small lungs, well-developed bones and muscles, and tolerable abundant adipose tissue." It can hardly be doubted that those who read the papers of Professors Bowditch and Beneke will be induced to examine things which before would have had for them no interest, and therefore to make and record observations in pathological anatomy which otherwise would have been lost.

The second difficulty referred to, viz., the want of means for making accurate records, is one that is yearly growing less. It behoves us to be modest in our predictions as to what may be accomplished in the future towards the solution of our Sphynx's riddle. We see as through a glass darkly, and, except through the glass, in nowise; but at least we have made such progress that what we do see we can to a great extent so record that our successors, yet unborn can also see: and it is owing to this fact that a part of the medical literature of the last quarter of the nineteenth century will be more valuable than all that has preceded it.

The word-pictures of disease traced by Hippocrates and Sydenham, or even those of Graves and Trousseau, interesting and valuable as they are, are not comparable with the records upon which the skilled clinical teacher of the present day relies. But how imperfect in many cases are even the best of these records as compared with what might be given with the resources which we have at our command. The temperature-chart has done away with the errors which necessarily follow attempts to compare the memory of sensations perceived last week with the sensations of to-day; and the balance and the burette enable us to estimate with some approach to precision the tissue-changes of our patient by the records of change in the excretions which they furnish

(b) Iles, "Mathematics in Evolution." *Pop. Sci. Monthly*, 1876, in page 207.

ut we must still trust to our memory, or to the imperfect escriptions of what others remember, when we attempt to ompare the results obtained on successive days by auscultion or percussion, although the phonograph and microhone strongly hint to us the possibility of either accurately eproducing the sounds of yesterday, or of translating them nto visible signs, perhaps something like the dot and dash ecord of the telegraph code, which could then be given to he press, and so compared with each other by readers at the ntipodes.

We are beginning to count the blood corpuscles, and to se photomicrography, but we do not yet apply the latter rocess to the former so as to enable every reader to count or himself.

The connexions of medicine with the physical sciences are early becoming closer, and the methods by which these iences have been brought to their present condition are hose by which progress has been, and is to be, made in therapeutics as well as in diagnosis or in physiological research. These methods turn mainly upon increasing the delicacy and accuracy of measurements: of expressing manifestations of force in terms of another force, or of dimension in space or time. The balance and the galvanometer, the microscope and the pendulum, the camera, the sphygmograph and the thermometer, are some of the means by which investigators, at the bedside and in the laboratory, are seeking to obtain records which shall be independent of their own sensations or personal equations; which shall be taken and used as expressing, not opinions, but facts; and with every addition to, or improvement in, these means of measurement and record, the field of observation widens, and new and more reliable materials are furnished for the application of logical and mathematical methods.

Upon the third difficulty which has been referred to, viz., our confused and defective terminology, I need not dwell. "Science," said Condillac, "is a language well made"; and though this is far from being the whole truth, it is an important part of it. In examining medical reports and statistics, it is necessary to bear constantly in mind that to understand many terms you must know what the individual writer means by them. When, for example, we find in such statistics a certain number of deaths attributed to gastroenteritis, or croup, or scrofula, we have to take into account the country, the period, and the individual author, in order to get even a fair presumption as to what is meant.

The three difficulties which have been referred to, although the most important, are by no means the only causes of the confusion and imperfection of our records.

Prominent among the minor troubles of the investigator are defective or misleading titles;—and in behalf of the readers and bibliographers of the future I would appeal to authors, and more especially to editors, to pay more attention than many of them do to the matter of titles and indexes. The men to whom your papers are most important, and who will make the best use of them provided they know of their existence, are for the most part hard workers, busy men, who have a right to demand that their literary table shall be provided with properly prepared materials, and not with shapeless lumps.

The editors of transactions of societies, whether these are sent to journals, or published in separate form, often commit numerous sins of omission in the matter of titles. The rule should be that every article which is worth printing is worth a distinct title, which should be as concise as a telegram, and be printed in a special type. If the author does not furnish such a title, it is the editor's business to make it, and he should not be satisfied with such headings as "Clinical Cases," "Difficult Labour," "A Remarkable Tumour," "Case of Wound, with Remarks." The four rules for the preparation of an article for a journal will then be:—1. Have something to say; 2. Say it; 3. Stop as soon as you have said it; 4. Give the paper a proper title.

Some societies and editors do not seem to appreciate fully their responsibility for the articles which they accept for publication—a responsibility which cannot be altogether avoided by any formal declaration disclaiming it. This is due to the fact that while the merits of a paper can usually be determined by examination, this is by no means always the case. In every country there are writers and speakers whose statements are received with very great distrust by those best acquainted with them. Supposing these statements to be true, the papers would be of much interest and

importance; but the editor should remember that a certain number of readers, and especially those in foreign countries, have no clue to the character of the author, beyond the fact that they find his works in good company. In medical literature, as in other departments, we find books and papers from men who are either constitutionally incapable of telling the simple literal truth as to their observations and experiments, although they may not write with fixed intention to deceive, or from men who seek to advertise themselves by deliberate falsehoods as to the result of their practice. Such men are usually appreciated at their true value in their immediate neighbourhood, and find it necessary to send their communications to distant journals and societies in order to secure publication.

I presume that you are all familiar with the peculiar feeling of distrust which is roused by too complete an explanation. The report of a case in which every symptom observed, and the effect of every remedy given, is fully accounted for, and in which no residual unexplained phenomena appear, is usually suspicious, for it implies either superficial observation, or suppression or distortion of some of the facts. A diagramatic representation is usually much plainer than a good photograph, but also of much less value as a basis for farther work.

No fact is more familiar to this audience than the vast extent of the field of the science of to-day—so vast that few may hope to master more than a small part of it, and yet so closely connected that even the small part cannot be fully grasped without some acquaintance with a much wider field.

But little over a hundred years ago, Haller in Göttingen was professor of anatomy, botany, physiology, surgery and obstetrics, and lecturer on medical jurisprudence. At the same time he was writing one review a week, and summing-up existing medical science in his Bibliothecæ. To-day any one of these branches requires all the time of the most energetic and learned of our contemporaries, but on the other hand the well-educated medical graduate of to-day could give Haller valuable instructions in each of the branches of which he was professor. It is also true, as I have pointed out, that our actual progress is by no means in proportion to the work done, nor as great as these merely quantitative statements would seem to make it.

Science has been termed "the topography of ignorance." "From a few elevated points we triangulate vast spaces, enclosing infinite unknown details. We cast the lead, and draw up a little sand from abysses we shall never reach with our dredges. If it is true that we understand ourselves but imperfectly in health, it is more signally manifest in disease, where natural actions imperfectly understood, disturbed in an obscure way by half-seen causes, are creeping and winding along in the dark toward their destined issue, sometimes using our remedies as safe stepping-stones, occasionally, it may be, stumbling over them as obstacles."(c)

In days of old, when the profession of medicine, or of a single medical specialty, was an inheritance in certain families, a large part of their knowledge, and the efficiency of their remedies was thought to depend upon these being kept a profound mystery. Among the precepts of magic there was no more significant one than that which declared that the communication of the formula destroyed its power, and that hence attempts to reveal the secret must always fail. We have changed all that. Every physician hastens to publish his discoveries and special knowledge, and a good many do the same by that which is not special, or which is not knowledge. For the individual, in a degree—for the nation or the race in a much greater degree—the literature produced is the most enduring memorial. The whole result of civilisation has been cynically defined as being roughly, "Three hundred million Chinese, two hundred million natives of India, two hundred million Europeans and North Americans, and a miscellaneous hundred million or two of Central Asians, Malays, South Sea Islanders, etc., and over and above all the rest the Library of the British Museum. This is the net result of an indefinitely long struggle between the forces of men and the weights of various kinds in the attempt to move which these forces display themselves."(d)

And thus in our great medical libraries each of the folios

(c) "Border Lines of Knowledge," etc., by O. W. Holmes, Boston, 1862, pages 7, 8.
(d) "Liberty, Equality, and Fraternity," by James Fitz James Stephen, New York, 1878, page 176.

or quaint little black-letter pamphlets which mark the first two centuries of printing, or of the cheap and dirty volumes of more modern days, with their scrofulous paper and abominable typography, represents to a great extent the life of one of our profession and the fruit of his labours, and it is by the fruit that we know him.

After stating that modern physicists have concluded that the sun is going out, that the earth is falling into the sun, and therefore that it and all things in it will be either fried or frozen, Professor Clifford concludes that "our interest lies so much with the past as may serve to guide our actions in the present, and with so much of the future as we may hope will be affected by our actions now. Beyond that we do not know and ought not to care. Does this seem to say, Let us eat and drink, for to-morrow we die? Not so, but rather, Let us take hands and help, for this day we are alive together." To this I join a verse from the Talmud which will remind you of the first aphorism of Hippocrates, and is none the worse for that: "The day is short, and work is great,—the reward is also great, and the master presses. It is not incumbent on thee to complete the work, but thou must not therefore cease from it."

AN ADDRESS ON THE

VALUE OF PATHOLOGICAL EXPERIMENTS.

Delivered at the Second General Meeting of the International Medical Congress, August 3, 1881.

By RUDOLPH VIRCHOW.

(*Concluded from page 145.*)

ANTIQUITY only exhibits one period at which a powerful commencement of the independent development of human anatomy was made. This was in the time of the Alexandrian School in the third century B.C., when Erasistratus and his followers, under the protection of the Ptolemies, first practised methodical dissection of the human body; and, although this school subsisted but for a brief period, it inflicted the first sensible shock on the humoro-pathological system. With a more exact knowledge of the nervous system, there grew up a new and stronger race of Solidists; the Empirics rose against the Dogmatists, and although soon subdued again, they left behind them as an abiding inheritance the idea that there is a certain limit to human consideration, that the right of the individual in the maintenance of the integrity of his body is superseded by death, and that the veil which conceals the mysteries of life cannot be raised without the forcible destruction of the connexion of the parts of the body. From this idea it is, when finally worked out, that the New Medicine has sprung. But for 1800 years after the Alexandrian School did the prevalence of the humoral pathology keep down all independent movement in medicine; and during this long period no positive advance in pathology took place. Bacon admirably says, "Quæ in natura fundata sunt, crescunt et augentur; quæ autem in Opinione, variantur, non augentur." The old humoral pathology was not susceptible of development, because it was founded not on nature, but on doctrines. However different the origins these have arisen from, Galenism is found intimately connected with orthodoxy, as also the Arabian teachers with Islamism, and those of the West with Christianity; and the powerful movement of the Reformation was required in order to rend the chains in which antiquated custom and hierarchical discipline held bound the opinions even of physicians. From Erasistratus to Vesalius, and finally to Morgagni, such immense progress took place that it could not remain concealed from even the dimmest vision. Not merely the outward shape, but the very nature of medicine had undergone a change. If after Vesalius, and even after Morgagni, humoral pathology was spoken of as still existing, and if I myself have been constrained to oppose Rokitansky, the last avowed humoro-pathologist—yet it must not be forgotten that this was no longer the Galenic or Hippocratic humoral pathology. The "four cardinal humours" had already been interred by Paracelsus, and the New Medicine can only recognise the actual fluids which stream through the vessels into the substance of the tissues.

Modern humoral pathology is actually hæmatopathology. Only in name does it agree with the humoral pathology of the ancients: in fact, it is something entirely different.

But hæmatopathology has also, fortunately, been superseded, and that again in a direction due to anatomical teaching. From the earliest, but very imperfect, investigations which Bichat commenced at the beginning of this century in so-called general or philosophical anatomy, down to the constantly increasing advances made at the present time, by means of the microscope, in the knowledge of the minuter occurrences in healthy and diseased life, attention has been more and more turned from the coarser conditions of entire regions and organs of the body to the structures of which these organs consist, and to the elements which constitute the centres of activity within the midst of these tissues. Immediately after Schwann had shown the signification of cells in the development of tissue, Johannes Müller and John Goodsir made the happiest applications of the new discovery to pathological processes; and on looking back at this period, that we ourselves have lived through, and which embraces little more than a generation, we may say with satisfaction that never did a time exist before in which so great a zeal in research, or anything like a comparable progress in knowledge and ability, have existed amongst physicians. The multiplication of working power, the constantly increasing rivalry in research, and the unmistakable importance of the problems to be solved—all these are facts of the most gratifying character, and we should be very ungrateful if we did not admit that they are in a great measure due to the improvements in education and the multiplication of laboratories.

No one can be more ready to admit the great worth of anatomical study in the development of medicine than one who has sought as part of the task of his life to assign to anatomy and histology the high position they deserve in the estimation of his contemporaries. Nothing can be farther from me than to oppose those who foresee the great benefits which will accrue to the future of medicine from the pursuit of these studies. Let the young men, certainly, who will after us have to secure the advance of medicine, learn from our example how advisable it is to regard anatomy as the true foundation of our science. Most surely, much of that which to us is obscure will in this way become clear.

But we must not allow ourselves to be forced into regarding this as the one permissible means. If experiments on living animals are entirely or in great part prohibited, it is probable that the same procedures which have now been commenced against vivisection, would also be attempted against mortisection, only then we should not have arrayed against us societies for the protection of animals, but societies for the protection of dead bodies, desecration of the corpse being then the cry thundered forth in place of the torture of animals. Under the flag which is now displayed on the part of animals, the campaign against the barbarian doctors would be preached in a much more aggressive manner. An appeal would be made to the feelings of the masses—those of the mother for the body of her child, and of the son for the beloved remains of his parents. It would be shown that the dissection of the human body brutalised manners and was contrary to Christianity, while for the treatment of disease it was useless; and it is possible that ignorant, timid, or self-sufficient physicians might present themselves as witnesses against our science. The mildest of our opponents might perhaps propose the compromise that we should again make the anatomy of animals the basis of our instruction—in short, that we should revert to the times before Mundinus and Erasistratus.

Such ideas are not the mere production of an alarmed fancy. The study of history teaches us sufficiently that a victorious fanaticism knows no limits. It will realise the fruits of its victory, and even when the leaders may be contented, the excited masses push on to the complete conclusion. We need not go back to antiquity to picture the condition of such minds. In no country at the present time are examples wanting, recognisable by the living eye, which, under the form of brotherhoods or associations—somewhat more moderate, it is true, than the societies against "the scientific torture of animals,"—are earnestly exerting themselves against the scientific examination of dead bodies. It requires only an emotional and excited agitation, like that now in operation against the "torture-chambers of science," to denounce the dissecting-rooms to the indignation of the people as places for the brutalising of students. Whoever will undertake to describe, with the same fanciful extravagance that is now employed in the accounts given of physiological laboratories, the dissection of a body, or even an anatomical theatre, will never want readers who turn away with shudders and horror at the misdeeds of the anatomists!

In vain will be the statement that not a single school of medicine has ever existed, which, without a fundamental knowledge of anatomy, has ever contributed to the progress of science and the art of healing. The homœopathists and the so-called nature-doctors, who are already in position to strengthen the ranks of the anti-vivisectors, will stand forth and exhibit their results. The scepticism which from time to time seizes hold of physicians themselves, and only too easily meets with support from those who have sought aid in vain from medical art for themselves or those belonging to them, will point out with scorn how often the physician is powerless in the face of disease. Therapeutics will be regarded as so much rubbish, and it will be held out, as it already has been in the petitions of the societies for the protection of animals, that hygiene may be substituted for therapeutics, and that the treatment of individual patients can be effected by sanitary observances! And it will be sought to arouse the belief that prophylaxis is not dependent upon anatomy and experiments.

A glance at those present in so large an assemblage of physicians as this shows into how many specialties the medicine of the present time has become divided. All these branches do not require in the same degree, and with the same continuousness, all the means of investigation and scientific preparation which are indispensable to medicine in its entirety. From time to time, therefore, a palpable onesidedness prevails in some of these branches. Self-sufficiency is believed in, and the rest of medicine is looked upon with indifference, or sometimes with a sort of assumed contempt. Even purely scientific work is not secure from this one-sidedness. On the contrary, human pride and the tendency to self-exaggeration operate upon those engaged in it more powerfully than with those employed in practical studies. We ourselves have witnessed how Organic Chemistry, with a one-sided employment of a very moderate scientific store, made the attempt, and truly not without temporary success, to prescribe her laws to Medicine; and several practical physicians, unmindful of the history of our science, sought for the power of healing in a new form of chemical medicine. Indeed, I have yet a lively recollection that when I first entered on a scientific career, the expectation of a purely physical form of biology was so strong, that every effort of morphological research was treated as antiquated.

We have not hereby been prevented continuing the pursuit of anatomical investigation with all our energies, and we are now in the fortunate position of finding it everywhere recognised, that every advance in minute anatomy is followed by an advance in physiological knowledge. The physiologists themselves have become more and more histologists; but no one would demand of them that physiology should be wholly resolved into histology, which would be to replace one form of one-sidedness by another. What is essential in common to all the branches of the great medical science is the *knowledge of life*; but this can as little be attained by the external contemplation of the living being as by the one-sided examination of the dead. It is attainable by no single study or specialty, but is far rather the general outcome of the acquisitions of all the branches of the science.

Whatever is obtainable by the mere external examination of living beings has been completely taught by the older medicine during thousands of years. Both the sick and the healthy have been observed with assiduous industry, and, in fact, most valuable material has been collected by the most sagacious modes; but nothing beyond "symptoms" was attained. All that was seen were the signs (*signa*) of an internal process which could not be perceived, and the possibility of the perception of which was despaired of from the first. Life itself, also standing beyond the sphere of observation, was an object of speculation. Clever formulæ were devised, which, according to the general mental bias of the individual or of the period, took a materialistic or spiritual form; but all agreed in regarding life itself as a transcendental and metaphysical problem. The actual knowledge of the practical physician commenced with symptomatology, for the disease itself was to all

appearance no less transcendental than life itself, of which it was the counterpart.

How, then, has it come to pass that Symptomatology, which little more than a generation since held so high a position, has so entirely lost consideration that at most universities it is no longer taught as a specialty? Have signs no longer a signification for the practitioner? Can he establish his diagnosis without a knowledge of the symptoms? Certainly not. But, for the scientific physician, symptoms have ceased to be the expression of a concealed power which is recognisable only in its outer workings. He searches for this power itself, and endeavours to find its seat, in the hope of therein fathoming its nature. Therefore the first question of the pathologist, as of the biologist, in general is, "Where?" That is the anatomical question; and whether we seek to discover the seat of the disease or of life with the knife of the anatomist or merely by the eye or the hand, whether we therefore dissect or only observe, the method of procedure is always anatomical. Thoroughly logical, then, was the title of "De Sedibus Morborum," given by the founder of pathological anatomy to his fundamental book, which originated a movement that in a few decades changed the whole face of the science.

This change has been accomplished most completely with respect to diseases of the eye. Who can avoid the conviction that the ophthalmology of the present day scarcely bears any resemblance to that of the last century? Who would rest satisfied with the symptoms of amaurosis? Who despairs of recognising the nature of glaucoma? Every oculist has at hand the means of studying the disease itself, and not merely its signs. Even anti-vivisectors acknowledge that ophthalmology is a fertile form of study; but they forget that every organ is not so favourably placed and constructed for observation as is the globe of the eye. Since the wonderful discovery of the ophthalmoscope, anatomical analysis can be carried, without the aid of the knife, so far into the constituent parts of the eye that we are enabled to examine the smallest textural portions of its fundus—nay, single cells or groups of cells—just as easily as in an artificial preparation of an eye that has been excised. But we should not forget what prolonged prior anatomical and physiological study was required for the interpretation of that which is now so conveniently seen. The structure, disposition, and function of each separate part had first to be laboriously made out, before it became possible to ascertain by a mere glance at the altered tissue what had really taken place; and no student will be able truly to understand the nature of the changes, who has not previously made himself thoroughly acquainted with the anatomy and physiology, and the possible pathological alterations, of each constituent part of the eye.

It is easy to object that all branches of medicine do not stand on the same level as ophthalmology, for that can never be the case. Just as it is easier to explore the ocean in its depths than the solid land, so will the most transparent organ of the body be the one most fitted for medical diagnosis and treatment. While a cysticercus at the hindmost part of the retina can always be seen without difficulty, it will always be found that a cysticercus in a muscle, or a trichina, can only be exhibited by means of a vivisection. It can never be expected that every medical specialty will attain the certainty of recognition and treatment that characterises diseases of the eye; but we should only seek for the attainable amount of this by applying the ophthalmological method in a corresponding manner to the other special branches. This method is the anatomical, or, as it has also been termed, the *localising* method.

With this, we have arrived at the point which indicates, as it were, the boundary between the Old and New Medicine. *The principle of modern medicine is localisation.* To those who are always asking, What good has modern science done to practical medicine? we may simply reply that every branch of medical practice has adapted itself to the principle of localisation—not merely in pathology, but also in therapeutics,—and that to the great benefit of the sick. It would be quite superfluous to seek for special examples of the utility of this new knowledge. Such examples abound, but we do not need them, as we can refer to the general characteristics of modern medicine. All those subjects which already, in earlier times, had a natural inclination to localisation, as surgery and dermatology, have, quite logically, continued to advance in the same sense. But those branches which had preserved from the old humoral pathology—a tendency to set forth general formulæ, have gradually abandoned the tradition that had become so dear to them; and it has become admitted more and more that, in truth, generalisation is nothing else than a *multiplication* of *foci*, and that the cure of a so-called general disease signifies the extinction of each separate centre. This is indeed a reform from head to foot, and he who has not grasped it cannot say that he has followed the advance of science with effect.

This idea of the general admissibility of the doctrine of the localisation of disease, and of the multiplication of the foci of disease in the same individual, stands, as was often objected to me when I commenced my career as a teacher, in direct opposition to the idea of the unity of disease, or, as expressed in the customary phrase, the *ens morbi*. My contemporaries still maintained much of this idea, and deemed the practitioner as falling into arbitrary and dangerous speculations when he in presence of a single case of disease regarded it as a multiple. To me, on the other hand, it seemed much rather that the practitioner had entered upon a fruitless and, for the individual patient, dangerous theorising (*schematismus*) if, in conformity with the opinions of this school, or of those he himself had formed, he assumed the unity of disease, and regulated his prognosis and therapeutics accordingly. In the meantime, these reflections, derived from medical practice, as to the *utility* of a certain mode of viewing a disease, decide nothing in regard to the *truth* of this, and yet it is this at which we seek to arrive. How is this to be established?

Everyone is agreed that disease presupposes life. No disease can occur in a dead body; and at death life and disease alike disappear. This reflection led the older physicians to form a conception of disease as of a self-animated or even soul-endowed nature, which took its place in the living body beside the vital principle. Many went so far as to define disease as a struggle between two combative principles, the innate life and an intrusive foreign nature. But all acknowledge life as the preliminary condition of disease. In the old School of Leyden the conception first acquired profundity. From Boerhaave came the proposition, which was placed by his pupil Gaubius in front of his "Handbook of General Pathology" (the first written on the subject, and which continued so long in repute), "*Morbus est vita præternaturam*"—disease is itself life, or, more exactly speaking, it is a part of life.

This conception displaced the unfortunate dualism which had so long lorded it over medicine, or at least it ought to have done away with the dualism between life and disease. If, nevertheless, it did not completely accomplish this, so that more than a century had to elapse before this persisting dissonance could be superseded, this lay in the difficulty of finding a satisfactory idea of life. And here the question could not be passed by, Where is the special seat of life? "*Ubi sedes vitæ?*" John Hunter fell back upon the old idea, already announced in the Mosaic formula, "For the life of the flesh is in the blood"; and Flourens believed that he had found its seat in the *nœud vital*, in the central nervous system, in the medulla oblongata. Both found themselves compelled to perform experiments on living animals for the elucidation of this difficult question. In this way the experimental method in the more strict sense began to form part of the practice of pathologists, and vivisection became a regular adjuvant to research.

In truth, the belief that life could only be learned from among the living themselves had long prevailed, but the exact period in ancient times when it was first acted upon could only with difficulty be determined. Only uncertain traditions concerning it survive. Zacharias Sylvius, a Rotterdam physician, who wrote the preface to the Dutch edition of Harvey's "Exercitationes," 1671, refers to the story of Democritus, whom the Abderites regarded as mad from his being constantly engaged in vivisections. The great Hippocrates, however, fully recognising his procedures, declared that it was the Abderites who were insane, and Democritus alone in his right senses. Probably the tale was invented at the expense of the Abderites, but it yet shows that vivisection had long "been in the air." Just as little can I decide whether it is true that the teachers of the Alexandrian School utilised the permission of their king to dissect criminals. Only one thing I may conclude from these narrations is that experiments upon animals must at that time have already been performed; for anyone who

conceived the idea of dissecting men must, especially at a period when the anatomy of animals formed the basis of medical study, assuredly have already performed vivisection on animals. In the school of the Empirics, which sprang out of the Alexandrian, and in which the autopsy was first taught as a chief source of knowledge, experiment also appears as an acknowledged claim; and in the famous formula which has been termed the tripod of the Empirics, and which served as a programme of the school, deliberately arranged experiment is expressly mentioned (φυσικὴ ἢ αὐτοσχεδὶς τήρησις). As there is no evidence as to the extent research on living animals was then carried, it would be of no avail to inquire what advantage ancient medicine derived from vivisection.

In fact, the first great and decided example of successful vivisection which is known in the history of medicine is due to William Harvey. The establishment of the doctrine of the circulation, which in its chief points was experimental, has entirely changed the basis of the direction of medical thought. Had we but this one example, it would suffice as a striking demonstration of the utility, and even the indispensability, of vivisection. Never was a doctrine sanctioned by the traditions of centuries and strengthened by every description of authority, so that in truth it constituted the centre of a powerful and generally received system, annihilated by so precipitous a fall. Fully appreciating the significance of such a man, Haller has already declared that his name is the second on the roll of medicine, counting backwards from Hippocrates. But it was a difficult step to take, to stand forth with a new and unheard-of doctrine, seizing hold of science in so revolutionary a manner. Long did Harvey hesitate whether he should publish his discovery, and when at last he carried his resolution into effect, the great vivisector exclaimed, "Utcunque sit, jam jacta est alea, spes mea in amantium veritatis et doctorum animorum candore sita." The purity of a truth-loving and educated spirit is still requisite at the present time to free Harvey from the reproaches of heartlessness or even of brutality in which our anti-vivisectors deal so liberally. This new doctrine cost many animals their lives. It began, as he himself says, "ex vivorum (experiendi causa) dissectione, arteriarum assertione disquisitione que multimoda." And yet was the least thing objected to him; for even kings were at that time so little tender-hearted, or, as our opponents would say, so brutalised, that Charles I. took pleasure in witnessing the experiments of his physician.

At the present time, after Malpighi had in the same century demonstrated on living animals the circulation in the capillaries, and after, in our own century, the knowledge of the existence of an actual capillary wall has been supplied, the doctrine of the circulation seems so self-evident, and has so entirely entered into general conception, that it now requires a specially instructed mind to enter into the ideas of the old physicians in respect to the local conditions governing the circulation. Whoever without such preparation peruses the medical classics, will only fall from one misunderstanding into another. The views concerning these local processes have undergone an entire change; and yet the circulation (but much rather the capillary than the general circulation) still stands in the foreground of pathological interest, perhaps almost more than it should do. The widely comprehensive doctrines of inflammation and new formation, within which almost the principal share of practical cases is comprised, are based upon experiments upon the capillary circulation, as also is the doctrine of the cure of local processes of disease of the most varied kind.

Even the bitterest opponents of vivisection acknowledge the services of Harvey, but they declare that nothing of any importance has been accomplished since his time by means of vivisection. They are not aware that that portion of the circulation which relates to the vital properties of the organs of circulation themselves was entirely untouched by Harvey. On what does the activity of the heart depend? What influence do the vessels exert in propelling and distributing the blood? What share falls to the arteries, what to the veins, what to the capillaries? All these questions are of the highest practical importance, and none of them can be examined into except by experiment on living animals. But Harvey could not investigate them, because in his time minute anatomy had not yet become developed. Who then knew anything about the nerves of the heart and vessels? Who then had any presentiment of what share in the active operations of the heart and vessels belongs to the nerves, and what to the constituents of the vessels, especially their minute muscles? Another interval of two hundred years had to elapse before Edward Weber, by experiments on the vagus in living animals, unveiled, in an unexpected and unheard-of manner, the secret of the innervation of the heart, and anticipated our now so much abused friend Claude Bernard, by showing on the living animal the influence of the sympathetic on the vessels of the head and neck.

Now only, and by the aid of numerous other allied experiments, are we able to understand the circulation in its particulars. The pulse, the highly prized object of the old symptomatology, now admits of interpretation. It is no longer for us the sign of this or that disease, but the sign of the existence or non-existence of definite activities, of strength or weakness, of the tension or relaxation of certain tissues. It is only now that we understand the action of the heart itself, and the influence of certain substances upon it, as for example the heart-poisons; and that not only in relation to valvular disease, to which the anti-vivisectionists alone allude with not very intelligible sneers, on account of its incurability, but also of febrile diseases and of parenchymatous and nervous changes, the symptoms, nature, and results of which we are enabled to survey with exactitude.

The length of time which elapsed between Harvey and the modern experiments on the innervation of the vascular apparatus is also explicable, that in this interval two entirely new studies had to be created, for both of which the discovery of the circulation furnished both an impulse and a preparation,—I mean physiology and general pathology, therefore, exactly those branches of study which are to be regarded as the chief supporters of the experimental method, and which were at first comprised under the name "Institutiones Medicæ." Hermann Boerhaave still combined them during his teaching, and even united them with practical medicine; but under his pupils the division of labour began, and the formal separation of these two branches took place. Haller was really the creator of physiology. His experiments were first directed towards the exploration of the vital properties of the separate parts of the body, or, as we should now say, of the various tissues. Among these properties he placed irritability, following the example of the eminent Glisson, who, it seems to me, has scarcely yet received sufficient honour in his own country. It would lead me too far, were I to attempt to describe the details of this memorable investigation, the understanding of which has been rendered very difficult by the insufficient clearness of the ideas attached to the terms "irritability" and "contractility." It will sufficiently answer our purpose to indicate that then, for the first time, nerves and muscles, the two highest developed, and therefore most energetic, parts of the economy were made the subjects of searching experiment in relation to their special actions. Contractility and sensibility appeared as the special tokens of vital activity. The question of the foundation of vital activity seemed herewith so closely approached, that Gaubius, who was then constructing his general pathology,(a) without more ado, indicated vital power as the cause of contraction.

From such beginnings was developed, at first in a very obscure and unproductive manner, and much disturbed by speculative vitalism, the doctrine of life in its modern form. It has required very prolonged and, for the most part, experimental labour to attain, in spite of all obstacles, great and practical results. Out of the idea of irritability, originally due to Glisson, contractility has gradually been evolved; and the opposition in which Haller placed irritability and sensibility to each other has been rectified by regarding contractility and sensibility as two forms of vital expression connected with various elements, subordinated to general irritability. In this sense, irritability and vitality are well-nigh identical. Both are properties of tissues, and, as such, are directly or indirectly accessible to observation and experiment.

And, in fact, experiments became now more directed to the tissues themselves. The discovery of electrical contraction by Galvani, the researches of A. vox. Humboldt on the irritation of muscle and nerve fibres, and many other contemporary investigations, bear witness to the changed direction of the new biology. The mysticism of the nature of life and disease,

(a) Gaubius, "Institute Path. Med.," page 72.

and the speculations on vital power, sank more and more into discredit, while from generation to generation medicine assumed more and more the character of true natural science. The obscurity which had so long prevailed, especially with respect to the nervous system, was dispersed under the combined action of anatomists and experimenters, and especially since Charles Bell taught the difference between nerves—hitherto considered as alike,—and opened the way to the investigation of the signification and properties of the various divisions of the central nervous system, work after work has appeared, spreading new light over this difficult and complicated subject. It would be impossible to notice all these productions on this occasion, and it would be superfluous to do so in such an assemblage of specially competent persons, many of whom have themselves laboured at this glorious work.

I will only prominently mention in a few words that one idea, the origin of which stretches far backwards, has always come out more clear and more victorious; and that is the idea of a *life proper to the individual parts*—the *vita propria*. Every new form of experiment that is contrived renders new parts accessible to the investigations of natural science, and with every step we become more clearly convinced that the great life-unity, in the usual sense, is a mere fiction arising from the observation that in the hierarchical organisation of the human body certain organs attain so high a development, and thereby so great an importance, that they have full right to the name of *vital organs;* and as among these organs the medulla oblongata possesses the highest importance, it may be easily understood how the idea has arisen that this may be the precise seat of life. But we now know that life is a collective action of all parts —the higher or vital, as well as the lower or less worthy; and that there is no *single* seat of life, but that every true elementary part, and especially every cell, is a seat of life. In biological as well as pathological research, also, we have arrived at a multiplication of foci: but it is obvious that the number of vital centres is much larger than that of disease centres ever can be; and therefore disease and life—or, to speak more precisely, diseased and healthy life—may very well co-exist in the same organism: invariably, however, in such a manner that disease always signifies an abridgment, a *minus* of healthy life. In this investigation we have again come upon the essence of disease that had so long disappeared; but truly not in its spiritual form, but as an entirely material *ens*, a real, corporeal thing—the *altered cell*.

Has all this proved useful? Was it worth while for this to give pain to and to sacrifice so many animals? Have we a just right to claim that the experimental method should still be permitted? We can answer all these questions confidently in the affirmative. It is not every experiment upon animals that is followed by the consequences which attended Galvani's—consequences which have not only led to a new and efficacious method of treating disease, electro-therapeutics, and disclosed a new and large province of vital processes, but have provided a vast series of most important technical arrangements—the first condition of the knowledge of the natural processes. But galvanism should prove even to limited and timid minds a striking and consolatory example that it is not from every result of a true observation of nature that its practical consequence will at once become prominent, and that notwithstanding it may possess great practical value. The cellular theory and the proof of the *vita propria seu cellulosa*, are in themselves very abstruse things, and they could not be utilised in practical medicine without further elucidation, and yet they have become the basis, and in some measure the security, for localising therapeutics; and they will certainly become more so from day to day when the materia medica has to a greater extent pursued the path which toxicology has long since followed with such excellent results.

How are we to expect any great results in the art of healing if experiments on animals are discontinued? For a long time past no remedy has met with so ready an acceptance and so wide a diffusion as chloral, the properties of which were in my Institute discovered and established by Professor O. Liebreich by means of experiments. How would it have been possible to acquire a knowledge of these properties without experiments? The animals' friends say, "Try these new remedies on yourselves!" and point to the "provings" of the homœopaths. But, apart from the fact that the "provings" of the homœopaths have never yet led to the recognition of a new remedy which could even be remotely compared with chloral, and that these "provings," even as regards medicines already well known, never meet the most moderate requirements of a scientific investigation, and should not therefore be offered as patterns,—surely no one would seriously desire that various bodies, possibly poisonous, should become the objects of self-experiment by physicians or other persons! This kind of morality, which prohibits experiments on animals, and advises their performance on one's own body or on persons who are ill, is in fact devoid of the primary foundations of intelligent consideration.

To prove the great importance of hygiene and prophylaxis would be somewhat superfluous; and if any class of men have been active in this direction it has been medical practitioners. Never have zealous hygienists been wanting among them, and whenever a great problem in prophylactics has required solution, you may then be certain to find medical men at work. We have been so much accustomed to this conjunction that we have come to always regard hygiene and prophylaxis as appertaining to medicine and no other science; but it is mere empty babbling to say that prophylaxis renders therapeutics, and to some extent medicine, superfluous. The procedures of this imperfect world are such that as long as there are men there will be certainly no want of sick; and we are nowise frightened at the threat that we shall be no longer employed. We are indispensable for the progress of hygiene, and still less can experiments on animals be done without. Shall hygienists be required to allow the influence of the various "causes"—cold and heat, dryness and moisture, dust and noxious gases, micrococci and bacteria —to operate upon their own persons, in order to verify the effects of these and formulate laws concerning them? Intelligent governments must perceive that it would be an act of folly to sacrifice men's lives only because a small number of persons regard it as immoral to take those of animals. Medical practitioners during the period of epidemics of all kinds, in their hospital work, in the country, in visiting the sick at night, and in operations and post-mortems, are more exposed than any other class of society; and it required the complete blindness of the animal-fanatic to also demand of them that they should test in their own persons the curative, poisonous, or indifferent effects of unknown substances, and also settle by means of self-observation the strength of permissible doses of medicinal substances.

The suppression of experiments upon animals is sought for in the names of humanity, morals, and religion; for, in point of fact, it is not merely vivisection that is in question, but the experimental method in general. And when vivisection is spoken of it is made to include all painful effects, even when no cutting has taken place; and in order to prevent any misunderstanding, not only physiological, but pathological and pharmacological experiments are expressly attacked. *Pain is the criterion, and anything which in the course of an experiment upon an animal inflicts pain is,* they say, *animal torture,* and so far immoral and contrary to religion. Such a definition of cruelty to animals applied to other occupations or people might give rise to strange consequences. Lovers of dogs who in training them often employ or allow to be employed cruel methods and painful punishments, might easily be brought into great danger, while training horses for certain purposes could not go on. A large portion of our domestic animals would have to go untrained in order that they might be spared pain; and we might perhaps get into the same condition as that brought about by the wild dogs of Turkey.

Some anti-vivisectors are at least so far logical, that they would wish also to see the slaughtering of animals prohibited. From the vegetarian point of view the opposition attains a kind of systematic appearance. Thus, Herr von Seefeld(b) calls for a vegetable diet and the prohibition of vivisection, but as he, as a vegetarian, does not require meat, he feels much disposed to make further concessions. He rejects hunting with the aim of pleasure, but believes that it cannot quite be dispensed with for defence. Others go still further, and sacrifice even war. With such persons it may be possible to argue; but principles have first to be cleared up.

The principle can scarcely be denied, that *to kill is more than to torture;* and a criminal code could hardly be found which punishes the intentional killing of a man less severely

(b) A. von Seefeld, "Altes und Neues über die vegetarianische Lebensweise." Hannover, 1880, s. 33.

than cruelty to a man. The position is well founded, that a man, who after any mal-treatment still retains his life, may yet attain a full enjoyment of existence. Extenuating circumstances may be admitted, even in murder; but, as a principle, the extremest injury is the most severely punished.

On the other hand, the anti-vivisectors regard the torturing worse than the killing of animals. Although they reject any painful or tormenting mode of killing even of cattle, they allow even highly organised animals to be killed or slaughtered, not only for the purpose of being eaten, but also on other purely subjective grounds. They indeed go so far as to demand that an animal which has outlived a vivisection should be killed, although it might still be capable of enjoying a long and happy life. Is there any logic or morality in this? What, then!—we may have the right to kill an animal on the ground of any ordinary object of utility, as the eating its flesh, the disposing of its skin, or grinding its bones for manure, and yet we are to have no right to undertake a scientific experiment which we have instituted on purely theoretical grounds, or for public utility, and in performing which we are in danger of acquiring disease? He who claims for himself the right to kill animals, has no right to prohibit physicians from performing vivisection on them as a means of investigation, or submitting them to other painful procedures.

It speaks for itself that we ought not to expect that an abuse of this right should go unpunished; for it is with such abuse, and not with the infliction of pain, that cruelty to animals actually first commences. If all infliction of pain is to be regarded as cruelty to animals, the veterinary surgeon would then be liable to punishment for an operation performed on an animal to secure its recovery. But cruelty should be regarded as punishable when animals are subjected to pain in a needless and aimless manner. Nothing, therefore, should be objected to the submission of every experimenter to inspection, but this certainly should not be conducted by a society for the protection of animals. Anyone who takes more interest in the domestic animals than in science, i.e., in the recognition of truth, cannot be a suitable person to exert official control over scientific procedures. Where would it lead to if an experimenter, who had instituted his investigation in good faith, found himself, perhaps during the very progress of the experiment, compelled to explain to some layman, or, after its completion, to a magistrate, why he had not chosen some other method or some other instrument, or even had not resorted to some other experiment?

No! Here we have to do with no question of objective right. As long as any owner of animals, according to his own judgment, is at full liberty to kill any of these, whether wild or tame, that he chooses, so long should experiments on living animals, made for scientific purposes, be permitted. As to the necessity of such experiments, the investigator himself can alone decide; while as to the choice of time, place, and the admission of strangers, he may have to make arrangements with the official inspector. But the carrying out of the experiments must be left in his hands. That is how we understand the expression "Freedom of Science."

It is objected to us that the outraged feelings of the owners of horses, dogs, and cats excite in them the fear that a similar fate may await their beloved animals, that has overtaken those in our scientific institutes. Here we can sympathise with them. We would force no one to hand over their pets to us, nor would we steal them: and if either of these things occurred, it is probable that in every country the intervention of the law might be successfully appealed to. But we must insist upon it that our power of disposal of the lives and being of animals we have come into the lawful possession of shall not be diminished; and that we shall not be represented *à priori* as devoid of moral feeling and as brutal barbarians, standing almost on the threshold of crime. The proof that moral earnestness has undergone diminution among the medical body of the present day is nowhere forthcoming; and the statement that Christianity is endangered by Christianity, is worthy of Abdera. The allegation that the medical student has become inwardly "brutalised" by dissection and vivisection is as unfounded as is the calumny that the morality of his teachers has sustained injury. But there is no ground for any fear for science itself. What Bacon says of the sun may be said of it: " Palatia et cloacas ingreditur, neque tamen polluitur."

GENERAL ADDRESS
ON THE
CONNEXION OF THE BIOLOGICAL SCIENCES
WITH MEDICINE.

By T. H. HUXLEY, LL.D.,
Secretary to the Royal Society, and Vice-President of the Congress.

———

THE great body of theoretical and practical knowledge which has been accumulated by the labours of some eighty generations, since the dawn of scientific thought in Europe, has no collective English name to which an objection may not be raised; and I use the term "medicine" as that which is least likely to be misunderstood; though, as everyone knows, the name is commonly applied, in a narrower sense, to one of the chief divisions of the totality of medical science.

Taken in this broad sense, "medicine" not merely denotes a kind of knowledge, but it comprehends the various applications of that knowledge to the alleviation of the sufferings, the repair of the injuries, and the conservation of the health of living beings. In fact, the practical aspect of medicine so far dominates over every other that the "healing art" is one of its most widely received synonyms. It is so difficult to think of medicine otherwise than as something which is necessarily connected with curative treatment, that we are apt to forget that there must be, and is, such a thing as a pure science of medicine—a "pathology" which has no more necessary subservience to practical ends than has zoology or botany.

The logical connexion between this purely scientific doctrine of disease, or pathology, and ordinary biology is easily traced. Living matter is characterised by its innate tendency to exhibit a definite series of the morphological and physiological phenomena which constitute organisation and life. Given a certain range of conditions, and these phenomena remain the same, within narrow limits, for each kind of living thing. They furnish the normal and typical characters of the species; and, as such, they are the subject-matter of ordinary biology.

Outside the range of these conditions, the normal course of the cycle of vital phenomena is disturbed, abnormal structure makes its appearance, or the proper character and mutual adjustment of the functions cease to be preserved. The extent and the importance of these deviations from the typical life may vary indefinitely. They may have no noticeable influence on the general well-being of the economy, or they may favour it. On the other hand, they may be of such a nature as to impede the activities of the organism, or even to involve its destruction.

In the first case, these perturbations are ranged under the wide and somewhat vague category of "variations"; in the second, they are called lesions, states of poisoning, or diseases; and, as morbid states, they lie within the province of pathology. No sharp line of demarcation can be drawn between the two classes of phenomena. No one can say where anatomical variations end and tumours begin, nor where modification of function, which may at first promote health, passes into disease. All that can be said is, that whatever change of structure or function is hurtful belongs to pathology. Hence it is obvious that pathology is a branch of biology; it is the morphology, the physiology, the distribution, the aetiology of abnormal life.

However obvious this conclusion may be now, it was nowise apparent in the infancy of medicine. For it is a peculiarity of the physical sciences, that they are independent in proportion as they are imperfect; and it is only as they advance that the bonds which really unite them all become apparent. Astronomy had no manifest connexion with terrestrial physics before the publication of the "Principia"; that of chemistry with physics is of still more modern revelation; that of physics and chemistry with physiology has been stoutly denied within the recollection of most of us, and perhaps still may be.

Or, to take a case which affords a closer parallel with that of medicine. Agriculture has been cultivated from the earliest times; and, from a remote antiquity, men have attained considerable practical skill in the cultivation of plants, and have empirically established many scientific truths concerning the conditions under which they flourish. But it is within the memory of many of us that chemistry, on the one hand, and vegetable physiology on the other, attained a stage of development such that they were able to furnish a sound basis for scientific agriculture.

Similarly, medicine took its rise in the practical needs of mankind. At first, studied without reference to any other branch of knowledge, it long maintained—indeed, still to some extent maintains—that independence. Historically, its connexion with the biological sciences has been slowly established, and the full extent and intimacy of that connexion are only now beginning to be apparent. I trust I have not been mistaken in supposing that an attempt to give a brief sketch of the steps by which a philosophical necessity has become an historical reality may not be devoid of interest, possibly of instruction, to the members of this great Congress, profoundly interested as all are in the scientific development of medicine.

The history of medicine is more complete and fuller than that of any other science, except, perhaps, astronomy; and if we follow back the long record as far as clear evidence lights us, we find ourselves taken to the early stages of the civilisation of Greece. The oldest hospitals were the temples of Æsculapius; to these Asclepeia, always erected on healthy sites, hard by fresh springs, and surrounded by shady groves, the sick and the maimed resorted to seek the aid of the god of health. Votive tablets or inscriptions recorded the symptoms, no less than the gratitude, of those who were healed; and from these primitive clinical records the half priestly, half philosophic caste of the Asclepiads compiled the data upon which the earliest generalisations of medicine, as an inductive science, were based.

In this state, pathology, like all the inductive sciences at their origin, was merely natural history; it registered the phenomena of disease, classified them, and ventured upon a prognosis wherever the observation of constant co-existences and sequences suggested a rational expectation of the like recurrence under similar circumstances.

Further than this it hardly went. In fact, in the then state of knowledge, and in the condition of philosophical speculation at that time, neither the causes of the morbid state nor the *rationale* of treatment were likely to be sought for as we seek for them now. The anger of a god was a sufficient reason for the existence of a malady, and a dream ample warranty for therapeutic measures; that a physical phenomenon must needs have a physical cause was not the implied or expressed axiom that it is to us moderns.

The great man whose name is inseparably connected with the foundation of medicine, Hippocrates, certainly knew very little—indeed, practically nothing—of anatomy or physiology; and he would probably have been perplexed, even to imagine the possibility of a connexion between the zoological studies of his contemporary, Democritus, and medicine. Nevertheless, in so far as he, and those who worked before and after him in the same spirit, ascertained, as matters of experience, that a wound or a luxation or a fever presented such and such symptoms, and that the return of the patient to health was facilitated by such and such measures, they established laws of nature, and began the construction of the science of pathology. All true science begins with empiricism—though all true science is such exactly in so far as it strives to pass out of the empirical stage into that of the deduction of empirical from more general truths. Thus, it is not wonderful that the early physicians had little or nothing to do with the development of biological science; and, on the other hand, that the early biologists did not much concern themselves with medicine. There is nothing to show that the Asclepiads took any prominent share in the work of founding anatomy, physiology, zoology, and botany. Rather do these seem to have sprung from the early philosophers, who were essentially natural philosophers, animated by the characteristically Greek thirst for knowledge as such. Pythagoras, Alcmæon, Democritus, Diogenes (of Apollonia), are all credited with anatomical and physiological investigation; and though Aristotle is said to have belonged to an Asclepiad family, and not improbably owed his taste for anatomical and zoological inquiries to the teachings of his father, the physician Nicomachus, the "Historia Animalium," and the treatise "De Partibus Animalium," are as free from any allusion to medicine as if they had issued from a modern biological laboratory.

It may be added, that it is not easy to see in what way it

could have benefited a physician of Alexander's time to know all that Aristotle knew on these subjects. His human anatomy was too rough to avail much in diagnosis, his physiology was too erroneous to supply data for pathological reasoning. But when the Alexandrian School, with Erasistratus and Herophilus at their head, turned to account the opportunities of studying human structure, afforded to them by the Ptolemies, the value of the large amount of accurate knowledge thus obtained to the surgeon for his operations, and to the physician for his diagnosis of internal disorders, became obvious, and a connexion was established between anatomy and medicine, which has ever become closer and closer. Since the revival of learning, surgery, medical diagnosis, and anatomy have gone hand in hand. Morgagni called his great work, " De Sedibus et Causis Morborum per Anatomen indagatis," and not only showed the way to search out the localities and the causes of disease by anatomy, but himself travelled wonderfully far upon the road. Bichat, discriminating the grosser constituents of the organs and parts of the body one from another, pointed out the direction which modern research must take; until, at length, histology, a science of yesterday, as it seems to many of us, has carried the work of Morgagni as far as the microscope can take us, and has extended the realm of pathological anatomy to the limits of the invisible world.

Thanks to the intimate alliance of morphology with medicine, the natural history of disease has, at the present day, attained a high degree of perfection. Accurate regional anatomy has rendered practicable the exploration of the most hidden parts of the organism, and the determination during life of morbid changes in them; anatomical and histological post-mortem investigations have supplied physicians with a clear basis upon which to rest the classification of disease, and with unerring tests of the accuracy or inaccuracy of their diagnoses.

If men could be satisfied with pure knowledge, the extreme precision with which, in these days, a sufferer may be told what is happening and what is likely to happen, even in the most recondite parts of his bodily frame, should be as satisfactory to the patient as it is to the scientific pathologist who gives him the information. But I am afraid it is not; and even the practising physician, while nowise understimating the regulative value of accurate diagnosis, must often lament that so much of his knowledge rather prevents him from doing wrong than helps him to do right.

A scorner of physic once said that nature and disease may be compared to two men fighting, the doctor to a blind man with a club, who strikes into the mêlée, sometimes hitting the disease, and sometimes hitting nature. The matter is not mended if you suppose the blind man's hearing to be so acute that he can register every stage of the struggle and pretty clearly predict how it will end. He had better not meddle at all until his eyes are opened, until he can see the exact position of the antagonists, and make sure of the effect of his blows. But that which it behoves the physician to see, not indeed with his bodily eye, but with clear intellectual vision, is a process, and the chain of causation involved in that process. Disease, as we have seen, is a perturbation of the normal activities of a living body; and it is, and must remain, unintelligible so long as we are ignorant of the nature of these normal activities. In other words, there could be no real science of pathology until the science of physiology had reached a degree of perfection unattained, and indeed unattainable, until quite recent times.

So far as medicine is concerned, I am not sure that physiology, such as it was down to the time of Harvey, might as well not have existed. Nay, it is perhaps no exaggeration to say that within the memory of living men, justly renowned practitioners of medicine and surgery knew less physiology than is now to be learned from the most elementary text-book; and, beyond a few broad facts, regarded what they did know as of extremely little practical importance. Nor am I disposed to blame them for this conclusion; physiology must be useless, or worse than useless, to pathology, so long as its fundamental conceptions are erroneous.

Harvey is often said to be the founder of modern physiology; and there can be no question that the elucidations of the functions of the heart, of the nature of the pulse, and of the course of the blood, put forth in the ever-memorable little essay " De Motu Cordis," directly worked a revolution in men's views of the nature and of the concatenation of some of the most important physiological processes among the higher animals; while, indirectly, their influence was perhaps even more remarkable.

But, though Harvey made this signal and perennially important contribution to the physiology of the moderns, his general conception of vital processes was essentially identical with that of the ancients; and, in the " Exercitationes de Generatione," and notably in the singular chapter " De Calido Innato," he shows himself a true son of Galen and of Aristotle.

For Harvey, the blood possesses powers superior to those of the elements; it is the seat of a soul which is not only vegetative, but also sensitive and motor. The blood maintains and fashions all parts of the body, " idque summâ cum providentia et intellectu, in finem certum agens, quasi ratiocinio quodam uteretur."

Here is the doctrine of the "pneuma," the product of the philosophical mould into which the animism of primitive men ran in Greece, in full force. Nor did its strength abate for long after Harvey's time. The same ingrained tendency of the human mind to suppose that a process is explained when it is ascribed to a power of which nothing is known except that it is the hypothetical agent of the process, gave rise in the next century to the animism of Stahl; and, later, to the doctrine of a vital principle, that "asylum ignorantiæ" of physiologists, which has so easily accounted for everything and explained nothing, down to our own times.

Now, the essence of modern, as contrasted with ancient, physiological science, appears to me to lie in its antagonism to animistic hypotheses and animistic phraseology. It offers physical explanations of vital phenomena, or frankly confesses that it has none to offer. And, so far as I know, the first person who gave expression to this modern view of physiology, who was bold enough to enunciate the proposition that vital phenomena, like all the other phenomena of the physical world, are, in ultimate analysis, resolvable into matter and motion, was René Descartes.

The fifty-four years of life of this most original and powerful thinker are widely overlapped on both sides by the eighty of Harvey, who survived his younger contemporary by seven years, and takes pleasure in acknowledging the French philosopher's appreciation of his great discovery.

In fact, Descartes accepted the doctrine of the circulation as propounded by " Hervæus, médecin d'Angleterre," and gave a full account of it in his first work—the famous " Discours de la Méthode"—which was published in 1637, only nine years after the exercitation "De Motu Cordis"; and, though differing from Harvey in some important points (in which, it may be noted in passing, Descartes was wrong and Harvey right), he always speaks of him with great respect. And so important does the subject seem to Descartes, that he returns to it in the "Traité des Passions," and in the "Traité de l'Homme."

It is easy to see that Harvey's work must have had a peculiar significance for the subtle thinker, to whom we owe both the spiritualistic and the materialistic philosophies of modern times. It was in the very year of its publication, 1628, that Descartes withdrew into that life of solitary investigation and meditation of which his philosophy was the fruit. And, as the course of his speculations led him to establish an absolute distinction of nature between the material and the mental worlds, he was logically compelled to seek for the explanation of the phenomena of the material world within itself; and having allotted the realm of thought to the soul, to see nothing but extension and motion in the rest of nature. Descartes uses "thought" as the equivalent of our modern term "consciousness." Thought is the function of the soul, and its only function. Our natural heat and all the movements of the body, says he, do not depend on the soul. Death does not take place from any fault of the soul, but only because some of the principal parts of the body become corrupted. The body of a living man differs from that of a dead man in the same way as a watch or other automaton (that is to say, a machine which moves of itself), when it is wound up and has in itself the physical principle of the movements which the mechanism is adapted to perform, differs from the same watch, or other machine, when it is broken and the physical principle of its movement no longer exists. All the actions which are common to us and the lower animals depend only on the conformation of our organs and the course which the animal spirits take in the brain, the nerves, and the muscles; in the same way as the movement of a watch is produced by nothing but the force of its spring and the figure of its wheels and other parts.

Descartes' treatise on Man is a sketch of human physiology in which a bold attempt is made to explain all the phenomena of life, except those of consciousness, by physical reasonings. To a mind turned in this direction, Harvey's exposition of the heart and vessels as a hydraulic mechanism must have been supremely welcome.

Descartes was not a mere philosophical theorist, but a hard-working dissector and experimenter, and he held the strongest opinion respecting the practical value of the new conception which he was introducing. He speaks of the importance of preserving health, and of the dependence of the mind on the body being so close that perhaps the only way of making men wiser and better than they are, is to be sought in medical science. "It is true," says he, "that as medicine is now practised, it contains little that is very useful; but, without any desire to depreciate, I am sure that there is no one, even among professional men, who will not declare that all we know is very little as compared with that which remains to be known; and that we might escape an infinity of diseases of the mind, no less than of the body, and even, perhaps, from the weakness of old age, if we had a sufficient knowledge of their causes, and of all the remedies with which nature has provided us.(a) So strongly impressed was Descartes with this, that he resolved to spend the rest of his life in trying to acquire such a knowledge of nature as would lead to the construction of a better medical doctrine.(b) The anti-Cartesians found material for cheap ridicule in these aspirations of the philosopher; and it is almost needless to say that, in the thirteen years which elapsed between the publication of the "Discours" and the death of Descartes, he did not contribute much to their realisation. But, for the next century, all progress in physiology took place along the lines which Descartes laid down.

The greatest physiological and pathological work of the seventeenth century—Borelli's treatise "De Motu Animalium"—is, to all intents and purposes, a development of Descartes' fundamental conception; and the same may be said of the physiology and pathology of Boerhaave, whose authority dominated in the medical world of the first half of the eighteenth century.

With the origin of modern chemistry, and of electrical science, in the latter half of the eighteenth century, aids in the analysis of the phenomena of life, of which Descartes could not have dreamed, were offered to the physiologist. And the greater part of the gigantic progress which has been made in the present century is a justification of the prevision of Descartes. For it consists, essentially, in a more and more complete resolution of the grosser organs of the living body into physico-chemical mechanisms.

" I shall try to explain our whole bodily machinery in such a way, that it will be no more necessary for us to suppose that the soul produces such movements as are not voluntary, than it is to think that there is in a clock a soul which causes it to show the hours."(c) These words of Descartes might be appropriately taken as a motto for any modern treatise on physiology.

But though, as I think, there is no doubt that Descartes was the first to propound the fundamental conception of the living body as a physical mechanism, which is the distinctive feature of modern, as contrasted with ancient physiology, he was misled by the natural temptation to carry out, in all its details, a parallel between the machines with which he was familiar, such as clocks and pieces of hydraulic apparatus, and the living machine. In all such machines there is a central source of power, and the parts of the machine are merely passive distributors of that power. The Cartesian school conceived of the living body as a machine of this kind; and herein they might have learned from Galen, who, whatever ill-use he may have made of the doctrine of "natural faculties," nevertheless had the great merit of perceiving that local forces play a great part in physiology.

The same truth was recognised by Glisson, but it was first prominently brought forward in the Hallerian doctrine of the "vis insita" of muscles. If muscle can contract without nerve, there is an end of the Cartesian mechanical explanation of its contraction by the influx of animal spirits.

(a) "Discours de la Méthode," 6e partie, ed. Cousin, page 193.
(b) Ibid., pages 198 and 211. (c) "De la Formation du Fœtus."

The discoveries of Trembley tended in the same direction. In the fresh water Hydra, no trace was to be found of that complicated machinery upon which the performance of the functions in the higher animals was supposed to depend. And yet the hydra moved, fed, grew, multiplied, and its fragments exhibited all the powers of the whole. And, finally, the work of Caspar F. Wolff,(d) by demonstrating the fact that the growth and development of both plants and animals take place antecedently to the existence of their grosser organs, and are, in fact, the causes and not the consequences of organisation (as then understood), sapped the foundations of the Cartesian physiology as a complete expression of vital phenomena.

For Wolff, the physical basis of life is a fluid, possessed of a "vis essentialis" and a "solidescibilitas," in virtue of which it gives rise to organisation; and, as he points out, this conclusion strikes at the root of the whole iatro-mechanical system.

In this country, the great authority of John Hunter exerted a similar influence; though it must be admitted that the too sibylline utterances which are the outcome of Hunter's struggles to define his conceptions are often susceptible of more than one interpretation. Nevertheless, on some points, Hunter is clear enough. For example, he is of opinion that "Spirit is only a property of matter" ("Introduction to Natural History," page 6), he is prepared to renounce animism (loc. cit., page 8), and his conception of life is so completely physical that he thinks of it as something which can exist in a state of combination in the food. "The aliment we take in has in it, in a fixed state, the real life; and this does not become active until it has got into the lungs; for there it is freed from its prison" (Observations on Physiology," page 113). He also thinks that, "It is more in accord with the general principles of the animal machine to suppose that none of its effects are produced from any mechanical principle whatever; and that every effect is produced from an action in the part—which action is produced by a stimulus upon the part which acts, or upon some other part with which this part sympathises so as to take up the whole action" (loc. cit., page 152).

And Hunter is as clear as Wolff, with whose work he was probably unacquainted, that "whatever life is, it most certainly does not depend upon structure or organisation" (loc. cit., page 114).

Of course it is impossible that Hunter could have intended to deny the existence of purely mechanical operations in the animal body. But while, with Borelli and Boerhaave, he looked upon absorption, nutrition, and secretion as operations effected by means of the small vessels, he differed from the mechanical physiologists, who regarded these operations as the result of the mechanical properties of the small vessels, such as the size, form, and disposition of their canals and apertures. Hunter, on the contrary, considers them to be the effect of properties of these vessels which are not mechanical, but vital. "The vessels," says he, "have more of the polypus in them than any other part of the body," and he talks of the "living and sensitive principles of the arteries," and even of the "dispositions or feelings of the arteries." "When the blood is good and genuine the sensations of the arteries, or the dispositions for sensation, are agreeable. . . . . It is then they dispose of the blood to the best advantage, increasing the growth of the whole, supplying any losses, keeping up a due succession, etc." (loc. cit., page 123).

If we follow Hunter's conceptions to their logical issue, the life of one of the higher animals is essentially the sum of the lives of all the vessels, each of which is a sort of physiological unit, answering to a polype; and, as health is the result of the normal "action of the vessels," so is disease an effect of their abnormal action. Hunter thus stands in thought, as in time, midway between Borelli on the one hand, and Bichat on the other.

The acute founder of general anatomy, in fact, outdoes Hunter in his desire to exclude physical reasonings from the realm of life. Except in the interpretation of the action of the sense organs, he will not allow physics to have anything to do with physiology.

"To apply the physical sciences to physiology is to explain the phenomena of living bodies by the laws of inert bodies. Now, this is a false principle, hence all its consequences are

(d) "Theoria Generationis," 1759.

marked with the same stamp. Let us leave to chemistry its affinity, to physics its elasticity and its gravity. Let us invoke for physiology only sensibility and contractility."(e)

Of all the unfortunate dicta of men of eminent ability, this seems one of the most unhappy, when we think of what the application of the methods and the data of physics and chemistry has done towards bringing physiology into its present state. It is not too much to say that one-half of a modern text-book of physiology consists of applied physics and chemistry; and that it is exactly in the exploration of the phenomena of sensibility and contractility that physics and chemistry have exerted the most potent influence.

Nevertheless, Bichat rendered a solid service to physiological progress by insisting upon the fact that what we call life, in one of the higher animals, is not an indivisible unitary archæus, dominating, from its central seat, the parts of the organism, but a compound result of the synthesis of the separate lives of those parts.

"All animals," says he, "are assemblages of different organs, each of which performs its function, and concurs, after its fashion, in the preservation of the whole. They are so many special machines in the general machine which constitutes the individual. But each of these special machines is itself compounded of many tissues of very different natures, which, in truth, constitute the elements of those organs" (loc. cit., lxxix.). "The conception of a proper vitality is applicable only to these simple tissues, and not to the organs themselves" (loc. cit., lxxxiv.).

And Bichat proceeds to make the obvious application of this doctrine of synthetic life, if I may so call it, to pathology. "Since diseases are only alterations of vital properties, and the properties of each tissue are distinct from those of the rest, it is evident that the diseases of each tissue must be different from those of the rest. Therefore, in any organ composed of different tissues, one may be diseased and the other remain healthy; and this is what happens in most cases" (loc. cit., lxxv.).

In a spirit of true prophecy, Bichat says, "we have arrived at an epoch in which pathological anatomy should start afresh." For as the analysis of the organs had led him to the tissues as the physiological units of the organism; so, in a succeeding generation, the analysis of the tissues led to the cell as the physiological element of the tissues. The contemporaneous study of development brought out the same result, and the zoologists and botanists, exploring the simplest and the lowest forms of animated beings, confirmed the great induction of the cell theory. Thus the apparently opposed views, which have been battling with one another ever since the middle of the last century, have proved to be each half a truth.

The proposition of Descartes, that the body of a living man is a machine, the actions of which are explicable by the known laws of matter and motion, is unquestionably largely true. But it is also true, that the living body is a synthesis of innumerable physiological elements, each of which may nearly be described in Wolff's words, as a fluid possessed of a " vis essentialis," and a " solidescibilitas "; or, in modern phrase, as protoplasm susceptible of structural metamorphosis and functional metabolism ; and that the only machinery, in the precise sence in which the Cartesian School understood mechanism, is that which co-ordinates and regulates these physiological units into an organic whole.

In fact, the body is a machine of the nature of an army, not of that of a watch, or of a hydraulic apparatus. Of this army, each cell is a soldier, an organ, a brigade, the central nervous system headquarters and field-telegraph. the alimentary and circulatory system the commissariat. Losses are made good by recruits born in camp, and the life of the individual is a campaign, conducted successfully for a number of years, but with certain defeat in the long run.

The efficacy of an army, at any given moment, depends on the health of the individual soldier, and on the perfection of the machinery by which he is led and brought into action at the proper time ; and therefore, if the analogy holds good, there can be only two kinds of diseases, the one dependent on abnormal states of the physiological units, the other on perturbation of the co-ordinating and alimentative machinery.

Hence, the establishment of the cell theory, in normal biology, was swiftly followed by a " cellular pathology," as its logical counterpart. I need not remind you how great an

(e) "Anatomie Générale," I., page liv.

instrument of investigation this doctrine has proved in the hands of the man of genius to whom its development is due, and who would probably be the last to forget that abnormal conditions of the co-ordinative and distributive machinery of the body are no less important factors of disease.

Henceforward, as it appears to me, the connexion of medicine with the biological sciences is clearly defined. Pure pathology is that branch of biology which defines the particular perturbation of cell life, or of the co-ordinating machinery, or of both, on which the phenomena of disease depend.

Those who are conversant with the present state of biology will hardly hesitate to admit that the conception of the life of one of the higher animals as the summation of the lives of a cell aggregate brought into harmonious action by a co-ordinative machinery formed by some of these cells, constitutes a permanent acquisition of physiological science. But the last form of the battle between the animistic and the physical views of life is seen in the contention whether the physical analysis of vital phenomena can be carried beyond this point or not.

There are some to whom living protoplasm is a substance, even such as Harvey conceived the blood to be, " summá cum providentia et intellectu in finem certum agens, quasi ratiocinio quodam ;" and who look, with as little favour as Bichat did, upon any attempt to apply the principles and the methods of physics and chemistry to the investigation of the vital processes of growth, metabolism, and contractility. They stand upon the ancient ways ; only, in accordance with that progress towards democracy which a great political writer has declared to be the fatal characteristic of modern times, they substitute a republic formed by a few billions of " animals " for the monarchy of the all-pervading " anima."

Others, on the contrary, supported by a robust faith in the universal applicability of the principles laid down by Descartes, and seeing that the actions called " vital " are, so far as we have any means of knowing, nothing but changes of place of particles of matter, look to molecular physics to achieve the analysis of the living protoplasm itself into a molecular mechanism. If there is any truth in the received doctrines of physics, that contrast between living and inert matter, on which Bichat lays so much stress, does not exist. In nature, nothing is at rest, nothing is amorphous ; the simplest particle of that which men in their blindness are pleased to call " brute matter " is a vast aggregate of molecular mechanisms, performing complicated movements of immense rapidity, and sensitively adjusting themselves to every change in the surrounding world. Living matter differs from other matter in degree and not in kind ; the microcosm repeats the macrocosm ; and one chain of causation connects the nebulous original of suns and planetary systems with the protoplasmic foundation of life and organisation.

From this point of view, pathology is the analogue of the theory of perturbations in astronomy ; and therapeutics resolves itself into the discovery of the means by which a system of forces competent to eliminate any given perturbation may be introduced into the economy. And, as pathology bases itself upon normal physiology, so therapeutics rests upon pharmacology, which is, strictly speaking, a part of the great biological topic of the influence of conditions on the living organism, and has no scientific foundation apart from physiology.

It appears to me that there is no more hopeful indication of the progress of medicine towards the ideal of Descartes than is to be derived from a comparison of the state of pharmacology, at the present day, with that which existed forty years ago. If we consider the knowledge positively acquired, in this short time, of the modus operandi of urari, of atropia, of physostigmin, of veratria, of casca, of strychnia, of bromide of potassium, of phosphorus, there can surely be no ground for doubting that, sooner or later, the pharmacologist will suppl the physician with the means of affecting, in any desired sense, the functions of any physiological element of the body. It will, in short, become possible to introduce into the economy a molecular mechanism, which, like a very cunningly contrived torpedo, shall find its way to some particular group of living elements, and cause an explosion among them, leaving the rest untouched.

The search for the explanation of diseased states in

modified cell life; the discovery of the important part played by parasitic organisms in the ætiology of disease; the elucidation of the action of medicaments by the methods and the data of experimental physiology;—appear to me to be the greatest steps which have ever been made towards the establishment of medicine on a scientific basis. I need hardly say they could not have been made except for the advance of normal biology.

There can be no question, then, as to the nature or the value of the connexion between medicine and the biological sciences. There can be no doubt that the future of pathology and therapeutics, and therefore that of practical medicine, depend upon the extent to which those who occupy themselves with these subjects are trained in the methods and impregnated with the fundamental truths of biology.

And, in conclusion, I venture to suggest that the collective sagacity of this Congress could occupy itself with no more important question than with this. How is medical education to be arranged, so that, without entangling the student in those details of the systematist which are valueless to him, he may be enabled to obtain a firm grasp of the great truths respecting animal and vegetable life, without which, notwithstanding all the progress of scientific medicine, he will still find himself an empiric?

SECTIONAL ADDRESSES.

Section of Anatomy.

INAUGURAL ADDRESS BY PROF. W. H. FLOWER, LL.D., F.R.S., F.R.C.S., etc.,
President of the Section.

"The Museum of the Royal College of Surgeons of England."

While thinking over various subjects for an address with which to open the business of the Section over which I have the honour to preside, it has occurred to me that the time which has been allotted by the arrangements of the Congress for the purpose may be made most useful to my hearers, if, instead of entering upon a discussion of any abstract question, I were to ask your attention to a subject upon which I may possibly be able to give a little information of practical use to members of the Congress during their visit to this city.

No class of persons can appreciate so fully the importance and value of museums as those whose occupation it is to study the form and relations of the various parts of the body, whether of plants, animals, or man.

Our science would make little progress if the objects of our inquiries, once used for examination or description, were then thrown aside, and those coming after were denied the opportunity of which we have availed ourselves. A museum is a register, in a permanent form, of facts suitable for examination, verification, and comparison one with another.

Hence, ever since serious attention has been awakened to the interest of anatomical study, museums have always been important adjuncts to their successful prosecution, and the preservation of the various structures of the body has occupied the attention of very many anatomists, since the time of the great Italian teachers of the early part of the seventeenth century, with whom apparently the art commenced.

We have in London, as you are all aware, a museum which stands, in some respects, in a peculiar position, differing perhaps from any in the world in its origin, its scope, its method of maintenance, and its relation to the profession and to the State, in which for very nearly twenty years, it has been my privilege to pass my days. It has occurred to me that a few words in explanation of the history, arrangement, and contents of that Museum, might add to the interest and profit of those visits which I trust everyone here will find time to pay to it during the meeting of the Congress.

The great mind of John Hunter, far in advance of his age —and, it may be, even of ours—saw at one glance the vast importance of biological science, and the best means to further its pursuit. To this end he founded his Museum,

and directed by his will that it should always be maintained in its integrity. Wherever civilised men are gathered together, there are now minds who feel what Hunter felt. The necessities of such minds have created in every country in Europe, and the enlightened parts of the New World, museums designed to serve in their different degrees the same functions as our Hunterian Collection. Such museums are evidently national needs; they have already come, though not by any means to the extent they will in future come, to be looked upon as an essential portion of the educational machinery of the State. Such museums are, in almost every capital of Europe, supported directly at the expense of the State, or are connected with some great educational institution dependent upon Government for aid. In England alone the need has been supplied, first, by a private individual, and, secondly, by a private or semi-private institution, composed of members of a single profession, with only occasional assistance from the State. In this country the State (and therefore every individual composing it) is indebted to John Hunter and the Royal College of Surgeons for relieving it of the burden which must otherwise have fallen upon it, of providing that portion of the national education afforded by a biological museum.

The period occupied by John Hunter in the formation of his collection was all comprised between thirty years—1763, the date of his return from service with the Army in Portugal, and 1793, that of his death. The labour which he accomplished during this time was something prodigious, as has often been recounted in various biographies and Hunterian "Orations." Notwithstanding all that has been written and said, it is impossible to do justice to his wonderful activity and industry. In nothing, however, were these qualities so conspicuous as in the formation of his Museum.

Public museums at that time scarcely existed. The British Museum was little more than a library and gallery of art; the small cabinet of natural history, reinforced by the old collection of the Royal Society, scarcely made any show. Anatomical specimens, even bones and teeth, were looked upon with disfavour. Some that had accidentally found their way into the collection were, even within the present century, treated as intruders, and turned out without much ceremony.

Teachers of anatomy were forming their own private collections, but these were all eclipsed by those of the two Hunters, William and John. That of the latter especially grew to such an extent as to become in some sort a national and public institution. He built a large room to contain it in Castle-street, at the back of his house in Leicester-square, and when finally arranged there, so much interest was taken in it that he found it necessary to open it to public inspection at certain stated times. Still it was maintained entirely at his own cost, and it is stated that by the time of his death he had spent upwards of £70,000 upon it. Whether this estimate be correct or not, his expenditure on it must have been very great, as, though he had for many years made one of the largest professional incomes in London, his museum was the sole property he left behind.

John Hunter was a very miscellaneous collector—minerals, coins, pictures, ancient coats of mail, weapons of various dates and nations, and other so-called "articles of virtu" engaged his attention. These, however, and his furniture and books, had to be sold to meet the most pressing needs of the family. What would be now called the "biological" part of his collection was kept intact during the six years which elapsed between his death and its purchase by the English Government in 1799. The preservation of the collection during this period is mainly due to the devotion of William Clift, Hunter's last assistant, whose services were retained for this purpose at a very small salary by the executors, Sir Everard Home and Dr. Matthew Baillie, and whose fidelity was rewarded by his being appointed the first "Conservator" of the collection after it came into the possession of the College of Surgeons.

The story of the negotiations with a Government whose interests and energies were then concentrated upon the great Continental war, and the answer of the Prime Minister, Pitt, when applied to on the subject—"What! buy preparations! Why, I have not money enough for gunpowder!"—are well known. These difficulties were, however, overcome, and, on the recommendation of a Committee of the House of Commons appointed to inquire into the subject, the sum agreed to by the executors, viz., £15,000, was voted for its purchase on June 13, 1799. Then came the question what was to be done with it. There was at that time no department of Government under the care of which such a collection could be placed. The condition of the British Museum has already been alluded to. The now flourishing and all-absorbing "Department of Science and Art" had not been invented. There was one body in London which might be supposed to have some special interest in the maintenance of such a collection—the venerable and dignified College of Physicians—but that body, it is commonly reported, demurred to accept it, on the ground of want of funds to meet the annual expense of its maintenance. With reference to this report, Dr. Pitman has been kind enough, in response to my inquiries, to examine the archives of the College, and finds that there is no record of any such offer having been made or refused. If any negotiations were entered into, they must, therefore, have been of a purely informal nature.

There was still another corporate body—a comparatively obscure one at that time—the Corporation of Surgeons, which had only separated itself some fifty-four years before from the old City Company of Barbers and Surgeons,(a) and although it had thrown off the connexion which restrained its members from assuming the position of cultivators of a liberal profession, it had as yet done little to raise itself in public estimation, and had few resources from which to provide for the expenses of such a collection. Nevertheless, the Court of the Corporation determined by an unanimous vote on December 23, 1799, to accept the Museum on the terms proposed by the Government, and almost simultaneously obtained a new charter, under which they became "The Royal College of Surgeons," a body accredited by Government to examine all persons wishing to practise surgery in the kingdom, and migrated from their old quarters in the City to the house in Lincoln's-inn-fields, round which the present establishment has grown up.

Thus, John Hunter's Museum, and the College of Surgeons of England, though of entirely independent origin, have had their fortunes inextricably intermixed, since the former became national property, and the latter took the title and position it now holds.

The College is still the principal examining body for those who practise surgery throughout the kingdom. It takes no part directly in professional education, though it exercises a considerable indirect influence by the manner of conducting its examinations, and by the curriculum it requires from candidates. Its revenues are mainly derived from the fees paid for the diplomas which it grants, which, for the last ten years, have averaged 383 a year. In former times these fees considerably exceeded the expenses of the comparatively slight examination required from candidates, and the surplus, besides defraying the current expenses of the Museum and Library, was devoted to the erection of the present buildings, and the acquisition of the freehold property and invested capital of the College. It says much for the personal disinterestedness of the eminent members of the surgical profession who have constituted the Court of Examiners, and who, until very lately, were practically the ruling body of the College, that they fixed their own remuneration at so low a rate as to permit an expenditure during the present century, upon the purposes just indicated, of a sum which cannot be estimated at less than £400,000. Now, owing to the more searching and practical character of the examinations, the expenses of conducting them have augmented to such an extent as to be scarcely more than covered by the payments of the candidates; and, but for the proceeds of the investments made under different circumstances, the College would not have the means of carrying on the scientific work it has undertaken.

The various professorships and lectureships that are attached to the College have grown up chiefly in conse-

(a) By an Act of Parliament, passed in the 18th year of the reign of George II., instituted, "An Act for making the Surgeons of London, and the Barbers of London, two separate and distinct Corporations," it was enacted that the union and incorporation of the Barbers and Surgeons of London, made by the Act of the 32nd year of King Henry VIII., should from and after the 24th day of June, 1745, be dissolved, and that each of the members of the said united Company who were freemen of the said Company, and admitted and approved surgeons within the rules of the said Company and their successors, should from thenceforth be made a separate and distinct Body Corporate and Commonalty Perpetual, which at all times thereafter were to be called by the name of "The Master, Governors, and Commonalty of the Art and Science of Surgeons of London." The first Charter of the Company dates from the first year of the reign of King Edward IV. (A.D. 1461).

quence of one of the conditions under which the Hunterian Collection was entrusted to it by Government—that a course of no less than twenty-four lectures shall be delivered annually, by some member of the College, upon comparative anatomy and other subjects, illustrated by the preparations. Other lectureships have been founded by private benefactions, but these are of limited number, or on special subjects, and are intended, not so much for the education of students, but rather as the means of introducing new discoveries or ideas to members of the profession and others interested in scientific pursuits, to all of whom they are freely open without payment.

Besides the Museum, the College has added to its means of benefiting its own members and the profession generally, a library containing every important work and periodical upon surgery, medicine, anatomy, and the collateral sciences.

During the first six years after the collection came into the possession of the College, it remained in the gallery in Castle-street, which had been built by Hunter for its reception; but in 1806, the lease of the premises having expired, it was removed temporarily to a house in Lincoln's-inn-fields, adjoining the College of Surgeons, while the building in which it was destined to be lodged was preparing for its reception. This building, towards the erection of which Parliament contributed the sum of £27,500, was completed and first opened to visitors in 1813.

The Museum was greatly enlarged entirely at the expense of the College in 1835, and a still more important addition, that of the great eastern hall, was completed in 1855. Towards the expense of this, Parliament contributed a further grant of £15,000, the whole of the rest of the expenses of the purchase of the site, the building, and the annual maintenance of the Museum, having been borne by the College.

In accepting the Hunterian Collection, the College of Surgeons undertook a heavy responsibility, weightier perhaps than was contemplated at the time. Although not required by the letter of the contract to do more than preserve Hunter's specimens, the College undertook the charge in the spirit of the founder, and thus made itself responsible for maintaining such a collection as should meet the requirements of the ever-expanding and vigorous young science to which it ministers. Hunter's Collection was held to be the nucleus of a national biological museum, and its preservation and augmentation by the College has certainly prevented the formation of such a collection by the State.

Hunter was no specialist, and even after eliminating the non-biological subjects before alluded to, a very miscellaneous collection remained; illustrations of life in all its aspects, in health and disease; specimens of botany, zoology, palæontology, anatomy, physiology, and every branch of pathology; preparations made according to all the methods then known; stuffed birds, mammals and reptiles, fossils, dried shells, corals, insects, and plants; bones and articulated skeletons; injected, dried, and varnished vascular preparations; dried preparations of hollow viscera; mercurial injections, dried and in spirit; vermilion injections; dissected preparations in spirit of both vegetable and animal structures, natural and morbid; undissected animals in spirit, showing external form, or awaiting leisure for examination; calculi and various animal concretions; even a collection of microscopic objects, prepared by one of the earliest English histologists, W. Hewson.

It is very difficult to compare the present Hunterian Museum, as it is still often called, although officially only recognised as the Museum of the Royal College of Surgeons of England, with any other existing collection, as its nature and the character of its contents have been determined by several accidental circumstances rather than by any very settled purpose. Originally a private collection, embracing a large variety of objects, it has been carried on and increased upon much the same plan as that designed by the founder, with modifications only to suit some of the requirements of advancing knowledge. The only portions of Hunter's biological collection which has been actually parted with, are the stuffed birds and beasts, which, with the sanction of the trustees, appointed by Government to see that the College performs its part of the contract as custodians of the collection, were transferred to the British Museum, and a considerable number of dried vascular preparations, which, having become useless in consequence of the deterioration in their condition, resulting from age and decay, have been replaced by others preserved by better methods. Of the various departments of which the Museum now consists, very few, in fact only the collection of illustrations of skin diseases, and the collection of surgical instruments, are not the direct continuation of series founded by John Hunter.

To find an analogous institution to the Museum of the College of Surgeons, in Paris, for instance, we should have to combine the collections of Comparative Anatomy and Anthropology at the Jardin des Plantes, and even a portion of the separate palæontological collection at that establishment, the collection of human anatomy of the Musée Orfila, and that of pathological anatomy of the Musée Dupuytren. If these were all brought together under one roof, and somewhat compressed and rearranged, we should have something in its nature resembling the Museum of which I am now speaking.

In this combination on one spot, and under one management, of so many diverse collections, we have a survival of a condition of scientific knowledge more characteristic certainly of the last century than of the one in which we live; but in this age of specialities, it is well perhaps to be reminded by such an institution of the essential unity of biological knowledge, and of the important illustrations which one branch of it may afford to another, especially when the detailed facts are to be combined for the purpose of philosophical generalisation.

In visiting the Museum, and in the comparison which may be instituted between it and others of its kind, it is important to recollect this origin and history, as they will account for many shortcomings. It must not be forgotten that to its comparative antiquity (for it is certainly the predecessor and prototype of all the anatomical museums of this country and of America, and to most of those on the Continent) is due many faults of construction and arrangement which should not be found in a building designed with the knowledge and experience of recent years. I have elsewhere pointed out what I consider the chief of these.(b)

Though the large size of the principal rooms allows of a fine coup d'œil, such a construction does not permit of that separation and distribution of the different series which is desirable for the purposes of study. Human anatomy, invertebrate zoology, and pathology, for instance, come into such near juxtaposition as to produce some confusion in the minds of strangers, though familiarity with the arrangement soon disperses the difficulties at first met with in finding the situation and limits of the particular department required. The narrowness and unprotected condition of the shelves in the galleries is also a radical defect now unfortunately irremediable. Furthermore, the indulgence of those who have the happiness to live elsewhere than in the absolute centre of a population of four millions of coal-burning people, must be asked for certain dusky results of such a situation, which no amount of care and expense can obviate.

I must now ask leave to be your guide to some of the contents of the Museum, as it is at present arranged, and will take the different branches of biology which are illustrated in it in some kind of order, beginning with the part which relates to life in a normal condition. Hunter's collections and observations were not limited to the animal kingdom. Wherever any physiological process could be illustrated by vegetable life, vegetables were pressed into the service, as may be seen in the physiological gallery, and by the Memoranda on Vegetation, left by him in MS., and printed by the College in 1860. In his collection were many portions of various recent plants, and a series, amounting to 184 in number, of fossil-woods, fruits, and impressions of stems and leaves. These specimens, with some additions made in former years (for since the great development of the parts of the Museum more essential to the general purposes of the institution, it has been necessary to restrict the growth of such branches as are more fully and advantageously illustrated elsewhere), are arranged in the large wall-case on the right-hand side (on going in) of the entrance door of the first or western hall.

The zoology of invertebrate animals largely attracted Hunter's attention. Many of the treasures collected in the famous voyages of Captain Cook came into his possession through his friend, Sir Joseph Banks. He purchased, when-

(b) Journal of Anatomy and Physiology, vol. ix., May, 1875.

ever opportunity offered, as at the sale of Mr. Ellis's famous collection of corals and zoophytes. In 1786, at the sale of the Duchess of Portland's museum, he bought, for fifteen guineas, the fine "Pentacrinus" now in the Museum, of which very few examples had then been found. Of insects, especially Lepidoptera, he had a large series. Of fossil invertebrates, as many as 2092 specimens are now recorded in the catalogue as Hunterian. The series of fossil cephalopods is remarkably rich.

Such invertebrated animals as are dissected, or illustrate any special anatomical fact, are arranged in the so-called physiological series in the gallery, to be described presently, but beyond these there remained a vast number of specimens only showing external form, which by selection and arrangement have been lately formed into a special zoological collection, intended to introduce the student to a general knowledge of the principal forms of animal life, and to the mode in which they are grouped. This series, arranged in the floor cases on the left side of the western Museum, includes selected specimens of nearly all the orders, and in many cases of the families, both of the living and extinct forms; illustrated both by their hard and imperishable parts, as the "corals" or stony skeletons of the Actinozoa, the shells of Mollusca, and the tegumentary structures of the Articulata, and by the softer and more destructible parts of the bodies preserved in spirit. The various groups are distinctly separated from each other and clearly named. Students who desire to pursue the study of any of the sections more deeply than the small selected series of exhibited specimens will allow, will find the remainder of the specimens mentioned in the catalogues arranged in drawers below the cases. The series does not extend beyond the Invertebrata, as the peculiarities of the remaining classes of the animal kingdom are abundantly illustrated in other parts of the Museum.

Although locally far removed, occupying one portion of the upper gallery of the middle Museum, a small but interesting special collection, illustrating the subject of helminthology, may be mentioned here. It was thought that the importance in a medical and social point of view of those animals which infest the interior of man and the principal domestic and other animals, justified a more extended exhibition of their modifications than could be assigned to any other group of animals of such inferior organisation, and by the aid of the well-known helminthologist, Dr. Spencer Cobbold, the present collection was arranged and catalogued in 1866; the materials being mostly already in the collection, though scattered in other series or hidden in the store-rooms. The collection contains upwards of two hundred specimens, and may still be somewhat extended. The intention is to show every parasitic animal which, under any circumstances, can affect the human body, and a selection of the principal types of those that inhabit the lower animals, especially such species as are associated with man. If increased beyond these limits, the collection would become interesting only to the student of detailed systematic zoology, and therefore not a legitimate object for our Museum.

I will pass next to the section of the Museum which is, perhaps, altogether the most characteristic, and is certainly the most eminently Hunterian. It was specially the creation of his mind, is still arranged almost exactly as he left it, and, notwithstanding the very numerous additions, still contains a larger proportion of Hunterian specimens than any other department. This is the collection which is called Physiological, because the specimens in it are classified mainly according to their supposed function. Physiology, as we know it now, is scarcely a subject which can be illustrated in a museum. The processes and actions which take place in the living body are not to be shown in bottles, but the organs through the medium of which physiological processes are performed, can be, and it is these which are illustrated in this collection. It is more truly a collection of comparative anatomy, or morphology as we should now call it. It shows the variations in form which the different organs undergo either in different species, or in the same species under different conditions, as age and sex or season. Many of these modifications clearly have relation to function, as we see in the difference of form and relative size of the compartments of the stomach of the young ruminant, which is nourished by milk, and the adult which feeds on grass, the periodic variations in the size of the testis in birds, etc. But in a vast number more we can see no special adaptation to purpose, but merely variation, apparently for variety's sake. Look, for instance, at all the differences of the form of the liver throughout the mammalian series, which, as far as we know, have no relation to its action as a secreting gland. Though of little interest to the physiologist, modifications of this kind are of the highest importance to the morphologist. They throw light upon one of the great biological problems, classification, which, when rightly interpreted, means nothing more or less than a statement of the order in which living beings have been evolved one from another. From such variations of form most precious indications of the relationship of one animal to another can be obtained, and the less these variations are related to adaptation to some particular function, the better they can be relied on for this purpose. But Hunter's ideas were far different. He tried to bring together analogous parts according to their uses—organs of progressive motion adapted for flying—eyes modified for seeing in water—eyes modified for seeing in air, and so forth. Practically, such a system could not be logically carried out. Too many modifications of form were found to occur, to which no special modification of function could be assigned; a compromise had to be made, and in the large number of cases the organs had to be arranged according to the affinities of the animals to which they belonged—brains of fishes, brains of birds, brains of mammals, etc. As the collection continues to advance, the classification according to homology is gradually superseding that according to analogy, with which it began.

This collection at present contains 6982 specimens mounted in bottles, of which 3745, or more than one-half, are Hunterian. It may be convenient to know that these are distinguished by the figures upon them which refer to the catalogue being painted in black. The specimens added since Hunter's time are lettered in red. The greater number of the former must be fully a century old, and being still in as perfect preservation as when first put up, afford a fair guarantee of the absolute permanence, with proper care, of specimens preserved in alcohol. The skill displayed in dissecting, injecting, and mounting the majority of these preparations, has scarcely ever been surpassed in modern times; and this collection alone, if it were all that Hunter had left, would be a grand monument to his industry and zeal for anatomical knowledge—as is its valuable and instructive descriptive catalogue, published in five volumes, and completed in the year 1840, a lasting evidence of the same qualities on the part of Mr. Clift's eminent successor in the conservatorship of the Museum, Professor Owen.

Many points in comparative anatomy can be illustrated quite as efficiently, and more economically, by dried preparations, which require neither spirit nor bottles to preserve them in. Though we have not attained in this country the art of making such preparations in the elegant and instructive manner pursued in several of the museums in Italy, notably Pisa, and though nearly all the original Hunterian dried preparations have perished long ago, or become partially useless, there will still be found some worthy of attention in the rail cases round the galleries which contain the spirit preparations. While speaking of the contents of these cases I would specially call attention to the series showing the modifications of the small bones of the ear throughout the mammalian class, arranged a few years ago by Mr. Alban Doran, one of the assistants in the Museum, which is probably not surpassed in extent or variety and method of arrangement anywhere else.

The histological collection is contained in a separate small room adjoining the physiological galleries, and consists of upwards of 12,000 specimens, illustrating the minute structure of the tissues of plants and animals, mostly prepared under the direction of Professor Quekett, the third Conservator of the Museum, who devoted the greater part of his life to this work. Since his death in 1861, it has been re-arranged and kept in order; but the additions have not been numerous, chiefly in consequence of the practical difficulties in exhibiting such a collection to visitors to a public museum.

Although the anatomy of man naturally takes its place among that of other species in the physiological series, the preparations illustrating it are chiefly confined to viscera—the details of regional anatomy, and of the arrangement and distribution of muscles, vessels, and nerves, not finding a natural place in the scheme upon which that department of

the Museum was organised. It was, however, a few years ago, thought desirable that human anatomy, in consideration of its great importance to our profession, should be exhibited on a much more extended scale than it had been hitherto, and that a ready demonstration should be afforded by means of permanent preparations of the structure of all parts of the human frame. To those who have already learnt their anatomy, and who wish to refresh their memory, or verify a fact about which some passing doubt may be felt, or those who are precluded by circumstances from visiting the dissecting-room, the preparations of this series must prove of great value. The series of dissections already made with this end, commenced by a former able assistant in the Museum, Dr. J. Bell Pettigrew, and carried on to their present perfection by Mr. W. Pearson, are arranged on shelves over the floor cases on the western side of the western Museum, contiguous to the series of human osteology, to which they form the natural sequel.

No portions of the structure of vertebrate animals can be preserved with greater facility than the bones and teeth. Moreover, the skeleton being the framework around which the rest of the body is built up, gives, more than any other system, an outline of the general organisation of the whole animal, and it has this special importance, that a large number of species—all those, in fact, which are not at present existing upon the earth—can be known to us by little beyond the form of the bones. Osteology has, therefore, always had many votaries as a special branch of study, and it is one which finds much favour in the eyes of curators of museums, from the satisfactory manner in which it can be illustrated by specimens. Hunter's osteological collection was considerable—quite in advance of any other in this country. The two small whales (*Balænoptera rostrata* and *Hyperoodon rostratus*) which formed part of it were almost the only skeletons of animals of their order which existed in any museum at the time of his death. This fact alone shows the marvellous change that has taken place within less than a century in the facilities for the study of comparative anatomy. How great the contrast to what may now be seen here in the College of Surgeons, in the British Museum, in Oxford, Cambridge, Edinburgh, Dublin, in a score or more of museums on the European continent, in America, even in Australia and New Zealand! Richly supplied osteological collections have sprung up in every considerable centre of scientific culture all over the world; but as ours was one of the first in point of time, we may also claim for it a high position in point of completeness. Others, such as that at the British Museum, the Jardin des Plantes at Paris, and the famous Leiden Collection, may be larger, but this is because the College Museum has been designedly limited rather to selected illustrations of all the most important modifications of structure, than to numerous examples of closely allied species, which may be perfectly necessary in a purely zoological museum. When important forms have become extinct, their characters are shown by their fossilised remains, which, though at present most illogically arranged in a distinct room apart from their existing allies, will soon be incorporated in the general osteological series, where alone they can find a reasonable position in an anatomical museum.

The value of a collection is not to be estimated only by the number of specimens it contains, nor by even their rarity or judicious selection, but also by the condition of the specimens, and the facility by which they may be made available for study and reference. On this head we claim to be somewhat in advance of other museums, on account of the improvements which have been made in late years in preparing and articulating entire skeletons, and displaying portions of the bony framework in an instructive manner. Formerly all the bones were rigidly fixed together, so that their articular surfaces, if not actually destroyed, were completely concealed; and no bone could possibly be removed and separately examined. The aim of a series of changes in the method of mounting skeletons introduced here, and now adopted more or less completely in many other museums (the details of which were carried out with great skill by our late able articulator, Mr. James Flower), has been to obviate all these difficulties and to make each bone, as far as possible, independent of all the rest, while preserving the general aspect and form of the entire skeleton.

Another improvement in the osteological series introduced

within the last twenty years has been the formation of a special collection designed to show the principal modifications of each individual element of the skeleton throughout the vertebrate classes, by placing the homologous bones of a number of different animals in juxtaposition. For convenience of comparison, the specimens of this series are all placed in corresponding positions, mounted on separate stands, and to each is attached a label bearing the name of the bone, and the animal to which it belongs. This series is especially instructive to the students of elementary osteology, and forms an introduction to the general series.

As in other departments of the Museum, the more nearly man is approached in structure, the more complete do the illustrations of anatomical modification become, and, as might be expected, the osteology of man is far more thoroughly shown than that of any other species. The specimens of human osteology (of which a revised catalogue, enumerating 1306 specimens, was published two years ago) begin by illustrations of the development of the bones; these are followed by the normal skeleton, exhibited under various aspects, then by individual variations, among which may be mentioned one of the most remarkable objects in the museum, the skeleton of the celebrated Irish giant, O'Brian, who died in London in 1783, and about the preservation of whose remains so many legends are told in the biographies of John Hunter. Finally, the special osteology of man or illustrations of the osteological characters of the various races of mankind. In this important subject Hunter was a long way in advance of most of his contemporaries, as the origin of his collection dates almost, if not quite, as far back as that of the founder of physical anthropology, the celebrated Blumenbach. The series has been greatly augmented of late years, and completely rearranged; and the splendid addition made to it last year by the purchase of the great private collection of the late Dr. Barnard Davis has brought it up in point of completeness to truly national importance.

As forming a transition from the department of normal anatomy and physiology to that of pathology, may next be mentioned the teratological series, or collection of congenital malformations of man and the lower animals, which necessarily forms part of every general biological museum. This difficult, mysterious, and, as far as the light it throws upon the workings of the laws of nature, still unsatisfactory subject, had considerable attraction for Hunter, and many of the specimens in the series form part of his Museum. It has been steadily, though not very rapidly, increasing ever since, and had the advantage, a few years ago, of being thoroughly revised, rearranged, and catalogued by Mr. B. T. Lowne. It is arranged in the upper gallery of the middle Museum.

The pathological series is the section of the Museum to the study of which, in the eyes of Hunter and his successors, all the others form an introduction. It occupies the whole of the two galleries and part of the ground floor of the western hall. As the Museum of the College differs from those attached to the various medical schools, in having no hospital or post-mortem room in connexion with it, from which to draw the supplies for completing this collection, it has been increased by the acquisition from time to time, when opportunity afforded, of various private collections, as those of Mr. Heaviside in 1829, Mr. Langstaff in 1835, Mr. Howship and Mr. Taunton in 1841, Mr. Liston in 1842, and Sir Astley Cooper in 1843—obtained by purchase; and the collections of Sir William Blizard in 1811, Sir Stephen Love Hamminck in 1851, and Dr. Peacock in 1876—presented to the College. Contributions of recent specimens are also constantly received from numerous individual donors, the acquisitions from this source having greatly increased of late years. The total number of specimens now in the catalogue amounts to 5148, of which 1672 are Hunterian. As in the physiological galleries, the latter are distinguished by their numbers being painted in black. The descriptive catalogue of this series, written by Sir James Paget, and published in five quarto volumes between the years 1846 and 1849, is one of the best-known and most valuable of all the publications of the College, and has always been looked upon as a model upon which other pathological catalogues should be formed. The additions made to the collection since that time have been so numerous that the necessity of a new catalogue has long been felt. Under these circumstances, it is a matter of great congratulation to all who are interested in the welfare of this valuable

collection, that the author of the original catalogue has undertaken, with the co-operation of Dr. Goodhart and Mr. Doran, to make a new one, in which the old descriptions will be revised, the new specimens incorporated in their appropriate places, and such changes introduced into the general arrangement as the advance of pathological knowledge and greater experience of the requirements of the Museum appear to necessitate. This great work, especially arduous for one so much engaged in professional avocations as Sir James Paget, is now far advanced. The prospect of its early completion will doubtless compensate the members of the Congress who will make an inspection of this part of the collection, for the transitional and somewhat disarranged condition in which they will find it on their present visit.

As adjuncts to the general pathological series are certain special collections, which have separate catalogues devoted to them. One, which will be examined with interest by those devoting themselves to aural pathology, is the series of preparations illustrative of diseases of the ear, formed by the late Mr. Joseph Toynbee, which came into possession of the College at his death in 1866. It is a large and probably unique collection of 824 specimens, illustrating all the known morbid conditions of the organ of hearing, such as could only have been brought together by one specially engaged for a considerable number of years in investigating this branch of surgery, and the value of which is greatly enhanced by a complete descriptive catalogue, published during Mr. Toynbee's lifetime. This series is arranged in part of the rail cases of the lower pathological gallery in the western Museum. The remainder of the same cases are devoted to the collection of urinary calculi and other concretions, salivary, biliary, and intestinal, both from man and various animals—probably the most complete and best arranged in the world. The careful chemical analysis and description of the whole of these specimens has been the work of Mr. Thomas Taylor.

In a corresponding position in the upper gallery of the same Museum is the dermatological collection, consisting of an extensive series of beautifully executed models, of actual specimens, casts, and drawings, illustrating the various affections of the skin. This collection was commenced in the year 1870, the whole of the specimens in it, the cases which contain them, and the catalogue describing them, having been presented to the College by Mr. Erasmus Wilson, at that time Professor of Dermatology in the College.

Lastly, must be mentioned a collection—for the reception of which a separate room, approached from the end of the eastern Museum, was devoted in 1870—of surgical instruments and appliances, which, though small at present, contains many instruments curious for their antiquity, or interesting for their associations; and doubtless, now that a convenient and appropriate locality has been established for their reception and preservation, it will be gradually augmented by additions of a similar nature. It is mainly to the interest taken in the subject which it illustrates by the late Sir William Fergusson that the establishment of this collection is due.

Such is the general outline of the history and contents of the Museum, which for eighty years the College of Surgeons has maintained for the benefit not only of its own members, but for that of the profession at large, and indeed of all who take any interest in biological science, whether the young student preparing for his examination, or the advanced worker, who has here found materials for many an important contribution by which the boundaries of knowledge have been materially enlarged. To all such it is freely open without any fee or charge. Even the written or personal introduction of members, still nominally required, is never asked for on the four open days from any intelligent or interested visitor; and on the one day of the week in which it is closed for cleaning, facilities are always given to those who are desirous of making special studies, and to the increasing number of lady students, whether artistic, scholastic, or medical. Artists continually resort to the museum, to find opportunities of studying the anatomy of man and animals, which no other place in London affords; and of late years it has been the means of a still wider diffusion of knowledge, by the visits which have been organised on summer Saturday afternoons by various associations of artisans, to whom a popular demonstration of some part of its contents is usually given on each occasion by the Conservator.

If the knowledge of organic nature is of any value to man—and this is a proposition which I am sure all who attend this Congress will admit, as on such knowledge the whole superstructure of their profession is built—there can be no question but that such an institution as I have here sketched out must be one of pure and simple benefit. Its maintenance has been a worthy object upon which the College has spent its care and its money, and whatever may be the changes which impending legislation may effect in the organisation of the profession, we may all hope that the great work begun by John Hunter, and carried on by those who, under the guidance and support of the Council of the College, have followed him in the care of the collection, may not be impaired or destroyed. Whether the whole of the charges of maintaining such a museum in all its parts on a continually extending scale should be the duty of one institution, like the College of Surgeons, or even of one profession, may be a question for future consideration; but, in the meantime, how easily could its preservation and future extension be rendered entirely independent of all the chances and changes of medical education and legislation, or even of Government assistance and interference! When we see the immense sums voluntarily provided every year in this country by donation and bequest; when we see, and see with pleasure and gratitude, through the length and breadth of the land, cathedrals, churches, chapels, colleges, schools, hospitals, and asylums founded, endowed, enlarged, and restored, may we not hope that an old and tried institution like ours will not be so entirely neglected as it has hitherto been by members of our profession in search of some means for the disposal of any surplus wealth they may possess? Few objects can be so surely productive of good, so little liable to abuse at any future time, as the preservation, augmentation, and maintenance of a Museum, in which the facts of the beautiful and wonderful world around us are displayed for the instruction of mankind.

SECTION OF MEDICINE.

ADDRESS BY SIR WILLIAM GULL, BART., M.D., D.C.L., LL.D., F.R.S.,
President of the Section.

GENTLEMEN, FRIENDS, AND COLLEAGUES,—I am deeply sensible of the honour conferred upon me in being called upon to preside over this Section, and I offer you my cordial thanks. Happily the duties will not be arduous, since the General Addresses which have been arranged and admirably allotted relieve me of the responsibility of attempting to develope before you the actual position of medicine, or the probable lines of its future progress. As the International Medical Congress assembles in England for the first time under the auspices of Queen Victoria, so I am reminded that three hundred years ago, under Queen Elizabeth, Bacon enunciated for the first time, in the simplest terms, the position of the student of Nature in relation to the work before him.

Prone as we mostly are to easy satisfaction on imperfect evidence, and to rest in the *experientia fallax*, it is something that we are all agreed in aim and means, and admit that there is but one source and test of knowledge, "the observation of the order of Nature." We have no principles, but facts; no eclecticism, but of these; and nothing touching the conditions of humanity is foreign to our consideration.

Anatomy, physiology, and pathology have an impersonal and scientific object. Their aim is wide and general. The facts with which they deal are subject to no deflection from affection. Great or small, they have all an equal value. Pathology even denies its name in the presence of that which is universal, merges into physiology, and sees that "whatever is, is right." But far otherwise is it with clinical medicine, where the welfare of the individual alone has to be considered. We call ourselves physicians, and cannot be too jealous of the title and of all that it includes; but we are *medici* or curers of disease. Hence, together with the highest duties which science imposes, there are the various personal claims of humanity, augmented by suffering and

charged with every disturbing element that weighs upon the heart of man; but at the same time for us with every high and quickening motive. These are warping influences, and to correct them we have often with effort to bring our clinical questions into relation with that which is impersonal and above passion.

It is an agreeable fancy on these occasions to suppose that civilisation may have been differentiated into its various nationalities, less for the strife of war, than that each nation might contribute, according to its genius, to the progress of the sciences. It may be utopian to see it thus. Yet a review of the past two or three centuries would suggest as much. That scientific congresses have met, and that they continue to meet, promise better things to come out of the social chaos; as the imagination realises organisation springing up amidst the strife of the elements in an early world.

To Italy and the South we owe the early development of anatomy. The illustrious names of Morgagni, Galvani, Scarpa, and others, many of whom have left their names for ever inscribed on our textures, bear early and continued witness of this. And although we Englishmen will ever be tenacious of vindicating for our Harvey the immortal honour of having first demonstrated the circulation of the blood, we equally admit that Italy was his teacher of anatomy. And no less did Italy lead the way in morbid anatomy, as testify the pages of Morgagni in his treatise " De Causis et Sedibus Morborum."

To Germany and the North we are largely indebted for analytical progress. Their profound investigations in chemistry, and their exhaustive researches into minute anatomy and histology, have gone far to solve the problems of organic composition and organic structure. I will not support my position by citing illustrious names. Happily, many whom I should have to mention are still among us; but biological science will never forget Leeuwenhoek and Ehrenberg, Berzelius and Liebig, nor the labours of the modern schools.

France, with her rare synthetic faculty, seems especially gifted for promoting the science of physiology. I have but to recall the name of Bichat, and to point to the refined investigations of Bernard, and to those of his successors of to-day. And with France I may join Switzerland, whose Haller gave the earliest and strongest impulse to the study of the laws of living things, as a separate science; though, as in the case of Harvey, his lamp was lighted abroad, in the famous school of Leyden.

The English genius is perhaps more fitted for the historical method and its obvious lessons. But perhaps I ought not to say obvious, for not rarely the English have been satisfied with records without inferences. There are, however, splendid instances of both; of the one in the museum of Hunter, and of the other in the works of Darwin.

But here you will be ready to exclaim, "Siste!" for who in the least acquainted with the progress of the biological sciences in different schools at the present time would venture to claim for either some special fitness over the rest for any line of pursuit, and when the spirit of each can say like Goethe's Natur-geist—

"In Lebensfluthen, in Thatensturm
Wall ich auf und ab
Webe hin und her!"

Some have prophesied that the advancement of the biological sciences will leave medicine a barren waste in their midst; but such a result, in the natural course of things, cannot happen. There is an indissoluble union between all the sciences, which, for medicine especially, human interest will ever strengthen. The past history and the present state of our profession give us abundant assurance of this. It is not too much to assert that the study of medicine will for all time attract a large proportion of the best thinkers and workers of the world. It has ever been so; and what has been, doubtless shall be in the time to come. Besides, almost every germ of scientific thought has sprung in some way from medicine; and I have only to remind you that some of the most illustrious physiologists and pathologists of to-day are members of our own profession. And if from the delicacy, intricacy, and the demands made upon all the powers of the intellect by the extent and character of their investigations, they have, as it were, turned aside from immediate clinical work, they are still so much in union with us, that we daily at the bedside avail ourselves of the results of their labours, and gratefully acknowledge that they are our ministering angels, ascending and descending upon the ladder of science in the furtherance of all good practice.

Clinical medicine, however, of itself affords opportunities for the study of pathology which are in some respects at least unique. Through it, and through it alone, we become acquainted with the first deviations from normal function. From such early beginnings we may trace the development of pathological processes until the organism is finally, and in different ways, overwhelmed by them. I need only suggest those chronic lesions which spring up from conditions *ab intra*. In the latter stages of these degenerative processes we are apt, without their history, to be so impressed with the more prominent mechanical results, that these would seem to us the original and essential conditions; as to the Nile-worshipper, the river is a power in itself.

It is well for the progress of clinical medicine that its lines of investigation are thus intimately interwoven with the more scientific departments. It saves us from the dangers of separatism, and our colleagues from those of pharisaism; and it quickens our observations where they might otherwise be thought insignificant. If we cannot weigh and measure the data before us, we may still advance the solution of some of the more difficult problems of our condition by critical and exact records. How much has been done in this field of late, especially in cerebral physiology, need not now be told. Every fact to the clinical physician has its value, though it may be of a different order to the phenomena of gravitation. A tone of the voice, the play of the features, the outline and carriage of the body, are to him as invariably related to the central conditions which they reveal as are the grosser facts of nature.

The work of the next few days, so far as it is foreshadowed by the list of promised papers, will raise some important pathological questions. You will be asked to consider peripheral lesions, having their origin in nerve-centres—lesions which have, for the most part, been hitherto chiefly considered primarily humoral and chemical, but now referred to "trophic changes of nerve-origin." On this point it may not be uninteresting to notice how "Solidism" is widely reasserting itself in the science of living things—not as an *à priori* system, but through the progress of our knowledge. The proximate conditions of pyrexia are no longer vaguely referred to nerve, but to definite nerve-centres; hyperæmia and inflammatory changes to sympathetic lesions; abnormal chemistry to the great respiratory centres; the strange conditions of Addison's disease, with its characteristic pigment, to the supra-renal bodies, themselves probably but nerve-centres, and related, at least by structure, to the system of the pituitary gland; epilepsy, supposed in Hippocratic times to be due to extraneous maleficent spiritual influences, is traceable to apparently trifling changes in a few grey nerve-cells. The specific fever-processes notoriously owe much of their character and intensity to the nervous system. Their relation to time, their occurrence only in warm-blooded animals, the great mortality they cause through nerve-exhaustion, and the immunity they leave behind them, indicate that, whatever may be the nature or mode of operation of their several poisons, it is by implication of nerve-elements that fever obtains its chief clinical characteristics.

Further, in the advance of "Solidism," what can interest us more than the recent investigations on contagia? Perhaps no more important step has been made in practical pathology than the proof that some at least of these contagia are organised solids. This discovery, which it has tried the patience, experimental skill, and scientific criticism of the best observers to establish, has brought us at length within view of that which has hitherto been so mysterious. To have been able to separate, though imperfectly, the contagious particles—to have come to the conclusion that no fever-poisons are soluble—is a hopeful preliminary towards forcing them to yield up the secret of their nature.

If "Solidism," as a theory of organic processes, wanted confirmation, we could point to nothing more striking than the present established views on putrefactive changes, and to the amazing fact that the normal textures and fluids of the body resist decomposition, unless invaded by microscopic organisms.

May we not hereafter find that all organic chemistry is the resultant of mechanical changes in organic solids—all

nature, in fact, as Newton asserted, but the Great First Cause? Of this we are admonished on all sides. Histology, physiology, pathology, clinical medicine, teach us more and more the supreme importance of *form* and *relation*.

Lesions extending from alteration of the bloodvessels will also come under consideration. Of course the more common facts relating to aneurism and valvular disease, or such as are thrombotic or embolic, need not be discussed; but there is a contribution which raises the question how far primary, general, arterial tension may be a starting-point at least in renal pathology.

The etiology of typhoid fever will be raised at one of our meetings. This cannot but enforce a rigid criticism of the infective processes, and of the differences between the states of simple pyrexia, septicæmia, and the specific fevers.

The pathology and treatment of gout, rheumatoid arthritis, and rheumatism, to which, in one form or another, the English seem rather especially prone, will also come up for discussion. Whether they have humoral sources has of late become more and more doubtful.

Of the pathology of acute rheumatism we may be said to know but little beyond its clinical records and its symptoms; but, unhappily, this has not always been sufficiently recognised, and too often a dangerous polypharmacy has rushed into the cure where science has not yet advanced her foot.

The forms of renal diseases, for a long time included, with little exception, under the term "Bright's disease," will undergo a further degree of analysis. It was a happy omen of this when they moved from the singular into the plural form, "Bright's diseases"; and we may hope now for a more methodical subdivision of them, making their clinical recognition more easy and their therapeutics more precise.

In the matter of diagnosis we have invited contributions on the pathognomonic and diagnostic value of the localisation of disease in the brain and spinal cord, which will be an occasion for a review of our knowledge of *cerebral* and *spinal mechanism*, and for further elucidating the pathology of the different conditions of blood, bloodvessels, and connective tissue concerned in the nutrition and diseases of these great nerve-centres. Brain-texture proper seems but little liable to primary disease. As the nervous lamina takes the lead in embryonic evolution, so it would seem that its equivalents in the adult maintain a degree of resistance to morbid change throughout life.

Time fails me to speak of all that we hope to undertake. Any one paragraph of our programme would more than consume the time at our disposal. It must not therefore be inferred that the importance attached to any one of the subjects is in proportion to the prominence given to it in this hasty review. The treatment of disease, for instance, is a subject too large and weighty to speak of in general terms. In some minor points it will come before us, as in a paper on the advantage of high altitudes in the treatment of pulmonary phthisis.

An organisation such as our own, which it has taken countless ages to evolve, must reasonably require incalculable time for its scientific analysis; and the same may be said of the infinite and varying conditions by which it is maintained, and upon which its existence constantly and immediately depends. At best we know but a few proximate facts, yet these in judicious hands have afforded a good harvest of practical results: what better fruit we may gather when science has penetrated deeper into the laws of our being, and all that affects it, it is impossible to forecast.

In the spirit of the exhortation given by the President in his address to-day, and in the slightly altered words of Bacon, with whom I began, let me conclude by saying, "It were a heaven upon earth to have the mind illumined by knowledge, to move in charity, and turn upon the poles of truth."

ELEPHANT'S MILK.—Prof. Doremus has analysed some milk obtained from an elephant that had suckled its calf for about a year. The milk approached cream in composition, but did not possess its consistency. It was pleasant in flavour and odour, and very superior in these respects to the milk of goats, and fully equal to cow's milk. The elephant-calf, when born on March 10, 1880, in Philadelphia, weighed 213½ lbs., and gained many hundred pounds on this milk in the course of a year.—*Boston Med. Jour.*, June 16.

TERMS OF SUBSCRIPTION.
(Free by post.)

British Islands	. . . .	*Twelve Months*	. £1 8	0
"		*Six*	" . 0 14	0
The Colonies and the United States of America	. . . }	*Twelve*	" . 1 10	0
"	"	*Six*	" . 0 15	0
India	. . . .	*Twelve*	" . 1 10	0
" *(vià Brindisi)*	. . .	"	" . 1 15	0
"	. . . .	*Six*	" . 0 15	0
" *(vià Brindisi)*	. . .	"	" . 0 17	6

Foreign Subscribers are requested to inform the Publishers of any remittance made through the agency of the Post-office.

Single Copies of the Journal can be obtained of all Booksellers and Newsmen, price Sixpence.

Cheques or Post-office Orders should be made payable to Mr. JAMES LUCAS, 11, *New Burlington-street, W.*

TERMS FOR ADVERTISEMENTS.

Seven lines (70 words)	. . . .	.£0 4 6
Each additional line (10 words)	. .	. 0 0 6
Half-column, or quarter-page	. .	. 1 5 0
Whole column, or half-page	. .	. 2 10 0
Whole page	. . .	. . 5 0 0

Births, Marriages, and Deaths are inserted Free of Charge.

THE MEDICAL TIMES AND GAZETTE *is published on Friday morning: Advertisements must therefore reach the Publishing Office not later than One o'clock on Thursday.*

Medical Times and Gazette.

SATURDAY, AUGUST 13, 1881.

ADDRESSES - IN - CHIEF.

WE place before our readers, this week, the remainder of Professor Virchow's Address, which will, we doubt not, be carefully read and studied. The promise that he would be present at, and take part in, the work of the Congress, was one of the early assurances that the meeting would certainly be a success. His pre-eminence as a scientific worker and pathologist is universally acknowledged; and he could not have chosen a happier subject for his address than the Value of Pathological Experiment. It is a subject on which he has won the full right to speak as one having authority; and he used the opportunity to make his address a most forcible and telling demonstration of the inestimable benefits that scientific medicine, and through it mankind, have gained by means of pathological experiment. His argument in favour of vivisection—so-called—was most masterly, and admirably well-sustained throughout; and his word-painting of the course of medical science strikingly clear and graphic. The fanatical anti-vivisectionists will not, probably, be converted by the address, if they even read it; but it can hardly fail to have effect on all who, though they have been led to join that movement, are not bigoted or strongly prejudiced. And it may help weak-kneed and agitation-fearing legislators to know that such a man as Virchow insists that the practice of vivisection is essential to the real and solid advance of medical science. The whole of the address is of great value to medical men, and we may, most of us, profit by well studying and thinking over Professor Virchow's declaration that life is the sum of the joint action of all parts, of the higher or vital ones, and as well of the lower and inferior. There is no one seat of life, but every really elementary part, especially every cell, is a seat of life. His address is one of the most marked and valuable fruits of the Congress.

The address on " Our Medical Literature," by Dr. Billings (of Washington), on Friday, the 5th, was listened to with great delight by a very full audience. The subject was a fresh one, and Dr. Billings handled it excellently well. His address was indeed begotten by wisdom out of fulness of knowledge, and was throughout lit up by flashes of wit and humour. We publish it at length, but we fear that, to those who can only read it, it loses some of its brilliancy and effect; for it was as admirably delivered as conceived. He dealt with medical literature at large—the medical literature which is the common property of the educated physicians of the world, which forms the intra- and inter-national bond of the medical profession of all civilised countries; and " by virtue of which," Dr. Billings said,' " we, who have come hither from the far West and the farther East, do not now meet, for the first time, as strangers, but as friends, having common interests, and, though of many nations, a common language, and whose thoughts are perhaps better known to each other than to some of our nearest neighbours." Dr. Billings remarks that it is usual to estimate that about one-thirtieth part of the whole mass of the world's literature belongs to medicine and its allied sciences; and he finds that this estimate corresponds very well to the results obtained from an examination of bibliographies and of the catalogues of the principal medical libraries. This mass of literature is now increasing at the rate of 1500 volumes and 2500 pamphlets annually, produced for the edification of the (about) 180,000 medical men scattered over the earth, " who, by a liberal construction of the phrase, may be said to be educated, that is, who have some kind of a diploma." Our readers may glean a great amount of curious and interesting information about " our medical literature " from Dr. Billings, about its rate of growth, its value, etc., in different countries and among the diverse nations; and much very useful instruction about the right and most fruitful mode of using libraries and library-catalogues. He is a little hard on the editors of transactions of societies, whether sent to journals or published separately. He says, most rightly, every article should have " a distinct title," and if the author does not furnish this, " it is the editor's business to make it." We fear the editor might in so doing get not seldom into hot water. We heartily endorse, however, and hope that all intending writers will ponder, his four rules for the preparation of an article for a journal:—" 1. Have something to say; 2. Say it; 3. Stop as soon as you have said it; 4. Give the paper a proper title."

We must, we fear, be content to place Professor Huxley's address—" On the Connexion of the Biological Sciences with Medicine "—in the hands of our readers without any comment or notice, except to commend it to their attention. They will find in it plenty to interest them, much to make them think, and something that many, or some, of them will not agree with. But the space at our disposal will not suffer us to say more about the address than that we are glad to find that Professor Huxley takes a very bright view of the future of our therapeutical knowledge and art. He thinks that some day, sooner or later, the physician will be armed with the means of affecting any function in any desired way. He predicts that it will become possible " to introduce into the economy a molecular mechanism which, like a cunningly contrived torpedo, shall find its way to some particular group of living elements, and cause an explosion among them, leaving the rest untouched." Who shall say, after this, that there are not poets among the scientists and physicists of the day?

The crowded state of our pages must be our excuse also for neither publishing nor saying aught about the extremely interesting and eloquent address, delivered at the request of the President of the Congress, by Professor Pasteur, in St. James's Hall, on Monday, the 9th. The address embodied the results of M. Pasteur's most recent researches in what has been called Animal Vaccination—results which promise to be of very great importance; but we cannot find room for the address now; and, moreover, notice of the researches have already appeared from time to time in our columns as they were made known in Paris. But we may give the address, ere long, as the most authoritative *resumé* possible of Professor Pasteur's long-continued labours on the nature of ferments, etc. We will note here, however, that the reception accorded to Professor Pasteur everywhere during the Congress must have been very gratifying to him as a proof of the high place he has won in the esteem of the profession in England.

THE WEEK.

TOPICS OF THE DAY.

Our contemporary, *Nature*, says:—"The accommodation for anatomical work at the Prosector's Rooms in the Zoological Society's Gardens, which has hitherto been somewhat limited, has lately been increased by the erection of three new working-rooms, intended for the use of students. These rooms are now finished, and are at present tenanted by a small long-vacation class from Cambridge, who, under the superintendence of Mr. T. T. Lister, the Demonstrator of Comparative Anatomy in that University, are studying practically the anatomy of the mammalia on the abundant material in that group provided for the Society's menagerie. It is to be hoped that when this class concludes its labours at the end of the month, other students may be found disposed to profit by the new facilities for work afforded them by the Zoological Society, and that thus the expense incurred in the erection of these new rooms may be fully justified by the increased scientific results reaped in the Regent's-park from the superabundant material at the disposal of Mr. Forbes."

At a recent meeting of the Guardians of the St. Saviour's Union, the Clerk reported that the Local Government Board, in a letter referring to the resolution of the Guardians to build a new workhouse on the land just acquired at Champion Hill, pointed out that, in the opinion of their inspectors, an infirmary, instead of a workhouse, should be erected on that site. The Board point out that the present infirmary at Newington affords more accommodation than is absolutely necessary for the whole sick poor of the union, and that it is besides unsuited for the purposes of an infirmary by reason of its construction. They consider that if a new infirmary were constructed at Champion Hill it would only be necessary to make provision for about 500 patients, and the existing infirmary, if used as a workhouse, would afford accommodation for a considerably larger number of inmates than it is at present certified for. The Board, therefore, urge the Guardians to re-consider their resolution. It was resolved that the letter should be discussed at a future meeting of the Board.

At the last meeting of the Metropolitan Asylums Board, the returns presented showed that there had been admitted to the several asylums during the past fortnight 303 patients—namely, 94 to the Atlas, 50 to Homerton, 26 to Stockwell, 74 to Fulham, and 59 to Deptford. In all, 47 had died, 137 had been transferred from acute wards to convalescent wards, 214 had been discharged, 644 remained under treatment in the general hospitals of the Managers, and 154 at Darenth Camp, being 798, as against 1032 a fortnight ago, making a decrease of 234. The fever returns showed an increase of scarlet, typhus, and enteric fever in the metropolis. A fortnight since there were 184 patients in the fever asylums; the present returns showed that the number had risen to 230. A return just issued by

the Local Government Board, dated July 18, 1881, states that out of the whole of the vestries and district boards of the metropolis, only two have themselves provided permanent accommodation for small-pox patients, six have provided temporary accommodation only, seven have arranged with other authorities to receive such patients, and no less than twenty-four have failed to provide any accommodation at all.

In answer to a question put by Baron H. de Worms in the House of Commons, the President of the Local Government Board maintained that no danger was to be apprehended from the small-pox hospital-ships at Greenwich. We hear, however, that it is positively stated that these vessels are only ninety yards from the shore, where a number of workmen are constantly employed, and that they are stationed higher up the river than the *Dreadnought* formerly was. It is also pointed out that there is no analogy between the two cases, the *Dreadnought* having been used as an ordinary hospital-ship, and not for the exclusive treatment of infectious disorders. Although the Thames Conservators and the Metropolitan Asylums Board originally recommended that the ships should be moored lower down the river, the Local Government Board, however, decided on placing them in their present position, solely, it is alleged, for the convenience of the medical staff.

INTERNATIONAL MEDICAL CONGRESS.—PROTEST IN FAVOUR OF EXPERIMENTS ON ANIMALS.

In addition to the resolution upon the subject of what is known as vivisection, but which we should prefer to call experiments on animals, passed at the general meeting of the Congress, the two following resolutions were agreed to at the meeting of Section 15—Materia Medica and Pharmacology—on the 8th inst. It was proposed by Professor Stockvis (of Amsterdam), and seconded by Professor Lauder Brunton—"That the Section resolves that, in their opinion, advancement of the science of the action of medicines in the present state of science cannot be obtained without experiments on lower animals." This resolution was warmly supported by the two physiologists named, by Professor Wood (of Philadelphia), Professor Dujardin-Beaumetz (of Paris), Professor Rossbach (of Würzburg), Professor Quinlan (of Dublin), and Dr. Farquharson, M.P. The second resolution was to the effect—"That the Council of the Section be instructed to transmit this resolution to the President of the International Congress, with a request to submit it to a general meeting of the Congress."

SMALL-POX HOSPITALS FOR THE METROPOLIS.

A very important and interesting Parliamentary return has just been issued, showing the number of hospitals, whether temporary or permanent, which have been provided for small-pox patients, under Section 37 of the Sanitary Act (1866), by the vestries and the district boards in the metropolis; the situation of such hospitals; the year in which they were established; the number of patients which they are capable of accommodating; and the actual number of patients therein on June 13, 1881. It appears from the return that only two of the authorities referred to have provided themselves with permanent hospital accommodation for small-pox patients under the powers conferred upon them by the Act. In six districts temporary accommodation only has been provided; seven of the boards have arranged with other authorities to receive small-pox patients; and no less than twenty-four of the vestries or district boards have failed to provide any accommodation whatever. The return shows that the total number of patients who can be received is 388, and that the number of patients actually under treatment on June 13 last was eighty. In several cases the authorities give as their reason for not taking action under the provisions of the Act that it would be impossible for them to do so in the present state of the law, as the same difficulties would occur as in the case of the Metropolitan Asylums Board and the Hampstead Hospital. Looking to the very little which has been done by the district boards, as shown by this return, and having regard to the fact, stated by the President of the Local Government Board in the recent debate on the subject in the House of Commons, that the district boards are not under the jurisdiction of the central board, it appears to be clear that some further legislation in the matter is urgently needed.

THE HARVEY TERCENTENARY MEMORIAL.

FOLKESTONE was en fête on Saturday last, when the statue to the memory of Harvey was unveiled. It will be remembered by our readers that a first public meeting was convened at the Town Hall, Folkestone, in the year 1871, to consider the propriety of erecting in his native town a suitable memorial to the immortal Harvey. That ten long years and an immense amount of labour on the part of the promoters should have been necessary before this work could be accomplished, is a matter for reflection. The old proverb says, "All's well that ends well," and so we will let this part of the proceedings alone. It must, however, have been gratifying that the ceremony of unveiling occurred in the presence of a more cosmopolitan gathering than could possibly have been secured had it not taken place during the meeting of the International Medical Congress in London this year. A special train, kindly and gratuitously placed at the disposal of the Memorial Committee by the South-Eastern Railway Company, conveyed a large company from London to Folkestone. The town was gaily decorated with flags of all nations, and an immense concourse of persons assembled to do honour to this occasion. The ceremony of unveiling was performed in the presence of the Mayor and Corporation of Folkestone, by Professor Owen, F.R.S., after which he gave an address, showing what influence Harvey's discovery had produced on medical science, and how vivisection was a necessary part of that science. The company then adjourned to the Town Hall to partake of a sumptuous collation with the Mayor and Corporation. The weather was beautifully fine, and the whole proceedings passed off with the greatest éclat. We cannot conclude this brief notice without congratulating Mr. G. Eastes on the successful accomplishment of a project which was started by him, mainly carried on by him, and to whose energy its success was so largely due.

THE DISTRIBUTION OF THE HOSPITAL SUNDAY FUND.

AT a meeting of the Council of the Hospital Sunday Fund, recently held at the Mansion House, under the presidency of the Lord Mayor, it was officially stated that the sum received amounted to £31,000 exclusive of the balance from last year. The Distribution Committee brought up a report recommending the payment of £27,402 to ninety hospitals, and four institutions which might be classed as hospitals; £2515 to fifty dispensaries, setting aside £610 for the purchase of surgical appliances during the twelve months. The awards to the general hospitals were apportioned as follows:—Charing-cross, £731; French (Lisle-street), £227; German, £675; Great Northern, £225; King's College, £1462; London, £2212; Metropolitan Free, £281; Poplar, £292; Royal Free, £518; St. George's, £1575; St. John and St. Elizabeth, £112; St. Mary's, 1012; Seamen's (Greenwich), £787; Middlesex, £1405; Tottenham Training Hospital, £281; University College, £810; West London, £309;

Westminster, £731. In moving the adoption of the report, the Bishop of London referred to the necessity for increased hospital accommodation in the suburbs to meet the wants of the growing population, and also to the need for proper hospital ambulances. Dr. Allon seconded the motion, which was spoken to by several members, and eventually agreed to unanimously.

ILLNESS OF DR. BROWNING.

WE learn with regret that Dr. B. Browning, Medical Officer of Health for Rotherhithe, is suffering from serious blood-poisoning, incurred in the discharge of his duties. Having caused the seizure, as totally unfit for human food, of a great number of American hams and sides of pork, he proceeded to examine them microscopically, and in so doing wounded and poisoned his hand. The meat was so putrid that he was compelled to use disinfectants, which obscured the minute structures, but he satisfied himself that the animals had been the subjects of, if they had not died of, pig-typhus, and he believes also that they were trichinised. The culprit got off with one month in gaol; while Dr. Browning has narrowly escaped permanent maiming.

THE LATE DR. OTIS.

DURING a discussion on Friday, in the Section of Military Surgery and Medicine, on the transport of sick and wounded in the field, Dr. Gori (of Amsterdam) made reference to the death of Dr. Otis, which drew forth the following remarks from the President, Surgeon-General Longmore:—"This seems to be a very fitting occasion, representatives as we are of the science and practice of military surgery in all countries, for us to express our profound regret at Surgeon Otis having been taken away from among us before he was able to complete the greatest of all his many valuable professional works, as he had hoped to do; and it seems also to be a fitting opportunity to convey to Surgeon-General Barnes, and, through him, to all the medical officers of the United States Army, our heartfelt sympathy with them on the great loss their medical service in particular, and at the same time military surgical science in all parts of the world, has sustained in the death of their great colleague. I say these few words in the presence of an eminent friend and fellow-labourer of Dr. Otis,—Dr. Billings, who occupies an important post in the Surgeon-General's Office at Washington, —and I beg to propose to the meeting that Dr. Billings be asked kindly to allow himself to be made the medium of communicating this, I may truly say, international expression of feeling—for I see plainly you all share with me in sentiments I have tried to express,—to the distinguished chief at the head of the Department, and to his colleagues, on his return to Washington." Dr. Billings, in reply, said—"In behalf of the Medical Department of the United States Army, of the Surgeon-General, and of the colleagues and friends of Dr. Otis, I desire to return thanks for, and to express the highest appreciation of, the eloquent tribute which Surgeon-General Longmore has paid to the memory of Dr. Otis. I shall not attempt to add to the eulogy which Surgeon-General Longmore has pronounced upon my friend and colleague; I can only say that I find I want words to express the emotion with which I have listened to it, and that I shall convey the message with which he has charged me, to the best of my ability. You will all, I am sure, be glad to know that before his death Dr. Otis had completed so much of the Surgical History of the War, upon which he was engaged, as relates to wounds of the extremities. There remains yet to be completed the account of the complications of wounds, such as gangrene, tetanus, septicæmia, etc. Another surgeon of the Army will be assigned to complete this history, and you can readily conceive how difficult he will find it to prepare a report which will be the continuation of, and be constantly compared with, the work of Dr. Otis."

THE FORTY-NINTH ANNUAL MEETING

OF THE

BRITISH MEDICAL ASSOCIATION.

HELD AT RYDE, AUGUST 8, 9, 10, AND 11.

(*From our Special Correspondent.*)

THE contrast is great. Yesterday we were driven from pillar to post by that gigantic assemblage, the International Medical Congress; to-day we are enjoying the fresh sea-breezes and watching the flight of the yachts as they slip past the winning-post,—for this is Regatta week, as well as the week of the British Medical Association at Ryde. The change is agreeable, and, to many, most welcome; for the work at the great Congress was too hard for anyone who had work to do, and the pace was too tremendous to last. Here the numbers are just as nearly as possible one to ten there; whilst the lightness of the work to be accomplished renders it easy to overtake it without tasking ourselves or others. And truly the place is well adapted for its purpose—land and sea alike may both be called under contribution to pleasure and instruction; and if the weather will only continue favourable, a pleasant meeting will be passed; whilst the outcome, if not so brilliant, will perhaps be not less substantial than that of the Congress.

The work, as usual, began with a short religious service, which was not so well attended as it might be, for few members had arrived by the time it was held. But the great event of the day is the annual general meeting, where grievances may be ventilated and redress sought. Fortunately, such discussions seldom occur: and then, beyond purely business matters, the address by the President is the chief feature of this the first general meeting. The President (Mr. Barrow), on this occasion, is particularly fitted for the post. He may be said to know every foot of the island, and everyone in it. Moreover, he has been Mayor of the borough for five years, is an excellent business man, with a clear and distinct voice, fitted to rule and to guide.

In his opening address, Mr. Barrow referred to those who had been called hence during the past year. Robert Céely (of Aylesbury), Randall Wilbraham Falconer, Alfred Hudson, aged seventy-two, William Robert Saunders, aged fifty, Henry Day (of Stafford), and George Rolleston (of Oxford). As for himself, he was most fully sensible of the honour conferred upon him by being elected President for the current year—an honour which any man might be proud of, and which he should ever look upon as the crowning event of his fifty years' professional career. "I think I may claim for our island towns equality, if not superiority, as to drainage, water-supply, and other sanitary appliances. So far as this locality is concerned, it will give our Surveyor much pleasure to accompany gentlemen to our waterworks, four miles distant, and to explain every particular in reference to the sanitary arrangements of the borough. I have little doubt that the surveyors in other towns will do their part." Mr. Barrow said he might, perhaps, qualify the last statement, after the somewhat sweeping criticisms by a Government medical inspector—to many of whose criticisms he did not subscribe. "I am quite prepared," said Mr. Barrow, "to prove a negative. As regards our water-supply, I think you will all agree with me that the analyses with which you will be supplied amply testify to its surpassing excellence. If, moreover, you will avail yourselves of our Surveyor's kind offer, he will explain our system of drainage; and having care-fully surveyed this, I believe you will come to the same conclusion as I have, that from the defects which are the main causes of zymotic diseases we are almost free. I beg, in the name of the medical profession of the island and of

the inhabitants generally, to offer you the heartiest welcome. (Applause.) Rest assured that our best endeavours have been and will continue to be, exerted to render the forty-ninth anniversary of our great Association as successful and agreeable as any that have preceded it. I feel—indeed, all who have worked, and are working with me, feel—the responsibility of the position we occupy, knowing that many have come here at personal inconvenience and loss, to gather up what fragments of knowledge they may—no less than to recruit energies after months of arduous labour and thought, hoping by these united means (as is the object of all practitioners) to return to their duties refreshed both in mind and body, better prepared to meet the ever-recurring and never-ceasing wants, and to relieve the sufferings of their fellow-men."

Among other things they have resolved on this year, is to appoint a Committee of Collective Research, with a fairly well-paid Secretary. This, probably, is intended to take the place of the scientific grants, about which nothing is this year said, and from which nothing has come of great importance, if we except Rutherford's researches on the bile. There was other important business, however, to be got through. Dr. Alfred Carpenter has resigned the post of Chairman of the Committee of Council (by far the most important in the Association), and has been elected a Vice-President for life; whilst Mr. Wheelhouse, of Leeds, assumes the chairmanship. No better selection could be made; Mr. Wheelhouse is not only a good and wise practitioner, but a shrewd man of business, who will undoubtedly manage the affairs of the Association as well as they can be managed. The only thing to be regretted is his distance from London, for matters are constantly occurring which demand the attention of the Chairman, and, anyhow you like, the journey from Leeds to London and back occupies an entire day.

The next thing to be arranged was the place of meeting for 1882, and, as had long been anticipated, an invitation of the most cordial kind was received from Worcester, where the Association was founded by Sir Charles Hastings; and that it will celebrate its jubilee in the place of its birth. It was also intimated that in all probability the meeting-place in 1883 would be Liverpool, and in 1884 Glasgow. Dr. Strange, of Worcester, was unanimously elected President for next year.

The great business of the second general meeting is, however, to listen to the Address in Medicine. The speaker this year was Dr. Bristowe, of St. Thomas's Hospital, and curiously enough he chose for his text the somewhat hackneyed topic of the Life and Doctrines of Hahnemann. He has made a careful study of the subject, and the address is very well worth reading, being both vivid and vivacious. Towards the conclusion, however, he entered on somewhat doubtful ground. He said that many homœopathic practitioners of the present day were men of culture and learning, and that, in his opinion, these gentlemen should be treated as such. Nor, as far as we could make out from a very imperfectly heard address, would he shrink from associating with or assisting any such men. No clamour was heard at first, though the conclusions were evidently unpalatable to many, and a vote of thanks was proposed by Dr. Davey (of Ryde). The seconder, however, Dr. Long Fox (of Bristol), took care to signify his dissent from certain portions of Dr. Bristowe's address, much to the satisfaction of many. Finally, the President pointed out, that though he had allowed Dr. Fox to proceed, it must be distinctly understood that any criticism of these addresses was out of order, the views expressed being those of the speaker alone, who was alone responsible for them.

In the afternoon, sectional work began. Dr. Long Fox, President of the Section of Medicine, gave a short address specially with reference to spinal disease. After which came an interesting discussion on distension and dilatation of the stomach, coupled with gastric catarrh, by Dr. W. Wade (of Birmingham). In Surgery, Mr. Coates (of Salisbury), the President of the Section, made some opening remarks with regard to piles and their treatment; whilst in Midwifery, Dr. Coghill discussed the mechanical treatment of uterine flexions and displacements.

What promised to be the most interesting of all, the discussion on animal vaccination, introduced by Mr. Ernest Hart, and in which Warlomont (of Brussels) and Martin (of Boston) were expected to take part, was postponed till Thursday.

THE INTERNATIONAL MEDICAL CONGRESS.

THE Medical Congress is over, and the multitude of physicians and surgeons lately gathered together in London from all parts of the civilised world have separated and dispersed, some to their homes, and some to a seaside gathering of a similar character in the pleasant town of Ryde. The total number of members inscribed on the roll of the Seventh International Congress has been 3210; and the Congress will be long remembered as by far the largest, and in every sense the most successful, meeting of the kind ever held. All has gone well, with a marvellously slight amount of friction, considering the magnitude of the undertaking, and for this success our heartiest acknowledgments are due to all who had the labour and responsibility of organising and managing the meeting; and are due most especially to the President of the Congress, Sir James Paget, and its Honorary Secretary-General, Mr. Mac Cormac, whose labours must have been enormous for long before, and during, the meeting. The Presidents and the Secretaries of Sections also deserve that their untiring attention to work, their assiduity and courtesy, should be especially acknowledged. That much real and lasting gain must result from all the labours of the Congress, we cannot doubt. It is impossible that so many eminent men of all civilised nations, of such varied intellectual gifts and temperament, training, and experience, can have come together to discuss prominent questions in the science and art of medicine without real advance and benefit. Some of the addresses also, general and sectional, will remain as landmarks of a period when stock was taken of recent gains, and whence new departures in advance will be dated.

On Thursday, the 4th, the third general meeting of the Congress was held in St. James's Hall, when the address prepared by the late Professor Maurice Reynaud (of Paris), on "Le Scepticisme en Médecine, au temps passé et au temps présent," was read by Dr. Féréol, his intimate friend. The fourth general meeting took place on the 5th inst., when Dr. Billings delivered his admirable address on "Our Medical Literature" to a very large and highly appreciative audience. The fifth general meeting did not take place till Monday, the 8th. On that day the general address was from Professor Volkmann, on "Modern Surgery," and in the course of his address he paid a high tribute to Professor Lister as the discoverer of the Antiseptic System—a system which has been very widely, and one may say enthusiastically, adopted in Germany, with the happiest results. On this day also, before Professor Volkmann's address, Professor Pasteur (of Paris) described at length, and with eloquence as well as precision, his researches and discoveries on the vaccination-like protection of animals from infectious diseases.

The final meeting of the Congress was held in St. James's Hall on the afternoon of Tuesday, August 8. The Great Hall was filled, and the first proceeding was the delivery of an address by Professor Huxley on "The Connexion of the Biological Sciences with Medicine," which will be found in full elsewhere in our columns. After the address, Mr. Mac Cormac read a short report of the work of the Congress, from which it appeared, inter alia, that 119 meetings of sections had been held, at which 464 written and 360 spoken communications had been made. Sir James Paget, the President, then submitted to the meeting resolutions which had been received from the Physiological and Ophthalmological Sections, promising that if any dissented from the first their names would be recorded. The resolution, which had been most carefully discussed and considered, sent by the Physiological Section, was in the following terms :—"That this Congress records its conviction that experiments upon living animals have proved of the utmost service to medicine, and are indispensable for its further progress; that, accordingly, while strongly deprecating the infliction of unnecessary pain, it is of opinion that, alike in the interest of man and of animals, it is not desirable to restrict competent persons in the performance of such experiments." This resolution was received with great applause, and was declared carried without a single dissentient—a unanimity of opinion which was probably partly due to Professor Virchow's address.

Sir James Paget then explained that the views of the Ophthalmological Section were about to be drawn up in due form by a small committee, and placed in the hands of the Executive Committee of the Congress. Meanwhile, the Section recommended that their resolutions should be adopted as acts of the Congress, in order that they might be forwarded through the Secretary-General to the President of the Board of Trade, the First Lord of the Admiralty, and the Secretary of State for Foreign Affairs, with an expression of the desire of the Congress that they should be favourably entertained and, if approved, be recommended for adoption by foreign governments. A resolution to this effect was also agreed to unanimously.

On the motion of Mr. Bowman, seconded by Professor Lister, medals of honour were next presented to the President of the last Congress, Professor Donders (of Utrecht) ; to the General Secretary, Dr. Guye (of Amsterdam) ; and to the readers of general addresses in the present Congress—Dr. Féréol (of Paris), Dr. Billings (of Washington), Professor Volkmann (of Halle), Professor Huxley (of London), and Professor Virchow (of Berlin). And it was resolved also that a medal should be sent to the widow of the lamented Dr. Maurice Reynaud, who had written, and was to have delivered, the address on "Le Scepticisme en Médecine, au temps passé et au temps présent," which had been read by his friend, Dr. Féréol.

Votes of thanks, at the instance of Professor Langenbeck, Professor Charcot, Professor Donders, Dr. Billings, and others, were then passed to Mr. Mac Cormac, Hon. Secretary-General, and to his assistants, Mr. Makins and Dr. Coxwell ; to others, medical and lay, who had helped to make the Congress so successful in every way ; and to Sir James Paget, President of the Congress. All these votes were very heartily passed by the meeting ; and Mr. Mac Cormac, on rising to express his thanks, was received with warm and richly deserved applause.

Sir James Paget, in bidding the members "Good-bye," stated that the Executive Committee would take into consideration the time and place of next meeting. They had received an invitation from the King of Spain to hold their next meeting in that country, but there was a desire on the part of many that one of the Scandinavian capitals should be selected.

SECTIONAL WORK.

THE business in the Section of Anatomy commenced on Thursday morning, the 4th inst., with an introductory address on "The Museum of the Royal College of Surgeons," by the President of the Section, Professor Flower, F.R.S. Amongst the audience we noticed many foreign anatomists of eminence, such as Kölliker, His, Braune, Hannover, Toldt, Caruccio, Rahl-Rückhardt, as well as nearly all the British members of the Council of the Section. The subsequent sectional meetings were regularly attended by most of these gentlemen, and the papers and discussions have been of considerable value and interest. After the introductory address a vote of thanks to Professor Flower was moved by Dr. Allen Thomson, and seconded in a few well-chosen sentences in English by Professor Kölliker. Professor His (of Leipzig) brought forward the very important proposition that "the number of embryos which have been described is sufficient for anatomists to determine what are the normal characters of the human embryo, and that probably in no normal embryo is there ever a free vesicular allantois."

Professor His described his embryonic preparations at some length, and showed some beautiful wax models and stereoscopic slides in illustration of his remarks.

Dr. Allen Thomson considered that Professor His's proposition was rather premature, inasmuch as some of the embryos mentioned by him were undoubtedly pathological, as most abortions must necessarily be ; and Dr. Thomson, as well as most of the other anatomists present, also thought that there was more variability in the amount of attachment of the allantois to the chorion than Professor His had stated. In fact, the general conclusion of the meeting seemed to be that further specimens must be carefully examined before such a general proposition as that of Professor His could be adopted.

The remainder of the sitting was devoted to a discussion on the characteristics of human crania in relation to race, and was introduced by Professor Turner in a paper " On the Cranial Characters of the Natives of the Admiralty Islands." The skulls described were eleven complete and one calvaria (all adults), seven males and five females ; they were smeared with a red pigment, and one had an artificial nose and eyes modelled in a black material. They had been obtained in March, 1875, by the scientific staff of the Challenger, and entrusted to Professor Turner for description. The crania were markedly dolicho-cephalic ; somewhat higher than broad ; and whilst the females were microcephalic, the males were mesocephalic, there being a difference of about 250 cubic centimetres between the two sexes. They approximated very nearly to the skulls obtained from the people inhabiting the coast line of New Guinea. In the subsequent discussion Professor Flower pointed out the increasing value of such complete cranial descriptions in reference to the determination of races in places where there has been but little, if any, admixture with foreign nations ; and Dr. Rabl-Rückhardt (of Berlin) gave a short account of forty-two skulls from New Britain, which had been collected during a German expedition to the Kerguelen Island. It was a point of interest that these skulls, although coming from an island much nearer to the Admiralty Islands than to Australia, bore a greater resemblance to the Australian type than to those described by Professor Turner. Professors Toldt (of Prague) and Lesshaft (of St. Petersburg) joined in a most interesting anthropological conversation, the latter referring especially to twenty-five Kalmuck skulls which he had examined.

On Friday, Professor Struthers described minutely a series of dry and wet specimens showing a supra-condyloid process. He showed that, although well known to every anatomist in its ordinary form, when it is also of great importance to the operating surgeon, it had been overlooked in its rudimentary condition, which he had found to exist normally in every human subject which he had examined. In these cases it is found as a band or bands of fibres beneath the brachialis anticus muscle. A striking instance of its hereditary transmission was next described, and the theory of descent referred to as the only explanation of its presence, occurring, as it does, so widely amongst mammalia, from the Ornithorhynchus paradoxus upwards to man, and in the latter no teleological explanation being available. Professor Flower pointed out that the very variability of this process in the mammalia was in favour of its being transmitted by descent. It may be casually remarked that in the subsequent discussion all the anatomists who spoke regarded the evolution theory as the only possible hypothesis for the explanation of the occurrence of this and similar structures ; no one even ventured on teleological argument.

Professor Lesshaft next read two papers—(1) On the Causes which determine the Shape of the Bones, illustrated by numerous specimens from man and the lower animals ; and (2) On the Position of the Stomach. He considered that this organ is placed more vertically than is generally supposed, but its oblique position, as shown in Dureg's model, made under the supervision of Luschka, was strenuously maintained by Professors His, Kölliker, and Braune, and by Mr. Holden, who all agreed that a vertical stomach only existed in the young child.

Dr. Laura (of Turin) read two papers on the Minute Structure of the Spinal Cord and Medulla Oblongata.

Professor Adamkiewicz (of Cracow) made a short communication of the minute vessels of the spinal cord ; and Professor Léon Tripier (of Lyons) showed some anatomical transparent preparations of sections of the limbs, and described his method of preparing and mounting them. These gentlemen exhibited their specimens and gave a further demonstration in the Museum in the afternoon.

On Saturday, the subject of Cranial Measurements was again brought forward by Professor Benedikt (of Vienna), who described a new method of measurement by means of an instrument which he had invented, and showed some drawings which he had made by this process. Professor Hannover (of Copenhagen) next gave a most lucid and interesting account, in English, of the Primordial Cartilage of the Human Skull, and showed several embryonic cartilaginous crania and some special preparations, demonstrating that Meckels' cartilages do not unite in the median line, as is generally supposed, but that they are separated by a slight interval and terminate in a hooked extremity ; and Professor Redfern made a few remarks on the insignificance of the question as to whether ossification is preceded by cartilage, or takes place in an original fibrous membrane. Another very important communication was read by Dr. Cunningham (of Edinburgh) on the importance of the Nerve Supply in determining the Homology of Muscles in different animals. He considered that attention should be given thereto, as well as to the mere attachments, but could not go so far as to accept the position of Dr. Ruge (of Heidelberg), who has recently asserted that the nerve-supply is an infallible guide in determining these questions. Professors Macalister, Kölliker, Struthers, Turner, and Mr. Forbes took part in the discussion, and showed that the segmentation of the primitive muscle masses was so very different in different animals that questions of homological relationship were very difficult to make certain of, and required great caution in handling, although their study was most interesting and captivating. Dr. Fesebeck, of Brunswick, gave a short description of some exquisite dissections which he has made to prove the independence of the small or motor portion of the fifth nerve ; and Dr. Howard pointed out the anatomical mechanism by which a post-oral passage may be secured for the entrance of air into the lungs in cases of threatened apnœa.

On resuming the business of the Section on Monday, Professor Kölliker gave an excellent resumé in English of his views on the formation of the embryonic mesoderm, as seen by him in the rabbit. In this animal he had clearly traced its derivation from the cells of the ectoderm, but thought that it might arise differently in different animals, and so in some cases be derived from the endoderm as described by some other embryologists. Even at the earliest periods the cells of the mesoderm resemble connective tissue corpuscles, and not epithelial cells, although subsequently in certain places they may be transformed into the latter.

Professors His, Schäfer, and Allen Thomson took part in a discussion ; after which, Professor Kölliker, in response to a request made by Professor Turner, explained his views of the formation of the chorda dorsalis from the mesoderm, and not from the endoderm, as is often supposed. Professor Kölliker exhibited some specimens of embryos in support of his views, and illustrated his communication by some remarkably clear drawings on the blackboard as he proceeded with his remarks. The Professor next made a communication on behalf of his son, Dr. Theodore Kölliker, "On the Human Intermaxillary Bone." Dr. Kölliker had demonstrated its separate existence in fœtuses of eight weeks old, but at the end of the ninth week it was always fused with the superior maxilla. The number of teeth in the intermaxillary bone was not constant. Mr. Fenwick then gave a clear account of the subcutaneous veins of the trunk, as described by him under the supervision of Professor Braune (of Leipzig). He stated that he had been obliged to make as many as 500 or 600 injections in order to fill the system completely. They might be arranged into three zones—an upper zone, running into the axillary vein ; a lower zone, into the femoral ; and an intermediate zone, destitute of valves,—emptying themselves indiscriminately into either of the other sets. The communication between the portal system and the epigastric veins, by means of Sappey's vein, in the round ligament of the liver, was also shown. Professor Braune referred to the pump-like action on the venous circulation, of the movements of the fascia at the points where the veins pass through, and to the arrangement of the valves at these points. The remainder of the session was occupied with a spirited discussion on Anatomical Teaching, introduced by Professor Struthers, who compared British and Continental schools with the object of stimulating the improvement of the former, which he regarded as deficient, except in respect to surgical anatomy ; and with another communication, by Professor Keen (of Philadelphia), on the advantages of a systematic use of the living subject in facilitating Anatomical Study.

On Tuesday, Mr. Knott (of Dublin) opened the proceedings with an exhaustive account of the cerebral blood sinuses and their variations ; those of forty-four skulls were carefully examined. Dr. Garson read a paper on Pelvic Measurements, with a view to determine which are the most important for the purpose of comparing the pelves of different races, and was of opinion that transverse measurements at the brim were to be preferred to the antero-posterior. The comparative measurements of the pelves of fourteen European females, five Australians, and thirteen Andamanese were given in illustration. Professors Turner, Braune, and Thane suggested other measurements as being likewise of great value. Dr. G. Rein (of St. Petersburg) communicated a paper on the Development of the Mammary Gland, in the course of which he took exception to Dr. Creighton's description of the surrounding fatty tissue taking any part in the formation of the parenchyma of the gland. Dr. Schedeff (of St. Petersburg) read a paper on the Origin of Anencephaly; and Professor Sapolini (of Milan) another on " A Thirteenth Cranial Nerve," for such he considered the origin of the portio intermedia of Wrisburg from the brain to be, and traced it into, the chorda tympani. The proceedings of the Section terminated with a demonstration by Professor Hannover I(of Copenhagen) of the Funiculus Sclerotica in the Human Eye.

Last week we mentioned the opening address in the Section of Physiology, which this week we print elsewhere in our columns, and we mentioned that immediately after the address a discussion on cerebral localisation was begun by Professor Goltz (of Strasburg)—a strong disbeliever, it may be added, in the localisation theory. Time, however, has begun to have its effect on his mind, and if he still maintains that every portion of the brain has the same function as every other portion, it is with a much less tenacious grasp than formerly. His speech was very long and, being delivered in German, intelligible to but a few. Though many were present well qualified to discuss the subject, the only other speakers were Panum (of Copenhagen) and Dr. Gerald Yeo (of King's College). In the afternoon the proceedings were of a more interesting character. Goltz had brought with him a dog which had been operated on, and which was supposed to illustrate his views, but we fear not very successfully. On the other hand, Ferrier showed two monkeys on which he had operated some time ago, and which, as far as the condition of two animals could, amply confirmed the views he has already enunciated. One he had long ago rendered hemiplegic, and from this hemiplegia it was gradually recovering, just as in man. One side had been completely paralysed, but the animal had recovered some power of the lower limb, so that it was able to walk about exactly as do recovering hemiplegics. But the upper extremity was beginning to pass into the rigid state, with the forearm bent on the arm, the hand on the wrist, and the fingers on the palm, just as is seen in man himself. The other monkey showed a condition still more interesting. The centre of hearing, which lies just below the fissure of Sylvius, constituting the so-called superior temporo-sphenoidal lobe, had been destroyed. The hearing had got worse and worse, so to speak, and, when shown, a pistol might be fired off close to the animal's ear without making it start in the slightest degree, though the other monkey showed the greatest excitement.

On Friday morning a discussion on the regulation of the heart's action was introduced by Dr. François Frank (of Paris) in a French address. He took the ordinary view with regard to the retardor and accelerator powers of the vagus and sympathetic respectively. He was followed by Mr. Gaskell, who gave the results of a long series of experiments made in Dr. Michael Foster's laboratory at Cambridge. From these he deduced the somewhat heretical doctrine that the vagus was essentially an accelerator nerve, even when producing what seemed to be a perfect standstill. He in turn was followed by Brown-Séquard, and others. In the afternoon there was a demonstration of many useful physiological instruments, some exhibited by a manufactory which has been started in Cambridge.

On Saturday there was no meeting in this Section.

Monday morning's sitting was introduced by a short discussion on the Structure of Muscular Fibre by Professor Rutherford. His most important conclusion was that 'the whole of a muscular element was contractile, the clear as well as the darker part. He was followed by Professor Haycroft (of Birmingham) on the same subject, who in

turn was succeeded by others. The second topic was that of the Structure of Cells, introduced by Dr. Klein, whose views, as illustrated in his "Histology," are now pretty well known. In the afternoon the time was occupied by Donders on the Sensation of Colour, and a demonstration of the Physico-Chemical Properties of the Lecithines by M. le Professeur Dastre.

On Friday, in the Section of Medicine, Dr. Althaus (of London) continued the discussion on "Syphilis as a Cause of Locomotor Ataxy," opened by the paper of Professor Erb the previous afternoon. Dr. Althaus could not agree with Professor Erb—(1) because he finds tabes described, as to symptoms, by Hippocrates, long before syphilis had appeared in Europe; (2) because syphilis imitates, does not cause, independent diseases; and (3) because drugs benefiting locomotor ataxy have no effect on syphilis, and iodide of potassium has no curative effect, merely preventing, in some cases, further increase. Professor Gairdner (of Glasgow) gave it as his impression that Professor Erb's statistics had been compiled under a personal bias; and Professor Lancereaux (of Paris) opposed his conclusions on the ground that syphilitic lesions are circumscribed, while those of locomotor ataxy are diffuse. After a few remarks from Dr. Banks (of Dublin), Dr. Zambaco (of Constantinople), and Professor Rosenstein (of Leyden), Professor Erb replied, opposing strongly the opinion of Professor Lancereaux as to the invariable circumscription of syphilitic lesions.

A full and exhaustive paper by Dr. Greenhow (of London) on "Addison's Disease," was then read by Dr. Ord. A short discussion took place by Professor Semmola, Professor Gairdner, Professor Paget (of Cambridge), Professor Zuelzer, Dr. de Mussy, Dr. Matterson, and Sir William Gull; but, as Professor Gairdner remarked, no one in London or the provinces could pretend to supplement Dr. Greenhow's paper.

On the Section resuming work in the afternoon, Dr. Clifford Allbutt read a short but important paper on "Scrofulous Neck," its causes and treatment. In the discussion, Mr. Frederick Treves (of London) pointed out that while undoubtedly the local causes are highly important, the element of heredity cannot be ignored. The cause of, the glandular swelling, he found, was generally inflammation of adenoid tissue, present in great quantity in the naso-pharyngeal tract; and the treatment he had found most successful in twenty cases was puncturing the glands with a smallish point of Pacquelin's thermo-cautery. Mr. Teale (of Leeds), who had co-operated with Dr. Clifford Allbutt in the treatment of his cases, confirmed the statements of the paper, and expressed his full satisfaction with the results of a removal of local causes and local surgical treatment.

Dr. Woakes (of London) then read a paper on the "Inferior Cervical Ganglion as a Correlating Nerve Centre." The paper, although of an abstruse character, had a markedly practical bearing. It was followed by an important and interesting paper by Dr. William Roberts (of Manchester) on "Bacteruria," worthy of more time than the exigencies of the Section allowed.

On Saturday the working of the Section began ominously. The day had been set apart specially for the discussion of certain questions connected with Bright's disease, but for some reason Dr. Jules Guérin (of Paris) was allowed to begin with a paper on the development of typhoid from cercaceous matter; and he began, and seemed determined to end, a lengthy pamphlet he had written on the subject. Twice the President suggested that the matter might be given in abstract, but Dr. Guérin was not to be disposed of so easily. Finally, however, after talking the better part of an hour, he consented to sit down, evidently considering himself an ill-used man.

Coming to the subject of Bright's disease, the first paper read was of a mixed character. It was by Dr. Garrod, and dealt with kidney-disease and eczema as associated with gout. There was nothing very new in it, but the analysis of a vast number of cases, which accompanied it, will no doubt prove useful when it appears. Dr. Grainger Stewart followed, dealing with the various modifications of the urine in the different forms of Bright's disease. This was both succinct and interesting. Next came Rosenstein (of Leyden), who spoke in German—his subject was the anatomical forms of Bright's disease; whilst Dr. George Johnson took the opportunity of applying his well-known cast theory to the subject of glomerulo-nephritis. After a few words from the President, Semmola (of Naples) spoke, dealing, however, rather with albuminuria than with Bright's disease; and he was succeeded by Stokers (of Amsterdam), who tried to reconcile some apparently conflicting views.

On Monday, August 8, the Section adjourned *en masse* till 11.30 a.m. to the Pathological Section, where an important discussion was to be opened by Sir William Gull on "Renal Disease in relation to Disturbance of the General Circulation."

On the reassembling of the Section, Mr. Jonathan Hutchinson read a paper on "Rheumatism, Gout, and Rheumatic Gout." Dr. Garrod opposed Mr. Hutchinson's views as constituting a distinct step backwards as to the differentiation of disease. Dr. Garrod then discussed eczema and renal disease as manifestations of the gouty diathesis, his observations being derived from 2500 cases. In rheumatoid arthritis there are no tophi, and while, no doubt, the children of gouty parents suffer from this disease, that is simply because they are the children of degenerate parents, and so are liable to this as to other diseases. Sir Robert Christison rarely sees gout in Scotland, while rheumatism is common. Gonorrhoeal rheumatism, Dr. Garrod considered allied to pyæmia, not to either gout or rheumatism. Dr. Roberts (of Manchester), who occupied the chair, continued the discussion, which was taken part in by Professor Stokvis, Dr. Maclagan, Dr. Dyce Duckworth, and others. In his reply, Mr. Hutchinson expressed satisfaction at the substantial agreement with his views. He did not hold that either gout became rheumatism, or rheumatism gout; but that they frequently mingle as do water and spirits. Lithate of soda he considered pathognomonic of gout; but many a person was gouty who showed no deposits. In gonorrhoeal rheumatism there is no tendency whatsoever to the production of pus.

In the afternoon, Professor Eulenburg read a paper on the "Graphic Representation of the Tendon Reflexes." Dr. Buzzard, who occupied the chair, asked Professor Eulenburg's opinion if the knee-phenomenon was really a reflex, considering the short period occupied by it. Professor Eulenburg believed from his experiments that it is not—an opinion concurred in by Dr. Waller (of London).

Dr. D'Espine (of Geneva) then read a paper on "Clinical Cardiography," some of the conclusions in which were opposed by Dr. Barr (of Liverpool).

A paper, by Dr. Bedard (of Paris), on "Local Thermometry," was, in his absence, held as read. Two papers were then read—one by Professor Lépine (of Lyons), on "Biliary Secretions in Morbid States"; the other, by Professor Zuelzer of Berlin), on the "Phosphor-Acids in Urine."

On Tuesday, August 9, the business of the Section was opened by a paper on "The Physical Examination of the Thorax" by Professor Austin Flint (of New York), followed by a paper on "Aphonic or Whispering Pectoriloquy in the Diagnosis of Pleuritic Effusions," by Dr. Douglas Powell (of London). The symptoms of whispering pectoriloquy Dr. Bacelli (of Rome) considers diagnostic of serous effusion into the pleura, and Dr. Powell finds this generally, but by no means invariably, true. Sir William Gull pointed out that as early as 1846 (in *Guy's Hospital Reports*) the importance and *rationale* of this phenomenon had been discussed by Dr. Addison. Dr. Ewald (of Berlin) concurred with Dr. Powell in finding whispering pectoriloquy by no means absolutely diagnostic of serous effusion, the only absolute sign being the serum in a Pravaz syringe used to puncture the chest. Dr. Powell, discussing Professor Flint's paper, remarked that many abnormal sounds believed to be pulmonic were in reality transmitted glottic sounds, *e.g.*, "bronchial breathing" in solidified lung. Professor D'Espine (of Geneva) wished to know Professor Flint's opinion as to the signs of a cavity. Dr. Mahomed (of London) spoke of the confused and undefined character of our nomenclature in physical examination, and urged the appointment by the Congress of a committee to consider and report on this point. Dr. Theodore Williams (of London) pointed out that the sounds given by different instruments differed, and thus, in adopting a common nomenclature, we would require to adopt a common instrument. In his reply, Professor Flint said he purposely avoided going into the *rationale* of lung sounds. "Bronchial breathing" was, he believed, glottic; but the point for us is to hear the sound, and by post-mortem examination verify the existing condition. In this way alone could we be free from fallacy. "Bronchial" and "cavernous" breathing he considered perfectly distinct. For

mediate auscultation he recommended Cameron's stethoscope, supplemented by immediate auscultation.

Sir William Gull proposed that the following committee be appointed to consider the nomenclature of physical signs, viz. : Dr. Ewald (of Berlin), Professor D'Espine (of Paris), Dr. Douglas Powell (of London), and Dr. Mahomed (of London), and Professor Austin Flint (of New York),—which resolution was carried unanimously.

A paper was then read by Dr. C. T. Williams (of London), on "The Treatment of Phthisis by Residence at High Altitudes," followed by a discussion, in which Dr. Norman Chevers (of London), Dr. Hermann Weber (of London), and Dr. Alan Herbert (of Paris) took part.

The Section dissolved at 1 p.m.

In the Section of Obstetric Medicine and Surgery, on Friday, August 6, the main subject of the morning was the operation known as "Battey's." The discussion was opened by Dr. Battey himself, in a communication which, by the author's candour, moderation, and simple desire to arrive at the truth, most favourably impressed the audience. Dr. Savage followed with a virtual reproduction of a pamphlet which it became our duty to criticise a few weeks ago. The discussion was opened by Dr. Priestley, who may be praised for the suavity of his compliments to the writers of the papers and the skill with which he trimmed his course between those who advocate and those who condemn the operation. Mr. Knowsley Thornton forcibly and clearly pointed out the danger of the operation, the very imperfect nature of many of the reports of cases in which it has been performed, and the consequent impossibility of yet determining under what conditions it should be recommended. Dr. Martin, of Berlin, contributed some fresh and valuable facts to the discussion, by briefly and plainly narrating his own experience of the operation; and Dr. Heywood Smith made suggestions as to one or two points in its *technique*. Mr. Lawson Tait then rose, distribute'd a printed sheet containing a list of the cases he had operated upon, and successfully appealed to some gentlemen in the audience (who had seen some of the cases) to confirm the truth of the statements made concerning those cases in the sheet. In this sheet, however, the result of the cases was only indicated by words such as "complete cure," "complete relief,"—terms the meaning of which may, in the minds of different persons, differ; and, will, in the present instance, differ according to what may have been expected from the operation. Results so stated will be entirely conclusive arguments only if we are sure that records have been accurately and completely kept, and if we thoroughly understand the meaning attached to the language used. That at least one of these conditions has not been fully complied with, was shown by an explanation Mr. Tait had to make. He had done two different operations on the same day; one patient had died, and the other recovered. He had forgotten which one it was that died, and which got well, and so had erroneously published a case as fatal which really was one of cure. It is clear from this that the records upon which Mr. Tait bases his statements cannot have been very carefully kept. Certain criticisms imputing a resort to the operation from pecuniary motives, he answered very effectively. The speech of Dr. Goodell, who followed, seemed hardly worthy of his high reputation. He quoted exceptional cases without any recognition of the fallacy of *post hoc ergo propter hoc*, to which his interpretation of them was very open, and spoke of the benefit to be derived in cases of dysmenorrhœa from the mode of treatment recently introduced by Dr. Weir Mitchell (for a condition of a different kind), without any attempt to point out the distinctive marks of such cases. Any harm which that speech might have done was neutralised by Mr. Spencer Wells, who narrated several cases showing the exact opposite to those of Dr. Goodell. The latter speaker (we suppose, by way of a joke) advocated the spaying of all insane women : had he been serious, he surely ought to have also recommended the corresponding operation in insane men! The speech of the morning, however, was made by Dr. Matthews Duncan, who began by expressing his opinion that the operation had been done far too often; and then, with crushing force, displayed the unscientific character of many of the statements and arguments advanced in support of the operation. First, t was recommended because it brought about the menopause. This, however—the very ground and basis of the operation—was not yet proved. Next, the statements made as to the importance and gravity of the nervous and reflex symptoms which called for this operation were enormously exaggerated; the words of women being taken for fact. He narrated a case, that of a lady, whose ovaries it had been proposed to remove on account of the intolerable agony they were supposed to cause her. During the week previous to the consultation with Dr. Duncan—a week in which her sufferings were said to have been indescribable—she had been out to dinner five times, and to the theatre three times! She was, in fact, a discontented woman—nothing more. He referred to assertions often made and implied, especially in American writings, that ovarian neuralgia and hysteria may cause death. In emphatic tones, he said : There is no such thing as death from these causes ; the statement is not true. Lastly, he referred to Mr. Tait's tables, in which he found that out of twenty-six cases of uterine fibroid in which the ovaries were removed, five died. Could anyone, he asked, show such a mortality from fibroids let alone ? Mr. Spencer Wells, commenting on the frequency with which certain surgeons thought it necessary to extirpate the ovaries, said that he himself, somehow, did not see the cases ; perhaps they all went to Birmingham. It is indeed an astounding thing that in a provincial town two surgeons should within ten years meet with more than one hundred cases in which this operation was absolutely necessary, while in the same time the greatest living authority on diseases of the ovary —a man of world-wide fame—found so few cases in which he could advise it that they could be counted on the fingers of one hand ! To give another illustration of the same thing, Dr. Battey, the introducer of this operation, to whom persons go from all parts for his opinion as to its advisa- bility, has in nine years met with sixteen cases in which he could advise it. But in Birmingham a larger number have presented themselves in as many months in the practice of each of two medical men !

Dr. Bantock added his voice to those who condemn the way in which the operation has been hitherto performed. An interesting bye-point was that both Mr. Spencer Wells and Dr. Pallen mentioned cases in which clitoridectomy had been performed for the cure of onanism ; without the slightest benefit.

The remainder of the time was occupied by papers by Dr. Graily Hewitt and Dr. Edis, bearing chiefly on the reflex effects of uterine disease. The discussion took place in the afternoon, when the attendance was but small. Communica- tions were also read, bearing upon the subject of uterine deviations, by Dr. P. F. Mundé (of New York), Dr. Beverley Cole (of San Francisco), and Dr. Verrier (of Paris).

On Saturday, the first subject down for consideration was the operation of extirpating the cancerous uterus, devised by Professor Freund. Dr. Freund was not present : therefore his paper was read by one of the secretaries. Drs. Martin (of Berlin), Hennig (of Leipsic), and Czerny (of Vienna) gave their experience of this operation, and of the methods for effecting the same thing practised by Schroeder, Billroth, and others. The results they brought forward were more favour- able than those previously known to British surgeons. Drs. Marion Sims and Wynn Williams described the mode they adopted to destroy malignant disease of the cervix, but brought forward no new point. Dr. Marcy (of Chicago) showed some new drainage-tubes, suitable for these as well as other cases. Mr. Spencer Wells pointed out how rarely we meet the cases requiring this operation—viz., those in which the disease is so far advanced as to be beyond re- moval by amputation or the caustic, and yet not so ex- tended as to involve more than the uterus. More general interest seemed to be aroused when the question of the operative treatment of laceration of the cervix was raised by Dr. Henry Bennett. This author thought the operation seldom called for and of little use. Dr. Playfair, in an animated speech, described how he at first had a strong prejudice against the operation, but had been converted by clinical experience, and now regarded it as one of the most important improvements of modern times. He stated, how- ever, his belief that it had been done very often without necessity ; and Dr. Goodell, who followed, candidly confessed that he had done it in many cases which now, with greater knowledge, he would let alone. Dr. Playfair described the cases in which its utility had been most striking—cases of cervical endometritis, easily curable by other means, but

constantly relapsing ; repair of the cervix, on the contrary, producing a permanent cure. There can be no doubt that the prejudice against this operation at one time felt by many English gynæcologists was excited by the exaggerated lan- guage in which its benefits were described by American writers. What has to be done is to point out exactly what are the cases in which the operation is required. Dr. Play- fair specified some such ; and we have no doubt his speech will greatly promote the adoption of the operation in this country. For their fertility of resource and inventive genius, for their industry of research and enthusiasm for their sub- ject, American gynæcologists command the admiration of the scientific world ; and if they would add to these a little greater exactness in their statements, and more caution before too hastily judging of results, their improvements would meet with more rapid acceptance.

As was stated last week, the real work in the Section of Diseases of Children was inaugurated by a discussion on the Treatment of Spinal Curvature, with especial reference to Sayre's method. Several interesting communications were read, after which the discussion was commenced. Mr. Arthur Barker (of London) generally spoke in its favour ; as did Dr. Oxley (of Liverpool) : this last gentleman mentioned some important points in carrying out the treatment, suggesting a means by which personal cleanliness might be largely attended to, even while the treatment was carried out in its entirety. Mr. Owen spoke in a more guarded manner, and, with Mr. Morgan, and other speakers, questioned both the value and the propriety of the extension, on which Professor Sayre seemed to set much value. Dr. Diver (of Kenley) was in favour of the entire plan. Mr. Bernard Roth thought it very useful in Pott's disease, but not in cases of lateral curvature. Mr. Reeves was in favour of the old method of treatment by spinal apparatus. Mr. Holmes summed up the arguments for and against, saying there appeared to be a general consensus of opinion that the method was a real and great advance in practical surgery. Professor Sayre (of New York), in the course of his remarks, drew especial attention to the fact that he had advocated suspension, not to overcome the angular projection, but to reduce the reflex muscular tension which was present in all cases of joint-disease, and largely contributed to it.

The real position of the so-called Rubeola, Rötheln, or German Measles, and its relation to scarlatina and measles, was the next subject, and gave rise to an interesting discus- sion. Dr. Cheadle (of London), in a careful paper, not only insisted that rötheln exists as a separate disease, but also that it might occur in a severe form which was little recognised, or classed as an exceptionally severe variety of common measles. Dr. Squire (of London) also believed in its separate identity ; he regarded it as self-protective, as distinct from measles as varicella from variola, contagious, and as occurring but once in the same person. Dr. Kassowitz (of Vienna) thought that if it had any special relationship with another exanthem, it was with measles rather than scarlet fever. Dr. Lewis Smith (of New York), Dr. Shuttleworth (of Lancaster), Drs. Fergus and Glaister (of Glasgow), Dr. D'Espine (of Geneva), Dr. Jacobi (of New York), all believed in the existence of this disease as a separate and distinct form, in which opinion Dr. West coincided. Mr. Howard Marsh (of London) introduced the subject of so- called "Surgical Scarlet Fever." M. Trélat (of Paris) and Dr. Riedinger (of Würzburg) both agreed with him that it was only a form of ordinary scarlet fever. Hereditary Syphilis as a cause of Rickets naturally gave rise to an animated debate. M. Parrot (of Paris), who first in this country enunciated this doctrine at the Pathological Society of London last year, has advanced in his views, so that he now teaches that syphilis is the cause of rickets. M. Parrot, however, found but one supporter for his views. On the other hand, Dr. Bouchut (of Paris) held that syphilis was not a direct factor, its influence (if any) being similar to that which other dyscrasiæ produce. M. Jules Guérin (of Paris) followed, and spoke strongly against the doctrine. Professor Ranke (of Munich) also ex- pressed his inability to accept it. Dr. Byers (of Belfast), Dr. Lee (of London), and Dr. Sansom (of London) followed in the same strain. Dr. Gibert (of Le Havre) said he was a convert to Parrot's views, malgré lui. The President thought that M. Parrot's conclusions were as yet "not proven."

M. Magitôt (of Paris) introduced the subject of Syphilitic

Teeth, by a paper in which "it was considered as a retrospective sign of infantile convulsions." He failed, on the one hand, to prove the absence of syphilis, while, on the other, no attempt was made to explain the reason of the convulsions. It appeared to us as though what he described, and what English surgeons know as "Hutchinson's teeth," were two very different lesions. Mr. Moore and Mr. Coleman (both of London) joined in the discussion.

The Pathology and Treatment of Genu Valgum gave rise to a long discussion. Dr. MacEwen (of Glasgow) advocated section of the femur above the condyles. In this manner the knee-joint was not interfered with; while the lower part of the femur, which was primarily at fault in a large proportion of the cases, was attacked at the seat of the pathological lesion causing the deformity. While Dr. Little (of London) believed that the use of instruments sufficed in all the milder forms, he thought that for the severer cases MacEwen's plan was the best. Mr. Brodhurst (of London) advocated tenotomy and instruments, and strongly disapproved of any operation which directly involved the bone. This was also Mr. Heary Baker's view. Most of the speakers seemed to think that, with proper instruments and time, operative measures were not called for during childhood while the bones are soft; and Mr. Holmes (London) also seemed to be of this opinion.

Diphtheria was taken in hand on Monday morning, August 8, and led, as might be expected, to considerable discussion. The conditions governing the occurrence of albuminuria, and of paralysis as attendant on it or as its sequela, were first discussed; and the nature and mode of propagation of its contagium were next brought up. Dr. John Abercrombie (of London) read a very carefully prepared paper on Diphtheritic Paralysis, which received the President's commendation. Dr. Jacobi seemed to think that the contagium was of a chemical nature, but his reasons for so doing did not transpire. Dr. Hubert Airey (of London), in a well-written paper, which was illustrated with charts, gave his reasons for believing that the contagium is carried by the wind. As regards the surgical treatment of croup and diphtheria, nothing very materially new transpired. Professor Buchanan (of Glasgow) read a short practical paper; and Mr. MacEwen advocated the use of tubes passed by the mouth into the larynx, instead of tracheotomy. Mr. Bird preferred dilators to the ordinary tube. Professor Ranke also spoke.

On the Surgical Treatment of Empyema there was a fairly unanimous opinion that aspiration ought to be tried before other means were resorted to. Dr. Gerhardt (of Würzburg) introduced the subject in a practical paper; but there was nothing very worthy of note in it. Among the speakers may be mentioned Dr. Jacobi, Dr. Lee, Mr. B. Cross (of Bristol), Mr. Parker (one of the Secretaries, of London), Mr. Holmes, and Dr. West.

Dr. Steffen (of Stettin) opened the debate on the Relationship of Chorea to Rheumatism. This was followed by others—from Dr. Octavius Sturges, who regards chorea as a psychic manifestation; from Dr. Mackenzie, who gave an analysis of all the cases which had been treated in the London Hospital during the past six years, showing a marked relationship between it and rheumatism—a view, moreover, sustained by Drs. Barlow and Warner, who also introduced a new element into the discussion. These gentlemen related some cases of rheumatism characterised by the occurrence of small subcutaneous nodules close to bones or tendons, without chorea; but they had observed these same nodules occurring in chorea without rheumatism, and hence concluded that as the nodules were common both to rheumatism and chorea, there must necessarily be a connexion between the rheumatism and the chorea. Want of time prevented the point being fully discussed; and, moreover, much shortened the debate on joint-disease, which immediately followed.

Two able papers, however, were read on "The Treatment of the Diseases of the Joints, with a view to the Prevention of Deformity," which will afford much matter for future thought —one by Professor Hueter (of Greifswald), and the other by Professor Ollier (of Lyons); while Mr. Morgan, Mr. Marsh, Mr. S. Bruton, and others took part in the rather brief discussion that followed.

The work in this Section was carried on with considerable spirit; all the time at the disposal of members—twenty-one hours—was fully occupied, and some papers had to be passed over for want of time. Upwards of 500 members inscribed their names in the book kept for the purpose, and if we refer back to the speakers, it will be conceded that most of those

who are best known in this department of practice took part in the work of the Section.

Dr. West(a) presided with all the ability which he is known to possess, both as a speaker and as an experienced president: not a little of the success is due to this fact. Mr. Holmes, the Surgical Vice-President, conducted the surgical debates.

In the Section of Mental Diseases, on Wednesday, August 3, the President (Dr. Lockhart Robertson) delivered his introductory address on "Lunacy in England," which will be published in full in our pages shortly.

He considered that the increase in the number of lunatics under treatment was due to no real invasion of lunacy, but to the greater diligence with which the insane were now sought out and secluded. He touched on the subjects of lunacy legislation, the management of county asylums, and of registered hospitals. While disapproving of the principle that anyone should derive profit from the detention of the insane, he was at the same time opposed to any interference of the law with the private asylums now existing. He disagreed with the action of the Commissioners of Lunacy in restricting the licences of houses for a few patients; in his opinion the results of home care, which had been so strongly advocated by Baron Mundy, of Moravia, were highly satisfactory. Dr. Robertson concluded by drawing attention to the numerous objects, comprising a large collection of brains of criminals, photographs of the insane, some fine microphotographs upon a very large scale of sections of the spinal cord, plans, drawings, and photographs of asylums and asylum requisites, which were on view in the rooms devoted to the Section.

On Thursday, August 4, Dr. Fournié (of Paris) read a paper on the Physiological Pathology of Hallucinations, in which he advocated the view, which met with general acceptance, that an hallucination was an act of over-vivid memory; and he explained his views as to the nature of the process in the brain on which this over-vivid memory depends.

Dr. Foville read a paper on Megalomania, which, he asserted, was of two kinds—in the first the delusions being transitory, incoherent, and absurd; while in the second they are persistent and systematised. The first variety occurs in general paralysis and in certain other conditions; the second forms a distinct species of chronic incurable insanity. Dr. Holler (of Vienna) described his Method of Preparing Large Sections of Human Brains for Microscopical Examination (a method resembling that of Dr. Sankey), and exhibited sections prepared by this means. Dr. Savage described some Changes produced in Nervous Tissue by Spirit Hardening, to which he attributed the appearances described as miliary sclerosis. Dr. Clouston then read his paper on Teaching of Psychiatric Medicine, in which he insisted on the importance of a knowledge of mental diseases, and the prime importance of this knowledge being gained by the student by actual face-to-face converse with patients. Well-marked cases should be selected, and their essential features pointed out; the student should actually draw up and sign certificates, should see and handle brains in which pathological changes are well marked, and should be taught to associate together in his mind mental symptoms and brain changes as necessary associates. Questions on mental diseases should be set at examinations, and at all examinations for honours psychiatric medicine should be an optional subject.

On Friday, August 5, the discussion of Dr. Clouston's paper on the teaching of psychiatric medicine was resumed. Dr. Hack Tuke animadverted on the attitude of the London University, which, while accepting an attendance of three months in a lunatic asylum in lieu of a similar attendance in a hospital, yet maintained so crowded a curriculum in other subjects that the concession had become a mockery.

(a) In our last week's number some printer's devil, no doubt a highly instructed product of a Schoolboard School, thinking that our simple "Dr. West" was not respectful enough, got at Churchill's "Directory" for a West with a satisfying Christian name, and a fitting array of initials to append. The result was that Dr. West or Charles West, M.D., known all the world over as a high authority on Diseases of Children, was made to give way as President of this Section to a rising young physician of London, who is not at present, at least, at all especially interested in the subject.

If a knowledge of mental diseases were made compulsory to candidates for degrees, the difficulty in the way of gaining clinical instruction would soon disappear. Dr. Macdonald (of New York) had had to overcome many prejudices in establishing a course of clinical instruction, but had found that the patients were much benefited by the change involved, and that the average quality of the certificates he now received was much higher than before. Professor Ball (of Paris) had found no want of interest taken in mental diseases by the students, nor any inferiority in the results of examinations on this as compared with other subjects. He insisted on the necessity of practical instruction by the exhibition of cases, and considered that the sentimental objection to the exhibition of cases of insanity for this purpose was absurd and detrimental to their true interests. Dr. E. Forbes Winslow stated that his class, which had originally consisted of from two to four students, now numbered between forty and fifty. He thought that attendance on the lectures should be compulsory. Dr. Maudsley, speaking as a member of the Senate of the London University, admitted and regretted the absence of mental diseases from the curriculum. He had brought the matter before the Senate, by whom it had been attentively considered, but the difficulty of getting clinical instruction for the students had been found insuperable. He reminded members of the great difference between Edinburgh, where there was one school controlled by one central authority, and an asylum within very easy reach, and London, where there were twelve or thirteen schools and no central authority. Everyone would admit the desirability of the clinical instruction of students, but he believed that it was not at present possible to provide it. Dr. Mould, whose asylum was distant nine miles from Owens College, had found no difficulty in getting students to come that distance for instruction. Dr. Clouston, in replying, considered that what could be done in Paris and New York could be done in London by sufficient enthusiasm and attention being directed to the subject, and that if the subject were made compulsory, even to the extent of a single question being set upon it in the medical examinations, great good would be done.

Professor Ball then read a paper on the occurrence of Mental Symptoms in certain cases of Paralysis Agitans, and gave abstracts of cases in which such symptoms had occurred. The mental aberration ranged from mere restlessness and irritability, to hallucinations, insanity of suspicion, suicidal tendencies, lypemania, and dementia; and the severity of the mental aberration bore no proportion to the severity of either the motor disturbance or the pain. Dr. Savage said that, in his experience, diseases of the nervous system terminating in intellectual disorders were more often associated with the sensory than with the motor tract, and in this respect the cases related by Professor Ball must be looked on as exceptional. He was aware of a few such cases, which he related in brief: one of insular sclerosis, passing through lypemania and excitement to dementia; and one of general paralysis supervening on essential paralysis. If, as Professor Ball thought, paralysis agitans was a neurosis, it ought to breed true, as in hysteria, melancholia, and other neuroses. Dr. Mercier thought that in every case of paralysis agitans there was intellectual defect; but that this defect, being of a purely negative character, was overlooked in consequence of the greater prominence of the physical symptoms. Dr. Ringrose Atkins (of Cork), Dr. Hack Tuke, Dr. Bucknill, and Dr. Huggard also took part in the discussion; and Dr. Ball replied to the various speakers.

Dr. Motet read a paper of great interest on mania following "shock" of various kinds, occurring during alcoholism, and showing the similarity of effect produced by traumatic fever, non-traumatic fever, or "artificial traumatism," and moral shock. In the discussion which followed, Drs. Ashe, Mercier, Maudsley (who suggested the existence of hereditary predisposition in the cases related by Dr. Motet), Clouston, and Benedikt took part. Papers by Drs. Beach and Shuttleworth on Idiocy were then read.

On Saturday, August 6, the discussion on the papers of Drs. Shuttleworth and Beach was opened by Dr. Huggard, who argued from the extreme malformations of the cranium deliberately produced by the parents among aboriginal tribes, without any consequent mental impairment on the part of the children so malformed, that when injuries are received during parturition, and are causes of mental defect subsequently appearing, such injuries must be suddenly produced. Further, that the respective deformities of brain

and of skull must not be considered as either causing the other, but as being both due to a common cause. Dr. Ireland believed that synostosis was not always the cause of microcephaly. the latter being evident in some cases with open fontanelles and ununited sutures; and he could not allow that hour-glass contraction of the uterus upon the cranium was a probable cause. The number of cases rendered idiotic by the use of the forceps was, he believed, very small; and many more were damaged by prolonged labour, whose mental defect might have been prevented by the use of the forceps. Dr. Delly took exception to the use of the terms "Mongolian" and "Kalmuck," as applied to idiots. Far from having the large, bold, open orbit and heavy jaw of the Mongolian races, idiots of this type had characters just the reverse. He did not think that the scapho-cephalic condition was due to compression during labour. Dr. Crochley Clapham and Dr. Hack Tuke also spoke.

Dr. Shuttleworth, in replying, said that of the various forms of cranial malformation the "Mongolian" type was comparatively common, pure microcephaly rare, and, in his experience, in the North of England cretinoid idiots were very rare. In cases of hydrocephaly, when active symptoms have subsided, great intellectual improvement may be effected by education. He believed that the deficiency in the occipital regions of the brain to which attention had been drawn was due to the anterior part of the brain being developed first, and the arrest of development occurring rather late. Dr. Fletcher Beach, in replying, admitted that high palates were not confined to idiots, but contended that when they occurred in them they proved the idiocy to be congenital.

Professor Tamburini then read, on Cerebral Localisation and Hallucinations, a brief but weighty paper, in which he brought forward certain facts and considerations in support of the hypothesis that hallucinations are due to disease of the sensory cortical centres. Professor Ferrier said that the labours of various workers in the field of localisation, while not agreeing as to the exact limitations of particular areas, yet determine, beyond question, the existence of distinct regions in which impressions are received, and that hallucinations occur from the morbid excitation of these sensory centres, just as convulsions occur from the morbid excitation of motor centres. He referred to the experiments previously shown in the physiological section, as proving to demonstration the existence of an auditory centre, and asserted the existence of similarly localised areas for sight, for tactile sensibility, for smell, and for taste. These facts of localisation once established, continued the Professor, will lend psychologists the most valuable assistance, and if this line of investigation is followed out, we shall arrive at a localisation both as to subjective and objective aspects which will be of enormous influence, and in time will become the basis of practical treatment both of nervous diseases and of insanity.

Dr. Benedikt (of Vienna) then read a paper on the Brains of Criminals, illustrated by forty-eight hemispheres of thirty criminals. From researches on these he claimed to have arrived at the positive result that the brains of criminals were distinguished from those of well-conducted people by the tendency of their fissures to run together. In great detail the connexions of the different fissures, and the relative frequency with which they occurred in his specimens and in more normal brains. After a few words from Dr. Maudsley and Dr. F. Beach, Dr. Crichton Browne asked if Dr. Benedikt was willing to submit to the test of picking out from one hundred brains of ordinary people the brains of twenty criminals mixed indiscriminately among them. He considered that the distinction alleged by Dr. Benedikt was merely this—that the brains were of a simple type, and that they differed in no recognisable respect from ordinary brains of inferior character and development. These views met with the general concurrence of the meeting.

Dr. Alexander Robertson (of Glasgow) read a paper on Unilateral Hallucinations and Localisation, in which he related many cases of hallucinations of the various senses, in each of which the morbid appearance was referred to one side, and he discussed the probable position of the nervous centres concerned in the disorder.

After a brief discussion, Dr. Hack Tuke read a paper on Mental Stupor, in which he sought, by an analysis of three cases of mental stupor, to show that this condition is allied to somnambulism, and that acute dementia should be considered as a variety of mental stupor combined with melancholia. In the discussion which followed, in which Dr. C. Browne, Dr. Clouston, Dr. Bonville Fox, and Dr. Mortimer Granville took part, the balance of opinion was against the views of Dr. Tuke.

On Monday, August 8, Professor Tamburini read a paper on Hypnotism, describing and illustrating by graphic tracings the surprising effect which the mere approach of the hand to the epigastrium and other parts of the body of patients in this condition had upon the frequency and depth of the respiratory act. On its conclusion, Dr. Gasquet said that the detail and scientific severity of Professor Tamburini's observations, which were a model of investigation, precluded discussion of the subject without serious study. Only when the paper appeared in the transactions could it be considered where these important facts would lead us. Dr. Rayner read a paper on Gout and Insanity, in which he drew attention to the several ways in which gout could affect the nervous system, and so produce insanity. For the purposes of this subject he divided gout into three forms—the retrocedent form, in which the gout after appearing was driven back into the system; the atonic form; and the restrained or intensive form, in which all the joints having been frequently affected, have at last lost their power of giving relief. He related cases of each form, spoke of the connexion between insanity and lead- and alcoholic-poisoning and gout, and stated that the recognition of gout in a case of insanity enabled us to give a much more hopeful prognosis. Finally, he believed that a protracted and mild form of gouty toxæmia caused hallucinations, a sudden and intense toxæmia produced epilepsy or acute mania, and a protracted and intense toxæmia caused general paralysis. Dr. Savage related a case in which the attack of gout was simultaneous with the sudden disappearance of suicidal mania. Having previously doubted the existence of suppressed gout, he had now become a convert. Dr. Crichton Browne said he believed that there was no essential or necessary connexion between gout and insanity, because tens of thousands of people suffer with gout without becoming insane; but when gout occurs in people in whom there is an hereditary predisposition to insanity or epilepsy, then the nervous disturbance always produced by the gouty attack may mount into actual insanity. He believed that many cases of melancholia attonita occurring in young girls with feeble circulation were associated with inherited gout, and such cases were much relieved by arsenic.

Dr. Lasègue demonstrated his views as to the various forms of Epileptic and Epileptoid Convulsion, in a speech which was admirably delivered and frequently applauded.

Dr. Bucknill then read a paper of great eloquence and learning on Testamentary Incapacity, criticising with great force the doctrine laid down by the late Lord Chief Justice of England in the case of Banks v. Goodfellow. An animated discussion of this paper concluded the business of the Section, after which cordial votes of thanks were tendered to the President, Dr. Lockhart Robertson, and the Secretaries, Drs. Savage and Gasquet. On Tuesday the members of the Section visited the Criminal Asylum at Broadmoor; and on the previous Sunday a party of them enjoyed the hospitality of Dr. Savage at the Bethlem Convalescent Home at Witley, near Godalming.

In the Section of Diseases of the Teeth, on Thursday, August 4, the subject for discussion was the Transplantation and Replantation of Teeth, communications being contributed by Dr. Magitôt (of Paris) and Dr. Finley Thompson (of London). Dr. Magitôt, who addressed the meeting in French, gave the results of 100 cases in which the operation of replantation had been undertaken for the cure of chronic alveolar periostitis. Minute particulars of each case were contained in the tables accompanying the paper, and the result claimed was that the disease in question was curable by replantation in 92 per cent. of the cases. A paper on the same subject was then read by Dr. Finley Thompson, who, having described and illustrated by diagrams the structure of the pericementum, the membrane on which the operation of replantation was wholly dependent for its success, showed that the existence of protoplasmic cells in this membrane at once established a *primâ facie* case in favour of the probability of union taking place between the alveolus and a replanted tooth. Dr. Thompson claimed

two advantages for replantation in extreme cases—one being the promptness of the relief it gave, the other that it did not require the continued services of the practitioner. The disadvantages were—first, the patient's repugnance to the operation, and the constant care required on his part for the first few days after its performance; and, secondly, the known danger attending extraction. Dr. Thompson concluded by stating that, of the eighty cases which had come under his notice, 88 per cent. were successful. The President having thanked Dr. Thompson for his paper on behalf of the Section, Mr. C. S. Tomes produced a tooth which had been the subject of unsuccessful replantation. Dr. Taft, of Cincinnati, then proceeded to open the discussion. He said that he had in his own practice confined the operation of replantation to very obstinate cases of alveolar abscess. He did not regard the periosteum as an indispensable element in the reunion of the tooth with its socket; but it was nevertheless important to injure it as little as possible. The discussion was continued by Mr. Coleman, who thought that Dr. Magitôt had brought success up to a point where replanting might be regarded as a legitimate operation; by Dr. W. H. Atkinson (of New York) who spoke in praise of individual histological research; by Mr. Balkwill, who attributed failure to absorption of the root caused by the scraping off of the periosteum preparatory to replantation; and by Dr. Joseph Izalai, who expressed a doubt as to the utility of the operation in cases of alveolar periostitis, and preferred treating such cases by disinfecting the pulp cavity. This was also the view of Mr. Spence Bate, who said that he was decidedly against replantation where inflammatory action was present to any large extent. After a proposal of Mr. S. J. Hutchinson to take the opinion of the meeting on certain questions connected with the subject had been rejected, the discussion was brought to a close by a few remarks from Mr. Browne Mason.

A paper was then read by Mr. Daniel Corbet (of Dublin), entitled, "Interrupted Second Dentition as a cause of Reflex Constitutional Disturbance," in which the importance of dental experience in many otherwise medical cases was especially insisted on.

In the afternoon sitting, which was poorly attended, papers by Dr. Arköry, of Buda-Pesth, Mr. Gaddes, and Mr. A. Coleman were read. Dr. Arköry's communication gave the results of experiments which he had made on dogs, with the object of discovering the relative influence of different agents as devitalisers of the tooth pulp. Briefly, his conclusions were that arsenious acid and pepsine are the only available agents; that neither acts except when in direct contact with the pulp; that arsenious acid is the more powerful, but at the same time by far the more dangerous of the two, and that in certain cases which he formulated pepsine should be used in preference. Mr. Gaddes' communication was a plea for the better instruction of army medical officers in dental surgery, and Mr. Coleman's was a most favourable record of the experience of the Dental Hospital of London in the use of anæsthetics.

At the sitting on Friday, the 5th inst., the subject for discussion was "Premature Wasting of the Alveoli (Rigg's Disease) and its Amenability to Treatment." Dr. W. H. Atkinson opened the discussion by reading a paper, in which he contended that the disease in question was due to debility, and that a vigorous removal of the dead bone, until living tissue was reached, was the true conservative treatment. Dr. Walker exhibited microscopical specimens and diagrams illustrating on the one hand the normal processes of bone-formation and bone-absorption, and on the other the abnormal processes of inflammation and recedence of the gum. The starting-point of the disease was shown to be a subacute inflammation in the periosteum, whence it passed to the bone; and the point of interest was to account for the great activity of this subacute process. Dr. Arköry detailed inquiries he had made to elucidate the pathology of "Rigg's disease," and described the forms of microzymes he had found in the course of his research. Similar remarks were contributed by Dr. Izalai; and Dr. J. M. Rigg then gave a brief account of his forty years' experience of the disease, which some of his New England friends had done him the honour to name after him. In the first stage only the margin of the gum was affected, but in the second stage the absorbents participated, pus was poured out, and the edge of the alveolar border began to break down. The only treatment was surgical—to remove with a firm but

90 per cent. of the cases would be radically and effectively cured. Mr. Walter Coffin described the treatment which his father had found successful, and which consisted in the mechanical removal of the diseased tissue, and the careful application of hydrate of phenol. The discussion was continued by Mr. Oakley Coles, who called attention to the general health as connected with the causation of the disease, and warned practitioners against a too localised treatment; and by Professor Shepard (of Harvard), who spoke strongly in favour of Dr. Rigg's treatment; and was brought to a close by a reply from Dr. Walker.

A paper was then read by Mr. J. Tomes, F.R.S., on "Dental Education," in which the history of dentistry in England and the passing of the Dentists Act were briefly described. The paper was received with much applause, and after remarks from Dr. Taft, Professor Shepard, and Professor Holländer, the Section adjourned.

In the afternoon the Section had a joint meeting with Section VII., in the rooms of the Antiquaries' Society (Dr. Charles West in the chair), to discuss the subject of "Erosion or Honeycombing of the Teeth." The discussion was opened by Dr. Magitôt, who, in a paper entitled "Honeycombed Teeth regarded as an Evidence of Infantile Convulsions," attempted to refute the hypothesis of Parrot, attributing the appearance in question to hereditary syphilis. The paper was profusely illustrated by models, specimens, and tabulated statistics. A lively discussion followed, in which Mr. Moon, Mr. C. S. Tomes, Dr. Dully, Dr. Blacke, Mr. Hayward, Dr. Parrot, Mr. Coleman, and Mr. Jonathan Hutchinson took part. The most important speech was that delivered by Mr. Hutchinson, who showed that he had never attributed the appearances described by M. Magitôt to syphilis, and admitted that there was some ground for M. Magitôt's conclusion. M. Magitôt replied, and the meeting adjourned.

On August 6 the chief paper was one by Mr. Arthur Underwood and Mr. W. J. Milles, entitled "An Investigation into the Effects of Organisms upon the Teeth and Alveolar Portion of the Jaw." It detailed the varieties of organisms most frequent in the mouth; the conditions favourable to their existence and proliferation; their chemical products; and the conditions which rendered their life impossible. It then went on to describe the effects of organisms upon enamel and upon dentine, the latter being demonstrated by contrasting the destruction of tissue—(a) in teeth subjected to the action of acids under aseptic conditions; (b) in teeth subjected to the action of germs under excessively septic conditions. The paper concluded with an account of the effects of organisms upon the surrounding tissues, and a brief resumé of the author's experience of the eucalyptus oil and iodoform employed in alveolar abscess, in dead roots, and in roots partially dead. After a brief acknowledgment from the President, Dr. Taft (of Cincinnati) said that the experiments were interesting, but looked in one direction only. It was, indeed, impossible to simulate out of the mouth and on dead tissues the changes which took place in the mouth during life. After remarks from Dr. W. H. Atkinson and Mr. S. J. Hutchinson, Mr. J. Tomes said that until they had some better explanation of caries than had been yet brought forward, the theory now advanced might, he thought, be accepted provisionally; while Mr. C. S. Tomes contended that the present researches were the first which had been rigorously made on the production of caries by septic organisms, and they had a practical bearing on the whole of the dentist's work. Mr. Coleman, Mr. Spence Bate, and the President also spoke.

Dr. Dean then read a paper on "Alveolar Abscess," in which he described the method of treatment which he had found most useful in practice.

This was followed by Dr. Norman Kingsley's paper on "Civilisation in its Relation to the Increasing Degeneracy of the Human Teeth." In the course of an eloquent address, Dr. Kingsley showed that civilisation was not responsible for the physical or other evils which follow in her path. These come from the neglect of, or the abuse of, the agencies, the resources, or the products of civilisation. The most alarming evil of civilisation at the present time, from a hygienic view, was the increase of nervous diseases, and coincident with this, and correlated to it (each influencing and in a measure causing the other), was the increasing deterioration of the teeth. In the discussion which followed, Dr. Kirby Beard gave a cordial support to this theory of the author, but M. Magitôt would not accept it without the production of statistics.

On Monday, August 8, the papers were of a very technical nature. Communications were read by Mr. Walter Coffin on "A Generalised Treatment of Irregularities of the Mouth"; by Dr. T. B. Gunning (of New York), on "The Causes of Irregularities of Position of the Teeth"; by Mr. Oakley Coles, on "The Origin and Treatment of certain Irregularities of the Teeth"; and by Dr. Izzlai (of Buda-Pesth), on "Carrabelli's 'Morden Prorsus.'" A brief discussion followed: after which, Mr. A. Coleman read a paper on "Erosion of the Teeth, or Decay by Denudation." He accurately described the disease, which is very different in its nature from ordinary caries, and gave a brief outline of the best treatment. A brief discussion took place, and the meeting adjourned.

The first paper on the last day of sitting was by Dr. Taft (of Cincinnati), on "Antral Abscess." The author described the antrum itself and the parts about it, then went on to deal with the treatment of antral abscess in its simple and complicated forms, considering also the influence of disease arising in this cavity upon other and neighbouring structures, instancing cerebral disease as one of the serious and even fatal maladies which might start from disease of the antrum. Mr. S. J. Hutchinson and Mr. C. S. Tomes having commented on this communication, Dr. Deutz read a paper, in which he suggested that the term caries be abandoned as inappropriate. Caries of the teeth was an affection totally distinct from caries of the bone, and the use of the same term for different diseases caused great perplexity not only to students, but to surgeons and practitioners who did not give a special study to dentistry. Dr. Atkinson combated the views of Dr. Deutz, contending that there was only a difference of degree between caries of the teeth and caries of the bone. Dr. Parmley Brown read an interesting paper on "Contour Restoration of the Superior Central Incisors," and illustrated by means of diagrams his treatment of caries in its several stages. An animated discussion followed, in which the following gentlemen took part:—Dr. Atkinson, Mr. Hutchinson, Dr. Rosenthal, and Mr. Stocken.

The business of this week being concluded, the President, Mr. E. Saunders, delivered a brief address, and after a very cordial vote of thanks had been passed to him, the Section rose.

In the Section of State Medicine, on Thursday morning, August 4, the members were engaged in the consideration of the means by which the spread of communicable diseases from one country to another might be prevented. Dr. Billings (of the United States) opened with a paper detailing the experience of his countrymen with regard to cholera and yellow fever. Dr. Sarell (of Constantinople) reported on the successful results of quarantine in checking the progress of cholera and the plague in South-Eastern Europe and Egypt. Inspector-General Lawson took up the question of yellow fever, and Professor Christie (late of Zanzibar) that of dengue. The latter advanced a theory as to some supposed relation between cholera and dengue, which was unanimously condemned as untenable, especially by Dr. Norman Chevers, and others who had had long experience of both diseases in India.

On Friday, August 5, the morning's sitting was occupied entirely with the question of the prevention of syphilis, papers being read by Drs. Castella (of Turin), Da Cunha Bellem (of Lisbon), Gihon (U.S.N.), Drysdale and Mr. H. Lee (of London), and Dr. Allbutt (of Leeds). The debate was taken up by Drs. Bell Taylor, Nevins, van Overbeek de Meyer, Krauss, Grosz de Czatar, Pacchiotti, Routh, and others. Drs. Bellem and Gihon advocated measures of repression so severe and interfering so constantly with every relation of life as to be justly considered impracticable even by those who most firmly believed in legislation as regards prostitution. The English speakers were either opposed to or incredulous as to the efficacy of the Contagious Diseases Acts, but Dr. Nevins astonished the meeting by asserting that he had never known an infant to die of congenital syphilis, and exhibited a glaring illustration of the misuse of statistics in assuming the deaths registered as such to represent the total mortality from the disease, and actually estimated its prevalence among seamen by the number of sailors afloat who died of or were disabled by it. Dr. Routh assured his foreign friends that, thanks to our higher morality, it was not so terrible or frequent a disease here as it was abroad, and maintained the limited efficacy of legislation. Professor delicate hand all the necrosed portions. By this treatment Pacchiotti, in a most eloquent harangue, urged on all, whether physicians, preachers, parents, or teachers, in public and private, to unite by precept and influence in a crusade against the plague-spot of society; and the other foreign members, admitting the inutility of legislation alone, still held it to be useful, and desired the inspection to be extended to soldiers and sailors. All, however, seemed to agree that the uncertainty of the diagnosis of communicable disease in the female was fatal to the real success of the Contagious Diseases Acts in preventing the spread of syphilis.

In the afternoon the Home Contagia, for the discussion of which no time had been found on the previous day, were taken up, in papers by Drs. De Chaumont; Stopford Taylor, Medical Officer of Health for Liverpool; and Page, Medical Officer of Health for Kendal. Dr. Taylor complained of the importation of typhus into Liverpool from Ireland. Dr. Grimshaw, Registrar-General for Ireland, rejoined by adducing cases of small-pox brought to Dublin from Liverpool, but complimented the authorities of the latter town on their arrangements, by which he had been able to trace the origin of infection of a case of small-pox in Dublin to New York, which the man had left just thirteen days before, passing through Liverpool on his way to Dublin. The importance of registration and medical inspection of emigrants in all cases, and of quarantine under some circumstances, was agreed on.

Dr. Page's paper elicited a discussion on the spread of scarlatina by children in schools, and the necessity for a longer isolation than is commonly enforced; and the feeling in favour of compulsory notification of all dangerous infectious disease was unanimous,—Dr. Grimshaw especially insisting that the first appearance of such in any town should be at once published, that the authorities of others might be put on their guard in time; urging very pertinently that by the time that the deaths have been reported by the Registrar-General the infection has been conveyed far and wide. He showed the fallacy of the argument against interference with the business of private individuals whose houses might be infected, drawn from the loss of trade, by proving from actual instances that the burden thrown on the rates in providing poor relief, in the erection of temporary hospitals, and other measures necessitated by epidemics, far exceeded any the most liberal compensation, or even the entire maintenance of the families first attacked, to say nothing of the private loss of wages, etc.

A member exhibited a disinfecting respirator, for the use of medical men in fever wards, which he considered to be more effectual and certainly more convenient than Dr. MacCormac's proposal to hold one's breath while in immediate contiguity with the patient.

On Saturday morning the relation between food and disease was gone into, Dr. Creighton giving the result of his observations on the pearl disease of cattle, which, contrary to the opinion once enunciated by Virchow, he believed to be truly a tubercular affection communicable to man by the use of milk from animals thus affected. Mr. E. Hart analysed a number of epidemics of scarlatina, diphtheria, and enteric fever, traceable to infected milk-supplies distinctly in twenty, and with more or less probability in thirty more; the number of cases of disease amounting to nearly 5000.

Mr. F. Vacher discussed the communication of specific and other diseases, directly and indirectly, by means of articles of food, whether diseased or putrid meat, or by milk, grocery, etc., which had been handled by persons affected with, or convalescent from, contagious affections. Dr. Ballard recounted the investigation by himself and Dr. Klein as to the outbreak of a peculiar acute specific disease attended by the presence of bacilli, and produced by the consumption of certain hams at Welbeck in 1880; and other gentlemen brought forward cases of sausage-poisoning and of trichinosis. In Dr. Tidy's cases of sausage-poisoning the poison was proved to be a crystalline alkaloid, analogous compounds being obtainable from the stomachs, etc., of persons dying of various diseases.

Later in the day, Dr. Alfred Carpenter entertained a large party at the Old Hall of Beddington, and conducted them over the Croydon Sewage Farm.

On Monday, August 8, Dr. Acland read a paper on International Conditions of Admissibility to Medical Practice, and Drs. Finkelburg (of Bonn) and Rabagliati (of Bradford) on the avoidance of errors in Medical Statistics, and on the

Classification and Nomenclature of Diseases. In the discussions which followed, Dr. van Overbeek de Meyer (of Utrecht) gave some remarkable results of the study of the physiological characteristics of different races as affecting the statistics of disease, from his observations on the two constituents of the Belgian population—the Flemings and the Walloons. Dr. Ezra Hunt (of New Jersey, U.S.A.) desired a classification of diseases for purposes of statistical inquiry, distinct from, though based on the same lines as, the recognised nomenclature of diseases. This should, he held, be simpler and less precise than the nomenclature, but should indicate what diseases were comprised under each of its more comprehensive heads, and should be as far as possible international. Dr. Grimshaw agreed with the last speaker, but deprecated too frequent changes in the statistical classification. The exhaustive nomenclature would change almost from year to year if keeping pace with the progress of pathological science—new diseases being identified, and old ones resolved into others; but if like perfection were attempted in the statistical tables it would be impossible to compare the sanitary condition of a people in one decade with that in a previous one, and the first aim of statistics be defeated. He would, however, approve of Dr. Hunt's suggestion for a definition of each group by an enumeration of the pathological states or minute diseases included from time to time, since this would be of great value for local inquiries and for checking statistics, while the rougher classification would remain intact for general conclusions as to the health of the population.

Dr. van Overbeek de Meyer then read a paper by his friend, Dr. van Capelle (of the Hague), on the Effect of the Legislation of 1875 in checking the spread of Rabies in the Netherlands. At that time the disease had attained such alarming proportions that severe enactments were promulgated, enforcing the slaughter of all affected animals, or of animals bitten by rabid dogs, with the muzzling for four months of all dogs within a certain distance of a place where a case had appeared. The result was a speedy falling off in the returns, those cases which have occurred since 1876 having been, with a very few exceptions, met with in the frontier provinces of Zeeland and Limburg, and therefore presumably imported from France or Germany. Even the exceptions were some of them only apparent, one having been recently brought from England, and another traced to Rotterdam. Dr. Dolan confirmed Dr. van Capelle's views as to the propagation of the disease exclusively by direct contagion, and never de novo, ridiculing the notion that it, any more than small-pox in man, could be induced by deprivation of sexual intercourse. He showed that of 950 cases reported in England in seven years, over 300 occurred in the counties of Lancashire, Cheshire, and the western part of Yorkshire, a district containing a large canine population but little under police inspection. In the same period only forty cases had been known in the whole metropolitan area, and none among packs of hounds, except when one had been bitten by a strange dog. He had drafted a Bill almost identical with the Act of the Belgian Chambers, which he intended pressing on our own Legislature, believing that, by such means, rabies, and with it hydrophobia, might be speedily stamped out. The meeting concurred with these speakers in urging international co-operation for the suppression of these diseases.

Dr. Colam, R.N., gave an account of a disease in some points resembling rabies, which had of late years appeared among the dogs of Greenland; but, as Dr. Dolan remarked, the only constant anatomical lesion observed by Dr. Colam, viz., extensive ulceration of the intestines, resembled rather that seen in distemper, a disease allied to typhoid.

On Tuesday, the discussion on Home Contagia (adjourned from Friday) was concluded.

THE CONGRESS MUSEUM.

[Second Notice.]

DURING the Congress, two American surgical instruments—or rather, machines—were shown, both worked on the lathe principle, and designed generally for the removal of necrosed bone; though Dr. Goodwillies' is specially intended for operations on the nasal and oral bones. Small saws, gouges, and drills are made to rotate very rapidly, and so to excise, closely and quickly, the exact amount of bone desired. The advantages of the machines in operating on exostoses and in limited caries are obvious; but we must hope to be provided ere long with a less cumbrous form of machine than either of these.

Of the other instruments, not many call for special notice. A "tumour-probe" of Dr. Kraus's will be found useful for removing small fragments from the interior of tumours; and Dr. Dudgeon's sphygmograph is a model of compactness and ingenuity.

Some painted transparencies of anatomical sections from Lyons were shown, which might be employed for demonstration.

Dr. Adamkiewicz (of Cracow) had some original drawings in colours and pen-and-ink of the vascular supply of the spinal cord, which deserve the highest praise. They prove that the large vessels enter by the anterior fissure, that each vein and artery passes into both sides of the cord, that the next important vessels form a plexus in the posterior cornua, and that the white matter is comparatively destitute of vessels.

A good wax-model illustrates an elaborate dissection of the superficial abdominal and thoracic veins, made in Leipzig, by Mr. Fenwick.

It appears unfortunate that M. Parrot has chosen to introduce fresh divisions into the life-history of syphilis, which is, perhaps, already too arbitrarily divided: in the bone-lesions alone he speaks of four periods, two of which are further divided into degrees. It is still more unfortunate that his casts of "syphilitic" teeth show what some would call simply varieties of carious or "honeycomb" disease; the only notched teeth being from the temporary set. Surely congenital syphilis cannot differ so much in Paris from that in London? M. Parrot relies, as corroborative signs of syphilis, upon craniotabes in all its forms, rickety bends of the long bones, splenic enlargement, and scars upon the buttocks and condyx; whilst lesions of the eye and ear do not seem to have any prominence. Some beautiful models and bones are used to illustrate this, but it requires much faith to accept a few small non-pigmented scars on a healthy-looking buttock, and a bending forwards and outwards of the tibiae and femora, as proofs of congenital syphilis.

The calculi which are shown as the results of nephrotomy, differ greatly in size. Dr. Patterson's, which were, so to speak, removed as an incident following upon incision for renal abscess, are uric acid calculi, measuring only one-eighth of an inch in diameter. A uric acid stone of Mr. Morris's measured half an inch across, and weighed thirty grains. Both these operations were successful, and, without doubt, saved the patients from the risk of speedy death. Mr. Couper's case, however, was a very different one, as the patient, a woman, was forty-seven years old, and the calculi were three brittle phosphatic ones—half an inch, two inches, and three inches in length.

The living specimens shown at the Museum have been of great interest, including several cases of myxoedema, Charcot's joint-disease, ruptured brachial plexus, and extreme forms of gout and rheumatism. By many these demonstrations have been valued as one of the best features of the Congress.

THE Medical Acts Commission met on the 29th and 30th ult., and also on the 1st inst. Mr. Charles Macnamara, Dr. F. Pocock, Dr. G. Y. Heath, Mr. Henry Morris, Professor Gairdner, Dr. Billings (U.S.A.), and Mr. Thomas Cooke were examined. There were present the Earl of Camperdown (chairman), the Bishop of Peterborough; the Right Hon. W. H. F. Cogan, the Master of the Rolls; Mr. Simon, C.B., Professor Huxley, Professor Turner, Mr. Bryce, M.P., and the Secretary. The Commission has now adjourned for the recess.

THE annual business meeting of the Social Science Association was recently held in Adam-street, Adelphi, Lord Denman presiding. Lord O'Hagan was elected President of the Association for the ensuing year, and the retiring President, Lord Reay, was elected a permanent Vice-President. The nominations of the Right Hon. J. T. Ball, LL.D., and of Lord Powerscourt, as Presidents of the Jurisprudence and Art Departments, were confirmed. Mr. Hastings, M.P., was re-elected President of the Council, and other officials and the standing committees of the Association were appointed. This year's Congress will be held at Dublin, from Monday, October 3, to Saturday, October 8, and the Board of Trinity College have granted the use of their buildings for the purposes of the meeting, which there is every reason to believe will be largely attended.

VITAL STATISTICS OF LONDON.

Week ending Saturday, August 6, 1881.

BIRTHS.

Births of Boys, 1129; Girls, 1113; Total, 2242.
Corrected weekly average in the 10 years 1871-80, 2530·1.

DEATHS.

	Males.	Females.	Total.
Deaths during the week	854	863	1717
Weekly average of the ten years 1871-80, corrected to increased population	876·2	802·4	1462·7
Deaths of people aged 80 and upwards	...	...	60

DEATHS IN SUB-DISTRICTS FROM EPIDEMICS.

	Enumerated Population, 1881 (unrevised).	Small-pox.	Measles.	Scarlet Fever.	Diphtheria.	Whooping-cough.	Typhus.	Enteric (or Typhoid) Fever.	Simple continued Fever.	Diarrhœa.
West	668998	5	11	8	1	...	8	1	...	51
North	905677	9	18	18	...	8	1	2	...	59
Central	261798	...	2	7	1	1	1	...	...	23
East	695530	2	10	7	...	7	...	8	1	64
South	1255576	22	19	17	...	6	...	3	1	62
Total	3814571	38	60	45	4	22	2	10	2	287

METEOROLOGY.

From Observations at the Greenwich Observatory.

Mean height of barometer	29·986 in.
Mean temperature	62·3°
Highest point of thermometer	89·4°
Lowest point of thermometer	45·5°
Mean dew-point temperature	57·6°
General direction of wind	S.W.
Whole amount of rain in the week	0·52 in.

BIRTHS and DEATHS Registered and METEOROLOGY during the Week ending Saturday, August 6, in the following large Towns:—

Cities and boroughs (Municipal boundaries except for London.)	Estimated Population to middle of the year 1881.*	Persons to an Acre. (1881.)	Births Registered during the week ending Aug. 6.	Deaths Registered during the week ending Aug. 6.	Temperature of Air (Fahr.) Highest during the Week.	Temperature of Air (Fahr.) Lowest during the Week.	Temperature of Air (Fahr.) Weekly Mean of Daily Mean Values.	Temp. of Air (Cent.) Weekly Mean of Daily Mean Values.	Rain Fall. In Inches.	Rain Fall. In Centimetres.
London	3829751	50·8	2242	1717	85·4	49·5	63·8	17·97	0·52	1·31
Brighton	107934	45·9	61	34	76·0	51·0	61·9	16·61	0·36	0·91
Portsmouth	128335	28·6	67	51	...	...	...	...	...	...
Norwich	88038	11·8	42	35	...	...	...	...	...	...
Plymouth	75292	54·0	44	14	71·7	49·6	60·1	15·62	1·09	2·67
Bristol	207140	46·5	132	71	78·5	47·5	59·7	15·39	0·70	1·76
Wolverhampton	75934	22·4	44	26	81·3	44·3	59·3	15·17	0·00	0·09
Birmingham	402986	47·9	283	147	...	...	...	...	...	...
Leicester	128120	38·5	85	71	...	...	...	...	...	...
Nottingham	188635	18·9	145	99	83·0	41·1	60·0	15·56	0·38	0·97
Liverpool	553985	106·3	346	290	77·0	50·4	59·6	15·34	0·72	1·83
Manchester	341289	79·5	237	144	...	...	...	...	...	...
Salford	177760	34·4	113	62	...	...	...	...	...	...
Oldham	112176	24·0	65	47	...	...	...	...	...	...
Bradford	184037	25·5	132	76	79·6	47·1	60·1	15·62	0·61	1·55
Leeds	310493	14·4	212	134	81·0	45·0	60·9	16·06	0·84	2·13
Sheffield	295621	14·5	226	110	83·0	44·0	61·2	16·22	0·27	0·69
Hull	155161	42·7	74	86	83·0	43·0	58·8	15·34	1·11	2·82
Sunderland	116754	42·2	99	65	88·0	48·0	62·8	17·12	1·19	3·02
Newcastle-on-Tyne	146675	27·1	88	63	...	...	...	...	...	...
Total of 20 large English Towns	7608775	38·0	4737	3342	88·0	41·1	60·8	16·01	0·65	1·65

* These figures are the numbers enumerated (but subject to revision) in April last, raised to the middle of 1881 by the addition of a quarter of a year's increase, calculated at the rate that prevailed between 1871 and 1881.

At the Royal Observatory, Greenwich, the mean reading of the barometer last week was 29·86 in. The lowest reading was 29·96 in. on Sunday, 31st ult., at noon, and the highest 30·16 in. on Thursday morning.

MEDICAL NEWS.

APPOINTMENTS.

BENNETT, FREDERICK JOSEPH, M.R.C.S. Eng., L.D.S. Eng.—Dental Surgeon to the St. Marylebone General Dispensary.

NAVAL, MILITARY, ETC., APPOINTMENTS.

ADMIRALTY.—Fleet-Surgeon Francis William Davis has been promoted to the rank of Deputy Inspector-General of Hospitals and Fleets in H.M. Fleet, with seniority of August 3, 1881. Fleet-Surgeon Martin Magill, M.D., has been placed on the retired list of his rank.

BIRTHS.

ALLEN.—On August 4, at 40, Wellington-square, Hastings, the wife of B. H. Allen, M.D., of a daughter.

BASHAM.—On July 30, at 70, St. George's-road, the wife of William Richard Basham, M.R.C.S., of a son.

BURROUGHS.—On August 1, at Maison Génet, St. Etienne, France, the wife of Hastings W. Burroughs, M.R.C.S., of a son.

DE CHAUMONT.—On August 5, at Woolston Lawn, Southampton, the wife of Professor F. de Chaumont, M.D., F.R.S., of a son.

HASSARD.—On July 15, at Kussowlie, Punjaub, the wife of Deputy Surgeon-General H. B. Hassard, of a daughter.

PHIPPS.—On August 8, at Clairville, Manchester, the wife of G. Constantine Phipps, M.D., F.R.C.S., of a daughter.

POPHAM.—On August 1, at R.M. Depôt, Walmer, Kent, the wife of T. D. Popham, M.D., R.N., of a son.

ROGERS.—On August 5, at 117, Old-street, Finsbury, E.C., the wife of J. F. Rogers, L.R.C.P., of a son.

SWINTON.—On August 3, at 26, Waterloo-place, Leamington, the wife of Thomas S. Swinton, M.R.C.S., of a daughter.

MARRIAGES.

AYLING—NELSON.—On August 3, at Regent's-park, Arthur H. W. Ayling, Esq., of 94A, Great Portland-street, only son of Dr. Ayling, to Grace Crighton, eldest daughter of James Crighton Nelson, Esq., of 9, St. Andrew's-place, Regent's-park.

CULBARD—McQUIE.—On August 4, at Blundellsands, near Liverpool, Arthur Dingwall Fordyce, only son of Dr. Culbard, of Lagrange, Denkeld, N.B., to Constance Gertrude, third daughter of P. E. McQuie, Esq., of Sunnyside, Blundellsands.

DALZEL—NASH.—On August 2, at Hove, William Frederick Blyth Dalzel, M.D., Surgeon-Major late Bengal Army, to Mary Ann, daughter of the late Thomas Nash, Esq.

FRANCIS—HALE.—On August 4, at Wells-street, Peregrine Charles Colton Francis, Esq., eldest son of the late Col. P. M. Francis, B.E., to Florence Clementine, daughter of R. Douglas Hale, M.D., of Harley-street, W.

HURLEY—WINTER.—On August 4, at Teddington, James Hurley, M.D., to Harriette Emily, second daughter of the late Silas Winter, Esq., R.N.

MACMAMARA—DOORLY.—On June 27, at Port of Spain, Trinidad, W.I., Rawdon Macnamara, Esq., Assistant Colonial Surgeon, to Annie Jane, second daughter of the late Major M. Doorly, of Sierra Leone.

PLUNKET—CUPISS.—On August 4, at Southampton, J. C. Plunket, Esq., second son of the late Hon. Patrick Plunket, of Dublin, to Alice, third daughter of Francis P. Cupiss, F.R.C.S., of St. Servan, France.

SUCKLING—JEROME.—On August 3, at Sutton Coldfield, Warwickshire, Cornelius William Suckling, M.B., of Queen's College, Birmingham, to Anna Maria, eldest daughter of the late John S. Jerome, Esq., of Holland House, Sutton Coldfield.

TAYLOR—COLE.—On July 30, at Louth, Lincolnshire, John Taylor, B.A., elder son of Dr. John Taylor, recently of Bayswater, London, to Effie Josephine Helen, younger daughter of the late James E. Cole, Esq., of Calcutta.

DEATHS.

ABBOTTS, MARY ANN, wife of William Abbotts, M.D., at 109, Abbey-road, N.W., on August 5.

ANDERSON, CHARLES BELL, son of J. Anderson, M.D., of 1, New Cross-road, S.E., on July 29, in his 20th year.

CLARKE, JANE WATT, wife of G. M. K. Clarke, L.R.C.P., M.R.C.S., formerly of Invercargill, New Zealand, at 28, Gerrard-street, Soho, W., on August 5, aged 86.

CROSSE, THOMAS HENRY, M.R.C.S., at Maida-hill, W., on August 2, in his 75th year.

KELLY, JOHN PRICE, Surgeon-Major (retired list, Bengal Army), at 49, The Gardens, Peckham-rye, on August 2, aged 61.

PERN, HARRIETTE, wife of Alfred Pern, M.R.C.S., at Botley, near South-ampton, on August 2, aged 38.

WHITE, AMELIA ELIZABETH, wife of John White, M.D., at 13, Beaufort-place East, Bath, on August 5, aged 67.

WILLIS, THOMAS, M.D., M.R.C.P., at 16, St. John's-terrace, Hove, on August 4, aged 77.

VACANCIES.

HECKMONDWIKE INDUSTRIAL CO-OPERATIVE SOCIETY (LIMITED).—Resident Medical Officer. Candidates must be duly registered, and possess a diploma or degree in surgery from the College of Surgeons of London, Edinburgh, or Dublin, or from one of the Universities, and a diploma, degree, or licence in medicine from a university or duly recognised licensing body of Great Britain or Ireland. Applications and testimonials, stating salary required, age, whether married or single, to be sent to the Heckmondwike Industrial Co-operative Society (Limited), Oak-street, Heckmondwike, on or before August 29.

LEITH HOSPITAL.—Assistant-Surgeon. Candidates must be duly qualified. Applications, with testimonials, to be sent to the Secretary, Mr. George V. Mann, 33, Bernard-street, Leith, from whom all particulars can be obtained.

MACCLESFIELD GENERAL INFIRMARY.—Senior House-Surgeon. Candidates must be doubly qualified and duly registered. Applications, with recent testimonials, to be addressed to the Chairman, House-Committee, Macclesfield Infirmary, on or before August 13.

NORTHAMPTON GENERAL INFIRMARY.—House-Surgeon. (For particulars see Advertisement.)

OWENS COLLEGE, MANCHESTER.—Demonstrator of Anatomy. (For particulars see Advertisement.)

WEST LONDON HOSPITAL, HAMMERSMITH.—House-Surgeon. Candidates must be registered under the Medical Act and unmarried. They are requested to send their applications and testimonials to R. J. Gilbert, Secretary and Superintendent, not later than August 20, and to attend the House-Committee at the Hospital on August 29, at 10.30 a.m.

As the Select Committee on the Artisans' and Labourers' Dwellings Improvement Act have been unable to complete their inquiries, Sir Richard Cross will, at the commencement of next session, move the re-appointment of the Committee.

ROYAL MEDICAL AND CHIRURGICAL SOCIETY.—The Library will be closed for one month from Monday, August 15, and will reopen on Thursday, September 15.

NOTES, QUERIES, AND REPLIES.

Be that questioneth much shall learn much.—Bacon.

Census of Victoria.—According to the Census taken on April 3, 1881, the whole population of Victoria on that date was 845,977, namely, 438,186 males and 407,791 females, exclusive of the Chinese, who number 11,835, and aborigines, 770.

The South and East Cornwall Hospital.—The foundation-stone of the new buildings to this institution was laid last week by the Earl of Mount-Edgcumbe. The old building was erected forty years ago, and has been twice enlarged, but the accommodation is insufficient to meet the requirements of the present time. The new building is estimated to cost £34,000, of which about £10,000 remains to be subscribed.

F. T.—§, No. 2. Sir Benjamin Brodie told the Commissioners on the Water-Supply of the Metropolis, in 1869, that, in judging of the comparative salubrity of waters, it was safer in the present condition of the science to rely on statistical facts than on chemical analysis.—"Statistics elicit relations of cause and effect on which you cannot deliberately experiment."

Presentation to a Philanthropist.—At Twickenham, last week, Miss Elizabeth Twining was presented with her portrait, in recognition of her many philanthropic acts for the relief of the sick and suffering, and the establishment and endowment of St. John's Hospital—a much needed institution in the locality, which was opened about two years since.

Healthy Dwellings for the Working Classes.—The thirty-ninth half-yearly meeting of the Improved Industrial Dwellings Company was held last week. The report showed the continued prosperity of the Company, which had nearly 4000 tenements, accommodating 19,000 persons. The sanitary condition of the dwellings was such that the death-rate averaged only 16·7, as against 23·14 in the metropolis generally, and 30 or 40 per thousand in low and crowded neighbourhoods.

Ingratitude.—
　　"God and the doctor we alike adore,
　　But only when in danger—not before:
　　The danger o'er, both are alike requited—
　　God is forgotten, and the doctor slighted."

COMMUNICATIONS have been received from—

THE REGISTRAR OF THE UNIVERSITY OF LONDON; THE SECRETARY OF THE MILITARY DEPARTMENT OF THE INDIAN OFFICE, London; Messrs. R. LEHMAN AND CO., London; Mr. T. ALLEN, Bristol; THE REGISTRAR OF APOTHECARIES' HALL, London; Mr. J. W. HAWARD, London; Mr. I. S. WOOD, London; THE SECRETARY OF THE ROYAL COLLEGE OF PHYSICIANS AND SURGEONS, Edinburgh; Dr. E. FOURNIÉ, Paris; Mr. MYERS, London; Mr. WARRINGTON, Harpenden; Messrs. SCHIEFFELIN AND CO., London; Mr. M. JUDGE, London; Dr. WILLOUGHBY, London; Mr. ESCHER, London; Dr. HERMAN, London; Dr. MERCIER, London; Dr. PHILPOT, London; Mr. H. MORRIS, London; Dr. LYELL, London; Mr. F. STEVENS, London; Mr. W. WATSON CHEYNE, London; Mr. G. H. PAGE, Dublin; THE SECRETARY OF THE INTERNATIONAL MEDICAL AND SANITARY EXHIBITION; Mr. J. CHATTO, London.

PERIODICALS AND NEWSPAPERS RECEIVED—

Lancet—British Medical Journal—Medical Press and Circular—Berliner Klinische Wochenschrift—Centralblatt für Chirurgie—Gazette des Hôpitaux—Gazette Médicale—Le Progrès Médic-l—Bulletin de l'Académie de Médecine—Pharmaceutical Journal—Wiener Medizinische Wochenschrift—Centralblatt für die Medizinischen Wissenschaften—Revue Médicale—Gazette Hebdomadaire—National Board of Health Bulletin, Washington—Nature—Deutsche Medicinal-Zeitung—Boston Medical and Surgical Journal—Oil and Drug News—Medical Inquirer—Centralblatt für Gynäkologie—Alienist and Neurologist—St. Louis Courier of Medicine—Bristol Mercury, August 1—Chemists' Journal—Therapeutic Gazette—Canada Lancet—Practitioner—Chicago Medical Review—Louisville Medical News.

THE FORTY-NINTH ANNUAL MEETING

OF THE

BRITISH MEDICAL ASSOCIATION,

HELD IN RYDE, AUGUST 9, 10, 11, AND 12, 1881.

PRESIDENT'S ADDRESS.

By BENJAMIN BARROW, F.R.C.S.,

Consulting Surgeon, Royal Isle of Wight Infirmary.

AFTER a graceful reference to the distinguished members of the Association who had died in the past year, and some reference to the objects of interest in the island, Mr. Barrow said that he proposed to show that the duties of our profession, and the honest and honourable performance of them, ought to command for the profession an equality, at the least, with every other, and to entitle them to the highest position in public esteem; and if this position had not been won, he would seek the causes of the failure. For these purposes he would pass in review, cursorily, the habits of medical men—the manner in which, both in ancient and in modern times, they had carried out their manifold duties. First, he spoke of the antiquity of the profession, and then of the excellent work excellently done by men of the past and being done by men of the present; dealing with his subject under two heads—the secular and the sacred. He conducted his hearers quickly from and through the far and misty past, down to our own days, and then proceeded to say:—

Having, I fear, already tried your patience, I must pass as quickly as possible over that portion of my subject which consists in a record of the many works which fall to the lot of the medical man; works often, too often, combated by the laity, sometimes not without the assistance of men from our own ranks. The work which the medical man has necessarily to carry on is sufficient to occupy his anxious thoughts, without having his time engaged in refuting charges and upholding in his public capacity those principles which he believes to be right, and which, as a law-abiding subject, he is bound to carry out.

Take, then, the temperance question, regarding which frequent assaults are made upon us, not only by the public, but by some of our abstaining friends. I respect every man who acts up to his principles; but no man has a right to accuse another of leading his patient to an immoral life because, in his judgment, some moderate stimulant is necessary, either to assist in the cure of disease or to maintain the standard of health. The man, I care not who he is, that scares the public by saying "stimulants are of no use in any class of case or disease," says that in proof of which he can produce no sound philosophic or scientific reasoning; he makes a declamation which I should have been sorry to carry out in my years of practice, and which is no sounder than that made by a man who once said "he cured all cases of cholera with salt." Medical men have been traduced on this subject most unfairly, most unscrupulously. Take away stimulants altogether from the treatment of disease, and I believe you take away one of the chief anchors of medical treatment. I know that stimulants were at one time too freely administered, and they may be so still in rare cases; but who dares to say that the prescriber did not so conscientiously, believing it was for the benefit of his patient? Beware of giving way to doctrines wholesale, which may be prejudicial to health and dangerous to life!

What shall I say of the anti-vaccinators, and of the advocates for the suppression of the Contagious Diseases Acts?

My opinion of revaccination I have already indirectly expressed. After years of research, it was found to answer the anticipations of its discoverer; it has borne the test of years, in spite of the criticisms of every class of man and woman, still holding its own valued place as the surest preventive against the most loathsome of diseases, one which is alike destructive of life, faculties, and health. Is it

VOL. II. 1881. No. 1625.

because, ever and anon, we have an outbreak of small-pox, a case of the disease or of death after vaccination, that therefore the operation is a useless one? All men may not be equally cautious in the lymph they use, and I am not sure but that vaccination is one of those minor operations which has not received the amount of attention which it commands.

The law of compulsory vaccination is faulty, in not being strict enough; for no man, whatever his own peculiar views may be, has a right to violate a law which has been framed for the protection of mankind at large, the breaking of which not only endangers his own life (which the law says he shall not jeopardise), but that of his neighbour. I trust that, if there be legislation, it will be to introduce clauses more stringent than at present exist. I hope there will not be found one man in our ranks who will countenance or support the most unphilosophical, unscientific cry which has ever been raised against a grand discovery.

What shall I say of the anti-contagionists? Of these I would speak only one degree less strongly than I have done of the anti-vaccinationists. Although the test of time has not been very extended, still there is evidence enough to prove that much good has been achieved, and that much disease and distress has been stayed. The argument used, that the Act legalises sin, is only one-sided. Because men and women will sin, are we, having a remedy at hand, not to apply it? Are we to leave men and women who sin, and, unrestrained by their sin, destroy the life, the health, and the happiness of a race still unborn? Shall we not strive to lessen the chances of "the iniquities of the fathers being visited upon the children," not for one but for many generations? I grieve that the cry against the Contagious Diseases Acts should receive the concurrence of any in our profession; I grieve more particularly because one, an old friend of my own, Dr. Nevins, has taken up this position—a position he strives to maintain by statistical reasonings which do not stand the ordeal of strict investigation.

Another class of oppositionists has still to be dealt with—the anti-vivisectionists. I have already told you that the great discovery of the lacteals by Asellius was made during the vivisection of a dog. What should we have known of the effects of poisons upon the coats of the stomach and intestines? what of the injury to, and destruction of, the nerve-centres? what of the treatment of diseases and injuries of bones, if our friends of to-day had sprung up half a century ago? How many more benefits might I not enumerate, accruing to the human race from the experiments upon animals—experiments not carried on from curiosity, but from a desire to add to the blessings of health! Scientific men are not such brutes as some would have the world believe; they carry on their researches with every regard to humanity. Let me ask, Will the anti-vivisectionists give up their fishing and shooting, their delicacies of crimped salmon, lobsters, and crabs? I trow not. The experiments carried on by the man of science are none so painful as the indulgences just described entail upon living animals.

Legislate for the total abolition of vivisection, and one of the levers for increasing our knowledge of the action of new remedies is taken away, and mankind must be the losers. Let me, in concluding this subject, add a paragraph from Darwin's answer to Professor Holmgren, who inquired what Darwin's opinion of vivisection was. He writes: "What improvements in medical practice may be directly attributed to physiological research, is a question which can be discussed only by those physiologists and medical practitioners who have studied the history of these subjects; but, as far as I can learn, the benefits are already great. However this may be, no one, unless he be grossly ignorant of what science has done for mankind, can entertain any doubt of the incalculable benefits which will hereafter be derived from physiology, not only by man, but by the lower orders. Look, for instance, at Pasteur's results in modifying the germs of the most malignant diseases from which, as it so happens, animals will in the first place receive more relief than man. Let it be remembered how many lives and what a fearful amount of suffering have been saved by the knowledge gained of parasitic worms through the experiments of Virchow and others on living animals. In the future, everyone will be astonished at the ingratitude shown, at least in England, to these benefactors of mankind. As for myself, permit me to assure you that I honour, and shall always honour, everyone who advances the noble science of physiology."

One word more on this subject. What would be the relation of human suffering saved by the knowledge gained by vivisection to that endured by animals who have been the victims of experiments?

Those who know anything of the matter, can but admit that they bear no comparison. Legislation cannot—it must not—be allowed to interfere with free scientific research.

I would commend the foregoing to the company of anti-vivisectionists at their next drawing-room assembly.

Two other subjects of controversy are still present to my mind—that of lady-doctors and lady-nurses, and the compulsory reporting of infectious cases. Of the last, I would say, that in my opinion no such obligation should be imposed upon the medical man who is the confidential adviser of the infected household, and under no state of things ought he to be forced to reveal the secrets of that house, be they what they may. The burthen of such revelation ought to be borne by the occupier of the house; to legislate in this direction would be legitimate, and much good would, I doubt not, follow.

The other subject presents many points of delicacy and difficulty. It is one, as you well know, which has given rise to much controversy; it is open to fair argument and differences of opinion. My own views, I believe, are opposed to those of a considerable number of men whose opinions I value; but I shall nevertheless express them freely in as few words as possible.

I am not over-squeamish, nor am I over-sensitive; but I almost shudder when I hear of things that ladies now do, or attempt to do; when I hear them talk—the old, the middle-aged, and the young,—speaking of things not sotto voce, but boldly and loudly, in society made up of both sexes. One can but blush, and feel that modesty, once inherent in the fairest of God's creation, is fast fading away. You, gentlemen, who know the delicacy of women's organisation, you must know that constitutionally they are unfitted for many of the duties which are required from both doctor and nurse. May not habit, may not the performance of duties which entail long watchings, much exhaustion of mind and body—may they not, will they not, so change that fine organisation, that sensitive nature of woman, as to render her dead to those higher feelings of love and sympathy which now make our homes so happy, so blessed? Will not the strain upon the delicately nurtured female have a prejudicial effect upon the babe still unborn? Will not England's glory fade without its modest sympathising women, and its race of stalwart youths and blooming maidens? You now, gentlemen, know my views as to the propriety of ladies becoming doctors or nurses.

Turning now for a moment from civil to military life, are not medical men found equally prominent in other relations to the State? Has not the battle-field told many a tale of heroism, the devotion of medical men, total abnegation of self, sacrifice of life, to save that of others? Has the State adequately rewarded these men—equally brave on land or water—for services rendered? Our profession can boast of many Porters. The one who died but [yesterday in Afghanistan lives in the memory of not only those who personally knew him, but of the United Kingdom at large. Neither are we wanting in men such as John Frederick M'Crea, lately graciously decorated by our beloved Queen with the Victoria Cross, for his conspicuous bravery in South Africa, who, in the midst of fire and shot, conveyed a wounded burgher to the shelter of a large ant-hill, then sought an ambulance for the relief of the wounded soldier, and, whilst thus engaged, was himself severely injured, but, nothing daunted, continued at his post, assisting to secure the safety of many more wounded and disabled soldiers. Thus, having done his duty, it was only left for him to dress his own wounds, having no medical brother to assist him. Is not the story an honour to our profession, a glory to our calling?

Let me now turn for a few brief moments to the second part of my argument—the sacred.

If I appear to any of my hearers to dwell unnecessarily upon, as it were, the religious portion, let me ask you to withhold a criticism prejudicial to my observations; for I cannot forget that the profession has been, and is, even to this day, by some people accused of being sceptical, and as denying the power of God in creation. I therefore venture humbly to crave your indulgence if I place prominently before you the thoughts which are uppermost in my mind, and which, from my knowledge of medical men, I believe to be present in theirs. As I have previously said, life is a tremendous reality, a serious responsibility. How can this be disputed? Are we not born by, and in, the image of the Almighty? Perfect in all our parts, endued with the finest organisation, can we doubt that we are born to show forth the glory of God in all our works? Can it be possible that there is one man in our ranks who denies, or even doubts, the existence of a God?

The study, or even the simple observation, of nature—whether it be the animate or the inanimate—ought to prove to the man of science, or the man of ordinary intellect, that all has been created and is preserved by one Almighty Power. If such be the 'case, is not life a serious responsibility—may I not say a sacred one?—and is not every man, be his calling what it may, bound to exercise his best powers to preserve not only his own life, but that of his fellow-men; to do his duty in that station unto which he has been called? Is not our calling a sacred one, being obliged, if we fail not in our duty, to go hither and thither, with or without other recompense, save that of a conscience void of reproach, and the feeling of satisfaction that we have succoured a suffering body; thus following in the steps of our Lord and Master? Is it possible to aspire or attain to a higher position than that of being instruments for good, under the guidance of the Great Healer?

That we have a right to aspire to such a height I have no doubt, though some may still be sceptical as to our calling, and may follow Dryden, who, with irreverent vigour, in verse declares:—

"Better to hunt in fields for health unbought,
Than fee the doctor for a nauseous draught;
The wise for cure on exercise depend;
God never made His work for man to mend."

Once again. Is not our calling sacred, if we consider our admittance into the domestic circle as a sacred position? Is not our intercourse with families a privilege, which must not be abused? Are we not often brought into contact with sin as well as suffering? Are we not entrusted, in confidence, with the cause of suffering, mental as well as bodily? Are we not sometimes, too, the happy medium of reconciliation between those most nearly related? Is it not often in our power to sever those ties which ought to be held the most sacred? If we fulfil properly the trust reposed in us, and treat domestic confidences with that silent judgment which becomes the honourable gentleman, I say confidently that we have the right, looking at all these calls upon our time and upon our hearts, to proclaim our profession as standing upon the highest grounds.

As the Hippocratic oath set forth how the honourable performance of our professional duties is to be carried out, so, I think, with equal force, do the words of Galen bring home to us the sacred view. If I failed to place before you the religious feelings which formed the predominant feature of his character, I should be doing a great injustice to his memory.

Remember, Galen was brought up in the darkness and polytheism of the Pagans; and yet, so fully had his anatomical researches impressed him with the conviction that the grand fabric of the human frame could only be the work of the all-wise, as well as all-powerful and beneficent, Being, that he gives vent to the following burst of religious feeling, worthy of a Christian of the nineteenth century, no less than of a Pagan of the second. He says: "In writing these books I compose a true and real hymn to that awful Being who made us all; and, in my opinion, true religion consists not so much in costly sacrifices and fragrant perfumes offered upon his altars, as in a thorough conviction impressed upon our minds, and an endeavour to produce a similar impression upon the minds of others, of His unerring wisdom, His resistless power, and His all-diffusive goodness. For His having arranged everything in that order and disposition which are best calculated for its preservation and continuation, and His having condescended to distribute His favours to all His works, is a manifest proof of His goodness, which calls loudly for our hymns and praises. His having found the means necessary for the establishment and preservation of this beautiful order and disposition, is as incontestable a proof of His wisdom as His having done whatever He pleased is of His omnipotence." Many similar examples abound throughout this great man's works, and show that a spirit of genuine piety directed all his thoughts. If the record of these sentiments be true, ought not the accusation of scepticism, even as regards men of old, to vanish from the minds of men? And if, as I contend, the same sentiments are still uppermost in the minds of medical men, ought they to be ever branded by the title of sceptics?

Gentlemen, I have thus endeavoured, imperfectly I know, to show why we deserve the esteem and respect of all men. If we are not so esteemed and respected, what is the cause? Does it rest in ourselves? I can but fear that to some extent this is the case. We have a censorious public to deal with, and, being in a measure their servants, we cannot throw them off; for, although they are not independent of us, still we are dependent upon them: there is mutual dependence, and there ought to be mutual confidence—indeed, there *must* be, if we are satisfactorily to do our duty. I advise the man who feels he has lost the confidence of his patient to retire immediately from attendance—he will be no loser by thus showing that he respects his own feelings. I say there must be confidence between the patient and the practitioner. How often is this broken by the innuendoes of one medical man in reference to another? Is there no jealousy, no backbiting between man and man living in close neighbourhood? Does that brotherly love exist between men which there ought to be, and which I think the very sacredness of our calling demands? How often do we hear it said, "Mr. A. says Mr. B. has treated me all wrong, has not understood my case at all." How glad, alas! is Mr. A. to write a prescription altogether different from what Mr. B. has done! Medical men must differ in opinion as to treatment; and this very difference is the greatest safeguard the public can have; but the difference of opinion and the treatment to be followed need not be made the subject of comment to the patient. The difference ought to be sacred, as between man and man; and I pray that the freer communication now possible, as I have expressed in a former portion of my address, may be the means of reconciling many men hitherto kept apart by only a partial knowledge of each other.

Again, how sadly do medical men arouse the astonishment of the public when called upon to give evidence in judicial inquiries; how diametrically opposed are the opinions advanced, without regard for their own character or for that of the profession: the opinion must be in favour of those on whose behalf each man is called to give evidence. Can we be surprised that the laity often accuse us of violating the principles of honour? In no class of cases is this brought more prominently before the public eye than in railway accidents. Is it impossible for medical men, before giving evidence in such cases, to come to some mutual understanding? I trust some way may be found to escape from the scandal by which, under the above circumstances, we are now surrounded. As long as these controversies last, just so long will it be before we attain to that position which we ought to hold in the estimation of the public.

How the backbitings, the jealousies, have existed for so long is marvellous, even in times gone by, in reference to the power, the prosperity, and dignity of one college of learning over another, and which, even to this day, are so far existing as to greatly impede, I fear, the cause of education, and the proof, by one combined examination, as to the fitness of men to be entrusted with the health and lives of their fellow-men. How different this from what Harvey anticipated, as expressed by the last Harveian Orator, Dr. Barclay, "how in the early days of the College of Physicians jealousies crept in, instead of that large-heartedness which Harvey hoped would guide the steps of the Fellows of the College."

Can we be surprised, then, that the public, being critical, should look doubtfully upon our profession, and refuse us that meed of just sympathy and position which we certainly deserve? Let us hope that a great future is in store for all our colleges and seats of learning, and that they may be pregnant of great results, both as regards the advance of science and the eligibility of those who are destined to go about doing good, following in the steps of their Great Master.

The avoidance of allowing patients to be participators in our differences and our jealousies, will go far to disabuse the minds of the public that medical men are always differing, always quarrelling, always standing upon etiquette. Now,

this brings me to a point upon which I desire to be explicit, for this word "etiquette" has been within the last few months frequently in the mouths of the public. I allude, as you all, I doubt not, have already surmised, to the subject of consultations—a subject upon which I think the public take a very erroneous view, and the profession are not altogether free from reprehension. Medical men are too apt to think that, because a patient or a patient's friends desire a second opinion, in the course of a long attendance, their skill is called in question; umbrage is taken, confidence lost, and for the future an uncomfortable feeling exists between the patient and the attendant. Gentlemen, this is wrong. Is there any one of us who, in case of a long and trying illness in one we love, does not seek advice of many men?—and why should not our patients?

The public are wrong in accusing medical men of standing upon etiquette, when they refuse to meet the practitioner (to wit, the homœopath) of a system of medicine entirely at variance with the ordinary routine. No one can, I think, deny that the homœopath stands upon very peculiar ground. He practises a system of medicine (although I have no belief in it); nevertheless, it is a *system*, and, if carried on in its purity, as laid down by the founder of the system, and as long as the homœopath adheres strictly thereto, I fail to see how he can be called a quack, or why he should be tabooed by the profession—as it were, cut off from a position amongst medical men, forbidden to gather together with them, and prevented from discussing publicly his system, and hearing the contrary from those practising legitimate medicine. The benefit would be mutual, and these discussions would be of benefit to the public, and an additional proof to them that their weal was uppermost in our minds. But I say he ought to be shunned, if he throws out the bait of practising both according to the ordinary system and homœopathically. He must either believe in one or the other; if he puts in practice the one he disbelieves, because the patient wishes it, he treats his patient for gain only; he fails in that honourable performance of his duty which is the boast and pride of our profession.

The combination cannot be carried out honourably. As regards consultation with the professed homœopath, I will give you the answer I have always made to such request— "I cannot accede to your wish; not out of any ill feeling towards the gentleman you desire me to meet, but because I cannot waste my own time, nor the time of the homœopath, nor rob you, or be a party to the robbery. If we meet, we cannot agree: you gain nothing for the fees you have thrown away." You, gentlemen, cannot, you must not, consult under any circumstances with the man who practises a system of medicine opposed to that which science and long usage have proved to be the only safe and secure one. If you once break this rule, you are ever after placed in a false position; you not only lose your self-respect, but you lose the respect of your patient, and of the whole profession. Let us hope that the faith of the public in a faulty and pernicious system is fast fading away.

The word "pernicious" may appear a harsh one, but, with the view I hold of the value of the infinitesimal, I can apply no other. A long and patient observation and noting of cases has brought clearly to my mind—it may not to yours—this important point, viz., that homœopathy having destroyed, to a great extent, the faith of the public in medicinal remedies, many practitioners have gone to the opposite extreme to please their patients in the administration of medicines; the non-administration of which, I hesitate not to say, retards in many cases recovery, and when that is achieved, the recovery (if I may call it so) in very many cases is only partial and temporary. The sequelæ of the class of disease which come under the title of zymotic are now much more serious and frequent than they were when medicinal remedies were efficiently and abundantly administered.

I have made rather a long digression from my original subject, but much that I have said in this digression was necessary to establish my plea that medical men only stand upon what the public call "etiquette" from a sense of what is due to themselves and to their patients.

Permit me now to draw my conclusions from what I have ventured (I hope without offence to any individual, present or absent) to place before you. I trust, moreover, that the sum and substance of my observations may have the effect which I greatly desire, of clearing away some of the clouds which surround the lay public, and that my observations may bring those who have hitherto looked upon our profession as a necessary evil, rather than a good, to believe at any rate that, although we may differ individually as to treatment of disease, we are not antagonistic collectively; that our feelings towards each other are brotherly; and that in the performance of our duty towards our patients and to the public we are actuated by true and honest motives, and the most honourable intentions. Gentlemen, a review of what I have already said cannot fail, I am bold enough to hope, to prove that our profession merits the highest consideration from the world at large, and that it stands upon the topmost pinnacle of fame.

Gentlemen, only a few words more, and I have done. Many thanks for your patient attention to my sayings, which I fear have been dull and uninteresting. I trust that no word has fallen from my lips, offensive to anyone here. I have spoken from the fulness of my heart, with but one desire, viz., that the high position in which our profession already stands may be maintained and increased, and secure for you, individually and collectively, that respect which, if honestly, honourably, and perseveringly carried on, your calling merits.

In conclusion, I would venture to say, Pray each morning before you commence your day's labour, which labour cannot be attended but by much anxiety, and at times by disappointment and sorrow, mingled happily, however, by some bright spots,—pray, I say, that you may be blessed by that Divine help, which can alone sustain you and carry you successfully through labours and anxieties of no mean order; and, when evening comes, pour forth thanksgivings that strength and knowledge have been given you to do your duty, in mitigating to some extent the sufferings of your fellow-men. These are the only sure and safe steps to a happy life and a prosperous career.

It only remains for me to assure you that I pray God may bless you in your everyday work, in yourselves and in your families; that you may leave the Island refreshed for future work. At any rate, carry with you the assurance that you have our heartiest prayers that God may speed you on your way, and that when He calls you hence, you may leave behind you "footprints" for good, so beautifully described in the following lines by our favourite American poet :—

> " Lives of great men all remind us
> We can make our lives sublime,
> And, departing, leave behind us
> Footprints on the sands of time.
>
> " Footprints, that perhaps another
> Sailing o'er life's solemn main,
> A forlorn and shipwrecked brother,
> Seeing, shall take heart again.
>
> " Let us, then, be up and doing,
> With a heart for any fate,
> Still achieving, still pursuing,
> Learn to labour and to wait."

ADDRESS IN MEDICINE.

By JOHN SYER BRISTOWE, M.D.,
Senior Physician to St. Thomas's Hospital.

MR. PRESIDENT AND GENTLEMEN,—There are few more interesting and curious studies than the history of medicine. Taking its origin in the very dawn of human existence, not in the instincts which lead men to obey the dictates of Nature, but in the sense of rebellion which the pains and penalties she inflicts engenders, it was cradled in the credulity and superstition, which are the first fruits of thought struggling for independence. It is not surprising, therefore, that in the earlier ages, when their origin and nature seemed alike mysterious, diseases should be attributed to the influence of stars and comets, to the malignity of demons, to the wrath of deities; and that their alleviation or cure should be sought in amulets and charms, in sacrifices and prayers. Nor is it surprising that in later times, when the knowledge of disease had advanced, and the influence of drugs had become recognised, a belief came to prevail that, for every morbific evil which Nature permitted to afflict mankind, she had provided an antidote. Nor, perhaps, is it to be wondered at that, even at the present time, in this enlightened age, not —crely among the lowly and the ignorant, but amongst the noble, the learned, and even the scientific, credulity and superstition in relation to the common enemy of mankind—disease—should still widely prevail; that diseases should still be attributed to supernatural causes, and to the spleen of an offended deity; that still amulets and charms, sacrifices and prayers, should be included in the popular materia medica; or that the belief should still be entertained (for which no scientific basis whatever exists) that diseases, which are the necessary correlatives of mortality, are mere puzzles, designed by Nature for the exercise of ingenuity in the discovery of remedies, which she has industriously hidden in the eternal rocks, and in the living things which people the face of the earth or clothe it with verdure.

It has been largely held, and is doubtless still believed, that the position of medicine as a science is a discredit to the age in which we live: and it may be freely admitted that, while the arts and sciences generally have been making rapid strides, medicine, in its primary and chief object—namely, the cure of diseases—has made but scanty and doubtful progress. But those who hold this view have given little real thought to the subject. In no small measure they are persons who have no acquaintance whatever with medicine, who judge of it by its failure to accomplish ends which are probably impossible of accomplishment, and who are themselves to a great extent credulous in the efficacy of measures and remedies whose use is an outrage on common sense. But largely they are persons who base their judgment on a false comparison of the progress of medicine with that of the exact sciences, and of the natural sciences on which alone scientific medicine is built. They forget that mathematics and geometry are (difficult, no doubt, but) comparatively simple sciences, which men may cultivate in the closet, apart from life and nature, and which the ancients, therefore, were as well able to investigate with success as ourselves. They forget that the physical sciences and chemistry, which deal only with the simple forces of nature and unliving matter, have only within the last hundred years made those gigantic strides which have raised them from the depths of empiricism and quackery to the marvellous position they now hold among our intellectual and effective possessions. They forget that the natural sciences, the sciences which deal with living nature—namely, botany, zoology, anatomy, physiology, and pathology—though long cultivated fitly and to little purpose, have only of late years made systematic progress; and that it is mainly within the present century that anatomy, physiology, and pathology have risen into the dignity of sciences, and have worked a very revolution in our knowledge and estimate of life, in both its normal and its abnormal conditions—of health and disease. And, lastly, they forget that the scientific treatment of disease can only be based on a scientific knowledge of the structure and functions of the healthy body, on a scientific knowledge of the causes and processes of diseases in it, and on a scientific study of the methods and means by which those morbid causes and processes can be prevented, counteracted, or destroyed; and that such a study is only now becoming possible.

I confess that to me it seems altogether Utopian and unreasonable to expect either that diseases shall ever be banished from the earth, or that even diseases generally shall become curable by therapeutical or any other treatment. All living things are foredoomed to die; and the more complicated their structure, and the higher and more multifarious their functions, the more liable are they to suffer from those changes of structure and derangements of function which constitute essential elements of disease. Moreover, the causes of disease abound, and form as much as we ourselves do an integral part of the economy of nature. Why should they cease to exist and act, and we survive? Again, assuming the persistence of diseases, what grounds of reason or experience have we to justify the belief that for disease an antidote or cure will sooner or later be discovered? The history of medicine raises no such hope. There is nothing in the nature of diseases themselves to render such a consummation probable. The immortality of mortal life is neither conceivable nor to be desired. Still less is there any reasonable or sufficient basis for the assumption that diseases, differing apparently from one another in their nature, and depending on causes which have no mutual connexion and act upon the system in various and independent ways, should all be amenable to treatment in accordance with one simple theory of therapeutics.

I am not presuming to question the benefits that medicine has conferred upon mankind; still less to deny the promise of greater things to come. I know that, in the past, many glimpses of therapeutical truth have from time to time been caught; and that veins of bright ore have here and there been discovered in the dreary waste of empiricism and charlatanism. I see that, at the present time, pathology and the investigation of the causes of disease are throwing fresh and unexpected light on the nature of diseases, and are leading us into new lines of successful practice, especially in relation to their prevention. And I cannot doubt that, as our knowledge of the processes and causes of disease extends, so will our power to prevent disease acquire a wider range, and attain more certainty of operation; and that here, more than in the direct treatment of disease, our future successes will be found. But neither can I doubt that the progress of this and cognate sciences, aided by well-devised experiments and careful observation of diseases, will lead both to the discovery of new remedies and to the more successful use of those we already employ.

I shall not pursue the subject of the potentialities of medicine, fascinating though it be. It is in the vagaries, and not in the science, of medicine, that for this hour my interest centres. I am not going to investigate or explain, how it is that systems of medical treatment of disease have originated, have played their part in the drama of human life, have given place to others, and yet (though henceforth discredited in the eyes of man) have left behind them relics which are still embodied in the therapeutical practice and theories of the present day. It is easy, however, to understand how, on the one hand, the vague beliefs, speculations, and errors—the growth of ages—should have gradually acquired form, and blended into creeds; and how, on the other hand, ingenious and self-reliant minds, speculating on the mysteries of nature, should have gradually evolved out of their inner consciousness elaborate systems in explanation, with nothing but their ingenuity to commend them. Thus it was that, in accordance with the first alternative, the Doctrine of Signatures gradually arose; thus it was that, in accordance with the second, Galen elaborated his celebrated hypothesis respecting the virtues and operations of medicines. It seems marvellous that such fantastic fictions as these were, should ever have been developed in the minds of men, and for ages have been accepted as true, and adopted in practice, not only by the ignorant and thoughtless, but by physicians of conspicuous ability and eminence.

But, gentlemen, the age of credulity is not yet passed; and doubtless, as long as humanity strives to unravel the secrets of nature, and to explain her actions, there will be men, and men too of cultivated intellects, who, in the search after truth, will be led astray by Wills-o'-the-Wisp, and who will end by making idols of the vain figments of their minds, by pulling down and worshipping the golden images they have themselves set up. Such a man, it seems to me, was Hahnemann, the notorious founder of homœopathy. It is of him, and of the sect he founded, that I propose to speak to-day.

Hahnemann became a medical man from choice, and pursued his studies in respectable schools and under fairly eminent teachers. He acquired some credit as a practitioner while yet young; though probably not more credit than many of his contemporaries, and many who have preceded and many who have followed him, have also obtained, whose names, nevertheless, have never emerged from obscurity. But he appears to have given his mind mainly to the study of chemistry, botany, and therapeutics; and certainly there is no evidence from his writings, or from any other source, that the study of disease itself had any interest for him. Though he had friends, he seems, like most physicians, to have failed in early life to make his profession lucrative; and either for this reason, or, as some assert, because he became dissatisfied with the methods and systems of treating disease then in vogue, he retired for a time from practice, and gave himself up to his favourite studies, and to the translation of French and English works relating to them into his mother-tongue. However this may be, many will sympathise with him now, as many doubtless would have sympathised with him then, in the dissatisfaction which, about this period, he undoubtedly felt with the chaotic state of therapeutical theory and practice at that time prevalent, and with the aspirations that sprang up within him to make order out of confusion, to discover some intelligible relation

between therapeutic agents and morbid processes, to systematise the curative treatment of disease. And many even of those who dissent most widely from his conclusions will still, I think, admire the tenacity, the energy, and the sublime bigotry he displayed in the development of that system, of which he was at once the creator and the apostle.

His system took its origin in those scholastic views of the nature of disease, of the nature of remedies, and of the influence of remedies on disease, which more or less have influenced the theory and practice of medicine from the earliest ages down to the present day. Looking upon diseases, not as what they are, but as mere assemblages of symptoms; and upon remedies, not as what they are, but as agents specially given by Providence with the one hand to cure the evils which He had scattered broadcast with the other; and guided by certain superficial relationships, easily observed, between the effects of certain morbid conditions and the effects of certain drugs; it was not unnatural for observant and thoughtful men to speculate on the hidden laws which might be supposed to underlie such relationships, and to generalise. Thus, some perceiving that constipation of the bowels was overcome by purgatives, diarrhœa by astringents, and that hæmorrhages were arrested by styptics, thought that in such facts they recognised the general therapeutical law that all diseases should be treated by their opposites (*contraria contrariibus curantur*): some noticing that coma was relieved by purgatives (that is, that affections of the head were favourably influenced by remedies acting on the bowels), that affections of internal organs were benefited by counter-irritants, and such like phenomena, originated the theory that disease was curable by remedies which were unlike in operation to themselves, the theory to which the term *allopathy* was given by Hahnemann : and, again, some observing that diarrhœa was often relieved by purgatives, that constipation was often best treated by remedies having a tendency to restrain the action of the bowels, that inflammation of the skin was frequently cured by the application of remedies which themselves tended to irritate the skin, were pioneers in the alleged discovery which Hahnemann proclaimed to the world in the legend *similia similibus curantur*, and under the name of *homœopathy*.

It is clear that, if one look only at some of the coarser phenomena of disease and effects of remedies, there is some warrant in fact for each of these three theories of treatment, but none for regarding one or other of them as of universal applicability. It is clear, too, that anyone arguing back from such facts as these to the hidden workings of diseases and remedies within the corporeal frame, and at the same time shutting his eyes to the phenomena of life as they exist actually, might bring himself to the belief that there were three modes, corresponding to those enumerated above, and three only, in which remedial agents could act upon the processes of disease—namely, one by acting in opposition to them (*antipathy*), one by acting in accordance with them (*homœopathy*), and one by acting heterogeneously to them (*allopathy*). But it is difficult to understand how anyone who has followed in any degree the advances during the present century of the natural sciences, and especially of those which relate to the structure and functions of the human body in health and disease, and to the etiology of disease, can see any plausibility in such speculations, any provisional hypothesis even, such as sometimes aids the advance of science—any meaning whatever in them.

How Hahnemann's special views of disease and its treatment originated, and how they underwent gradual development, until they found exact expression in his "Organon," the bible of homœopathy, I shall not attempt to discuss. The "Organon" itself, however, is a remarkable work, very interesting also, and very entertaining; for it comprises not only the quintessence of his labours, but reveals the character of the man, as in a mirror, with all his strength and all his weakness, all his wisdom and all his folly.

He was a physician who had a supreme contempt for pathology, and on the whole for etiology. He inveighs over and over again against the absurdity of those who endeavour to discover, in morbid phenomena within the body, an explanation of the symptoms which persons who are ill present. He says: "We may well conceive that every malady implies a change in the interior of the organism, but this change can only be surmised obscurely and fallaciously from the symptoms; it can never be recognised infallibly in its complete reality. The invisible changes wrought by the malady within the organism, and the changes perceptible to our senses (that is to say, in some of the symptoms), together form a complete image of the malady; but that image is only visible in its entirety to the eye of the Creator. It is the totality of the symptoms which alone constitute the part of it accessible to the doctors; but it is likewise in the totality of the symptoms that we find everything that is needful to know in order to cure." To Hahnemann it is a matter of no moment whether ascites depends on cirrhosis of the liver, or tubercle of the peritoneum; whether an attack of constipation and colic arises from lead-poisoning or from a cancerous stricture; whether a paralytic seizure is the outcome of hysteria, or is due to some material lesion of the brain. In each case, to him, what is the condition of things within is an idle speculation; the symptoms of which the patient complains comprise all that the medical man need know; and to treat those according to the true laws of homœopathy is to cure the disease. But he goes further; for, not satisfied with stigmatising all pathological investigations as mere pedantry and foolishness, he actually objects to all attempts on the part of systematic writers and practical physicians to distinguish and classify diseases. Speaking of pathology in the past, he says: "It created arbitrarily the object of cure—namely, the malady. Men decided authoritatively what are the number of diseases, what their form, and what their genera. Good God!" says he, "the infinity of diseases which nature excites in man, exposed as he is to so many different influences, under conditions never to be determined beforehand, and infinitely varied, is reduced to such an extent by pathology, that there remains only a handful of them, furnished according to its whim." Elsewhere he observes, "We may also pass over in silence the fact that persons have tried to reduce the number of maladies—those infinitely varied deviations from the state of health—to a limited list of denominations, and to give the definite descriptions (which vary, nevertheless, according to different pathological views), in order to afford a ready indication of medical treatment for each form of illness that is artificially defined in therapeutics." And again he says, in reference to the causes of disease (which he regards as innumerable): "Thence come an infinite number of heterogeneous diseases, which are so different from one another that (to speak strictly) any case of illness appears only once, and (if we except the few diseases which originate in a miasm always of the same kind, or which arise from the same cause) every man who becomes affected suffers from a special malady, to which no specific name can be given, and which has never existed in the same manner as in the present case, in the particular individual and under existing circumstances, and will never be reproduced in exactly the same form."

From these quotations, we may fairly gather what his views of the nature of disease were. In the first place, he admitted that diseases originated in causes; but these causes were innumerable, and operated in innumerable combinations, and hence (excepting in the cases of miasmatic affection, and some few specific fevers of which he could not deny the existence, and enumerated) were barren subjects of investigation, and as indications for treatment worthless, if not misleading. Indeed, in one place, speaking of intestinal worms (which we regard as causes of disease), he denies that they are causes of disease at all; and says that when they irritate, they irritate simply from the fact that they are themselves suffering, together with their host, of some malady under which their host labours; professing (in accordance with his preconceived views) to imagine some hidden cause, rather than to acknowledge that as the cause, which offered itself in a visible and tangible form to his senses. For him, I should think, preventive medicine, which deals specially with the causes of disease, and has been successful only in proportion to its knowledge of them, would have been a delusion and a snare. In the second place, pathology, and more especially morbid anatomy, had no meaning for him. All the laborious investigations conducted in our deadhouses, which we fondly imagine to add to our knowledge of disease, and to which (in association with clinical study) we attribute most of the advances that have been made in medicine of late years—such as the differentiation of kidney-diseases, the recognition of supra-renal maladies, the discovery of the condition known as embolism, the exact recognition of the nature of tumours, the discoveries which have been made in regard

to the diseases of the nervous system—would be looked upon by him with contempt. For what, in the third place, have such investigations and such knowledge to do with diseases as he understood them? His diseases, as I have shown, were, with a few exceptions, simply groups of symptoms—mosaics of which the component pieces admitted of endless rearrangement. Intermittent fever constituted one of the cases in which he recognised the operation of a definite cause; but, notwithstanding this, intermittent fevers were themselves innumerable, and each case that came before him was an independent disease.

I do not wish to misinterpret his views. He recognises, I admit, the existence of morbific causes; but he seems to liken them to the impulse which propels a ball, and to think that with their initial impulse all their specific influence ceases. Nor does he deny the existence of pathological changes in the interior of the body; but he says that we cannot detect them,—that, as a matter of fact, they are correlated with the symptoms which patients present, and together with this are common manifestations of the same disease,—and that in the symptoms alone we have a sufficient indication of the nature of the disease and of the treatment to be adopted for its cure.

Of course, in all this there is much that is true, and much that is specious. Were it not so, his theories would long ago have been abandoned; for it is in the mixture of truth and verisimilitude with error that gives error currency. But how much of wild speculation, how much of absolute ignorance of the matters which he proposes to teach, how much obstinate shutting of his senses to the truths of nature!

Hahnemann's views of the nature of disease were doubtless subservient to his views of the curative operation of drugs. And it is on his therapeutical views, if on anything, that his reputation must depend. He says, in his introduction: "All human maladies have up to the present time been cured, not in accordance with reasonings founded on nature and experience, but in accordance with hypotheses arbitrarily devised, such as (amongst others) the law of palliatives, *contraria contrariis*. Yet it was from this opposite side that the true method of cure was arrived at. It is based on the following principle: to cure gently, promptly, certainly, and durably, we must select, in every case of sickness, a medicine which produces of itself a similar affection to that which it is intended to cure. No one up to the present time has taught this homœopathic method; no one has yet practised it." And he goes on to add that all the maladies that had heretofore been cured had been cured by homœopathic remedies. Let us see exactly what the nature of his teaching is. He seems to start from the fascinating belief that all symptoms of disease, and therefore from his point of view all diseases, are curable. He seems also to have adopted the belief (already adverted to) that for all diseases nature has provided a cure. And he holds that the only proper and efficient cure for any assemblage of symptoms is a remedy which is capable itself of causing in a healthy person an identical assemblage of symptoms.

Stated generally, his views are as follows:—The innumerable diseases which afflict mankind, and which arise out of natural causes, consist, for the purposes of the physician, of groups of symptoms: the innumerable remedial agents which exist in nature, locked up in the animal and vegetable kingdoms, and in the inorganic world, are themselves the causes of a parallel basis of artificial diseases, which again, for the purpose of the therapeutist, consist of groups of symptoms. In order to cure any natural disease that may come before us, it is necessary to administer that particular remedial agent which is capable of producing identical symptoms with it; and, of course, this must be given in a suitable dose, for, if in too minute a dose, it leaves a residuum of the original disease uncured—if in too large a dose, it cures the disease, but induces after-effects of its own. And, further, inasmuch as we are not yet acquainted with the specific virtues of all remedies, and inasmuch, therefore, as for a large number of diseases the most suitable homœopathic remedy has not yet been discovered, we must in such a case select a remedy the effect of which approximates to the symptoms of the disease, by which means we shall cure a certain area, so to speak, of the primary disease, but we shall leave a new disease behind, compounded of the, as yet, uncured symptoms of the old disease, and the supernumerary symptoms due to the drug itself, which new disease must be treated *de novo* on homœopathic principles. How curious, how ingenious, how interesting the whole thing is! How excellent, if true! And has it not the simplicity of truth in it? The entire range of diseases, the entire range of therapeutics, converted into Chinese puzzles; the phenomena of diseases and the effect of drugs upon them treated as algebraical equations! It is impossible to conceive of any physician working daily by the bedside of patients, and in the dead-house, and seeing diseases as they are, forming such a system, except as a joke. It could only have been, as in fact it was, the serious work of a visionary, who had thrown off the trammels of fact, and, allowing his imagination to run riot, mistook its fantastic figments for a revelation from heaven.

That Hahnemann believed in himself and in the absolute truth of all that he taught, is beyond dispute. He was a prophet, not only to his followers, but in his own eyes. All other systems of therapeutics but his were folly, and all who pursued them were fools. That he had training, and ability, and the power of reasoning, is abundantly clear. He saw through the prevalent therapeutical absurdities and impositions of the day; he laughed to scorn the complicated and loathsome nostrums which, even at that time, disgraced the pharmacopœias; and he exposed with no little skill and success the emptiness and worthlessness of most of the therapeutical systems which then and theretofore had prevailed in the medical schools; and then he invented and proclaimed a system of his own at least as empty and as worthless as any that had gone before. In this, I suppose, there is nothing very strange; for it is only the broadest intellects (and his was an essentially narrow one) which are capable of treating the offspring of their own brains with the same impartiality they manifest in other cases. But, under the circumstances, it will be interesting to consider, however briefly, the character of the therapeutical facts and arguments which he himself alleges in support of his doctrines, and the methods of investigation which he taught and practised.

In the first place, in order to prove the truth of his assertion, that all cures, which had heretofore been effected by drugs, were effected in virtue of their homœopathic action, he ransacks the writings of his predecessors; and, while omitting to quote (probably, in his opinion, as absolutely worthless) any of the multitude of recorded cases in which cures had been attributed to remedies which could in no sense be regarded as homœopathic, he quotes a number of at least equally worthless cases, in which he thinks he recognises the curative influence of unconsciously applied homœopathic treatment. The following are two of his quotations:—"The English sweating disease, at its beginning more deadly than the plague itself, and which, according to Willis, destroyed ninety-nine patients out of every hundred, could not be overcome until doctors had learnt to treat the sick with sudorific remedies; from that moment, as Sennert remarks, few persons died of it." Again, "Albus informs us that the high temperature of an acute fever, with 130 beats of the pulse in a minute, was much reduced by a hot bath of 100 degrees of Fahrenheit, and that the beats of the pulse consequently sank to 110." I have no doubt the quotations he gives here are essentially accurate. But, surely it is well known that all the older physicians claimed to have discovered, towards the close of any epidemic fever, no matter what its virulence, the true method of curing it, which discovery coincided in time with the rational disappearance of the disease. Many men have thought and declared that they had cured plague, and cholera, and typhus under similar circumstances by remedies, some of which may even have been homœopathic. Does anyone believe that such asserted cures of these incurable diseases ever took place? Is there any sufficient reason to admit that the sweating disease was ever more amenable to treatment than this? or that it was, in fact, ever cured by sudorifics, or any other remedies? And, as regards the case of the reduction of temperature by the bath, Hahnemann fails entirely to see that the patient's temperature was much higher than that of the bath; that the bath was relatively cold to him; that it relieved him by reducing his temperature; and that the treatment was not only not homœopathic, but essentially antipathic; that the case, if it proves anything, proves the efficiency of one of those very methods against which he pours out the vials of his wrath. These are simply samples. I could run through the whole series of them, and show that, while a large number of them were merely loose and untrustworthy statements of supposed facts, nearly all of them prove nothing whatever, to my unbiassed

mind, in response to those homœopathic principles which they are assumed to support. Naturally, the recently introduced inoculation of cow-pox as a preventive of variola is adduced by him as a homœopathic remedy against the latter disease. He fails to observe that it is preventive alone; and that, so far from acting as a cure of small-pox, it aborts when applied to a variolous patient, while his disease runs its course wholly uninfluenced by it.

In the second place, as regards his own homœopathic observations, these, as given in his "Organon," are not very numerous. For the most part, he there lays down the law oracularly, and quotes the more or less questionable and loose statements of other authors in support of his opinions. There are two or three observations, however, apparently his own, or at any rate confirmed by his own experience, which are really interesting. He speaks, as I have before pointed out, of intermittent fevers as being innumerable, and derides the blind pathology which makes of these one disease; and proceeds: "Pathology feigns this in order to give pleasure to her dear sister Therapeutics, who, excepting antimony and sal-ammoniac, has, as a rule, no other remedy against intermittent fevers than cinchona, with which it treats them according to a fixed method, as if they were all identical! It is true," he continues, "that these fevers can be suppressed by enormous doses of cinchona—that is to say, that their periodical recurrence is overcome by it; but those who are affected with intermittents for which this remedy is unsuitable are not cured by it, but remain continually ill, and worse than they were before. And this is what the vulgar art of medicine calls a cure!" He regards cinchona, and mentions it elsewhere, as a homœopathic remedy for ague attended with certain groups of symptoms. Homœopathic, forsooth! when the most striking therapeutical fact concerning quinine is that it lowers temperatures; while the most striking clinical feature of ague is the extraordinary rise of temperature which attends its paroxysmal attacks. But fancy ague, which (Hahnemann notwithstanding) is in all its forms identically the same disease, being homœopathic to quinine in one case, and allopathic or antipathic in another; being in one case curable by quinine administered in infinitesimal quantities, and in another aggravated by the same remedy in large doses! I do not know what the present views of homœopathic practitioners may be as to the relations of quinine and ague, but I appeal to everyone of experience besides as to whether ague ever succumbs to the use of infinitesimal doses of quinine; and whether, in the large majority of cases, it does not yield with no ill consequence (due to the drug) to quinine in large quantities? What is the experience of our Indian colleagues in this matter? Again, he speaks over and over again of itch, a disease with which he seems to have been familiar, and which he assumes to be an affection pervading the whole organism, but attended, as small-pox is, with a rash; and in reference to it, he insists upon the folly of endeavouring to cure this skin-disease by local applications, a procedure which, he says, has the effect of aggravating the constitutional disorder; and he teaches that the disease is only to be cured by the internal administration of sulphur in homœopathic doses. Now, it is pretty certain that Hahnemann did not very clearly distinguish itch from many other forms of cutaneous eruption; still, many of his cases of itch were true itch, no doubt. But what can practical men think of the insight into diseases, of the power of observation, of that man who discovers that to destroy the local phenomena of itch is to aggravate the patient's illness; that itch itself is even curable by any internal remedy whatever? No doubt he was not aware that itch is due to the burrowing of parasites in the skin; but if he had been, it would have made no difference to him, for he would have argued of them and of their relation to itch, as I have already shown that he argues of intestinal parasites and the symptoms of disease which are usually attributed to their presence.

But, in the third place, before medicines can be employed homœopathically, their collective effect must of course be ascertained and tabulated, and, before cases of disease can be treated homœopathically, their symptoms must all be accurately determined and tabulated, in order that the appropriate, or at any rate the most appropriate, remedy may be selected for each. We cannot, therefore, quarrel with Hahnemann for requiring that drugs shall be carefully tested or proved, and that cases shall be carefully and accurately recorded. But what does he mean by proving of medicine, and what by testing of cases? Most men accustomed to scientific investigations would say that, in order to determine the precise potential characteristics of any unknown agency, it should be interrogated, and cross-examined, and tested from all points of view ; that, if a drug, its chemical properties should be determined, and its action on the living and on the dead, in health and in disease, should be exhaustively ascertained. That is not Hahnemann's notion at all. Drugs being, in his view, agencies which impart disease, must be tested only on the healthy body, in order to determine, in accordance with homœopathic requirements, what natural diseases their effects simulate. And the method of procedure is, that the experimenter, and those who act under his direction, shall take regulated doses of the drugs they wish to examine, and thus note in each case accurately every phenomenon which developes itself during some period, determined more or less arbitrarily, after the reception of the drug. The results to the uneducated eye look, perhaps, fair and reasonable. But we must admit the truth of the homœopathic view of the relations between medicines and diseases before we can admit the special value of investigations conducted only on the healthy body; and, as regards the method of investigation which he teaches, can anything be better calculated to promote self-deception? Think of the innumerable phenomena which a hypochondriacal old man, a youthful enthusiast in experimental research, or a credulous lecturer, would find under such circumstances arising from inconceivable doses of the most inert substances—the itching at this joint, the aching at that, the variation in the pulse, the watering of the eyes, the noise in the ears, the muscular startings, the eructations, the swellings in the bowels, and many other matters of the same kind. What pictures of the mimicry of disease may be thus produced and varied, *ad infinitum;* of what innumerable pictures of the kind (comprising here and there, doubtless, accurate and valuable observations) is the homœopathic literature on the processes of drugs made up! The recording of cases, according to Hahnemann's directions, is of a piece with the proving of medicines. He tells us to listen carefully to the account the patient gives of himself, to hear all that the friends and others about the patient say concerning him, and to note down everything accurately, and in tabular form. You are not to interrupt. And then, when the recitals have been completed, you are permitted to ask certain questions, the character of which he carefully specifies. But you are never to suggest anything to the patient; and you are never, so far as I can make out, to cross-examine him. Imagine the picture of her condition that a garrulous old lady would give under such conditions! Imagine the innumerable histories of diseases you would get, in which everything accessory and unimportant would be recorded, and everything really distinctive and important for diagnosis and treatment, as we understand them, omitted! I am not prepared to say the method is a wrong one from the homœopathic point of view, in which diseases as objects of medical treatment are regarded only as an assemblage of symptoms, and in which the interconnexion of symptoms is comparatively unimportant. But what a caricature of scientific case-taking it reveals to us! What an unpractical condition of mind it manifests in him who elaborated it! What light it throws on his curious incapacity for exact scientific observation! How like his method is to that of an industrious newly appointed clinical clerk! How utterly opposed to the procedure of the experienced scientific physician!

Perhaps the most astonishing feature of homœopathy, as Hahnemann bequeathed it to us, is his hypothesis of infinitesimal doses. He discovered, from the results of his experiments and practice, that, when once the true homœopathic remedy for any disease, or rather collection of symptoms, had been ascertained, it was needful, in order at the same time to secure the full effect of the drug and to obviate any ill effects it might leave of its use, to reduce the doses of it to an inconceivable minuteness. The millionth, the billionth, the trillionth of a grain were gigantic quantities compared with some of those which finally he found it best to administer. It has been calculated that a drop from the lake of Geneva, through the waters of which a single grain of medicine had been diffused, would contain one of his ordinary doses; and that a drop from a mass of water similarly treated long enough to filtrate the whole solar system, would contain as large a dose as is furnished by some of these extreme attenuations! When we laugh at these infinitesimal doses,

the retort is often made that we ourselves use small doses ; and calculations are flung at us, showing how excessively minute must be the amount of any potent drug administered by the stomach which reaches the organ wherein it induces specific effects, and how absolutely inappreciable must be the bulk of odorous particles which not only affect the sense of smell, but even provoke coryza, sickness, and faintness. Wherein, then, is the absurdity of the Hahnemannic dosage? But this is not a retort that Hahnemann would have made ; and, indeed, it is one that could only rise to the lips of degenerate followers of his. It is not the amount of any drug which reaches any one part of the organism which is in question, but the amount of it which has to be administered for a dose. And it cannot be denied that the smallest doses employed by us, even such as Dr. Ringer recommends, are gross indeed compared with those of Hahnemann. Where we give a drop or the hundredth part of a grain, he would have given the millionth or the billionth part of that quantity at the very most, and, probably millions of billions less than that. Moreover, the principles underlying the two cases are wholly dissimilar.

The limit in the efficacy of infinitesimal doses involved the violation of his theory. It was, indeed, I think, the natural outcome of it. The mystical powers, which for him resided in drugs, bore no quantitative relation to the ponderable element with which they were associated. They are contained in them, much as the genies in the fisherman's story in the "Arabian Nights" are contained in the leaden bottle which was fished up from the bottom of the sea. It is easy, then, if not inevitable, for him to imagine that the power of drugs became more and more developed in proportion as the grosser matters which environed them were removed. It is easy, too, from another point of view, for a vaguely mathematical mind like his (which had already dealt with diseases as if they were algebraical equations) to conceive that, just as mathematics becomes a more and more potent instrument, according as the encumbrances of arithmetical and ordinary algebraical præcipe are thrown aside, and one comes that deal, as in the differential calculus, with the mere ratios which survive in quantities which have been reduced to zero, so medicine would become a more and more potent art, according as the coarser portions of drugs and of diseases are eliminated for consideration, and we have only to do with the relations or ratios (if I may so express it) between drugs attenuated to nothing, and diseases reduced to mere groups of intangible subjective phenomena! One may, I think, follow Hahnemann's lines of thought; one may trace, I think, without much difficulty, the steps by which his system acquired its full development, and culminated at length in the doctrine of infinitesimal doses. The author of homœopathy himself carried homœopathy to its logical consequences: and was there ever a more amazing *reductio ad absurdam?*

I intended, gentlemen, when I first thought of preparing the address, to divert no inconsiderable portion of it to the consideration of some of the modern developments of homœopathy. But the time at my disposal is insufficient for that purpose; and I shall content myself with only one or two remarks upon the subject. It is only natural that, amongst the many followers of Hahnemann, some, though believing in the essential truth and value of his teachings, have ventured, within certain limits, to think for themselves; and that hence subsects, or a tending to the formation of subsects, should have arisen. It is hardly possible, for example, that all homœopaths, who have received a medical education, should accept Hahnemann's views of the nature of diseases; and many at the present day do, I believe, acquiesce in the teachings of modern pathology. It is hardly possible, again, that every homœopath should believe fully in the efficacy of the infinitely little doses which Hahnemann contended were the most efficacious, or should believe in the potential effect of the shakings of his preparations, to which, in fact, he largely attributed the development of curative energy in them. Hence the change with some is much larger than Hahnemann could have sanctioned. Then, again, was it to be expected that any thinking man could admit that remedies cured because they produced identical effect with them (and, indeed, unless one assumes that remedies act like Pharaoh's lean kine, and then die of a surfeit, it is difficult, to say the least, to imagine Hahnemann's process of cure in progress)? And hence has arisen an hypothesis with respect to the influence of minute doses in the cure of diseases, which is fully as ingenious as Hahnemann's own, and is probably just as true, but which has the theoretical disadvantage for homœopaths of converting homœopathy into antipathy! It is to the effect that all medicines have opposite effects, according as they are given in large or in small doses, and that when, as the consequence of proving on the healthy person, a drug is found to excite the symptoms of a disease, it cures that disease by its opposition to it when given in small doses. I shall not stop to consider the propriety or plausibility of these and other like innovations in orthodox homœopathy; and I leave those who advocate them to reconcile them as best they may with the teachings of their founder; neither shall I quarrel with the homœopaths who choose to maintain that these only represent successive stages in the progressive development of homœopathy. To me, I confess, they seem in direct contravention of homœopathic principles, and fraught with ultimate disaster to the homœopathic cause.

It is perhaps the most difficult thing in the whole practice of medicine to determine, in disease, whether the drugs which we are giving are directly influencing it for good. This difficulty is specially great when, as sometimes happens even to ourselves, we are, from ignorance of the essential nature of the disease we are treating, or from failure to form an accurate diagnosis, compelled to treat, as Hahnemann only treated, groups of symptoms. It is true that even the most accurate observers constantly deceive themselves. It was mainly by treating diseases simply in groups of symptoms, that Hahnemann deceived himself from first to last. And it is mainly thus that homœopathic practitioners continue to deceive themselves down to the present time. When they can show that, by remedies acting homœopathically, they can cure habitually definite diseases which by other means we cure uncertainly or fail to cure altogether, or can cut short or render less fatal than they are the fevers that tend to run a definite course, it will be time for us to make homœopathy a serious study. For tetanus, for epilepsy, for hydrophobia, typical homœopathic remedies exist. Was ever tetanus, epilepsy, or hydrophobia cured by homœopathy? They profess to ward off and to cure scarlet fever, by what they hold to be its homœopathic antagonist—belladonna. Is scarlet fever less frequent or less fatal in the families of homœopaths than amongst the general population? What evidence is there which we can accept, that any internal inflammation, any internal growth, any specific fever, has ever been cured, or even ameliorated, by homœopathic remedies? Of course, affirmative assertions will be made; of course, statistical evidence will be forthcoming. But mere assertions, and mere statistics, which are simply tabulated assertions, are not evidence which a man professing scientific caution would accept in such a case. Nevertheless, did homœopathy possess one tittle of the curative power which Hahnemann claimed for it, it must long before now have commended the homage of even its most inveterate enemies. For it must be recollected that the claims of homœopathy are not to equality of results with those of orthodox medicine, but that they are to alleviate and cure diseases over which we have little or no control; to relieve where we hurt, to save life where we kill.

So far, gentlemen, I have discussed only on homœopathy as a science and an art. I wish to add a few words on homœopathists as men, and as members of our common profession.

That a very strong feeling of hostility should have arisen early between orthodox practitioners and homœopathists, is not to be wondered at, when we consider, on the one hand, the arrogance and intolerance which Hahnemann displayed, at any rate in his writings, and on the other hand, the contempt which experienced physicians felt and freely expressed for him and his whimsical doctrines. Nor is it to be wondered at, that the variance should still be maintained, for homœopathy is still a protest against the best traditions of orthodox clinical medicine, and there is a natural tendency among us still to look upon homœopathic practitioners as knaves or fools; but surely this view is a wholly untenable one.

That all homœopathists are honest men, is more than I would venture to repeat; but that in large proportion they are honest, is entirely beyond dispute. It is quite impossible that a large sect should have arisen, homœopathic schools and hospitals have been established, periodicals devoted to homœopathic medicines be maintained, and a whole

literature in relation to it have been created, if it were all merely to support a conscious imposture. No, gentlemen; the whole history of the movement and its present position are amply sufficient to prove that those, at any rate, who take the intellectual lead in it are men who believe in the doctrines they profess, and in their mission; and who practise their profession with as much honesty of purpose, and with as much confidence in their power to benefit their patients, as we do. That all homœopathic practitioners are men of ability and education it would be absurd to maintain; but it is absolutely certain that many men of ability and learning are contained within their ranks. If you care to dive into homœopathic literature, you will find in it (however much you may differ from the views therein inculcated) plenty of literary ability; and I have perused many papers by homœopaths, on philosophical and other subjects unconnected with homœopathy, which have proved the authors to be men of thought and culture, and from which I have derived pleasure and profit. Again, I will not pretend that even a considerable proportion of homœopaths are deeply versed in the medical sciences; yet they have all been educated in orthodox schools of medicine, and have passed the examinations of recognised licensing boards; so that it must be allowed that they have acquired sufficient knowledge to qualify themselves for practice, and some among them possess high medical attainments.

But it may be replied, If these men are honest and educated, and at the same time duly qualified practitioners in medicine, how can they believe, and how can they practise, such a palpable imposition as homœopathy? Well, gentlemen, it is very difficult to account for the beliefs and vagaries of the human intellect. It is only occasionally that our convictions are the result of conscious reasoning. For the most part they arise in the mind, and take possession of it, we know not how or why; and our reasonings in regard to them (if we reason at all) are merely special pleadings prompted by the very convictions they seem to us to determine—in other words, they are not the foundations of our beliefs at all, but exhalations from them. It is not surprising, therefore, that, even on matters of supreme importance, irreconcilable differences of opinion prevail, aye, even amongst men of high integrity and cultivated intellect. And if we desire to live broad and unselfish lives, we must be slow to condemn all those who entertain convictions which to us seem foolish or mischievous and logically untenable, or to refuse to co-operate with them.

There are few, even of the best among us, who have not weak points in intellect or character. And it would be deplorable indeed if, for example, those of us who look at spiritualism as one of the grossest follies of the times in which we live, were to scout the distinguished chemists and the great writers who devoutly believe in it; or were to refuse to do homage to the conspicuous abilities and high character of a great judge, because, throwing off the judicial impartiality which befits a judge, and acting under the influence of prejudice, emotion, and ignorance, he has made himself the leader of all the hysterical sentimentalism of the day in a crusade against experimental physiology in the land of Harvey and of Hunter! The remarks just made apply especially to beliefs in relation to those matters which are incapable of exact scientific proof, and in which the feelings are largely involved—pre-eminently, therefore, to religion, to politics, and to medicine.

I ask you, gentlemen, to forbear with me if I push my argument to the logical conclusion, and venture now to express an opinion which is opposed to the opinion which many, perhaps most, of you entertain. I do not ask you to agree with it; still less do I ask you to adopt it. But I ask you to consider it: and I am content to believe that, if it be just, it will ultimately prevail. It is that, when homœopathists are honest, and well-informed, and legally qualified practitioners of medicine, they should be dealt with as if they were honest and well-informed and qualified. I shall not discuss the question whether we can, with propriety or with benefit to our patients, meet homœopaths in consultation. I could, however, I think, adduce strong reasons in favour of the morality of acting thus, and for the belief that good to the patient would generally ensue under such circumstances. I shall not consider at length whether the dignity of the profession would be compromised by habitual dealing with homœopathists. But I may observe that it is more conducive to the maintenance of true dignity to treat with respect and consideration, and as if they were honest, those whose opinions differ from ours, than to make broad our phylacteries and enlarge the borders of our garments, and wrap ourselves up, in regard to them, in pharisaic pride. I appeal, gentlemen, in support of my contention, to other considerations. It has been held, that to break down the barriers that at present separate us from homœopathists would be to allow the poison of [quackery to leaven the mass of orthodox medicine. But who that has any trust in his profession, any scientific instinct, any faith in the ultimate triumph of truth, can entertain any such fear? All the best physicians of old times, all the greatest names in medicine of the present day, are with us; and we know that as a body we are honest seekers after truth. What have we to fear from homœopathy? Bigots are made martyrs by persecution; false sects acquire form and momentum and importance mainly through the opposition they provoke. When persecution ceases, would-be martyrs sink into insignificance; in the absence of the stimulus of active opposition, sects tend to undergo disintegration and to disappear. The rise and spread of homœopathy have been largely due to the strong antagonism it has evoked from the schools of orthodox medicine, and to the isolation which has thus been imposed on its disciples. If false, as we believe it to be, its doom will be sealed when active antagonism and enforced isolation no longer raise it into fictitious importance. At any rate, breadth of view and liberality of conduct are the fitting characteristics of men of science.

THE LONDON HOSPITAL.—Mrs. Elizabeth Letheby has left a sum of £1000 to form a scholarship or prize, to be awarded annually to the student, in the medical school of the London Hospital, who shows himself most proficient in chemistry. Such scholarship is to be known as the "Dr. Letheby Prize," in memory of her husband, who was for many years Professor of Chemistry at the London Hospital.

THE APOTHECARIES' HALL OF IRELAND.—At the annual meeting of the General Council of the Apothecaries' Hall of Ireland, convened by authority of the Act of Incorporation, on Monday, August 1, 1881, the following were elected office-bearers for the ensuing year:—*Governor :* Thomas Collins. *Deputy-Governor :* Robert Montgomery. *Court of Directors and Examiners :* Edward H. Bolland, John Evans, Arthur Harvey, Charles Holmes, Charles Henry Leet, Charles Frederick Moore, Henry P. Nolan, Jerome O'Flaherty, Edward J. O'Neill, Sir George B. Owens, John Ryan, James Shaw, George Wyse. *Examiners in Arts :* Henry Colpoys Tweedy, M.D., ex-Scholar Trin. Coll. Dub. ; George Y. Dixon, B.A. Univ. Dub. *Representative on the General Medical Council :* Thomas Collins. *Secretary :* Chas. Henry Leete.

REMARKABLE ATTEMPT AT SUICIDE.—The *Progrès Médical,* July 30, gives an account of a man who, after a domestic quarrel, seized a poignard, ten centimetres in length, and placing it vertically at the top of his head, drove it by help of a hammer into the cranium as far as the hilt. Finding that he had not caused death as he intended, he summoned a doctor in order to have the instrument removed. This, notwithstanding all the force that two persons could employ, was found impossible, and the removal could only be effected by taking him to a workshop and putting some machinery in motion for its extraction; the force employed being sufficient to raise him a little from the ground, on to which he fell again when the poignard was withdrawn. He all along retained his senses and power of movement, and accompanied the doctor to his carriage after the operation had succeeded. The blade of the poignard was found somewhat curved towards its point, it having struck against the occipital fossa, and become impacted. In fear of possible consequences, the patient was placed in one of M. Péan's wards at the St. Louis for a week, when he was discharged, not having meanwhile exhibited any inflammatory or paralytic symptoms.

CORYZA.—The following mixture has been found useful at the commencement of a cold :—Carbolic acid crystals 5 parts, rectified spirit of wine 15, liquor ammonia 5, distilled water 10 parts. A few drops are let fall on blotting-paper and inhaled at a distance through the nose and mouth.— *Union Méd.,* July 30.

THE INTERNATIONAL MEDICAL CONGRESS.

SECTION OF MENTAL DISEASES.
ADDRESS BY
C. LOCKHART ROBERTSON, M.D. CANTAB., F.R.C.P., *President of the Section.*

GENTLEMEN,—In now opening the Eighth Section of this great International Medical Congress, and in offering to the alienists of Europe and America our cordial welcome to London, I must ask leave to explain to you that it is only by the accident of official position as Senior Physician to the Lord Chancellor, who, under the Royal prerogative, has in England the guardianship of all lunatics and persons of unsound mind, that I occupy to-day this presidential chair. But for the desire of the Executive Committee thus to recognise the paramount authority of the Lord Chancellor in our department of medicine, I cannot doubt that the place I now fill would have been allotted to our most distinguished English writer on lunacy, Dr. J. C. Bucknill, one of the Vice-Presidents of this Congress, whose writings and whose name are a household word in all the asylums where the English tongue is spoken. Called from my official position rather than on personal fitness to preside in this Section, I may the more venture to ask at your hands a generous interpretation of my efforts, so to guide your deliberations here that they may advance the science and practice of this department of medicine in which we are all enrolled.

I think I shall best use this occasion by laying before you a brief statement of the present condition of the insane in England, and[of the manner and method of their care and treatment. In the German tongue the word *Irren-Wesen* exactly expresses the subject of this address.

The number of the insane in England of whom we have official cognisance is about 71,000, being in the ratio of 27·9 per 10,000, or 1 in 350, of the population. Of these no less than 63,500 are paupers chargeable to the rates and maintained at the cost of the community. The remaining 7600 are private patients, whose means vary from £50 to £50,000 a year, much the larger number being nearer £50, for insanity necessarily tends by arresting the power of production to the impoverishment of its subjects. Thus, of the total of the insane in England, 90 per cent. are paupers maintained at the public cost, and 10 per cent. only are kept by their own resources.

There has, since the passing of the Lunacy Act of 1845, been a great yearly increase in the registered numbers of the insane—an increase chiefly, if not solely, among the pauper class,—which admits of satisfactory explanation, as I have elsewhere(a) endeavoured to show, with accepting the popular fallacy of an increase of insanity; a theory which, if carried to its logical conclusion, leads us to the result that as the registered lunatics in 1845 were as 1 to 800 of the population, while in 1880 they stand, as I have just stated, as 1 to 350, therefore lunacy in England has more than doubled during the last thirty years—which is a manifest fallacy. I only regret that my present limits preclude farther reference to this interesting problem.(b)

I have prepared a table which exhibits the number of the insane in England, with their place of residence and their proportion to the population in the decenniums 1860, 1870, and 1880. This table shows that the total registered number of the insane has risen from 38,000 in 1860, to 71,000 in 1880, and the ratio to the population from 19·1 per 10,000 to 27·9. It is evident from my figures that this increase is

(a) "The Alleged Increase of Lunacy" (*Journal of Mental Science,* April, 1869) ; "A Farther Note on the Alleged Increase of Lunacy" (*Journal of Mental Science,* January, 1871).
(b) In the Report of the Scotch Commissioners in Lunacy for 1880, this question of the apparent increase of insanity is ably discussed and dealt with in a careful statistical inquiry. I can only here give their conclusion :—"We have frequently pointed out that the difference in these rates of increase is not necessarily due to an increasing amount of mental disease, but is probably due in a large measure to what is only an increasing readiness to place persons as lunatics in establishments."

mainly in the pauper class. The private patients in 1860 numbered 5900, in 1880 they were 7500, and their ratio to the population 2·5 and 2·9 respectively, an increase of 0·4 only as compared with the increase of 8·8 among the pauper lunatics on each 10,000 of the population.

Table I. gives the distribution per cent. of the 71,000 registered lunatics in England and Wales, and I have here contrasted the same with that of the 10,000 lunatics registered in Scotland.

TABLE I. — *Showing the Distribution per Cent. of all Lunatics in England and Wales, and in Scotland, in 1880 (January 1).*

	DISTRIBUTION PER CENT.					
	In England and Wales.			In Scotland.		
	Private.	Pauper.	Total.	Private.	Pauper.	Total.
In public asylums * ...	5·0	56·5	61·5	14·6	61·0	75·6
In private asylums† ...	5·0	1·5	6·5	1·6	None.	1·6
In workhouses‡	None.	23·0	23·0	None.	7·0	7·0
In private dwellings§ ...	0·5	8·5	9·0	1·1	14·7	15·8
Total	...	...	100	...	...	100

* Including county and district asylums and Scotch parochial asylums; lunatic hospitals and Scotch chartered asylums; naval, military, and East India asylums; idiot asylums; Broadmoor Criminal Asylum; and Perth Prison wards.
† Including provincial and metropolitan licensed houses.
‡ Including the metropolitan district asylums.
§ Including 338 Chancery lunatics residing in the private houses of " the committee of the person."

Table I. is interesting as contrasting the total distribution of lunacy in England with that of Scotland. In England 61·5 per cent. of the lunacy of the country is maintained in the public asylums. In Scotland it reaches 75·6 per cent., while on the other hand the proportion of patients in private asylums is 6·5 per cent. in England as against 1·6 in Scotland. In England 9 per cent. only of all lunatics are placed for care in private dwellings; in Scotland the proportion rises to 15·8. In England we have 23 per cent. in workhouses; in Scotland there are only 7 per cent.

Table II. gives the relative distribution per cent. of private and pauper lunatics respectively in England and Wales, and in Scotland.

TABLE II. — *Showing the Distribution per Cent. on their several Numbers of the Private and Pauper Lunatics respectively in England and Wales; and in Scotland, in 1880.*

	DISTRIBUTION PER CENT.			
Where maintained.	In England and Wales.		In Scotland.	
	Private.	Pauper.	Private.	Pauper.
In public asylums	49·0	63·0	84·0	72·7
In private asylums	43·0	1·6	9·5	None.
In workhouses	None.	26·0	None.	8·5
In private dwellings	8·0	9·4	6·5	17·8
Total	100	100	100	100

Table II. brings strikingly before us the existing difference in the method and treatment of the insane in the two kingdoms. In England 43 per cent. of the private patients are in private asylums, while in Scotland the proportion is 9·5 only. The public asylums, on the other hand, have 84 of the Scotch private patients under treatment as against 49 in England. In England, owing to the traditional preference of the Court of Chancery for private dwellings for the care of its wards, we find the proportion of patients so placed stands as 8 to 6·5 in Scotland, while with pauper lunatics these figures are reversed, the proportion in England being 9·4 as contrasted with 17·8 in Scotland.

I. PUBLIC ASYLUMS.

There are 43,700 patients in the public asylums of England, or 60·5 per cent. of the whole lunacy of the country. Of these 40,000 are pauper lunatics, and 3700 are private patients. The former are maintained in the county and borough asylums; the latter are divided between these and the registered lunatic hospitals.

(a.) *County and Borough Asylums.* — The county and borough asylums of England, (o) sixty in number, contain 40,000 beds, varying from 2000 to 250. They have been built and are administered under the provisions of the Lunacy Act of 1845. The average cost per bed has been under £200; the weekly maintenance of each patient is 10s., to which must be added the interest on the cost of construction and the yearly repairs of the asylum, which are borne by the county rate, bringing the yearly cost for each pauper lunatic maintained in the county asylums to nearly £40.

The government of the English county asylums is entrusted, by the Lunacy Act, 1845, to a committee of the justices of the peace, under the control of the Secretary of State for the Home Department. The administration is in the hands of the resident medical superintendent. A yearly inspection of the asylum is made by the Commissioners in Lunacy, and a yearly medical and financial report is presented by the committee and medical superintendent to the quarter sessions, and published.

The proportion of cures (discharged recovered) in the county and borough asylums in the last decennium, 1870–80, was 40·28 per cent. on the admissions, and the mortality 10·59 on the mean population. In Scotland, during the same period, the recoveries were 41·6, and the deaths 8. The only private patients admissible under the statute are those bordering on pauperism, and whom the law requires, as to classification and diet, clothing, etc., to be treated as the paupers. Herein the English county asylums differ from those on the continent of Europe and in America, where alike, and, I think, most wisely, special and often excellent provision exists for the care and treatment of private patients. At the public asylums near Rouen, at Rome, at Munich, and at Utica in the States, I have seen extremely good accommodation provided for private patients.

In Mr. Dillwyn's Lunacy Law Amendment Bill, 1881, which was read a second time on May 25, but has since been withdrawn for this session, there was a clause (Section 4) enabling the visitors of county asylums to provide there suitable accommodation, by additional buildings or otherwise, for private patients. I regard this proposal as one of the most important reforms, since the Lunacy Act of 1845, in the treatment of the insane of the middle-class, providing as it would for the small ratepayers, at a cost within their means, such care and treatment as they cannot obtain in the cheaper private asylums, where the accommodation and comfort are absolutely below that of the paupers in county asylums, not to refer to the superior acquirements of the medical superintendents of the latter.

I do not feel called upon from this chair (nor does time admit) to enforce and illustrate the now incontestable superiority of public asylums, even in a financial point, for the curative treatment of the insane poor as contrasted with the private licensed houses to which, before the Act of 1845, they were farmed out by their respective parishes. "Our present business is to affirm that poor lunatics ought to be maintained at the public charge. I entertain myself a very decided opinion that none of any class should be received for profit; but all, I hope, will agree that paupers, at any rate, should not be the objects of financial speculation." These words, spoken by Lord Shaftesbury in the House of Commons when he introduced the Lunacy Act of 1845 (the Magna Charta of the insane poor), settled this question once for all. Whose voice will speak similar words of comfort and healing to the insane of the upper and middle classes, and declare with authority which shall no longer be questioned, "that all insane captives whose freedom would not

(c) A return was ordered by the House of Commons to be printed, August 14, 1878, of the cost of construction of each of the county asylums, the number of beds, the annual and weekly maintenance rate, the percentage of recoveries, deaths, etc. Unfortunately it has been, as regards England, carelessly prepared, and no abstract or summary of its contents or averages is given. It is impossible to make out clearly in which asylums the yearly repairs are included in the total cost of construction, and in which they are omitted. The quarter sessions of Warwickshire have made no return at all! In contrast, in the same Parliamentary paper, stand the clear tables and summary relating to the public asylums of Scotland. From the English return we can only gather an approximate estimate of the cost of construction, amount of land, salaries, cures, etc., no averages being given.

be dangerous should be liberated, and those who remain be surrounded with every safeguard of disinterestedness, humanity, and public responsibility"?

In here recording the success which has attended the Act of 1845—a success that led my friend Dr. Paget, in his Harveian Oration, to call the sight of one of our English county asylums "the most blessed manifestation of true civilisation that the world can present,"—I cannot refrain from adding a word of tribute to the memory of my revered friend John Conolly, whose work of freeing the insane from mechanical restraint, and of thereby founding our English school of psychological medicine, preceded the legislation promoted by the Earl of Shaftesbury, and insured the success of these enactments.(d)

Dr. Conolly's four annual reports of the County Lunatic Asylum at Hanwell for 1839, '40, 41, '42, still form the groundwork of our treatment of the insane poor in the English county asylums, while these asylums themselves—whose fame, I may be permitted to say, based as it is on the successful application of the English non-restraint system, has gone forth into the whole civilised world, and brought rescue to the most suffering and degraded of our race—stand throughout this fair land imperishable monuments of the statesman to whom they owe their origin, and of the physician who asserted the great principle on which the treatment within their walls is founded.

"The system as now established," he writes, "will form no unimportant chapter in the history of medicine in relation to disorders of the mind. It has been carried into practical effect in an intellectual and practical age, unostentatiously, gradually, and carefully, and is, I trust, destined to endure as long as science continues to be pursued with a love of truth and a regard for the welfare of man."(e)

We have made arrangements whereby you will have the opportunity of visiting and inspecting two of the best of the English county asylums—that for Sussex at Hayward's Heath, and for Surrey at Brookwood,—as also the four great metropolitan asylums with a joint population of 6600 lunatics, at Hanwell, Colney Hatch, Banstead, and Wandsworth. There has since the Lunacy Act of 1845 been a steady increase in the number of pauper lunatics placed in the county asylums. In 1860 the proportion was 57 per cent., in 1870 it rose to 61 per cent., and in 1880 it was nearly 65 per cent. of their number. I think this continued increase is the most injurious alike to insane poor and to the due administration of the county asylums. The accumulation in such large numbers of harmless and incurable lunatics in these costly asylums is, moreover, a needless burden on the rates.

I think we may now, with an experience of thirty-five years, assert that the utmost limits within which the county asylum can benefit or is needed for the treatment of the insane poor is 50 per cent. of their number,(f) and that a

further accumulation of lunatics there serves no practical purpose, and hence is an unjustifiable waste of public money. The workhouses contain 16,500 pauper lunatics, or 26 per cent. of their number. A recent statute facilitates the adaptation of wards in the county workhouses(g) for the reception of lunatics; and if these arrangements were properly carried out, I think another 14 per cent., or 40 per cent. of the incurable and harmless pauper lunatics and idiots, might be provided for in the workhouses. That this is no fancy estimate I may quote the parish of Brighton, long distinguished for its wise and liberal administration of the Poor-law, which has already 36 per cent. of its insane poor in the workhouse wards, and 55 per cent. only in the county asylum. The transfer of twenty chronic cases—no impossible feat—from Hayward's Heath to the Brighton workhouse wards would at once bring the Brighton statistics up to my ideal standard for the distribution of pauper lunatics —viz., in county asylums, 50 per cent.; in workhouse wards, 40 per cent.; leaving 10 per cent. for care in private dwellings.

(b.) *Lunatic Hospitals (Middle-class Public Asylums).*— Besides the county asylums for the insane poor, we have in England fifteen lunatic hospitals, including the idiot asylums at Earlswood and Lancaster, where the principle of hospital treatment followed in the county asylums is applied to the insane of the upper and middle class with the most satisfactory results.

The following table gives a list of these asylums, with the date of their foundation, their present accommodation (number of beds), and their average weekly cost of maintenance :—

TABLE III.—*The Registered Lunatic Hospitals (Middle-class Asylums) in England, with the Date of their Foundation, the Number of Beds, and the Average Weekly Cost of Maintenance in 1880.*

Name and site of asylum. (Registered hospital.)	Date of foundation.	Number of beds.	Average weekly cost.*
			£ s. d.
Bethlem Royal Hospital	1400	300	1 11 7
St. Luke's Hospital	1751	300	0 19 3
York Lunatic Hospital	1777	180	1 1 1
Friends' Retreat, York	1796	150	1 13 6
Wonford House, Exeter	1801	100	1 11 0
Lincoln Lunatic Hospital	1890	60	1 3 3
Bethel Hospital, Norwich	1825	70	0 15 3
Warneford Asylum, Oxford	1826	70	1 2 7
St. Andrew's Hospital, Northampton	1836	300	1 10 1
Cheadle Asylum, Manchester	1849	180	2 3 0
The Coppice, Nottingham	1859	70	1 10 4
Coton Hill, Stafford	1854	150	1 13 10
Barnwood House, Gloucester	1860	110	1 14 3
Earlswood Idiot Asylum	1847	570	0 18 3
Albert Idiot Asylum, Lancaster	1864	350	0 14 0

* The fabric charges are not included in these figures. Another 5s. a week must be added to complete this estimated weekly cost of maintenance.

These asylums have nearly 3000 beds, and the average weekly cost of maintenance is £1 10s., or, including the fabric account, £1 15s.

There are 7828 private lunatics registered in England, who are thus distributed :—

In registered hospitals	2702 or 36 per cent.	In public asylums 49 p. c.
In county asylums	484 or 6 "	
In State asylums	553 or 7 "	
In private asylums	3406 or 43 "	
In private dwellings	676 or 8 "	

(d) "In June, 1839, Dr. Conolly was appointed Resident Physician at Hanwell. In September he had abolished all mechanical restraints. The experiment was a trying one, for this great Asylum contained 800 patients. But the experiment succeeded ; and continued experience proved incontestably that in a well-ordered asylum the use even of the straitwaistcoat might be entirely discarded. Dr. Conolly went further than this. He maintained that such restraints are in all cases positively injurious; that their use is utterly inconsistent with a good system of treatment; and that, on the contrary, the absence of all such restraints is naturally and necessarily associated with treatment such as that of lunatics ought to be—one which substitutes mental for bodily control, and is governed in all its details by the purpose of preventing mental excitement, or of soothing it before it bursts out into violence. He urged this with feeling and persuasive eloquence, and gave in proof of it the results of his own experiment at Hanwell. For, from the time that all mechanical restraints were abolished, the occurrence of frantic behaviour among the lunatics became less and less frequent. Thus did the experiments of Charlesworth and Conolly confirm the principles of treatment inaugurated by Daquin and Pinel; and prove that the best guide to the treatment of lunatics is to be found in the dictates of an enlightened and refined benevolence. And so the progress of science, by way of experiment, has led men to rules of practice nearer and nearer to the teachings of Christianity. To my eyes a pauper lunatic asylum, such as may now be seen in our English counties, with its pleasant grounds, its airy and cleanly wards, its many comforts, and wise and kindly superintendence, provided for those whose lot it is to bear the double burden of poverty and mental derangement—I say this sight is to me the most blessed manifestation of true civilisation that the world can present."—The Harveian Oration, 1886, by George E. Paget, M.D. Cantab., Regius Professor of Medicine in the University of Cambridge.

(e) "The Treatment of the Insane without Mechanical Restraint," by John Conolly, M.D. Edin., D.C L. London: Smith, Elder, and Co., 1856.

(f) There is a unanimous concurrence of opinion on the part of the lunacy officials and the visiting justices that the grant from the Consolidated Fund of 4s. a week made by Lord Beaconsfield's Government in 1874 for every pauper lunatic detained in the county asylums has led to a needless increase in the admission there of aged lunatics and idiot chil-

dren, who were and can with equal facility be kept in the workhouses. This grant has risen year by year, and in the estimates of 1881-82 is placed at £485,000. Instead of relieving the landed interest, as this ill-considered attempt to shift part of their burden on the fundholders was intended, it has actually increased the county rate by the forced enlargements and extension of the county asylums. The editor of the *Times* in 1874 and 1876 allowed me at some length to direct attention to this yearly increasing misdirection of the public funds. It is to be hoped that when the heavy local taxation of England is readjusted, this outlet of wasteful expenditure may not be overlooked.

(g) The success of the Metropolitan District Asylums at Leavesden, Caterham, and Darenth, which contain 4470 chronic lunatics maintained at the rate of 7s. a week, shows how, even in so difficult a place as London, the treatment of chronic and harmless pauper lunatic in workhouse wards is to be accomplished, with a large saving to the ratepayers and a relief to the crowded wards of the county asylums, which are thus made available for the curative treatment of acute and recent cases.

The existing lunatic hospitals, or middle-class public asylums, thus already receive 36 per cent. of all the private patients. The advocates of this method of treatment of the insane, as opposed to the private asylum system, may now fairly say that by thus providing for the care and treatment of 36 per cent. of the private lunatics they have demonstrated the practicability of this method as applicable to the other 43 per cent. now in private asylums.

They can also appeal to the official statistics to show their superiority as regards results over the private asylums. In the last decennium 1870-80 the average recoveries per cent. on the admissions in the registered hospitals was 46·84; in the metropolitan private asylums it was 30·5; and in the provincial private asylums 34·7. The mean annual mortality during the same period was in the registered hospitals 8·12; in the metropolitan private asylums it rose to 11·01, and in the provincial private asylums it was 8·61. They may, moreover, point to Scotland and say, that while in England 49 per cent. of the private patients only are provided for in public asylums, 84 per cent. are so cared for in Scotland. What has been accomplished in Scotland may surely be done in England. And certainly, as their strong and final argument, they may challenge a comparison of these asylums, conducted at half the cost, with the best of the private asylums in England. We have made arrangements for your visiting Bethlem(h) and St. Luke's in London, and also the middle-class asylum, St. Andrew's Hospital, Northampton. I should very much like you to see St. Andrew's Hospital, which now contains 300 private patients of the upper and middle classes, from whose payments it derives a revenue of £40,000 a year, of which £10,000 was saved last year for further extensions. It would be difficult to overpraise the power of organisation which has enabled Mr. Bayley, the medical superintendent, to achieve this great result in the last ten years only. I can from frequent visitation speak of the order and comfort which reign throughout this asylum.

Mr. Dillwyn's Select Committee, in their Report (March 28, 1878), suggested "that legislative facilities should be afforded by enlargement of the powers of the magistrates or otherwise, for the extension of the public asylum system for private patients, and in his Lunacy Law Amendment Bill, 1881, read a second time in May, Section 1 enables the justices to provide asylums for the separate use of private lunatics in like manner as the county pauper asylums were built. There can be no doubt, after the experience I have just related of St. Andrew's Hospital, Northampton, that, especially in the populous Home Counties, where no public provision for private lunatics exists, several such asylums, with 300 beds, might be built on the credit of the rates, and would in thirty years repay the capital and interest sunk out of the profits, and without, therefore, costing the ratepayers one penny. This clause alone would have made of Mr. Dillwyn's Bill a great gift to the insane of the upper and middle class.(i) I cannot but regret that so valuable a measure had to be withdrawn from want of time. It is already a well-worn complaint that home legislation is in England sadly impeded by the weary Irish agitation and debates.

Another method of providing public asylum accommodation for private patients was laid by me before Mr. Dillwyn's Select Committee, in a "Memorandum on the Establishment of Three State Asylums for Chancery Lunatics," signed by Dr. Bucknill, Dr. Crichton Browne, and myself. The insane wards of the Court of Chancery pay upwards of £100,000 a year for care and treatment in private asylums. Certainly no loss could be incurred by the Treasury in advancing funds to build these asylums, where the yearly profits would, as at St. Andrew's Hospital, insure the regular repayment of capital and interest. As the Court of Chancery controls in every detail the expenditure of the income of its insane wards, it is not an unreasonable demand to require that Court to provide fit public asylum accommodation, and such as the visitors deem necessary for the Chancery patients now placed in private asylums, in the selection of which their official visitors have no voice, and over the conduct and management of which they exercise no control.

<hr/>

(h) In the *Journal of Mental Science* for July, 1876, there is a very interesting sketch of the history of Bethlem Hospital since 1400, by Dr. Hack Tuke.

(i) I brought this whole subject before the Brighton Medical Society in 1862, in a paper "On the Want of a Middle-class Asylum in Sussex," subsequently inserted in the *Journal of Mental Science* for January, 1863.

II. PRIVATE ASYLUMS.

There are 3400, or 43 per cent., of the private patients in England confined in private asylums, of whom 1850 or 54 per cent. are in the thirty-five metropolitan licensed houses which are under the sole control and direction of the Commissioners in Lunacy, who diligently visit them six times a year. The remaining 1550, or 46 per cent., are in the sixty-one provincial licensed houses which are under the jurisdiction of the justices in quarter sessions, but are inspected twice a year by the Lunacy Commissioners. I cannot—even did I so desire—avoid in an address like the present stating to you my opinion of this method of treatment of the insane. The tenor of my remarks when referring to the extension of the lunatic hospitals (middle-class asylums) has already shown the direction towards which my opinions and feelings tend. John Stuart Mill, the strenuous advocate of freedom of contract, nevertheless, in his "Political Economy," in treating of this subject, observes that "insane persons should everywhere be regarded as proper objects of the care of the State," and, in quoting this authority, I must add, from long personal observation, my opinion that it would be for the interests of the insane of the upper and middle class to be treated as are the paupers in public asylums, where no questions of self-interest can arise, and where the physician's remuneration is a fixed salary, and not the difference between the payments made by his patients for board and lodging, and the sums he may expend on their maintenance. "Is there not," writes Dr. Maudsley, "sufficient reason to believe that proper medical supervision and proper medical treatment might be equally well, if not better, secured by dissociating the medical element entirely from all questions of profit and loss, and allowing it the unfettered exercise of its healing function? Eminent and accomplished physicians would then engage in this branch of practice, who now avoid it because it involves so many disagreeable necessities."

Probably all not directly interested in this system, and many who, to their own regret, are so, will concur that if the work had to be begun anew the idea of licensed private asylums for the treatment of the insane of the upper and middle class would be by every authority in the State as definitely condemned as was in 1845 the practice of farming out the insane poor to lay speculators in lunacy. It is, however, a different matter dealing with an established system, and I am not of those who call for the suppression of all private asylums. The friends of many patients in England distinctly prefer them to public asylums, and some patients who have had experience of both contrast the personal consideration and study of their little wants which they receive in private asylums with the discipline and drill of the public institutions. I see no reason why private asylums should not continue to exist side by side with the public middle-class asylums. Time and competition will show which system shall ultimately gain the approval of the public. I am glad to find this opinion supported by Dr. Arthur Mitchell, Commissioner in Lunacy for Scotland, in his evidence before the Parliamentary Committee of 1877.

"I think," he said, "there should be no legislation tending to the suppression of private asylums. I would let the principles of free trade settle the matter. If the public have confidence in private asylums, and encourage them, I would let private asylums exist. I would give them no privileges, and would simply take care that the inspection and control over them are sufficient."

The verdict of public opinion in Scotland has been definitely against the private asylum system. While in England 31·5 per cent. of the private patients are confined in private asylums, the proportion in Scotland falls to 9·5.

If private asylums are to continue there should be entire freedom of trade in the business. The Lunacy Commissioners have for many years placed endless impediments in the way of licensing new and small asylums in the metropolitan district. I entirely differ from this policy, and I think that small asylums for four or six patients licensed to medical men would tend to lessen the existing evils of the larger private asylums. The monopoly which the Commissioners have established in the metropolitan district has certainly not raised the asylums there to a higher standard than those of the provinces, where free trade in lunacy prevails. I am tempted to say that it has had the contrary effect.

III. The Insane in Private Dwellings.

Further reform in the treatment of the insane is not merely a question of whether and how they shall be detained in public or private asylums, but rather whether and when they should be placed in asylums at all, and when and how they shall be liberated from their imprisonment and restored to the freedom of private life. This is the reform in lunacy treatment which is beginning at last to take hold on the public mind in England, and has received a new impulse by the recent publication of an essay by Dr. Bucknill, " On the Care of the Insane and their Legal Control."(k)

It is more than twenty years ago since the question of the needless sequestration of the insane was first raised in England by my friend Baron Jaromir Mundy, of Moravia. He spoke then to dull and heedless ears. I remember well I thought him an amiable enthusiast, and I said there was no fit or proper treatment for the insane to be found out of the walls of an asylum. I have since learnt a wiser experience. Well might he say on leaving us, " Arbores serit diligens agricola quarum fructus nunquam aspiciet." I am very glad to have this great opportunity of doing honour to the zeal and far-seeing wisdom of the first preacher of this new crusade : would he were here with us to-day to accept my formal adherence to his cause.

There is, I believe, for a large number of the incurable insane a better lot in store than to drag on their weary days in asylum confinement—

> "The staring eye glazed o'er with sapless days,
> The slow mechanic pacings to and fro,
> The set gray life and apathetic end."

In my evidence before Mr. Dillwyn's Select Committee in 1877 I was examined at some length on this question, and I stated that but for my experience as Lord Chancellor's Visitor, and if I had not personally watched their cases, I could never have believed that patients who were such confirmed lunatics could be treated in private families in the way that Chancery lunatics are. I also said that one-third of the Chancery patients were already so treated out of asylums, and I added that I was of opinion that one-third of the present inmates of the private asylums might be placed in family treatment with safety. In support of this opinion I put in this table :—

TABLE IV.—*Showing the Proportion per Cent. in Asylums and in Private Dwellings of the Chancery Lunatics and of the Private Patients (Lunatics, not Paupers) under the Commissioners in Lunacy in England and Wales and in Scotland.*

	Proportion per Cent.	
	In lunatic asylums.	Under home treatment in private dwellings.
Chancery lunatics	65·4	34·6
English private lunatics	94·1	5·9
Scotch private lunatics	93·8	6·1

This table deserves your attention. If 34·6 per cent. of the Chancery lunatics is successfully treated in private dwellings, while only 65·4 per cent. are in asylums, it is evident that of the private patients under the Commissioners, of whom 94 per cent. are in asylums, some 30 per cent. are there needlessly, and hence wrongly confined. I see instances of such cases every visit I pay to the private asylums.

Another convert to his cause, made by Baron Mundy, is one of the distinguished Vice-Presidents of this Section, Dr. Henry Maudsley, who, in 1867, in the first edition of his work on the "Physiology and Pathology of the Mind," strenuously condemns the indiscriminate sequestration of the insane in asylums, observing—"The principle which guides the present practice is, that an insane person, by the simple warrant of his insanity, should be shut up in an asylum, the exceptions being made of particular cases. This I hold to be an erroneous principle. The true principle to guide our practice should be this : that no one, sane or insane, should ever be entirely deprived of his liberty,

(k) Macmillan and Co. (London, 1880), second edition.

unless for his own protection, or for the protection of society."

Dr. Maudsley (to strengthen his argument) pointed to the condition of the numerous Chancery patients in England who are living in private houses. "I have," he writes, " the best authority for saying that their condition is eminently satisfactory, and such as it is impossible it could be in the best asylum," and he concluded an elaborate defence of this method of cure with this remark :—"I cannot but think that future progress in the improvement of the treatment of the insane lies in the direction of lessening the sequestration, and increasing the liberty of them. Many chronic insane, incurable and harmless, will be allowed to spend the remaining days of their sorrowful pilgrimage in private families, having the comforts of family life, and the priceless blessing of the utmost freedom that is compatible with their proper care."

In his recent essay on "The Care of the Insane," Dr. Bucknill has a chapter entitled " Household Harmony "—

> " After many moody thoughts,
> At last by notes of household harmony
> They quite forgot their loss of liberty."

I give you therefrom his final and weighty conclusions in his own words :—" It is not merely the happy change which takes place in confirmed lunatics when they are judiciously removed from the dreary detention of the asylum into domestic life; it is the efficiency of the domestic treatment of lunacy during the whole course of the disease which constitutes its greatest value, and of this the author's fullest and latest experience has convinced him that the curative influences of asylums have been vastly overrated, and that those of isolated treatment in domestic care have been greatly undervalued."

What I have hitherto said under this section applies to the home treatment of private patients. The treatment of pauper lunatics in private dwellings is another part of this question, and in which important financial results are involved. The system takes its origin from Gheel, and has been adopted in Scotland with great success. No less than 14·7 per cent. of the insane poor in Scotland are placed in private dwellings under the official inspection of the Lunacy Board. Dr. Arthur Mitchell's evidence before Mr. Dillwyn's Select Committee, and the several annual reports of the Scotch Commissioners, give details of this method of treatment, which my limits only allow me now to refer you to. Financially the cost of this treatment does not reach 1s. a day; in the county asylums (including the cost of the fabric) it is not less than 2s.—a difference of 100 per cent. in expenditure.

With regard to 6000 pauper lunatics, or 8·5 per cent. of their number, are registered as living with relatives, or boarded in private dwellings under the authority of the boards of guardians, whose medical officers visit the patients every quarter and make returns to the visitors of the county asylums, to the Lunacy Commissioners, to the Local Government Board. None of these authorities, however, take much notice of the returns, and little or nothing is known of the condition, care, or treatment of these 6000 pauper lunatics. Any further amendment of the Lunacy Law should certainly, in some way, bring them within the cognisance and inspection of the Lunacy Commissioners, as is done in Scotland.

A successful effort further to extend this system in England is related by Dr. S. W. D. Williams, the Medical Superintendent of the Sussex County Asylum, Hayward's Heath, in his evidence before Mr. Dillwyn's Select Committee, and also in a paper, " Our Overcrowded Lunatic Asylums," published by him in the *Journal of Mental Science* for January, 1872. My limits compel me to be satisfied with this brief reference to the important questions included in this third section of my address, "The Insane in Private Dwellings."

IV. The English Lunacy Law.

Lastly, I would say a few words on the Lunacy Law of England, which, setting aside the special statutes, dating from King Edward II., regulating the proceedings in Chancery, are the result of the legislation of 1845, and consist chiefly of Acts amending other Acts. They form a large volume, which has been carefully edited by Mr. Fry.(l) A

(l) "The Lunacy Acts: containing the Statutes relating to Private Lunatics, Pauper Lunatics, Criminal Lunatics, Commissions of Lunacy, Public and Private Asylums, and the Commissioners in Lunacy; with an Introductory Commentary, etc." By Danby P. Fry, of Lincoln's-inn, barrister-at-law. Second edition. London, 1877.

Bill for the general consolidation and amendment of these several statutes is an urgent need. The Government of Lord Beaconsfield announced in Her Majesty's speech from the throne on the opening of Parliament in February, 1880, that such a measure was in preparation ; and although the political necessities of the Irish question have this year unfortunately absorbed all the energies and time of the Government, we have assurance in the extreme solicitude which the Lord Chancellor on all occasions so markedly shows for the welfare of the insane that the Government will be prepared to give the question of Lunacy Law reform their early and careful attention. I am disposed to think that previous to such legislation a Royal Commission should be issued to investigate and report on the working in detail of the Lunacy Law, and to make suggestions for its consolidation and amendment.

It is exactly twenty-one years since a Parliamentary Committee reported to the House "On the Operation of the Acts of Parliament and Regulations for the Care and Treatment of Lunatics and their Property." Many changes have passed over this department of medicine since the date of that report, and the temporary amendments of the Lunacy Law of 1845, which resulted therefrom, have almost served their purpose. The chief of these enactments of the Lunacy Acts Amendment Act, 1862, passed the following year, and embodied the various suggestions of the Lunacy Commissioners, based on their experience of the working of the Act of 1845, and from an official point of view was a valuable contribution to the Lunacy Law, but it failed to give effect to many of the recommendations of the Select Committee of 1860. In the same year passed the Lunacy Regulation Act, 1862, which led to considerable amendment of the proceedings in Chancery. The important requisite, however, of a cheap and speedy method of placing the property of lunatics under the guardianship of the Lord Chancellor has yet to be attained. One of the most experienced officials in Chancery, Master Barlow, in his evidence before Mr. Dillwyn's Committee, in 1877, said :—"I am a great advocate for a great reform in Lunacy (Chancery) proceedings; I would facilitate the business of the procedure in the office, and shorten it in such a way as to reduce the costs."

After the evidence given by Dr. Arthur Mitchell before Mr. Dillwyn's Select Committee of 1877, it is evident that, in the consolidation and amendment of the English lunacy laws, the Scottish lunacy law and practice must be carefully considered. It is in Scotland alone that the whole lunacy of the kingdom is under the control and cognisance of the Lunacy Board.(m)

Again, the relation of the Lunacy Commissioners to the county asylums under the county financial boards (whose advent is nigh at hand) is a difficult question, the final solution of which will influence for good or evil the future of these asylums. Herein also falls the question I have before referred to of the annual Parliamentary grant for pauper lunatics maintained in asylums, and reaching now to half a million a year. Is the central Government to check, through the distribution of this grant, the county boards; or are they to retain the same authority over the county asylums as is now exercised by the justices in quarter sessions? The whole future efficiency of the English county asylums depends upon the right adjustment of the relative control given to the local authorities through the new county boards, and to the central Government through the Commissioners in Lunacy.

There is also for consideration, as in contrast with the lunacy laws of Scotland, the divided jurisdiction of the Local Government Board and the Commissioners in Lunacy over pauper lunatics in workhouses, of whom 17,000, or 26 per cent. of their number, are there and in the metropolitan district asylums under the control of the Local Government Board, with the merest shadow of inspection by the Lunacy Commissioners. Again, to what extent is the credit of the ratepayers to be used in the establishment of public asylums for private patients? I have already said how much I desire to see the public asylum system, as now existing in the registered lunatic hospitals, extended, more particularly in the Home Counties, by this method. Then the wide question of official asylum inspection. Is the present amount of it enough, and the method of it sufficient for the needs and protection of the insane, or does the Lunacy Commission require both extension and remodelling?

These are but a few examples of the difficulties besetting the question before us of the consolidation and amendment of the English Lunacy Law, and which lead me to the opinion that the whole subject, now ripe for solution, requires skilful and scientific sifting by a Royal Commission, previous to any consolidating and amending Act being laid before Parliament. I am glad to have this occasion to express my personal confidence in the ability, industry, and integrity with which the existing Lunacy Law is administered by the Commissioners. If I were disposed to criticise their policy, I should say that they trust too much to their one remedial agent, the extension of the county asylums, for meeting all the requirements and exigencies of the insane poor, while as regards the private asylums, with 56 per cent. of the private asylum population under their sole control in the metropolitan district, they have from the first, since 1845, been content to enforce the remedying of immediate shortcomings rather than endeavoured to place before the proprietors any standard of excellence to which they must attain.

In concluding my remarks on the last section of my subject—the Lunacy Law of England,—I would say that no mere amending Act like that of 1862, embodying simply the further suggestions of the Lunacy Commissioners, will satisfy the requirements of the medical profession or of the public. In the evidence taken before Mr. Dillwyn's Select Committee in 1877 will be found many suggestions for the further amendment of the Lunacy Law of an important character, one or two of which Mr. Dillwyn embodied in his Lunacy Law Amendment Bill of this year, which, as I have already said, has been withdrawn. It is impossible for any private member of Parliament, actuated though he be by an earnest desire to remedy grave evils, to deal with so wide and complicated a question as the consolidation and amendment of the English Lunacy Law. No one is more fully aware of this impossibility than is Mr. Dillwyn, and no member of the House is prepared more heartily to support the Government in passing a wide and comprehensive measure of Lunacy Law Reform.

SECTION OF MATERIA MEDICA AND PHARMACOLOGY.

ADDRESS BY PROFESSOR FRASER, F.R.S.,
President of the Section.

GENTLEMEN,—The section whose work we inaugurate to-day is devoted to the subjects of Materia Medica and Pharmacology. The occasion of our meeting is one on which we have every reason to congratulate ourselves. The International Medical Congress meets in this country for the first time, and affords an opportunity which has never before been equalled in Great Britain for personal intercourse and exchange of ideas between men from every country in which the study of medicine and of the science of life occupies an intelligent position.

The vastness of this study, the many subjects of separate interest which it includes, and the unfortunate limitations in the power of the human intellect, have necessitated its subdivision into many departments, one group of which has been consigned to the charge of this Section.

I have purposely used the word "group," as the title of our section shows that it embraces not one but several subjects. The words "Materia Medica" no doubt imply a description of the agents used in the treatment of disease; but this description is not restricted to the physical proportion of these agents, for it includes also their actions and their uses in disease. The department of materia medica encroaches, therefore, on the one side upon the science of physiology, and, on the other, upon the art of treating disease; while it concerns itself at the same time with physics, chemistry, botany, and zoology.

This "many-sidedness" has led to the introduction of special terms applicable to the chief subdivisions, and as each subdivision deals with questions which are distinct in themselves, it has become individualised not only by a separate designation, but also, in great measure, by forming an independent subject of study and investigation.

(m) I may be pardoned if I venture here to refer to the annual reports of the Commissioners in Lunacy for Scotland as containing an amount of well-directed statistical information regarding the lunacy of the kingdom which we search for in vain elsewhere.

The introduction into the title of our Section of the word "Pharmacology" illustrates the necessity which has now arisen for this subdivision. To this word we no longer assign the old significance which it bore as a mere synonym of materia medica. It now implies the science of the action of remedies, and it accordingly deals with the modifications produced in healthy conditions by the operation of substances capable of producing modification. The methods of investigation which it requires are totally distinct from those followed in the study of either pharmacy or pharmacognosy, and so it is that the specialist in this subject may have but little knowledge of pharmacy or pharmacognosy, and may never concern himself with the investigation of their problems. On the other hand, as pharmacology constitutes the chief bases for the application of remedies in disease, it closely allies itself to therapeutics, and constitutes the most important connecting link between materia medica and the art of medicine.

In this Section we cannot with propriety concern ourselves with therapeutics. It is so inseparably related to the etiology and pathology of disease that the advantages to be gained by a subdivision of medicine into separate departments would be annulled were our Section to deal with it as a separate subject. The remaining subdivisions of materia medica are those to which our attention may best be devoted. To each of them, however, an equal amount of attention would not be appropriate. It will, I think, be generally admitted that, on account of some of the considerations I have referred to, and while fully recognising their practical utility and importance, pharmacy and pharmacognosy are probably sufficiently represented in our programme by the proposed discussion on an international pharmacopœia. In this discussion the section are to have the advantage of an expression of opinion from Professor Eulenburg (of Greifswald), and I hope also from several of the distinguished pharmacists who are now conducting an International Congress in this city with a success we must try to emulate, and many of whom, I am glad to say, are to favour us with their co-operation as extraordinary members.

Our programme chiefly contains subjects for discussion which are drawn from pharmacology, and I trust that the consideration of the various important subjects that have been selected for discussion, and of the facts that are to be laid before us in other communications, will justify the Council in their selection, and will result in some addition being made to the rapidly increasing data upon which the science of pharmacology is now being founded.

It is clearly appreciated by all who are actively interested in the progress of pharmacology, that it is essentially an experimental science, and that its advancement can be obtained only by the application of the experimental method. This method, indeed, is as old as science itself; and although it has been the instrument by which all true progress in medicine has been achieved, during a long period in the history of medicine it had been distorted by the importation of metaphysical phantasies, and dominated by the contending theories of the schools. From data of the most insufficient description, theories were evolved of wide application; and in no department of medical knowledge was this more strikingly manifested than in pharmacology and therapeutics.

Fanciful resemblances between medicines and pathological products or normal structures were considered sufficient to explain the effects of the medicines, or to indicate the conditions of disease in which they should be applied. The resemblance between the white spots on the leaves of Pulmonaria officinalis and the morbid product tubercle led to the use of this plant in diseases of the lungs; the colour of the common carrot formed an indication for the administration of the carrot in jaundice; and the heart-like shape of the fruit of Limocarpus anacardium, and the reniform shape of the fruit of Anacardium occidentale, were considered sufficient characters for the administration of the one in diseases of the heart, and of the other in diseases of the kidneys. The doctrine of "Signatures," which prevailed for many years, and was accountable for these and many other absurdities, now mainly possesses the interest of affording an example of the ever-existing desire for guiding principles in the application of remedies—a desire which found satisfaction also in the systems of Paracelsus, Stahl, Brown, and Rasori.

These and all other systems that have been propounded erred in the insufficiency of the facts on which they were constructed. The knowledge of the age in which each of them was introduced lent for a time a plausible support in their favour, but it was insufficient to disprove them. Each in turn, however, was discarded as knowledge advanced and supplied the data required for refutation.

This knowledge was the fruit of observation. In its crudest form, observation restricted itself to the noting of the symptoms of disease, and of the changes produced in those symptoms by treatment. It is exemplified in the writings of Hippocrates, Theophrastus, Celsus, and Aretæus; and, in the present day, in the records of so-called experience. The general symptoms of a disease were ascertained, the changes produced by the administration of remedies were observed, and the result was preserved as a guide for the treatment of other cases. An experiment, in fact, was performed; but the experiment was one in which the conditions are complex, and the causes of fallacy numerous.

In the early history of medicine, when the normal conditions of life were unknown, and when the conceptions of disease were, in most cases, mere fancies of the imagination, erroneous doctrines and applications inevitably resulted from the restricted employment of this method of observation. Even at the present time, its employment is surrounded by difficulties and fallacies of a similar description. Notwithstanding the remarkable advancements in biological science that have followed the application of the methods of research inaugurated by Bacon and Galileo, the normal composition and functions of the component parts of the body, and much less their abnormal conditions in disease, are in very few, if in any, instances thoroughly understood. The labour of years has resulted in proving but too distinctly their complexity, and perhaps, above all, in making it apparent that much is unknown. The mere separation of the symptoms of disease from the mental or moral reactions of the individual is even, in many instances, a matter of difficulty. It is far from being an easy task to estimate the effects produced upon the patient by the remedy that has been administered, not only on account of the nature of the problem, but also because of the tendency—too often irresistible—on the part of the observer to confound sequences with consequences. Experience has, in all ages, supplied proofs that the aphorism, Sublatâ causâ, tollitur effectus, is in the art of medicine little more than a disappointing mockery.

That experimental method which deals with problems of so great complexity as those with which crude observation is concerned having failed to produce results which satisfied the generous aspirations that have at all times formed the incentive to medical investigation, a new development was fortunately given to the study of the effects of remedies, by the introduction of an experimental method in which the conditions are more simple and controllable than in those forming the basis of so-called experience. The introduction of this method is due to Bichat, and by its subsequent applications by Magendie pharmacology was originated as the science we now recognise. Bichat represents a transition state, in which metaphysical conceptions were mingled with the results of experiment. Magendie more clearly recognised the danger of adopting theories in the existing imperfections of knowledge, and devoted himself to the supplementing of these imperfections by experiments on living animals. The advantages of such experiments he early illustrated by his investigation on the upas poison, and afterwards by a research on the then newly-discovered alkaloid, strychnia. The results of these researches enabled him to lay the foundation for the doctrine that remedies exert their actions upon special structures—a doctrine which was afterwards further developed and illustrated in the classic researches of his pupil, Claude Bernard.

Magendie's epoch-making investigations inaugurated the present century. The value of his method was quickly appreciated, and adopted in Germany, Italy, and Britain. It, however, necessitated experiments on living animals, and it is curious to observe that even in his day the embarrassments which sentimental opposition has succeeded in raising to the progress of pharmacology in this country were not unknown in France. To this subject Claude Bernard makes some reference in the biographical notice of Magendie which forms the introductory chapter of his work on the "Effects of Poisonous and Medicinal Substances."

He there furnishes us with an argument against the views of those who oppose experiments on living animals, which has the special interest of having been written, apparently, chiefly in defence of experimenters in this country; where, as he rightly supposes, prejudices are most strongly developed and stated. As all science must be founded on experiment, so the science of life, he remarks, necessitates vivisection, because the phenomena of life occurs only in living beings; but experiments on living beings, governed and inspired by a true scientific spirit, do not deserve the reproach of cruelty, any more than the vivisections of the surgeon prompted by the idea of saving the life of his patient.

On this subject, however, I propose afterwards to make some further remarks; but, before doing so, I would briefly refer to the results that have already been obtained by the experimental study of pharmacology during the present century.

By the experimental method, I do not refer to that which is associated with the name of Hippocrates, which searches for truth by means of experiments of a complicated description, in which the data are in a great measure unknown and almost entirely beyond the control of the experimenter. It would, at the same time, be impossible to assert that by observation of the effects of remedies upon patients much advantage and many valuable results have not been gained. A large number of remedies have been introduced, even although their physiological action was entirely unknown, and several of these yet retain their position as valuable means of treating disease. On the other hand, the greatest number of them have certainly been discarded as knowledge advanced, and not a few retain their position simply because other and more trustworthy reasons for their employment have been brought to light.

This light has been derived from the experimental method, which, while it does not neglect crude observations, endeavours, as far as possible, to simplify the conditions of the experiment, by using as the subjects of experiment animals in whom the conditions admit of being controlled. A certainty is thus given to the results which could not otherwise be obtained, and applications to disease acquire a prominence which is in striking contrast to the ephemeral and fleeting opinions which are derived from the empirical method. Magendie's research on strychnia may be cited as an illustration of this. He demonstrated the action of this substance upon the spinal cord by experiments upon the lower animals so thoroughly that subsequent investigations have added but little to his results. He also recognised the advantage that might be expected from its administration in disease, and proposed its application in cases of paralysis. This application was first effected by Fouquier, and since that time strychnia has retained its position as a remedy for paralysis.

Since that time, also, the method has been applied to the investigation of a large number of active substances, with results of the highest importance to humanity. Rational explanations have been discovered for previously observed therapeutic facts, and it has become possible to apply many known remedies with judgment and confidence. Previously unknown therapeutical actions have been brought to light, and symptoms of disease which before were beyond control can now be alleviated by the production of definite remedial actions.

To the members of this section it must seem almost a superfluous task to recall examples in support of these statements. Let me content myself by instancing merely the action of ergot on the bloodvessels; of aconite, digitalis, and a host of other substances upon the heart; of nitrite of amyl upon the blood tension; and of the large groups of substances which act as emetics, diaphoretics, cathartics, diuretics, and cholagogues. Many of the examples I have cited will be considered with detail in the discussions and papers which are to engage the attention of the section, and I now do no more than refer to them in illustration of the great benefit which pharmacology, and therefore therapeutics, has derived from the adoption of the experimental method.

I may further illustrate the value of the results obtained by this method, and, I might even say, the necessity for pursuing it, by considering for one moment the action of digitalis and of anæsthetics.

The former substance was introduced into practice by Drs. Cullen and W. Thormic. Towards the end of the last century, and therefore answering to the inauguration of the experimental method and to the foundation of pharmacology as a science, it was introduced as a remedy for dropsy; and on the applications which were made of it for the treatment of that disease, a slowing action upon the cardiac movements was observed, which led to its acquiring the reputation of a cardiac sedative. Numerous observations were made on man by the originators of its application, by Dr. Sanders, and by many other physicians, in which special attention was paid to its effects upon the circulation; but no further light was thrown upon its remarkable properties, with the unimportant exception that in some cases it was found to excite the circulation. It was not until the experimental method was applied in its investigation—in the first instance by Claude Bernard, and subsequently by Dybkowsky, Pelikon, Meyer, Boehm, and Schmiedeberg—that the true action of digitalis upon the circulation was discovered. It was shown that the effects upon the circulation were not in any exact sense sedative, but, on the contrary, stimulant and tonic, rendering the action of the heart more powerful, and increasing the tension in the bloodvessels. The indications for its use in disease were thereby revolutionised, and at the same time rendered more exact, and the striking benefits which are now afforded by the use of this substance in most diseases were made available to humanity.

The introduction of anæsthetics into medical practice has certainly produced more benefit than that of any class of substances. The insensibility which they produce is a condition which can be readily established by the most crude method of experiment, as it requires merely the exhibition of the substance and the observation of the effect; and this simple process of investigation is that by which their introduction was effected. Following upon this introduction and the wide extension of their employment, however, it was soon found that insensibility was not their only effect. They produced insensibility, but they also produced other actions, which assumed a grave importance, as they were occasionally sufficient to destroy life. The nature of these additional actions became, therefore, a matter of interest, for upon them apparently depended many questions governing the indications for the use of anæsthetics and the treatment which should be adopted in order to avert or counteract their dangerous effects. No sufficient light, however, could be thrown upon them by the simple experiments which were sufficient to prove that these substances produce insensibility. By observing the phenomena presented by a patient in the anæsthetic condition, the mechanism by which the dangerous effects were caused could not be revealed. It could not even be determined whether death were produced by an action upon the brain, or upon the heart, or upon the respiration. The necessity for extending the investigation of their action to lower animals, in whom the experimental conditions could be controlled and varied, became obvious; and the researches which have already been undertaken by Hermann, Bert, Ferguson, Coates, and McKendrick have furnished much information with regard to those difficulties that could not be solved by mere observation of effects in human beings. They have provided indications for forming an opinion of the relative dangerousness of many anæsthetics, of the class of cases in which each should be specially avoided, and of the means by which their dangerous actions may best be counteracted; and it is needless to remark that, if results of such importance can be obtained by no other means than by experiments upon the lower animals, the performance of such experiments is an imperative duty.

I have already defined pharmacology as the science of the action of remedies, and pointed out that, like every other science, it must be founded upon experiment, while, from the nature of its problems, the experiments must be performed upon living beings. These propositions are generally recognised by those who are engaged in the study of the means of treating disease; and, upon their application the present condition of medical art and science is dependent. Embarrassment and difficulties have, however, been encountered in the application of the last proposition, which, fortunately, have not assumed an equal importance in every country. In Britain, however, they have assumed an importance which constitutes a crisis in the history of pharmacology. Exaggerated and erroneous statements of the horrors of experiments on the lower animals, and ignorant assertions regarding the history of medical progress, have raised a sentimental clamour before which a representative Government has found itself powerless. An Act has been passed, imposing restrictions of the most harassing description upon those who are engaged in pharmacological and physiological research, and relegating to officials who are utterly ignorant of the subject the duty of deciding what investigations shall be undertaken. Under this Act, no one is permitted to perform an experiment upon a living vertebrate animal who is not furnished with a licence from the Home Secretary, who is all-powerful to grant or refuse licences at his pleasure. I need not say that the imposition of the degrading restrictions contained in this Act was opposed by the indignant remonstrances of the profession. It was characterised as unjust to the profession, detrimental to the interests of society, and an obstruction to the progress of knowledge. The Act was, however, passed, and now, according to the law of this country, "any person may inflict any pain short of torture on any domestic animal, and any torture he pleases on any non-domestic animal," but he cannot inflict the most trifling injury upon any animal, whether domestic or wild, so long as his object is a scientific one, unless he is first furnished with a licence.

On the passing of the Act, I believe an assurance was given by the then Secretary of State that it was not the intention of the Legislature to prevent altogether scientific research by means of experiments upon animals; and that as well as other assurances and modifications of the Act as it was first introduced, had some effect in calming indignation and in lessening opposition. I cannot help thinking that this opposition was too easily lessened, and that the bribe of a few unimportant compromises induced the profession to submit but too readily to the imposition of an unjust Act, which their knowledge assured them could only be followed by injury to medical science, instead of continuing the uncompromising opposition which was so ably advocated by Mr. Lowe.

Pharmacologists and physiologists have now had some experience of the Act, and I do not think any other opinion will be expressed than that it has impeded the development of their sciences, and rendered the prosecution of these sciences so difficult and harassing that original investigation is now almost impossible in the country of Harvey, Bell, Reid, and Christison. It is true that during the first few years immediately succeeding the passing of the Act some consideration was shown to the interests of science and the aspirations of investigators, for permission was generally given for the conducting of experiments. Legislation, however, originating in hysterical clamour is not likely to remain uninfluenced by subsequent manifestations of the same disease. There is, indeed, no malady in which firm opposition is more likely to be beneficial, and in which even the slightest exhibition of indulgent compromise is more likely to produce more frequent or more uncontrollable manifestations. The passing of the Act was largely due to compromise; the subsequent history of the operations of the Act proves that in place of appeasing clamour, this compromise has served as a strong incentive to its continuance. Investigators to whom the Home Office has afforded the necessary licences for performing experiments have been assailed with unbridled invective, and influence is being brought to bear upon the Secretary of State to cause him to interpret the Act as one for the entire suppression of experiments on animals. How effectively this influence has operated, or how hazardous it is to place the progress of a science entirely at the mercy of a State official, utterly ignorant of its aims and triumphs, is now being exemplified. In several instances in which the objects were of the highest interest, and in which the importance of the results could not be predicted, the Government has constituted itself the supreme arbiter of science, and has ventured to decide that certain experiments were not required, and should not be performed. I do not make this statement unadvisedly. The instances are within my own knowledge, and in one of them I have the best of reasons for knowing the facts, as only the other day I experienced the mortification of being refused a licence. In this case, permission was requested for performing a few experiments on rabbits and frogs with a reputed poison used by the natives of Borneo to anoint their arrows. If this be an active substance, it is impossible to predict what advantages

might be gained from its use in the treatment of disease; but, apart from this, it is surely important to discover, in the interest of travellers, whether it really possesses toxic properties, and, if it do possess such properties, what are their characteristics, and what is the best method of counteracting its effects. I am obliged to conclude, however, that those who are now authorised to decide such questions for us entertain a different opinion, and consider that these objects and the interests of science are insufficient to justify the most trivial infliction of pain upon rabbits and frogs. That the infliction of pain would be only trivial will, I think, be apparent when I state that the only operation for which permission was requested was the subcutaneous injection of the poison; for the question of the possible infliction of pain by the action of the supposed poison does not arise, as the substance might, without any infringement of the Act, be placed in the stomach or in contact with any absorbent surface, provided no wound was inflicted. The absurd position has now been assumed by the State that an operation implying merely such a wound as can be produced by a needle-point is not justifiable, so long as it is performed for the purpose of acquiring knowledge and in the hope of benefiting the human race.

To us the matter bears a most serious aspect. To us it is as clear as the light of day that the action of remedies cannot be ascertained otherwise than by experiments on the lower animals. If this method of research be denied to us, what means are we to adopt for increasing the resources of our art? How are the rich treasures which the enterprise of travellers and the never-ceasing discoveries of chemists place at our disposal to be applied, as hitherto they have in so many instances been most beneficially applied, to the treatment of disease? How are we to discover antidotes to the poisonous action of toxic agents? Experiments on man with substances regarding whose properties no knowledge exists will ever be repugnant to medical science; and on that account, as well as because of their entire insufficiency, they cannot be adopted as substitutes for experiments on the lower animals.

Is, then, the progress of pharmacology to be brought to a termination, and the treatment of disease to lapse into the former irrationalism, so distasteful to present aspirations, which are anxiously striving to attain exactitude in the art of medicine?

So far as this country is concerned, this result must inevitably occur unless we obtain our knowledge entirely from other countries, or unless the freedom of research is again asserted among us.

I believe the latter alternative is not impossible to be attained. Much of the clamour that has been raised against experiments on animals is the outcome of erroneous information and sentimental prejudice, and many who are now taking part in this clamour would cease to do so were their erroneous impressions removed. Let them endeavour to appreciate the problems we have to solve, let them realise the incentives that urge us to increase our knowledge, let them consider that each advancement is a gain for humanity, and in place of lending themselves to obstruction and obloquy, they will repay our exertions with commendation.

It is stated that Alderman Sir Sydney Waterlow (the Treasurer of St. Bartholomew's Hospital) has received from Mr. Charles Kettlewell, of Armadale Castle, Island of Skye (a governor of the Hospital), a communication offering the sum of £10,000 for the erection of a convalescent home for St. Bartholomew's Hospital, as a memorial to his late brother, who died of fever in Naples. The offer is conditional upon a suitable site being found within a reasonable time.

GERMAN STUDENTS IN THE SUMMER SESSION OF 1881.—Berlin, 3924 (730 medical); Bonn, 1070 (187); Breslau, 1380 (295); Erlangen, 462 (90); Freiburg, no returns; Giessen, 462 (60); Göttingen, 1002 (151); Greifswald, 644 (316); Halle, 1293 (190); Heidelberg, 825 (147); Jena, 608 (85); Kiel, 344 (119); Königsberg, 841 (175); Leipzig, 3183 (457); Marburg, 701 (158); Munich, 1824 (434); Rostock, 197 (44); Strasburg, 770 (171); Tübingen, 1230 (164); Würzburg 969 (454); total, 21,569 students, 4494 of the number being medical students. Of the 21,569 students, 20,418 were Germans and 1131 foreigners; and of the 4494 medical students, 4197 were Germans and 297 foreigners.—*Deutsche Med. Woch.*, No. 30.

TERMS OF SUBSCRIPTION.
(*Free by post.*)

British Islands	*Twelve Months*	.	£1	8	0
„ „	*Six* „	.	0	14	0
The Colonies and the United }	*Twelve* „	.	1	10	0
States of America . . . }					
„ „ „ . .	*Six* „	.	0	15	0
India „ „ . .	*Twelve* „	.	1	10	0
„ (*vià Brindisi*) . . .	„	.	1	15	0
„ „	*Six* „	.	0	15	0
„ (*vià Brindisi*) . . .	„	.	0	17	6

Foreign Subscribers are requested to inform the Publishers of any remittance made through the agency of the Post-office.

Single Copies of the Journal can be obtained of all Booksellers and Newsmen, price Sixpence.

Cheques or Post-office Orders should be made payable to Mr. JAMES LUCAS, 11, New Burlington-street, W.

TERMS FOR ADVERTISEMENTS.

Seven lines (70 words)	.£0	4	6
Each additional line (10 words) . .	. 0	0	6
Half-column, or quarter-page . .	. 1	5	0
Whole column, or half-page . .	. 2	10	0
Whole page	. 5	0	0

Births, Marriages, and Deaths are inserted Free of Charge.

THE MEDICAL TIMES AND GAZETTE *is published on Friday morning: Advertisements must therefore reach the Publishing Office not later than One o'clock on Thursday.*

Medical Times and Gazette.

SATURDAY, AUGUST 20, 1881.

THE RYDE MEETING.

THE annual gathering of the British Medical Association came so immediately upon the close of the Congress, when medical men might well have, for a while, felt utterly wearied of hearing of the science and art of medicine, that no one could have been surprised had it turned out a somewhat small and almost dull meeting—a *succès d'estime*, perhaps, but nothing more. It has, however, proved a very well attended, very animated, satisfactory, and successful meeting. The charming seaside resort, Ryde, where the meeting was held, was itself a great attraction after "the dust and din and steam of town," and of the Congress. The weather was, on the whole, very favourable. Some of our Continental and American brethren of distinction were happy to take the opportunity of watching a little of the working of the Association, and at the same time seeing a well-known little British watering-place *en fête*, and the work provided was quite enough in quantity and quality to give a satisfying appearance and tone of business to the whole proceedings.

Even the orators of the occasion—the President, and those who gave the addresses-in-chief—seem, happily, to have recognised generally that it would be well not to make any very serious demands on the attention and powers of their audiences—that the occasion was one for light and elegant repasts rather than solid food; and accordingly the addresses, while excellent in their way, have, with the exception of Dr. Coghill's, been general rather than learned and scientific in character and tone. The President, Mr. Barrow, gave a slight and brief sketch of the origin and history of Medicine, and of the labours of eminent medical men in the past and present times, and stated the opinions he had arrived at during his long and honourable career on some of the burning questions of the day; Dr. Bristowe, who gave the Address in Medicine, took for his theme Hahnemann and the system founded and taught by him; and Mr. Hutchinson, in his Address

in Surgery, while treating principally of specialism, also touched on homœopathy. Dr. Bristowe has, as all would expect, no belief in homœopathy; he spoke of it as being still, in its most modern form, "a protest against the best traditions of orthodox clinical medicine," and he reminded his hearers that "all the best physicians of old times, all the greatest names in medicine of the present day, are with us: all science is on our side"; but he protested against our looking upon homœopathic practitioners as knaves or fools. And this protest is hardly needed in these days. We are quite ready to recognise, with him, that they may be, and not seldom are, "honest, well-informed, and legally qualified medical men"; but when he goes on to speak in favour of our "co-operating" with them, it is quite another thing. Mr. Barrow, who also spoke on this matter, would not "taboo" the homœopathic practitioner, but he would not meet him in consultation. He holds that we may not, "under any circumstances consult with the man who practises a system of medicine opposed to that which science and long usage have proved to be the only safe and secure one." Mr. Hutchinson more nearly agreed, we believe, with Dr. Bristowe. This renewal of discussion regarding our behaviour towards professed homœopaths was due, no doubt, in great part, at least, to the controversy and excitement connected with the last illness of the late Lord Beaconsfield, though probably in no small degree also to the spread of what is called "toleration," but which is sometimes only a fine name for indifferentism and selfishness. No discussion on the addresses is permitted, but Dr. Bristowe's opinion as to co-operation with homœopaths was not allowed to pass without a protest, and evidently did not find much favour. It seems clear, however, that after such expressions of opinion from men like Dr. Bristowe and Mr. Hutchinson, further discussion has become necessary, and perhaps some fresh action. Indeed, it was resolved at a meeting of the Council, held on the day when Mr. Hutchinson's address was delivered, that the whole subject shall be taken up at their October meeting.

DR. KOCH'S DEMONSTRATIONS ON THE GERM THEORY.

AMONG the many interesting facts brought forward and the discussions held during the Congress, none surpassed, if indeed any equalled, the work done by Dr. Robert Koch (of Berlin), whose name is no doubt familiar to many of our readers through the Sydenham Society's translation of his book on Traumatic Infective Diseases, which was published last year. At great trouble and expense, Dr. Koch brought over his apparatus and assistants from Berlin in order that those interested in infective disease might not only read, but actually see and judge for themselves, of the reality of the facts recorded. His demonstrations were given in the Physiological Laboratory at King's College, on Saturday, August 6, and Monday, August 8, and were, as far as possible, on account of the impossibility of showing them to a number of men at one time, limited to those who have been and are, actually working at the subject. Among those present were Professors Pasteur, Lister, Burdon-Sanderson, Chauveau, De Wahl, etc.

[Dr. Koch first brought forward some new methods of cultivation, which surpass in beauty and simplicity, as well as in usefulness, anything that has yet been done in this way. He began to study the growth of pigment bacteria on boiled potatoes, and soon observed that as the organisms were there growing on a firm substratum they did not become mixed up with each other or with accidental contaminations, and he could always find a spot where the bacterium was pure. He could then inoculate another potato from this spot, and obtain the organism pure. Any organism introduced accidentally grew only where it fell, and thus a pure cultivation from a pure part was always possible; on the other hand, if these organisms had been growing in a fluid, the introduction of another form would have rendered them impure for ever. Dr. Koch exhibited specimens of *micrococcus prodigiosus* which produces a red pigment, and also of the bacillus which causes blue pus, and that which causes blue milk. Other forms of bacilli were shown which microscopically were indistinguishable, but which could be at once separated from each other by differences in their mode of growth on solid substances. The advantages of a solid rather than a liquid cultivating material being thus apparent, Dr. Koch next turned his attention to the solidification of other cultivating materials, such as would nourish pathogenic bacteria, and he found that by the addition of gelatine to the fluid, used in the proportion of 3 or 4 per cent., a solid cultivating material was obtained, whose power of nourishing organisms was not in any way interfered with by the presence of the gelatine.

Some of this material, being rendered fluid by heating and spread out on a slide, was allowed to solidify, and then bacteria could be sown on it, and their mode of growth watched with a low power of the microscope. Thus, a minute quantity of dry earth was scattered over such a slide, and in a few hours development could be seen to be accruing around almost every particle. In this particular specimen seven different sorts of bacilli were present; many of these could not have been distinguished from each other by the microscope, but a difference was at once observed between their mode of growth on the solid substance, some forming round balls, others growing out in a star-shaped manner, others growing in a fine network, etc.

In the same way the number and nature of the organisms present in any given quantity of air could be estimated. A broad shallow vessel was filled with the gelatine mixture and exposed for a given time to the air. At every point where an organism fell on it, growth occurred, and thus the number and nature of the organisms present could be at once ascertained. But, further, as each organism was a pure cultivation, pure flasks could be inoculated from each variety, and thus its further life-history and pathogenic characters could be investigated.

Similarly with water. The material in a test-tube having been rendered fluid, a given quantity of water was shaken up with it till solidification occurred. At every point where an organism was present in the water, development occurred, and thus the number and nature of the organisms present in a given specimen could be at once ascertained.

Dr. Koch also exhibited some of his pathogenic bacteria. Animals which had been killed with anthrax were shown. The fatal nature of the poison was demonstrated; the constant presence of the *bacillus anthracis*, its mode of growth in the gelatine substance, and its virulent properties after being grown in it, were all made apparent. The bacillus of mouse septicæmia, which is described in his work, was shown in a similar manner. For several months this organism had been cultivated in gelatine blood serum, forming a fine cloudy mass and retaining its form and other characteristics. A minute drop of this was placed under the skin of a mouse. This animal died in forty-eight hours; and in its blood were numerous bacilli. Another mouse inoculated from this blood also died. In gelatine inoculated with this blood these organisms developed; and after further cultivations with this, the minutest drop killed another mouse. Septicæmia was shown in pigeons, rabbits, mice, etc., due to a minute bacillus of peculiar form, resembling in appearance the organism of the "*choléra des poules*" of Pasteur. The same sort of proof was given with regard to this organism as in the former case. And lastly, a beautiful form of erysipelas was shown in the ear of rabbits, caused by the inoculation of the rod-shaped bacillus of the septicæmia of mice; this sometimes, though not always, killed the animals.

The importance of these experiments can scarcely be estimated at present, but there is no doubt that they show a great advance, and no work has more tended to throw light on the complicated subject of pathogenic bacteria than that of Dr. Koch. Dr. Koch lays great stress on the value of microphotography as essential to an accurate record of facts; and the photographs which he showed on Friday were certainly very fine examples of what can be done in this way.

THE WEEK.

TOPICS OF THE DAY.

THE condition of the river Thames between Greenwich and Gravesend has become so offensive from sewer contamination that the large shipping firms of the port of London, and the inhabitants of the riverside parishes, are taking united and vigorous action with a view of providing a remedy. Within the last few days 10,000 signatures have been appended to the following petition to be presented to the House of Commons:—"The water of the Thames for miles above and below the metropolitan outfall is so highly charged with sewage that it has become a serious nuisance, and even danger, to those engaged on the banks or afloat on its surface. The evil is yearly increasing, and requires immediate remedy. Your petitioners, therefore, pray that some steps may be taken to relieve the Thames of the sewage of London." The petition is being extensively signed by the district boards and vestries of parishes abutting on the Thames, by the General commanding the troops at Woolwich, and the officers comprising the Sanitary Committee of the garrison, together with many heads of departments in the Royal Arsenal. It is stated that large quantities of black mud, or sewage deposit, have accumulated on both sides of the river above and below the outfall sewer at Crossness, while the vessels on their passage daily plough through ten inches of diluted sewage, emitting a stench extremely annoying to all on board. Recently, at the Woolwich Local Board of Health, the district representative at the Metropolitan Board of Works admitted that the complaints had been recognised by the latter Board, and that the members had been down to the southern outfall and had discussed remedial measures, whilst Sir Joseph Bazalgette had been instructed to prepare plans for extension works, to be considered by the Metropolitan Board after the autumn recess. The fact was that the main drainage system, though adequate for the requirements of the metropolis at the time of its construction twenty years ago, was not so now. It has been arranged that a deputation, to be introduced by Sir Charles Mills, M.P., shall wait upon the Local Government Board on the subject.

The first annual report of Mr. H. W. Hoffman, the Inspector of Retreats licensed for the admission of habitual drunkards under the Act of 1879, has been presented to the Home Office, and is anything but satisfactory. Only two retreats, up to the present time, have been opened under the Act—one near Stroud, Gloucestershire, and the other at Cannock, Staffordshire. The report says:—"The short time during which the Act has been in operation is hardly sufficient to enable me to speak confidently as to the results at present. I am unable to point out a single case where a permanent cure has been effected, but I can refer to several cases in which I think some good has resulted, and I am able to say that, as a rule, the general health of the patient has improved during their residence in these retreats." The Inspector believes that, with a few amendments which experience will dictate, the Act will justify the expectations of its promoters, but the licensees of the retreats have had many difficulties to contend with, and there has been some hesitation in laying out money on the establishments, the licences of which the justices might refuse to renew at the end of thirteen months, and where they are working under an Act which may cease at the expiration of ten years. The general condition of both of the retreats opened is stated to have been good as regards sanitary matters, and very fair as regards comfort, and the patients seemed in the main to be satisfied with their treatment. In the hope of being able to give a more encouraging account of the number of retreats licensed under the Act, and to gain a little more time for observation upon those established, Mr. Hoffman delayed the presentation of his report. However, not only have no fresh applications for licences been received, but one even of the two retreats now reported on has ceased to exist since April last, in consequence of the licensee having decided not to seek a renewal of his licence. There is, nevertheless, a rumour that the opening of three new retreats is contemplated.

The following resolutions were passed by the American delegates to the International Medical Congress, before separating, after the close of that great meeting :—" Resolved —That we highly appreciate the privilege we have enjoyed of attending this Congress, which has been, in every sense, a great success. That we offer our thanks to the officers of the Congress for the manner in which they have organised and conducted its meetings, and also to the corporations, societies, and individuals of whose unbounded hospitalities we have had such ample experience; and that we shall always preserve the most pleasant and grateful memories of the uniform courtesy and kindness which we have received, and which will strengthen the ties of friendship which exist between the United States and the mother-country. Montrose A. Pallen, Chairman; Henry O. Marcy, Secretary; Austin Flint, President of Committee; Joseph C. Hutchison, D. W. Yandell, Robert Battey, Moses Gunn, Beverley Cole, Henry J. Bigelow—Committee."

It is announced that the sum of £930 only has up to the present time been received for the fund which was formed to present a testimonial to Dr. William Farr, C.B., F.R.S., on his retirement from the post which for so long a time he had worthily filled in the office of the Registrar-General. This sum has been temporarily invested, and as at least twelve months have elapsed since the inauguration of the movement, it is not intended to keep open the list after the amount has reached £1000. This latter sum it is proposed, at the request of Dr. Farr, to invest for the purpose of supplementing the small provision he has been enabled to make for his family.

A Board of Trade return, recently issued, shows that the mortality in the British mercantile marine service was last year considerably greater than during 1879. The number of deaths from all causes was 4100, against 3692 in 1879—an increase, which, even making allowance for a probable increase of tonnage consequent upon a slight recovery in trade, seems far too large to be in proportion. The tabulated statistics disclose the fact that 675 more sailors were "drowned by wreck" in 1880 than in the previous year, the respective totals being 1655 and 978. Fatal accidents, other than by wreck, were almost precisely the same, while mortality from disease was considerably less than in 1879, which would appear to have been an exceptionally unhealthy year. Out of the 4100 sailors who lost their lives last year in the British mercantile marine, only 17 are returned as having died through natural causes; it should, however, be mentioned that deaths through various specified diseases are

excluded from this category, of which fevers were the most fatal, and next lung complaints and diseases of the heart.

After a long interval, during which it would appear nothing important has been done, the Lower Thames Valley Sewerage Scheme has once more cropped up. A deputation from the Sewerage Board of Kingston-on-Thames, headed by Sir Thomas Nelson, recently had an interview with Mr. Dodson, President of the Local Government Board, Mr. Hibbert, M.P., and Sir John Lambert, for the purpose of asking the present Government to support them in getting passed into law a sewerage scheme for the Thames Valley, prepared by Mr. Hawksley, C.E. The scheme, if sanctioned, was to lay down twenty-six miles of iron piping from Kingston, viâ Battersea, Camberwell, New Cross, Deptford, Woolwich, and so on to the mouth of the Thames. The promoters would not, however, make an effort unless they were backed by the Government. They had, they explained, already tried a private Bill, but had been threatened with surcharges. Mr. Dodson exhibited, as usual, an eminent talent for saying little and doing nothing : his department, he observed, greatly sympathised with the deputation, but their best plan was to proceed to file a Bill, which the Government would carefully consider, and see what support could be given to the scheme. Sir Thomas Nelson said such a course would be impossible, as they would immediately be met with a Bill being filed against them. Mr. Dodson could only recommend them to consult counsel on the subject; meanwhile, he promised that any plan left with him should have the most careful consideration.

ROYAL COLLEGE OF SURGEONS OF ENGLAND.

AT the ordinary meeting of the Council of the Royal College of Surgeons, held on Thursday, the 11th inst., the resignation of Mr. John Marshall, F.R.S., of his office as a member of the Court of Examiners, was accepted. The vacancy thus created will not be filled before the meeting of the Council in October next, and no nominations for it have yet been made; but we understand that Mr. John Croft will very probably be a candidate for the office. Mr. Croft has lately been elected to the Special Chair of Clinical Surgery created at St. Thomas's Hospital, having taught Practical Surgery there for many years. He has been examiner in surgery at the Royal College of Physicians.

UNIVERSITY COLLEGE, LIVERPOOL.

THE Medical Faculty of University College have issued their prospectus for the session 1881-82. The opening meeting will be held on October 3, when the Right Hon. the Earl of Derby, President of University College, will take the chair and distribute the prizes. The introductory address will be delivered by Oliver Lodge, Esq., D.Sc. Lond., the recently appointed Professor of Experimental Physics. The site selected for the College buildings is that now occupied by the Ashton-street Lunatic Asylum. The close proximity of the new College to the School of Medicine (of which it will really form a part), its central position and healthy elevation, render the selection of this spot the most suitable, probably, that could be obtained. An effort is also being made to secure some financial advantages from the City Council in favour of the College. The City Council is asked to purchase the buildings and area, and to let them to the College on a lease of seventy-five years at a nominal rent. The example of Nottingham is quoted as a precedent for this. It should also be mentioned that Mr. G. H. Rendall, Fellow and Assistant Tutor of Trinity College, Cambridge, has been appointed Principal of the College.

METROPOLITAN WATER-SUPPLY.

THE Local Government Board have recently addressed a circular letter to the vestries and district boards in the metropolis, in which they state that, in a report made to them by Lieutenant-Colonel Bolton, the Water Examiner under the Metropolis Water Act, 1871, their attention has been drawn to the serious deterioration which water frequently undergoes after delivery, by being kept in impure cisterns. The Board, referring to the general importance of the remarks made by Colonel Bolton on the subject, desire that they should be brought under the serious consideration of the sanitary authorities, and, with that end in view, they forward in their circular letter some extracts from his reports, which have more than once been noticed in our pages. The matter is of vital importance, as it affects the health and well-being of every householder and his family.

THE LATE MR. JAMES LUKE, F.R.C.S., F.R.S.

WE regret to have to record the death, at the age of eighty-two, of Mr. James Luke, F.R.C.S., F.R.S., which took place on August 15, at his residence, Fingest Grove, High Wycombe, Bucks. Mr. Luke became a Member of the Royal College of Surgeons on September 6, 1822, and a Fellow on December 11, 1843. He was elected a Member of the Council in 1846, and of the Court of Examiners in 1851. He was in 1852 the first chairman of the Board of Examiners in Midwifery, and again filled that office in 1861. His last service to the College was in 1865, when he became a member of the Board of Examiners in Dental Surgery. He was President of the College in 1853 and again in 1862, and delivered the Hunterian Oration in 1852. He had retired from practice for many years before his death. He was for many years one of the best known surgeons on the staff of the London Hospital, to which institution he became, on his retirement from active service, Consulting Surgeon in 1863. We hope to more fully notice his life and work.

THE SUMMONS AGAINST THE GRAND JUNCTION WATERWORKS COMPANY.

THE adjourned summons against the Grand Junction Waterworks Company for the non-supply of water to Mr. Hull, poulterer, of Swallow-place, Oxford-street, has been heard and decided by Mr. Newton at the Marlborough-street Police-court. The particulars of this case we published a few weeks back. Mr. Newton now said he was of opinion that Mr. Hull had made out his case, as it was clear from the evidence that for some time—namely, from the 16th to the 23rd of a month—there was a total failure of the water-supply. Counsel for the Company had taken an objection that the complaint was not well founded, because Mr. Hull had not paid the water-rate in advance, as required by the Act of Parliament; but he (Mr. Newton) did not see anything to that effect in the section of the Act under which the summons was taken out. It was proved before him that Mr. Hull had recently rebuilt his premises, and that there had not been any assessment made on the new building. Mr. Hull could not pay a rate which had not been made. After considering the whole case, he (Mr. Newton) could come to no other conclusion than to order the Company to pay a penalty of £10, with £5 costs. Mr. Poland, on behalf of the Company, said he should have to ask for a case to be stated for the opinion of the Court above—a course of which Mr. Newton approved. Another case against the same Company, that of Messrs. Jay, of Regent-street, was then proceeded with, but, after some evidence had been given, it was, by the consent of all parties concerned, adjourned for six weeks.

QUARANTINE IN LIVERPOOL.

AN endeavour is being made by Dr. Taylor, the Medical Officer of Health, to bring to a practical issue in Liverpool the observations made at the International Medical Congress by Dr. Billings and Dr. Lawson in regard to quarantine and ships affected with yellow fever. Dr. Taylor concurs with the opinion of these authorities, and considers the present quarantine laws as obsolete. He recommends the management of quarantine to be put into the hands of the Local Government Board. The vessels then could be disinfected at once, and allowed to proceed to sea.

THE PARIS WEEKLY RETURN.

THE number of deaths for the thirtieth and thirty-first weeks combined (July 22 to August 4) was 2317 (1245 males and 1072 females) ; and among these there were from typhoid fever 45, small-pox 38, measles 50, scarlatina 23, pertussis 9, diphtheria and croup 90, dysentery 75, erysipelas 14, and puerperal infections 8. There were also 86 deaths from tubercular and acute meningitis, 32 from acute bronchitis, 123 from pneumonia, 483 from infantile athrepsia (175 of the infants having been wholly or partially suckled), and 84 violent deaths. While the deaths in the thirtieth week amounted to 1259, they sank to 1058 in the thirty-first week—a decrease, therefore, of more than 200, greatly due to the abatement of the very high temperature. Epidemic diseases participated in the diminution, for typhoid fever sank from 26 in the thirtieth to 19 in the thirty-first week, diphtheria from 49 to 41, and measles and scarlatina each a few deaths. Small-pox alone remained the same (19) in both weeks. Although the deaths from athrepsia (often termed "cholera of infants" or "choleeine") diminished from 257 to 226, they are still very numerous as compared with the weekly number (60 to 80) registered during the prevalence of only moderate temperatures. Amelioration in the thirty-first week is especially notable in the decrease of deaths from cerebro-spinal diseases from 127 to 74, those of the circulation from 61 to 46, and of meningitis from 54 to 34. The sudden deaths also diminished from 56 to 28. The births for the two weeks amounted to 2346—viz., 1243 males (956 legitimate and 287 illegitimate), and 1103 females (828 legitimate and 275 illegitimate) ; 184 children (111 males and 73 females) were born dead, or died within twenty-four hours.

DEATH OF PROFESSOR SPIEGELBERG.

WE regret to hear of the death of Professor Spiegelberg, of Breslau. He was known to all obstetricians as one of the editors of the *Archiv für Gynäkologie*, and also by his voluminous and able work on Midwifery.

"A PREDICTION VERIFIED."—Under this title, Surgeon Sternberg, of the United States Army, relates that he had received a minute quantity of dried blood containing *bacillus anthracis*, which was sent by Prof. Burdon Sanderson to Prof. Newell Martin, of Johns Hopkins Hospital, with the statement that it was seven or eight years old, adding, "I have no doubt that you will find, if worked up with salt solution, and injected into a mouse, you will have the spleen, after from twenty-four to thirty-six hours, enlarged and infiltrated with bacillus." The material weighed about a sixth of a grain, and after being added to a little salt solution a few minims were injected beneath the skin of a mouse on June 4. In twenty-four hours the mouse was dead, and at the autopsy the spleen was found to contain the bacillus in considerable numbers, resembling exactly the bacillus of milzbrand or anthrax, as photographed by Koch in the *Beiträge s. Biologie d. Pflanzen*, Band 2.—*Philadelphia Med. Times,* June 18.

INTERNATIONAL MEDICAL CONGRESS.

SECTIONAL WORK.

THE discussions held in the Pathological Section were of special interest and importance. The meeting on Wednesday, August 3, was very well attended, and was opened by a short, but suggestive, address by the President, Dr. Wilks, which is already in our readers' hands. After this had been delivered, Dr. Malherbe (of Nantes) read two papers treating on Tumours. In the discussion which followed, some suggestive observations were made on the importance of a reconsideration of the terms applied to tumours, and of the adoption of a sort of international nomenclature.

On Thursday, a most interesting discussion on Tubercle was opened by Dr. Grancher (of Paris). He was followed by Mr. Treves, who held that tubercle has nothing specific about it, but is merely a peculiar form of inflammation. There is never a deposit of tubercle *per se*; there is always, in the first instance, a proliferation of the cellular tissue. At no place can it be said that here inflammation ends and the deposit of tubercle begins. The giant-cell indicates the first step to tubercle, and is merely a coagulation of the lymph in the lymph-canals. These views as to the nature of giant-cells were not accepted by any of the other speakers. Dr. Creighton pointed out that they could be found in the placenta of the pig, and that they were vasoformative structures, and indicated some special difficulty in the formation of vessels. Professor Virchow thought that it was unscientific to define tubercle as a form of inflammation. He held that tubercle was often a new deposit in an inflamed tissue, and often in a tissue unaffected with inflammation. Virchow had demonstrated that the giant-cells were really cells, and not lymph coagula; for if a concentrated solution be first added to the cell, and then a dilute solution, the wall of the cell becomes separated from its contents, and it is then seen as a distinct membrane. Further, all the intermediate stages can be traced between cells with single nuclei and the typical multi-nucleated giant-cell. Professor Virchow did not agree with Dr. Creighton as to the origin of *Perlsucht*. He had not been able to produce the disease in animals, as Dr. Creighton had done, simply by feeding them with the infected material. In such cases he had often found that the submaxillary and cervical glands became enlarged, but not the mesenteric, and he did not think that this could be explained by infection. But surely enlargement of these glands would imply that infection had occurred through the mouth, just as surely as enlargement of the mesenteric glands would imply infection by the food swallowed. Dr. Wilson Fox also spoke, but merely on the matter of nomenclature—not on the subject of tubercle.

The most interesting days were Friday and Saturday, when the discussions on the Germ Theory were held, and on Friday the room was crowded till near the end of the sitting. The discussion was opened by Mr. Lister, who uttered a much-needed word of warning against the tendency of the present day to exaggerate the importance of micro-organisms. He referred to the constant occurrence of micro-organisms in acute abscesses, and stated that he felt inclined to accept Mr. Watson Cheyne's view that very often these organisms were accidental concomitants, rather than Dr. Ogston's view that they were always the cause of the abscess—that, in fact, suppuration does not occur without the presence of organisms. Mr. Lister pointed out that many inflammations and suppurations were caused through the nervous system "by sympathy," and that they might also be due to some chemical irritant; he also alluded to the fact of counter-irritation as a cure of inflammation, to show that it could hardly be effectual if micro-organisms were always the cause. Dr. Bastian followed, and took up the old story of spontaneous generation. He asserted that wherever tissues were deprived of vitality or had their vital power lowered, organisms could originate spontaneously, and that if a portion of the brain were removed from an animal, and placed in a solution of chromic acid, organisms developed in its interior. These facts were answered by Mr. Watson Cheyne, who pointed out that he and others had removed

large portions of organs and tissues from animals, and kept them for days in flasks containing cultivating infusions without any development of organisms whatever. He further referred to his views on the relation of micrococci to acute abscesses, and supported them by stating, among other things, that an acute abscess containing micrococci may be produced by the subcutaneous injection of croton oil, that large quantities of micrococci taken from aseptic wounds may be introduced subcutaneously without any abscess resulting, etc. He held that they entered the abscess from the blood after its formation, as the result of the lowered resisting power of the living body. The speech of M. Pasteur was characterised by a most amusing episode. He said that he had not understood Dr. Bastian's speech, but he had been told that he advocated the spontaneous generation of organisms. Turning to Dr. Bastian he asked if this were true. Receiving no negative reply after waiting a little, he raised his hands to heaven and exclaimed, "Mon Dieu! mon Dieu! est-ce que nous sommes encore là? Mais, mon Dieu, ce n'est pas possible!" and then, in a vigorous speech, he proceeded to demolish Dr. Bastian's arguments. The debate was carried on on Saturday by Dr. Fokker (of Gröningen), Professor Béchamp (of Lille), Professor Klebs (of Prague), Dr. Vandyke Carter, who brought forward some very interesting facts with regard to the spirillum of relapsing fever; and Professor Hueter (of Greifswald). We must not omit here to refer to the remarkable exhibition of microphotographs given on Friday afternoon by Dr. Koch to a crowded and enthusiastic audience.

On Monday and Tuesday the interest in this Section seemed to have almost subsided, only a comparatively small audience being present to hear the debate on Renal Disease, which was opened by Sir William Gull, and discussed by Dr. Lanceraeux, Dr. George Johnson, Dr. Sutton, Dr. Saundby, and other speakers. On Tuesday, only a few stragglers were present to see the beautiful sections of the medulla and pons exhibited by Professor Pierret and others. Dr. Dreschfeld also gave a most interesting and remarkable account of a case of primary lateral sclerosis.

The Surgical Section met in the Library of the University of London, Burlington-gardens, a large and handsome room, which, however, presented one great disadvantage in its very bad acoustic qualities. This was to some extent remedied on the second day of the Congress by putting up a plain deal sounding-board, but even then speakers with a rapid articulation or an indistinct voice were very imperfectly heard, except by those in the immediate vicinity of the tribune and in the middle of the room. Notwithstanding this, however, the meetings were largely attended, and it seems generally allowed that Section V. was one of the most successful among the many successful gatherings. Not that the interest displayed was uniform, for at one or two of the afternoon sittings the attendance was thin, but some of the meetings were very large, numbering sometimes as many as three hundred, and the discussions were well maintained and of considerable interest. Mr. Erichsen's business-like habits and firm though gentle rule insured the maintenance of order and decorum; and as the result of holding a sitting during the lunch hour on two occasions, and working hard in the afternoon, the whole of the large amount of work set out upon the programme was, contrary to expectation, accomplished.

It is not necessary to refer again to the short but interesting introductory address of the President (Mr. Erichsen). It was delivered before a full audience, on the afternoon of Wednesday, August 3; and as the material to be dealt with was so large, it was determined to proceed at once to attack one of the main subjects for discussion. That selected was "The Forms of Aneurism in which Treatment by Esmarch's Elastic Bandage is applicable, and the method by which a cure is effected by its action." This was introduced in a concise and descriptive paper by Walter Reid, M.D., R.N., which was followed by a scientific disquisition by Mr. A. Pearce Gould, on the manner in which coagulation actually occurs during this and other forms of treatment. The only other speakers on this question were Mr. Bryant and Mr. Oliver Pemberton, the former recounting his belief in certain dangers which are to be feared, founded on the treatment of two or three cases; and the latter giving a description of a single case which had terminated fatally. It was clear that there would have been a fuller discussion if time had allowed, but the hour for adjournment had already been reached, and it did not seem wise to devote any further time to this interesting subject.

On Thursday, August 4, a large audience collected in the morning to hear Mr. Spencer Wells introduce the subject of the "Recent Advances in the Surgical Treatment of Intraperitoneal Tumours." Mr. Wells gave a very brief *résumé* of what has been done of late years in this direction; and when he had finished, Mr. Lawson Tait read an account of the wonderful success that he has been recently fortunate enough to obtain at Birmingham without the use of antiseptic means. A short paper was afterwards read by Dr. de Zwaan (of the Hague) on a new modification of Péan's operation for Extirpation of the Uterus. A large number of speakers joined in the debate, which principally hinged upon the question whether antiseptic measures, in the present acceptation of the word, were for the benefit of the patient, or whether their adoption did not produce actual injury. A striking feature of the morning was the appearance of Dr. Keith (of Edinburgh), who was greeted with loud cheers. His assertion of the fact that he has given up the employment of antiseptics because he found his results were better without them, was received with very different feelings by the two parties, and, as will be seen, received an answer or explanation from Mr. Lister on a subsequent occasion. Very various were the opinions expressed, and it was difficult, if not impossible, to decide the general feeling of the meeting, but we fancy the majority of the speakers were rather disposed to agree with Dr. Keith, at least as far as ovariotomy is concerned. If space permitted, we should gladly touch upon the appropriate remarks of Professor Volkmann and others, but we must be content with enumerating the names of the speakers :—Professor Czerny (of Heidelberg), Dr. Marcy (of Boston), Mr. Knowsley Thornton, Dr. Martin (of Berlin), Dr. Keith (of Edinburgh), Dr. Nelson (of Chicago), Professor Volkmann (of Halle), Dr. Marion Sims, Dr. Battey (of Georgia), Mr. Bantock, Dr. Dunlap (of Ohio), and Dr. Heywood Smith.

At one o'clock Mr. Erichsen gave up the chair to Professor Bennett, the genial Vice-President from Dublin, who, with the assistance of one of the three Secretaries, presided over the discussion of the following papers:—Cases of Gastrostomy, by R. J. Pye-Smith, F.R.C.S. (of Sheffield); Note on Strangulated Hernia, by D. Mollière, M.D. (of Lyons); on the Cure of Hernia in reference to Parents and the Profession, by W. D. Spanton, M.R.C.S. (of Hanley); on the Cure of Hernia by the Antiseptic Use of Animal Ligatures, by Henry O. Marcy, M.D. (of New York).

At the short afternoon sitting, a subject akin to that of the morning was dealt with, though time did not permit of its discussion; it was "The Diagnosis of certain Diseases of the Kidney admitting of Surgical Treatment, and the Operations that may be practised for their Relief or Cure." Professor Czerny's paper, describing his wide experience of thirteen cases, was highly interesting and well delivered. Other papers followed—by Mr. Morrant Baker, describing three cases; by Mr. Barker, propounding certain questions for consideration; by Mr. Lucas, describing a case; and by Mr. Barwell, describing another. Some remarks were then made by Dr. Martin (of Berlin), which brought to a conclusion a day of distinctly hard and, it may be hoped, valuable work.

Friday morning was fixed for the discussion of a subject which is at the present time one of great interest to the profession, viz., "Recent Advances in the Methods of Extracting Stone from the Bladder of the Male," and the notice that Sir Henry Thompson and Professor Bigelow were expected to speak drew together a large audience. Sir Henry Thompson was quite at his best, and read his paper with great animation. He gave Professor Bigelow high praise for the innovations which he has introduced into lithotrity, while pointing out what he considers disadvantages in his instruments, and pleading for the merits of Clover's apparatus for emptying the bladder; he also touched on sundry other recent improvements and suggestions. Professor Bigelow gave a most interesting description of his inventions and their application, and insisted on the great advantages of his method of performing lithotrity. Papers were then read by Dr. Anger (of Paris) on a Method of performing Lithotomy with the Actual Cautery, and by Mr. Reginald Harrison on Bigelow's Operation. Speakers then followed in rapid succession, most of whom were loud in their praises of lithotrity at one sitting, though some of the seniors appeared to be disposed to dwell on the older methods

of procedure. The discussion was carried on by Dr. George Buchanan (of Glasgow), Professor Spence (of Edinburgh), Mr. Walter Coulson, Professor Pirrie (of Aberdeen), Mr. Teevan, Dr. Reliquet (of Paris), Mr. Clover, Mr. Berkeley Hill, Mr. Buckston Browne, Mr. Lund (of Manchester), and Mr. T. P. Teale (of Leeds). The sitting was again continued during the lunch hour, and papers by Dr. Otis (of New York) on the subject of the morning's discussion, and Dr. Adolf Fischer (of Buda-Pesth) on "Partial Resection of the Urinary Bladder," were listened to by a not very considerable audience. To this prolongation of the morning's debate, and its intrinsic interest, was probably due the fact that the commencement of Dr. Gross's paper on "The Relation between Adenoma, Sarcoma, and Carcinoma of the Mammary Gland in the Female: their Diagnosis in the Earlier Stages of the Disease, and the Results of their Treatment by Operation," was not so well attended as the merits of the communication deserved. Dr. Gross, as was pointed out in a remarkably lucid and well-delivered speech by Mr. Butlin, seems to see an order and arrangement amongst mammary tumours which some of us find it difficult to appreciate; he advocates a very free removal of the mamma in all malignant cases, and the systematic investigation, if not the clearing out, of axillary glands, whether perceptible before the axilla is opened or not—a plan which several English surgeons have for some time been in the habit of pursuing. Dr. Semmola (of Naples) and Mr. Banks (of Liverpool) made some remarks on the subject; and the meeting then took up two of the promiscuous papers—one, by Dr. Vincent (of Lyons) on "Laparatomy and Cystorrhaphy," and another by Dr. Mazzoni (of Rome) on "Perineal Calculi."

The fifth meeting of the Section again proved attractive, and, notwithstanding that it was Saturday morning, a lively discussion took place. The subject was, "The Forms of Disease by which different Joint Structures may be affected primarily, and the Comparative Value of Early and Late Resection in Articular Disease." The tendency of the debate is well summed up by a remark made to us by a foreign surgeon—"We foreigners are astonished to find all the Englishmen objecting to our advocacy of early excision, and yet we thought that we were only following the teaching of the English school." The papers read on the subject were by Professor Ollier (of Lyons), Professor Kocher (of Berne), Dr. Newman (of Stamford)—a case, and Dr. Sayre (of New York). The speakers were Mr. Croft, Mr. Howard Marsh, Mr. T. P. Teale (of Leeds), Mr. Treves, Professor Redfern (of Belfast), Dr. Barton (of Dublin), Professor Küster (of Berlin), Mr. Bryant, Mr. Christopher Heath, and Mr. Macnamara. The remaining time was occupied in reading the following papers:—"The Cure of White Swelling by Electrolysis," by Professor Agnello d'Ambrosio (of Naples); "Reduction of Unreduced Dislocation of the Humerus," by Professor Kocher (of Berne); "The Treatment of Fractured Femur," by Mr. Rushton Parker (of Liverpool); and two unannounced communications—"De la Mégéthométrie," by Dr. de l'Aulnoit, and "On Deformities of the Tibia," by Dr. Cuignet (both of Lille).

On Monday, the 8th, a very large audience attended to hear the debate of the subject appointed to be discussed in the morning, viz. :—"The Causes of Failure in obtaining Primary Union in Operation Wounds, and on the methods best calculated to secure it." Mr. Savory opened the discussion with his usual eloquence and ability, and, much in the manner of his Cork address, confessed himself reluctantly obliged to occupy the position of a Cassandra with regard to the engrossing question of antiseptic surgery. This gave the keynote to the debate. Mr. Gamgee in sonorous tones sounded the praises of rest and pressure. Professor Humphry had passed over this preliminary ground, and was just reaching the question of germs, when the fatal call-bell sounded, and he was about to obey the warning, but the cheers of the meeting procured him a few minutes' grace to deal with these malignant organisms. Professor Verneuil propounded views with which we find it hard to sympathise; he spoke of dangers to be deduced from attempting to obtain primary union in some cases, which we thought were somewhat problematical; he also returned to the subject of antiseptics at the end of his speech, and this was afterwards never lost sight of. We regret that want of space forbids us to do more than mention the modifications of "Listerism" described by Professor Esmarch, the dry dressings of Dr. Greene, the sage remarks of Professor Volkmann, etc., but the interest shown may be gathered from the following list of speakers :—Professor

Volkmann (of Halle), Professor Esmarch (of Kiel), Mr. Lund (of Manchester), Dr. Greene (of Portland, U.S.A.), Mr. Hardie (of Manchester), Dr. Barton (of Dublin), Dr. Martin (of Boston, U.S.A.), Mr. Gant (of London), and Professor Létievant (of Lyons). The President had given notice that Mr. Lister would conclude the debate at a quarter to one, and at that time the room was crowded, and the Professor was greeted with great applause. He first dealt with the remarks of Dr. Keith, and pointed out how the surgery of the abdomen differs from that of other regions with reference to antiseptics—first, on account of the high vitality of the parts and the great absorbing power of the peritoneum, and secondly, because the vast absorbing surface exposed might be expected, d priori, to offer objections to the use of such an irritant as carbolic acid. He was, therefore, long ago prepared for the results obtained by Mr. Lawson Tait and Dr. Keith; but he pointed out the revolution that the adoption of antiseptic means during the performance of ovariotomy had accomplished in less healthy institutions than our Edinburgh and London hospitals, and in the hands of less skilled operators than the gentlemen referred to. He insisted that the comparison of ovariotomy with other operations cannot fairly be made, and then turned to the results of his own observations on the tendency of blood-serum and blood-clot to putrefy, which he showed was much less than was generally supposed. He scarcely hoped that many of the precautions he now uses will be dispensed with; but if the time should ever come when it was proved to demonstration that no floating particles were present in the air which could cause putrefaction, he would heartily join in the now well-known exclamation, "Fort mit dem Spray!" Mr. Lister could not compress his remarks into the fifteen minutes usually allowed; he was accordingly granted a little grace, and the meeting did not rise till about twenty minutes past one. The interest in the work of the Section culminated in this important debate. The attendance afterwards was fluctuating and never large. The following papers were read at the afternoon sitting:—"Eversion of the Great Toe," by Professor Reverdin (of Geneva); "Rotary Lateral Curvature," by Dr. Sayre (of New York), on which Mr. Barwell made some remarks; "Resection of the Larynx," by Professor Caselli (of Reggio Emilia); "On the Permanent Retention of the Œsophageal Bougie," by Dr. Krishaber (of Paris); "On Intra-nasal and Intra-oral Extirpation of the Bones of the Nose and Mouth by means of the Surgical Engine," by Dr. Goodwillie (of New York); "Removal of the Entire Tongue by Scissors," by Mr. Walter Whitehead (of Manchester), to which Mr. Lund added some remarks; "A Case of Rupture of the Brachial Plexus," by Mr. Banks (of Liverpool); and lastly, a description, by Dr. Adolf Fischer (of Buda-Pesth), of two New Irrigators, one for the nose and the other for the male urethra.

On Tuesday, the 9th, the last subject for discussion—"The Modifications of Syphilis in the Tuberculous, Gouty, and other Constitutions"—was introduced by Professor Verneuil in a paper which was perhaps more impressive than convincing. Mr. Hutchinson, who followed, stated that he had not met with any definite hybrid of syphilis and struma, tubercle, or gout; nor had he been able to recognise any modification of syphilis by those affections. He thought, however, that the idiosyncrasies of patients were accountable for many variations of the disease. The only other speakers were Professor E. H. Bennett (of Dublin), Dr. Henri Petit (of Paris), and Dr. Drysdale.

A few short papers were read after this; and Dr. Martin (of Boston), who had on the previous day been called to order for wandering from the subject of debate, was now allowed to describe his method of treating synovitis by means of the india-rubber bandage; and then Mr. Erichsen made a few valedictory remarks, and the Section separated.

The business of the Ophthalmological Section was conducted by allotting to each day a special subject, relating to which papers were read and discussions followed; the remaining papers being taken in order after the several discussions. By this means the whole of the work before the Section was satisfactorily accomplished. On Thursday, the first morning of meeting, the subject of the Antiseptic Method in Eye Surgery was introduced in a paper by Professor Horner (of Zurich), who considered, after a careful analysis of all the cases of eyes lost from primary suppuration after cataract extraction, that the average percentage, which according to present statistics amounts to 4·8, can be materially diminished by a strict use of antiseptic precautions. The measures recommended were prophylactic antiseptic precautions, and antiseptic dressing; and by these means he had succeeded in reducing the percentage to 1·5. Dr. Reymond (of Turin), in a paper on the same subject, insisted strongly on the thorough carrying out of the method, and on the careful application of the dressing; otherwise the operation was liable to be followed by various complications in the healing of the wound. Among 350 cases treated in this manner there had been seven cases of primary sloughing of cornea, four patients having removed the dressing themselves on the third day. As bearing on the subject of infection, a paper was read by Professor Leber (of Göttingen), detailing the results of a series of experiments as to the action of foreign bodies introduced into the interior of the eye, and from which he concluded that the destructive suppurative inflammation which followed resulted from the presence of germs introduced by the foreign body. Inasmuch, however, as foreign substances absolutely clean, but which are capable of chemical change, still excite a certain degree of inflammation, the action of the germs introduced from without probably results from the formation of certain chemical substances which act in exciting inflammation. The papers read on this subject were concluded by one from Dr. Emmert (of Berne), dealing statistically with the frequency of ophthalmia neonatorum and other suppurating diseases of the eye at different periods of the year.

The discussion was opened by Dr. De Wecker (of Paris), who, whilst a strong supporter of antiseptic measures, had not in his adoption of them found results exactly constant with regard to the percentage of suppurations, even when the operation was practised under exactly the same conditions. Other operators considered the method only advisable in certain cases when surroundings or local conditions of patient demanded it; whilst Dr. Knapp disbelieved that the suppuration resulted from infection, but rather from injury to the cornea during the operation.

In summing up the discussion, Professor Horner gave his statistics, showing that the operations on which his conclusions were based ranged over fourteen years, and that improvement was progressive, being greatest in the last years, the most recent percentage being as low as 1·1. The remainder of the morning sitting was occupied with papers—by Dr. Landolt (of Paris), on Motor Affections of the Eye, insisting upon the importance of investigating the monocular and binocular field of fixation in all cases of paralytic and nonparalytic strabismus; by Dr. Abadie (of Paris), who, believing the Muscular Insufficiency in Myopia to be intimately associated with its increase, recommended a partial tenotomy of the external rectus; and by Dr. Javal (of Paris), who described and exhibited the practical working of his Instruments for the subjective and objective determination of Astigmatism. By the ophthalmometer of Javal and Schiötz the degree of corneal astigmatism is at once, and with great readiness, determined, whilst the entire refraction is ascertained subjectively by the optometer, consisting of two revolving discs fitted with spherical and cylindrical lenses.

On Friday, the subject of the nature of Sympathetic Ophthalmia, and the mode of its transmission, was opened in a paper by Professor Snellen (of Utrecht). The pathology of this disease still remains an open question, two theories being advanced to explain it—the one that of reflected nerve action, and the other that of extension of diseased action by nerve-continuity from one eye to the other. The former must be rejected. According to Snellen, two important anatomical changes are present—the dilatation of the posterior lymph spaces, and plastic inflammation of the uveal tract,—both factors being necessary for the induction of the sympathetic inflammation. The lymph-spaces are the most probable channel of communication, and especially those which have been demonstrated as existing around the optic nerve. As to the substantial inflammatory constituent thus conveyed, it has been suggested by Leber and others to be parasitic in nature, and Snellen accepts that possible explanation of the granular masses visible in the structures of the altered eye. The subject was continued in a paper by Dr. Brailey, who described the pathological changes found in the uveitis of sympathetic inflammation. These characteristics, consisting of lymphoid cellular infiltration into all the uveal tract, are nearly always recognisable in both eyes, even when the disease begins in the sympathising eye as serous iritis and keratitis. Although the disease is not characterised by structural change in optic or ciliary nerves, Brailey inclines to the theory of direct transmission rather than of reflex action. Dr. Poncet (of Cluny) described the changes found in an eye in which sympathetic ophthalmia followed after optico-ciliary neurotomy, in which the peripheral ends of the ciliary nerves were compressed by a dense fibrous mass, the nerves being the seat of interstitial sclerosis, and suggested that terminal neuritis exists in those cases in which enucleation does not prevent sympathetic mischief.

The discussion was opened by Dr. Mooren (of Düsseldorf), the reflex character of the affection receiving no support from any speaker. Dr. Grünhagen (of Königsberg) referred, however, to a remarkable experiment, the results of which he ascribed to the influence of the vaso-motor nerves. After cauterising the centre of one cornea in an animal, the anterior chamber in *both* eyes became partially and rapidly filled with pus and a fibrinous fluid which coagulated on removal from the eye. These results had not been obtained in his experiments, that the influence is conveyed by the vaginal sheath of the optic nerve. The discussion, which was briefly replied to by Professor Snellen, was followed by two papers on Colour-Blindness—one by Dr. Libbrecht (of Ghent), with practical observations on the examination of railway servants and seamen; and the other by Dr. Ole Bull (of Christiania), describing a new method of examining and numerically expressing the colour-perception by first obtaining the four principal colours of an equal intensity, and from these deriving six graduated fainter tints by mixing the principal colours with grey on a Maxwell's disc. The meeting concluded with a paper by Mr. Eales (of Birmingham), describing a form of recurring Retinal and Vitreous Hæmorrhages in young men, which he believed to be due to an inherited vaso-motor neurosis.

On Saturday, Professor Leber introduced the subject of the relation between optic neuritis and intracranial disease. This form of optic neuritis is in all respects a true inflammation, altogether distinct and different from the hyperæmia and other lesions of venous stasis. The optic nerve acts as the path of transmission between the brain and the eye. Dr. Bouchut followed with a paper on the Relation between Ophthalmoscopic Conditions and Intracranial Disease, in which he maintained that all the important diseases of the brain and cord, as well as the serious diathetic diseases, may be recognised by ophthalmoscopic examination. To this method he applies the term cerebroscopy. The discussion which followed was a prolonged one, the conclusions arrived at by most of the speakers being the same as that advanced in the opening paper, that optic neuritis is a true inflammation. Professor Leber, in reply, considered that the inflammation was propagated from the brain; and where no meningitis existed, such as in the case of a tumour at a distance from the optic nerve, explained it by exudation of fluid into the vaginal space, exciting inflammation. He agreed also with the opinion of Pinot regarding the possibility of a lymphatic inflammation leading to serous-fluid exudation into ventricles and vaginal space.

Monday and Tuesday mornings were chiefly devoted to the consideration of the Pathology and Treatment of Glaucoma, a subject, the discussion of which evoked very considerable interest, and a numerous audience. On Monday, Dr. Weber (of Darmstadt) described in an interesting paper the pathological changes preceding and causing glaucoma. The invariable antecedent is a progressive contraction of the outlets of the intra-ocular fluids. The path of outlet of the fluids from the eye is from the vitreous to the posterior chamber, through the pupil into the anterior chamber, out at its periphery; any obstruction at any point in this path causes retention of fluid behind it, such obstruction being the first factor in the causation of glaucoma. The changes preceding glaucoma are most commonly disturbances of the general circulation, which diminish the difference between the arterial and venous pressure; such vascular disturbances may result from general nervous conditions. Local morbid changes of circulation, of nerve-function, and of tissue may contribute to the development of the disease. On this subject Mr. Priestley Smith made a brief communication, in which, after restating his theory that the obstruction in the path of the excretory fluids consists of a gradual enlargement of the lens by age, encroaching on the circumlental space, he gave the results of an examination of a series of lens of different ages, with respect to their weight and volume, and found that the lens increases in weight and volume with the advance of life.

Dr. Angelucci (of Rome), in an investigation on the Development of the Canals of Schlemm and Fontana, concluded that the cause of glaucoma is not to be found in the closure of Fontana's space, but in sclerosis of all the membranes of the eye, and chiefly of the bloodvessels. The discussion which followed these papers was short. With respect to the theory of Priestley Smith, Professor Leber had been unsuccessful in establishing a permanent tension in the vitreous in living animals by injection of fluid, and believed that glaucoma might come on in different ways. Dr. Brailey also objected that his examination and measurements of glaucomatous lenses after removal showed them to be distinctly below the average size. A paper by Knapp followed on the Results obtained from the Peripheral Division of the Capsule in Cataract Extraction. In 5 per cent. the eye was lost, or there was only perception of light.

The business of the Section terminated on Tuesday by a consideration of the treatment of glaucoma, with especial reference to the operation of sclerotomy. Dr. de Wecker reviewed the subject in an able paper. He considers the more or less complete action of myotics to be an excellent indication for the operation, inasmuch as it is indispensable for its success that there should be a perfect contraction of the pupil under myotics, this forming the only guarantee against entanglement of the iris in the wound. He concluded by enumerating the conditions requiring sclerotomy, viz., the hæmorrhagic, congenital, premonitory, absolute, and chronic simple varieties of glaucoma, and unsuccessful iridectomy. Mr. Bader, in a communication on the same subject, contended that this operation is superior to iridectomy; and that, to obtain the most perfect success, it is desirable to maintain a staphyloma of the conjunctiva, with or without prolapse of iris. To confirm this opinion, he exhibited four successful cases of different varieties of glaucoma which had been treated in this manner. Dr. Abadie's paper recommended sclerotomy in cases of increased ocular tension with anterior chamber of full depth, and especially in certain forms of hydrophthalmos. In the discussion which followed, the merits of the various operations were debated. Mr. Power had performed Hancock's operation extensively with considerable success; but preferred iridectomy to sclerotomy, and objected to the doctrine of the desirability of a prolapse of the iris in sclerotomy as being dangerous. That the operation of sclerotomy is not entirely innocent was shown by Knapp (of New York), who mentioned a case of intra-ocular suppuration following its employment. Before adjudging the merits of the different operations, wider scope and larger statistics are required, to enable general conclusions to be framed as to their application.

Papers were read by Dr. Pagenstecher (of Wiesbaden), on a New Operation for Ptosis, by passing a thread through the tissues of the lid between the supra-orbital margin above and the ciliary margin below; by Dr. George Martin, on Occlusion of the Pupil; and by Dr. Stevens, on Oculo-neural Reflex Irritation. This concluded the work of the Section, and formed the last of a series of highly successful meetings.

Before separating, the members of the Section passed a hearty vote of thanks to Mr. Bowman for presiding, and to the Secretaries (Mr. Nettleship and Dr. Brailey).

Among the instruments and specimens which were on exhibition during the days of meeting were the ophthalmometer and optometer of Dr. Javal, a registering perimeter of Dr. Stevens, a new instrument for the operation of closed pupil by Dr. Howe, a chromoptometer for the examination of railway servants by Dr. Parinaud; microscopic specimens of tuberculosis of the eye by Dr. Hirschberg and Mr. Story, and others by Mr. Nettleship, Dr. Brailey, and Mr. Gunn.

In the Section of Obstetric Medicine and Surgery, on Monday, August 8, the greater part of the morning was occupied in the discussion opened by papers from Dr. Robert Barnes and Dr. More Madden, "On the Treatment of Post-partum Hæmorrhage." The discussion was a somewhat barren one, many speakers going over the same ground as their predecessors. Drs. Montbrun, Winckel (of Dresden), Beverley Cole (of San Francisco), Byrne (of Dublin), Matthews Duncan, Playfair, Budin (of Paris), Pallen (of New York), Edis, and others, spoke. Dr. Matthews Duncan declared that the injection of perchloride of iron was a more dangerous thing than post-partum hæmorrhage; that contraction of the uterus, not styptics, was the thing required to arrest hæmorrhage. Dr. Playfair regarded the iron injection as a thing which might lead to septic infection. He urged the importance of attention to the third stage of labour in order to prevent hæmorrhage; and in this received strong support from Dr. Jones Morris, a general practitioner from Wales, who described the mode in which he managed the third stage of labour, and his happy freedom from post-partum hæmorrhage. Dr. Rothe spoke as to the danger of the iron, and mentioned a case in which it had led to peritonitis. Dr. Byrne, of Dublin, on the contrary, warmly advocated its use. The President, Dr. McClintock, said he regarded the iron injection as a remedy which was dangerous, but justifiable in very bad cases. He had, however, known it fail. He expressed a decided opinion that chloroform predisposed to hæmorrhage; and in this was supported by Dr. Barnes. On the whole, the general opinion seemed to be that Dr. McClintock's position with regard to the iron injection was the right one. Dr. George Roper's paper, on "Trismus and Tetany of the Uterus in Labour," with a short, but interesting and useful, discussion which it led to, filled up the morning. In the afternoon sitting some more papers were read, but the discussions presented no feature of interest.

The first subject for discussion on the last day of the sittings was that of Antiseptics in Midwifery. Professor Spiegelberg, who was to have opened it, was unfortunately absent, but his paper was read by one of the secretaries. Professor Winckel (of Dresden), who followed, gave an account of the results which had followed in his country, from insisting upon the observance of antiseptic precautions by midwives. Dr. Fancourt Barnes contributed his experience of antiseptic midwifery at the British Lying-in Hospital. Professor Tarnier described the system of management at the Paris Maternity, an institution where, as is known, the results are exceedingly good. Drs. Reid, Edis, and others also took part in the discussion. A communication of the highest value was then made by Dr. Mouat, one of the medical inspectors to the Local Government Board, who presented a return of the child-bed mortality in the workhouse infirmaries of England and Wales during a period of ten years. These statistics embraced a total of 87,726 deliveries, and the mortality was about one in 114. Dr. Mouat's figures confirm the calculations of Dr. Matthews Duncan, Dr. McClintock, and others, as to the usual puerperal mortality, and add to the scepticism with which we receive accounts from outdoor maternity charities, in which the death-rate is returned at one in a thousand or thereabouts. The figures obtained from workhouse infirmaries have this advantage: that the patients being in the workhouse from poverty, and being kept there till they are not merely well enough to get about, but able to get their living, the termination of each case is known; and puerperal diseases and deaths cannot be overlooked. Professor Halbertsma next advocated his view that puerperal eclampsia is in most cases due to compression of the ureters; a theory which, as Dr. Barnes pointed out, was held by Dr. Lever. Professor Halbertsma, however, extended it, by supposing that distension of the ureters destroyed their peristaltic action, and so the effects of pressure persisted after delivery; and thus he explained the occurrence of post-partum convulsions. After this, Dr. Eustache drew a comparison between embryotomy and Cæsarian section, greatly to the advantage of the latter, but based on the extraordinary assumption that the maternal mortality from craniotomy was 50 per cent.! Dr. Barnes, in commenting on the paper, said that his craniotomy mortality was either about 1 per cent. or nothing at all; and the views of Dr. Eustache were well combated by Dr. Meyer, a Swedish physician. For some unexplained reason, Dr. Barnes wound up the Section at half-past twelve, although three more papers, one of them an important one, remained to be read. The Section was a marked success; the discussions and the social intercourse must have greatly promoted mutual understanding, removed misconceptions, and enlarged the knowledge of its members, and the genial courtesy of the President made the meetings pleasant as well as profitable.

The meetings of the Section of Military Surgery and Medicine were remarkable on account of the great importance and practical character of the papers brought forward for discussion, and the variety, and even conflict, of the opinions expressed by *authorities* upon particular subjects, such diversity of opinions being probably the result of service under varying and peculiar circumstances in different parts of the world.

On Thursday, the 4th inst., after the address by Surgeon-General Longmore, C.B., the President, papers were read

bearing upon the question of the feasibility of the application of the antiseptic method to the treatment of the wounded in the field—by Dr. Lilburne, Deputy Inspector-General, R.N., "On Antiseptic Treatment of Wounds in the Field"; Dr. Port (of Munich), on "Antiseptic Treatment of Wounds in the Field"; Surgeon-General Dr. Beck (of the 14th German Army Corps), on "Antiseptic Dressing of Wounds"; and Surgeon-Major Melladew, Royal Horse Guards, on "Lessons of the Late Russo-Turkish War"; and a discussion followed.

Professor Esmarch contended that the question was—where should the antiseptic method begin, where could the first antiseptic dressing be applied? On the battle-field itself, he thought, a genuine antiseptic dressing, Listerian in all its details, in its precautions, would be impossible. It should be an axiom, *Non nocere.* The brilliant experience of his Russian colleagues had fully confirmed his previously expressed opinion, that a very large number even of the most severely wounded cases ran an aseptic course when they had not been disturbed or uselessly examined by the introduction of a dirty finger or probe; therefore every attempt to maintain the asepticity of the wound should be made. The wound should be protected from hurtfulness of transport by a covering of some antiseptic material. On this principle had the Professor constructed his dressing pad, which he showed and demonstrated. Every soldier provided with such a pad could dress his wound quite independently of the surgeon.

Surgeon-Major Melladew, in his paper, referred to the statistics of Bergmann, Reyher, and Cammerer, which conclusively showed that wherever honest attempts were made to act in the spirit of antisepticism, there the results were successful and complete. The dictum of Professor Esmarch, that the "Schwerpunct" of antiseptic treatment is on the battle-field itself, and that of Professor Nussbaum, "that the fate of the wounded man is in the hands of the surgeon who first attends him," had been amply illustrated in the late Russo-Turkish war. He advised early closure of the wound (without disturbance) by a firm pad overlaid by cotton-wool or other antiseptic material; and mentioned various antiseptic materials and modes of application, and showed an antiseptic pad to be carried by each soldier sewn in the breast of his tunic just below the collar-bone, where it would form a soft cushion.

Dr. Gori (of Amsterdam) said the value of antisepticism on the field of battle could only be decided by experience, but the question as to what details of Listerism were absolutely essential, should be studied in time of peace. The wound should be touched only with aseptic, and covered quickly with antiseptic, material; Protection from evils of transport by antiseptic covering was the essential part of the first dressing. Dr. Gori recommended the "compresses antiseptiques" of Messrs. Schaffhausen, a combination of Guérin's cotton-wadding with Lister's gauze and a piece of protective paper. How to preserve an antiseptic dressing was the desideratum of military surgery.

Surgeon-General Mouat, V.C., said he had practised antiseptic treatment as long ago as 1840 in India. He spoke highly of the antiseptic properties of creasote: it rapidly destroyed maggots; it had been used with success in general field-hospital in Crimea after the attack on the Redan, June 18. Condy's fluid had proved very serviceable in New Zealand, in 1864-65. Dr. Mouat did not think Listerism applicable to the field; and was in favour of simple antiseptic solutions, cleanliness, and pure air.

Dr. Reyher quoted the vastly superior results gained by Listerism in the Russo-Turkish War of 1877, as contrasted with the statistics of the Prussian campaign of 1870-71. Of seven primary resections of shoulder-joint, all had recovered; of nine primary resections of elbow, only one had died. Similar success had resulted from his operations on the lower extremity.

Professor Longmore concluded the discussion by stating that there seemed a general consensus of opinion that there were almost insuperable difficulties to overcome in the application of Listerism to the first line of surgical assistance, but that it was the goal that all military surgeons should have in view. Listerism would be feasible in the stationary hospitals. The great want was a dressing that could be carried on the person of the soldier, and that would not deteriorate by keeping or by exposure. The simpler it could be, the better.

On Friday, Professor Esmarch read a very interesting and valuable paper " On the Treatment of Injuries of Bloodvessels in the Field." Professor Esmarch showed an extremely ingenious adaptation and application of the ordinary trousers-suspenders of the soldier for the purpose of arresting hæmorrhage ; and a discussion followed, in which many members of the Section took part. Papers were also read on important questions of Transport of Sick and Wounded Troops in time of War, by Dr. Gori, by Dr. Cunha Bellem (of Lisbon), and by Dr. Ash ; and some remarks were made on the subject.

Dr. Fagan showed a splint for injuries of spine, pelvis, and lower extremities, by him termed the "Transport Splint"; and Dr. Ennes (of Lisbon) read a paper on the Disinfection of the Battle-field, in which he strongly advocated cremation.

On Saturday, Surgeon-General Maclean, C.B., Professor of Military Medicine, Netley, communicated a most important and valuable paper "On the Prevalence of Enteric Fever among Young Soldiers in India : its Causes and the most Rational Means of Prevention."

Monday and Tuesday were devoted—(1) to a discussion on the influence of the Contagious Diseases Acts upon the prevalence of venereal affections among the troops serving in the United Kingdom, opened by Inspector-General Lawson ; (2) important communications by Surgeon-General Longmore and Dr. Kirker, R.N., on the Wounds and Effects produced by the Cylindro-conoidal Bullets ; (3) a valuable and interesting paper by Sir Joseph Fayrer, upon Insolation or Sunstroke among troops in quarters or on the line of march in tropical countries.

In response to the kind invitation of Surgeon-General Longmore, Surgeon-General Fasson, and officers of the Army Medical Department, Aldershot, a number of the military and naval officers attending the International Medical Congress, visited Aldershot on Wednesday last, for the purpose of witnessing the drill, training, and practical working in the field of the bearer companies of the Army Hospital Corps. The party left Waterloo Station by the 10.15 a.m. train, under the guidance of Surgeon Myers, of the Coldstream Guards, whose uniform courtesy and ceaseless activity were frequently referred to and warmly acknowledged by the various distinguished representatives of foreign powers. Amongst them we noticed Surgeon-General Lommer, of the Prussian War Department ; Surgeon-General Coler, Surgeon-General Roth, of the Saxon Army ; Dr. C. Smith, the delegate from Norway ; Inspector-General Dr. Landa, of Spain ; Medical Director Dr. Browne, of Washington, as the representative of the United States Navy ; Dr. Cunha Bellem and Dr. Ennes, of Portugal ; Surgeon-Major Malladew, Royal Horse Guards, whose linguistic attainments were invaluable ; Brigade-Surgeon Becher, Dr. Starcke, Mr. MacKellar, Dr. Sommerbrodt, Dr. Jankowski, Dr. Port (of Munich), and many others.

On arrival at the South Camp the party was met by Surgeon-Major Hoyle with waggonettes, provided by the courtesy of the officers of the Army Medical Department, and immediately driven to the head-quarters of the medical staff. Here they were received by the principal medical officers of the Aldershot Camp, Surgeon-General Fasson, C.B., and Deputy Surgeon-General Madden, C.B. The bearer companies were already drawn up on parade under the command of Surgeon-Major Sandford Moore, assisted by Surgeons Bradford and Croft. After an inspection of the lines, the men of the Army Hospital Corps were put through a few simple evolutions, and, preceded by their band, marched past the saluting point, winding up with a general salute. Stretcher drill succeeded, the various movements of which were executed with a quiet, steady earnestness that much impressed the spectators. The bearers seemed to act with great gentleness and tenderness of manner, as if actually dealing with wounded men, the "dummies"—men told off from the ranks to do duty as "wounded"—admirably feigning limpness and utter helplessness. After stretcher drill came the transport of wounded by means of litters and cacolets borne by mules. The visitors now adjourned to some open ground adjoining the Cambridge Hospital. Here a singular spectacle presented itself. Some sixty men, told off from the 95th to posture as wounded, were lying on the field in all directions, each man having attached to a breast-button of his tunic a ticket explanatory of the nature of his supposed injury,

such as "compound fracture of thigh," "flesh wound of arm," "wound of shoulder," etc. Here, the same earnestness of purpose remarked in the stretcher drill was again apparent ; there was no "scamping," no hurrying of work, no sign of make-believe. Every operation was conducted as if actually occurring on the battle-field ; but there was, of course, a stillness utterly foreign to the battle-field,—it lacked the roar of cannon, the rattle of musketry, the smoke, the groans, the cries for water, the dying and the dead, to complete the stern, grim reality of war. The cases were so arranged as to illustrate the numerous modes of application of the triangular bandages of Professor Esmarch, and in every case coming under our observation the bandages had been neatly and deftly applied, and evidently by practised hands. In gunshot fractures of thigh with hæmorrhage, a tourniquet had been accurately applied, and the limb fixed, the rifle of the wounded man being used as a long outside splint. The first dressing done, the man was carefully lifted on to the stretcher, his knapsack serving as a pillow, and at the word of command carried off to the ambulance waggon. The realism of the acting of the wound was still kept up : a man shot in the right arm in handing a comrade's kit into the waggon, used solely the left arm, and carefully guarded the right from injury. The unusual and interesting character of the sight naturally attracted many spectators, including large numbers of ladies, and some combatant officers ; two of whom, recently returned from active service (one from Afghanistan, the other from the Transvaal), watched the proceedings with evident interest. There were present also Surgeons-Major Paterson and Barker (of the Cambridge Hospital), Surgeon-Major Gasteen, and Surgeon Grier, whom our readers will remember as having recently received the Albert Medal for distinguished gallantry in having, for the time, saved the life of an officer suffering from diphtheria, by clearing an obstructed tracheotomy-tube by suction with his mouth. The wounded all picked up, the parade-ground was revisited. There a transformation had been effected ; the men with gunshot fractures of thigh, disencumbered of their splints, had now fallen in ; and the many gravely wounded were serving as models to illustrate the application of various extemporised materials. An inspection of the field panniers, and contents of the medical and surgical store waggons, concluded the parade.

The visitors were most hospitably entertained at luncheon by the officers of the Army Medical Department, and afterwards an inspection was made of the Women's and Cambridge Hospitals. Their condition left nothing to be desired. The visitors were lavish in their praise of the practical character of the operations they had witnessed, and of the generous hospitality they had enjoyed.

MULTIPLICITY OF MEDICAL WRITINGS.—Using the "Index Medicus" as a guide, we find that in the world last year 11,700 doctors thought they had something new to say, or some new way of saying something old. Mostly were they moved by vanity, and surely the outcome is vexation of spirit. What the end of all this is to be is not easy to perceive. In fifty years more, if things go on, our unfortunate descendants may witness 20,000 doctors, with vehement haste, yearly urging their pens in eager rivalry for fortune.—*Philadelphia Med. Times*, July 2.

HYPODERMIC INJECTIONS OF MORPHIA.—Dr. Dujardin-Beaumetz employs one gramme of chlorhydrate of morphia dissolved in fifty grammes of cherry-laurel water, a gramme containing two centigrammes of the salt. He begins by injecting from five to ten milligrammes in cases of lesion of the aorta (contraction or insufficiency), to relieve dyspnœa, attacks of angina, cardiac pain, and the symptoms of cerebral anæmia, such as vertigo and lipothymia. The injection may be made in the dorsal surface of the forearm, the walls of the abdomen, or, better still, in the vicinity of the pain. If the morphia is ill tolerated and induces vomiting, the following solution may be used :—Chlorhydrate of morphia, ten centigrammes ; neutral sulphate of atropia, one centigramme ; and cherry-laurel water, twenty grammes. A gramme of this contains half a centigramme of morphia and half a milligramme of atropia, and the whole syringeful may be injected. More favourable results are often obtained from this than from morphia alone. Before any of these injections are used, we should be certain that the kidneys act regularly.—*Union Méd.*, July 26.

THE FORTY-NINTH ANNUAL MEETING
OF THE
BRITISH MEDICAL ASSOCIATION.
HELD AT RYDE, AUGUST 8, 9, 10, AND 11.

(From our Special Correspondent.)

IT is astonishing what a number of small errors anyone may fall into, who is not gifted with the ubiquity of Sir Boyle Roche's bird; and this is especially the case where one trusts to programmes which may be varied from day to day. Thus, last week I spoke of a discussion of uterine flexions, introduced by Dr. Coghill, as taking place on Wednesday, but it still headed the list of the day's work on Thursday morning; and on Friday I found among the *agenda* the sums to be voted for research, which I thought had been permanently put on one side. The first public business of importance on Thursday was, however, the third general meeting, at which the report of the Parliamentary Bills Committee was read, certain portions of which gave rise to keen discussion, and to some conduct which might, without saying too much, be described as disorderly. In fact, we have never, even when the great question of the admission of women was debated, seen so much warmth of feeling and excitement shown as at the recent meeting. The point in connexion with the Parliamentary report which excited most discontent was the proposal to render the registration of infectious diseases compulsory. A Bill to this end has been introduced into the House of Commons by Mr. George Hastings, at the instance of the Social Science Association, which proposes to impose the duty of notification directly upon the medical man in attendance. The Parliamentary Bills Committee, therefore, recommend that early next session a Bill should be introduced, on the part of the Association, carrying out the views on this subject which the Association have already endorsed. Mr. Sibley and Dr. Ransome proposed the adoption of the report, but Mr. Michael, Q.C., moved, as an amendment, that it should be an instruction to the Committee to support Mr. Hastings' Bill; and a very warm discussion ensued, the opposition to the amendment being led by Dr. Fitzpatrick (of Dublin), who, in a long harangue, protested against such responsibility being thrown on a medical man's shoulders. Many other speeches followed, and the amendment was speedily lost when put to the vote. When, however, the President came to the original motion, no division could at first be got, the purport of the Committee's report having been misunderstood, nor was the tumult appeased—some calling for one thing, some for another, some for the views of the Committee—until Mr. Sibley had assured the meeting that the view of the Committee was simply this: that the medical man should be bound to report the nature of the case to the parent or guardian of the sick person, leaving the responsibility of communicating with the authorities to rest on their shoulders, not on his. With this explanation the resolution for receiving and adopting the report and reappointing the Committee was promptly carried.

Then followed the chief business of the morning, viz., the Address in Surgery, delivered by Mr. Jonathan Hutchinson. The first part of the address might almost be described as an *apologia pro domo sud*, for it dealt with specialties, and especially those in which Mr. Hutchinson has attained such eminence. He pointed out that whilst ophthalmic surgery had, long ago, become a specialty, certain of its methods were rapidly reverting to the condition of general subjects, being largely employed in scientific medicine. Other specialties were not so soon or so readily recognised as ophthalmology; and he alluded to what took place some five-and-twenty years ago, when the Hospital for Stone was instituted, and a kind of protest was signed by all the chief hospital surgeons in London, he himself among the rest. He declared that he would sign no such protest now, and he thought that many others were of the same opinion as he.

By a somewhat curious coincidence, Mr. Hutchinson had resolved upon saying something about homœopathy and homœopaths, but finding that this subject had already been touched upon by Dr. Bristowe on the previous day, he would have passed it by, had not the meeting insisted on hearing his views, which were nearly identical with those of Dr. Bristowe. Mr. Hutchinson's address will, however, probably appear shortly in your pages.

The question of Vivisection has been a good deal discussed recently, in consequence, to a great extent, of the action taken by the present Home Secretary. In the time of Sir Richard Cross matters went on tolerably smoothly, but since Sir W. Vernon Harcourt came into office he has apparently endeavoured to prove that men of science can look for very little consideration at his hands. The obstacles and difficulties which have been put in the way of any research being carried out, however important, have been such as to prevent men from attempting anything in this direction. At the International Medical Congress, general resolutions were passed, condemning this state of things; and something similar was proposed at Ryde by Professor Humphry, only the last-named gentleman limited his resolution, in effect, to deprecating any farther prohibition of what is commonly called vivisection. When speaking, however, he ably met all the arguments used against vivisection, and justified the practice in a very effective and well-delivered speech, which was thoroughly well received and applauded by his audience. Thoughtful men will agree with him in this respect, that any attempt to renew an agitation for legalised vivisection might end disastrously for science. Many well-meaning but ill-informed people, knowing nothing of what they speak, are violently opposed to any experiments on living animals, and deliberately state that they would prefer man to suffer rather than that his sufferings should be alleviated by knowledge acquired in such a manner. Nor should it be forgotten that medical men have been to blame for the evil odour which animal experimentation has acquired. Operations on living beings were at one time in some places too lightly regarded, and too much prominence was perhaps given to them as a means of education. And the present seems no well-chosen time for a renewal of agitation which might end in the total abolition of animal experimentation, in hands however skilled, and for objects however important. At all events, Professor Humphry's motion was carried with a single dissentient voice, and surely this gentleman deserves credit for the courage of his opinions.

On Thursday afternoon the Section of Medicine was chiefly engaged with Nervous Diseases; whilst in Surgery some very good remarks were made introductory to a discussion on the subject of Resection of the Knee-joint in early life, by Mr. W. Stokes (of Dublin). But the chief attraction lay in the Public Health Section, where a discussion of Animal Vaccination was begun by Mr. Ernest Hart, in which Dr. Warlomont (of Brussels) and Dr. Martin (of Boston) were expected to take part. Unfortunately, Dr. Warlomont was unable to be present, but Dr. Martin spoke with that weight and authority which his long and extensive experience enables him to bring to bear on the subject.

Mr. Hart first of all alluded to the great difficulty which had been encountered in getting successive Governments to take up the subject of animal vaccination. At last, however, in June, 1880, Mr. Dodson announced that the Government had taken the matter into consideration, and were prepared to undertake the supply of animal lymph as well as that of long humanisation. This concession has, unfortunately, not resulted in anything practical up to the present, since the Board, a year after Mr. Dodson's promise, still reply to inquirers that their arrangements for the supply of animal lymph are not completed. It is difficult to understand why so long a delay has been allowed to take place; but it would be unprofitable, as well as vexatious, to inquire minutely into the causes, since we all know how slow Government offices are to move. There are two chief questions in connexion with this subject, to which it may be well to direct attention for a few moments—viz., the practicability of animal vaccination, and its efficiency.

It has been argued that, however useful and valuable animal lymph may be, its cultivation is a matter of difficulty; that the keeping up of the stock on a series of animals is liable to interruptions; that the lymph does not keep well—and similar objections. It is undoubtedly true that, like everything else requiring care, a certain amount of skill and patience is required for the successful cultivation of calf-lymph; but those who have acquired the dexterity necessary for the operation will state that they have no difficulty in keeping up their stocks, and that they are now using lymph obtained by an unbroken series of transmissions through several hundreds of animals. As regards the keeping qualities of calf-lymph, it is generally admitted that, preserved in tubes, its efficacy soon becomes impaired; and all cultivators recommend its collection on points as being the most certain method. As to the efficiency of animal vaccination, there can be but little question. Attempts have been made to compare the ordinary current calf-lymph vaccinations with those performed with human lymph from arm to arm by a specially skilled vaccinator of the highest repute. Fairly compared, animal lymph shows equal, if not superior, insertion-results to that derived from the arms of infants, and as regards its prophylactic power against variola there are undeniable proofs of the decided advantage which it possesses in this respect. That the lymph manifests greater results on the human system than current lymph, simply shows its greater vaccinal power; and in ordinary cases the constitutional disturbance is no more intense than typically perfect vaccination ought to be. Dr. Carsten (of the Hague) has shown that at Amsterdam during the last six years there has been but one failure out of a total of 14,849 insertions.

There was but one other point to which Mr. Hart especially referred, and that was the undoubted advantage which animal vaccination possesses in its freedom from the suspicion of being concerned in the possible inoculation of syphilis into the human body. If for no other reason than this, its use ought to be encouraged. On the subject of the possible inoculation of syphilis, a variety of opinions have been expressed in this country and abroad, and it could serve no useful purpose to attempt to discuss them at the present moment. But, however much opinions on this point may differ, there is a general agreement in recommending the cultivation and official recognition of calf-lymph as a means of calming the apprehensions (however ill-founded) of parents as to the qualities of the virus used. The counter-objection, that calf-lymph may be the means of inoculating the vaccinee with animal diseases, hardly needs serious discussion.

This, together with the reading of several allied papers, and the discussion which followed, occupied the greater part of the afternoon; and in the evening came the annual dinner, for which there were issued, for the first time, two kinds of tickets—one entitling to wine and dinner, the other to dinner and aerated waters only.

As Friday is the last day of work at the Association meeting, everyone is afoot betimes, the last general address being delivered at ten o'clock. On this occasion the subject chosen was Obstetrics, the lecturer being Dr. Coghill (of Ventnor), formerly, if I recollect aright, assistant for a time to Professor Simpson, and one of the candidates for the Edinburgh chair of Midwifery on the decease of that lamented physician. At all events, Dr. Coghill is fully master of his subject, and elected—what is not a very easy task—to give some account of the various advances in obstetric medicine since the last obstetric address was given, some three years ago. The first portion of the address, and perhaps in one way the most interesting, referred to the advances which had been made in our knowledge of uterine and ovarian physiology; the second dealt with midwifery, properly so-called; whilst in the latter portion other parts of a wide subject were dealt with. The papers read in the various sections were of the most varied kind. In Medicine, a paper on Jaundice had been promised by Dr. Brunton, to be followed by a discussion; in Surgery, a discussion on the Early Recognition and Treatment of Spinal Caries was introduced by a paper from Mr. Edmund Owen; whilst in the Health Section the two most important and interesting papers were—one by Dr. Beveridge (of Aberdeen), on a Peculiar Outbreak of Disease in connexion with the Supply of Milk; and one by Dr. A. P. Stewart, on the all-important question of Convalescent Homes for Scarlatinal Patients.

Finally, at half-past one, came the concluding general meeting, about which a word must be said. The chief business on this occasion was the receiving and adopting of two reports—one from the Habitual Drunkards' Reformation Committee, and the other from the Medical Reform Committee. The substance of the former was that a body should be formed and enrolled, under the Limited Liability Act, for the purpose of establishing a model reformatory, to be called a Dalrymple Home. With the aims of those who have thus sought the reclamation of persons most sincerely to be pitied, your journal has ever sympathised; but it is doubtful whether their success is likely to be brilliant, if we are to take the published results of last year's attempts as any criterion.

At all events, it is clear that they are actuated by the purest benevolence, and certainly deserve to succeed.

The next discussion gave rise to the other somewhat disorderly discussion to which I have alluded. The outcome of the report of the Medical Reform Committee was embodied in the Bill backed by Sir Trevor Lawrence, Mr. Horncastle, and Dr. Farquharson, and there was one clause in it which specially roused the ire of the meeting. This was in reference to the suppression of the two Apothecaries' Halls and the Glasgow Faculty as examining bodies, and the extinction of their representation on the Medical Council. The Scotch and Irish bodies had but few representatives present, but there were many sturdy supporters of the Apothecaries' Hall of London; nevertheless, the clause was allowed to pass in the long run. After all, it does not greatly matter; the whole business is now before the Royal Commission, and Sir William Jenner has clearly indicated what course that body is likely to take, nor is it probable that it will be greatly moved by any such opposition as that which has been seen up to the present time.

The last business was the voting of scientific grants, or rather of £300, to be allotted as the Grants Committee think best. As I have already hinted, nothing very great has come of these as yet. The afternoon was to have been devoted to a garden party given by the President and Mrs. Barrow, but the weather by this time was fairly broken, and, as is too often the case, a more uncomfortable afternoon for an al fresco meeting could not well be imagined. In fact, all through the meeting we sadly missed the brilliant weather which last year saluted us at Cambridge. It is not, however, to be supposed that the meeting was dull, languid, or disagreeable. There was a quiet enjoyment on all sides, in marked contradistinction to the affairé appearance of those engaged in the actual work of the London Congress. The hospitality shown, especially by the President, was unbounded, and contributed not a little to the success of the meeting. The numbers as registered amounted to more than four hundred, but at no time were there many more than three hundred present, as some had departed before others had entered an appearance. At all events, most of the members of the Association and the visitors will, I think, be able to look back on the Ryde meeting with pleasure and gratification.

GENERAL CORRESPONDENCE.

THE INDIAN MEDICAL SERVICE AND PROPOSED MEMORIAL TO THE ARMY MEDICAL OFFICERS.

LETTER FROM DR. A. DUNCAN.

[To the Editor of the Medical Times and Gazette.]

SIR,—My fellow medical officers of the Indian Army will hardly credit me when I inform them that, by the decision of the committee at Whitehall, the proposed memorial to the memory of the army medical officers who fell in the campaigns in Afghanistan and Zululand is to be confined to the officers of the Army Medical Department, and has not any reference to the memory of the officers of the Indian Medical Service; yet such is the case. Now, sir, as far as I have been able to gather, twelve medical officers lost their lives from wounds received in action, or from disease contracted during the campaign whilst serving their country in Afghanistan: of these, six belonged to the Indian Army.

The Indian Medical Defence Fund has done good service in pointing out how, under the specious guise of amalgamation, the military branch of the Indian Medical Service has been absolutely ruined. It has, however, been reserved for the committee of the proposed memorial to show to the officers of the Indian Service that, notwithstanding this amalgamation of the two services under one Surgeon-General —always, be it remarked, belonging to the Army Medical Department—a memorial, which should have been common to all medical officers who fell in the campaign in Afghanistan, has been reserved exclusively for those of the Army Medical Department. I would suggest, through the medium of your columns, that a committee be formed in India for erecting likewise a memorial to these surgeons of the Indian Army who lost their lives whilst serving their country in Afghanistan.

ANDREW DUNCAN, M.D., B.S. Lond., F.R.C.S.
(Surgeon late attached to 8th Bengal Cavalry.)
8, Henrietta-street, Covent-garden, August 16.

VITAL STATISTICS OF LONDON.

Week ending Saturday, August 13, 1881.

BIRTHS.

Births of Boys, 1286; Girls, 1191; Total, 2477.
Corrected weekly average in the 10 years 1871-80, 2490·1.

DEATHS.

	Males.	Females.	Total.
Deaths during the week	805	773	1578
Weekly average of the ten years 1871-80, corrected to increased population ...	869·4	785·5	1654·9
Deaths of people aged 80 and upwards ...			47

DEATHS IN SUB-DISTRICTS FROM EPIDEMICS.

	Enumerated Population, 1881 (unrevised)	Small-pox.	Measles.	Scarlet Fever.	Diphtheria.	Whooping-cough.	Typhus.	Enteric (or Typhoid) Fever.	Simple continued Fever.	Diarrhœa.
West ...	662995	6	7	3	2	3	...	6	...	40
North ...	905677	5	15	14	3	5	...	1	...	51
Central ...	361793	1	3	6	2	1	...	1	...	16
East ...	692580	5	7	9	4	4	...	3	...	37
South ...	1965676	12	16	25	4	11	3	6	1	66
Total ...	3814571	29	48	57	15	22	3	17	1	210

METEOROLOGY.

From Observations at the Greenwich Observatory.

Mean height of barometer ...	...	...	...	...	29·845 in.
Mean temperature ...	...	...	...	...	59·0°
Highest point of thermometer	...	...	...	...	73·7°
Lowest point of thermometer	...	...	...	...	47·6°
Mean dew-point temperature	...	...	...	...	54·4°
General direction of wind ...	...	...	...	...	S.W.
Whole amount of rain in the week	...	...	...	...	1·76 in.

BIRTHS and DEATHS Registered and METEOROLOGY during the
Week ending Saturday, August 13, in the following large Towns:—

Cities and boroughs (Municipal boundaries except for London.)	Estimated Population to middle of the year 1881.*	Persons to an Acre. (1881.)	Births Registered during the week ending Aug. 13.	Deaths Registered during the week ending Aug. 13.	Temperature of Air (Fahr.) Highest during the Week.	Temperature of Air (Fahr.) Lowest during the Week.	Temperature of Air (Fahr.) Weekly Mean of Daily Mean Values.	Temp. of Air (Cent.) Weekly Mean of Daily Mean Values.	Rain Fall. In Inches.	Rain Fall. In Centimetres.
London ...	3829751	50·8	2477	1578	78·7	47·5	59·0	15·00	1·76	4·47
Brighton ...	107934	45·9	56	47	75·0	48·5	60·8	16·01	1·04	2·64
Portsmouth ...	128835	28·6	95	54	...	...	...	...	...	...
Norwich ...	88038	11·5	36	31	...	...	...	...	...	...
Plymouth ...	76282	54·0	37	27	68·5	48·8	58·1	14·50	0·76	1·93
Bristol ...	207140	46·5	136	80	67·1	42·7	56·7	13·72	1·85	4·70
Wolverhampton ...	75934	22·4	44	25	66·3	45·3	54·5	12·50	1·32	3·35
Birmingham ...	402256	47·9	291	162	...	...	...	...	...	...
Leicester ...	123120	38·5	96	81	70·3	44·0	55·0	12·78	1·88	4·78
Nottingham ...	189235	18·9	142	94	73·2	44·4	56·8	13·78	0·78	1·98
Liverpool ...	553898	106·3	398	258	...	...	...	...	...	...
Manchester ...	341269	79·5	217	122	...	...	...	...	...	...
Salford ...	177760	34·4	137	74	...	...	...	...	...	...
Oldham ...	112176	24·0	65	37	...	...	...	...	...	...
Bradford ...	184037	25·5	116	52	67·6	47·6	56·4	13·55	0·35	0·89
Leeds ...	310490	14·4	214	156	68·0	47·0	56·5	13·61	0·41	1·04
Sheffield ...	285621	14·5	241	107	70·0	46·0	55·9	13·24	0·59	1·50
Hull ...	155181	42·7	122	67	72·0	44·0	54·3	12·39	1·04	2·64
Sunderland ...	116756	42·2	100	54	74·0	47·0	57·8	14·34	0·44	1·12
Newcastle-on-Tyne	145675	27·1	111	55	...	...	...	...	...	...
Total of 20 large English Towns ...	7606775	38·0	5153	3167	78·7	42·7	56·8	13·78	1·02	2·59

* These figures are the numbers enumerated (but subject to revision) in
April last, raised to the middle of 1881 by the addition of a quarter of a
year's increase, calculated at the rate that prevailed between 1871 and 1881.

At the Royal Observatory, Greenwich, the mean reading
of the barometer last week was 29·65 in. The highest reading
was 30·02 in. at the beginning of the week, and the lowest
29·40 in. on Monday evening.

MEDICAL NEWS.

APOTHECARIES' HALL, LONDON.—The following gentle-
men passed their examination in the Science and Practice of
Medicine, and received certificates to practise, on Thursday,
August 4 :—

Cook, Augustus Henry, Hampstead, N.W.
Conway, John, Broomfield, Maidstone.
Davies, John, New Mills, Manaford.
Duncan, David, Chester-le-Street.
Hart, William Hamilton, 19, Trinity-square, S.E.
Hatton, Edwin Fullarton, Peterborough, Canada.
Lipscomb, Arthur Augustus, Forest-hill, S.E.
Russell, Michael William, 29, Alfred-place, W.C.
Sen, Rajani Kaula, Baldhara, Bengal.
Voisey, Clement Bernard, Manchester.

And on the 11th :—

Clegg, John Hague, 25, Canonbury-square, N.
Goulden, James Henry Oswald, Stockport.
Mark, Leonard Portal, 62, Pall-mall, S.W.
Minchinton, Henry James, Brixham, South Devon.
Pollard, Joseph, 17, Welbeck-street, W.
Pounds, Thomas Henderson, Chatham.
Scott, Bernard, Brighton.
Voss, Francis Henry Vivian, 26, Clapton-square.

The following gentlemen also on August 4 passed their
primary professional examination :—

Batt, Richard Bush Drury, St. Bartholomew's Hospital.
Miller, James, St. Thomas's Hospital.
Rogers, Harry Cornelius Edwin, University College.

And on the 11th :—

Fowler, Charles Owen, University College.
Smith, John, Charing-cross Hospital.
Underwood, John Charles, Guy's Hospital.

APPOINTMENTS.

EDWARD LEEDS, M.A., M.B. Oxon.—Physician to the Seamen's Infirmary,
Ramsgate, in place of T. A. Henderson, M.D., deceased.

BIRTHS.

BRUNTON.—On August 12, at 50, Welbeck-street, W., the wife of T. Lauder
Brunton, M.D., F.R.S., of a daughter.
GILBERT-SMITH.—On August 12, at 68, Harley-street, Cavendish-square,
the wife of T. Gilbert-Smith, M.D., of a son.
HARDWICKE.—On August 12, at Purton Lodge, Sheffield, the wife of
Herbert Junius Hardwicke, M.D., F.R.C.S., of a son.
INSTONE.—On August 16, at 35, The Avenue, Bedford Park, Chiswick,
the wife of R. Vaughan Instone, M.R.C.S., L.S.A., of a son, stillborn.
KEYWORTH.—On August 3, at Wem, Shropshire, the wife of George
Hawson Keyworth, M.B., of a son.
ODLING.—On August 8, at Shiraz, Persia, the wife of T. F. Odling,
M.R.C.S., of a son.
PHILPOT.—On August 11, at 24, Redcliffe-gardens, S.W., the wife of J.
Henry Philpot, M.D., of 96, South Eaton-place, S.W., of a son.
PORTER.—On July 11, at Royapettah, Madras, the wife of Surgeon-Major
A. Porter, of a son.
ROWLAND.—On August 8, at Gloucester House, Malvern Wells, the wife
of H. Mortimer Rowland, M.D., of a daughter.

MARRIAGES.

BOULTER—STEELE.—On August 11, at Dublin, Harold Baxter Boulter,
F.R.C.S., to Dorothea Anna Georgina, eldest daughter of George
Vandeleur Steele, Esq., formerly of Skerke, Queen's County, Ireland.
COMYN—OWEN.—On August 10, at Woolwich, J. Sarsfield Comyn, M.B.,
Surgeon-Major Army Medical Department, to Sophia Agnes, second
daughter of Colonel Owen, Royal Artillery.
COOK—SHEPHEARD.—On August 9, at Hampstead, Augustus Henry Cook,
M.R.C.S., L.S.A., second son of William Henry Cook, M.D., of Aber-
crombie Villa, Hampstead, to Ellen Neville, only daughter of the late
Rev. Henry Shepheard, M.A., of Ambleside, Westmoreland.
GRIFFIN—LUCAS.—On August 12, at Kensington-park, Charles Thomas
Griffin, M.R.C.S., of Hewshetts, Ceylon, and youngest son of William
Griffin, M.D., of Ledbury, to Catharine Agnes, widow of the late Richard
Jago Lucas, Esq.
HOLT—BROATCH.—On August 13, at Piccadilly, James W. Holt, Esq., of
Aigburth, Liverpool, to Clara, eldest daughter of James Broatch,
L.F.P.S., of Glasgow.
JOTHAM—LAXTON.—On August 16, at Clifton, Frederick Charles, younger
son of the late G. W. Jotham, M.R.C.S., of Kidderminster, to Mary
Catherine Anne, only daughter of Henry Laxton, M.R.C.S., of Clifton.
MACKENZIE—COWAN.—On August 11, at Edinburgh, William Scobie
Mackenzie, L.R.C.P., of Normanton, to Susannah Hathaway, daughter
of the late Alexander Cowan, Esq.
NANKIVELL—THRELFALL.—On August 9, at Lytham, Lancashire, Frank
Nankivell, M.D., of Broadhayes, Bournemouth, youngest son of T. H.
Nankivell, M.R.C.S., of Bootham, York, to Margaret, second daughter
of the late Thomas Threlfall, Esq., of Edenfield, Lytham.
PARKES—FOSTER.—On August 9, at Wandsworth, Louis Ooltman Parkes,
M.B., to Lucy, elder daughter of the late Peter Le Neve Foster, M.A.,
of Wandsworth.
PHILLIPS—JOHNSTON.—On August 13, at South Hampstead, Stephen
Thomas Phillips, L.R.C.P., of Wellington, Hereford, to Mary Stuart,
eldest daughter of John Johnston, Esq., of Mansfield-road, Haverstock-
hill, N.W.

SMITH—MOORE-MILLER.—On August 11, at Wickham, Hants, Edmund Philip Bowden Smith, Esq., Commissariat Staff, to Kate Mary, eldest daughter of J. W. Moore-Miller, M.D., J.P., of Southsea.

THOMPSON—FRASER.—On August 11, at Walthamstow, Harold Thompson, M.R.C.S., of Wellington-square, Oxford, to Fanny, twin daughter of John Fraser, Esq., of Leyton, Essex.

WILLIAMSON — WALKER.—On August 16, at New Beckenham, Kent, William Herbert Williamson, M.D., of Aberdeen, to Amelia, eldest daughter of Joseph Walker, M.D., of 22, Grosvenor-street, Grosvenor-square, and Wolverton, Beckenham.

WOODHEAD—ERSKINE.—At Eldercroft, Peebles, on the 17th inst., by the Rev. John McMurtrie, M.A., of St. Bernard's, Edinburgh, German Sims Woodhead, M.D., M.R.C.P.E., Demonstrator of Pathology, University of Edinburgh, to Harriett Elizabeth St. Clair Erskine, second daughter of James Yates, Esq., of Victoria, Vancouver's Island, British Columbia.

DEATHS.

HOLMAN, H. MARTIN, M.D., at Hurstpierpoint, on August 9, aged 60.

LUKE, JAMES, F.R.C.S., F.R.S., at Fingest Grove, Wycombe, Buckinghamshire, on August 15, aged 82.

ODLING.—The wife of T. F. Odling, M.R.C.S., at Shiraz, Persia, on August 13, aged 31.

SHEPHERD, CHARLES DUNCAN, only child of C. C. Shepherd, M.B., at the General Hospital, Barbadoes, W.I., on July 19, aged 10 months.

SPENCER, WILLIAM EDWARD, eldest son of W. H. Spencer, M.D., at 5, Lansdown-place, Clifton, on August 12, aged 21.

VACANCIES.

BIRMINGHAM FRIENDLY SOCIETIES' MEDICAL INSTITUTION. — Medical Officer. (For particulars see Advertisement.)

BRIGHTON AND HOVE DISPENSARY.—Resident House-Surgeon. (For particulars see Advertisement.)

CHILDREN'S HOSPITAL, BIRMINGHAM.—Assistant Resident Medical Officer. Candidates must be duly registered. Applications, with testimonials and certificate of registration, to be sent to the Secretary, Children's Hospital, Steelhouse-lane, Birmingham, not later than August 31.

NORTHAMPTON GENERAL INFIRMARY.—House-Surgeon. (For particulars see Advertisement.)

SWANSEA HOSPITAL.—Resident Medical Officer. Candidates must be registered both in medicine and surgery. Applications, with testimonials, to be sent to the Secretary, not later than August 23.

WORCESTER GENERAL INFIRMARY.—House-Surgeon. (For particulars see Advertisement.)

UNION AND PAROCHIAL MEDICAL SERVICE.

, The area of each district is stated in acres. The population is computed according to the census of 1871.

RESIGNATIONS.

Nantwich Union.—The Tarporley District is vacant by the death of Dr. Beller: area, 14,987; population 4807; salary £44 per annum.

Poplar and Stepney Sick Asylum.—Mr. Denis Walshe has resigned the office of Assistant Medical Officer.

Thame Union.—Mr. A. Newington has resigned the Waterperry District: area 2557; population 302; salary £15 per annum.

Wantage Union.—Mr. R. G. M. Colman has resigned the Ilsley District: area 19,047; population 3584; salary £75 per annum.

Westhampnett Union.—Dr. N. E. Cresswell has resigned the Manhood District: area, 17,455; population 3507; salary £190 per annum.

APPOINTMENTS.

Crediton Union.—William J. C. Nourse, L.R.C.P. Edin., L.R.C.S. Edin., L.S.A., to the Morchard Bishop District.

Faringdon Union.—George F. P. Nixon, L.R.C.S. Ire., L.A.H. Dub., to the Shrivenham District.

Hatfield Union.—Thomas W. Thomson, M.R.C.S. Eng., L.R.C.P. Edin., L.S.A., to the First District.

Melton Mowbray Union.—Richard Johnston, F.R.C.S.I., L.R.C.P., to the Wymondham District.

Newton Abbot Union.—George F. Symons, M.R.C.S. Eng., L.S.A., to the Kingskerswell District.

Penistone Union.—Charles Bewley, M.R.C.S. Eng., to the Silkstone District.

Strand Union.—William Jones, L.R.C.P. Edin., L.R.C.S. Edin., L.S.A. Lond., to the Workhouse.

West Derby Union.—Henry Wilson, M.R.C.S. Eng., L.S.A., to the Wavertree District.

York Union.—William Preston, B.M. and M.C. Edin., to the Fifth District.

NOTES, QUERIES, AND REPLIES.

Be that questioneth much shall learn much.—*Bacon.*

A Juryman on Infanticide.—The remark of the foreman of a jury on two inquests recently held by Mr. Langham, touching the death of children found dead, is not unworthy of attention. He said, "That in some of these cases there seemed to be a little amount of laxity in continuing the investigations to find the culpable parties. The same stereotyped evidence was given in nearly every case, and child-murder was committed with impunity."

O. E. F.—Up to the end of last year nearly a thousand members of the Metropolitan Police Force had availed themselves of the instruction given at the Ambulance classes held under the auspices of the Order of St. John of Jerusalem, and nearly seven hundred had obtained certificates of proficiency.

Gascoigne, O.A.—The Hospital Saturday collection at Oldham this year realised £989 19s. 9d. for the benefit of the Infirmary, against £869 10s. 6d. last year.

A Practical Suggestion.—Referring to the recent railway accident at Blackburn, a correspondent suggests that, in addition to the course of instruction afforded by the Order of St. John of Jerusalem Society, a proportion of ambulance litters and material should be always available for use in case of emergency at all our large railway-stations. That these appliances and material should be inspected periodically, and the railway officials and servants, or a proportion of them, practised in the use of them.

Retributive Justice.—A cloth manufacturer, of Batley, has been sentenced at the Leeds Assizes to a year's imprisonment on a charge of manslaughter of four of his workmen who had died from the effects of injuries received by a boiler explosion on his premises in January last. It appears the defendant had frequently been warned as to the dangerous condition of the boiler. The relatives of one of the deceased have also brought an action against him for damages.

Doctors at Hong-kong.—According to the Governor of the colony, the Chinese are gradually elbowing the Europeans out of Hong-kong. In reference to the doctors, he states that in 1876 there were 198 Chinese doctors, but now (January, 1880) there are 383. The Chinese medical men appear to have a firm belief in the benefit of vaccination, for the Governor observes that they have taken the matter out of the hands of the hospital doctors, and vaccinated the people by thousands.

Jerry-Building : Threatening a Surveyor.—A builder of Willesden has been charged at the Edgware Petty Sessions by the Willesden Local Board with contravening their by-laws by neglecting to put in concrete foundations, using macadam slop in lieu of mortar, and rotten bricks, in the construction of certain houses being erected in the Melville-road, Harlesden. The evidence was to the effect that the notice of the Local Board had been totally disregarded, and the buildings were disgraceful, and would be unfit for habitation. The mortar in the walls smelt offensively, and contained 9½ per cent. of organic matter, animal and vegetable. The defendant was fined £10. The defendant was then charged with using threatening language towards the Surveyor to the Willesden Local Board, who had given evidence in the previous case, which Dr. Danford Thomas, the Medical Officer, corroborated. The defendant was also fined 20s., and ordered to find two sureties of £25 each to keep the peace.

COMMUNICATIONS have been received from—

Dr. ANDERSON, London; THE REGISTRAR OF APOTHECARIES' HALL, London; Messrs. A. AND M. ZIMMERMANN, London; Messrs. DOMEIER AND Co., London; Dr. R. G. DAUNT, London; Mr. MARK H. JUDGE, London; THE LOCAL GOVERNMENT BOARD, London; Mr. E. J. GODLEE, London; Dr. HIRSLIN, London; Dr. W. ALEXANDER, London; Mr. J. CHATTO, London; Dr. J. MITCHELL BRUCE, London; THE SECRETARY OF THE BREAD REFORM LEAGUE, London; Mr. W. WATSON CHEYNE, London; Dr. ANDREW DUNCAN, Bengal Medical Service; Mr. BECHER, London; THE SECRETARY OF THE LONDON HOSPITAL, London; Mr. F. STEVENS, London; THE SECRETARY OF THE ROYAL POLYTECHNIC INSTITUTION, London.

BOOKS, ETC., RECEIVED:—

Health Preservation, by Richard Herring—Small-pox and Vaccination in London, by Charles T. Pearce—Report of the Borough of Newcastle-upon-Tyne for 1880—Hastings and St. Leonards-on-Sea—On the Physiological and Therapeutic Properties of Mineral Waters, by Paul Kilian, M.D.—Report on the Health of the Metropolitan Police Force during the Year 1880—Beiträge zur klinischen und operativen Glaucombehandlung, von Dr. Med. Albert Mooren—Report on the Health of the Borough of Birmingham for the Quarter ending July 2, 1881—Report on the Sanitary Condition of the Parish of St. Mary, Islington, during the Year 1880—British Botany, by Charles Cardale Babington, M.A., etc.—Parasitic Diseases of the Skin, by James Startin —Indigestion and Biliousness, by J. Milner Fothergill, M.D.—Surgery for Dental Students, by Arthur S. Underwood, M.R.C.S., L.D.S.E.— The Sanitary and Constructive Supervision of Dwellings, by Lewis Angell, M.Inst.C.E.—Annual Report of the Convalescent Home of the Victoria Hospital for Children, Churchfields, Margate—Bread Reform League : Advantages of Wheat and Whole-meal Breads—Annual Report of the Victoria Hospital for Children, Queen's-road, Chelsea—Sixtieth Report of the *Dreadnought* Seamen's Hospital, Greenwich—What to do in Cases of Poisoning, by William Murrell, M.D., M.R.C.P.—Annual Report for the Gloucestershire Combined Sanitary District for the Year 1880—The Floating Matter of the Air, by John Tyndall, F.R.S.—Annals of Chemical Medicine, vol. ii., by J. L. W. Thudichum, M.D.—Dental Surgery and Pathology, by A. Coleman, L.R.C.P.—The Sanitary Chronicles of the Parish of St. Marylebone during June, 1881—La Contrattilità dei Capillari in Relazione ai Due Gas dello Scambio Materiale.

PERIODICALS AND NEWSPAPERS RECEIVED:—

Lancet—British Medical Journal—Medical Press and Circular—Berliner Klinische Wochenschrift—Centralblatt für Chirurgie—Gazette des Hopitaux—Gazette Médicale—Le Progrès Médical—Bulletin de l'Académie de Médecine—Pharmaceutical Journal—Wiener Medizinische Wochenschrift—Centralblatt für die Medizinischen Wissenschaften—Revue Médicale—Gazette Hebdomadaire—National Board of Health Bulletin, Washington—Nature—Deutsche Medicinal-Zeitung—Oil and Drug News—Louisville Medical News—Boston Journal of Chemistry—L'Imparziale Médicale—Utica Morning Herald—Vaccination Inquirer —Revista de Medicina—Dublin Journal of Medical Science—New York Medical Journal, etc.—Philadelphia Medical Times—El Observador Medico—Revue de Chirurgie—Archives of Medicine—Maryland Medical Journal—Journal of the British Dental Association—Students' Journal and Hospital Gazette—Canadian Journal of Medical Science—Charity Record.

THE FORTY-NINTH ANNUAL MEETING

OF THE

BRITISH MEDICAL ASSOCIATION.

HELD AT RYDE, AUGUST 8, 9, 10, AND 11.

ADDRESS IN SURGERY.

By JONATHAN HUTCHINSON, F.R.C.S.,

Professor of Surgery and Pathology, Royal College of Surgeons;
Senior Surgeon to the London Hospital and Hospital for Skin Diseases;
Consulting Surgeon, Royal London Ophthalmic Hospital.

MR. PRESIDENT AND GENTLEMEN,—As we are most of us fresh from a long week's carnival of medical science, I feel sure that you will not desire that I should on the present occasion address you on any subject directly connected with surgical practice. The very successful and industrious Congress which concluded yesterday has had its numberless section meetings, in which most of us have taken some part; and, if I do not misinterpret the general feeling, it is a longing for a little rest as regards the matters in the discussion of which we have so recently and so fully engaged. I purpose, therefore, to employ the hour which you have done me the honour to entrust to me, in bringing under your consideration certain general topics having reference to surgical ethics, surgical education, and, lastly, the best means of advancing the clinical knowledge of disease.

Five-and-twenty years ago, the surgeons of the metropolis were alarmed—I might almost say scandalised—by a proposal to open a hospital for the treatment of stone and diseases of the bladder. A memorial was got up, and signed first by the ever-respected name of Brodie, and then by almost the whole of those then connected with the general hospitals. This memorial severely condemned the multiplication of special institutions, and with particular vigour denounced the one in contemplation. Amongst the names at its foot, mine may be found. I am not ashamed of having signed it then, but I unhesitatingly say that I would sign no such memorial now. Nor can I believe that many of those who then did so would now differ from my present conclusions. Not that the facts then stated have been materially changed, but others have been added. Year by year we have seen more clearly that, in large communities, special hospitals will develope, and that it is beyond the power of the profession to prevent them. But we have seen more than this: we have seen that they are clearly a gain to the public; not an unmixed gain—for what gain is unmixed?—but still a gain. Even at the time when the memorial to which I have referred was written, it was a matter of necessity to admit that diseases of the eye constituted an exception, and some thought that orthopædic institutions should also be permitted. Since then, I suppose that those for diseases of women, for diseases of children, and perhaps for diseases of the skin, have justified themselves.

The final triumph of ovariotomy did not result from any new discovery. There had been many pioneers. The instruments and the modes of practice which had been devised by others were those which were still employed; but these, in the hands of able surgeons, who gave their whole time and energy to this one subject, and who had, above all, the power of excluding from their special institutions those sources of evil from which a general hospital can never be wholly free—attained for this operation its present proud position. Let us note carefully the two elements of success. It may be that Listerian or some equivalent precautions may in the future make the wards of a general hospital as safe a place in which to open the peritoneal cavity as is a private home or a special hospital; but, even if this be done, they can never supply the familiarity with detail which comes only from constant practice. We must never forget that our profession exists, not for the benefit of ourselves, still less of any special class amongst us, but for our patients; and that its institutions must be so managed, or so modified,

that they shall best serve their permanent interests. Nor can I think that there is any real difficulty in making the two coincide. Let the profession set its face, not against specialisms as a whole, but rather against those institutions which are conducted in a narrow spirit. Let it insist upon open elections of officers, free admission of students and practitioners; above all, let it encourage the formation of special departments in our general hospitals, since it is clearly here that they can best be made useful in the education of the student.

These general principles of conduct being granted, I would not oppose the beginning of any speciality, however detailed. Already the comprehensive department of eye-diseases is submitting to some process of natural subdivision, and it will not be long before we shall have in our large cities those who devote themselves chiefly to operations on the eye, those who attend specially to its diseases properly so-called, and those who rectify its congenital or acquired defects by means of optical aids. It by no means follows that because a man is a good operator for cataract, he will be equally familiar with the details of astigmatism. It is impossible to question the fact that the great discoveries in ophthalmology have been made by specialists, and sometimes by those who had devoted their attention chiefly to special branches of that department. Let it be understood that I am not arguing in favour of the promotion of subdivisions of surgical labour, but rather to the effect that, when they come naturally, we should not oppose them. Let us have charity for the various motives by which different men are urged to different courses; let us hold high our standard, inscribed "for the good of all," and allow to natural energy a full and free development. Let us not waste our time in opposing, but seek rather to employ and use.

I rank amongst the gains from the detailed cultivation of special branches of medical pursuit, that it has a definite tendency to destroy specialisms as such, and add their conquered territory to the general possessions. Whilst it does this to a large extent, it also at the same time creates new departments before unthought of, into which science pushes its way, and gives its help towards the mitigation of man's many disabilities of man.

Witness what has been done in ophthalmology; how discoveries one after the other have been made, which have been at once added to the knowledge of the general physician. Note how the ophthalmoscope has taken its place with the stethoscope as an indispensable aid to the physician in the diagnosis of disease. The knowledge of diseases of the eye has indeed rapidly attained in the profession at large, and not alone amongst specialists, a very high degree of perfection. I do not hesitate to assert that there are few departments of practice so well and widely appreciated, and few which more definitely attract the attention of students. Nor do the gains to the public from this increase of general knowledge represent the whole gain; for the study of eye-disease must be claimed as especially useful as a training in the art of precise observation. No student masters it who does not become in so doing much better fitted for other fields of clinical research. This study is indeed, in relation to other branches of surgery, almost what mathematics is in general education. We have but to reflect on such facts as these, and next try to recall what the ignorance of eye-disease was less than a century ago, and what the position held by the oculist and the spectacle-vendor, and we shall be able to estimate a part of the debt which we owe to specialists.

There was a time when diseases of the skin were regarded by the higher class of surgeons with feelings almost allied to contempt. They were repulsive alike in the portrait, and in the person of the patient. They required no operations; and a knowledge of the use of arsenic, and of the constituents of a few ointments and lotions, was held to be all that was needed for their treatment. Then followed a period during the early cultivation of the speciality, when to outsiders it seemed as if it offered only an arena for endless wrangles as to schemes of classification, and for ingenuity in the devising of new names, and affixing to them a countless variety of unclassical adjectives. I am not quite sure that this era has even yet wholly passed away. It may be that there yet lingers a feeling of prejudice to this speciality amongst some who should know better. With the majority, however, and especially amongst our rising pathologists, a wholly different conviction is rapidly superseding such feelings. We are learning to care little about names, and to seek knowledge as to the nature of things; and those who do this in earnest rapidly find out that, of all the departments of pathological and clinical research, there is none which offers such rich and varied attractions as does dermatology. The simple facts that a morbid process in the integument is, from its beginning to its ending, exposed to view, that the aid of the lens may be brought to bear upon it while yet *in situ*, and that the histologist is in very many instances not obliged to wait the death of his patient before he is allowed to gratify his thirst for knowledge of ultimate details, largely justify my assertion. But it is not upon them solely that I rely, when I assert that diseases of the skin ought to be regarded as fundamental in professional education. Many illustrations which they afford, of the changes in vascular supply and its results; of the influence of the several parts of the nervous system in the production of disease; of the laws of inheritance; of the numberless varieties in the inflammatory process in connexion with diathesis, idiosyncrasy, and special forms of poisoning; are far beyond those afforded by any other department—varied and instructive. Above all, we find in dermatology the most remarkable and conclusive proofs of the direct connexion between morbid causes and their effects. I cannot doubt that, possessing these advantages, skin-diseases must in the future be accepted as not only of the utmost interest for themselves, but as invaluable to the physician and pathologist in the elucidation of the phenomena of diseased action, as met with in regions and organs less open to inspection. I by no means claim for this insight into the educational value of a knowledge of skin-diseases that it is wholly of modern growth. It was recognised long ago by the Paris physicians; and the work done by Anthony Todd Thompson, by Jenner, Gull, and above all by Addison, attest to its partial recognition amongst ourselves. But its growth is only recent, and never had dermatology such an army of workers who are not specialists as it at present claims amongst the younger physicians and surgeons, not only in London, but in all parts of the world. In their hands, it is certain before long to assume that foremost place which I claim for it as its natural position.

Let us remember, respecting a large majority of the maladies which it has been the fashion, in some sort, to stigmatise as "skin-diseases," that nothing is more certain than that they belong mainly to other departments of pathology. Herpes is a neuritis which simply chances to display some of its symptoms on the skin. Morphœa is an affection of the vaso-motor nerve, leading to changes in bones, muscles, and joints, as well as to those which, from occurring externally, first attracted attention, and still almost monopolise it. In the study of ringworm, we may engage, if we will, in the most interesting investigations as to the laws of life in minute vegetable organisms. Leprosy offers us a dietetic problem of at least equal interest with those which concern gout and rickets. In psoriasis and its allies, we study a heritable peculiarity of health or of skin which shows its effects through a whole life, and is influenced for better or worse in ways that are curiously instructive. Who can doubt the power of drugs who has seen arsenic cause herpes or cure pemphigus? The polymorphism of syphilis is a fact to claim the permanent wonder of all who are well instructed in pathological speculation.

We listened, with delight, last week, to the eloquent words in which, in his opening address, Sir James Paget enforced the duty of charity amongst ourselves. It is in this spirit, I think, that we should meet the various questions which open out in connexion with the medical education of women; and that, also, as to consultation with those who, whilst educated amongst us, have openly professed their adoption of peculiar doctrines. I fear that I am here venturing upon ice that is very thin indeed; and I must proceed either with great boldness or extreme caution. I shall prefer the latter. Let me say, then, that the profession of medicine always has offered, probably always will offer, peculiar attractions to those who, with weak principles, and still weaker consciences, desire to make profit by trading on the credulity of their patients. The thing is so exceedingly easy to do. Our real knowledge of disease in many of its departments is very vague, and our knowledge of therapeutics still less certain. There is room on all sides for differences of opinion, scope for the introduction of new theories and the

employment of high-sounding epithets. The fatal facilities thus afforded to the charlatan have naturally made the well-principled professors of physic very vigilant in guarding our ranks against the introduction of quackery. We wish to be honest, and we wish to associate with none but those who are so. There lived, now more than a century ago, a talented and learned enthusiast, who thought—sincerely, I have little doubt—that he saw his way to an immense reform in the use of drugs. That reform was needed, we all admit. He noticed a few common facts, such as the marvellous subdivision of which odorous substances are susceptible; the change of effect, or even reversal, which accrues from change in the dose of a drug; and that, respecting some few medicines, it was true that they seemed to produce in large doses just what they tended to repress in small ones. I am not here to apologise for Hahnemann. His facts were few, his reasoning illogical, his ignorance of the natural progress of disease, and its tendencies to spontaneous recovery, such as would be utterly disgraceful in the present day. Whatever foundation we may grant for his theories, he certainly pushed them to the wildest lengths. His self-confidence, had it been properly balanced, might have become almost sublime.

If, however, we may find theme for marvel in the presumptuous self-sufficiency of this would-be reformer, I do not think that we need seek far for the explanation of the success of his teaching. It inculcated faith in drugs, but it changed their form, and gave us cleanly globules and tasteless fluids for the bolus, pill, and potion then in vogue. It supplied a theory of cure, as well as its means; and to the intelligent, but, at the same time, not specially trained, its theory sounded at least as good as those of orthodox physic. The love of novelty conspired with a cheerful faith in the possibility of progress, and with delight in escape from the disagreeableness of the old methods, to draw converts to the new creed. Those converts were not the ignorant, nor were they the poor. No wonder that some from our own ranks should have thought they saw their interest in adopting the new method, and equally little that most of those who observed their conduct held the motives of the man who put "homœopath" on his door to below and self-seeking. In nineteen cases out of twenty, probably, the verdict was right; but when the flat went forth that a homœopath must be either a fool or a knave, I doubt whether the modesty of nature was not somewhat overstepped. There are fools and fools; and we are guilty alike of unkindness and unfairness if we widen that disrespectful epithet overmuch and apply it too freely. There is such a combination of weak power for the estimation of facts, with enthusiastic optimism as regards possible progress, which, whilst it in no degree establishes a claim to wisdom, yet scarcely brings its possessor into the category of fools. Amongst the laity, of those who became homœopaths, most were of this character, and some, probably, of those who seceded from our own ranks.

I fear that it may be thought that I am travelling very far from the proper subject of an address on surgery. I also much fear that I may be misunderstood. What, it will be asked, has homœopathy to do with surgery? and why introduce the question of consultations with homœopaths by such a lengthy prelude? Now, it is precisely because homœopathy has nothing to do with surgery that it becomes of interest to us to settle the question in dispute. The circumstances of Lord Beaconsfield's illness are fresh in the memory of us all. We did honour to Sir William Jenner for his stern and manly refusal to have anything to do with what he thought quackery. We sympathised with Dr. Quain in his perception that the occasion had arrived for the sacrifice of sentiment and the performance of a disagreeable duty. But what particularly struck me in the transaction, and what constitutes my chief reason for mentioning it now, was the reason alleged by Sir William Jenner why he could not meet Dr. Kidd. It was not that he felt compelled on principle to decline all intercourse with the heterodox, but that the patient could not possibly be a gainer by a conference between those who held such different opinions respecting the principles of therapeutics. It is clear that, had it been the aid of a surgeon that was needed, no such reason would have been valid. Homœopaths have not as yet succeeded in developing any new system of surgery. The knife and the catheter are the same to them that they are to us, and are used on the same indications. I never myself wittingly consulted with a homœopath; but I believe that I have, without knowing it at the time, several times met them, and I never yet encountered the slightest difference of opinion. The surgeon, then, cannot possibly feel that he is in any way serving the interest of his patient when he refuses to meet his weak-minded doctor. On the contrary, it may easily be the fact that he knows that it would be the greatest possible kindness if he would go without an hour's delay. To "Boycott" a quack on principle is one thing; to attend to the interests of the quack's patient may be another. Hence the duties of surgeons in this matter, and especially of those engaged in consultation practice, have always been very difficult. The obvious incongruity which exists in the case of a physician is not present to the surgeon; his temptations are both more frequent and stronger, and his sources of inward strength are also fewer. He refuses neither for his own good, nor the patient's good, but in obedience to professional rule. With a few exceptions, this rule has been, I believe, honourably upheld by the consulting surgeons of England. There have, however, been some exceptions, and there have been difficulties and annoyances without number. We cannot possibly, in our profession, have one rule for the peer and another for the tradesman. I avow my deliberate conviction that Dr. Quain, and those whose counsel he sought, interpreted the obligations of our profession correctly. We enjoy a law-established monopoly in the art of healing, and we must be very careful how we stint or refuse our services when they are demanded. If, in consultation, it be found that the opinion of the consultant is not that of the consulter, and if the latter be not willing to waive his own, then the proper course of conduct is clear. But such inability to act in concert should not be assumed on light grounds surely, or hearsay evidence. Unless the previous knowledge be very special, it should be established at the bedside in each individual case. I am speaking of formal consultations only, not of social intercourse. We know well how to accord and refuse professional honour. If a man be guilty of non-professional conduct, we can blackball him at a society, and avoid his company in social life. We enter upon a course of conduct which needs a wholly different justification if we refuse to meet and confer with him when the life of a third person is concerned. Here I confess that it seems to me that the claims of the public should stand first, and that if a man's name is on the "Medical Register" we ought to meet him, so long as the consultations result in that which we deem most for the patient's advantage. Whenever they do not, our duty is clear, and we should readily know how to perform it. Many advantages would, I think, result, if we were to leave with the licensing bodies the responsibility of decision as to who are to be admitted to the privileges of formal consultation, and who excluded. To do so would save at once much loss of time and of temper, and avoid frequently recurring complexities. It would encourage honesty and openness of conduct, and remove temptation to the secret perpetration of that which is known to be against the professional rule. But, above all, I would urge that it seems to be almost a matter of justice to the third party, our patients, who have surely a right to assume that, when a duly qualified man is employed, they can obtain, in consultation with him, if wished, the aid of any other who possesses the same diploma. That we run the risk of fostering homœopathy by according to its disciples the courtesy of professional consultation, I do not for a moment believe. It has hitherto been fostered by opposition. Let us have more confidence in the vital energy of truth, and let us venture to let the wheat and the tares grow together till the harvest. We believe that its principal theory is absurd, and much of its practice ridiculous; but, at the same time, we are prepared to admit that gleams of a fruitful suggestion may be occasionally discerned in its discussions, and we can surely afford to leave it as a whole to itself, and let it develope to its natural end.(a)

I will pass to a less distasteful topic, and proceed to make some suggestions as to the possible improvement in our

methods of clinical teaching. It must be noted, in the first place, as a great defect in our English system that it makes no provision for retaining the services of good clinical teachers. It trains them, and then casts them adrift. The early period at which our surgeons and physicians retire from hospital work is a matter of amazement to our foreign confrères, and few can doubt that the evil is on the increase. Either by the bribery of private practice or the gentle compulsion of a retirement rule, we induce our best teachers to desist from work in public just at the time when their services are of most value to the student. The names of Paget, Jenner, Erichsen, Gull, and Bowman will occur to us all in illustration of what I assert. Not only do our customs make the early retirement of successful men a matter of necessity, but they often cramp their usefulness to the student during the latter part of the period of their tenure of office, and also hinder their services to science in other directions. Success in our profession means absorption of the whole time and whole mental energy in attention to private practice. No individual surgeon can help himself; he is in the meshes of the social net, and escape is hopeless. It is a change of custom which must effect the reform, and surely such a change is urgently required. It might come, I think, very suitably in some such form as this. Let there be constituted a rank of pure consultants, whose fees shall be so modified as to enable them to make the same incomes that they now do, with a third of the personal labour. Let election to such grade be by their respective colleges. Let us no longer leave the time and the energies of our foremost minds at the mercy of any wealthy man who, however trivial may be his ailment, determines to have "the best advice," just as he would seek the most expensive jeweller or buy the most costly wine. They are surely too valuable for that. By the plan which I suggest, leisure would be left to them for study and for teaching, and they would be retained in their proper sphere of public work. Such consultants, having voluntarily restricted their spheres of observation of disease in private, would find it necessary, in order alike to sustain reputation and keep abreast with progress, to retain their public appointments, and to continue to teach. The gain would be a great one to medical education, and also, I think, to the public interest. The evil to which I refer is an increasing one, and it exists to a far greater extent in London than in any other capital.

A large part of the education of students may very suitably be done by young professors. Age adds but little to the ability to deal well with the facts of anatomy and physiology, and it may even detract from it. When, however, we come to the knowledge of disease at the bedside, and the correct estimation of its various symptoms, then experience must tell. Without it there can never be that trust on the part of the student or that free power of illustration, from facts which have been personally observed on the part of the teacher, which are essential to success.

Yet it is precisely this clinical teaching which is of most importance to the student, and in which, if I mistake not, our modern system is most at disadvantage. Apprenticeships have been abandoned, and few that remember their inconveniences can wish to revert to them. Yet they had their uses, and those not trivial ones. They unquestionably often secured to the student a clinical and practical training which is now but too often missed. Permit me to make for your consideration a suggestion of a plan by which possibly most of their advantages might be retained, and others which they did not always possess secured. Let us endeavour to widen the basis of medical teaching, and to enlist, as responsible partakers in this all-important work, a large section of the profession. This might be done if our examining boards were to recognise as private teachers all fellows of their respective colleges, all possessors of diplomas of the higher class, all medical officers of hospitals and dispensaries, indeed, all who could bring proof of the possession of special opportunities or qualifications for clinical teaching. Let it be required of every student that he should bring, in addition to those now required, certificates from two, three, or more of these registered teachers that he had been—in a real and bonâ fide manner, under their personal supervision—instructed in practical matters, and that he was in their opinion qualified for a diploma. Make such certificates necessary, but let them not modify in the least the curriculum of the school or the test-examination. To prevent these certificates from being signed in a perfunctory manner, let it be the rule to inform those who

(a) These paragraphs concerning consultation with homœopaths did not form part of the address, as given at Ryde. They had been written out for delivery, but, on the evening before, I learnt that the same subject had been far more ably dealt with by Dr. Bristowe in his Address on Medicine. The explanation of our having selected the same subject is easily given. Dr. Bristowe dealt with the whole subject, whilst I have spoken only as to the inexpediency of continuing to refuse formal consultations. I have reinstated these paragraphs, in consequence of a general request that they should appear when the address was printed.

signed them of the results obtained by their *protégés*, and if in the course of a five years' period the proportion of rejections should be more than an average, let the name of the teacher concerned be for the next five years removed from the list of those privileged to sign. This plan would, I think, work well in many ways. It would add to the value of the higher diplomas, and increase the number of those who seek them. It would encourage in those registered as private teachers the endeavour to keep well instructed in the knowledge of the day; whilst its advantages to the student —by bringing him into closer personal contact with those interested in his success—are obvious.

How various are the qualifications which are to be desired in the medical practitioner! He should be a gentleman of good manners and address; skilled alike in the principles of biology and in the knowledge of character; able to visualise at short notice the details of human anatomy; and he should carry in his memory, ready for prompt use, the best recipes for a thousand varying forms of ill-health. If we measure his responsibilities by the possibilities of his usefulness and the risks of his failure, they are very great indeed. It may be true that the greater part of his duties are routine and easy of performance, but he may, at a moment's notice, be called upon to deal with the unusual and difficult. Regarded from this point of view, the amount of knowledge required of him is enormous—greater, probably, than that necessary in any other avocation. It is, further, steadily on the increase; every fresh discovery brings with it something fresh for the general surgeon to master and retain in memory. Hence many of the increasing difficulties in surgical education; hence unquestionably the increasing ratio of plucks to passes at our examining boards. It is not that examiners are more strict, students less able, or teachers less zealous; but simply that the thing to be taught has grown in bulk, and become year by year more and more difficult of attainment within the allotted period. There is nothing whatever to discourage us in the fact; much, indeed, to tend in the opposite direction. But we must boldly meet the changed and everchanging circumstances. An extension of the period of study, a well-considered limitation of its subjects, and, lastly, a careful development of its methods, are the three measures which severally suggest themselves. The last is, of course, approved by all, and is too obviously desirable to need comment; but concerning each of the others there is room for much debate. As to the extension of the compulsory period of study, such proposals may, I think, be dismissed with the remark that the practice of liberal rejection of candidates imperfectly qualified really amounts to the same thing, and attains its end with more justice to the diligent and able. In the future, it may perhaps come to be considered a great credit to pass the first time, and no disgrace to be referred. Careful men, appreciating the necessities of the case, will probably voluntarily lengthen their period of study. Were the period compulsorily fixed at five or six years instead of four, the careless would still, as now, idle till near the end of it. I cannot but think, therefore, that the practice of early examination, with its necessary result of many rejections, works, on the whole, better than would any which should make an undiscriminating demand for longer time.

It is impossible not to regard without the utmost jealousy any proposal that the subjects of professional study should be reduced. So far from its being desirable to strike out botany and comparative anatomy, we might prefer to see added, if possible, a good knowledge, not only of the anatomy and functions, but also of the diseases of both plants and animals. It is from a broad education in these directions that we may hope for future advance. Having said this, however, we must hasten to admit that a large majority of the profession are to be trained, not so much as biologists, nor even as pathologists, but as practitioners. In our surgical education there is much that is valuable, very much indeed that is of the greatest possible interest, concerning which it still cannot be said that it is essential. It is certainly the duty of both teacher and examiner to draw a strong and clear distinction between essential and non-essential acquirements. Howsoever the latter may fare, the public has a right to demand at our hands that the former shall be in as complete possession as possible. It is no comfort to the glaucoma patient, who has been treated by lotions and leeches until he is blind, to know that his surgeon is a good anatomist; nor will the most excellent knowledge of histology avail to save a practitioner from something

in its nature not unlike manslaughter, who believes that he ought to wait for tympanites and stercoraceous vomiting as the chief symptoms of strangulated hernia. It is common sense and practical knowledge of common things that we mainly want. I well recollect an anecdote, which was told to me when a boy, respecting a smart young farm-labourer in my father's employ. This young fellow had incurred the wrath of a half-witted young woman in the village, who, in revenge, said of him: "He can whistle fairly, and he can sing pretty well, but he can't plough straight." This homethrust so rankled in his breast that his accomplishments became annoyances to him, and he finally left the neighbourhood, unable to bear up under the frequent reminders as to what "daft Meg" had said. The distinction between the essential and the ornamental was here so strongly emphasised that, although the latter was not in the least depreciated, it stood as less than nothing in comparison with the former. So surely it ought to be with us. Respecting the essential, examiners might perhaps do well to leave nothing to chance, but, regardless of time to make sure, so far as is possible, that the candidate possesses a really sound knowledge of them. It by no means follows that a candidate who knows what to do in traumatic gangrene is equally up to the mark in reference to purulent ophthalmia; nor does a good knowledge of the latter imply ability to treat prostatic retention with success. Yet these are all equally essential, and they stand pretty much in the same relation to the duties of a surgeon as does straight ploughing to a farm-labourer.

We may reasonably hope that improved methods of instruction, and the application of common sense to our plans of teaching, will do away with the need for any material curtailment of the scope of study. The means provided for the education of students may be classed under three heads. —teachers, books, and museums. Of the two former I do not propose to say much, but the last is an attractive topic which I cannot pass. The change which followed on the introduction of printing, in reference to the value of oral instruction, has often been the subject of comment. At the present time this change is complete, and no discoverer or propounder of new doctrines would ever think of bringing his observations before the public in any other way than by the aid of the printing-press. He does not expect his hearers to come and listen to his professor's lecture, but he embodies his opinions in a book, and thus sends them broadcast over the world. If, in the first instance, he read a paper or give a lecture, it is that it may be printed afterwards. The professor of the present day is, for the most part, an exalted development of the tutor, and his duties are almost as much to ascertain that his pupils do really learn from books as to teach them from his chair. Few, indeed, are there who can attract hearers from outside their allotted classes. Nearly all have themselves published books, and their success, in nine cases out of ten, depends far more on their willingness to adapt themselves to the existing state of things as regards the students' requirements—to advise, supervise, and question—than upon their abilities in the lines of original research. For the latter, the vocation is elsewhere. I am speaking, of course, of the professors and teachers in our colleges and schools of medicine. They have become the expositors of books, not of their own original and unwritten opinions. It is, I think, not improbable that another development is at hand, which will yet further diminish the importance of our chairs, and of oral instruction in general. I allude to the creation of students' museums. The museum, hitherto, has existed chiefly as an appendage to the chair. Our examining boards have required that teachers of anatomy, physiology, and pathology should possess or create a museum of specimens from which to select illustrations for lectures. In many instances, these collections have not even been made accessible to students; and in none, until quite recently, has encouragement been given to the student to regard the museum as a place in which he ought to work. In one of our largest European capitals, possessing a flourishing medical school, there was, I believe, until very recently— and I am not sure that things are materially changed now —no museum which a student could enter without the most troublesome formalities. In several other continental cities possessing medical schools, the creation of a pathological collection, worthy the name of museum, is a matter of exceedingly recent date. I claim it as a distinguishing feature of our own country—one, however, which I willingly share with our Scandinavian relations,—that our museums have for long been numerous and good; and I further assert that it is amongst the most valuable proofs of life in the scientific spirit which we can show, that they are constantly growing and improving. In no country, however, have we as yet seen the full development of museums as means of medical education; and, if I am not much mistaken, these institutions are destined in the future to assume an importance of which we have as yet scarcely dreamed. Well managed, it will be found that the museum may be made to combine the advantages of dissecting-room, ward, lecture-theatre, and book in one, and that it can supply permanently, at all times and to all comers, opportunities which are for the most part accessible elsewhere only at special times and to a privileged few. I do not mean that dissected preparations or models can ever supersede or rival work done *proprid manu* with forceps and scalpel, but they may be made to assist it, to prepare for it, and to supplement it with most excellent results. Hitherto our museums, whether medical or in connexion with general knowledge, have been far too miscellaneous. Huge crowded collections of material, some of it of the greatest value, and some of it very little, have jostled together in a more or less orderly kind of confusion, through which only the well-instructed can find their way. They have been by the majority visited rather as places of wonderment, or perhaps of bewilderment, than for systematic instruction. Now, museums ought to be as legible as books; and, when they are made so, they will be eagerly read. The very most that can be said of our very best, as yet, is that they have approached somewhat to the character of cyclopædias, from which fragmentary information upon all sorts of subjects may be obtained by those who know how to search for it. For students' purposes, something of a different kind is required—something much less voluminous, at once more concise and more consecutive: in fact, to pursue the comparison, more of the nature of a *handbook*. A students' museum should contain those things which a student wants, and those only. They should be well arranged, with plenty of space; and well labelled, not merely with a name, but a description. There should be nothing to distract attention, and everything to favour study. Anatomy should be illustrated by dissected preparations, casts, drawings, and diagrams; and these should be kept in juxtaposition; and from anatomy to pathological change the steps should be direct and clear. Side by side with the normal joint should be the diseased joint; with the specimens illustrating the precise position of the epiphyses, those showing their detachment by violence. No knowledge should be taken for granted in the learner, and as far as possible everything should be demonstrated. I must not go further into detail. Let me conclude what I have to say on this topic by the remark that we ought to have museums for educational purposes, distinct and wholly separate from those which are designed as magazines of facts deposited for the use of original investigators. The two objects are different; and not unfrequently that which is essential to the completeness of the one is useless and cumbersome to the other. In speaking of students, hitherto, I have been thinking of those who have not passed their examinations: but it is the boast of our profession that it possesses countless students of another grade, who have no longer the fear of the examiner before them, but who recognise the fact that even a lifetime is too short to acquire a fair familiarity with the facts of pathology, and who, however long their lives may be, will remain in the position of pupils. For these also—for these, perhaps, especially—museums ought to be provided; and here, again, I make bold to assert that nothing in the least adequate to the wants of the case has as yet been attempted. Our grandsons, if not our sons, will smile at the *dilettante* manner in which we have been content to hunt for the truth in matters of clinical research. We so often treat disease—at any rate, in its less common forms—as if it were sent merely that we should write papers about it, and discuss its nature in more or less detail, and with more or less seriousness, according to the humour of the hour. I do not speak now of the more practical section of the profession—men engaged in the daily and hourly discharge of arduous duties, in the conscientious endeavour to apply well-known rules to the treatment of disease, and only exceptionally concerned in the pursuit of new knowledge. I speak rather of the more ambitious amongst us—and, thank Heaven, they are now very nume-

rous—men who attend societies, compile statistics, collect specimens, and write papers. Of these I assert—may I be permitted to claim for myself a humble position amongst them, and say, of us?—that we are far too ready to yield to the temptation of thinking that disease was made for the physician, and not the physician for disease. We investigate it in the same spirit that an amateur geologist brings to his problems—as a thing which may agreeably exercise our ingenuity and train our minds, upon which we may perhaps base our reputations, and out of which there may perhaps come some good for mankind. We claim to lay aside our work when we are tired of it, and to vote its too urgent pursuit a bore, forgetting that such investigations are to us a matter of the most urgent professional duty, and to our clients one of life and death.

That I may not seem to loose an unaimed shaft, I will take an example, and it shall be one in which almost the whole of the English profession, to some extent, is concerned. The Museum of the Royal College of Surgeons, the Hunterian Collection, with its fifty years' additions, is without a rival in the world. It is a noble museum, and has been nobly cared for by a succession of curators, who have made their names famous in science by work done within its walls. It may seem a bold thing to charge against an institution so foremost, that its arrangements are inadequate to the wants of the present day. Amongst the wants of the medical profession at the present time, and amongst those wants which alone a national museum is fitted to supply, is the fullest possible information respecting the symptoms of disease. It is not enough that we illustrate its final results, that we keep in bottles or otherwise the documents which demonstrate its ultimate conditions: we need a pathology of the living as well as of the dead; and everything that human contrivance can do to elucidate this should be attempted. Here we must mark a huge hiatus in the arrangements of our College. There is little or no attempt to illustrate the effects of either disease or injury in the living, and an exceedingly meagre attempt to show what has been done in reference to instruments for surgical treatment. The modeller's art, of which such beautiful examples from Paris have recently been shown to us in the Congress Museum, is at our College "unknown and like esteemed." I must correct myself; for there is, in a topmost gallery, a small collection of models, the gift of our present President. These, however, are only a little series selected from the magnificent array of similar objects to be seen in the St. Louis Museum at Paris. It is imperfect and ill-shown, and the College makes no effort to add to it. A museum adapted to the wants of the practitioner should supplement the hospital, whenever possible, in the display of the outward characters of disease. Nothing in the whole range of diseases of the eye and skin or other external parts, nothing that a speculum can show, or a modeller delineate, should escape it; the common and the rare should alike be there, and the practitioner should be able to resort to its galleries when in doubt as to diagnosis, or desiring to recapitulate his knowledge, with confidence that he will there see all that can be shown. Nothing less than completeness should be the aim, and from all sources copies should be procured where the original cannot be had—the photographer, the modeller, and the artist being employed without regard to expense.

If a surgeon were now to go to our museum and ask to see models which would help him in the diagnosis of the different forms of chancre, or in the recognition of such sores on unusual parts of the body, I fear that he would be disappointed. He might find an unequalled collection of prehistoric skulls, and the skeleton of a splendid whale, but little or nothing in reference to the practical object of the diagnosis of surgical disease. Yet, in proof that it is possible to give such aid, I again appeal to the St. Louis Collection.

Let it not be thought that I speak in disparagement of anthropology or comparative anatomy. It is a proud boast of our profession that its members have been foremost in these pursuits, and long may it be sustained. In their liberal cultivation, we follow the example of the founder of our museum, and keep up its most cherished traditions. But surgery has widened much since Hunter's time, and its special cultivation now asserts claims which did not then exist. And these claims are, I cannot but think, primary in such an institution; and, whatever it leaves undone, it should first attend to the duty of giving all that it can possibly give to the elucidation of human disease and the means of its relief. I cannot, however, believe that a liberal development in the new direction would necessitate any curtailment in the old. Let but a proper appeal be made to the profession, the public, and the Government, and means would surely be forthcoming which would enable our National Museum of Surgery so to devèlope itself, that no surgeon should ever spend a day in London without a visit to its collection, and none should pass through its rooms without obtaining information which would be of the utmost value to his patients.

There is yet another kind of museum which is, I think, a desideratum, and which I have no doubt the future will possess: I refer to a museum-hospital, in which living persons, the subjects of chronic and incurable diseases of an unusual kind, should be collected and encouraged to remain, with, of course, every attention to their comforts, for long periods; every facility being offered for their inspection by all members of the profession. From such hospitals I would wholly exclude common cases, such as are useful, nay, essential, in the training of the student, and would collect only those likely to be instructive to advanced practitioners. Each case should be carefully studied by competent authorities, and described in an accessible catalogue. A visit to such an institution would be invaluable to the man engaged in busy general practice, and its growing records would become rich mines of information to the clinical investigator. Rare maladies are not to be regarded as mere objects of scientific curiosity, but should be utilised to the utmost, and made, if practicable, familiar to all; for in them often lies the key to the interpretation of other pathological phenomena which are common enough. Let us cease from dilettantism, and try to economise our resources. When we do so, surely we shall find that there is a better way of dealing with examples of myxœdema, of Addison's disease, of Charcot's joints, and morphœa, than by relegating them to the wards of a union asylum, where they will be seen by none. I mention these merely as examples; there are many others concerning which it is equally true that, if opportunities were afforded for their collection together, under conditions of facility for research and inspection, great help would be given both to medical education and to the progress of clinical knowledge.

I should be very sorry if what I have said, perhaps too plainly, as to what appear to me to be defects in our existing arrangements for the promotion of surgical knowledge, should have left the impression that I am in any degree a dissatisfied complainer. I hope that I yield to none in thankful appreciation of what has been accomplished in the past. But surely the fulness of the harvest which we have been permitted to reap should prompt us to increased diligence in putting in seed for the next. We have every reason to feel encouraged and hopeful, but let us not allow the sentiment of confidence to lull us into sloth.

The chemist and the empirical seeker after new drugs may, I suppose, share the pleasure which must come from the knowledge of how iodide of potassium has made curable a whole phalanx of maladies before hopeless, and not the less full of misery because often accompanied by the bitterness of self-reproach. The operating surgeon may remember the triumphs of ovariotomy, which has restored in health hundreds of mothers to their families. If we could bring together in one place those who, thanks to the ingenuity and industry of Von Gräfe, have been by iridectomy saved from blindness through glaucoma, and are now enjoying the blessing of sight, they would crowd this large hall, and leave no standing room. The abstruse optical researches of Young, Helmholtz, and Donders have borne fruit in the fact that thousands all over the world, whose sight was comparatively useless, now enjoyed it in almost full perfection. The purely practical man may rejoice in remembering how much Sayre's jacket and Martin's bandage have done, and are daily doing, for the mitigation of suffering and the cure of diseases which rendered life a burden. The application of the germ theory to the treatment of wounds, has, I doubt not, had for one of its results, amongst many others, that at the present moment there live, scattered in very distant places, many thousands of able-bodied men, the fathers of families, now earning their children's bread, who but for it would long ago have been in their graves. It is true that we as yet see no hope of a cure for cancer, but the pathological doctrine, which is rapidly gaining ground, that many

forms are local, and that the pre-cancerous stage should be vigilantly recognised and vigorously treated, is already saving many from becoming its victims.

A few weeks ago, visiting a renowned cathedral, I found inscribed on its floor at long distances apart, three remarkable words—Credo, Spero, Amo. I am not ignorant of the special meaning which in such association was meant to attach to these words, nor would I now for one moment attempt to employ them in a different sense, if I thought it would give pain to the tenderest conscience in this room. But indeed they are words of the widest bearing, and refer to feelings and attainments which lie at the very basis of all human character. We become what we are, we effect what we do, in virtue of what we love, what we believe, and what we hope. I have ventured to censure as a weakness to which those who work in pursuit of a more intimate knowledge of disease are very liable, a spirit of dilettantism, a willingness to be contented with half results. For that weakness, the cure rests in the Amo. He who intensely loves will sympathise with the miseries which afflict his fellow-men, and will be ever zealous for their relief. Nor will he fail to use every opportunity of becoming familiar with the reality of those miseries, and thus warm his sympathies and increase his love. Next comes the Credo. Do we heartily believe, in respect to the advancement of the happiness of man, in the value of the discovery of scientific truth? From the Credo to the Spero in this instance the step is very easy, for they are almost phases of the same sentiment.

I have just enumerated very briefly a very few of the countless encouragements to hope which those conversant with the history of our profession may easily find in the records of the last half-century. Can any doubt that they are but an earnest of far greater triumphs to come? The work that is before us spreads out in a sort of three-fold division. We have to apply in the best practicable manner our present knowledge for the benefit of those around us; we have to do our best to increase that knowledge; and thirdly, we have to find the best means for transferring it to the new generation which will soon succeed to our duties. Medical practice, the advancement of the knowledge of the nature of disease, and the training of our sons—such are our three great spheres of duty. Some of us work in one, some in another, most of us to some extent in all. Let us all seek to love the great final object at which we aim, to believe in the means which we are employing, and to hope confidently of their results.

IODOFORM IN THE VULVITIS OF CHILDREN.—Prof. Parrot applies iodoform by means of a badger's-hair pencil at whatever stage the aphthæ may be in, covering the parts affected with a thick layer of iodoform without previous cleansing, and then applying a little charpie. This dressing is repeated every twenty-four hours until amendment takes place, which it usually does very rapidly. Even after the first application it is rare not to find a considerable improvement. The ulcerated parts look as clean as if they had been carefully washed. Their borders sink and their cavities fill up, and when they are not very extensive they are not easily distinguished from the surrounding parts. The changes take place rapidly, and lead to the speedy disappearance of vulvular or perineal breaches of surface. —Gaz. des Hop., August 9.

CASTRATION FOR MASTURBATION.—Dr. Folsom, writing to the Michigan Medical News, says that Dr. Josiah Crosby, in 1843, with the assistance of Dr. Folsom and another medical student, and with the consent of the patient and his father, castrated a young man for approaching dementia from masturbation. The patient was twenty-two years of age, intelligent and educated. He had ceased to leave the house or mix in society, and did not wish to see anyone. He had been medically treated by various physicians to no purpose. The operation completely cured him and restored him to usefulness, and he afterwards became an active man of business. Dr. Folsom believes that this was the only treatment that could have saved him, and he thinks that there are many such cases who can be cured in no other way. Superintendents of insane asylums especially, he says, should, with the consent of the patients' friends, castrate hopeless cases of dementia from masturbation.—New York Med. Record, July 16.

THE INTERNATIONAL MEDICAL CONGRESS.

SECTION OF PHYSIOLOGY.

ADDRESS BY PROF. MICHAEL FOSTER, F.R.S.,
President of the Section.

GENTLEMEN,—In seeking some words with which to welcome from this chair-my brother physiologists to their part in this gathering of the medicine-men of all nations, my choice has fallen on the story of the share which the country in which we have this year assembled has taken in the past in building up our science of physiology. Such a step might seem to savour of national egotism were the end which I had in view that of magnifying the labours of British physiologists, but our meeting here to-day is in itself a proof that the true worker, wherever he may happen to draw his breath, belongs to all lands; and in attempting to recall to your minds to-day the services of those who laboured in the past in Great Britain, I trust I shall appear in the eyes of our foreign guests merely as a cicerone striving to render a visit the more interesting by weaving connexions between the present and the past.

At the head, both in chronological order and in point of worth, of the roll of British physiologists comes a name concerning which I may begin and at the same time end by simply naming it. It would ill become me to waste your time by attempting to tell the more than twice-told tale of William Harvey. May I not simply say that his renown is a statue of solid real metal, which the blows directed against it from time to time in the present, as in the past, have not so much as dented or tarnished, but simply polished and made bright?

In any country the giving birth to a great man may be followed by two opposite effects. On the one hand, his example and influence may stir up his fellows to increased activity; on the other hand, the making of him, like powerful tetanus in a muscle, seems often to lead to national fatigue, and the land which bore him appears for a while unable to produce his like. This, indeed, would appear to be Nature's method of making science truly international. In her series of great men she continually changes the venue from land to land. As in calling forth Harvey to succeed Vesalius she shifted the scene from Italy, where the latter at least did his chief work, to England, where the former lived and laboured; so, to find the next truly great man after Harvey, we must cross the Channel and pass to France, to Italy, to Leyden, or to Berne, according to the views we hold as to exactly on whose shoulders the mantle of Harvey fell.

Happily, in England the national exhaustion was not so great but that Harvey's direct influence was manifest in his being succeeded, not so much, as might be expected, by feeble imitators and still more feeble cavillers, as by men who, if not of the first rank, were yet of notable worth, and by their sound work showed themselves worthy to follow in his footsteps. For in the years which followed immediately after Harvey the anatomical and physiological mind of England was by no means idle. During the middle and latter thirds of the seventeenth century there were several centres of scientific activity in more or less close union. First and foremost is the Society which, beginning with modest beginnings, has waxed in strength and usefulness as years have rolled on, and which for this long while has been the large-minded nurse of British science—I mean the Royal Society. Closely connected with this mother society, and, indeed, in genetic relation with it, was a gathering of earnest, active men, whose home was the University of Oxford. Nor was the sister University of Cambridge at that time wholly idle. More strictly professional in activity, but none the less zealous in the promotion of real science, was the College of Physicians of London. Lastly, but not least, it was a feature especially of the latter part of the time of which I am speaking, that, in spite of the difficulties of loco-motion, a large number of men scattered all over the country

were active members of the republic of science, in continual communication with each other, and with the centres of which I have just spoken. Physicians resident in country towns, enlightened surgeons and apothecaries, and educated gentlemen of leisure, many of these sought recreation in the pursuit of knowledge, and their contributions to science, sometimes of no little value, may be found in the *Philosophical Transactions* or other publications.

Among the men, after Harvey (belonging to these several centres), who added to physiological science, I might mention first Francis Glisson, whose name has been handed down to us in "Glisson's capsule," and whose chief work, "Anatomia Hepatis," was published in 1654, a quarter of a century after Harvey's great work. Appointed Regius Professor of Physics in the University of Cambridge in 1636, almost immediately after taking his medical degree, he appears to have practised at Cambridge and Colchester, but from 1650 onwards, to his death at eighty-one years of age in 1677, to have lived chiefly in London. His reputation during his life and after his death was very great, his works passing through several editions—and deservedly so, for no one can read his writings without feeling that he was a strong man of great knowledge, with a clear head and logical mind. Unfortunately, he was greatly enamoured of dialectic formalities. He begins his work on the liver with a prolix discussion on anatomy in general, and he has so written his other great work, "De Ventriculo et Intestinis," that his views are largely unintelligible, unless the reader have first waded through an elaborate treatise, "De Vita Naturæ." Yet whoever has courage to disinter the truths which Glisson has to tell from the definitions and syllogisms and long-winded verbal discussions in which they are buried, will, I think, be willing to admit that, apart from the more strictly anatomical credit which is due to his careful descriptions of the liver and alimentary canal, he deserves mention for having laid hold of an important physiological idea. Not only was he, so far as I know, the first to introduce that phrase irritability, which in Haller's hands was made to teach so much, and which is now one of our household words, but in the chapter where he is treating of the fibres of the stomach and intestines, he shows that he had grasped the important truth of independent muscular irritability. "From these instances," says he, "it is sufficiently clear that fibres [muscles] can, without any aid of the senses, perceive an irritation, and conformably move themselves." He, moreover, clearly distinguished between contraction and relaxation, and by means of an experiment which is almost the exact antitype of the modern plethysmograph, he satisfied himself that the arm does not increase, but rather decreases in bulk, when its muscles are even violently contracted, and concludes "that the fibres shorten themselves by their own vital movement, and have no need at all of any copious afflux of spirits, whether animal or vital, by which they are inflated in order that they may be shortened."

But these were views put forward by an old man of eighty with one foot in the grave. Had they come to him in his early life, when the enthusiasm of youth would have permitted him to preach and push them, the doctrine of muscular power might have been saved the waste of near a hundred years.

Leaving on one side Glisson's temporary, Wharton, of anatomical, rather than physiological worth, as well as some others, let me pass from the University of Cambridge to that of Oxford, which a company of able, zealous men, in part founders of the Royal Society, were making a centre of scientific activity.

Conspicuous in this company was the brilliant Thomas Willis, who in 1660 was appointed Sedleian Professor of Natural Philosophy, but who in 1666 moved to London, where, till his death in 1675, he was busily engaged in a successful and lucrative practice.

The great reputation which Willis achieved in his own time, leaving on one side his purely medical works, rested on a basis partly anatomical, partly physiological. In the first place, in his work "Cerebri Anatome" he gave a more complete account than had yet appeared of the anatomy of the brain and cranial nerves; an account, moreover, embodying many new discoveries. In the second place, he was bold enough to develope a physiological and psychological theory of the functions of the whole nervous system.

The value of the anatomical work is undoubted. The phrases circulus Willisii and nervus accessorius Willisii, which are still current words among us, give but slight hints of the many contributions to our knowledge of the anatomy of the brain and cranial nerves which the world owes to Willis's works. But there would seem to be a sort of contradiction between the nature of this part of his work and the character of the man himself. Report speaks of Thomas Willis as a man of versatile parts, of a nature averse to patient anatomical investigation. He himself states that in many of the details of his work he was largely assisted by a man of a very different stamp, the patient, careful, clearheaded Richard Lower (of whom I have presently to speak); and ill-natured critics of the time insisted that the many anatomical discoveries disclosed in Willis's name came in reality from the hand and mind of Lower. It is not worth our while to attempt to sift this question now; all the more so since both Willis's acknowledgment of Lower's help was free and ungrudging, and Lower, so far as I know, never took occasion publicly to reproach the master whom he evidently so much loved. But this may be observed, that the theories of Willis have not, like his anatomy, stood the test of time. His descriptions of the brain and nerves, with the additions and corrections of Vieussens, who followed him a little later in the same century, served as the basis of teaching till recent times (indeed, Charles Bell speaks of the system of Willis as being current in his day). But his guesses as to the functions of the parts of the brain proved no solid addition to knowledge, and his theory of the *anima brutorum* pervading the whole of the bodies of all animals, though it may be interpreted as foreshadowing the modern doctrine of the life of the tissues, was unable to make way against the gathering force of the mechanical doctrines of the Cartesian philosophy. Willis, in fact, as many have done before and since, grappled with a subject too big for him, and attempted to solve problems for whose solution the world was not yet ripe. Yet the talent of the man is seen even in his failure. He appears to have laid hold of the idea of reflex action; and if anyone is inclined to smile when he learns that Willis thought the cerebellum was the seat of involuntary, as the cerebrum of voluntary, actions, he will do well to read the author's guesses as to the functions of the corpora quadrigemina, corpora striata, corpus callosum, cerebral convolutions, and the like—for he will find that these are not so far unlike other guesses about the same things which have been published in the journals of our own time.

The next two names which I have to mention illustrate a feature peculiar almost to England. In the rest of the learned world progress in science is for the most part distinctly professional; discoveries are made by members of the professoriate. In England it is a matter of notoriety that some of the most important steps have been due not to accredited professors, but to free lances in science; to men of business, lawyers, clergymen, and men of fortune. I have spoken of Glisson, the professor at Cambridge, and of Willis, the professor at Oxford, but after them the University professoriate, as far as physiology is concerned, became dumb. If you read the roll of the regius and other professors in the old universities you will find merely a long list of men, respectable it may be in their way, but whose names are unknown to physiological science. This feature, which appears so strange to men of other lands, is partly due to the anomaly that the great metropolitan heart of England—London—never had a university, and, indeed, till quite recently, was without even the beginning of one. Hence arose a divorce between metropolitan activity and the old-established seats of learning. From its very beginning, the Royal Society—the Invisible College, as Boyle called it—has performed the higher functions of a university, and the very essence of the life of that body always has been that it gathers into its fold all manner of folk, demanding only that they shall have the desire and the power to advance knowledge.

At all events, whatever be the cause, the next contributions brought by England to physiological science came through hands not professional, not even medical.

The great work of Harvey remained incomplete by reason of the lack of true ideas as to the uses of the lungs. A clear conception of the nutritive mechanism of the body, of which Harvey's discovery was the keystone, was still impossible so long as men, even though they had given up the idea of cardiac refrigeration, continued shackled with the view that the mere mechanical movement of the lungs was the be-all and end-all of the respiratory act. Although the great Vesalius, in one of those passages which make us feel how near the

father of modern anatomy came to being also the father of modern physiology, shows that he once, at least, was drawing near to the truth; though many afterwards similarly touched the coast; although Van Helmont, by his discovery that gas silvestre or carbonic anhydride rendered respiration fruitless, formally began the chemical theory of respiration: I may, I think, venture to assert, without fear of being reproached with national vanity, that it was reserved for a group of Englishmen, all more or less contemporaries, all more or less friends, two only of whom were doctors, and none of whom were professors, to lay the first foundation of our real knowledge concerning the nature of breathing. I do not neglect the importance of the anatomical labours of the great Malpighi, whose work on the lungs was published about the same time (1661), nor do I forget that a little later (1680) the clear logical mind of Borelli led him in this, as in so many other vexed questions of the animal economy, far into the truth; but the latter had the advantage of already knowing what had been done by the men of whom I speak.

Concerning one of these—Robert Boyle—the sagacious natural philosopher (who, though for a while he took up his abode at Oxford, was not bred at that university), who was for so long one of the pillars of the Royal Society, who busied himself with anatomy only in so far as he busied himself with all parts of natural knowledge, who touched nothing which he did not throw light on; to whom even more than to any of his fellows must be given the credit of having established, by experiment itself, the pre-eminence of what we know as the Experimental Method, whose name is praised even if his works be not read by all men,—I need say little here. It will be enough if I remind you that his simple experiments showing that air, and fresh air, was necessary for the respiration and life of aquatic, as well as of terrestrial animals, that the respiratory value of air varied according as it was rarefied by the vacuum Boylianum or condensed by pressure, and that air already breathed became unfit for further respiratory use, mark the point at which the older view, that the chief use of the respiratory movements was to favour the circulation of the blood, began to be recognised as clearly untenable.

Tending even more strongly in the same direction was the classic experiment of Robert Hook, who, in his early days the assistant first of Willis and then of Boyle, afterwards curator and experimenter, and subsequently Secretary to the Royal Society, was for many years a prime mover in English science. Mathematician, physicist, chemist, engineer, microscopist, physiologist, virtuoso, and city surveyor, some might perhaps be tempted to call him Jack-of-all-trades and master of none; yet he was a man of almost unbounded fertility and vast energy. We may forgive him his unlucky opposition to Newton, and overlook both the petulant quarrelsomeness which engaged him in conflict with nearly all his friends in turn, and the miserly niggardliness which, after leading him during his life into perpetual squabbles over a few pounds, left him at his death with much riches stored up,—when we call to mind his many and varied contributions to science. In 1662 he was appointed Curator to the Royal Society at a salary of £50 a year on the understanding that he should "furnish the Society every day they meete with three or four considerable experiments," and for many years he was always ready with "considerable experiments" of one kind or another, sometimes mechanical, sometimes physical, sometimes physiological.

For it was a feature of the Royal Society at that time that the Fellows thought much of seeing with their own eyes the "considerable experiments" which were brought before them to serve as a basis for new scientific views: they were not then content with hearing an account, still less with hearing an abstract of an account, of experiments performed elsewhere. A no less striking feature of the Society was the catholic feeling of all the Fellows towards all branches of learning. Each one was interested in results gained on other lines of research than his own, and differentiation of study had not yet proceeded so far as to prevent each one from appreciating the labours of all the rest. Not the medical Fellows alone, but nearly all of them, were concerned in the progress of physiological inquiry, took part in physiological discussions, and witnessed physiological experiments. When "an anatomy" from the gallows at Tyburn had been obtained, a circular was despatched to the Fellows, stating when and where and by whom the dissection would be performed; and the Society's bills contained items for animals to be experimented on. These men, who, in various branches, were making the Society looked up to throughout the world as the centre of the new philosophy, had no doubt whatever that the true knowledge of life and disease was henceforward to be won by careful, repeated experiments. They had not yet learnt that it was wrong to kill an animal in pursuit of truth, though right to-kill it for the sake of food or in pursuit of sport; and were their irascible curator to revisit to-day the scenes of his former labours, great, I imagine, would be his indignation and scathing his words when he learnt that his philosophical experiments had been made penal by Act of Parliament—by an Act of Parliament the passing of which, and indeed the passing of some of the harsher clauses of which, had been the work of men who actually bore the title of Fellows of his old Society.

Of the many "considerable" physiological experiments which Hook performed before this Society, I will content myself with reminding you of one, and only one. Years before, Vesalius had performed artificial respiration, and traced its effects on the movements of the heart and the blood; but Hook did something more than merely repeat Vesalius's experiment. He showed, by an ingenious experiment—viz., by keeping the lungs distended with a brisk current of air passing through them—that the central fact of respiration was the effect of the air on the blood, and not the movement of the lungs—a demonstration which I venture to regard as a cardinal fact in the history of respiration. Only a knowledge of the chemistry of the blood-changes was necessary to make the theory of breathing approximately complete. And that also was, though imperfectly, supplied by the labours of two other Englishmen, Hook's contemporaries—Richard Lower and John Mayow.

To Lower I have already referred in speaking of Thomas Willis. At first the pupil, afterwards the coadjutor, and during their lifetimes the attached personal friend of that brilliant physician, Lower was a man of very different mould. Patient, unassuming, industrious, clear-headed, fertile in ideas and methods, and yet withal accurate and exact, he had in him all the making of the great man of science. Had he remained in the academic repose of Oxford, devoted, without distractions, to his researches, it is difficult to say whither he might not have reached. Unhappily, Willis persuaded him to move with him to London, where, especially after his master's death, his talents soon gained him an extensive practice. He became the most noted physician in London and Westminster. "No man's name was more cried up at Court than his," and the powers of mind which might have made him a second Harvey, were used for the immediate benefit of his patients and himself.

Of even such work as he did, we cannot take the full measure, since it is now impossible to unravel out his share in the work which is ascribed to Willis, but his independent volume, the "Tractatus de Corde" (1669), shows the metal of the man. As a piece of careful anatomical work, made alive with physiological suggestions, it may even at the present day be read, not only with pleasure but with profit. And the story of the transfusion of blood, which at the time made so great a stir, shows at least how skilful an experimenter he was. When the decayed clergyman, Arthur Coga, for the reward of a guinea, allowed Lower and King to inject into his veins, through silver pipes and common quills, ten ounces of blood from a sheep, he showed a confidence in the operators greater than which could not be given to the modern master of experimental physiology, Carl Ludwig, with all the ingenious safeguards at his command. When, however, we strive to appreciate the genetic and historic moment of Lower's work, we must, I think, admit that his chief contribution to physiology was certainly not the transfusion of blood, not the aid he gave to Willis, not even his careful cardiac anatomy, with its physiological deductions, but the notable, well-directed experiments by which he demonstrated, once for all, that the change of colour from venous to arterial blood was due not to any fermentation in the heart, not to the extinction of the claret hue by the action of the veins, but simply and solely to the passage of air through the pulmonary walls, and its admixture, or, as we should say now, its absorption, by the blood; that the change in the lungs was identical with that which takes place when the surface of a venous clot becomes florid by exposure to the air. "How much they err," says he, "who deny altogether this commerce of the air with the blood. For without it

it would be possible for one to live as wholesomely in the foul atmosphere of a prison as in the midst of pleasant groves; for wherever fire can fitly burn, there we too can fitly breathe." I take it that if we try to throw ourselves back into the ideas of the times of which I am speaking, this clear experimental proof of the essential fact of respiration must appear to us an epoch-making step. One thing was lacking in Lower's exposition: he did not appear to have recognised the true nature of the converse change from arterial to venous blood; the process of tissue oxidation was unknown to him. He speaks of the air as escaping from the blood in its passage through the tissues, and transpiring through the pores of the body. At least he leaves us uncertain as to what he thought was the exact function of the air thus gained and lost by the blood. In the very same year, however, in which Lower's "Tractatus" appeared, there was published a little work in which the world had a glimpse of the true meaning of those mysterious changes from purple to scarlet, and scarlet to purple, the full understanding of which had to be deferred for near a hundred years.

Among Lower's friends and contemporaries at Oxford was one John Mayow, of whom it may be said that the more one reads of what he wrote, the more one is astonished at his penetrative intellect. Striking out for himself a new path, his meditations led him in a way to forestall the discoveries which made resplendent the latter half and closing years of the next century. I believe all those who have read with care Mayow's treatises "De Sal Nitro et Spiritu Nitro-æreo" and "De Respiratione," have become convinced that under cover of the phrase "spiritus nitro-æreus" he laid his hand, so to speak, on that mysterious element which, nearly a hundred years later, Priestley and Lavoisier taught us to call oxygen; nay, more, that he had formed, if not a wholly clear, yet at all events an approximately correct, conception of the part which this great agent plays, not only in the special pulmonary respiration, but in the life of all the tissues. He saw that it was this nitro-aërial constituent of the atmosphere, and not the whole body of air, which passed into the blood in the lungs, and that hence this constituent was deficient in the expired breath. He saw, moreover, that the change from arterial to venous blood in the tissues was due to the same nitro-aërial spirit escaping from the blood and mingling with the elements of the flesh, he even saw that the energy of the living machine was the issue of the struggle between the same spirit and the sulphurous particles of the body, or, as we say now, was set free in the oxidation of the combustible elements of the tissue. In reading an old author writing in distant times we are apt to fall into the error of two errors; on the one hand, the strangeness of his terminology may lead us to overlook the truth and correctness of his ideas; on the other hand, we are equally apt to read into his old words conceptions wholly of our own time. Making every allowance for the latter source of error, it would, I venture to think, still be found that Mayow's work, translated into modern phrases, would represent with wonderful nearness those views of respiration on which we pride ourselves to-day.

"Vir ingeniosus neque mathematicam ignosus," says Haller, in speaking of Mayow, and a perusal of the little tract, "De Motu Musculari," will, I imagine, convince the reader that while Mayow went far beyond Borelli in comprehending the chemical basis of muscular contraction, he anticipated in part the mechanical interpretations of muscular action for which the great Italian mathematician justly became celebrated.

Nearly the whole, indeed, of the little which John Mayow wrote is marked with accurate observation, experimental acumen, and original conceptions. Had he lived like the great Haller himself, to a ripe old age, one page of the history of physiology might have been very different from what it is. "Juvenis," to quote Haller again, "in hypotheses pronior." He was not spared to work out the many hypotheses which were seething in his brain. Carried off at the early age of thirty-three, his name not yet inscribed in the roll of the College of Physicians, the world had to wait many years till other minds took up his broken work.

Did time and opportunity permit, much more might be said, possibly not without profit, concerning these men, at whose lives and works I have thus rapidly glanced, and, indeed, concerning others whom I have not so much as mentioned; but I trust I have already said enough to show that at a time when physiologists were far from abundant on the Continent, when the chief physiological impulses there were coming from the philosopher Descartes, the anatomist Malpighi, and the mathematician Borelli, when the greater European names in biology (Stenon, Bellini, Graaf, Redi, Ruysch, Swammerdam, Leeuwenhoek, Vieussens, and others) were those of anatomists, naturalists, or physicians rather than physiologists, pure experimental physiology was being pursued with diligence and success in England. But with the departure of this group of men, the *venue* of our science was once more changed. I have already said that after Glisson the University of Cambridge in matters physiological became dumb. So also, with Willis and Lower, Boyle and Mayow, the book of Oxford physiology was closed. Not only so, but for awhile the whole of England became, as far as our subject is concerned, sterile. She produced naturalists like Grew and Lister, she gave birth to successful, indeed distinguished, physicians, and to some worthy anatomists, but the institutes of medicine were for a while neglected.

The school of mathematical physiologists, who, incited by the example of Borelli and the influence of Newton, fancied that the calculus alone could solve the mysteries of the living body, made a stir in their day, without really advancing our science, and the works of the versatile Jacobite Pitcairne, of Keil, and Jurin are justly forgotten. A little later on, the first Monro began the long series of Scottish celebrities; but he was an anatomist rather than a physiologist. Indeed, in the early part of the eighteenth century the centre of physiological activity was at Leyden, where the brilliant, fascinating Boerhaave was making a school of world-wide reputation.

Boerhaave passed away, and Haller became his intellectual successor. The eighteenth century ran more than half its course with scarcely a sign of physiological activity in England, save one. And this came not from the older universities, for they, leaving their old catholic sympathies were wrapping themselves in narrower studies,—not from the wigged leaders of the College of Physicians, for they were wasting time and talents in fruitless discussions of the doctrines of the schools,—not indeed from the profession at all, but, after a truly English fashion, from the sister calling of religion.

As you pass up the Thames from London towards Oxford, you come, a little beyond Richmond, to the first obstruction to navigation, in the shape of Teddington Locks. In the early part of the eighteenth century the minister of the adjoining hamlet of Teddington was the Rev. Stephen Hales, also rector of Farringdon in Hampshire, a man of varied accomplishment, of great practical ingenuity, and a master in the art of experimental investigation. Early fascinated with the mysteries, which fascinate so many of us even to-day, of muscular contraction, dissatisfied with current interpretations, as well as with the calculations of Borelli and the succeeding school of iatro-mathematicians, he turned his attention seriously to physiological experiments. In his statical essays, which formed the "Imprimatur" of the Royal Society, the first volume in 1726.27, the second in 1732-33, after relating researches into vegetable statics, the movement of sap, etc., which, though of prime importance in vegetable physiology, need not detain us here, he proceeds to relate his experiments on the pressure of blood in the arteries and veins of horses, sheep, and dogs. Save that his methods were somewhat rough, that he measured pressure, not by a mercury manometer, though strangely enough he employed this in determining the force of inspiration and expiration, but by the height of the column of blood itself, that with characteristic ingenuity he used as flexible tube to connect the cannula with his manometer, the actual trachea of a goose, instead of that rigid and yet flexible artificial trachea which we nowadays construct out of caoutchouc and rings of glass, his research is a piece of quite modern work, the prototype and original of those valuable memoirs on vascular dynamics which have appeared from time to time from the laboratory at Leipsig.

I do not think I am exaggerating matters when I affirm that, next to Harvey's discovery, a correct appreciation of blood-pressure is the keystone to the physiology of the vascular system, and indirectly of the rest of physiology and of pathology as well. Pull out from the web of our system of physiology the strand marked blood-pressure, you pull out also all that is suggested by the phrase vaso-motor, and

leave the rest of the fabric a confused and tangled heap. If so, then how much is due to Stephen Hales, for he surely first opened the way in this weighty matter! In strong contrast with the labours of Keil, Jurin, and others of the iatro-mathematic class, is his work. They, like some other mathematicians, fascinated with the very operations of their calculus, were content with such data as were at hand, and often, indeed, careless about them. In consequence, their labours were sterile. To Stephen Hales the living organism was not simply a pretty field for mathematical exercises, but a crowd of problems to be solved first by diligent observation, and then, and then only, by calculation. He was an experimental philosopher, in the truest sense of the word. As you read his works you feel that the experiments were not made, as experiments sometimes are, for the sake of the experiment, but simply that he might push further into the secrets of Nature. His reflections and deductions are as weighty as his operations were ingenious. There is one passage in particular where he is descanting on the great variation of blood-pressure, not only in different kinds of animals, but in the same kind, and in the same individual at divers times, and under differing circumstances, in which he says (page 31, third ed.) : " Even in the same animal the force of the blood is continually varying according to many circumstances ; for the healthy state of animals is not confined to the scanty limits of one determinate degree of vital vigour in the blood ; but the all-wise Framer of these admirable machines has so ordered it as that their healthy state shall not be disturbed by every little variation of this force, but has made it consistent with a very considerable latitude in the variation of it." Does not this sentence clearly show that Hales had completely freed himself from the animistic doctrines to which so many of his predecessors, and indeed contemporaries, were attached, and how far, on the other hand, he had pushed beyond the Cartesian ideas of a mechanism worked by a central force, and how fully he had entered into those conceptions of the animal body as an exquisitely adapted, self-regulating machine, which 'we prize, and justly prize, as our leading views of to-day? As a clergyman, and therefore not brought up to a familiarity with the dissecting-knife and the operation-room, he was naturally averse to anatomical procedures. As a man of kindly humane nature, indeed as one of England's earliest and best philanthropists, he felt a repugnance—as, indeed, who does not ?—to dabbling in the blood of living animals. "The disagreeableness of the work," he says, " did long discourage me from engaging in it ; but I was, on the other hand, spurred on by the hopes that we might thereby get some further insight into the animal economy." And further insight he did get, as indeed everyone must get who works in Hales' spirit. No doubt ever crossed his mind as to the beneficial character of his labours, and I take it that could we now question him as to how he thought he had best served mankind, he would answer that it was not so much by his having been the chief means of introducing ventilation into our then wretched English gaols, though he invented a ventilator for the purpose—great as has been the suffering thus saved—not so much by any of his many other similar practical inventions, as by the indirect results of his hydraulic and other theoretic researches.

Hales' essays are indeed, even to-day, a mine of delightful observations and reflections. He not only exactly measured the amount of blood-pressure under varying circumstances, the capacity of the heart, the diameter of bloodvessels, and the like, and from his several data made his calculation and drew his conclusions ; by an ingenious method he measured the rate of flow of blood in the capillaries in the abdominal muscles and lungs of a frog. He knew how to keep blood fluid with saline solutions, got a clear insight into the nature of secretion, studied the form of muscles at rest and contraction, and speculated that what we now call a nervous impulse, but which was then spoken of as the animal spirits, might possibly be an electric change. And though he accepted the current view that the heat of the body was produced by the friction of the blood in the capillaries, he was not wholly content with this, but speaks of the mutually vibrating action of solids and fluids as an independent cause of animal heat, in a way which makes us feel that, had the chemistry of the time been as advanced as were the physics, many weary years of error and ignorance might have been saved our science.

Stephen Hales was a clergyman, and though his works

found acceptance with the medical profession and with the general learned public, he had in England no successor. While, abroad, Haller was making a name and founding a school, Great Britain was for the most part silent. Save from some little activity north of the Tweed, where the second Monro succeeded his father, for some scattered memoirs in the *Edinburgh Medical Essays*—notably one by Stevenson, on "Animal Heat,"—and for the elaborate work of the ingenious but misdirected Robert Whytt, little or nothing was doing in this country. The chemist Black, at Edinburgh, moved on the theory of respiration a step by demonstrating the presence of carbonic acid in expired air, but further discoveries yet to come were necessary to make the value of that step apparent.

The next physiological light was to come from a body which had hitherto had little opportunity of contributing to science. In the eighteenth century the barber-surgeons rose in power and influence as they became simply surgeons. And while the professoriate of England had wholly, and the doctorate largely, deserted the path of physiological and experimental inquiry, the genius of a surgeon, in spite of the difficulties of an imperfect education, was drawing directly from Nature the inspiration of new physiological ideas. For I venture to think I am right in claiming John Hunter as physiological rather than anatomical in the bent of his mind. True, he busied himself, as we all know, with structures rather than with apparatus, with dissections much more than with experiments, but in reality he cared little for morphology, for the laws of animal form. He sought to know the details of animal structure, because he thought to learn from them the secrets of animal function—his guiding idea in amassing what has since become the great Hunterian Museum, being that the parts of animals should speak for themselves as to their use and work.

So much from nearly every point of view has been so often said of John Hunter, that I will to-day content myself with dwelling for a moment on what, especially to our foreign brethren, may appear a contradiction between, on the one hand, the immense influence which he has exercised over both the physiologists and the profession in general in this country, and the reverence in which his memory is held by us, and on the other, the small amount of definite gain to the broad truths of physiology which in the general history of the science is usually attached to his name.

The reason, I would suggest, may be found in the reflection that John Hunter was emphatically a man whose ideas outran the knowledge of his age. Not only was he himself somewhat meanly provided at the start with such general knowledge of nature as existed at the time, but he had to struggle with the imperfections of the physical, and especially of the chemical, learning of the day. So long as he busied himself with special and superficial problems which could be solved by the help of direct observation and experiment, or by the comparison of animal forms, he was happy and successful; but his genius was ever pushing him forward towards higher generalisations concerning the nature of vital processes, and then he found himself at cross purposes with the chemical and physical teaching of the age. What he heard from his brother chemists and physicists often hindered instead of helping him. Hampered by this, he often was led by instinct to conclusions for which he could give no explicit satisfactory reasons; still more often he failed to clothe his conceptions in intelligible forms, because neither chemistry nor physics could give him the terms he needed.

Let any of us to-day throw himself back a hundred years, and try to fancy what his thoughts about the animal frame would be, if the composition of water were as yet uncertain, if the existence and nature of oxygen were unknown, and all the manifold processes of oxidation wrapped in obscurity and confusion,—if he were without the guide of the doctrine of conservation of energy. If we do this, and thus put ourselves somewhat at John Hunter's standpoint, when we read in his works that one of his fundamental ideas was that there were three kinds of matter—common matter, vegetable matter, and animal matter—the latter being, as he said, "a second remove from the first,"—that he believed all vegetables to be formed out of water, and was consequently led to the view that water, though to appearance the simplest substance in existence, "must be of itself a compound of every species of matter into which we find it capable of being converted," we should not laugh at his

views as being absurd, but rather ask ourselves whither his ideas were tending, and how they would read translated into modern phrases.

And I venture to urge that when an adequate translation of Hunter's obscure and rugged diction is carefully made, it will be found that in reality he was stretching out his hand for those doctrines of protoplasm which form the basis of our teaching to-day. We have cast away the animistic conceptions of old. Descartes has been justified of his intellectual children to the extent that we have been shown how in large measure the phenomena of life are the results of the working of an exquisite machinery; but we have not driven animism wholly out of doors, we have but swept it into the corner of the tissues, into the cell. We are still, after Hunter's fashion, obliged to admit an as yet impassable gulf between the characters of that protoplasmic matter which we call living, and of that common matter which we call dead. Before the problem we stand as helpless as he did before other lesser ones which we seem to have solved, and possibly our gropings towards its solution may appear to our successors as strange as his do to us.

Some of us may have visions of a possible molecular interpretation of the change from dead food to living flesh. In Hunter's mind also, lying hid behind his vitalistic expressions, there were like conceptions. He too speculated, as we do now, that the phenomena of life might be due to "just a peculiar arrangement of the most simple particles."

Indeed, when we read Hunter, thus translating him as we go, it is most striking to note how many of his views adapt themselves at once to modern conceptions, and I cannot but think that we underrate rather than over-estimate the influence which his labours have had in preparing a ready acceptance for the doctrines which we now teach.

I cannot leave John Hunter without saying a word concerning his friend and fellow-worker, William Hewson. Born in 1739, dying of a dissection wound in 1774, in his thirty-fifth year, while his work, so to speak, was just beginning, this gentle teacher of anatomy left behind him the record of labours which, if they be considered as epoch-making, afford a distinct contribution to knowledge, and are of such quality as to make every reader of them sincerely deplore his untimely loss. His memoir on the lymphatics, and that on the red corpuscles of the blood, in which he first pointed out that these were discs, and not spheres, as Leeuwenhoek thought, are perhaps, though admirable in their way, anatomical rather than physiological; while in his essay on the "Properties of Blood," published first in the *Philosophical Transactions* for 1770, and afterwards in a separate form in 1771 and 1772, he gave the first sound account of the coagulation of the blood, showing much more clearly than had been done before that the phenomena were due to a solidification in the liquor sanguinis, anticipating Johannes Müller in his proof that coagulation was independent of the red corpuscles, recording many discoveries which have had to be rediscovered more than once again.

John Hunter, I have said, failed to see his way because he was without the lamp of adequate chemical and physical knowledge. The physiologists of the nineteenth century are distinguished from those of the eighteenth century by this mark above all others—that the former got to know, while the latter remained ignorant of, the nature of the process of oxidation. While the western world was in throes with the labour of a new order of things, social and political, an immortal Frenchman, in the centre of the convulsions, was quietly preparing a scientific revolution, no less far-reaching in its results. If we think over what every tyro in physiology knows now, and dwell on the promise of what we are about to know, comparing the physiology of to-day with that of John Hunter, we must, I think, confess that even the work of William Harvey was less momentous in its results than the exquisite demonstration by the great Lavoisier of the true nature of respiration, so great were the clouds of darkness which that discovery rolled away.

And England may justly be proud that she too had a hand in that glorious work, for Lavoisier's path was prepared for him by the labours of an Englishman—an Englishman who, as in so many cases before, was no member of the University professoriate; no Fellow of the College of Physicians; no member even of the medical profession, but, like his forerunner Stephen Hales, a minister of religion, though a minister of an irregular, often persecuted cult. I think I am not saying too much when I assert that Joseph

Priestley, when in 1771 he showed that air rendered unfit for respiration by being breathed, or through combustion taking place in it, became under the influence of living plants once more fit for breathing; and still more when, in 1774, he atoned for his previous advocacy of phlogiston by the discovery of oxygen, won for himself the right of being called a physiological worthy.

Having reached the nineteenth century, and drawn near to matters which have been the subject of bitter controversies, well remembered, and indeed shared in, by members whom we are delighted to see able to take part in our Congress to-day, my words may fitly come to an end. But I cannot close without saying at least a word concerning three English physiologists of the first half of our century whom not ourselves only, but the whole brotherhood delights to honour.

Thomas Young I need only name, for though for some time an active member of the medical profession, though physiology owns him as one of her chiefs, on account of his admirable labours on vision, though his counsel and criticisms were of frequent value to his friends more directly engaged in physiological research, he was one of those many men whom the profession has given to sciences other than our own, and he is remembered not so much as a physiologist as the Natural Philosopher of his time.

When I mention the name of Charles Bell it is not to revive the controversies of which I just spoke, nor will I attempt here to distribute the exact meed of praise to him, to Magendie, and Johannes Müller respectively, in the all-important matter of sensory and motor nerves. I take it that all who have gone into the story are willing to admit at least this, that Charles Bell was the first to lay hold of the truth, and the first to afford approximative, though not complete, proof that sensory and motor impulses pass along different fibres, and travel to and from the spinal cord by different spinal roots. That, and that only, being admitted, the issue in 1811, though for private distribution only, of the one hundred copies of the "New Idea of an Anatomy of the Brain," becomes at once an epoch in the physiology of the central nervous system. With the subsequent firm experimental establishment of Bell's idea, the understanding of the central nervous system stepped at once from a platform which was not so very different from that of Willis, to a platform which, in its main features, is the one on which we stand to-day.

But the story of Charles Bell's great achievement, while it gives rise to congratulation, contains a warning. A careful study of his works compels one to confess that good fortune had no small share in his success. As things turned out, in one leading conception of his new idea he was right; but as one reads his memoirs, one feels that he might have gone wrong in a way which would have been impossible for the other men of whom I have spoken—Priestley and Hunter, Hayles, Boyle, and Harvey. We all know that he brought forward striking experimental proof of the distinct functions of the anterior and posterior roots of spinal nerves. We also all know that later on he refused to employ the experimental method, and relied exclusively on deductions from anatomical data, and the teachings of pathological cases. In his paper "On the Nervous Circle which connects the Voluntary Muscles of the Brain," after stating his theorem that each muscle is connected with the brain by both motor and sensory fibres, he goes on to state an imaginary experiment by which this might be proved, but warns the reader that the fibres of the nerve must be stimulated outside their origin from the central nervous system before they become mixed. And he continues thus:—"To expose these nerves near their origins, and before any filament of a sensitive nerve mingles with them, requires the operator to cut deep; to break up the bones, and to divide the bloodvessels. All such experiments are much better omitted; they can never lead to satisfactory conclusions." And again, a little later on, we find these words:—"I feel a hesitation when I reason upon any other ground than on the facts of anatomy. Experiments are more apt to be misinterpreted, and the very circumstance of a motor and sensitive nerve being generally combined together, affords a pregnant source of error."

I suppose we are all willing to admit the justice of these remarks. An anatomical fact, clear and unmistakable, is more to be trusted than the result of a complicated experiment, with a multitude of varying factors, all of which must be appreciated before the outcome is correctly interpreted. He who makes an experiment, be it on a living animal or on a dead weight, without valuing the possibilities of error, makes a bad experiment, or rather no true experiment at all. And undoubtedly our science has again and again suffered, I may say is continually suffering, from deductions rashly made from so-called experiments badly conceived and rashly carried out. But, passing on one side the reflection that the so-called facts of anatomy, when they are pushed far enough, often become dim and uncertain, and have themselves to be verified by experiment, the true philosopher, I venture to think, will reply that in the long run the difficulties of an experiment are in a way the measure of its value; that, being overcome by care and diligence, they in the end bring the greatest rewards; and that he who would enter into Nature's secrets must be prepared not to turn back at such rebuffs as at a slough of despond, until he has thoroughly satisfied himself that their amendment is above his might, that there is no path by that way. I imagine that Stephen Hales, revisiting the earth and reading Charles Bell's sentence, would have been tempted to say, "I, as a clergyman, with temptations to devote myself to other studies, have felt equally with, if not more than yourself, the repugnance to experimenting on living animals; I, as mathematician and physicist, trained in severer studies than those which have occupied you, have felt and seen as clearly, if not more clearly, than you the possible errors which the subtle fluctuations of the living flame must introduce into all physiological work; but, so far from discouraging me, these obstacles stimulated me to exacter efforts; the cognisance of them saved me from possible errors, and led me to place the physics of the circulation on a basis such as they had never had before my time."

And, indeed, the Nemesis which ever follows after errors—be they even errors committed with the best intentions, or in spite of the greatest care—overtook Charles Bell. We justly honour him as the author of the distinction between motor and sensory fibres; but that was only a part of the whole system of his new idea. That was the part which he submitted to the touchstone of experiment; that is the part which has remained, and which continues to this day, more and more abounding at once in scientific fruits and in practical benefit to mankind. The rest of his views (his nervous circles, his paths within the cerebral-spinal axis, his respiratory nervous system)—and if rumour be true, it was on these that he most prided himself—he refused to submit to experiment. And what has become of them? Are they not forgotten, or remembered only as stumbling-blocks, and rocks of offence? Nay, more, he maintained that the anterior and posterior columns, as the continuations of the anterior and posterior roots, were engaged exclusively in conveying motor and sensory impulses respectively; and, though at first his anatomical data led him to look at the cerebellum as the origin of the latter, he subsequently satisfied himself that he could trace both right up to the cerebrum. It is not, I venture to think, too much to say that the chief effect of this view has been to serve as a stumbling-block and hindrance to further inquiry. He further insisted that in the midst of the general sensori-motor nervous system there was intercalated a special nervous mechanism, of independent distribution and function, a nervous mechanism of respiration. The reader of Charles Bell's papers (where he is treating of the independence of the respiratory function) cannot but feel that, with his genius, had he not forsaken the path of experiment, he must almost inevitably, in struggling to understand the respiratory nerves, have come upon that doctrine of reflex action which was destined at once to complement, and at the same time to swallow up, the doctrine of motor and sensory fibres.

That Charles Bell accomplished as much as he did, shows how valuable are the lessons which may be learnt as simple but careful deductions from anatomical data : that he failed to accomplish more, warns us no less clearly that the teachings of anatomical deductions need to be verified or guarded by experimental research.

The mention of the word reflex action brings me to the last Englishman whom I will name to-day. And here, too, I will not attempt to revive bitter controversies, which in the memory of many living seem only just to have calmed down. I think you will agree with me that even when we have dwelt as strongly as possible on the insight expressed in the works of various anatomists and physiologists, from

Descartes downwards, where they have insisted on the independence from cerebral action of certain movements (and among these are certainly prominent several of the names which I have mentioned to-day—Willis, Boyle, Hales, and especially Robert Whytt); when we have enlarged as much as possible on the views of Prochaska and the experiments of Johannes Müller, there still remains the fact that the doctrine of reflex action became firmly established as a definite part of physiological and medical teaching largely by the labours of Marshall Hall. It was his numerous researches, and perhaps even more his enthusiastic, ingenious advocacy, and the skill with which he applied the results of the new doctrine to the practical art of healing, which brought about a revolution in our conceptions of the nervous system.

Marshall Hall may well serve as the near-point of this brief historic sketch. Names coming after him are too near the mind's eye to be brought satisfactorily into mental focus. Rather than attempt to speak of the work of men since his time, many of whom are happily still with us, I would prefer to indulge, for the few minutes still left to me, in a few reflections, which must, I think, force themselves on every English physiologist who is led to compare the present and the past.

I have, I venture to think, already said enough to show that in physiology, as well as in other sciences, certainly during the seventeenth, and though to a less extent during the eighteenth century, England held its own against other countries as regards productiveness both in quality and quantity. In the first third of the nineteenth century the three names on which I have just dwelt—Bell, Young, and Marshall Hall—present an equally satisfactory contribution from English minds to physiological science.

But we Englishmen are, I imagine, the first to admit that in the middle third, which has gone, and the latter third, which is passing, of this nineteenth century, Great Britain has not left on the physiological record a mark commensurate with the number, the intelligence, and the activity of its inhabitants. One reason is not far to seek. Across the Channel we find that the pursuit of learning is in the hands of a distinct professoriate, whose acknowledged academic function is to carry on research, and indeed the well-being of the professoriate may be taken in the several countries as the measure of scientific fruitfulness. In proportion as the universities in a country are numerous and well cared for, so that the rivalry between them becomes an incitement to labour, without leading to a commercial system of outbidding, we find research active and fruitful.

In England, leaving out for the present the other components of the United Kingdom, we have—or rather had—but two universities, those of Cambridge and Oxford; and these, as we have seen, as far as physiological science is concerned, late in the seventeenth century folded their hands for sleep.

The College of Physicians, so long as the field of science was limited and the bonds between it and the Royal Society continued close, had, more or less, an academic function, and the labours of Harvey, Glisson, Willis, and Lower were all carried on with the help or sympathy of the College. But as science widened and became differentiated, as the demands of practice became more exacting, the College lost its hold on physiological inquiry, its efforts were directed exclusively to disease, its speculative activities were wasted in the doctrines of the schools, and in the long gap from Richard Lower to Thomas Young and Marshall Hall no distinctly physiological voice of weighty tones spoke from the College hall, no name of prominent physiological worth was inscribed on the College roll.

The names of Hunter, Hewson, Bell, and many others of less moment which I might mention, suggest the reflection that the various medical schools which, at the end of the eighteenth and especially during the present century, have sprung into existence in London, might be considered as supplying the place of a university. And, indeed, had they been less numerous, they might have performed an academic function—they might have afforded homes for professed physiologists. With the ever-widening field of physiological research it has become year by year less and less possible for men to serve with success it and some other master at the same time. Men of genius, like Hunter and Bell, did so, it is true, and men like them may do it once more; but with each succeeding decade the task becomes more difficult, and

what has been is less likely to be again. As the present century has advanced it has become more and more clear that in England, as abroad, a physiologist must devote his whole life to his work. But the various competing, and in many cases small, medical schools of the metropolis were unable to afford independent physiological careers. During the middle third of the century, while Alison, Reid, and Goodsir were all professors, there was as a matter of fact one, and only one, professor of physiology in England. And it is no weak argument in support of the view which I am urging, that whatever little revival of physiology there may be in these later days, is in great measure due to him, the one real professor of physiology. Though after his earlier active years he ceased to publish much in his own name, William Sharpey had a hand in nearly every physiological work of any moment which this country produced from the fourth decade onward; his genial sympathy encouraging younger men to effort; his wide knowledge and marvellous sagacity saving many of them from error. It is idle to speculate on "the might have been," but we may at least venture so far into probabilities as to surmise that such men as Wharton Jones, whose early works were so full of grasp and insight; William Bowman, whose labours on muscle and on the kidney are still classic works, known and read of all instructed physiologists; Carpenter, whose writings have been the early physiological nature of so many of us, and others whom I need not name, would have devoted the whole of their lives instead of fragments of time, to our science. Had such been the case the nineteenth century would, I venture to think, have had no reason to be ashamed of English physiology.

At the present day careers are opening up, and a fair amount of useful work is, I trust, being done, or rather perhaps would be done had not in this country physiology fallen upon evil days of a kind unknown in the eighteenth or any other century. A zeal, not according to knowledge, has, whatever commendable impulses may have nurtured it, given rise to legislative action, which has gone far to cripple physiological research in this country. Our science has been made the subject of what the highest legal authority stated in the House of Lords to be a *penal Act*. We are liable at any moment in our inquiries to be arrested by legal prohibitions, we are hampered by licences and certificates. When we enter upon any research we do not know how far we may go before we have to crave permission to proceed, laying bare our immature ideas before those who are, in our humble opinion, unfit to judge them; and we often find our suit refused. We sigh in our bondage, like the Israelites of old; we are asked to make bricks when they have taken away from us our straw. One good fruit of the present Congress may be this, that our foreign brethren, seeing our straits, will go home determined in their respective countries to resist to the utmost all attempts to put the physiological inquirer in chains. For we surely are all agreed that experiment is the chief weapon with which we can fight against the powers of darkness of the mysteries of life. This is written in letters which he who runs may read, over all the brief story which I have ventured to tell to-day. What was true in the days of Willis is true now, and I may fitly close with the very same words with which he ends the preface to the "Cerebri Anatome":—

"Nam aut hac via scilicet per vulnera et mortes per Anatomiam et quasi Cæsareo partu, in lucem prodibit verit as aut semper latebit." "For either in this way—namely, through death and wounds, through dissection and, as it were, by a Cæsarian operation—will truth be brought to light, or otherwise will lie for ever hid."

COD-LIVER OIL.—Mr. Fairthorne suggests a new method for the administration of cod-liver oil, which consists in adding about one part of tomato or walnut catsup to four of the oil, the mixture being well shaken up before being taken. He very pertinently remarks that taking an ordinary emulsion of cod-liver oil is like eating cod fish or lobster with a dressing of sugar and gum. He has found this mixture to agree much better with many persons than any other form which they have tried. This he attributes to the association of such condiments as are generally employed as additions to food, and which experience has shown best to bring into operation those digestive faculties of the stomach which might otherwise remain dormant.—*Boston Jour.*, June 23 (from *Amer. Jour. of Pharmacy*).

REPORTS OF HOSPITAL PRACTICE

IN

MEDICINE AND SURGERY.

KING'S COLLEGE HOSPITAL.

For the notes of these cases we are indebted to Mr. W. J. Penny, Surgical Registrar, King's College Hospital.]

CASE OF RETRO-PHARYNGEAL ABSCESS POINTING IN THE PHARYNX, BUT OPENED BY AN INCISION BEHIND THE STERNO-MASTOID—CURE.

(Under the care of Mr. W. WATSON CHEYNE.)

Alfred B., aged forty-two, compositor, was admitted into hospital on April 25, complaining of dysphagia and dyspnœa. Previous history good; no specific history. About five weeks before admission, without any assignable cause, the patient noticed pain in the back of his neck, and after a few days experienced some difficulty in breathing and swallowing. This difficulty gradually increased for rather more than a fortnight, and since that time, he said, it got rather better. The patient was first seen by Mr. Cheyne on April 23, but he would not come into the hospital until the 25th, during which time, he said, his symptoms slightly subsided.

When admitted he still complained of great difficulty in breathing and swallowing, fluids only being taken; his voice was also very thick and indistinct. On examining the throat, the fauces were found much inflamed, and a swelling the size of a walnut could be seen at the back of the pharynx; this felt tense and compressible, and fluctuation could be made out in it. No swelling could be felt from the outside. The right side of the face was rather more flushed than the left, and the right pupil rather more contracted. He perpetually expectorated a quantity of tenacious muco-purulent fluid.

Operation (April 25).—Chloroform was very carefully administered, great difficulty being experienced, owing to the obstruction to the respiration, which became very stertorous. Mr. Cheyne, observing the usual antiseptic precautions, made an incision about two inches long at the posterior border of the sterno-mastoid, the incision commencing about one inch below the mastoid process; the deep cervical fascia was carefully divided, and by the finger and forceps the soft tissues were pushed aside, and a channel burrowed to the back of the pharynx. The wall of the abscess was then broken down, and about one ounce and a half of pus (free from odour) escaped. Immediately the breathing became natural. Mr. Cheyne then carefully examined the vertebræ with his finger, but could feel nothing abnormal. A large-sized drainage-tube, about four inches in length, was then introduced, some salicylic cream (composed of one part salicylic acid to five of a 5 per cent. solution of carbolic acid in glycerine) smeared over the surrounding hair, and the usual antiseptic dressings applied.

April 26.—Patient had a very good night, his breathing being much easier. Talked naturally. Fauces not so inflamed. The swelling in the pharynx was much smaller. Sputum copious, viscid, muco-purulent, slightly tinged with blood. Dressed; free discharge, sanguineo-serous, quite free from odour. Temperature, morning 99·6°, evening 99·4°; pulse 96.

27th.—Talked naturally. Swelling still smaller. Right side of face continued slightly flushed, and right pupil more contracted than the left. Dressed; free discharge; tube projected, and was shortened in consequence. Temperature, morning 98·2°, evening 98·6°; pulse 96.

28th.—Very little discharge; dressed. Pupils more equal. Temperature, morning 98·8°, evening 99·8°; pulse 84.

30th.—Very little discharge; dressed. Pupils equal, and contracted equally. Right side of face still slightly flushed. Very little swelling left in the pharynx, and that was quite hard.

After this date the patient progressed favourably, and was discharged cured on May 18, the wound being then quite healed.

Remarks.—The usual mode of opening retro-pharyngeal abscess is very unsatisfactory, and, unless great care be taken, it is dangerous. The advantage of having an opening at the side of the neck is of course evident, by thus avoiding the immediate dangers of the operation and the existence of a putrid cavity afterwards. The mode of treatment carried out in this case is advantageous in that the abscess can be treated antiseptically, and a free drainage is obtained. These points are of greatest importance when the abscess is connected with diseased vertebræ. The operation is a very simple one. As soon as the deep fascia at the posterior border of the sterno-mastoid is divided, the finger can be passed round the transverse processes of the vertebræ, and, by keeping it close to the front of the vertebræ, the vessels are pushed forwards, and the wall of the abscess is soon reached, without danger to the numerous important structures in the vicinity.

The operation was first performed by Mr. Chiene, of Edinburgh, in April, 1877, in a case of disease of the upper cervical vertebræ, with the most satisfactory results. (See British Medical Journal, vol. ii. for 1877.)

REMOVAL OF A MASS OF SCIRRHUS FROM THE AXILLA—LIGATURE OF THE AXILLARY VEIN—RECOVERY.

(Under the care of Mr. W. WATSON CHEYNE.)

Maria S., aged thirty-four, admitted into King's College Hospital, April 12, 1881.

Previous History.—Twelve months before admission, the left mamma and axillary glands were excised for scirrhus. Six months afterwards the patient noticed a hard lump, the size of a pea, in the cicatrix; this has gradually increased in size up to her admission. No other illness.

On admission, patient looked fairly healthy; in the centre of the cicatrix was a hard swelling, the size of a filbert; this was movable on the deeper parts, but seemed to extend upwards under the pectoralis major. The pectoralis was prominent, and there was a diffuse hardness to be felt which moved with the muscle. There was no œdema or pain, and the glands above the clavicle were not implicated. It was therefore thought proper to attempt the removal of the growth.

Operation (April 12).—The patient being chloroformed, a transverse elliptical incision was made so as to enclose the nodule in the cicatrix. On removing this, another nodule was felt at the edge of the pectoralis major; and on passing the finger upwards beneath the muscle, several masses of scirrhus were felt, extending as high up as the clavicle, and adherent to the pectoralis major. There seemed to be no swelling beneath the pectoralis minor, and the finger passed behind the mass at the upper part felt the artery and nerves between it and the thorax. A vertical incision through the skin was therefore made at right angles to the former, extending as high as the clavicle, and the pectoralis major was also divided in the same line. Mr. Cheyne then proceeded to remove the growths, and the portion of muscle adherent to them. At the upper part the axillary vein was found to be involved in the mass, and to be drawn forward away from the artery and nerves; the vein was ligatured above and below, and the intermediate portion removed with the mass. The cephalic vein was also divided and tied. The divided portions of the pectoralis major were then brought together with catgut stitches. Two large drainage-tubes were introduced, one into the axilla, the other across the chest; and a smaller one into the clavicular end of the vertical incision. A small horsehair drain was also introduced. The margins of the incision were then brought together with lead buttons and silver wire, the edges stitched with silver wire and silk sutures, and the usual antiseptic dressings applied. Very little difference was observed between the two arms after the operation.

April 14.—Patient had a good night, but complained of some shooting pains in the clavicular region. Wound dressed; copious sero-sanguineous discharge; looking remarkably well. There was no œdema of the arm, the only difference noticed being slight puffiness of the left hand, and slight prominence of one of the veins on the dorsum of the hand. The left hand also felt rather numb. Temperature, morning 100·2°, evening 101°; pulse, morning 116, evening 108.

15th.—Patient slept well, and took her food well, but complained of the shooting pains between her shoulders, and the numbness of the hand. Copious, sanguineo-serous discharge; dressed; looked well; no inflammation; hand less puffy. Three wire sutures removed. Temperature, morning 100·2°, evening 101°; pulse, morning 98, evening 96.

16th.—Felt well; no œdema of arm, and all puffiness of

hand gone; dressed; much less discharge; all stitches removed, incisions having healed. All the drainage-tubes shortened, and the horse-hair drain lessened. Temperature, morning 100·6°, evening 101·4°; pulse 104.

17th.—Dressed; looking well. Temperature, morning 100·2°, evening 100°; pulse 108.

19th.—Dressed.

21st.—Dressed; all tubes removed.

22nd.—There being some accumulation of discharge, another tube was introduced at the clavicular end of the incision.

24th.—Another tube introduced into axilla.

25th.—Much less discharge.

Since this dressing, the wound progressed favourably. It was dressed on April 26, 28, May 2, 6, when the tubes were again removed. And on May 11, as the wounds were quite superficial, a dressing of boracic lint was substituted for the carbolic gauze dressing, and the patient was discharged.

Remarks.—The point of interest in this case is the removal of the upper part of the axillary vein. The slight amount of œdema which followed is certainly surprising. The result seems only explicable on the supposition that a collateral venous return had already been established, owing to the difficulty which the blood must have experienced in passing through a vein which was altered in position and pressed on by a mass of scirrhus. Probably also the fact that in the former operation the contents of the axilla had been cleared out, and numerous veins tied, had something to do with the result. The absence of phlebitis is not, of course, a thing to be wondered at, seeing that the wound remained aseptic and free from inflammatory disturbance from first to last.

' PHYSICIANS AND DRUGGISTS IN PHILADELPHIA.—The Philadelphia correspondent of the *Boston Journal* (June 30) states that at the annual meeting of the Medico-Legal Society of that city much discussion took place as to the various points at issue between physicians and druggists. Several members of the Society have taken to dispensing their own medicines in consequence of the extortionate charges made by druggists and the frequency of adulteration. Dr. Peltz, in an address upon the subject, stated that very little reliance could be placed upon the purity of the drugs and the proper mode of preparation employed by the greater number of pharmacists of the city, while their charges were so excessive as to be almost prohibitive. As to the property in prescriptions, the practice of a physician was described, and approved of by those present, who reserved all the prescriptions which he wrote for those consulting him, and handed them over to a graduate in pharmacy, who, after dispensing them and forwarding the medicines to the patients, returned the prescriptions to the physician.

JUBILEE OF THE "BULLETIN DE THÉRAPEUTIQUE."—In their number for July 15, the Editorial Committee (Profs. Bouchardat, Le Fort, and Potain, and Dr. Dujardin-Beaumetz) of the *Bulletin de Thérapeutique* sing their song of joyfulness at the continued and uninterrupted success of their journal during a period of half a century, having now completed its one-hundredth volume. The first number was published by Miquel, July 15, 1831, and although the attempt seemed then a bold one, it was at once crowned with success. In the struggle which followed the fall of the doctrines of Broussais, pathological anatomy reigned supreme, and it became necessary to affirm that the great end of medicine was the cure of diseases. This was what Miquel did by founding a journal exclusively devoted to therapeutics, in which might be received, accumulated, and co-ordinated all the facts bearing upon the treatment of medical and surgical diseases, enabling them by this publicity to be submitted to renewed investigations. Miquel dying sixteen years afterwards, his work was successfully carried on by Debout, Brichetean, Gauchet, Dolbeau, and the present editors, who exclaim, "It is not without a deep sense of pride that we contemplate this unique collection of a hundred volumes, wherein are found all the facts observed relating to medical and surgical therapeutics during fifty years, whether in France or abroad, accumulated under such different directors, without their ever departing for an instant from the line of probity and honour traced by the founder."

TERMS OF SUBSCRIPTION.
(*Free by post.*)

British Islands	Twelve Months	. £1 8 0
"	Six "	. 0 14 0
The Colonies and the United } States of America }	Twelve "	. 1 10 0
" "	Six "	. 0 15 0
India	Twelve "	. 1 10 0
" (viâ Brindisi)	"	. 1 15 0
"	Six "	. 0 15 0
" (viâ Brindisi)	"	. 0 17 6

Foreign Subscribers are requested to inform the Publishers of any remittance made through the agency of the Post-office.

Single Copies of the Journal can be obtained of all Booksellers and Newsmen, price Sixpence.

Cheques or Post-office Orders should be made payable to Mr. JAMES LUCAS, 11, New Burlington-street, W.

TERMS FOR ADVERTISEMENTS.

Seven lines (70 words)	. .	£0 4 6
Each additional line (10 words)	.	0 0 6
Half-column, or quarter-page	.	1 5 0
Whole column, or half-page	.	2 10 0
Whole page	. . .	5 0 0

Births, Marriages, and Deaths are inserted Free of Charge.

THE MEDICAL TIMES AND GAZETTE *is published on Friday morning: Advertisements must therefore reach the Publishing Office not later than One o'clock on Thursday.*

Medical Times and Gazette.

SATURDAY, AUGUST 27, 1881.

MR. HUTCHINSON'S ADDRESS.

WE this week place in full in the hands of our readers the address delivered by Mr. Hutchinson at Ryde. It is entitled, as usual, "The Address in Surgery," though anything but surgery is the theme of it. Mr. Hutchinson, remembering that medical men had just had a surfeit of science and art, surgical and medical, very wisely avoided these matters, so far as practice and science are concerned, and instead laid before his hearers some thoughts on surgical ethics, surgical education, and on the best means of advancing the clinical knowledge of disease. All these matters are subjects of very great interest and importance; upon each and all of them very much can be said; and certainly the profession will be very glad to hear Mr. Hutchinson's thoughts about them. His address is eminently suggestive; it is full of opinions, thoughts, suggestions, propositions, etc., that are sure to meet with much and careful consideration, and nearly as sure, some of them at least, to excite not a little criticism, if not opposition. The subject first dealt with is that of specialism—that is, special hospitals and specialties. He would not oppose the beginning of any specialty, however detailed; and for two reasons. First, opposition is useless: we cannot prevent the establishment of special hospitals, or the development of specialties in practice. And secondly, because they are a gain. The first reason is philosophical. Accept the inevitable, Mr. Hutchinson says; but he does not stop there, he wisely adds—employ and use it. Insist that special hospitals shall not be close boroughs; insist upon open elections of officers, and free admissions of students and practitioners; and above all, insist upon, or at least encourage, the formation and development of special departments in our general hospitals. As to the gains from the "detailed cultivation" of special branches of medical and surgical practice, Mr. Hutchinson points to the immense advances made in ophthalmology, in dermatology, and in other departments of practice since educated members of the profession began to make them respectively the special subjects of clinical cultivation and scientific research. And he more than suggested that we shall have yet greater subdivisions of the great field of labour than any we have yet seen; for, special cultivation of branches of practice " creates new departments before unthought of, into which science pushes its way," and gives marked help towards the mitigation of the diseases and disabilities of man. Mr. Hutchinson adds, with just a suspicion of maliciousness—if one can suspect him of such a thing—that he ranks among the gains from detailed cultivation of this kind that it "has a definite tendency to destroy specialisms as such, and add their conquered territory to the general possessions."

Thus far, Mr. Hutchinson's opinions and arguments will meet, no doubt, with general acceptance. He next takes up a very delicate subject, and treads on very tender ground. He proceeds to speak and to argue in favour of consultations " with those who, whilst educated amongst us, have openly professed their adoption of peculiar principles "—i.e., with homœopaths; and our readers will find in our pages the paragraphs concerning this matter which were omitted from his address when it was delivered at Ryde. He does not deal with the whole subject of homœopathy, as Dr. Bristowe did ; and the position he takes up in speaking of " the inexpediency of continuing to refuse formal consultations " with homœopaths is less untenable, we think, than is Dr. Bristowe's. The latter mercilessly exposes the follies and weaknesses of homœopathy, and denounces it as a palpable imposture ; and then says, " I shall not discuss the question whether we can with propriety, or with benefit to our patients, meet homœopaths in consultation," and adds, " I could, however, I think, adduce strong reasons in favour of the morality of acting thus, and for the belief that good to the patient would generally ensue under such circumstances." While Mr. Hutchinson grounds his argument for such consultations mainly, if not entirely, on the probable benefit to the patient. He does not in the least defend or palliate homœopathy. Speaking of Hahnemann, he says : "his facts were few, his reasoning illogical, his ignorance of the natural progress of disease, and its tendencies to spontaneous recovery, such as would be utterly disgraceful in the present day," and so on ; but he is tender toward human weaknesses and temptations ; and he speaks of the fostering tendencies of opposition (a dangerous argument). He rests, however, as we have said, his plea on our duty to the public. "We enjoy a law-established monopoly in the art of healing, and we must be very careful how we stint or refuse our services when they are demanded." We should not assume an irreconcilable difference of opinion ; but unless the existence of such difference is established by previous special knowledge, it should be established at the bedside. It seems to him that the claims of the public should stand first, and that if a man's name is on the Medical Register (Dr. Bristowe also would require this) we ought to meet him, so long as the consultations result in that which we deem most for the patient's advantage. " Whenever they do not, our duty is clear, and we should readily know how to perform it."

We cannot enter further into this subject now, and we have left ourselves neither time nor space for the consideration of Mr. Hutchinson's other and very important themes. Much more has to be said and considered, however, before the question raised by Dr. Bristowe and Mr. Hutchinson can be settled ; but, in parting from the subject for the present, we will remind our readers that, in 1851, Sir Benjamin Brodie wrote :—" To join with homœopathists in attendance on cases of either medical or surgical disease, would be neither

wise nor honest. The object of a medical consultation is the good of the patient ; and we cannot suppose that any such result can arise from the interchange of opinions, where the views entertained, or professed to be entertained, by one of the parties as to the nature and treatment of disease, are wholly unintelligible to the other."

SEWAGE-FARMING.

THE best mode of dealing with our sewage is a question still undecided, and steadily growing more and more urgent. Shall we simply throw it away, or shall we utilise it ? If the latter, by what method ? Injunctions against the pollution of rivers are being issued on all sides, and it becomes daily more important that the rival claims of the irrigationists and precipitationists to the possession of the best methods of so depurating sewage as to permit of its discharge into our natural watercourses, ;without detriment to their subsequent employment as sources of water-supply for drinking and domestic use, should, if possible, be determined. In strictly correct language, however, there is no such thing as a precipitation process, all ammonia compounds being soluble ; and the dispute resolves itself, on impartial examination, into the question whether the organic matters can be intercepted and removed more completely and more profitably by filtration through the soil and by the agency of growing vegetation, or by means of chemical reagents, as charcoal, lime, etc. We are strongly inclined to think most favourably of irrigation—i.e., of direct utilisation, and through it depuration,—but it must be admitted that the effluent waters from Sillar's (the A B C) and General Scott's processes are nearly as pure as those from well-managed sewage farms, and though not actually potable, may be safely discharged into running streams of moderate size, and there left to the oxidising influences of air and water. It may be granted also, for argument's sake, that there may be places where land is not available for irrigation, as in the environs of rapidly growing, and especially of manufacturing, towns, though even there the expense of conducting the sewage by one or more culverts some distance into the country would involve merely an initial, and by no means a ruinous, outlay. The success of all so-called precipitation schemes, viewed as commercial undertakings, depends on the finding of a ready sale for their products, labour and cost of carriage being as important factors in the result as the actual manurial or market value of the manufactured article. In irrigation, on the other hand, there is absolutely no expenditure on machinery, chemicals, or carriage to be set against the proceeds ; the cost of labour is but small, or rather is nil, since it corresponds to the ultimate employment of the manure by the purchaser in other methods ; and the profits are immediate, and unaffected by any accidental contingencies. These are facts which cannot be denied. The objections commonly urged against irrigation are of a different kind, and are, we think, founded on ignorance or misconception.

The chief of these is the popular fear that the diffusion of sewage over extensive areas will give rise to emanations of the same noxious character as those which are well known to be produced in closed or open sewers, and especially to the propagation of enteric fever and other zymotic diseases ; or that, at the least, a nuisance will be created, leading to the deterioration in value of adjoining property. Another objection, which was persistently urged by the late Mr. Alfred Smee, is that the health of animals pastured on sewage farms must suffer in some way, and their flesh and milk be, therefore, rendered more or less unwholesome. That this objection has any solid foundation whatever has yet to be proved ; and though it may be conceded, as a mere possibility, that the ova of *tænia* might be found on the fodder of a sewage farm, and thus be swallowed by the cattle, it is absurd to suppose that crude organic matter can be taken up unchanged into the vegetable tissues. Lastly, there is the apprehension that the soil may be incapable of getting rid of such a volume of fluid as is employed in irrigation, and may be converted into a fetid swamp.

All these objections are completely refuted by the experience of the Local Board of Health of Croydon, extending over twenty years, whose sewage farm at Beddington, the members of the late Congress had, through the kindness of Dr. Alfred Carpenter, an opportunity of visiting. The degree of success already achieved there is the more satisfactory since the work has hitherto been carried on under the most unfavourable circumstances; the soil being poor, heavy, and ill adapted for irrigation, and the land, until the present year, held on lease at an exorbitant rental. No attempt has been made to exclude the rainfall or storm waters from the higher districts from the sewage; while the same false economy has led the managers to the rejection from their scheme of all market-gardening (a most profitable form of sewage culture), and to stint to the lowest possible figure their outlay on farm buildings, labour, and even the necessary means of irrigation. Besides, the Committee of Management includes neither scientific men nor practical agriculturists. Yet their success has been so encouraging that they have purchased the freehold of the estate, and are about to carry out considerable improvements, erecting new buildings and substituting concrete culverts for the larger ditches which required constant cleansing by manual labour.

The total area of the farm is 540 acres, but of these only 450 are regularly irrigated. On these is poured daily the sewage of about 68,000 persons, averaging in dry weather 2,000,000 gallons, but rising, when the rainfall is added, to sometimes twice that volume, with no further treatment than a coarse straining to separate sticks, rags, paper, and such solid masses. The sewage is conveyed to every part of the estate by a system of channels and feeders, and turned on to each field in order for twelve to twenty-four hours at a time. The smallest trenches are dammed at intervals by boards, to distribute the flow over the land. After having been thus filtered through one field, it is conducted in like manner to a second or a third before it is allowed to pass into the river Wandle.

The effluent water is clear and devoid of taste and smell, and numbers of young fish may be seen in the conduit by which it leaves the farm. Even in parts actually submerged to the depth of an inch or more, no odour is perceptible; none anywhere, in fact, save in the neighbourhood of an uncleansed ditch, and there not to be compared with the stench arising from the turning over of an ordinary dunghill.

In short, it may be now taken as proved that sewage in a state of minute subdivision and of intimate contact with fresh earth does not undergo the septic changes to which it is prone in mass. On this depends the sanitary success of the earth-closet; but the sewage farm presents this advantage: that while the growing vegetation, constantly removing organic matter from the land, keeps it from becoming surcharged therewith, it at the same time avoids that prolonged, and therefore complete and destructive, oxidation of the organic matter which detracts so much from the fertilising power of the earth from the closet.

The principal crop, as on all sewage farms, is Italian rye-grass, a plant whose powers of absorption are enormous. On common pastures it yields two crops in a season; here it is cut seven times, each crop averaging fifty to sixty tons, and worth £5 to £6 per acre. It is mostly used as green fodder, but there is no reason why it should not be made into hay, which would find a ready sale. Mangel-wurzel is also largely

grown. These crops are specially suited for sewage culture, but none need be excluded, and good fields of wheat may now be seen on land which has not been irrigated since the corn was sown. The cattle kept on the farm are fattened for the butcher solely on its produce at the rate of four head per acre, ordinary pastures supporting not more than one. This is a most important fact in relation to the problem of our meat supply.

The question of the influence of sewage farms on the health of the surrounding population has also been conclusively settled by the farm under consideration. The population of the adjacent town of Croydon has risen in the past decade from 53,000 to 77,000, and the birth-rate, which always entails a proportionate mortality, is unusually high, yet the death-rate of Croydon has steadily decreased, until for several years it has not exceeded 16 per 1000—that of London being 22. In Beddington it is only 14 in a population of 5000, many of whom unwittingly drink the effluent water, as is shown by the rise in the nearest wells which follows each irrigation. In the very midst of the farm stands the Orphan Asylum, and the visitors had an opportunity of bearing witness to the healthy appearance of the girls—165 in number. About one death has occurred yearly from phthisis or tubercular disease; there has not been a fatal case of any zymotic disease.

All opposition in the neighbourhood has been disarmed by experience, and the value of property in Beddington has doubled in the last ten years, the proximity of the sewage farm not having deterred the wealthy citizens of London from erecting their villas around. All claims for compensation made against the projectors of similar schemes have therefore no foundation in fact, and should be strenuously opposed.

Sewage farms are on sanitary grounds unobjectionable; they offer a complete solution of the problem of how to dispose of town sewage, and commercially they are a proved success. Great as is the profit derived from their extraordinary productiveness, which would amply justify the investment in them, of larger capital than has hitherto been bestowed upon them, it would be still greater if rain and surface waters were excluded from the sewage and conveyed by separate channels to the nearest rivers. "It would also be wise in future to utilise the sewage of towns on small areas at the outfalls from their own particular watersheds, or as near as practicable, rather than to concentrate it so as to make greater depôts, which from their very magnitude are more difficult to be disposed of." Such is the advice of Dr. Carpenter, whose long attention to the subject gives weight to his opinion.

THE WEEK.

TOPICS OF THE DAY.

THE deputation which we last week announced was to be introduced to the President of the Local Government Board by Sir C. Mills, M.P., duly waited upon that gentleman for the purpose of directing attention to the pollution of the lower reaches of the Thames, occasioned by the sewage outfalls at Barking and Crossness, and the urgent necessity for some legislative measure to abate the nuisance, and thereby improve the sanitary condition of the riparian districts. Amongst those who attended were—Dr. Jessett, Medical Officer of Health for Erith; Captain Gillett, of the *Warspite*; Mr. Bailey, of the East and West India Docks; and Mr. Edward Kimber, a member of the Plumstead Sanitary Authority. Mr. Bailey, in introducing the question, drew particular attention to the largely increasing deposits of mud in the India Docks, which he attributed almost entirely to the discharge of sewage matter from the outfalls. Captain

Gillett said that at certain times, more especially in July, the surface of the river became slate-coloured, instead of retaining its usual muddy hue. In reply, Mr. Dodson said he had listened with great interest to the remarks of the various speakers. It had been stated that nausea and sickness were occasioned in consequence of the offensive state of the river, but there had been no direct complaints of ill-health arising from the nuisance. He should like to know if it was the fact that there was more illness among those resident on the banks, or among men employed on the river, than there was formerly. The deputation appeared to be unable to answer this inquiry, but Captain Gillett explained that in former years cases of typhoid fever had occurred on board the *Warspite*, which were attributed to the pollution of the river. With the usual stereotyped promises from Mr. Dodson, the deputation concluded the interview, and withdrew.

Rather curiously, the annual report of the Conservators of the Thames for the year 1880 was made public on the same day that the deputation, as above reported, waited upon Mr. Dodson. It states that, with the object of preventing pollution, the Conservators have caused a rigid inspection to be maintained over the river, and likewise over the tributaries within ten miles of the Thames. The sewage works at the various places above the intakes of the water companies having been completed, the sewage formerly discharged directly into the river has been diverted. Occasionally some defect in the action of these works is discovered, when steps are immediately taken, by legal proceedings if necessary, to cause the defect to be remedied. On the tributaries many offensive and injurious discharges have been stopped, and several local authorities and other persons are now under the notices required to be given by the Conservancy Acts, to discontinue the flow of sewage and of other offensive and injurious matter into the affluents of the Thames. During hot weather, when there has been little rainfall, complaints of the pollution of the river within and below the metropolitan district frequently reach the Conservators. The pollution thus complained of is indicated by the offensive odour and highly discoloured state of the water. The report further observes that it must be remembered that Kingston and Richmond, and other places below the intakes of the water companies, still pass their sewage into the river, the penalties for their doing so having been suspended by the Legislature, to give time for overcoming the difficulties of carrying out a complete sewage system for this district; and although the discharges from these places may in some degree affect the purity of the river near the metropolis, it can hardly be doubted that the chief cause of the polluted state of the river within and below the metropolis arises from the discharge at the outfalls and storm outlets of the Metropolitan Board of Works, in whose district ordinary sewage is excepted from the provisions of the purification sections of the Conservancy Acts.

The Corporation of Brighton, a short time since, decided to erect a large sanatorium at the cost of about £15,000 on a site near the parochial cemetery on the north-east side of the town; but, being pressed by the Board of Guardians to give immediate relief to the workhouse infirmary, they have within the past few weeks erected, at the cost of £5000, a large wooden building, which will be used as a sanatorium, upon a part of the site already referred to. The structure consists of three blocks of buildings; the centre block will be used for administrative purposes, and on each side of this are elongated wards, one block being for male, and the other for female, patients. Only the end walls of the buildings are constructed of masonry, but all the necessary offices have been substantially erected, and, when

recently inspected by the Mayor and several members of the Town Council, the opinion was freely expressed that the building will meet all the requirements of the town for many years to come.

A meeting of the Commons Preservation Society was recently held at the private residence of the President, Lord Mount-Temple, when a large number of influential members attended. A letter, heartily approving the Society's aims and the manner in which these are persevering enforced, was sent by the Right Hon. Henry Fawcett, M.P., a vice-president of the Society. Speeches were made and resolutions were passed in support of the cause which this influential body advocates with great earnestness and practical effort. The work, as one of the speakers impressively observed, is one that, once done, is accomplished for ever, and if not done now can never be done hereafter. It was remarked, as a matter on which the Society and the public may fairly congratulate themselves, that not only is the present Government, as a whole, friendly to the objects in view, but it is also well represented in the list of vice-presidents and on the general committee. It may suffice to mention the names of Mr. Fawcett, Sir Charles Dilke, Earl Granville, and Sir William Harcourt, as proof that the preservation of open spaces is now authoritatively recognised as a national benefit and necessity.

At a recent representative meeting of prominent townsmen, held at Southampton, under the presidency of the Mayor, it was unanimously resolved to confirm the accepted invitation by the British Association at Swansea, to hold next year's meetings at Southampton, which was selected in competition with Leicester, Southport, and Nottingham. The financial difficulties in which the town of Swansea had become involved through the expenditure for affording the necessary accommodation were fully considered, and the forty gentlemen present subscribed and guaranteed a sum of about £350 to form the nucleus of £1500, the maximum sum required. It was announced that the whole of the large public companies had promised their warmest support. One of the reasons given for the selection of Southampton was its contiguity to Osborne, which would enable Prince Leopold, the President of the Association, to attend. The arrangements are now in the hands of an influential local committee, and a deputation will proceed to York upon the occasion of the Association's meeting of this year, to renew the invitation on the part of the town.

At the last meeting of the Metropolitan Asylums Board, authority was given for the defence of certain actions brought against the Managers; and a letter written by the Local Government Board to several ratepayers in London-fields was read, regretting that the ratepayers should have taken alarm at the establishment of a station in George-street, London-fields, for the ambulances employed in the removal of small-pox patients to the hospital-ships now moored off Greenwich. The Board pointed out that it was necessary that some place should be selected as a depôt for the ambulances, and the spot chosen was the most convenient one for the purpose; in fact, it was very doubtful whether any other premises could be obtained. They had also caused the station to be visited by their inspector, who had inquired into the arrangements made for preventing the spread of contagion; and from the information received they believed that no danger would arise, and the regulations being much more strict than previously, the effect would be an increase of safety to the public. The Board believed there would be no real danger to the neighbouring population, and impressed upon the public the desirability of promoting vaccination and revaccination. Official returns were presented, showing a decrease of 234 small-pox cases under treatment, as compared with the return at the previous meeting, and the Board then adjourned for the recess until September 3.

THE HONORARY SECRETARY-GENERAL OF THE INTERNATIONAL MEDICAL CONGRESS.

WE are informed that the Prime Minister has signified to Mr. Mac Cormac Her Majesty's gracious intention of conferring upon him the honour of knighthood, in recognition of his long-continued, laborious, and eminently successful work in arranging and managing in all ways the late International Medical Congress. We heartily congratulate Mr. Mac Cormac on receiving an honour so exceptionally well-deserved; and we feel sure that all our brethren will agree with him in regarding the distinction thus conferred upon him as also a recognition of the labours of his able assistants, and of the important position of the medical profession.

THE PARIS WEEKLY RETURN.

THE number of deaths for the thirty-second week, terminating August 11, 1881, was 1138 (625 males and 513 females), and among these there were from typhoid fever 38, small-pox 25, measles 18, scarlatina 11, pertussis 8, diphtheria and croup 34, dysentery 3, erysipelas 4, and puerperal infections 7. There were also 44 deaths from tubercular and acute meningitis, 12 from acute bronchitis, 43 from pneumonia, 184 from infantile athrepsia (53 of the infants having been wholly or partially suckled), and 47 violent deaths. The amelioration noted for the preceding week has not continued, the number of deaths having increased by 80, these being principally due to diseases of the cerebro-spinal apparatus and circulatory systems, the deaths from typhoid also increasing from 19 to 38, and the sudden deaths from 28 to 47. The number of admissions for typhoid also increased from 50 to 87, while the number of cases treated à domicile has also almost doubled, so that it is to be feared that the number of deaths from it will continue to increase rather than decrease. The births for the week amounted to 1163, viz., 620 males (457 legitimate and 163 illegitimate) and 543 females (389 legitimate and 154 illegitimate); 101 children (55 males and 46 females) were born dead or died within twenty-four hours.

THE ETIOLOGY AND ANATOMY OF ENDOMETRITIS.

DR. KARL RUGE, in a contribution to the Zeitschrift für Geburtshülfe und Gynäkologie describes the morbid anatomy of endometritis. He distinguishes three forms of the disease—the interstitial, the glandular, and the mixed form. The interstitial form is characterised by general thickening and softening of the uterine lining membrane, due to the infiltration of the tissue with small round cells; the vessels are enlarged and tortuous, the glands unaffected. The glandular form is marked by increase in the gland tissue; the glands are widened, and diverticula branch from them in all directions; the membrane looks finely cystic or sieve-like, and is greatly thickened. In the mixed form these changes may either be combined, or they may be found quite separate and distinct at different parts of the same uterus. The interstitial form histologically approaches sarcoma; the glandular form is allied to adenoma. The interstitial form may occur at any age; the glandular form is more common in the later years of sexual life. Child-bearing is a predisposing cause for each kind; the twenty-six cases examined by Dr. Ruge, excluding three who had no children, had had on an average six children each. Dr. Ruge's "interstitial" form seems to us identical with that described by Olshausen under the name of "chronic hyperplastic endometritis." If so, it is a pity that writers cannot agree to give the same name to the same thing. As

Dr. Ruge quotes Olshausen, he is aware of that author's work, and doubtless has good reason for inventing a new name; but he does not state the reason for discarding Olshausen's term.

NEGLECTED INQUIRIES.

WE have more than once called the attention of medical men to the importance of giving notice to the Registrar of any change of address. But, further, they will do well to take note of the fact that, by the 14th Section of the Medical Act, they are liable to have their names erased from the Register if they omit to answer the Registrar's inquiries in regard to their addresses. The following excerpt from the inquiry form shows how careful they should be to answer these inquiries. All that is required of them is to state in the form whether the printed address (cut out of the Register and pasted on the form) is correct, or, if not, to correct it. The duty is easy and clear; yet it is to be feared many practitioners have neglected it, and consequently, unless they communicate with the Registrar, incurred the risk of finding, in the next edition of the Register, that their names have been removed from it.

Important Notice.—" Every registered medical practitioner should be careful to send to the branch registrar, by whom he was originally registered, immediate notice of any change in his address, *and also to answer any inquiries that may be sent to him by the Registrar in regard thereto*, in order that his correct address may be duly inserted in the Medical Register; otherwise, by Section 14 of the 'Medical Act (1858),' such practitioner is liable to have his name erased from the Medical Register, and thus, by Sections 31 to 37 of the said Act, to lose the right to hold certain appointments, to sign valid certificates, or to recover, in any court of law, charges for professional aid, advice, and visits, and the cost of any medicines or other medical or surgical appliances rendered or supplied by him to his patients." Alterations or corrections in answer to this inquiry should be sent to the Registrar of the General Medical Council and of the Branch Medical Council for England, to the following address :—W. J. C. Miller, Medical Council Office, 315, Oxford-street, London, W.

Form to be returned signed, and, if necessary, corrected.

Name.	Address.	Date and place of registration.	Qualifications.

INTERNATIONAL MEDICAL AND SANITARY EXHIBITION, 1881.

THE Medical and Sanitary Exhibition, organised by the Committee of the Parkes Museum, was open for the last time on Saturday, August 13, when the number of visitors, exclusive of season-ticket holders, was 1221—making a total of 24,333 visitors for the four weeks during which the Exhibition has been open, allowing only for one visit by each season-ticket holder. The exhibitors generally have expressed themselves as well satisfied with the result of the Exhibition, some going so far as to say that they had done an exceptional amount of business, owing to the fact that a very large proportion of the visitors had been either medical men, architects, or engineers. The closing of the Exhibition was taken advantage of by the St. John Ambulance Association, to give a demonstration of ambulance practice, and during the afternoon a large number of the visitors assembled in the conservatory to witness the practice, which was conducted by Major Duncan, Mr. Cantlie (of Charing-cross Hospital), Mr. Furley, Dr. Crookshank, and Surgeon-Major Baker. Prizes were competed for by squads of the Grenadier Guards, the Finsbury Rifles, and the Metropolitan Police. Mr. John Eric Erichsen (the Chairman), Dr. Poore, Dr. Steele, Mr. George Godwin, Mr. Rogers Field, and other members of the Exhibition Committee, were present during the day. It is expected that the prizes which have been awarded will be distributed at the annual meeting of the Parkes Museum in the autumn.

LAPAROTOMY DURING PREGNANCY.

PROFESSOR SCHROEDER, of Berlin, in a communication to the *Zeitschrift für Geburtshülfe und Gynäkologie*, gives his experience of ovariotomy during pregnancy, and of the complication of pregnancy with uterine fibroids, including a case in which he removed two myomata by abdominal section during pregnancy. The first subject we need not refer to, as upon it Mr. Spencer Wells's (whose paper Professor Schroeder does not seem to have read) much larger experience has been put before the profession. But the latter operation, removal of uterine fibroids, involves, of course, much more interference with the uterus than the extirpation of an ovarian cyst, and the cases in which it has been done during pregnancy are few, if there are any. In Professor Schroeder's case, the main tumour reached to the ribs, and grew by a broad pedicle from the right side of the uterus. The omentum was connected to the tumour by many very vascular adhesions. The tumour was so closely squeezed in between the uterus below and to the left, and the liver above and to the right, that the incision had to be prolonged almost to the ensiform cartilage. The pedicle was tied with a double ligature, and the tumour removed. Two other small subserous fibroids were then removed. Twenty-four sutures were required to close the abdominal wound. Several other fibroids, which it was not practicable to remove, were left untouched. The patient recovered without interruption, and was delivered of a living child five months after the operation.

BROMIDE OF POTASSIUM IN HÆMOPTYSIS.—Dr. Frans Heller relates (in the *Allg. Wien. Med. Zeit.*, July 26) the remarkable success which attended the use of this remedy in an attack of hæmoptysis occurring in a case of phthisis, and in which the subcutaneous injection of ergotine had been tried with but little effect. There was a good deal of fever, with sleeplessness and persistent cough. A gramme and a half of the bromide was administered three times a day in sugared water. The relief of the hæmoptysis and of the congestion of the lung was almost immediate, and in a short time the patient was well enough to leave for a warmer climate.

CASE OF DIABETES INSIPIDUS.—M. Duguet has been treating a case of simple polyuria occurring in a woman, the details of which have been published in the *Gaz. des Hop.* by M. Duplaix. Notwithstanding the abundance of the urine (eight litres), and the quantity of liquid constantly taken by the patient, no sugar has ever been found, the urea has always been in its normal proportion, and a density of 1010 has never been attained. It became necessary to ascertain the cause of this polyuria, and diabetes mellitus being excluded, the hypotheses of renal sclerosis and diabetes insipidus remained. In favour of the first there was the age of the patient (fifty-six), as well as prior lumbar pains and some disturbance of vision, which had continued for some time; but, on the other hand, none of the important signs of interstitial nephritis were present, amid others the *bruit de galop* of the heart. Nor did the stomach, the eyes, or the encephalon present any of the ordinary accidents of renal sclerosis. Moreover, in that affection the polyuria would be capricious and bear no relation with the amount of fluid drank, which is contrary to what is observed in the present case. If to this we add that there is intense polydipsia in direct proportion to the polyuria, with a total absence of albumen, the diagnosis of diabetes insipidus would seem to be established.—*Rev. Méd.*, July 16.

INTERNATIONAL MEDICAL CONGRESS.

SECTIONAL WORK.

IN the Sub-section for Diseases of the Throat, the Chairman (Dr. George Johnson), after a cordial welcome to the members, made a few remarks on the great advantage which had accrued to general medicine from the introduction of the laryngoscope, and then called upon Signor Manuel Garcia to give his account of "The Invention of the Laryngoscope." Signor Garcia said that, while investigating the mode in which the voice was produced, the idea occurred to him that it would throw the greatest possible light on the subject could he only succeed in seeing the vocal apparatus actually at work; and he described how it suddenly flashed across his mind that, by a suitable arrangement of mirrors, this might be accomplished. He immediately applied to Charrière, of Paris, who gave him a dentist's mirror, by means of which and a reflector he was enabled to get his first view of his own larynx. Signor Garcia's address was received with much enthusiasm.

Dr. Rumbold (of St. Louis) read a paper on the use of the Spray-Producer in making Applications to the Superior Portion of the Respiratory Tracts. He dwelt on the importance of removing morbid secretions from, and applying remedies to, every portion of the affected surface without causing the least irritation, and stated that, in his opinion, the spray-producer was the only instrument which fulfilled these indications.

The discussion on the important subject of the Local Treatment of Diphtheria was opened by Dr. Morell Mackenzie, whose conclusions seemed to meet with general approval. He advised ice in the first stage, and steam inhalations when the false membrane begins to separate. Solvents, such as lime-water and lactic acid, and antiseptics, of which chloral hydrate is the most certain, may be used; but he stated that of late years he had relied solely on the application of varnishes, so as to exclude air from the false membrane. He employed one part of tolu dissolved in five of ether. Caustics were said to be always injurious, whilst astringents are useless and sometimes hurtful. The only speaker who advocated the opposite plan of treatment was Dr. Meyer (of Copenhagen), who read, for Dr. Nix, a Danish general practitioner, a paper in which scraping off the false membrane and free cauterisation of the raw surface was strongly advised. In his reply, Dr. Mackenzie stated that this plan had been tried in England, in 1856-57, with disastrous results.

Professor Krishaber (of Paris), who opened the discussion on the "Pathology of Laryngeal Phthisis," pointed out that the lesions depend upon a local tuberculosis, even when at the post-mortem the presence of tubercles in the tissue of the larynx can no longer be demonstrated. He was of opinion that tubercular laryngitis presents such well-marked characters that its diagnosis, with the aid of the laryngoscope, is very easy. Professor Rossbach (of Würzburg) considered it impossible to recognise laryngoscopically the deposition of tubercles in the larynx before or during the period of ulceration, and he spoke of the difficulty in distinguishing between tubercular and syphilitic ulceration unless there were signs of pulmonary consumption, though the different behaviour of the two to iodide of potassium would assist in the differentiation. Dr. Fränkel (of Berlin) did not agree with the latter statement, as he had seen undoubted phthisical laryngitis improve under the use of the iodide. There was considerable difference of opinion as to the existence of primary laryngeal tubercle; those who believed in its existence said that it was always eventually complicated by pulmonary lesions. There was a general agreement that the disease was not to be regarded as an incurable one, and that success in the treatment of pulmonary phthisis ought to stimulate further efforts to cure laryngeal phthisis.

Professor Gerhardt (of Würzburg) drew attention to the fact that the question of nervous disorders of the larynx, which, a short time ago, seemed fully solved, had assumed at the present time a wholly new aspect in consequence of recent researches, referring especially to the doubtful innervation of the crico-thyroid muscle, and to the proclivity of the abductor fibres of the recurrent nerve to disease both of central and peripheral origin, in cases in which apparently the whole of the nerve was involved. Professor Lefferts (of New York) proposed a new classification of these cases. As a practical outcome of this discussion it may be broadly stated that paralysis of the abductors points to organic disease, whereas paralysis of the adductors is usually of functional origin.

Professor Schnitzler (of Vienna) and Dr. Elsberg (of New York) contributed papers on "Neuroses of Sensation of the Pharynx and Larynx,"—that of the latter being read in his absence by Dr. Morell Mackenzie. The brief space at our disposal prevents us from doing more than allude to this complicated and difficult subject.

Professor Rossbach (of Würzburg) made some valuable and practical remarks on the formation of Mucus in the Larynx and Trachea, and he stated that it depended exclusively upon peripheral nerve-cells situated within the mucous membrane itself. He gave a list of means of augmenting or diminishing the flow.

Dr. Bayer's (of Brussels) paper on the "Influence of the Female Sexual Apparatus on the Vocal Organ and Formation of Voice" was a carefully thought-out treatise on the interdependence of the two. In the discussion which followed, Dr. Fränkel (of Berlin) and Dr. Semon insisted upon the importance of not giving too hopeful a prognosis, as cure of disease of the generative system was not invariably followed by a disappearance of the aphonia, etc., which appeared to be dependent on the former.

Dr. Fauvel (of Paris) and Professor Burow (of Königsberg) introduced the discussion on "Indications for Extra- or Intra-Laryngeal Treatment of Growths in the Larynx," and a very animated debate followed. After alluding to the curious difference existing between surgeons and laryngologists on this question, Professor Burow declared emphatically that every benign laryngeal tumour ought, if possible, to be removed per vias naturales; and only if an experienced laryngologist has established the inexpediency of this method may the extra-laryngeal be adopted. Dr. Semon pointed out that, in view of the grave dangers liable to accrue from the use of intra-laryngeal instruments by the inexperienced, the removal of laryngeal growths must necessarily be limited to the specialist; and this was generally agreed to. The outcome of this discussion was to support the view of the gentlemen who read the introductory papers, namely, that the intra-laryngeal method should be employed if possible; some of the speakers made a partial exception, insomuch that they recommended thyrotomy in certain cases.

Dr. Koch (of Luxemburg) and Dr. Hering (of Warsaw) opened the discussion on the "Results of the Mechanical Treatment of Laryngeal Stenosis." The former spoke of the importance of seeing that the morbid process was at an end before adopting any method of dilatation. Dr. Hering's statistics comprised 100 cases, and his paper was of a most systematic and complete character. He insisted on the fact that comparatively unfavourable results of this plan of treatment were to be explained by want of patience, perseverance, and energy of either surgeon or patient.

Dr. Foulis (of Glasgow) in opening the discussion on the "Indications for the Complete or Partial Extirpation of the Larynx," based his remarks on the result of an examination of all the recorded cases, a chart of which, completed after the plan in Dr. Morell Mackenzie's work, was brought before the meeting. The surgeons advocated a more general employment of this procedure than seemed desirable to the laryngologists. The interest of the debate was much increased by the participation in it of Professor Czerny (of Heidelberg), whose experiments on dogs first demonstrated the possibility of the performance of this operation.

Professor Voltolini (of Breslau), as the originator of the method, very appropriately introduced the subject of the Employment of the Galvano-cautery in the Nose, Pharynx, and Larynx, the other introductory paper being read by Professor Solis Cohen (of Philadelphia). Great stress was laid on the necessity of employing the proper kind of battery and instruments. The method was highly commended for use in the nose and pharynx; in the larynx the dangers attending its use more than counterbalanced the advantages claimed for it by its more enthusiastic admirers. Dr. Foulis claimed for the actual cautery the advantages of cheapness and readiness of application.

"Adenoid Vegetations in the Vault of the Pharynx," which are of interest both to the laryngologist and otologist, were the subject of a valuable paper by Dr. Meyer (of Copenhagen), who was the earliest observer to insist on the importance of these growths. He drew attention to the universality of their occurrence, their almost exclusive limitation to youth, and the unsatisfactory result of an expectant plan of treatment. Among operations for their removal, those are to be deprecated where neither the finger nor the eye guides the cutting instrument. Dr. Loewenberg (of Paris), in his introductory paper, pointed out the combination of suppression of nasal respiration and nasal voice, generally accompanied by ear-trouble, as characteristic of this complaint. The discussion turned chiefly on the question of treatment—cutting instruments, the galvano-cautery, and the finger-nail being recommended by different speakers.

The "Nature and Treatment of Ozæna" was introduced by Dr. Fränkel (of Berlin) and Dr. Fournié (of Paris) in very able and instructive papers. The chief points elicited were—that ozæna is a symptom of many different diseases; that a complete cure is hardly to be expected; that, as regards treatment, the best results have been obtained by freeing of the nasal cavity from secretions by means of the syringe or douche, and by the employment of Gottstein's tampon. Michel's plan of syringing was recommended to be adopted as less liable to cause ear-trouble.

Demonstrations of patients and instruments were given on two afternoons at the Hospital for Diseases of the Throat and Chest, Golden-square. Among the more important instruments shown were a set of tracheotomy tubes, by Professor Krishaber; a curious relation was stated to exist between the diameter of the trachea and the height of the body; apparatus for heating the actual cautery, by Dr. Foulis; galvano-caustic loop and mode of removing adenoid growths, by Dr. Michel; mouth dilator, by Dr. Fränkel; india-rubber tampon, to be filled with water for dilatation of laryngeal stenosis, by Dr. Tornwaldt; battery for galvano-cautery, by Professor Voltolini; galvano-caustic trachea-tome, by Professor Caselli; instruments for removal of adenoid vegetations in pharynx, etc., by Dr. Meyer; and a surgical instrument for the removal of exostoses, etc., by Dr. Goodwillie.

SECTION OF DISEASES OF THE SKIN.—There has probably never been a more representative meeting of the workers in dermatology than that of this Section, which met under Mr. Erasmus Wilson, President of the Royal College of Surgeons. Whether we consider the number of rare and interesting cases brought together, the papers and discussions in the Section, or the enormous series of drawings and specimens in the museum, we cannot but regard this Congress as having materially contributed to the advancement of dermatology.

No less than seven cases of Leprosy were exhibited, four by Mr. Hutchinson, two by Dr. Radcliffe Crocker, and one by Mr. James Startin. Of Mr. Hutchinson's cases, one showed recovery from everything but the lesion of the ulnar nerve, and the others phases of the fully developed tubercular form of the disease. Mr. Startin's case was complicated with syphilis; the ulnar nerves were very large, but the anæsthesia was incomplete, and there was some hyperæsthesia. Dr. Radcliffe Crocker's cases were two boys of nine—one from the West, the other from the East Indies. In one of them the disease did not appear till after he had been six months in England, and had had an attack of ague in Essex; the disease was of three years' duration, and the ulnar nerves had been stretched, but without any effect on the paralysis and anæsthesia. In the museum this disease held an important place: drawings, photographs, wax models, and specimens were shown by Mr. Hutchinson (from Guy's Hospital), by the Royal College of Surgeons of Ireland, Dr. Anderson (of Japan), and Dr. de Wahl (of Dorpat). While Dr. Abrahams' microscopical demonstrations were most interesting, of which the micro-organisms of Hansen may be specially mentioned.

Three cases of Diffused Scleroderma were brought forward by Dr. Colcott Fox, Mr. Gaskoin, and Dr. Stowers. The last-named gentleman read a description of his interesting case in the Section.

Circumscribed Scleroderma or Morphœa was copiously

illustrated, bringing out many interesting points of occasional occurrence, such as symmetry, pigmentation, and ulceration. Cases were shown by Mr. Morrant Baker, Dr. Radcliffe Crocker, Dr. Fox, Mr. Gaskoin, and Dr. Stephen Mackenzie. Its unilateral distribution in the course of nerves was abundantly demonstrated by two cases of Mr. Baker's, drawings of Mr. Hutchinson's, and models from Guy's Hospital.

Of Xanthelasma Planum there was one case by Dr. Radcliffe Crocker, on the eyelids of a man with diabetes insipidus; and two cases of Xanthelasma Tuberosum. A girl of five years, shown by Mr. Startin, in whom symmetrical groups of tubercles had existed for two years in the gluteal cleft, the points of the elbows, and the popliteal spaces; she was quite healthy, but her sister has similar tubercles in the popliteal spaces. Mr. Gaskoin also had a case of a man with tubercles in groups upon the backs of the hands, forearms, elbows, and knees. In all the living cases hepatic disease was absent.

Lupus Erythematosus, in anticipation of the discussion announced upon it, was largely represented both by numerous drawings belonging to Mr. Hutchinson, and by cases by the same gentleman, by Dr. Stephen Mackenzie, Mr. Morrant Baker, and Mr. Malcolm Morris—so that all the features of the disease could be studied. Of especial interest were Mr. Morris's two cases, one showing the stage-before loss of substance occurred, which Hebra first described as seborrhœa congestiva, and the other a woman in whom the disease had gradually involved the whole body, leaving large tracts of cicatrisation. The discussion upon the subject was opened by Professor Kaposi, who enunciated his well-known views in favour of its being inflammatory rather than a new growth, and also set forth for discussion—1. If inflammatory, what kind of inflammation is it, since it leads to cicatrisation? 2. What are the local conditions? 3. What remote causes lie at the bottom of the disease? 4. If his division into discoid and aggregated corresponds to this form of lupus. Dr. Veiel, Professor Simon, the President, Dr. Vidal, Dr. Unna, and Dr. Thin, continued the discussion; but on the whole it was disappointing. There was much force in Dr. Unna's remark that in acute cases, and at the beginning, it resembled an inflammation; but in proportion to its duration it resembled a neoplasm.

Mr. Morrant Baker's three cases of True Prurigo were the prelude to an important paper on this disease; the truth of his remarks and the genuineness of his cases being acknowledged unequivocally by Professor Kaposi, Mr. Hans Hebra, and others of our German confrères. The two former also remarked that Hebra himself latterly did not insist upon all cases coming up to the standard of the terrible portrait he drew, while they were, when treated early, less obstinate than he formerly supposed. These admissions, and the living evidence he brought, made Mr. Baker's paper one of the most interesting in the Section to English dermatologists.

On the other hand, the cases of Urticaria Pigmentosa were new to foreigners, and were consequently of great interest to them. Four were shown—two by Dr. S. Mackenzie, one by Dr. Cavafy, and one by Dr. Fox. The last was the one his brother first described as xanthelasmoidea, and was interesting, as nearly all the flat tubercles had undergone involution. Dr. Liveing also showed a case which deserved the name urticaria pigmentosa more than those usually ranged under that title, since the wheals were transitory or at most of a few weeks' duration, and left only pigmentary deposit in their site.

Other defects of pigmentation received important illustration. Of the hair, Mr. Hutchinson showed a unique case of a girl aged eight: three years previously she had had an attack of pityriasis rubra; this was followed by complete loss of hair, and on its regeneration it was quite white. The eyebrows and lashes remained of their natural dark-brown colour, except a small tuft on one eyelid. The wholeskin was said to be several shades fairer than before the attack. Dr. Sangster had a case of alopecia areata in which the hair was said to have turned white in tufts before falling off, thus completely reversing the usual order of things. Leucoderma with typical characters was seen in a case of Mr. Hutchinson's —a girl of sixteen years; while Mr. Morrant Baker showed a girl of ten years in whom pigmentation preceded bleaching (this was similar to one brought to the Clinical Society a year ago by Dr. Crocker). The occurrence of this sequence has often been denied.

Mr. Malcolm Morris contributed a case of a Pigmented Papilloma growing on the cicatrix consequent on the removal of a pigmented nævus; and lastly, Dr. Crocker showed a woman with deep pigmentation left by lichen planus. He also showed cases of this disease, both with papules and infiltrations: Mr. Morris and Dr. Mackenzie also bringing cases.

Single examples of disease, interesting either from their rarity or from the evidence they afforded on disputed points, were—a case of keloid of ten years' duration on the site of a blister, undergoing involution, by Dr. Dyce Duckworth; elephantiasis Arabum of the arm and hand, with ulceration of the hand, consequent upon inflammatory blocking of the lymphatics, by Mr. M. Baker; epithelioma developing upon an old syphilitic lesion, by Dr. Liveing; recurrent pruriginous herpetic eruption, by Mr. Hutchinson (the original of one of the portraits of skin diseases by the New Sydenham Society); a case of a minute papular syphilide affecting the hair-follicles, indistinguishable, as regards the eruption, from lichen scrofulosorum, but covering the limbs, and in a woman of forty-three, by Dr. Radcliffe Crocker (Professor Kaposi said he had seen true lichen scrofulosorum in adults as old); a case of congenital papillary mole in a man of twenty, unilaterally distributed upon the scrotum, penis, and inner part of the thigh in groups and patches, evidently in the course of nerves, and leading Mr. Hutchinson, whose case it was, to suggest the possibility of its being due to intra-uterine herpes. He showed drawings of somewhat similar cases. His very interesting drawings of lesions from iodide of potassium and gangrene following vaccinia and varicella, bromide eruption, and herpes, would have been more appalling but for the extreme rarity of such occurrences. Paget's disease of the nipple—the malignant papillary dermatitis of Thin—was demonstrated by a well-marked case of Dr. Fox's, a drawing of Dr. Macnaughton Jones's, and two specimens of breasts removed for consequent cancer by Mr. George Lawson.

The above by no means fully represent the drawings and specimens illustrating dermatology, contributed by public institutions and private enterprise, but want of space prevents further notice of them.

The publication of the abstracts renders it unnecessary to allude in detail to all the papers.

Professor Oscar Simon drew attention to the frequency of Balanitis in cases of Diabetes Mellitus, and how it had, in his practice, led to the discovery of previously unsuspected diabetes. This concurrence he ascribed to a fungus of the same nature as that Haller discovered in diabetic urine. Fungus spores have also been discovered in non-diabetic balanitis, however; but Professor Simon says never mycelium, as in diabetic cases.

Dr. Sangster's cases—one which would clinically be called papilloma of the scalp, the other which he regarded as neurotic excoriation—gave rise to much discussion as to their pathology. In the first, Dr. Sangster, supported by Mr. Butlin, considered the tumour to be a sarcoma; while Kaposi thought it inflammatory; and Thin, allied to rodent ulcer. The second was shown to the meeting, together with drawings, and was generally considered to be self-induced, though perhaps in a subject whose skin easily resented slight injuries. Dr. Sangster, however, ably defended his position.

Dr. Angelucci's views that Micrococci which can be cultivated into Bacteria caused the scales of psoriasis, papular eczema, and the changes of molluscum contagiosum, received support only from Dr. Thin, and that merely as regards molluscum.

Dr. Behrends' paper on Vaccinal Eruptions was interesting. Acquitting vaccinia of any but an indirect influence on their production, he stated that the eruptions themselves were not peculiar to vaccination, which acted like irritating ingesta only on predisposed subjects, while the eruptions were mild and of short duration.

Dr. Liveing's paper ably supported the neurotic theory of Alopecia Areata, but was energetically opposed by Professor Hardy and Dr. Vidal, who related cases that the theory of contagion alone explained satisfactorily. These, and the cases of the late Dr. Hillier, where there was an outbreak in a school, show that there are still two sides to this vexed question, apart from the doubtful evidence of the microscope, and that neither theory quite fits all cases. Dr. Thin stated that he had found micrococci in the affected hair-follicles, and that in his hands sulphur was invariably and speedily curative, exciting the envy of many who had hitherto tried that remedy in vain.

Professor Schwimmer's paper on Leukoplakia Buccalis described the disease that Mr. Hulke first brought under the notice of the profession under the name of ichthyosis linguæ, and confirmed his observation that it was often non-specific, though syphilis, excessive smoking, and irritation of the alimentary canal predisposed to it. Local treatment, with ⅓ per cent. solution of hydrarg. bichlor., or 1 per cent. solution of chromic acid, were the best remedies, and often averted the otherwise almost inevitable epithelioma. Mr. Morrant Baker concurred with Professor Schwimmer, and preferred his name to such misleading appellations as ichthyosis, psoriasis, tylosis linguæ, etc. Some good drawings of this affection were exhibited in the museum by Mr. Davies Colley, Dr. Goodhart, etc.

Dr. Unna (of Hamburg) read a critical and historical essay on the Sweat Secretion, contending that sweat was secreted not only from the coil, but from the duct along its whole course, the vessels of the papillary layer contributing fluid which was conveyed along the epithelial spaces of the rete to that part of the duct, and that the sweat, therefore, was a mixture of fluids, the best theory of its secretion being one founded on a vaso-motor and musculo-motor hypothesis, which explains the action of the involuntary muscles of the gland, and such phenomena as fatty mucoid pigmented and "cold" sweat.

Dr. Thin showed and described a case of Congenital Abnormality in the Hair Production of the Scalp in a girl, in which the hair was rough, crisp, and brittle, breaking off at an inch or less from the scalp when firmly rubbed. The hairs showed variations in thickness in the shaft, and there was epithelial accumulation at the mouth of the follicles, so that Professor Kaposi thought it was analogous to keratosis (so-called "lichen pilaris") of other parts of the body.

Dr. Vidal read a paper on the lesions produced by a new fungus (Microsporon anomœon), and gave an oral account of Lymphadénie of the Skin.

Dr. Verrier's paper was on the influence of climate, difference of race, and mode of life on the development and character of Parasitic Diseases of the Hairy Scalp.

Dr. Rasori (of Rome) read a paper on General Inflammation of the Sweat-glands following the prolonged internal administration of pilocarpine.

Dr. Walter Smith related a case of the occurrence of Dipterous Larvæ beneath the human skin.

The work of the Section was brought to a close by a short paper by the President on Dermato-Therapœia, in which the advantages of the benzoated oxide of zinc ointment in the treatment of eczema were brought forward.

Before the meeting broke up, Dr. Bulkley (of New York) proposed, and Dr. S. Mackenzie seconded, that an international committee should be appointed to agree upon a uniform nomenclature for skin diseases, and ultimately a classification. This was passed nem. con., and the President nominated Dr. Liveing, Dr. Bulkley, Professor Kaposi, and two others, with power to add to their number.

On reviewing the solid advantages to dermatology that accrue from this meeting, we must reckon the enormous assemblage of living cases, specimens, and drawings, which enabled men in a week to form a conception of rare diseases that it would take many years of ordinary experience to attain. This was especially the case as regards leprosy, xanthelasma, urticaria pigmentosa, and lupus; and, from drawings, iodide and bromide rashes, and gangrenous terminations of inflammation of the skin. Further, we must now add—thanks to Mr. Morrant Baker—prurigo to our list of English diseases; while our foreign brethren will carry home in their minds the picture of urticaria pigmentosa. Last, but not least, we may place the fact of our being brought face to face with men who have been hitherto only names to us, and whose writings will henceforth be more real and interesting now that they are clothed with the living personality of the authors with whom we have been so closely associated during the week of the International Congress of 1881.

In the Aural Section, the first subject for discussion was "On the Value of Operations in which the Tympanic Membrane is Incised." A paper on this subject was read by Dr. Paquet (of Lille), who claims for his operation the advantage of being able to maintain a permanent opening in the membrana tym-

pani; the operation not only incises the membrane, but divides the tensor tympani muscle at the same time.

The discussion was opened by Dr. Guye (of Amsterdam). He divides the cases in which myringodectomy may be performed into four classes: 1. In acute inflammation, with pus in the tympanic cavity; 2. In subacute or chronic inflammation, with mucous accumulation; 3. Chronic proliferous catarrh with nervous symptoms, such as vertigo or tinnitus; 4. In certain anomalous cases. As an illustration of such, he mentioned two cases of acute catarrh, attended with great pain, but where, owing to the patency of the Eustachian tube, fluid secreted escaped into the pharynx. Dr. Loewenberg (of Paris) advocated the operation also in inflammation of the mastoid cells, as a means of cutting short the inflammation and relieving the distressing pain. Many of the members spoke in favour of the operation in the first two classes of cases. Mr. Dalby pointed out that the point of greatest interest was, to determine in what cases in group 3 myringodectomy could be performed with advantage to the patient.

No satisfactory information was obtained as to the benefit of section of the tensor tympani muscle, few of the members appearing to have had any experience of the operation.

On Thursday, Dr. Cassells read the abstract of his paper on "The Ætiology of Aural Exostoses." The chief points of his paper were these: an exostosis is a new growth; a hyperostosis, a hyperplasm. An exostosis appears before complete ossification of the meatus; a hyperostosis is never seen till after complete ossification. They differ from each other in origin, site, shape, structure, and number. He prefers the gouge for the removal of exostosis, the drill for hyperostosis. Dr. Guye believes that multiple hyperostoses never completely occlude the meatus, for as soon as the tumours touch one another, they cease to grow—thus leaving a central passage for the escape of secretion.

Dr. Knapp related the result of his examination of 250 skulls of the mound-builders; he found exostosis in 44 cases. The condition was supposed to be due to the habit of carrying foreign bodies in the meatus.

On Friday the subject of discussion was, "On Loss of Hearing where the External and Middle Ears are Healthy." The papers read on this subject were: "Nerve Lesion—Deafness," by Dr. Gellé (of Paris); "Physical Diagnosis of Affections of the Acoustic Apparatus, with Healthy Middle and Outer Ears," by Dr. Lucae (of Berlin); "On certain Conditions of the Eyes as a Cause of Loss of Hearing by Reflex Irritation," by Dr. Stevens.

In connexion with this subject, Dr. Knapp related the result of his experiments on the loss of vision and hearing caused by large doses of quinine. In both the loss was temporary. The objective symptoms in the ear were negative; in the eye he found that the arteries of the retina almost disappeared, the veins were scarcely traceable, and the disc looked atrophied. The field of vision was narrowed on the inner side; light and colour perception diminished. The return of sensibility to light passed from the centre to the periphery. Mr. Dalby said he could not doubt that large doses of quinine, long continued, did produce impairment of hearing; while Dr. Jones (of Chicago) stated that he had never seen a case of permanent impairment of hearing resulting from large doses of quinine.

On Monday, Dr. Fournié read a paper, "On the Functions of the Eustachian Tube." He believes that one of the essential functions of the tube is to prevent unpleasant resonance of external and internal noises, and that the muscles which are usually considered dilators are in reality obliterators of the tube; farther, that the tube is shut by the tensor and levator palati muscles, and opened by the palato-pharyngeus muscles, and palato-glossus. Dr. Rumball did not agree with the conclusions of Dr. Fournié, but believed that the generally accepted views as to the action of the pharyngeal muscles were correct; and farther, he holds that the air in the tympanic cavity is always in a state of slight rarefaction.

Dr. Knapp next read a paper on "The Cotton-Wool Pellet as an Artificial Drumhead." Its advantages are—1. It improves the hearing; 2. It protects the tympanic cavity from the noxious influence of the atmosphere; 3. It promotes a healthy condition of the cavity by absorbing the morbid secretions. He believes it improves the hearing, sometimes by bracing up the stapes on the fenestra ovales.

Dr. Woakes read a paper on "Paretic Deafness." The chief points he lays stress on in the diagnosis of this affection are—the negative symptoms, as regards the ear; the positive, as regards the palate and faucial regions. In a paper "On the

Action of Syphilis on the Ear," Dr. Pierce (of Manchester) noticed that the effects of congenital and acquired syphilis on the ear are less observed than its effects on the eye, teeth, skin, etc. He discussed the question whether the obstinate symptoms of aural syphilis are due to a periostitis of the parts, or to a proliferous form of inflammation of the mucous membrane. His summary of the characteristics of acquired and congenital syphilis affecting the ear is as follows:—1. The extreme degree of deafness manifested early in the progress of the disease. 2. The rapidity of the progress, and the absence of pain. 3. The early and extreme loss of hearing for the tuning-fork over the vertex. 4. Constancy of the tinnitus. 5. Frequency of simultaneous inner-ear symptoms. 6. Less complete recovery than in simple catarrh.

Dr. Barr next read a paper on " Caseous Accumulations in the Middle Ear, regarded as a Probable Cause of Miliary Tubercle." Papers were also read, by Dr. MacBride, "On some Difficulties presented in the Diagnosis, Prognosis, and Treatment of a certain form of Middle-Ear Deafness"; and by Mr. Arthur Kinsey, " On the Prevention of Dumbness in those Cases where it follows Loss of Hearing."

There was an extra meeting on Tuesday afternoon, when the following papers were read :—" A Fluid Artificial Membrana Tympani," by Dr. Michelle ; "On the way Sound-Waves reach the Auditory Apparatus," by Dr. Sapolini (of Milan) ; and " On the Advantages of Nasal Inspection in some Cases of Difficult Catherisation of the Eustachian Tube," by Dr. Loewenberg. The meeting terminated with a vote of thanks to the President, and to the two Secretaries.

In the Section of Materia Medica and Pharmacology, on Friday, August 5, the members were chiefly engaged in a discussion on the introduction of an International Pharmacopœia. The debate was introduced by Professor Eulenburg (of Greifswald), and sustained by Drs. Gille (of Brussels), Waldheim (of Vienna), Mehu (of Paris), Brunnengräber (of Geneva), Stockvis (of Amsterdam), Goddefroy (of Vienna), Mr. Schacht (of Clifton), Dr. Prosser James, Mr. Carteighe, M. Petit (of Paris), Mr. Greenish, Professor Bentley, Dr. Rawdon Macnamara, Mr. Andrews (of London), Dr. Churton, and the President. It will be gathered from this list of speakers that the subject was thoroughly handled. In his introductory paper, Professor Eulenburg gave, first, a brief historical sketch of the efforts made in the direction of securing a Universal Pharmacopœia at previous meetings of the Congress in 1875, 1877, and 1879, and at the Pharmaceutical Congress at St. Petersburg in 1874. At present there existed an international committee on the subject, but with limited and ill-defined powers. The first proposal therefore was to augment this committee by the addition to its number of medical and pharmaceutical experts, and to relieve it of all duties but those of creating a pharmacopœia. Secondly, the following points were suggested as a basis—(a.) Ought not the language to be Latin, at least for the names of remedies ? (b.) All scales should be on the decimal system. (c.) The nomenclature (botanical, chemical, etc.) should be uniform. (d.) Should the arrangement be alphabetical or systematic ? (e.) The remedies admitted should be limited in number by their importance and value. Supplements might contain remedies of local value. (f.) Uniform regulations should be adopted as to tests and degree of purity required, and as to maximum doses. Lastly, if such a pharmacopœia were drawn up, the therapeutists of each country ought to strive to have their respective national pharmacopœias approximated to the international standard.

Mr. G. F. Schacht, of Clifton, Vice-President of the Pharmaceutical Society of Great Britain, urged the Congress to accept the conclusions at which the International Pharmaceutical Congress had just arrived after anxious deliberation. The most important of these resolutions was that for the present they should give up the project of a universal pharmacopœia as being impracticable, and confine themselves to the equalisation of the preparations of the most potent drugs used in general practice. This work might be undertaken immediately, and form the nucleus of future efforts in the desired direction.

After a lengthened discussion, the following resolution was agreed to :—" That this Section confirms the resolutions passed at previous International Medical Congresses as to the utility of a Universal Pharmacopœia, but is of opinion that it is necessary at once to appoint a committee, consisting of two delegates from every country represented at

this Congress, which shall co-operate with a committee appointed by the International Pharmaceutical Congress to prepare a compilation in which the strength of all potent drugs and their preparations is equalised." The following are the names of this committee, as far as provisionally chosen :—Great Britain—Professors Fraser and Lauder Brunton ; France — Professors Dujardin-Beaumetz and Vulpian ; Germany—Professors Rossbach and Eulenburg ; Austria—Professor Schroff ; Russia—Professors Botkin and Dogiel ; Holland—Professors Stockvis and Fokker ; Switzerland—Professor Prevost ; and the United States—Professors Wood and Flint.

At the same sitting, Professor Plugge read an interesting paper on the alkaloids known as Aconitia. M. Petit, Mr. Carteighe, and the President took part in discussion that followed upon the subject ; and the general consensus appeared to be that, inasmuch as the alkaloids derived from *Aconitum napellus* and from *Aconitum ferox* respectively are by no means of equal strength, it is highly desirable that a tincture of the former root should be ordered, and not any preparation of the active principle.

On Saturday, August 6, two subjects of importance occupied the meeting of the Section—namely, Physiological Antagonism, and the Action and Uses of Pilocarpin and Jaborandi. The discussion on the former subject was opened by a paper of great excellence from the pen of Professor Wood (of Philadelphia). All functional activity being the result of molecular movements in living protoplasm, all active remedies must either chemically unite with the protoplasm, or alter the character of these movements. We might expect to find forces antagonistic in their action on the organism, as we find them everywhere in nature. Most substances, indeed, which quicken molecular action at first, end by arresting it. Dr. Wood referred to Professor Prevost's distinction between antidotism and antagonism, a physiological antidote relieving symptoms that cause death, whilst a physiological antagonist acts in direct opposition to some other substance (chloral and strychnia). The treatment of disease by antagonism is as much possible as the antagonistic treatment of poisoning. But inasmuch as the action of a "disease" poison is complex and obscure, we have, as a rule, to fall back on antidotal treatment (i.e., the treatment of symptoms), and wait for the elimination or destruction of the disease-poison. Bearing in mind the distinction between antagonism and antidotism, the mixed falsity and truth of *similia similibus curantur* is seen. "Allopathy" is no more true than "homœopathy," but the law of antagonism is of wide applicability in therapeutics, and its range must continually increase.

A very desultory conversation followed, in which therapeutical principles of every nature were fully expressed.

A paper on Pilocarpin was read by Dr. William Squire (of London), which dealt very fully with the physiological action, and especially with the therapeutical applications, of the new remedy. Dr. Squire prefers to use the muriate of pilocarpin in simple solution, one grain to fifteen minims of water for hypodermic injection, one grain to four ounces of water for internal use—one-third of a grain being the largest, and one-fifteenth of a grain the smallest dose required. A full dose should be given at once. The principal use of pilocarpin is in some cases of diphtheria and the different kinds of Bright's disease. Dr. Huchard (of Paris) recommended great caution in the use of pilocarpin in Bright's disease when the heart was threatening to give way. He had observed the greatest benefit from its employment in polyuria, and a certain amount of good in cases of sweating in phthisis. Dr. Jacobi (of New York) said that perspiration without introduction of water into the system being dangerous, it is necessary in Bright's disease to combine the use of pilocarpin with injections of water per rectum. Dr. Jacobi also indicated the class of diphtheritic cases in which pilocarpin was of some value. Professor Quinlan (of Dublin) did not fear so much the action of pilocarpin as a cardiac depressant. Mr. Gerard and Mr. Martindale spoke on pilocarpin from the pharmaceutical point of view.

On Monday, August 8, the attention of the Section was fairly divided between the consideration of a series of important resolutions upon the subject of Experiments on Animals and the discussion of several papers of considerable interest. We have already referred, under the head of " News " last week, to the former matter. Whilst the remarks that fell from English therapeutists chiefly took the form of indignant protests against the indifference of the Government to the interests of science, the foreign members naturally gave expression rather to astonishment at the existence of such a state of affairs in "free" England. The speech of Professor Wood (of Philadelphia) was at once encouraging and highly suggestive, giving, as he did, an account of the way in which the anti-vivisection movement was met and utterly defeated in one of the States. By almost incredible labour the leading scientists of Pennsylvania "got at" the doctor of every member of the Legislature, and of the editor of every newspaper and magazine in the country ; and common sense, enlightened by a plain statement of the truth, and as to the danger of the movement prevailed. It appears highly probably that advantage may be taken of the complete medical organisation in this country to secure, if possible, the same end.

Professor Dujardin-Beaumetz (of Paris) then opened a discussion upon Absorbent Remedies. Starting from the normal nutrition of a cell, which consists of a dual process of integration and disintegration, the Professor described the three normal methods of disintegration—viz., return to the embryonic state, fatty-granular degeneration, and fibroid substitution. Absorbent remedies favour these processes, either mechanically (compression, etc.), by evulsion (blisters, etc.), through the nutrition (galvanism, etc.), by surgical means, or, lastly, by absorbent medicines (mercury and iodide of potassium par excellence). Whilst the value of mercury and iodine was unquestionable, no satisfactory explanation of their mode of action had been offered.

Dr. Mitchell Bruce continued the discussion. Limiting his remarks to mercury and its action upon the solid growths of syphilis, he pointed out, first, that mercury accelerated only a natural process, which alone was frequently sufficient to remove specific disease. In studying the effect of mercury as clinically observed, the nature of this natural process was readily appreciated, for it was found that mercury hastened the disintegrating factor of nutrition or metabolism throughout the whole body ; and if the other factor, the upbuilding or "integrating" process, were not supported by abundant nourishment, a condition of body was produced which closely resembled the effects of starvation as seen in London, characterised by erythema, œdema, stomatitis, and great debility. The next question was, Why did acceleration of general nutrition lead to the disappearance of syphilitic growths ?—and this question the speaker sought to answer by the fact that these growths were the youngest or most embryonal in the body, and consequently those in which nutrition was most sensitive and most easily impaired. With respect to the exact modus operandi of mercury on cells, Dr. Bruce suggested that, being a substance which was freely absorbed, incorporated, and excreted by cell-substance, mercury had the power of increasing the activity of the cell-life, in other words, of exercising the cells; and that this simple stimulation, or "wear and tear" of the cells, might suffice to explain the action of mercury on them without recourse to a "poisonous" or "virulent influence."

Dr. Matthew Hay (of Edinburgh) then read a paper of much value on Saline Purgatives, in which he described a series of experiments on the precise manner of action of salines in the production of purgation. The paper was attentively listened to throughout; and Professor Wood and others took part in the remarks which it elicited.

Dr. Waterman (of Indianapolis) next read a paper on Colchicum as an Antipyretic. In general terms he described the remarkable powers which colchicum had exhibited in his hands over the production of the body-heat, and gave this drug the very first place amongst antipyretics in sthenic fevers. This paper met with a considerable amount of criticism.

Tuesday, August 9, was chiefly occupied in this Section with the subject of the Action of Medicines upon the Circulation, introduced by a paper by Professor Boehm (of Marburg). This paper was of the most elaborate and exhaustive description, discussing the various influences that affect the heart, the bloodvessels, or the whole circulatory apparatus, and analysing as far as possible the precise manner in which such effect was produced. Mr. Gaskell followed with a paper on the Action of various Poisons, especially Atropia, upon the Heart of the Frog ; and Dr. Gibson (of Edinburgh) with a paper upon the Physiological Action of Duboisia on the Circulation. Dr. Murrell, Professor Stookvis, and others supported the debate. A few remarks by the President brought the business of the Section to an end.

WOOL-SORTERS' DISEASE.

The following report of Professor Brown, the Professional Officer of the Veterinary Department of the Privy Council Office, has been presented to Parliament :—

"Referring to the report of Mr. John Spears, of the Local Government Board, on the subject of the wool-sorters' disease (anthrax), and the questions in the House of Commons as to the intention of the Privy Council in regard of legislation for the prevention of anthrax among animals in this country, arising from the use of the refuse of wool manufactures for manure, I have the honour to submit the following points for the consideration of the Lord President :—

"1. The inquiry recently conducted by Mr. Spears at Bradford has established the fact that the wool-sorters' disease, which was first observed forty-three years ago, when the import of mohair commenced, is a form of anthrax, a disease which is due to the presence of a microscopic plant, the Bacillus anthracis, in the fluids of the body.

"2. Anthrax is essentially an affection of the lower animals, but is as readily communicable to man as to the lower animals by the introduction of the spores of the Bacillus anthracis into the blood.

"3. Anthrax, in the form of splenic fever, has long been known in this kingdom as a disease which occurs occasionally among farm stock. The affection does not, however, spread to any extent by contagion, and, as a rule, does not extend beyond the farm on which the outbreak occurs. The disease is more virulent in some parts of Ireland than it is here, and on the Continent it sometimes prevails extensively. The Siberian plague, which is now rife in Russia, is one of the most virulent and fatal forms of this disorder. It may be remarked that anthrax is one of the diseases which are distinguished by periods of excessive prevalence and decline.

"4. It may be accepted as a fact that the use of wool, hair, and other substances, from animals which have died of anthrax, in agriculture or manufactures, is attended with danger to men and animals.

"5. So far as animals are concerned, the risk of the communication of anthrax through the agency of the refuse of wool factories used as manure is comparatively slight, and might be further diminished by limiting the use of such refuse to arable land.

"In this connexion the most important thing seems to be the adoption of means to make farmers aware of the danger which attends the employment of the refuse of wool mills as top dressing for pastures. It can hardly be imagined that the refuse would be used for this purpose if it were known that the risk of introducing anthrax would be incurred thereby. It has been suggested that the sale of wool-bags and the refuse of wool factories should be prevented ; but the measure could hardly be justified on the evidence which has been adduced as to the injury which such substances are likely to cause. I am not aware of any outbreak of anthrax having been traced to the use of wool-bags for any purpose, and there is only one instance recorded of the appearance of the disease under circumstances which afforded reasonable ground for concluding that it was due to the use of sewage mixed with wool refuse on land where cattle were grazing.

"A more serious aspect of the question is the danger to which the wool-sorters are exposed, owing to the mixture in the bales of wool of inferior sorts of wool, some of which have undoubtedly been clipped from the skins of animals which have died of anthrax. Mr. Spears suggests that in preference to a total prohibition of the importation of this inferior wool, which would continue to be imported even if it were prohibited, it should be imported separately, in such a form that it could be dealt with on landing by being disinfected or otherwise treated as might be found necessary to render it harmless.

"While agreeing with Mr. Spears in his view of the desirability of an arrangement of this sort, I may be permitted to point out that legislation could not prevent the foreign exporter from mixing the inferior with the best quality of wool; and in order to detect this fraud it would be necessary to sort the wool while in charge of the Customs—a proceeding which would merely divert the risk of disease from the workers in the factory to the examining officers (who at the same time must be skilled wool-sorters) in the custom-houses. It may, however, be assumed that all illegally mixed wool would be confiscated and destroyed, and the loss to the importer would in time have a deterrent effect.

"The examination of wool and hair at the place of landing would necessitate the appointment of special officers, as the officers of Customs could not undertake the work; indeed, they do not possess the necessary technical knowledge, even if they could devote the time which would be required, for the efficient performance of the duty."

FROM ABROAD.

THE CARLSBAD WATERS TREATMENT.

IN a paper read at the Philadelphia Medical Society (*Phil. Med. Times*, May 7), Dr. Bruen, after admitting the value of the Carlsbad salt (especially when administered highly diluted whilst fasting), observes that it does not represent the waters as they issue from their natural sources. It is, indeed, after all, only Glauber's salt; while the waters, in addition, also contain (in the pint) thirteen grains of carbonate of sodium and two of sulphate of sodium, besides a fair amount of chloride of sodium, some carbonate of lime and magnesium, with free carbonic acid, at a temperature varying from 122° to 166° F. Speaking from personal experience at Carlsbad, he says that the cases resorting thither may be divided into three classes—1. Enlargement of the liver and spleen, as a consequence of repeated congestions, induced by chronic dyspepsia or chronic malarial disease; interstitial hepatitis, or the primary stage of cirrhosis, especially when jaundice and insufficient intestinal digestion persist; and the cases of chronic indigestion with deficient assimilation, whether or not constipation be a prominent symptom. 2. Cases of chronic rheumatism or gout. 3. Cases of the gouty state, or those obscure cases attended with renal congestion or inactivity, as evidenced by the passage of a deficient amount of urine of low specific gravity, usually associated with deficient vaso-motor tonus. These cases are subject to transient attacks of headache as hysterical nervousness.

The springs differ from each other chiefly in temperature and in the amount of carbonic acid. Patients usually rise at six, and spend about two hours at the springs, taking at fifteen minutes' interval three or four ounces of the water. Beginners usually indulge in from twelve to sixteen ounces a day, and the amount is often carried up to twenty-four or thirty ounces. Exercise is taken while drinking the waters. A strict diet is necessary for the success of "the cure," and consists of a light breakfast of eggs, bread, and coffee, with meat (steak or chicken) at noon; the same meal being repeated in the evening. No one under treatment must venture on a *table-d'hôte*, or even a more liberal meal. Early hours and moderate exercise are insisted on. Most persons experience a laxative action, although some require compound liquorice powder to obtain motions. Without exception, individuals experience the most profound exhaustion, and extreme anæmia usually ensues. The urine is usually notably increased, and is sometimes of a blackish-green colour, the stools also being often greenish. Notwithstanding these effects, the treatment is continued for three or four weeks, when the patient is sent to Ischl, St. Moritz, or some other springs, the waters of which contain iron, and then the blood crasis is restored. In persons weakened by previous long sickness, recuperation is very slow; and Dr. Bruen believes that often the treatment is pushed too far in such cases. Sir Henry Thompson believes that as good an effect is produced by six to eight ounces of the water daily for six or seven weeks as by the usual three-weeks course of larger doses. In serious cases a repetition of the course every three or four months is desirable if the patient's strength will bear it, and too much must not be expected from a single course. Dr. Bruen believes that the restriction placed on articles of diet contributes much to the favourable results. Thus, alcohol or fermented liquors must either be relinquished or given only in the most diluted and purest form; sugar, fatty matters, butter, cream, and fruits are proscribed; while vegetables and good fish are unattainable.

The "after-cure" consists in sending the patient to some mountainous resort possessing a ferruginous spring, two places being just now in vogue—viz., Ischl in the Tyrol, and St. Moritz in the Engadine. Dr. Bruen gives the preference to Ischl on account of its equable climate, good hotels, and interesting adjacent country. At St. Moritz the climate is variable, and there is but one month in which it is really comfortable—viz., July or August, as the case may be; and even then the temperature may vary fifteen or twenty degrees. The climate is too cold (60° to 65° Fahr.) for anæmic people, while the hotel accommodation and the drainage are both bad. The waters are, however, good, and containing only a small proportion of iron, are well digested; and baths consisting of the same water, heated as required, are very agreeable and exhilarating. As a careful reparative diet is of high importance, and is not obtainable in this locality, Dr. Bruen believes it preferable after the "cure" to return home, even at the cost of having to repair to Carlsbad a second time.

MEDICO-LEGAL EXPERTS.

Medical practitioners and the public of the United States are as dissatisfied with the present state of medical expertism as we are in this country; and, indeed, still more so, for not only is there a discreditable and purchasable class of practitioners there who thrust themselves forward, assuming the title of experts; but the judges and juries seem to attach as much importance to their testimony as they do to that of witnesses who have made the subjects in question the business of their lifetime. The "war of experts," as it is termed, disgraces almost every trial of importance, and as yet no means has been tried for the removal of the scandal. Dr. Reese, Professor of Medical Jurisprudence in the University of Philadelphia, sets forth the existing grievances in the *Philadelphia Med. Times* of April 23, and states that, in his opinion, they are only to be remedied by the adoption of some modification of the system which prevails in Prussia. Each American State should appoint, by the agency of the judges of its Supreme Court, as the most independent tribunal existing, one or more thoroughly educated practical physicians, properly trained in medical jurisprudence, and designated as State Medical Experts. There should be skilled witnesses for the prosecution, and should sit as assessors with the judges, and should be able to undertake any examinations that may be required. The accused would, of course, be enabled to employ experts in defence.

In the *Boston Med. Journal* (July 7), Dr. Walter Channing proposes that a measure, formerly advocated by Dr. Draper, should become law, as giving the best chance of removing the present evils, which he vividly depicts. He thinks it all-important that some kind and period of experience should be necessary to render it possible for a physician to appear in court as an expert, and to this end proposes this clause: "No medical practitioner shall be regarded as competent to appear as an expert in court unless he can clearly show that he has had a continuous experience of at least ten years in the active practice of the branch of medical science in which he is called to testify." Dr. Draper's measure, which it is proposed to legalise, is as follows:—

"Section 1. In any action, suit, or proceeding, civil or criminal, in which the testimony of a medical expert witness is desired by the parties, they may at any time before the trial file a written agreement that such witness shall be summoned, designating him by name if agreed upon. As soon as may be after the service of the subpœna, the witness shall make such examination of the case as may, in his judgment, be necessary and practicable, and he shall attend, as commanded in the subpœna, and answer such questions as may be put to him in relation to the case. 2. If no person is designated by the agreement of the parties, the court, or any judge thereof in chambers, or in vacation, shall designate a proper person, learned in the science of medicine, to be summoned as such expert-witness. If the parties do not agree that a medical expert shall be summoned in the case, the court, upon motion of either party, and upon hearing, may determine the question and may designate the person to be summoned. (Section 3 provides for payment of the experts.) 4. In any case, the court, upon its own motion, or for cause shown, may order more than one and not exceeding three persons to be summoned as medical expert witnesses. 5. In any criminal proceeding the defendant may call and examine other medical expert witnesses in addition to those hereinbefore provided for, but at his own cost, and in such case other medical expert witnesses may be called on behalf of the commonwealth."

HOW TO USE THE BROMIDES.

In a paper read at the American Neurological Association (*New York Med. Record*, July 2), Dr. Beard laid down the following propositions:—1. The object generally is to produce a definite effect—bromisation in a greater or lesser degree. In a certain sense it is a disease artificially produced; but in most cases mild effects are all that is needed. 2. To induce bromisation it is usually advantageous to give immense doses—as a drachm or more. Doses of fifteen or twenty grains might be given for some time without producing symptoms of any kind. In some cases 100 grains taken in one or two tumblers of water are all that is required to break up an attack of hysteria or headache, or to prevent sea-sickness. 3. These immense doses should be given only for a short time, except in epilepsy or epileptoid conditions. The cumulative effects must be constantly borne in mind. Sometimes a single large dose is sufficient to produce bromisation, which may occur within twenty minutes. 4. Bromides, when used long and frequently, should be given in alternation or in combination with tonics—bromides one week, and tonics the next, is a good rule. 5. It is advantageous to use a number of the bromides in combination. 6. While bromides are administered the patient must be kept continuously under observation. Dr. Hammond observed that he prefers the bromide of sodium, if any of the salts are employed; but of late he has been using pure bromine (bromine ʒj. ad aq. ʒviij.; teaspoonful well diluted with water), and thus avoided acne and the ulceration caused by the salts. Dr. Jewell had also used pure bromine with good results in cases in which the alkaline bases were not tolerated; and Dr. Seguin regards the bromine as the really efficient agent.

BOYLSTON PRIZE QUESTIONS.—The following are proposed for 1882:—1. Sewer-gas, so-called (the gas found in sewers): what are its physiological and pathological effects on animals and plants? ($300.) 2. The therapeutic value of food administered against or beyond the patient's appetite and inclination? ($200.) For 1883:—1. Measles, German measles, and their counterfeits. ($200.) 2. The differential diagnosis of abdominal tumours, especially those connected with the genito-urinary organs. ($200.) The Editor of the *Boston Med. Journal* (June 23), commenting on the fact of the two last prizes having been carried away by Drs. Page and Cheyne, of London, observes that while formerly the obtaining a Bolyston Prize was considered a necessary step in the career of any ambitious Boston physician, the home competitors have of late been fewer, and last year not a single dissertation was sent in from Boston. For Dr. Shattuck's prize at the Massachusetts Medical Society also no essay has been sent in.

WALKING WITH A FRACTURED PATELLA.—Dr. Trésoret relates (*Gaz. des Hop.*, August 11) the case of a robust countryman, forty-five years of age, who, on crossing a railway, fell down and struck his left knee against some stones. The violent pain which ensued disenabled him from rising for some minutes; after when, however, he managed to walk two kilometres, amidst great suffering, and with his leg in a state of forced extension, any attempt at flexion greatly increasing his pain and exposing him to falls. Next day he walked thirteen kilometres in great pain, and from that time continued his labours in the fields. Three weeks later, a swelling n the pre-patellar region led him to examine the knee, and to come to the conclusion that the patella was broken; but he did not apply for advice until more than two months after the accident. When Dr. Trésoret saw him, an indolent hygroma about the size of an egg existed in front of the patella, which was treated first by blister and then by puncture. The walls of the cyst being very flaccid, a transverse fracture of the patella at the junction of its lower with its middle third was readily detected—a fibrous callus uniting the two fragments so closely that it measured only some lines in breadth. An iodine injection was thrown into the cyst, and at the time of the report, a month afterwards, all pain and tumefaction having disappeared, the patient was regarded as cured.

MEDICAL NEWS.

UNIVERSITY OF LONDON.—The following are the names of candidates who passed the recent examinations at this University:—

FIRST M.B. EXAMINATION.

ENTIRE EXAMINATION.

First Division.—Robert Black, London and Sussex County Hospitals; Edward John Cave, St. Bartholomew's Hospital; Louis Albert Dunn, Guy's Hospital; Edward Gordon, Owens College; William Ayton Gostling, B.Sc., University College; Arthur Grayling, St. George's Hospital; Wheelton Hind, Guy's Hospital; William Henry Horrocks, University College; Walter Hull, St. Thomas's Hospital; John Harvey Jones, Owens College; Laurie Asher Lawrence, St. Bartholomew's Hospital; Albert Martin, Guy's Hospital; Sydney Sargent Merrifield, King's College; George Victor Peres, University College; Frances Helen Prideaux, London School of Medicine for Women; Ernest Septimus Reynolds, Owens College; Edmund Wilkinson Roughton, St. Bartholomew's Hospital; Mary Ann Dacomb Scharlieb, Madras Medical College and London School of Medicine for Women; Thomas William Shore, B.Sc., St. Bartholomew's Hospital; James Henry Targett, Guy's Hospital; Theodore Thomson, University of Aberdeen and University College; William Thorburn, B.Sc., Owens College; Thomas Wilson, University College; Frederick Womack, B.Sc., St. Bartholomew's Hospital.

Second Division.—Charles Frederick Bailey, St. Bartholomew's Hospital; Frederick William Bennett, Owens College; William Jones Black, Owens College; Arthur Thomas Bown, St. George's Hospital; William Henry Brown, University College; Frederick Foord Caiger, St. Thomas's Hospital; Matthew Carnelley, Guy's Hospital; John Howard Champ, Guy's Hospital; Edmund Percival Cockey, St. Mary's Hospital; Robert Cuff, Guy's Hospital; Wm. Dudley, Queen's Hospital, Birmingham; William Arnold Evans, Owens College; Willmott Henderson Evans, B.Sc., University College; John Fletcher, Manchester School of Medicine; Wm. Wadham Floyer, Guy's Hospital; John Philip Glover, St. Thomas's Hospital; Charles David Green, St. Thomas's Hospital; Joseph Langton Brewer, St. Bartholomew's Hospital; George William Hill, St. Mary's and St. George's Hospitals; Frederick Knight, University College; James Maugham, Liverpool School of Medicine and Guy's Hospital; Charles Harvig Lono Meyer, Guy's Hospital; Herbert Meyrick Nelson, Milton, St. Thomas's Hospital; Michael O'Kane, Guy's Hospital; Frederick John Paley, St. Bartholomew's Hospital; Maurice Parry-Jones, Guy's Hospital; John Joseph Powell, University College; Thomas Sydney Short, King's College; Druce John Slater, St. Bartholomew's Hospital; Herbert Ritchie Spencer, University College; Emily Tomlinson, London School of Medicine for Women; Alfred Jefferis Turner, University College; Alfred Mason Vann, King's College; Edwin James Wenyon, B.A., B.Sc., Guy's Hospital.

EXCLUDING PHYSIOLOGY.

Second Division.—Charles Gross, Guy's Hospital; Herbert Wheatley Hart, Westminster Hospital; William Herbert Lister Marriner, St. Thomas's Hospital; Henry Shillito, Birmingham School; Alfred Tilly, St. Mary's Hospital.

PHYSIOLOGY ONLY.

First Division.—Harry Lord Richards Dent, King's College.

Second Division.—Robert Fortescue Fox, London Hospital; Robert Parry, Guy's Hospital; Charles Ernest Richmond, Owens College.

ROYAL COLLEGE OF PHYSICIANS AND SURGEONS, EDINBURGH.—DOUBLE QUALIFICATION.—The following gentlemen passed their First Professional Examination during the July sittings of the examiners:—

James Hayward Hough, Cambridge; Charles Thomas Duce, Wednesbury; George Brown, co. Tipperary; Ronald Angus Daniel, Wexford; Thomas Leslie Crooke, Sheffield; Cornelius Buckley, co. Cork; John Cundill Wood, Sunderland; Simon Vincent Daly, Cork; Robert Walter Mackinstry, Monaghan; David Lloyd, Warwickshire; Thomas Frederic Watkin Rowlands, Wales; Thomas Galland Charls Hesk, Derbyshire; Henry Bolingbroke Seymour Curll, Australia; John Hanson, Norfolk; Alex. Macrae Bremner, Ross-shire; John Adolph Albrecht, Lancashire; John Walter Burbidge, London; Thomas Williams, Anglesea; Ernest Offord Stuart, co. Kent; John Salter Gettinge, Staffordshire; Arthur Hawkyard, Yorkshire; Henry Arthur Lowndo, Bombay; Winton Dixon, Yorkshire; Joseph Spilsbury Smith, Sierra Leone; Edward Ellis, Yorkshire; John William Irvine, California; William Cæsar Hamilton, East Lothian; Robert Lowry Dickson, co. Fermanagh; John Greenhalgh, Lancashire; Thomas Edwards, Birmingham; Ernest Westbrook, London; Robt. Grant Adamson, Aberdeen; Robt. Ashburner, Ulverston; Maurice Cussen, Kerry; Henry J. Thornton, Margate; Edward Hodges Soggin Phillips, Limerick.

And the following gentlemen passed their Final Examination, and were admitted L.R.C.P. Edinburgh and L.R.C.S. Edinburgh:—

William Bain, Caithness; Francis Edward Cane, Kilkenny; Charles Thomas Duce, Wednesbury; Robert Baird, co. Mayo; John Muirhead Watson, Lanark; Thomas Arthur Wise, Bilston, Stafford; William Richards Parry-Jones, Anglesea; Kenneth Alexander James McKenzie, Manitoba; Dugald Christie, Glencoe; William Robert Turner, Tuam; James Armstrong, Dumfriesshire; Michael Carmody, co. Limerick; Charles Pope, Yorkshire; Arthur William Egerton Brydges Barrett, Bath; George Hollies, Worcestershire; Arthur George Eyre Naylor, Calcutta; Edward Murray Laffan, Cork; Elisha Hodkinson Monks, Wigan; William James Spence, Darlington; George Pearce Baldwin, Wolverhampton; St. David Gynlais Walters, Ystradgynlais; Albert Victor Wheeler, Dublin; Arthur Ewen Yates, Calcutta; William Kyd Aitken, Edinburgh; William Bradshaw Paulin, Halifax, Nova Scotia; John Nagle Jeffries, co. Cork; James Henry Ferguson, Bolton-le-Moors; Frederic Theodore Underhill, Staffordshire; Basil Ronald, Calcutta; Thomas Guillaume Munyard, Paris; David Lloyd, Warwickshire; Arthur

Woolledge Aldrich, Mildenhall, Suffolk; James Hunter Dryden, Edinburgh; Richard Francis Walsh, co. Cork; James Patrick Casey, co. Limerick; Andrew Stewart, Greenock; James Garry, co. Clare; William Charles Griffiths, Llangranog; James Dunlop Dunlop, Edinburgh; James Joseph Taylor, Newcastleton; Arthur Kimberley Scattergood, Leeds; Francis Joseph Power, Cork; Peter Dunlop, co. Down.

ROYAL COLLEGE OF SURGEONS, EDINBURGH.

During the July sittings of the Examiners, the following gentleman passed his First Professional Examination :—

Ralph Barry Stoney, Roscommon.

And the following gentlemen passed their Final Examination, and were admitted Licentiates of the College :—

George Andreas Berry, Edinburgh; Alexander Matthew Moore, Devon; Robert Smith, co. Kerry; Charles William Sharples, London; Thomas Andrew Dickson, Whitehaven; Patrick Richard Dennehy, co. Tipperary; Thomas Wm. Shepherd, Somersetshire; John Leonard Aherne, Limerick; Richard George Minchin, King's County.

The following gentlemen passed their First Professional Examination for the Licence in Dental Surgery of the College :—

Matthew Finlayson, Alloa; David Monroe, Edinburgh; John James Bailey, Longton; Thomas Mansell, Hanley; John Sedgwick Spain, Dover; Henry Blandy, Chesterfield.

And the following gentlemen passed their Final Examination, and were admitted Licentiates in Dental Surgery :—

John James Bailey, Longton; Thomas Mansell, Hanley; John Sedgwick Spain, Dover; Robert Peel Thomson, Dublin.

ROYAL COLLEGE OF SURGEONS IN IRELAND.

At the quarterly examination for the Letters Testimonial, held on July 25 and following days, the undermentioned gentlemen were successful; and, having taken the declaration and signed the roll, were admitted Licentiates of the College, viz. :—

Louis E. Anderson, Thomas A. Baldwin, George V. Byrne, Thomas E. Cahill, James Coane, William J. Corbett, Charles E. Donning, Henry J. Dixon, Robert J. Fayle, Alexander J. Fleming, William Henry Johnson, G. Hunt, John M. Kennedy, William Kenny, Frederick W. Kidd, Thomas Magner, Vincent J. Magrane, Bernard Maguire, William L. McCormack, James A. Morris, Richard M'Nugent, Charles Parsons, Henry R. Peyton, Frederick Robinson, William S. Scott, Patrick de B. Skerrett, Thomas J. Stafford, James A. Swann, Maurice J. Treston, John Tuthill, William D. Waterhouse, and Miles E. Wilkinson.

APOTHECARIES' HALL, LONDON.

The following gentlemen passed their examination in the Science and Practice of Medicine, and received certificates to practise, on Thursday, August 18 :—

Grün, Edward Ferdinand, Osborn Villas, Putney.
Longman, Arthur, Andover, Hants.
Rees, John, Maesteg, South Wales.
Webster, George Leonard, 85, Portadown-road, W.

The following gentlemen also on the same day passed their primary professional examination :—

Bruce, Robert Marston, St. Thomas's Hospital.
Thomas, John Henry, London Hospital.
Treadwell, Oliver F. N., St. Thomas's Hospital.
Walker, Joseph, Liverpool Royal Infirmary.

APPOINTMENTS.

*** The Editor will thank gentlemen to forward to the Publishing-office, as early as possible, information as to all new Appointments that take place.

BARTON, TRAVERS B., A.B., M.D., L.R.C.S.I., L.M.—Surgeon to the County Donegal Hospital, Lifford, vice R. Little, F.R.C.S.I., deceased.

BIRTHS.

O'BRIEN.—On August 22, at 2, Victoria-terrace, Heavitree, near Exeter, the wife of Surgeon-Major T. M. O'Brien, Army Medical Department, of a daughter.

PAUL.—On August 22, at Loughborough, the wife of Reginald Paul, M.R.C.S., of a daughter.

ROBINSON.—On July 18, at Mercara, Coorg, Southern India, the wife of Surgeon Mark Robinson, Indian Medical Department, 40th Regt. M.N.I., of a son.

MARRIAGES.

ARMSTRONG—MACVICAR.—On August 18, at East Barkwith, Lincolnshire, Benjamin Armstrong, M.D., to Florence, youngest daughter of John Young Macvicar, Esq., of Barkwith House, Wragby.

CUTFIELD—FINCHAM.—On August 22, at Bishopsgate, Arthur Cutfield, B.A., B.Sc., M.R.C.S., to Agnes Mary Hulme, daughter of the late Frederick Fincham, Esq., of Manchester.

GUMPERT—BOECKER.—On August 18, at Manchester, E. Gumpert, M.D., of Manchester, to Matilda, youngest daughter of the late Dr. W. Boecker, of Bonn.

LAWFORD—LAWFORD.—On August 23, at Highgate Rise, Charles Harcourt Leftwich, M.R.C.S., of New Cross-road, Hatcham, to Ada Elizabeth, daughter of the late John E. Lawford, Esq., of Highgate Rise.

O'NEILL—NORTON.—On August 15, at Cliftonville, Margate, John Gregg O'Neill, M.B., to Emily Elizabeth, youngest daughter of the late Hon. James Norton, M.L.C., of Elswick, Sydney, N.S.W.

PYE-SMITH—GILL.—On August 20, at Plymouth, Rutherford John Pye-Smith, F.R.C.S., of Sheffield, to Emily Barbara, fourth daughter of John Edgcumbe Gill, Esq., of Plymouth.

DEATHS.

HAWKINS, THOMAS HENRY, M.D., F.R.C.S., formerly of Newbury, Berks, at Adelaide, South Australia, on July 2, aged 43.

HETT, J. C. W., M.D., of 42, Westbourne-terrace, Hyde-park, London, at the Balmoral Hotel, Edinburgh, on August 19, aged 69.

SHETTLE, B. C., M.D., of London-street, Reading, at the residence of his eldest son, on August 11, aged 87.

VIGERS, CATHERINE, wife of Harman Vigers, Esq., and fifth daughter of J. G. Davey, M.D., at Clevedon, Somerset, on August 18, aged 32.

VACANCIES.

In the following list the nature of the office vacant, the qualifications required in the candidate, the person to whom application should be made and the day of election (as far as known) are stated in succession.

BIRMINGHAM FRIENDLY SOCIETIES' MEDICAL INSTITUTION.—Resident Medical Officer. Candidates must be legally qualified practitioners, registered under the Medical Act, over thirty years of age, and married. They must produce their diplomas, certificates, and licences to the Committee. Applications, stating age, and enclosing recent testimonials as to qualifications and character, to be sent to Frederick Girling, 5, Cowper-street, Summer-lane, Birmingham, on or before September 15, marked " Medical."

CHILDREN'S HOSPITAL, BIRMINGHAM.—Assistant Resident Medical Officer. Candidates must be duly registered. Applications, with testimonials and certificate of registration, to be sent to the Secretary, Children's Hospital, Steelhouse-lane, Birmingham, not later than August 31.

KNIGHTON UNION.—District Medical Officer and Medical Officer of Health. Candidates must be legally qualified medical practitioners. Applications, accompanied by recent testimonials, to be sent to Edwin H. Deacon, Clerk to the Guardians, not later than September 1.

LIVERPOOL NORTHERN HOSPITAL.—Assistant House-Surgeon. Candidates must possess a medical and surgical qualification from one or more British colleges or institutions recognised under the Medical Act. Applications and testimonials to be addressed to the Chairman of the Committee, not later than September 12.

ROYAL FREE HOSPITAL, GRAY'S-INN-ROAD.—Junior Resident Medical Officer. (For particulars see Advertisement.)

ROYAL UNITED HOSPITAL, BATH.—House-Surgeon. (For particulars see Advertisement.)

WEST KENT GENERAL HOSPITAL, MAIDSTONE.—House-Surgeon. (For particulars see Advertisement.)

WORCESTER GENERAL INFIRMARY.—House-Surgeon. (For particulars see Advertisement.)

UNION AND PAROCHIAL MEDICAL SERVICE.

*** The area of each district is stated in acres. The population in computed according to the census of 1871.

RESIGNATIONS.

Reading Union.—Mr. Oded Lovsley has resigned the St. Giles District : area 9416 ; population 14,241 ; salary £125 per annum.

Headington Union.—Mr. A. S. L. Newington has resigned the Wheatley District : area 19,677 ; population 4359 ; salary £80 per annum.

Pickering Union.—The Pickering District and the Workhouse are vacant by the death of Dr. William Smith Scholefield : population 6221 ; salary £43 per annum ; salary for Workhouse £18 per annum.

Sedbergh Union.—Mr. T. Beaufoy Green has resigned the Sedbergh District and the Workhouse : area 32,081 ; population 2897 ; salary £15 per annum ; salary for Workhouse £15 per annum.

Wirral Union.—The Eastham District is vacant by the death of Mr. R. A. Jackson : area 7899 ; population 3000 ; salary £30 per annum.

APPOINTMENTS.

Banbury Union.—Frederick W. Fowke, L.R.C.P. Edin., M.R.C.S. Eng., L.S.A., to the Chipping Warden District.

Dewsbury Union.—James Turton, M.R.C.S. Eng., L.S.A., to the Heckmondwike District.

Keynsham Union.—F. M. Page, L.R.C.P. Edin., L.R.C.S. Edin., to the Bilton District.

Pembroke Union.—William Murray, M.B. Dub., M.R.C.S. Eng., to the First District.

Staines Union.—Edward J. Parrott, M.R.C.S. Eng ; L.R.C.P. Lond., to the Crauford District.

THE ROYAL COLLEGE OF SURGEONS OF ENGLAND.

CLINICAL EXAMINATIONS.—At the pass examination for the diploma of membership of the Royal College of Surgeons, which was brought to a close on the 29th ult., the following were the clinical cases selected from the metropolitan hospitals, viz. :—Abscess in the thigh, syphilitic testicle, division of muscles of the forearm and of the ulnar nerve, lymphadenoma, hydrocele, syphilitic periostitis of the fibula, congenital nævus in the forehead, and fractured humerus involving the musculo-spiral nerve in the callus, fracture of the radius (Colles'), inguinal hernia; atrophy of the testicle, hydrocele ; fractured thigh, syphilitic ulcer of the tongue, undescended testis, fatty tumour of the back, syphilitic eruption, large hydrocele, hæmorrhoids and scrotal hernia, tinea, epididymitis (double), strumous lymphatic glands, caries of the cervical vertebræ, spinal curvature, dislocation of the shoulder and abscess in the arm, fractured skull, paralysis of the left facial nerve; syphilis, roseola; strumous disease of the os calcis, tertiary syphilis of the urethra; epithelioma of the tongue, enlarged cervical glands; glandular tumour (? malignant), hydrosarcocele; strabismus, depressed fracture of the skull, locomotor affection of lower limbs; epithelioma linguæ, nodes in the head, hæmorrhoids and double hernia, hydrocele of the cord, malignant glandular tumour of the neck, scrofulous glands of the neck; ulcers of the leg, displacement of the great toe, bunion; sclerosis of the tibia, tertiary ulcer of the leg, warty growth on the skin of the foot, hæmatoma of the inguinal region, abdominal tumour.

MEDICAL LICENCES.—At the recent pass examination for membership of the Royal College of Surgeons, the following recognised licences were held by some of the candidates, exempting them from an examination in medicine, viz.:—L.S.A., 44; M.B. Edin., 6; L.R.C.P. Edin., 5; M.B. and C.M. Aber., 2; M.D. Kingston, Canada, 1; M.D. Paris, 1; M.D. Queen's Univ., Ire., 1; L.K.Q.C.P. Ire., 1; L.R.C.P. Lond., 1; M.B. Toronto, 2; M.B. and L.R.C.P. Edin., 1; M.B. Durh., 2; etc.

THE GERMAN NATURALISTS AND PHYSICIANS.—The fifty-fourth meeting of this body will be held this year at Salzburg, from September 17 to 24. It has been resolved to reduce the general addresses from three to two, in order to give more time for sectional work.

TREATMENT OF GONORRHŒA.—Prof. Ashhurst, in a clinical lecture delivered at the Hospital of the University of Pennsylvania, said that in a simple uncomplicated case of gonorrhœa he did not think internal medicines were requisite. When there is very painful scalding, relief is obtainable from the following mixture, which should be taken in divided doses within the twenty-four hours:—Linseed tea one pint, bicarbonate of soda a teaspoonful, and sweet spirits of nitre a tablespoonful. In the local treatment of the early stages he injects, every three or four hours, two syringefuls of argent. nitr. gr. ij., vini opii gt. xx.-xxx., aq. rosar. ℥viij. In the second stage he employs the following injection, in which a double decomposition takes place:—Liq. plumb. acet. ℥vj., zinc. sulph. ℈j., aquæ ʒij. If the discharge still continues, he recommends sulphate of copper one or two grains to the ounce. Later on, when it has become gleet, he has found tannic acid, weak at first, but gradually increased up to ʒj. ad ℥j., very effective. Glycerite of tannin may also be locally employed by means of a piece of cotton dipped into it, and put in at the end of a probe. When a slight stricture is present, a bougie should be passed to effect gradual dilatation, or a little mercurial ointment may be put on its end. —*New York Med. Record*, June 25.

APPOINTMENTS FOR THE WEEK.

August 27. *Saturday* (*this day*).

Operations at St. Bartholomew's, 1½ p.m.; King's College, 1½ p.m.; Royal Free, 2 p.m.; Royal London Ophthalmic, 11 a.m.; Royal Westminster Ophthalmic, 1½ p.m.; St. Thomas's, 1½ p.m.; London, 2 p.m.

29. *Monday*.

Operations at the Metropolitan Free, 2 p.m.; St. Mark's Hospital for Diseases of the Rectum, 2 p.m.; Royal London Ophthalmic, 11 a.m.; Royal Westminster Ophthalmic, 1½ p.m.

30. *Tuesday*.

Operations at Guy's, 1½ p.m.; Westminster, 2 p.m.; Royal London Ophthalmic, 11 a.m.; Royal Westminster Ophthalmic, 1½ p.m.; West London, 3 p.m.

31. *Wednesday*.

Operations at University College, 2 p.m.; St. Mary's, 1¼ p.m.; Middlesex, 1 p.m.; London, 2 p.m.; St. Bartholomew's, 1½ p.m.; Great Northern, 2 p.m.; Samaritan, 2½ p.m.; King's College (by Mr. Lister), 2 p.m.; Royal London Ophthalmic, 11 a.m.; Royal Westminster Ophthalmic, 1½ p.m.; St. Thomas's, 1½ p.m.; St. Peter's Hospital for Stone, 2 p.m.; National Orthopædic, Great Portland-street, 10 a.m.

September 1. *Thursday*.

Operations at St. George's, 1 p.m.; Central London Ophthalmic, 1 p.m.; Royal Orthopædic, 2 p.m.; University College, 2 p.m.; Royal London Ophthalmic, 11 a.m.; Royal Westminster Ophthalmic, 1½ p.m.; Hospital for Diseases of the Throat, 2 p.m.; Hospital for Women, 2 p.m.; Charing-cross, 2 p.m.; London, 2 p.m.; North-West London, 2½ p.m.

2. *Friday*.

Operations at Central London Ophthalmic, 2 p.m.; Royal London Ophthalmic, 11 a.m.; South London Ophthalmic, 2 p.m.; Royal Westminster Ophthalmic, 1½ p.m.; St. George's (ophthalmic operations), 1¼ p.m.; Guy's, 1½ p.m.; St. Thomas's (ophthalmic operations), 2 p.m.

VITAL STATISTICS OF LONDON.

Week ending Saturday, August 20, 1881.

BIRTHS.

Births of Boys, 1244; Girls, 1288; Total, 2532.
Corrected weekly average in the 10 years 1871-80, 2590·4.

DEATHS.

	Males.	Females.	Total.
Deaths during the week	765	709	1474
Weekly average of the ten years 1871-80, corrected to increased population ...	839·0	763·5	1602·5
Deaths of people aged 80 and upwards ...	...	...	42

DEATHS IN SUB-DISTRICTS FROM EPIDEMICS.

	Enumerated Population, 1881 (unrevised).	Small-pox.	Measles.	Scarlet Fever.	Diphtheria.	Whooping-cough.	Typhus.	Enteric (or Typhoid) Fever.	Simple continued Fever.	Diarrhœa.
West	668993	1	7	3	2	1	...	4	1	28
North ...	905677	9	14	16	4	7	...	4	...	32
Central ...	281793	2	4	4	1	3	...	1	...	8
East	692530	7	10	7	1	7	...	1	1	29
South	1265378	19	23	21	1	10	2	5	...	44
Total	3814571	38	58	51	9	28	2	15	2	141

METEOROLOGY.

From Observations at the Greenwich Observatory.

Mean height of barometer	29·523 in.
Mean temperature	56·1°
Highest point of thermometer	72·1°
Lowest point of thermometer	48·0°
Mean dew-point temperature	53·5°
General direction of wind	W.S.W.
Whole amount of rain in the week	0·25 in.

BIRTHS and DEATHS Registered and METEOROLOGY during the Week ending Saturday, August 20, in the following large Towns:—

Cities and boroughs (Municipal boundaries except for London.)	Estimated Population to middle of the year 1881.*	Persons to an Acre. (1881.)	Births Registered during the week ending Aug. 20.	Deaths Registered during the week ending Aug. 20.	Temperature of Air (Fahr.) Highest during the Week.	Temperature of Air (Fahr.) Lowest during the Week.	Temperature of Air (Fahr.) Weekly Mean of Daily Mean Values	Temp. of Air (Cent.) Weekly Mean of Daily Mean Values.	Rain Fall. In Inches.	Rain Fall. In Centimetres.
London	3829751	50·8	2532	1474	72·1	48·0	58·1	14·50	0·25	0·63
Brighton	107934	45·9	72	39	72·0	49·0	59·0	15·00	0·59	1·50
Portsmouth ...	128335	28·6	80	51	...	...	...	...	...	...
Norwich	88038	11·8	38	31	...	...	...	...	...	...
Plymouth	75262	54·0	46	20	67·7	48·5	57·2	14·00	0·46	1·17
Bristol	207140	46·5	141	71	67·8	47·5	55·4	13·00	0·99	2·51
Wolverhampton ...	75934	22·4	50	43	68·5	45·0	53·4	11·89	0·77	1·96
Birmingham ...	402296	47·9	269	154	...	...	...	...	...	...
Leicester	123120	38·5	95	88	69·5	44·2	55·2	12·89	0·74	1·88
Nottingham ...	188035	18·9	157	115	71·9	43·8	55·7	13·17	0·66	1·68
Liverpool	553988	106·3	392	296	65·3	50·1	54·7	12·61	0·66	1·68
Manchester ...	341269	79·5	221	153	...	...	...	...	...	...
Salford	177760	34·4	125	83	...	...	...	...	...	...
Oldham	112176	24·0	80	45	...	...	...	...	...	...
Bradford	184037	25·5	109	60	64·1	48·0	55·0	12·78	0·71	1·80
Leeds	310490	14·4	198	115	...	...	...	...	...	...
Sheffield	285621	14·5	205	123	71·0	49·0	57·3	14·06	0·77	1·96
Hull	155161	42·7	120	93	67·0	46·0	55·2	12·89	1·82	4·62
Sunderland ...	116753	42·2	70	37	...	...	...	...	...	...
Newcastle-on-Tyne	145675	27·1	97	78	...	...	...	...	...	...
Total of 20 large English Towns ...	7608775	38·0	5097	3169	72·1	43·8	56·0	13·33	0·77	1·96

* These figures are the numbers enumerated (but subject to revision) in April last, raised to the middle of 1881 by the addition of a quarter of a year's increase, calculated at the rate that prevailed between 1871 and 1881.

At the Royal Observatory, Greenwich, the mean reading of the barometer last week was 29·52 in. The lowest reading was 29·29 both on Wednesday and Friday, and the highest 29·78 on Saturday afternoon.

NOTES, QUERIES, AND REPLIES.

Ye that questioneth much shall learn much.—Bacon.

Too Good to be True?—Snake Poison.

TO THE EDITOR OF THE MEDICAL TIMES AND GAZETTE.

Sir,—The journals of Rio de Janeiro give news which has rarely been exceeded in interest. Permanganate of potassa is the infallible antidote to the poison of serpents. The discoverer is a Brazilian physician—Dr. John Baptist de Lacerda—attached to the National Museum of Natural History of Rio de Janeiro. Repeated successful experiments, positive and negative, have been performed by him in the presence of His Majesty the Emperor Peter II., first scientist and first *littérateur* of the Empire; and there is said to be no doubt felt in Rio as to the thorough truth of the discovery. I am not aware of the doses in which the permanganate is applied, and if it is employed by hypodermic injection or by the mouth. It is a curious coincidence that *Lacerta* (Latin form of Lacerda) signifies lizard, and the lizard is one of the great enemies of snakes, fighting them and swallowing them entire. During the fight the lizard pauses to eat the leaves of a certain plant, which renders it proof against the venom.
I am, &c.,

RICHARD GUMBLETON DAUNT, M.D. Edin.
Campinas, San Paulo, Brazil, July 19.

Benevolence.—The late Dr. Thomas Radford, of Higher Broughton, Manchester, has bequeathed to St. Mary's Hospital, Manchester, £900, free of legacy duty, to be applied under the direction of the Medical Committee in the purchase of casts, models, or wet obstetrical preparations for the purpose [of adding to and enriching the Radford Museum at the aforesaid Hospital.——Lady Harriet M. Scott Bentinck has given donations to the following institutions, namely:—£1000 to the Royal Hospital for Diseases of the Chest, City-road, and the like sum to St. Mary's Hospital, Paddington; also £700 to the North-Eastern Hospital for Children, Hackney-road; and £9000 towards the expenses of the University College Hospital.

Medical Advancement of Learning.—Lord Bacon's words were—"Medicine is a science which hath been, as we have said, more professed than laboured, and yet more laboured than advanced; the labour having been, in my judgment, rather in circle than in progression. For I find much iteration and small progression."

A Jealous Authority.—It will be remembered that the authorities of the University of Oxford took active measures as to the sanitary condition of the lodging-houses after the death of a student from diphtheria, due, it was alleged, to the insanitary condition of his lodgings, and that subsequently the University authorities issued orders to the lodging-house keepers (whose houses they have had inspected) to conform to the rules laid down, and in the case of those supplied with well-water to have it analysed by the University analyst. These orders have apparently offended the susceptibilities of the Local Board, and the University has, in consequence, received a notice that any alterations in sanitary arrangements must be entrusted to the Board, but the University can refuse to license lodging-houses where the regulations considered necessary are not complied with.

The Temperance Movement.—A coffee-tavern, said to be the largest and most comprehensive of its kind in the kingdom, was opened at Woolwich last week. It has cost nearly £10,000, and is situated close to the Arsenal station of the North Kent Railway. It has three classes of dining-rooms, library, reading and recreation rooms, and a large public hall, capable of seating 1000 persons. A special feature of the scheme is the bedroom floor, where accommodation is provided for a number of single men lodgers.

Baby Farming and a Registrar of Births and Deaths.—There were circumstances connected with a baby-farming case that came before Mr. Bridge, the Southwark police magistrate, a few days since, which should be noticed. A woman was summoned for infringing the Infant Life Preservation Act by taking charge of children without having previously obtained a licence. No ill-treatment or insufficiency of food was alleged, although several children in the defendant's care had, it appeared, died; but the vitiated air of the small room occupied by the children and their foster-parent, it was considered, had contributed more than anything else to their death. A fine of £5 was imposed, with the alternative of two months' imprisonment. But the special feature of the case was that the Registrar of Births and Deaths for the district, who is a chemist (and the woman resided in the same locality), had issued an order for the burial of the children, though no certificate as to the cause of death had been given. The magistrate described this as "very irregular." Moreover, this Registrar had supplied the defendant with medicines for the children; and the magistrate very properly recommended the inspector to report the Registrar's conduct to the Local Government Board.

Casualties in London Thoroughfares.—According to Sir E. Henderson's report for the year 1880, just issued, the fatal accidents in the streets increased from 124 in 1879 to 187 in 1880, while the number of persons more or less seriously injured through being knocked down or run over rose from 2950 in the former year to 3359 in the latter. These numbers refer only to cases which were brought to the knowledge of the police, but do not represent the total numbers of fatalities and casualties.

The Commons Preservation Society.—The good work accomplished by this Society during the past few years, in the preservation from spoliation of commons and open spaces in the interests of the public weal, is worthy of notice and commendation. It appears that considerable success has attended the action of the Society during the past session. There have been no less than twenty different proposals to take portions of commons for railway purposes, which, if they had been adopted or carried, would have deprived the public of the right to no less than eight hundred acres of recreation ground. The Society has successfully contested the confiscation clauses of these Bills, and deserves the generous support of the public in its praiseworthy endeavours in their behalf.

Urban and Rural Sanitary Works.—A plan for the efficient drainage of Margate has been approved at an estimated cost of £44,000.——At the Royal Naval Barracks, Sheerness, extensive alterations in the sick-bay arrangements have just been completed, and commodious and comfortable wards are ready for the reception of patients. The whole of the wing facing the sea is now used for sick-bay purposes, and, in the event of an outbreak of infectious disease, it could be isolated from the rest of the establishment.——A scheme of sewerage and sewage disposal is to be carried out at Burgess Hill, Sussex.——The Urban Sanitary Authority of Watford, Herts, are about to modify the present arrangements on their sewage farm by the introduction of intermittent filtration in combination with wide irrigation.——Public baths are to be erected at Wigan on a site fronting the Free Library, at an estimated cost of £5000 for the building.——The Tottenham Local Board of Health have decided on a comprehensive scheme for dealing with the storm water of the Woodlands and Harringay-park Estates, and to construct a swimming bath.——The Local Board of Cottingham, near Hull, have approved plans for the drainage of New Cottingham.——The Matlock (Bath) Local Board have opened negotiations with the Matlock Waterworks Company for the transfer to the Board, as Urban Sanitary Authority, of their works, plant, and undertaking.——Waterworks have just been opened at Corstorphine, near Edinburgh. For many years the want of water had been severely felt. The water is obtained from the Edinburgh and District Water Trust.——The Metropolitan Board of Works Money Bill, recently introduced to Parliament, provides powers to borrow, *inter alia*, the following sums, namely:—For the purpose of main drainage and sewerage, £100,000; in respect to the new Hackney-commons, £34,200, and £100,000 for "minor improvements," and contributions to local improvements; for parks, commons, and open spaces, £15,000; to be expended in street improvements, £1,500,000, and £200,000 is required in connexion with artisans' dwellings; in addition, the Bill provides powers to advance loans to vestries and district boards to the extent of £200,000; to boards of guardians, £150,000; to the Managers of the Metropolitan Asylums, £50,000. The actual amount of the Board's borrowing powers provided by the Bill is £4,526,394.——The Water Commissioners of Stirling are about to construct an additional reservoir on the Touch Hills, at an estimated cost of £15,000.

COMMUNICATIONS have been received from—
The Secretary of the New Sydenham Society, London; Mr. F. Livens, Bournemouth; The Registrar of the Apothecaries' Hall, London; The "Liverpool Journal of Commerce"; Mr. J. Chatto, London; The Town Clerk of Hastings; Dr. W. H. Pearse, Plymouth; Dr. Radcliffe Crocker, London; Dr. F. de Havilland Hall, London; Mr. Bucher, London; The Secretary of the London Company, Wrexham; Professor Lépine, Lyons; Mr. Lawson Tait, Birmingham.

BOOKS, ETC., RECEIVED—
Joint Diseases of the Lower Extremity, by A. B. Judson, M.D.—Index Catalogue of the Library of the Surgeon-General's Office, U.S. Army—Hip Disease, by A. B. Judson, M.D. New York—The Climate of the Undercliffe, Isle of Wight, by J. L. Whitehead, M.D.—The New Sydenham Society's Lexicon of Medicine and the Allied Sciences, by Henry Power, M.B., and Leonard W. Sedgwick, M.D.—Annual Report of the Parish of St. Mary Abbotts, Kensington, for the Year 1880—Annual Report of the Borough of Huddersfield for the Year 1880—La Infezione Palustre nello Stato Presente della Scienza, pel Dott. Carlo Girone—Notes on Two Classes of Locomotor Ataxy, by A. Davidson, M.D.—On Vaccination Penalties, by Lord Clifton—Davos Platz, by Alfred Wise, M.D.—Notes on Midwifery, by J. J. Reynolds, M.R.C.S.

PERIODICALS AND NEWSPAPERS RECEIVED—
Lancet—British Medical Journal—Medical Press and Circular—Berliner Klinische Wochenschrift—Centralblatt für Chirurgie—Gazette des Hôpitaux—Gazette Médicale—Le Progrès Médical—Bulletin de l'Académie de Médecine—Pharmaceutical Journal—Wiener Medizinische Wochenschrift—Centralblatt für die Medizinischen Wissenschaften—Revue Médicale—Gazette Hebdomadaire—National Board of Health Bulletin—Washington—Nature—Deutsche Medicinal-Zeitung—Boston Medical and Surgical Journal—Australian Medical Journal—Scientific Roll—Centralblatt für Gynäkologie—Louisville Medical News—Martin's Chemists' and Druggists' Bulletin—Northern Evening Express, August 10—Monthly Index—Oil and Drug News—Physician and Surgeon—Detroit Lancet—The American—Morningside Mirror—Union Medica—Weekblad—Tijdschrift voor Geneeskunde—Occasional Notes—Revue d'Hygiène.

INTERNATIONAL MEDICAL CONGRESS.—We learn that Mr. Barraud's picture of this subject, for which all the leading visitors to England sat, will be published in November. Mr. Barraud has been requested to wait until the middle of October before closing his sittings, as many eminent English members of the Congress will not be able to sit before that month.

THE FORTY-NINTH ANNUAL MEETING
OF THE
BRITISH MEDICAL ASSOCIATION.
HELD AT RYDE, AUGUST 8, 9, 10, AND 11.

ADDRESS IN OBSTETRIC MEDICINE.
By J. G. SINCLAIR COGHILL, M.D., F.R.C.P.E.,
Interim Lecturer on Midwifery in the University of Edinburgh ;
late Lecturer on General Pathology in the Edinburgh Medical School ;
Hon. Visiting Physician, Royal National Hospital, Ventnor.

IN rising to deliver the Address in Obstetric Medicine, I must confess I do so with very mingled feelings. In the first place let me say how deeply sensible I am of the great honour paid me, and, through me, to my professional brethren in the Isle of Wight, in being invited by the President and Council of our Association to occupy so distinguished a position—one which circumstances, to which I need not further refer, render peculiarly gratifying—one for which I am more indebted to your kindness than to my own merit. This feeling of pleasure, however, is only equalled by the deep sense of responsibility which a duty so onerous necessarily involves—intensified, as it must be, by the recollection of the eminent obstetricians who have addressed you on former occasions. I have been reminded that the first to deliver this address was a provincial physician, the late Dr. Thomas Radford of Manchester, a worthy exponent of the great obstetric school. With affectionate remembrance, I next recall my old master, the great Simpson, who, if not the creator of modern gynæcology, was at least the author of its renaissance. Again, the ancient glories of the Dublin school have been worthily represented before you by the late Dr. Beatty, at Newcastle, in 1869. I cannot forget that you have listened to Dr. Matthews Duncan, whose contributions to obstetric literature are such models of the application of the exact method to the investigation of scientific questions. More recently, at Manchester again, you have been privileged to hear one eminent indeed among us—one who has done so much to extend the principles, and to precise the practice of our art—to rear obstetric pathology on the sound basis of its physiological equivalents, and who has striven so eloquently to elevate obstetric medicine to its true position in the medical sisterhood—I refer to Dr. Robert Barnes.

In seeking for a subject on which to address you, I find myself in a position of some difficulty. I have no great discovery in obstetrics to announce to you ; I am unable to indicate any new point of departure in our art ; I cannot invite you to tread with me on scientific pastures new. I must, therefore, be content to fill a much more humble rôle. Nevertheless, such topics as do suggest themselves are neither wanting in number nor in variety ; and they possess that interest which attaches to questions of vital importance, not only to us as physicians, but to humanity at large. In obstetric medicine, there are principles still in process of development, problems yet unsolved, methods not yet determined, mysteries still unravelled, results anticipated but not realised. That the Address in Obstetric Medicine is only delivered at irregular intervals of years, shows plainly enough the position assigned to it in the Medical Trilogy, and seems also to indicate the character which such an address ought to assume. I believe, therefore, I shall most usefully discharge the duty assigned me, if I follow this indication, and give my address to some extent a general character, by directing your attention to a few considerations in connexion with the claims, intrinsic and relative, of obstetric medicine to increased recognition and cultivation, and the directions in which its development should be encouraged ; and, further, to sketch, in form of retrospect, a few of the principal points of progress which have marked its annals during the past triennium. The rapid advances which obstetric medicine has so recently made, and the corresponding changes in pathological views and modes of treatment, render my task by no means easy. I must, therefore, bespeak your indulgence for the imperfect manner in which it may be accomplished.

Obstetric medicine comprehends obstetrics proper, gynæcology, and pædiatrics ; such is the terminology which represents our old familiar terms : midwifery, and diseases of women, and diseases of children. These Greek derivatives are cumbersome in form, uncouth in sound, and want the ready ring of household words. I humbly submit that we have been especially unhappy in our nomenclature, and I hope some more than usually scholarly obstetrist will take up the subject for serious reform. If we are to retain these terms, why not use obstetrics as the generic term, and substitute tocology for obstetrics proper or midwifery ? I make this suggestion as my little contribution to the much-needed reform. I bear in mind, however, that, in a rapidly advancing science, we must be cautious in changing our nomenclature ; for change of name with changing doctrine does not necessarily imply progress.

The tendency of modern medicine to cultivation in a great variety of special branches, although favourable to the attainment of technical skill when such is necessary, is in some respects to be deprecated. It is an inclination apt to interfere with the grand ideal unity of medicine as an art based on general principles, and tends to interrupt the harmonious continuity of its scientific development. Obstetric medicine, however, deals exclusively with the special set of organs and functions which distinguish women only, which dominate in a special manner all their other organic conditions, and which present special phenomena without parallel even in the other sex. The sexual system in women constitutes, in fact, a true imperium in imperio. Its functions are so important, and the phenomena, normal and morbid, which they present, are themselves so intrinsically specific in character, and in the nature of the influences they exert over the other organic systems, as to make their study necessarily a specialty in the widest and best sense of that much-abused term. Special qualifications, mental and physical, are requisite for practice in this wide field. Physical energy and powers of endurance, moral courage, rapidity of thought, and readiness of resource in presence of unexpected difficulties immediately involving human life, are more imperatively demanded in this than in either of the sister branches of the healing art. But the unity of our common profession, as much as the interests of those whose physical health and moral well-being are confided to our care, alike require that the obstetrician, to the culture of the physician and the surgeon, should add something more—the culture of his own special department. The more he qualifies himself in the sister branches, the more thoroughly and scientifically will he cultivate his own ; since we cannot arrive at an exact knowledge of the state of any one organ, or organic system, without taking into account the state of all the rest in their absolute and related conditions. The mutual relations, indeed, of obstetrics, medicine, and surgery, are so intimate, that no discovery or progress is possible in one without largely influencing the others. We must ever bear in mind that their special pathologies have a common basis in one general pathology.

Considering that to the vast majority of the profession, especially in the earlier part of their career, when their professional character and status is being made, obstetric practice in its several branches forms the bulk as well as the most anxious and engrossing part of their work, it seems incredible that the provision for teaching gynæcology particularly, both systematic and clinical, in our medical schools and hospitals should still be so limited and imperfect. The very subjects which will occupy a man's attention at a time when the character of his work may perchance determine professional success, are, in the course of his education, either made optional or left to chance, while other less essential subjects are forced upon him ; and he thus enters on his labours imperfectly prepared, or, it may be, profoundly ignorant of all practical acquaintance with what will form a large share of them. Familiarity with the practice of obstetric and gynæcological details can only acquired by demonstration. It is very much easier amputate a limb or to pass a catheter, from a description of these operations read out of a book, than to determine the nature of an uterine flexion by means of the sound, or to get a good view of the cervix by means of the speculum. A gynæcological clinique, with ample service, should be established in connexion with all our hospitals; and this is the more necessary, that the opportunity for such technical instruction afforded by old system of apprenticeship is much less freely taken advantage of in the present day. The marked progress of obstetric medicine in America, and its splendid achievements, are no doubt due to some extent to the absence of old-world traditions, but much more to the full recognition of its importance, and to the ample provision made everywhere for its clinical as well as for its scientific cultivation.

If the progress of obstetric medicine is to be satisfactory, if it is to become less empirical and more and more scientific, in the study of pathology must be sought the means of determining the principles on which a rational system of therapeutics is to be founded. It is in a complete knowledge of the anatomy and physiology of the female sexual system that the foundations of uterine pathology must be laid. The elements of this pathology must naturally be sought for in connexion with the special physiological conditions which distinguish the female sex. The sexual system dominates the other organic systems in woman. Her nature is altogether more emotional than man's. His nature is objective, and is reflected externally; woman's nature is subjective, and is reflected internally. The sexual system in man does not attain this organic supremacy, therefore he escapes the innumerable referred, sympathetic, or reflex disturbances to which woman is liable from her physical and mental constitution, through the action and reaction of her sexual system. There is a constant provision going on in her system for the conception and nutrition of a new being, necessitating an organic mobility which in her involves the gravest contingencies.

Menstruation and pregnancy, although strictly physiological in design and general issue, are yet conditions of such extreme organic tension that they may pass, by almost imperceptible degrees, into the domain of pathology. They are essentially physiological, but at the same time potentially pathological. The growth of the human body, although continuous until the adult term is reached, presents certain marked developmental crises which occur at regular epochs, when additional nutritive force seems to be determined to certain organs, in connexion with which special functions are thereby established. These cycles of development, as well as their corresponding functions, appear to follow with a limited margin the figure seven and its multiples, and may have led to this numeral being invested with a *quasi* sacred character, and its being brought into prominence as a measure of time and otherwise. The first cycle of seven years corresponds to the period of the first dentition, and to a marked epoch in the development of the cerebrum. The second cycle of seven years marks the attainment of puberty in woman, by the establishment of the process or function of ovulation, as shown by the appearance of the catamenia. Twenty-eight days may be assumed as the average menstrual cycle; while its duration until the climacteric or menopause is reached, at or about the forty-ninth year, corresponds to the completion of the seventh cycle from birth, or the fifth cycle of seven years after puberty, including the whole period of menstrual activity. Pregnancy, again, lasting about 280 days, covers a period of ten catamenial cycles of twenty-eight days. The appearance of the menstrual phenomena proclaims that a new organ, with its system, for the purpose of reproduction, has attained its development. In this periodic function, the nervous and vascular systems are largely concerned. It is characterised by a condition of increased vascular tension or hyperæmia, which, if not relieved by menstrual expenditure, or pregnancy, or subsequently by lactation, may not only lead to uterine and ovarian disease, but also to grave disorders of the general health. Another source of uterine troubles, in connexion with this function, is to be looked for in excessive, as well as in imperfect, sexual congress. Faulty habits of life again, excess of animal food and stimulants, neglect of bodily exercise, mental fatigue—indeed, all causes which tend to increase either vascular or nervous tension—tend to disease by exaggerating or perverting normal conditions. To these, we must add another order of causation incidental

to the condition of pregnancy, to the process of parturition, and to the puerperal state—none being more frequent or grave than those presented as a result of imperfect or interrupted puerperal convalescence. The body, in which the occurrence of conception marks such an organic revolution, which for so many months is the seat of the remarkable changes culminating in delivery, must be in a state of great organic instability, oscillating narrowly between the confines of health and disease.

Obstetric medicine, indeed, offers to the scientific student problems of the most complex and wonderful nature—problems more easily followed and unravelled than many presented by the other departments of medicine. What more extraordinary than the genetic force evoked by the contact and fusion of the male and female fecundating elements in the act of conception? What more remarkable than the forces or changes which determine the periodicity of the special functions in women? What more interesting than the reflex nervous phenomena developed through the cerebro-spinal system, in connexion with ovario-uterine disorders? Obstetric physicians, indeed, more than any others, have constantly to take into account, and to become familiar with, reflex conditions. The abundant organic connexions of the nerves of the sexual apparatus in women with those of the cerebro-spinal and sympathetic systems, permit the play of the emotional or psychical element as an influencing or disturbing power in relation to the functions of the uterine system. This association is full of interest as a potential factor in its morbid manifestations. The explanation of the protean phenomena of the various forms of hysteria and hystero-epilepsy—the "hysteria major" of Charcot—is to be found in this connexion. The controlling centre of nerve-action in the genital apparatus was long held to reside in the ovaries; but both clinical experience and actual observation have latterly tended to depose them from that position. The survival—nay, even initiation—of sexual desire and pareunia, after removal of both organs in the operation of ovariotomy, affords satisfactory clinical proof that at least the primary sexual nervous centre must be looked for elsewhere. The discovery by Goltz and Frensburg of a nervous centre of sexual power opposite the fourth lumbar spine seems to determine this interesting point, and throws considerable light on hitherto obscure and apparently anomalous phenomena. It is known in the East that castration, performed on the male adult after the exercise of the sexual organs has developed their full power, still leaves the individual capable of the formality of coitus—that is, of erection and orgasm without emission. Eunuchs of this class are accordingly a much less valuable commodity than those castrated in early life or completely mutilated. The explanation is, of course, that the sexual nerve-centre in the spinal cord, having been developed under functional activity, remains active, although part of the sexual apparatus—formerly credited with the essential control of the whole phenomena—has been eliminated. A parallel is afforded by what takes place when a limb, such as the arm or leg, has been amputated *in utero* or blighted *in ovo*. In this case the portion of the spinal cord corresponding to the nerve-supply of the absent limb remains in its *embryonic* form, undeveloped; but, when the limb has been removed in adult life, the activity of its nerve-centre remains, and sensations and pains continue to be consciously interpreted as coming from the side of the absent member.

There has undoubtedly been latterly a great revival of the former view of the importance of the nervous system in relation to the functions of the other organic systems of the body. More extended researches in microscopic anatomy have greatly tended to this result. The terminations of the nerves have been traced much further than when I published my "Lectures on the Peripheral Nervous System" in 1859. Klein in this country, and Frankenhäuser, Kehrer, Koch, Spiegelberg, and others, have shown that there exists a much more intimate organic continuity between the ultimate nerve-terminations and the other tissue-elements, especially the epithelial, the important bearings of which, both on physiological and pathological processes, cannot be overlooked in its clinical relations. I believe, further—and strict physiological analogy permits the deduction as legitimate—that nerve-force may even be discharged free into and affect the fluid contents of the animal cells, and in the same manner influence the blood itself, which, in every sense and purpose, is a living tissue endowed with the highest organic and functional mobilit

It is, perhaps, through this presumed neuro-vascular association that we may find the channel by which maternal impressions are conveyed to the fœtus; and it is more reasonable to suppose that the contents of the bloodvessels are in this manner directly affected by nerve-force, than merely by the contraction and dilatation of their walls. I am not aware that this idea has ever been previously suggested, and I offer it with due reserve. The uterus receives the greater part of its nervous supply from the hypogastric branches of the posterior mesenteric ganglion, and partly also from the sacral plexus. The important observations of Patenka of St. Petersburg show that these also include the coats of the uterine bloodvessels in their distribution. According to the experiments of Basch and Hofmann, electrical irritation of the hypogastric nerves causes contraction of the circular muscular fibres, under which the uterus descends and the os opens; while, under similar excitation of the sacral plexus, the longitudinal muscular fibres contract and the os uteri closes. These latter observations settle definitely the previous but contradictory views of Spiegelberg and of Frankenhäuser, the former of whom denied motor power to the hypogastrics, and the latter to the sacrals. The cervix uteri is peculiarly rich in its nerve-supply, as might be expected from its exalted sensibility and active functions. As has been pointed out by Dr. Braxton Hicks, the uterus is the only organ in the body whose main nervous supply is derived from the sympathetic, to which we have such access, and which can be so freely handled and examined. It is, indeed, a great example of the decentralisation of that system. Dr. Reimann of Vienna found that the uterus separated from the cerebro-spinal axis, and also when removed from the body, responded to irritation by peristaltic and rhythmical movements of the whole organ, even when only a portion of it had been irritated; that also, removed from the body, but maintained at its normal temperature, it exhibited systolic movements for an hour after the death of the animal. The uterus has then an independent ganglionic system connected with, and therefore influenced by and reacting through, the cerebro-spinal system, but organically related to and derived from the sympathetic. The arrangement and distribution of the uterine bloodvessels are peculiar to that organ, as shown by the investigations of Rouget and Snow Beck. The arterial and venous systems freely anastomose, and seem more dependent on the contractility of the permeated tissues than on the elasticity of their own walls for propelling the blood. Hence the effect of general debility, or, on the other hand, of hyperæmia, in causing or favouring uterine congestion and hæmorrhage. This anatomical peculiarity of the uterine vascular system has important bearings on the occurrence and treatment of parturient and other forms of uterine hæmorrhage.

The great importance of the mucous lining of the uterus, so varied in its structural differentiation, with its elaborate glandular apparatus and great functional activity, must not be overlooked in this connexion. The uterine nerves have been traced into the epithelial cells lining its free surface; placing it, therefore, in organic solidarity with distant surfaces, where we know one of its periodic phenomena may be manifested vicariously through reflex action; for vicarious function is simply referred or reflex function. And we must remember that pathological liability is always in relation to complexity of structure and activity of function. More recent studies of the changes in the uterine mucous membrane, induced by menstruation and conception, have thrown considerable light on the physiological relations of this important structure, especially in relation to ovulation, to conception, to the duration of pregnancy, and to the pathology of one form at least of dysmenorrhœa. Maericke observed, from portions of the uterine mucosa removed by means of a curette during the pre-menstrual, menstrual, and post-menstrual periods, that in every instance the true or deeper layer of the epithelial lining was completely preserved. If the mucous membrane of the uterus were entirely destroyed during menstruation, it would be a pathological process, no longer a physiological one. It would, indeed, be contrary to all analogy for an elaborate structure to be reproduced, except from histogenic elements left behind for the purpose. Kundrat's investigations show that, for several days before the appearance of the catamenial flow, and probably preceding the discharge of the ovum, the mucous surface is swollen, loose and almost diffluent, and covered with a

whitish or bloody mucus. It is freely injected in parts, and in many instances it is found coloured a deep red. It appears that the uterus is prepared for the reception of the ovum a certain time before the rupture of the Graafian vesicle. The menstrual flow follows, and is caused by the retrograde changes in the surface of the mucous membrane, of the nature of fatty degeneration, which follows the death of the ovum. The impregnated ovum belongs, then, not to a menstruation just past, but to one just prevented by fecundation. In the light of the latest researches, each menstruation simply means the death and extrusion of an unimpregnated ovum, and of the materials prepared in utero in anticipation of conception.

Let us now turn to the subject of obstetrics proper, or midwifery. Recent progress in this branch of medicine has consisted more in an extended knowledge of the mechanism of parturition, and in greater precision in the choice of methods and times for interference, than in new means of treatment in operative midwifery, or in novelties in instrumental aids to labour. Exact methods of research have been successfully applied to the elucidation of many interesting and important questions in connexion with pregnancy, parturition, and the puerperal state. Among the most urgent questions that present themselves in this category is the prophylaxis of post-partum hæmorrhage, and of puerperal fever—the two great opprobria of obstetrics, and on the latter of which the antiseptic teaching of Lister has already begun to exert an important influence. The mechanism of parturition, the nature and the amount of the force exerted in that process, and the postural relations of the fœtus and maternal passages, have engaged the attention and have received adequate treatment at the hands of Ribemont, Schultze, Küneke, Schrœder, Haughton, Matthews Duncan, and Hart.

A speculative theory has been lately broached by Dr. Mortimer Granville, suggesting the predetermination of sex by intention. He endeavours to show that the sex of children is determined by the relative ardency of parents. " A preponderance of impulse on the part of the male produces female offspring; while excess on the part of the female parent produces male progeny." But I am sure we have all known families with a large proportion of sons, in which the mothers were physically fragile and sexually apathetic. It is long since the observation was made, that the sex of the older parent prevailed in the progeny in some proportion to the disparity of age. This latter explanation is more in harmony with the law of nature which has determined the relative proportion of the sexes, and seeks to maintain it by providing for the replacement of the sex of that parent of more precarious survivorship—that is, the elder.

An extremely interesting and valuable communication with reference to the time and mode of separating the fœtus and umbilical cord has been made by Ribemont, in a recent number of Les Archives de Tocologie, which shows satisfactorily the great influence of the " thoracic aspiration " of the fœtus on the umbilical circulation before its ligature. This was first pointed out by Budin; but is denied, among others, by Schücking. Determined by the manometer, it was found that—1. Tardy ligature of the cord benefits the child by increasing the quantity of blood which is required for the establishment of the third circulation—that is, the fœtal pulmonary. 2. The immediate ligature of the cord deprives the infant of a quantity of blood, larger or smaller in proportion to the time of ligature; and it especially deprives it of necessary blood if the ligature has been applied before the child has breathed. 3. The early ligature of the cord thus compels the abstraction of the blood necessary to establish the pulmonary circulation from the general circulation. The result is a diminution of the arterial tension equal to one-third of the initial tension. 4. The cause of the penetration of the blood into the pulmonary circulatory system of the child is the " thoracic inspiration." This is proved by the constant superiority of the pressure of the blood in the umbilical arteries to that in the umbilical vein. Again, the thoracic respiration is observed to produce considerable oscillations in the tension of the arterial and venous blood. The uterine contractions are utterly insufficient to force any blood along the umbilical vein when the arterial pulsations of the cord have ceased. 5. Thoracic aspiration causes the *sufficient* and *necessary* amount of blood to enter the pulmonary vessels—*sufficient*, because, under these circumstances, the tension in the arterial system does not fall; *necessary*, because the arterial tension in the umbilical cord of a newly born child is never seen to rise after tardy ligature of the cord. Professor W. T. Lusk, of New York, in corroborating Ribemont's views, says that, in children born pale and anæmic, and suffering from syncope, late ligation of the cord furnishes an invaluable means of restoring the equilibrium of the fœtal circulation.

An interesting communication of Dr. Langdon Down, on the obstetrical aspects of idiocy, shows that this condition is due more to prolonged labour than to timely and judicious operative delivery. Of 2000 cases, 24 per cent. were first-born; only 2 per cent. twins; twice as many male children as female; while, contrary to previous views, only 3 per cent. were forceps cases. In this connexion, I may refer to the recent outcry as to a supposed diminution in the size of "the heads of the people," inferring gradual racial degeneracy. The hatters, however, soon settled the question by pointing out that the saleable sizes of hats had certainly become smaller, but that this was due to the change of fashion, which led to hats being worn on the very top of the head instead of over the ears. Analogy forbids the supposition. Heads are probably still enlarging with increasing mental cultivation, as shown probably also in the increasing difficulty of parturition. We know that the armour of former times is much too small for modern heroes.

Dr. Lebert, of Nice, and Dr. Ortega have followed up the views of Grisolle, published in 1850, as to the deleterious effects of pregnancy on phthisical females. It is still a popular belief that child-bearing arrests pulmonary consumption and improves the health of the mother. Lebert's observations support the view of the aggravation of phthisis by pregnancy, but show that the effects of the labour itself are much more prejudicial to the mother. Of thirty-three phthisical girls who returned to their first labours. Ortega has had ninety-five cases under observation. Of these, only thirteen bore more than one child; more than one-third aborted, or were prematurely confined; only eleven out of sixty-four children were suckled by their mothers, and these soon showed signs of insufficient nutrition, and died. Ortega holds that pregnancy hastens the evolution of phthisis, and that delivery is rapidly followed by the death of the mother. I have no doubt of the correctness of these views, which are pointedly borne out by the Registrar-General's Report for 1879, according to which only two women died of phthisis during pregnancy, while no fewer than 222 died of phthisis after delivery, not classed as due to accidents of childbirth, or metria. I believe, however, the stage of the disease is an important element; and that marriage, when conception can be avoided, from its stimulus to the nervous and nutritive systems, has a beneficial effect on the general health, and through it on the tendency to pulmonary trouble.

As bearing on the subject of the general prophylaxis of childbirth by the anticipation of parturient difficulties, the investigations of Aschfeld of Leipzig on craniometry are extremely interesting. Aschfeld has ascertained the size of the child in utero in 250 cases, by applying one limb of Baudelocque's pelvimeter to the occiput per vaginam, and the other to the breech as outlined in the contracted fundus externally. In one most important series of observations, he gives the exact relative proportions between the length of the child and the two transverse diameters of the head. I have no doubt that pelvimetry with craniometry are destined to become important elements of scientific obstetric management. Attention also has again been drawn to the facility (first pointed out especially by Wiegand) with which the position of the fœtus and the point of placental insertion can be determined by examination through the maternal walls, and its position rectified, if need be, by external manipulation before and even during labour. Lobat, who has more recently devoted attention to this matter, lays down the following points:—1. Version by external manipulation is possible in certain cases during labour. 2. When the position of the fœtus is transverse, and the placenta is inserted near the os uteri, cephalic version by external manipulation renders the hæmorrhage less severe. 3. When cephalic version is impossible, pelvic version should be resorted to. 4. Dr. Pinard's eutocic bandage is not always necessary to retain the changed fœtal attitude. This is a modified form of binder to retain the head on the brim after

version. A head-presentation may thus be secured weeks before delivery.

The intense interest taken by the profession in the discussions on post-partum hæmorrhage, in the Association meeting of 1879; and on the forceps, at the Obstetrical Society of London more recently, shows how earnestly attention is devoted to questions bearing so directly on the safety and expedition of labour. The great debate on the forceps, in the Obstetrical Society, must be regarded as one of the most valuable contributions to practical midwifery of our time. Dr. Barnes, in his able opening, stated the advantages of the forceps over its alternatives, ergot, turning, and craniotomy, and formulated the conditions or indications for its employment in a manner that the subsequent discussion only tended to confirm. The statistics brought forward on that occasion show what influence on human life changes in choice of means and times for interference may exert. Collins performed craniotomy in one out of 211 cases, and used forceps in one in 607; Ramsbottom performed craniotomy once in 802 cases, and used forceps once in 670; Dr. Robert Lee, up to 1863, performed craniotomy in 116, and used forceps in 53 cases only. Contrast this with the other extreme of Johnston, who performed craniotomy in the proportion of one in 231, and delivered with forceps one in 10½! This experience is a perfect demonstration of a true method erroneously applied, for the resulting mortality more than neutralised the conservative intention of his method.

In connexion with operative midwifery, I must refer to the latest addition to the already formidable obstetric armamentarium—the basilyst, invented by my old friend, Professor Alexander Simpson of Edinburgh. It is constructed on the principle of a terebrator, and designed by a combined perforating and cutting action to break up the base of the skull as a substitute for the cephalotribe, the cranioclast, or the perforator and crotchet. It is declared by its author to be for this purpose *the* instrument of the future.

I would now direct your attention to the subject of post-partum hæmorrhage, and rather in relation to its prophylaxis than to its treatment. It is, as we well know, one of the gravest of parturient contingencies, whether regarded with reference to immediate danger to life, or to its more remote effects as a starting point of subsequent pathological conditions. I doubt much whether this last aspect of the results of post-partum hæmorrhage has received adequate recognition at the hands of gynæcologists. In 1876 it was computed that 1038 lives were lost from this cause; in 1879, the Registrar-General's Report gives 497 deaths from flooding, by far the largest item under the head "Child-birth," but there were 206 deaths from placenta prævia, 39 from retained placenta, 58 from abortion, and 49 from miscarriage. That this form of hæmorrhage is a largely preventable occurrence, is now very generally acknowledged. In the discussion on the subject, at the meeting in Cork, Dr. More Madden expressed the opinion that " with the advancement of our art such cases had gradually become less frequent, and would probably be altogether unknown in the more perfect obstetric practice of the future." In a large experience, both in hospital and private practice, he had seen only two fatal cases. Dr. Fleetwood Churchill, in 2547 cases in his private practice, has " never known hæmorrhage to occur when firm grasping was applied to the uterus immediately after the child was born, causing it to contract rapidly and expel the placenta into the vagina "; thus in twenty years he " never had to extract the placenta by hand." I have found also from my own experience, now stretching over more than a quarter of a century, that post-partum hæmorrhage is largely, if not entirely, preventable in otherwise normal labour, and also that, under ordinary circumstances, the smaller the amount of puerperal loss, the quicker and more satisfactory the convalescence. My attention, indeed, has been much drawn to this subject, because eight of the most active years of my professional life were spent in an eastern subtropical climate where this accident was extremely common and fatal to European women. It has been well remarked in relation to post-partum hæmorrhage, that where labour is conscientiously and intelligently supervised such cases should be few. As Dr. Farr puts it, " The mothers' lives lost are at their most valuable age, and skill can do more here in averting danger and death than in other operations." The prophylaxis, however, should be remote as well as immediate. The incidence of this form of flooding, in nearly every case, depends on the management of the second and third stages of labour; but the preventive measures should commence long before its occurrence is imminent. The management of the labour itself is only one part of the prophylactic scheme. The predisposing conditions very often present themselves during pregnancy, and their treatment should form part of a general training of the system to prepare the mother for the approaching ordeal of parturition. These predisposing causes exist in the opposite general states of plethora and of anæmia. In the first-named, the hyperæmia incidental to pregnancy is exaggerated, and the extreme vascular tension resulting supplies the necessary condition. On the other hand, in the anæmic state the uterine muscle partakes of the general malnutrition and consequent want of tone, and, readily exhausted by the parturient efforts, it refuses to contract after delivery and close the placental vascular orifices. I know no condition which illustrates more thoroughly the influence of the luxurious habits of civilised life in giving a morbific liability to a normal process, than in the instance of post-partum hæmorrhage; nor one in which the indications both for prevention and treatment are more plainly afforded by the study of natural conditions and processes. In the carefully recorded practice of Dr. Swayne, of Bristol, he states 3½ per cent. of his post-partum hæmorrhage cases occurred among poor, and 6 per cent. among rich patients. These observations on the prophylaxis of post-partum hæmorrhage, which I have selected as the largest mortality item and the type of the preventable accidents of childbirth, lead us fitly to the consideration of the subject in this connexion, above all others of most importance to us and to humanity—viz., general puerperal prophylaxis. The scientific development of surgery is conservative, that of medicine preventive, that of obstetrics ought to and must obey the same law. The question of puerperal fever, or septicæmia, is one of the most urgent that suggests itself in the whole range of obstetrics; it is the great source of death in childbed. It results from septic influences operating from within or from without, and therefore largely preventable in the light of modern antiseptic treatment. I say "largely," because puerperal circumstances present, so far, inseparable difficulties in the way of complete antiseptic precautions. It would not suffice, as has been suggested by an enthusiastic disciple of Lister, to arrange for "the nebulous carbolic reception of the new-born babe," nor would puerperal safety be secured by using an antiseptic apron extending from the umbilicus to the knees of the puerpera.

To show the importance of this subject, I would invite you to consider with me the value we are to attach to the statistics from which we derive our information as to the extent and variation in the rate of puerperal mortality, and endeavour to ascertain what light they throw on the subject.

Parturition may be physiological in design, but in general result the combined influences of civilised life have unquestionably rendered it largely pathological. As Dr. Edis well puts it—" In the present state of obstetric science, a certain number of deaths from divers causes are inevitable;" but "we must bear in mind that we are not dealing with the data of some mysterious disease that baffles our art and bids defiance to our efforts, but with the records of what should be the performance of a mere physiological function." When we reflect for a moment on the number of women who are delivered annually in this country, on the significant proportion of them to whom that event is fatal; when we consider the delicate balance there is between the healthy and morbid aspects of the process, we cannot fail to be struck with the vast influence which even the apparently most insignificant precautions may exert over the result, and the urgent call there is for inquiry into the causes of this enormous mortality, and the possible means of its diminution. If self-preservation is the first law of nature, surely our first duty is to inquire what is the extent of the mortality of child-bearing, and what are the means available for its reduction or prevention. The amount of puerperal mortality may be fairly regarded as the measure of progress or otherwise of obstetrics, quite as much as the balance to credit is of the success of a commercial undertaking. According to Merriman's well-known table—

For the 20 years ending 1680, 1 in 44 mothers delivered died.
　　　　　　　　　　1700, 1 in 58

For the 20 years ending 1740, 1 in 71 mothers delivered died.
　　" 　　　" 　　1760, 1 in 77 　　" 　　"
　　" 　　　" 　　1780, 1 in 82 　　" 　　"
　　" 　　　" 　　1800, 1 in 100 　　" 　　"
　　" 　　　" 　　1820, 1 in 107 　　" 　　"

In 1879, according to the Registrar-General's Return, it was only 1 in 353. The vital statistics furnished by the State are more valuable in relation to midwifery than to medicine or surgery. The number of registered births fairly represent the number of deliveries, and the maternal deaths the ratio of mortality. With respect to medical and surgical cases, we only learn from the returns how many die from a particular disease, or after a certain operation, but we do not learn the number of cases of which these are the results. These two departments of medicine, therefore, are incapable, approximately even, much less exactly, of estimating the success or failure of treatment.

The phenomena of disease are so unstable and complicated in themselves, and are so susceptible of variation from a variety of influences, that the numerical method as applied to the elucidation of medical problems, in the form of so-called vital statistics, is open to many inherent sources of fallacy. It is impossible, for the most part, to get that accuracy and equality of observation which is requisite with reference to each particular event of the aggregate numerical expression or total. It is quite otherwise in the domain of physical science. The numerical as a subordinate instrument of the inductive method has a great fascination for a particular order of minds; and, if employed with preconceived views, the figures, by some mysterious process of unconscious cerebration, seem to lend themselves, or are at least capable of being so adapted, as to appear to establish the desired doctrine. The profession has more than once seen two able statists arrive at diametrically opposite views from the use of the same body of figures, while a third party has stepped forward and declared himself satisfied that both numerical arrangements supported yet another proposition! In such cases, the true facts lie between the extremes. It has been said by a distinguished political economist that you can prove anything with the same figures. Still, however, according to another great authority on the subject, "statistics do offer a test by which the impressions of unrecorded and limited experience are corrected."

The puerperal statistics published by the Registrar-General, as at present available, are only unfortunately of comparative value. They do not furnish sufficiently absolute data from which to deduce inferences for purposes of exact comparison. They are hence open to the various sources of fallacy notoriously inherent in the purely numerical method of investigation. In the first place, we have no information that all the puerperal convalescences from which the fatal cases were recorded were an equal or sufficient time under the observation of the reporters. Next, the information is derived from returns furnished by medical men, and also by midwives; the relative number of each employed can only be roughly computed at one-third of the former and two-thirds of the latter. It is evident that the materials furnished by these two widely different classes of reporters will be of correspondingly different degrees of reliability, more especially when we have the discrimination of the two great divisions of puerperal mortality—viz., metria and accidents of childbirth—left entirely to their discretion. Another source of fallacy arises from the opprobrium which notoriously attaches to the accoucheur or midwife in puerperal cases of unfortunate issue. Obstetric human nature must be very different from the ordinary variety if it is unable to resist, even unconsciously, the instinctive tendency there is to refer the result to causes other than that with which it is really concerned. Again, with the spread of education and intelligence among the laity, registration has been year by year becoming more efficiently carried out; and, at the same time, increasing professional knowledge and efficiency, while diminishing the absolute amount of puerperal mortality, are leading steadily towards a more exact recognition of its nature, and consequently of its fuller registration. To illustrate this last proposition, I might refer to the Registrar-General's Abstract, where we find that deaths registered under the head of "Causes ill-defined tabulated is as essential to the value of statistics for scientific purposes as the capacity and trustworthiness of the reporters. If we are to compare different sets of puerperal mortality statistics, we must see that the items stated are reported and observed under the identical conditions. One of the most important of these is, as I have already remarked, that the whole puerperal convalescence has been under observation for the same given period. This, however, is by no means the case even in those collected from lying-in hospitals; certainly it is not the case in the outdoor practice of maternity charities, and still less in those furnished to the Registrar-General. The conclusion, therefore, is forced on us, that these various classes of puerperal statistics can only be used each separately for comparison of its own data from year to year; and that, while the Registrar-General's Reports are in themselves interesting, and afford material for general comparison, they do not supply such an accurate, detailed, definite, and uniformly derived body of facts as will serve for the basis of a scientific inquiry, such as is desiderated for our purpose.

The endeavour to ascertain by statistics what might be considered a conventional standard or reasonable rate of puerperal mortality has been made from time to time by some of our greatest obstetric authorities; but the results are imperfect, and, from their wide range of difference, unsatisfactory. Dr. Farr estimates it at 1 in 190; Dr. Matthews Duncan, at 1 in 120 to 100; Dr. McClintock, at 1 in 105. These calculations, however, are based on very unequal data. They include the result of practice in lying-in hospitals, outdoor maternity charities, and private practice both at home and in the colonies, besides the practice of obstetric and gynæcological specialists, which necessarily include elements of special morbidity. This was evidently and notoriously the case in Simpson's practice, which showed a mortality of 1 in 50. In order to obtain a true standard ratio, which shall be an attainable ideal, we should take the experience of a sufficient number of men in general class practice, partly urban and partly rural, in this country alone. With this view, then, I have collated the last eight lists of consecutive cases of this character, without selection, which have been published in the *Lancet* and the *British Medical Journal* :—

Dr. Cooper Rose	1,250 cases,	2 deaths,	= 1 in 625·
Mr. George Rigden	5,882 cases,	12 deaths (6 non-puerperal)	= 1 in 487·1
Mr. Godson	3,213 cases,	8 deaths,	= 1 in 402·3
Dr. Whalley	2,200 cases,	7 deaths,	= 1 in 314·2
Dr. Newham	1,000 cases,	4 deaths (3 non-puerperal),	= 1 in 250·
Dr. Swayne	1,049 cases,	4 deaths (1 non-puerperal),	= 1 in 212·2
Dr. H. Veale	818 cases,	4 deaths (2 non-puerperal),	= 1 in 204·5
Mr. Plaister	800 cases,	4 deaths (2 non-puerperal),	= 1 in 200·
	16,022 cases,	**47 deaths (15 non-puerperal),**	**= 1 in 340·6**

The total number of cases is 16,022, with 47 deaths, or a mortality equal to 1 in 340·9; or, deducting the 15 deaths from non-puerperal causes, a mortality of 1 in 500·6—say 500. This I take to be a fair standard of death in childbed under the best average conditions on the part of the locality, of the patient, and of the attendant. The inference I draw from the comparison between this ratio and all less favourable, is that the difference between them represents the amount of preventable mortality. I cannot better illustrate this proposition than by pointing out the difference between the puerperal mortality of the nearly equal populations of London and the North-west of England Registration Districts. In the former, for the year 1879, it amounted to 372 only, while in the latter it was 687. In this same year, if the puerperal mortality of London were in proportion to that of England and Wales, it would have amounted to 406·4, instead of 372 as stated. According to the Registrar-General's Report, the average puerperal mortality for the thirty-three years from 1847 to 1879 inclusive, was at the rate of 4·9 per 1000 of births registered, which is a rate of 1 in 244. The maximum rate was, in 1874, 6·9 per 1000, or 1 in 143; the minimum in 1874, 3·7 per 1000, or 1 in 271. In 1873, the year preceding the maximum, it was 1 in 200. In 1874, there were 1644 more deaths registered under the head "Metria" than in 1873—the full numbers being 3108 and 1644, or 132 and 58 per 1,000,000 respectively. It is most satisfactory to note that the death-rate in childbed has steadily decreased during the five years including and following

1874—when it was 6·9 per 1000.
_____ 1875   ..   6   ..

1876—when it was 4·7 per 1000.
1877—   ,,   3·9   ,,
1878—   ,,   3·7   ,,

In 1879, it had risen to 3·8 per 1000, or 1 in 268; but this slight fluctuation detracts very slightly from this satisfactory record.

The figures which have just engaged our attention speak plainly enough. They show what amount of change for the better is taking place year by year in the bill of puerperal mortality; they also show what can be done. This mortality has two great sources indicated in the Registrar-General's headings, viz., "Childbirth," and "Metria." The former is largely preventable by increased attention and skill on the part of the attendant; the latter by the adoption of those antiseptic precautions with which modern science has already accomplished so much. We must remember that the heavy death-rate is only part of the puerperal penalty paid. We are apt to forget the fate of too many of the survivors, who leave the lying-in chamber for the last time, physically disabled, and incapable of again discharging the great function of womanhood. It was my intention to have referred in some detail to the antiseptic measures already adopted in some of the great maternity hospitals abroad; for instance, those carried out with such distinguished success by Professor von Weber in the great Landes Gebäranstalt in Prague, where the death-rate has been actually reduced to ·36 per cent. But the inexorable hand of time warns me to turn to another part of my subject.

We shall now, gentlemen, turn our attention for a short space to the subject of gynæcology.

From their greater organic mobility, women react much more than men to their environment. They are more affected physically by the conditions under which they live; and in no respect are the continuous influences of civilised life more apparent than in the effect they have had of modifying or disturbing the sexual functions in women, and so increasing their morbid liabilities. The higher the civilisation, the more delicate the human product, seems to be a law of social development. The diseases of women naturally arrange themselves round the two great distinguishing functions of their sex. We have one group characterised by disturbances of the function of menstruation, accompanied by, or dependent upon, organic changes in the ovaries, in which the essential phenomena of ovulation are initiated, or in the uterine mucous membrane where they are principally manifested. Another group consists of morbid conditions arising in connexion with the reproductive function—conception, pregnancy, parturition. All healthy women living in normal conjugal relations during the greater part of the period of menstrual activity should bear children. It follows, therefore, that, when this has not occurred, or when child-bearing is suspended, morbid conditions, either original or acquired, are present in the sexual apparatus. A heavy puerperal mortality, as I have elsewhere shown, is but part of the penalty the gentler sex pay for the precarious privileges of maternity. Far too many of them rise from the perils of childbed crippled in health and sexually disabled, perhaps for ever. In how many families do parental anxieties centre round an only child ?

The diseases of women form so numerous and important a class, that even if we are not, as physicians and surgeons, called upon to treat them ourselves, yet we ought to be able to recognise them, if only to exclude them as powerful factors in other ailments. Gynæcology is a comparatively modern study. There is no department of medicine in which so much remains to be done, notwithstanding what has already been accomplished within the comparatively short time since its revival. This progress, however, unfortunately, has been much more rapid than satisfactory. Perhaps in this respect it has only reflected the character of every new and rapidly extending branch of knowledge. In none has progress been so much from the side of experiment and empiricism. The pathology of uterine affections is still obscure, and requires further investigation as a basis for more and greater precision in treatment. The physiology even of the genital apparatus in women is still capable of much elucidation. No class of diseases present themselves in such protean shapes, obscuring diagnosis and baffling ordinary treatment, as those which engage the attention of the obstetric physician. They are indeterminate in form and progress; they run no regular course; they are very rarely uncomplicated; and in nearly all of them there are neurotic elements which add vastly to the difficulties of the situation. The progress of gynæcology so far has been marked by distinct periods of development, which unfortunately correspond less to advances in physiology and pathology, than to the application of new means of physical investigation and the introduction of therapeutic novelties largely mechanical in character. The progress which might have resulted from these experiments in diagnosis and therapeutic resources has been greatly retarded by too hasty generalisation from isolated and imperfectly observed and recorded facts; hence, narrow views, erroneous theory, and empirical practice, if not worse, have followed one another in a sequence which would be amusing were it not very serious in some of its aspects. The memory of this generation is carried back to an almost prehistoric time, as far as gynæcology is concerned, when diseases of the womb were either altogether ignored or held to be beyond the province of legitimate medicine. The period when the importance of uterine disease began to dawn was yet one of darkness. Prolapsus and leucorrhœa were the presiding pathological conditions: vaginal plugs and injections composed the therapeutics. Next came the speculum or ocular period, disclosing inflammations and ulcerations of the cervix, with caustics and scarifications as their treatment. Then came the distinction - anatomical, physiological, and pathological—between the cervix and body of the uterus, developing intra-uterine medication, to the extent even of pyrotechnics in the form of a sound at a red heat. The uterine sound inaugurated a new era—that of mechanics—in uterine pathology and treatment. All ailments were obscured in versions and flexions of the womb, which mechanical appliances could alone relieve and cure. The cervix again became the object of attention. Dysmenorrhœa and sterility were referred to peculiarities in its configuration and to stricture of its canal, which could only be removed by slitting it up. Next the clitoris, as the subject of clitoridectomy, to cure certain reflex troubles, had fortunately only a brief, inglorious reign. The ovaries, in turn, long credited with the highest pathological honours, are now apparently doomed to general extirpation unless they cease to trouble. The female perineum also, always an object of solicitude to obstetricians, has quite recently been elevated by certain American gynæcologists into a position of eminence in relation to the causation of uterine difficulties, displacements, and such like, almost as great as that accorded by another school to the cervix uteri; indeed, lacerations of the former are made to share with lacerations of the latter in all the pathological honours. According to this school, "the perineal body is a great factor in co-ordinating all the parts within the pelvic cavity." An old acquaintance has again turned up with a new face, in the lacerated puerperal cervix, which, to use the words of one of the latest authorities, "should be stitched up, however alight the laceration." A distinguished American gynæcologist, writing me lately about sundry professional matters in his department, says, in characteristic style, with reference to this procedure and that of oöphoreotomy : "Battey's operation is a formidable one, and rarely resorted to as compared with the trifling one of sewing up a lacerated cervix uteri, which seems greatly to occupy some American gynæcologists at present. The frequency of this operation by some has been equalled, in our day, only by the frequency with which the cervix used to be slit as a cure-all. The field is a wide one, and I daresay many old slits will be repaired. Our great master, Simpson, has left behind him a few. The pendulum swings. Time alone will bring the verdict. We are too near the period to speak plainly and judge intelligently about it." The lesson to be learned from all this is, that scientific method has been faulty or wanting, our art has been advancing experimentally in narrow grooves without unity or comprehensiveness of design, our observations have been partial, and our treatment speculative where not empirical. In fact, our therapeutics have had no foundation in sound pathology. Improved methods of investigation, and refinements in physical diagnosis, have had, unfortunately, the effect of drawing attention from general conditions, in which a large proportion of local troubles have their origin. They have elevated into importance objective symptoms at the expense of subjective. Objective symptoms have the merit of accessibility and exactness; they are easily recorded and readily compared. They are, in a word,

more definite. Subjective symptoms ought not, however, to be ignored. They afford information and evidence of changes experienced and felt by the patient preceding those capable of objective recognition. We should not forget that all the knowledge that constitutes the inheritance of modern medicine was thus alone derived. This exclusive study of objective symptoms has undoubtedly had a most injurious effect on the dignity, character, and progress of gynæcology. There has been far too great attention paid to local treatment. The use of instruments for diagnosis and treatment, and direct personal medication, have been greatly overdone. The *nimia diligentia* has been too rampant. I cannot help recalling to your mind the remark of the late Sir John Forbes, in his classic work on "Nature *versus* Art in Disease," about "over-active perturbative treatment and mischievous polypharmacy." I am not sure that many of us are capable of realising the effort that is necessary to enable a virtuous (or indeed any) woman to submit to the painful ordeal of local examination and manipulation, or the gradual deterioration of delicacy which in too many its frequent repetition tends to accomplish. When I read of a gynæcologist who states that he has made a vaginal examination by speculum "almost daily for two years," I cannot help thinking that the moral deterioration has extended also to the medical attendant. When we read of an uterine sound being used with such force as to bend it, we remember that it should not be used with much more force than necessary to pass a catheter into a male bladder. Another gynæcologist recommends the approximate determination of the volume and shape of the uterus being ascertained by a bimanual examination "before sounding"! Another recommends the sound, and yet another, tents for cervical dilatation, to be passed through the speculum! I cannot do better than quote, in this connexion, what appeared a few days ago in one of our medical journals from the editorial pen, under the title of "Uterine Therapeutics" :—"There are few things more characteristic of an untutored intellect than the propensity to ' discover' unlooked-for and startling phenomena as associated with common-place and trivial causes. Speaking generally, it is a case in which either the intelligence or the veracity is open to the gravest suspicion. That a pernicious and demoralising amount of interference with the genital apparatus of females is chargeable against certain practitioners is likewise a proposition, to the truth of which, we are sorry to believe, assent will be accorded by the best men in the ranks of the profession." I trust I shall not be misunderstood in thus expressing myself. I do so, because I feel keenly all that concerns the dignity of that department of medicine with which I have identified myself. As I have said on a previous occasion, I deprecate in the strongest terms the *nimia diligentia* in the treatment of uterine diseases generally. I am strongly of opinion that an endeavour should always be made in the first place to correct the local trouble by treatment directed to correct the general health when affected, and only when this unaided has failed, should local treatment involving manual or operative interference with the parts be attempted. Generally speaking, the speculum should never be used, unless local medication, first by the patient herself, have failed to arrest the abnormal discharges and relieve the local symptoms. The sound should never be introduced unless there be presumptive evidence of uterine flexion, displacement, subinvolution, or the reverse. And, finally, let me say, mechanical treatment of every kind should certainly be withheld in all cases until relief by rest, position, and local medication has failed to be afforded. The diagnosis in all cases should be inductive—under no circumstances either speculative or experimental.

Time will not admit of my doing more, before leaving the subject of gynæcology, than referring very briefly to one or two of the more recent contributions to the science and art of gynæcology. One of the most valuable is Dr. Hart's (of Edinburgh) investigations into the anatomy of the pelvis and its contents. They shed most valuable light on the physical relations of the uterus and its appendages, especially with reference to the mechanism by which it is supported and maintained *in situ*, and its bearings on displacement of that organ. He shows that the womb is more dependent on the support of the pubic and sacral oblique planes of the pelvic fasciæ, which form a true pelvic floor, than on its so-called ligaments. Prolapsus is caused by the pubic portion slipping past the sacral portion. The pubic layer is triangular, and has comparatively loose attachments, and the uterus lies anteverted (inclined forward) on it. The sacral layer is quadrilateral in outline, and has strong bony attachments. Prolapsus is caused not so much by the weight of the uterus, as by laceration or thinning of the anterior edge of the sacral layer, the plane allowing the relaxed pubic segment to slip past. Increased weight of the uterus does not initiate the movement, but must of course exaggerate it. There are three primary factors in the movement, viz.—(a) loss of apposition of the pubic and sacral portions, in most cases started by perineal laceration; (b) loss of "tone" in the anterior triangle or pubic plane; (c) intra-abdominal pressure. It is on such a basis as this that a system of mechanical therapeutics should be founded.

It has been remarked that the tendency of gynæcology is becoming more and more surgical.' Indeed, the operations with which the names of Spencer Wells and Thomas Keith are so gloriously identified must be regarded as common ground. It is not so very long since the operation of ovariotomy was pronounced by the unanimous voice of the profession practically as well as theoretically justifiable. The same question can hardly yet be answered in the affirmative with reference to the operation first introduced in America by Dr. Battey, of Rome, Georgia, under the name of normal ovariotomy or oöphorectomy, as a remedy for neurasthenic and other troubles having their origin in ovarian irritation. It has since been extensively repeated in America, on the Continent, and in this country. Call the result what they may, "simply reaching the climacteric earlier than usual," "attaining premature sexual senescence," or "anticipating menstrual senescence," it is a grave matter, under any circumstances, literally to unsex a woman by an operation dangerous to life, which may even fail to relieve, for what, as far as can be ascertained, is a purely functional derangement. Nothing but conditions immediately threatening life or reason can justify such a proceeding, the necessity for which must always constitute an opprobrium in our art. It seems to me that the systematic treatment of neurasthenic disorders practised with such success by Dr. Weir Mitchell of Philadelphia, and recently brought to the notice of the profession by Professor Playfair with such a corroborative record of success, offers an alternative to Battey's operation of the most promising kind. Dr. Weir Mitchell's book was brought to me about four years ago by a lady whose sister had been restored to health under the treatment. Skilled nursing is the great difficulty in connexion with carrying out the system successfully.

The operation introduced in America, by Dr. Emmett, of stitching up lacerations of the cervix uteri, has already gained extensive acceptance on the Continent. This accident is alleged to cause eversions of the os uteri, endometritis, leucorrhœa, sterility, abortion, to disturb involution, and to prevent the cure of displacements and flexions of the womb. Verily, a grave catalogue! This accident must certainly be more frequent in its occurrence and more serious in its effects elsewhere than in this country. Dr. Pallen, of New York, says he has operated on 900 cases in six years, in only 200 of which, however, was there interference with the generative functions, or other symptom, produced. It is very rare to find a multiparous cervix in any other than a dilapidated condition with more or less laceration. I have often found, as no doubt all of you have, a hard fissure on one or other side of the cervix, causing pain on pressure, but at once relieved by free scarification, as one would treat a rectal or other fissure.

The name of Dr. Emmett is also associated with another most valuable but very much simpler contribution to uterine therapeutics, in what is known as the "hot vaginal douche." Of this, Dr. Dudley, of Chicago, says, "in uterine therapeutics, the value of the hot-water douche is perhaps greater than that of all other topical applications combined;" and I heartily endorse the opinion. It should be used as hot as can be borne for twenty to thirty minutes at a time. It can be tolerated comfortably by the vagina at a temperature which the hand cannot bear. It acts by first dilating the arterioles, followed by the tonic result of contraction, which continues for some time. The mucous membrane becomes blanched, the calibre of the vagina diminished, and the surfaces astringed. The whole pelvic circulation is thus influenced and relieved through the vagina. It has also secondarily the valuable effect of removing the restlessness and insomnia of nervous women. Drs. Windelband, of Vienna, and Lombe Atthill, of Dublin, recommend it in post-partum hæmorrhage.

My last reference is to the diseases of children, and it must necessarily be a very brief one.

The association of the diseases of women and children is entirely conventional. There is no essential relation between them. The diseases of children constitute in themselves an entirely new and independent departure from the domain of general pathology. The subjects embraced under the general term pædiatrics form a group so characteristic and inter-related, and otherwise so distinct from either obstetrics or gynæcology, that they merit separate treatment. I trust the time is not far distant when they will attain the dignity of a separate section at our annual meetings. In the meantime, it will be impossible for me to do more than reiterate the assertion of their claims to independant consideration. I would, however, draw your attention for a moment to what I believe to be one of the most interesting aspects of children's diseases. It is their constitutional nature as derived by inheritance. The prevention of disease is now wisely held to be the highest object of medical science, and at no period of life is it so easy to interrupt the hereditary sequence of morbid influences, and prevent their subsequent development. A large proportion of the diseases of adult life result from the environment of the individual, his habits as regards food, stimulants, and exercise, unequal strain on the organic system, the effects of the complex and anomalous conditions of civilised life, in addition to those from specific infections, and other essentially morbid influences. But these conditions not only affect the individuals immediately exposed to them, developing types of humanity more or less physically retrograde, but they produce in the offspring marked diathetic states from their transmission. We accordingly, in infancy, meet with numerous temperamental developments, and diatheses of hereditary origin. They give a distinct complexion to, and largely influence, the character and progress of acquired disease. We are also called upon to treat their corresponding cachexiæ or characteristic morbid developments, which constitute in themselves so many distinct morbid entities or diseases. To a great extent, fortunately, many of these inherited diatheses and their cachexiæ are capable of cure, and all of them of amelioration. The vegetative activity and developmental mobility of youth lend themselves readily to the influences—hygienic, nutritive, and therapeutic—which may be skilfully brought to bear upon them. It is impossible to overestimate the importance of these considerations in relation to the pathology and therapeutics of children's diseases. They certainly have not met with that recognition to which their pathological value entitles them, and I refer to them merely to point out what a field there is here presented to the student of pædiatrics for independant and original research.

RADICAL CURE OF HYDROCELE.—In a lecture on Hydrocele (New York Med. Record, July 16), Prof. Ashhurst, of Philadelphia, observes that although many other injections are used, and that too with greater or less success, he has found in his experience that, although not invariably followed by a permanent cure, iodine, of all things, can be the most relied upon when used as advocated by Prof. Syme—that is, by injecting the undiluted tincture and allowing it to remain.

ILLEGAL PRACTICE IN FRANCE.—An interne of one of the hospitals in Paris having attended upon a lady at the request of one of the Professors of the Faculty, brought an action against his patient for the recovery of his fees after he had procured his doctor's diploma. The court rejected his claim, declaring that any commission of this kind given by a professor to a student to take charge of a patient could not dispense with the possession of a diploma. One of the evils country practitioners have to contend with in France is the furnishing of advice and medicine by the religious bodies. When any of these are proceeded against, the fines inflicted by the local magistracy are usually only nominal. In a recent case, however, death resulted from the administration of a medical substance by the superior of the Sisters of Port d'Envaux. She was convicted of the illegal practice of pharmacy, and of having caused homicide by imprudence, and was fined 500 fr., and sentenced to pay the expenses amounting to 15,000 fr.

ORIGINAL COMMUNICATIONS.

INSTANCES OF THE

EVOLUTION OF EPIDEMICS AND THE ALLIANCES OF SOME DISEASES.

By WILLIAM H. PEARSE, M.D. Edin.,
Senior Physician to the Plymouth Public Dispensary; late of the Government Emigration Service.

DURING many voyages, made in medical charge of emigrants, from England to Australia, and from Calcutta to the West Indies, I was accustomed to record every case of disease which showed, however slight

The voyage from England to Australia embraces from 50° N. latitude to about 50° S. latitude, crossing the equator and both tropics. The last six weeks of such a voyage is chiefly in from 45° to 50° S. latitude, and in the prevailing westerly gales. Thus, in such a voyage, the systems of the people are, in a period of three months, exposed to extreme differences of external physical conditions.

The voyage from Calcutta to the West Indies is tropical, save for about three weeks, when it is in latitudes of from 23° 30′ S. to 35° S., being the period of rounding the "Cape."

Although in both voyages the course is at once southward, and to warmer latitudes, it is not the less true that much "shock" or depression happens to the people on, and for some days after, sailing; and this is as true and marked on leaving the warm region of Bengal for the Bay of Bengal, as it is of leaving the soil of England for the Channel.

The people in both voyages are of the poorer classes, and who have never before been accustomed to travel, or been exposed to acclimatising influences. The mental or nerve energy and bodily condition of such people must be considered low. The sudden "change" from the shore to the sea involves a depression or "shock." We have, therefore, in such voyages, man placed in well-defined, experimental conditions —for voyages present a so-far limited and known range of physical conditions; and in the changes of climate and physical surroundings therein involved there is a somewhat near parallel to the greater season changes which belong to different latitudes of the earth and to different periods of the year; and which, in the present state of our knowledge, seem to be the main occasions of the appearance of epidemic deviations.

I propose now to state shortly some phenomena which presented.

CHOLERA.—The coolie emigrant ship Alnwick Castle embarked 479 souls at Calcutta on October 28, 1861. Temperature, 8 a.m., 75°. The health of the people in depôt prior to embarkation had been good. We reached the Sandheads (mouth of the river), on October 31; the equator on November 11; the southern tropic on November 26. On November 27, when in 25° 32′ S. lat., and 57° 15′ E. long., having been thirty-one days on board, and twenty-seven days at sea, wholly free from communication with the shore or boats, a case unmistakably choleraic occurred:—

Sagoor, male, aged thirty. 9.30 a.m., had two motions (not seen); copious vomiting; skin cold; no pulse (at wrist); voice good; pain and cramp in abdomen and toes. 10 a.m.: No pulse (at wrist); body warm, extremities cold. Noon: Body warm, arms warm. 8 p.m.: Warm; no cramps; passed urine; one stinking, congy-like motion.

The aspect of this man at 9.30 a.m. was strikingly choleraic —cold, collapsed, and cramped. No case like it had occurred in depôt prior to embarkation, or during the thirty-one days since embarkation. What cause could be sought for such a case?

We had two kinds of water on board—Calcutta tank square (which is taken from the Hooghly) in casks, and Normandy's distilled water. I made it a constant rule that no cask-water should be issued direct from the casks; but such cask-water, prior to issue, was invariably pumped from the casks into an iron tank. In the concussion of pumping from the casks into the tank the water lost much of the offensive smell of cask-water. Calcutta water, taken from the iron tank, had been issued wholly to the people on six days for

cooking, and for seven days wholly for drinking, since we sailed. On all other occasions Normandy's distilled water had been issued. No result to the health of the people had become apparent from this interchange of waters. But on the morning of November 27, by a neglect, and for the first time, water had been issued, both for drinking and cooking, direct from the casks. Within two hours the choleraic case happened.

Certain questions arise in medical theory:—First, Did he imbibe a stray cholera-germ, so-called? or, secondly, may we assume that the choleraic type evolved from the change to water of a somewhat different physical state from that to which he was habituated, just as a fatal cholera has often shown in India after taking Seidlitz or Epsom salts? Thirdly, May we not fairly lean to the view that there was no specific poison or cause, but rather that the system of the native of India (in this age and time) naturally tends, from slight depressions or small losses of the entirety of habituated physical surroundings, to those directions of loss of vital power or "energy," whose after-symptoms are those known as cholera? that what we approximatively call "shock" or "depressing influences" may, in the native of India, lead to cholera, quite apart from any "specific" poison? As an illustration of this principle, I may quote the following case:—In 1867 I was in charge of about a thousand natives in the Trinidad Depôt in Calcutta. Every day during ten days, I spent many hours amongst the people; there was no cholera. At 9 a.m. on September 3, I found a man, aged thirty, in cholera, and who died in the afternoon. I found him lying where he had slept, in the passage-way of one of the sheds, where he had been exposed during the night to the draught and cold. No other case followed, either in depôt or amongst the 532 people I embarked on September 7, four days after. The "weather had been very hot and calm for some days," with "several nights of great heat and calm," followed on September 2 by "cool N.E. wind and rain." The night of September 2 was calm and hot, but in the early morning of the 3rd came N.E. wind and fall of temperature. It must be remembered that it is often "cold" to our feelings in the tropics far beyond what the thermometer may show.

This isolated case in a large community of natives, coincident with a sudden change towards cooler weather and depressions, and having shown in a man who, beyond the rest of the community, was exposed to cold night influences, though not a "crucial instance," yet points towards the proposition that cholera may occur or evolve in the native from "depressing influences" or "shock" (these are temporary hypothetical terms), wholly independent of "specific" poison.

I may illustrate the potent influence of change of water in producing diarrhœa. The coolie emigrant ship Arabia, with 404 souls, from Calcutta to Demerara, put into St. Helena on February 28, 1863. The daily cases of diarrhœa for a week prior to, and for a week after, the use of the new and changed water were as follow:—

PRIOR TO ST. HELENA.			AFTER ST. HELENA.		
Date.	Lowest night temperature.	Number of new cases of diarrhœa.	Date.	Lowest night temperature.	Number of new cases of diarrhœa.
Feb. 21 ...	69°	2	Feb. 28...	76°	11
,, 22 ...	71	7	Mar. 1...	75·5	10
,, 23 ...	71	2	,, 2...	75	7
,, 24 ...	71	1	,, 3...	76	5
,, 25 ...	72	1	,, 4...	76	4
,, 26 ...	74	2	,, 5...	...	4
,, 27 ...	74	1	,, 6...	77	6

No one will suppose that the clean mountain spring water of St. Helena contained any poison, or special purgative quality; it was the change from the habituated circumstances of the people, in relation with physical conditions of water—however slight the change—which disturbed the corelations of the system. In what exact way a change to a pure spring water from an habituated river or distilled water produced diarrhœa, the present state of our knowledge does not show us; nor does the instance of evolved cholera in the ship Alnwick Castle, associated with changed water, show us the "form"(a) or nature

(a) See Bacon's "Advancement of Learning" for the great need of this term.

of the phenomena in that case; not the less, such examples tend to point to wider generalisations than any single "cause" or "poison," but rather to a view which sees certain groups of those phenomena, known as diseases, as the developed or evolved "contained variabilities" of the system, and apt to appear on "shock" or after certain changes in habituated physical conditions, including food. One may fairly ask, as I strongly felt at the time, Is it not likely that an epidemic of cholera would have happened in the ship *Alnwick Castle* had the cask-water been similarly issued earlier in the voyage?

MEASLES.—The iron ship, *Oasis*, 1116 tons, embarked at Calcutta, on September 2, 1865, 446 souls, viz., 370 adults, 43 children from one to ten years, and 33 infants under one year. We cleared the Sand-heads on September 6. On September 21, noon temperature 85·7°, lowest night temperature 80°, in lat. 9° N., and twenty days from embarkation, the first case of measles occurred in a European apprentice. On the 22nd he had "copious eruption of well-marked measles."(b) After the attack he was isolated in a cabin which was separated by an iron bulkhead from the emigrants' deck. Prior to the attack he had been for a week in constant intercourse with the emigrants. Our three weeks at sea had been in trying weather, beating down the Bay against the S.W. monsoon. There followed amongst the native emigrants, on September 28, 3° N. lat., a case, a girl, aged six years, "covered with raised fine points (of eruption), no vesicles; somewhat, perhaps, concentric; hot, dry skin; tongue coated, no red papillæ (on tongue); short breath; eruption all gone on the 30th." At the time I viewed this case as one of measles.

Between these two cases of measles—viz., on September 25 and 26—two other cases of febrile disease, with eruption on the skin (vesicular), had shown in two women. Were all these four cases measles? The first case was well marked in type.

The ship left the S.W. monsoon on September 30, in 0° 30′ N. lat., the wind on October 1 being S.S.E., with a fall of temperature of from 2·5° to 3·5°. Crossed the equator on October 4; temperature 78·5°; wind S.S.E. No case allied to the above occurred during the succeeding eleven weeks of the voyage.

That the course of such cases of measles does not conform to the prevailing type of measles as seen in Europe, does not preclude their absolute and near alliance to measles. To illustrate this variation of type of measles, this "form" of "variability," I will abstract below the complete record of an epidemic of measles which showed in the ship *Alumbagh*, of 1100 tons, from Plymouth to Melbourne, with 412 souls, including 86 children under twelve years, of whom 54 were under seven years. Measles prevailed during the voyage from 38° N. lat., to about 100° E. long., 44° S. lat. Sailed July 31, 1870. The first case showed on August 7. There were twenty-four cases. None were fatal.

Period of Ailing.—The period of ailing, prior to the appearance of the eruption, was one day in eleven cases, two days in eleven cases, three days in one case.

Temperature of Cases.—In no case did the temperature reach 104°; in two cases it was over 108°; in six cases, over 102°; in seven cases, over 101°; in six cases, over 100°; in two cases, over 99°.

This *Alumbagh* epidemic illustrates the variation of type of measles under the changing physical environments of a voyage; or, as it may, perhaps, be better expressed, it illustrates the tendency of the prevailing rates or order of deviation of the system into diseased rates, to be modified by changed physical environment.

Four cases occurred in depôt in Calcutta about one thousand people on September 5, 1867 (a case had shown about twelve days earlier). We embarked in ship *Liverpool*, on September 7; on September 23, in about 1° N. lat., 90° E. long., sixteen days from embarkation, two children showed measles. One other case showed in the fourth week, in about 6° S. lat., 96° E. long. No case like measles appeared afterwards during the remaining ten weeks of the voyage, and among 530 people, including over forty children under ten years.

Thus, then, in the ship *Oasis*, measles appeared twenty days after embarkation; in the ship *Alumbagh*, seven days

(b) Where inverted commas are used, I have copied, word for word, from my note-books.

after sailing; in the ship *Liverpool*, sixteen days after embarkation.

Measles.—Ship "Alumbagh."—Continuance of Disease.

Period of promonitory ailing.	Average days.	Commencement of ailing to normal temperature.	Average days.	Eruption out.	Average days.	Highest temperature.
3 days		10 days		6 days		108°
2 „	2	9 „	8	5 „	4	103
1 day		9 „		7 „		102·
2 days		6 „		7 „		102
1 day	1·5	6 „	5·23	2 or 3 days...	3·28	102
1 „		5 „		3 days... ...		102
2 days		5 „		3 „		102·
1 day		5 „		3 „		101
1 „		5 „		4 „		101
2 days		7 „		4 „		101
2 „	1·57	5 „	5	3 „	2·71	101
1 day		3 „		3 „		101
3 days		6 „		1 day		101
1 day		5 „		3 days... ...		101·
2 days		5 „		3 „		100·
1 „		5 „		2 „		100
1 day	1·5	5 „	5	3 „	2·83	100
1 „		4 „		3 „		100
1 day		4 „		2 „		100·
1 „	1·5	4 „	5	1 or 3 days.	2	99
1 „		4 „		3 days... ...		99
Average, 1·55 days.		Average, 5·34 days.		Average, 2·95 days.		...

Measles.—Ship "Alumbagh."—Temperatures below Normal.

Name.	Sex.	Age.	Highest temperature.	Day of disease.	Lowest temperature.	Day of disease.
Williams...	M.	3	100·8°	3rd	98·7°	5th
West	F.	1	100·3	3rd	97·7	5th
Parsons	F.	5	102·6	3rd	{97·3 / 98·3}	4th / 5th
Williams...	F.	7	102·3	2nd	98	3rd
J. Wright	M.	4	99·5	4th	97·8	6th
R. Wright	M.	4	100·3	2nd	97·4	4th
Callaghan	F.	5	102·3	1st	97·8	5thr
Noble	M.	5	102·3	3rd	97·8	5th

SMALL-POX OR CHICKEN-POX.—The ship *Arabia* embarked at Calcutta 404 souls, including twenty under twelve years, on January 7, 1863. On January 27, in 11° S. lat., 80° E. long., twenty-one days on board, a boy, aged thirteen, showed an eruptive disease, either small-pox or chicken-pox; three other cases showed two days after, on January 29.

My notes for the four cases state—"Three of the four cases have good old small-pox marks; one was never vaccinated or inoculated. The spots in all the cases very much alike—watery (in early stage)—and on abdomen, chest, and arms; about twenty-four spots on abdomen and chest."

There were eight cases in all, occurring from January 27, 11° S. lat., 80° E. long., lowest night temperature 80·5°, to February 16, 36° S. lat., 20° E. long., lowest night temperature 72·5°:—Six males, of ages 12, 13, 16, 16, 18, 40; two females, of ages 20 and 28.

My note-book at the time recorded—"February 3 : Five cases of *pustular* eruption put into hospital (ship's hospital) as supposed small-pox."

My notes at the time record the various cases:—"Permessur, spots, four days out and full; Ramdeen .... six days, maturating; Jagoor .... six days, maturating ; Seemoty . . . three days, some pitting." This last case, "Seemoty," was the one free from old inoculation or small-pox marks.

Such cases may be modified small-pox or chicken-pox; at the time I felt such were modified small-pox.

From the date of embarkation to that of the first discovered case was twenty-one days. Some minds will view this interval as one of "incubation"; other minds will tend to a wider hypothesis—that the epidemic was an evolution, that one of the "contained variabilities" or contained capacities for febrile rates developed with the changing environment in a certain proportion of the people.

We see, also, that with 404 souls on board, of whom 20 were under twelve years, in the fact of the disease not spreading, some great force of co-ordination or acclimatisation must have been in action coincident with the changing latitudes and climates—changes, it appears to me, parallel to season-changes in countries, and which are so closely associated with the cessation of epidemics.

Ague showed in a man on the first burst of the westerly gales, after leaving the Southern Tropic, in the ship *Elisa*, Plymouth to Adelaide, 1856. He had not suffered ague for over twenty-five years previously. In the same latitude I had ague in 1868, not having had an attack in the interval since 1865, at which latter date I was in Bengal.

Erysipelas.—I have seen a case evolve after a scalp-wound, when off the Cape, nine or ten weeks from England, none other having shown in the ship before.

Where were the so-called malaria, or poisons, or germs? I fail to see how the hypothesis of evolution can be excluded from a scientific or philosophical method of viewing such phenomena.

Query, Whooping-Cough?—The iron ship *Oasis*, of 1100 tons, embarked 294 men, 76 women, 31 boys under ten, 12 girls under ten, and 33 infants (total, 446 souls), on September 2, 1865. The period was along with and after the Orissa famine. The people were very feeble; there was much chronic diarrhœa and a general prevalence of chronic cough, also intermittent or remittent fever, of varying duration of from three, four, five, or six days—such "fever" being often associated with diarrhœa or bronchial attacks.

On October 21, in 24° S. lat., 56° E. long. (the lowest night temperature having fallen during the week ending October 21, from 73° to 63°), the first sound of whooping-cough was heard on board, in a boy aged seven years, having embarked fifty days previously and been at sea forty-seven days.

My notes at the time state:—

Seventh Week.—October 21 (last day of seventh week): Male, aged seven; whooping-cough.

Eighth Week.—October 27: Female, aged five; whooping-cough.

Ninth and Tenth Weeks.—November 6: Buchla, female, aged two; whooping-cough (the whooping fairly heard). November 10: Moncar, male, aged one; whooping-cough; a few moist râles; skin hot. November 11: Male, aged eight; whooping-cough.

Eleventh Week.—November 16: Seeburty, female, aged eighteen; whooping-cough; bronchitis; every night for four nights past had "tup," *i.e.*, fever.(c) November 17: Kubotore, female, aged eighteen; whooping-cough; very hot at 8 p.m. November 18: Very hot at 3 p.m.; pulse at 8 p.m. very fast; cool at noon.

Thirteenth Week.—November 28: Male, aged sixteen; whooping-cough; cool. Jugarthy, female, aged twenty-five; whooping-cough.

	Lowest night temperature of week.	Whooping-cough. No. of cases.	Place.
Last day of 7th week to 24° S. lat., 56° E. long....	63°	1	{24° S. lat. {56° E. long.
8th week, ending Oct. 26 ...	59	. 1	{26° S. lat. {49° E. long.
9th „ „ Nov. 4 ...	56	1	Off Cape.
10th „ „ „ 11 ...	—	1	Table Bay.
11th „ „ „ 18 ...	—	3	To 29° S. lat.
13th „ „ Dec. 2 ...	—	2	{13° S. lat. {16° W. long.
15th „ „ „ 16 ...	—	1	Equator.

Note made at the time:—

"November 17.—Some cases of fever (that is, at night); great heat, high pulse. Most of these complain of much cough (bronchial râles are found); the heat is less in the morning; one has a whoop with her cough; others show the same heat at 8 p.m., but have a diarrhœa."

"November 29.—Whooping-cough shows mostly as whooping-cough, bronchitis, and remittent fever in one."

Kubotore, female, aged eighteen. "Severe heat; severe cough; high pulse; sonorous and moist râles. About four days after the attack, which she called fever, she whooped."

Seeburty, female, aged eighteen. "Whooping-cough and bronchitis; a kind of remittent fever. Very hot every night; very high pulse."

Whether these ten cases be held to be specifically one with whooping-cough or not, the cases are suggestive, and show that new localisations of phenomena evolved, coincident

(c) "Tup" is the common word for feverish states, agues, etc.

with the fall of temperature, on emerging from the southern tropic into higher latitudes. A changing type from the previous prevailing fever and bronchitis took place with changed physical environment, and this new type showed an epidemic form.

A similar phenomenon was seen in the ship *Liverpool*, which embarked 329 men, 159 women, 22 boys, 13 girls, and 9 infants, on September 7, 1867, at Calcutta. On October 3, when in about 5° S. lat., 96° E. long., and when twenty-seven days on board, a female child, aged two years, was heard to whoop. A second time, in the fifteenth week of the voyage, the sound of whooping was heard.

In the ship *Hougoumont*, Plymouth to Adelaide, 1866, with 335 souls, on August 14, in 38° S. lat., 0° 4' E. long., and when sixty-seven days at sea, a boy, aged two, showed whooping-cough. My notes, made at the time, state:—

"Ryan, male, aged two. (August 14, 1866.) Whooping-cough: cool skin, distinct whoop; became dull and feverish four days ago for a day or two, since then has been fretful; eats well." This was "the first sound of whooping-cough which had been heard on board. The elder brother had lately had measles."

August 17.—Ryan, male, aged two. "Has cough; skin cool; cheerful; coughs seldom; whoop very slight."

Affinities of, or Merging of, Scarlet Fever and Measles; or Comparative Symptomatology.

The ship *Hougoumont*, Plymouth to Adelaide, 1866, having on board 147 men, 137 women, 25 boys, 21 girls, 5 infants—equal to 335 souls—experienced an epidemic of measles; the number of cases of measles, in successive weeks, were—

Ship "Hougoumont," 1866.

Weeks	Place.	Measles.	Scarlet fever.	Sore-throat.	"Colds."	Diarrhœa.	Whooping-cough.
1	Plymouth to 46° N. L., 7° W.	2	...	...	3	3	...
2	To 31° N., 15° W.	2	...	1	3	1	...
3	To 15 N., 25 W.	...	...	2	4	5	...
4	To 3 N., 24 W.	1	...	3	4	3	...
5	To 2 N., 26 W.	...	...	3	11	5	...
6	To 10 S., 34 W.	...	1	3	1	6	...
7	To 16 S., 36 W.	4	...	2	0	5	...
8	To 33 S., 35 W.	3	...	3	2	0	...
9	To 41 S., 11 W.	3	...	1	0	0	...
10	To 41 S., 5 E.	1	...	1	0	0	1
11	To 43 S., 74 E.	1	1	5	5	0	...
12	To 41 S., 84 E.	...	...	1	3	7	...
13	To 44 S., 96 E.	...	...	1	3	0	...
14	To 35 S., 139 E.	...	...	1	1	4	...

I have included in this table all the cases of measles, scarlet fever (?), whooping-cough (?), and also those cases of generally prevalent "colds"; which latter seem to be of a common order of change, from the normal rates of health, with a great variety of so-called different diseases. These symptoms—"colds"—have local manifestations, which vary in different voyages, and also in different cases, in different periods of the same voyage; such "colds," generally commencing with a shivering and depression, and variously, in "pains in the bones," headache, feeling of general weakness, slight cough, etc.

In this voyage, 28 cases of measles occurred; none died. Of the total 28 cases, 17 were under twelve years, 11 were over twelve years. Very great variety and degrees of intensity of symptoms showed. The average duration of cases, from the first ailing, to cheerfulness and recovery, was five days. Diarrhœa was noted in 10 cases; bronchial effusion, hoarseness, or croupy cough, in 12; 8 of the cases were in persons over fourteen years, 14 were under six years. Symptoms were more severe in older than in younger patients. The eruption was generally deep red, raised, and crescentic; it often showed in the first twenty-four hours of ailing. Except a single gentle aperient to any who were costive, no medicine was given. Cold water as a drink; free admission of air, without draught; warmth; and whatever food the patient would take—was the treatment.

But the interest of the voyage is mostly in the alliances which were shown between measles, scarlet fever, sore-throat, etc.

However important it may be to group symptoms, and to define "diseases," yet there exists the greater and more prevailing "form" of their common alliances; and this voyage presented phenomena of what Bacon termed "travelling instances," *e.g.*, in the sixth week the first case *like* scarlet fever occurred, and in the eleventh week the second and only other of the same type.

In the sixth week, July 17, 1866, Dunn, a male, aged twenty-four, had sore-throat on 16th. On the 17th "eruption over chest of fine red spots, less dark than that of any of the cases of measles, and not crescentic. The measles eruption in other cases has been very distinct, concentric, livid."

18th.—₆ p.m. : "Pulse 148; copious reddish eruption in symmetrical patches on thorax (not on sternum) and limbs."

July 19.—"Pulse 130; copious eruption; tongue clean; throat not painful."

In the eleventh week, on August 19, in 41° S. lat., 18° E. long., a boy, aged six years, presented (*like*) scarlet fever. He was dull on the 17th; rash came out on the 18th, red, rough; a skin like scarlet fever. "19th: Cheerful; rash out; tonsils swollen, white spots on both."

Both these cases had well-marked scarlet fever skin and sore-throat. Of the twenty-eight cases of measles, one only had sore-throat; and he had copious and well-marked eruption of measles.

Thus the type, both of skin and throat, of these two cases was nearer to scarlet fever than to measles.

Of the epidemic of "sore-throat," which went along with that of the measles, there were twenty-nine cases. Of these twenty-nine, seven were under twenty years of age, two under seventeen. None under ten years showed "sore-throat."

The character of the "sore-throat" was redness and white spots on one or both tonsils; ulcerated-like patches on back of pharynx; and in a few, severe white ulceration of the tonsils. As a general rule, the early symptoms were slight, and not complained of until the throat became affected; in others, severe earlier symptoms existed. The duration of the cases till health returned was usually three or four days; a few cases continued six or seven days. The cases were most numerous in the tenth and eleventh weeks, when the measles had almost ceased.

I cannot but think it very important, in respect to philosophical method, that one should view these three several "diseases"—measles, scarlet fever, and sore-throat—as of *one order of change* and of *one series*.

Although the experience of this voyage does not *prove* the evolution of scarlet fever and whooping-cough, yet it carries to me the deep conviction that, in viewing the phenomena of the normal rates or state of the human system (in the class of fevers or "colds"), the alliances of so-called different diseases have a greater place in nature, or in their "form," than have their "specific" differences.

I find in my notes, made at the time, as follows :—"Sore-throat cases now more frequent among the adults ; not many or any cases of measles " . . . . "the two diseases are, *to a certain degree*, allied " . . . . "diarrhœa now showing : this diarrhœa is an affection of the whole system, and is not different from the measles, sore-throat, etc." Although it is necessary, and philosophically just, to lean to the view that scarlet fever, measles, whooping-cough, cholera, etc., are "specifically" (whatever that term may mean) different, yet it may be equally just to seek a wider and deeper "form" common to them all; and the variations of type of disease which I have shown in the ship *Hougoumont* are "travelling instances," which, like the abnormal deviations of animal structure, open to our view the law or order of relationship and evolution.

The conditions of health or the prevailing normal rates are in absolute corelation with prevailing physical environment. Epidemic deviations are grandly associated with "season changes," or often with yet wider physical corelations in recurrent periods of varying duration. Voyages such as these under consideration may be viewed as large experimental trials on communities under changing physical corelations ; and the more so in that the environment of the sea-clime is so physically different from that environment under which the people had hitherto lived. "Climate," says Dr. Haughton ("Lectures on Physical Geography"), may be defined as the *complex effect* of external conditions of heat, moisture (etc.), upon the life of plants and animals. This complex, but very intelligible, idea explains how it happens that the surroundings of each plant or animal, in its own country, are such that it is with extreme difficulty, in many cases, that it can be removed and successfully *acclimatised* in another country, where the surroundings are somewhat different."

(*To be continued.*)

REPORTS OF HOSPITAL PRACTICE
IN
MEDICINE AND SURGERY.

MANCHESTER ROYAL INFIRMARY.

MULTIPLE SYPHILOMATA—PARALYSIS OF THE MUSCULI CRICO-ARYTENOIDEI POSTICI—RAPID RECOVERY.

(Under the care of Dr. DRESCHFELD.)

B. M., a married woman, aged forty-two, was admitted on May 6, 1881, suffering from some tumours in her face and neck, and excessive difficulty in breathing.

She is stated to have always enjoyed good health till twelve months ago, when she suffered from sore throat, which, however, soon subsided. Three months ago she noticed some swelling over the right lower jaw, which increased, and was soon followed by other swellings in the neck ; she at the same time experienced difficulty in opening the mouth, in swallowing, and in breathing ; the latter had become so severe, especially on exertion, that she was frightened of suffocation. She has been married twenty-three years, and has had three children, of whom only one is alive ; one was still-born ; and the other died, seven years old, from some acute disease. There is no history of syphilis. The menstruation ceased three years ago.

Present Condition.—Patient is thin and emaciated ; there is a large, firm tumour over the right lower jaw, passing upwards underneath the masseter muscle ; the skin is movable, and close examination of the tumour from the inside of the mouth shows it to be connected with the lower jaw, springing probably from the periosteum. Another small tumour is found on the right side of the thyroid cartilage, separate from the thyroid gland, of firm consistence, and closely connected with the thyroid cartilage, with which it moves. A number (five or six) of enlarged glands are felt beneath the symphysis of the lower jaw. No other tumours are seen on the surface of the body.

The patient cannot open the mouth 'wide, owing to the tumour on the lower jaw. There is seen a small round ulcer, with sharply cut edges, on the left side of the palate. Deglutition is difficult. On passing an œsophagus bougie, a slight resistance is felt in the lower portion of the pharynx ; the bougie can, however, be passed into the stomach when once this resistance is overcome. The tongue is clean ; appetite good; bowels regular. The other abdominal organs show nothing abnormal on examination.

The circulatory system is normal ; the pulse weak and easily compressible. The physical examination of the lungs shows nothing but extensive bronchial catarrh ; on auscultation the left lung seems to admit air somewhat less freely than the right. On percussion, however, nothing is detected to indicate pressure on a bronchus. There is a little frothy sputum. When the patient is sitting quiet or lying down, the breathing is fairly normal; on walking or running, excessive inspiratory dyspnœa comes on, with engorgement of the veins in the neck and dusky appearance of face and neck. The laryngoscopic examination shows almost complete paralysis of the abductors of the vocal cords; during deep inspiration the vocal cords are drawn closely together. Adduction of the cords is well performed, and the voice of the patient is but little affected.

Owing to the very excessive dyspnœa, the patient was at once subjected to an energetic anti-syphilitic treatment (daily inunction and twenty grains of iodide of potassium *pro dos.*), under which she markedly and rapidly improved ; the tumours soon decreased ; the dyspnœa disappeared, and the general condition of the patient so much improved, that she was made an out-patient on June 3, when the following entry into the case-book was made by Mr. J. W. Bentley, clinical clerk :—"The patient's condition has very much mproved ; she has gained flesh and feels herself able to ollow her work again. The tumour on the lower jaw has quite disappeared; that near the thyroid gland is much smaller; the enlarged lymphatic glands have also much diminished. She can now open her mouth well, swallow with ease, has no longer any difficulty of breathing on walking or running, and suffers very little from her cough. On laryngoscopic examination it is seen that both vocal cords move with inspiration and expiration; on inspiration the left cord moves less than the right."

The patient attended the out-patient room of the Manchester Royal Infirmary till the beginning of August, when she was discharged free from any symptoms whatever.

Remarks (by Dr. Dreschfeld).—From the above given brief account it will be seen that we had to do here with a case of paralysis of the abductors of the vocal cords. Cases of this description are now found to be—since attention has been drawn to them by Morell Mackenzie, Ziemssen, Riegel, Semon, and others—not so rare as at first supposed. They are chiefly characterised by the inspiratory dyspnœa, especially on exertion, the stridulous breathing during sleep, and the absence of any great amount of hoarseness; whilst laryngoscopically they are easily recognised by the approximation of the vocal cords during inspiration. The causes of this affection are very various, sometimes central, sometimes peripheric, and here again affecting primarily either the nerves or the crico-arytænoid muscles themselves. In the above case the most probable cause was a syphilitic tumour or infiltration situated between the larynx and œsophagus, pressing upon the muscles and causing their paralysis, or on the nerves going to the muscles. This view is based on the facts that the patient had difficulty of swallowing, that on the introduction of the œsophageal sound a distinct resistance was felt at the corresponding point, that several distinct tumours were seen in the neighbourhood, and that the symptoms quickly subsided on the energetic anti-syphilitic treatment which was adopted.

CASE OF MULTIPLE SYPHILOMATA — SPONTANEOUS FRACTURE OF CLAVICLE AND OF A RIB, ETC. — RAPID IMPROVEMENT UNDER TREATMENT.

(Under the care of Dr. DRESCHFELD.)

Peter M., aged thirty-six, single, labourer, was admitted into the Infirmary on February 12, 1881, when the following notes were taken by Mr. R. Maguire, Clinical Clerk:— Patient served in the Army until ten years ago, in China, Africa, and Japan. Since then he has been an ironworker's labourer; has been exposed to many hardships; has not been very temperate; he contracted syphilis sixteen years ago, but beyond a sore-throat has not had any other syphilitic symptoms. About two years ago he began to suffer from pains in the limbs, which continued off and on for eighteen months. Six months ago a tumour appeared on the right clavicle, and he suffered from stiffness of the left side of neck; he was also unable to move the left arm, from pain and contraction in the left shoulder. Six or seven weeks ago, another tumour appeared on the back below the scapula, and another on the right side of the head, which gave a great deal of pain.

Present Condition.—Patient is very much emaciated, and has a worn expression of countenance. Finger-nails are clubbed. On the knees are numerous copper-coloured marks. On the scalp, immediately above and about two inches from right ear, is a small swelling, soft, giving an almost fluctuating feel, and the edges of the bone round it are raised. Over the right clavicle, about half an inch from the sterno-clavicular articulation, is a somewhat globular swelling, of the size of an orange. When this is handled, it gives rise to a sense of crepitation, as in fractures, and loose spicula of bone can be felt. The broken end of the clavicle can be distinctly perceived on moving the arm. There is no pain in the tumour, and the patient had never any injury to it. On the left side of the neck, along the posterior border of the sterno-mastoid muscle, is a smooth, hard swelling beneath the muscle; the muscle itself seems infiltrated and hardened. The left shoulder is in a state of partial anchylosis, and allows only of a very limited movement of the arm. The shoulder muscles are neither atrophied nor swollen, and there is very little pain on passive movement of the shoulder. Posteriorly, over the ninth rib, there is a soft, badly defined elastic swelling, which gives rise, both on palpation and auscultation, to distinct crepitations. The ninth rib can

be felt through this emphysematous swelling as thickened, but no fractured ends can be made out. The lymphatic glands of the body are enlarged and hard, especially in the inguinal and posterior cervical regions. The physical examination of the mouth and throat shows on the tip of the tongue a small hard ulcer, with slightly raised edges and greyish floor. The examination of the chest organs shows extensive bronchial catarrh; behind, over the swelling, the crepitations of the subcutaneous emphysema are heard. The liver is very much enlarged, reaching as far down as the umbilicus in the middle, and its surface is smooth; its lower margin, somewhat blunt, can be felt distinctly. The spleen is not enlarged. The urine, of normal colour and specific gravity, contains neither albumen nor sugar. The nervous system and special-sense organs show no symptoms of any disease.

Treatment.—The patient was at once put under a strong anti-syphilitic treatment; he received daily inunctions of mercury in the way described by Sigmund, and twenty-grain doses of iodide of potassium. Under this treatment the symptoms speedily disappeared. The syphilitic nodes on head and clavicle and rib disappeared; the fractured ends of the clavicle could be very distinctly felt; the emphysema over the fractured rib behind also disappeared. The anchylosis yielded perfectly, and the liver diminished considerably in size. On March 3 the mercurial inunctions were stopped, as the patient felt so much better, having gained fifteen pounds since his admission. On March 8 the clavicle was put up in the usual way, the fractured ends being brought into close apposition. On March 14 the patient was sent to the Convalescent Hospital at Cheadle; and returned to the out-patient room on May 3, reporting himself quite cured. On examination, it was found that the fractured ends of the clavicle had undergone union, though the line of union was oblique, and the fractured parts not quite in the same plane. Of the syphilitic lesions, there remained only an enlarged liver; all the other tumours had disappeared.

Remarks (by Dr. Dreschfeld).—The case is chiefly interesting on account of its rare complications—namely, the spontaneous fractures and the arthritis. As for the spontaneous fractures, they are of very rare occurrence in syphilis, and, when they do occur, are usually attributable to necrosis. In this case, however, we had simply a periostitis and osteitis (without either caries or necrosis), and yet spontaneous fractures of the clavicle and of one rib took place. As for the arthritis of the left shoulder-joint, which had already produced partial anchylosis, there can be little doubt, from the rapidity with which it disappeared under a purely antisyphilitic treatment, that it was of syphilitic nature. This complication, though very rare, has been several times observed and described, and I may refer to Lancereaux ("Traité de Syphilis," page 202) for further cases.

PLIABLE IODOFORM.—Dr. Fowler makes a pliable mass for iodoform by mixing it with isinglass and glycerine. The isinglass is reduced to a jelly by steam, and enough glycerine added to give it consistency and pliability. The proportions are as follow:—Iodoform ʒj., isinglass ℥viij., glycerine ʒiv.—*New York Med. Record,* July 9.

PROLONGED RETENTION OF A DEAD FŒTUS.—Prof. Depaul presented at the Académie de Médecine a specimen of a fœtus which was expelled after a pregnancy that had lasted between ten and eleven months. A young woman, who had already borne a child, ceased menstruating after September 8, and she was delivered on August 14 of a child, which had died at the fifth month, and was expelled without the membranes having been ruptured, and exhibiting no signs of putrefaction. It is the first time that a pregnancy has occurred in Prof. Depaul's practice which has been prolonged between ten and eleven months, the fœtus not being expelled for from five to six months after its death. The mother neither during her pregnancy, nor since her delivery, has presented any symptom of a morbid character whatever. This case, he observed, was only one to be added to many others proving that a fœtus dead in utero may sojourn therein for several months, providing that the membranes remained intact, without any injury to the mother. The macerated fœtus on this occasion did not exhale the slightest smell of putrefaction, although it had remained in contact with air and water during twenty-four hours.—*Union Méd.,*

TERMS OF SUBSCRIPTION.
(Free by post.)

British Islands	Twelve Months	.	£1	8	0
" " " "	Six	"	.	0	14	0
The Colonies and the United } States of America . . . }	Twelve	"	.	1	10	0
" " "	Six	"	.	0	15	0
India " " "	Twelve	"	.	1	10	0
" (viâ Brindisi) . . .	"	"	.	1	15	0
" " " . . .	Six	"	.	0	15	0
" (viâ Brindisi) . . .	"	"	.	0	17	6

Foreign Subscribers are requested to inform the Publishers of any remittance made through the agency of the Post-office.

Single Copies of the Journal can be obtained of all Booksellers and Newsmen, price Sixpence.

Cheques or Post-office Orders should be made payable to Mr. JAMES LUCAS, 11, New Burlington-street, W.

TERMS FOR ADVERTISEMENTS.

Seven lines (70 words) .	.	.	.£0	4	6
Each additional line (10 words)	.	.	0	0	6
Half-column, or quarter-page	.	.	1	5	0
Whole column, or half-page	.	.	2	10	0
Whole page	.	.	5	0	0

Births, Marriages, and Deaths are inserted Free of Charge.

THE MEDICAL TIMES AND GAZETTE *is published on Friday morning: Advertisements must therefore reach the Publishing Office not later than One o'clock on Thursday.*

Medical Times and Gazette.

SATURDAY, SEPTEMBER 3, 1881.

THE INDIAN MEDICAL SERVICE.

THE report just issued of the Executive Committee of the Indian Medical Service Defence Fund may be considered as, on the whole, a satisfactory one. It will be remembered that the Association was formed last year for the purpose of obtaining redress for various very grave grievances arising out of the reorganisation of the Indian Medical Service, and that the measures of redress advocated by the Committee were, shortly, as follows:—1. That the Military Surgeons-General in India shall be nominated alternately from the British and Indian Services. 2. Compensation to be granted to the senior Surgeons-Major for reduction in the number of administrative posts. 3. Equalisation of relative Army rank with the Army Medical Department, and extension of the new grade of Brigade-Surgeon to the Indian Service. 4. Improved scale of pensions. 5. Abolition of examination for promotion to the rank of Surgeon-Major. 6. Improved rates of invalid pension. 7. Abolition or modification of the system of "unemployed pay" for junior officers. 8. An increased number of good service pensions. 9. Honorary rank on retirement after twenty years' service. 10. Honorary promotion to the rank of Deputy Surgeon-General of all officers appointed Queen's Honorary Physician or Queen's Honorary Surgeon. 11. Increase in the number of decorations and honorary rewards. The Committee report that of these objects the following have been either fully or partially secured:—The relative Army rank of officers of the Indian Service has been equalised with that of the Army Medical Department; and the new grade of Brigade-Surgeon has been extended to the Indian Service; an improved scale of pensions has been granted; the examination for promotion to the rank of Surgeon-Major has been abolished or modified; the grievance of "unemployed pay" has been, we suppose, lessened; honorary rank on retirement after twenty years' service, and the honorary promo-

tion of all officers appointed Q.H.P. or Q.H.S., have been granted or promised. On these points, which include the grievances summarised under heads 3, 4, 5, 7, 9, and 10 of the list given above, the Committee are of opinion that the Government have granted as much as could be reasonably expected, though it will be observed that in the communication which we publish to-day, from an Indian officer, the subjects of "unemployed pay" and of examination for promotion to the rank of Surgeon-Major are spoken of as still existing grievances. With regard to grievance number one, the Committee remark that no definite or satisfactory reply has as yet been elicited from the Government on the subject; but that "a somewhat ambiguous explanation has been offered, that it was never intended that Indian officers should be permanently debarred from filling the post of Military Surgeon-General in each presidency, and that such promotion, therefore, is open to specially qualified officers of either service." This is cold comfort; and the Committee observe that one, if not two, vacancies will occur within the next year, and they hope the Government of India will—if only as a matter of policy—avail itself of the opportunity to prove that the "Instruction" published in the Army Circulars of January 30, 1880, was issued in good faith, and was not intended to remain a dead letter.

Then, with regard to grievance the second, a very real and substantial grievance, the Committee cannot report or give hope of any gain whatever. The authorities, home and Indian, in face of the protective clauses of the Acts of 1858 and 1860, reduced the number of appointments in the administrative rank, thereby setting aside the guaranteed rights of the senior Surgeons-Major regarding promotion, and they refuse compensation of any kind to the officers whose prospects have been so seriously injured. The Committee have been informed that, "in a dispatch not yet published," the Secretary of State admits the retardation of promotion, and the supersession by their juniors to which the senior Surgeons-Major have been subjected, but argues that a full set-off has been received by them in the beneficial change made affecting the Service as a whole. This view the Committee of course do not accept. They reply, "The hybrid position of Brigade-Surgeon, entailing increased responsibilities, but conferring no extra military rank or additional pay, is assuredly no compensation for men, ten of whom would now have been Deputy Surgeons-General had there been no reduction in the guaranteed number of that rank been made." The gain to the whole Service from the changes made may be great, but the senior Surgeons-Major must be far above average human nature if they can look upon that as a full compensation for their own losses as regards promotion, pay, and pension. With respect to the grievance as to the rates of invalid pensions, a medical officer of the Indian Service, if compelled by ill-health to retire prematurely, is still treated less liberally than an officer of the Army Medical Department under like circumstances; and to this point the Committee have again called the attention of the Secretary of State. There remain only grievances 8 and 11 to notice, and with regard to these the Committee say— "The Government of India have promised that an increased number of good service pensions shall henceforth be allotted to the Indian Medical Service, and that the claims of its members for honorary rewards and decorations shall be more carefully regarded in the future." What this "promise" is worth remains to be seen. Authorities, governors, and governments change, and promises made by one government, in one set of circumstances, may be very lightly regarded in new circumstances and by other men.

Still, much has been done to mend matters as regards the Indian Medical Service since the promulgation of the startling G.G.O., No. 13, of January 2, 1880; and the Executive Committee of the Defence Fund—men who have gained high distinction in the Service, who are proud of it, and jealous for its fame and prosperity—say, " the Service as a whole has greatly benefited from the changes effected during the last eighteen months, inasmuch that, with the exception of the senior Surgeons Major, the pecuniary prospects of every member of the Service, from the Surgeons-General with the Government, to the youngest cadet at Netley, have been materially improved." In these circumstances the Executive, " believing that the existence of their organisation is to a certain extent inconsistent with the good feeling and confidence which ought to exist between a Government and its officers," thought the Committee might be dissolved; but it has been strongly represented to them that the Service has no official representative in this country, and that it would, therefore, be especially inopportune to dissolve at a time when a scheme for the unification of the British and Indian Medical Services is under consideration. It has consequently been decided to keep the Association together for the present, but in a passive form—" the machinery of their organisation will be maintained intact, but thrown out of gear." We think the final decision of the Committee is a right one, though we entirely agree with them in holding that anything like an organised agitation in or in connexion with one of the public services is an evil; justifiable in some circumstances, and notably in those which called the Indian Medical Defence Fund into existence; but to be discontinued the moment its objects have been secured, or it has become perfectly clear that might will continue to count itself as right. The Government determined to reorganise the Indian Medical Service, and in so doing to disregard certain rights that had been guaranteed by Act of Parliament. The determination was carried out, and circumstances have combined to render any chance of influencing the Government through the House of Commons more than usually hopeless.

But some of the shortcomings of the new organisation of the Service have been remedied, and much of the mischief done by the inconsiderate and blundering way in which the scheme was promulgated has been repaired; and the Committee are wise in being content with the possible, and in not continuing to kick against the pricks when it has been made clear the kicking will not benefit anybody; and they are wise also in retaining machinery that can be promptly put in action should need again arise. Owing to the promptness, the all but unanimity, and the strength of the agitation raised by the earliest revealings of the Government scheme for " reforming " the Indian Medical Service, such amendments have been made in it, by alteration and addition, that the Service is fast regaining its old prestige and popularity. We are glad to learn that, at the entrance examination just held, twenty-nine candidates for commissions in the Service competed for ten vacancies; that twenty-seven of the candidates passed; and that the list of those obtaining appointments is distinguished by an absence of the Indian-like names that appeared so frequently in the two or three preceding lists. It is now again recognised that the honoured old Indian Medical Service offers a highly attractive career to eligible British candidates; though it is still second in attractiveness to the Army Medical Department.

THE ADDRESS IN OBSTETRIC MEDICINE.

Dr. Sinclair Coghill's Address in Obstetric Medicine at Ryde had the distinction of being the only one of the three addresses given which dealt directly and exclusively with its own special topic. This accidental singularity, however, was its least merit, for Dr. Coghill's thoughtful and scholarly oration demands, and will repay, the attention of the profession. The subject of it, as defined by its author, was " the claims, intrinsic and relative, of obstetric medicine to increased recognition and cultivation, and the directions in which its development should be encouraged." After some general remarks, in which he pointed out the importance of this special study, and the qualifications required for practice in this field, Dr. Coghill gave a practical bearing to the broad truisms he had been bringing to the attention of the audience by commenting on the deficiencies in the obstetric and gynæcological training of our English medical schools. " Considering," he said, " that to the vast majority of the profession. . . . . obstetric practice in its several branches forms the bulk as well as the most anxious and engrossing part of their work, it seems incredible that the provision for teaching gynæcology particularly, both systematic and clinical, in our medical schools and hospitals, should still be so limited and imperfect. . . . Familiarity with the practice of obstetric and gynæcological details can only be acquired by demonstration. . . . A gynæcological clinique, with ample service, should be established in connexion with all our hospitals. . . . The marked progress of obstetric medicine in America, and its splendid achievements, are no doubt due, to some extent, to the absence of old-world traditions." Now, as to the abstract *desirability* of the systematic and complete gynæcological training of every student, we imagine that few differences of opinion will exist. But its *practicability* is quite another matter. To teach gynæcology a supply of patients is needed; and in diseases of this kind that public demonstration of morbid phenomena which is the most useful part of clinical teaching is so peculiarly painful to female delicacy, that most Englishwomen would go through a great deal, and make great sacrifices, rather than submit to it. In this department experience has shown that a large number of patients, and a large amount of teaching, are incompatibles. The teacher who is in charge of a gynæcological department has therefore to steer between two evils: if he does not teach, the students suffer; if he uses the patients too much for teaching, they will not come to him. The " old-world traditions" of modesty, or, as some enthusiasts might call it, prudery, are still very prevalent in England, whatever may be the case in America; and they are found, not only in patients, but even in physicians and surgeons.

Passing from the standpoint of the student to that of the specialist, Dr. Coghill remarked on the direction in which progress in obstetric science is to be hoped for. " If the progress of obstetric medicine is to be satisfactory, if it is to become less empirical and more and more scientific, in the study of pathology must be sought the means of determining the principles on which a rational system of therapeutics is to be founded. It is in a complete knowledge of the anatomy and physiology of the female sexual system that the foundations of uterine pathology must be laid." The great principle that the orator here enunciated applies to every branch of our science, and not merely to obstetrics; but obstetricians, whose duties to their patients forbid them from actively prosecuting the anatomical investigations even of healthy, much more of morbid structures, perhaps need more than others to be reminded of the fundamental importance of such researches.

Dr. Coghill then briefly passed in review certain recent advances in obstetric science. He touched on that most difficult subject, the reflex symptoms of uterine disease, as to which little is certainly known, and much that is exceedingly mischievous has been written. He broached an ingenious suggestion to explain the supposed influence of maternal impressions upon the fœtus. "I believe . . . . that nerve-force may even be discharged free into, and affect-the fluid contents of the animal cells, and in the same manner influence the blood itself, which, in every sense and purpose, is a living tissue endowed with the highest organic, and functional mobility. It is, perhaps, through this presumed neuro-vascular association that we may find the channel by which maternal impressions are conveyed to the fœtus; and it is more reasonable to suppose that the contents of the bloodvessels are in this manner directly affected by nerve-force, than merely by the contraction and dilatation of their walls." In referring to recent investigations into the innervation of the female genital organs, Dr. Coghill makes a statement which we read with some surprise: "The cervix uteri is particularly rich in its nerve-supply, as might be expected from its exalted sensibility and active functions." "Exalted sensibility" is a quality scarcely attributable to a structure which can be cut and cauterised without producing appreciable suffering; nor should we have judged the functions of the cervix uteri to especially deserve the epithet "active." The changes which the lining membrane of the uterus undergoes during menstruation; Dr. Mortimer Granville's theory of the predetermination of sex by intention, with which Dr. Coghill's experience does not accord; the influence of the thoracic aspiration of the fœtus upon the umbilical circulation; the effect of prolonged labour in producing idiocy, as shown by the researches of Dr. Langdon Down—were next referred to. The orator then drew attention to the views of Lebert, Ortega, and Grisolle, as to the deleterious effect of pregnancy upon phthisical women. There is a popular belief that pregnancy is beneficial in phthisical women. Dr. Coghill, with the authors he quoted, holds the reverse. The grain of truth underlying the error he believes to be "that marriage, when conception can be avoided, from its stimulus to the nervous and nutritive systems, has a beneficial effect on the general health, and through it on the tendency to pulmonary trouble."

Coming to midwifery proper, the speaker made a prediction in which we are sure he is right: "I have no doubt that pelvimetry with craniometry are destined to become important elements in scientific obstetric management." It is, indeed, obvious that, had we the means in every case of labour to determine at the commencement of the process the exact dimensions of the pelvis and of the fœtal head, the choice of means by which aid should be given to the delivery would be made with the same precision, and certainty of a satisfactory result, as the oculist's selection of a pair of spectacles for defective accommodation. Post-partum hæmorrhage, puerperal fever, the use of the forceps, and puerperal mortality, were then touched on by the orator. His conclusion as to the average mortality of childbirth differs from the estimate given by some eminent men who have carefully studied the subject. One in five hundred, Dr. Coghill thinks a fair standard of deaths in childbed. In getting at this he adopts what we take to be an error—that is, he deducts from the result given by statistics the deaths which are described as "non-puerperal." Dr. Coghill himself says—a "source of fallacy arises from the opprobrium which notoriously attaches to the accoucheur or midwife in puerperal cases of unfortunate issue. Obstetric human nature must be very different from the ordinary variety if it is able to resist, even unconsciously, the instinctive tendency there is to refer the result to causes other than that with which it is really concerned." This fallacy tends to make the reported obstetric mortality lower than the actual; and to allow deaths which the reporter could not help connecting with childbirth, to be explained away by calling them "non-puerperal," is to add to the amount of error which this fallacy produces. It is very difficult, indeed, often impossible, to say that the

occurrence of a death in childbed has not been influenced by the incidents of parturition. The only true way of separating the mortality of childbed from the mortality in childbed, is, as Dr. Matthews Duncan has pointed out, to take the gross mortality in childbed, and deduct from it the average death-rate among non-parturient women at the same age and during the same period of time.

Dr. Coghill's remarks upon gynæcology were wise and weighty, but they were chiefly of the nature of criticism, and therefore, although only too true, do not call for detailed comment. The fault which he found with modern gynæcology is this: "There has been far too great attention paid to local treatment. The use of instruments for diagnosis and treatment, and direct personal medication, has been greatly overdone. The *nimia diligentia* has been too rampant." He gave instances in illustration of this fault. But it does not follow that because certain persons use instruments without necessity, therefore the instruments are to be condemned. What is wanted for the progress of gynæcology, is not general denunciation of the misdeeds of individual practitioners, or even of particular schools of practice, but more accurate definition of the circumstances under which instrumental interference is required, and the kind and degree of benefit it is capable of effecting.

THE WEEK.

TOPICS OF THE DAY.

THE case of "Chambers and others v. the Metropolitan Asylums District Board" was recently heard by Mr. Justice Cave and Mr. Justice Kay, sitting as a Divisional Court, in the Queen's Bench Division of the High Court of Justice. The application was for an interlocutory injunction to restrain the defendants from sending any more patients into the Fulham Small-pox Hospital until the hearing of the action. A large number of affidavits were filed on each side. There were three plaintiffs—Mr. Chambers, the lessee of Lilliebridge Grounds, who alleged that his business was being destroyed by the maintenance of the Hospital; Colonel Gunter, the owner of land round the Hospital; and Mr. Pickersgill, whose daughter had suffered from the disease. The plaintiffs' affidavit included several from the medical officers of the district, and from other resident physicians. These affidavits alleged that the Hospital was a centre of contagion, and that the district had never been free from the disease when there were patients in the Hospital. Plans were produced, which purported to give the number of small-pox cases that had occurred within radii of a quarter of a mile, half a mile, three-quarters of a mile, and one mile, and which showed an enormous proportion of cases near the Hospital. The defendants filed affidavits from the physicians of the Hospital and others to show that it was very carefully managed, and that the cases of small-pox near the Hospital could be traced to various other causes. One medical officer went so far as to say he would have no hesitation in taking a residence adjoining the Hospital. Their Lordships, during the course of the argument, remarked that it would be a most serious matter to stay the working of a great public institution, and the plaintiffs must show the most pressing necessity for an interim injunction. To try on the motion thoroughly would really be to try the action itself, and, as at present they could only get affidavit evidence, that was a most undesirable course. They suggested that the defendants might very well undertake not to send into the Hospital any patients from outside districts until the hearing of the cause. It appeared, however, that the defendants had not power to enter into such an arrangement without the consent of the Local Government Board, and eventually it was suggested that the matter should stand over for three weeks, to enable the decision of Mr. Dodson to be taken.—Sir Hardinge Giffard, who appeared for the defendants, promising that he would advise the Local Government Board to agree to the undertaking advised by their Lordships.

Almost the first place visited by Her Majesty on her arrival in Edinburgh was the Royal Infirmary. In the afternoon of the day of her arrival, the Queen, accompanied by the Princess Beatrice and the Duke of Connaught, went to this institution, where the Lord Provost, the treasurer, a number of the Infirmary managers, several professors, and others had already assembled. The Royal party were received by the Lord Provost, who conducted Her Majesty through the building. On arriving at the end of the corridor, overlooking the Medical Hospital, the Queen named the ward lying to the south (Dr. Muirhead's) the Albert Ward. Returning to the Surgical Hospital, the party were conducted through wards Nos. 10, 11, and 12 by Dr. Joseph Bell. One of these wards received the name of the Victoria Ward. Her Majesty manifested great interest in the patients, and spoke to several of them. Before leaving, the Royal party inscribed their names in an album in the managers' room, and subsequently paid a visit to the Albert Ward.

Just before the prorogation of Parliament, Mr. Causton inquired of the President of the Local Government Board, in reference to the statement contained in the report of the Conservators of the river Thames that Kingston and Richmond, and other places below the intakes of the water companies still pass their sewage into the Thames, whether any, and if any, what, steps were being taken to remedy the evil. In reply, Mr. Dodson recapitulated the well-known story that in 1878 a joint board was formed, called the Lower Thames Valley Main Sewerage Board, for the purpose of providing for the disposal of the sewage of these as well as other places; that in 1879 they brought in a Bill for this purpose, which was unfortunately thrown out on the second reading. Further, that last year they proposed another scheme, which, after a long inquiry, the Local Government board were unable to approve, and that recently the joint Board have proposed another scheme for consideration. We hear a great deal of the law's delay, but it is a question whether in any civilised country, other than our own, so much delay would have been permitted in carrying out a work of the importance of the one now inquired into.

The town of Eastbourne, profiting by recent example, has been holding an exhibition of sanitary appliances. The originators were Mr. Rodda, a gentleman who takes an active interest in the welfare of the town, and Mr. Schmidt, the building surveyor. It was organised under the patronage of the Duke of Devonshire, by a council of local gentlemen, the president being Dr. Jeffery, who is chairman of the Local Board. The exhibition was of considerable extent, and was held in the pavilion in Devonshire Park, and in a temporary annexe constructed near at hand. The object of the show was announced to be the advancement of sanitary science and building construction, and the exhibits admitted were in conformity with these views. Many articles of interest were transferred from the late medical and sanitary exhibition at South Kensington, and a series of lectures in the afternoon and evening were delivered by Dr. Alfred Carpenter, Professor Kerr, Mr. E. C. Robins, Dr. H. D. Ellis, Mr. Schmidt, and other gentlemen, who are held to be authorities in sanitary matters.

According to the report of the Registrar-General for Scotland for the month of June last, there were registered in the eight principal towns the births of 3781 children, and the deaths of 2102 persons. Allowing for increase of popula-

tion this latter number is 367 under the June average for the last ten years. A comparison of the deaths registered in the eight towns shows that during the month under notice the annual mortality was at the rate of 15 deaths per 1000 persons in Perth, 17 in Dundee and in Aberdeen, 18 in Greenock, 21 in Edinburgh and in Leith, and 23 in Glasgow and in Paisley. The miasmatic order of the zymotic class of diseases caused 293 deaths, and constituted 13·9 per cent. of the whole mortality. In Edinburgh scarlet fever and whooping-cough were prevalent, and in Leith 8 deaths were attributed to typhus fever. Whooping-cough was altogether responsible for 60 deaths, diarrhœa for 48, scarlet fever for 42, measles for 38, croup for 14, and small-pox for 1. The diseases from inflammatory affections of the respiratory organs (not including consumption, whooping-cough, or croup) amounted to 405, or 19·3 per cent. Those from consumption alone numbered 280, or 13·3 per cent. A widow died at ninety years of age, and a shawl-weaver (a male) at ninety-two.

An important Local Government Board inquiry was recently conducted by Captain Hildyard, one of the Board's inspectors, at Henley-on-Thames, as to the sanitary condition of the town. The inquiry was instituted on account of certain statements made in a memorial to the Local Government Board by Mr. Owthwaite, asserting that the town had no system of drainage, that in winter time cellars and underground rooms were constantly under water; further, the memorialists alleged that the refuse from cesspools drained into the Thames, and that the authorities should no longer allow this, as the waterworks system of the London companies was thereby placed in great jeopardy. After hearing a great number of witnesses, the inquiry was adjourned by mutual consent until October 6 next.

One of the many evil effects of the prolonged and reiterated time-absorbing discussions and struggles in Parliament on the Irish Land Bill has been to block the progress of several important Acts affecting the welfare of this country, and much inconvenience has been the result. Amongst the Bills thus retarded was the Local Loans Bill, owing to the failure of which the Public Works Loan Commissioners have been unable to meet the demands made upon them by several local authorities. At Sittingbourne, for instance, a large infectious hospital is in course of construction by the joint sanitary boards of the district, the cost of which, it was arranged, should be met by a loan from the Commissioners, and the stoppage of supplies has caused the utmost inconvenience. At the adjoining town of Milton, the authorities, who are carrying out sewerage and waterworks improvements, have been placed in a similar dilemma by the non-receipt of an expected loan, and have had to make arrangements for a temporary advance from another source to pay the contractors.

The following particulars, elicited at an inquest recently held by the Birmingham Deputy-Coroner, confirm much that has already been written on the subject of false burial certificates. The body of an infant which had been sent for burial as still-born to the sextoness of All Saints' Church was about to be buried on the simple certificate of a midwife, who described the child as still-born, though it was evidently born alive, and who certified that she was present at the birth, though she did not arrive at the house until nearly two hours after. It transpired that the sextoness, a very illiterate woman, had been in the habit of burying children described as still-born, on the certificate merely of the midwife, and she kept no list of such burials. In the present case, the body, which had been four days in the house of the sextoness, was in an advanced stage of decomposition, but the medical evidence was conclusive as to the child having lived; death was attributed to suffocation. The Coroner animadverted strongly upon the conduct of the midwife, whose certificate contained two false statements, and pointed out the danger resulting from such a laxity of system. The jury, in returning a verdict of "Accidental death," called the attention of the vicar and churchwardens of the church to the irregular manner in which the burial of still-born children was carried out at All Saints', and strongly censured the midwife for giving a false certificate.

It is rumoured that the extension works contemplated by the Metropolitan Board, in respect to the main drainage of the metropolis, do not include any plan for carrying the outfalls further down the river. It has been proposed that Sir Joseph Bazalgette should prepare plans for an enlargement of the reservoirs at Barking and Crossness, but the proposal remains in abeyance until the Board reassembles in the course of a few weeks.

A joint deputation from the Society of Medical Officers of Health and the British Medical Association recently had an interview with Mr. Dodson, M.P., and Mr. Hibbert, M.P., at the office of the Local Government Board, to ask for a reform of the present insecurity in the tenure of office of extra-metropolitan medical officers of health, in consequence of their liability to periodical re-election. The deputation asked that the Local Government Board should exercise the compulsory powers for which they applied to Parliament, and obtained in the Public Health Act, 1875, to put medical officers of health on the same footing in regard to the tenure of their office as Poor-law medical officers. Mr. Dodson, in reply, expressed his sense of the hardship which must fall upon medical officers in cases where they gave up their private practice for the public service, and then found their careers as public officers of health cut short, with no alternative but to return to private practice. The policy of the Board had been to encourage fixity of tenure so as to induce men of standing to take such posts; but they could only encourage that in combined districts, where the districts themselves were large and the salary was remunerative. Thus far Mr. Dodson's talk was of the usual official platitude type—though it is wonderful that "the good of the public" was not made more of; but the real feeling of the Minister spoke out when he added that he "preferred to leave matters in local hands." Of course the observations of the deputation will "receive the most careful attention of himself and his colleagues."

An important question of liability has been brought before the County Court Judge of Dover. Dr. Simpson, the Public Vaccinator and Medical Officer to the Dover Board of Guardians, claimed £35 18s. 6d. for vaccinating 481 children. The correctness of the claim was not disputed by the Guardians; but they stated that though Dr. Simpson was appointed Vaccination Officer on November 21, 1879, the Local Government Board had failed to confirm the appointment until May 18, 1881. During this period the Medical Officer continued to perform the duties of vaccination officer, for which, however, they declined to hold themselves responsible or to sanction payment, contending that Dr. Simpson had not been properly authorised. The Judge reserved his decision until the next Court, but remarked that in the meantime he would undertake to communicate privately with the Secretary to the Local Government Board upon a matter which he considered of great public importance. But for Dr. Simpson having persevered in his duties, as instanced by his having vaccinated those 481 children, they would probably have gone unvaccinated, and the danger of the spread of a most malignant disease would have been very much increased. In the meantime he advised that a representation should also be made by the Board of Guardians to the Local Government

Board, and gave full permission for the use of his name, and a statement of his opinion that the claim of the medical officer ought to be admitted.

THE LONDON WATER-SUPPLY FOR THE MONTHS OF JUNE AND JULY.

THE report of the Water Examiners on the supply delivered by the metropolitan companies during the month of June last showed that the state of the water in the Thames, where several of the intakes are situated, was good in quality during the whole of that month, and the same remark applied to the water in the river Lea. If there was apparently some danger on the score of quantity, there appeared to have been none on that of quality. The following is extracted from the report (made for the water companies) by Messrs. Crookes, Odling, and Tidy, on the composition and quality of daily samples of the water supplied to London, from May 20 to June 30, 1881:—"Judged by our daily examinations, the water supplied to London is, in our opinion, whether considered as to its efficient filtration, or as to its proper aëration, or as to its purity and wholesomeness, unimpeachable. The result of our six months' work, and the examination during this period of 1127 samples, enable us to state that, as an excellent drinking supply, it leaves nothing to be desired." Dr. Frankland's report for the month of June was not quite so laudatory, but satisfactory. He remarked that the water drawn from the Thames by the Chelsea, West Middlesex, Southwark, Grand Junction, and Lambeth Companies, although still of very much better quality than the average water from that source, was rather inferior to the May samples. This deterioration was most marked in the case of the Southwark Company's water. With the exception of that distributed by the Grand Junction Company, all the Thames water was efficiently filtered before delivery. For July, Colonel Bolton reports that the state of the water in the Thames at Hampton, Moulsey, and Sunbury (where the intakes of the West Middlesex, Grand Junction, Southwark and Vauxhall, Lambeth, Chelsea, and East London Companies are situated) was good in quality during the whole month, as was also water in the river Lea. Dr. Frankland states that, "taking the average amount of organic impurity contained in a given volume of the Kent Company's water during the nine years ending December, 1876, as unity, the proportional amount contained in an equal volume of water supplied by each of the metropolitan water companies and by the Tottenham Local Board of Health was—Kent, 1·5; Colne Valley, 1·6; New River, 1·7; Tottenham, 1·8; East London, 2·2; West Middlesex, 2·3; Chelsea, 3·0; Grand Junction, 3·1; Lambeth, 3·2; Southwark, 3·5. The supplies of the West Middlesex, Grand Junction, and Lambeth Companies were slightly turbid from inefficient filtration. The Lea water distributed by the New River and East London Companies was efficiently filtered: the New River Company's water was, in point of chemical purity, second to none but the best of the deep-well waters, and that of the East London Company was superior to any of the Thames waters. Colonel Bolton again draws attention to the grievous way in which the condition of domestic water-receptacles—cisterns, tanks, and butts—is neglected; and observes that the purest water in the world would be poisoned by being stored in uncared-for and filthy places.

THE NIGHTINGALE FUND, 1880.

FROM the report of the Nursing School at St. Thomas's Hospital for the year 1880, it appears that on January 1 there were 34 probationer nurses in the School, and that 39 were admitted during the year. Of this total of 73, as many as 16 resigned or were discharged as unsuitable for the work; 25 completed their year's training and received appointments; and there remained in the School, on December 31, 32; of whom 12 were special or lady probationers, and 20 nurse probationers. It will be noted that the proportion of candidates who fail from some cause or another after trial is very large; and in the report it is stated that "while the number of candidates of the gentlewoman class is far greater than can be admitted, those who are well qualified are few," but we do not gather what proportion, if any, of the 16 who failed during the year 1880 were "of the gentlewoman class." The practical training and instruction given to the probationers is, as is well known, good—i.e., they work in the wards as assistant-nurses, and thus learn by daily practice how to nurse, in the full meaning of the term; and they are instructed by the "home-sister" in the values of weights and measures, in reading prescriptions, and in preparing for operations, in bandaging, etc. But we venture to more than doubt the wisdom and advisability of their being instructed in the "classification of medicines, their origin and uses; elementary anatomy, physiology, and chemistry;" or even in "Domville's Glossary of Medical Terms and Abbreviations"; and still more of the "nine lectures on medical subjects, and seven clinical," by Dr. Bristowe; "seventeen lectures on anatomy and surgical subjects, and eleven clinical lectures," by Mr. Croft; and "twelve lectures on the chemistry of food and drink," by Dr. Bernays. And when we find that "the expenses of training hospital nurses"—i.e., of turning out twenty-five such nurses in the year—amounted to £1432 (besides £62 odd for "clothing of probationers" and £139 for "advertisements, printing, books, secretary's and clerk's salary, and petty cash"), we cannot but think that a hospital nurse trained in St. Thomas's School is a rather costly article. Moreover, as the balance of receipts for 1879 was £1389, and for 1880 £1272, and the proportion of failures, from various causes, is so large as has been stated, it may be questioned whether some reform is not needed to make the School as fruitful as it might and should be.

THE ROYAL UNIVERSITY OF IRELAND.

THE Standing Committee met this week, under the Presidency of the Right Hon. Lord O'Hagan, Vice-Chancellor of the University. They had under consideration the revision of the scheme rendered necessary by the recent Act of Parliament; and we are informed that they agreed to recommend to the Senate that the Matriculation Examination shall be held this year on Tuesday, December 6, and following days; and that candidates be required to send in their names to the secretaries on or before October 15.

EXPERIMENTS ON LIVING ANIMALS.

THE report of Mr. W. Thornley Stoker, the Inspector for Ireland under the Vivisection Act, has lately been issued as a Parliamentary paper. There appear to be seven registered places and six licences in Ireland. One of the licences only has a special licence for experiments without anaesthetics. The inspector writes:—"I have to report that I have carefully considered the nature and bearing of all the experiments performed under the Act, and that I am of opinion that they have been free from any appreciable sufferings, and have all been of a character useful to science, and tending to increase our knowledge of disease and to improve its treatment. The total number of experiments made was thirty-four; of these twenty-four were performed under the licence, and ten under certificate C, which was the only certificate allowed during the year. I have every reason to believe that those persons holding licences and certificates have rigidly adhered to their conditions as regards the use of anaesthetics."

THE PARIS WEEKLY RETURN.

THE number of deaths for the thirty-third week, terminating August 18, 1881, was 1024 (540 males and 484 females), and among these there were from typhoid fever 50, small-pox 14, measles 10, scarlatina 14, pertussis 5, croup and diphtheria 44, erysipelas 9, and puerperal infections 6. There were also 34 deaths from tubercular and acute meningitis, 17 from acute bronchitis, 43 from pneumonia, 196 from infantile athrepsia (74 of the children having been wholly or partially suckled), and 21 violent deaths. The number of deaths has diminished since the preceding week by 114, but epidemic diseases, taken generally, have not contributed to this diminution, for while the deaths from measles and small-pox are fewer, those from typhoid and scarlatina have sensibly increased. The fear expressed last week of an increased number of deaths from typhoid, owing to the greater number of hospital admissions and cases in private practice, have been realised, for while the deaths were 19 in the thirty-first week, and 38 in the thirty-second, they have reached 50 in the present week. The births for the week amounted to 1123, viz., 574 males (428 legitimate and 146 illegitimate) and 549 females (408 legitimate and 141 illegitimate); 77 children (41 males and 36 females) were born dead or died within twenty-four hours.

THE ARMY MEDICAL SERVICE.

THE following is a list, in order of merit, of the twenty-five candidates who were successful for appointments as surgeons in Her Majesty's British Medical Service at the competitive examination held in London on the 15th ult., with the number of marks obtained by each:—

	Marks		Marks
N. M. Reid	2390	J. W. Jerome	1920
W. H. P. Lewis	2235	W. W. Pike	1875
W. Dick	2296	M. E. Fitzgerald	1870
F. J. Jencken	2141	L. H. Trueditt	1870
H. O. Stuart	2125	J. M. Irwin	1870
F. H. Treherne	2105	P. J. Nealon	1850
S. F. Lougheed	2100	E. O. Wight	1840
J. C. Haslett	2075	W. A. Morris	1825
H. J. Barratt	2065	F. H. M. Burton	1810
H. E. R. James	2025	J. Heath	1805
H. O. Trevor	1990	C. E. Nichol	1805
A. F. Russell	1985	J. D. T. Reckitt	1805
E. J. Fayle	1971		

THE INDIAN MEDICAL SERVICE.

THE following is the list of the candidates who were successful at the competitive examination held on the 15th ult. for Her Majesty's Indian Medical Service. Twenty-nine candidates competed for ten appointments. Twenty-seven were reported qualified.

	Marks		Marks
L. T. Young	2702	John Smyth	2175
J. B. Gibbons	2610	R. B. Roe	2125
D. St. J. Grant	2410	H. Greany	2015
G. J. Shand	2360	J. Kernan	1965
D. J. Crawford	2225	E. P. Youngerman	1795

OPENING THE OESOPHAGUS.

THERE is an interesting case of stricture, probably epitheliomatous, now in the wards of the London Hospital, and it is proposed to perform the rare operation of oesophagostomy on Tuesday next at two o'clock. As the patient, a young woman, is rapidly wasting, and as the attempt to pass bougies or to swallow brings on severe dyspnœa, the operation of opening the stomach was suggested, but it appears to the surgeon under whose charge the patient is that the neglected method of making an opening in the gullet in these cases will be the more correct and less dangerous proceeding in the first instance. The patient can be at once nourished through the opening, and subsequently, in non-malignant cases, the stricture may be dilated from above or below, and, should this endeavour succeed, the œsophageal opening may be closed. Should circumstances in any particular case demand it, gastrostomy can be resorted to after the preliminary and much less dangerous œsophagostomy has had a fair trial. The modern operation of excising the diseased part is a very severe proceeding, and in the very few cases in which it has been performed, the result has not been encouraging.

THE METROPOLITAN FISH-SUPPLY.

THE leading recommendations of the Special Committee appointed by the Court of Common Council to inquire into the metropolitan fish-supply, briefly summarised, are as follows :—The rates for the carriage of fish to London operate prejudicially, and should be revised. The present approaches to Billingsgate Market are absolutely inefficient, and though the market there has been enlarged and reconstructed, additional market accommodation is absolutely necessary. One wholesale market is calculated to meet the requirements of the trade and the interests of the public, and it should be at the waterside. There should be ample and sufficient approaches from all parts of the metropolis to the site of any wholesale fish market. Should the Court concur in the opinion that the market should be at the waterside, two sites are suggested for consideration—one at Blackfriars-bridge, and the other by the addition of the present Custom House to the site of Billingsgate. The St. Katharine Docks site is not recommended. If the Court should be of opinion that an inland market for railway-borne fish is also required, a site in Farringdon-road, north of Charterhouse-street, or the site of the present Farringdon Market, is suggested. There should be a wholesale, semi-wholesale, and retail market, all under one roof, with no restrictions as to the hours of business, and an official salesman of fish should be appointed. A numerously attended meeting was recently held at Cannon-street Wharf, under the presidency of Mr. Daniel Tallerman, to consider a scheme for the more speedy transmission of fish by rail to Billingsgate Market. The following resolution was unanimously adopted :—" That this meeting is of opinion that the Cannon-street Wharf, connected as it is with the South-Eastern Railway, and through that with the other railway systems, presents evident facilities for the delivery of land-borne fish into Billingsgate by river ; and the subject is worthy of consideration by the Corporation of London."

PAROTITIS AS A COMPLICATION OF OVARIOTOMY.

DR. MÖBICKE, in a communication to the *Zeitschrift für Geburtshülfe und Gynäkologie*, narrates five cases in which inflammation of the parotid gland followed ovariotomy, and in four of them went on to suppuration. He refers to the well-known connexion between inflammation of the testis and of the parotid gland, and quotes cases from other authors in which affections of the female genitals—swelling of the labia, vulvo-vaginal catarrh, swelling and pain in the breasts, swelling and pain of the ovary—came on in the course of mumps. He thinks these instances point to a connexion between the parotid gland and the ovary, similar to that which exists between the parotid gland and the testicle. In support of this view he further states that he has never seen parotitis follow any other operation on the female genitals, although the operations of this kind (which he has done far exceed in number his ovariotomies. In one of his cases there was the possible source of fallacy, that some children suffering from mumps were in the hospital at the time, and a nurse caught

the disease. But the ovariotomy case was kept separate from the other patients, had her special nurse, and no other patients in the hospital caught the disease. The criticism, that parotitis is not uncommon in the course of the acute infectious diseases (typhus, scarlatina, etc.), and in pyæmia, he anticipates by saying that his patients were not suffering from any of these diseases; nor was the inflammation so acute or so dangerous as is the pyæmic form. In time of occurrence and in frequency it closely resembled the orchitis which complicates mumps. The parotitis came on five times out of 200 cases of ovariotomy, and began from the third to the seventh day after the operation. Orchitis in mumps is said to occur once in sixty cases, and to come on, as a rule, about the sixth day.

THE SOCIAL SCIENCE CONGRESS.

THE following is a list of Presidents for the Social Science Congress, to be held in Dublin, October 3 to 8, 1881 :— President of the Association—Lord O'Hagan, Lord Chancellor of Ireland ; Jurisprudence—J. T. Ball, ex-Lord Chancellor of Ireland ; Education—Sir Patrick Joseph Keenan, Resident Commissioner of National Education ; Health—Charles Cameron, M.D., M.P. for Glasgow ; Economy and Trade— Mr. Goldwin Smith ; Art—Viscount Powerscourt. Dr. Mouat, late Inspector-General of Prisons in India, will be the Chairman of the Repression of Crime Section.

UNCERTIFIED DEATHS IN THE PARISH OF ST. MARY, NEWINGTON.

REFERRING to the subject of uncertified deaths, Dr. W. T. Iliff, the Medical Officer of Health for the parish of St. Mary, Newington, in his report for the year 1879, remarks that during that period, out of a total of 2664 deaths, there were no less than 79 uncertified, or nearly one in every 34. Of this number 49 died under five years of age (39 not arriving at one year), and 17 beyond sixty. The assumed causes of death were, on the whole, natural, though one, "disease of the throat " at the age of forty, and another, "inflammation of the bowels" at the age of fifty-nine, would certainly appear to have required some investigation. So far as Dr. Iliff could ascertain, every case was reported to the coroner's officer, and many through him to the coroner, who is the authority legally appointed to take cognisance of suspicious deaths; and as this system of investigation, on the whole, seems to work well, the proposition to make the medical officer of health responsible for the inquiries, must, Dr. Iliff thinks, clash with the coroner's duties if thoroughly performed. But he believes the best plan would be to select the coroner's officer from a class of better educated men, and to provide that *every* case of uncertified death after due inquiry should be reported to the coroner, and his certificate alone should be the registrar's authority for registering the death. Further, it should be a misdemeanour, punishable by law, to bury any corpse without the production of the registrar's certificate, as at present a large number are so buried.

TRANSMISSION OF TUBERCULOSIS BY VACCINE.

AT the meeting of the Academy of Sciences on August 1, M. Toussaint communicated some important results of his investigations into the microbial nature of tuberculosis. He had already succeeded, as Klebs and Cohnheim have, in cultivating these organisms, and had found that two drops of the liquid of the fourth artificial cultivation, inoculated into pigs, rendered them speedily and completely tuberculous. He then vaccinated a cow in an advanced stage of tuberculosis with lymph absolutely pure. The vesicles progressed normally, and with the lymph obtained from them he vaccinated different animals, all of whom subsequently became tuberculous. The significance of these experiments can scarcely be overrated, for though a judicious vaccinator would not use lymph taken from a child who exhibited already evidence of the disease, the chances of cows in whom spontaneous vaccinia may appear, and whose lymph would at the present time be eagerly sought after, being, like so many of their species, tuberculous, are great; and it would seem, in consequence, that the dangers of animal vaccination may be greater than those of human, which are supposed to be avoided by having recourse to the cow. As many who fully believe in the existence] of a tuberculous microbion have failed in their attempt to cultivate it, we shall at the earliest opportunity give the details of M. Toussaint's methods.

THE ROYAL EDINBURGH ASYLUM FOR THE INSANE.

THE annual report of the Royal Edinburgh Asylum for the Insane, for the year 1880, appears to foreshadow a change in the constitution of that institution. It seems to have occurred to the managers that it is scarcely just to ask the friends of the wealthier inmates to contribute towards the support of the pauper patients by paying large fees, and thereby relieving the parochial rates; and Dr. T. S. Clouston, the Physician-Superintendent, calls attention to the fact that the number of pauper patients admitted during the past year was greater than ever before, and has nearly stopped the admission of private patients at the low rates of board, by taking up all the space that used to be available for such cases. A suggestion has been thrown out by one of the visiting Commissioners that an economical auxiliary asylum should be built close by for incurables, and this suggestion Dr. Clouston endorses. The general history of the institution presents no feature of novelty; it records the fact that each year sees a larger number of patients under treatment than during the one preceding, the total number in 1880 having been 1168, or thirty-three in excess of the total of 1879. Since his last report Dr. Clouston has paid a visit to America, and taken the opportunity of visiting some of the very newest asylums in the United States. He remarks that it will be satisfactory to the friends of the Royal Edinburgh Asylum to learn that recent improvements in that institution bring it fully abreast of the most recent ideas of construction in modern hospitals for the insane; whilst, with regard to the question of expense, it is a great deal more economical than the American institutions.

THE NATURE OF SNAKE-POISONS.

M. GAUTIER read before the Academy of Medicine, at the séance of July 26 last, an account of his researches into the nature of snake-poisons, especially that of the cobra (Naja tripudians). He has succeeded in isolating them, and finds them to have nothing in common with ferments, but to be chemical bodies of definite composition and considerable stability, acting with an energy proportioned to the quantity employed; and but slightly impaired by subjection to a temperature of 125° C. (258° Fahr.) for several hours. Having dissolved a milligramme of the poison in several drops of water, he inoculated rabbits and birds, who invariably died in a few minutes, the heart remaining in systole and muscular contractility being abolished. He then employed like doses, but mixed with various reputed alexipharmics, for half an hour to an hour before injection. Perchloride of iron, and essential oils of thyme, mint, etc., he found to be quite inert. Tannin, nitrate of silver, and liquid ammonia delayed but did not avert the fatal termination. The alkaline carbonates were also useless. But—and here lies the great interest of his experiments—although the poison seems to be of the nature of an alkaloid, it has in its crude state an acid

reaction, and a quantity of caustic potash or soda just sufficient to neutralise this acidity rendered it absolutely inert. He also verified the fact that the poison may be taken into the digestive canal with impunity. Subsequent neutralisation of the alkali with an acid did not restore the energy of the poison, which would seem to point to decomposition rather than mere neutralisation by the potash. He failed to prevent death by subcutaneous injection of alkaline solutions, but he has certainly opened a new path for further experiment which may lead to great results.

ON THE INDIAN MEDICAL SERVICE.

(From an Indian Correspondent.)

THE new scale of Pension Rules promulgated with the dispatch of Her Majesty's Secretary of State for India, dated April 14, 1881, will be hailed by the members, both present and future, of Her Majesty's Indian Medical Service. The pensionary scale now (and retrospective from January 1, 1881) is, after seventeen years' service, with an allowance of furlough of one year and eight months, £292 a year, instead of (after the same, and with the same amount of leave) £290. The next rate gives, after twenty years' service, with an allowance of furlough of two years, £365; according to the old rules, there was no separate pension for this length of service, but after twenty-one years' service, with an allowance of two years' furlough, the pension was £292, and the rate of £365 a year was not reached till after twenty-four years' service. This term of service is dropped as to rates of pension; but after twenty-five years' service, with an allowance of furlough of three years, the pension is now £500 a year. According to the old Rules, after twenty-seven years' service, with three years' furlough, a pension of £456 a year was granted; and, after thirty years' service, with four years of furlough, a pension of £550; while, according to the new scale, the intermediate rate of pension is dropped, and the pension for thirty years' service, with four years of furlough, is raised to £700 a year. For administrative medical officers, provided they serve for five years in their respective grades, with an allowance of leave, six months on medical certificate, or four months on private affairs, there are pensions (extra pensions) of £350 and £250 a year respectively for Surgeons-General and Deputy Surgeons-General.

The above scale is a fairly liberal one, but not too liberal, taking into count the pension scales of the sister service, the members of which may have a term of home service, while their brethren of the Indian Service have to serve the whole time in India. There are some other grievances not yet removed, which may be mentioned here in the hope that they also will ere long be things of the past. I allude, in the first place, to the scale of what is called "Unemployed pay." This is really an anomaly when the officers are actually employed; and there seems to be no reason why medical officers of the Indian Service, whilst employed, but without appointments, should receive less pay than in the British Service. But if an officer is bond fide unemployed it would then be quite a different matter. This is a hardship which specially affects the junior members of the Service, who for three and four years, and even longer, receive the "unemployed pay," which under five years' service is only 286 rs. and 10 annas. If the officer has passed the lower standard examination in Hindostani, he should at once draw his full pay, in whatever capacity he is employed. Without an appointment, as it is, he has to run the chance of being moved about from place to place, and this, though he travels at the "public expense," costs him no small portion of his small pay, especially if he be married. Another point to which it is desirable to invite attention is the matter of "travelling expenses." The members of the British Medical Service, when travelling on duty or proceeding on or returning from sick leave, do so at the public expense, while those of the Indian Service are at a disadvantage in this respect: they have either to travel at their own expense, or they pay for second-class and travel first-class, which generally saves them half the railway fare; but if the travelling be by road, which is more generally the case, and which is the more expensive mode of the two, they have to pay all the costs themselves.

It would be a good thing if the Indian Medical Service were divided into a civil and a military department, promotions to the administrative grades for the military being from among officers who have elected to serve and have served in a military capacity, and similarly for those in the civil branch or department. For the Indian Military Medical Service there should be none of the "unification" or departmentalisation which has gone such a long way to render the Queen's service unpopular. In the opinion of most competent critics the experiment of that system has proved a signal failure, and nobody but its authors and a few advocates expected it to be otherwise. The present condition of the medical officers is unsatisfactory, as they are in a destitute condition, having no regiments, no messes, no home; and being, or liable to be, knocked about from pillar to post, and back again from post to pillar, there is nothing to induce them to think well of the Service. The combatant officers, and the men too, dislike the arrangement, by which they have no fixed doctor of their own. New men are told off and changed so frequently that there is no such thing as their having "a family attendant"; this being so, the medical man can know little of the previous histories of cases, and by being only "attached" until an unknown day, he cannot be expected to take anything like deep interest in everybody belonging to the regiment, nor the latter in him, as would have been the case had the medical officers formed part and parcel of regiments.

FROM ABROAD.

PRIZES AND PRIZE-QUESTIONS AT THE ACADÉMIE DE MÉDECINE.

AT the public annual meeting of the Académie de Médecine, held August 2 (*Union Médicale*, August 4), Dr. Bergeron, the Annual Secretary, read his report upon the prizes that have been decreed. This is an interesting but lengthy document, occupying more than twenty pages of the *Bulletin*, in which the reasons that have actuated the various committees of the prizes in making their awards are set forth; but our space will only allow of our enumerating the bare results. 1. The Academy prize of 1000 fr. (subject, the Reciprocal Influence of Diseases of the Heart and those of the Liver) has been adjudged to M. Rendu, *professeur agrégé* of the Faculté and Physician of the Tenon Hospital. 2. The Civrieux prize of 1500 fr. (the Influence exerted by the Nervous System in Diseases of the Heart) is accorded to Dr. Liégeois, a physician of Bainville-aux-Saules in the Vosges. Speaking of the essays sent in in competition for this prize, Prof. Peter, the reporter of the committee, says—"I cannot avoid making the remark that at least two out of the three essays sent in demonstrate that the young medical generation in France, as everywhere else, is carried away by an irresistible current—the current of physiologism. Three experiments are made on the same subject, with three discordant results, and the young physiologist hastens to apply the result of one of the experiments to the pathological case upon which he is engaged. It speaks for itself that he chooses the experimental result which tallies best with his personal theories. And this is called young medicine, physiological and pathogenic medicine, as opposed to the old medicine of observation, now regarded as obsolete and empirical!" 3. The Capuron prize (the Influence of Coxofemoral Dislocation on the Conformation of the Pelvis) was not adjudged, an "encouragement" of 500 fr. being, however, awarded to Dr. Verrier, of Paris, for his essay on the subject. 4. The Barbier prize of 7000 fr. for the discovery of a Cure of Diseases usually regarded as Incurable (hydrophobia, cancer, epilepsy, scrofula, typhus, cholera, etc.) is of course unawarded; but "encouragements" have been decreed for four essays which seem to bear no relation

whatever to the prize-subject.—2000 fr. are given to Surgeon-Major Delorme for a memoir on "Ligature of Arteries of the Palm"; 1000 fr. to Dr. Masse, of Bordeaux, for his work, "The Influence of the Attitude of the Limbs on their Articulations"; 1000 fr. to Dr. Christian Smith, of Brussels, for his clinical manual on Affections of the Urinary Organs; and 1000 fr. to Dr. Burow, medical naval officer of the first class, for his work "On the Fever termed Inflammatory Bilious of Guiana." 5. For the Godard prize of 1500 fr., for the best work on Internal Pathology, no less than fifteen works were sent in, most of which, in the opinion of the committee, were characterised by sufficient originality or indicated sufficient scientific progress to deserve the prize. Some of them, however, were of sufficient interest to entitle them to a "recompense." Therefore, 600 fr. were awarded to Dr. Grasset, of Montpellier, for his works on the Localisations of Cerebral Diseases and Diseases of the Nervous System; 400 fr. to Dr. Damaschino, *professeur agrégé* of the Faculty, for his Diseases of the Digestive Organs; 250 fr. to Dr. Marvaud, Physician to the Bey's Hospital, Algiers, for his Thermometrical and Clinical Observations on the principal forms of Fever observed in the military hospitals of Algeria; and 250 fr. to Drs. Brissaud and Josias, of Paris, on Scrofulous Gummata and their Tubercular Nature. 6. The Desportes prize of 2000 fr., for the best work on Practical Therapeutics, is adjudged to Prof. Fonssagrives, of Montpellier, for his book entitled "A Treatise on Applied Therapeutics." 7. The Buignet annual prize of 1500 fr., offered for the best printed or manuscript work on the Applications of Physics or Chemistry to Medical Science, is given to Drs. Beauregard and Galippe for their Guide to the Student and Practitioner in Micrography. A "very honourable mention" is also decreed to Dr. Budal for his Influence of the Diameter of the Pupil and of the Diffusion Circles on the Acuity of Vision; and an "honourable mention" to Dr. Chapuis for his work on the Influence of Fatty Bodies on the Absorption of Arsenic. 8. The Falret prize of 1500 fr. (Insanity designated by the names Circular Insanity, Insanity of Double or Alternating Forms) is divided between Dr. Ritti, Physician to the Charenton, and Dr. Mordret, Medical Superintendent of the Asile de la Surthe at Mans. 9. The Huguier prize of 2000 fr., for the best printed or manuscript work on the Diseases of Women, and especially their Surgical Treatment, is awarded to Dr. Petit, the Assistant Librarian of the Académie de Médecine.

The prize questions for 1882 announced are as follow:—
1. The Academy prize of 1000 fr., "Generalised Arterial Atheroma, and its Influence on the Nutrition of Organs." 2. The Portal prize of 2000 fr., "The Lymphatic System in the Pathological Point of View." 3. The Civrieux prize of 2000 fr., "The Causes of Locomotor Ataxy." 4. The Capuron prize of 2000 fr., "The Normal and Pathological Conditions of the Lochia." 5. The Barbier prize of 4000 fr. for the discovery of a Cure of Diseases usually reputed as Incurable. 6. The Godard prize of 1500 fr. for the best work on Internal Pathology. 7. The Desportes prize of 2000 fr. for the best work on Practical Medical Therapeutics. 8. The Buignet prize of 1500 fr. will be given for the best printed or manuscript work on the Applications of Physics or Chemistry to Medical Science. 9. The Orfila prize of 4000 fr., "Veratrine, Sabadilline, Black Hellebore, and White Varaire." 10. The Itard triennial prize of 3000 fr. for the best work or memoir on Practical Medicine or Applied Therapeutics. 11. The Falret prize of 1500 fr., "Vertigo with Delirium." 12. The Saint Lager prize of 1500 fr. for the Experimental Production of Bronchocele by the administration to animals of substances extracted from the waters of localities in which goître prevails endemically. 13. M. and Madame Victor St. Paul have offered a sum of 25,000 fr. as a prize to be decreed to the person who discovers a Remedy for Diphtheria, the sovereign efficacy of which is acknowledged by the Academy. In the meantime, the interest of this sum is to be given biennially to persons whose works and researches on diphtheria may seem to the Academy to merit such recompense. 14. The prize of 1000 fr., in relation to the hygiene of infancy, "Weaning and its comparative investigation in different regions of France." All essays or works, written in French or Latin, and accompanied by a sealed envelope, containing the authors' names and addresses, must be sent to the Academy before July 1, 1882.

THE INOCULATION OF TUBERCLE.

In a paper read at the Académie de Médecine, Drs. Krishaber and Dieulafoy (*Gazette Hebdomadaire*, August 26), after endeavouring to explain some of the causes of the discrepancies in the results reported by different observers, state that the series of experiments which they have undertaken have been performed on the monkey as being the animal which nearest approaches to man, and which, like him, is also liable to attacks of spontaneous tuberculosis. But public opinion on this last point has been somewhat exaggerated, for their inquiries at the various zoological gardens of Europe and at private aperies have convinced the authors that the proportion of monkeys so attacked is not considerable, and that much depends upon the condition of life which they lead.

The investigations of MM. Dieulafoy and Krishaber have been made on 40 monkeys, 16 of these having been inoculated and 24 kept for purposes of comparison. The 16 inoculated monkeys were divided into four groups, and of the 3 constituting the first group 1 died, having caseous glands, and the other 2 survived, 1 of them having resisted two other inoculations. The 13 other monkeys, distributed into three other groups (with the exception of 2 who died accidentally immediately after the inoculation), all died from tuberculosis in a lapse of time varying from 34 to 218 days. The inoculations were made with different tubercular products—grey granulations, pulmonary parenchyma infiltrated with grey tubercle, and caseous deposits. The most rapid results were obtained by means of grey granulations: of 4 animals inoculated at the same time, 3 died the same day. To sum up, of the 16 inoculated monkeys (2 of which cannot be counted, having died accidentally), 12 died tuberculous, constituting a proportion of 86 per cent., while of the 24 non-inoculated animals, 5 only died of spontaneous tuberculosis, that is 21 per cent. From these experiments the authors of the paper believe that they are justified in concluding:—1. Tubercle taken from man and inoculated on monkeys has caused the death of the animals experimented upon at the rate of about 9 out of 10, exhibiting lesions analogous to those of the human species. 2. The degree of nocuity of the inoculations has varied according to the matter employed in the experiments, tubercular granulations proving most rapidly transmissible, while the pulmonary parenchyma was less infectant. 3. Two of the monkeys were refractory to inoculation, which was repeated several times on one of them. 4. Inoculated tubercle has proved four times more fatal to monkeys than spontaneous tubercle. The communication is referred to a committee to report upon, and its authors are also about to communicate to the Academy the results of their inoculations of non-tubercular matters.

OBSTETRICAL INSTRUCTION AT VIENNA.—Dr. Dixon, in a letter to the *Boston Med. Jour.* for June 30, describing the great value of the obstetrical teaching for advanced students at the Vienna General Hospital, says that Prof. Braun's assistant, Dr. Powlik, undertakes what is called a "touch" course, that lasts a month, during which, for an additional fee of twenty-two dollars, each student has the opportunity of examining four women a day. First, a thorough external examination of the abdomen is made by palpation and auscultation, the student reporting upon the position of the child or the presence of twins, his diagnosis being subjected to the criticism of Dr. Powlik and of three other students. Especial stress is laid upon making out the position by grasping the child's neck between the thumb and fingers of the right hand, and by deep pressure (not sufficient to be at all painful to the woman) distinctly feeling the chin of the child, which, by approximating the thumb and fingers underneath the neck, can be easily grasped, and in most cases readily moved from side to side. This point, I think, has never been described by any writer. The diagnosis is then confirmed by an examination per vaginam, the women, most of whom are in their eighth or ninth month, being first examined by Dr. Powlik. "If this 'touch' course should be attempted to any extent at our lying-in hospitals," Dr. Dixon adds, "the probable result would be a depopulation of the hospitals in a very short time, as in our cities there are many places where women can be confined with good care, while at Vienna the General Hospital is about the only place for them."

On Cancer, its Allies, and other Tumours, with special reference to their Medical and Surgical Treatment. By F. ALBERT PURCELL, M.D., M.R.C.S. London: J. and A. Churchill. 1881. Pp. 311.

WE shall probably best criticise this work by allowing it to speak for itself; the reader will then be able to gather whether he is likely to discover in it a particularly pure specimen of the Queen's English, or any startling novelties in the direction of pathology or therapeutics. We will accordingly content ourselves with two or three quotations, in which we have accurately followed not only the words, but the punctuation of the author.

"With implicit faith in the statement coming from such a man as Professor Clay, without prejudiced scepticism and with earnest determination to test the remedy, impressed, then, with these views, fortified with a consciousness of the clinical investigation, which was made during a period of twelve months by Professor Clay, we placed all the cases the most suitable for the treatment on to the Chian turpentine, keeping each specimen of the drug supplied us (for we had many sent to us from all sides) distinctly labelled, and the one allotted to the case selected for its exhibition was duly noted, so that if a relief of the disease or an approaching tendency to cure was reported, we were in a position to record which and from whence the specimen came."

We would commend this sentence to the Board School authorities as a test of the capabilities of their *alumni* in the act of parsing. But take another—

"Sarcoma may be defined to be a tumour of connective tissue origin, formed generally of embryonic tissue and without alveolar structure, composed of round, or fusiform, or giant cells, and these are packed in a more or less abundant basis; the vessels are often mere fissures between the cells, and the cells increase in number by division. The new tissue often traversed by fibrous tissue, and not uncommonly exhibiting a delicate reticulated structure, or of fusiform or spindle cells, arranged in the form of trabeculæ, which interlace, join, and cross each other at various angles. Sometimes, mixed with these two forms, there occur stellate cells in a viscid or hyaline basis, or hyaline cartilage may be found forming either a kind of framework through the growth or perhaps a large portion of its bulk."

Surely, however, it is scarcely necessary to multiply examples; and when it is added that the author recommends for the hardening of tumours "a solution of chromic acid (20 per cent.)," enough will have been said to enable the reader to form a judgment as to whether Dr. Purcell is justified in the hope he thus expresses in his preface—

"The results of my experience are here recorded; and the views that I have propounded, and those that I have adopted from other authors, may, I hope, contribute in some measure to the insight of so distressing a malady."

Dysmenorrhœa, its Pathology and Treatment. By HEYWOOD SMITH, M.A., M.D. Oxon., Physician to the Hospital for Women and to the British Lying-in Hospital; author of "Practical Gynæcology." London: J. and A. Churchill. 1881.

WE cannot think that the author has in this book done himself justice. One who has been for some years a chief member of the staff of a large special hospital, the largest of its kind in this country, could not fail, if he were only to carefully and faithfully record his experience, to produce a work which would demand and receive attentive study from the profession. But Dr. Heywood Smith appears to have, for some reason, imposed upon himself a limit of space which prevents him from treating his subject in any but a most bald and brief manner. We constantly, when we think we are coming to some interesting information, are told that to give it would extend the work beyond its original scope. The author simply expounds his ideas upon the different parts of his subject in a general, *ex cathedrâ* manner, much in the style of a lecturer addressing junior students or nurses. The latter comparison is the more appropriate, for the book abounds with references to the social aspects of the subject, which, of course, are of great interest to women, but have no bearing on the scientific side of the questions. There is nowhere any summary of experience or statement of reasons; the author gives his opinion, and that is all.

There are some features of the book which, to our thinking, are very objectionable. One is, the excessive activity of the local treatment recommended. There is scarcely a disease for which the knife, caustic, tent, leeches, or pessary is not advised. In some instances we believe that if the patients had full knowledge, before the treatment was begun, of its risk, uncertainty, and disagreeable character, they would deliberately prefer to put up with their malady. One of the author's operations is new, viz., cutting through the utero-sacral ligaments for retroflexion. He performed it on January 20 of this year; but the result is not stated in this book, nor have we seen it elsewhere. We fail to see what good this operation could effect; but if the patient was cured, theoretical criticism must be silent. Therefore, we hope the author will not fail to publish a full account of the case, as soon as he has watched the patient long enough to know the result.

Another point is the very great influence which the author constantly ascribes to the sexual feelings, and the acts resulting therefrom. He goes so far as to say (page 7) that "the sexual sensations and functions constitute that for which they" (the sexual organs), "and indeed *the whole woman*, are formed . . . . the most important factor in the entire range of causation of such diseases" (the italics are ours). Of this teaching we will only say, that we can scarcely conceive anything which would more surely lower our profession in the estimation of the public, diminish its usefulness, and repel the best class of minds from its ranks, than for our young men to be sent into practice with such notions as these in their heads. We cannot believe that the author is alive to the full meaning of these sentences. We may mention that he recommends clitoridectomy. "Clitoridectomy, though from ill-judged performance avoided by most gynæcologists, affords in some cases the only prospect of cure, but that it does produce such an effect, I and others have sufficient testimony" (page 32). We had thought the contrary was the generally received opinion. If Dr. Heywood Smith would publish the facts which lead him to think as he does, he would do more good than by writing about the sexual functions in a way more dogmatic than correct.

There is one point upon which the author lays more stress than is usual, and in which we quite agree with him, and that is, the importance of constipation as a cause of dysmenorrhœa.

Although we cannot call this a good book, still it is an improvement upon "Practical Gynæcology."

MUZZLING DOGS IN RELATION TO HYDROPHOBIA.— In Italy, where the muzzling of dogs is continuous, the mean number of deaths from hydrophobia occurring annually is 19. In 1879 there was the exceptionally large number of 30 deaths. But what are 30 deaths from hydrophobia for a whole kingdom, when in a single city like Paris, where muzzling does not exist, there were as many as 80 deaths from this cause in 1879?—*Lyon Méd.*, August 21.

RESORCINE belongs to the class of bodies called *phenols*, to which carbolic acid belongs. In chemical composition they resemble alcohols. It was originally obtained by fusing certain resins, as gum ammoniacum or galbanum, with caustic potash, extracting it from the fused mass by acetifying with sulphuric acid and shaking with ether, and then purifying by distillation. It crystallises in colourless plates or columns, and dissolves readily in water, alcohol, or ether. It is not poisonous in moderate doses, and from twenty-five to thirty grains are required to produce marked effects. It has been found to reduce the temperature in febrile affections, but its effect is of short duration, and unpleasant after-effects have been noticed. Andeer finds that it possesses the power of stopping decay, and 1 per cent. of chemically pure resorcine will stop the development of fungi and mould. In every degree of concentration it coagulates albumen, and precipitates it from solution, on which account it may be used as a caustic to remove unhealthy tissue. In crystals it cauterises as powerfully as lunar caustic. Dr. Koller prophesies a great future for resorcine, which, he says, will be the disinfectant and antiseptic of the physician, the chemist, and the druggist. It is, however, too powerful a reagent to be taken internally in an unlimited amount.—*Phil. Med. Times.*

THE RYDE ADDRESSES AND HOMŒOPATHY.

LETTER FROM DR. J. H. CLARKE.

[To the Editor of the Medical Times and Gazette.]

SIR,—Some time ago you were kind enough to publish a letter of mine, correcting some inaccuracies in one of your leading articles. I now ask you to repeat the favour. Speaking of Dr. Bristowe's address, in your leader on Mr. Hutchinson's, in your last issue, you say he (Dr. Bristowe) "mercilessly exposes the follies and weaknesses of homœopathy, and denounces it as a palpable imposture." This seems to me a generalisation very unfair both to Dr. Bristowe and to homœopathy. I have read the address with care and delight—one can enjoy a worthy opponent who tries to be fair,—and I find in it no want of mercy, and nothing that can be construed into a "denunciation of homœopathy as a palpable imposture." Dr. Bristowe is mistaken on many points of fact. He gives a different account of the origin of Hahnemann's idea from Mr. Hutchinson's,—and neither account is correct. But at any rate he does his best to be fair. He allows there is some truth in the idea, as also does Mr. Hutchinson. The denunciations, in both addresses, of Hahnemann's pathology apply as much to the then orthodox pathology as to his, and not at all to that of the homœopathists of the present day. Happily, his system of practice is based on more enduring ground than his pathology.

I cannot think you have been more successful in generalising fairly Mr. Hutchinson's remarks on this head than you have Dr. Bristowe's.

With regard to your concluding quotation from Sir B. Brodie, I have an interesting comment. In my possession is a letter written by that surgeon to a late eminent and well-known homœopathist about a case regarding which they had been in consultation. No difficulty arose, and the patient was benefited. Perhaps had Sir Benjamin been living now, he would be as little inclined to endorse the words you quote as he would to sign again a memorial against special hospitals.

If your remarks had occurred in a less scrupulous journal I should not have noticed them, but believing you are not of those who would condemn a prisoner without hearing his defence, I have ventured to trouble you a second time.

I am, &c.,   JOHN H. CLARKE, M.D.
15, St. George's-terrace, Gloucester-road, S.W., August 29.

[Our correspondent is clearly mistaken on certain points. We deny the existence of any law of similars. It may be possible that a certain drug may cure a certain disease, and that the same drug may, when given to a healthy individual, produce certain symptoms not unlike those which have been produced by disease. But these are clearly instances far too few on which to found any induction. Listening to Dr. Bristowe and Mr. Hutchinson, we distinctly understood them to speak on behalf of certain qualified practitioners who were also homœopaths; but in no sense to contend for the truth of homœopathy. —ED. Med. Times and Gas.]

ROYAL COLLEGE OF SURGEONS.—The Library and Museum of this institution were closed on Wednesday last, for the annual cleaning and re-arrangement, and will not be re-opened till Monday, October 3.

LARGE CALCULUS.—Dr. Morton exhibited to the Philadelphia Academy of Surgery a calculus weighing four ounces and a half, and measuring six inches and a half in circumference, which he had removed by a transverse vaginal incision from the bladder of a lady seventy-nine years of age. She had presented symptoms of vesical disease for forty years, but had never allowed an examination to be made. The stone was so large that it could not be turned in the bladder. After its removal, silver sutures were introduced, and the patient made a rapid recovery.—*Phil. Med. Times*, June 18.

REPORTS OF SOCIETIES.

THE OBSTETRICAL SOCIETY OF LONDON.

WEDNESDAY, JULY 6.

Dr. MATTHEWS DUNCAN, President, in the Chair.

Dr. FANCOURT BARNES showed an instrument designed by Dr. C. Duncan, of Rome, to measure the amount of flexion existing in anteflexion or retroflexion of the uterus.

Dr. POPE showed an anencephalous fœtus. It was the first of twins, and an arm and funis presented.

Dr. GODSON showed for Dr. Cronk two specimens.—1. A malformed heart with transposition of great vessels; 2. Cystic degeneration of umbilical cord, which measured five inches in its greatest circumference. Dr. Godson showed also, for Mr. W. A. Thomson, a pocket case of instruments in the form of a cigar-case, made by Messrs. Arnold.

A report by Drs. Galabin, J. Williams, and Cleveland was read on a specimen shown by Dr. Cleveland at the May meeting. The fleshy substance had a central canal and a smooth orifice like the uterus, and was two inches and a half long. The whole of its structure was that of uterine decidua. The committee considered that it was the entire decidua from the unimpregnated side of a double uterus, and thought it most probable that the body only was double, the cervix single.

Dr. CARTER asked whether there had been an opportunity of verifying the condition of the uterus.

Dr. GALABIN understood that Dr. Cleveland hoped to do so at a future time.

NON-ENCAPSULED FIBROIDS RESEMBLING RETAINED PLACENTA.

Dr. JAMES BRAITHWAITE read a paper on non-encapsuled fibroids resembling retained placenta. Two cases were related. In the first, unexpected hæmorrhage occurred ten days after delivery, and a ragged mass was felt within the uterus, which at first seemed to resemble placenta, but was tough in its deeper parts, and an integral part of the uterine wall. A great part was detached from the uterine wall, and removed in portions by scissors. Dr. Galabin reported on the growth that it showed no evidence of cancer, but was highly nucleated, and contained large muscular fibres, resembling the tissue sometimes seen in soft, rapidly growing fibres. The patient did well. In the second case, four days after an abortion at three months, hæmorrhage occurred, and a ragged mass was felt within the uterus. The os was dilated with tents, and the growth removed by seizing a portion at a time, and crushing it with strong forceps. On microscopic examination it was found to consist of very loose fibroid tissue.

Dr. EDIS had met with a similar case, in which, after a miscarriage at the fourth month, a mass, at first suspected to be placenta, turned out to be a submucous fibroid, encapsuled in the tissue of the uterus.

Dr. HERMAN mentioned a case which had been under his care at the London Hospital, in which there was a large abdominal tumour, shown by autopsy to be malignant. The uterine cavity was dilated, and contained a growth of loose stringy texture. The patient at first thought herself pregnant, and a medical man, who was sent for, took the case for one of placenta prævia.

Dr. ROPER gave further details as to a patient who was aged twenty-eight, married six years, and who believed herself pregnant for the first time. The history was like that of pregnancy, but flooding came on at the seventh month. The case was supposed to be one of placenta prævia, and Dr. Roper was summoned in the middle of the night. The os uteri admitted two fingers, and a mass like placenta could be felt. There was a loud bruit in each iliac region. Labour did not come on. Many months later the patient died rather suddenly, and at the autopsy the case was found to be one of medullary cancer, which seemed to have commenced outside the uterus.

Dr. FANCOURT BARNES had distinctly heard the sound called placental souffle in Dr. Roper's case. He should like to hear some explanation of these sounds.

Dr. HEYWOOD SMITH did not consider that the intra-uterine growths described quite answered to the ordinary characteristics of fibroids, especially as regarded their regularity of surface and tendency to break down. Having regard to Dr. Galabin's report, he thought that they approximated rather to a malignant character.

Dr. GALABIN thought that there was nothing actually malignant in the specimen he examined for Dr. Braithwaite. He thought the growth might possibly recur, because the tissue was so highly nucleated. It contained also large thin-walled vascular spaces.

A CASE OF PREGNANCY COMPLICATED BY CANCER OF THE CERVIX UTERI, FOLLOWED BY PYÆMIA, ASSOCIATED WITH SYMPTOMS SIMULATING DIPHTHERIA.

Dr. GALABIN related a case of pregnancy complicated by cancer of the cervix uteri, followed by pyæmia associated with symptoms simulating diphtheria. The author saw the patient, aged thirty-four, the mother of five children, in consultation with Dr. R. U. Wallace. She was then nearly six months pregnant, and the whole circuit of the os was involved in firm cancerous growth. There was a laceration, however, on the left side, apparently antecedent to the cancer, which seemed to reach the outer limit of the growth. The author was at first inclined to recommend Cæsarian section at the seventh month, but the patient refused her consent to this. Eventually she came into Guy's Hospital for the induction of labour. Dr. Braxton Hicks examined her, and advised the trial of Barnes' bags to dilate the cervix. These were employed after labour had been started at six and a half months' pregnancy by means of an elastic bougie. Dilatation of the os was effected up to a little more than two inches laterally, but the os remained of a horseshoe shape. The hand could not be introduced for version. Perforation and cephalotripsy were performed, but the flattened head did not readily enter the cervix. It was extracted, however, by gradually stretching it out by means of Barnes' craniotomy forceps. The operation occupied altogether less than an hour. For some days after delivery pulse and temperature were extremely variable, ranging from a normal value up to a somewhat high level. On the fifth day the throat became inflamed, and on the tenth an adherent membrane was seen upon the pharynx, while at the same time some albumen appeared in the urine. Dr. F. Taylor saw the patient, and diagnosed the condition as being almost certainly diphtheria. She died on the eighteenth day. At the autopsy, pus was found in the veins near the cervix, and pyæmic abscesses in the lungs. The membrane on the pharynx contained a mycelium fungus; and Dr. Goodhart, who made the examination, considered it to be merely a thrush. The author was rather inclined to consider that it was of a pseudo-diphtheritic character, secondary to the pyæmia, and analogous to the membrane seen upon the pharynx in some epidemics of virulent puerperal septicæmia. Microscopic sections were shown of the membrane in situ, of the growth in the cervix, and of the kidneys, which showed some tubal nephritis, but no granular degeneration.

Dr. HERMAN expressed his opinion that the therapeutic means in these cases which offered the greatest hope of benefit to the mother, were (1) the induction of abortion at the earliest possible period, and (2) the removal of as much of the diseased tissues as could safely be cut or burnt away.

Dr. ROPER said that when such a case came under notice only at the seventh or eighth month of pregnancy, the only alternative was between delivery per vias naturales after induction of labour, and Cæsarian section. But in the early months he believed that the production of abortion was the proper treatment.

Dr. GODSON mentioned a case which occurred at the City of London Lying-in Hospital during a severe endemic of puerperal fever, in which the symptoms were almost identical with those of Dr. Galabin's patient. She was almost the only woman who recovered,—which tended strongly to prove that the disease was septic, and not the thrush of a moribund woman, spoken of by Dr. Goodhart.

Dr. EDIS thought the question very important, whether the whole circuit of the cervix was involved in cancer. In a case in which about two-thirds of the cervix were involved, he had delivered a living child by forceps, but the mother ultimately died from pyæmia. If the whole circumference were involved in a patient at full term, he thought Cæsarian section the best treatment.

Dr. GALABIN said that his case was one in which he should have considered the induction of abortion indicated, if he had seen the patient at an earlier stage. He should feel some hesitation in making extensive incisions through a cancerous cervix, for fear both of hæmorrhage, and septic absorption afterwards. The actual operation had proved easier than he expected, although followed by a fatal result.

DISSECTION OF A MALFORMED CHILD.

Mr. LENTON HEATH read this paper. The child lived to the end of the sixth week, dying then from hydrocephalus. The frontal bones showed craniotabes. The forearms on both sides were absent, the appearances presented by the stumps being very similar to those cases described as being due to intra-uterine amputation; but dissection proved that this had not occurred, but that there was an abnormal development of the lower end of both humeri. The acetabula were absent, and the lower limbs also much deformed.

Dr. ROPES considered intra-uterine amputation to be an exceedingly rare phenomenon, most of such alleged cases being the result of arrest of development, and not of amputation.

Mr. POWDRELL mentioned the case of a female child, having a similar deformity, which he had delivered at full term. Development had ceased at the lower end of the right humerus, but on the left hand were two thumbs. He hoped to show the child at a future meeting.

Dr. HERMAN asked whether, in Mr. Heath's case, the condition of the hip-joints resembled that which occasioned the so-called " congenital dislocation of the hip."

MEDICAL NEWS.

UNIVERSITY OF LONDON.—The following are the names of the candidates who have passed the recent Honours Examinations:—

FIRST M.B. EXAMINATION.

ANATOMY.

First Class.—Frances Helen Prideaux (Exhibition and Gold Medal), London School of Medicine for Women; Edwin James Wenyon, B.A., B.Sc. (Gold Medal), Guy's Hospital.

Second Class.—James Henry Targett, Guy's Hospital; Albert Martin, Guy's Hospital.

Third Class.—Sydney Sargent Merrifield, King's College.

PHYSIOLOGY AND HISTOLOGY.

First Class.—William Thorburn, B.Sc. (Exhibition and Gold Medal), Owens College; Wheelton Hind, Guy's Hospital, and Alfred Jefferis Turner, [University College, *equal*; Ernest Septimus Reynolds, Owens College, and Theodore Thomson, University of Aberdeen and University College, *equal*.

Second Class.—Frederick Knight, University College.

Third Class.—William Henry Horrocks, University College, and James Henry Targett, Guy's Hospital, *equal*; Thomas William Shore, B.Sc., St. Bartholomew's Hospital; Edwin James Wenyon, Guy's Hospital; Edward John Cave, St. Bartholomew's Hospital.

MATERIA MEDICA AND PHARMACEUTICAL CHEMISTRY.

First Class.—Alfred Mason Vann (Exhibition and Gold Medal), King's College; Sydney Sargent Merrifield, King's College; Mary Ann Dacomb Scharlieb, Madras Medical College and London School of Medicine.

Second Class.—William Ayton Gostling, University College, and Thos. William Shore, St. Bartholomew's Hospital, *equal*.

Third Class.—Charles Frederick Bailey, St. Bartholomew's Hospital; Frederick Knight, University College, and Thomas Sydney Short, King's College, *equal*; Edward John Cave, St. Bartholomew's Hospital.

ORGANIC CHEMISTRY.(a)

First Class.—Wheelton Hind (Exhibition and Gold Medal), Guy's Hospital; *William Thorburn, Owens College.

Second Class.—James Henry Targett, Guy's Hospital; Charles Hartvig Lomø Meyer, Guy's Hospital, and Emily Tomlinson, London School of Medicine for Women, *equal*.

FIRST B.SC. AND PRELIMINARY (M.B.) CONJOINTLY.

INORGANIC CHEMISTRY.

First Class.—Thomas M. Morgan (First B.Sc.), [disqualified by age for Exhibition,] private study.

Second Class.—Henry Stroud (First B.Sc.), Owens College.

Third Class.—Evan William Small (First B.Sc.), Christ's College, Cambridge; Walter Collingwood Williams (First B.Sc.), Sir Josiah Mason's College, Birmingham; Evan Evans (First Sci.), University College of Wales; Charles Caldecott (Prel. Sci.), Guy's Hospital; Mark Robinson Wright (First B.Sc.), private study and Firth College, Sheffield; Letitia Caroline Bernard (Prel. Sci.), London School of Medicine for Women.

EXPERIMENTAL PHYSICS.

First Class.—Henry Stroud (First B.Sc.), [Arnott Exhibition and Medal,] Owens College.

Second Class.—Alice Mitchell (First B.Sc.), Bedford College; William Maddock Bayliss (Prel. Sci.), University College; Walter Collingwood Williams (First B.Sc.), Sir Josiah Mason's College, Birmingham.

(a) The candidate whose name is preceded by an asterisk (*) obtained the number of marks qualifying for a medal.

Third Class.—John Waddell (First B.Sc.), Dalhousie College, Nova Scotia, and Mark Robinson Wright (First B.Sc.), private study and Firth College, Sheffield, *equal*; John Molony (First B.Sc.), St. Joseph's College, Clapham; Henry Langhorne Orchard (First B.Sc.), private study; Henry Sydney Maudslay (Prel. Sci.), Christ's College, Cambridge, and Lewis Eric Shore (First B.Sc.), Hartley Institution, Southampton, *equal*; Frank Hichens (Prel. Sci.), London Hospital and Epsom College.

BOTANY.

First Class.—Roger N. Goodman (Prel. Sci.), [Exhibition,] St. John's College, Cambridge; Henry John Webb (Prel. Sci.), University College; Arthur Everitt Shipley (First B.Sc.), Christ's College, Cambridge.

Second Class.—Wm. Leonard Braddon (Prel. Sci.), Guy's Hospital, and Mary Isabella Webb (First B. Sc.), Bedford College, *equal*; Wm. Maddock Bayliss (Prel. Sci.), University College; Eustace Frederick Bright (Prel. Sci.), University College; Alice Mitchell (First B. Sc.), Bedford College.

Third Class.—Ernest Paul A. Mariette (Prel. Sci.), King's College, and Edward Gaved Stocker (Prel. Sci.), University and Regent's-park Colleges, *equal*; Annie Besant (Prel. Sci.), private tuition; Walter George Spencer (Prel. Sci.), private study.

ZOOLOGY.

First Class.—Wm. Maddock Bayliss (Prel. Sci.), [Exhibition,] University College; Samuel Cromwell Jones (First B. Sc.), University College, Wales, and University College, London.

Second Class.—Henry Selby Green (Prel. Sci.), University College; Eustace Frederick Bright (Prel. Sci.), University College.

Third Class.—Edward Gavid Stocker (Prel. Sci.), University and Regent's-park Colleges; Henry Stroud (First B. Sc.), Owens College; Brian Mailland (Prel. Sci.), Owens College; John Ross Bradford (Prel. Sci.), University College.

APOTHECARIES' HALL, LONDON.—The following gentlemen passed their examination in the Science and Practice of Medicine, and received certificates to practise, on Thursday, August 25 :—

> Benson, Ernest Walter, Merton, Surrey.
> Harris, Walter Thomas, Ipplepen Vicarage, Devon.

The following gentleman also on the same day passed his primary professional examination:—

> Turner, Alfred James, Charing-cross Hospital.

APPOINTMENTS.

. The Editor will thank gentlemen to forward to the Publishing-office, as early as possible, information as to all new Appointments that take place.

ACLAND, T. D., M.B. Oxon., M.R.C.S., L.R.C.P.—House-Surgeon to St. Thomas's Hospital.

BUTLER, H. P., M.R.C.S., L.R.C.P.—Resident Accoucheur at St. Thomas's Hospital.

CARPENTER, A. B., B.A. Oxon., M.R.C.S., L.R.C.P.—Assistant House-Physician to St. Thomas's Hospital.

CLEGG, WALTER H., M.R.C.S. Eng., L.R.C.P. Lond.—Senior 'Resident Surgeon to the North Staffordshire Infirmary, Hartshill, Stoke-on-Trent, *vice* George Russell, M.B., etc., resigned.

COXWELL, C. F., B.A., M.B. Cantab., M.R.C.S.—House-Physician to St Thomas's Hospital.

HOLBERTON, H. N., M.R.C.S., L.R.C.P.—Assistant House-Physician to St. Thomas's Hospital.

MARLOW, F., M.R.C.S., L.S.A.—House-Surgeon to St. Thomas's Hospital.

SAVILL, J. D., M.R.C.S., L.S.A.—House-Physician to St. Thomas s Hospital.

WELLS, A. E., M.R.C.S.—Assistant-Surgeon to St. Thomas's Hospital.

NAVAL, MILITARY, ETC., APPOINTMENTS.

ADMIRALTY.—The following qualified candidates for the Naval Medical Service have been appointed Surgeons in H.M.'s Fleet with seniority of August 25, 1881 :—Matthew Digan; Ernest Edward Bray; John Leonard Aherne, B.A.; Joseph Anderson, M.D.; Edward James Biden; Samuel Cairns Browne; Charles Henry Wheeler, M.D.; Edward Goffe Swan; William Eames; Arthur William Egerton Brydges Barrett; Charles William Sharples; Robert William Anderson; John Ottley.

BIRTHS.

KINGSTON.—On August 21, at 3, Sussex-terrace, Plymouth, the wife of C. Albert Kingston, M.D., of a daughter.

MARTIN.—On August 20, the wife of Henry A. Martin, M.D., late A.M.D., The Lodge, East Cosham, Hants, of a daughter.

PAUL.—On August 24, at Tochieneal House, Cullen, Banffshire, the wife of Deputy-Surgeon-General J. L. Paul, of a daughter.

PLAYFAIR.—On August 26, at 25, Rutland-street, Edinburgh, the wife of John Playfair, M.B., F.R.C.P., of a daughter.

WOODMAN.—On August 26, at 5, Prospect-terrace, Ramsgate, the wife of Samuel Woodman, F.R.C.S., of a son.

MARRIAGES.

BRITTAN—ROBINSON.—On August 26, at St. Martin's-the-Less, London, Frederick Brittan, M.D., of Victoria-square, Clifton, Bristol, to Eliza Alice, youngest daughter of the late Richard Robinson, Esq., of Richmond Cottage, Clifton.

CARPENTER—HADY.—On August 25, at Havant, Sidney, eldest son of H. T. Carpenter, Esq., of Upper Clapton, to Emma Leonard, widow of the late Lieutenant S. Hardy, R.H.A., and daughter of H. Downs, M.D., Deputy Inspector-General, of Tiverton.

CASH—BRIGHT.—On August 24, at Torquay, Theodore Cash, M.D., of London, to Margaret Sophia, youngest daughter of the Right Hon. John Bright, of Rochdale.

CRICHELL—SNAPE.—On August 23, at Wiveliscombe, Somerset, William John Chichell, Esq., to Emily Lucy, eldest daughter of Charles Snape, M.D., of Lambrooke House, Wiveliscombe.

COGAN—LESLIE.—On August 9, at Slindon, Sussex, Surgeon-Major Michael Cogan, A.M.D., to Violet, eldest daughter of Charles Leslie, Esq., of Balquhain.

DE LÉRY—ROWAND.—On August 11, at Quebec, Canada, William Henri Brouage Chaussegros de Léry, eldest son of the late Hon. Alexandre René Chaussegros de Léry, to Kate, daughter of A. Rowand, M.D., of Quebec.

DENNY—GUPPY.—On August 24, at Falmouth, Richard Denny, Esq., Lieutenant and Adjutant Royal Marines L.I., to Mary, eldest daughter of T. S. Guppy, M.D., of Falmouth.

FULLER—DALTON.—On August 22, at Newhaven, Sussex, Thomas Fuller, Esq., of H.M. Customs, Newhaven, to Lily, only daughter of Dr. Dalton, of Newhaven.

HAWKINS—GREEN.—On August 25, at Redland, Bristol, Walter R. T. Hawkins, M.R.C.S., to Sarah Elizabeth, daughter of the late Thomas Green, M.D., of 7, Berkeley-square, Bristol.

LUNN—NORTHCOTT.—On August 25, at Ealing, John R. Lunn, L.R.C.P., M.R.C.S., L.S.A., to Ida Maund de P., second daughter of W. C. Northcott, M.A., of Rochester House, Little Ealing.

MACKERN—KIDD.—On August 24, at Kidbrook, Blackheath, John Mackern, M.B., to Louie, second daughter of Joseph Kidd, M.D., of Brooklands, Blackheath.

MOBERLY—BOWDEN.—On August 26, at Birchanger, Essex, Herbert J. R. Moberly, Surgeon A.M.D., to Clara Adeline Sophia, elder daughter of late Henry Bowden, Esq.

TWINING—CROSS.—On August 24, at Leeds, John Harrington Twining, B.A., of Dinnington, son of Edwd. Twining, M.R.C.S., of Walthamstow, Essex, to Gertrude, second daughter of George Cross, Esq., of Clarendon-road, Leeds.

DEATHS.

BRADLEY, W. H., Retired Deputy Inspector-General of Hospitals, late of H.M. Indian Forces, at Castle Green, Sandgate, on August 22.

COWAN, J. M., M.D., late of the Hon. East India Company's Service, at Queen's Hotel, Upper Norwood, on August 24.

PRALL, SAMUEL, M.D., F.R.C.S., of Town Malling, at Broadstairs, on August 28, aged 48.

SKAE, F. W. A., M.D., L.R.C.S., F.R.C.S., Commissioner in Lunacy for New Zealand, at Wellington, New Zealand, on June 25, aged 39.

WELDON, ANNE, wife of Walter Weldon, F.R.S., at Rede Hall, Burstow, Surrey, on August 27, in her 53rd year.

VACANCIES.

BATH GENERAL OR MINERAL WATER HOSPITAL.—Resident Medical Officer. (For particulars see Advertisement.)

BIRMINGHAM FRIENDLY SOCIETIES' MEDICAL INSTITUTION.—Resident Medical Officer. Candidates must be legally qualified practitioners, registered under the Medical Act, over thirty years of age, and married. They must produce their diplomas, certificates, and licences to the Committee. Applications, stating age, and enclosing recent testimonials as to qualifications and character, to be sent to Frederick Girling, 5, Cowper-street, Summer-lane, Birmingham, on or before September 15, marked "Medical."

LIVERPOOL NORTHERN HOSPITAL.—Assistant House-Surgeon. Candidates must possess a medical and surgical qualification from one or more British colleges or institutions recognised under the Medical Act. Applications and testimonials to be addressed to the Chairman of the Committee, not later than September 1.

NORTHUMBERLAND COUNTY LUNATIC ASYLUM, MORPETH.—Assistant Medical Officer. (For particulars see Advertisement.)

ROYAL ISLE OF WIGHT INFIRMARY.—House-Surgeon and Secretary. Candidates are requested to send their testimonials, not later than September 12, to the Secretary, Isle of Wight Infirmary, Ryde.

ROYAL UNITED HOSPITAL, BATH.—House-Surgeon. Candidates must be M.R.C.S., and registered. Diplomas and testimonials of professional capacity and moral character to be sent to the Secretary, on or before September 7.

UNION AND PAROCHIAL MEDICAL SERVICE.

*** The area of each district is stated in acres. The population is computed according to the census of 1871.

RESIGNATIONS.

Battle Union.—Mr. F. H. Corbyn has resigned the Fifth District: area 4590; population 875; salary £36 per annum.

Bury Union.—The Pilkington District is vacant by the death of Mr. John Telford: area 5468; population 11,943; salary £50 per annum.

Ticehurst Union.—The Hurst Green and Robertsbridge Districts are vacant by the resignation of Mr. F. H. Corbyn. Hurst Green: area 3601; population 864; salary £40 per annum. Robertsbridge: area 6421; population 9080; salary £40 per annum.

APPOINTMENTS.

Berwick-on-Tweed Union.—John A. Macdonald, F.C.C.S. Edin., L.R.C.P. Edin., M.D. Irc., to the Berwick District.

Nottingham Union.—George B. Powell, L.R.C.P. Edin., L.R.C.S. Edin., L.A.H. Dub., to the Third District.

OUR FUTURE DOCTORS.

OUR FUTURE DOCTORS.—Judging from the large number of gentlemen now undergoing their preliminary examinations in Arts, etc., at Burlington House, for the diploma of Fellow and Member of the Royal College of Surgeons, there need be no fear of any scarcity of medical men in the immediate future. Some 650 candidates are now going through the ordeal; those who prove successful will be able to enter on their professional studies in the ensuing October.

VITAL STATISTICS OF LONDON.

Week ending Saturday, August 27, 1881.

BIRTHS.

Births of Boys, 1209; Girls, 1184; Total, 2393.
Corrected weekly average in the 10 years 1871-80, 2590·4.

DEATHS.

	Males.	Females.	Total.
Deaths during the week	696	646	1342
Weekly average of the ten years 1871-80, corrected to increased population ...	801·8	729·9	1531·7
Deaths of people aged 90 and upwards ...	...	...	43

DEATHS IN SUB-DISTRICTS FROM EPIDEMICS.

	Enumerated Population, 1881 (unrevised).	Small-pox.	Measles.	Scarlet Fever.	Diphtheria.	Whooping-cough.	Typhus.	Enteric (or Typhoid) Fever.	Simple continued Fever.	Diarrhœa.
West ...	668998	6	3	9	5	1	...	...	...	15
North ...	905677	5	5	7	3	12	...	5	...	19
Central ...	281798	...	4	6	1	1	...	...	...	8
East ...	692580	2	11	9	2	5	1	5	...	28
South ...	1265673	21	10	22	5	8	...	2	2	47
Total ...	3814571	36	33	53	16	27	1	12	2	117

METEOROLOGY.

From Observations at the Greenwich Observatory.

Mean height of barometer	29·535 in.
Mean temperature	58·0°
Highest point of thermometer	71·4°
Lowest point of thermometer	47·0°
Mean dew-point temperature	53·7°
General direction of wind	S.W.
Whole amount of rain in the week	1·43 in.

BIRTHS and DEATHS Registered and METEOROLOGY during the Week ending Saturday, August 27, in the following large Towns:—

Cities and boroughs (Municipal boundaries except for London.)	Estimated Population to middle of the year 1881.[*]	Persons to an Acre. (1881.)	Births Registered during the week ending Aug. 27.	Deaths Registered during the week ending Aug. 27.	Temperature of Air (Fahr.) Highest during the Week.	Lowest during the Week.	Weekly Mean of Daily Highest Values.	Weekly Mean of Daily Mean Values.	Temp. of Air (Cent.)	Rain Fall. In Inches.	In Centimetres.
London ...	3829751	50·8	2303	1342	71·4	47·0	56·1	13·39		1·43	3·63
Brighton ...	107934	45·9	54	43	68·4	50·4	58·4	14·66		1·57	3·99
Portsmouth ...	128336	29·6	83	38	...	...	...	...		...	...
Norwich ...	88038	11·8	68	28	...	...	...	...		...	...
Plymouth ...	75262	54·0	48	21	65·8	49·2	57·5	14·17		1·38	3·51
Bristol ...	207140	45·5	132	63	66·2	48·2	55·9	13·23		2·41	6·12
Wolverhampton ...	75034	22·4	48	22	64·4	46·0	54·0	12·22		1·55	3·94
Birmingham ...	402296	47·9	275	185	...	...	...	...		...	...
Leicester ...	123120	38·5	90	43	...	...	...	...		...	...
Nottingham ...	188035	18·9	133	63	68·0	49·2	54·6	12·56		2·54	6·45
Liverpool ...	553985	106·3	360	256	62·9	47·4	53·5	11·95		1·43	3·63
Manchester ...	341289	79·5	211	138	...	...	...	...		...	...
Salford ...	177760	34·4	93	60	...	...	...	...		...	...
Oldham ...	112176	24·0	94	44	...	...	...	...		...	...
Bradford ...	184037	25·5	106	57	64·0	45·6	53·4	11·89		2·28	5·79
Leeds ...	310490	14·4	207	98	64·0	45·0	53·6	12·01		2·36	5·99
Sheffield ...	285621	14·5	184	96	65·0	45·5	54·1	12·23		2·03	5·16
Hull ...	155161	42·7	105	95	...	...	...	...		...	...
Sunderland ...	116758	42·2	63	34	67·0	44·0	53·5	11·95		2·45	6·22
Newcastle-on-Tyne	145675	27·1	100	65	...	...	...	...		...	...
Total of 20 large English Towns ...	7605775	38·0	4847	2756	71·4	42·2	53·0	12·16		1·95	4·95

[*] These figures are the numbers enumerated (but subject to revision) in April last, raised to the middle of 1881 by the addition of a quarter of a year's increase, calculated at the rate that prevailed between 1871 and 1881.

At the Royal Observatory, Greenwich, the mean reading of the barometer last week was 29·54 in. The highest reading was 29·76 in. at the beginning of the week, and the lowest 29·27 in on Friday at noon.

NOTES, QUERIES, AND REPLIES.

He that questioneth much shall learn much.—Bacon.

INTERNATIONAL MEDICAL CONGRESS.

TO THE EDITOR OF THE MEDICAL TIMES AND GAZETTE.

SIR,—Will you allow me to ask Dr. McClintock through your journal to verify the reference to the exact words, as given as a quotation in his address, that, "according to Dr. Aveling" . . . . '*His* [Harvey's] *was the first book on Midwifery written by an Englishman and printed in our own language,*'" as reported in the *Medical Times and Gazette* for August 6, 1881. Also his authority for his statement, on the following page, that "*Dr. John Arbuthnot . . . . was an eminent accoucheur in his day,*" and for the poetical quotation,

"Arbuthnot's soft obstetric hand."

I am, &c.,

16, Bloomsbury-street, W.C., August 23. E. NOCK.

M.B., M.A., Ryde.—Mr. Benjamin Barrow, President of the Association was admitted a Member of the College, June 27, 1836 and a Fellow November 18, 1861. He married a daughter of his old teacher, Mr. S. E. Stanley, Surgeon to St. Bartholomew's Hospital, twice President of the Royal College of Surgeons.

Dwellings for the Working Classes.—The Peabody trustees have purchased from the Metropolitan Board of Works the site of Peartree-court, situate between Clerkenwell Close and Farringdon-road, for the purpose of erecting dwellings under the Artisans' and Labourers' Dwellings Act, and they also propose to effect certain improvements adjacent thereto.

The International Medical Congress and Women Doctors.—"A Fellow of the Royal College of Surgeons of England," writes to a morning contemporary as to the denial to the published statement, "that at a preliminary meeting of the Executive Committee of the (late) International Medical Congress, the majority were rather in favour of admitting women doctors; when they were overruled by Sir William Jenner declaring he was empowered to remove the name of the Queen as patron of the Congress if ladies were invited." "On further inquiry," the writer adds, "I learn that what Sir William Jenner really said was, 'if any lady medical practitioner was allowed to be present at a medical meeting he would walk out of the room, and that if invitations were sent to qualified medical women he would induce the Queen to remove her name as patron of the Congress.' I give this on the authority of one of the Committee present, and I challenge Sir William Jenner to deny his having made a statement to this effect."

A District Board of Health, Southgate.—This village has hitherto been under the jurisdiction of the Board of Health of Edmonton, but by a recent decision of the Committees of both Lords and Commons, the preamble of a Separation Bill was confirmed. Under the Act passed the election of a board for the new district thus made terminated on the 20th ult. in the return, by a considerable majority, of the nine nominees of the separationists, who are the largest landowners in the district.

Noteworthy.—The Local Board of Eastbourne have got a clause in their Bill whereby they are enabled not only to regulate the junction of house-drains with the sewer, but to go inside the house and see that it is constructed on sanitary principles, without which permission will not be given for occupation.

A Hospital Milk Contractor.—The Governors of the Devon and Exeter Hospital last week commenced a prosecution against the contractor for the supply of milk to the Hospital. It appears that, during the year, the Committee pay about £400 for milk, which is supposed to be of the best quality. Suspicion was, however, aroused that the milk was below what it should be. On an analysis, it was found that a great deal of cream had been taken from the milk. When the case was brought on for hearing before the magistrates, a technical objection was taken that the prosecution was in the name of the person who had caused the analysis to be made—an objection which the bench held was fatal to the present proceedings, and the summons was dismissed.

Babies.—We do not see that there is a single word to be said in favour of baby-shows. There is no use or value in them, so far as the ordinary purposes of exhibition go. Their mothers are, we believe, nursing-mothers chiefly, and such shows are positively harmful in some senses, besides being useless and degrading.

A Volunteer Surgeon.—A mass of useful and interesting information is to be found in the Statistical Memoirs of the United States Sanitary Commission—"Investigations in the Military and Anthropological Statistics of American Soldiers," by Benjamin A. Gould, Ph.Dr.—not only concerning the health of camps and the relations of military life to sanitary questions, but also concerning the stature, form, constitution, vigour, and physical development of the men distributed according to the national and local subdivisions under which the soldiers constituting the Volunteer army of the North are classified.

A. Wallace P., Surrey.—The principle of respecting private property was upheld by Parliament in the Act for the Preservation of Metropolitan Commons, which was passed in 1866. The obligation to compensate for individual rights which may be interfered with for the general good is disputable.

S. J. G.—At the period referred to, 3000 persons in every million living died annually of the disease. Macaulay's description of the ravages of the disease is thus:—"The small-pox was always present, filling the churchyards with corpses, leaving on those whose lives it spared the hideous traces of its power, turning the babe into a changeling at which the mother shuddered, and making the eyes and cheeks of the betrothed maiden objects of horror to the lover."

Modern Therapy.—Sir W. Gull. He has a way of wording truths so picturesquely that they sound new. He said that the strength of modern therapeutics lies in the clearer perception that we now have of the great truth that diseases are but perverted life-processes, and have not only a beginning, but a period of culmination and decline. The effects of disease may be for a third or fourth generation, but the laws of health are for a thousand.

Templar.—The *abuse* of alcohol in Sweden seems to have begun during the last century, and in spite of the united efforts of physicians and legislators, matters have reached a point that Dr. Magnus Huss ("Ueber die endemischen Krankheiten") said, "The Swedish nation is menaced with incalculable evil. . . . . No measures can be too strong. It is better to save at any price than have to say, 'It is too late.'"

Cookery and Hospital Nurses.—The authorities of St. Thomas's Hospital are about to take a practical step in the promotion of the comfort of their patients. A class will commence on Tuesday, September 6, of nurses belonging to the Hospital at the National Training School for Cookery, Exhibition-road, South Kensington, to receive instruction in the details of sick-room cookery. This is one of the first of such classes that has been sent out from a hospital.

COMMUNICATIONS have been received from—

THE SECRETARY OF THE ZODONE COMPANY, Wrexham; THE LOCAL GOVERNMENT BOARD, London; THE SECRETARY OF THE WAR OFFICE, London; THE REGISTRAR OF THE APOTHECARIES' HALL, London; Mr. C. BOOTH, London; Dr. HERMAN, London; THE REGISTRAR OF THE UNIVERSITY OF LONDON; THE SECRETARY OF THE NIGHTINGALE FUND, London; Mr. J. CHATTO, London; Mr. M. BECHER, London; Dr. F. E. WILLOUGHBY, London; Dr. JOHN H. CLARKE, London; THE MILITARY SECRETARY OF THE INDIA OFFICE.

BOOKS, ETC., RECEIVED—

On the Study of Cancer in Relation to its Cure—The Uses of Country Hospitals, by G. W. Rigden—Deaf-Mutism, by Dr. Arthur Hartmann—Operative Surgery, by Stephen Smith, A.M., M.D.

PERIODICALS AND NEWSPAPERS RECEIVED—

Lancet—British Medical Journal—Medical Press and Circular—Berliner Klinische Wochenschrift—Centralblatt für Chirurgie—Gazette des Hopitaux—Gazette Médicale—Le Progrès Médical—Bulletin de l'Académie de Médecine—Pharmaceutical Journal—Wiener Medizinische Wochenschrift—Centralblatt für die Medizinischen Wissenschaften—Revue Médicale—Gazette Hebdomadaire—National Board of Health Bulletin, Washington—Nature—Deutsche Medicinal-Zeitung—Boston Medical and Surgical Journal—Louisville Medical News—The American—Occasional Notes—The Western Medical Reporter—The Church of England Pulpit, etc.—La Independencia Médica—Maryland Medical Journal—Oil and Drug News—La Presse Médicale—The Kensington News, August 30—Archives of Laryngology—St. Louis Courier of Medicine—Italian Times—National Anti-Compulsory Vaccination Reporter—Edinburgh Medical Journal—Leisure Hour—Friendly Greetings—Boy's Own Paper—Girl's Own Paper—Sunday at Home—Students' Journal and Hospital Gazette—Philadelphia Medical Times—Washington National Board of Health Bulletin—Weekblad—Monthly Homœopathic Review—North Carolina Medical Journal—Veterinarian.

APPOINTMENTS FOR THE WEEK.

September 3. Saturday (this day).

Operations at St. Bartholomew's, 1½ p.m.; King's College, 1½ p.m.; Royal Free, 2 p.m.; Royal London Ophthalmic, 11 a.m.; Royal Westminster Ophthalmic, 1½ p.m.; St. Thomas's, 1½ p.m.; London, 2 p.m.

5. *Monday.*

Operations at the Metropolitan Free, 2 p.m.; St. Mark's Hospital for Diseases of the Rectum, 2 p.m.; Royal London Ophthalmic, 11 a.m.; Royal Westminster Ophthalmic, 1½ p.m.

6. *Tuesday.*

Operations at Guy's, 1½ p.m.; Westminster, 2 p.m.; Royal London Ophthalmic, 11 a.m.; Royal Westminster Ophthalmic, 1½ p.m.; West London, 3 p.m.

7. *Wednesday.*

Operations at University College, 2 p.m.; St. Mary's, 1¼ p.m.; Middlesex, 1 p.m.; London, 2 p.m.; St. Bartholomew's, 1½ p.m.; Great Northern, 2 p.m.; Samaritan, 2½ p.m.; King's College (by Mr. Lister), 2 p.m.; Royal London Ophthalmic, 11 a.m.; Royal Westminster Ophthalmic, 1½ p.m.; St. Thomas's, 1½ p.m.; St. Peter's Hospital for Stone, 2 p.m.; National Orthopædic, Great Portland-street, 10 a.m.

8. *Thursday.*

Operations at St. George's, 1 p.m.; Central London Ophthalmic, 1 p.m.; Royal Orthopædic, 2 p.m.; University College, 2 p.m.; Royal London Ophthalmic, 11 a.m.; Royal Westminster Ophthalmic, 1½ p.m.; Hospital for Diseases of the Throat, 2 p.m.; Hospital for Women, 2 p.m.; Charing-cross, 2 p.m.; London, 2 p.m.; North-West London, 2½ p.m.

9. *Friday.*

Operations at Central London Ophthalmic, 2 p.m.; Royal London Ophthalmic, 11 a.m.; South London Ophthalmic, 2 p.m.; Royal Westminster Ophthalmic, 1½ p.m.; St. George's (ophthalmic operations), 1¼ p.m.; Guy's, 1½ p.m.; St. Thomas's (ophthalmic operations), 2 p.m.

THE STUDENTS' NUMBER

OF THE

MEDICAL TIMES AND GAZETTE

FOR

1881-82.

IN accordance with old-established custom and undeniable convenience, this number of the *Medical Times and Gazette* is for the most part specially devoted to the supply of needful information to parents, guardians, and intending medical students old enough to judge for themselves as to what course they must pursue in seeking to enter the medical profession. It is not often, however, that such inquirers are left entirely to such guidance. Everyone knows, or his friends know, some medical practitioner who is, as a rule, most willing to give aid and assistance where often it is sadly needed; for very many circumstances which cannot here be indicated enter into the questions to be determined, with regard to an intending student of medicine. Foremost amongst these is the selection of a school, which, however, is often practically determined by convenience, or even by the question of fees; but the amount of money to be paid is not in reality the most important point to be settled. Large fees no more predicate good teaching and training than a smaller sum means that the teaching is wholly bad. More important than fees—in many cases, at least—is the character of the school for industry or idleness, for expensive or economical (which does not of necessity imply slovenly) habits; in short, what constitutes the whole tone of a school. For the character of a medical school is only less important than that which pervades a public school, after which parents so anxiously inquire. Matters of this kind cannot be discussed in books papers, or advertisements, though in certain respects they are even more important in a medical than in a public school. In the former the students are only kept in restraint during a few hours in the day, whereas in the latter the supervision is more or less constant.

In seeking the advice of medical men, however, the inquirer must never forget that there is a strong *esprit de corps* among the different schools, aided or unaided, as to what is necessary to be done by the intending student, where the last to condemn, were it not that it arises in a way which is hardly creditable to the various hospital and school authorities themselves. Such things as allied hospital sports, cricket and football clubs, and so on, are now gradually breaking down the walls of separation which formerly existed between different schools, and which were on purpose kept up by making all schools self-sufficing, and still more by the positive discouragement even now given to students passing from one school to another.

We purpose, therefore, to lay before our readers as fully as possible the materials whereby they may arrive at a sound judgment for themselves, aided or unaided, as to what is necessary to be done by the intending student, where the knowledge demanded of the pupil at his qualifying examinations may be obtained, and at what cost. Moreover, as in the meantime the requirements of the various qualifying bodies as regards attendance on classes, etc., differ among themselves, we have given, as fully as need be, the various rules and regulations enforced by each of these.

I.—PRELIMINARY EDUCATION.

—

REGISTRATION AS A MEDICAL STUDENT.

IT is universally conceded that the establishment and enforcement of an examination in matters of ordinary education has done much to raise the status of the medical practitioner. It has especially tended to elevate him above the dull level which he formerly occupied, and to raise him in the social scale. Moreover, it has at once choked off (if we may use the expression) a great number of men obviously unfitted for the profession at the very commencement of their would-be career, and induced them to turn their attention to other occupations better suited to the bent of their genius. All are agreed, we repeat, as to the utility of this examination, but all are *not* of the same mind as to its scope and purport. In these utilitarian days the test of all things is, too often, Will it pay? And to this end many would have the future medical practitioner trained up, so to speak, from his very cradle, with a view to his ultimate destination in life. How often such intentions are frustrated we need hardly say; and it is a terrible thing to contemplate a mind cramped and confined in a single groove through life. Rather we would seek in preliminary education what will give breadth and power to the character and intellect

in the shape of that tincture of letters which is useful to all men, and to none more than to the medical practitioner. The General Medical Council have duly provided for this by insisting that every examination which they will recognise shall comprehend the following subjects:—1. English Language, including grammar and composition.(a) 2. English History. 3. Modern Geography. 4. Latin, including translation from the original and grammar. 5. Elements of Mathematics, comprising—(a) Arithmetic, including vulgar and decimal fractions; (β) Algebra, including simple equations; (γ) Geometry, including the first two books of Euclid, or the subjects thereof. 6. Elementary Mechanics of solids and fluids, comprising the elements of statics, dynamics, and hydrostatics.(b) 7. One of the following optional subjects:—(a) Greek, (β) French, (γ) German, (δ) Italian, (ε) any other modern language, (ζ) Logic, (η) Botany, (θ) Elementary Chemistry.

(a) The General Medical Council will not consider any examination in English language sufficient that does not fully test the ability of the candidate (1) to write sentences in correct English on a given theme, attention being paid to spelling and punctuation as well as to composition; (2) to write correctly from dictation; (3) to explain the grammatical construction of sentences; (4) to point out the grammatical errors in sentences ungrammatically composed, and to explain their nature; and (5) to give the derivation and definition of English words in common use.

(b) This subject may be passed either as Preliminary, or before or at the First Professional Examination.

A

Some bodies specially insist on Greek; and care should be taken to comply with this demand, if possible, at the time of the Preliminary Examination, even when it is possible to postpone it to a later season, which in all probability will be found not to be so convenient.

We would specially impress on all who seek to attain to the higher grades of the profession—to take a degree in Arts, if possible, before entering on their strictly professional studies; and this can be done nowadays at Cambridge much more easily than would be supposed. At all events, whether attained with ease or not, a degree in Arts gives a stamp to a man which is of unspeakable value to him in after life.

Two examining bodies disregard the possession of a degree in Arts. Thus, the University of London will only accept its own Matriculation Examination, whilst the Royal College of Physicians include in their examination for the membership questions in Greek, Latin, French, and German. Otherwise there is an increasing tendency to accept the certificates of any respectable institution whose examinations comprehend the subjects insisted on by the General Medical Council. This body now accepts the *testamur* of any one of the following certificates about to be enumerated; and generally speaking, what is accepted by the Medical Council will be accepted elsewhere, with the exceptions above mentioned. The Royal College of Surgeons of England, who formerly held an examination in preliminary education of their own, have now abandoned the plan, and expect all those seeking its diploma to come provided with a certificate of competency in the various subjects deemed necessary by the Medical Council. The following is the list of bodies whose testimonials of proficiency are received and acknowledged by the Medical Council:—

EXAMINING BODIES WHOSE EXAMINATIONS FULFIL THE CONDITIONS OF THE MEDICAL COUNCIL AS REGARDS PRELIMINARY EDUCATION.

I.—*Universities in the United Kingdom.*

Oxford.—Junior Local Examinations, certificate to include Latin and Mathematics, and also one of the following optional subjects:—Greek, French, German, Natural Philosophy, including mechanics, hydrostatics, and pneumatics. Senior Local Examinations, certificate to include Latin and Mathematics; Responsions; Moderations; Examination for a degree in Arts.

Cambridge.—Junior Local Examinations, certificate to include Latin and Mathematics, and also one of the following optional subjects:—Greek, French, German, Natural Philosophy, including the elements of statics and hydrostatics. Senior Local Examinations, certificate to include Latin and Mathematics; Higher Local Examinations; Previous Examination; Examination for a degree in Arts.

Durham.—Junior Local Examinations, certificate to include Latin and Mathematics, and also one of the following optional subjects:—Greek, French, German, Natural Philosophy, including mechanics, hydrostatics, and pneumatics. Senior Local Examinations, certificate to include Latin and Mathematics; Registration Examination for medical students; Examination for students at the end of their first year; Examination for a degree in Arts.

London.—Matriculation Examination; Preliminary Scientific (M.B.) Examination; Examination for a degree in Arts or Science.

Edinburgh.—Local Examinations (Junior certificate), certificate to include English Literature, Arithmetic, Algebra, Geometry, and also one of the following optional subjects:—Greek, French, German, Natural Philosophy; Local Examinations (Senior certificate), certificate to include English Literature, Arithmetic, Algebra, Geometry, Latin, and also one of the following optional subjects:—Greek, French, German, Natural Philosophy; Preliminary Examination for graduation in Science or Medicine and Surgery; Examination for a degree in Arts.

Aberdeen.—Local Examinations (Honours certificate), certificate to include English Literature, Arithmetic, Algebra, Geometry, Latin, and also one of the following optional subjects:—Greek, French, German, Natural Philosophy; Preliminary Examination for graduation in Medicine or Surgery; Examination for a degree in Arts.

Glasgow.—Local Examinations (Senior certificate), certificate to include English Literature, Arithmetic, Algebra, Geometry, Latin, and also one of the following optional subjects:—Greek, French, German, Natural Philosophy; Preliminary Examination for graduation in Medicine or Surgery; Examination for a degree in Arts.

St. Andrews.—Local Examinations (Honours certificate), certificate to include English Literature, Arithmetic, Algebra, Geometry, Latin, and also one of the following optional subjects:—Greek, French, German, Natural Philosophy; Preliminary Examination for graduation in Medicine or Surgery; Examination for a degree in Arts.

Dublin.—Public Entrance Examination; Examination for a degree in Arts.

Queen's University (Ireland).—Local Examinations for Men and Women, certificate to include all the subjects required by the General Medical Council as set forth in Recommendation 4; Entrance or Matriculation Examination; Previous Examination for B.A. degree; Examination for a degree in Arts.

Oxford and Cambridge Schools' Examination Board.(c)—Certificate to include—Arithmetic (including vulgar and decimal fractions), Algebra (including simple equations), Geometry (including the first two books of Euclid), Latin (including translation and grammar); also one of these optional subjects:—Greek, French, German, mechanical division of Natural Philosophy.

II.—*Other Bodies named in Schedule (A) to the Medical Act.*

Apothecaries' Society of London.—Examination in Arts.

Royal College of Physicians and Surgeons, Edinburgh.—Preliminary Examination in General Education, conducted by a Board appointed by these two Colleges combined.

Faculty of Physicians and Surgeons of Glasgow.—Preliminary Examination in General Education.

Royal College of Surgeons in Ireland.—Preliminary Examination; certificate to include Mathematics.

Apothecaries' Hall of Ireland.—Preliminary Examination in General Education.

III.—*Examining Bodies in the United Kingdom not included in Schedule (A) to the Medical Act* (1858).

College of Preceptors.—Examination for a First or Second Class Certificate, provided that, in the case of the latter, the candidate has passed in the First or Second Division, and has taken Algebra, Euclid, Latin, and a modern language.

Examiners for Commissions and Appointments in Her Majesty's Service, Military, Naval, and Civil.—Certificate, including all the subjects required by the Council's 4th Recommendation.

IV.—*Indian, Colonial, and Foreign Universities and Colleges.*

Universities of Calcutta, Madras, and Bombay.—Entrance Examination; certificate to include Latin.

Universities of M'Gill College, Montreal; Bishop's College, Montreal; Toronto; Trinity College, Toronto; Queen's College, Kingston; Victoria College, Upper Canada; Fredericton, New Brunswick; Halifax, Nova Scotia; Melbourne; Sydney; Adelaide; Medical College, Halifax, Nova Scotia; Michigan College of Medicine.—Matriculation Examination.

University of Manitoba.—Previous Examination.

University of King's College, Nova Scotia.—Matriculation Examination; Responsions.

Tasmanian Council of Education.—Examination for the degree of Associate of Arts; certificate to include Latin and Mathematics.

University of the Cape of Good Hope.—Matriculation Examination; Examination for a degree in Arts.

University of Otago.—Preliminary Examination.

University of New Zealand.—Entrance Examination.

Christ's College, Canterbury, New Zealand.—Voluntary Examinations; certificate to include all the subjects required by the Council's 4th Recommendation.

Codrington College, Barbadoes.—English Certificate for Students of two years' standing, and Latin Certificate, or "Testamur."

Ceylon Medical College.—Preliminary Examination (Primary Class).

Germany and other Continental Countries.—Gymnasial Abiturienten Examen in Germany, and the corresponding Entrance Examination to the Universities in other continental countries.

We have already pointed out that the University of London insists on all its would-be members passing its own Matriculation Examination. This is somewhat stiff; but, if fairly passed, it gives a man a certain standing, which is always of value. Moreover—and *this is very important*—the University counts no medical study until this examination has been passed, so that even if a man has gone right through a complete medical curriculum, and should yet desire the University of London degree, he would have to go back to the very beginning over again to attain the object of his ambition.

UNIVERSITY OF LONDON.—The following are the particulars relating to the Matriculation Examination:—

Matriculation.—There shall be two examinations for Matriculation in each year—one commencing on the second Monday in January, and the other on the third Monday in June.(d)

No candidate shall be admitted to the Matriculation Examination unless he have produced a certificate(e) showing that he has completed his sixteenth year. This certificate shall be transmitted to the Registrar at least *fourteen days* before the commencement of the examination. A fee of £2 shall be paid at matriculation. No candidate shall be admitted to the examination unless he have previously paid this fee to the Registrar.(f) The examination shall be conducted

(c) The *English* is provided for by the following resolution of the Executive Committee:—"That, as every candidate for the certificate of the Oxford and Cambridge Schools' Examination Board is required to answer questions in such a manner as to satisfy the examiners that he has an adequate knowledge of English Grammar and Orthography, this shall be held as conforming to the requirements of the Medical Council in reference to English Language."

(d) These examinations may be held, not only at the University of London, but also, under special arrangement, in other parts of the United Kingdom, or in the colonies.

(e) A certificate from the Registrar-General in London, or from the Superintendent Registrar of the district, or a certified copy of the baptismal register, is required in *every case in which it can possibly be obtained*. In other cases the best evidence procurable is admitted. The certificate of each candidate is returned to him when he inscribes his name on the Register of the University. Information respecting the time for doing this will be sent to each candidate when the receipt of his certificate of age is acknowledged.

(f) The fee must be paid when the candidate inscribes his name on the Register of the University.

by means of printed papers; but the examiners shall not be precluded from putting, for the purpose of ascertaining the competence of the candidates to pass, *vivâ voce* questions to any candidate in the subjects in which they are appointed to examine. Candidates shall not be approved by the examiners unless they have shown a competent knowledge in each of the following subjects, according to the details specified under the several heads:—1. Latin. 2. Any two(g) of the following languages: Greek, French, German, and either Sanskrit or Arabic.(h) 3. The English ,Language, English History, and Modern Geography. 4. Mathematics. 5. Natural Philosophy. 6. Chemistry.

The following are the particulars relating to the foregoing subjects of examination for the year 1882:—

Languages.—In Latin the following authors have been selected:— January, 1882—*Horace:* Odes, Books I. and II. June—*Livy:* Book II. The paper in Latin shall contain passages to be translated into English, with questions in history and geography arising out of the subjects of the book selected. Short and easy passages shall also be set for translation from other books not so selected. A separate paper shall be set containing questions in Latin grammar, with simple and easy sentences of English to be translated into Latin.(i) In Greek(k):—January, 1882—*Xenophon:* Anabasis, Book VI. June—*Homer:* Iliad, Book XVIII. The paper in Greek shall contain passages to be translated into English, with questions in grammar,(l) and with questions in history and geography arising out of the subjects of the book selected. Short and easy passages shall also be set for translations from other books not so selected. French—The paper in French shall contain passages for translation into English, and questions in grammar, limited to the Accidence. German—The paper in German shall contain passages for translation into English, and questions in grammar, limited (except when German is taken as an alternative for Greek) to the Accidence. Sanskrit; Arabic—The paper in Sanskrit and the paper in Arabic shall contain passages for translation into English, and questions in grammar. The English Language, English History, and Modern Geography—Orthography; writing from dictation; the grammatical structure of the language. History of England to the end of the seventeenth century; with questions in modern geography.

Mathematics.—Arithmetic: The ordinary rules of arithmetic; Vulgar and Decimal Fractions; Extraction of the Square Root. Algebra: Addition, Subtraction, Multiplication, and Division of Algebraical Quantities; Proportion; Arithmetical and Geometrical Progression; Simple Equations. Geometry: The First Four Books of Euclid, or the subjects thereof.

Natural Philosophy.(m)—Mechanics: Composition and Resolution of Statical Forces; Simple Machines (Mechanical Powers)—Ratio of the Power to the weight in each; Centre of Gravity; General Laws of Motion, with the chief experiments by which they may be illustrated; Law of the Motion of Falling Bodies. Hydrostatics, Hydraulics, and Pneumatics: Pressure of Liquids and Gases, its equal diffusion and variation with the depth; Specific Gravity, and modes of determining it; the Barometer, the Syphon, the Common Pump and Forcing Pump, and the Air Pump. Optics: Laws of Reflection and Refraction; formation of Images by Mirrors and Simple Lenses. Heat: its Sources; Expansion; Thermometers —relations between different Scales in common use; difference between Temperature and Quantity of Heat; Specific and Latent Heat—Calorimeters; Liquefaction; Ebullition; Evaporation; Conduction; Convection; Radiation.

Chemistry.—Chemistry of the Non-metallic Elements, including their compounds as enumerated below, their chief physical and chemical characters, their preparation, and their characteristic tests. Oxygen, Hydrogen, Carbon, Nitrogen; Chlorine, Bromine, Iodine, Fluorine; Sulphur, Phosphorus, Silicon. Combining Proportions by weight and by volume; General Nature of Acids, Bases, and Salts; Symbols and Nomenclature. The Atmosphere - its constitution; effects of Animal and Vegetable Life upon its composition. Combustion; structure and properties of Flame; nature and composition of ordinary fuel. Water: Chemical peculiarities of Natural Waters, such as rain-water, river-water, spring-water, seawater. Carbonic Acid; Carbonic Oxide; Oxides and Acids of Nitrogen; Ammonia; Olefiant Gas; Marsh Gas; Sulphurous and Sulphuric Acids, Sulphuretted Hydrogen. Hydrochloric Acid, Phosphoric Acid, and Phosphuretted Hydrogen; Silica.

ENTRANCE ON PROFESSIONAL STUDIES.

In all cases the period of medical studies is supposed to extend over four years, or more exactly forty-five months; and in Scottish universities this is rigidly enforced, but in England the curriculum is so arranged in all hospital schools, that three winter and two summer sessions' attendance suffices for school work. This leaves an odd year, which may be spent in attendance on a hospital which has no school attached, provided it complies with certain conditions, or with a private medical man holding certain appointments. This extra-scholastic period may likewise be spent—and is usually best spent, especially by those seeking the higher qualifications—in clinical work in the school to which the student belongs, after he has completed his stated curriculum. But the odd year may also be taken before entering on school life, thus to a certain

(g) No credit will be given for more than two of these languages.
(h) Candidates who desire to be examined in either Sanskrit or Arabic must give at least *two calendar months'* notice to the Registrar, and must mention the other optional language which they select.
(i) Special stress is laid on accuracy in the answers to the grammar questions, and on the correct rendering of English into Latin.
(k) Candidates may substitute German for Greek.
(l) Special stress is laid on accuracy in the answers to the questions in Greek grammar.
(m) The questions in Natural Philosophy will be of a strictly elementary character.

extent simulating the ancient system of apprenticeship. The last-mentioned plan is not yet entirely disused, and there are some who would like to see it revived. And though with this view we are not altogether in accord, we freely admit that something of the kind is highly necessary before a man enters on the duties of his profession on his own account. Under the old system, a student learned something of the aspect of drugs and of their properties; and he was taught to read, write, and compound a prescription. Nowadays, he learns little or nothing of all this. Every hospital has its own pharmacopoeia, and, for the purpose of saving time, prescriptions are ordinarily, and as far as possible, written in accordance with this. But the knowledge thus conveyed to the student, except he refer directly and on all occasions to the book in question, is infinitesimal; whilst to the style of hospital dispensing the same remark applies. It must be said, however, that the period assigned to apprenticeship, which was commonly five years, was far too long; and one year spent in this way, after a student has passed through his curriculum, will do as much good, if not more, than the five under the old system. It is quite true that a student who has served some kind of an apprenticeship starts on his curriculum with certain advantages not possessed by those who come more directly from a school; but they do not, as a rule, long maintain this lead; and, too frequently, they have to submit to that most tedious, troublesome, and disagreeable of tasks—the unlearning of many things, more especially with regard to the true methods of study and investigation. For our own part, we vastly prefer students to come to us with a good fair mental culture of the broadest kind, and something more than a smattering of Physics, Chemistry, Botany, and Zoology. But of this we shall speak in our next section.

REGISTRATION.

As soon as the student has passed his preliminary examination, and provided he desires to enter on his studies at once, so as to make time count, he ought to register his certificate at the office of the General Medical Council, 315, Oxford-street, W., or at that of the Branch Registrar in Scotland (Archibald Inglis, 33, Albany-street, Edinburgh), or in Ireland (W. E. Steele, 35, Dawson-street, Dublin), as the case may be, which will save him all further trouble as regards preliminary education. This is necessary, if the student desires to spend the first year with a general practitioner or at a country hospital, so as to enable the time thus spent to be included in the period of medical study. But when the student begins by entering a medical school, he must register the actual commencement of his hospital studies as being likewise the date of the commencement of medical studies. In London everyone used to register at the College of Surgeons; but that plan has been abandoned. It is now the practice for the return required by the General Medical Council to be sent in by the school authorities. *All registration must in any case take place within fifteen days of the beginning of medical studies,* at whatever time that may be, no time previous to this counting.

II.—SCIENTIFIC EDUCATION.

As matters now stand, instruction in medical and scientific knowledge is, during the student's first year, inextricably mixed, as far as the latter subjects are in most schools taught at all. Thus, on entering a school, the student is set to work at once on Chemistry, Anatomy, and Physiology; whilst in summer, Botany, Practical Chemistry, and Materia Medica are taught simultaneously. It would be far better if the student came to the study of medicine ready prepared in the scientific subjects already named, for the strictly scientific subjects clash with the purely medical, and are never greatly relished by the student, whilst Physics and Zoology are hardly ever efficiently taught in a purely medical school. Great inducements are now being held out by the College of Physicians for students thus to master certain branches before entering on their professional education. Thus, in Botany, Chemistry, Pharmacy, and Materia Medica, no regular class certificates are required, but only certificates of having received instruction, which anyone may give. This scheme is founded on the so-called Conjoint Scheme, so that it will in all probability be adopted by other licensing bodies. In most large public schools, science is now well taught—sometimes much better than in medical schools: the teachers are specially selected for their scientific acquirements and their powers of communicating instruction, and not in accordance with hospital rules, by which too often the round stick is found in the square hole, and a capital teacher of Medicine or Surgery is allowed to waste in working at a most uncongenial subject. At such a school as Epsom, Physics, Chemistry, Botany, and Zoology are now well and efficiently taught, and a boy on leaving should have little difficulty in passing the greater part of his First Examination at the College of Physicians, which may be done immediately after registration.

The University of London, as usual, takes its own course independently of all others, and holds a special Preliminary Scientific Examination of its own. We would again urge on all intending graduates to get this over as soon as possible, for with much sadness we have often seen men grinding at these preliminary subjects at a period of their career when they should have been engaged in strictly professional work. But there is no use trying to "fluke" through this examination; it as just as well to recognise at once that no one has a chance of passing whose knowledge is not good and accurate. It is in fact the *pons asinorum* of the London degree, and usually thins in a woful manner the ranks of the would-be candidates. The following is a synopsis of the regulations and of the subjects on which the questions are put:—

Preliminary Scientific (M.B.) Examination.

No candidate shall be admitted to this examination (which takes place on the third Monday of July) until he shall have completed his seventeenth year, and shall have either passed the Matriculation Examination or taken a degree in Arts in one of the Universities of Sydney, Melbourne, Calcutta, or Madras (provided that Latin was one of the subjects in which he passed); nor unless he have given notice of his intention to the Registrar at least *fourteen days* before the commencement of the examination.

The fee for this examination shall be £5.

No candidate shall be admitted to the examination unless he have previously paid this fee to the Registrar.(n) If, after payment of his fee, a candidate withdraws his name, or fails to present himself at the examination, or fails to pass it, the fee shall not be returned to him; but he shall be allowed to enter for any *two* subsequent Preliminary Scientific (M.B.) Examinations without the payment of any additional fee, provided that he give notice to the Registrar at least *fourteen days* before the commencement of the examination; such notice, in respect to the privilege aforesaid, being considered equivalent to entry.

Candidates shall be examined in the following subjects(o):—

Inorganic Chemistry.

Differences between mechanical mixture, solution, and chemical combination; outlines of crystallography; formation of crystals; dimorphism; isomorphism; conditions on which the melting-point and the boiling-point of a substance depend; difference between elementary and compound substances; laws of chemical combination; equivalent weights of the elements; multiple proportions; the atomic theory; atomic value (quantivalence); molecules; molecular weights; relation between the density of a gas and its molecular weight; abnormal densities; Avogadro's hypothesis; combination of gases by volume; compound radicals; atomic and molecular combination. Meaning of chemical symbols, formulæ, and equations; calculation of quantities by weight and by volume; chemical changes, and the conditions under which they occur; combination; decomposition; double decomposition; nature of acids, bases, and salts; capacity of saturation of acids and bases; nomenclature. Relation between atomic weight and specific heat; Faraday's electrolytic law; principles of spectrum analysis; diffusion of gases. Hydrogen, chlorine, bromine, iodine, fluorine; the combination of the last four elements with hydrogen. Oxygen; ozone; water and peroxide of hydrogen; the oxides and oxyacids of chlorine; chlorates and hypochlorites. Sulphur; sulphuretted hydrogen; the oxides of sulphur; sulphuric acid and the sulphates; sulphurous acid and the sulphites; chlorosulphuric acid. Nitrogen; the atmosphere and its relations to animal and vegetable life; ammonia; ammonium and its salts; the oxides of nitrogen; nitric acid and nitrates; nitrous acid and nitrites. Phosphorus; phosphoretted hydrogen; the oxides of phosphorus; phosphoric acid and the phosphates; chloride and oxychloride of phosphorus. Arsenic and its oxides; arseniuretted hydrogen; arsenious acid and its salts; arsenic acid and its salts; the sulphides of arsenic; detection of arsenic. Antimony, its oxides and sulphides; antimoniuretted hydrogen; chlorides of antimony; compounds of antimonic oxide; detection of antimony. Boron; boracic acid and the borates. Carbon; carbonic oxide and carbonic acid; the carbonates; carbon oxysulphide; sulphocarbonic acid; marsh-gas; ethylene; combustion; structure of flame; coal-gas; Davy lamp; principles of illumination. Silicon; siliciuretted hydrogen; silicon chloride; silicon chloroform; silica and the silicates. Potassium; sodium; silver. Calcium; strontium; barium. Aluminium. Magnesium; zinc; cadmium. Lead. Manganese; iron; cobalt; nickel; chromium. Bismuth; copper; mercury; gold; tin. Platinum. The chief compounds of these metals with the more important acid radicals; the detection of these metals and their compounds, in powder or in solution.

Experimental Physics.

[Candidates will be expected to show a general acquaintance with the methods and apparatus by which the leading principles of Physics as enumerated below can be illustrated and applied.]

Units of measurement. The laws of motion considered experimentally. The chief forces of nature. The general properties of solids, liquids, and gases. The nature, intensity, and transmission of fluid pressure in general. The pressure of liquids in equilibrium under the action of gravity. The equilibrium of solids floating or entirely immersed in gravitating fluids. The specific gravities of substances, with the ordinary modes of determining them. Measurement of the pressure of the atmosphere and of the elastic force of gases. Diffusion of liquids and gases. Definition of work and energy; conservation and transmutation of energy.

Acoustics.—Production and mode of propagation of sound; intensity, pitch and quality. Velocity of sound in air. Influence of temperature and density. Velocity of sound in other media. Laws of reflection and refraction. Nature of musical sounds. Longitudinal vibrations of rods and of columns of air. Transverse vibrations of strings; variation in their rate of vibration by changes in their tension, length, thickness, and substance.

Heat.—Definitions of heat and temperature. Construction of instruments for the measurement of temperature. Expansion of solids, liquids, and gases under heat. Change of state; tension of vapours; latent heat. Radiant heat; its reflection refraction, and absorption. Conduction; definition of thermal conductivity. Convection. Specific heat; mechanical equivalent of heat.

Magnetism.—Properties of magnets; induction—magnetic relations of iron and steel. Terrestrial magnetism.

Electricity.—Two electrical states, and their mutual relations. Conduction and insulation. Induction. Electric attraction and repulsion. Distribution and accumulation of electricity on conductors. Electric discharge. Voltaic electricity; the various batteries. Electro-motive force, strength of currents, resistance; Ohm's law. Heating and chemical effects of electric currents; action between currents and magnets; electro-magnetism. Induced currents; magneto-electricity. Thermo-electricity.

Optics.—Laws of propagation of light; measurement of velocity of light; photometry. Laws of reflection and refraction of light. Reflection at plane and at spherical surfaces. Refraction at plane and at spherical surfaces. Refraction through lenses, including the formation of images. Chromatic dispersion.

Botany and Vegetable Physiology.(p)

Structure, functions, and life-history of simple unicellular plants, such as *Protococcus* and *Saccharomyces* (yeast), as types of vegetable life. Structure, functions, and life-history of *Penicillium*, *Mucor*, or some other simple fungus. Structure, functions, and life-history of *Chara* or *Nitella*. Morphology, histology, and history of the reproduction of a fern. Morphology and histology of a flowering plant; structure of a flower; homologies of leaves and floral organs; histology of ordinary vegetable tissues, such as epidermis, parenchyma, fibro-vascular tissue, and their arrangement in the stem and leaves. General principles of vegetable nutrition; food of plants; action of green parts of plants; nature and flow of sap. Growth of a flowering plant; formation of wood and bark; nature of cambium. Reproduction of a flowering plant; structure of ovule; methods of fertilisation; development of ovule into seed; distinctive characters of gymnosperms. Distinctive characters of the principal British natural orders, viz.,—*Dicotyledons*, Ranunculaceæ, Cruciferæ, Caryophylleæ, Leguminosæ, Rosaceæ, Umbelliferæ, Compositæ, Scrophulariaceæ, Labiatæ, Amentaceæ; *Monocotyledons*, Orchideæ, Liliaceæ, Cyperaceæ, Gramineæ; *Acotyledons*, Filices, Musci, Lichens, Algæ, Fungi. (Description in technical language of specimens of flowering plants to be provided by the examiners.) Derivation and meaning of the following terms, and demonstration of their application on specimens (provided by the examiners):—Thalamifloral, calycifloral, corollifloral; hypogynous, perigynous, epigynous; monandrous, diandrous, etc.; individual, variety, species, genus, order, class, kingdom.

Zoology.

General structure and life-history of the following animals, as types of some of the principal divisions of the animal kingdom:—Amœba, paramœcium, hydra, tænia, leech, mussel, snail, centipede, insect, lobster, frog. Comparative structure of the digestive apparatus (including the teeth) in the dog, sheep, pig, and rabbit. Comparative structure and actions of the circulating and respiratory organs in the animals enumerated in the first paragraph, and also in each of the vertebrated classes. Essential structure of secretory organs; principal varieties in the structure of the liver and kidney. General plan of the nervous system in mollusca, arthrozoa, and vertebrata. Proportionate development of the spinal cord and of the several encephalic centres in the ascending series of vertebrata. Respective functions of those centres. Modes of reflex action. Outlines of the comparative history of embryonic development in frog, bird, and mammal.

(n) The fee must be paid when the candidate inscribes his name on the Register of the University. Information respecting the time for doing this will be sent to each candidate with the acknowledgment of his notice.

(o) Candidates who shall pass in all the subjects of the Preliminary Scientific (M.B.) Examination, and shall also pass *at the same time* in the Pure Mathematics of the first B.Sc. examination, or who shall have previously passed the first B.A. examination, shall be admissible to the second B Sc. examination.—The attention of such candidates is directed to the fact that, under the new regulations for the B.Sc. degree, this degree may be obtained by passing at the second B.Sc. examination in the three biological subjects only.

(p) Candidates for this and other botanical examinations are expected to bring with them a pocket-lens or simple microscope of two powers, and also a sharp penknife.

III.—PROFESSIONAL EDUCATION.

It is clear that the main object sought to be attained by every scheme of medical education should be the preparation of the student for the duties of professional life. But it is equally clear that, with the short time at our disposal, it is impossible to do more than lay a solid foundation for the future acquisition of knowledge. It is not possible for a student during his short scholastic career to see every form of disease and to master the mode of treating it. Were it so, clinical Medicine and Surgery might well be the only subjects taught; but much must be taken for granted which has never been seen—hence the necessity for systematic books and lectures. For the same reason, bedside teaching should as much as possible assume the shape of training in method, especially as regards the various steps to be taken in coming to a correct diagnosis; whilst experience, or the guidance of others, direct or indirect, must teach the best means of remedying the diseased condition. But before entering on the practice of his profession the young medical man must procure some form of qualification which will admit him to registration as a medical practitioner. At the present time there are no fewer than nineteen bodies whose diploma or licence entitles the owner to registration. Moreover, the value of these various qualifications, as indicated by the curriculum demanded and the character of the examination, is far from being uniform. Hence it is that a great cry has gone out for uniformity as regards the lowest grade of requirement, leaving all questions as to higher degrees and every form of honours examination to be dealt with much as now. Should it be resolved to adopt that as a principle of reform, uniformity of curriculum and education will probably be obtained by some form of Conjoint Board scheme, or—which would be more feasible—by the establishment of a final State Examination for admission to the Medical Register. Meanwhile, however, the different licensing bodies exist, and exact very different amounts of class attendance, hospital practice, and even years of study. Hence it is that we must enter on the rules and regulations of the various licensing bodies in some detail, counselling the student to make his course of professional study as broad and comprehensive as possible, lest at any time he should change his mind and seek another diploma in addition to, or instead of, that he had originally in view.

The following is a list of the various licensing bodies, with the regulations attaching to each:—

(A.)
REGULATIONS OF BODIES GRANTING THE DEGREE OF DOCTOR OF MEDICINE.

1. UNIVERSITY OF OXFORD.

DEGREES IN MEDICINE.

Every student in Medicine is required to have passed all the examinations for the degree of B.A., and to reckon the time of his medical study from the final examination for Arts.

1. Candidates for the degree of B.M. are required to pass two examinations, each of which is held yearly in the end of the summer or Trinity Term, due notice being given, in the usual manner, by the Regius Professor of Medicine.

The subjects of the first examination are Human Anatomy and Physiology, Comparative Anatomy and Physiology to a certain extent, and those parts of Mechanical Philosophy, Botany, and Chemistry which illustrate Medicine. The subjects of the second examination are the Theory and Practice of Medicine (including Diseases of Women and Children), the Materia Medica, Therapeutics, Pathology, the Principles of Surgery and Midwifery, Medical Jurisprudence, and General Hygiene. Every candidate at this second examination is to be examined in two of the ancient authors, Hippocrates, Aretæus, Galen, and Celsus; or in one of those four, and in some more modern author approved by the Regius Professor,

as Morgagni, for instance, Sydenham, or Boerhaave, or some German or French medical author.

Before a candidate is admitted to the first of these two examinations, he must have spent two years in professional studies after having passed the examinations required for the degree of B.A., unless he was placed in the first or second class in the School of Natural Science, in which case, if he received from the public examiners a special certificate of his attainments in Physics, Mechanical Philosophy, Chemistry, or Botany, he may be admitted to this examination at once, and need not then be examined again in any science specified in such certificate. Nor, indeed, is he, by recent decree, re-examined in Physics or Chemistry if he has passed the Natural Science school. If he bring evidence of a first or second class in Biology, he may be admitted in the same way. But he is equally examined, nevertheless, in every case, in Anatomy and Physiology.

Before a candidate is admitted to the second examination, he must have completed sixteen terms from the date of the same testamur, and two years from the date of his testamur in the first medical examination, and must deliver to the Regius Professor satisfactory evidence of his attendance at some first-class hospital.

No one from another University can be incorporated as a graduate in Medicine without passing these two examinations, as well as having previously passed all examinations for the B.A. degree at his own University.

An examination in Preventive Medicine is held annually. Candidates must have taken the degree of B.M. at Oxford.

2. A Bachelor of Medicine wishing to proceed to the degree of Doctor is required to read publicly within the precincts of the Schools, in the presence of the Regius Professor, a dissertation composed by himself on some medical subject approved by the Professor, and to deliver to him a copy of it.

A student deciding to graduate in Medicine should proceed as follows:—1. To enter a college or hall or become an unattached student by applying to the "Delegates of Unattached Students." 2. To pass the requisite examinations in Arts. 3. After passing the requisite examination for the degree of B.A., to spend two years in study(a) prior to a scientific examination for the degree of Bachelor of Medicine; and two years more prior to the final or practical examination for the same degree. These four years of medical study may be spent either out of or in Oxford, at a first-class hospital. This degree confers the licence to practise. For the degree of Doctor in Medicine a dissertation has to be publicly read three years after the B.M.

2. UNIVERSITY OF CAMBRIDGE.

Cambridge is a better place for the purely scientific than for the student of medicine; nevertheless, even for the latter it offers many and great advantages during the earlier portion of the medical curriculum. A student may live as cheaply as in London, and there are a vast number of science scholarships to help him on his way. Nor should the advantages of a University life be neglected or overlooked.

REGULATIONS FOR DEGREES IN MEDICINE AND SURGERY.

Degree of Bachelor of Medicine.—Before a student can become a Bachelor of Medicine he must have resided nine terms (three academical years) in the University as a member of a college or as a non-collegiate student, and have graduated in Arts, or have passed the Previous Examination. This may be passed in the first term of residence, or through the "Local Examinations," or the "Oxford and Cambridge School Board Examinations," *before* coming up to the University. By the last course, time is saved, and the student is able, in his first October term, to join the Natural Science and Medical classes at the commencement of the several courses and at the commencement of the academical year.

Five years of medical study are required, unless the student has graduated with honours as Bachelor of Arts, in which case four years of medical study are deemed sufficient.

There are three examinations for M.B.

The first examination is in—1. Chemistry and other branches of Physics; 2. Botany. Before presenting himself for it the student must have attended lectures on Chemistry, including manipulations, and on Botany.

The second examination is in—1. Elements of Comparative Anatomy; 2. Human Anatomy and Physiology; 3. Pharmacy.

(a) If he have taken the higher honours in the Natural Science School, he may go in for the first M.B. examination on the first opportunity.

The student must have completed two years of medical study; and must also produce certificates of attendance on lectures on the Elements of Comparative Anatomy, on Human Anatomy and Physiology, and on Pharmacy; and of one year's hospital practice, and of one season's dissections.

The third examination is in—1. Pathology and Practice of Physic; 2. Clinical Medicine; 3. Medical Jurisprudence; 4. Principles of Surgery; and 5. Midwifery. The candidate must have completed the course of medical study, and must produce certificates of attendance on one course of lectures on each of the following subjects:—Pathological Anatomy, Principles and Practice of Physic, Clinical Medicine, Clinical Surgery, Medical Jurisprudence, and Midwifery, with attendance on ten cases of Midwifery; and of having attended the medical practice of a hospital during three years, and the surgical practice during one year; and of having been clinical clerk for six months at a recognised hospital, or of having had special charge of hospital, dispensary, or union patients under a qualified medical practitioner; and of having acquired proficiency in Vaccination.

The third examination is divided into two parts—one including Midwifery and the Principles of Surgery, the other Pathology and the Practice of Medicine and Medical Jurisprudence; and candidates are allowed to enter the two parts of the examination at separate times.

After the third examination an Act has to be kept, which consists in reading an original thesis, followed by a *vivâ voce* examination on the subject of the thesis, as well as on other subjects of the Faculty.

The Degree of Doctor of Medicine may be taken three years after M.B. An Act has to be kept, with *vivâ voce* examinations and an essay has to be written extempore. A Master of Arts of four years' standing can proceed direct to M.D. provided he produces the same certificates and passes the same examinations as for M.B.

Degree of Master in Surgery.—The candidate must have passed all the examinations for the degree of M.B., and must produce certificates of having attended a second course of lectures on Human Anatomy, one course of lectures on the Principles and Practice of Surgery, one year's clinical surgical lectures, a second season of dissections, three years' surgical practice of a recognised hospital, and of having been House-Surgeon or Dresser for six months. The subjects of the examination are—1. Surgical Anatomy; 2. Pathology and the Principles and Practice of Surgery; 3. Clinical Surgery.

All the examinations for medical degrees take place in the Michaelmas and Easter Terms.

For additional information respecting graduation in Cambridge, see the "Student's Handbook to the University" and the "Student's Guide to the University," published by Messrs. Deighton, Cambridge, price 1s. 6d. each.

---

3. UNIVERSITY OF LONDON.(a)

BACHELOR OF MEDICINE.

This University grants degrees both in Medicine and Surgery, and certificates in subjects relating to Public Health. Those available for young students are the Bachelorships of Medicine and Surgery.

Every candidate for the degree of Bachelor of Medicine shall be required—

1. To have passed the matriculation examination in this University (unless he has taken a degree in Arts in one of the Universities of Sydney, Melbourne, Calcutta, or Madras, and Latin was one of the subjects in which he passed).

2. To have passed the preliminary scientific examination (see page 302). (Candidates for the degree of M.B. are strongly recommended by the Senate to pass the preliminary scientific examination before commencing their regular medical studies.)

3. To have been engaged in his professional studies during four years subsequently to matriculation or graduation in Arts, at one or more of the medical institutions or schools recognised by this University; one year, at least, of the four to have been spent in one or more of the recognised institutions or schools in the United Kingdom.

4. To pass two examinations in Medicine.

FIRST M.B. EXAMINATION.

The first M.B. examination shall take place once in each year, and shall commence on the last Monday in July.

No candidate shall be admitted to this examination unless

he have passed the preliminary scientific examination at least one year previously, and have produced certificates to the following effect:—

1. Of having completed his nineteenth year.

2. Of having, subsequently to having passed the matriculation examination or taken a degree in Arts in one of the before-named universities, been a student during two years at one or more of the medical institutions or schools recognised by this University; and of having attended a course of lectures on each of three of the subjects in the following list:—Descriptive and Surgical Anatomy, Histology and Physiology, Pathological Anatomy, Materia Medica and Pharmacy, General Pathology, General Therapeutics, Forensic Medicine, Hygiene, Obstetric Medicine and Diseases peculiar to Women and Infants, Surgery, Medicine.

3. Of having, subsequently to having passed the matriculation examination or taken a degree in Arts, dissected during two winter sessions.

4. Of having, subsequently to having passed the matriculation examination or taken a degree in Arts, attended a course of Practical Chemistry, comprehending practical exercises in conducting the more important processes of general and pharmaceutical Chemistry; in applying tests for discovering the adulteration of articles of the Materia Medica, and the presence and nature of poisons; and in the examination of mineral waters, animal secretions, urinary deposits, calculi, etc.

5. Of having attended to Practical Pharmacy, and of having acquired a practical knowledge of the preparation of medicines.

The fee for this examination shall be £5.

Candidates shall be examined in the following subjects:—Anatomy, Physiology and Histology (candidates may be required to show their acquaintance with such parts of Comparative Anatomy and Physiology as are included in the Examination in Zoology at the preliminary scientific examination),(b) Materia Medica and Pharmaceutical Chemistry, Organic Chemistry.

SECOND M.B. EXAMINATION.(c)

No candidate shall be admitted to the second M.B. examination within two academical years of the time of his passing the first examination, nor unless he have produced certificates to the following effect:—

1. Of having passed the first M.B. examination.

2. Of having, subsequently to having passed the first M.B. examination, attended a course of lectures on each of two of the subjects comprehended in the list given above, and for which the candidate had not presented certificates at the first M.B. examination.

3. Of having conducted at least twenty labours. (Certificates on this subject will be received from any legally qualified practitioner in medicine.)

4. Of having attended the surgical practice of a recognised hospital or hospitals during two years, with clinical instruction and lectures on Clinical Surgery.

5. Of having attended the medical practice of a recognised hospital or hospitals during two years, with clinical instruction on and lectures on Clinical Medicine. N.B.—The student's attendance on the surgical and on the medical hospital practice may commence at any date after his passing the preliminary scientific examination, and may be comprised either within the same year or within different years; provided that in every case his attendance on surgical and medical hospital practice be continued for at least eighteen months subsequently to his passing the first M.B. examination. Attendance during three months in the wards of a lunatic asylum recognised by the University, with clinical instruction, may be substituted for a like period of attendance on medical hospital practice.(d)

6. Of having, after having attended surgical and medical

(b) Any candidate shall be allowed, if he so prefer, to postpone his examination in Physiology and Histology from the first M.B. examination at which he presents himself for examination in the remaining subjects until the first M.B. examination in the next or any subsequent year; but such candidate shall not be admitted to compete for honours on either occasion; and he shall not be admitted as a candidate at the second M.B. examination until after the lapse of at least twelve months from the time of his passing the examination in Physiology and Histology.

(c) Any candidate for the second M.B. examination who has passed the first M.B. examination under the former regulations will be required to have also passed the examination in Physiology at some previous first M.B. examination carried on under the present regulations; at which examination he shall not be allowed to compete for honours.

(d) The Senate regard it as highly desirable that candidates for the degree of M.B. should practically acquaint themselves with the different forms of insanity by attendance in a lunatic asylum.

hospital practice for at least twelve months subsequently to passing the first M.B. examination, attended to Practical Medicine, Surgery, or Obstetric Medicine, with special charge of patients, in a hospital, infirmary, dispensary, or parochial union, during six months, such attendance not to be counted as part of either the surgical or the medical hospital practical work prescribed in Clauses 4 and 5.

7. Of having acquired proficiency in vaccination. (Certificates on this subject will be received only from the authorised vaccinators appointed by the Privy Council.)

The candidate shall also produce a certificate of moral character from a teacher in the last school or institution at which he has studied, as far as the teacher's opportunity of knowledge has extended.

The fee for this examination shall be £5.

Candidates shall be examined in the following subjects:— GENERAL PATHOLOGY, GENERAL THERAPEUTICS AND HYGIENE, SURGERY, MEDICINE, OBSTETRIC MEDICINE, FORENSIC MEDICINE.

The examinations shall include questions in Surgical and Medical Anatomy, Pathological Anatomy, and Pathological Chemistry.

BACHELOR OF SURGERY.

No candidate shall be admitted to the examination for the degree of Bachelor of Surgery unless he have produced certificates to the following effect:—

1. Of having passed the second examination for the degree of Bachelor of Medicine in this University.

2. Of having attended a course of instruction in Operative Surgery, and of having operated on the dead subject.

The fee for this examination shall be £5.

Candidates are examined in Surgical Anatomy and surgical operations, by printed papers; examination, and report on cases, of surgical patients; performance of surgical operations upon the dead subject; application of surgical apparatus; vivâ voce interrogation.

MASTER IN SURGERY.

No candidate shall be admitted to this examination unless he have produced certificates to the following effect:—

1. Of having taken the degree of Bachelor of Surgery(e) in this University.

2. Of having attended, subsequently to having taken the degree of Bachelor of Surgery in this University—a. To Clinical or Practical Surgery during two years in a hospital or medical institution recognised by this University. b. Or to Clinical or Practical Surgery during one year in a hospital or medical institution recognised by this University; and of having been engaged during three years in the practice of his profession. s. Or of having been engaged during five years in the practice of his profession, either before or after taking the degree of Bachelor of Surgery in this University. (One year of attendance on Clinical or Practical Surgery, or two years of practice, will be dispensed with in the case of those candidates who at the B.S. examination have been placed in the first division.)

3. Of moral character, signed by two persons.

The fee for the degree of Master in Surgery shall be £5.

Candidates shall be examined in the following subjects:— LOGIC AND PSYCHOLOGY.

Names, notions, and propositions. Syllogism. Induction and subsidiary operations. The senses. The intellect. The will, including the theory of moral obligation.

Any candidate who has taken the degree either of B.A., B.Sc. (if including Branch IX.), or M.D. in this University, is exempted from this part of the examination; and any candidate who has passed the second M.B. examination may at any subsequent M.S. examination present himself for Logic and Psychology alone, if he so prefer; thereby gaining exemption, if he should pass, from examination in that subject when he presents himself to be examined for the degree of Master in Surgery.

The subjects of examination are—Logic and Psychology; a commentary on a case in Surgery, by printed papers; Surgical Anatomy and Surgery, by printed papers; examination and report on cases of surgical patients in the wards of a hospital; dissection of a surgical region or performance of surgical operations; vivâ voce interrogation.

(e) Candidates who have obtained the degree of Bachelor of Medicine previously to 1866 will be admitted to the examination for the degree of Master in Surgery without having taken the degree of Bachelor in Surgery; and in the case of such candidates, the attendance on surgical practice may commence from the date of the M.B. degree.

DOCTOR OF MEDICINE.

No candidate shall be admitted to this examination unless he have produced certificates to the following effect:—

1. Of having passed the second examination for the degree of Bachelor of Medicine in this University.

2. Of having attended, subsequently to having taken the degree of Bachelor of Medicine in this University—s. To Clinical or Practical Medicine during two years in a hospital or medical institution recognised by this University. b. Or to Clinical or Practical Medicine during one year in a hospital or medical institution recognised by this University; and of having been engaged during three years in the practice of his profession. s. Or of having been engaged during five years in the practice of his profession, either before or after taking the degree of Bachelor of Medicine in this University. (One year of attendance on Clinical or Practical Medicine, or two years of practice, will be dispensed with in the case of those candidates who at the second M.B. examination have been placed in the first division.)

3. Of moral character, signed by two persons.

The fee for the degree of Doctor of Medicine shall be £5.(f)

Candidates shall be examined in the following subjects:— LOGIC AND PSYCHOLOGY.

Names, notions, and propositions. Syllogism. Induction and subsidiary operations. The senses. The intellect. The will, including the theory of moral obligation.

Any candidate who has taken the degree either of B.A., B.Sc. (if including Branch IX.), or M.S. in this University, is exempted from this part of the examination; and any candidate who has passed the second M.B. examination may at any subsequent M.D. examination present himself for Logic and Psychology alone, if he so prefer; thereby gaining exemption, if he should pass, from examination in that subject when he presents himself to be examined for the degree of Doctor of Medicine.

The subjects of examination are—Logic and Psychology; a commentary on a case of Medicine or Obstetric Medicine, at the option of the candidate, by printed papers; Medicine, by printed papers; examination and report on cases of medical patients in the wards of a hospital; vivâ voce interrogation and demonstration from specimens and preparations.

4. UNIVERSITY OF DURHAM.

FACULTY OF MEDICINE.

There are two licences and three degrees conferred—viz., a Licence in Medicine and a Licence in Surgery, and the degrees of Bachelor in Medicine, Master in Surgery, Doctor in Medicine.

Attendance at the College of Medicine for one year is considered equivalent to one year of residence at Durham for the degree of B.A.

A certificate of proficiency in Sanitary Science is also awarded.

REGULATIONS FOR LICENCES AND DEGREES.

I. The *Licence in Medicine* may be obtained by candidates of not less than twenty-one years of age, who can produce certificates of age, of registration in the books of the General Council of Medical Education and Registration, of good moral conduct, and of attendance on such lectures and hospital practice as the Warden and Senate require.

Each candidate must have been engaged in medical and surgical study for four years after registration as a student in Medicine. One of the four years must have been spent at the University of Durham College of Medicine, Newcastle-upon-Tyne, and the other three either at the same place, or at one or more of the schools recognised by the licensing bodies named in Schedule (A) of the Medical Act of 1858 (see Medical Register).

The course of attendance on lectures and hospital practice above mentioned is the same as that required by the Royal College of Surgeons of England, together with the following extra courses:—

Botany and Therapeutics, one course, three months each; Public Health and Medicine, one course, six months each; Medical Hospital Practice and Clinical Lectures on Medicine, one winter and one summer session each.

There are two professional examinations: the first, held twice yearly, viz., in October and April; the second, twice

(f) This fee will continue to be £10 to all such as, having taken their M.B. degree under the former regulations, shall not have paid the fee of £5 at the Preliminary Scientific Examination.

yearly, in December and June. The subjects of the primary examination are Anatomy, Physiology, Botany, and Chemistry; and those of the final are Medicine, Surgery, Pathology, Materia Medica and Therapeutics, Midwifery and Diseases of Women and Children, Medical Jurisprudence, and Public Health.

Candidates for the first examination, for which they should present themselves at the end of their second winter session, must produce certificates of registration, of attendance on two courses of lectures on Anatomy, on one of Physiology, on one of Theoretical and on one of Practical Chemistry, and on one of Botany, of twelve months' Dissection, and of attendance on a course of Practical Physiology of not less than thirty demonstrations.

Candidates for the second examination must produce certificates of age, of good moral conduct, and of attendance on the remainder of the prescribed course of medical and surgical study and hospital practice as indicated above.

II. For the *Licence in Surgery* the regulations are the same as those for the Licence in Medicine. The second examination is directed more particularly to Surgery, and it may be passed at the same time as the second examination for the Licence in Medicine.

The dates of the examinations for the licences are the same as for the degrees.

III. For the *Degree of Bachelor in Medicine*, every candidate must be not less than twenty-one years of age, and must produce certificates of age, of registration as a student in Medicine in the books of the General Medical Council, of good moral conduct, and of attendance on such lectures and hospital practice as the Warden and Senate require.

In addition to the certificate of registration, the candidate must produce one or other of the following certificates:— (a) A certificate of graduation in Arts at one of the following Universities, viz.:—Oxford, Cambridge, Durham, Dublin, London, Queen's (Ireland), Edinburgh, Glasgow, St. Andrews, Aberdeen, Calcutta, Madras, Bombay, the McGill College (Montreal), and Queen's College (Kingston); or (b) a certificate of having passed the preliminary or extra-professional examination for graduation in Medicine at one of the following Universities, viz.:—London, Edinburgh, Glasgow, St. Andrews, Aberdeen, and Queen's (Ireland); or (c) a certificate of having passed the preliminary examination in Arts qualifying for the membership of the Royal College of Physicians of London; or (d) a certificate of having passed the preliminary examination in Arts for the degrees in Medicine of the University of Durham. This examination is held twice yearly, in April and September, at the same time as the registration examination. The next examination will commence on September 20, 1881, and will include the following subjects, viz.:—Necessary subjects: Greek—Xenophon's Anabasis, Book II.; Euclid—Books III. and IV. Optional subjects (of which two only must be taken): Latin—Cicero's De Amicitiâ; French—Sainte-Beuve's M. Daru; German—Freytag's Der Staat Friedrich's des Grossen; Mechanics, Hydrostatics, and Pneumatics; English History—Before the Norman Conquest. Another examination will commence on April 18, 1882.

Application for admission must be made at least one month before the examination. The fee will be £1.

Candidates who, at the commencement of their professional education, passed the Arts examination for registration only, may pass in the extra subjects required, either before or after presenting themselves for the first examination for the degree, but must do so before presenting themselves for the second examination.

For the curriculum required see Section I. It is necessary that one of the four years of professional education shall be spent in attendance at the College of Medicine, Newcastle-upon-Tyne. During the year so spent, the candidate must attend at least two courses of lectures in the winter session and two in the summer session, together with the class and test examinations held in connexion with those classes, and must also attend medical and surgical hospital practice and clinical lectures on Medicine and Surgery at the Infirmary. Candidates may fulfil this portion of the curriculum at any time before they present themselves for the second examination for the degree. They are not required to reside at Durham. They may spend the other three years of the curriculum either at Newcastle-upon-Tyne, or at one or more of the schools recognised by the licensing bodies named in Schedule (A) of the Medical Act, 1858.

There are two professional examinations—the first being held twice yearly, viz., in October and April; and the second twice yearly, in June and December. The subjects of the first examination are—Anatomy, Physiology, Chemistry, and Botany.

The subjects of the second examination are Medicine, Surgery, Midwifery and Diseases of Women and Children, Pathology, Medical Jurisprudence, Materia Medica and Therapeutics, and Public Health.

The first examination will commence on October 10, 1881, and on April 24, 1882. The second examination will commence on December 5, 1881, and on June 19, 1882.

The successful candidates for the first and second examinations for the degree of Bachelor in Medicine will be arranged in three classes, the first and second, honour, according to merit, and the third or pass in alphabetical order.

N.B.—Candidates, who have completed part of their curriculum elsewhere, may pass their first examination previous to entering at Newcastle, and are recommended to commence their year of residence at Newcastle at the beginning of the winter session.

IV. For the degree of *Doctor in Medicine*, candidates must be of not less than twenty-four years of age, must have obtained the degree of Bachelor in Medicine, and must have been engaged for at least two years subsequently to the date of acquirement of the degree of Bachelor in Medicine, in attendance on the practice of a recognised hospital, or in the Military or Naval Services, or in medical and surgical practice.

Each candidate must write an essay, based on original research or observation, on some medical subject, selected by himself and approved by the Professor of Medicine, and must pass an examination thereon, and must be prepared to answer questions on the other subjects of his curriculum so far as they are related to the subject of the essay. A gold medal will be awarded to the candidate who presents the best essay (provided that the essay is judged to be of sufficient merit). The successful candidate will be permitted to publish his essay. Candidates, for their essays, must use folio ruled paper, according to pattern, to be obtained of the Secretary of the College of Medicine. The essays will be retained by the Faculty of Medicine.

V. *For the Degree of Master in Surgery*, candidates must have passed the examination for the degree of Bachelor in Medicine, and must have attended one course of lectures on Operative Surgery. Each candidate will have an additional paper on Surgery, and will have to perform operations on the dead body, and to explain the use of instruments.

The examinations for the licences and degrees above-named are conducted at the College of Medicine, and in the Infirmary at Newcastle. Candidates are examined:—1. By printed papers of questions; 2. Practically; 3. *Viva voce.*

Every candidate who intends to present himself for any of the above-named examinations must give at least twenty-eight days' notice to the Registrar of the College, and must, at the same time, send the fee, £5, and the necessary certificates. If, after payment of the fee, a candidate withdraw his name, or fail to present himself at the examination, or fail to pass it, he shall not receive back the fee, but shall be allowed to enter for one subsequent examination of the same kind without the payment of any additional fee.

The Degree of Doctor of Medicine, for Medical Practitioners of Fifteen Years' Standing, without Residence.—The Warden and Senate of the University of Durham, with the view of affording to practitioners of fifteen years' standing an opportunity of obtaining the degree of Doctor of Medicine, have instituted a special examination, under the following regulations:—

1. That the candidate shall be registered by the General Council of Medical Education and Registration of the United Kingdom.

2. That the candidate shall have been in the active practice of his profession for fifteen years as a qualified practitioner.

3. That the candidate shall not be under forty years of age.

4. That the candidate shall produce a certificate of moral character from three registered members of the Medical profession.

5. That if the candidate shall not have passed, previous to his professional examination (in virtue of which he has been placed on the Register), an examination in Arts, he shall be required to pass an examination in Classics and Mathematics. The subjects for this examination shall be as follows:—*a.* An English essay. (A short essay on some subject to be specified at the time of the examination.) *b.* Arithmetic. *c.* Euclid—

Books I. and II. *d.* Latin—Translation from Virgil, Æneid, Books I. and II., together with grammatical questions. *e.* One of the following subjects:—(i.) Greek—Translation from Xenophon's Memorabilia, Books I. and II., with grammatical questions. (ii.) French—Translation from Voltaire's "Charles XII.," with grammatical questions. (iii.) German—Translation from Goethe's "Dichtung und Wahrheit," Book I., with grammatical questions. (iv.) Elements of Mechanics, Pneumatics, and Hydrostatics. (v.) Some treatise on Moral, Political, or Metaphysical Philosophy.

6. That if the candidate shall have passed, previous to his professional examination (in virtue of which he has been placed on the Register), a preliminary examination, he shall be required to translate into English passages in any of the parts specified below of any one of the Latin authors mentioned—Cæsar, "De 'Bello Gallico," first three books.(a) The candidate shall have an opportunity of showing proficiency in Greek, Moral Philosophy, or some modern Language.(b)

7. That the candidate shall be required to pass an examination in the following subjects:—*a.* Principles and Practice of Medicine, including Psychological Medicine and Hygiene. *b.* Principles and Practice of Surgery. *c.* Midwifery, and Diseases peculiar to Women and Children. *d.* Pathology, medical and surgical. *e.* Anatomy, medical and surgical. *f.* Medical Jurisprudence and Toxicology. *g.* Therapeutics.

8. That the fee shall be £52 10s.

9. That if the candidate shall fail to satisfy the examiners the sum of £21 shall be retained; but that if he shall again offer himself for the examination the sum of £42 only shall then be required.

An examination, in accordance with the above regulations, will commence on December 5, 1881, and on June 19, 1882, in the College of Medicine, Newcastle-upon-Tyne.

Gentlemen intending to offer themselves as candidates are requested to forward their names to Dr. Luke Armstrong, Registrar of the University of Durham College of Medicine, Newcastle-upon-Tyne, on or before November 1, 1881, or May 1, 1882, together with the fee and the before-mentioned certificates.

FEES.

For registration examination, £1; extraordinary registration examination, £2; preliminary Arts examination for degrees, £1; registration, 5s.; public examination in Medicine or in Surgery, each £5; a Licence in Medicine, £3; a Licence in Surgery, £3; a degree of Master in Surgery, £6; a degree of Bachelor in Medicine, £6; a degree of Doctor in Medicine, £5, and for practitioners of fifteen years' standing, £52 10s.; a certificate in Sanitary Science, £5 5s., and for Medical Officers of Health, £10 10s.

The Registrar or Secretary will be happy to give any information either to students or their friends. Applications with regard to examinations should be made to the Registrar, Dr. Luke Armstrong, Clayton-street West, Newcastle-upon-Tyne; all others to the Secretary, Mr. H. E. Armstrong, 6, Wentworth-place, Newcastle-upon-Tyne.

SCOTTISH UNIVERSITIES.

5. UNIVERSITY OF ST. ANDREWS.

ORDINARY DEGREES.

THE degrees in Medicine granted by the University of St. Andrews are those of Bachelor of Medicine (M.B.), Master in Surgery (C.M.), and Doctor of Medicine (M.D.).

The preliminary examination and professional curriculum and examinations for these degrees are generally the same as those of the Universities of Edinburgh, Aberdeen, and Glasgow. The following regulations, however, for candidates for the degrees of Bachelor of Medicine and Master in Surgery present some difference:—

No one shall be received as a candidate for the degree of Bachelor of Medicine or Master in Surgery unless two years at least of his four years of medical and surgical study shall have been in one or more of the following universities and colleges, viz.:—The University of St. Andrews; the University of Glasgow; the University of Aberdeen; the University

(a) The candidate may choose for himself any one of the three above-named authors on whose works he is to be examined.
(b) For these subjects no extra marks are awarded.

of Edinburgh; the University of Oxford; the University of Cambridge; Trinity College, Dublin; Queen's College, Belfast; Queen's College, Cork; and Queen's College, Galway.

The remaining years of medical and surgical study may be either in one or more of the universities and colleges above specified, or in the hospital schools of London, or in the School of the College of Surgeons in Dublin, or under such private teachers of medicine as may from time to time receive recognition from the University Court.

Attendance on the lectures of any private teacher in Edinburgh, Glasgow, or Aberdeen shall not be reckoned for graduation in St. Andrews if the fee for such lectures be of less amount than is charged for the like course of lectures in the University of Edinburgh, of Glasgow, or of Aberdeen, according as the teacher lectures in Edinburgh, Glasgow, or Aberdeen.

Fees for Graduation.—For the degree of Bachelor of Medicine £5 5s. in respect of each of the three divisions of the examination on professional subjects; and if the candidate desires to be admitted to the degree of Bachelor of Medicine only, he shall not, on admission thereto, be required to pay any further fee in addition to the £15 15s. so paid by him; but if he desires to be admitted to the degree of Master in Surgery also, he shall, on being admitted to such degree pay a further fee of £5 5s.; and every candidate for the degree of Doctor of Medicine, who has previously obtained the degree of Bachelor of Medicine, shall pay, in addition to the fees paid by him as a candidate for the degree of Bachelor of Medicine, a fee of £5 5s., exclusive of any stamp duty which may for the time be exigible.

SPECIAL DEGREES.

The degree of Doctor of Medicine may be conferred by the University of St. Andrews on any registered medical practitioner above the age of forty years, whose professional position and experience are such as, in the estimation of the University, entitle him to that degree, and who shall, on examination, satisfy the medical examiners of the sufficiency of his professional knowledge; provided always, that degrees shall not be conferred under this section to a greater number than ten in any one year.

Regulations regarding the Examination of Registered Medical Practitioners above the Age of Forty Years.—The examinations are held yearly, towards the end of April. The graduation fee is £52 10s. Candidates, whose certificates are approved of by the Medical Faculty, are enrolled for examination in order of application, provided they have complied with the under-mentioned regulations as to certificates and deposit. Candidates for graduation shall lodge, with the Professor of Medicine, the following certificates and deposit, along with their application for admission to examination:—1. Certificate of age from parish registrar, or by affidavit before a magistrate. 2. At least three certificates from medical men, of such acknowledged reputation in the profession, or of such standing in the medical schools, as shall satisfy the Senatus of the professional position and experience of the candidate. 3. A certain portion (viz., £10 10s.) of the graduation fee shall be forfeited should the candidate fail to appear at the time appointed for examination, or should he fail to graduate. 4. The examination shall be conducted in writing and *vivâ voce*, and shall include the following subjects:—(1) Materia Medica and General Therapeutics; (2) Medical Jurisprudence; (3) Practice of Medicine and Pathology; (4) Surgery; (5) Midwifery, and Diseases of Women and Children.

6. UNIVERSITY OF EDINBURGH.

This University grants degrees in Medicine, Surgery, and Science (including Health).

No one is admitted to the degree of Bachelor of Medicine or Master in Surgery who has not been engaged in medical and surgical study for four years—the medical session of each year, or *annus medicus*, being constituted by at least two courses of not less than one hundred lectures each, or by one such course, and two courses of not less than fifty lectures each; with the exception of the Clinical Courses, in which lectures are to be given at least twice a week during the prescribed periods.

Every candidate for the degrees of M.B. and C.M. must give sufficient evidence by certificates—

1. That he has studied each of the following departments of medical science—viz., Anatomy, Chemistry, Materia Medica, Institutes of Medicine or Physiology, Practice of Medicine, Surgery, Midwifery and the Diseases peculiar to Women and Children (two courses of Midwifery of three

months each being reckoned equivalent to a six months' course, provided different departments of Obstetric Medicine be taught in each of the courses), General Pathology (or, in schools where there is no such course, a three months' course of lectures on Morbid Anatomy, together with a supplemental course of Practice of Medicine or Clinical Medicine), during courses including not less than one hundred lectures; Practical Anatomy, a course of the same duration as those of not less than one hundred lectures above described; Practical Chemistry, three months; Practical Midwifery, three months at a midwifery hospital, or a certificate of attendance on six cases from a registered medical practitioner; Clinical Medicine, Clinical Surgery, courses of the same duration as those of not less than one hundred lectures above prescribed, or two courses of three months' lectures being given at least twice a week; Medical Jurisprudence, Botany, Natural History (including Zoology), during courses including not less than fifty lectures.

2. That he has attended for at least two years the medical and surgical practice of a general hospital which accommodates not fewer than eighty patients, and possesses a distinct staff of physicians and surgeons.

3. That he has been engaged, for at least six months, by apprenticeship or otherwise, in compounding and dispensing drugs at the laboratory of a hospital, dispensary, member of a surgical college or faculty, licentiate of the London or Dublin Society of Apothecaries, or a member of the Pharmaceutical Society of Great Britain.

4. That he has attended for at least six months, by apprenticeship or otherwise, the out-practice of a hospital, or the practice of a dispensary, physician, surgeon, or member of the London or Dublin Society of Apothecaries.

The studies of candidates for the degrees of Bachelor of Medicine and Master in Surgery are subject to the following regulations :—.

1. One of the four years of medical and surgical study required must be in the University of Edinburgh.

2. Another of such four years of medical and surgical study must be either in the University of Edinburgh, or in some other university entitled to give the degree of Doctor of Medicine.

3. Attendance during at least six winter months on the medical or surgical practice of a general hospital which accommodates at least eighty patients, and, during the same period, on a course of Practical Anatomy, may be reckoned as one of such four years, and to that extent shall be held equivalent to one year's attendance on courses of lectures as above prescribed.

4. One year's attendance on the lectures of teachers of Medicine in the hospital schools of London, or in the school of the College of Surgeons in Dublin, or of such teachers of Medicine in Edinburgh or elsewhere as shall from time to time be recognised by the University Court, may be reckoned as one of such four years, and to that extent shall be held as attendance on courses of lectures as above prescribed.

5. Candidates may, to the extent of four of the departments of medical study required, attend in such year or years of their medical and surgical studies, as may be most convenient to them, the lectures of the extra-academical teachers of Medicine specified in the foregoing Sub-section 4. Students of Medicine in the London Schools and in the School of the College of Surgeons in Dublin can obtain there two anni medici out of the four required for the Edinburgh degree in Medicine. Courses of lectures in these schools are regarded as equivalent to lectures on the corresponding subjects in this University, except Materia Medica and Midwifery, which, being only three months' courses in them, are not equivalent. One annus medicus may be constituted by attendance on Practical Anatomy and Hospital Practice during the winter session. Another annus medicus by attending either (a) Full Winter courses on any two of the following subjects :—Anatomy, Physiology, Chemistry, Pathology, Surgery, Medicine, Clinical Surgery, Clinical Medicine; or (b) on one such course and three months' courses on any two of the following subjects—Botany, Practical Chemistry, Natural History, Medical Jurisprudence. If the student selects the arrangement prescribed in (a), certificates of attendance on either a third winter course, or a third three months' course, will also be accepted by this University. The other subjects, and the additional courses, not given in London or Dublin, required for the degrees of the University, will have to be attended at this University. In provincial schools, where there are no lecturers recognised by the University Court, a candidate can have only one annus medicus, and this is constituted by attendance on a qualified hospital along with a course of Practical Anatomy.

6. All candidates not students of the University availing themselves of the permission to attend the lectures of extra-academical teachers in Edinburgh must, at the commencement of each year of such attendance, enrol their names in a book to be kept by the University for that purpose, paying a fee of the same amount as the matriculation fee paid by students of the University, and having, in respect of such payment, a right to the use of the library of the University.

7. The fee for attendance on the lectures of an extra-academical teacher in Edinburgh, with a view to graduation, must be of the same amount as that exigible by medical professors in the University. (The fee must be paid at the commencement of the course.)

8. No teacher is recognised who is at the same time a teacher of more than one of the prescribed branches of study, except in those cases where professors in the University are at liberty to teach two branches.

9. It is not necessary for any teacher, attendance on whose lectures was recognised before 1881 for the purposes of graduation in the University, to obtain a new recognition from the University Court; and attendance on the lectures of every such teacher will continue to be recognised as heretofore.

10. It is in the power of the University Court, if they shall see cause, at any time to withdraw or suspend the recognition of any teacher or teachers.

Every candidate must deliver, before March 31 of the year in which he proposes to graduate, to the Dean of the Faculty of Medicine—

1. A declaration, in his own handwriting, that he has completed his twenty-first year (or that he will have done so on or before the day of graduation), and that he will not be, on the day of graduation, under articles of apprenticeship to any surgeon or other master.

2. A statement of his studies, as well in Literature and Philosophy as in Medicine, accompanied with proper certificates.

Each candidate is examined, both in writing and vivâ voce—first, on Chemistry, Botany, and Natural History; secondly, on Anatomy, Institutes of Medicine, Materia Medica (including Practical Pharmacy), and Pathology; thirdly, on Surgery, Practice of Medicine, Midwifery, and Medical Jurisprudence; fourthly, clinically on Medicine and on Surgery in a Hospital. The examinations on Anatomy, Chemistry, Institutes of Medicine, Botany, Natural History, Materia Medica, and Pathology are conducted, as far as possible, by demonstrations of objects placed before the candidates.

The degree of Doctor of Medicine may be conferred on any candidate who has obtained the degree of Bachelor of Medicine, and is of the age of twenty-four years, and produces a certificate of having been engaged, subsequently to his having received the degree of Bachelor of Medicine, for at least two years in attendance on a hospital, or in the Military or Naval Medical Services, or in medical and surgical practice: provided always that the degree of Doctor of Medicine shall not be conferred on any person, unless he be a graduate of Arts in one of the universities of England, Scotland, or Ireland, or of such other universities as are above specified, or unless he shall, before or at the time of his obtaining the degree of Bachelor of Medicine, or thereafter, have passed a satisfactory examination in Greek, and in Logic or Moral Philosophy, and in one at least of the following subjects—namely, French, German, higher Mathematics, and Natural Philosophy; and provided also that the candidate for the degree of Doctor of Medicine shall submit to the Medical Faculty a thesis, certified by him to have been composed by himself, and which shall be approved by the Faculty, on any branch of knowledge comprised in the professional examinations for the degree of Bachelor of Medicine, which he may have made a subject of study after having received that degree. The candidate must lodge his thesis with the Dean on or before April 30 of the year in which he proposes to graduate. No thesis will be approved by the Medical Faculty which does not contain either the results of original observations in Practical Medicine, Surgery, Midwifery, or some of the sciences embraced in the curriculum for the Bachelor's degree; or else a full digest and critical exposition of the opinions and researches of others on the subject selected by the candidate, accompanied by precise references to the publications quoted, so that due verification may be facilitated.

Candidates, settled for a period of years in foreign parts, who have complied with all the regulations for the degree of M.D. (under the new statutes), but who cannot appear personally to receive the degree, may, on satisfying the Senatus to that effect, by production of sufficient official testimonials, have the degree conferred on them in absence.

NOTICES TO CANDIDATES FOR GRADUATION IN MEDICINE.

1. An annus medicus is constituted by at least two winter courses of one hundred lectures each, or by one such course, and two summer courses of fifty lectures each, all being duly certified.

2. Four anni medici are required for graduates in Medicine. Two at least of these years must be passed at a university which grants degrees in Medicine, one of the two being at Edinburgh.

3. One or two of the anni medici may be taken at qualified extra-academical schools, in the manner stated in the succeeding paragraph :

4. In University College, in King's College, in the hospital schools of London, in the extra-academical School of Edinburgh, in the School of the College of Surgeons of Dublin, and in certain medical schools where at least two lecturers have been qualified by the University Court, a candidate may make two anni medici—one of which must be constituted by hospital attendance and Practical Anatomy, and the other by at least two courses of one hundred lectures, or one such course, and two courses of fifty lectures. The classes at these schools only qualify to the extent of four, and one of the four must be Practical Anatomy.

5. In provincial schools where there are no lecturers qualified by the University Court, a candidate can make one annus medicus only, and this is constituted by attendance on a qualified hospital, along with a course of Practical Anatomy.

The Fees are—For the degree of M.B., three Examinations, £5 5s. each, £15 15s.; for the degree of C.M., £5 5s. additional; for the degree of M.D., £5 5s. additional to that for M.B., exclusive of £10 Government stamp.

The fees for C.M. and M.D. are required to be paid on or before July 15.

Note.—Total fees and stamp for graduating as M.D. only, by regulations, for students commencing before February, 1881, £25.

N.B.—The above fees include all charges for the diplomas.

RIGHTS OF THE MEDICAL GRADUATES OF SCOTLAND ACCORDING TO THE MEDICAL ACT.

Before the passing of the Medical Act of 1858, the degree of Doctor of Medicine granted by the universities of Scotland (as the possessor underwent a complete education and examination in all departments of Physic and Surgery), qualified the graduate to practise every branch of the medical profession throughout Scotland. One principal purpose of the Medical

Act was to extend local rights of practice over the whole of her Majesty's dominions. But according to the hitherto accepted reading of a dubious clause in the Act, no one can practise both Medicine and Surgery without possessing two distinct diplomas—one for Medicine, and another for Surgery. The universities were thus compelled, in justice to their graduates, to give them the additional title of Master in Surgery, not as implying any additional study or examination, but as declaring more distinctly their qualifications, and to permit registration as regularly qualified practitioners in the whole field of their professional education. The Secretary for War some time ago issued an order that candidates for admission into the Medical Service of the Army should obtain their qualifications in Physic and Surgery from two different sources; the effect of which would have been to prevent any one university from qualifying for this purpose. The Scottish Universities' Commissioners, recognising the serious evils of such a system, followed up a remonstrance which had been offered on the part of the University of Edinburgh, and obtained the rescinding of all restrictions in the source of qualification. Consequently, any single university in Scotland can now qualify candidates for the military service as well as for any other public medical service in the country.

The Medical Faculty have resolved that the written and oral examinations on Chemistry, Botany, and Natural History, in October, 1881, and April, 1882, shall be restricted in the following manner:—

1. *Chemistry.*—Classification of elements; general laws of chemical combination and action, as illustrated in the simpler compounds of the more commonly occurring elements; symbolic notation. Preparation and properties of the non-metallic elements and their chief compounds. Classification and general properties of acids, bases, and salts—electrolysis of salts. Oxygen, ozone, oxidation, and reduction. Hydrogen, water, peroxide of hydrogen, chlorine, hydrochloric acid, hypochlorites, chlorates, perchlorites, bromine, hydrobromic acid, bromates, iodine, hydriodic acid, iodates, periodates, fluorine, hydrofluoric acid. Sulphur, sulphuretted hydrogen, oxides of sulphur, sulphites, sulphates, hyposulphites, chlorides of sulphur, chloride of sulphuryl, nitrogen, the atmosphere, oxides of nitrogen, nitrates, nitrites, ammonia, ammonia salts, phosphorus, oxides of phosphorus, chlorides and oxychloride of phosphorus, phosphates, phosphites, hypophosphites, boron, boracic acid, borates, fluoride of boron, silicon, silica, silicates, chloride of silicon, fluoride of silicon, hydrofluosilicic acid. Carbon, oxides of carbon, carbonates, phosgene. Classification of carbon compounds. Marsh gas and its homologues. Methylic and ethylic alcohols and ethers. Methylamine, dimethylamine, trimethylamine, tetramethylammonium. Formic and acetic acids, aldehyde, acetone, olefiant gas, oxalic acid, lactic acid, tartaric acid, citric acid. Fats and oils, saponification, glycerine, cellulose, sugars, starch. Products of distillation of wood and of coal. Coal-gas, coal-tar, benzol, benzoic acid, oil of bitter almonds, hydrocyanic acid, cyanides, cyanates, sulphocyanates, urea. The following metals, their oxides, sulphides, and more important salts :—Potassium, sodium, magnesium, calcium, strontium, barium, aluminium, zinc, cadmium, manganese, chromium, iron, nickel, cobalt, bismuth, lead, copper, mercury, silver, tin, gold, platinum, antimony, arsenic. Simple qualitative analysis. [*The examination in analysis is conducted practically.*]

2. *Botany.*—Candidates to be examined on the following subjects :— A. Structural Botany : (*a.*) Histology—Structural elements, their general character, chemical and anatomical. General structure of roots, stems, and leaves. (*b.*) Organography—General characters and modes of arrangement of the nutritive and reproductive organs, root, stem, leaf, floral envelopes, stamen, pistil, fruit, and seed. Vernation, phyllotaxis, inflorescence, arrangement and insertion of floral parts, placentation. B. Physiological Botany : (*a.*) Nutrition—Absorption, elaboration of organic out of inorganic material, digestion, metastasis, respiration, movement of the sap, growth. (*b.*) Reproduction—Fertilisation and embryogeny in phanerogamia, and the higher cryptogamia; germination; asexual reproduction or gemmation. C. Systematic Botany : The candidate may be asked to define given sub-kingdoms, divisions, classes, series, or sub-classes, or to refer given plants to such groups. He may also be examined on any of the following natural orders :—Ranunculaceæ, Papaveraceæ, Cruciferæ, Violaceæ, Caryophyllaceæ, Malvaceæ, Leguminosæ, Rosaceæ, Onagraceæ, Umbelliferæ, Dipsacaceæ, Compositæ, Valerianaceæ, Campanulaceæ (including Lobeliaceæ), Primulaceæ, Solanaceæ (including Atropaceæ), Scrophulariaceæ, Labiatæ, Polygonaceæ, Coniferæ, Liliaceæ, Amaryllidaceæ, Iridaceæ, Orchidaceæ, Graminaceæ, Filices, Musci.

3. *Zoology and Comparative Anatomy.*—The general characters of the animal kingdom, and the general structure and organisation of animals; principles of zoological classification; general plan of structure, and physiology of the types : Protozoa, Porifera, Cœlenterata, Echinodermata, Vermes, Articulata, Mollusca, and Vertebrata. The special distinctive characters of the following groups, with a knowledge of familiar examples of each, and the conditions and circumstances under which they occur (candidates will be required to refer any specimens shown to them by the examiner for this purpose to their respective groups) :—Rhizopoda, Infusoria; Porifera silicea, calcarea; Zoantharia, Alcyonaria, Hydrozoa, Echinidea, Asteridea, Crinoidea; Platyelmia, Nematelmia, Annelida; Crustacea, Arachnida, Myriapoda, Insecta; Lamellibranchiata, Gastropoda, Cephalopoda; Pisces, Amphibia, Reptilia, Aves, Mammalia.

ARRANGEMENTS FOR THE PRELIMINARY EXAMINATIONS IN GENERAL EDUCATION.

The preliminary examinations in general education are held in the Upper Library Hall, and students matriculated for the academic year are admitted on presenting their matriculation tickets at the door. Students matriculated for the summer only and non-matriculated students pay a fee of 10s. each, and are admitted on showing their receipts. Those who

pay the fee in March will be admitted to the examination in October without further payment. Payment in October does not exempt from payment in March. The academic year is reckoned from November 1 to November 1.

Candidates are required to enter their names *in full*, and at the same time to mention the subject or subjects in which they offer themselves for examination. They are also required to state whether they have appeared for any preliminary or professional examinations at this University.

Any candidate who cannot appear personally at the time fixed to enter his name and pay the fee, must complete the schedule required for the purpose, and transmit it with an order for the fee to the Clerk of the University.

In conformity with Section I. of the Statutes, examinations on the preliminary branches of extra-professional education will take place on Tuesday, Wednesday, Thursday, and Friday, October 4, 5, 6, and 7, 1881; and on Tuesday, Wednesday, Thursday, and Friday, March 14, 15, 16, and 17, 1882.

Examination on Tuesdays.—Arithmetic, 9 to 11 a.m.; Mathematics (Euclid, Algebra), 11.30 a.m. to 1.30 p.m.; and Higher Mathematics, 2 to 4 p.m.

Examination on Wednesdays.—English, 9 to 11 a.m.; Natural Philosophy, 11.30 a.m. to 1.30 p.m. Mechanics, 2 to 4 p.m.

Examination on Thursdays.—Latin, 9 to 11 a.m.; Logic, 11.30 a.m. to 1.30 p.m.; Moral Philosophy, 2 to 4 p.m.

Examination on Fridays.—Greek, 9 to 11 a.m.; French, 11.30 a.m. to 1.30 p.m.; German, 2 to 4 p.m.

7. UNIVERSITY OF GLASGOW.—FACULTY OF MEDICINE.

Three medical degrees are conferred by this University, viz. :—Bachelor of Medicine (M.B.), Master in Surgery (C.M.), and Doctor of Medicine (M.D.); all of which are recognised by the Medical Act as qualifying for practice throughout the British dominions.

The degree of Bachelor of Medicine may be obtained by candidates of the age of twenty-one years who have complied with the regulations as to education and examination. The degree of Master in Surgery is only conferred upon those who at the same time obtain the Bachelorship of Medicine; and the degree of Doctor of Medicine may be conferred on candidates of not less than twenty-four years of age who have obtained the Bachelorship two or more years previously, and have fulfilled certain conditions to be afterwards mentioned.

The medical curriculum is as nearly as possible the same as that in the University of Edinburgh.

By an order of Her Majesty in Council, dated August 13, 1877, the following are the arrangements for Professional Examinations :—

1. Every candidate for the degrees of Bachelor of Medicine and Master in Surgery shall be examined both in writing and *vivâ voce*—first on Chemistry, Botany, and Natural History; second, on Anatomy and Physiology; third, on Regional Anatomy, Materia Medica and Pharmacy, and Pathology; and fourth, on Surgery, Clinical Surgery, Medicine, Clinical Medicine, Therapeutics, Midwifery, and Medical Jurisprudence. The Examination in Chemistry shall include Practical Chemistry; and the Examinations in Anatomy and Physiology shall include Practical Anatomy, Histology, and Practical Physiology; and the Examination in Surgery shall include Operative Surgery.

2. Students may appear for examination in the first of the foregoing divisions of subjects who have completed their attendance on the required courses during one winter and two summer sessions, or during one summer and two winter sessions.

3. Students who have passed the first examination may appear for examination in the second division of subjects after having completed their attendance on the requisite courses (including those of the subjects of examination), and after the lapse of two winter and three summer sessions, or of three winter and two summer sessions, from the time of the commencement of their studies.

4. Students who have passed the two previous examinations may appear for examination in the third division of subjects at any of the terms fixed for examinations by the Senate, after the conclusion of the third winter's session of attendance upon medical classes (including those of the required subjects).

5. Students who have passed the examinations in the

subjects of the three previous divisions may appear for examination in the subjects of the fourth division at the first term for the final examination after the conclusion of their curriculum of study.

DEGREE OF DOCTOR OF MEDICINE.

The degree of Doctor of Medicine may be conferred on any candidate who shall produce evidence—a, that he is not less than twenty-four years of age; b, that he has obtained the Bachelorship two or more years previously; c, that he possesses a degree in Arts, or has, in addition to the preliminary examination in general education required for the Bachelorship, also passed an examination in Greek, and Logic or Moral Philosophy, together with any one of the other optional subjects included in the second part of the subjects of general education; d, that he has been engaged in professional study or avocation for two years after having obtained the Bachelorship. He must also lodge an inaugural dissertation, certified by him to have been composed by himself, on any subject included in the branches of knowledge embraced in the professional curriculum. Theses for the degree of M.D. must be lodged with Mr. Moir, the Assistant Clerk of Senate, on or before March 20, June 20, or October 20. No thesis will be approved unless it gives evidence of original observation, or, if it deals with the researches of others, gives a full statement of the literature of the question, with accurate references and critical investigation of the views or facts cited; mere compilations will in no case be accepted.

The fees for degrees are the same as in Edinburgh.

The Examinations in General Education take place twice yearly—viz., in October and March. The examinations for session 1881-82 will be held on Wednesday, Thursday, Friday, and Saturday, October 5, 6, 7, and 8, 1881, and Wednesday, Thursday, Friday, and Saturday, March 29, 30, and 31, and April 1, 1882. Those who intend to present themselves for either of these examinations are required to send in their names to the Assistant Clerk of Senate on or before September 21 or March 15. Those who are not matriculated students of the University pay a fee of 10s. on first entering their names for this examination.

The Professional Examinations are held at the following periods, viz.:—The first, second, and third in October and April (in 1881-82, beginning on October 11 and April 7); and the fourth in June and July (beginning on June 9, 1882).

---

8. UNIVERSITY OF ABERDEEN.

The following are the degrees in Medicine granted by this University—namely, Bachelor of Medicine (M.B.), Master in Surgery (C.M.), and Doctor of Medicine (M.D.).

The preliminary examination and professional curriculum, and examination for the degrees of M.B., C.M., and M.D., being in conformity with the Ordinances of the Scotch Universities Commissioners, are nearly the same as those of the Universities of Edinburgh, Glasgow, and St. Andrews.

The studies of candidates for the degrees of Bachelor of Medicine and Master in Surgery are subject to these regulations:—

One at least of the four years of medical and surgical study must be in the University of Aberdeen.

Another of such four years must be either in this University or in some other University entitled to give the degree of Doctor of Medicine.

FEES FOR GRADUATION.

1. Each candidate for the degree of M.B. shall pay a fee of £5 5s. in respect of each of the three professional examinations.

2. If the candidate desires to be admitted to the degree of Bachelor of Medicine only, he shall not, on admission thereto, be required to pay any further fee in addition to the £15 15s. so paid by him; but if he desires to be admitted to the degree of Master in Surgery also, he shall, on being admitted to such degree, pay a further fee of £5 5s.

3. And every candidate for the degree of Doctor of Medicine shall pay, in addition to the fees paid by him for the degree of Bachelor of Medicine, a fee of £5 5s., exclusive of any stamp duty which may for the time be exigible.

EXEMPTION FROM THE FOREGOING REGULATIONS.

Students who shall have begun their medical studies before the first Tuesday of November, 1861, are entitled to appear for examination for the degree of M.D. after four years' study, two of which must have been at the University of Aberdeen.

IRISH UNIVERSITIES.

9. UNIVERSITY OF DUBLIN.

DEGREES AND LICENCES IN MEDICINE AND SURGERY.

THE degrees and licences in Medicine, Surgery, and Midwifery granted by the University are—1. Bachelor of Medicine; 2. Doctor of Medicine; 3. Bachelor in Surgery; 4. Master in Surgery; 5. Master in Obstetric Science; and Licences in Medicine, Surgery, and Obstetric Science. Besides these degrees and licences, the University also grants a qualification in State Medicine.

UNIVERSITY DEGREES.

1. *Bachelor in Medicine.*—A candidate for the degree of Bachelor in Medicine must be a graduate in Arts, and may obtain the degree of Bachelor in Medicine at the same commencements as those at which he receives his degree of B.A., or at any subsequent commencements, provided the requisite medical education shall have been completed, and the necessary examinations passed. The medical education of a Bachelor in Medicine is of four years' duration, and comprises attendance on one course of lectures on each of the following subjects:—Winter: Anatomy, Practical Anatomy, Theoretical and Operative Surgery, Chemistry, Institutes of Medicine (Physiology), Practice of Medicine, Midwifery. Summer: Botany, Institutes of Medicine (Practical Histology), Comparative Anatomy, Pharmacology and Therapeutics, Medical Jurisprudence, Practical Chemistry. Term Courses: Michaelmas Term—Heat; Hilary Term—Electricity and Magnetism. Six months' Dissections are also required.

Hospital attendance includes—1. Three courses of nine months' attendance on the clinical lectures of Sir Patrick Dun's or other metropolitan hospital recognised by the Board of Trinity College. 2. A certificate of personal attendance on fever cases, with names and dates of cases. The following hospitals, in addition to Sir Patrick Dun's Hospital, are recognised by the Board:—Meath Hospital, House of Industry Hospitals, Dr. Steevens' Hospital, Jervis-street Infirmary, City of Dublin Hospital, Mercer's Hospital, St. Vincent's Hospital, Adelaide Hospital, Mater Misericordiæ Hospital, St. Mark's Ophthalmic Hospital, the National Eye and Ear Infirmary. Students who shall have diligently attended the practice of a recognised county infirmary for two years previous to the commencement of their metropolitan medical studies are allowed, on special application to the Board of Trinity College, to count those two years as equivalent to one year spent in a recognised metropolitan hospital. N.B.—The recognition of these schools and hospitals is conditional on their students being furnished with *bonâ fide* certificates of an amount of regular attendance equivalent to that required by the University—viz., three-fourths of the entire number of lectures in each course.

The qualifying course of Practical Midwifery consists of six months' instruction, including clinical lectures. Certificates of Practical Midwifery are received from (1) the Rotunda Hospital, (2) the Coombe Hospital, (3) Sir Patrick Dun's Hospital Maternity, and (4) Dr. Steevens' Hospital Maternity.

DEGREE EXAMINATIONS.

1. *Bachelor in Medicine.*—The candidate for the M.B. examination must have previously passed the Previous Medical Examination in all the subjects; and have lodged with the Medical Registrar, on a certain day to be duly advertised before the examination, certificates of attendance upon all the courses of study prescribed in the preceding curriculum. Candidates are then required to pass a final examination in the following subjects:—Physiological Anatomy, Practice of Medicine, Surgery, Midwifery, Medical Jurisprudence, Institutes of Medicine (Pathology and Hygiene), Therapeutics. The fee for the *Licet ad Examinandum* is £5. The fee for the degree of M.B. is £11.

2. *Doctor in Medicine.*—A Doctor in Medicine must be a Bachelor in Medicine of three years' standing, or have been qualified to take the degree of Bachelor in Medicine for three years. He must also read a thesis publicly before the Regius Professor of Physic, or must undergo an examination before the Regius Professor of Physic, according to regulations to be approved by the Provost and Senior Fellows. Total amount of fees for this degree, £13.

3. *Bachelor in Surgery.*—A Bachelor in Surgery must be a Bachelor in Arts, and have spent four years in the study of Surgery and Anatomy. He must also have passed the M.B.

examination, before presenting himself at the B.Ch. examination, having previously completed the prescribed curriculum of study. The curriculum comprises the following, in addition to the complete course for the degree of Bachelor in Medicine:—Operative Surgery, one course; Dissections, two courses; Ophthalmic Surgery, one course. Candidates are required to perform surgical operations on the dead subject, and will also be examined in Bandaging and Minor Surgery, and in Surgical Pathology. Candidates for the degree of Bachelor in Surgery, who have already passed the examination for the degree of Bachelor in Medicine, will be examined in Anatomy and Surgery only. Fee for the *Liceat ad Examinandum*, £5. Fee for the degree of Bachelor in Surgery, £5.

4. *Master in Surgery.*—A Master in Surgery must be a Bachelor in Surgery of three years' standing, or have been qualified to take the degree of Bachelor in Surgery for three years; and must read a thesis publicly before the Regius Professor of Surgery, or undergo an examination before the Regius Professor, according to Regulations to be approved by the Provost and Senior Fellows. Fee for the degree of Master in Surgery, £11.

5. *Master in Obstetric Science.*—A Master in Obstetric Science must have passed the M.B. and B.Ch. examinations, and produce certificates of having completed the following curriculum:—1. One winter course in Midwifery. 2. Six months' practice in a recognised lying-in hospital or maternity. 3. A summer course in Obstetric Medicine and Surgery. 4. Two months' practice in the Cow-pock Institution. Existing graduates in Medicine, of the standing of M.D., are entitled to present themselves for examination without complying with Regulations 3 and 4. Fee for the degree of Master in Obstetric Science, £5.

UNIVERSITY LICENCES.

Candidates for the licences in Medicine, Surgery, or Obstetric Science must be matriculated in Medicine, and must have completed two years in Arts, and four years in Medical studies.

1. *Licentiate in Medicine.*—The medical course and examination necessary for the licence in Medicine are the same as for the degree of M.B. A Licentiate in Medicine, on completing his course in Arts, and proceeding to the Degree of B.A., may become a Bachelor in Medicine on paying the degree fees without further examination in Medicine. Fee for the *Liceat ad Examinandum*, £5. Fee for the licence in Medicine, £5.

2. *Licentiate in Surgery.*—The surgical course and examination necessary for the licence in Surgery are the same as for the degree of Bachelor in Surgery. Fee for the *Liceat ad Examinandum*, £5. Fee for the licence in Surgery, £5.

3. *Licentiate in Obstetric Science.*—The course and examination for the licence in Obstetric Science are the same as for the degree in Obstetric Science. Fee for the licence in Obstetric Science, £5.

10. QUEEN'S UNIVERSITY IN IRELAND.

We still continue to print the regulations of the Queen's University in Ireland, though that has been abolished, and the Royal Irish University has taken its place. We do so because the Queen's Colleges still give their allegiance to the Queen's University, and the Royal University is not yet in working order.

This University confers the degrees of M.D. and M.Ch., and a diploma in Midwifery. Students who wish to obtain the degrees or diploma of the Queen's University must be matriculated students of one of the Queen's Colleges at Belfast, Cork, or Galway, and must pursue the courses of study prescribed by the Senate of the University.

Each candidate for the degree of Doctor in Medicine or Master in Surgery is required—1. To have passed in one of the Colleges of the Queen's University the entrance examination in Arts, and to have been admitted a matriculated student of the University. 2. To have attended in one of the Queen's Colleges lectures on one modern continental language for six months, and lectures on Natural Philosophy for six months. 3. To have also attended, in some one of the Queen's Colleges, at least two of the courses of lectures marked below with an asterisk. For the remainder of the courses, authenticated certificates will be received from the professors or lecturers in universities, colleges, or schools recognised by the Senate of the Queen's University in Ireland. 4. To pass the University examinations—the first and second University examinations, and the degree examination. The curriculum

extends over at least four years, and is divided into periods of at least two years each. Candidates are recommended to pass the matriculation examination prior to entering on the second period. It is recommended that the first period shall comprise attendance on the following courses of medical lectures:—*Chemistry; *Botany, with Herborisations for practical study, and Zoology; *Anatomy and Physiology; *Practical Anatomy; *Materia Medica and Pharmacy. And that the second period shall comprise attendance on the following courses of medical lectures:—Anatomy and Physiology (second course), Practical Anatomy (second course), *Theory and Practice of Surgery, *Midwifery, *Theory and Practice of Medicine, *Medical Jurisprudence. In addition to the above courses of lectures, candidates shall have attended during either the first or second period, a course of lectures on a modern continental language (in one of the colleges of the University), and Experimental Physics (in one of the colleges of the University). Also, during the first period—Practical Chemistry, (in a recognised laboratory), and medico-chirurgical hospital (recognised by the Senate) containing at least sixty beds, together with the clinical lectures therein delivered, at least two each week—a winter session of six months. And during the second period—Practical Midwifery, at a recognised midwifery hospital, with the clinical lectures therein delivered, for a period of three months, or of having attended a midwifery dispensary for the same period, or of having attended ten cases of labour under the superintendence of the medical officer of any hospital or dispensary where cases of labour are treated; medico-chirurgical hospital (recognised by the Senate) containing at least sixty beds, together with the clinical lectures therein delivered, eighteen months, including either three winter sessions of six months each, or two winter sessions of six months each, and two summer sessions of three months each. Medical examinations are held in June, and in September and October. The June examinations are pass examinations. Both honour and pass examinations are held in September. Each candidate for examination in June must forward to the Secretary, on or before May 20, notice of his intention to offer himself as a candidate, along with his certificates; and each candidate for examination in September must forward similar notice along with his certificates, before August 20.

(B.)

BODIES GIVING LICENCES OR OTHER FORMS OF QUALIFICATION NOT BEING DEGREES IN MEDICINE.

A.—England.

1. THE ROYAL COLLEGE OF PHYSICIANS, LONDON.

The following very important modifications have been made in the regulations for the Licence of this great body. They have reference to all students beginning their studies after March, 1880.

THE Licence of this College is a qualification to practise Medicine, Surgery, and Midwifery, and is recognised by the Poor-law Board as a qualification in Surgery as well as in Medicine.

The College will, under its charter, grant licences to practise Physic, including therein the practice of Medicine, Surgery, and Midwifery (which licences are not to extend to make the Licentiates Members of the Corporation), to persons who shall conform to the following by-laws.

I.—Every candidate for the College licence (except when otherwise provided by the by-laws) who shall commence professional study after March 25, 1880, will be required, at the times prescribed in Section II. for the respective examinations, to produce satisfactory evidence:—

1. Of having passed, before the commencement of professional study, one of the preliminary examinations on subjects of general education recognised by the General Medical Council.

2. Of having been registered as a medical student in the manner prescribed by the General Medical Council, at least forty-five months previously to admission to the third or final examination, unless specially exempted. *Note A.*—Professional studies commenced before registration, except in the cases of Chemistry, Materia Medica, Botany, and Pharmacy, will not be recognised.

3. Of having been engaged in professional studies at least forty-five months, during which not less than three winter sessions and two summer sessions shall have been passed at one or more of the medical schools recognised by the College. One winter session and two summer sessions

may be passed in one or more of the following ways:—a. Attending the practice of a hospital, infirmary, or other institution duly recognised as affording satisfactory opportunities for professional study. b. Receiving instruction as a pupil of a legally qualified practitioner having opportunities of imparting a practical knowledge of Medicine, Surgery, or Midwifery. c. Attending lectures on one or more of the required subjects of professional study at a duly recognised place of instruction.

4. Of having received instruction in Chemistry, including Chemical Physics, meaning thereby heat, light, and electricity.

5. Of having received instruction in Practical Chemistry.

6. Of having received instruction in Materia Medica.

7. Of having received instruction in Botany.

8. Of having received instruction in Practical Pharmacy. Note B.—By this is meant instruction in Practical Pharmacy by a registered medical practitioner, or by a member of the Pharmaceutical Society of Great Britain, or in a public hospital, infirmary, or dispensary.

9. Of having attended a course of lectures on Anatomy.

10. Of having performed Dissections during not less than twelve months.

11. Of having attended a course of lectures on General Anatomy and Physiology.

12. Of having attended a separate practical course of General Anatomy and Physiology.

13. Of having attended a course of lectures on the Principles and Practice of Medicine.

14. Of having attended a course of lectures on the Principles and Practice of Surgery.

15. Of having attended a course of lectures on Midwifery and Diseases peculiar to Women. A certificate must also be produced of attendance on not less than twenty labours, which certificate must be signed by one or more legally qualified practitioners.

16. Of having undergone systematic practical instruction in the departments of Medicine, Surgery, and Obstetric Medicine. Note C.—Under this clause the candidate will be required to show that he has been personally exercised in practical details, such as—(1) The application of anatomical facts to the investigation of disease; (2) the methods of examining various organs in order to detect the evidence of disease or the effects of accidents; (3) the employment of instruments used in diagnosis and treatment; (4) the examination of normal and diseased structures, whether recent or in a museum; (5) the chemical examination of morbid products; (6) operations on the dead body; (7) post-mortem examinations.

17. Of instruction and proficiency in the practice of vaccination. Note D.—The certificate must be such as will qualify the holder to contract as a public vaccinator under the regulations, at the time in force, of the Local Government Board.

18. Of having attended a course of lectures on Pathological Anatomy.

19. Of having attended demonstrations in the post-mortem room during the whole period of attendance on clinical lectures (see Clause 22).

20. Of having attended a course of lectures on Forensic Medicine.

21. Of having attended, at a recognised hospital or hospitals, the practice of Medicine and Surgery during three winter and two summer sessions. Note E.—No metropolitan hospital is recognised which contains less than 150, and no provincial or colonial hospital which contains less than 100 patients. A three months' course of clinical instruction in the wards of a recognised lunatic hospital or asylum may be substituted for the same period of attendance in the medical wards of a general hospital.

22. Of having attended during nine months clinical lectures on Medicine, and also during nine months clinical lectures on Surgery; and of having been engaged during a period of three months in the clinical study of Diseases peculiar to Women.

23. Of having discharged the duties of a medical clinical clerk during six months, and of a surgical dresser during other six months. Note F.—These duties may be discharged at a general hospital, infirmary, or dispensary, or parochial or union infirmary, duly recognised for this purpose, or in such other manner as shall afford sufficient opportunity for the acquirement of practical knowledge.

The certificates of attendance on the several courses of lectures must include evidence that the student has attended examinations in each course.

II.—Professional Examinations.—There are three professional examinations, called herein the First Examination, the Second Examination, and the Third or Final Examination, each being partly written, partly oral, and partly practical. These examinations will be held in the months of February, April, July, October, and December, unless otherwise appointed.

The First Examination.—The subjects of the First Examination are—Chemistry and Chemical Physics, meaning thereby heat, light, and electricity; Materia Medica, Medical Botany, and Pharmacy; Osteology. (Schedules indicating the range of subjects in the examinations, in Chemistry and in Materia Medica, Medical Botany, and Pharmacy, may be obtained together with the regulations.) A candidate will be admitted to the First Examination on producing evidence of having been registered as a medical student by the General Medical Council, and of having complied with the regulations prescribed in Section I., Clauses 4, 5, 6, 7, and 8. The fee for admission to the First Examination is £5 5s., being part of the entire fee for the licence; and if a candidate be rejected, he will be required to pay an additional fee of £3 3s. before re-admission to the examination. A candidate rejected in the First Examination will not be re-admitted to examination until after the lapse of three months from the date of rejection.

The Second Examination.—The subjects of the Second Examination are Anatomy and Physiology. (A schedule indicating the range of subjects in the examination in Physiology may be obtained with the regulations.) A candidate will be admitted to the Second Examination on producing evidence of having passed the First Examination, of having completed, subsequently to registration as a medical student, eighteen months of professional study at a recognised medical school or schools, and of having complied with the Regulations prescribed in Section I., Clauses 9, 10, 11, and 12. The fee for admission to the Second Examination is £5 5s., being part of the entire fee for the licence; and if a candidate be rejected, he will be required to pay an additional fee of £3 3s. before re-admission to the examination. A candidate rejected in the Second Examination will not be re-admitted to examination until after the lapse of not less than three months from the date of rejection.

The Third or Final Examination.—The College does not admit to the Third or Final Examination any candidate (not exempted from registration) whose name has not been entered in the Medical Students' Register at least forty-five months, nor till the expiration of two years after the passing of the Second Examination. The subjects of the Final Examination are—Medical Anatomy and Pathology (including Morbid Anatomy), and the Principles and Practice of Medicine; Surgical Anatomy and Pathology (including Morbid Anatomy), and the Principles and Practice of Surgery; Midwifery, and Diseases peculiar to Women. Forensic Medicine, Public Health, and Therapeutics are subjects included in the Final Examination. A candidate will be admitted to the third or Final Examination on producing evidence—(1) Of being twenty-one years of age; (2) of moral character; (3) of having passed the Second Examination; (4) of having studied Medicine, Surgery, and Midwifery in accordance with the regulations prescribed in Section I., Clauses 3 and 13 to 23. The fee for admission to the Third or Final Examination is £5 5s., being part of the entire fee for the licence, and if a candidate be rejected, he will be required to pay an additional fee of £3 3s. before re-admission to the examination. A candidate rejected in the Third or Final Examination will not be re-admitted to examination until after the lapse of six months from the date of rejection.

The fee for the licence is £15 15s.

Any candidate who shall produce satisfactory evidence of having passed an examination on any of the subjects of the First Examination, conducted at a university in the United Kingdom, in India, or in a British colony, will be exempt from re-examination on those subjects in which he has passed.

Any candidate who shall produce satisfactory evidence of having passed an examination on Anatomy and Physiology, conducted by the Royal College of Surgeons of England, or the Royal College of Surgeons of Edinburgh, or the Royal College of Surgeons in Ireland, or the Faculty of Physicians and Surgeons of Glasgow, after a course of study and an examination satisfactory to the College, will be exempt from re-examination on those subjects.

Any candidate who shall produce satisfactory evidence of having passed an examination on Anatomy and Physiology required for a degree in Medicine or Surgery at a university in the United Kingdom, in India, or in a British colony, after a course of study and an examination satisfactory to the College, will be exempt from re-examination on those subjects.

Any candidate who shall have obtained a degree in Surgery at a university in the United Kingdom, after a course of study and an examination satisfactory to the College, will be exempt from re-examination on Surgical Anatomy and Pathology, including Morbid Anatomy, and on the Principles and Practice of Surgery.

Any candidate who shall have passed the examination on Surgery conducted by the Royal College of Surgeons of England, or the Royal College of Surgeons of Edinburgh, or the Royal College of Surgeons in Ireland, or the Faculty of Physicians and Surgeons of Glasgow, after a course of study and an examination satisfactory to the College, will be exempt from re-examination on Surgical Anatomy and Pathology, including Morbid Anatomy, and on the Principles and Practice of Surgery.

Any candidate who shall have obtained a foreign qualification which entitles him to practise Medicine or Surgery in the country where such qualification has been conferred, after a course of study and an examination equivalent to those required by the regulations of the College, shall, on production of satisfactory evidence as to age, moral character, and proficiency in vaccination, be admissible to the Pass Examination, and shall be exempt from re-examination on such subjects as shall in each case be considered by the Censors' Board to be unnecessary.

2. THE ROYAL COLLEGE OF SURGEONS, ENGLAND.

By far the most important qualification in this country is that of the Royal College of Surgeons of England, inasmuch as almost all English and many Scottish and Irish students become candidates for the Membership of that body. The College consists of two grades—Fellows and Members. The Fellowship is still partly honorary, sometimes being conferred on Members of a certain standing, but is now only obtainable by examination. The Membership is the qualification sought by students leaving their hospitals, hence the importance of the following regulations :—

SECTION I.

This Section refers to Preliminary Education (see page 300).

SECTION II. *Professional Education.*

I. Professional studies prior to the date at which the candidate shall have passed an examination in general knowledge are not recognised.

II. The following will be considered as the commencement of professional education :—

1. Attendance on the practice of a hospital or other public institution recognised by this College for that purpose.
2. Instruction as the pupil of a legally qualified surgeon holding the appointment of surgeon to a hospital, general dispensary, or union workhouse, or where such opportunities of practical instruction are afforded as shall be satisfactory to the Council.
3. Attendance on lectures on Anatomy, Physiology, or Chemistry, by lecturers recognised by this College.

III. Candidates, prior to their admission to the first or primary examination on Anatomy and Physiology, will be required to produce the following certificates, viz. :—

1. Of having passed, prior to the commencement of professional study, a recognised preliminary examination as required by Section I.
2. Of having attended lectures on Anatomy during two winter sessions.
3. Of having performed Dissections during not less than two winter sessions.
4. Of having attended lectures on General Anatomy and Physiology during one winter session.
5. Of having attended a practical course of General Anatomy and Physiology during another winter or a summer session, consisting of not less than thirty meetings of the class.
Note A.—By the practical course referred to in Clause 5, it is meant that the learners themselves shall, individually, be engaged in the necessary experiments, manipulations, etc. ; but it is not hereby intended that the learners shall perform vivisections.
Note B.—The certificates of attendance on the several courses of lectures must include evidence that the student has attended the practical instructions and examinations of his teacher in each course.

IV. Candidates, prior to their admission to the second or pass examination on Surgical Anatomy and the Principles and Practice of Surgery and Medicine, will be required to produce the following certificates, viz. :—

1. Of being twenty-one years of age.
2. Of having been engaged, subsequently to the date of passing the preliminary examination, during four years, or during a period extending over not less than four winter and four summer sessions, in the acquirement of professional knowledge.
3. Of having attended lectures on Surgery during one winter session.
4. Of having attended a course of Practical Surgery during a period occupying not less than six months prior or subsequent to the course required by the preceding Clause 3.
Note C.—The course of Practical Surgery referred to in Clause 4 is intended to embrace instruction in which each pupil shall be exercised in practical details, such as in the application of anatomical facts to surgery, on the living person, or on the dead body. The methods of proceeding and the manipulations necessary in order to detect the effects of diseases and accidents, on the living person, or on the dead body. The performance, where practicable, of the operations of surgery on the dead body. The use of surgical apparatus. The examination of diseased structures, as illustrated in the contents of a museum of morbid anatomy, and otherwise.
5. Of having attended one course of lectures on each of the following subjects, viz.:—Chemistry, Materia Medica, Medicine, Forensic Medicine, Midwifery (with practical instruction, and a certificate of having personally conducted not less than ten labours) ; Pathological Anatomy during not less than three months.
Note D.—The course of lectures on Chemistry included in Clause 5 will not be required in the case of a candidate who shall have passed a satisfactory examination in this subject in his preliminary examination.
6. Of having studied Practical Pharmacy during three months.
7. Of having attended a three months' course of Practical Chemistry (with manipulations), in its application to medical study.
8. Of instruction and proficiency in the practice of Vaccination.
Note E.—The certificate of instruction in Vaccination must be such as will qualify its holder to contract as a public vaccinator under the regulations at the time in force of the Local Government Board :—
Note F.—The certificates of attendance on the several courses of lectures must include evidence that the student has attended the practical instructions and examinations of his teacher in each course.
9. Of having attended, at a recognised hospital or hospitals, the practice of Surgery during three winter(a) and two summer(b) sessions.

(a) The winter session comprises a period of six months, and, in England, commences on October 1, and terminates on March 31.
(b) The summer session comprises a period of three months, and, in England, commences on May 1, and terminates on July 31.

10. Of having been individually engaged, at least twice in each week, in the observation and examination of patients at a recognised hospital or hospitals, under the direction of a recognised teacher, during not less than three months.
Note G.—It is intended that the candidate should receive the instruction required by Clause 10 at an early period of his attendance at the hospital.
11. Of having, subsequently to the first winter session of attendance on surgical hospital practice, attended, at a recognised hospital or hospitals, clinical lectures on Surgery during two winter and two summer sessions.
12. Of having been a dresser at a recognised hospital, or of having, subsequently to the completion of one year's professional education, taken charge of patients under the superintendence of a surgeon during not less than six months, at a hospital, general dispensary, or parochial or union infirmary recognised for this purpose, or in such other similar manner as, in the opinion of the Council, shall afford sufficient opportunity for the acquirement of Practical Surgery.
13. Of having attended, during the whole period of attendance on surgical hospital practice (see Clause 9), demonstrations in the post-mortem rooms of a recognised hospital.
14. Of having attended, at a recognised hospital or hospitals, the practice of Medicine, and clinical lectures on Medicine, during one winter and one summer session.
N.B.—Blank forms of the required certificates may be obtained on application to the Secretary, and all necessary certificates will be retained at the College.

SECTION III.

I. Certificates will not be received on more than one branch of science from one and the same lecturer; but Anatomy and Dissections will be considered as one branch of science.

II. Certificates will not be recognised from any hospital in the United Kingdom unless the surgeons thereto be members of one of the legally constituted Colleges of Surgeons in the United Kingdom ; nor from any school of Anatomy and Physiology or Midwifery, unless the teachers in such school be members of some legally constituted College of Physicians or Surgeons in the United Kingdom ; nor from any school of Surgery, unless the teachers in such school be members of one of the legally constituted Colleges of Surgeons in the United Kingdom.

III. No metropolitan hospital will be recognised by this College which contains less than 150, and no provincial or colonial hospital which contains less than 100 patients.

IV. The recognition of colonial hospitals and schools is governed by the same regulations, with respect to number of patients and to courses of lectures, as apply to the recognition of provincial hospitals and schools in England.

V. Certificates of attendance upon the practice of a recognised provincial or colonial hospital, unconnected with, or not in convenient proximity to, a recognised medical school, will not be received for more than one winter and one summer session of the hospital attendance required by the regulations of this College ; and in such cases clinical lectures will not be necessary, but a certificate of having acted as dresser for a period of at least six months will be required.

VI. Those candidates who shall have pursued the whole of their studies in Scotland or Ireland will be admitted to examination upon the production of the several certificates required respectively by the College of Surgeons of Edinburgh, the Faculty of Physicians and Surgeons of Glasgow, and the College of Surgeons in Ireland, from candidates for their diploma, together with a certificate of instruction and proficiency in the practice of vaccination, and satisfactory evidence of having been occupied, subsequently to the date of passing the preliminary examination, at least four years, or during a period extending over four winter and four summer sessions, in the acquirement of professional knowledge ; and in the case of candidates who shall have pursued the whole of their studies at recognised foreign or colonial universities, upon the production of the several certificates required for their degree by the authorities of such universities, together with a certificate of instruction and proficiency in the practice of vaccination, and satisfactory evidence of having been occupied, subsequently to the date of passing the preliminary examination, at least four years, or during a period extending over four winter and four summer sessions, in the acquirement of professional knowledge.

VII. Members or licentiates of any legally constituted College of Surgeons in the United Kingdom, and graduates in Surgery of any University recognised for this purpose by this College, will be admitted to examination on producing their diploma, licence, or degree, together with proof of being twenty-one years of age, a certificate of instruction and proficiency in the practice of vaccination, and satisfactory evidence of having been occupied, subsequently to the date of passing the preliminary examination, at least four years, or during a period extending over four winter and four summer sessions, in the acquirement of professional knowledge.

VIII. Graduates in Medicine of any legally constituted

College or University recognised for this purpose by this College will be admitted to examination on adducing, together with their diploma or degree, proof of being twenty-one years of age, a certificate of instruction and proficiency in the practice of vaccination, and satisfactory evidence of having been occupied, subsequently to the date of passing the preliminary examination, at least four years, or during a period extending over four winter and four summer sessions, in the acquirement of professional knowledge.

SECTION IV.—*Professional Examination.*

This examination is divided into two parts.

1. The first or primary examination, on Anatomy and Physiology, is partly written and partly demonstrative on the recently dissected subject, and on prepared parts of the human body.

2. The second, or pass examination, on Surgical Anatomy and the Principles and Practice of Surgery and Medicine,(c) is partly written, partly oral, and partly on the practical use of surgical apparatus, and the practical examination of patients.

3. The primary examinations are held in the months of January, April, May, July, and November, and the pass examinations generally in the ensuing week. respectively.(d)

4. Candidates will not be admitted to the primary examination until after the termination of the second winter session of their attendance at a recognised school or schools; nor to the pass, or surgical examination, until after the termination of the fourth year of their professional education.

5. The fee of £5 5s., paid prior to the first admission to the primary examination, is retained whether the candidate pass or fail to pass the examination, but is allowed as part of the whole fee of £22(e) payable for the diploma. A candidate, after failure at any primary examination, is required, on admission to any subsequent primary examination, to pay a further fee of £3 3s., which is retained, whether he pass or fail to pass the examination, and which further fee is not allowed as part of the whole fee of £22 for the diploma.

6. The fee of £16 15s. is payable prior to each admission to the pass examination; but on each occasion of failure the balance of £11 10s. is returned to the candidate.

7. A candidate having entered his name for either the primary or pass examination, who shall fail to attend the meeting of the Court for which he shall have received a card, will not be allowed to present himself for examination within a period of three months from the date at which he shall have so failed to attend.

8. A candidate referred on the primary examination is required, prior to his admission to re-examination, to produce a certificate of his performance of dissections during not less than three months subsequently to the date of his reference.(d)

9. A candidate referred on the primary examination, who shall not obtain more than half of the total minimum number of marks, is not re-admitted to examination until after the lapse of six months, and is then required to produce, in conformity with the foregoing paragraph 8, a certificate of the performance of dissections during not less than three months subsequently to the date of his reference.(d)

10. A candidate referred on the pass examination is required, prior to his admission to re-examination, to produce a certificate of at least six months' further attendance on the surgical practice of a recognised hospital, together with lectures on Clinical Surgery, subsequently to the date of his reference.(d)

The certificate of qualification in Midwifery is practically in abeyance, there being no Board of Examiners.

3. SOCIETY OF APOTHECARIES (ENGLAND).

Every candidate for a certificate of qualification to practise as an apothecary will be required to produce testimonials:— 1. Of having passed a preliminary examination in Arts, as a test of general education, of twenty-one years. 3. Of good moral conduct. 4. A certificate of three months' Practical Pharmacy from some recognised hospital or dispensary, or from a qualified medical practitioner. 5. Of having pursued a course of medical study in conformity with the regulations of the Court.

Course of Study.—Every candidate must attend the following lectures and medical practice: each winter session to consist of not less than six months, to commence on the 1st and not later than the 15th of October; each summer

(c) Candidates can claim exemption from examination in Medicine under the following conditions, viz.:—(1.) The production by the candidate of a degree, diploma, or licence in Medicine entitling him to register under the Medical Act of 1858; or a degree, diploma, or licence in Medicine of a colonial or foreign university approved by the Council of the College. (2.) A declaration by the candidate, prior to his admission to the final examination for Membership or Fellowship, that it is his intention to obtain either of the medical qualifications mentioned in the foregoing paragraph, in which case the diploma of the College will not be issued to him until he shall produce either the said medical qualification or proof of having passed the several examinations entitling him to receive the same.

(d) The required certificates, whether for the primary or pass examination, must be forwarded through the post not less than ten clear days prior to the date of each examination; except in the case of a referred candidate whose term of additional study will not expire until the date of the examination, in which case a written application must be sent by him in lieu of the certificates, such certificates to be produced the day before the examination.

(e) This sum of £22 is exclusive of the fee of £2 paid for the preliminary examination.

session to commence on the 1st and not later than the 15th of May.

First Year.—Winter Session: Chemistry; Anatomy and Physiology, including Dissections and Demonstrations. Summer Session: Botany; Materia Medica and Therapeutics; Practical Chemistry.

Second Year.—Winter Session(a): Anatomy and Physiology, including Dissections and Demonstrations; Clinical Medical Practice. Summer Session: Midwifery and Diseases of Women and Children; Forensic Medicine and Toxicology; Clinical Medical Practice.

Third Year.—Winter Session: Clinical Medical Lectures; Morbid Anatomy; Pathology and Clinical Medical Practice. Summer Session: Practical Midwifery and Vaccination; Morbid Anatomy Clinical Medical Practice.

No certificates of lectures, or of anatomical instructions delivered in private to particular students apart from the ordinary classes of recognised public medical schools, can be received by the Court of Examiners.

SYLLABUS OF SUBJECTS FOR EXAMINATION.

1. *The English Language.*—The leading features of its history; its structure and grammar; English composition.

2. *The Latin Language.*—January Examination: Livy—Book I., caps. 1. to xii. April Examination: Horace—Odes, Book IV. September Examination: Cicero—First Catiline Oration. Re-translation of easy sentences. Grammatical questions will be introduced into the Latin paper, and each candidate will be expected to give satisfactory answers to these.

3. *Mathematics.*—The ordinary rules of arithmetic. Vulgar and Decimal Fractions. Addition, Subtraction, Multiplication, and Division of Algebraical Quantities. Simple Equations. The First Two Books of Euclid.

4. (a) *Greek.*—Homer: Iliad, Book I. Grammatical questions. (b) *French.*—Voltaire: Histoire de Charles XII. Translation from English into French. Grammatical questions. (c) *German.*—Lessing: Minna Von Barnhelm. Translation from English into German. Grammatical questions. (d) *Natural Philosophy.*—Mechanics. Hydrostatics and Pneumatics.

Professional Examinations.—The Court of Examiners meet in the Hall every Wednesday and Thursday, where candidates are required to attend at 4.30 p.m. Every candidate intending to offer himself for examination must give seven days' notice previous to the day of examination, and must at the same time deposit all the required certificates, with the fee, at the office of the Beadle, where attendance is given daily, from ten to four o'clock; Saturdays, ten to two.

The certificates being found correct, a card to admit the candidate will be sent, stating the day and hour of examination.

The examination of candidates is divided into two parts, and is conducted partly in writing and partly *viva voce.*

The first examination which may be passed after the second winter session, embraces the following subjects:—Physicians' Prescriptions and Pharmacy; Anatomy and Physiology, including an examination on the living subject; General and Practical Chemistry; Materia Medica and Botany; Histology.

Testimonials required of Candidates for the First Examination. —Of having passed an examination in Arts, recognised by the Medical Council; of having completed the curriculum of study to the close of the second winter session; of having attended three months' Practical Pharmacy; and of good moral conduct. Any candidate who presents himself for the first examination and is rejected may be admitted to re-examination at the expiration of three calendar months.

The Second Examination.—At the termination of the medical studies: Principles and Practice of Medicine, Pathology and Therapeutics; Midwifery, including the diseases of women and children; Forensic Medicine and Toxicology; Microscopical Pathology.

Certificates required of Candidates for the Second or Pass Examination.—Of having completed four years' medical study, including the period spent at the Hospital; of being twenty-one years of age; and of good moral conduct. Of having passed the first examination. Of having completed the prescribed curriculum of study according to the schedule, including a personal attendance of twenty cases of Midwifery, (a certificate of which will be received from any registered practitioner); and of having received instruction in practical Vaccination, and vaccinated not less than twenty cases (this certificate must be obtained from a public vaccinator recognised by the Local Government Board). Of having served the office of clinical clerk at a recognised hospital during the period of six weeks, at least. Of having been examined at the class examinations instituted by the various lecturers and professors

(a) One course of Principles and Practice of Medicine, and one on the Principles and Practice of Surgery. The latter may be taken at the student's convenience after the second year.

of their respective medical schools and colleges. By the 22nd section of the Act of Parliament of 1815, no rejected candidate for the licence can be re-examined until the expiration of six calendar months from his former examination.

Modified Examinations.—1. All graduates in Medicine of British universities will be admitted to a clinical and practical examination in the practice of Medicine, Pathology, and Midwifery. 2. Licentiates of the Royal College of Physicians, London; of the Royal College of Physicians, Edinburgh; of the Royal Colleges of Physicians and Surgeons, Edinburgh; of the King and Queen's College of Physicians, Ireland; of the Faculty of Physicians and Surgeons, Glasgow; and of the Apothecaries' Hall, Dublin, will be admitted to a clinical and practical examination in the Practice of Medicine, Pathology, Midwifery, Forensic Medicine, and Toxicology. 3. Any candidate who has passed his first examination for the Licence of the King and Queen's College of Physicians, Ireland; the joint Licence of the Royal Colleges of Physicians and Surgeons, Edinburgh; or for the single Licence of the College of Physicians, Edinburgh; the Licence of the Faculty of Physicians and Surgeons, Glasgow; the first professional examination for the degree of M.B., or Master in Surgery, in the Universities of Oxford, Cambridge, London, or Durham; or the second part of the professional examination for the degree of M.B., or Master in Surgery in the Universities of Edinburgh, Aberdeen, St. Andrews, and Glasgow; or the second examination for medical and surgical degrees in the Irish universities; or the first examination for the Licence of the Apothecaries' Company, Dublin; or the first and second examinations of the Royal College of Physicians of London, will be admitted to a single examination in Anatomy and Materia Medica (to those candidates who have not undergone an examination in those subjects), Practice of Medicine (including Clinical Medicine), Pathology, Therapeutics, Midwifery, Forensic Medicine, and Toxicology, which examination will be partly written and partly *vivâ voce.* 4. Members of the Royal College of Surgeons, England; Licentiates of the Royal College of Surgeons, Edinburgh; and Licentiates of the Royal College of Surgeons, Ireland; and all candidates who have passed the first anatomical examination of the Royal College of Surgeons, London; the Royal College of Surgeons, Edinburgh; and the Royal College of Surgeons, Ireland, will have to undergo the two examinations, but will be exempt from writing on Anatomy and Physiology only, in their first examination.

The examination of candidates for certificates of qualification to act as Assistant in compounding and dispensing medicines will be as follows:—In translating physicians' prescriptions; in the British Pharmacopoeia; in Pharmacy, Pharmaceutical Chemistry, Materia Medica, and Medical Botany.

By Section 22 of the Act of Parliament, no rejected candidate as an Assistant can be re-examined until the expiration of three calendar months from his former examination.

Fees.—For a certificate of qualification to practise, £6 6s., half of which is retained in case of rejection, to be accounted for at a subsequent examination. For the first examination, £3 3s., which sum is retained in case of rejection, and accounted for subsequently; for the second examination, £3 3s.; for an Assistant's certificate, £2 2s., which sum is retained in case of rejection, and accounted for subsequently.

Prizes are annually offered for proficiency in the knowledge of Materia Medica and Pharmaceutical Chemistry. The prizes consist of a gold medal awarded to the candidate who distinguishes himself the most in the examination; and a silver medal and a book or books to the candidate who does so in the next degree. Also two prizes for proficiency in the knowledge of Botany, consisting of a gold medal to the candidate who distinguishes himself the most in the examination; and a silver medal and a book or books to the candidate who does so in the next degree.

B.—Scotland.

In Scotland, besides the Universities, there are three licensing bodies, viz.:—

4. ROYAL COLLEGE OF PHYSICIANS, EDINBURGH;
5. ROYAL COLLEGE OF SURGEONS, EDINBURGH;
6. FACULTY OF PHYSICIANS AND SURGEONS OF GLASGOW.

The first alone can give a qualification in Medicine; the two latter can give only a surgical qualification. Each of the

surgical bodies has, however, most sensibly joined with the College of Physicians, so that a candidate can, by a single set of examinations, acquire a qualification both in Medicine and Surgery. For this reason, and as the greater must include the less, we shall only give the rules applying to these conjoint examinations. These are so nearly identical, that one set of regulations will suffice.

The Royal College of Physicians and the Royal College of Surgeons, Edinburgh, and the Royal College of Physicians of Edinburgh and the Faculty of Physicians and Surgeons of Glasgow, while they continue to give their diplomas separately under separate regulations, have made arrangements by which, after one series of examinations, the student may obtain two separate licences—one in Medicine, and one in Surgery.

The general principle of this joint examination is, that it is conducted by a board in which each body is represented, the object being to give to students facilities for obtaining from two separate bodies, and at less expense, a double qualification in Medicine and in Surgery. Students passing these examinations successfully will be enabled to register two qualifications under the Medical Act—viz., Licentiate of the Royal College of Physicians and Licentiate of the Royal College of Surgeons, Edinburgh; and Licentiate of the Royal College of Physicians of Edinburgh and Licentiate of the Faculty of Physicians and Surgeons of Glasgow.

Candidates for these qualifications commencing professional study on or after October 1, 1866, must have been engaged in professional study during forty-five months after registration as students, and in actual attendance at a university or recognised school of medicine during not less than four winter sessions or three winter sessions and two summer sessions, and must have completed the following curriculum:—

1. Anatomy, two courses of lectures in distinct sessions, six months each.
2. Practical Anatomy, twelve months.
3. Chemistry, one course of lectures, six months.
4. Practical or Analytical Chemistry, one course, three months.
5. Physiology, not less than fifty lectures.
6. Practice of Medicine, one course of lectures, six months.
7. Clinical Medicine, extending to six months.
8. Another course of Practice of Medicine, or of Clinical Medicine, at the option of the candidate.
9. Principles and Practice of Surgery, one course of lectures, six months.
10. Clinical Surgery extending to six months.
11. Another course of Surgery, or of Clinical Surgery, at the option of the candidate.
12. Materia Medica, one course of lectures, three months.
13. Midwifery, one course of lectures, three months.
14. Practical Midwifery, attendance on at least six cases of labour.
15. Medical Jurisprudence, one course of lectures, three months.
16. Pathological Anatomy, instruction in the post-mortem rooms of a recognised hospital, three months.
17. Practical Pharmacy, instruction, three months.
18. General Hospital, attendance on the practice of a public general hospital, containing on an average not less than eighty patients, twenty-four months.
19. Proficiency in Vaccination, certified by a public vaccinator or a registered practitioner.

[Attendance for six months on the practice of a public dispensary, or certificate of having been engaged for six months as visiting assistant to a registered practitioner.—Edinburgh.]

Students are strongly recommended to avail themselves of any opportunities they may possess of studying Ophthalmic and Mental Diseases, Natural History, Comparative Anatomy, and Practical Physiology, in addition to what is required in the curriculum.

The examinations are conducted partly in writing and partly orally. Recent dissections, anatomical specimens, chemical tests, articles of the materia medica, the microscope, surgical and obstetrical apparatus, and pathological specimens, are employed at the discretion of the examiners. Candidates at the second examination are subjected in the hospital to a practical clinical examination in Medicine and Surgery.

Candidates for the double qualification who have passed the examination in Anatomy, Physiology, and Chemistry of one or other of the licensing bodies enumerated in Schedule (A) of the Medical Act, on complying with the regulations in other respects, are admissible to the second professional examination. No candidate is exempted from examination in any of the subjects of the second examination. No candidate shall be admissible to examination who has been rejected by any other licensing board within the three preceding months.

C.—Ireland.

7. KING AND QUEEN'S COLLEGE OF PHYSICIANS IN IRELAND.(a)

This body consists of Fellows, Members, and Licentiates.

THE LICENCE IN MEDICINE.

The regulations relating to Licentiates are as follows:—Candidates must produce—1. Evidence of having been engaged in the study of Medicine for four years. 2. A certificate of having passed the preliminary examination of one of the recognised licensing corporations before the termination of the second year of medical study. 3. Certificates of having studied at a school or schools recognised by the College, the following subjects, viz.:—Practical Anatomy, two courses; and Physiology or Institutes of Medicine, Botany, Chemistry, Practical Chemistry, Materia Medica, Practice of Medicine and Pathology, Surgery, Midwifery, Medical Jurisprudence, one course each. 4. Certificates of having attended a medico-chirurgical hospital in which regular courses of clinical lectures are delivered, together with clinical instruction, for twenty-seven months. 5. Of having been in attendance during at least three months on a clinical hospital which contains wards for the treatment of infectious fevers, and of having daily recorded observations on at least five cases of fever.(b) 6. Of having attended Practical Midwifery and Diseases of Women for six months at a lying-in hospital or maternity recognised by the College ; or, where such hospital attendance cannot have been obtained during any period of the student's course of study, of having been engaged in Practical Midwifery under the supervision of a registered practitioner holding public appointments; the certificate in either case to state that not less than twenty labour cases have been actually attended. 6. Certificates of character from two registered physicians or surgeons.

A candidate who has already obtained a medical or surgical qualification recognised by the College is only required to produce his diploma or certificate of registration, a certificate of Practical Midwifery, evidence of the study of fever, and testimonials as to character.

Examination for the Licence in Medicine.—The examination consists of two parts. The subjects of the first part, or previous examination, are—Anatomy, Physiology, Chemistry, and Materia Medica. The subjects of the second part, or final examination, are—Practice of Medicine, Medical Jurisprudence, Midwifery, Clinical Medicine, Pathology, Hygiene, and Therapeutics.

Examinations in the first part are held quarterly, in January, April, July, and October. Examinations in the final or second part are held monthly (except in August and September) in the week following the first Friday of each month.

All candidates for the second or final examination (with the exception below specified) (c) are examined in the Practice of Medicine at the bedside in one of the hospitals of Dublin, and in the College by means of printed questions and orally in all the subjects of examination.

Candidates qualified as follows are required to undergo the *second part* of the professional examination *only*, viz.:— 1. Graduates in Medicine of a university in the United Kingdom, or of any foreign university approved by the College. 2. Fellows, Members, and Licentiates of the Royal College of Physicians of London or Edinburgh, who have been admitted upon examination. 3. Graduates or Licentiates in Surgery. 4. Candidates who, having completed the curriculum above mentioned, have passed the previous professional examination or examinations of any of the licensing corporations in the United Kingdom.

THE LICENCE IN MIDWIFERY.

Candidates already qualified in Medicine or Surgery may apply for permission to be examined for the Licence in Mid-

(a) No return.
(b) This rule to be enforced in the case of all candidates after January 1, 1881.
(c) Candidates who are registered practitioners of five years' standing are exempted from the written portion of the examination.

wifery. The certificates required to be lodged are the same as those required from *qualified* candidates for the Licence to practise Medicine. Examinations, by printed questions and orally, for the Licence in Midwifery are conducted on the Thursday following the first Friday of each month except August and September.

Fees.—Fee for the licence in Medicine, £15 15s. Fee for licences in Medicine and Midwifery, if taken out within an interval of a month, £16 16s. Fee for the licence in Midwifery, £3 3s.

MEMBERSHIP.

The qualification of Member is conferred only on those already Licentiates of some standing; consequently it does not fall within the scope of our abstract of regulations.

FELLOWSHIP.

The election for Fellowship takes place twice a year, viz., on the first Friday in April and on St. Luke's Day (October 18). Candidates (who must be Members of the College of one year's standing) must be proposed and seconded three months previously. Fee £35, and £25 stamp duty.

8. ROYAL COLLEGE OF SURGEONS, IRELAND. (d)

This body grants two qualifications—that of Fellow, and Letters Testimonial equivalent to a Licentiateship. The regulations relating to the latter are as follows:—

Candidates for the Letters Testimonial of the College may present themselves either at a Special or at a Stated Examination, as follows:—

SPECIAL EXAMINATIONS.

Every registered pupil shall be admitted, upon payment of a special fee of £5 5s., to a Special Examination for Letters Testimonial, if he shall have laid before the Council the following documents:—

a. A receipt showing that he has lodged, in addition to his registration and special fees, a sum of £21 in the Bank of Ireland, to the credit of the President, and for the use of the College.

b. A certificate that he has passed a preliminary examination, conducted by a board recognised by the General Medical Council, into the curriculum of which the Greek language enters as a compulsory subject.

c. A certificate showing that he has been engaged in the study of his profession for not less than four years.

d. Certificates of attendance during three years at a hospital recognised by the Council, where clinical instruction is given.

e. Certificates of attendance on three courses of lectures on Anatomy and Physiology ; three courses of lectures on the Theory and Practice of Surgery ; and of the performance of three courses of Dissections, accompanied by demonstrations; also certificates of attendance on two courses of lectures on Chemistry, or one course of lectures on General and one on Practical Chemistry; one course of lectures on Materia Medica; one course of lectures on the Practice of Medicine; one course of lectures on Midwifery; one course of lectures on Medical Jurisprudence; and one course of lectures on Botany.

N.B.—The subjects for examination, and the mode of carrying these out, for a Special Examination, will be the same as those hereinafter laid down for the Stated Examinations, and any rejected candidate will only be entitled to receive back £15 15s. of the fees lodged by him.

VACCINATION.—NEW ORDINANCE OF COUNCIL.

On and after August 1, 1879, no candidate for letters testimonial shall be admitted to examination without producing a certificate of attendance for one month at the Cow-pock Institution, or some other institution to be approved of by this Council, under the instruction of a public vaccinator specially recognised by this College for the purpose, and that he is practically acquainted with vaccination.

STATED EXAMINATIONS.

1st. Stated Examinations shall be held in the months of April, July, and November, commencing on dates of which due notice shall be given beforehand by the Council of the College, and to which *candidates cannot be admitted unless they be registered pupils*, and at which they shall be divided into two classes—Junior and Senior.

(d) No return.

2nd. The Junior Class shall produce certificates of having passed a preliminary examination conducted by a board recognised by the General Medical Council, into the curriculum of which the Greek language enters as a compulsory subject; and of having attended three courses of lectures on Anatomy and Physiology; three courses of lectures on Practical Anatomy, with dissections; two courses of lectures on Chemistry; one course of lectures on Materia Medica; one course of lectures on Botany; and one course of lectures on Forensic Medicine.

3rd. This class shall be examined in Anatomy, Histology, Physiology, Materia Medica, and Chemistry.

4th. The fee for this examination shall be £5 5s., in addition to the registration fee of £5 5s.—not to be returned in case of rejection, but to be allowed the candidate in case he presents himself a second time for examination.

5th. The Senior Class shall produce certificates of having attended three courses of lectures on the Theory and Practice of Surgery, one course of lectures on the Practice of Medicine, and one course of lectures on Midwifery; also certificates of attendance at a recognised hospital for three winter and three summer sessions.

6th. This class shall be examined in Surgery, Operative Surgery and Surgical Appliances, Practice of Medicine, Medical Jurisprudence, and Prescriptions.

7th. The fee for the Senior Class Examination shall be £15 15s., returnable to the candidate in case of rejection.

8th. Both of these examinations shall be conducted partly by written and partly by oral questions.

9th. In addition to the foregoing fees, a fee of £1 1s. is to be paid to the Registrar on handing each licentiate his diploma.

10th. Every candidate rejected at any of the Stated Examinations, on applying for re-examination, shall be required to pay to the College, in addition to the regular fees, the sum of £2 2s. to reimburse the College the necessary expense of his re-examination.

This body also grants a diploma in Midwifery, for which the following are the regulations:—

Qualifications of Candidates for the Diploma in Midwifery.—Any Fellow or Licentiate of the College shall be admitted to an examination for the diploma in Midwifery upon laying before the Council the following documents:—*a.* A certificate showing that he has attended one course of lectures on Midwifery and Diseases of Women and Children, delivered by a professor or lecturer in some School of Medicine or Surgery recognised by the Council. *b.* A certificate showing that he has attended, during a period of six months, the practice of a lying-in hospital recognised by the Council; or the practice of a dispensary for lying-in women and children recognised by the Council and devoted to this branch of Surgery alone. *c.* A certificate showing that he has conducted thirty labour cases, at least.

Fees to be paid by Candidates for the Diploma in Midwifery.—The candidate pays £1 1s. for the Midwifery diploma, provided he takes it out within one month from the date of his letters testimonial; after that date the fee will be £3 3s.

9. THE APOTHECARIES' HALL OF IRELAND.

This body grants a licence to practise, on the following conditions:—

1. Of having passed an examination in Arts before one of the recognised public boards previously to entering on professional study.

2. Of having been registered in the Students' Medical Register.

3. Of being at least twenty-one years of age, and of good moral character.

4. Of pupilage to a qualified apothecary, or of having been otherwise engaged in practical pharmacy for a period of twelve months subsequent to having passed the examination in Arts.

5. Of having spent four years, or forty-five months, in professional study from the date of registration in the Students' Register.

6. Of having attended the following courses, viz.:—Chemistry, during one winter session; Anatomy and Physiology, during one winter session; Demonstrations and Dissections, during two winter sessions; Botany and Natural History, during one summer session; Practical Chemistry (in a recognised laboratory), during three months; Materia Medica, during three months; Principles and Practice of Medicine and Therapeutics, during one winter session; Midwifery and Diseases of Women and Children, during six months; Practical Midwifery at a recognised hospital (attendance upon twenty cases); Surgery, during one winter session; Forensic Medicine, during one summer session; instruction in the practice of Vaccination.

7. Of having attended, at a recognised hospital or hospitals, the practice of Medicine and clinical lectures on Medicine, during two winter and two summer sessions; also the practice of Surgery and clinical lectures on Surgery, during one winter and one summer session.

8. Of practical study, with care of patients, as apprentice pupil, assistant, clinical clerk, or dresser, in hospital, dispensary, or with a registered practitioner.

9. Of having performed the operation of vaccination successfully under a recognised public vaccinator.

The examination for the licence to practise is divided into two parts:—The first part comprehends Chemistry, Botany, Anatomy, Physiology, Materia Medica, and Pharmacy; the second—Medicine, Surgery, Pathology, Therapeutics, Midwifery, Forensic Medicine, and Hygiene.

The professional examinations will be held quarterly, and will commence on the first and second Mondays in the months of January, April, July, and October.

ENTRANCE SCHOLARSHIPS.

The following is a list of Entrance Scholarships given at the various London hospitals:—

St. Bartholomew's Hospital.—Two open Scholarships in Science, each £130 for one year; subjects—Physics, Chemistry, Botany, and Zoology. Also one of £50 in Preliminary Education; and one in Science, likewise £50.

Charing-cross Hospital.—Two Entrance Scholarships, £30 and £30. Subjects—compulsory: English, Latin, French or German, Mathematics; optional (one only may be selected): Chemistry, Mechanics, German or French. The subjects and authors will be the same as those chosen for the London Matriculation of the preceding June.

Guy's Hospital.—Two of £131 5s.—one in Preliminary Education (subjects—Classics, Mathematics, Modern Languages), the other in Science (subjects—Chemistry, Physics, Botany, and Zoology).

London Hospital.—Two Entrance Science Scholarships, £60 and £40 (subjects—Physics, Botany, Zoology, Inorganic Chemistry); and two Buxton Scholarships, £30 and £20—Preliminary Education.

King's College.—Two Warneford Scholarships (of £25 each annually for two years)—General Literature and Science; two Clothworkers' Company Scholarships (one of £50 and one of £25 per annum), each tenable for two years—Science; two Sambrooke Scholarships (one of £30 and one of £40)—Literature and Science.

St. Mary's Hospital.—Two Entrance Scholarships, £150 and £100—Natural Science.

Middlesex Hospital.—Two Entrance Scholarships, £25 and £20 annually, tenable for two years.

St. Thomas's Hospital.—Two (£100 and £60) Entrance Science Scholarships—Chemistry and Physics, with either Botany or Zoology at the option of candidates.

University College.—Three Entrance Scholarships of the respective values of £100, £60, and £40 per annum. Subjects of examination the same as those of the Preliminary Scientific Examination of the University of London.

Westminster Hospital.—Two Entrance Scholarships, each of £40 annually. Subjects—Latin, Mathematics, French or German, and Chemistry and Natural Philosophy.

"CEASING TO ATTEND" LECTURES.—In an account in the *Indian Medical Gazette* for July of the opening of the forty-seventh session of the Calcutta Medical College, it is stated that, in his report on the previous session, Brigade-Surgeon Dr. Coates stated that the number of students who "ceased to attend" reached the large figure of fifty-three. Dr. Coates had ascertained that the causes of these cessations were a family law-suit, the death of a relative or guardian, but most of all the marriages of sisters and the debts thus incurred. Fees are in future to be demanded in advance, in order if possible to reduce the number of desertions. "If excessive expenditure on marriage ceremonies is really responsible for ruining the career of so many young men—and after reading an interesting chapter on the subject in a work by Baboo Shib Chunder Bose, entitled 'The Hindoos as they are,' we are inclined to conclude that such is the case—then the sooner reform is introduced in this respect the better."

LONDON HOSPITALS AND MEDICAL SCHOOLS.

ST. BARTHOLOMEW'S HOSPITAL.

MEDICAL AND SURGICAL STAFF.

Consulting Physicians.
Sir G. Burrows, Bart., D.C.L., F.R.S., Dr. Farre, Dr. Harris, Dr. Martin.

Consulting Surgeons—Sir J. Paget, Bart., D.C.L., F.R.S., Mr. Holden.

Physicians.	*Surgeons.*
Dr. Andrew.	Mr. Savory, F.R.S.
Dr. Southey.	Mr. Thomas Smith.
Dr. Church.	Mr. Willett.
Dr. Gee.	Mr. Langton.

Assistant-Physicians.	*Assistant-Surgeons.*
Dr. Duckworth.	Mr. Morrant Baker.
Dr. Hensley.	Mr. Marsh.
Dr. Brunton, F.R.S.	Mr. Butlin.
Dr. Legg.	Mr. Walsham.

| *Physician-Accoucheur.* | |
| Dr. Matthews Duncan. | *Ophthalmic Surgeons.* |

| *Assistant Physician-Accoucheur.* | Mr. Power. |
| Dr. Godson. | Mr. Vernon. |

Casualty Physicians—Dr. Nall, Dr. P. Kidd, Dr. Tooth.
Dental Surgeon—Mr. Coleman.
Assistant Dental Surgeons—Mr. Lyons, Mr. Ewbank.
Administrator of Chloroform—Mr. Mills.
Medical Registrar—Dr. S. West.
Surgical Registrars—Mr. Macready, Mr. Cripps.

LECTURERS.

Botany—Rev. George Henslow.
Chemistry and Practical Chemistry—Dr. Russell.
Clinical Medicine—Dr. Andrew, Dr. Southey, Dr. Church, and Dr. Gee.
Clinical Surgery—Mr. Savory, Mr. Thomas Smith, Mr. Willett, Mr. Langton.
Comparative Anatomy—Dr. Moore.
Dental Anatomy and Surgery—Mr. Coleman.
Descriptive and Surgical Anatomy—Mr. Langton and Mr. Marsh.
Public Health and Hygiene—Dr. Thorne.
Forensic Medicine—Dr. Southey.
General Anatomy and Physiology—Mr. Morrant Baker.
Histology—Dr. Klein.
Materia Medica—Dr. Brunton.
Medicine — Dr. Andrew and Dr. Gee.
Mental Diseases—Dr. Claye Shaw.
Midwifery and the Diseases of Women and Children—Dr. Matthews Duncan.
Ophthalmic Medicine and Surgery—Mr. Power.
Pathological Anatomy—Dr. Legg.
Surgery—Mr. Savory.

DEMONSTRATORS.

Chemistry—Dr. Armstrong.
Diseases of the Ear—Mr. Langton.
Diseases of the Eye—Mr. Vernon.
Diseases of the Larynx—Dr. Brunton.
Diseases of the Skin—Mr. Baker.
Mechanical and Natural Philosophy—Mr. Macalister.
Morbid Anatomy—Dr. Moore.
Orthopædic Surgery—Mr. Willett.
Practical Anatomy and Operative Surgery—Mr. Bruce Clarke, Mr. Edwards, and Mr. Lockwood.
Practical Physiology—Dr. V. Harris.
Practical Surgery—Mr. Butlin and Mr. Walsham.

Medical Tutor—Dr. S. West.

This Hospital comprises a service of 710 beds, of which 676 are in the Hospital in Smithfield, and 34 are for convalescent patients at Lauderdale House, Highgate.

SCHOLARSHIPS AND PRIZES.

Open Scholarships in Science, founded 1873; subjects of examination :—Physics, Chemistry, Botany, and Zoology. These scholarships, of the value of £150 each, tenable for one year, will be competed for on September 26 and following days.

Preliminary Scientific Exhibition, founded 1873; subjects of examination—Physics, Chemistry, Botany, and Zoology. This exhibition, of the value of £50, is awarded in October.

Lawrence Scholarship and Gold Medal, of the value of £40, founded in 1878, by the family of the late Sir W. Lawrence.

Brackenbury Scholarship in Medicine, and Brackenbury Scholarship in Surgery, founded in 1875 by the will of the late Miss Hannah Brackenbury, who left £2000 for this purpose.

Senior Scholarship of the value of £30—Anatomy, Physiology, and Chemistry.

Junior Scholarships of the value of £50, £30, and £20 are awarded after an examination in the subjects of study of the first year at the end of the summer and winter sessions.

The Jeaffreson Exhibition, of the value of £50, is awarded at the commencement of each winter session, after open competition, on the same days as the Science Scholarships in Class Ics, Mathematics, and Modern Languages.

The Wix Prize is awarded for the best essay on the following subject :—"The Religio Medici of Sir T. Browne."

Bentley Prize : subject of examination—Bishop Butler's Analogy.

Bentley Prizes (two), for the best report of Surgical and Medical Cases occurring in the wards of the Hospital during the previous year. It is expected that the reports will comprise the histories, progress, treatment, and results of not less than twelve cases, with observations thereupon.

Foster Prize : subject of examination—Practical Anatomy, senior.

Treasurer's Prize : subject of examination—Practical Anatomy, junior.

The Kirkes Gold Medal : subject of examination—Clinical Medicine.

FEES.

Whole fee for attendance on lectures and hospital practice £138 12s., payable by instalments—first winter £42, first summer £48 6s., second summer £48 6s.—or a single payment

of £131 5s. Payment in either of these ways entitles to a perpetual ticket.

A College for resident students exists in connexion with the Hospital; Warden, Dr. Norman Moore, from whom students will obtain information respecting rooms in the College, or will be advised regarding residence out of the Hospital.

All communications to be addressed to the Warden of the College, St. Bartholomew's Hospital, E.C.

CHARING-CROSS HOSPITAL.

MEDICAL AND SURGICAL STAFF.

Consulting Physician—Sir Joseph Fayrer, M.D., K.C.S.I., F.R.S., F.R.C.P.
Consulting Surgeons—Mr. E. Canton, F.R.C.S., and Mr. F. Hird, F.R.C.S.

Physicians.	*Surgeons.*
Dr. A. J. Pollock.	Mr. R. Barwell.
Dr. A. Silver.	Mr. E. Bellamy.
Dr. T. H. Green.	Mr. J. Astley Bloxam.

Assistant-Physicians.	*Assistant-Surgeons.*
Dr. J. Mitchell Bruce.	Mr. J. Cantlie.
Dr. W. B. Houghton.	Mr. J. H. Morgan.
Dr. Robert Smith.	Mr. H. R. Whitehead.
Dr. D. Colquhoun.	

| *Physician-Accoucheur.* | *Dental Surgeon.* |
| Dr. J. Watt Black. | Mr. John Fairbank. |

Physician for Skin Diseases.	*Chloroformists.*
Dr. A. Sangster.	Mr. Woodhouse Braine.
	Mr. G. H. Bailey.

| *Medical Registrar.* | *Surgical Registrar.* |
| Mr. A. Leahy. | Mr. Hayward Whitehead. |

LECTURERS AND TEACHERS.

Anatomy—Mr. Edward Bellamy.
Minor Surgery—Mr. James Cantlie.
Botany—Dr. D. Colquhoun.
Chemistry & Practical Chemistry—Mr. C. W. Heaton ; Demonstrator, Mr. J. J. Broadbent.
Clinical Medicine—Dr. Pollock, Dr. Silver, and Dr. Green.
Clinical Surgery—Mr. Barwell, Mr. Bellamy, and Mr. Bloxam.
Ophthalmic Surgery—the Staff of the Royal Westminster Ophthalmic Hospital.
Comparative Anatomy—Mr. W. A. Forbes.
Demonstrations and Dissections—Mr. James Cantlie.
Dental Surgery — Mr. John Fairbank.
Diseases of Children — Dr. D. Colquhoun.
Forensic Medicine — Dr. W. B. Houghton.
Physics—Mr. Nelson.
Materia Medica and Therapeutics—Dr. J. Mitchell Bruce.
Mental Diseases—Dr. L. S. Forbes Winslow.
Operative Surgery — Mr. J. A. Bloxam.
Pathology and Morbid Anatomy—Dr. T. Henry Green.
Physiology, Theoretical—Dr. Alexander Silver.
Physiology, Practical—Dr. Wolfenden.
Principles and Practice of Medicine—Dr. A. J. Pollock.
Principles and Practice of Midwifery and Diseases of Women—Dr. J. Watt Black.
Principles and Practice of Surgery—Mr. R. Barwell.
Public Health—Mr. C. W. Heaton and Mr. W. Eassie.
Skin Diseases—Dr. A. Sangster.
Surgical Pathology — Mr. J. H. Morgan.

SCHOLARSHIPS, MEDALS, AND PRIZES.

Two Entrance Scholarships, of the value of £60 and £30 respectively, tenable for one year, will be awarded annually in October, after a competitive examination in the following subjects :—Compulsory : English, Latin, French or German, Mathematics. Optional (only one of which may be selected) : Chemistry, Mechanics, German or French. The subjects (as regards extent and the authors selected) will be the same as those chosen for the Matriculation Examination of the University of London in the June immediately preceding. Candidates must give notice of their intention to compete on or before Saturday, September 17, 1881. The successful candidates will be required to enter for their medical education at Charing-cross Hospital.

The Llewellyn Scholarship of £25 is open to all matriculated students who have just completed their second academical year. The examination is held at the end of the second summer session, and includes the following subjects :—Descriptive and Surgical Anatomy, Physiology, Materia Medica, Medicine, Surgery, Midwifery.

The Golding Scholarship of £15 is open to all matriculated students who have just completed their first academical year. The examination is held at the end of the first summer session, and includes the following subjects :—Descriptive Anatomy, Physiology, Materia Medica, and Chemistry.

The Pereira Prize of £5 is open to all matriculated students who shall have completed their third academical year. It is awarded to the author of the best Clinical Reports of Cases in the Hospital during the preceding year, Medical and Surgical Cases being selected in alternate years.

Each candidate must produce a certificate of good conduct from the Dean of the Medical School, at the time of giving in his name as a competitor ; and the names of the candidates for Scholarships are to be delivered to the Librarian one week before the first day of the examination.

The Governors' Clinical Gold Medal.—The competition for this medal is open to matriculated students who shall have completed, at the end of the current session, their attendance on the Medical and Surgical Practice of the Hospital. Candidates are examined on the subjects of Clinical Lectures delivered during the session, and on Medical and Surgical Cases in the wards of the Hospital.

Silver Medals.—Silver Medals are awarded in all the classes.

Bronze Medals.—Where two sessions' attendance on a course are required, a Bronze Medal is awarded in the junior class, in addition to the Silver one in the senior class.

Certificates of Honour are awarded to both senior and junior students who, not being the most proficient, have yet attained a marked degree of excellence.

FEES.

Total fees, £91 7s., payable by instalments, if entered for the full period of study—October (on joining), £29 8s., including matriculation fee; May (following), £18 18s.; October, £18 18s. May, £15 15s.; October, £10 10s. Dental Students: October (on joining), £22 2s., including matriculation fee; October (following), £20—total, £42 2s.

Students are admitted to the Medical and Surgical Practice for the full period required by the University of London, the Royal College of Physicians, the Royal College of Surgeons, and the Society of Apothecaries (including the clinical courses in both departments), on payment of £31 10s. Non-matriculated students are admitted on payment of the following fees:—Either Medical or Surgical Practice (including the clinical lectures): Three months, £6 6s.; six months, £10 10s.; twelve months, £15 15s.; full period, £21. Both Medical and Surgical Practice (including the clinical lectures): Three months, £10 10s.; six months, £15 15s.; twelve months, £21; full period, £31 10s. For a longer period, £5 5s. for each additional winter, and £3 3s. for each additional summer session.

For further particulars apply to the Dean, at the Hospital.

ST. GEORGE'S HOSPITAL.

MEDICAL AND SURGICAL STAFF.

Consulting Physicians—Dr. Wilson, Dr. Pitman, Dr. Ogle.

Consulting Surgeons.

Mr. Cæsar Hawkins, F.R.S., Mr. Prescott Hewett, F.R.S., Mr. Pollock, Mr. H. Lee.

Physicians.	Surgeons.
Dr. Barclay.	Mr. Holmes.
Dr. Wadham.	Mr. Rouse.
Dr. Dickinson.	Mr. Pick.
Dr. Whipham.	Mr. Haward.
Assistant-Physicians.	*Assistant-Surgeons.*
Dr. Cavafy.	Mr. Bennett.
Dr. Watney.	Mr. Dent.

Obstetric Physician—Dr. Barnes.
Assistant Obstetric Physician—Dr. Champneys.
Ophthalmic Surgeon—Mr. Brudenell Carter.
Assistant Ophthalmic Surgeon—Mr. Frost.
Aural Surgeon—Mr. Dalby.　　*Dental Surgeon*—Mr. A. Winterbottcm.

LECTURERS.—WINTER SESSION.

Chemistry & Physics—Mr. Donkin.	Ophthalmic Surgery—Mr. Brudenell Carter.
Clinical Lectures on Diseases of Women—Dr. Barnes.	Pathology—Dr. Whipham.
Clinical Medicine—Drs. Wadham and Whipham.	Physiological Chemistry—Dr. Wm. Ewart.
Clinical Surgery—Messrs. Rouse and Pick.	Physiology and General Anatomy—Dr. Watney and Mr. Dent.
Descriptive and Surgical Anatomy—Mr. Pick.	Principles and Practice of Physic—Drs. Barclay and Dickinson.
Histology—Mr. Bennett.	Principles and Practice of Surgery—Messrs. Holmes and Rouse.
Morbid Anatomy—Dr. Owen.	

SUMMER SESSION.

Aural Surgery—Mr. Dalby.	Med. Jurisprudence—Dr. Wadham.
Botany—	Midwifery and Diseases of Women and Children—Dr. Barnes.
Clinical Demonstrations of Diseases of the Skin—Dr. Cavafy.	Practical Chemistry—Mr. Donkin.
Clinical Medicine—Dr. Dickinson.	Practical Medicine—Dr. Whipham.
Clinical Surgery—Mr. Holmes.	Practical Surgery—Messrs. Bennett and Dent.
Comparative Anatomy—Dr. Bralley.	Psychological Medicine—Dr. Blandford.
Dental Surgery—Mr. Winterbottom.	
Materia Medica—Dr. Owen.	

EXHIBITIONS AND PRIZES.

The William Brown Exhibition, of £100 per annum, tenable for two years, to be competed for by perpetual pupils who have recently obtained their diploma.

The William Brown Exhibition, of £40 per annum, tenable for three years, to be competed for by students during their fourth year of study.

The Brackenbury Prizes of £35 each in Medicine and Surgery, awarded annually after a competitive examination.

The Treasurer's Clinical Prize of £10 10s., the gift of the Duke of Westminster, to be competed for annually.

Sir Charles Clarke's Prize for Good Conduct: The interest of £300 Consols, to be awarded annually to the student of the Hospital, "who, by reason of his general good conduct during the preceding year, should be considered the most deserving."

The Thompson Medal: A silver medal to be awarded annually for the best clinical report of Medical and Surgical Cases observed in the Hospital during the preceding twelve months.

Sir Benjamin Brodie's Clinical Prize in Surgery will be awarded to the pupil of the Hospital who shall have delivered to the Surgeons the best report of not more than twelve surgical cases which have occurred in the Hospital during the preceding twelve months.

Dr. Acland's Clinical Prize in Medicine will be awarded to the pupil of the Hospital who shall produce the best report of not more than twelve medical cases which have occurred in the Hospital during the preceding twelve months.

The Henry Charles Johnson Memorial Prize in Anatomy will be awarded to that pupil who shall, in the judgment of the Medical School Committee, exhibit the greatest proficiency in Practical Anatomy.

General Proficiency Prizes: To pupils in their first year, £10 10s.; to pupils in their second year, £10 10s.; to pupils in their third year, £10 10s.

FEES.

Perpetual pupils pay £45 in their first year, £45 in their second year, and £40 in their third year of study, or £125 on entrance.

Gentlemen are admitted to the hospital practice and lectures required for the licensing bodies on payment of the following fees—viz., £45 for the first year of study, £45 for the second year of study, and £20 for each of the two succeeding years. These are not perpetual pupils.

Dental pupils are admitted to the required courses on payment of £30 for their first year, and £25 for their second year, including Practical Chemistry.

Pupils may also enter to the hospital practice and lectures separately.

For further particulars apply to Dr. Wadham, Dean of the School.

GUY'S HOSPITAL.

MEDICAL AND SURGICAL STAFF.

Consulting Physicians—Sir William Gull, Bart., Dr. G. Owen Rees.
Consulting Obstetric Physician—Dr. Henry Oldham.
Consulting Surgeons—Mr. E. Cock, Mr. Birkett.

Physicians.	Surgeons.
Dr. S. Wilks.	Mr. Thomas Bryant.
Dr. F. W. Pavy.	Mr. Arthur Durham.
Dr. W. Moxon.	Mr. H. G. Howse.
Dr. C. Hilton Fagge.	Mr. N. Davies-Colley.
Assistant-Physicians.	*Assistant-Surgeons.*
Dr. P. H. Pye-Smith.	Mr. R. Clement Lucas.
Dr. Frederick Taylor.	Mr. C. H. Golding-Bird.
Dr. J. F. Goodhart.	Mr. W. H. A. Jacobson.
Obstetric Physician.	*Ophthalmic Surgeons.*
Dr. J. Braxton Hicks.	Mr. G. Bader.
	Mr. C. Higgens, *Asst.*
Assistant Obstetric Physician.	*Dental Surgeon.*
Dr. A. L. Galabin.	Mr. H. Moon.
Medical Registrar.	*Aural Surgeon.*
Dr. Mahomed.	Mr. W. Laidlaw Purves.
Curator of the Museum.	*Surgical Registrar.*
Dr. Fagge.	Mr. C. J. Symonds.

Dean—Dr. F. Taylor.

WINTER COURSES.—LECTURES.

Anatomy, Descriptive and Surgical—Mr. Howse and Mr. Davies-Colley.	Clinical Lectures on Midwifery and Diseases of Women—Dr. Braxton Hicks.
Chemistry — Dr. Debus and Dr. Stevenson.	Experimental Physics—Prof. A. W. Reinold.
Clinical Medicine—Dr. Wilks, Dr. Pavy, Dr. Moxon, and Dr. Fagge.	Medicine—Dr. Wilks and Dr. Pavy.
Clinical Surgery—Mr. Bryant, Mr. Durham. Mr. Howse, and Mr. Davies-Colley.	Physiology—Dr. Pye-Smith.
	Surgery — Mr. Bryant and Mr. Arthur Durham.

DEMONSTRATIONS.

Cutaneous Diseases — Dr. Pye-Smith.	Practical Anatomy—Mr. R. E. Carrington and Dr. Horrocks.
Morbid Anatomy—Dr. Fagge and Dr. Goodhart.	Practical Physiology—Mr. Golding-Bird.

Practical Surgery—Mr. Lucas.

SUMMER COURSES.—LECTURES.

Botany—Mr. Bettany.	Hygiene—Dr. F. Taylor.
Clinical Medicine—Dr. Fagge, Dr. Pye-Smith, Dr. F. Taylor, and Dr. Goodhart.	Materia Medica and Therapeutics—Dr. Moxon.
	Medical Jurisprudence—Dr. Stevenson.
Clinical Surgery—Mr. Davies-Colley, Mr. Clement Lucas, Mr. Golding-Bird, and Mr. Jacobson.	Mental Diseases—Dr. Savage.
Clinical Lectures on Diseases of Women—Dr. A. L. Galabin.	Midwifery and Diseases of Women—Dr. Braxton Hicks and Dr. Galabin.
Comparative Anatomy & Zoology—	Ophthalmic Surgery—Mr. Bader.
Dental Surgery—Mr. Moon.	Pathology—Dr. Fagge.

DEMONSTRATIONS.

Morbid Histology—Mr. Jacobson.	Practical Chemistry—Dr. Debus.
	Operative Surgery—Mr. Lucas.

This Hospital contains 695 beds.

OPEN SCHOLARSHIPS.

An open Scholarship of the value of £131 5s. in Classics, Mathematics, and Modern Languages.

An open Scholarship of the value of £131 5s. in Science.

PRIZES.

For First Year's Students—At the end of the summer session, in Anatomy, Physiology, Chemistry, Materia Medica, Botany, and Comparative Anatomy: Prizes, £50, £35, and £10 10s. (presented by one of the Governors).

For Second Year's Students.—In the winter session, the Michael Harris Prize of £10 in Anatomy. Summer session, examination in Anatomy and Physiology: The Sands-Cox Scholarship of £15 per annum, tenable for three years—subject, Physiology.

For Third Year's Students.—Medical and Surgical Anatomy, Operative and Minor Surgery, Midwifery, Therapeutics: First Prize £25, Second Prize £10.

For Fourth Year's Students.—Summer session, examination in Medicine, Surgery, and Medical Jurisprudence: Prizes, £15 and £10.

For Senior Students.—The Treasurer's Gold Medal for Clinical Medicine; the Treasurer's Gold Medal for Clinical Surgery; the Gurney Hoare Prize of £25 for Clinical Medicine and Surgery. The Bassay Scholarship of £31 10s. for Pathology.

FEES.

The fees for hospital practice and lectures are as follows:— A perpetual ticket may be obtained—(1.) By the payment of

B

£131 5s. on entrance. (2.) By two payments of £66, at the commencement of the first winter session and the following summer session. (3.) By the payment of three annual instalments, at the commencement of the sessional year: First year £50; second year, £50; third year, £37 10s. Materials used in practical courses are charged extra.

For further information apply to the Dean, Dr. F. Taylor.

KING'S COLLEGE HOSPITAL.

MEDICAL AND SURGICAL STAFF.

Consulting Physicians—Sir Thos. Watson, Bart., M.D., Dr. George Budd, Dr. Arthur Farre, Dr. W. A. Guy, Dr. W. O. Priestley, Dr. A. B. Garrod.

Physicians.	*Surgeons.*
Dr. George Johnson.	Mr. John Wood.
Dr. Lionel S. Beale.	Mr. Joseph Lister.
Dr. Alfred B. Duffin.	Mr. Henry Smith.
Dr. William Playfair.	Mr. H. Royes Bell.
Dr. J. Burney Yeo.	
Dr. T. C. Hayes.	*Assistant-Surgeons.*
Dr. David Ferrier.	Mr. William Rose.
	Mr. W. W. Cheyne.
Assistant-Physicians.	
Dr. E. B. Baxter.	*Dental Surgeon.*
Dr. John Curnow.	Mr. S. Hamilton Cartwright.

Ophthalmic Surgeon—Mr. M. M. McHardy.
Aural Surgeon—Dr. Urban Pritchard.
Vaccinator—Mr. R. W. Dunn.
Pathological Registrar—Mr. A. B. Barrow.
Chloroformist—Mr. Charles Moss.
Sambrooke Registrars—Mr. V. Matthews, Mr. Hugh Smith, and Mr. W. J. Penny.

PROFESSORS.

Anatomy, Descriptive and Surgical—Dr. John Curnow.
Botany—Mr. Robert Bentley.
Chemistry and Practical Chemistry—Mr. C. L. Bloxam; Mr. J. M. Thomson, Demonstrator; Mr C. S. Johnson, Assist.-Demonstrator.
Clinical Medicine—Dr. G. Johnson.
Clinical Surgery—Mr. John Wood.
Comparative Anatomy—Mr. F. Jeffrey Bell.
Dental Surgery—Mr. S. Hamilton Cartwright.
Forensic Medicine—Dr. D. Ferrier.
Hygiene—Dr. Charles Kelly.
Materia Medica and Therapeutics—Dr. E. B. Baxter.
Ophthalmology—Mr.M.M.McHardy

Obstetric Medicine, and the Diseases of Women and Children—Dr. W. Playfair.
Pathological Anatomy—Dr. A. B. Duffin.
Physiology and Practical Physiology—Dr. Gerald F. Yeo; Mr. J. W. Groves.
Psychological Medicine—Dr. Edgar Sheppard.
Principles and Practice of Medicine—Dr. L. S. Beale.
Principles and Practice of Surgery—Mr. Henry Smith.
Surgery and Practical Surgery—Mr. Henry Smith; Mr. H. Royes Bell, Mr. W. Rose, and Mr. W. W. Cheyne, Demonstrators.

Dean of the Faculty—Professor Bentley.
Sub-Dean and Medical Tutor—Dr. N. I. C. Tirard.

SCHOLARSHIPS, EXHIBITIONS, AND PRIZES.

Warneford Scholarships: "For the encouragement of the previous education of medical students," two scholarships of £25 per annum each, to be held for three years; and, "for the encouragement of resident medical students," one scholarship of £25 per annum, to be held for two years.

Medical Scholarships: The following are given every year to matriculated students of this department :—1. One of £40, to be held for two years, open to students of the third and fourth years; 2. One of £30, for one year, open to students of the second year; 3. One of £30, for one year, open to students of the first year.

Daniell Scholarship: £20, tenable for two years; is open to every student of the College who has worked in the laboratory for at least six months.

Sambrooke Registrarships: Two of £50 every year.

Science Exhibitions: Two annually; one of £50 and one of £25 per annum, each tenable for two years, for proficiency in Mathematics, Mechanics, Physics, Chemistry, Botany, and Zoology.

Sambrooke Exhibitions: Two annually, one of £50, and one of £40, for proficiency in English, Elementary Physics, Inorganic Chemistry, Botany, Zoology, Mathematics, and Languages.

Leathes Prizes: Bible and Prayer-book, annually, to two matriculated medical students.

Warneford Prizes: £40 is expended annually in the purchase of medals and books as prizes to two matriculated medical students.

Class Prizes are awarded annually of the value of £3 in each subject of study.

Two Medical Clinical Prizes, one of £3 for the winter session, and the other of £2 for the summer session, and two Surgical Clinical Prizes of the same value, are given annually for attendance at the Hospital.

Todd Medical Clinical Prize: This prize was founded in memory of the late Dr. Todd, and is awarded annually. It consists of a bronze medal and books to the value of £4 4s.

Tanner Prize: Of the value of £10 in each year, for proficiency in the study of Obstetric Medicine, and in Diseases of Women and Children.

FEES.

The fees for perpetual attendance amount to £125 if paid in one sum on entrance; or £130 if paid in two instalments—viz., £70 on entrance and £60 at the commencement of the second winter session; or £135 if paid in three instalments—viz., £60 on entrance, £50 at the beginning of the second winter session, and £25 at the beginning of the third winter session. Students are, however, recommended to add to the

above the fee for attendance on the medical tutor's class for one year—viz., £3 3s.; or, in the case of those preparing for the Preliminary Scientific Examination of the University of London, £5 5s.

For further information apply to Professor Bentley, Dean of the Medical Faculty.

LONDON HOSPITAL AND MEDICAL COLLEGE.

MEDICAL AND SURGICAL STAFF.

Consulting Physician—Dr. Herbert Davies and Dr. Ramskill.
Consulting Surgeons—Mr. Luke, F.R.S., and Mr. Curling, F.R.S.

Physicians.

Dr. Andrew Clark.	Dr. Sutton.
Dr. Langdon Down.	Dr. Fenwick.
Dr. Hughlings-Jackson, F.R.S.	Dr. Stephen Mackenzie.

Dr. A. E. Sansom.

Assistant-Physicians.

Dr. F. Charlewood Turner.	Dr. F. Warner.
Dr. Gilbart Smith.	Dr. C. H. Ralfe.

Surgeons.

Mr. Hutchinson.	Mr. Jas. Adams.
Mr. Couper.	Mr. Waren Tay.
Mr. Rivington.	Mr. McCarthy.

Assistant-Surgeon—Mr. Reeves and Mr. Fredk. Treves.
Obstetric Physician—Dr. Palfrey.
Assistant Obstetric Physician—Dr. G. E. Herman.
Surgeon-Dentist—Mr. Ashley Barrett.
Surgeons to the Ophthalmic Department—Mr. James Adams and Mr. Waren Tay.
Surgeon to the Aural Department—Mr. A. Gardiner Brown.
Physician to the Skin Department—Dr. Stephen Mackenzie.

LECTURES.

Anatomy and Pathology of the Tooth—Mr. Ashley Barrett.
Botany—Mr. Warner.
Chemistry—Dr. C. Meymott Tidy.
Comparative Anatomy.
Descriptive and Surgical Anatomy—Mr. Walter Rivington.
Diseases of the Throat and Use of the Laryngoscope—Dr. Morell Mackenzie.
Forensic Medicine—1. Toxicology, Mr. J. R. D. Rodgers; 2. Medical Jurisprudence and Public Health, Dr. C. Meymott Tidy.
Materia Medica and General Therapeutics—Dr M. Prosser James.
Midwifery and Diseases of Women—Dr. James Palfrey.

Medicine—Dr. Stephen Mackenzie.
Pathology and Demonstrations of Morbid Anatomy—Dr. H. G. Sutton.
Practical Anatomy—Mr. Frederick Treves.
Practical Chemistry—Dr. C. Meymott Tidy.
Practical Histology, and Use of the Microscope—Mr. McCarthy.
Physiology and General Anatomy—Mr. McCarthy.
Ophthalmic Surgery—Mr.J.Couper.
Operative Surgery—Mr. J. Adams.
Practical Surgery—Mr. Reeves.
Surgery—Mr. Jas. Adams.
Aural Surgery—Mr. A. Gardiner Brown.

Warden—Mr. Munro Scott.

SCHOLARSHIPS AND PRIZES.

Ten scholarships will be offered for competition during the ensuing winter and summer sessions.

Two Entrance Scholarships in Natural Science, of the value of £60 and £40 respectively, will be offered for competition at the end of September. The subjects will be Physics, Botany, Zoology, and Inorganic Chemistry.

The two Buxton Scholarships will be awarded in October to the students who distinguish themselves most in the subjects appointed by the General Council of Medical Education and Registration as the subjects of the preliminary examinations. 1. A scholarship, value £3), to the student placed first in the examination. 2. A scholarship, value £10, to the student placed second in the examination.

A Scholarship, value £30, will be awarded to the first-year student who shall pass in March, 1881, the best examination in Human Anatomy and Physiology.

A Scholarship, value £25, will be awarded to the first-year or second-year student who shall pass at the end of the winter session the best examination in Anatomy, Physiology, and Chemistry.

A Hospital Scholarship, value £30, for proficiency and zeal in Clinical Medicine.

A Hospital Scholarship, value £30, for proficiency and zeal in Clinical Surgery.

A Hospital Scholarship, value £30, for proficiency and zeal in Obstetrics (awarded at the end of June, 1881).

The Letheby Prize, value (at least) £35, for proficiency in Chemistry.

The Duckworth-Nelson Prize, value £10, will be awarded by competition biennially, and will be open to all students. The subjects of examination will be Practical Medicine and Surgery.

Money prizes, to the value of £60 per annum, are awarded by the House Committee to the most meritorious of the Dressers in the out-patient rooms who have passed their first College examination.

The Hospital contains nearly 800 beds, and the number of in-patients last year amounted to 6312, exclusive of 532 remaining under treatment at the commencement of the year.

Owing to the great size of the Hospital, the appointments are necessarily numerous and most valuable. They are all free to full students without additional fee.

The resident appointments consist of five House-Physicians, four House-Surgeoncies, and one Accoucheurship, each being tenable for six months, and renewable for two further periods of three months each. The holders of these appointments are provided with board and lodging free of expense. Two Dressers and two Maternity Assistants also reside in the Hospital.

Attached to the Pathological Department of the London

Hospital is a laboratory, under the supervision of Dr. Sutton, which contains a large number of microscopic sections, carefully indexed and recorded. This important addition is entirely due to the liberality of the Hospital authorities, and was made a part of the new "Grocers' Wing."

FEES.

Perpetual fee for attendance on all the lectures with two years' Practical Anatomy, and for attendance on medical and surgical practice, qualifying for examination at most of the medical and surgical boards, £94 10s. if paid in one sum, or £105 in three instalments of £47 5s., £42, and £15 15s., at the commencement of the first, second, and third years respectively; composition fee for gentlemen entering at or before the beginning of their second winter session, their first year having been spent at a recognised medical school elsewhere, £73 10s. if paid in one sum, or £78 15s. in two instalments of £47 5s. and £31 10s.; perpetual fee for lectures alone, £52 10s.; perpetual fee for hospital practice alone, £52 10s. Extra fees: Practical Chemistry (for apparatus, etc.), £2 2s.; Practical Physiology do., £1 1s.; subscription to the library (compulsory), £1 1s.

Students in Arts of Universities where residence is required, who have attended lectures in Anatomy, Physiology, Chemistry, Botany, or Comparative Anatomy, and have obtained signatures for such attendance, fulfilling the requirements of the Examining Boards, may become pupils of the London Hospital, eligible for all hospital appointments, on payment of the fee of £52 10s. for practice at the Hospital. This payment does not give the right to signatures for courses of lectures at the Medical College.

Students who have passed the Preliminary Scientific Examination at the University of London, and have obtained signatures for lectures on Botany, Zoology, Chemistry, and Practical Chemistry, shall have the fees for the same, amounting to £18 18s., remitted on entering as full students at the London Hospital; and students who have attended the above courses elsewhere, and have obtained signatures for the same previous to their entrance at the London Hospital, shall also have these fees remitted, provided they pass the Preliminary Scientific Examination within eighteen months of their entry as full students.

Communications should be addressed to Mr. Munro Scott, the Warden, at the London Hospital Medical College, Turner-street, Mile-end, London, E.

ST. MARY'S HOSPITAL.

MEDICAL OFFICERS.

Consulting Medical Officers.
Sir James Alderson, M.D., F.R.S., Dr. Chambers, Mr. Lane, Mr. Spencer Smith, Mr. White Cooper.

Physicians.	*Surgeons.*
Dr. Handfield Jones, F.R.S.	Mr. Haynes Walton.
Dr. Sieveking.	Mr. James R. Lane.
Dr. Broadbent.	Mr. Norton.

Surgeons in charge of Out-Patients.
Mr. Edmund Owen.
Mr. Herbert W. Page.
Mr. Pye.

Physicians in charge of Out-Patients.
Dr. Cheadle.
Dr. Shepherd.
Dr. David Lees.

Assistant-Surgeon.
Mr. Pepper.

Physician-Accoucheur—Dr. Alfred Meadows.
Assistant Physician-Accoucheur—Dr. Wiltshire.
In charge of the Department for Diseases of the Skin—Dr. Cheadle, Mr. Malcolm Morris.
Surgeon in charge of the Ophthalmic Department—Mr. Haynes Walton.
Surgeon in charge of the Department for Diseases of the Throat—Mr. Norton.
Aural Surgeon—Mr. G. Field.
Surgeon-Dentist—Mr. Howard Hayward.
Post-mortem Examinations—Dr. Henderson.
Instructor in Vaccination—Mr W. A. Sumner.

LECTURES.—WINTER SESSION.

Anatomy—Mr. Owen.	Dental Surgery—Mr. Howard Hayward.
Clinical Medicine—Dr. Handfield Jones, Dr. Sieveking, and Dr. Broadbent.	Medicine—Dr. Broadbent and Dr. Cheadle.
Clinical Surgery — Mr. Haynes Walton, Mr. J. R. Lane, and Mr. Norton.	Physiology—Mr. Pye.
Chemistry and Natural Philosophy —Dr. C. R. A. Wright.	Practical Physiology—Mr. Pepper.
Pathology—Dr. Shepherd.	Practical Surgery—Mr. Herbert W. Page.
	Surgery—Mr. James R Lane and Mr. Norton.

SUMMER SESSION.

Aural Surgery—Mr. G. Field.	Materia Medica—Dr. Lees.
Botany—Rev. J. M. Crombie.	Midwifery—Dr. Meadows and Dr. Wiltshire.
Comparative Anatomy—Mr. St. George Mivart, F.R.S.	Ophthalmic Surgery—Mr. Anderson Critchett.
Diseases of the Skin—Dr. Cheadle and Mr. Malcolm Morris.	Practical Chemistry—Dr. C. R. A. Wright.
Medical Jurisprudence—Dr. Randall	

The Hospital contains 190 beds—88 medical, and 102 surgical. There are special departments for the Diseases of Women and Children, and for Diseases of the Eye, the Ear, the Skin, and the Throat.

SCHOLARSHIPS, PRIZES, ETC.

Two Scholarships in Natural Science, tenable for three years, the first of a total value of £150, the second of a total value of £105. These are awarded by open competitive examination at the commencement of the winter session.

A Scholarship in Anatomy, of the annual value of £30, is offered for competition amongst those students who have completed their second or third winter session; and a Scholarship in Pathology, of the value of £40 (the holder of which is styled Assistant-Curator), for those students who have completed their third winter session.

Examinations for prizes are held at the termination of each session in the various classes for students of the first, second, and third year.

Two Prosectors are appointed annually, who each receive a certificate and £5 for their services in the dissecting-room.

FEES.

The entrance fee may be paid in instalments by arrangement with the Dean of the School. Students who have kept the two years' course at the University of Cambridge are admitted as perpetual pupils on payment of £72 9s., and those who have kept a portion of the course elsewhere at a proportionate reduction. A fee of £1 1s. is required to be paid to the library and reading-room. Instruction in vaccination can be obtained; fee £1 1s.

Further information may be obtained from Dr. Shepherd, Dean of the School; or from the Registrar, at the Hospital.

MIDDLESEX HOSPITAL.

MEDICAL AND SURGICAL STAFF.

Consulting Physicians—Dr. A. P. Stewart, Dr. Goodfellow, Dr. Henry Thompson, Dr. Greenhow, F.R.S.
Consulting Surgeons—Mr. Shaw, Mr. Nunn.
Consulting Dental Surgeon—Mr. Tomes, F.R.S.

Physicians.	*Surgeons.*
Dr. Cayley.	Mr. Hulke, F.R.S.
Dr. Sidney Coupland.	Mr. Lawson.
Dr. Douglas Powell.	Mr. Morris.

Assistant-Physicians.	*Assistant-Surgeons.*
Dr. David Finlay.	Mr. Andrew Clark.
Dr. J. K. Fowler.	Mr. Robert Lyell.
Dr. C. Y. Biss.	

Obstetric Physician—Dr. Hall Davis.
Physician to Skin Department—Dr. Robert Liveing.
Assistant Obstetric Physician—Dr. Arthur Edis.
Ophthalmic Surgeon—Mr. William Lang.
Aural Surgeon—Mr. Arthur Hensman.
Dental Surgeon—Mr. Turner.
Assistant Dental Surgeon—Mr. Storer Bennett.
Curator of Museum and Pathologist—Dr. J. K. Fowler.
Registrars—Dr. J. W. Browne and Mr. Sidney Phillips.
Resident Medical Officer—Mr. R. A. Fardon.
Chloroformist—Mr. G. Everitt Norton.

LECTURES.—WINTER SESSION.

Chemistry—Mr. Wm. Foster.	Physiology and General Anatomy—Mr. B. Thompson Lowne.
Clinical Lectures on Medicine and Surgery—The Physicians and Surgeons.	Practical Demonstrations on Diseases of the Eye—Mr. Lang.
Clinical Lectures on Diseases of Women and Children—Dr. J. Hall Davis.	Practical Surgery — Mr. Andrew Clark.
Descriptive and Surgical Anatomy —Mr. Hensman.	Principles and Practice of Medicine —Dr. Cayley.
Pathological Anatomy—Dr. Coupland.	Principles and Practice of Surgery —Mr. Henry Morris.

SUMMER SESSION.

Botany—Dr. Biss.	Diseases of the Skin—Dr. Robert Liveing.
Clinical Lectures on Medicine and Surgery—The Physicians and Surgeons.	Practical Demonstrations on Diseases of Women and Children—Dr. Arthur Edis.
Clinical Lectures on Diseases of the Eye—Mr. Lang.	Practical Demonstrations on Diseases of the Larynx and Ear—Mr. Hensman.
Comparative Anatomy and Zoology —Dr. Thorowgood.	Practical Physiology and Histology —Mr. B. Thompson Lowne.
Materia Medica and Therapeutics—Dr. Thorowgood.	Practical Chemistry — Mr. Wm. Foster.
Medical Jurisprudence—Dr. D. W. Finlay.	Psychological Medicine—Mr. Henry Case, Supt. Leavesden Asylum.
Midwifery and Diseases of Women and Children — Dr. J. Hall Davis.	Public Health—Dr. D. W. Finlay.

This Hospital contains 310 beds, of which 190 are for surgical and 120 for medical cases. There is a special department for Cancer cases, affording accommodation for thirty-three in-patients, whose period of residence in the Hospital is unlimited. Wards are also appropriated for the reception of cases of Uterine Disease and of Syphilis, and beds are set apart for patients from Diseases of the Eye. There are special out-patient departments for Diseases of the Skin, the Throat, the Eye and Ear.

PRIZES AND SCHOLARSHIPS.

Two Entrance Scholarships of the annual value of £25 and £20, tenable for two years, are afforded for competition at the commencement of the winter session.

A Science Scholarship of the value of £50 will be offered for competition at the commencement of the winter session 1881-82. The successful candidate will be required to become a general student of the school. Examination in Inorganic Chemistry, Botany and Vegetable Physiology, Zoology, and Experimental Physics. The schedule of these subjects will be that of the Preliminary Scientific Examination of the University of London, and there will be a practical examination in the first three.

Two Broderip Scholarships of the annual value of £30 and £10, tenable for two years, and a clinical prize of £10 10s., are annually awarded to those students who pass the most satisfactory examination at the bedside, and in the post-mortem room.

The Murray Scholarship is open to all general students, and will next be awarded in 1883. Examinations in Medicine, Surgery, and Midwifery.

The Governors' Prize of £21 is awarded annually to the student who shall have most distinguished himself during his three years' curriculum.

FEES.

The fee for attendance on the hospital practice and lectures required by the Colleges of Physicians and Surgeons and the Society of Apothecaries is £90 if paid in advance, or £40 on entrance, £35 at the beginning of the second winter session, £20 at the beginning of the third winter session, and £5 at the beginning of the fourth winter.

Dental students who intend to become Licentiates in Dental Surgery of the Royal College of Surgeons are admitted to attend the requisite courses of lectures and hospital practice on payment of a fee of £42, either in one payment or by instalments of £30 on entrance, and £15 at the beginning of the second winter session.

ST. THOMAS'S HOSPITAL.

MEDICAL AND SURGICAL STAFF.

Honorary Consulting Physicians—Dr. Barker, Sir J. Risdon Bennett, Dr. Peacock.

Honorary Consulting Surgeons—Mr. F. Le Gros Clark, Mr. Simon, C.B.

Consulting Ophthalmic Surgeon—R. Liebreich, Esq.

Physicians.
Dr. Bristowe.
Dr. Stone.
Dr. Ord.
Dr. Harley.

Obstetric Physician.
Dr. Gervis.

Assistant-Physicians.
Dr. Payne.
Dr. Sharkey.
(Vacancy.)

Assistant Obstetric Physician.
Dr. Cory.

Resident Assistant-Physician.
Dr. Gulliver.

Surgeons.
Mr. Sydney Jones.
Mr. Croft.
Mr. Mac Cormac.
Mr. Mason.

Ophthalmic Surgeon.
Mr. Nettleship.

Assistant-Surgeons.
Mr. W. W. Wagstaffe.
Mr. A. O. MacKellar.
Mr. H. H. Clutton.
Mr. W. Anderson.

Dental Surgeon.
Mr. J. W. Elliott.

Assistant Dental Surgeon.
Mr. W. G. Ranger.

Resident Assistant-Surgeon.
Mr. B. Pitts.

Anæsthetist—Mr. S. Osborn.
Electrician—Mr. Kilner, M.B
Demonstrators of Morbid Anatomy—Dr. Reid and Dr. Sharkey.
Analytical Chemist of the Hospital—Dr. Albert J. Bernays.
Curator to the Museum—Mr. C. Stewart.
Apothecary—Mr. Plowman.
Medical Registrar—Mr. G. Gulliver, M.B.
Surgical Registrar—Mr. W. H. Battle.
Secretary to the Medical School—Dr. Gillespie. *Dean*—Dr. Ord.

LECTURES AND DEMONSTRATIONS.

Medicine—Dr. Bristowe and Dr. Ord.
Clinical Medicine—Dr. Bristowe, Dr. Stone, Dr. Ord, and Dr. Harley.
Obstetric Clinical Medicine—Dr. Gervis.
Surgery—Mr. Sydney Jones and Mr. Mac Cormac.
Clinical Surgery—Mr. S. Jones, Mr. Croft, Mr. Mac Cormac, and Mr. Mason. Special Course : Mr. Croft.
Descriptive Anatomy—Dr. Reid and Mr. Anderson.
General Anatomy and Physiology —Dr. John Harley.
Practical Physiology – Dr. T. C. Charles.

Ophthalmic Surgery—Mr. Nettleship.
Chemistry and Practical Chemistry —Dr. Bernays.
Midwifery and the Diseases of Women and Children—Dr. Gervis.
Physics and Natural Philosophy—Dr. Stone.
Materia Medica and Therapeutics—Dr. Stone.
Forensic Medicine—Dr. Payne and Dr. Cory.
Pathological Anatomy—Dr. Payne and Dr. Sharkey.
Botany—Mr. A. W. Bennett.
Comparative Anatomy — Mr. C. Stewart.
Mental Diseases—Dr. H. Rayner.
State Medicine—Dr. A. Carpenter.

TEACHERS OF PRACTICAL SUBJECTS AND DEMONSTRATORS.

Practical Chemistry—Dr. Bernays.
Practical and Manipulative Surgery —Mr. Mason and Mr. MacKellar.
Demonstrations in Anatomy—Dr. Reid, Mr. Anderson, Mr. Taylor, Mr. Haslam, and Assistants.
Demonstrations in Microscopical Anatomy—Mr. Rainey.
Demonstrations of Morbid Anatomy —Dr. Reid and Dr. Sharkey.

Demonstrations in Physiology—Mr. Hutton.
Demonstrations in Practical Physiology—Mr. R. P. Smith.
Diseases of the Eye—Mr. Nettleship.
Diseases of the Skin—Dr. Payne.
Diseases of the Throat—Vacancy.
Diseases of the Ear—Mr. Clutton.
Diseases of the Teeth—Mr. J. W. Elliott and Mr. W. G. Ranger.

PRIZES AND APPOINTMENTS.

Entrance Scholarships of £100 and £50, awarded after an examination in Physics and Chemistry, with either Botany or Zoology, whichever the candidate may choose.

First Year's Prizes.—Winter : The Wm. Tite Scholarship of £20 ; College Prizes—£20 and £10. Summer Prizes : £15 and £10.

Second Year's Prizes.—Winter : The College Scholarship of £42, tenable for two years ; College Prizes—£20 and £10. Summer Prizes : £15 and £10.

Third Year's Prizes.—Winter : £30, £15, and £10. Summer : £15 and £10. The Cheselden Medal, awarded after a special examination in Surgical Anatomy and Surgery. The Mead Medal, awarded after a special examination in Practical Medicine and Hygiene. The Solly Medal, biennially, with a prize of at least £10 10s., for a collection of surgical reports. The Treasurer's Gold Medal, for general proficiency during the entire course of study. The Grainger Testimonial Prize, of the value of £20, will be awarded biennially to the third or fourth year's students for a physiological essay, to be illustrated by preparations.

The Dresserships and the Clinical and Obstetrical Clerkships are open to students who have passed the primary examination at the Royal College of Surgeons, without extra charge.

FEES.

Gentlemen are informed that the admission fees to practice and to all the lectures may be paid in one of three ways, entitling to unlimited attendance—1st, £125, paid on entrance, entitle a student to unlimited attendance ; 2nd, £130 in two payments, of £70 on entrance and £60 at beginning of next year ; 3rd, by three instalments, of £60 the first year, £50 the second, and £30 the third. Special arrangements are made for students entering in second or subsequent years, and for Dental students ; and separate entries may be made to any course of lectures, or to the hospital practice.

There are special departments for Diseases of the Eye, Diseases of Women and Children, Vaccination, Diseases of the skin, Diseases of the Teeth, and Mental Diseases.

For further information, apply to Dr. Gillespie, Secretary to the Medical School, St. Thomas's Hospital, London, S.E.

UNIVERSITY COLLEGE HOSPITAL.

MEDICAL AND SURGICAL STAFF.

Consulting-Physicians.
Dr. Walter H. Walshe.
Dr J. Russell Reynolds
Sir William Jenner, Bart.

Physicians.
Dr. Wilson Fox.
Dr. Sydney Ringer.
Dr. H. Charlton Bastian.
Dr. F. T. Roberts.

Obstetric Physician.
Dr. Graily Hewitt.

Physician to the Skin Department.
Dr. Radcliffe Crocker.

Assistant-Physicians.
Dr. W. R. Gowers.
Dr. G. V. Poore.
Dr. T. Barlow.

Assistant Obstetric Physician.
Dr. John Williams.

Consulting-Surgeons.
Mr. Richard Quain.
Mr. J. Eric Erichsen.
Sir Henry Thompson.

Surgeons.
Mr. Marshall.
Mr. Berkeley Hill.
Mr. Christopher Heath.

Assistant-Surgeons.
Mr. Marcus Beck.
Mr. A. Barker.
Mr. R. J. Godlee.

Ophthalmic Surgeon.
Mr. J. F. Streatfeild.

Assistant Ophthalmic Surgeon.
Mr. J. Tweedy.

Dental Surgeon.
Mr. G. A. Ibbetson.

Assistant Professors of Clinical Medicine—Dr. W. R. Gowers and Dr. T. Barlow.
Assistant Professors of Clinical Surgery—Mr. Marcus Beck and Mr. A. Barker.
Assistant Professor of Midwifery—Dr. John Williams.
Surgical Registrar—
Resident Medical Officer—Mr. J. W. Bond, M.B., B.S.

LECTURES.—WINTER SESSION.

Chemistry—Dr. Williamson.
Clinical Medicine—Dr. W. Fox, Dr. S. Ringer, Dr. Bastian, Dr. Roberts, Dr. Barlow, Dr. Gowers.
Clinical Midwifery—Dr. G. Hewitt, Dr. John Williams.
Clinical Surgery—Mr. Erichsen, Mr. Marshall, Mr. B. Hill, Sir H. Thompson, Mr. C. Heath, Mr. Streatfeild, Mr. Beck, Mr. Barker.
Dental Surgery—Mr. Ibbetson.
Surgery—Mr. Marshall.
Skin Diseases—Dr. R. Crocker.

Descriptive Anatomy—Mr. Thane ; Demonstrations—Mr. Rickman J. Godlee, Dr. A. G. Silcock, Mr. B. Pollard, Mr. H. R. Woolbert, Mr. A. Kempe, Mr. W. C. Wilkinson.
Medicine—Dr. Sydney Ringer.
Practical Surgery—Mr. B. Hill, Mr. M. Beck, Mr. A. A. Barker.
Physiology and General Anatomy —Dr. E. Sanderson, Mr. Schäfer.
Zoology and Comparative Anatomy —Mr. E. R. Lankester.

SUMMER SESSION.

Botany—Professor Oliver.
Forensic Medicine—Dr. G. V. Poore.
Histology and Practical Physiology —Dr. B. Sanderson. Mr. Schäfer.
Hygiene—Dr. Corfield.
Materia Medica—Dr. F. T. Roberts.
Midwifery—Dr. Graily Hewitt, Dr. John Williams.
Operative Surgery—Mr. M. Beck.

Morbid Anatomy and Pathology—Dr. H. C. Bastian.
Natural Philosophy—Prof. G. C. Foster.
Ophthalmic Surgery — Mr. John Tweedy.
Practical Chemistry—Dr. Williamson.
Practical Pharmacy—Mr. Gerrard.

SCHOLARSHIPS AND EXHIBITIONS.

The Atkinson-Morley Surgical Scholarship, £45 per annum, tenable for three years, is awarded every year for proficiency in the theory and practice of Surgery.

The Atchison Scholarship, value about £55, tenable for two years, for general proficiency.

The Sharpey Physiological Scholarship, of about £70 a year, for proficiency in Biological Science.

The Filliter Prize of £30, for proficiency in Pathological Anatomy.

Dr. Fellowes' Clinical Medals, one gold and one silver, each winter and summer session, and certificates of honour, for reports and observations on the Medical Cases of the Hospital.

The Liston Gold Medal, and certificates of honour, for reports and observations on the Surgical Cases in the Hospital.

The Alexander Bruce Gold Medal, for Pathology and Surgery.

The Cluff Memorial Prize, awarded every other year for proficiency in Anatomy, Physiology, and Chemistry.

Gold and silver Medals, as well as certificates of honour, are awarded as class prizes.

The Jews' Commemoration Scholarship of £15 a year, tenable for two years, for general proficiency in the Faculty of Arts or of Science, for students of one year's standing; the Tuffnell Scholarship, £100, tenable for two years, for proficiency in Chemistry; and the Clothworkers' Exhibition for Chemistry and Physics, of £30 a year, tenable for two years, may be held by students who, after obtaining it, enter the Medical Faculty.

The Morris Bursary of £25, tenable for two years.

ENTRANCE EXHIBITIONS.

Three Entrance Exhibitions, of the respective value of £100, £60, and £40 per annum; subject—Science, as in London Preliminary Scientific Examination.

FEES.

For the lectures and hospital practice for the licences of the Royal College of Physicians, Society of Apothecaries, and M.R.C.S., £131 5s. if paid in one sum; or first year, £63; second year, £52 10s.; third year, £21.

Further information and detailed prospectuses may be obtained from the College, Gower-street, W.C.

WESTMINSTER HOSPITAL.

HOSPITAL STAFF.

Consulting Physician—Mr. Radcliffe.
Consulting Surgeons — Mr. Barnard Holt, Mr. Holthouse.

Physicians.	Surgeons.
Dr. Fincham.	Mr. Cowell.
Dr. Sturges.	Mr. Richard Davy.
Dr. Allchin.	Mr. Macnamara.

Assistant-Physicians.	Assistant-Surgeons.
Dr. Horatio Donkin.	Mr. T. Cooke.
Dr. De Havilland Hall.	Mr. T. Bond.
Dr. Hughes Bennett.	Mr Gould.

Obstetric Physician—Dr. Potter.
Assistant Obstetric Physician—Dr. Grigg.
Dental Surgeon—Dr. Walker.
Aural Surgeon—Mr. Keene.
Surgeon in charge of the Ophthalmic Department—Mr. Cowell.
Surgeon in charge of the Orthopaedic Department—Mr. R. Davy.
Surgeon in charge of the Skin Department—Mr Bond.
Physician in charge of the Throat Department—Dr. Hall.

LECTURERS.

Anatomy—Mr. A. Pearce Gould; Demonstrator, Mr. Black.
Aural Surgery—Mr. Keene.
Botany—Mr. Worsley-Benison.
Chemistry—Dr. Dupré.
Clinical Medicine — Dr. Radcliffe, Dr. Fincham, Dr. Sturges, Dr. Allchin.
Clinical Surgery—Mr. Holt, Mr. Holthouse, Mr. Cowell, Mr. Davy, Mr. Macnamara.
Comparative Anatomy—Dr. Leslie Ogilvie.
Dental Surgery—Dr. Walker.
Diseases of the Skin—Mr. Bond.
Experimental Physics—Dr. George Ogilvie.
Forensic Medicine and Hygiene—Mr. Bond, Dr. Dupré.

Materia Medica and Therapeutics—Dr. Murrell.
Medicine — Dr. Fincham, Dr. Sturges.
Midwifery and Diseases of Women—Dr. Potter.
Ophthalmic Surgery—Mr. Cowell.
Pathology and Morbid Anatomy—Dr. Allchin.
Physiology—Dr. Allchin.
Practical Chemistry—Dr. Dupré.
Practical Surgery — Mr. Richard Davy.
Practical Physiology and Histology—Mr. North.
Psychological Medicine — Dr. Sutherland.
Surgery — Mr. Cowell, Mr. Macnamara.

Treasurer of the School—Mr. Cowell.
Sub-Dean—Mr. Gould.
Pathologist and Curator of the Museum.—Dr. Hebb.
Dean of the School—Dr. Allchin.
Tutors—Dr. De Havilland Hall and Mr. Black.

In addition to the practice of the Hospital, which contains 201 beds, and has lately been enlarged and improved, the general students of this school are admitted to the practice of the Royal Westminster Ophthalmic Hospital, and to that of the National Hospital for Epilepsy and Paralysis.

PRIZES.

Entrance Scholarships (next October): The Fence, £40 a year for two years; and one other, value £40. Subjects—Latin, Mathematics, French or German, Chemistry, and Natural Philosophy. The Latin books the same as the June examination of the University of London Matriculation—Livy, Book II.

There are also an Exhibition, value £10 10s, for first year's men; a Scholarship in Anatomy and Physiology, value £21, for second year's men; Prizes for Clinical Medicine and Surgery of £5 each; the Frederic Bird Medal and Prize, value £15; the Chadwick Prize for general proficiency, value £21; numerous dresserships and clerkships; the posts of Pathologist and Curator of the Museum, with £52 10s. a year; Medical and Surgical Registrar, each with £40 a year; and of House-Physician (two), House-Surgeon, Resident Obstetric Assistant, Assistant House-Surgeon, Physician's Assistant, Surgeon's Assistant, Ophthalmic Assistant, and Assistant in the Skin Department.

FEES.

The entry fee to lectures and hospital practice required by the College of Physicians and Surgeons and the Society of Apothecaries may be paid in one sum of £100; in two payments of £52 10s. each, at the commencement of the first two years; or in five payments of £23 each, at the commencement of the first five sessions. The fees for Dental Students are £50 in one sum, or £32 10s. and £20 respectively at the commencement of each academic year.

Full particulars as to the preliminary scientific and tutorial classes, the courses of lectures and mode of instruction, will be found in the published Calendar, and any further information may be obtained by personal application to Dr. Allchin, the Dean of the School, or to Mr. Gould, the Sub-Dean.

PROVINCIAL MEDICAL SCHOOLS.

OXFORD.

THERE is no School of Medicine at Oxford.

CAMBRIDGE.

The following is a list of the classes and lectures in the Cambridge University School of Medicine:—

WINTER COURSES.

Anatomy—Professor Humphry and the Demonstrator (Mr. Hill).	Medicine—Professor Paget.
Superintendence of Dissections by the Professor of Anatomy and Demonstrators.	Physics—Professor Lord Rayleigh.
	Practical Chemistry — Professor Liveing and Mr. Hicks.
Anatomy and Physiology—Professor Humphry.	Physiology—Dr. Michael Foster.
Chemistry—Professor Liveing.	Zoology and Comparative Anatomy —Professor Newton, also by Mr. Balfour. Demonstrations by the Demonstrator.
Materia Medica—Professor Latham.	

SUMMER COURSES.

Botany—Professor Babington.	Human Osteology—Prof. Humphry or an Assistant.
Chemistry and Practical Chemistry — Professor Liveing and Mr. Hicks.	Pathology—Dr. Bradbury.
	Practical Physiology—Dr. Michael Foster or his Assistant.
Comparative Anatomy, Dissections by the Demonstrator.	Practical Histology—Mr. Hill.

ADDENBROOKE'S HOSPITAL, CAMBRIDGE.

This Hospital contains 120 beds.

MEDICAL AND SURGICAL STAFF.

Physicians.	Surgeons.
Dr. Paget.	Mr. Humphry.
Dr. Latham.	Mr. Carver.
Dr. Bradbury.	Mr. Wallis.
	Mr. Wherry.

Fees for attendance upon the practice (medical and surgical), £15 15s. for an unlimited period; £10 10s. for one year; £8 8s. for six months.

DOWNING COLLEGE, CAMBRIDGE.

Every alternate year an election to a Fellowship takes place, the holder of which must be engaged in the active pursuit of the studies of Law or Medicine. These Fellowships are of the annual value of £300, and are tenable for twelve years. They are not vacated by marriage, and the Fellows are not required to reside. Foundation Scholarships of £50 per annum (in some cases with rooms and commons) are offered annually for distinction in Natural Science, tenable until the B.A. degree, and in case of special merit for three years longer. Minor Scholarships of £40 to £70 per annum, tenable until their holders are of standing to compete for a Foundation Scholarship, are offered each year for competition before entrance, and one or more of these is awarded for proficiency in Natural Science.

THE QUEEN'S COLLEGE, BIRMINGHAM.

WINTER SESSION.

Chemistry—Dr. A. Bostock Hill.	Medicine—Professor Foster.
Demonstrations on Practical Anatomy—Mr. Bennett May and Mr. Henry Eales.	Pathology—Professor Rickards.
	Physiology — Professors Norris, Bartleet, and Carter.
Descriptive and Surgical Anatomy —Professor Thomas.	Surgery — Professors Pemberton and Furneaux Jordan.

SUMMER SESSION.

Botany—Professor Hinds.	Forensic Medicine and Toxicology —Profs. J. St. S. Wilders and Hill.
Dental Mechanics—Prof. C. Sims.	
Dental Metallurgy—Professor A. Bostock Hill.	Midwifery — Professors Clay and Bassett.
Dental Anatomy and Physiology—Professor F. K. Batchelor.	Ophthalmic Surgery — Professor Solomon.
Dental Surgery—Prof. Howkins.	Practical Chemistry—Professor A. Bostock Hill.
Diseases of Women and Children—Professors Berry and B.C. Jordan.	Operative Surgery—Professors Pemberton and Jordan.
Materia Medica—Professor Sawyer.	

Honorary Curator of Museum—Dr. A. H. Carter.
Medical Tutor—Mr. C. W. Suckling.

SCHOLARSHIPS AND PRIZES.

The Sands Cox Prize.—A prize of the value of £20 is given annually in the Medical Department, in accordance with the Act of Parliament, "in commemoration of the exertions of Mr. William Sands Cox in founding and supporting the College. This prize is open to students who have completed their curriculum, and is awarded after examination in Medicine, Surgery, and Midwifery. Every candidate is required to produce a certificate of good conduct from the Warden. The examination for this prize will be held in the third week in March

The Ingleby Scholarships.—Two Ingleby Scholarships, founded in memory of the late Dr. Ingleby, formerly Professor of Midwifery in this School, will be awarded annually, after examination in Obstetric Medicine and Surgery and Diseases of Women and Children. These scholarships are open to students who have completed the first two years of their curriculum in this College.

Class Prizes.—Medals and certificates of honour are awarded annually in each class after examination.

THE GENERAL AND QUEEN'S HOSPITALS, BIRMINGHAM.

GENERAL HOSPITAL STAFF.

Consulting Physician—Dr. Bell Fletcher.
Consulting Surgeon—Mr. D. W. Crompton.

Physicians.
Dr. Russell.
Dr. Wade.
Dr. Foster.
Dr. Rickards.

Surgeons.
Mr. Alfred Baker.
Mr. Oliver Pemberton.
Mr. T. H. Bartleet.
Mr. Robert Jolly.

Assistant-Physicians.
Dr. R. Saundby.
Dr. Simon.

Assistant-Surgeons.
Mr. W. G. Archer.
Mr. T. F. Chavasse.

Obstetrical Medical Officer—Dr. Edward Malins.
Resident Medical Officer—Dr. H. Malet.
Resident Surgeon and Surgical Tutor—Mr. H. G. Lowe.
Registrar and Pathologist—Dr. Berling.

QUEEN'S HOSPITAL STAFF.

Consulting Surgeon—Mr. Gamgee.

Physicians.
Dr. Heslop.
Dr. Sawyer.
Dr. Carter.
Dr. Hunt.

Surgeons.
Mr. West.
Mr. Furneaux Jordan.
Mr. J. St. S. Wilders.
Mr. Bennett May.

Obstetric Surgeon—Mr. John Clay.
Ophthalmic Surgeon—Mr. Priestley Smith.
Dental Surgeon—Mr. Charles Sims.
House-Physicians—Mr. Orchard and Mr. Vinrace.
House-Surgeons—Mr. Clarke and Mr. Bendall.

PHYSICIAN PRIZES.

The following prizes will be given annually:—Senior Medical Prizes, for third or fourth year students First Prize, £5 5s. Senior Surgical Prizes : First Prize, £5 5s. Junior Medical Prizes, for second year students : First Prize, £3 3s. Junior Surgical Prizes: First Prize, £3 3s. Midwifery Prize, £4 4s.

The examination for the above-mentioned prizes will be conducted by the Clinical Board, and, together with various resident hospital appointments, will be open for competition to all students registered by the Clinical Board.

BRISTOL SCHOOL OF MEDICINE.

COURSES OF LECTURES.—WINTER SESSION.

Chemistry—Mr. Thomas Coomber.
Descriptive and Surgical Anatomy—Mr. F. Richardson Cross.
Medicine—Dr. William H. Spencer and Dr. E. Markham Skerritt.

Surgery—Mr. Nelson C. Dobson.
Physiology—Dr. R. S. Smith.
Practical Anatomy—Demonstrator : Mr. William H. Harsant.
Hygiene—Mr. David Davies.

SUMMER SESSION.

Botany—Mr. Adolph Leipner.
Comparative Anatomy—Professor W. J. Sollas.
Materia Medica and Therapeutics—Dr. John E. Shaw.
Medical Jurisprudence—Dr. Reginald Eager and Dr. Alfred J. Harrison.
Midwifery and Diseases of Women—Dr. Joseph G. Swayne and Dr. A. E. Aust-Lawrence.

Operative Surgery and Surgical Pathology—Mr. V. Powell Keall.
Pathology and Morbid Anatomy—Dr. William H. Spencer and Dr. E. Markham Skerritt.
Practical Chemistry—Mr. Thomas Coomber.
Practical Physiology and Histology —Mr. George F. Atchley.
Practical Surgery—Mr. Arthur W. Prichard.

BRISTOL ROYAL INFIRMARY.

MEDICAL AND SURGICAL STAFF.

Honorary and Consulting Physicians—Dr. Alexander Fairbrother, Dr. Frederick Brittan, and Dr. Edward Long Fox.
Honorary and Consulting Surgeons—Mr. John Harrison and Mr. Augustin Prichard.

Physicians.
Dr. William H. Spencer.
Dr. R. Shingleton Smith.

Dr. Henry Waldo.
Dr. John E. Shaw.

Surgeons.
Mr. Edmund C. Board.
Mr. Christopher H. Dowson.

Mr. Arthur W. Prichard.
Mr. F. Richardson Cross.

Mr. J. Greig Smith.

Assistant-Surgeon.—Mr. William H. Harsant.
House-Physician—Mr. C. S. Watson.
House-Surgeon—Mr. A. A. Landon.
Medical Superintendent—Mr. J. H. Lee Macintire.

This Infirmary was founded in the year 1735, and is one of the largest provincial hospitals in England. It contains 250 beds.

PRIZES.

Suple's Medical Prize, consisting of a gold medal of the value of £5 5s., about £7 7s. in money, is given annually to the successful candidate

---

in an examination held by the Physicians. The examination comprises reports of cases in the medical wards, and the preparation of morbid specimens illustrative of disease, accompanied, if possible, by microscopic and chemical illustrations, besides written replies to questions in Medicine.

Suple's Surgical Prize corresponds in value and character to the medical one described above. In this case the examination is conducted by the Surgeons, and comprises surgical subjects only.

Clark's Prize.—The interest of £500, bequeathed by the late Henry Clark, Esq., Consulting Surgeon to the Infirmary, will be given annually to the most successful student of the third year at the examination held at the Medical School, provided he has attended his hospital practice at the Bristol Royal Infirmary, and can produce certificates of good moral character.

Tibbits' Memorial Prize.—A prize of about £12 12s., founded by public subscription in memory of the late E. W. Tibbits, Esq., Surgeon to the Infirmary, will be awarded annually after a competitive examination.

Crosby Leonard's Prize.—The interest of £300 will be awarded annually for the best reports of Surgical Cases.

Pathological Prize.—The Pathological Clerk at the expiration of his term of office will receive a prize of the value of £3 3s. if his duties have been performed to the satisfaction of the Faculty.

FEES.

An entrance fee of £2 2s. to the Infirmary, and subscription of £1 1s. per annum to the Library. Medical or Surgical Practice, £7 7s. for six months, £12 12s. for one year, £21 perpetual ; Medical and Surgical Practice together, in one payment, £21 for one year, £36 15s. perpetual. The above fees include Clinical Lectures. Clinical Clerkship, £5 5s. for six months, £8 8s. for one year ; Dressership, £6 6s. for each six months; Obstetric Clerkship, £3 3s. for each three months

All fees are paid to the Secretary, at the Infirmary.

BRISTOL GENERAL HOSPITAL.

MEDICAL AND SURGICAL STAFF.

Honorary and Consulting Surgeons—Mr. Robert W. Coe, Mr. W. Michell Clarke, Dr. Henry Marshall.
Honorary and Consulting Physician-Accoucheur—Dr. Joseph G. Swayne.

Physicians.
Dr. George F. Burder.
Dr. E. Markham Skerritt.
Dr. Alfred J. Harrison.

Surgeons.
Mr. F. Poole Lansdown.
Mr. George F. Atchley.
Mr. Nelson C. Dobson.
Mr. William F. Keall.

Physician-Accoucheur.
Dr. A. E. Aust-Lawrence.

House-Surgeon.
Mr. Charles F. Pickering.

Physician's Assistant.
Mr. Bryden.

Assistant House-Surgeon.
Mr. E. M. Knapp.

Dentist—Mr. Thomas C. Parson.

SCHOLARSHIPS AND PRIZES.

Martyn Memorial Entrance Scholarship.—This scholarship, of the value of £20, founded by public subscription, in memory of the late Dr. Samuel Martyn, Physician to the Hospital, is awarded annually at the commencement of the winter session, after a competitive examination in subjects of general education.

Clarke Scholarship.—A Surgical Scholarship of £15, founded by H. M. Clarke, Esq., of London, is awarded annually, at the end of the winter session, after an examination in Surgery.

Sanders Scholarship.—A scholarship, founded by the late John Nash Sanders, Esq., and consisting of the interest of £500, is awarded annually, at the end of the winter session, after examinations in Medicine, Surgery, and Diseases of Women.

Lady Haberfield Prize.—This prize, founded by the late Lady Haberfield and consisting of the interest of £1000, is awarded annually, at the end of the winter session, after examinations in Medicine, Surgery, and Diseases of Women.

The Martyn Memorial Scholarship and the Lady Haberfield Prize, when not awarded as above, are available for the remuneration of a Museum Curator, to be appointed from amongst the students after a competitive examination in subjects bearing upon the duties of the office.

The rules relating to the several scholarships may be had on application.

FEES.

Medical or Surgical Practice, £6 for six months ; £10 for one year ; £20 perpetual. Entrance fee for Clinical Clerk or Dresser, £5 5s. for six months. Entrance fee for Obstetric Clerk, £3 3s. for three months. Library fee, £1 1s. per annum. Resident pupils (including board, lodging, and washing) £100 for the first year, £50 for each subsequent year ; or for five years, with apprenticeship to the Hospital, £250.

Further particulars respecting the Infirmary may be known on application to the Dean of the Infirmary Faculty ; respecting the Hospital, on application to Dr. Harrison, or to the House-Surgeon, at the Hospital. Information regarding the Medical School will be afforded by the Honorary Secretary of the School, E. Markham Skerritt, M.D., Medical School, University College, Tyndall's Park, Bristol.

UNIVERSITY OF DURHAM COLLEGE OF MEDICINE.

The winter session will be opened on Monday, October 3.

The Infirmary contains 230 beds. There are special wards set apart for Diseases of the Eye, for Lock Cases (male and female), and for Children.

Clinical lectures are delivered by the Physicians and Surgeons in rotation three times a week. Pathological demonstrations are given as opportunity offers by the Pathologist. Practical Midwifery can be studied at the Newcastle Lying-in Hospital, where there is an outdoor practice of about 500 cases annually, available for students without fee.

SCHOLARSHIPS, ETC.

A University of Durham Scholarship, of the value of £25 a year for four years, for proficiency in Arts, awarded annually to perpetual students in their first year.

The Dickinson Scholarship, value £15 annually, for Medicine, Surgery, Midwifery, and Pathology.

The Tulloch Scholarship, value £20 annually, for Anatomy, Physiology, and Chemistry.

The Charlton Scholarship, value £25 annually, for Medicine.

The Gibb Scholarship, value £25 annually, for Pathology.

At the end of each session a silver medal and certificate of honour are awarded in each of the regular classes.

An Assistant Curator of the Museum is appointed annually from among the senior students, and receives an honorarium of £12 for the year.

Assistant Demonstrators of Anatomy, and Assistants to the Lecturer on Practical Physiology, are appointed yearly.

Four times in the year, two Resident Medical Assistants, two Resident Surgical Assistants, three Non-resident Clinical Clerks, and sixteen Non-resident Dressers (eight for the In-patients, and eight for the Out-patient Department), are nominated by the Medical Board, and, if approved, are appointed by the House Committee for three months.

Assistants in the Pathological Department, and two Assistants to the Dental Surgeon, are appointed in March and October.

FEES FOR HOSPITAL PRACTICE AND LECTURES.

1. A composition ticket for the complete course of lectures at the College may be obtained (1) by the payment of £52 10s. on entrance; (2) by two payments of £28 7s. at the commencement of the first and second winter sessions; (3) by the payment of three annual instalments, each of £21, at the commencement of the sessional year. The classes of Chemistry and of Practical Physiology are excepted from the number of classes that may be attended in perpetuity by perpetual students.

2. Fees for attendance on Hospital Practice:—Three months, £5 5s.; six months, £8 8s.; one year, £12 12s.; perpetual, £26 5s.; or by instalments at the commencement of the sessional year, viz.:—First year, £12 12s.; second year, £10 10s.; third year, £6 6s.; or by two instalments, viz.:—First year, £14 14s.; second year, £12 12s.

3. Single courses of lectures or tutorial classes (except the course on Chemistry), £4 4s.; Chemistry, £5 5s.

A fee of 10s. is required for the use of the College Library, from students attending the College for one year only, and a fee of 15s. from those attending for a longer period; and £1 1s. caution-money, to be returned at the end of the session, is required for the use of apparatus in the chemical laboratories, and 5s. caution-money for the use of bones.

Further particulars may be obtained from Dr. Luke Armstrong, Registrar, Clayton-street West; or Mr. Henry E. Armstrong, Secretary, 6, Wentworth-place, Newcastle-upon-Tyne.

NEWCASTLE-UPON-TYNE INFIRMARY.

MEDICAL AND SURGICAL STAFF.

Physicians.	Surgeons.
Dr. Phillipson.	Dr. Arnison.
Dr. Drummond.	Dr. Armstrong.
Dr. Oliver.	Dr. Hume.
	Mr. Page.

Assistant-Surgeons—Mr. G. E. Williamson and Mr. T. A. Dodd.

LIVERPOOL SCHOOL OF MEDICINE.

PROFESSORS AND LECTURERS.

Medicine—Dr. A. T. H. Waters.	Clinical Medicine—Dr. A. T. H. Waters, Dr. T. R. Glynn, and Dr. A. Davidson.
Surgery—Mr. Rushton Parker.	
Anatomy—Mr. W. Mitchell Banks.	
Physiology—Dr. Richard Caton.	Clinical Surgery—Messrs. R. R. Bickersteth, Reginald Harrison, and W. Mitchell Banks.
Pathology—Dr. A. Davidson.	
Ophthalmology—Mr. T. S. Walker.	
Chemistry—Dr. J. C. Brown.	Diseases of Children—Dr. R. Gee.
Experimental Physics—Dr. O. J. Lodge.	Materia Medica—Dr. W. Carter.
Midwifery and Gynæcology—Dr. J. Wallace.	Medical Jurisprudence—Dr. Ewing Whittle.
	Botany—Dr. George Shearer.

Comparative Anatomy—Dr. E. H. Dickinson.

DEMONSTRATORS.

Histology and Practical Physiology—Mr. F. T. Paul.	Practical Anatomy — Dr. Hyla Greaves.

ROYAL INFIRMARY, LIVERPOOL.

Consulting Physician—Dr. Turnbull.
Consulting Surgeon—Mr. Hakes.

Physicians.	Surgeons.
Dr. Waters.	Mr. Bickersteth.
Dr. Glynn.	Mr. Harrison.
Dr. Davidson.	Mr. Banks.

Obstetric Physician—Dr. Wallace.
Assistant-Surgeon—Mr. Parker.　　Pathologist—Mr. Paul.
Dental Surgeon—Mr. Phillip.
Surgeon to the Lock Hospital—Mr. McOheane, Mr. F. W. Lowndes.

The Infirmary contains nearly 300 beds. There are special wards for the treatment of Uterine and other Diseases of Women.

The Lock Hospital, adjoining the Infirmary, contains sixty beds.

SCHOLARSHIPS AND PRIZES.

Roger Lyon Jones Scholarships.—Two Lyon Jones Scholarships (£21 for two years) will be awarded in October to the applicants who have taken highest place at the matriculation examination of the London University, on condition that they become composition ticket-holders of the School. A third Lyon Jones Scholarship (£21 for two years) is awarded to second-year students for proficiency in Anatomy, Physiology, Chemistry, Botany, Materia Medica, and Practical Chemistry.

A Lyon Jones Gold Medal will be awarded to the senior student who passes the best examination in Medicine, Surgery, Pathology, and Midwifery, provided a sufficiently high standard of merit be attained.

Torr Medal.—A gold medal for Anatomy and Physiology, presented by Mr. John Torr, M.P., is awarded to the first student in the second year subjects.

Bligh Medal.—This gold medal, which is presented annually by Dr. John Bligh, Liverpool (also for the encouragement of the study of Anatomy and Physiology), is awarded to the first student in the first-year subjects.

Many other medals and prizes are also awarded.

FEES.

Composition Fee.—A payment of £63 on entrance or in two equal instalments (one-half on entrance, and the remainder within twelve months), entitles the student to attendance on all the lectures and demonstrations required for the Membership of the Royal College of Surgeons, the Licence of the College of Physicians and the Apothecaries' Society.

Library.—All medical students on registering are required to pay an annual fee of 10s. 6d. to the library and reading-room, or a perpetual fee of £1 1s.

The perpetual Hospital fee (£33 12s.) and the School composition fee for lectures required by the licensing bodies (£52 10s.) amount together to £96 12s. In addition to this must be reckoned Vaccination fee (£1 1s.), Dissecting-room expenses (roughly estimated at £3 3s.), and a summer course of Practical Anatomy, which, though not absolutely essential, is generally taken (£2 2s.), in all amounting to £6 6s. The total expenses of the education necessary to procure a medical and surgical qualification thus amount to somewhat over £100.

For prospectuses and all further information, apply to the Dean of the Medical Faculty, Dr. Caton, 184, Abercromby-square, Liverpool.

LIVERPOOL NORTHERN HOSPITAL.

MEDICAL AND SURGICAL STAFF.

Physicians—Dr. E. H. Dickinson and Dr. R. Caton.
Surgeons—Mr. Manifold, Mr. Pusey, and Dr. MoF. Campbell.
House-Physician—Mr. C. Shears.
House-Surgeon—Mr. G. G. Hamilton.
Assistant House-Surgeon—Mr. W. R. Parker.

The Hospital contains 146 beds (including special Children's Ward).

Fees for hospital practice and clinical lectures—Perpetual, £26 5s.; one year, £10 10s.; six months, £7 7s.; three months, £4 4s. Students can enter to Medical or Surgical Practice separately on payment of half the above fees. Practical Pharmacy, £2 2s. for three months.

Attendance on the practice of this Hospital qualifies for all the examining boards.

For further particulars, apply to the House-Surgeon.

LIVERPOOL ROYAL SOUTHERN HOSPITAL.

MEDICAL AND SURGICAL STAFF.

Physicians—Dr. Cameron, Dr. Carter, Dr. Williams.
Consulting Surgeons—Mr. Minshall, Mr. Higginson, and Dr. Nottingham.
Surgeons—Mr. Hamilton, Dr. Little, Mr. Paul.
Senior House-Surgeon—Mr. Davies.
Junior House-Surgeon—Mr. Chisholm and Dr. Davison.

There are 200 beds in this Hospital.

Clinical lectures given by the Physicians and Surgeons during the winter and summer sessions. Clinical clerkships and dresserships open to all students. Special wards for Accidents and Diseases of Children. Rooms for a limited number of resident students.

Fees for hospital practice and clinical lectures—Perpetual, £26 5s.; one year, £10 10s.; six months, £7 7s.; three months £4 4s.

The practice of the Hospital is recognised by all the examining bodies. Further information can be obtained from the Senior House-Surgeon.

VICTORIA UNIVERSITY, MANCHESTER (MEDICAL DEPARTMENT).

PROFESSORS AND LECTURERS.—WINTER SESSION.

Chemistry—Dr. Henry F. Roscoe.
Comparative Anatomy—Dr. Milnes Marshall.
Descriptive and Practical Anatomy —Dr. Morrison Watson.
General Pathology and Morbid Anatomy—Dr. Julius Dreschfeld.
Hospital Instruction — Physicians and Surgeons to Royal Infirmary.
Clinical Medicine — Dr. William Roberts.

Principles and Practice of Medicine —Dr. J. R. Morgan.
Organic Chemistry—Mr. C. Schorlemmer.
Physiology and Histology — Dr. Arthur Gamgee.
Surgery—Mr. Edward Lund.
Practical Surgery — Mr. Thomas Jones.
Surgical Pathology—Mr. Alfred H. Young.

SUMMER SESSION.

Botany—Mr. W. C. Williamson.
Diseases of Children—Dr. Henry Ashby.
Embryology—Dr. Milnes Marshall.
Hygiene and Public Health—Dr. Arthur Ransome.
Materia Medica and Therapeutics— Dr. Leech.
Medical Jurisprudence—Mr. C. J. Cullingworth.
Mental Diseases—Mr. G. H. Mould.

Midwifery and Diseases of Women —Dr. J. Thorburn.
Operative Surgery — Mr. Thomas Jones.
Ophthalmology—Dr. D. Little.
Practical Chemistry—Dr. Henry E. Roscoe.
Practical Morbid Histology—Dr. J. Dreschfeld.
Practical Physiology and Histology —Dr. Arthur Gamgee.

Demonstrators in Anatomy—Mr. A. Fraser and Mr. J. Macdonald Brown.
Registrar—Mr. J. Holme Nicholson.
Dean of the Medical School—Professor Gamgee, M.D., F.R.S.

SCHOLARSHIPS AND PRIZES.

A Turner Scholarship of £25 for fourth year's students. Prizes in books or instruments varying from £3 3s. to £5 5s. will be offered for competition in the several classes.

Platt Physiological Scholarships.—Two Scholarships of £50 each, tenable for two years, one of which is offered annually, are open to the competition of all students of the College who shall have studied Physiology in the College laboratory during one entire session, and whose age on January 1 preceding the examination shall not be under eighteen nor over twenty-five years.

Platt Exhibitions, value £15 each, are offered for competition in the senior and junior classes of Physiology respectively.

Dumville Surgical Prize, value £20: The prize will consist of books or surgical instruments at the option of the winner.

Dauntesey Medical Scholarship.—The Scholarship is of the value of about £100, and is tenable for one year.

Gilchrist Scholarships.—Three of £40 each, tenable for three years, one of which is annually awarded to the candidate who shall stand highest at the Matriculation Examination of the University of London in June, provided he pass in the honours division, and failing such, two of £25 each will be given to the two candidates who stand highest in the first division.

FEES.

A composition fee, of £63, payable in two sums of £31 10s. each at the commencement of the first and second years of studentship, admits to the four years' course of study. Students desirous of repeating attendances on any class after the expiration of the four years' course, will be allowed to do so on paying for each class attended one-third of the fee payable by students who do not compound. A student, however, who desires to continue his study of Practical Anatomy beyond two sessions, will be required to pay at the rate of £2 2s. for a three months' or £3 3s. for a six months' course.

Extra fees are charged for attendance on the practical classes in Botany and in Comparative Anatomy, and for Operative Surgery. Tutorial classes are held in Anatomy and Physiology (fee £2 2s.), and in Chemistry, Zoology, and Botany (fee 10s. 6d. for each class).

A charge of £1 1s. is also made for the chemicals used in the class of Practical Chemistry.

MANCHESTER ROYAL INFIRMARY.

MEDICAL AND SURGICAL STAFF.

Consulting Physicians—Dr. R. F. Ainsworth, Dr. Frank Renaud, Dr. T. H. Watts, and Dr. Henry Browne.
Consulting Surgeon — Mr. George Bowring.

Physicians.
Dr. William Roberts.
Dr. Henry Simpson.
Dr. John E. Morgan.
Dr. Daniel J. Leech.

Surgeons.
Mr F. A. Heath.
Mr. Edward Lund.
Mr. Walter Whitehead.
Mr. Thomas Jones.

Assistant-Physicians.
Dr. Julius Dreschfeld.
Dr. James Ross.

Assistant-Surgeons.
Mr. James Hardie.
Mr. F. Armitage Southam.

Obstetric Physician.
Dr. John Thorburn.

Ophthalmic Surgeon.
Dr. Little.

Dental Surgeon—Mr. G. W. Smith.
Resident Medical Officer—Dr. Graham Steell.
Resident Surgical Officer—Mr. C. H. Howlett.

Medical Supt. of the Royal Lunatic Hospital at Cheadle—Mr. G. W. Mould.
Medical and Surgical Registrar—Mr. G. A. Wright.
Pathological Registrar—Mr. A. H. Young.
General Superintendent and Secretary—Mr. W. L. Saunder.

STUDENTS' FEES.

Medical Practice.—Three months, £4 4s. ; six months, £8 8s. ; twelve months, £12 12s. ; full period required by the examining board, £18 18s.

Surgical Practice.—Three months, £6 6s. ; six months, £9 9s. ; twelve months, £18 18s. ; full period required by the examining board, £31 10s.

Composition Fee.—The fees for the full period required by the examining boards of both medical and surgical practice may be paid by a composition fee of £42 on entrance, or by two instalments of £22 each at an interval of twelve months.

In addition to the practice of the Infirmary, the Monsall Fever Hospital and the Barnes Convalescent Home will also be open, under certain regulations, to students for the purposes of instruction.

SHEFFIELD SCHOOL OF MEDICINE.

LECTURERS.—WINTER SESSION.

Anatomy, Descriptive and Surgical —Mr. E. Skinner. Mr. Snell
Clinical Surgery—The Surgeons of the Infirmary and Public Hospital and Dispensary.
Clinical Medicine—The Physicians of the Infirmary and Public Hospital and Dispensary.
Physiology - Dr. Dyson and Mr. W. D. James.

Chemistry—Mr. Allen.
Demonstrations of Anatomy—Mr. R. J. Pye-Smith, Dr. Davison.
Principles and Practice of Medicine — Dr. Bartolomé, Dr. Banham, Dr. W. R. Thomas.
Principles and Practice of Surgery— Mr. W. F. Favell, Mr. A. Jackson.
Lecturer on Diseases of the Eye— Mr. Snell.

SUMMER SESSION.

Botany—Mr. Birks.
Demonstrations of Pathology and Microscopy—The House-Surgeon (at the Infirmary).
Demonstrations of Operative Surgery—Mr. Favell.
Demonstrations of Practical Histology and Physiology—Vacant.
Practical Chemistry—Mr. Allen.

Materia Medica and Therapeutics —Dr. Young.
Medical Jurisprudence and Toxicology—Mr. Harrison, Mr. Bell.
Midwifery and Diseases of Women —Dr. Hime.
Practical Surgery—The House-Surgeon (at the Infirmary).
Public Medicine—Dr. Drew.

SHEFFIELD GENERAL INFIRMARY.

MEDICAL AND SURGICAL STAFF.

Physicians.
Dr. Bartolomé.
Dr. Law.
Dr. Banham.

Surgeons.
Mr. Barber.
Mr. Favell.
Mr. Jackson.

Ophthalmic Surgeon—Mr. Snell.
House-Surgeon—Dr. S. John Wright.
The Infirmary contains 180 beds for in-patients.

PUBLIC HOSPITAL AND DISPENSARY.

Physicians.
Dr. H. J. Branson.
Dr. Dyson.
Dr. W. R. Thomas.

Surgeons.
Dr. Keeling.
Mr. Thorpe.
Mr. Pye-smith.

House-Surgeon—Mr. Willey.

This Hospital contains 112 beds. Recognised by the Royal College of Surgeons.

FEES.

One fee admits to the Infirmary and the Public Hospital and Dispensary. For the summer session, £3s 3s. ; for the winter session, £6 6s. for Medicine, and the same for Surgery.

SHEFFIELD HOSPITAL FOR DISEASES OF WOMEN.

MEDICAL OFFICERS.

Dr. Keeling, Dr. Hime, Mr. Woolhouse, Mr. R. Favell.

FEES.

Anatomy and Physiology, first course, £6 6s. ; second course, £4 4s. Practice of Medicine, first course, £4 4s. ; second course, £2 2s. Practice of Surgery, first course, £4 4s. Chemistry, first course, £4 4s. Midwifery and Diseases of Women, first course, £3 3s. Materia Medica, first course, £3 3s. Medical Jurisprudence, first course, £3 3s. Botany, first course, £3 3s. Practical Chemistry, first course, £3 3s. Practical Physiology, £3 3s. Practical Surgery, £3 3s. These fees include demonstrations, but not Tutor's fee, which is £2 2s.

Perpetual fee for attendance on all the lectures required by the Royal College of Surgeons and the Apothecaries' Hall, £45.

All further information may be obtained on application to the Hon. Secretary, Arthur Jackson, Wilkinson-street, Sheffield.

LEEDS SCHOOL OF MEDICINE.

CLASSES AND LECTURES.

Descriptive Anatomy—Mr. John A. Nunneley, Mr. Edmund Robinson, and Mr. A. F. McGill.

Demonstrator of Anatomy—Mr. A. W. M. Robson; assisted by Dr. J. B. Hellier and Mr. R. N. Hartley.

Demonstrator in Physiology and Pathological Histology—Dr. R. H. Jacob.

Physiology and General Anatomy—Mr. Chas. J. Wright and Mr. John Horsfall.

Practical Physiology and Histology—Mr. James Walker.

Chemistry (at the Yorkshire College)—Prof. T. E. Thorpe.

Practical Chemistry (at the Yorkshire College)—Prof. T. E. Thorpe.

Botany (at the Yorkshire College)—Prof. L. C. Miall.

Materia Medica and Therapeutics—Dr. Thomas Churton.

Pathology and Morbid Anatomy—Mr. A. W. M. Robson.

Medicine—Dr. T. Clifford Allbutt and Dr. John Edwin Eddison.

Clinical Medicine—Dr. T. Clifford Allbutt, Dr. John Edwin Eddison, and Dr. Thomas Churton.

Surgery and Practical Surgery—Mr. T. R. Jessop, and Mr. Edward Atkinson.

Clinical Surgery—Mr. C. G. Wheelhouse, Mr. T. P. Teale, Mr. T. R. Jessop, and Mr. Edward Atkinson.

Comparative Anatomy and Zoology (at the Philosophical Hall)—Prof. L. C. Miall.

Midwifery—Mr. W. N. Price, and Dr. James Braithwaite.

Forensic Medicine—Mr. Thomas Scattergood.

Mental Diseases—Dr. H. C. Major.

Resident Curator—Mr. Frederick Greenwood.

LEEDS GENERAL INFIRMARY.

MEDICAL AND SURGICAL STAFF.

Consulting Physician—Dr. Charles Chadwick.
Consulting Surgeon—Mr. Samuel Hey.

Physicians.	Surgeons.
Dr. T. Clifford Allbutt.	Mr. C. G. Wheelhouse.
Dr. John Edwin Eddison.	Mr. T. Pridgin Teale.
Dr. T. Churton.	Mr. T. R. Jessop.
	Mr. Edward Atkinson.

Surgeons to the Ophthalmic and Aural Department.
Mr. John A. Nunneley and Mr. R. P. Oglesby.
Dental Surgeon—Mr. T. Carter.

SCHOLARSHIPS AND PRIZES.

The Hardwick Clinical Prize.—Candidates for this prize must be in attendance on the lectures of the Leeds School of Medicine, and must have completed their first year's course there. They must be in registered attendance upon the medical practice of the Hospital, and have served the office of Clinical Clerk, or be holding that office at the time of competition. The prize is given annually for the best set of reports of medical cases in the Hospital during the winter session, subject to such regulations as may be laid down at the commencement of the session. Its value is £10 in money. Should the funds admit, a second prize may be given.

The Surgeons' Clinical Prizes.—Three prizes of the value of £3, £5, and £8 in money are offered annually by the Surgeons of the Hospital, subject to conditions similar to those relating to the Hardwick Prize.

The Thorp Prize in Forensic Medicine.—A prize of £20 (founded by a former Lecturer and present honorary member of the Council) is awarded at the close of each summer session, in one or more sums, subject to such regulations as may be made from time to time, of which due notice will be given.

Competitive Class Examinations.—At the close of each session, competitive examinations are held, when silver and bronze medals, books, and certificates of honour are awarded according to merit; but in no cases will prizes be awarded unless a reasonable standard of merit has been attained.

FEES.

The fees for school lectures, and for hospital practice (which includes clinical lectures) are distinct, and are paid separately.

Students may enter for single courses of lectures, or pay a composition fee. All students, however, must pay an entrance fee of £1 1s., which confers the privilege of using the library and reading-room.

The composition fee is £52 10s., if paid in one sum on entrance; or £27 6s. on entrance, and the same amount at the expiration of twelve months.

This composition fee, when the payment is completed, entitles a student to attend all the school lectures required for the examinations for the licence of the Royal College of Physicians of London, the membership of the Royal College of Surgeons of England, and the licence of the Society of Apothecaries.

The fee of 10s. 6d. is charged to students attending the demonstrations of Morbid Histology, for the use of reagents and apparatus.

Fees for medical practice and clinical lectures:—One summer session, £6 6s.; one winter session, £7 7s.; twelve months, £12 12s.; eighteen months, £15 15s.; three years, £21; perpetual, £26 5s.

The fees for surgical practice and clinical lectures:—One summer session, £6 6s.; one winter session, £7 7s.; twelve months, £12 12s.; eighteen months, £15 15s.; three years, £21; perpetual, £26 5s.

Instruction in vaccination, as required by the College of Surgeons and by the Poor-law Board, is given by one of the Public Vaccinators—fee £1 1s.

All further information may be obtained from the Honorary Secretary, Mr. John Horsfall, Hillary House, Leeds.

SCHOOLS AND HOSPITALS IN SCOTLAND.

UNIVERSITY OF EDINBURGH.—FACULTY OF MEDICINE.

SESSION 1881-82.

Principal—Sir Alexander Grant, Bart., LL.D.

THE session will be opened on Tuesday, October 25, 1881.

WINTER SESSION.

*Anatomy—Prof. Turner.

*Anatomical Demonstrations—Prof. Turner.

Botany—Prof. Dickson.

Chemistry—Prof. Crum Brown.

Clinical Medicine—Profs. Maclagan, Grainger Stewart, and T. R. Fraser. (Prof. Simpson on Diseases of Women.)

Clinical Surgery—Prof. Annandale.

General Pathology—Prof. Greenfield

Institutes of Medicine or Physiology—Prof. Rutherford.

Materia Medica—Prof. T. R. Fraser.

*Midwifery and Diseases of Women and Children—Prof. Simpson.

Natural History—Prof. Sir C. Wyville Thomson.

*Practice of Physic—Prof. Grainger Stewart.

*Surgery—Prof. Spence.

WINTER AND SUMMER SESSION.

*Anatomical Demonstrations—Prof. Turner.

Bandaging and Surgical Appliances—Prof. Spence.

*Operative Surgery—Prof. Spence.

*Obstetrical and Gynæcological Operations—Prof. Simpson.

Practical Physiology, including Histology, Chemical Physiology, and Experimental Physiology—Prof. Rutherford.

Practical Anatomy—Prof. Turner.

Practical Chemistry—Prof. Crum Brown.

* In University New Buildings.

SUMMER SESSION.

Practical Instruction in Mental Diseases at an Asylum — Dr. Clouston, Lecturer.

Practical Natural History — Prof. Sir C. Wyville Thomson.

Practical Morbid Anatomy and Pathology—Prof. Greenfield.

Practical Botany—Prof. Dickson.

Vegetable Histology—Prof. Dickson.

Tutorial Class of Clinical Medicine in the Wards of the Royal Infirmary by the Clinical Tutor, Dr. Jas. Murdoch Brown.

During the summer session lectures will be given on the following subjects :—

Anatomical Demonstrations—Prof. Turner.

Botany—Prof. Dickson.

Chemistry—Prof. Crum Brown.

Clinical Medicine—Profs. Maclagan, Grainger Stewart, and T. R. Fraser. (Prof. Simpson on Diseases of Women.)

Clinical Surgery—Prof. C. Annandale

Mental Diseases, with Practical Instruction at Morningside Asylum —Dr. Clouston, Lecturer.

Medical Jurisprudence—Prof. Maclagan.

Natural History — Prof. Sir C. Wyville Thomson.

Obstetrical and Gynæcological Operations—Prof. Simpson.

Information relative to matriculation and the curricula of study for degrees, examinations, etc., will be found in the University Calendar, and may be obtained on application to the Secretary at the College.

A list of fees is given on the next page.

During the summer session the following means are afforded for practical instruction :—

The *Dissecting Rooms* are open daily, under the Superintendence of the Professor, assisted by D. J. Cunningham, M.D., and other assistants.

The *Royal Edinburgh Asylum* is open to members of the class of Medical Psychology exclusively for practical instruction in Mental Diseases by the Physician-Superintendent, Dr. Clouston.

Chemical Laboratories.—The laboratory for instruction in Analytical Chemistry and for chemical investigation, under the superintendence of the Professor, assisted by R. M. Morrison, D.Sc., John Gibson, Ph.D., and Leonard Dobbin, Ph.D., is open from ten to four. The Laboratory for Instruction in Practical Chemistry, under the superintendence of the Professor, assisted by A. P. Aitken, M.A., D.Sc.

The *Physiological Laboratory* is open daily for physiological investigation, under the superintendence of the Professor, assisted by J. P. Anderson Stuart, M.B.

The *Physical Laboratory* is open daily from ten to three, under the superintendence of Professor Tait.

The *Medical Jurisprudence Laboratory* is also open daily from ten to three, under the superintendence of the Professor, assisted by James Allan Gray, M.D.

The practice of Obstetrical and Gynæcological Operations is carried out in the Obstetrical Museum, under the superintendence of the Professor, assisted by David B. Hart, M.D.

The *Natural History Laboratory* is open daily, under the superintendence of the Professor, Sir C. Wyville Thomson, assisted by Wm. A. Herdman, D.Sc.

The *Natural History Museum* in the Museum of Science and Art, Chambers-street, is accessible to the students attending the Natural History Class.

The *Royal Botanic Garden, Herbarium, and Museum* are open daily.

MEDICAL FELLOWSHIPS, SCHOLARSHIPS, BURSARIES, ETC.

Fellowships.

The Falconer Memorial Fellowship, value £100, tenable for two years. It is for the encouragement of the study of Palæontology and Geology, and is open to graduates in Science or Medicine of the University of not more than three years' standing.

The Syme Surgical Fellowship, value about £100, tenable for two years, open to competition among Bachelors of Medicine of not more than three years' standing, who shall present the best thesis on a surgical subject, giving evidence of original research.

The Leckie-Mactier Fellowship, consisting of the free annual proceeds of £2000, open to competition to Bachelors of Medicine of not more than three years' standing. The Fellowship to be tenable for three years, and the next award will be in November, 1882. The examination will comprise written reports and commentaries on three medical cases, three surgical cases, and one gynæcological case in the University wards in the Royal Infirmary; a written examination in Midwifery, Medical Jurisprudence, and Public Health; and an oral examination in Medicine, Surgery, Midwifery, Medical Jurisprudence, and Public Health.

Scholarships.

The Sibbald Scholarship, value about £40, tenable for four years.

A Hope Prize Scholarship, value about £30, will be awarded in March, 1881, to the most distinguished junior student in the chemical laboratory during the winter session.

The Thomson Scholarship, of the value of £40 yearly, tenable for four years, will be awarded in October, 1882; the subjects of examination, Botany, Zoology, and Elementary Mechanics. Candidates to be matriculated students about to commence their first winter session in the Medical Faculty; a preference to be given to candidates of the names of Thomson or Traquair, or to natives of the town or county of Dumfries, or of the city of Edinburgh.

Vans Dunlop Scholarships: Six scholarships, of the annual value of £100, tenable for four years—one to be awarded in March, 1881, to the candidate who, at the preliminary examination in March or the preceding October, shall have obtained the highest total number of marks required to enable him to appear for a professional examination; one in July, 1881, to the candidate who obtains the highest marks in Botany, Zoology, Chemistry, and Anatomy; one in March, 1881, for the highest marks in Physiology and Surgery; the other three to be awarded to the students who, at the end of the third winter session, shall obtain the highest number of marks in an examination, specially conducted for the purpose, on Anatomy, Physiology, Materia Medica, and Pathology—one scholarship, to be awarded in April, 1881, another in April, 1882, the third in April, 1883, and so on in each successive year.

The Vans Dunlop Scholarships in Chemistry and Chemical Pharmacy, and in Natural History, including Botany and Geology.—These Scholarships are of the value of about £100, and are tenable for three years.

The Coldstream Memorial Medical Missionary Scholarship, consisting of the free annual proceeds of at least £400, is open to students of Medicine who intend to prosecute their studies in the University of Edinburgh, and who propose to devote their lives to the calling of a Medical Missionary. The Scholarship is tenable for four years, and the next award may be made in October, 1883.

The Buchanan Scholarship, consisting of the annual proceeds of £1000, will be awarded yearly, on the day of medical graduation, for proficiency in Midwifery and Gynæcology. The award will be based upon the results of competitive examinations in the class of Midwifery and Diseases of Women and Children, upon the character of the records kept of cases treated in the gynæcological section of the class of Clinical Medicine, and upon the appearance made by the candidate at the final graduation examination.

Bursaries.

The Abercromby Bursary of £20, tenable for four years, is open to students who have been brought up in Heriot's Hospital during their medical curriculum.

The Sibbald Bursaries are open to the sons of duly registered medical men practising, or who may have practised in Scotland, and to the sons of parents who are, or who may have been, householders in Edinburgh. They are of the value of £30 each, tenable for four years, and available for the Faculty either of Arts, Law, Medicine, or Divinity.

Eight Thomson Bursaries, value £25 each, tenable for four years; one to be competed for each March and October, at the preliminary examinations required from candidates for graduation in Medicine. Candidates shall be those about to commence their medical curriculum, who shall attend the said preliminary examination, and who shall pass in a sufficient number of subjects to enable them to appear for a professional examination; a preference to be given to candidates of the names of Thomson or Traquair, or to natives of the town or county of Dumfries, or of the city of Edinburgh. Information as to the Thomson Bursaries and Scholarship may be got from Messrs. Traquair, Dickson, and Maclaren, W.S., 11, Hill-street, Edinburgh.

Four Grierson Bursaries of £20 a year.

One Tyndall-Bruce Bursary of £25, tenable for one year, to be competed for by students who have reached the end of their third winter session—subjects of examination, to be Materia Medica and Pathology. Competitors for the above bursaries must have studied the subjects of examination at the University of Edinburgh; and these are not to be held along with any other bursary or fellowship.

Two Dr. John Aitken Carlyle's Medical Bursaries, of the value of £25 each, tenable for one year, to be awarded at the end of each winter session—one to a first year's student for proficiency shown in the ordinary class examinations in Anatomy and Chemistry; one to a second year's student for proficiency shown in the ordinary class examinations in Anatomy and Physiology.

Two Mackenzie Bursaries, consisting of the proceeds of £1000, to be awarded annually—one to the student in the junior class of Practical Anatomy, and one to the student in the senior class of Practical Anatomy, who shall respectively display the greatest industry and skill in their Practical Anatomy work during the winter session.

Prizes.

The Ettles Medical Prize is awarded annually to the graduate in Medicine whom the Medical Faculty may consider the most distinguished of the year. Value about £40. The Beaney Prize will be awarded annually to the candidate for the degrees of M.B. and C.M. who, after having attended, within the University, courses of Anatomy, Surgery, and Clinical Surgery, qualifying for graduation, shall obtain the highest number of marks in those subjects during his examination for these degrees. Value about £40.

The Hope Chemistry Prize, open to all students of the University of not more than twenty-five years of age, who have worked for eight months, or for two summer sessions, in the Chemical Laboratory of the University. Value £100.

The Neil Arnott Prize, of about £40, is awarded to the candidate who shall pass with the greatest distinction the ordinary examination in Natural Philosophy for the degree of M.A. Candidates must have been medical students of this University during either a summer or a winter session, and the successful candidate must continue a medical student of this University during the winter session. No student can appear for examination after the completion of his third *annus medicus*; no candidate shall be allowed to offer himself more than once.

The Ellis Prize for the best essay "On the Respiration of Plants as distinguished from their Nutrition," is open to students or graduates of five years' standing. Value, proceeds of the sum of £500 accumulated for three years.

The Goodsir Memorial Prize of £60 is awarded triennially for the best essay containing results of original investigations in Anatomy or in Experimental Physiology.

The Wightman Prize is awarded to the student of the class of Clinical Medicine who shall write the best report and commentary on cases treated in the University clinical wards during the academic year.

The Cameron Prize, consisting of the free income of £2000, to be given yearly to the member of the medical profession who shall be adjudged to have made the most valuable addition to Practical Therapeutics during the year preceding the award.

The Medical Faculty Prizes.—Gold medals are given on the day of graduation to Doctors of Medicine whose theses are deemed worthy of that honour.

Lectureship.

The Swiney Lectureship on Geology, value £144, tenable for five years, is open to Doctors of Medicine of the University of Edinburgh. It is in the patronage of the trustees of the British Museum.

MINIMUM COST OF ATTENDING THE MEDICAL CLASSES, WITH THE ORDER OF STUDY.

Whilst there is no authorised order of study, the usual course is given below—Preliminary Examination in Arts to be taken in the month of March or October, before entering medical classes. By order of the General Medical Council, all medical students require to be registered as such within fifteen days after the commencement of the session. Students are recommended to commence their medical studies by attending the summer session.

First Summer Session.—Preliminary examination fee, 10s.; matriculation fee, 10s.; Botany (garden fee, 5s.), £4 4s.; Natural History, £4 4s.; total, £9 8s.

First Winter Session.—Matriculation (for whole year), £1; Anatomy, £4 4s.; Practical Anatomy, £3 3s.; Chemistry, £4 4s.; hospital, £6 6s. (perpetual ticket, £10); total, £18 17s.

Second Summer Session.—Botany or Natural History, if not attended previously; Practical Chemistry, £3 3s.; examination in Botany, Natural History, and Chemistry, in October following,(a) £5 5s.; total, £8 8s.

Second Winter Session.—Matriculation, £1; Institutes of Medicine, £4 4s.; Surgery, £4 4s.; hospital, £6 6s.; examination in Botany, Natural History, and Chemistry, in April, if not previously passed; total, £15 14s.

Third Summer Session.—Practical Pharmacy, £3 3s.; hospital; total, £3 3s.

Third Winter Session.—Matriculation, £1; Materia Medica, £4 4s.; Pathology, £4 4s.; Clinical Surgery, £4 4s.; hospital; examination in Anatomy, Physiology, Materia Medica, Pathology, in April or July, £5 5s.; total, £18 17s.

Fourth Summer Session.—Medical Jurisprudence, £4 4s.; outdoor dispensary, £2 2s.; hospital and clinical lectures; total, £6 6s.

Fourth Winter Session.—Matriculation, £1; Practice of Medicine, £4 4s.; Midwifery, £4 4s.; Practical Midwifery, £1 1s.; Clinical Medicine, £4 4s.; Vaccination, £1 1s.; outdoor dispensary, £1 1s.; hospital; total, £16 15s.

Fifth Summer Session.—Hospital; final examination for M.B. and C.M., £10 10s.; total minimum expenses for M.B. and C.M., £107 18s.

Only one course of instruction on each subject is here stated, that being the minimum.

Fees for Degrees.—Examination in Botany, Chemistry, chemical testing, and Natural History, £5 5s.; examination in Anatomy, Institutes of Medicine, Materia Medica, Pathology, £5 5s.; final examination in Surgery, Midwifery, Practice of Physic, Clinical Medicine, Clinical Surgery, Medical Jurisprudence, and prescriptions, during last summer session, £5 5s.; total fees for M.B. diploma, £15 15s. Additional fee for C.M. diploma, £5 5s.; additional fee for M.D. diploma, £5 5s.; Government stamp-duty (for M.D. only), £10.

Note.—Total fees and stamp for graduating as M.D. only, by regulations for students commencing before February, 1861' £25.

N.B.—The above fees include all charges for the diplomas.

Further information as to the classes, courses of lectures, etc., may be obtained on application to Thomas R. Fraser, M.D., Dean of the Faculty of Medicine; or from the University Calendar, published by James Thin, Edinburgh.

The new buildings intended for the Faculty of Medicine to the University are now sufficiently advanced to admit of the departments of Surgery, of Practice of Physic, and of Midwifery being removed there for the ensuing winter session, in addition to the department of Anatomy, which was carried on there during the past session.

ROYAL INFIRMARY, EDINBURGH.

In this Hospital a portion of the beds is set apart for clinical instruction by the Professors of the University of Edinburgh.

(a) For those who have certificates for two summer sessions and one winter session, and who have attended two courses during each of these three sessions.

Courses of Clinical Medicine and Surgery are also given by the ordinary Physicians and Surgeons. Special instruction is given in the Medical Department on Diseases of Women, Physical Diagnosis, etc., and in the Surgical Department on Diseases of the Eye. Separate wards are devoted to fever, venereal diseases, diseases of women, diseases of the eye; also to cases of incidental delirium or insanity. Post-mortem examinations are conducted in the Anatomical Theatre by the Pathologist, who also gives practical instruction in Pathological Anatomy and Histology.

MEDICAL DEPARTMENT.

Consulting Physician—Dr. D. R. Haldane.
Consulting Physician for Diseases of Women—Dr. Alex. Keiller.
Professors of Clinical Medicine—Dr. Maclagan, Dr. Alex. R. Simpson, Dr. Grainger Stewart, Dr. Thos. R. Fraser.
Extra Physician and Lecturer on the Diseases peculiar to Women— Dr. Angus Macdonald.
Ordinary Physicians and Lecturers on Clinical Medicine—Dr. G. W. Balfour, Dr. Claud Muirhead, Dr. David J. Brakenridge.
Assistant-Physicians—Dr. John Wyllie, Dr. J. O. Affleck, Dr. Andrew Smart.

SURGICAL DEPARTMENT.

Consulting Surgeons—Dr. Dunsmure, Dr. J. D. Gillespie.
Professor of Surgery—Mr. Spence.
Ordinary Acting Surgeons—Mr. Joseph Bell, Dr. John Duncan, Mr. John Chiene.
Professor of Clinical Surgery—Mr. Annandale.
Ophthalmic Surgeons—Mr. Walker, Dr. D. A. Robertson.
Extra Surgeon for Treatment of Ovarian Diseases—Dr. Thomas Keith.
Extra Acting Surgeon—Dr. P. H. Watson.
Assistant-Surgeons—Dr. Alex. G. Miller, Dr. P. H. Maclaren, Dr. John Smith.
Dental Surgeon—Dr. John Smith.
Pathologist—Mr. D. J. Hamilton.

HOSPITAL TICKETS.

Perpetual, in one payment, £12; annual, £6 6s.; half-yearly, £4 4s.; quarterly, £2 2s. Separate payments, amounting to £12 12s., entitle the student to a perpetual ticket.

SCHOOL OF MEDICINE, EDINBURGH.

On October 3 the Practical Anatomy Rooms and Chemical Laboratories will be opened. On October 24 the inaugural address will be delivered by Dr. A. G. Miller, at 11 a.m. The courses of lectures will be commenced — winter session, October 25; summer session, May 1.

WINTER SESSION.

Anatomy: Practical Anatomy, Course of Lectures, Course of Demonstrations—Mr. J. Symington and Mr. Charles W. Cathcart.
Chemistry: Lectures, Practical Chemistry, Analytical Chemistry —Dr. Stevenson Macadam, Mr. J. Falconer King, Mr. Ivison Macadam, Dr. Drinkwater, and Mr. Buchanan.
Practice of Physic—Dr. John Wyllie, Dr. J. O. Affleck, and Dr. Byrom Bramwell.
Surgery—Dr. P. Heron Watson, Mr. Chiene, Mr. Duncan, and Dr. A. G. Miller.
Midwifery and Diseases of Women and Children — Dr. Angus Macdonald and Dr. Charles Bell.
Institutes of Medicine or Physiology—Dr. James and Mr. James Hunter.
Clinical Medicine (Royal Infirmary) —Drs. G. W. Balfour, Claud Muirhead, and Brakenridge. Dr. Angus Macdonald (Diseases of Women).
Clinical Surgery (Royal Infirmary)— Mr. Joseph Bell.

Medical Jurisprudence and Public Health—Dr. Littlejohn.
Materia Medica and Therapeutics— Dr. Francis W. Moinet and Dr. William Craig.
Practical Materia Medica, including Practical Pharmacy — Dr. Wm. Craig.
Pathology and Morbid Anatomy— Dr. Bryan Waller and Dr. J. B. Buist.
Systematic and Practical Pathology —Dr. D. J. Hamilton.
Natural History, Zoology, and Comparative Anatomy—Dr. Andrew Wilson.
Diseases of the Ear — Dr. Kirk Duncanson.
Diseases of the Eye — Dr. John Robertson.
Vaccination (Royal Dispensary)— Dr. Husband.
Diseases of Children—Dr. James Andrew and Dr. Carmichael.
Practical Midwifery — Dr. Angus Macdonald and Dr. Charles Bell.
Practical Gynaecology—Dr. Halliday Croom.

SUMMER SESSION.

Anatomy: Practical Anatomy, Course of Demonstrations—Mr. J. Symington and Mr. C.W. Cathcart.
Chemistry: Practical Chemistry, Analytical Chemistry—Dr. Stevenson Macadam, Mr. J. Falconer King, Mr. Ivison Macadam, Dr. Drinkwater, and Mr. Buchanan.
Materia Medica and Therapeutics— Dr. Francis W. Moinet and Dr. William Craig.
Practical Materia Medica, including Practical Pharmacy—Dr. W. Craig.

Midwifery and Diseases of Women and Children—Dr. Keiller, Dr. Underhill, Dr. Halliday Croom, and Dr. Charles Bell.
Medical Jurisprudence and Public Health—Dr. Littlejohn.
Clinical Medicine (Royal Infirmary) —Drs. Geo. W. Balfour, Claud Muirhead, and Brakenridge. Dr. Angus Macdonald (for Diseases of Women).
Clinical Surgery (Royal Infirmary) —Mr. Joseph Bell.

SUMMER SESSION—continued.

Practical Physiology—Dr. James and Mr. James Hunter.
Practical Pathology—Dr. Bryan Waller and Dr. J. B. Buist.
Natural History, Zoology, and Comparative Anatomy—Dr. Andrew Wilson.
Diseases of the Eye — Dr. Argyll Robertson and Dr. J. Robertson.
Practical Medicine and Diagnosis— Dr. Byrom Bramwell.
Medical Anatomy and Physical Diagnosis—Dr. George A. Gibson.
Diseases of the Ear—Dr. Kirk Duncanson and Dr. McBride.

Vaccination—Dr. Husband.
Diseases of Children—Dr. James Andrew and Dr. Carmichael.
Practical Midwifery—Dr. Keiller and Dr. Charles Bell.
Insanity—Dr. J. Batty Tuke.
Diseases of the Skin—Dr. Allan Jamieson.
Operative and Practical Surgery— Dr. P. Heron Watson.
Surgical Anatomy and Operative Surgery—Mr. Chiene.
Practical Surgery—Mr. Duncan.
Operative Surgery and Surgical Anatomy—Dr. G. A. Miller.

The lectures qualify for the University of Edinburgh and the other Universities; the Royal Colleges of Physicians and Surgeons of Edinburgh, London, and Dublin, and the other medical and public Boards.

FEES.

For a first course of lectures, £3 5s.; for a second, £2 4s.; perpetual, £5 5s. To those who have already attended a first course in Edinburgh the perpetual fee is £2 4s. Practical Anatomy (six months' course), £3 3s. Course of Demonstrations, £2 2s.; perpetual, £4 4s.; Practical Anatomy, with course of Demonstrations, £4 4s. Practical Chemistry, £3 3s.; Analytical Chemistry, £2 a month, £5 for three months, or £10 for six months. Practical Materia Medica (including Practical Pharmacy), Diseases of the Ear, Diseases of the Skin, and Diseases of Children, each £2 2s. Vaccination, £1 1s. For summer courses of Clinical Surgery and Clinical Medicine, each £2 4s.; Practical Anatomy (including Anatomical Demonstrations), Operative Surgery, and Medical Anatomy and Physical Diagnosis, each £2 2s.; Insanity, £1 1s.

The minimum cost of the education in this School of Medicine for the double qualification of Physician and Surgeon from the Royal College of Physicians and Surgeons, including the fees for the joint examination, is £95, which is payable by yearly instalments during the period of study; whilst the minimum cost for the single qualification of either Physician or Surgeon, including the fee for examination, is £85.

Much valuable information with regard to the Edinburgh Medical School is contained in a small volume entitled "The University Calendar," published by James Thin, of 55, South Bridge, Edinburgh.

UNIVERSITY OF GLASGOW.—FACULTY OF MEDICINE.

LECTURES AND CLASSES.—WINTER SESSION.

Anatomy, Junior; Anatomy, Senior; Practical Anatomy—Prof. Cleland and Demonstrators.
Chemistry, Chemical Laboratory —Prof. Ferguson.
Clinical Medicine—Prof. McCall Anderson.
Clinical Surgery — Prof. George Buchanan.

Materia Medica—Prof. Charteris.
Midwifery—Prof. Leishman.
Pathology—The Pathologists of the Infirmaries.
Physiology—Physiological Laboratory; Prof McKendrick.
Practice of Physic—Prof. Gairdner.
Surgery—Prof Macleod.
Zoology—Professor Young.

SUMMER SESSION.

Botany, Botanical Demonstrations —Prof. Bayley Balfour.
Clinical Medicine—Prof. McCall Anderson.
Clinical Surgery—Prof. Buchanan.
Embryology and Demonstrations on Anatomy, Elementary Anatomy, Practical Anatomy—Prof. Cleland and Demonstrators.
Forensic Medicine—Prof. Simpson.
Operative Surgery—Prof. Macleod.

Practice of Medicine—Prof. Gairdner.
Practical Chemistry, Organic Chemistry, Chemical Laboratory— Prof. Ferguson.
Practical Materia Medica — Prof. Charteris.
Practical Physiology—Prof. McKendrick.
Zoological Laboratory — Professor Young.
Insanity—Dr. Yellowlees.

CLASS FEES.

Fee for each course, £3 3s., except lectures on the Eye, for which the fee is £1 1s.

In addition to the University courses, the following Hospitals and Dispensaries afford ample means for practical instruction in the various departments of Medicine and Surgery:—

WESTERN INFIRMARY.

This Hospital contains beds for medical and surgical patients, with wards for skin diseases and for diseases of women.

MEDICAL AND SURGICAL STAFF.

Physicians.	Surgeons.
Prof. W. T. Gairdner.	Prof. George H. B. Macleod.
Prof. T. McCall Anderson.	Prof. George Buchanan.
Dr. James Finlayson.	Dr. Alexander Patterson.
Dr. Gavin P. Tennent.	Dr. Hector C. Cameron.

Diseases of Women—Prof. W. Leishman.
Dispensary Physicians—Dr. Joseph Coats, Dr. D. C. McVail, and Dr. S. Gemmell.
Extra Dispensary Physician—Dr. Wm. G. Dun.
Dispensary Surgeons—Dr. J. G. Lyon, Dr. D. N. Knox, and Dr. J. Christie.
Extra Dispensary Surgeon—Dr. J. C. Renton.
Pathologist—Dr. Joseph Coats.
Consulti·Physician-Accoucheur—Professor Leishman, M.D.
Outdoor Phy·'nana-Accoucheur—Dr. Robert Kirk, Dr. W. L. Reid, and Dr. Murdoch Cameron.
Dispensary Surgeon for Diseases of the Ear—Thomas Barr, M.D.
Pathological Chemist—Dr. David Newman.
Dental Surgeon—Mr. James Rankin Brownlie.
Medical Superintendent—Dr. Alexander.
Lady Superintendent—Miss E. Clyde.
Secretary—Henry Johnston, 11, Bothwell-street.

The hour of visit is 9 a.m.

FEES.

The fees for admission to the practice of this Infirmary are
—First year, £10 10s.; second year, £10 10s.; afterwards
free. The fees for clinical lectures are included in the foregoing.

ANDERSON'S COLLEGE, GLASGOW.—FACULTY OF MEDICINE.

The winter session begins on Tuesday, October 25, 1881,
and closes on Friday, March 31, 1882; and the summer
session begins on the first Tuesday of May, and closes about
the middle of July.

WINTER SESSION.

Chemistry—Professor Dittmar.
Surgery—Professor Dunlop.
Junior Anatomy, Senior Anatomy, Practical Anatomy—Professor A. M. Buchanan and Demonstrator.
Institutes of Medicine (Physiology) and Practical Physiology—Professor Barlow.
Materia Medica—Professor Morton.

Practice of Medicine – Professor Gemmell.
Ophthalmic Medicine and Surgery and Clinical Instruction at Ophthalmic Institution—Dr. J. R. Wolfe.
Dental Mechanics and Metallurgy —Mr. W. S. Woodburn.

SUMMER SESSION.

Botany—Professor Wilson.
Operative Surgery—Prof. Dunlop.
Surgical Anatomy, Dissection, Osteology—Prof. A. M. Buchanan and Demonstrator.
Practical Medical Chemistry—Prof. Dittmar.
Midwifery—Prof. A. Wallace.
Public Health—Dr. James Christie.

Medical Jurisprudence—Professor Alex. Lindsay.
Ophthalmic Medicine and Surgery and Clinical Instruction at Ophthalmic Institution—Dr. J. R. Wolfe.
Aural Surgery—Dr. Thomas Barr.
Dental Anatomy—Mr. David Taylor.
Dental Surgery—Mr. J.R.Brownlie.

CLASS FEES.

For each of the above courses of lectures (Anatomy and
Dental lectures excepted), first session, £2 2s.; second session,
£1 1s.; afterwards free.

Anatomy Class Fees.—First session (including Practical Anatomy), £4 4s.; second session (including Practical Anatomy),
£4 4s.; third session, and perpetual, £1 1s.; summer fee
(including Practical Anatomy), £1 11s. 6d.; Osteology, £1 1s.

Dental Fees.—£2 2s. each course.

Students who have attended classes at other schools, but
who desire to pursue their studies at Anderson's College, will
be admitted to such classes as they may have attended elsewhere at the reduced fees.

Royal Infirmary.—*Fees.*—Hospital practice and clinical instruction, first year, £10 10s.; second year, £10 10s.; afterwards free. Six months, £6 6s.; three months, £4 4s.
Vaccination fee, £1 1s.

Dental Hospital.—Fee for the two years' hospital practice
required by the curriculum for the Dental Licence, £10 10s.

Ophthalmic Institution.—Students of Anderson's College are
admitted to the practice of this Institution on paying a matriculation fee of 5s.

The fees for all the lectures and hosp practice required
of candidates for the diplomas of Physician and Surgeon
amount to £48. This is not payable in one sum, but students
simply fee their classes as they take them out.

GLASGOW ROYAL INFIRMARY SCHOOL OF MEDICINE.

The winter session commences on October 27, and the
summer session on May 4. Lectures are delivered on the
subjects necessary for qualifying, and extra courses are given
on practical subjects now required by examining boards.
During summer, lectures on Insanity will be given by Dr.
A. Robertson, and the City Asylum under his charge is
free to students of this School.

Anatomy—Mr. H. E. Clark.
Chemistry—Dr. John Clark.
Clinical Medicine and Clinical Surgery—The Physicians of Hospital.
Dental Surgery—Dr. J. C. Woodburn.
Diseases of the Ear—Dr. Macfie.
Diseases of the Eye—Mr. H. E. Clark.
Forensic Medicine—Mr. Glaister.
Materia Medica—Dr. John Dougall.

Medicine—Dr. J. W. Anderson.
Mental Diseases—Dr. A. Robertson.
Midwifery—Dr. J. Stirton.
Pathology—Dr. D. Foulis.
Physiology—Dr. W. J. Fleming.
Practical Physiology and Operative Surgery—Dr. Fleming and Dr. Macewen.
Surgery—Dr. W. Macewen.

The Royal Infirmary contains 532 beds. Of these 214 are
for medical and 318 for surgical cases, with special wards for
the treatment of venereal disease in males and diseases of
women. Diseases of the ear and throat and eye are specially
treated at the outdoor department.

MEDICAL AND SURGICAL STAFF.

Physicians.
Dr. Perry.
Dr. Maclaren.
Dr. Wood Smith.
Dr. Charteris.

Physician for Diseases of Women.
Dr. Stirton.

Surgeons.
Dr. Morton.
Dr. Macewen.
Dr. R. Watson.
Dr. Dunlop.
Mr. Clark.

Dispensary Physicians.
Dr. Mather.
Dr. Lawrie.

Aural Surgeon—Dr. Macfie.

Extra Dispensary Physicians.
Dr. J. W. Anderson.
Dr. Weir.
Dr. Dougall.

Dispensary Surgeons.
Dr. Lothian.
Dr. Foulis.

Extra Dispensary Surgeons.
Dr. Whitson.
Dr. Fleming.
Dr. Barlow.

Vaccinator.
Dr. Tannahill.

Pathologist.
Dr. Foulis.

Diseases of the Throat.
Dr. Eben Watson.

Dental Surgeon—Dr. J. C. Woodburn.

APPOINTMENTS.

There are five Physicians' and five Surgeons' Assistants, who
are boarded and lodged in the Hospital at the rate of £25 per
annum, and who perform all the duties of House-Physicians
and House-Surgeons. These appointments are held for twelve
months—six in the medical, and six in the surgical wards—
and are open to those students of the Infirmary who have
passed all their examinations except the last, or who have a
qualification in Medicine or Surgery.

Clinical Assistants, Dressers, and Dispensary Clerks are
selected from the students without any additional fee; and
from the large number of accident cases and cases of acute
disease received into the wards, these appointments are numerous, and invaluable to the student. The number of capital
operations last year was ninety. The total number of operations was 649. Attendance at the Dispensary for the treatment of out-patients, and admission to the Pathological
Museum, are also free.

FEES.

For each course of lectures, first session, £2 2s; second
ditto, and perpetual, £1 1s.

The Anatomy Class fees are—first session, £4 4s.; second
ditto, £4 4s.; afterwards, £1 11s. 6d. per annum for Practical
Anatomy.

HOSPITAL FEE.

The fee for perpetual attendance on the practice of the
Infirmary and on the courses of clinical instruction and
lectures is £21.

Prospectuses can be obtained from Dr. Thomas, the Superintendent of the Hospital.

UNIVERSITY OF ABERDEEN.—FACULTY OF MEDICINE.

LECTURES.—WINTER SESSION.

Anatomy—Professor Struthers.
Chemistry—Professor Brazier.
Institutes of Medicine—Professor W. Stirling.
Materia Medica—Prof. Davidson.
Medical Logic and Medical Jurisprudence—Professor Ogston.
Midwifery and Diseases of Women and Children—Prof. Stephenson.

Practical Anatomy and Demonstrations—Professor Struthers and Assistants.
Practice of Medicine — Professor Smith-Shand.
Surgery—Professor Pirrie.
Natural History—Professor Cossar-Ewart.

SUMMER SESSION.

Botany—Professor Trail.
Practical Pharmacy—Prof. Davidson and Assistant.
Practical Midwifery and Gynaecology, and Clinical Diseases of Children—Professor Stephenson.
Practical Chemistry—Prof. Brazier.

Practical Anatomy and Demonstrations—Professor Struthers and Assistants.
Practical Physiology — Professor Stirling.
Natural History—Professor Cossar-Ewart.

The Anatomical Course in summer includes instruction in
Histology and in the use of the microscope; and instruction
in Osteology for beginners.

FEES.
Matriculation fee (including all dues) for the winter and summer session, £1; for the summer session alone, 10s.

Pathological Anatomy, Dr. Rodger, £2 2s. Practical Ophthalmology, Dr. A. D. Davidson. Practical Toxicology, Dr. F. Ogston, jun. Dental Surgery (in summer), Dr. Williamson.

The regulations relative to the registration of students of Medicine, and the granting of degrees in Medicine and Surgery, may be had of Professor Brazier, Secretary of the Faculty of Medicine.

Full information regarding the classes and degrees in the Faculties of Arts, Law, and Divinity, and in regard to Bursaries and Scholarships, will be found in the University Calendar, published by Messrs. Wyllie and Son, Union-street, Aberdeen, by post 2s. 2d.

ABERDEEN ROYAL INFIRMARY.

The Aberdeen Royal Infirmary contains about 200 beds.

MEDICAL AND SURGICAL STAFF.

Consulting Physician—Dr. A Harvey.
Consulting Surgeon—Professor W. Pirrie.

Physicians.	*Surgeons.*
Dr. J. W. F. Smith-Shand.	Mr. A. Ogston.
Dr. R. Beveridge.	Mr. J. O. Will.
Dr. Angus Fraser.	Mr. R. J. Garden.
	Mr. John Hall.

Resident Assistant-Physicians.　*Resident Assistant-Surgeon.*
Mr. E. W. Robertson.　Mr. George Shirres.

Ophthalmic Surgeon—Dr. Alex. D. Davidson.
Dental Surgeon—Dr. W. H. Williamson.
Chloroformist—Dr. P. B. Smith.
Resident Superintendent and Apothecary—Dr. R. Rattray.
Pathologist and Curator of Museum—Dr. J. Rodger.
Treasurer and Secretary—Mr. W. Carnie.

UNIVERSITY OF ST. ANDREWS.

There is no proper Faculty of Medicine in this University, but it is possible for the student to make an *annus medicus* by attendance on certain of the courses—as Natural History, Professor Nicholson, M.D.; Chemistry, Professor Heddle, M.D.; and Anatomy and Medicine, Professor Pettigrew, M.D.

SCHOOLS AND HOSPITALS IN IRELAND.

UNIVERSITY OF DUBLIN.—SCHOOL OF PHYSIC.

THE School of Physic is under the conjoint superintendence of the University authorities and those of the King and Queen's College of Physicians.

LECTURES AND CLASSES.

Anatomy and Surgery—Dr. Alexander Macalister.	Medical Jurisprudence—Dr. Robert Travers.
Botany—Dr. E. Percival Wright.	Midwifery—Sir Edward B. Sinclair.
Chemistry—Dr. J. E. Reynolds.	Natural Philosophy—Mr. Fitzgerald.
Comparative Anatomy—Dr. Alexander Macalister.	Operative Surgery—Dr. Richard G. Butcher.
Institutes of Medicine—Dr. J. M. Purser.	Practice of Medicine—Dr. W. Moore.
Materia Medica and Pharmacy—Vacant.	Surgery—Dr. Edward H. Bennett.
	University Anatomist—Dr. Thomas E. Little.

Winter Session, 1881-82.—The winter session commences on October 1. Lectures will commence on November 1. The dissecting-room will be opened on October 1.

SCHOLARSHIPS AND PRIZES.

Two Medical Scholars are elected annually, by the Board of Trinity College, at an examination held at the end of June—subject to conditions stated in the College Calendar. Each scholarship is worth £20 per annum, and is tenable for two years.

A Travelling Prize in Medicine and Surgery is offered in each alternate year, subject to certain conditions; the value of each prize is £100. Particulars may be obtained from the Medical Registrar.

SIR PATRICK DUN'S HOSPITAL.

MEDICAL AND SURGICAL STAFF.

Consulting Physician—Dr. Alfred Hudson.
Consulting Surgeon—Dr. W. Colles.

Clinical Physicians.	*Clinical Surgeons.*
Dr. John Malet Purser.	Dr. Thomas E. Little.
Dr. William Moore.	Dr. Edward H. Bennett.
	Dr. Alexander Macalister.

Midwifery Physician.　*Lecturer in Operative Surgery.*
Sir Edward B. Sinclair.　Dr. Richard G. Butcher.

Resident Surgeon—Dr. John Barton.

FEES.

Clinical Lectures and Hospital Attendance.—The payment of £3 3s. to the Hospital entitles any student to attend the clinic of the Hospital for twelve months, and to attend the lectures delivered by Dr. R. G. Butcher, University Lecturer in Operative Surgery. Students who have taken out the degrees of Bachelor in Medicine and Master in Surgery in Trinity College are entitled to attend the Hospital as perpetual free pupils. In addition to the Hospital fee, the payment of a fee of £6 6s. is required for the privilege of attending the clinical lectures. Total fees for Hospital and lectures for twelve months, £12 12s.

Practical Midwifery.—Students desirous of entering for twelve months' instruction in Practical Midwifery are required to pay a maternity fee of £3 3s. each. Students of Trinity College are not liable to any other payment for instruction in Practical Midwifery. Other students are required to pay £3 3s. each to the King's Professor for twelve months' practical instruction, in addition to the Hospital maternity fee. Students who have paid the Hospital maternity fee are entitled to attend the demonstrations in Obstetric Surgery given by the King's Professor. Total fees for College Students, £3 3s. total fees for Externs, £6 6s.

PRIZES.

Clinical Medals.—The Governors of the Hospital award a Silver Clinical Medal in Medicine to the student who shall pass the best examination on the medical cases treated in the Hospital during the year; and a Silver Clinical Medal in Surgery to the student who shall pass the best examination on the surgical cases treated in the Hospital during the year.

QUEEN'S COLLEGE, BELFAST.(a)

The lectures will commence on Tuesday, November 2.

Anatomy and Physiology—Dr. P. Redfern.	Natural Philosophy—Dr. J. R. Everett.
Chemistry—Dr. E. A. Letts.	Practice of Medicine—Dr. James Cuming.
Materia Medica—Dr. J. S. Reid.	
Medical Jurisprudence—Dr. J. F. Hodges.	Practice of Surgery—Dr. A. Gordon.
Midwifery—Dr. R. F. Dill.	Zoology and Botany—Dr. R. O. Cunningham.

The demonstrations in Anatomy are delivered by Dr. Anderson. The lectures in Midwifery and in Medical Jurisprudence, and the courses of Botany and Practical Chemistry, and a second course of Experimental Physics, will commence in May.

FEES.

Anatomy and Physiology—First course, £3; each subsequent course, £2. Anatomical Demonstrations and Practical Anatomy—each course, £3. Practical Chemistry, £3. Other medical lectures—first course, £2; each subsequent course, £1.

SCHOLARSHIPS.

Two Medical Scholarships are awarded to the students of each year of the medical course. The examinations commence on October 21.

BELFAST GENERAL HOSPITAL.

FEES.

Clinical Instruction—A winter session, £5 5s. A summer session, £2 2s. Perpetual fee, payable in one sum of £10 10s., or two instalments of £5 5s. each on entering for the first and second years. Hospital fee, 10s. 6d. each winter or summer session.

BELFAST LYING-IN HOSPITAL.

Fee for the session, £2 2s.

QUEEN'S COLLEGE, GALWAY.—FACULTY OF MEDICINE.(a)

LECTURES.

Anatomy and Physiology, and Practical Anatomy—Dr. J. P. Pye.	Medical Jurisprudence—Dr. R. J. Kinkead.
Botany and Zoology—Dr. A. G. Melville.	Midwifery and Diseases of Women and Children—Dr. R. J. Kinkead.
Chemistry—Dr. T. H. Rowney.	Natural Philosophy—Dr. Joseph Larmor.
Logic and Mental Philosophy—Dr. T. W. Moffett.	Practice of Medicine—Dr. John I. Lynham.
Materia Medica—Dr. N. W. Colahan.	
Practice of Surgery—Dr. J. V. Browne.	

The County Galway Infirmary, Town, and Fever Hospitals are in the immediate vicinity of the Queen's College.

SCHOLARSHIPS AND EXHIBITIONS.

Eight Scholarships of the value of £25 each, and Exhibitions varying in value from £12 to £16, are appropriated to students pursuing the course for the degree of M.D.

FEES.

Anatomy and Physiology, £3 first session; afterwards £2. Practical Anatomy, £3; Practical Chemistry, £3; Operative Surgery, £3; other classes, £1 for each course extending over one term only, £2 for each course extending over more than one term, and £1 for each re-attendance on the same. Hospitals, £4 4s.

For further information, application may be made to Professor Curtis, M.A., LL.D., Registrar.

(a) No return.

QUEEN'S COLLEGE, CORK.—FACULTY OF MEDICINE.

LECTURERS.

Anatomy and Physiology—Dr. J. J. Charles.
Chemistry and Practical Chemistry—Dr. Maxwell Simpson.
Materia Medica—Dr. M. O'Keefe.
Midwifery—Dr. H. Macnaughton Jones.
Natural Philosophy—Prof. John England.

Practical Anatomy—The Professor, assisted by Demonstrators.
Practice of Medicine—Dr. D. C. O'Connor.
Practice of Surgery—Dr. Stephen O'Sullivan.
Zoology and Botany—Professor A. Leith Adams.

SCHOLARSHIPS.

Eight Scholarships are awarded to students in Medicine, if qualified—viz., two scholarships of £25 each to students commencing their first, second, third, and fourth years. Clinical Medicine and Surgery at the North and South Infirmaries, and Clinical Midwifery at the Lying-in Hospital.

THE ADELAIDE MEDICAL AND SURGICAL HOSPITALS, PETER-STREET, DUBLIN.

MEDICAL AND SURGICAL STAFF.

Physicians.
Dr. Henry H. Head.
Dr. James Little.

Surgeons.
Mr. John K. Barton.
Mr. Benjamin Wills Richardson.
Mr. Kendal Franks.

Physician and Pathologist.
Dr. Richd. Purefoy.

Ophthalmic Surgeon.
Dr. Rosborough Swanzy.

Obstetric Physician.
Dr. Walter G. Smith.

Dental Surgeon.
Dr. R. Theodore Stack.

Further particulars can be obtained from Mr. Richardson, 22, Ely-place, or any other member of the medical staff.

ST. VINCENT'S HOSPITAL, DUBLIN.(a)

HOSPITAL STAFF.

Physicians.
Dr. Francis J. B. Quinlan.
Dr. Robert Cryan.

Surgeons.
Mr. Edward D. Mapother.
Mr. M. J. Kehoe.

Gynæcologist—Dr. J. A. Byrne.
Ophthalmic Surgeon—Mr. M. D. Redmond.
Surgeon-Dentist—Mr. William J. Doherty.
Apothecaries—Mr. C. T. Boland and Mr. J. McArdle.

FEES.

Winter and summer session, £12 12s.; separately, £8 8s. and £5 5s.

Further particulars may be learned on application to the Secretary, Dr. Quinlan, 29, Lower Fitzwilliam-street, Dublin, or at the Hospital during the hours of attendance.

DR. STEEVENS' HOSPITAL, DUBLIN.

MEDICAL AND SURGICAL STAFF.

Consulting Physicians—Dr. H. Freke and Dr. Grimshaw.
Consulting Surgeons—Mr. S. G. Wilmot and Mr. G. H. Porter.

Physicians.
Dr. H. J. Tweedy.
Dr. R. A. Hayes.
Obstetric Physician.
Dr. A. Duke.

Surgeons.
Mr. W. Colles.
Mr. E. Hamilton.
Mr. R. M'Donnell.

Surgeon-Dentist.
Mr. J. A. Baker.

Resident Surgeon.
Mr. T. Myles.

FEES.

Hospital Practice, nine months, £12 12s.; ditto, six months, £8 8s.

Further particulars may be learned from the Resident Surgeon at the Hospital; or from Dr. R. A. Hayes, Hon. Sec., 32, Merrion-square South.

JERVIS-STREET HOSPITAL, DUBLIN.

MEDICAL AND SURGICAL STAFF.

Physicians.
Dr. Stephen M. MacSwiney. | Dr. William Martin.

Surgeons.
Dr. J. Stannus Hughes.
Mr. J. K. Forrest.
Mr. Austin Meldon.

Mr. James Edward Kelly.
Dr. W. Stoker.
Dr. J. J. Cranny.

Dr. Robert MacDonnell.

This Hospital, which is at present being rebuilt upon an extensive scale, is most central in situation. From its proximity to the quays and principal factories it presents unrivalled opportunities to the students of seeing every form of surgical injury. An extensive Dispensary for out-door patients is attached to the Hospital, at which the students are allowed to perform minor operations, under the guidance of the Surgeon on duty, and are rendered familiar with the details of dispensary practice.

Instruction is given by the Physician and Surgeon on duty

(a) No return.

on alternate mornings, between nine and eleven o'clock, at the bedside, when the nature, progress, and treatment of each case are explained. Two clinical lectures are delivered each week on the most important cases under treatment, when pathological specimens are exhibited. Surgical instruments and appliances of all kinds are constantly made the subject of special instruction.

Surgical Operations are performed on Saturday mornings, at ten o'clock, except in cases of emergency, when due notice is given, if possible.

Practical Pharmacy is taught under the superintendence of the Apothecary.

Resident Pupils and Dressers are selected from among the most attentive of the advanced students, without payment of any additional fee. Two Interns are appointed each half-year, and are provided with apartments, etc., free of expense. Special Certificates are given to the Resident Pupils and Dressers who have performed their respective duties to the satisfaction of the Physicians and Surgeons.

Certificates of attendance are recognised by all the licensing bodies and examining boards in the United Kingdom.

CARMICHAEL SCHOOL OF MEDICINE, DUBLIN.

WINTER SESSION.

Systematic Anatomy—Dr. Heuston.
Practical Anatomy — Dr. Loftie Stoney.
Chemistry—Dr. Tichborne.
Midwifery—Drs. Jennings and Macan.

Surgery—Messrs. Barton and Corley.
Ophthalmic Surgery—Dr. C. E. Fitzgerald.
Practice of Medicine—Dr. Moore.
Physiology—Dr. Harvey.

SUMMER SESSION.

Botany—Dr. McNab.
Materia Medica—Dr. Duffey.
Medical Jurisprudence—Mr. H. A. Auchinleck.

Midwifery — Drs. Jennings and Macan.
Pathology—Dr. Woodhouse.
Practical Physiology—Dr. Harvey.
Practical Chemistry—Dr. Tichborne.

SCHOLARSHIPS AND PRIZES.

Prizes to the value of £67 on the foundation of the late Richard Carmichael, Esq., and the Mayne and Carmichael Scholarships, value £15 each, are awarded annually.

For further particulars apply to the Registrar at the School.

CATHOLIC UNIVERSITY SCHOOL OF MEDICINE, CECILIA-STREET, DUBLIN.

LECTURES AND CLASSES.

Anatomy and Physiology — Dr. Hayden and Dr. Nixon (locum tenens).
Anatomical Demonstrations — The Professors of Anatomy and Physiology.
Botany—Dr. Sigerson.
Chemistry—Dr. Campbell.
Dissections — Messrs. Redmond, Kehoe, McDonnell, McCullagh, McArdle, and Chance.
Medical Jurisprudence—Dr. MacSwiney.

Materia Medica—Dr. Quinlan.
Natural Philosophy—The Very Rev. Dr. Molloy.
Pathology—Dr. Lyons.
Practical Chemistry—Dr. Campbell.
Theory and Practice of Medicine—Dr. Lyons.
Theory and Practice of Midwifery—Dr. Byrne.
Theory and Practice of Surgery—Mr. Hayes.
Ophthalmology—(Vacant.)
Institutes of Medicine—Dr. Nixon.

PRIZES AND EXHIBITIONS.

At the termination of the winter session, public examinations will be held, when, in addition to prizes in each class, a Gold Medal will be awarded for the subjects mentioned in the School prospectuses.

At the termination of the summer session the University Exhibition (£90) will be awarded in addition to the usual prizes in each class.

FEES.

For each course £3 3s., excepting Dissections and Practical Chemistry, which are £5 5s. A reduction of one-sixth is made to perpetual pupils paying the entire of their fees in advance, or in two instalments at the commencement of the first and second years of their course. Parents and guardians are recommended to forward all fees directly, by cheque or order, to the Registrar, Professor Campbell, 161, Rathgar-road, or at the School.

Further particulars may be learned from any of the Professors; from the Secretary, Professor Campbell, 161, Rathgar-road; or on application at the School.

CITY OF DUBLIN HOSPITAL, UPPER BAGGOT-STREET.(a)

Consulting Physicians—Dr. James Apjohn and Dr. Alfred Hudson.
Consulting Surgeon—Mr. Joliffe T. Tufnell.
Physicians—Dr. Hawtrey Benson and Dr. J. Magee Finny.

Surgeons—Mr. Henry Gray Croly, Mr. William I. Wheeler, and Dr. Henry Fitzgibbon.

Ophthalmic and Aural Surgeon—Dr. Loftie Stoney.
Gynæcologist—Dr. Arthur V. Macan.

(a) No return.

Fees.—Nine months' hospital attendance, £12 12s.; six months, £8 8s.; three months, £5 5s.

For further particulars apply to Mr. Wheeler, 27, Lower Fitzwilliam-street.

MATER MISERICORDIÆ HOSPITAL, ECCLES-STREET, DUBLIN.(a)

MEDICAL AND SURGICAL STAFF.

Physicians.
Dr. John Hughes.
Dr. Thomas Hayden.
Dr. Christopher J. Nixon.

Assistant-Physician.
Dr. Joseph M. Redmond.

Consulting Surgeon.
Mr. Francis R. Cruise.

Surgeons.
Mr. Patrick J. Hayes.
Mr. Charles Coppinger.
Mr. Malachi Kilgariff.

Assistant-Surgeon—Mr. Kennedy.
Obstetric Physician—Dr. T. M. Madden.
House-Surgeon—Mr. Robert Browne.

This Hospital contains 250 beds, including fifty beds for fever and other contagious diseases.

Certificates of attendance upon this Hospital are recognised by all the licensing bodies in the United Kingdom.

PRIZES.

Two Clinical prizes (the "Leonard Prizes") of £15 each, one medical and one surgical, will be given at the end of the winter session.

Fee for nine months, £12 12s.; six winter months, £8 8s.; three summer months, £5 5s.

Further particulars may be learned by application to Dr. Nixon, Secretary to the Medical Board, 32, Upper Merrion-street, or to any of the other medical officers.

MEATH HOSPITAL AND COUNTY DUBLIN INFIRMARY.(a)

MEDICAL AND SURGICAL STAFF.

Physicians.
Dr. Arthur Wynne Foot. | Dr. John William Moore.

Surgeons.
Mr. George H. Porter. | Mr. Rawdon Macnamara.
Mr. James H. Wharton. | Mr. Lambert H. Ormsby.
Mr. Philip Crampton Smyly. | Mr. William J. Hepburn.

The ensuing winter session will commence on October 1, and the course of clinical lectures on the first Monday in November.

Clinical lectures, of which four will be delivered weekly, and instructions in Medicine and Surgery, will be given on alternate days.

The Physicians and Surgeons on duty will visit the Hospital at 9 a.m., so as to allow the members of the class to be in attendance at their respective Schools of Medicine at 11 a.m.

The Hospital, which contains 120 beds for the reception of medical and surgical cases, and to which an extensive dispensary (open daily), lending library, and physical laboratory are attached, is within a few minutes' walk of the University, the Royal College of Surgeons, the Carmichael College of Medicine and Surgery, and the Ledwich School of Medicine.

An additional ward has been erected for the reception of children, in which the pupils will have an opportunity of studying that highly important subject—infantile disease.

Certificates of attendance at this Hospital are recognised by all the universities, colleges, and licensing bodies in the United Kingdom.

Prizes will be given at the termination of the winter course to the best answerers in their respective classes.

The office of Resident Pupil is open to pupils as well as apprentices.

Further information may be obtained on application to W. J. Hepburn, Esq., Hon. Sec., 53, York-street, Dublin; or at the Hospital.

MERCER'S HOSPITAL, WILLIAM-STREET, DUBLIN.

STAFF.

Physicians—Dr. T. P. Mason and Dr. George F. Duffey.
Surgeons—Mr. E. S. O'Grady, Mr. Alcock Nixon, and Mr. M. A. Ward.

This Hospital, one of the first founded in Dublin, is situated in a central position, and is in close proximity to the Schools of the Royal College of Surgeons, the Carmichael College of Medicine and Surgery, Catholic University, and the Ledwich.

Fees for the winter and summer session (nine months) £12 12s.; for the six winter months, £8 8s.; for the three summer months, £5 5s.

Further information can be obtained from any of the medical officers of the Hospital, or from Dr. James Shaw, Secretary to the medical staff.

(a) No return.

ROYAL COLLEGE OF SURGEONS IN IRELAND. SCHOOL OF SURGERY.(a)

LECTURES.—WINTER SESSION.

Anatomy and Physiology — Dr. Mapother.
Descriptive Anatomy—Dr. Bevan and Mr. Thornley Stoker.
Midwifery—Dr. Roe.

Surgery—Mr. J. Stannus Hughes and Mr. Stokes.
Practice of Medicine—Dr. James Little.
Chemistry—Dr. Cameron.

SUMMER SESSION.

Materia Medica—Mr. Macnamara.
Medical Jurisprudence—Dr. Davy.
Botany—Dr. Minchin.
Practical Chemistry—Dr. Cameron.

Midwifery—Dr. Roe.
Hygiene—Dr. Cameron.
Ophthalmic and Aural Surgery—Mr. Swanzy.

A public course of lectures on Comparative Anatomy will be delivered by the Professor of Anatomy and Physiology, at the commencement of the session, and additional lectures on the same subject will be delivered during the winter.

The dissections are under the direction of the Professor of Anatomy, assisted by the demonstrators, who will daily attend to give instruction and to assist the students.

The fee for each course of lectures is £3 3s., excepting Descriptive Anatomy, which is £8 8s., Practical Chemistry, which is £5 5s., and Ophthalmic and Aural Surgery and Hygiene, which are free.

A composition fee of £56 17s. 6d. is taken as payment in full for all lectures and dissections required for the diploma in Surgery.

RICHMOND, WHITWORTH, AND HARDWICKE HOSPITALS.

MEDICAL AND SURGICAL STAFF.

Physicians.
Dr. J. T. Banks.
Dr. R. G. M'Dowel.
Dr. S. Gordon.
Dr. R. D. Lyons.

Surgeons.
Mr. William Stokes.
Mr. William Thomson.
Mr. W. Thornley Stoker.
Mr. A. Corley.

Consulting Obstetric Surgeon—Dr. Kidd.
Assistant Physician—Dr. Reuben J. Harvey.
Ophthalmic Surgeon—Dr. Charles E. Fitzgerald.

Clinical instruction will commence on October 1. These Hospitals contain 312 beds—110 for surgical cases, 82 for medical cases, and 120 for fever and other epidemic diseases. Premiums will be awarded in Clinical Medicine and Surgery. The Richmond Institution for the Insane, containing over 1200 patients, adjoins these Hospitals.

FEES.

For the winter and summer session (nine months), £12 12s.; for the six winter months, £8 8s.; for the three summer months, £5 5s. Resident clinical clerks, £21 for the winter session, £15 15s. for the summer session, including certificate of attendance.

Application to be made to Dr. Gordon, 13, Hume-street, or to Mr. Stokes, 5, Merrion-square North, Dublin.

LEDWICH SCHOOL OF ANATOMY, MEDICINE, AND SURGERY, PETER-STREET, DUBLIN(a).

COURSES OF LECTURES.

Anatomy, Physiology & Pathology, etc.—Mr. T. P. Mason, Mr. A. Ward, and Mr. T. Mason.
Forensic Medicine and Hygiene—Dr. R. Travers.
Institutes of Medicine—Mr. Ledwich.
Materia Medica and Therapeutics—Dr. Purefoy.
Midwifery and Diseases of Women and Children—Dr. S. A. Mason.
Theory of Chemistry, Practical Chemistry, & Natural Philosophy—Dr. Lepper.

Ophthalmic Surgery—Mr. Benson.
Surgical and Descriptive Anatomy, Demonstrations, and Dissections—Mr. Mason, Mr. Glanville, Mr. Ward, Mr. Robinson, Mr. Nixon, Mr. Porter, Mr. Kennedy, Mr. Baxter, Mr. Madden, Mr. R. Ledwich, Mr. Knight, Mr. Gaffney, Mr. Donnelly, Mr. Neill, and Mr. O'C. T. Delahoy.
Theory and Practice of Surgery—Mr. Wharton and Mr. Kelly.
Theory and Practice of Medicine—Dr. Foot.

The fee for each of the above courses will be £3 3s.

A course of operations to be performed by the students, under the superintendence of the lecturers (subjects, etc., included), £5 5s.

Further information may be obtained from any of the lecturers; from Mr. T. P. Mason, 92, Harcourt-street, and Mr. M. A. Ward, 9, Rathmines-road, Joint Secretaries; or from Mr. F. A. Nixon, 33, Harcourt-street, Registrar.

SEX IN CANINE RABIES.—As the proportion of male dogs which become the subjects of rabies very much exceeds that of bitches, M. Voiteller proposes that the tax on dogs shall be double that on bitches. During the years 1876-79 of 1475 mad dogs, 1302 were male dogs, and only 173 bitches

(a) No return.

TABLE OF FEES FOR HOSPITAL LECTURES AND ATTENDANCE.

(The letter "i." denotes Single Course; "ii.," Two Courses, Perpetual or Unlimited Attendance.)

	St. Bartholomew's.	Charing Cross.	St. George's.	Guy's.	King's College.	London.	St. Mary's.	Middlesex.	St. Thomas's.
Anatomy . .	i. £9 9s. ii. £13 2s. 6d.	1st yr. £4 4s. 2nd yr. £2 2s.	i. £7 7s. ii. £8 18s. 6d.	i. £7 7s.	i. £9 9s. ii. £19 19s. (inc. Pr. An.)	i. £5 5s. ii. £8 8s.	i. £7 17s. 6d.	i. £3 3s. ii. £13 12s.	i. £7 7s. ii. £10 10s.
Demonst. and Dissections .	i. £7 7s.	1st yr. £3 3s. 2nd yr. £3 3s.	i. £3 3s.	i. £7 7s.	i. £6 6s. ii. £9 9s.	i. £5 5s. ii. £8 8s.	i. £1 15s.	i. £3 3s. ii. £3 3s.	3 mos. £4 4s. 6 mos. £6 6s. ii. £10 10s.
Theoret. Physiology	i. £9 9s. ii. £13 2s. 6d.	£4 4s. 2nd yr. £2 2s.	i. £7 7s. ii. £8 18s. 6d.	i. £7 7s.	i. £4 4s. ii. £11 11s.	i. £4 4s. ii. £6 6s.	i. £4 4s.	i. £3 3s. ii. £3 3s.	i. £7 7s. ii. £10 10s.
Practical Physiology . .	i. £7 7s.	£4 4s.	i. £3 3s.	i. £7 7s.	i. £6 6s. ii. £8 8s.	i. £3 3s. ii. £4 4s.	...	i. £4 4s.	i. £6 6s.
Histology . .	i. £2 12s. 6d.	...	i. £3 3s.	...	...	i. £3 3s.	i. £4 4s.	...	...
Chemistry . .	i. £5 16s. 6d. ii. £9 9s.	i. £5 5s.	i. £6 6s. ii. £7 17s. 6d.	i. £7 7s.	i. £8 8s. ii. £11 11s.	i. £7 7s. ii. £10 10s.	i. £6 16s. 6d.	i. £6 6s. ii. £8 8s.	i. £7 7s. ii. £10 10s.
Practical Chemistry	i. £3 3s.	i. £4 4s.	i. £4 4s.	i. £7 7s.	i. £6 6s. ii. £8 8s.	i. £5 5s.	i. £4 4s.	i. £3 3s.	i. £6 6s.
Botany . . .	i. £4 4s. ii. £5 5s.	i. £3 3s.	i. £3 13s. 6d. ii. £4 14s. 6d.	i. £5 5s.	i. £3 3s. ii. £6 6s.	i. £3 3s. ii. £4 4s.	i. £4 4s.	i. £3 3s.	i. £4 4s. ii. £5 5s.
Com. Anatomy	i. £2 12s. 6d. ii. £4 4s.	i. £3 3s.	£4 4s.	i. £5 5s.	i. £4 4s. ii. £6 6s.	i. £3 3s. ii. £4 4s.	i. £2 12s. 6d.	i. £3 3s.	i. £4 4s. ii. £5 5s.
Medicine. . .	i. £6 16s. 6d. ii. £9 9s.	1st c. £4 4s. 2nd c. £2 2s.	i. £7 7s. ii. £8 18s. 6d.	i. £7 7s.	i. £3 3s. ii. £9 9s.	i. £5 5s. ii. £6 6s.	i. £5 5s.	i. £3 3s. ii. £3 3s.	i. £6 6s. ii. £10 10s.
Practical Med.	...	...	i. £4 4s.	...	...	...	...	...	...
Surgery . . .	i. £6 16s. 6d. ii. £9 9s.	1st c. £4 4s. 2nd c. £2 2s.	i. £7 7s. ii. £8 18s. 6d.	i. £7 7s.	i. £3 3s. ii. £9 9s.	i. £5 5s. ii. £6 6s.	i. £5 5s.	i. £3 3s. ii. £3 3s.	i. £7 7s. ii. £10 10s.
Practical Surgery	i. £6 16s. 6d. ii. £9 9s.	...	i. £4 4s.	i. (Op.) £7 7s. (Prac.) £4 4s.	i. £3 3s. ii. £5 5s.	i. £6 6s.	...	i. £6 6s.	i. £6 6s.
Operative Surg.	£5 5s.	...	£2 2s.	...	...	i. £6 6s.	i. £4 4s.	i. £5 5s.	i. £5 5s.
Midwifery . .	i. £6 16s. 6d. ii. £7 17s. 6d.	i. £3 3s.	i. £4 14s. 6d. ii. £5 15s. 6d.	i. £7 7s.	i. £5 5s. ii. £6 6s.	i. £4 4s. ii. £6 6s.	i. £5 5s.	i. £4 4s. ii. £5 5s.	i. £5 5s. ii. £6 6s.
Pathology . .	i. £2 12s. 6d. ii. £4 4s.	i. £3 3s.	i. £3 3s.	i. (Dem.) £7 7s. (Lect.) £3 3s.	i. £3 3s. ii. £4 4s.	i. £3 3s. ii. £6 6s.	i. £4 4s.	i. £4 4s. ii. £5 5s.	} i. £6 6s.
Path. Anatomy	...	...	...	...	...	...	...	...	
Materia Medica	i. £6 16s. 6d. ii. £7 17s. 6d.	i. £3 3s.	i. £4 14s. 6d. ii. £5 15s. 6d.	i. £5 5s.	i. £5 5s. ii. £6 6s.	i. £3 3s. ii. £4 4s.	i. £5 5s.	i. £4 4s. ii. £5 5s.	i. £4 4s. ii. £5 5s.
Forensic Medicine	i. £4 4s. ii. £5 5s.	i. £3 3s.	i. £4 14s. 6d. ii. £5 15s. 6d.	i. £5 5s.	i. £5 5s. ii. £6 6s.	i. £3 3s. ii. £4 4s.	} i. £4 4s.	i. £4 4s. ii. £5 5s.	i. £4 4s. ii. £5 5s.
Public Health .	i. £2 12s. 6d.	£1 1s.	...	£3 3s.	...	...		i. £3 3s.	ii. £3 3s.
Ophth. Surgery	i. £2 12s. 6d. ii. £4 4s.	...	...	...	...	i. £2 2s. ii. £3 3s.	i. £2 12s. 6d.	...	ii. £3 3s.
Aural Surgery .	...	...	...	...	...	i. £2 2s. ii. £3 3s.	i. £2 12s. 6d.	...	...
Dental Surgery .	i. £2 12s. 6d. ii. £4 4s.	...	...	...	...	£2 2s.	i. £2 12s. 6d.	...	Dental Free. { i. £2 2s. ii. £3 3s.
Mental Dis. .	i. £2 12s. 6d. ii. £4 4s.	...	...	£3 3s.	...	...	...	i. £3 3s.	i. £2 2s. ii. £3 3s.
Library . . .	1 year, 10s.	£1 1s.	Each winter, 10s. 6d.	...	£1 1s.	£1 1s.	£1 1s.	£1 1s.	£1 1s.
Hospital Practice	*Medical.* 3 mos. £10 10s. 6 mos. £15 15s. 2 yrs. £23 12s. 6d. Unlimited, £33 1s 6d. *Surgical.* 3 mos. £12 1s. 6d. 6 mos. £19 19s. 12 mos. £26 5s. Unlimited, £33 1s. 6d.	*Med. or Surg.* 3 mos. £6 6s. 6 mos. £10 10s. 12 mos. £18 12s. Full period £21. *Med. and Surg.* 2 mos. £10 10s. 12 mos. £31 Full period, £31 10s.	*Med. or Surg.* 6 mos. £10 10s. 2 yrs. £21 Perp. £31 10s. *Med. and Surg.* 2 yrs. £42 Perp. £63	*Med. or Surg.* 3 mos. £10 10s. 6 mos. £15 15s. 1 yr. £24 3s. Perp. £31 10s. *Med. and Surg.* 3 mos. £15 15s. 6 mos. £34 3s. 1 yr. £31 10s. Perp. £47 5s.	*Med. or Surg.* 1 sum. £5 5s. 1 win. £9 9s. 1 yr. £12 12s. Perp. £31 10s. *Med. and Surg.* 1 sum. £8 8s. 1 win. £14 14s. 1 yr. £18 18s. Perp. £43	Perp. £52 10s. *Medical.* 6 mos. *£10 10/ 12 ,, †£15 15/ Unlim. †£26 5/ *Surgical.* 6 mos. 1£10 10/ 12 mos. £15 15s. 18 ,, ||£31 Unlim. §£26 5/ *Obstetric.* 1 year £4 4/ Incl. Lec. £6 6/ *Dental.* Gen fee £10 10/	Full period, £46 14s. 6d. *Medical.* 6 mos. £6 6s. 18 mos. £19 19s. Perp. £26 5s. *Surgical.* 6 mos. £7 17s. 6d. 18 mos. £11 11s. 12 mos. £36 5s. Perp. £36 17s.	*Med. or Surg.* Perp. £15 15s. 1 yr. £8 8s. 9 mos. £5 5s. 12 mos.£40 *Med. and Surg.* Perp. £95 5s., or £10 10s. at beginning of 1st and 2nd years, and 25 5s. each subsequent year. 6 mos. £7 7s.	*Med. and Surg.* 3 mos. £15 6 mos. £26 9 mos. £35 12 mos.£40 Perp. £55 Midwif.£55/ Ophthal. £2 2/

* Including three months' Clinical Clerkship.   † Including six months' Clinical Clerkship.
‡ Including three months' Dresserership.   ‡ Including six months' Dresserership. || Including nine months' Dresserership.

We have endeavoured to make this table as complete and correct as possible, but from imperfect returns and deficient information, *perfect accuracy cannot be vouched for.*

Many classes which to outside students are chargeable in heavy sums are gratuitous to the regular students of the various schools.

Totals cannot here be given for the same reason, and because many classes are extra.

Information as to the mode of paying fees, and their amount, is appended to the notice of each school.

TABLE OF FEES FOR HOSPITAL LECTURES AND ATTENDANCE.

(The letter "i." denotes Single Course ; "ii.," Two Courses, Perpetual or Unlimited Attendance.)

	UNIVERSITY COLLEGE.	WESTMINSTER.	OWENS COLL., MANCHESTER.	QUEEN'S COLL. BIRMINGHAM.	LEEDS.*	LIVERPOOL.	BRISTOL.	NEWCASTLE.*	SHEFFIELD.
Anatomy	i. £11 11s.	1st c. £6 6s.+ subs. o. £3 3s.+	i. £5 5s.	i. £6 6s.	i. £6 6s.	2 cs. ea. £5 5s.; 3, £3 12s. 6d.	i. £5 5s. ii. £8 8s.	i. £4 4s.	1 c. £4 4s. 2 c. £3 2s.
	ii. with 3 yrs. Pract.								
Demonst. and Dissections	Anatomy, £16 16s.	3 mos. £5 5s.; 6 mos. £8 8s.	6 mos. £3 3s. 3 mos. £2 2s.	i. £5 5s.	...	i. £3 3s.	...	...	In above.
Physiology	i. £8 8s. ii. £10 10s.	1st c. £6 6s. subs. c. £2 2s.	i. (Junior and Senior) ea. £2 12s. 6d.	i. £6 6s.	i. £6 6s.	1 & 2 cs. each £5 5s.; 3, £3 12s. 6d.	i. £5 5s. ii. £8 8s.	i. £4 4s.	1 c. £3 3s. 2 c. £2 2s.
Practical Physiology	i. £8 8s. add. c. £2 2s.	c. £7 7s.; either division, £3 3s.	i. £5 5s.	...	i. £6 6s.	£5 5s.	i. £3 3s. ii. £5 5s.	...	i. £3 3s.
Histology Morbid Hist.	£4 4s.	...	£2 2s.	...	...	...	...	...	...
Chemistry	i. £7 7s. ii. £9 9s.	1st c. £6 6s. subs. cs. £2 2s.	i. £6 6s. Org. i. £3 10s.	i. £5 5s.	i. £4 4s.	1 c. £5 5s.; 2 and 3, each £2 12s. 6d.	i. £5 5s. ii. £7 7s.	i. £5 5s.	i. £4 4s.
Practical Chemistry	i. £5 5s. sec. c. £3 3s.	1 c. £4 4s.	i. £4 4s.	i. £4 4s.	i. £3 3s.	i. £4 4s.	i. £3 3s. ii. £5 5s.	...	i. £3 3s.
Botany	i. £3 13s. 9d. ii. £5 5s.	1 c. £4 4s. 2 cs. £5 5s.	i. £2 12s. 6d.	i. £4 4s.	i. £4 4s.	1 c. £4 4s.; 2 and 3, each £2 2s.	i. £5 5s.	i. £4 4s.	i. £3 3s.
Com. Anatomy	i. £6 6s. ii. £8 8s.	1 c. £3 3s. 2 cs. £5 5s.	i. £2 12s. 6d.	i. £3 3s.	i. £1 1s.	1 c. £3 3s.; 2, £2 2s.; 3, £1 1s.	i. £4 4s.	...	...
Medicine	i. £9 9s. ii. £11 11s.	1st c. £6 6s. subs. c. £2 2s.	i. £5 5s.	i. £6 6s.	i. £5 5s.	1 and 2 c. each £5 5s.; 3, £3 12s. 6d.	i. £5 5s. ii. £8 8s.	i. £4 4s.	1 c. £4 4s. 2 c. £2 2s.
Practical Med.	...	...	...	...	...	...	...	...	...
Surgery	i. £7 7s. ii. £8 8s.	1st c. £6 6s. subs. c. £2 2s.	i. £5 5s.	i. £6 6s.	i. £5 5s.	1 c. £5 5s. 2 & 3, ea. £1 1s.	i. £5 5s. ii. £8 8s.	i. £4 4s.	i. £4 4s.
Practical Surgery	i. £5 5s. sec. c. £4 4s.	1st c. £4 4s. subs. c. £2 2s.	i. £4 4s.	...	...	1 c. £4 4s.	i. £4 4s. ii. £6 6s.	...	i. £3 3s.
Surgical Path. Operative Surg.	... £5 5s.	... sp. c. £4 4s.	£4 4s. £4 4s.	...	...	... £2 2s.	...	...	...
Midwifery	i. £6 6s. ii. £7 7s.	1 c. £4 4s. 2 cs. £5 5s.	2 ses. £5 5s.	i. £5 5s.	i. £4 4s.	1 c. £5 5s.; 2 &3, ea. £3 13s. 6d.	i. £4 4s. ii. £6 6s.	i. £4 4s.	i. £3 3s.
Pathology	i. £6 6s. ii. £7 7s.	1 c. £3 3s. 2 cs. £4 4s.	i. £4 4s.	...	i. £3 3s.	1 c. £3 3s.; 2 and 3, each £1 11s. 6d.	i. £3 3s. ii. £4 4s.	i. £4 4s.	...
Dis. of Children Materia Medica	... i. £6 6s. ii. £7 7s.	... 1 c. £3 3s. 2 cs. £4 4s.	£2 2s. i. £4 4s.	... i. £4 4s.	... i. £4 4s.	1 c. £4 4s.; 2 &3, each £3 2s.	i. £4 4s. ii. £5 5s.	... i. £4 4s.	... i. £3 3s.
Forensic Medicine	i. £5 5s. ii. £6 6s.	1 c. £3 3s. 2 cs. £4 4s.	...	i. £4 4s.	i. £4 4s.	1 c. £4 4s.; 2 &3, each £3 2s.	i. £5 5s.	i. £4 4s.	i. £3 3s.
Med. Juris. and Hygiene	...	...	i. £4 4s.	...	...	...	...	...	...
Ophth. Surgery	i. £2 2s.	i. £1 1s.	i. £3 3s.	i. £3 3s.	...	i. £1 1s.	...	...	...
Dental Surgery	i. £2 2s.	i. £2 2s.	...	i. £3 3s.	...	i. £3 3s.	...	...	...
Embryology: Lec. & Prac.	...	...	£5 5s.	...	...	...	...	...	...
Mental Dis.	...	i. £1 1s.	...	...	...	...	...	...	...
Public Health	i. £2 2s.	i. £1 1s.	...	...	£1 1s.	i. 10s. 6d.	£1 1s.	...	...
Library	...	£1 1s.	...	...	...	ii. £1 1s.	...	...	...
Hospital Practice	Med. and Surg. Perp. £36 15s. 1 yr. £15 15s. 6 mos. £10 10s.	Med. or Surg. 6 mos. £8 8s. 6 mos. £10 10s. Each subsequt 6 mos. £5 5s.	Royal Infirm. Full perp. £49; or 2 instalments, £22	General and Queen's Hospitals. 4 yrs. £49, or 1 sum. £6 6s. 12 mo. £12 12s. 18 mo. £15 15s. 3 yrs. £21 6 mos. £14	Infirmary. Med. or Surg. Perp. £33 12s. Medical. 12 mo. £12 12s. 18 mo. £15 15s. Perp. £26 15s.	Royal Infirm. Perp. £63 12s. Medical. 3 mos. £3 3s. 6 mos. £5 5s. 12 mos. £6 6s. Surgical. 3 mos. £4 4s. 6 mos. £6 6s. 12 mos. £8 8s.	Royal Infirm. Medical. 6 mos. £8 1 yr. £15 18 mos. £23 Perp. £30 Surgical. 1 yr. £12 12s. 2 yrs. £21 3 yrs. £26 5s. General Hos. Med. or Surg. 6 mos. £8 12 mos. £10 Perp. £25	Infirmary. 3 mos. £4 4s. 6 mos. £6 6s. 12 mos. £7 7s. Perp. £17 17s., or 1st year, £7 7s.; 2nd year, £6 6s.; 3rd yr. £5 5s.	Gen. Infirm., or Public Hos. sum. ses. £3 3s. win. ses. £6 6s.
	Practical Pharmacy. 3 mo. £5 5s.	3 yrs. £31 9s. Med. and Surg. 3 mos. £10 10s. 6 mos. £14 14s. Each subseqnt 6 mos. £7 7s. 3 yrs. £36 5s.	Medical. 3 mos. £4 4s. 6 mos. £8 8s. 12 mo. £12 12s. Full period, £18 18s. Surgical. 3 mos. £6 6s. 6 mos. £9 9s. 12 mo. £18 18s. Full p. £31 10s.						

* No returns.   + With two years' Practical Anatomy, £15 15s.   ‡ Including tutorial classes.

We have endeavoured to make this table as complete and correct as possible, but from imperfect returns and deficient information, *perfect accuracy cannot be vouched for.*

Many classes which to outside students are chargeable in heavy sums are gratuitous to the regular students of the various schools.

Totals cannot here be given for the same reason, and because many classes are extra.

Information as to the mode of paying fees, and their amount, is appended to the notice of each school.

THE STUDENT BEGINNING TO WORK.

TO STUDENTS.

IN the annual number in which we give the information as to the medical schools and examining bodies which students want, it has long been our custom to address to them some words of advice which we have hoped might help them to spend their student-time to the best advantage. From that custom we see no reason for departing.

In every profession there are certain qualities of mind and habits of work which give a man entering that calling a peculiar fitness for it, and therefore a greater chance of success in it; and which, on that account, those who belong to it will do well to cultivate. It is certainly so in Medicine; and we shall now try and point out to the student the method in which he should try to educate himself if he wishes to become a skilful and successful practitioner.

All medical knowledge that is worth anything is of the kind that logicians call *real*, as distinguished from symbolical. It is acquaintance with *things*, not recollection of words. This truth is the first great lesson that we would wish stamped on the mind of the youth who is beginning to study medicine.

Let us illustrate the application of this principle. When the student has entered the school he has chosen, he will find anatomy the thing first set before him to be learned. Now, if he think that learning a book by heart is the way to master this science, he may, perhaps, succeed in getting through examinations, but he will never know anatomy; and the getting of this parrot-like facility of using anatomical phrases in an appropriate manner, he will find an arid, weary, and profitless labour. The real work for him to do, is to learn the *body*, not the book. Let him at once secure a part for dissection: he cannot begin too soon. Let him also get a set of bones: these will occupy him until his part is ready. Let him never attempt to learn about a structure of the body without having the thing by him, that he may look at it and handle it. It should be his object, not to get the words of the book into his memory, but to get the image of the thing itself imprinted on his mind's eye. If he has done this, he will be able to stand the ordeal of any examination table: and the words of the book will become to him living realities, full of interest, and stimulating to thought. Learnt in the one way, anatomy will be dry and repulsive; in the other, the student will find in it an absorbing, never-failing attraction. And not merely let him dissect much, but let him aim at dissecting *well*. Every year surgery is advancing; more and more diseased conditions are made amenable to surgical treatment, and surgical success largely depends upon manual dexterity. Not only is this true of surgery, but in medicine also, for skill in the use of instruments of precision is becoming indispensable to the scientific physician. Now, the dissecting-room is a great practice field in which the student may learn to use his hands. The man who cannot make a neat dissection is not to be trusted to use a knife among the delicate structures of the eye.

The same method of work should be carried out in the other branches of science with which the student has to become acquainted. Chemistry should be learned in the laboratory; the beginner should make a point of seeing for himself every reaction, and thus of verifying by experiment, so far as he has the means, every statement contained in his text-book. Materia medica should be studied in the museum and in the dispensary, where the learner can familiarise himself with the smell, colour, taste, and behaviour of the drugs he is hereafter to prescribe. The man who has learnt the properties of drugs in this way will not be found ordering incompatible combinations, or making nauseous drugs still more repulsive by injudicious mixtures. There is much of physiology which he must learn by reading; but the histological and chemical part of it he may become practically acquainted with. Unfortunately, politicians who have weakly yielded to the clamour of hysterical sentiment have made it impossible for him, except by going abroad, to learn in any way than from books those parts of physiological science that have been ascertained by experiment.

It would seem almost superfluous to dwell on the importance of learning surgery and medicine by practice in preference to print, were it not that there are only too many who put their trust in books, and who, even when they get into practice, although they see much disease, yet do not take any pains to carefully observe nature. *Tota ars medicinæ est in observationibus* is an old, true, but often forgotten, aphorism. A great writer has said that there are more false facts than false theories in medicine. The false facts here meant are not so much the deliberate mis-statements of charlatans (for they do no permanent mischief), but the loose observations of well-informed and conscientious men, who, having read things in books, then went to the bedside only able to see what they expected to see; who were not accustomed to carefully watch and record natural phenomena, and who subsequently, in perfect good faith in the accuracy both of their observation and memory, made statements founded on inexact observation and treacherous recollection, but given weight and importance, and therefore the power of misleading others, by the respectability of their authors. The old question of Pontius Pilate, "What is truth?" should always be in the mind of the student. He should remember that medicine is not like law or theology: doubtful questions cannot here be settled once and for all by a judicial decision or an Œcumenical Council. While paying to the instruction of his teachers the respect due to seniority, experience, and to knowledge, he should never forget that they, like all men, are liable to error, and that they are only safe guides so long as they draw their knowledge from the great book which is open alike to him and to them—the book of nature. Everything he is told, everything he reads, he should test at the bedside. He should lose no opportunity of seeing practice; every dressership and clinical clerkship that he can get he should take, and throw his whole energy into the thorough discharge of its practical duties; and he should *take notes*. There is no more valuable aid to accurate observation than the habit of recording such observations at the time they are made. This custom has a value quite independent of its worth as an aid to memory. When we have to write a thing down, we are forced to distinctly formulate the idea in our mind. "Writing," said Lord Bacon, "maketh an exact man"; and in one whose life is to be given to science, precision both in mental conception and in verbal utterance is of the first importance.

The great statesman who at present rules over the British Empire has more than once expressed his opinion that there is no profession whose influence will in the future so much increase as that of the medical. With this forecast we agree. But its realisation will depend upon the spirit in which each individual member of that profession learns and practises his art. The future of medicine is in the hands of those who to-day are students; some of whom, a generation hence, will be its leaders. The way in which the profession will be viewed by those outside it will depend on the amount of accurate knowledge which it can show. The medical man will be valued by the public in proportion as they see that what he says is the truth—we mean, the truth in the largest sense of the word, not merely the opposite of falsehood, but actual correspondence of statements with fact. One who would do this must be sure of the facts, and he must also bear in mind how much there is that he does not know. Dogmatism about that which is uncertain, and multiplication of directions concerning things which are unimportant, although for a time they may look like knowledge, yet are soon found out, and lead to distrust and contempt. The power of seeing, when face to face with disease, that which is essential; skill in eliciting facts from the laity, and making them understand what is wanted, and why; expertness in using the senses both to observe morbid phenomena, and do what is necessary for their relief—these are attainments which can never be learned from books. They are gained only at the bedside, and learned best by making mistakes. Errors at the hospital will be corrected for the student by those who are older and wiser, before they can lead to serious harm; but a blunder afterwards will injure both patient and practitioner.

The medical profession, as a means of mental discipline, is in one respect above all others. In theology, in law, in classical study, for instance, excellence lies mainly in mastering that which has been done in the past. But it is the privilege of the student of medicine, not merely to learn what is already known, but to find out more. To seek truth from nature, and to apply truth for the benefit of his fellows—these are the functions of the medical man. The more clearly and steadfastly he keeps these ends before him, the more will he find his profession an ennobling one, and the higher place will he take in the esteem of his professional brethren, and the grateful regard of all educated men and women.

THE MEDICAL STUDENT'S PROSPECTS.

A DISCUSSION on future prospects may not prove very interesting to commencing students: for it may be taken for granted, in a large proportion of the cases, that the question of prospects has already been settled some way or other to their own entire satisfaction, before they decided upon entering on a medical career. But to parents and guardians the question must be one of great importance; while to those who are just about finishing their studies the question will be uppermost in their minds, presenting itself perhaps as —" What particular subject shall I take up?" or "Where shall I settle down?" This question, though it applies only to those who have completed their studies, is, nevertheless, more intimately connected with the period of study than is at first sight apparent, and hence it is eminently a subject for consideration in this number of the journal, which is dedicated to students.

For the future of the medical student, or rather of the medical man, depends not a little on circumstances which in themselves may seem trivial. Thus, accident more than design—want of opportunity, perhaps, more than want of ability—may prevent a student from passing his matriculation examination at the right moment; or he may have selected the Preliminary Examination at the College of Surgeons, which does not admit him to the further examinations at the University of London: thus his chances of graduating in London are at once knocked on the head by what at one time may have been regarded as a circumstance of little or no moment. The student must now either retrace his steps, and take an additional year in order to make up for the lost opportunity; or he must enter one of the Scotch or provincial Universities; or forego the satisfaction of graduating. This little omission assumes very different proportions when, in later life, the possession of a medical degree renders a candidate eligible for an appointment for which, without one, he would, *ipso facto*, be ineligible. The same applies

to all the higher qualifications, and especially to the Fellowship of the College of Surgeons.

Thus, speaking broadly, the future of the medical student depends largely on the diplomas or degrees with which he begins life; or, to put it better, the possession of the higher qualifications opens up lines of practice which are closed to those not so provided, although they do not by any means always testify to a man's special fitness for the practical exercise of his profession. It will be seen, therefore, that the student should, from the very first, aim at the maximum instead of the minimum of qualifications; for he can never foresee how they will prove of use to him, or what advancement may be lost for the want of them. It is far too much the custom with some students to pride themselves on the possession of a *practical knowledge* of their profession, and to affect to despise the scientific and theoretical knowledge, without which, nevertheless, real success is very difficult, not to say impossible, of attainment.

Next to the possession of first-class diplomas, the young Medicus should direct his thoughts to the resident appointments in the various hospitals. For while theoretical knowledge is very valuable, it is in its practical application to everyday life and its requirements that distinction is to be sought. After holding the house-surgeoncy and the house-physiciancy at his own hospital, much useful experience may be got by going to one or other of the special hospitals which abound. It will be obvious to the simplest understanding that a few months spent, say, in a children's hospital, or in a hospital for diseases of women, or in a hospital for the treatment of special diseases, will add greatly to a man's clinical knowledge of his profession—added knowledge which will prove of the highest value in whatever line of practice he may decide on. Moreover, it is while holding such appointments as these that the opportunities occur for developing any special powers or aptitudes which may decide a man as to the line of practice he shall definitely take up.

With these few preliminary remarks, we may now pass on to consider the prospects of the medical man. Such a course of study and subsequent work as we have foreshadowed often decides the future of men whose private means render them independent of practice for a few years. These drift, as it were, with the current, living on what they have, working for more knowledge, and content to await, it may be for years, any adequate return for the outlay which they must necessarily make. For such men our remarks are hardly applicable; we address ourselves rather to those who with the least possible outlay desire to commence a practice which shall be at once remunerative. It would be ridiculous, of course, to make believe that the possession of a competence does not immensely simplify the question we are considering, whatever line of practice is adopted. On the other hand, in many cases it is very mischievous, by removing one of the great incentives to work in a profession which, more than any other, requires *personal qualities* even still more than the possession of money. For in this respect our profession differs from all others—the services rendered must be personal; they cannot efficiently be rendered by a substitute. The higher the class of practice, the more personal do these services become: they are not so much the services of the doctor as of the individual; less a question of the actual present (a diagnosis) than a personal opinion of the probable future (a prognosis). Hence the importance of the preliminary studies, as well as of the hospital appointments to which we have alluded.

The usual division of medical men into consultants and general practitioners is becoming every day less and less marked. The higher education which is now afforded in the medical schools, no less than the multiplication of hospitals, not in London only, but also in the provinces—of special as well as general hospitals,—is fast levelling the once well-defined consultant, by elevating the general practitioner, on whose want of education and experience and opportunities he (the consultant) once flourished. Even the line of demarcation between medicine and surgery is no longer so well defined as formerly, and it is only at the extremes that it is well marked. All this again shows the necessity of a lengthened curriculum, supplemented by hospital appointments, in order to fit the medical man for the duties which may await him in practice.

This extended education is all the more necessary nowadays, in view of the large number of medical men who have to be provided for our wide-reaching colonies. And here a few words may be said on the advantages offered by the colonies. First and foremost, their extent, as compared with the mother-country, is immense; and we have full evidence of their vitality in their rapid growth in all directions. Well-educated medical men are a first necessity in such places, and can always be sure of lucrative employment. Then for many men a more genial climate than our own is absolutely necessary: for such men, the endless extent of our colonial empire allows ample choice in almost any latitude. The demand for medical men for the colonies is sure to increase, and we cannot do better than draw the attention of young surgeons, who are untrammelled by family ties or a too strong love of the old country, to the many openings which are constantly presenting themselves. But here again success depends, even more than in England, on personal qualities and on the possession of a wide-reaching education. When far away from brother practitioners, with nothing to rely upon but one's own knowledge, the experience gained while holding hospital appointments will prove invaluable when the surgeon is suddenly brought face to face with a serious case; while confidence on his part, and a ready practical knowledge, will command the confidence of the patient and his friends.

It may be asked, How can these colonial appointments be obtained? We confess the answer is not always an easy one. Some are to be obtained through the Colonial Office; and there is another way which is not very difficult, and which most often leads to success: that is, to go out and look for them. After the hard work of a prolonged curriculum, both rest and renovation become necessary; and a good way of obtaining these is to act for a few months as surgeon in some of the large ocean-going steamships. In this manner, while a small stipend is being earned and the health renovated, the man, during his voyages, is brought in contact with those who can give him valuable information; while those who may be interested in securing a medical man for some inland town, are brought face to face with one who is in search of such an opportunity to establish himself.

Apart, moreover, from any such advantages or opportunities, travelling about the world improves a man and enlarges his mind, and thus renders him better suited for any position which he may subsequently obtain.

The Services (Army and Navy) both offer advantages for a certain class of men. The life is that of a gentleman, and those who are already accustomed to its usages will find in either service associates with whom it will always be a pleasure to come in contact. The pay is certain, though it is small; and there is also a pension for those who by service care to earn it. In times of war there is excitement and adventure enough; but during the "piping times of peace" official routine must at last become monotonous even to the most long-suffering.

A few of the more fortunate men may rise to positions of distinction, but we fear it is the result of accident or seniority rather than of merit. At all times and on all occasions red tape is the order of the day, and very little, if any, allowance is made for special attainments or special aptitudes outside that of always seeming to be satisfied with the official inevitable.

One of the great features of the present day is the multiplication of special subjects, and of special hospitals for the study of them. It is generally thought that a special subject more quickly leads to practice than does general medicine or surgery, and hence many men no sooner qualify than they seek to attach themselves to some special hospital. This course we unhesitatingly condemn, for the successful practice of one special branch can only be carried on by those who are first good generalists, and who understand the relation of special parts with the remaining whole.

For the large majority of medical men, that which is very well called "general practice" is not only the best, it is the only line open to them. Given the personal qualities, a man may here find an immense field open to him; while the fact that he is brought in contact with all kinds of disease—medical as well as surgical—will keep him far more au courant with the details of his profession than would be possible were he devoting himself to any one of the so-called special branches of practice. For while the specialist has little chance of seeing general practice, it is in general practice that nearly all the special cases are first met with. Here again is it seen how invaluable a broad, sound education must prove to the medical man, enabling the general practitioner, as it does, to at once recognise disease in any of the special organs, even if he should not feel inclined to undertake the responsibility of its treatment.

A somewhat newer line of practice is opening for the more contemplative members of our profession—we mean the appointment of health officer. For these, special studies are essential, after the usual examinations have been passed. There can be little doubt, we think, that these appointments will constantly grow in importance; for as population tends to aggregate itself, so will disease, unless preventive medicine steps in and insists on a due regard of the natural laws which govern health and ward off disease.

Thus there is no lack of occupation for medical men—for those whose efforts are devoted to the cure of disease, as well as for those whose tastes lead them to do battle with the enemies which cause disease. For all there is work, which will bring its material reward. How great that reward shall be, and whether it shall be coupled with social distinction and public recognition, will depend entirely on the man.

The medical profession differs from its two fellows, the clerical and the legal professions, in not having any great public offices to which any and all its members may legitimately look forward. There is no Archbishop's mitre, and there is no Woolsack—each conferring high social status and precedence quite beyond the duties of the office. But the legitimate exercise of our profession nevertheless brings with it, besides its material reward, an immense personal satisfaction, and places those who need our skill under obligations which nothing can shake off. The more independently we can work, the greater will be our influence over our patients; the more thoroughly we understand ourselves, the greater our power over disease. Our social distinctions and precedence will then follow in due course.

ROYAL HOSPITAL FOR SICK CHILDREN, MEADOWSIDE HOUSE, EDINBURGH.

Consulting Physicians—Professor Sir Robert Christison, Bart., Drs. Charles Wilson, Graham Weir, and George W. Balfour.

Consulting Surgeon—Professor Spence.

Pathologist—Vacant.

Ordinary Physicians—Drs. Dunsmure, Andrew, Underhill, Cunynghame.

Extra Physicians—Drs. Carmichael and Playfair.

Surgeon-Dentist—Dr. Smith.

Ophthalmic Surgeon—Dr. Argyll Robertson.

Resident Physician—Dr. J. W. B. Hodsdon.

Honorary Secretary—Mr. John Henry, 20, St. Andrew-square.

Hon. Treasurer—R. S. Wyld, LL.D., 19, Inverleith-row.

DEGREES IN SCIENCE IN
THE DEPARTMENT OF PUBLIC HEALTH.

UNIVERSITY OF CAMBRIDGE.
EXAMINATION IN STATE MEDICINE.

AN examination in so much of State Medicine as is comprised in the functions of Officers of Health will be held in Cambridge, beginning on the first Tuesday in October, and ending on the following Friday.

Any person whose name is on the Medical Register of the United Kingdom may present himself for this examination provided he is in his twenty-fourth year. The examination will be in two parts, and will be oral and practical as well as in writing.

Part I. will comprise :—Physics and Chemistry. The principles of Chemistry, and methods of analysis with especial reference to analyses of air and water. Application of the microscope. The laws of heat, and the principles of pneumatics, hydrostatics, and hydraulics, with especial reference to ventilation, water-supply, drainage, construction of dwellings, disposal of sewage and refuse, and sanitary engineering in general. Statistical methods.

Part II. will comprise :—Laws of the realm relating to Public Health. Origin, propagation, pathology, and prevention of epidemic and infectious diseases. Effects of overcrowding, vitiated air, impure water, and bad or insufficient food. Unhealthy occupations, and the diseases to which they give rise. Water-supply and drainage in reference to health. Nuisances injurious to health. Distribution of diseases within the United Kingdom, and effects of soil, season, and climate.

Candidates may present themselves for either part separately, or for both together, at their option ; but the result of the examination in the case of any candidate will not be published until he has passed to the satisfaction of the examiners in both parts. Every candidate will be required to pay a fee of £4 4s. before admission to each part of the examination. Every candidate who has passed both parts of the examination to the satisfaction of the examiners will receive a certificate testifying to his competent knowledge of what is required for the duties of a Medical Officer of Health.

All applications for admission to this examination, or for information respecting it, should be addressed to Professor Liveing, Cambridge.

Candidates who desire to present themselves for examination in October next must send in their applications and transmit the fees on or before September 28.

UNIVERSITY OF LONDON.(a)
EXAMINATION IN SUBJECTS RELATING TO PUBLIC HEALTH.

A special examination shall be held once in every year in subjects relating to Public Health, and shall commence on the second Monday in December.

No candidate shall be admitted to this examination unless he shall have passed the second examination for the degree of Bachelor of Medicine in this University at least one year previously ; nor unless he shall have given notice of his intention to the Registrar at least two calendar months before the commencement of the examination.

Candidates shall be examined in the following subjects :—

1. Chemistry and Microscopy, as regards the examination of air, water, and food.

2. Meteorology as regards general knowledge of meteorological conditions, and the reading and correction of instruments.

3. Geology, as regards general knowledge of rocks, their conformation and chemical composition, and their relation to underground water, and to drainage and sources of water-supply.

4. Physics and Sanitary Apparatus. The laws of heat, mechanics, pneumatics, hydrostatics, and hydraulics, in relation (for sanitary purposes) to the construction of dwellings, and to the principles of warming, ventilation, drainage and water-supply, and to forms of apparatus for these and other sanitary uses. And the reading of plans, sections, scales, etc., in regard of sanitary constructions and appliances.

5. Vital Statistics, as regards the methods employed for determining the health of a community ; birth-rate ; death-rate ; disease-rate ; life-tables ; duration and expectancy of life. Present amount of mortality at the various ages, and its

(a) No return.

causes in different classes and communities. Practical statistics of armies, navies, civil professions, asylums, hospitals, dispensaries, lying-in establishments, prisons, indoor and outdoor paupers, friendly societies, sick clubs, medical and surgical practice, towns.

6. Hygiene, including the causation and prevention of disease, in which branch of examination reference shall be had to such matters as the following :—

Parentage, as influencing the individual expectation of health ; temperaments ; morbid diatheses ; congenital diseases and malformations ; effects of close inter-breeding. Special liabilities of the health at particular periods of life ; physical regimen of different ages. Earth and climate and changes of season in their bearing on the health of populations ; dampness of soil ; malaria. Conditions of healthy nourishment : dietaries and dietetic habits ; stimulants and narcotics in popular use ; dietetic privation, excesses, and errors, as respectively causing disease ; drinking-water, and the conditions which make water unfit for drinking ; adulterations of food. Conditions of healthy lodgment : ventilation and warming, and the removal of refuse-matters, in their respective relations to health ; filth as a cause of disease ; sanitary regimen of towns and villages ; "nuisances" (as defined by law) with regard to the sanitary bearing and the removal of each ; trade-processes causing offensive effluvia ; common lodging-houses and tenement houses. Conditions of healthy activity : work, over-work, rest, and recreation ; occupations of different sorts in relation to the health of persons engaged in them—e.g., factory work in general, occupations which produce irritative lung-disease, occupations which promote heart-disease, occupations which deal with poisons, etc. Hygiene of particular establishments and particular classes of population ; factories and workplaces ; schools ; workhouses ; asylums ; hospitals ; prisons. Disease as distributed in England : classifications of diseases for various purposes of medical inquiry ; excesses of particular diseases and injuries at particular places and at particular times. Particular diseases, as regards their intimate nature, causation, and preventability : e.g., enteric fever, cholera, typhus, small-pox, scarlatina, diphtheria, erysipelas, pyæmia, tubercular diseases, rheumatism, ague, cretinism, ophthalmia, pertigo, venereal diseases, scurvy, neptism, leprosy, insanity. Processes of contagion in different diseases ; incubation in each case ; particular dangers of infection—at schools, workplaces, etc., and from laundries, dairies, etc. Disinfectants and establishments for disinfection. Quarantine. Hospitals for infectious disease. Conveyance of the sick. Vaccination : existing knowledge as to its protectiveness ; revaccination ; precautions which vaccination requires ; arrangements for public vaccination in town and country ; natural cow-pox. Prostitution as regards the public health. Disease of domestic animals in relation to the health of man : rabies ; farcy and glanders ; anthrax ; parasites, especially trichina and the tæniadæ ; aphtha ; tubercle ; meat and milk of diseased animals. Diseases of the vegetable kingdom, and failures of vegetable crops, in relation to the health of man ; famine-diseases. Poisons in manufacture and commercial and domestic use—e.g., arsenic, lead, phosphorus, mercury ; poisonous pigments.

7. Sanitary Law, as regards the leading purposes of the following statutes, and the constitution and modes of procedure of the respective authorities, and any existing orders, regulations, or model by-laws of the Local Government Board in sanitary matters. The Public Health Act, 1875. The Vaccination Acts. The Rivers' Pollution Prevention Act, 1876. The Sale of Food and Drugs Act, 1875. The Artisans and Labourers' Dwellings Improvement Act, 1875. The Acts regulating the medical profession. The Acts regulating the practice of pharmacy. The Acts relating to factories and workplaces. The Acts relating to the detention and care of lunatics.

UNIVERSITY OF DURHAM.
STATE MEDICINE.

The Warden and Senate of the University of Durham, in recognition of the importance that medical officers of health, or those seeking appointments as such, should possess a proof of their special acquirements, have instituted examinations in State Medicine, by which the successful candidates will be entitled to receive a certificate of proficiency in Sanitary Science.

For the certificate of proficiency in Sanitary Science :—
1. That the candidate shall be a registered medical practitioner. 2. That the candidate shall have attended one course of lectures on Public Health at the College of Medicine, Newcastle-upon-Tyne, extending over one winter session. 3. That the candidate shall be required to pass an examination on the following subjects :—

1. Physics.—Laws of light, heat, hydro-dynamics, and pneumatics.

2. Chemistry.—As applied to the detection of noxious gases and atmospheric impurities ; analysis of air and water.

3. Sanitary Legislation.—Knowledge of the Acts of Parliament in force for the preservation and protection of health.

4. Vital Statistics.—Rates of births, deaths, and marriages ; methods of calculation, classification, and tabulation of returns of sickness and mortality ; data and conclusions deducible therefrom.

5. Meteorology, Climatology, and Geographical Distribution of Diseases in the United Kingdom.

6. Sanitary Medicine, more especially in relation to epidemic, endemic, epizootic, and communicable diseases; diseases attributable to heat, cold, or damp; insufficiency or impurity of air, food, or drink; habitation, occupation, over-exertion, intemperance, heredity; preventive measures—vaccination, isolation, disinfection; the regulation of noxious and offensive manufactures and trades; the removal of nuisances.

7. Practical Hygiene, in reference to site, materials, construction, lighting, ventilation, warmth, dryness, water-supply and refuse-disposal of dwellings, schools, hospitals, and other buildings of public and private resort; action with respect to nuisances and outbreaks of disease. Other duties of a Medical Officer of Health.

The examination shall be by written papers, practical and *vivâ voce*, and will commence on October 10, 1881, and on April 24, 1882.

UNIVERSITY OF EDINBURGH.

In consequence of the great demand which now exists for Medical Officers of Health, and the importance to the public of some means of ascertaining that members of the medical profession have specially studied the subject of Public Health, Science Degrees in the Department of Public Health have been instituted by the University of Edinburgh under the following conditions:—

1. Candidates for graduation in Science in the Department of Public Health must be graduates in Medicine of a British University, or of such foreign or colonial Universities as may be specially recognised by the University Court.

2. He must be matriculated for the year in which he appears for examination or graduation.

3. Candidates who have not passed an *annus medicus* in the University of Edinburgh must, before presenting themselves for examination, have attended as matriculated students in the University at least two courses of instruction, scientific or professional, bearing on the subjects of the examinations.

4. There are two examinations for the degree of Bachelor of Science in the Department of Public Health. Candidates who have passed the first examination may proceed to the second, immediately or at any subsequent Medical or Science examination.

5. Candidates must produce evidence that, either during their medical studies or subsequently, they have attended a course of lectures in which instruction was given on Public Health, and that they have studied Analytical Chemistry practically for three months with a recognised teacher.

6. The examinations are written, oral, and practical, and are conducted by University examiners selected by the University Court.

7. The subjects of the examinations for the degree of Bachelor of Science in the Department of Public Health are as follows:—

FIRST EXAMINATION.

1. *Chemistry.*—Analysis of air, detection of gaseous emanations and other impurities in the atmosphere; analysis of waters for domestic use, and determination of the nature and amount of their mineral and organic constituents; detection, chemical and microscopical, of adulterations in articles of food and drink, and in drugs: practical examination, including at least two analytical researches.

2. *Physics.*—Hydraulics and hydrostatics, in reference to water-supply, drainage, and sewerage; pneumatics, in reference to warming and ventilation; meteorology, and methods of making meteorological observations; mensuration and mechanical drawing in reference to the plans and sections of public and private buildings, mines, waterworks, and sewers. The candidate will be expected to make figured sketches from models, and to have such a knowledge of mechanical drawing as will enable him fully to understand engineering plans, sections, and elevations.

3. *Sanitary Law.*—Knowledge of the leading sanitary Acts of Parliament.

4. *Vital Statistics.*—Knowledge of statistical methods and data in reference to population, births, marriages, and deaths.

Examination.—First day: Chemistry and Physics. Second day: Sanitary Law and Vital Statistics.

An oral examination and an examination in practical chemistry in the laboratory will take place a few days after the written examination.

SECOND EXAMINATION.

1. *Medicine.*—Origin, nature, and propagation of epidemic and contagious diseases; prevention of contagion and infection; endemic diseases and the geographical distribution of disease; insalubrious trades; overcrowding; epizootics, including pathological changes.

2. *Practical Sanitation.*—Duties of a Health Officer in reference to water-supply; insalubrious dwellings and public buildings; removal and disposal of sewage and other refuse and impurities; cemeteries; nuisances from manufactories, etc.: bad or insufficient supplies of food; outbreaks of zymotic diseases; quarantine; disinfectants and deodorisers; construction of permanent and temporary hospitals.

The written examinations will take place in April, 1882. Candidates who intend to present themselves for examination are required to lodge with the Secretary of the Senatus proof of their being eligible, and to pay the fee on or before March 1.

DOCTOR OF SCIENCE.

A Bachelor of Science in the Department of Public Health may, after the lapse of one year, proceed to the degree of Doctor in the same department on producing evidence that he has been engaged in practical sanitation since he received the degree of Bachelor of Science, and on presenting a thesis on some subject embraced in the Department of Public Health. Every such thesis must be certified by the candidate to have been composed by himself, and must be approved of by the examiners.

The candidate for the degree of D.Sc. must lodge his thesis with the Dean of the Medical Faculty on or before January 31 in the year in which he proposes to graduate. No thesis will be approved which does not contain either the results of original observations on some subject embraced in the examination for B.Sc., or else a full digest and critical exposition of the opinions and researches of others on the subject selected by the candidate, accompanied by precise references to the various publications quoted, so that due verification may be facilitated.

The fees for the degrees in Science in the Department of Public Health shall be—For the First B.Sc. in Public Health examination, £5 5s.; for the Second B.Sc. in Public Health examination, £5 5s.; for the degree of D.Sc. in Public Health £5 5s.

The following are recommended as books to be studied in preparation for the above examinations:—E. Parkes' "Practical Hygiene"; George Wilson's "Handbook of Hygiene"; Edwd. Smith's "Manual for Public Officers of Health" and "Handbook for Inspectors of Nuisances"; Michael, Corfield, and Wanklyn's "Manual of Public Health," edited by E. Hart; Eassie's "Healthy Houses"; Baldwin Latham's "Sanitary Engineering"; Fleeming Jenkin's "Healthy Houses"; Henry Law's "Rudiments of Civil Engineering"; George Monro's "The Public Health (Scotland) Act"; Alexander Buchan's "Introductory Text-book of Meteorology."

UNIVERSITY OF GLASGOW.

THE QUALIFICATION IN PUBLIC HEALTH.

A special examination will be held once in every year in subjects relating to Public Health, and will commence on the second Tuesday in April. The examination will consist of two divisions, viz.:—First Division, embracing Physics, Chemistry, Meteorology, Geographical Distribution of Diseases. Second Diembracing State Medicine, vision, Sanitary Law, Vital Statistics. Fee for each division of the examination, £4 4s.

ROYAL COLLEGE OF PHYSICIANS OF EDINBURGH.

GENERAL REGULATIONS.

Candidates shall be already on the Medical Register, and be entered there as possessing a qualification in Medicine. Candidates shall not, in the meantime, be required to attend any special courses of instruction; but their attention is directed particularly to courses of lectures on State Medicine, and to the practice of Analytical Chemistry. Candidates shall be subjected to two examinations. Such examinations may be taken simultaneously, or with an interval not exceeding twelve months. The examinations shall be written, oral, and practical. The examinations shall be held in the Physicians' Hall, or elsewhere if found more convenient. Rejected candidates shall not be admitted for re-examination till after the expiry of six months. Fees will not be returned, except in the case mentioned in the paragraph relating to fees given below.

EXAMINATIONS.

I. The First Examination shall embrace — 1. Physics: Especially pneumatics, hydrostatics, hydraulics, and engineering in relation to sanitary operations, including a knowledge of architectural and other plans, sections, etc. 2. Chemistry: Especially analysis of air, water, food, including the biology of putrefaction and allied processes. 3. Meteorology: Including climate, topographical and seasonal influences in relation to health and disease.

II. The Second Examination shall embrace—1. Epidemiology and Endemiology: Including the corresponding departments in the diseases of animals and plants; contagious diseases; diseases of periods of life, professions, trades, seasons, and climates. 2. Practical Hygiene: Duties of a health officer; food; water-supply; sewerage and drainage; construction of hospitals, public buildings, dwellings: manufactories; cemeteries; nuisances. 3. Sanitary Law and Vital Statistics.

Meetings for both examinations shall be held annually in April and October. The first examination shall be held on the second Tuesday of the month, and shall occupy two days; the second examination on the immediately succeeding Thursday of the same week, and shall occupy two days. Candidates may enter for both examinations in the same week, or for one only. The examinations must be passed in their order, first and second. Candidates must appear for the second examination not later than twelve months after having passed the first. A candidate remitted at his second examination will be allowed to come up again after a further period of six months; but if he then fail to pass, he will be required again to undergo the first as well as the second examination before obtaining the certificate.

FEES.

No one shall be recognised as a candidate till he has paid the fee for the first examination. The fees for examinations must be paid at least a week before the day of examination. The whole charges by the College for the certificate amount to £10 10s. The fee for the first examination is £3 3s.; the fee for the second examination is £3 3s.; the fee payable before receiving the certificate is £4 4s. Candidates forfeit the fee for the examination which they have been unsuccessful in passing. If a candidate who has offered himself for both examinations fail to pass the first, he shall not be allowed to present himself for the second, and his fee for the second shall be returned to him.

DENTAL SURGERY.

REGULATIONS RELATING TO THE DIPLOMA IN DENTAL SURGERY.

ROYAL COLLEGE OF SURGEONS OF ENGLAND.

EDUCATION.

CANDIDATES are required to produce the following certificates :—

1. Of being twenty-one years of age.
2. Of having been engaged during four years in the acquirement of professional knowledge.
3. Of having attended, at a school or schools recognised by this College, not less than one of each of the following courses of lectures, delivered by lecturers recognised by this College, namely:—Anatomy, Physiology, Surgery, Medicine, Chemistry, and Materia Medica.
4. Of having attended a second winter course of lectures on Anatomy, or a course of not less than twenty lectures on the Anatomy of the Head and Neck, delivered by lecturers recognised by this College.
5. Of having performed dissections at a recognised school during not less than nine months.
6. Of having completed a course of chemical manipulation, under the superintendence of a teacher or lecturer recognised by this College.
7. Of having attended, at a recognised hospital or hospitals in the United Kingdom, the practice of Surgery and clinical lectures on Surgery during two winter sessions.
8. Of having attended, at a recognised school, two courses of lectures upon each of the following subjects, viz. :—Dental Anatomy and Physiology (human and comparative), Dental Surgery, Dental Mechanics, and one course of lectures on Metallurgy, by lecturers recognised by this College.

9. Of having been engaged, during a period of not less than three years, in acquiring a practical familiarity with the details of Mechanical Dentistry, under the instruction of a competent practitioner. In the case of qualified surgeons, evidence of a period of not less than two instead of three years of such instruction will be sufficient.

10. Of having attended at a recognised dental hospital, or in the dental department of a recognised general hospital, the practice of Dental Surgery during the period of two years.

[Note.—All candidates who commenced their professional education on or after July 22, 1878, are, in addition to the certificates enumerated in the foregoing clauses, required to produce a certificate of having, prior to such commencement, passed the preliminary examination in general knowledge for the diploma of Member of the College, or an examination recognised as equivalent to that examination.]

Candidates who were in practice as dentists, or who had commenced their education as dentists prior to September, 1859—the date of the Charter—and who are unable to produce the certificates required by the foregoing regulations, shall furnish the Board of Examiners with a certificate of moral and professional character, signed by two members of this College, together with answers to the following inquiries:— Name, age, and professional address. If in practice as a dentist, the date of the commencement thereof. Whether member or licentiate of any College of Physicians or Surgeons of the United Kingdom; and, if so, of what College. Whether graduate of any University in the United Kingdom; and, if so, of what University; and whether graduate in Arts or Medicine. The date or dates of any such diploma, licence, or degree. Whether member of any learned or scientific society; and, if so, of what. Whether his practice as a dentist is carried on in connexion with any other business; and, if so, with what business. Whether since July 22, 1876, he has employed advertisements or public notices of any kind in connexion with the practice of his profession. The particulars of professional education, medical or special. The Board of Examiners will determine whether the evidence of character and education produced by a candidate be such as to entitle him to examination.

N.B.—In the case of candidates in practice or educated in Scotland or Ireland, the certificate of moral and professional character may be signed by two Licentiates of the Royal College of Surgeons of Edinburgh, or of the Faculty of Physicians and Surgeons of Glasgow, or of the Royal College of Surgeons in Ireland, as the case may be.

EXAMINATION.

The examination is partly written and partly oral. The written examination comprises general Anatomy and Physiology, and general Pathology and Surgery, with especial reference to the practice of the dental profession. The oral practical examination comprises the several subjects included in the curriculum of professional education, and is conducted by the use of preparations, casts, drawings, etc. Members of the College, in the written examination, will only have to answer those questions set by the section of the Board consisting of persons skilled in Dental Surgery; and in the oral examination will be examined only by that section. A candidate whose qualifications shall be found insufficient will be referred back to his studies, and will not be admitted to re-examination within the period of six months, unless the Board shall otherwise determine. Examinations will be held in January and June. The fee for the diploma is £10 10s., over and above any stamp duty.

[Note.—A ticket of admission to the museum, to the library, and to the College lectures will be presented to each candidate on his obtaining the diploma.]

DENTAL HOSPITAL OF LONDON MEDICAL SCHOOL.

HOSPITAL STAFF.

Consulting Physician—Sir Thomas Watson, Bart., M.D.
Consulting Surgeon—Mr. Christopher Heath.
Consulting Dental Surgeons—Mr. S. Cartwright and Mr. John Tomes.

Dental Surgeons.

Mr. Fox.	Mr. Coleman.
Mr. Medwin.	Mr. Moon.
Mr. Gregson.	Mr. A. Hill.

Assistant Dental Surgeons.

Mr. F. Canton.	Mr. R. Woodhouse.
Mr. A. S. Underwood.	Mr. Storer Bennett.
Mr. D. Hepburn.	Mr. S. J. Hutchinson.

Chloroformists—Mr. Clover, Mr. Braine, and Mr. Bailey.
Medical Tutor—Mr. Morton Smale.
Demonstrators—Mr. Claude Rogers and Mr. John Askary.
House-Surgeon—Mr. Herbert Blackmore.
Assistant House-Surgeon—Mr. Arthur Curle.

The winter session will commence on Monday, October 3.

LECTURES.—WINTER SESSION.
Mechanical Dentistry—Dr. Walker.

LECTURES.—SUMMER SESSION.
Dental Surgery and Pathology—Mr. Alfred Coleman.
Dental Anatomy and Physiology (Human and Comparative)—Mr. C. S. Tomes.
Metallurgy in its Application to Dental Purposes—Mr. Louis.

SCHOLARSHIPS AND PRIZES.
The Saunders Scholarship of £20 per annum, and Prizes, are open for competition.

FEES.
Fee for two years' hospital practice required by the curriculum, £15 15s. Fees for lectures and practice, £31 10s. Additional fees for a general hospital for the two years to fulfil the requirements of the curriculum vary from £40 to £50.

For further particulars, apply to Mr. T. F. Ken Underwood, Dean.

NATIONAL DENTAL HOSPITAL AND COLLEGE.

The winter session will commence on October 3.

HOSPITAL STAFF.

Dental Surgeons.	*Assistant Dental Surgeons.*
Mr. G. Williams.	Mr. W. G. Weiss.
Mr. A. P. Canton.	Mr. G. Hammond.
Mr. H. T. K. Kempton.	Mr. G. A. Williams.
Mr. Harry Rose.	Mr. W. R. Humby.
Mr. F. Henri Weiss.	Mr. Thomas Gaddes.
	Mr. A. Smith.

LECTURERS.

Dental Anatomy and Physiology—Mr. Thomas Gaddes.	Deformities of the Mouth — Mr. Oakley Coles.
Dental Mechanics—Mr. Harry Rose.	Demonstrator of Dental Mechanics—Mr. W. R. Humby.
Dental Surgery and Pathology—Vacant.	Operative Dental Surgery — Dr. Thompson.
Dental Metallurgy—Mr. A. Tribe.	Arts and Literature—Rev. H. R. Belcher, M.A.
Elements of Histology—Mr. Thomas Gaddes.	

FEE.
The fee for hospital practice and lectures required by the curriculum is £25 4s.

Special arrangements for the education of dental students are made at Charing-cross and Middlesex Hospitals.

PHARMACEUTICAL CHEMISTRY.

PHARMACEUTICAL SOCIETY OF GREAT BRITAIN SCHOOL OF PHARMACY.

THE session will commence on October 3, 1881, and extend to July 29, 1882.

Lectures on Chemistry and Pharmacy will be delivered by Professor Redwood on Monday, Tuesday, and Wednesday mornings at nine o'clock, commencing on Monday, October 3. The course consists of sixty lectures, comprising an exposition of the leading principles and doctrines of the science of Chemistry, and of those branches of allied physical science, the applications of which are involved in the highest qualifications required for the practice of Pharmacy. There will be two of these courses during the session—the course which commences in October and ends in February being repeated in the following five months. Each course will be complete in itself, and will include a description of all the most important chemical and Galenical preparations used in medicine, which will be fully illustrated with experiments, diagrams, and specimens.

Lectures on Botany and Materia Medica by Professor Bentley, on Thursday, Friday, and Saturday mornings at nine o'clock, commencing Friday, October 7. During the session two courses of lectures will be delivered, each consisting of sixty lectures. The first course, extending from October to the end of February, will comprise Botany and Materia Medica, with especial reference to Structural Botany, and the use of the microscope in distinguishing the various drugs; and the second course, which commences in March and extends to the end of July, will also comprise Botany and Materia Medica, with especial reference to Systematic and Practical Botany. Each course will be complete in itself,

although each will have a definite object in view. The portion of the second course on Systematic and Practical Botany, consisting of twenty lectures, commences in May and ends in July. Separate entries may be made for this portion.

The Laboratories for the study of Practical Chemistry will be opened on Monday, October 3, at 10 a.m., under the direction of Professor Attfield. The Laboratories are fitted up with every convenience for the study of the principles of Chemistry by personal experiment. They are specially designed for the study of Pharmacy, but are also well adapted for the acquirement of a knowledge of Chemistry in its application to manufactures, analysis, and original research. There is no general class for simultaneous instruction, each student following an independent course of study always determined by his previous knowledge; pupils can therefore enter for any period at any date. A complete course of instruction, including the higher branches of Quantitative Analysis, occupies ten full months, and dates from the day of entry to that day twelvemonth. The Laboratories are open from ten o'clock in the morning until five in the afternoon daily, except on Saturdays, when they are closed at two o'clock. Vacation months, August and September.

Prospectuses and further particulars may be had of the Professors or their assistants, 17, Bloomsbury-square, W.C.

EDUCATIONAL VACCINATING STATIONS.

IN order to provide for the granting of those special certificates of proficiency in vaccination which are required to be part of the medical qualification for entering into contracts for the performance of Public Vaccination, or for acting as deputy to a contractor, the following arrangements are made:—

1. The Vaccinating Stations enumerated in the subjoined list are open, under certain specific conditions, for the purposes of teaching and examination.

2. The Public Vaccinators officiating at these stations are authorised to give the required certificate of proficiency in vaccination to persons whom they have sufficiently instructed therein; and

3. The Public Vaccinators whose names in the subjoined list are printed in italic letters are also authorised to give such certificates, after satisfactory examination, to persons whom they have not themselves instructed:—

LONDON.—Principal Station—Victoria Hall, Lancaster-street, Friar-street, Blackfriars-road : *Dr. Robert Cory*, who attends on Tuesday and Thursday, at 1 p.m. North-west Stations—Marylebone General Dispensary, 77, Welbeck-street : Mr. William A. Sumner, on Tuesday, at 2 p.m.; Hall of the Working-Men's Christian Association, Omega-place, Alpha-road : Mr. William A. Sumner, on Wednesday, at 10 a.m. West Station—9, St. George's-road, Pimlico, S.W. : Mr. Edward Lowe Webb, on Thursday, at 10 a.m. East Station—Eastern Dispensary, Leman-street : Mr. Charles T. Blackman, on Wednesday, at 11 a.m. North Station—Tottenham-court Chapel, Tottenham-court-road : Mr. William Edwin Grindley Pearse, on Monday and Wednesday, at 1 p.m. South-west Station—2, Regent-place, Horseferry-road : Mr. William Edwin Grindley Pearse, on Tuesday, at 2 p.m. Strand Station—14, Russell-street, Covent-garden : Mr. Robert William Dunn, on Thursday, at 11 a.m. South-east Station—Vestry Hall, St. John's, Horselydown : Mr. John Gittins, on Monday, at 2 p.m. St. Thomas's Hospital : Dr. Robert Cory, on Wednesday, at 11.30 a.m.

BIRMINGHAM.—At the School-room, 27, Old Meeting-street, Worcester-street, on Monday, at 11 a.m.; the Assembly Rooms, 103, Constitution-hill, opposite Bond-street, on Tuesday, at 11 a.m.; the Wesleyan Methodist Infant School-room, Monument-road, on Wednesday, at 11 a.m.; the Wesleyan School-room, Peel-street, Winson-green-road, on Wednesday, at 2 p.m.; and "The British Workman" Reading Rooms, Sherborne-street, near Grosvenor-street, on Thursday, at 11 a.m. : *Dr. Edmund Robinson.*

BRISTOL.—The Public Vaccination Station, Peter-street : *Mr. Henry Lawrence*, on Wednesday, at 10 a.m.

EXETER.—Odd Fellows' Hall, Bamfyld-street : *Mr. Charles H. Roper*, on Thursday, at 3 p.m.

LEEDS.—Reed-street : *Mr. Frederick Holmes*, on Tuesday, at 2.30 p.m.

LIVERPOOL.—St. Mary's School-room, Edgehill, West Derby : *Mr. Roper Parker*, on Thursday, at 2.30 p.m.

MANCHESTER.—72, Rochdale-road : *Mr. Ellis Southern Guest*, on Monday, at 3 p.m.

NEWCASTLE-UPON-TYNE.—The Central Vaccination Station, 21, Nun-street : *Mr. John Hawthorn*, on Wednesday, at 3 p.m.

SHEFFIELD.—The Public Vaccination Station, Townshend-street : *Mr. William Skinner*, on Tuesday, at 8 p.m.

EDINBURGH.—The Royal Dispensary : *Dr. William Husband*, on Wednesday and Saturday, at 12. The New Town Dispensary : Dr. James O. Affleck, on Wednesday and Saturday, at 1.

GLASGOW.—The Hall of the Faculty of Physicians and Surgeons : *Dr. Hugh Thomson*, on Monday, at 12. The Royal Infirmary : Dr. Robert Dunlop Tannahill, on Monday and Thursday, at 12. The Western Infirmary : Dr. David Caldwell McVail, on Monday, at 1 p.m.

Candidates for the Certificate by Examination are recommended to communicate some days beforehand with the Examiner at whose station they propose to attend.

The Association for the Supply of Pure Vaccine Lymph, which are the sole agents for Dr. Warlomont's calf vaccine, have their Depôt at 5, Hemming's-row, Charing-cross, London, W.C. Mr. Edward Darke is Secretary.

SPECIAL INSTRUCTION.

SCHOOLS AND OTHER PLACES OF GENERAL AND SPECIAL INSTRUCTION.

BESIDES the regular Schools with their various departments, there are many other institutions—devoted, some of them, to special purposes—where students and practitioners may acquire a sound knowledge of various subjects which hardly enter into the ordinary curriculum. We have already indicated that in the plan of studies the student may avail himself of a year at the beginning or at the end for such purposes. If at the beginning, we could not do better than advise him to take a session at the Royal School of Mines (now the Natural Science Department at South Kensington), studying especially Chemistry and Natural History, the value of which we have already indicated. If he takes the year at the end, then such special studies as Eye Diseases, Skin Diseases, Lunacy, Diseases of Women and Children, may well engage his attention. These may, as a rule, be studied in connexion with his school ; or, if a wider field is desired, in some one or other of the following institutions :—

Preliminary.

ROYAL SCHOOL OF MINES.(a)
Department of Science and Art.

During the thirty-first session, 1881-82, which will commence on October 3, the following courses of lectures and practical demonstrations will be given :—

Applied Mechanics—Mr. Goodeve.	Metallurgy — Mr. W. Chandler
Chemistry—Dr. E. Frankland.	Roberts.
Geology—Mr. John W. Judd.	Biology—Professor T. H. Huxley.
Mining—Mr. W. W. Smyth.	Physics—Dr. Frederick Guthrie.

The lecture fees for students desirous of becoming Associates are £30 in one sum, on entrance, or two annual payments of £20, exclusive of the laboratories. Tickets to separate courses of lectures are issued at £3 and £4 each. Officers in the Queen's service, her Majesty's Consuls, Acting Mining Agents and Managers, may obtain tickets at reduced prices. Science teachers are also admitted to the lectures at reduced fees. For a prospectus and information apply to the Secretary, Natural Science Department, South Kensington, S.W.

SOUTH LONDON SCHOOL OF CHEMISTRY AND PHARMACY,(a)
325, Kennington-road, and Central Public Laboratory, Kennington-cross, S.E.—Director—Dr. Muter.

THIRTEENTH SESSION—1881-82.

Daily lectures in Classics, Chemistry, Physics, Botany, Materia Medica, and Pharmacy. Laboratory open for Practical Chemistry from ten till five. Special instruction for Medical Officers of Health in Water, Air, Gas, and Food Analysis. For fees, etc., apply to W. Baxter, Secretary, Laboratory, Kennington-cross, S.E.

LONDON SCHOOL OF MEDICINE FOR WOMEN,
30, Henrietta-street, Brunswick-square, W.C.

LECTURERS.

Anatomy — Mr. Ottley, University College, and Mr. Albert Leahy, Charing-cross Hospital.	Hygiene—Drs. Sophia Jex Blake and Edith Pechey.
Physiology—Mr. Schäfer, F.R.S., University College.	Surgery—Mr. A. T. Norton, St. Mary's Hospital.
Chemistry—Mr. Heaton, Charing-cross Hospital.	Clinical Surgery—Mr. F. J. Gant, Royal Free Hospital, and Mr. W. Rose, Royal Free Hospital.
Botany—Dr. P. H. Stokoe.	Ophthalmic Surgery—Mr. Critchett, Middlesex Hospital, and Mr. Jas. Adams, Royal Ophthalmic Hospital.
Materia Medica—Dr. T. J. Maclagan.	
Practice of Medicine—Dr. H. Donkin, Westminster Hospital, and Mrs. Garrett-Anderson, M.D.	
Midwifery and Diseases of Women —Dr. Ford Anderson and Dr. Louisa Atkins.	Minor Surgery—Mr. James Shuter, M.B., Royal Free Hospital.
Forensic Medicine — Dr. Dupré, F.R.S., Westminster Hospital, and Mr. T. Bond, Westminster Hospital.	Tutorial Class for Auscultation and Percussion—Dr. Samuel West, Royal Free Hospital.
Clinical Medicine—Dr. Cockle, Royal Free Hospital, and Dr. Allen Sturge, Royal Free Hospital.	Pathology—Dr. Allen Sturge, Royal Free Hospital.
	Mental Pathology — Dr. Sankey, University College.
	Comparative Anatomy—Dr. Murie, Middlesex Hospital.

Dean of the School—Mr. A. T. Norton, St. Mary's Hospital.

The Winter Session of 1881-82 will commence on October 3, and will comprise classes in Anatomy, Physiology, Chemistry, Practice of Medicine, Midwifery and Diseases of Women, and Practical Anatomy with Demonstrations. Clinical Instruction will be given at the Royal Free Hospital, and will include lectures on Clinical Medicine, Clinical Surgery, Hospital attendance, and Pathological Demonstrations. Separate cliniques are held for the treatment of the Diseases of Women under Dr. W. Hayes, and for Ophthalmic Surgery under Mr. Grosvenor Mackinlay. Dressers, Clinical Clerks, and a Pathological Registrar will be selected from among the senior students. An Entrance Scholarship, value £30, is competed for annually.

Fees for ordinary curriculum of non-clinical lectures £80, or £40 the first year, £30 the second, and £15 the third. Fees for clinical instruction and lectures for four years £45, or £20 the first year, £15 the second year, and £15 the third, the fourth being free. Apply for information to the Dean, or to the Hon. Sec., Mrs. Thorne.

(a) No return.

LONDON.

General Hospitals.

GREAT NORTHERN HOSPITAL,
Caledonian-road.

Consulting Surgeon—Mr. F. Le Gros Clark, F.R.S.
Physicians—Dr. Cholmeley, Dr. R. Bridges, Dr. Cook, Dr. Burnet, Dr. Clifford Beale.
Obstetric Physician—Dr. Gustavus C. P. Murray.
Diseases of the Eye—Mr. W. H. Lyell.
Surgeons—Mr. Gay, Mr. W. Adams, Mr. W. Spencer Watson, Mr. W. H. Cripps, Mr. J. Macready.
Aural Surgeon—Mr. A. E. Cumberbatch.
Dental Surgeon—Mr. E. Keen.
Chloroformist—Mr. G. Easten.　House-Surgeon—Mr. A. Wharry.
Junior Resident Medical Officer—Mr. N. S. Webber.
Dispenser—Mr. J. W. Burgess.

SEAMEN'S HOSPITAL (late Dreadnought), GREENWICH, S.E.
Consulting Physician—Dr. George Budd, F.R.S.
Visiting Physicians—Drs. John Curnow, F.R.C.P., and R. E. Carrington.
Visiting Surgeon—Mr. G. Robertson Tanner, F.R.C.S.
Medical Officer, Well-street Dispensary—Mr. G. H. Makins, F.R.C.S.
Principal Medical Officer—Mr. W. Johnson Smith, F.R.C.S.
Secretary—Mr. W. Thomas Evans.

Special Hospitals.

CITY OF LONDON HOSPITAL FOR DISEASES OF THE CHEST,
Victoria-park.

Honorary Consulting Physician—Sir J. Risdon Bennett, M.D., F.R.S.
Consulting Physicians—Dr. T. B. Peacock, Dr. E. L. Birkett, and Dr. J. Andrew.
Consulting Surgeon—Mr. John Eric Erichsen.
Physicians—Dr. J. C. Thorowgood, Dr. A. B. Shepherd, Dr. Eustace Smith, Dr. J. B. Berkart.
Assistant-Physicians—Dr. J. H. Fothergill, Dr. Samuel West, Dr. G. A. Heron, Dr. V. D. Harris, Dr. J. A. Ormerod, and Dr. B. Clifford Beale.
Resident Medical Officer—Dr. Laurence Humphry.

HOSPITAL FOR CONSUMPTION AND DISEASES OF THE CHEST,
BROMPTON. (Number of beds, 192.)

Consulting Physicians—Dr. C. J. B. Williams, Dr. W. H. Walshe, and Dr. Richard Quain.
Consulting Surgeon—Prof. John Marshall.
Physicians—Dr. Jas. E. Pollock, Dr. B. Symes Thompson, Dr. C. Theodore Williams, Dr. R. Douglas Powell, Dr. John Tatham, and Dr. Reginald E. Thompson.
Assistant-Physicians—Dr. T. H. Green, Dr. J. Mitchell Bruce, Dr. William Ewart, Dr. J. Kingston Fowler, Dr. Percy Kidd, and Dr. Cecil Y. Biss.
Pathologist—Dr. William Ewart.
Dental Surgeon—Mr. Charles J. Noble.
Resident Medical Officer—Mr. Frederick J. Hicks, M.B., M.A., F.C.S.
Honorary Secretary—Sir Philip Rose, Bart.
Secretary—Mr. Henry Dobbin.

The clinical practice of this Hospital is open to students of Medicine and practitioners. Fee for three months, £3 3s. ; six months, £5 5s. ; perpetual, £10 10s.
A course of clinical instruction in Auscultation will be given by the medical officers.
Certificates of attendance on the medical practice of this Hospital are recognised by the University of London, the Apothecaries' Society, and by the Army, Navy, and Indian Boards.

THE HOSPITAL FOR SICK CHILDREN,
48 and 49, Great Ormond-street, W.C., and Cromwell House, Highgate.

Physicians—Dr. Dickinson, Dr. Gee, and Dr. W. B. Cheadle.	Surgeons—Mr. Thomas Smith and Mr. Howard Marsh.
Assistant-Physicians — Dr. S. J. Lee, Dr. O. Sturges, Dr. Thomas Barlow, Dr. D. B. Lees, Dr. Bridges.	Assistant-Surgeons — Mr. Edmund Owen and Mr. J. H. Morgan.
	Surgeon-Dentist—Mr. Alex. Cartwright.

Secretary—Samuel Whitford.

120 beds. In-patients, 1880, 1047. Out-patients attending, 14,512. The practice of the Hospital, in both in- and out-patient departments, is open at nine every morning.

BELGRAVE HOSPITAL FOR CHILDREN,
79, Gloucester-street, Warwick-square, S.W.

HONORARY MEDICAL STAFF.

Physicians—Dr. W. Hope and Dr. W. Ewart.
Surgeons—Mr. W. Bennett and Mr. C. Dent.
House-Surgeon—Mr. H. P. Dunn.

EAST LONDON HOSPITAL FOR CHILDREN AND DISPENSARY FOR WOMEN,
Shadwell, E.

Consulting Physicians—Dr. Barnes and Dr. Andrew Clark.	Consulting Ophthalmic Surgeon—Mr. George Cowell.
Physicians—Dr. Eustace Smith and Dr. Horatio B. Donkin.	Surgeons—Mr. A. Cæsar and Mr. H. A. Reeves.
Assistant-Physicians—Dr. Warner and Dr. Crocker.	Assistant-Surgeon — Mr. R. W. Parker.
Administrator of Anæsthetics—Mr. Thomas Bird.	House-Surgeon — Mr. J. Scott Battams.
Consulting Surgeon—Mr. B. Shillitoe.	

Secretary—Ashton Warner.

EVELINA HOSPITAL FOR SICK CHILDREN,
Southwark-bridge-road.
Consulting Physician—Dr. W. S. Playfair.
Consulting Surgeon—Mr. Prescott G. Hewett.

Physicians — Dr. E. Buchanan Baxter and Dr. Fredk. Taylor.
Physicians to Out-Patients — Dr. N. I. C. Tirard and Dr. Jas. Goodhart.
Surgeons—Mr. W. Morrant Baker and Mr. H. G. Howse.
Surgeon to Out-Patients—Mr. R. Clement Lucas.
Ophthalmic Surgeon—Dr. W. A. Brailey.
Dental Surgeon—Mr. Isidore Lyons.
House-Surgeon — Dr. W. Hale White.

Secretary—Mr. Thos. Sands Chapman.

VICTORIA HOSPITAL FOR CHILDREN,
Queen's-road, Chelsea ; and Churchfields, Margate.

Physicians—Dr. Julian Evans and Dr. T. Ridge Jones.
Physicians to Out-Patients — Dr. Grigg, Dr. W. H. Allchin, Dr. A. Venn, Dr. T. Colcott Fox.
Surgeon to Out-Patients—Mr. F. Churchill.
Surgeon—Mr. George Cowell.
Assistant-Surgeon—Mr. Walter Pye.
Dental-Surgeon—Mr. Risdon.
Assistant Dental Surgeon — Mr. Francis Fox.
Registrar—Mr. Dawson Williams.
House-Surgeon—Mr. W. C. Chaffey.

Secretary—Captain Blount, R.N.

THE ROYAL HOSPITAL FOR CHILDREN AND WOMEN,
Waterloo-bridge-road.
Consulting Physicians—Dr. Samuel Wilks and Dr. John Williams.
Consulting Surgeon—Mr. J. Cooper Forster.

Physicians—Dr. William Park, Dr. George Roper, and Dr. Edwin Burrell.
Surgeon—Mr. Edwin Canton.
Surgeon-Dentist—Mr. Walter Whitehouse.
Resident Medical Officer — Mr. Edmund Overman Day.

Secretary—Mr. R. G. Keatin.

HOSPITAL FOR WOMEN,
Soho-square, W.
Physicians—Dr. Protheroe Smith, Dr. Heywood Smith, Dr. Carter.
Surgeon—Mr. Henry A. Reeves.
Assistant-Physicians—Dr. R. T. Smith, Dr. Holland, Dr. Mansell-Moullin.
Surgeon-Dentist—Mr. Frederic Canton.
Administrator of Anæsthetics—Mr. Thomas Bird.
Pathologist and Curator of Museum—Dr. H. S. Gabbett.
Secretary—David Cannon.

QUEEN CHARLOTTE'S LYING-IN HOSPITAL,
191, Marylebone-road, London, N.W.
Physicians to the In-patients—Dr. Wm. Hope and Dr. W. C. Grigg.
Physician to the Out-patients—Dr. Percy Boulton.
House-Physician—Mr. Norman Dalton.

BRITISH LYING-IN HOSPITAL,
Endell-street, St. Giles's, W.C.
Consulting Physician—Dr. Priestley.
Consulting Surgeon—T. Spencer Wells, F.R.C.S.
Physicians—Dr. Heywood Smith and Dr. Fancourt Barnes.
Matron—Miss Freeman.
Secretary—FitzRoy Gardner, Esq.

LONDON FEVER HOSPITAL, ISLINGTON.
Consulting Physicians—Dr. A. Tweedie, Dr. Broadbent, and Dr. G. Buchanan.
Consulting Surgeon—Mr. W. S. Savory, F.R.C.S.
Physicians — Dr. Cayley and Dr. F. A. Mahomed.
Resident Medical Officer—Dr. W. Tonge Smith.
Secretary—Mr. Charles Finn.

ROYAL WESTMINSTER OPHTHALMIC HOSPITAL,
King William-street, Charing-cross.
The Hospital contains thirteen wards with fifty beds, and the patients (10,000 new cases annually) are seen daily at 1 p.m., and operations performed at 3 p.m. The following are the days of attendance of the Surgical Staff :—Monday and Friday, Mr. Power ; Monday and Thursday, Mr. Macnamara ; Tuesday and Saturday, Mr. Bouse ; Wednesday and Saturday, Mr. Cowell. Assistant-Surgeons: Monday, Wednesday, and Friday, Mr. Henry Juler ; Tuesday and Thursday, Mr. Hayward Whitehead. The practice of the Hospital is open to students. Fees—for six months, £3 3s. ; perpetual, £5 5s.
Secretary—Mr. Geo. C. Farrant.

ROYAL LONDON OPHTHALMIC HOSPITAL,
Bloomfield-street, Moorfields, E.C.
Consulting Surgeons—Mr. J Dixon, Mr. G. Critchett, Mr. W. Bowman, and Mr. J. Hutchinson.
Surgeons—Messrs. Wordsworth, Streatfeild, J. W. Hulke, G. Lawson, J. Couper, Waren Tay, J Adams, J. Tweedy, and R. Lyell.
House-Surgeons—Messrs. W. A. Milles and W. A. Fitzgerald.

ST. PETER'S HOSPITAL FOR STONE AND GENITO-URINARY DISEASES,(a)
54, Berners-street, W.
Surgeons—Mr. Walter J. Coulson and Mr. W. F. Teevan.
Assistant-Surgeon—Mr. F. R. Heycock.
House Surgeon—Mr. J. Whitehouse.
Secretary—R. G. Salmond.

(a) No return.

CENTRAL LONDON THROAT AND EAR HOSPITAL,
Gray's-inn-road, W.C.
Consulting Surgeon—Mr. Sydney Jones, F.R.C.S.
Surgeons—Mr. Lennox Browne, Dr. Llewellyn Thomas.
Assistant-Surgeons—Mr. G. R. Stell, Mr. Francis G. Hamilton, Mr. Arthur Orwin.
Defects of Speech—Mr. William Van Praagh.
Dental Surgeon—Mr. George Wallis.
Chloroformist—Dr. James Murray.
Registrar and Pathologist—Dr. J. Dundas Grant.
Secretary—Mr. Richard Kershaw.

HOSPITAL FOR DISEASES OF THE THROAT AND CHEST,(a)
Golden-street, W.
Consulting Physician—Dr. Billing, M.D.
Outpost—7, Newington-butts, S.E.
Physicians—Dr. Morell-Mackenzie, Dr Semple, Dr. Prosser James.
Dr. W. MacNeill Whistler, and Dr. F. Semon.
Surgeons—Mr. Edward Woakes and Mr. W. R. H. Stewart.
Dental Surgeon—Mr Oakley Coles.
Resident Medical Officer—Mr. T. Mark Hovell.

HOSPITAL FOR DISEASES OF THE SKIN,
51, Stamford-street, Blackfriars, S.E.
Surgeons—Mr. Jonathan Hutchinson and Mr. Waren Tay.
Assistant-Surgeons—Mr. Wyndham Cottle and Dr. E. Buchanan Baxter.
Secretary—F. G. Reynolds.

BRITISH HOSPITAL FOR DISEASES OF THE SKIN,(a)
West Branch, Great Marlborough-street, W. ; East Branch, Finsbury-square, E.C. ; and South Branch, Newington-butts, S.E.
Surgeons—Mr. Balmanno Squire and Mr. George Gaskoin.
Secretary—Mr. F. G. Reynolds.

ST. LUKE'S HOSPITAL FOR LUNATICS,(a)
Old-street, E.C.
Physicians—Dr. Henry Monro and Dr. William Wood.
Surgeon—Mr. Alfred Willett.
Resident Medical Superintendent—Dr. George Mickley.

NATIONAL HOSPITAL FOR THE PARALYSED AND EPILEPTIC,
23, 24, and 25, Queen-square, Bloomsbury.
Physicians—Drs. Ramskill, Radcliffe, Hughlings-Jackson, Buzzard.
Physicians for Out-patients—Drs. Charlton Bastian, Gowers, Ferrier.
Assistant-Physicians—Drs. Ormerod and Horrocks.
Surgeon—W. Adams, F.R.C.S.
Resident Medical Officer and Registrar—C. E. Beevor, M.B. Lond.

PROVINCIAL.

NORFOLK AND NORWICH HOSPITAL.
Physicians—Dr. Eade, Dr. Bateman, and Dr. Taylor.
Surgeons—Mr. Cadge, Mr. Crosse, and Mr. Williams.
Assistant-Surgeons—Dr. Beverley and Mr. Robinson.
Resident Medical Officer—Mr. D. D. Day.

[GENERAL INFIRMARY, NORTHAMPTON.
Physician—Dr. Buzzard.
Surgeons—Mr. Kirby Smith and Mr. G. H. Percival.
House-Surgeons—Vacant.
Resident Medical Officer—Mr. E. J. Morley.

WOLVERHAMPTON AND STAFFORDSHIRE GENERAL HOSPITAL,(a)
Medical Officers—Dr. Millington, Dr. Totherick, Dr. Joseph Hunt, Mr. Vincent Jackson, Mr. J. O'B. Kough, Mr. F. Manby.
Fees for hospital practice—For one year, £10 10s. ; perpetual, £21. Some members of the honorary staff receive resident pupils. For further particulars apply to Dr. Joseph Hunt (Honorary Secretary to the Medical Committee), Darlington-street, Wolverhampton.

THE ROYAL DISPENSARY, EDINBURGH.(a)
Consulting Physician—Professor Sanders.
Consulting Surgeon—Professor Spence.
Consulting Physician-Accoucheurs—Dr. Keiller and Dr. Bell.
Medical Officers—Dr. Linton, Dr. W. Husband, Dr. James Andrew, Dr. D. Wilson, Dr. F. W. Moinet, Dr. A. J. Sinclair, Dr. Cotterill, Dr. Waller, and Dr. Jamieson.
Midwifery Department—Dr. Andrew.
Vaccination—Dr. Husband.
Apothecary—Mr. J. Nicol.
Secretary to Medical Officers—Dr. Andrew.

GLASGOW HOSPITAL AND DISPENSARY FOR DISEASES OF THE EAR,
239 and 241, Buchanan-street.
HONORARY MEDICAL STAFF.
Senior Consulting Physician—Dr. P. Stewart.
Senior Consulting Surgeon—Dr. James Morton.
Consulting Dental Surgeon—Dr. J. Edwin Woodburn.
Consulting Surgeon for Throat Diseases—Dr. David Foulis.
Dr. A. K. Irwine, Dr. A. L. Kelly, Dr. J. Gardiner.
Aural Surgeon and Lecturer on Aural Surgery—Dr. James P. Cassells.
Clinical Assistants—Messrs. Robertson and Violette.

(a) No return.

EDINBURGH DISPENSARY FOR DISEASES OF THE EAR,
6, Cambridge-street, Lothian-road.
Surgeon—Dr. J. J. Kirk Duncan son.
Annual patients, 500.　Open Mondays and Thursdays, 12 noon.

GLASGOW EYE INFIRMARY,
170, Berkeley-street, and 75, Charlotte-street.
Consulting Surgeon—Dr. George Buchanan.
Surgeons—Drs. Thomas Reid, Thos. S. Meighan, and Henry E. Clark.
Assistant-Surgeons—Drs. J. Crawford Renton, D. N. Knox, and
Johnston Macfie.
Resident Surgeon—George Hunter.
Secretary—George Black, 88, West Regent-street.

ROTUNDA HOSPITALS, DUBLIN.(a)
Master—Dr. Lombe Atthill.
Assistant-Physicians—Dr. Alex. Duke and Dr. Andrew Horne.
Pathologist—Dr. G. F. Duffey.

ST. MARK'S OPHTHALMIC HOSPITAL AND DISPENSARY FOR
DISEASES OF THE EYE AND EAR,
Lincoln-place, Dublin.
Attending Surgeons—John B. Story, M.B., M.Ch., F.R.C.S.I., and
Arthur H. Benson, M.B.T.C.D., F.R.C.S.I.
Resident Surgeon—Stewart Davis, M.B., B.Ch., T.C.D.

THE PUBLIC SERVICES.

ARMY MEDICAL DEPARTMENT.

No candidate to exceed the age of twenty-eight years on
appointment as a Surgeon on probation.

He must be registered under the Medical Act in force at
the time of his appointment, as possessing two diplomas or
licences recognised by the General Medical Council—one to
practise Medicine, and the other Surgery—in Great Britain
and Ireland.

Candidates will be examined by the Examining Board in
Anatomy and Physiology; Surgery; Medicine, including
therapeutics, and the diseases of women and children; Chemistry and Pharmacy, and a practical knowledge of drugs.

The ranks and rates of pay of Officers will be as follows :—

		£	s.	d.
Surgeon-General	daily	2	15	0
After 25 years' service	,,	—		
,, 30 years' service	,,	—		
,, 35 years' service	,,	—		
At Head-quarters	yearly	1,300	0	0
Deputy Surgeon-general	daily	2	0	0
After 25 years' service	,,	—		
,, 30 years' service	,,	—		
,, 35 years' service	,,	—		
At Head-quarters	yearly	900	0	0
Brigade Surgeon	daily	1	10	0
After 5 years in the rank	,,	1	13	0
At Head-quarters	yearly	750	0	0
Surgeon-Major	daily	1	0	0
After 15 years' service	,,	1	2	6
,, 5 years' service as such	,,	—		
,, 20 years' service	,,	1	5	0
,, 25 years' service	,,	1	7	6
At Head-quarters	yearly	650	0	0
Surgeon	,,	200	0	0
After 5 years' service	,,	250	0	0
,, 10 years' service	daily	0	15	0
Surgeon on probation	,,	0	8	0

The rates of gratuity, retired pay, or half-pay, for Medical
Officers of the Army will be as follows :—

		£	s.	d.
Surgeon and Surgeon-Major :				
After 10 years' service	gratuity	1,250	0	0
,, 15 years' service	,,	1,800	0	0
,, 18 years' service	,,	2,500	0	0
Surgeon-Major :				
After 12 years' service	daily	—		
,, 15 years' service	,,	—		
,, 20 years' service	,,	1	0	0
,, 25 years' service	,,	1	2	6
,, 30 years' service	,,	1	5	0
Brigade-Surgeon :				
After 20 years' service	,,	1	7	6
,, 30 years' service	,,	1	10	0

(a) No return.

		£	s.	d.
Deputy Surgeon-General	daily	1	15	0
After 20 years' service	,,	—		
,, 25 years' service	,,	—		
,, 30 years' service	,,	—		
Surgeon-General	,,	2	0	0
After 20 years' service	,,	—		
,, 25 years' service	,,	—		
,, 30 years' service	,,	—		
Temporary Half-pay:				
A Medical Officer, under 5 years' service	,,	£0	6	0
,, ,, after 5 years' service	,,	0	8	0
,, ,, 10 years' service	,,	0	10	0
,, ,, 15 years' service	,,	0	13	6

Candidates for commissions in the Army proceed to the
Army Medical School at Netley to go through a course of
study after passing the examination in London.

INDIAN MEDICAL DEPARTMENT.

The rules for admission to the above department are
identical with those for the Army Medical Department. The
rates of pay are as follows :—

	Years' service	Per mensem.		
		R.	A.	P.
Brigade-Surgeon		(not yet fixed.)		
Surgeon-Major	25	888	12	0
,, ,,	20	852	3	7
,, ,,	15	677	6	11
,, ,,	12	640	14	6
Surgeon	10	410	9	5
,, ,,	6	392	5	2
,, ,,	5	304	14	2
,, ,,	under 5	286	10	0

The salaries of the principal administrative and military
appointments are :—

		Rs. per mensem.
Surgeon-General, Bengal		2700
,, ,, Madras		2500
,, ,, Bombay		2500
Deputy Surgeon-General { two at		2250
{ others at		1800
Brigade-Surgeon		(not yet fixed.)
Surgeon-Major of 20 years' service and upwards in charge of Native Regiments		1000
Surgeon-Major in charge of ditto		800
Surgeon above 5 years' full-pay service in charge of ditto		600
Surgeon under 5 years' ditto		450

Candidates for commissions in the Indian Medical Service
proceed to the Medical School at Netley to go through a
course of study after passing the examination in London.

The following are the regulations for the examination of
candidates for the appointment of Surgeon in Her Majesty's
Service, in the Indian Medical Service (with the exception of
Hindustani), and in the Navy :—

All natural-born subjects of Her Majesty, between twenty-
two and twenty-eight years of age at the date of the examination, and of sound bodily health, may be candidates. They
may be married or unmarried. They must possess a diploma
in Surgery, or a licence to practise it, as well as a degree in
Medicine, or a licence to practise it, in Great Britain or Ireland,
as well as a certificate of registration.

Candidates are examined in the following compulsory subjects, and the highest number of marks attainable will be
distributed as follows :—a. Anatomy and Physiology, 1000
marks ; b. Surgery, 1000 ; c. Medicine, including Therapeutics,
the Diseases of Women and Children, 1000 ; d. Chemistry and
Pharmacy, and a practical knowledge of drugs, 100 marks.
(The examination in Medicine and Surgery will be in part
practical, and will include operations on the dead body, the
application of surgical apparatus, and the examination of
medical and surgical patients at the bedside.)

The eligibility of each candidate for the Indian Medical
Service will be determined by the result of the examinations
in these subjects only.

Candidates, who desire it, will be examined in French,
German, and Hindustani, Comparative Anatomy, Zoology,
Natural Philosophy, Physical Geography, and Botany, with
special reference to Materia Medica.

The number of marks gained in these subjects will be added to the total number of marks obtained in the obligatory part of the examination by candidates who shall have been found qualified for admission, and whose position on the list of successful competitors will thus be improved in proportion to their knowledge of modern languages and natural sciences.

The maximum number of marks allotted to the voluntary subjects will be as follows:—French, German, and Hindustani (150 each), 450; Natural Science, 300.

After passing the preliminary examination, candidates will be required to attend one entire course of practical instruction at the Army Medical School, before being admitted to examination for a commission, on—(1) Hygiene, (2) Clinical and Military Medicine, (3) Clinical and Military Surgery, (4) Pathology of Diseases and Injuries incident to Military Service.

(These courses are to be of not less than four months' duration; but candidates who have already gone through a course at Netley as candidates for the Army or Navy Medical Service may, if thought desirable, be exempted from attending the school a second time.)

During the period of his residence at the Army Medical School, each candidate will receive an allowance of 8s. per diem, with quarters, or, when quarters are not provided, with the usual lodging and fuel and light allowances of subalterns, to cover all costs of maintenance; and he will be required to provide himself with uniform—viz., the regulation undress uniform of a Surgeon of the British Service, but without the sword.

At the conclusion of the course, candidates will be required to pass an examination on the subjects taught in the School. The examination will be conducted by the Professors of the School.

(The Director-General, or any medical officer deputed by him, may be present and take part in the examination. If the candidate give satisfactory evidence of being qualified for the practical duties of an Army Medical Officer, he will be eligible for a commission as Surgeon.)

The examinations for admission to the Indian Medical Service usually take place twice a year, viz., in February and in August.

ARMY MEDICAL SCHOOL.

President of the Senate.—Sir William M. Muir, K.C.B., M.D., Director-General of the Army Medical Department.

Members of the Senate.—Surgeon-General Sir Joseph Fayrer, M.D., K.C.S.I., F.R.S., Physician to the Council of India; the Principal Medical Officer, Royal Victoria Hospital (*ex officio*); and the Professors of the Army Medical School.

Professors.—Surgeon-General T. Longmore, C.B. (half-pay), Professor of Military Surgery; Inspector-General W. C. Maclean, M.D., C.B., Professor of Military Medicine; William Aitken, M.D., F.R.S., Professor of Pathology; Surgeon-Major F. S. B. F. De Chaumont, M.D., F.R.S. (half-pay), Professor of Military Hygiene.

Assistant-Professors.—Surgeons-Major R. Tobin (Military Surgery), H. E. L. Veale, M.D. (Military Medicine); Surgeon-Major J. L. Notter, M.D. (Military Hygiene); and Surgeon-Major J. P. H. Boileau, M.D. (Pathology).

Surgeons on probation for the British Army and medical candidates for commissions in the Queen's Indian Service proceed to Netley after passing the examination in London. At Netley they attend the medical and surgical practice of the Royal Victoria Hospital, and learn the system and arrangements of military hospitals. During four months they attend the lectures given by the Professors and Assistant-Professors, and go through a course of practical instruction in the hygienic laboratory and microscopical room.

NAVAL MEDICAL DEPARTMENT.

The rules for admission to this branch of the public service are, as nearly as possible, identical with those laid down for the Army, but the rates of full pay and half-pay are about 7 per cent. higher, retired pay being calculated on the Army scale.

Candidates for commissions in the Navy proceed to Haslar Hospital to go through a course of study after passing the examination in London.

The foregoing is a brief summary of the main points to be considered by students in choosing a career in the public services. All details and information are procurable on application (by letter) to the Secretaries of the different departments.

THE INTRODUCTORIES.

The following are the days and hours of the various Introductory Lectures, with the names of the respective lecturers:—

Hospital.	Date.	Lecturer.	Hour.
St. George's	Mon. Oct. 3.	Mr. J. W. Haward	4 p.m.
King's College	„	Sir John Lubbock	4 p.m.
Middlesex	„	Dr. Douglas Powell	—
St. Mary's	„	Mr. G. P. Field	—
St. Thomas's	Sat. Oct. 1.	Dr. Bernays	3 p.m.
University College	Mon. Oct. 3.	Dr. G. V. Poore	3 p.m.
Westminster	„	Mr. Bond	3 p.m.

TERMS OF SUBSCRIPTION.
(*Free by post.*)

British Islands	. . . . .	Twelve Months	.	£1 8 0
„ „	. . . . .	Six „		0 14 0
The Colonies and the United }		Twelve „		1 10 0
States of America }				
„ „ „	. . .	Six „		0 15 0
India	. . . . .	Twelve „		1 10 0
„ (viâ Brindisi)	. . .	„		1 15 0
„ „	. . . . .	Six „		0 15 0
„ (viâ Brindisi)	. . .	„		0 17 6

Foreign Subscribers are requested to inform the Publishers of any remittance made through the agency of the Post-office.

Single Copies of the Journal can be obtained of all Booksellers and Newsmen, price Sixpence.

Cheques or Post-office Orders should be made payable to Mr. James Lucas, 11, New Burlington-street, W.

TERMS FOR ADVERTISEMENTS.

Seven lines (70 words)	. . .	.	£0 4 6
Each additional line (10 words)	.	.	0 0 6
Half-column, or quarter-page	.	.	1 5 0
Whole column, or half-page	.	.	2 10 0
Whole page	. . .	.	5 0 0

Births, Marriages, and Deaths are inserted Free of Charge.

The Medical Times and Gazette *is published on Friday morning: Advertisements must therefore reach the Publishing Office not later than One o'clock on Thursday.*

Medical Times and Gazette.

SATURDAY, SEPTEMBER 10, 1881.

TO CORRESPONDENTS.

We beg to return our best thanks to the Registrars and Secretaries of the various Universities, Colleges, and Schools, for their prompt replies to our Circular, and for the trouble they have taken in supplying the latest Regulations of the Institutions with which they are connected.

As this number is almost entirely devoted to matter mainly concerning Students, many important communications and contributions unavoidably stand over.

We have here given everything of importance for the entering Student to know; for any further details he should apply for a prospectus to the authorities of the School he may select.

THE WEEK.

TOPICS OF THE DAY.

THE Lord Mayor has summoned a special meeting of the Court of Common Council for the purpose of taking into consideration the report of the Committee with regard to the fish supply, and respecting the destruction of fish at Billingsgate in consequence of the alleged insufficient accommodation. It is stated that the salesmen, poulterers, and other tradesmen of Leadenhall Market are moving in support of their brethren of Billingsgate. They consider that the present position of the latter market is most suitable for the requirements of the fish trade, and they urge on the Corporation the importance of Billingsgate to Leadenhall. The majority of fishmongers and dealers are, they say, likewise poulterers, and the close proximity of the two markets enables the trade to transact their business with all possible facility and despatch; and finally, they say, "Any removal of Billingsgate Market would ruin the trade of our (Leadenhall Market." We do not observe that they say anything about the public.

The fiftieth meeting of the British Association has recently been held at York—a most appropriate arrangement, when it is remembered that it was in that city, half a century ago, its first meeting was held. The chairman for the present year is Sir John Lubbock; and amongst a long list of distinguished presidents and vice-presidents of sections it will be sufficient for us to mention that Professor A. W. Williamson is president, and Mr. F. A. Abel and Professor Thorpe are vice-presidents, of the Chemical Science Section, Professor Flower presides over the department of Anthropology, and Professor J. S. Burdon Sanderson over the department of Anatomy and Physiology. The address delivered by Professor Williamson at the opening of the Chemical Section was on the growth of the Atomic Theory; after which papers of a technical nature were read by Professor Thorpe, Mr. W. Weldon, Mr. Lowthian Bell, and others. Professor Burdon Sanderson, in opening his section, chose for his subject the discoveries of the past half-century relating to Animal Motion. The meeting of the Congress has been very well attended, and its operations have secured an average amount of interest.

Economy in public expenditure is no doubt a highly praiseworthy virtue, but it may be overstrained; and when it is indulged in at the expense of efficiency, it becomes something very like a vice. The Middlesex magistrates are well known to keep a jealous watch upon the outlays connected with the coroners' courts under their jurisdiction; and, judging by the complaint elicited at a recent inquest, they would appear to have carried their economy decidedly too far. In the case referred to, Dr. Diplock was holding an inquiry at 231, Brompton-road, Kensington, concerning the lamented death of Mr. Charles F. C. Foxon, M.R.C.S., aged forty-nine, a greatly esteemed practitioner, who was found dead in his own house. Before the proceedings commenced, Mr. Pollard, who had been called in to attend the deceased, complained of the time which had elapsed between the death of Mr. Foxon and the receipt of the coroner's warrant authorising the examination of the body. The decomposition which had set in was so extensive that it had been impossible to make a thoroughly efficient examination. In his own justification, Dr. Diplock explained that since the abolition of his officer's travelling expenses by the Middlesex magistrates, he had been obliged to depend upon the post for information, etc.,—hence the delay. The magistrates, he observed, had reduced the fees in connexion with coroner's courts as much as possible, though he was bound to say it had resulted in a very small saving to the public. Economy of this character certainly imperils the efficiency of the inquiry, and, as Mr. Pollard is reported to have said, entails great inconvenience on medical witnesses; but in this instance Mr. Pollard was able to state that he found, from the examination of the body of the deceased, that death was due to fatty degeneration of the heart, and a verdict to that effect was accordingly returned.

The eighth annual collection of the Metropolitan Hospital Saturday Fund took place on Saturday last. The usual means were resorted to for securing contributions from pedestrians in various parts of London, but as these donations but rarely come out of the pockets of the "workingman" proper, it is difficult to discover on what principle this open-air collecting is adopted by the committee of an avowed "working man's" movement. The results will be published in due course.

CHANGES IN THE MEDICAL SCHOOLS.

THE following are the principal changes which have taken place in the London Medical Schools since our last "Students' Number" was issued:—At St. Bartholomew's, Mr. Holden has retired by reason of seniority. His place has been filled by the promotion of Mr. Langton to the rank of Surgeon, and the appointment of Mr. Walsham as Assistant-Surgeon. Charing-cross has had to mourn the deaths of two of its most promising members, Dr. Pearson Irvine and Mr. Amphlett. Dr. R. Smith has been consequently appointed Assistant-Physician, and Mr. Morgan Assistant-Surgeon. The staff of St. George's has been strengthened by the appointment of Dr. F. H. Champneys as Assistant Obstetric Physician and Lecturer on Midwifery. The deplorable course of action of the Treasurer and Governors of Guy's Hospital has resulted in the retirement of their Senior Physician, Dr. Habershon, and their Senior Surgeon, Mr. Cooper Forster. Dr. Hilton Fagge has become Physician, and Mr. Davies-Colley Surgeon, in the room of these gentlemen. Dr. E. B. Aveling has ceased to be connected with the London Hospital school. At St. Mary's Hospital, Mr. Anderson Critchett has been appointed Ophthalmic Surgeon, in the place of Mr. Haynes Walton, who has resigned. Dr. Robert King has retired from the staff of the Middlesex Hospital: Dr. Douglas Powell has consequently become Physician; and Dr. C. Y. Biss has been appointed Assistant-Physician. Mr. G. Critchett has ceased to be Ophthalmic Surgeon, and has been succeeded by Mr. W. Lang. At University College, Mr. John Tweedy has been appointed to the chair of Ophthalmic Surgery vacated by Professor Wharton Jones.

THE FULHAM SMALL-POX HOSPITAL.

THE case of Chambers v. the Managers of the Metropolitan Asylums District came on again on the 5th inst., before Mr. Justice Cave and Mr. Justice Kay, sitting as a Court of the Queen's Bench Division of the High Court of Justice. It will be remembered that the object of the plaintiffs was to obtain an interlocutory injunction restraining the defendants from using their Hospital at Fulham as a hospital for patients 'suffering from small-pox or other contagious diseases, and the plaintiffs came to the Divisional Court on August 25, by way of appeal from a decision of Mr. Justice Bowen. The Court then suggested that the defendants should undertake not to send into the Hospital any cases from outside districts until the cause could be heard out. But the defendants had no power to accept the proposal without the consent of the Local Government Board, and the case was adjourned in order to give time for consultation with that body. At the further hearing, on Monday this week, it appeared that no arrangement had been arrived at, and the arguments for and against the issue of an injunction were therefore resumed.

Finally, their Lordships, after expressing great regret that no arrangement had been come to between the parties, said that, as they were compelled to decide the case, they granted an injunction restraining the defendants, until the hearing, from bringing in patients to the Hospital from any district lying beyond a radius of one mile from the Hospital. This injunction would be without any prejudice to any question in the cause.

THE PARIS WEEKLY RETURN.

THE number of deaths for the thirty-fourth week, terminating August 25, 1881, was 995 (532 males and 463 females), and among these there were from typhoid fever 38, small-pox 12, measles 19, scarlatina 8, pertussis 7, diphtheria and croup 39, dysentery 2, erysipelas 7, and puerperal infections 7. There were also 37 deaths from tubercular and acute meningitis, 20 from acute bronchitis, 43 from pneumonia, 173 from infantile athrepsia (64 of the children having been wholly or partially suckled), and 48 violent deaths. The number of deaths continues to decrease, and although the mortality for this week is not much less than for the preceding (25), yet the fact that the decrease bears chiefly on epidemic diseases is satisfactory, as these are the chief characteristic signs of the public health. Thus typhoid fever has declined from 50 to 38, and diphtheria from 44 to 39. As is always the case, the number of deaths from athrepsia diminishes with the diminution of the temperature; it has diminished from 196 in the thirty-third week to 178 in the thirty-fourth. The births for the week amounted to 1136, viz., 609 males (475 legitimate and 134 illegitimate) and 527 females (398 legitimate and 129 illegitimate); 80 children (42 males and 38 females) were born dead or died within twenty-four hours.

MEDICAL NEWS.

BIRTHS.

HODSON.—On July 31, at Taraghar Sanitarium, near Ajmere, Rajpootana, India, the wife of Robert Doveton Hodson, Surgeon Army Medical Department, of a son.
WAKLEY.—On August 30, at Heathlands, Long Cross, Surrey, the wife of James G. Wakley, M.D., of a daughter.
NOAD.—On September 9, at Chesham Lodge, Lower Norwood, the wife of Henry Carden Noad, L.B.C.P., M.R.C.S., of a son.
EVANS.—On September 3, at 11, Crescent-place, Clapham-common, the wife of Lewis Evans, L.R.C.P., of a son, stillborn.
VARDON.—On September 5, at Lennox Lodge, South Hayling, Hants, the wife of Evelyn F. Vardon, M.D., of a daughter.

MARRIAGES.

OWENS—HOOLEY.—On September 1, at Long Stratton, Norfolk, Charles A. Owens, M.D., of Long Stratton, to Marion Isabella, only daughter of the Rev. S. Outler Hooley, vicar of Tharston.
HUME—CHAMBERS.—On August 23, at Hampstead, Frederick Henry Hume, M.R.C.S., of Islington, to Edith Jane, eldest daughter of Charles Chambers, Esq., late of Finchley.
WILLIAMS—CHAMPNEYS.—On August 30, at Cold Norton, Essex, Joseph Williams, M.D., of Holmhurst, Twickenham, to Georgiana Maria, widow of the late T. H. Walpole Champneys, Esq.
MACDERMOTT—SCOTT.—On September 1, at Crediton, Devon, Ralph MacDermott, M.B., M.R.C.S., of Petworth, Sussex, to Eva, second surviving daughter of H. G. Scott, Esq., of Masuri, N.W.P. India.
NORTH—ST. JOHN.—On August 2, at Trichinopoly, Madras Presidency, John North, Surgeon 6th Regiment M.N.I., to Annie Elphinstone, eldest daughter of Major F. C. St. John, 30th Regiment M.N.I.
HOWARD—PLAYER.—On August 25, at South Kensington, Heston Clark Howard, M.R.C.S., of 102, Lansdowne-road, S.W., to Annie Lucette Player.

DEATHS.

BILLING, ARCHIBALD, M.D., F.R.S., at 34, Park-lane, on September 2, in his 91st year.
ROSS, INNES JAMES, M.B., C.M., at sea, by the foundering of the Union Royal Mail steamship Teuton, aged 26.
GRIFFITH, R. C., M.R.C.S., at 90, Gower-street, on September 5, aged 90.
LLOYD, FRANCES HARRIETT, wife of Robert W. Lloyd, M.D., at Lambeth, on September 6, aged 33.
JORDISON, ROBERT BIRKS, M.R.C.S., L.S.A., at South Akendon, Essex, on September 3, aged 69.
HARDWARE, F. C., M.D., Bengal Medical Service, at 22, Chester-street, Edinburgh, on September 3.
STENS, E. S., M.D., at 18, Charles-street, Grosvenor-square, on August 28, aged 76.

VITAL STATISTICS OF LONDON.

Week ending Saturday, September 3, 1881.

BIRTHS.

Births of Boys, 1185; Girls, 1173; Total, 2358.
Corrected weekly average in the 10 years 1871-80, 2507·9.

DEATHS.

	Males.	Females.	Total.
Deaths during the week	632	558	1190
Weekly average of the ten years 1871-80, corrected to increased population ...	763·1	716·9	1480·0
Deaths of people aged 80 and upwards	...	...	43

DEATHS IN SUB-DISTRICTS FROM EPIDEMICS.

	Enumerated Population, 1881 (unrevised)	Small-pox.	Measles.	Scarlet Fever.	Diphtheria.	Whooping-cough.	Typhus.	Enteric (or Typhoid) Fever.	Simple continued Fever.	Diarrhœa.
West	669993	6	12	3	...	4	...	1	...	6
North	905677	7	7	11	3	1	...	1	...	11
Central	261793	...	1	3	2	3	...	2	...	3
East	692530	7	7	9	...	5	1	3	...	8
South	1265575	7	8	14	3	5	...	6	...	28
Total	3814571	34	35	40	8	18	1	13	...	57

METEOROLOGY.

From Observations at the Greenwich Observatory.

Mean height of barometer ...	...	...	...	...	29·983 in.
Mean temperature ...	...	...	...	...	54·5°
Highest point of thermometer	...	...	...	...	69·7°
Lowest point of thermometer	...	...	...	...	43·1°
Mean dew-point temperature	...	...	...	...	51·0°
General direction of wind ...	...	...	...	...	S.S.W., N., & N.N.W
Whole amount of rain in the week	...	...	...	...	0·36 in.

BIRTHS and DEATHS Registered and METEOROLOGY during the Week ending Saturday, Sept. 3, in the following large Towns:—

Cities and boroughs (Municipal boundaries except for London.)	Estimated Population to middle of the year 1881.*	Persons to an Acre.	Births Registered during the week ending Sept. 3.	Deaths Registered during the week ending Sept. 3.	Temperature of Air (Fahr.) Highest during the Week.		Temperature of Air (Fahr.) Lowest during the Week.	Temperature of Air (Fahr.) Weekly Mean of Daily Mean Values.	Temp. of Air (Cent.) Weekly Mean of Daily Mean Values.	Rain Fall. In Inches.	Rain Fall. In Centimetres.
London ...	3829751	50·8	235*	1190	69·7	43·1		54·5	12·50	0·36	0·91
Brighton ...	107934	45·9	5·0	27	68·0	45·8	54·2		12·33	0·57	1·45
Portsmouth ...	128335	28·6	65	33	...	...	...		...	...	...
Norwich ...	88038	11·8	52	23	...	...	...		...	...	...
Plymouth ...	75282	54·0	54	22	67·0	44·5	54·1		12·28	0·50	1·27
Bristol ...	207140	46·5	138	73	66·0	43·5	52·8		11·56	0·44	1·12
Wolverhampton ...	75934	22·4	42	26	64·5	46·6	51·4		10·78	0·84	2·13
Birmingham ...	402296	47·9	268	110	...	...	...		...	...	...
Leicester ...	123120	38·5	92	60	66·0	40·0	52·4		11·33	0·36	0·91
Nottingham ...	188035	18·9	134	71	68·8	38·0	52·8		11·56	0·69	1·75
Liverpool ...	553938	108·2	402	241	...	...	...		...	...	...
Manchester ...	341269	79·5	269	127	...	...	...		...	...	...
Salford ...	177760	34·4	155	62	...	...	...		...	...	...
Oldham ...	112176	24·0	76	33	...	...	...		...	...	...
Bradford ...	184037	25·5	96	62	...	...	...		...	...	...
Leeds ...	310490	14·4	202	106	62·0	46·0	52·5		11·39	0·40	1·02
Sheffield ...	285621	14·5	189	111	67·0	45·0	52·2		11·92	1·03	2·62
Hull ...	155151	42·7	110	74	67·0	43·0	52·3		11·24	1·27	3·23
Sunderland ...	116755	42·2	53	53	68·0	45·0	51·2		10·67	0·59	1·50
Newcastle-on-Tyne	145675	27·1	77	50	...	...	...		...	...	...
Total of 20 large English Towns...	7608775	38·0	4927	2542	69·7	38·0	52·8		11·56	0·64	1·63

* These figures are the numbers enumerated (but subject to revision) in April last, raised to the middle of 1881 by the addition of a quarter of a year's increase, calculated at the rate that prevailed between 1871 and 1881.

At the Royal Observatory, Greenwich, the mean reading of the barometer last week was 29·88 in. The lowest reading was 29·65 in. on Tuesday morning, and the highest 30·03 in. on Wednesday evening.

ORIGINAL LECTURES.

———◆———

THE "BRADSHAWE" LECTURE ON NERVOUS AFFECTIONS OF THE HAND.

Delivered at the Royal College of Physicians of London on August 18, 1881.

By GEORGE VIVIAN POORE, M.D., F.R.C.P.,

Professor of Medical Jurisprudence, University College; Assistant-Physician to University College Hospital, etc.

———

MR. PRESIDENT AND GENTLEMEN,—Before beginning to discuss the subject which I have chosen for the first Bradshawe Lecture, I feel that a few words about him in whose memory this lecture was founded will not be unacceptable.

William Woode Bradshawe studied medicine at the Westminster and Middlesex Hospitals, and became M.D. of Erlangen and M.R.C.S. in 1833, and an Extra-Licentiate of this College in 1841. About this time he was practising at Andover, and married there a widow lady, whose means were sufficient to render him practically independent of his profession. He subsequently moved from Andover to Reading, where he continued to reside till his death on August 18, 1866. He appears to have made use of his ease and leisure for the cultivation of his mind. He entered at New Inn Hall, Oxford, and ultimately became M.A. and D.C.L. He was elected a Fellow of the Royal College of Surgeons in 1854, and became a Member of this College in 1859. Dr. Bradshawe's professional writings comprised papers on the use of cod-liver oil, on narcotics, and on abdominal abscess. He also wrote upon matters of general interest, and was an occasional contributor to the magazines. Of his domestic character the best evidence is the reverence shown for his memory by his widow. This lady, who survived him fourteen years, bequeathed to this College, and also to the College of Surgeons, £1000 for the endowment of a lecture upon some subject connected with physic or surgery, to be called the "Bradshawe" Lecture, and to be delivered annually upon August 18, the anniversary of the death of William Woode Bradshawe. The already existing endowed lectures of this College have been of great service to scientific medicine, and it will be a satisfaction to Mrs. Bradshawe's relatives to know that by founding this lecture, which I have the honour to inaugurate, our munificent benefactress has conferred what cannot but be of permanent benefit to the profession of medicine, and indirectly to the public. It is unfortunate that by the terms of the will the date for the delivery of the lecture has been rigidly fixed for what is nearly the middle of the medical vacation. I feel deeply the honour and responsibility of being called upon to deliver the first "Bradshawe" Lecture, and, although I dare not question the judgment of our President, I am very conscious that, in spite of every effort, I can barely hope to justify the choice which he has made.

I have chosen for my subject the "Nervous Affections of the Hand," because I have enjoyed somewhat unusual opportunities of studying them, and the reflections and suggestions which I shall have the honour of making have been prompted by the study of 160 cases which I have seen during the past ten years. I have thought it best to proceed methodically, but in the course of an hour I can do little more than open the subject and lay down some fundamental principles, and I trust to be able to find some future opportunity of completing what I have to say.

For a thorough understanding of the nervous affections of the hand a knowledge of the nervous relations of the hand is necessary. That form of the manifestation of nerve-force which we call *the will* seems, in its passage to the upper limb, to be in some way intimately connected with certain parts of the brain-crust on either side of the fissure of Rolando in the

so-called ascending frontal and ascending parietal convolutions. This area of grey matter lies below the area which influences the lower limb, above that connected with the face, and behind that which seems to influence movements of the head and eye. Of the upper limb area itself, the fore part seems to control extension movements; the middle part, mainly in front of the fissure of Rolando, seems to control adduction, abduction, flexion, pronation, and supination; while the hinder part, entirely behind the fissure of Rolando, is said to control the special movements of the hand. Hitzig, Ferrier, and their followers, have shown that stimulation of these convolutions produces movement in the opposite upper limb, and clinical and pathological observations are daily confirming the teaching of these physiologists. From these convolutions, the will, on its way to the upper limb, seems to pass through the corpus striatum of the same side; thence along the lower layers of the crus cerebri, through the pons, to the anterior pyramid of the medulla oblongata. At this point the fibres forming the will-path divide. The greater part cross over to reach the opposite side of the spinal cord, while the smaller portion proceed direct to the same side of the spinal cord. The crossed fibres occupy in the cord the hinder central portion of the lateral column, while the direct fibres lie close to the edge of the anterior fissure. Between the fourth cervical and first dorsal nerves is the cervical enlargement of the spinal cord, and here those fibres which seem to originate in the grey matter of the brain presumably form connexions with the grey matter of the enlargement, and, issuing from the cord with the anterior efferent roots, they join the afferent posterior roots, and leave the spinal canal to form the brachial plexus. The brachial plexus is a complicated interlacement of nerves. (A schema, made of coloured wools, showing the complex arrangement of the fibres, was here shown.) The plexus is formed by the fifth, sixth, seventh, and eighth cervical and the first dorsal nerves, and I have assumed that wherever these nerves effect a junction there is a complete interchange of fibres. The practical fact to be remembered is, that the motor and sensory branches of the median and musculo-spiral have relations possibly with the whole of the cervical enlargement, whereas the motor and sensory branches of the musculo-cutaneous represent, as it were, not more than the upper three-fifths, and the motor and sensory branches of the ulnar not more than the lower two-fifths of the cervical enlargement. These speculations, founded upon coarse anatomical facts, receive a large amount of confirmation from the recent experiments of Professors Ferrier and Gerald Yeo. These gentlemen noted the muscles which were made to contract when each of the anterior roots of the nerves forming the brachial plexus of the monkey was stimulated. The result of their experiments was shortly this. No ulnar movement occurred when any of the roots above the eighth cervical were stimulated; no musculo-cutaneous movement followed stimulation of any roots below the fifth cervical; but both median and musculo-spiral movement followed stimulation of the fifth, sixth, seventh, and eighth cervical nerves. These experiments, therefore, bear out the speculation already made, that the median and musculo-spiral have a wide origin from the cervical enlargement, while the musculo-cutaneous is limited to the upper and the ulnar to the lower end. One of the effects of such an interlacement of fibres as is found in the brachial plexus is necessarily to scatter, as it were, the influence of the motor cells of the spinal cord, so that the cells of a particular level have a widely diffused action on the muscles of the limb. We may conclude (1) that as many muscles receive their innervation through the cells corresponding with more than one nerve-root, the function of these muscles will remain, in some degree, as long as any of the cells are intact from which any nervous influence is derived; (2) that when the motor cells in a limited area are destroyed the abolition of function is extremely limited, while impairment of function is far more extended.

We are thus enabled to explain what takes place when, at a certain level in the cord, the motor cells in the front horn are destroyed, as in the disease which it is now the fashion to call "anterior poliomyelitis," but which has long been known as infantile or spinal paralysis. In this disease we constantly find, after the acute stage has subsided, a few paralysed muscles surrounded by others which are merely paretic. The paralysed muscles probably derived their entire motor power through the cells which have been destroyed; while the paretic muscles were probably dependent upon the destroyed cells for only part of their motor power. Let us suppose that the motor cells at the level of the first dorsal nerve have been destroyed. We should expect to find in such a case a complete paralysis of some muscles in the hand, while certain muscles supplied by nerves into which fibres of the first dorsal penetrate would be to a greater or less extent weakened. The improvement which always takes place in the paretic muscles in anterior poliomyelitis is probably due to the fact that the power lost is in time compensated by an increased conduction of force through fibres of another colour. The coexistence in infantile paralysis of paralysed and merely weakened muscles is a fact of much practical importance.

Clinical observation has led Remak to think that the motor cells in the cervical enlargement are arranged in functional groups. The group for the deltoid, biceps, brachialis anticus, and supinators he places in the upper part, and that for the extensors of the digits and the intrinsic muscles of the hand in the middle part of the cervical enlargement. A study of the brachial plexus seems to render it unlikely that any limited lesion of the cord would cause complete paralysis of any considerable group of muscles; the structure of the plexus seems designed, among other things, to prevent such a catastrophe. On the other hand, it is likely that a lesion occurring at any of the junctions of the plexus might cause curious combinations of muscular paralysis; and, indeed, Hoedemaker, who has recorded two cases of Erb's paralysis (deltoid, biceps, brachialis anticus, and supinators), is inclined to place the lesion, not in the spinal cord, but at the point of junction of the fifth and sixth cervical nerves; and the fact that faradisation of a spot in the neck close to this point causes simultaneous contraction of the muscles concerned in Erb's paralysis is in favour of Hoedemaker's theory.

The junctions of the nerves are of importance in another connexion. It is well known that inflammatory action occurring in a nerve may travel in either direction along the nerve-trunk, and thus an ascending neuritis may strike a junction, and seriously impair the function of other nerves emanating from that junction: records of such occurrences are tolerably common. Weir Mitchell gives the history of Stephen Warner, who was shot through the left chest by a bullet. Three days later the movements of the arm below the shoulder were perfect, the pectoral muscles being alone paralysed. Shortly there ensued a neuralgia which spread to the median region of the arm and hand, and was soon followed by wasting and weakness of the flexors of the forearm and hand. Mitchell thinks that the external anterior thoracic nerve had been wounded, and that neuritis travelling along this nerve reached the external cord of the plexus, and involved the musculo-cutaneous and median trunks, which were distinctly tender. Duchenne, Putzel, Cæsar Boeck, and others have recorded similar cases. Inflammation once set up in a nerve seems to have a potentiality for evil not unlike that of a clot in an artery or vein.

It must not be forgotten that the nerves of the brachial plexus, as they issue from the spinal canal, form connexions with the sympathetic chiefly by branches from the inferior cervical ganglion. The many trophic changes occurring in the upper limb in consequence of nerve lesions give importance to this connexion between the nerves of sensation and muscle-motion and those of vessel-motion.

It is not necessary to dwell upon the origin and distribution of the nerves of the arm and hand. A few words may be said, however, upon the effect of paralysis of these nerves on the attitude and movement of the hand. When the median is paralysed we get an abolition of pronation and grasp (except in the ring and little fingers); the near Phalanges can still be flexed by the interossei, and owing to the unopposed action of these same muscles the mid and far phalanges are liable to be over-extended and curved backwards. It is the median nerve which confers what may be called the human functions on the thumb, and when it is paralysed the thumb cannot be abducted or opposed; the first and second metacarpal bones lie in the same plane, the thumb looks directly forwards, and we get what Duchenne called the "ape's hand." In paralysis of the musculo-spiral we get loss of supination and extension, which is total in the wrist and thumb, and partial in the fingers—i.e., the near phalanges cannot be extended, but the mid and far phalanges can still be extended by the interossei. The ulnar 's the nerve par excellence of delicate manipulation.

It supplies all the intrinsic muscles of the hand, except the two outer lumbricales, the opponens, abductor, and outer head of the short flexor of the thumb. All the ulnar muscles acting together give a conical shape to the hand, like that observed in tetany. When the ulnar is paralysed, sewing, writing, and all delicate manipulation become impossible. The patient cannot move the fingers to and fro in the same plane. The mid and far phalanges cannot be extended, nor the near phalanges flexed, and the patient cannot make a billiard bridge. After a time, the hand, by the unopposed action of the flexors and extensors of the fingers, becomes "clawed"—i.e., the near phalanges are extended, while the mid and far phalanges are flexed. I need not specify the well-known areas in the hand which cease to feel when either of these nerves is paralysed. I will merely say that motor function is always more easily abolished than sensory function; that, in cases of recovery from damage, sensation invariably returns before motion; and that occasionally sensation will return in a nerve area, notwithstanding the continued severance of the nerve-trunk. It must be remembered that anastomoses of the sensory branches of the three nerves of the hand exist on the back and palm, and on the pulps and along the edges of the digits, and that MM. Arloing and Tripier have proved that the "persistence of sensibility" in nerve-areas after division of the nerve itself is due to the conduction of sensory impressions (by means of these anastomoses) through the trunks of nerves which remain entire.

There are some purely mechanical conditions in the hand which are liable to lead to misconceptions as to the power of certain muscles. The fingers and the wrist-joint each have their own flexor and extensor muscles, which act independently of each other; and it is obvious that the state of the wrist-joint, whether flexed or extended, must influence the tautness or slackness of those tendons which, having no attachment to the wrist, pass over it to flex or extend the fingers. When the wrist is in an extreme degree of flexion or extension, those tendons which run over the convex side of the joint are taut, while those which run over the concavity are slack; and this tautness or slackness of the extensor or flexor tendons of the fingers is, be it observed, quite independent of any action on the part of the extensor or flexor muscles of the fingers. The fingers can be extended with greater ease and completeness with the wrist flexed than with the wrist extended; and, indeed, when the wrist is fully extended, a complete extension of the fingers can scarcely be accomplished, and the attempt causes great fatigue-pain in the palm, owing to the efforts of the interossei and lumbricales. The cause of this difficulty is clear enough. When the wrist is fully extended, the tendons of the extensors of the fingers are slack, and this has to be overcome before extension of the near phalanges can begin. Hence part of the difficulty. At the same time, the flexor tendons are taut, and tend, quite mechanically, to flex the mid and far phalanges. This is a second obstacle to complete extension of the fingers with the wrist extended. It is the interossei and lumbricales combined which extend the two end phalanges, and the lumbricales seem especially designed to overcome the obstacle offered to complete extension of the fingers by extension of the wrist. These muscles arise from the tendons of the flexor profundus, and are inserted with the interossei into the aponeurotic expansion on the back of the mid phalanges. When, therefore, they contract, they tend, by one and the same action, to slacken the far ends of the flexor tendons and to tighten the far ends of the extensor tendons. They thus permit extension by their action on the flexor tendons, and actively produce it by their action on the extensors. I am not aware that this view of the action of the lumbricales has been previously stated. The interossei and lumbricales have also the power of moving the fingers from side to side; but it must be remembered that, as the tendons of the extensors radiate to a slight extent from the wrist-joint, the fingers tend to separate from each other during the full action of the extensor communis digitorum. This may be mistaken for true interosseal action.

We are now in a position to discuss the effects of diseases at various points of the nervous system upon the form and functions of the hand. Beginning at the highest point, we will consider first the effect of diseases of the brain-crust. There seems to be no doubt that a lesion of the upper-limb convolutions in one half of the brain is capable of causing trouble in the upper limb of the opposite side, and what are called "brachial monoplegias" have been reported tolerably often. They are most common in tubercular meningitis and syphilis, which, when it attacks the brain, often affects the cortex. According to Landouzy, who has studied the subject of cortical paralyses, these paralyses are characterised by the following peculiarities :—1. They are partial and limited to any extent—i.e., we may have paralysis of only one limb, or of part of one limb. 2. They are very often incomplete—i.e., weaknesses rather than palsies. 3. They are often transitory. 4. They are variable—i.e., the area of the paralysis tends to get smaller or larger.

Landouzy has collected over one hundred cases from various sources which seem to support the theory that motor functions are localised in particular convolutions. Among them, however, are not many cases of arm palsy, and of these most were hemiplegic in the first instance.

In a case of congenital absence of the right hand recorded by Gowers, the right ascending parietal convolution at its middle third was found to be smaller than its fellow on the left side, measuring transversely only ·35 in. as against ·65 in.

In a case of congenital absence of the right hand which I lately had an opportunity of seeing, by the courtesy of my friend Mr. Barwell, in the Cripples' Home, Marylebone, there was a very noticeable inequality in the size of the two halves of the skull, that opposite to the absent hand being very much the smaller. A diagram made from measurements taken with a cyrtometer showed this clearly, but the difference was far more apparent to the eye than the diagram would lead one to suppose.

In another case of congenital absence of one hand which I saw a few weeks since at Andover, the head appeared to be perfectly symmetrical, but I had no opportunity of measuring it.

Hahn has recorded the case of a young man of twenty who had a weakness of the first three fingers of the right hand, for which he sought advice on August 11. He then became epileptic, and died comatose on August 30, without any extension of the paralysis. Post-mortem a part of the cortex of the left hemisphere "towards its hinder third" was found hardened and of a yellowish colour over an extent of 2 in. by 1 in.

Cotard in 1868 recorded the case of an old woman in whom an old paralysis of the left arm was found to correspond post-mortem with an atrophy of the convolutions at the upper end of the right fissure of Rolando.

Bourdon, Rosenthal, Ringrose Atkins, and others, have put similar instances upon record, so that the fact of the connexion of certain convolutions with the upper limb may be regarded as clinically established.

I have only had one case in which I have had reason to suspect a cortical lesion, and in this the hand was mainly affected. A gentleman, aged thirty-eight, actively engaged in literary pursuits, was much occupied in looking over many hundred examination papers. In order to get through this work by a certain time, he sat up at nights and goaded his brain with tea, coffee, and other stimulants. He was "taken ill," and his queer state attracting the attention of his friends, I was sent for about thirty-six hours after the attack. The right hand was distinctly paretic. The patient could move the right leg well enough, but he afterwards stated that when first attacked there was a difficulty in moving the leg. The right side of the face drooped perceptibly. Speech was unaffected. The patient was quietly delirious, but answered some questions fairly well, and knew me perfectly. He had pain in the left side of the head, and was possessed by a fixed delusion that an insect had taken possession of his left frontal sinus, and was trying to work its way into his nose. (He had studied anatomy.) The urine contained a trace of sugar. In a week or so he was practically well enough to go a long voyage alone. There is now, ten years and a half after the attack, not a trace of paralysis about him except that his handwriting is not so firm as it was. I believe this to have been a congestion of an overworked cortex, possibly accompanied by a minute hæmorrhage.

When, instead of the cortex, the corpus striatum is affected, we are confronted with an ordinary case of hemiplegia, which need not be discussed. In ordinary cases the hand suffers more than the leg, and is the slowest to improve.

There are two results of hemiplegia which mainly affect the hand, and which call for some special attention—these are contraction and spasm.

Late contraction or contracture is an almost constant phenomenon after hemiplegia; its completeness is usually proportionate to the completeness with which the limb is cut off from the will, and it is generally ascribed to a degenerative process descending along the path of the will. This degeneration is best marked after lesions of the corpora striata, and is said by Isidore Straus not to occur after lesions of the cortex; others, however, hold a different opinion. This degeneration follows the course of all nerve-degenerations, and travels slowly down the course of the extinct function. Its descent is completed in about two months, and then the contraction of the hand approaches its maximum. Ordinarily (in two-thirds of the cases) the contracted limb is in an attitude of flexion and pronation. As far as the hand is concerned, the attitude is an exaggeration of the cadaveric position—the fingers and thumbs being flexed upon the palm. It is probably due to the extinction of the will, and the abandonment of the limb to reflex stimuli reaching it through the cord, and the consequent tonic contraction of the stronger group of muscles. As a rule, the muscles do not waste, and respond to faradism, as in health. The contracted flexors can be made to contract still more by electric stimulation, showing that their contraction is not complete. The cadaveric position of the hand is similarly due, probably, to the tonic contraction of the stronger group of muscles in the interval between death and the dying out of muscular irritability. The "cadaveric position" is assumed, even though the force of gravity may tend to counteract it. I cannot believe that the late contraction of a hemiplegic arm is due to irritation, inflammation, or any form of discharge emanating from the brain. I have said that there is no wasting or degeneration of the muscles of a hemiplegic limb. The reason of this is, I believe, that sensory impressions made upon the palsied limb produce their effect upon the muscles and vessels of the limb through the spinal cord; and that this exercise of spinal function, independent of the will, serves to maintain the healthy nutrition of the limb. The case is very different, as we shall see, when a limb is cut off from both brain function and spinal function.

An apparent exception to this rule, that hemiplegic limbs do not waste, is met with in brain paralyses occurring in early life before development is complete. The wasting in these cases is apparent only, and is due to the fact that the sound limb, which is exercised, grows faster than the palsied limb, and, as it were, leaves its fellow behind in the developmental race. The practical lesson to be learnt from this fact is that, if we would prevent that distortion of the body which must result from an unequal growth and an unequal use of the two sides, the palsied limbs of children must be stimulated and exercised artificially and methodically until growth has finished. It is well to bear in mind that the amount of palsy or contraction in a hemiplegic limb may vary in degree from a maximum which those who run may read, to a minimum which leaves only a trifling degree of contraction of the flexor muscles, or a little unsteadiness in the performance of delicate manipulative acts. I have seen some eight or nine cases in which a functional trouble, such as a writing difficulty, was distinctly due to what I may be pardoned for speaking of as the dregs of a long antecedent, and perhaps forgotten, hemiplegia. Hemiplegia is not very uncommon in early life, and one must ever be watchful in after-life for the trifling effects of it.

Another, though rarer, result of brain lesion is spasm. I shall deal exclusively with chronic spasms occurring some time after the paralysing lesion, such as have been spoken of as post-hemiplegic spasm, spastic contraction, and athetosis. These three forms dovetail into each other, and I think it will be profitable to consider them together. These spasms vary immensely in extent. 1. They may affect all four limbs and the face, such cases being common enough in idiot asylums. Dr. Claye Shaw drew attention to them in 1873, and quite recently, through the kindness of Dr. Langdon Down and Dr. Grabham, I have been able to inspect several such cases at Normansfield and Earlswood. The movements are almost continuous, varying in form, in the same case, within certain limits; and they are increased by attempts at voluntary acts. They are congenital or begun very early in life. The intelligence is usually not much impaired, and in idiot asylums these patients rank high in the cale of intelligence. This general spasm is common, it is said, in first-born children; and very often some accident has befallen them during birth, so that they have been thought to be stillborn and have been recovered by artificial respiration, etc. Several of these children at Normansfield had an exaggerated knee-jerk when the patellar tendon was struck. In some cases there is contraction of the limbs as well as spasm. 2. In other cases this form of spasm follows an attack of hemiplegia. It is then limited to the paralysed limbs, and the arm is usually worse than the leg. Gowers has recorded one case in which there was late rigidity of the arm and spasm of the leg. 3. In cases of paraplegia from a limited lesion in the cord, with consequent degeneration in the lateral columns, there is liable to supervene a rigid state of the legs, and if voluntary power return to any extent there is a spastic spasm on attempting to move. It is in these cases that we get the most marked exaggerated knee-jerk and ankle-clonus.

Now, it seems probable that the mechanism of all these varieties of spasm is similar. In all the forms there is some amount of voluntary power, and in all there is some severance of the muscles from the will. In all, probably, there is more or less descending degeneration along the path of the will, and of this the existence of exaggerated knee-jerk is probably an evidence. Ankle-clonus and knee-jerk are probably due to a heightening of the spinal function (reflex or not), and it is certain that phenomena of this class are most easily observed in the legs, whose reflex functions are more highly developed than those of the arms. In these conditions of the cord, muscles are in such a state that when stretched they contract visibly. This is certainly only an exaggerated normal condition. Sir Charles Bell, in his classical treatise on the hand, pointed out that every voluntary movement implied not only an active contraction of the muscles which produce the movement, but also a regulated contraction of the antagonist muscles in order to check the movement and to prevent its being too jerky and sudden. Now, this check movement of a muscle is possibly provoked by the mere act of stretching, such as must necessarily occur in the extensors of a joint when the flexors are made to contract actively. These movements, provoked by stretching, if not true reflex movements, are in some way dependent upon the spinal cord, and in certain diseased conditions they apparently become so exaggerated as not merely to check the movements dictated by a weakened will-power, but even to cause movement in an opposite direction.

For the production of steady motion there must be a proper balance between the amount of muscular contraction caused by the will (the influence of which reaches the muscle, be it remembered, from both sides of the brain, by the crossed and the direct will-path), and the contraction caused by reflex influences and the mere stretching of the muscles. In the cases which I have been discussing, one or other of the will-paths is certainly more or less blocked at its source or throughout its whole length; certain spinal functions are exaggerated, the balance of power is upset, and disorderly movement results.

It is interesting to note that these spasms occur most frequently in children, in whom all reflex phenomena are but little under control. Of the seven cases which I have seen, six were congenital, or followed a hemiplegia occurring in childhood. In these children the functions of the spinal cord develope with the development of the child, while the brain-damage hinders the development of the controlling influence, and thus we get the balance of power very greatly upset.

In one of my cases of spasm, which came on seven years after a hemiplegic attack, caused by a blow on the head at the age of twenty-six, the spasm which affected the hemiplegic (right) arm, and to a less extent the leg, was in the arm of a very violent character, quite unlike the so-called athetotic spasm, and was moreover fixed and invariable in its form. The wrist was bent, and the hand violently twisted to a position of extreme pronation. There was in this case, however, evidence of a paralysis of the lower branches of the musculo-spiral, superadded, as it were, to the hemiplegia. There was a characteristic prominence on the back of the wrist, impaired sensibility in the radial area on the back of the hand, and the extensors of the wrist and fingers gave degenerative reactions. The paralysis of the extensors and supinators in this case was probably quite independent of the brain lesion, and I believe it served,

if not to start the spasm, at all even's to give it its determinate and fixed character. I have observed similar facts in at least two other cases.

Finally, I believe that the prime factor in all these forms of chronic spasm is the cutting off of the full influence of the will from the muscles, and their abandonment to other influences over which the patient has no control; that they are due, not to any active discharge from the brain, but are brought about rather because the brain fails to discharge its normal amount of voluntary stimulus to the muscles. I need not say that I do not mean to apply these remarks to transient convulsions of an epileptic type.

In one class of idiots there is observed a peculiarity of the hand which is worthy of mention, and which is said to be diagnostic of their mental condition. I saw several of these cases at Earlswood and Normansfield. The skin of the hand is soft, wrinkled like a washerwoman's, and looking too big for the hand, and the finger-tips are tapering and conical. These idiots are often the youngest children of large families. They have a fair amount of intelligence, are singularly imitative, and have the eyes obliquely set, like a Chinaman. The head is round. They never acquire a handicraft, though they are often musical. There is a high arch to the palate, the tongue is fissured, and they usually die of tubercle before puberty.

Before leaving the subject of the influence of brain lesions on the hand, I must mention a case of a child in whom was found a glioma as big as a small egg, growing from the left lobe of the cerebellum, and largely occupying the fourth ventricle. In this case, which was under my care at the Royal Hospital for Children in the autumn of 1878, there was observed the characteristic tetanic rigid condition of the limbs usually seen in cases of cerebellar tumour in children. For the last month of life the child was continuously in a state of opisthotonus with the legs extended and rigid, the left toes strongly flexed, and the right toes strongly extended; no rigidity about the jaws. As to the upper limbs, the arms were powerfully rotated inwards so that the backs of the extended elbows looked outwards and a little forwards, while the hands with the fists clenched were so strongly pronated that the palms looked almost directly forwards.

In dealing with those spinal lesions which cause troubles in the upper limbs I shall try to avoid the repetition of well-understood facts.

The best understood spinal lesion is probably that which is characterised by "inflammation" of the front horns with destruction of its motor cells. This disease, well known as infantile, spinal, or essential paralysis, or anterior poliomyelitis, begins with a sharp febrile attack. The area of the paralysis is at first extensive, but gradually gets smaller as the patient recovers, leaving one limb, or part of one limb only, paralysed, and finally, in typical cases, a small group of paralysed muscles is surrounded by a larger group of muscles which are merely weak. The reason for this I have already tried to explain. The paralysed muscles being cut off from every physiological stimulus, whether direct or reflex (the motor cells being apparently the path for both forms of stimulation), rapidly waste and degenerate. Sensation is perfect, or, more often, the skin is over-sensitive. There are no trophic lesions, but the affected limb is always cold, and very often blue and congested. The paralysed muscles, tested with electricity, give the degenerative reactions, and sometimes, in cases which are recovering, we may find muscles, lately paralysed, but paralysed no longer, which also give the degenerative reactions. This curious fact has been noticed also in some cases of lead-palsy.

In the following case this phenomenon was observed:—Walter B., a schoolboy of sixteen, was seen by me on the 3rd of this month. Three months ago, after a game of play, he had been seized with a typical attack of this disease, and at first nearly every muscle of his body was paralysed, and he was in a state of great danger. In a day or two he began to improve, and has steadily progressed. At present the legs are weak, but he can walk upon them fairly well. Both arms are still partially paralysed, and their condition is almost symmetrical, but the right is rather the worse. On both sides he can move the shoulders, flex the elbows, and extend the wrist to some extent. He can flex the left wrist and digits, but not the right, and on both sides there is paralysis of the triceps and of the interossei. The scapular muscles, biceps, and supinators on both sides respond to faradism, as do also the abductor and opponens of the left thumb. The flexors and extensors of the wrists and digits, and the interossei on both sides, as well as the right abductor and opponens, give degenerative reactions, although some of these muscles (the extensor of the wrist on both sides and the left extensors and flexors of the fingers) respond to the will and are no longer paralysed.

I should mention also that I have seen hopelessly paralysed muscles which formerly gave degenerative reactions, begin, after months of patient treatment, to respond to faradism, but nevertheless continue to remain as hopelessly paralysed as before. Thus, in this disease, under certain exceptional circumstances, we may find non-paralysed muscles giving degenerative reactions; while muscles hopelessly and incurably paralysed may respond normally to electricity.

The following case of complete paralysis of one arm is of exceptional interest from the point of view of diagnosis.

Mrs. L., aged twenty-four, consulted me on August 12, 1880, by the advice of Dr. C. Daniel, of Epsom. A fortnight previously the patient, who was pregnant, being heated by exercise, had sat with her back to an open window and had fallen asleep. Two days later she was seized with pain on the left side of the neck and scalp. There was vomiting, and the temperature rose to 102° F. There was noticed some want of power in the left arm; and after the pain subsided (in thirty-six hours) it was found to be completely paralysed, sensation remaining perfect. When first seen every movement of the arm caused pain, and there were pain and tenderness, but no swelling, up the left side of the neck. The left arm was absolutely powerless. The deltoid and pectoral muscles, and every muscle of the upper limb supplied by the brachial plexus, with the exception of the rhomboids, was paralysed, and gave degenerative reactions; sensation was perfect. There was no trophic change or change of colour, and there was no tendency for the arm to become cold. The pain soon left her. In December she was confined with a healthy child. The general health has steadily improved, and the patient has gained weight, but in spite of a daily, methodical, and most efficient galvanisation of the muscles, which I have myself seen performed upon several occasions, and the administration of mercury, strychnine, iodides, and arsenic, there has not been as yet, though a twelvemonth has elapsed since the attack, any tangible improvement in the power of the limb, which is still absolutely useless. The arm has not wasted as much as might have been expected, because of the constant galvanisation to which it has been subjected. There has been no difficulty in maintaining the temperature, no trophic change, and no tendency to contraction or deformity, for the very good reason that no muscles are capable of contracting. I have been in considerable doubt as to the diagnosis of this case. The early pain, the tenderness up the side of the neck, the absence of lividity, the ease with which the temperature has been maintained, and the fact that there has been no diminution of the area of the paralysis, have inclined me to think that this is not a case of anterior poliomyelitis, but possibly a compression of the anterior nerve-roots by a rheumatic thickening of the meninges. Two physicians who are equally eminent for their investigation of nervous diseases have seen this patient with me: the first, in January, thought with me that the motor cells were not affected; the second, in July, with the knowledge that no improvement had taken place in eleven months, considered the case to be one of anterior poliomyelitis. I confess I am still in doubt. It is needless to say that the diagnosis of motor cell (?) or nerve-root (?) is of great importance for prognosis. The regeneration of a motor cell is inconceivable, while the power of regeneration of conducting fibres seems almost unlimited.

For the sake of comparison with these cases, I will now bring forward a case of absolute paralysis of the right arm from a bruise of the brachial plexus.

In March, 1877, Miss F. W., aged fifty, fell down a flight of steps, alighting on her right shoulder. Shortly after the accident, the arm was devoid of motion and sensation from the shoulder downwards. When I saw her, three months later, the arm was much wasted; the deltoid, triceps, biceps, and all the other muscles of the limb gave degenerative reactions. The limb was absolutely useless, and sensation was entirely wanting below the middle of the forearm, and impaired elsewhere. On scratching the forearm, it was

noticed that vascular reaction occurred far more readily on the sensitive than on the insensitive part. The galvanic current, applied to the sensitive parts, caused an immediate uniform redness, but on the insensitive parts it slowly produced an irregular patchy redness, like a lichenous rash. The fingers were scurfy and bulbous at the tips, and the patient complained that they got hot at night. Galvanisation was efficiently and methodically applied to the arm by the patient's sister. By November, sensation had returned down to the finger-tips (imperfectly). The wrist was movable; the hand clawed and paralysed; the nails furrowed and white. During the winter the hand was covered with chilblains. In April, 1878, the arm was well, but the intrinsic muscles of the hand remained paralysed; the nails were a dead white. In July, 1878, the motion and sensation of the hand were still impaired, and the muscles of the hand gave degenerative reactions. In June, 1879, the intrinsic muscles of the hand responded to faradism. There were glazy spots at the roots of the finger-nails; nails harsh, hard, and grooved. In June, 1880, the hand was fairly useful, though still liable to chilblains, and the sensation still imperfect. I have a water-colour drawing of the hand at this time. In a letter dated August, 1881, this patient writes: "It is really quite a natural colour. Nails of thumb, first and third fingers well; and the others much better. Performance on the piano quite grand; I can reach an octave, but cannot strike it without holding the thumb. The thumb and first finger are the worst parts, as the thumb will not go out quite far enough, and the first finger is inclined to bend back. The chilblains last winter were nothing to what they were before."

This case is one of surpassing interest, and is most instructive from the point of view of nerve pathology. First, as to the time of duration of the symptoms. The accident happened in March, 1877, and in August, 1881, her recovery, though still progressing, is yet not complete, so that it has already been protracted over a period of nearly four years and a half. During the whole of this time there has been a steady, slow, evenly progressing recovery, so that her improvement was recognisable from month to month. Recovery has taken place in a regular order: sensation returned first, and always preceded the return of motion; and muscles situated nearest to the trunk recovered before those which were more distant from it. At present two muscles of the hand, the abductor of the thumb, and the first dorsal interosseous, alone remain paralysed. From what is known of nervous degeneration and regeneration one could hardly have expected the course of events to have been otherwise. The injury in this case was severe. The nerve-trunks were probably bruised and torn by the head of the humerus, so that immediately after the accident they were completely "blocked" to upward sensory impressions or downward motor stimuli. A disused nerve degenerates along the line of function, and the motor nerves in this case rapidly degenerated from the point of blocking down to their terminations, for no stimulation could possibly reach them either directly from the brain or be reflected to them through the spinal cord. Accordingly, within a month or so after her accident, it is probable that each motor nerve had been converted into a degenerated cord some three-quarters of a yard long, as incapable of conducting stimuli as the skin, fat, or connective tissue. Now, as the degeneration of a nerve takes place from trunk to end, so its regeneration takes place in the same direction, for there can be no regeneration unless physiological or artificial stimuli reach the point to be regenerated. Motor stimuli, both direct and reflex, impinging against the block, gradually induce molecular regeneration and the power of conducting stimuli, and thus little by little, as the stimuli are able to travel further, we get a complete regeneration of the nerves (a process which in this patient has already taken four and a half years). It is quite inconceivable that the stimulus which seems necessary for the regeneration of a nerve should be able to pass by any unregenerated portion. One might as well expect the makers of a well to begin their work in the middle. Just as a well has to be tediously bored, so is a degenerated motor nerve slowly opened for the traffic of stimuli from above. Provided stimuli can reach the nerve the power of regeneration seems almost unlimited, and, indeed, when pieces are cut out of a nerve-trunk the severed ends seem capable of worming their way, as it were, towards each other, and eventually effecting a junction in spite of every adverse circumstance. It seems probable that the bulbous ends in amputation stumps must be looked upon as an overgrowth due to the arrival of stimuli in the stump of the nerve, which are unable to produce their proper physiological effect. Bulbous nerve-ends, according to Weir Mitchell, are physiological rather than pathological, and are almost invariably present in stumps.

The earlier return of sensation in all cases of nerve-injury is due to the following facts :—1. That the sensory branches from the periphery to the obstruction are not deprived of their natural stimuli, and presumably do not entirely degenerate, and are consequently ready to resume their full functions directly the obstruction on the up-path is removed. 2. That in the parts above the block the incidence of impression of various kinds probably serves to keep up in some degree the healthy condition of the nerve; it is, in short, next to impossible to deprive a sensory nerve of its natural stimuli. 3. That, owing to the anastomoses which exist between sensory nerve branches, impressions have the power, to some extent, of choosing the path of least resistance. Hence, happily, it results that sensory impressions, so important for the nutrition of the limb, are able to produce their physiological effects in spite of very serious injuries.

A few words as to the trophic troubles observed in this patient. These were of three kinds :—1. Muscle-wasting. 2. A sluggishness or absence of vascular reaction when the skin was stimulated. 3. Scurfiness of the skin, loss of nails, and a tendency to chilblains.

Why does it happen that muscles paralysed from a brain-lesion scarcely waste at all, while those paralysed from destruction of the motor cells of the cord, or from injury to a nerve-trunk, rapidly waste and degenerate? Because, in the first case, physiological stimuli still reach it through the cord, while in the second case it is completely cut off from every source of physiological stimulation. So long as a muscle be stimulated it will maintain its size, no matter whether the stimulus come to it from the brain along the will-path, or from the surface or deep parts along the path of reflected impressions, or be artificially applied to it by means of a galvanic battery. If, on the other hand, a muscle be cut off from all sources of stimulation, it will waste. I do not, of course, mean to say that there may not be other causes for muscle-wasting, but I have never encountered an exception to the rule I have enunciated.

With regard to the trophic changes, I speak with less confidence, but I must express my absolute disbelief in the existence of special trophic nerves; and we clearly ought to exhaust every possible explanation before we proceed to do what is far too common in nerve pathology, viz., to give "to airy nothings a local habitation and a name." I believe that tissue-changes other than muscle-wasting are often due to the cutting off from the vessels which supply those tissues those physiological stimuli which produce the contraction and dilatation of the vessels, and thus exercise a local control over them. Every paralysed limb is deprived of one important aid to circulation, viz., the muscular contraction, which is a material aid to the circulation, especially in driving the blood towards the heart. Every paralysed limb must therefore be at a nutritive disadvantage, but yet in hemiplegic limbs whose connexions with the spinal cord are normal, no trophic changes usually occur, except a little congestion. When the motor cells of the cord are alone destroyed, no trophic changes occur. When a mixed nerve is destroyed, trophic changes are very liable to occur to some extent. When the posterior roots and sensory paths of the cord are damaged, trophic changes often occur, as witness the joint affections and occasional zones of locomotor ataxy. When a purely sensory nerve, such as the fifth, is damaged, trophic changes are common, but not invariable; their occurrence, according to some, depending upon the implication or otherwise of the Gasserian ganglion.

Now, in the case we have been considering there were trophic changes. There was impaired vascular reaction on stimulating the insensitive parts of the limb, and it is tolerably certain that cutaneous impressions were not reflected to the vaso-motor nerves of the limb. The local circulation was therefore cut off from the stimulus of muscular motion and from the stimulus of cutaneous impressions. It must not be forgotten, however, that impressions made upon one limb seem capable of being reflected to the vessels of the other, so that impressions made upon the left arm and other parts of the body were probably able to reach the paralysed limb. This fact is very suggestive of the importance which it is in the animal economy that cutaneous impressions should reach the vaso-motor nerves. A sensory impression is felt, if I may be allowed the expression—(1) by the brain; (2) by the muscles, being reflected to them by the spinal cord; (3) by the vessels being reflected to them by the cord or the ganglia on the posterior nerve-roots. It must be remembered that conceivably any one of these paths for sensory impressions may be blocked, while the other two may remain open; that any two may conceivably be blocked; or that all three may be blocked. The question is very complicated and very difficult to study. The dependence of nutrition upon a due connexion between the sensory and vaso-motor nerves combined with muscular motion seems to me extremely likely. Its absolute proof or disproof seems almost impossible.

I have to express my thanks to my friend Dr. Harrington Sainsbury for much assistance in looking up foreign authorities.

ON THE

DISCOVERIES OF THE PAST HALF-CENTURY RELATING TO ANIMAL MOTION.

Opening Address delivered to the Department of Anatomy and Physiology of the British Association.

By J. BURDON-SANDERSON, M.D., LL.D., F.R.S.,
Professor of Physiology in University College, London.

THE two great branches of Biology with which we concern ourselves in this section, Animal Morphology and Physiology, are most intimately related to each other. This arises from their having one subject of study—the living animal organism. The difference between them lies in this, that whereas the studies of the anatomist lead him to fix his attention on the organism itself, to us physiologists it, and the organs of which it is made up, serve only as *vestigia*, by means of which we investigate the vital processes of which they are alike the causes and consequences.

To illustrate this I will first ask you to imagine for a moment that you have before you one of those melancholy remainders of what was once an animal—to wit, a rabbit,—which one sees exposed in the shops of poulterers. We have no hesitation in recognising that remainder as being in a certain sense a rabbit; but it is a very miserable vestige of what was a few days ago enjoying life in some wood or warren, or more likely on the sand-hills near Ostend. We may call it a rabbit if we like, but it is only a remainder—not the thing itself.

The anatomical preparation which I have in imagination placed before you, although it has lost its inside and its outside, its integument and its viscera, still retains the parts for which the rest existed. The final cause of an animal, whether human or other, is muscular action, because it is by means of its muscles that it maintains its external relations. It is by our muscles exclusively that we act on each other. The articulate sounds by which I am addressing you are but the results of complicated combinations of muscular contractions; and so are the scarcely appreciable changes in your countenances, by which I am able to judge how much, or how little, what I am saying interests you.

Consequently, the main problems of physiology relate to muscular action, or, as I have called it, animal motion. They may be divided into two—namely (1) In what does muscular action consist?—that is, what is the process of which it is the effect or outcome? and (2) How are the motions of our bodies co-ordinated or regulated? It is unnecessary to occupy time in showing that, excluding those higher intellectual processes which, as they leave no traceable marks behind them, are beyond the reach of our methods of investigation, these two questions comprise all others concerning animal motion. I will therefore proceed at once to the first of them—that of the process of muscular contraction.

The years which immediately followed the origin of the British Association exceeded any earlier period of equal length in the number and importance of the new facts in morphology and in physiology which were brought to light; for it was during that period that Johannes Müller, Schwann, Henle, and, in this country, Sharpey, Bowman, and Marshall Hall, accomplished their productive labours. But it was introductory to a much greater epoch. It would give you a true idea of the nature of the great advance which took place about the middle of this century if I were to define it as the epoch of the death of "vitalism." Before that time even the greatest biologist—e.g., J. Müller—recognised that the knowledge they possessed both of vital and physical phenomena was insufficient to refer both to a common measure. The method, therefore, was to study the processes of life in relation to each other only. Since that time it has become fundamental in our science not to regard any vital process as understood at all, unless it can be brought into relation with physical standards, and the methods of physiology have been based exclusively on this principle. Let us inquire for a moment what causes have conduced to the change.

The most efficient cause was the progress which had been made in physics and chemistry, and particularly those investigations which led to the establishment of the doctrine of the Conservation of Energy. In the application of this great principle to physiology, the men to whom we are indebted are, first and foremost, J. R. Mayer, of whom I shall say more immediately; and secondly, to the great physiologists, still living and working among us, who were the pupils of J. Müller—viz., Helmholtz, Ludwig, Du Bois-Reymond, and Brücke.

As regards the subject which is first to occupy our attention, that of the *process* of muscular contraction, J. R. Mayer occupies so leading a position that a large proportion of the researches which have been done since the new era, which he had so important a share in establishing, may be rightly considered as the working out of principles enunciated in his treatise(a) on the relation between organic motion and exchange of material. The most important of these were, as expressed in his own words—(1) "That the chemical force contained in the ingested food and in the inhaled oxygen is the source of the motion and heat which are the two products of animal life; and (2) that these products vary in amount with the chemical process which produces them." Whatever may be the claims of Mayer to be regarded as a great discoverer in physics, there can be no doubt that as a physiologist he deserves the highest place that we can give him, for at a time when the notion of the correlation of different modes of motion was as yet very unfamiliar to the physicist, he boldly applied it to the phenomena of animal life, and thus reunited physiology with natural philosophy, from which it had been rightly, because unavoidably, severed by the vitalists of an earlier period.

Let me first endeavour shortly to explain how Mayer himself applied the principle just enunciated, and then how it has been developed experimentally since his time.

The fundamental notion is this: the animal body resembles, as regards the work it does and the heat it produces, a steam-engine, in which fuel is continually being used on the one hand, and work is being done and heat produced on the other. The using of fuel is the chemical process, which, in the animal body, as in the steam-engine, is a process of oxidation. Heat and work are the useful products; for as, in the higher animals, the body can only work at a constant temperature of about 100° F., heat may be so regarded.

Having previously determined the heat and work severally producible by the combustion of a given weight of carbon, from his own experiments and from those of earlier physicists, Mayer calculated that if the oxidation of carbon is assumed to represent approximately the oxidation process of the body, the quantity of carbon actually burnt in a day is far more than sufficient to account for the day's work, and that of the material expended in the body not more than one-fifth was used in the doing of work, the remaining four-fifths being partly used, partly wasted, in heat-production.

Having thus shown that the principles of the correlation of process and product hold good, so far as its truth could then be tested, as regards the whole organism, Mayer proceeded to inquire into its applicability to the particular organ whose function it is "to transform chemical difference into mechanical effect"—namely, muscle. Although, he said, a muscle acts under the direction of the will, it does not derive its power of acting from the will, any more than a steamboat derives its power of motion from the helmsman. Again (and this was of more importance, as being more directly opposed to the prevalent vitalism), a muscle, like the steamboat, uses in the doing of work not the material

of its own structure or mechanism, but the fuel—i.e., the nutriment—which it derives directly from the blood which flows through its capillaries. "The muscle is the instrument by which the transformation of force is accomplished, not the material which is itself transformed." This principle he exemplified in several ways, showing that if the muscle of our bodies worked, as was formerly supposed, at the expense of their own substance, their whole material would be used up in a few weeks, and that in the case of the heart, a muscle which works at a much greater rate than any other, it would be expended in as many days—a result which necessarily involved the absurd hypothesis that the muscular fibres of our hearts are so frequently disintegrated and reintegrated that we get new hearts once a week.

On such considerations Mayer founded the prevision, that, as soon as experimental methods should become sufficiently perfect to render it possible to determine with precision the limits of the chemical process either in the whole animal body or in a single muscle during a given period, and to measure the production of heat and the work done during the same period, the result would show a quantitative correlation between them.

If the time at our disposal permitted, I should like to give a short account of the succession of laborious investigations by which these previsions have been verified. Begun by Bidder and Schmidt in 1851,(b) continued by Pettenkofer and Voit,(c) and by the agricultural physiologists(d) with reference to herbivora, they are not yet by any means completed. I must content myself with saying that by these experiments the first and second parts of this great subject, namely, the limits of the chemical process of animal life and its relation to animal motion under different conditions—have been satisfactorily worked out, but that the quantitative relations of heat-production are as yet only insufficiently determined.

Let me sum up in as few words as possible how far what we have now learnt by experiment justifies Mayer's anticipations, and how it falls short of or exceeds them. First of all, we are as certain as of any physical fact that the animal body in doing work does not use its own material—that, as Mayer says, the oil to his lamp of life is food; but in addition to this we know what he was unaware of, that what is used is not only not the living protoplasm itself, but is a kind of material which widely differs from it in chemical properties. In what may be called commercial physiology—i.e., in the literature of trade puffs—one still meets with the assumption that the material basis of muscular motion is nitrogenous; but by many methods of proof it has been shown that the true "Oel in der Flamme des Lebens" is not proteid substance, but sugar, or sugar-producing material. The discovery of this fundamental truth we owe first to Bernard (1850-56), who brought to light the fact that such material plays an important part in the nutrition of every living tissue; secondly, to Voit (1866), who in elaborate experiments on carnivorous animals, during periods of rest and exertion, showed that, in comparing those conditions, no relation whatever shows itself between the quantity of proteid material (flesh) consumed, and the amount of work done; and finally, to Frankland, Fick, and his associate Wislicenus, as to the work-yielding value of different constituents of food, and as to the actual expenditure of material in man during severe exertion. The subjects of experiment used by the two last-mentioned physiologists were themselves. The work done was the mountain ascent from Interlaken to the summit of the Faulhorn. The result was to prove that the quantity of material used was proportional to the work done, and that that material was such as to yield water and carbonic acid exclusively.

The investigators to whom I have just referred aimed at proving the correlation of process and product for the whole animal organism. The other mode of inquiry proposed by Mayer, the verification of his principle in respect of the work-doing mechanism—that is to say, in respect of muscle taken separately—has been pursued with equal perseverance during the last twenty years, and with greater success; for in experimenting on a separate organ, which has no other functions excepting those which are in question, it is pos-

(a) J. R. Mayer, "Die organische Bewegung in ihrem Zusammenhange mit dem Stoffwechsel : ein Beitrag zur Naturkunde," Heilbronn, 1845.

(b) Bidder and Schmidt, "Die Verdauungssäfte und der Stoffwechsel," Leipzig, 1852.
(c) Pettenkofer and Voit, Zeitschr. f. Biologie, passim, 1866-80.
(d) Henneberg and Stohmann, "Beiträge zur Begründung einer rationellen Fütterung der Wiederkäuer," Brunswick and Göttingen, 1860-70.

sible to eliminate uncertainties which are unavoidable when the conditions of the problem are more complicated. Before I attempt to sketch the results of these experiments, I must ask your attention for a moment to the discoveries made since Mayer's epoch, concerning a closely related subject—that of the Process of Respiration.

I wish that I had time to go back to the great discovery of Priestley (1776), that the essential facts in the process of respiration are the giving off of fixed air, as he called it, and the taking in of dephlogisticated air, and to relate to you the beautiful experiments by which he proved it ; and then to pass on to Lavoisier (1777), who, on the other side of the Channel, made independently what was substantially the same discovery a little after Priestley, and added others of even greater moment. According to Lavoisier, the chemical process of respiration is a slow combustion which has its seat in the lungs. At the time that Mayer wrote, this doctrine still maintained its ascendency, although the investigations of Magnus (1838) had already proved its fallacy. Mayer himself knew that the blood possessed the property of conveying oxygen from the lungs to the capillaries, and of conveying carbonic acid gas from the capillaries to the lungs, which was sufficient to exclude the doctrine of Lavoisier. Our present knowledge of the subject was attained by two methods—viz., first, the investigation of the properties of the colouring matter of the blood, since called "hæmoglobin," the initial step in which was made by Professor Stokes in 1862 ; and secondly, the application of the mercurial air-pump as a means of determining the relations of oxygen and carbonic acid gas to the living blood and tissues. The last is a matter of such importance in relation to our subject that I shall ask your special attention to it. Suppose that I have a barometer of which the tube, instead of being of the ordinary form, is expanded at the top into a large bulb of one or two litres capacity, and that, by means of some suitable contrivance, I am able to introduce, in such a way as to lose no time and to preclude the possibility of contact with air, a fluid ounce of blood from the artery of a living animal into the vacuous space—what would happen ? Instantly the quantity of blood would be converted into froth, which would occupy the whole of the large bulb. The colour of the froth would at first be scarlet, but would speedily change to crimson. It would soon subside, and we should then have the cavity which was before vacuous occupied by the blood and its gases—namely, the oxygen, carbonic acid gas, and nitrogen previously contained in it. And if we had the means (which actually exist in the gas-pump) of separating the gaseous mixture from the liquid, and of renewing the vacuum, we should be able to determine (1) the total quantity of gases which the blood yields, and (2) by analysis, the proportion of each gas.

Now, with reference to the blood, by the application of the "blood-pump," as it is called, we have learnt a great many facts relating to the nature of respiration, particularly that the difference of venous from arterial blood depends not on the presence of "effete matter," as used to be thought, but on the less amount of oxygen held by its colouring matter, and that the blood which flows back to the heart from different organs, and at different times, differs in the amount of oxygen and of carbonic acid gas it yields, according to the activity of the chemical processes which have their seat in the living tissues from which it flows.(e) But this is not all that the blood-pump has done for us. By applying it not merely to the blood, but to the tissues, we have learnt that the doctrine of Lavoisier was wrong, not merely as regards the place, but as regards the nature of the essential process in respiration. The fundamental fact which is thus brought to light is this : that although living tissues are constantly and freely supplied with oxygen, and are in fact constantly tearing it from the hæmoglobin which holds it, yet they themselves yield no oxygen to the vacuum. In other words, the oxygen which living protoplasm seizes upon with such energy that the blood which flows by it is compelled to yield it up, becomes so entirely part of the living material itself that it cannot be separated even by the vacuum. It is in this way only that we can understand the seeming paradox that the oxygen, which is conveyed in abundance to every recess of our bodies by the blood-stream, is nowhere to be found. Notwithstand-

(e) Ludwig's first important research on this subject was published in 1857.

ing that no oxidation-product is formed, it becomes latent in every bit of living protoplasm ; stored up in quantity proportional to its potential activity—i.e., to the work, internal or external, it has to do.

Thus you see that the process of tissue-respiration—in other words, the relation of living protoplasm to oxygen—is very different from what Mayer, who localised oxidation in the capillaries, believed it to be. And this difference has a good deal to do with the relation of Process to Product in muscle. Let us now revert to the experiments on this subject which we are to take as exemplifications of the truth of Mayer's forecasts.

The living muscle of a frog is placed in a closed chamber, which is vacuous—i.e., contains only aqueous vapour. The chamber is so arranged that the muscle can be made to contract as often as necessary. At the end of a certain period it is found that the chamber now contains carbonic acid gas in quantity corresponding to the number of contractions the muscle has performed. The water which it has also given off cannot of course be estimated. Where do these two products come from ? The answer is plain. The muscle has been living all the time, for it has been doing work, and (as we shall see immediately) producing heat. What has it been living on ? Evidently on stored material. If so, of what nature ? If we look for the answer to the muscle, we shall find that it contains both proteid and sugar-producing material, but which is expended in contraction we are not informed. There is, however, a way out of the difficulty. We have seen that the only chemical products which are given off during contraction are carbonic acid gas and water. It is clear, therefore, that the material on which it feeds must be something which yields, when oxidised, these products, and these only. The materials which are stored in muscle are—oxygen, and sugar or something resembling it in chemical composition.

And now we come to the last point I have to bring before you in connexion with this part of my subject. I have assumed up to this moment that heat is always produced when a muscle does work. Most people will be ready to admit, as evidence of this, the familiar fact that we warm ourselves by exertion. This is in reality no proof at all. The proof is obtained when a muscle being set to contract, it is observed that at each contraction it becomes warmer. In such an experiment, if the heat-capacity of muscle is known, the weight of the particular muscle, and the increase of temperature, we have the quantity of heat produced.

If you determine these data in respect of a series of contractions, arranging the experiments so that the work done in each contraction is measured, and immediately thereupon reconverted into heat, the result gives you the total product of the oxidation process in heat.

If you repeat the same experiment in such a way that the work done in each contraction is not so reconverted, the result is less by the quantity of heat corresponding to the work done. The results of these two experiments have been found by Professor Fick to cover each other very exactly. I have stated them in a table,(f) in which we have the realisation, as regards a single muscle, of the following forecast of Mayer's as regards the whole animal organism. "Convert into heat," he said, "by friction or otherwise, the mechanical product yielded by an animal in a given time, add thereto the heat produced in the body directly during the same period, and you will have the total quantity of heat which corresponds to the chemical processes." We have seen that this is realisable as regards muscle, but it is not even yet within reach of experimental verification as regards the whole animal.

I now proceed abruptly (for the time at our disposal does not admit of our spending it on transitions) to the consideration of the other great question concerning vital motion—namely, the question how the actions of the muscles of an animal are so regulated and co-ordinated as to determine the combined movements, whether rhythmical or voluntary, of the whole body.

As everyone knows who has read the "Lay Sermons," the

(f) RELATION OF PRODUCT AND PROCESS IN MUSCLE.
(Result of one of Fick's experiments.)

Mechanical product	...	...	...	6670 gramme millimetres.
Its heat-value	...	...	...	15·6 milligramme units.
Heat produced	...	...	...	39·0 "
Total product reckoned as heat	...	...	54·6 "

nature and meaning of these often unintentional but always adapted motions, which constitute so large a part of our bodily activity, was understood by Descartes early in the seventeenth century. Without saying anything as to his direct influence on his contemporaries and successors, there can be no doubt that the appearance of Descartes was coincident with a great epoch—an epoch of great men and great achievements in the acquirement of man's intellectual mastery over nature. When he interpreted the unconscious closing of the eyelids on the approach of external objects, the acts of coughing, sneezing, and the like, as mechanical and reflected processes, he neither knew in what part of the nervous system the mechanisms concerned were situated, nor how they acted.(g) It was not until a hundred years after that Whytt and Hales made the fundamental experiments on beheaded frogs, by which they showed that the involuntary motions which such preparations execute cease when the whole of the spinal cord is destroyed—that if the back part of the cord is destroyed, the motions of the hind limbs, if the fore part, those of the fore limbs, cease. It was in 1751 that Dr.Whytt published in Edinburgh his work on the involuntary motions of animals. After this, the next great step was made within the recollection of living physiologists: a period to which, as it coincided with the event which we are now commemorating—the origin of the British Association,—I will now ask your special attention.

Exactly forty-nine years ago, Dr. Marshall Hall communicated to the Zoological Society of London the first account of his experiments on the reflex function of the spinal cord. The facts which he had observed, and the conclusions he drew from them, were entirely new to him, and entirely new to the physiologists to whom his communication was addressed. Nor can there be any reason why the anticipation of his fundamental discovery by Dr. Whytt should be held to diminish his merit as an original investigator. In the face of historical fact it is impossible to regard him as the discoverer of the "reflex function of the spinal cord," but we do not the less owe him gratitude for the application he made of the knowledge he had gained by experiments on animals to the study of disease. For no one who is acquainted with the development of the branch of practical medicine which relates to the progress of the central nervous system will hesitate in attributing the rapid progress which has been made in the diagnosis and treatment of these diseases, to the impulse given by Dr. Marshall Hall to the study of nervous pathology.

In the mind of Dr. Marshall Hall the word "reflex" had a very restricted meaning. The term "excito-motory function," which he also used, stood in his mind for a group of phenomena of which it was the sole characteristic that a sensory impression produced a motor response. During the thirty years which have elapsed since his death, the development of meaning of the word "reflex" has been comparable to that of a plant from a seed. The original conception of reflex action has undergone, not only expansion, but also modification, so that in its wider sense it may be regarded as the empirical development of the philosophical views of the animal mechanism promulgated by Descartes. Not that the work of the past thirty years by which the physiology of the nervous system has been constituted can be attributed for a moment to the direct influence of Descartes.

The real epoch-maker here was Johannes Müller. There can be no doubt that Descartes' physiological speculations were well known to him, and that his large acquaintance with the thought and work of his predecessors conduced, with his own powers of observation, to make him the great man that he was; but to imagine that his ideas of the mechanism of the nervous system were inspired, or the investigations by which, contemporaneously with Dr. Marshall Hall, he demonstrated the fundamental facts of reflex action, were suggested by the animal automatism of Descartes, seems to me wholly improbable.

I propose, by way of conclusion, to attempt to illustrate the nature of reflex action in the larger sense, or, as I should prefer to call it, the Automatic Action of Centres, by a single example—that of the nervous mechanism by which the circulation is regulated.

The same year that J. R. Mayer published his memorable essay, it was discovered by E. H. Weber that, in the vagus nerve, which springs from the medulla oblongata and proceeds therefrom to the heart, there exist channels of influence by which the medulla acts on that wonderful muscular mechanism. Almost at the same time with this, a series of discoveries(h) were made relating to the circulation, which, taken together, must be regarded as of equal importance with the original discovery of Harvey. First, it was found by Henle that the arterial bloodvessels by which blood is distributed to brain, nerve, muscle, gland, and other organs, are provided with muscular walls like those of the heart itself, by the contraction or dilatation of which the supply is increased or diminished according to the requirements of the particular organ. Secondly, it was discovered simultaneously, but independently, by Brown-Séquard and Augustus Waller, that these arteries are connected by nervous channels of influence with the brain and spinal cord, just as the heart is. Thirdly, it was demonstrated by Bernard that what might be called the heart-managing channels spring from a small spot of grey substance in the medulla oblongata, which we now call the "heart-centre"; and a little later by Schiff, that the artery-regulating channels spring from a similar head-central office, also situated in the medulla oblongata, but higher up, and from subordinate centres in the spinal cord.

If I had the whole day at my disposal, and your patience were inexhaustible, I might attempt to give an outline of the issues to which these five discoveries have led. As it is, I must limit myself to a brief discussion of their relations to each other, in order that we may learn something from them as to the nature of automatic action.

Sir Isaac Newton, who, although he knew nothing about the structure of nerves, made some shrewd forecasts about their action, attributed to those which are connected with muscles an alterative function. He thought that by means of motor nerves the brain could determine either relaxation or contraction of muscles. Now, as regards ordinary muscles, we know that this is not the case. We can will only the shortening of a muscle, not its lengthening. When Brown-Séquard discovered the function of the motor nerves of the bloodvessels, he assumed that the same limitation was applicable to it as to that of muscular nerves in general. It was soon found, however, that this assumption was not true in all cases—that there were certain instances in which, when the vascular nerves were interfered with, dilatation of the bloodvessels, consequent on relaxation of their muscles, took place; and that, in fact, the nervous mechanism by which the circulation is regulated is a highly complicated one, of which the best that we can say is that it is perfectly adapted to its purpose. For while every organ is supplied with muscular arteries, and every artery with vascular nerves, the influence which these transmit is here relaxing, there constricting, according (1) to the function which the organ is subject to discharge; and (2) the degree of its activity at the time. At the same time the whole mechanism is controlled by one and the same central office, the locality of which we can determine with exactitude by

(g) Descartes' scheme of the central nervous mechanism comprised all the parts which we now regard as essential to "reflex action." Sensory nerves were represented by threads (fliats), which connected all parts of the body to the brain ("Œuvres," par V. Cousin, vol. iv., page 359); motor nerves by tubes which extended from the brain to the muscles; "motor centres" by "pores" which were arranged on the internal surface of the ventricular cavity of the brain and guarded the entrance to the motor tubes. This cavity was supposed to be kept constantly charged with "animal spirits" furnished to it from the heart by arteries specially destined for the purpose. Any "incitation" of the surface of the body by an external object which affects the organs of sense, does so, according to Descartes, by producing a motion at the incited part. This is communicated to the pore by the thread, and causes it to open, the consequence of which is that the "animal spirit" contained in the ventricular cavity enters the tube, and is conveyed by it to the various muscles with which it is connected, so as to produce the appropriate motions. The whole system, although it was placed under the supervision of the "âme raisonnable," which had its office in the pineal gland, was capable of working independently. As instances of this mechanism, Descartes gives the withdrawal of the foot on the approach of hot objects, the actions of swallowing, yawning, coughing, etc. As it is necessary that, in the performance of these complicated motions, the muscles concerned should contract in succession, provision is made for this in the construction of the systems of tubes which represent the motor nerves. The weakness of the scheme lies in the absence of fact basis. Neither threads nor pores nor tubes have any existence.

(h) The dates of the discoveries relating to this subject here referred to are as follows:—Muscular structure of arteries, Henle, 1841; function of cardiac vagus, E. H. Weber, 1845; constricting nerves of arteries, Brown-Séquard, 1852, Aug. Waller, 1853; cardiac centre, Bernard, 1858; vascular centre, Schiff, 1856; dilating nerves, Schiff, 1854; Eckhard, 1864; Lovén, 1866. Of the more recent researches by which the further elucidation of this mechanism by which the distribution of blood is adapted to the requirements of each organ, the most important are those of Ludwig and his pupils and of Heidenhain.

experiment on the living animal, notwithstanding that its structure affords no indication whatever of its fitness for the function it is destined to fulfil. To judge of the complicated nature of this function we need only consider that in no single organ of the body is the supply of blood required always the same. The brain is, during one hour, hard at work, during the next hour asleep; the muscles are, at one moment, in severe exercise, the next in complete repose; the liver, which before a meal is inactive, during the process of digestion is turgid with blood, and busily engaged in the chemical work which belongs to it. For all these vicissitudes the tract of grey substance which we call the *vascular centre* has to provide. Like a skilful steward of the animal household, it has, so to speak, to exercise perfect and unfailing foresight, in order that the nutritive material which serves as the oil of life for the maintenance of each vital process may not be wanting. The fact that this wonderful function is localised in a particular bit of grey substance is what is meant by the expression "automatic action of a centre."

But up to this point we have looked at the subject from one side only.

No state ever existed of which the administration was exclusively executive—no Government which was, if I may be excused the expression, absolutely absolute. If in the animal organism we impose on a centre the responsibility of governing a particular mechanism or process independently of direction from above, we must give that centre the means of being itself influenced by what is going on in all parts of its area of government. In other words, it is essential that there should be channels of information passing inwards, as that there should be channels of influence passing outwards. Now, what is the nature of these channels of information? Experiment has taught us not merely with reference to the regulation of the circulation, but with reference to all other automatic mechanisms, that they are as various in their adaptation as the outgoing channels of influence. Thus the vascular centre in the medulla oblongata is so cognisant of the chemical condition of the blood which flows through it, that if too much carbonic acid gas is contained in it, the centre acts on information of the fact, so as to increase the velocity of the blood-stream, and so promote the arterialisation of the blood. Still more strikingly is this adaptation seen in the arrangement by which the balance of pressure and resistance in the bloodvessels is regulated. The heart, that wonderful muscular machine by which the circulation is maintained, is connected with the centre, as if by two telegraph wires—one of which is a channel of influence, the other of information. By the latter the engineer who has charge of that machine sends information to headquarters whenever the strain on his machine is excessive, the certain response to which is relaxation of the arteries and diminution of pressure. By the former he is enabled to adapt its rate of working to the work it has to do.

If Dr. Whytt, instead of cutting off the head of his frog, had removed only its brain—i.e., the organ of thought and consciousness—he would have been more astonished than he actually was at the result; for a frog so conditioned exhibits, as regards its bodily movements, as perfect adaptiveness as a normal frog. But very little careful observation is sufficient to show the difference. Being incapable of the simplest mental acts, this true animal automaton has no notion of requiring food or of seeking it, has no motive for moving from the place it happens to occupy, emits no utterance of pleasure or distress. Its life processes continue so long as material remains, and are regulated mechanically.

To understand this all that is necessary is to extend the considerations which have been suggested to us in our very cursory study of the nervous mechanism by which the working of the heart and of arteries is governed, to those of locomotion and voice. Both of these we know, on experimental evidence similar to that which enables us to localise the vascular centre, to be regulated by a centre of the same kind. If the behaviour of the brainless frog is so natural that even the careful and intelligent observer finds it difficult to attribute it to anything less than intelligence, let us ask ourselves whether the chief reason of the difficulty does not lie in this—that the motions in question are habitually performed intelligently and consciously. Regarded as mere mechanisms, those of locomotion are no doubt more complicated than those of respiration and circulation; but the

difference is one of degree, not of kind. And if the respiratory movements are so controlled and regulated by the automatic centre which governs them that they adapt themselves perfectly to the varying requirements of the organism, there is no reason why we should hesitate in attributing to the centres which preside over locomotion powers which are somewhat more extended. But perhaps the question has already presented itself to your minds, What does all this come to? Admitting that we are able to prove (1) that in the animal body Product is always proportional to Process, and, (2) as I have endeavoured to show you in the second part of my discourse, that Descartes' dream of animal automatism has been realised, what have we learnt thereby? Is it true that the work of the last generation is worth more than that of preceding ones?

If I only desired to convince you that during the last half-century there has been a greater accession of knowledge about the function of the living organism than during the previous one, I might arrange here in a small heap at one end of the table the physiological works of the Hunters, Spallanzani, Fontana, Thomas Young, Benjamin Brodie, Charles Bell, and others, and then proceed to cover the rest of it with the records of original research on physiological subjects since 1831, I should find that, even if I included only genuine work, I should have to heap my table up to the ceiling. But I apprehend this would not give us a true answer to our question. Although, etymologically, Science and Knowledge mean the same thing, their real meaning is different. By science, we mean, first of all, that knowledge which enables us to sort the things known according to their true relations. On this ground we call Haller the father of physiology, because, regardless of existing theories, he brought together into a system all that was then known by observation or experiment as to the processes of the living body. But in the "Elementa Physiologiæ" we have rather that out of which science springs, than science itself. Science can hardly be said to begin until we have by experiment acquired such a knowledge of the relation between events and their antecedents, between processes and their products, that in our own sphere we are able to forecast the operations of nature, even when they lie beyond the reach of direct observation. I would accordingly claim for physiology a place in the sisterhood of the sciences, not because so large a number of new facts have been brought to light, but because she has in her measure acquired that gift of prevision which has been long enjoyed by the higher branches of natural philosophy. In illustration of this, I have endeavoured to show you that every step of the laborious investigations undertaken during the last thirty years as to the process of nutrition, has been inspired by the previsions of J. R. Mayer, and that what we have learnt with so much labour by experiments on animals is but the realisation of conceptions which existed two hundred years ago in the mind of Descartes as to the mechanism of the nervous system. If I wanted another example I might find it in the previsions of Dr. Thomas Young as to the mechanism of the circulation, which for thirty years were utterly disregarded, until, at the epoch to which I have so often adverted, they received their full justification from the experimental investigations of Ludwig.

But perhaps it will occur to some one that if physiology founds her claim to be regarded as a science on her power of anticipating the results of her own experiments, it is unnecessary to make experiments at all. Although this objection has been frequently heard lately from certain persons who call themselves philosophers, it is not very likely to be made seriously here. The answer is, that it is contrary to experience. Although we work in the certainty that every experimental result will come out in accordance with great principles (such as the principle that every plant or animal is both, as regards form and function, the outcome of its past and present conditions, and that in every vital process the same relations obtain between expenditure and product as hold outside of the organism), these principles do little more for us than indicate the direction in which we are to proceed. The history of science teaches us that a general principle is like a ripe seed, which may remain useless and inactive for an indefinite period, until the conditions favourable to its germination come into existence. Thus the conditions for which the theory of animal automatism of Descartes had to wait two centuries, were (1) the acquirement of an adequate knowledge of the structure of the animal organism, and (2) the development of the sciences of physics and chemistry ; for at no earlier moment were these sciences competent to furnish either the knowledge or the methods necessary for its experimental realisation : and for a reason precisely similar, Young's theory of the circulation was disregarded for thirty years.

I trust that the examples I have placed before you to-day may have been sufficient to show that the investigators who are now working with such earnestness in all parts of the world for the advance of physiology, have before them a definite and well-understood purpose, that purpose being to acquire an exact knowledge of the chemical and physical processes of animal life, and of the self-acting machinery by which they are regulated for the general good of the organism. The more singly and straightforwardly we direct our efforts to these ends, the sooner we shall attain to the still higher purpose—the effectual application of our knowledge for the increase of human happiness.

The Science of Physiology has already afforded her aid to the Art of Medicine in furnishing her with a vast store of knowledge obtained by the experimental investigation of the action of remedies and of the causes of disease. These investigations are now being carried on in all parts of the world with great diligence, so that we may confidently anticipate that during the next generation the progress of pathology will be as rapid as that of physiology has been in the past, and that as time goes on the practice of medicine will gradually come more and more under the influence of scientific knowledge. That this change is already in progress we have abundant evidence. We need make no effort to hasten the process, for we may be quite sure that, as soon as Science is competent to dictate, Art will be ready to obey.

HYRTL'S "LEHRBUCH DER ANATOMIE DES MENSCHEN."—In his preface to his new edition, Prof. Hyrtl observes that the fact is unprecedented of a work on anatomy having undergone fifteen editions and seven translations in thirty-four years; and he attributes much of its success to the careful manner in which each edition has been brought up to the period of its publication.—*Allg. Wien. Med. Zeit.*, August 16.

CHOLERA STATISTICS IN AUSTRIA.—In the *Wiener Med. Woch.* of July 30, Herr Krafft, of the Statistical Bureau, furnishes the particulars of the outbreaks of cholera that have occurred in Austria. Without going into the details which he supplies, we may state that there have been five distinct visitations, viz. :—First, that of 1831-32, with 182,331 deaths (being 0·77 per cent. of the whole population in 1831, and 0·37 in 1832); second, that of 1847-51, with 290,800 deaths, or 0·47 of the population in 1847, 0·61 in 1848, 0·28 in 1849, 0·21 in 1850, and 0·05 in 1851; third, that of 1854-55, with 158,072 deaths, or 0·02 of the population in 1854, and 0·84 in 1855; fourth, that of 1866, with 165,292 deaths, or 0·84 of the population; fifth, that of 1872-73, with 127,705 deaths, or 0·10 of the population in 1872, and 0·51 in 1873.

THE POSITION OF THE NEGRO IN THE DARWINIAN HYPOTHESIS.—A writer in the *Louisville Med. News*, August 13, commenting upon some muscular anomalies described by Dr. Cilley, of the Ohio Medical College, refers to the fact that rudimentary organs are much oftener found in the negro than in whites. Thus, with regard to the *plantaris* and *psoas parvus* muscles, the former, as a rule, seems better developed in the African ; and while the latter is, according to Theile, present only in one of twenty in white subjects, it is found at least in one of six negro subjects, and well developed. So too the *lineæ transversæ* in the aponeurosis of the external oblique are much more conspicuous in the black, the aponeurosis being in general thicker and coarser. Indeed, the general coarseness of structure observed in the negro is a fact apparent to all who have dissected subjects of both races. "These observations, taken together with the flattened cranium and nose, thick lips, and prognathous jaws of the unmixed African, and the scanty development of the calf-muscles, which anyone may observe in the negro children who run bare-legged in the streets, would seem to indicate that in going from the Caucasian to the negro we approach more nearly the Darwinian progeniture of man, and we believe that a careful study of the comparative anatomy of the races would elicit some important facts bearing upon this interesting subject."

ORIGINAL COMMUNICATIONS.

INSTANCES OF THE

EVOLUTION OF EPIDEMICS AND THE ALLIANCES OF SOME DISEASES.

By WILLIAM H. PEARSE, M.D. Edin.,

Senior Physician to the Plymouth Public Dispensary; late of the Government Emigration Service.

(*Concluded from page 292.*)

I PROCEED to group some phenomena, under the hypothetical term, "shock," which illustrate the first deviations out of health, coincident with changed habitat from the land to the sea, and from tropical to higher latitudes, and in the hope that they may be suggestive of a right method of viewing the greater phenomena of epidemics in general.

On Shock on Changed Physical Environment, and the Evolution of Epidemics.

Taking as an example that deviation of health to which natives of India are most liable—viz., intermittent fever—the following table shows the influence of *changed* physical conditions on the evolution of this disease :—

Intermittent, etc., Fever.

				Ship Alnwick Castle.	Ship Arabia.	Ship Oasis.
1st week	...	...	...	250	17	15
2nd "	...	...	...	20	14	9
3rd "	...	...	...	14	3	6
4th "	...	...	...	17	5	10
Total for 1st month	...	301	39	39
5th week	...	...	...	6	3	3
6th "	...	...	...	14	6	2
7th "	...	...	...	10	3	2
8th "	...	...	...	3	6	0
Total for 2nd month	...	33	18	7

Bowel Complaints.

1st week	...	...	...	26	67	22
2nd "	...	...	...	34	38	20
3rd "	...	...	...	27	15	34
4th "	...	...	...	53	19	20
Total for 1st month	...	140	139	96
5th week	...	...	...	21	12	15
6th "	...	...	...	11	25	9
7th "	...	...	...	21	13	7
8th "	...	...	...	27	35	4
Total for 2nd month	...	80	88	35
9th week	...	...	...	11	15	5
10th "	...	...	...	17	10	11
11th "	...	...	...	11	1	5
12th "	...	...	...	5	0	8
Total for 3rd month	...	44	26	29

The first effect of a *change* to the sea, on the systems of a people who had been habitated in an Indian climate and soil, etc., was an outbreak of their most accustomed deviations—diseases—viz., intermittent fever and bowel complaints.

Similarly, the ship *Liverpool*, from Calcutta to Trinidad, West Indies, experienced an outbreak of severe sloughing ulcers. Seven cases developed in the first week ; seven in the second week ; none showed in the four following weeks. The cases were vast and rapid sloughs, extending generally from small previously existing sores. It need hardly be said that the change from the land to the sea is, in its *first* influence, a shock or depression to the system.

The power of changed physical conditions as the occasion for the evolution of disease is well shown when people on a voyage suddenly enter the westerly wind and colder regions after a passage through the tropics.(a)

The iron ship *Accrington*, of 2000 tons, embarked in Southampton, in June, 1862, for Melbourne, 43 men, 336 women, 27 boys, and 30 girls under twelve years of age.

(a) These westerly wind latitudes, which extend over latitudes from about 23° or 30° N. or S., to about 70° N. or S. lat., receive that stratum of air which, ascending at the equator, is over the tropics the *upper stratum* of air. (See Maury's "Physical Geography of the Sea.")

An outbreak of sore-throat happened, whose weekly returns are as follow :—

Weeks.	Dates.	Places.	Sore-throat.
1	To June 11 ...	Southampton	...
2	To June 18 ...	Channel	...
3	To June 25 ...	Tropics	1
4	To July 2 ...	North Tropics...	8
5	To July 9 ...	Equator	...
6	To July 16 ...	Passed South Tropic	7
7	To July 23 }	80° to 40° S. lat.	{ 2
8	To July 30 }		{ ...
9	To Aug. 6 ...	40° to 44° S. lat. ; Cape to St. Paul's...	17
10	To Aug. 13 ...	40° to 44° S. lat.	19
11	To Aug. 20 ...	40° S. lat.	27
12	To Aug. 27 ...	Melbourne	5

Almost without exception, the affections of the throat occurred in young and healthy single women. The general course of the cases was the same. At my morning visit the girl would say that she noticed no change in her health till the previous evening, when a severe shivering had come on, followed during the night by great heat of body and sore-throat. On examination, I should find the pulse fast, skin hot; tonsils red, swollen, and thickly studded with dirty-looking whitish specks. By the second evening, in almost all cases, heat, fast pulse, and pain had disappeared, and the patient was again passing rapidly to health. One case only did not thus rapidly recover—Morrish, male, aged seventeen, on the seventh day was as follows :—"Fauces natural colour, few spots on tonsils ; is pale, weak, sweats on nose and upper lip ; pulse 120 ; pain in abdomen ; aching of limbs ; tongue soft, large, and tremulous."

The marked commencement of the epidemic was in 12° S. lat., with the thermometer gradually falling, and with the greater tonic influences or shock of the wind when a ship is "braced up," than when sailing before the wind.

This epidemic illustrates two general facts :—1. The latent or contained capacity of the system for epidemic evolutions. 2. That the epidemic was coincident or corelated with changed and "depressing" physical or vito-physical environment. We shall surely not seek any "specific" poison or germ cause. Such epidemics of sore-throat are often experienced in the same latitudes on similar voyages.

Continuous throughout the voyage were cases of insidious bronchitis affecting the smaller air-tubes. On taking a deep breath, small moist rĳles were heard at the lower and back parts of the lungs, but without noticeable dulness on percussion. Such local changes were coincident with shivering, aching of limbs, general dulness of mind and energy, tremulous tongue, and some acceleration of pulse. The weekly return of such cases was about as follows :—1, 2, 3, 2, 3, 3, 3, 3, 4, 4, 0, 2.

Were they "fever" or were they "bronchitis"? Were these cases—of, say, bronchial colds or fever—of one primary course with the sore-throat cases. I have seldom made a voyage without seeing cases of bronchial colds," with associated "fever"-like malaise. In one ship, the *Star of the South,* of 1200 tons, from Liverpool to Melbourne, many young men and women died. The cases, during the earlier weeks of the voyage, presented only a trifling amount of small crepitation at the lower and back parts of the lungs ; the patient would be indisposed some days, but rarely confined to bed. As the voyage progressed, cases assumed a more serious aspect : the simple malaise had all the appearance of fever ; many died. Cases were more numerous, and of the worse type, in those who slept near deck openings. This epidemic established in my mind the conviction that "fever" and "epidemic bronchitis" were sometimes of one nature and order, and that the distinctions which our definitions give of disease (of the great "fever" group) do not exist on a wider view of nature.(b)

The ship *Accrington* presented a series of cases, which I entered as "colds"; their weekly numbers were 1, 0, 0, 3, 0, 1, 0, 3, 10, 2, 0, 1. The symptoms in these cases were sometimes well-marked shivering, followed by a little lassitude or aching of limbs ; in others, the aching of limbs and

(b) I am unable to fill in the exact numbers and detail of the ship *Star of the South* (1857). What I have written above is what I wrote many years ago, when I had access to my "journals" of the voyage. On re-applying for use of my journals to the Colonial Office, I received a reply (February 24, 1881) to the effect that the journals had been destroyed.

general dulness, coming on without marked shivering, would hang about the patient several days.

In the various instances I have adduced, shall we look for some "poison" or "germ" as the cause of the epidemic outbreaks of intermittent fever, diarrhœa, sore-throat, ulcers "bronchial fevers," "colds," etc.?

It appears to me far more philosophical to say that, with the altered physical and vito-physical existences or environment (whose corelations and whose correlations(c) with vital "energy" are so almost wholly unknown in their exact relation to life) involved in a change from the land to the sea, or from a tropical to a higher latitude, the body loses some of its accustomed and necessary corelations ; deviations of rate and loss of conserving power happen ; and disease, of varied degrees and types, naturally appears or evolves.

It is more than probable that a practice based on a narrow germ or poison theory has had a bad influence, leading us to excessive ventilation, and to the adopting of depressing influences, where a protective and conserving method was the true one.

It appears to me that the facts and experiences I have adduced, and the ideas which flow from them, have a very wide application to the phenomena of epidemics in great countries and communities—*e.g.*, the Rev. Dr. Haughton, in his "Lectures on Physical Geography," writing of the N.E. monsoon (the trade wind), which follows in Ceylon the S.W. monsoon, and which is a dry wind, and a vast *change* from the moist S.W. monsoon, says :—"The land wind (N.E.) is a dry chilling wind, and you instinctively feel that it is dangerous . . . . at night it is still more dangerous, and sitting even for a short time after dark in a verandah in this wind is to be avoided . . . . . it brings with it colds of all sorts, fevers, agues, and dysentery. Cholera, too, comes with the N.E. monsoon, during which it is more frequent than with the S.W. (monsoon)."

It must be plain that, under such conditions, the wise physician would seek to conserve the vital "energy" of the body by warmth, rest, diet, and perhaps also by some powerful co-ordinators of the vital correlations (quinine, arsenic, alcohol, etc.), rather than to be battling against hypothetical "poisons," "germs," etc. As pointing to general natural tendencies towards disease in their relation or corelation to general climatic changes, I may refer to cholera in India. From Drs. Lewis and Cuningham's Reports it appears that the heat-curve rises in Calcutta from 65° in January (lowest of the year) to 85° in April ; the cholera-curve rises with it. The cholera-wave, however, subsides earlier than the heat-wave. A second rise of the cholera-wave is in November, coincident with a fall of temperature in October and November of from 85° to 75°. Thus the earliest extreme of heat, and at the winter season the earliest extreme of cold, are two annual points of increase of cholera. Sir Ranald Martin also showed from the experience of the General Hospital, Calcutta, that the highest admissions from cholera were for the hot season (in May), and for the cold season (in November), the admissions in November being higher than in any months excepting April, May, and June.

Gradations of Type.—I have already adduced instances of the evolution, and also of the non-specific type, of epidemic diseases under changing physical environment. I will further adduce one other voyage as illustrating the gradation of type of disease. The ship *Tarquin* sailed from Plymouth for Adelaide on August 20, 1864, having on board 62 married couples, 105 single men, 49 single women, 21 boys, 23 girls, and 13 infants.

The following table gives the history of the voyage. It seems just to class the scarlet fever, the sore-throat of various kinds, the "colds," the bronchitis, and diarrhœa, as of one order. This is not *proved* by the fact of association, but the impression was ever being suggested to my mind when I was in daily presence of the phenomena. Even in one family, one member showed malignant scarlet fever, with eruption, sore-throat, and long-continued brain symptoms ; another showed sore-throat only ; another, slight sore-throat, with lassitude ; and another, the slightest sore-throat, but with lassitude, shivering, "aching of bones" etc. If such varied appearances exist, where are we to draw the line of a "specific" difference between the most severe case and the "cold" only? Many practitioners will see no

(c) I use the "corelation" in the sense of Darwin ; and "correlation" in the sense of Grove.

| Weeks, No. ... ... | 1. | 2. | 3. | 4. | 5. | 6. | 7. | 8. | 9. | 10. | 11. | 12. | 13. | 14. | 15. |
| Weeks ending ... | Aug. 27. | Sept. 4. | Sept. 11. | Sept. 18. | Sept. 25. | Oct. 2. | Oct. 9. | Oct. 16. | Oct. 23. | Oct. 30. | Nov. 6. | Nov. 13. | Nov. 20. | Nov. 27. | Dec. 4. |
Places		Tropic			Equator		Tropic			Cape		St. Paul's			Adelaide.
Scarlet fever with eruption:															
Throat affected	2	1	...	...	...	1	1	1	1	...	...	...	...	...	...
Throat not affected	...	...	...	1	...	...	1	...	...	...	...	...	...	...	...
Severe affection of tonsils, with severe general symptoms ...	...	1	...	...	...	1	...	1	...	1	...	...	...	...	...
Dirty-brown tonsils, and severe general symptoms	...	...	...	1	...	...	...	...	...	...	...	...	...	2	...
Jagged tonsils, and non-severe general symptoms	...	...	...	...	2	...	1	...	...	...	1	1	1	...	...
White specks on tonsils, and non-severe general symptoms	...	...	...	1	...	...	...	...	...	3	...	...	...	...	...
Patchy back of pharynx	...	...	...	...	...	...	...	6	...	...	...	...	...	...	1
Red pillars of tonsils and swollen uvula	...	...	...	...	...	1	1	...	...	1	...	3	1	2	...
First, some form of sore-throat, bronchitis following	...	...	...	...	1*	...	...	1*	...	...	...	3*	...	...	...
First, some form of sore-throat, diarrhœa following... ...	...	...	...	...	...	...	...	...	...	...	1*	...	...	...	...
"Aching bones," "Can't keep heat in me," after shivering...	...	...	...	...	2	...	...	3	2	...	...	3	...	1	2
These latter ending in bronchitis ...	...	...	...	...	...	...	...	...	2	2	...	...	...	4	...

Those marked * are included amongst the other cases of sore-throat.

difficulty in the alliance of the malignant scarlet fever cases and the varied sore-throat cases, but the type merged as markedly into the less defined "colds."

If the varied facts I have adduced establish the evolution of certain epidemic types of disease, and if the prevailing types of certain great classes of disease change with altered environment, we must then relinquish the doctrine of the "specific" as a final doctrine, and rather seek a wider "form" and generalisation, and which "form," embracing a wider view and greater time, shall include those facts which have given birth to the doctrine of the "specific," and we shall lean to a view which regards epidemics as latent "contained variabilities" of the body and of race made manifest by changed physical corelations.

Co-ordination.—Just as we have seen the evolution of disease, with changed latitudes and "climate," so further was seen the phenomenon of the arrest of epidemics with changing climate. Not viewing epidemics as "entities," having fixed and definitive qualities, there exists an almost à priori presumption that the deviations of the systems rates (epidemics) which evolve on certain, and especially on the first, changes of climate to the sea, would cease or modify with longer continued and thus habituated "climate" of the voyages; but I will state some facts. The ship Tarquin, having on board 335 souls, showed a case of small-pox, the first day after leaving Plymouth for Adelaide. The case was severe and confluent. None followed during a voyage of fifteen weeks. The man was separated from the other people to the utmost of my power. Many were successfully vaccinated during successive weeks.

The ship Oasis, Calcutta to Demerara, sailed September 2, 1865, with 446 souls. No case of measles occurred during the eleven weeks, after crossing the Line in the fourth week.

In the ship Arabia, Calcutta to Demerara, no cases of small-pox or chicken-pox occurred during the last five weeks of the voyage, when west of the "Cape."

The most complete co-ordination we know of is, that when the system has once passed through certain changes—say, e.g., scarlet fever—the body's capacity for that change is (in the main) exhausted for the future. Absolutely fixed amounts of change are not essential for the exhaustion of this latent capacity; thus, vaccination co-ordinates against small-pox.

"Acclimatisation," or the gradual corelation of the system to its environment (a true and actual correlation in fact), has a great place in the "form" of co-ordination; to this head will belong the "glaring instance" that negroes can undergo, with perfect enjoyment of health, the heaviest field labour in the deltas of Guiana, and the yet more "glaring instance" that the aborigines of Australia cannot take scarlet fever. The Rev. G. Taplin, missionary to the South Australian aborigines, says that measles is extremely rare among them; "this is remarkable when we remember the devastation caused by this disease in Polynesia. I have never known a case of scarlet fever among the aborigines, although it was very prevalent some years ago among the whites, and there is

reason to believe that a great deal of clothing from houses infected by the disease was given to the natives."

Certain vegetable products and mineral elements—quinine, opium, alcohol, arsenic, etc.—seem also co-ordinators against some fevers.

The instances I have given, from voyages, can only be stated as "arrests of epidemic disease," or the co-ordination of the system against epidemic rates with change of "climate."(d)

The instances I have cited, under the word "co-ordination," will serve to show the vast relations which epidemic phenomena have to the entirety of physical existences. The relations are cosmic: no mind has yet arisen which has grasped the facts and grouped them, as Coleridge says, with "illuminating idea," into a harmonious generalisation.

Just as the astronomer reaches the laws of all motion in the universe by the study of the movements of simple bodies; and as the chemist reaches universal laws by the analogies of the simplest changes; so, in the far more difficult and complex domain of the Organic, light may be reached from simple and common facts, if they be viewed in a right method.

There cannot be two systems in the organic universe. The "unity of method" which the astronomer holds, in the movements of the spheres; the unity of method which the chemist holds (since the days of Lavoisier and Dalton and Grove), the method of the correlation and continuity of all force and action, must be extended absolutely to organic phenomena: we are thus led to view epidemics as natural deviations and evolutions, in true determinated series and corelation with physical external changes, and with vito-physical changes, within the body.

The facts of the germ and poison theories will form minor parts of a grander theory of evolution.

Be this as it may, the facts I have stated, both of the apparent evolution of epidemics and of the apparent co-ordination against epidemic rates, will, I hope, be of value. Whatever generalisation may eventually arise, it can only be of value in so far as it conforms to the unity and simplicity of nature.

It may be that the so-far isolated and experimental phenomena of voyages may help us to a right method, just as the comparative philologist finds the key to a world of languages in the study of a single dialect.

Herschel says(e)—"As far as our experience has hitherto gone, every advance toward generality has been, at the same time, a step toward simplification." And again (par. 10)—"We must never forget that it is principles, not phenomena—laws ('forms'), not insulated independent facts—which are the objects of inquiry to the natural philosopher." "As truth is single and consistent with itself, a principle may be as completely and as plainly elucidated by the most simple and familiar fact as by the most imposing and uncommon phenomenon."

(d) The word "climate" must be held to embrace all the physical existences, and their correlations, of the earth's atmosphere, of whose exact relation to life so little is yet known.
(e) Herschel, "Preliminary Discourse," par. 398.

REPORTS OF HOSPITAL PRACTICE
IN
MEDICINE AND SURGERY.

MIDDLESEX HOSPITAL.

CASE OF HYSTERICAL CONTRACTURE.
(Under the care of Dr. FINLAY.)

MARGARET D., aged twelve, was admitted to Seymour ward on July 14, 1880. She was the child of healthy parents, and had five brothers and sisters, all healthy. Her own previous history was devoid of importance, except that in the month of November, 1879, she had suffered from a mild attack of rheumatism. Shortly after this date she fell against a cart, striking the left side of her abdomen. This was followed by pain and swelling of the same side, and obstinate constipation. In spite of treatment the constipation and swelling increased, the urine was thick and scanty, and she frequently went two or three days without passing any at all. There was no history of fits, and she had never menstruated. She had been told that she had a "cancerous tumour" in her abdomen.

On admission she is described as a well-nourished, bright-looking girl, with ruddy complexion, complaining of constipation, swelling of the abdomen with pain and tenderness, and inability to move the left leg. She describes the pain to be like "needles running through her side," and refers it chiefly to the left iliac region, where tenderness on pressure appears to be very excessive. The belly is prominent, measuring twenty-eight inches in girth at the level of the umbilicus; it moves tolerably freely with respiration. It is slightly more prominent on the left than on the right side; there is no ascitic wave nor enlargement of cutaneous veins, and the resonance over it is everywhere tympanitic. The left leg and foot are rigidly extended and adducted, the toes being flexed; and any attempt to move the leg or foot is apparently productive of great pain, both in the leg and in the abdomen. There is no wasting, both legs being equal in size; cutaneous sensibility is unimpaired, and faradic contractility somewhat diminished; percussion over the spine causes no pain. In the chest percussion and breath-sounds are everywhere normal; but there is a faint systolic murmur heard over the præcordia, most marked at the heart's apex. The urine has a specific gravity of 1010, is neutral and free from albumen. The temperature is 99·8°; pulse 98; respirations 26.

Shortly after admission she had two enemata, after which her bowels were freely opened, slightly after the first, and more copiously after the second; the motions were formed and dark in colour. Evening temperature 98·6°; pulse 84.

Next day (15th) she said she was unable to pass water, and had been shivering in the night; seventeen ounces of clear urine were drawn off by the catheter. The condition of affairs was pretty obvious, but as no very complete examination of the abdomen could be made, owing to the apparent tenderness when it was touched even lightly, the patient was put under the influence of chloroform, when the swelling of the abdomen at once subsided, the girth being now found to be twenty-four inches and a half. The rigidity of the leg also disappeared, and it could be freely moved about in all directions. As she came out of the anæsthetic condition the belly visibly swelled up, and the leg returned to its rigid state. In the evening it was observed that when she was asleep both leg and abdomen were perfectly normal in appearance. She was ordered a cold shower-bath every morning, and to have the leg and abdomen faradised daily.

This treatment was continued, with the addition of an occasional enema and aperient pill, till the 27th, when she was again anæsthetised, the left leg bandaged on a McIntyre splint, with the knee flexed and the foot placed in the natural position, and kept so. The splint was then slung. She slept well the following night, and experienced no discomfort from the altered position of the leg. Next day the splint was removed, and the leg at once returned to its former state.

On August 2 it was noted that she could bend her left a little, but could not evert the foot. The abdomen remained as before, but she could keep herself more upright in moving about the ward than she had done at the time of admission.

On August 5 the improvement was still more marked; and on the 16th the notes stated that the abdomen was much less tender, although still distended, and she could flex the knee-joint more. On the day following the girth of the abdomen was twenty-seven inches, her bowels in the meantime having been well opened.

On the 21st she could bend her knee almost to a right angle, and on September 2 she was able to go into the garden.

On September 28 the child could walk perfectly upright, and with but slight turning-in of the left foot; and on October 8 she was discharged able to walk perfectly well, the abdomen being soft and free from tenderness, and the turning-in of the left foot scarcely noticeable.

During all the time of her stay in hospital she had housemedicine or other aperient or enemata about every other day.

Remarks.—The foregoing case is a well-marked instance of hysterical contracture, the appearances of which are figured by Professor Charcot in his "Lectures on Diseases of the Nervous System" (New Sydenham Society's translation, page 294). Among the more noteworthy points in the present case may be remarked the absence of anæsthesia or analgesia, and of convulsive attacks either previously or subsequently to the appearance of the contracture, and the gradual progress towards recovery. The last point is perhaps the most interesting; for recovery, when it does take place in such cases, seems usually to occur suddenly under the influence of some strong mental emotion.

MANCHESTER ROYAL INFIRMARY.

PARALYSIS OF THE ABDUCTORS OF THE VOCAL CORDS IN A PATIENT AFFECTED WITH LOCOMOTOR ATAXY.
(Under the care of Dr. MORGAN.)
[We are indebted to Dr. STELL, Resident Medical Officer, for this case.]

J. G., clogmaker, married, had contracted syphilis sixteen years ago, which speedily yielded to treatment. He enjoyed good health till three years before admission, when he suffered from numbness in the left hand, gnawing and shooting pain in the left shoulder. This was followed by pain in the back of the neck. He noticed also that he could not stand with his eyes closed, and had often experienced shooting pains in the legs. He had already been told by his medical man that he was suffering from locomotor ataxy. Two years ago his walking and the pains in his legs became worse, and he was unable to see distant objects with the right eye. These symptoms persisted more or less; his gait became very awkward, and he began to suffer from a sensation of tightness round the chest.

He was admitted into the Infirmary on April 1, 1881, presenting the characteristic features of locomotor ataxy, and the following is a brief outline of the patient's condition on May 7, when I saw him:—Patient is well built, healthy looking. Lower Extremities: Characteristic ataxic walk; no atrophy of limbs; no paralysis; cutaneous sensibility slightly blunted and delayed; sense for pain and for temperature normal; muscular sense deficient; cutaneous reflexes normal; tendon reflexes absent. Upper Extremities: Slight ataxy—cannot execute delicate movements, such as buttoning his coat; muscular sense affected; no paralysis; no atrophy; cutaneous sensibility slightly impaired and markedly delayed; no other abnormalities. There is no pain in the head; no vertigo; no oculo-motor paralysis; Argyll Robertson's symptom is present; no optic neuritis; no affection of facial or trigeminal nerve. The speech of the patient is not affected; his voice is clear, not husky. He experiences, on walking, slight dyspnœa; during sleep, his breathing is accompanied by a loud stridor, of which the patients in the beds close by complain very much. Laryngoscopic examination shows marked paralysis of the abductors on inspiration, while the adductors are not affected. There are no other symptoms pointing to any other portion of the pneumogastric being affected. There have never been any gastric crises. The pulse is normal. The bladder and rectum are not affected; the urine, of normal colour, reaction, and quantity, contains neither albumen nor sugar.

The temperature is normal. The patient stayed in the hospital from April 1 to May 12, his symptoms remaining unchanged.

Remarks (by Dr. Dreschfeld).—The paralysis of the abductors of the cord in this case is either an independent or idiopathic affection, or a complication of the locomotor ataxy from which the patient suffers. In idiopathic cases the affection produces much more distressing symptoms, runs, as a rule, a rapid course, and the symptoms do not remain stationary for any length of time. The paralysis is much more likely, therefore, in this case to be due to a central cause, probably in the nucleus of the pneumogastric, and the laryngeal affection to be closely connected with the primary disease. Paralysis of the vocal cords (whether of abductors or of adductors) is, however, but rarely seen in ataxia. Eulenburg ("Nervenkrankheiten," page 150) mentions it as a complication. I have, however, not been able to find any case in which the ataxy was associated with paralysis of the abductors of the cord. Burow (*Berl. Klin. Wochenschrift*, 1879, No. 33 and 34) has tabulated all the cases (thirty-six in number) recorded up to then; and Mackenzie ("Diseases of the Throat and Nose," page 452) gives the further literature of the cases; but amongst all these cases I do not find a single one in which locomotor ataxy formed the primary disease. Mackenzie (*loc. cit.*, page 426) quotes a case of Charcot's, in which paralysis of the cords complicated ataxy, producing so-called "laryngeal crisis." On referring, however, to the case in the *Gazette des Hopitaux*, 1879, No. 1), I find that the laryngoscopic examination in that case was made by Krishaber, who believed the case to be one of spasm of the adductors of the cord, instead of paralysis of the abductors. Charcot's case, however, bears somewhat on the case given above, as showing the implication of the laryngeal nerves in locomotor ataxy.

TERMS OF SUBSCRIPTION.

(Free by post.)

British Islands	. . . .	*Twelve Months*	.	£1 8	0
" "	. .	*Six*	"	. 0 14	0
The Colonies and the United States of America	}	*Twelve*	"	. 1 10	0
" " "	.	*Six*	"	. 0 15	0
India " "	.	*Twelve*	"	. 1 10	0
" (*viâ Brindisi*)	.	"	"	. 1 15	0
" "	.	*Six*	"	. 0 15	0
" (*viâ Brindisi*)	.	"	"	. 0 17	6

Foreign Subscribers are requested to inform the Publishers of any remittance made through the agency of the Post-office.

Single Copies of the Journal can be obtained of all Booksellers and Newsmen, price Sixpence.

Cheques or Post-office Orders should be made payable to Mr JAMES LUCAS, 11, *New Burlington-street, W.*

TERMS FOR ADVERTISEMENTS.

Seven lines (70 words)	.	.	.£0 4	6
Each additional line (10 words)	.	.	0 0	6
Half-column, or quarter-page	.	.	1 5	0
Whole column, or half-page	.	.	2 10	0
Whole page	.	.	5 0	0

Births, Marriages, and Deaths are inserted Free of Charge.

THE MEDICAL TIMES AND GAZETTE *is published on Friday morning: Advertisements must therefore reach the Publishing Office not later than One o'clock on Thursday.*

Medical Times and Gazette.

SATURDAY, SEPTEMBER 17, 1881.

HAHNEMANN, HOMŒOPATHY, AND HOMŒOPATHS.

No ONE has failed to notice the somewhat singular prominence given, at the recent meeting of the British Medical Association, to a subject which had been for years tabooed. Even the events connected with the death of the Earl of Beaconsfield were hardly in themselves sufficient to account for the stir all at once made in connexion with the recognition of homœopaths; and suspicious ones found an opening for the suggestion that the word had been passed round once more to raise the dread spectre with a view to its being laid for ever. It is perfectly well known that many professing homœopaths have, by various ways, been enabled to enter the ranks of the British Medical Association, and office-bearers could hardly help taking to heart the anomalous position of men thus belonging to an Association in whose bosom homœopathy was held to be an accursed thing. It would have hardly been worth while to recall these memories—for memories they are—until further action had been taken, but in the meantime the tone of certain of the homœopathic publications is that of conquerors all round—a tone which is probably premature, certainly unpleasant, and thoroughly misleading. It is for these reasons, and whilst the whole matter may be said to be within the region of calm conferred by time, and that Gallio-like indifference which with many passes for breadth of view, that we again venture to say a few words on a subject which to us is thoroughly hackneyed. Homœopathic writers are fond of complaining that those whom they call allopaths have never taken the trouble to study their system. Heaven knows the labour of doing so is tedious, but a sufficient number of our craft have had the courage to wade through the mass of verbiage and windy observation which it contains, and by which it is overlaid, to be able to judge of it, so that it is in vain that any such cry should be raised at the present moment.

Putting all these matters on one side, then, it seems to us that the questions at issue, and which, whether ignorantly or on purpose, have been constantly mixed up, may be classed under the three headings we have roughly indicated by the heading of our article.

First, we should say what no homœopath will surely deny, the law, as it is called, of "similars" must be taken as the keystone of their whole system. Some would have it that this is a law valid, to all intents and purposes, as the law of gravitation. These say, "*Similia similibus curantur*"—roughly in English, "Like cures like." Others, not quite so bold, only say that the so-called law helps them in the selection of their remedies. If there is any such law it ought to be discussed in exactly the same way as we would a question of astronomy, altogether independently of its alleged discoverer.

Secondly, as we have just said, the application of this law may with advantage be considered altogether independently of the character and teaching of its reputed discoverer. But many believers in the law of similars will not do this. They will persist in introducing the personality of Hahnemann, and thus lay themselves open to scathing rejoinder.

Thirdly, there are few homœopaths among us at the present day who are purely Hahnemannians. They have learned more and must know more than he did. Surely homœopathy cannot be the only thing which does not advance. Practically, therefore, we have, as a profession, and as social beings, to deal with those men who are around us and mix with us in various capacities, and to whom alone, it is well to note, the words of the various speakers at Ryde had reference. Homœopaths were freely spoken of; not a word was said in support of what may be called Hahnemannism or of Homœopathy.

Well, then, as regards this supposed law of similars. Two modes of investigating it are open to us. First, we may adopt the *à priori* method, the weakness of which in most cases we are quite willing to admit, but which in this case is of unusual strength. According to the homœopathic ———— the efficacy of a remedy increases more and mo from the *simile* to the *similior*, and even to the *simillimum*, but the moment that the last becomes, instead of like, identical, it only intensifies the mischief. *A priori*, we should say such a law has much inherent improbability in it. But, secondly, we may test the law by its applications to particular instances; and here it is to be remembered that the burden of proof rests with those who advocate its general applicability, rather than with those who deny it. Still, tried in this way, we make bold to say that it entirely fails. There is not a single remedy—except among those which act only locally, as by irritating the skin or the bowels—which produces the same effect as does disease, and at best the resemblance between the effects of the two is of the most superficial and remote description. We say that the burden of proof remains with the homœopaths when they assert that this superficial similarity is any guide or key to the selection of a remedy for any form of disease, though we by no means deny that certain substances may be useful in certain cases, whatever the degree of similarity or dissimilarity in the symptoms produced by them and by the disease. The proof and test of the value of a remedy in a given form of disease is experience, and experience only. That the physiological effects of a drug, as ascertained by experiment and observation, are of incontestable value as an aid to its application in practical medicine, no one will seek to deny; but not so the fancies, fads, and whims of an individual who, after taking a certain dose of it, sits down deliberately to record all the abnormal sensations which may crop up in his mind whilst under its supposed effects. No; there are symptoms and symptoms, whether produced by drugs or by disease. But, under any circumstances, the effects of a drug, and its efficacy in the treatment of disease, must be tested at the bedside; and here the vast majority of our professional brethren say that the law of similars has failed in their hands when fully and duly tried in that bright light which beats around the bedside in a fully equipped and active medical school, where no work can escape acute and jealous criticism. Furthermore, if such a thing as disproof were possible in these matters, it was effected by a member of our profession, whose experiments, made with the utmost care, were published years ago, but the results of which have been studiously ignored by the younger and more ardent votaries of the law of similars. These experiments were made on healthy young men, and had reference to a certain number of the most notable remedies we possess; but in no instance where these were given in notable doses were any effects produced at all similar or even analogous to the diseases for which they were supposed to be specifics. So much for the so-called law of similars, which, as we allege, tried by whatever test you will, does not exist; nor even where it has a seeming existence is it of any value as a practical guide to the cure of disease.

Next as to Hahnemann himself. We have always thought that it was a misfortune for any system to be indelibly associated with the name of its founder. To take a kindred mystery, if we might use the word, few know even the name of the founder of what is called Hydropathy. Few who use water as a means of cure now adhere to the modes or the modes of treatment practised in days gone by at the first institute of the kind, but for many Hahnemannism and Homœopathy have remained identical. In our way of thinking, any elaborate inquiry into the views of Hahnemann are needless, but one or two main facts stand forth prominent in the history of his life. In the first place, Hahnemann had a very poor medical training. He took to real medicine late in life, and honourably maintained himself by means of his classical knowledge during the earlier period of his medical areer. The loss of an early and good professional training

is to medical men unspeakable, for we have ever found that those who take to medicine by way of second thoughts and with preconceived ideas are ever more prone to be led astray by will-o'-the-wisps in the shape of vain doctrine, —to seek for a ready way to knowledge by means of hypotheses, or even more pure imaginings, than by that hard work which clinical and pathological medicine imply. Then Hahnemann, mystic as he was by nature and training, had the misfortune to be persecuted for his beliefs—first by exclusion from the pages of *Hufeland's Journal*, and latterly and more distinctly for dispensing remedies without being duly qualified by law to do so. It is to this last fact, so they say, that is due Hahnemann's recourse to exceedingly small doses, such as could be easily transmitted by letter, as he was in the habit of doing. In this direction his progress was rapid. From small doses he speedily came to those which may be described as infinitesimal, invoking as his main argument the well-known fact that substances in different quantities do not produce the same effects, and further calling in the mystic doctrine of dynamisation, whereby he pretended that shaking or agitation imparted greater energy to the material particles the smaller they became. These two—*infinitesimal doses* and *dynamisation*—we take to be the prime errors of Hahnemannism. They need not of necessity have anything to do with the law of similars: they are an excrescence on the application of that so-called law, and have constituted the chief difficulty as regards the intercourse between ordinary and homœopathic practitioners; and it is not easy to see how men taking such doctrines as guides to practice can be well received by those who think both a delusion and a snare.

This leads us to our third point. There are many men, who, whilst believing in the law of similars, neither use infinitesimal doses nor believe in dynamisation. They are, in many instances, clever, well-educated men, and, as we have already said, it is with men that we have to deal. We cannot see that it would be possible for us to meet in consultation a man who insisted only on the application of our skill in diagnosis, and persisted thereafter in treating the mutual patient with some inert substance dynamised by the thirtieth or fiftieth dilution. But we can easily see that it would be possible to meet a man who merely says, I have found this rule of similars a help to aid and guide me in the selection of an appropriate remedy in any given case. We repeat again—there is Hahnemannism and there is Homœopathy.

ROSES, EUNUCHS, AND MONKS.

ALL knowledge, it has been shown, may be resolved into the recognition of resemblances and differences. Therefore the consideration of the points of likeness between things not obviously alike, and not generally put side by side, cannot be uninstructive. There does not seem much, and, superficially viewed, of course there is not any, likeness between the so-called queen of flowers and the most despised of human creatures; nor again, between the latter and the recluse whom at one time all Christendom regarded as the highest type of humanity. But, scientifically, there is a close analogy, and upon this analogy we propose to offer some remarks.

The rose, as everyone is aware, in a wild state is a small flower, with very little smell, and by no means one of the handsomest members of the floral family. The rose we are accustomed to look at with admiration, and whose odour we inhale with so much delight, is the product of cultivation, which has succeeded in changing its sepals and stamens into petals. In other words, changes, which we consider improve its beauty, have been produced in it at the expense of its reproductive organs.

Centuries ago, it was a customary thing to deprive youths of the power of propagating their species, for the purpose of preserving and further developing their admired soprano voices. Just as we rob the rose of its reproductive function for the sake of procuring smell, colour, and size of flower, and, by careful selection of the specimens to be submitted to this process, do actually get a result of great value and beauty, so the experts of the middle ages, by judicious choice of the subject from whom they removed the parts essential to generation, produced that marvellous quality and compass of voice for which the *evirati* were valued. Scientifically, both are monstrosities.

We have passed from vegetable to human pathology. Let us now go a step further, into the realm of mental phenomena. The monk, by a rigorous self-discipline, stamps out all thought of the joys of family life, puts from him all cares of fatherhood, and thus, dwarfing one side of his nature, develops in excess another: attains an emotional exaltation, a vividness of realisation of the things unseen, which cannot be attained among the anxieties, struggles, and disappointments of the outer world: a state of strong feeling which is communicable, by burning words and speaking gestures, to others less fervid, and the possession of which has made the lives and writings of such men—St. Bernard, for instance—among the most precious possessions of the world.

But, by maiming and dwarfing one set of faculties, we do not always get a result which is desirable. The deprivation of one function is not an advantage to the individual. Eunuchs have not always beautiful soprano voices, and the corruptions of monastic life have been often enough described. Whether the sexless rose will always be as much admired as it is, we will not discuss. Examined closely, with the aid of a magnifying glass, the barren repetition of petals does not present anything like the variety of beauty offered by the stamens, pistil, anthers, and pollen of the perfect flower. In diversity of form, delicacy of texture, and sweetness of colour, the natural state of the plant is superior to the monotonous uniformity of the blossom which is the result of the gardener's interference.

As we have said, it is not every eunuch in whom a fine soprano voice exists; and even then a more informed and cultivated taste prefers the resonant natural harmony of the manly bass or tenor to the artificial treble: so that were the question considered solely upon musical grounds, the production of *evirati* would not now be considered worth the trouble. And when we think also of the degradation of character, of the imperfect development both of mind and body, which we know to be the result of sexual nullity, no one can regret the abandonment of the practice. In the countries which at present lead the van of civilisation, the tendency is to regard monastic institutions as evil. In Protestant countries this is a matter of course. But even in Catholic countries, where the historic Church that claims to be "holy, catholic, and apostolic" is most revered, the religious communities of celibates have been put down and scattered by the strong arm of the law. And this is not because the Catholic ideal of religious perfection is dissented from, or not understood, or not valued, but because it has been found by the experience of generations that for one spirit that soars above the mass of mankind, the monasteries produce scores who only differ from the average in the greater ignorance, stupidity, idleness, and selfishness, that are the result in a commonplace individual of the absence of the healthy stimulus to toil that family cares and burdens give, and of the want of objects capable of inspiring unselfish affection.

In short, roses, eunuchs, and monks are alike in this—that they are imperfect, maimed, deficient. The deprivation of the reproductive function generally only produces a monstrosity, a defective specimen, but sometimes the result is rare, beautiful, and precious; the force ordinarily given to the reproduction of the species being turned to something else.

Mr. Herbert Spencer has laid down the general law that the higher the degree of evolution, the lower the reproductive power; and hence follows the speculation that the human race will die out—that, as its perfection progresses, reproductive power will fail. Whether the artificial changes we have referred to be improvements or not, they are such as, if imitated, would lead to the extinction of the type. Those who admire them may justify their preference by classing them with those changes in the organism which, by making it more complex, capable of more varied function, render it also more liable to be put out of gear. Were we to pursue this subject into another of its branches, we might point to social organisms, to Egypt, to Assyria, to Greece, to Rome, as instances in which high civilisation has led to national decay and death, and inquire whether the changes in the habits and customs of nations which high civilisation and aggregation in large cities bring with them have any analogy with the development of double roses. But to do so would take us into historical researches hardly fitting these columns; to say nothing of the differences between a flower and a nation. But there are analogies: we leave it to our readers' meditations to trace them.

THE WEEK.

TOPICS OF THE DAY.

EXTENSIVE preparations are being made in Dublin for the forthcoming meeting of the Social Science Congress, to be held there early next month. According to the present programme, on the evening of Monday, October 3, Lord O'Hagan, as President, will deliver the inaugural address in the Exhibition Palace. The next day, at ten o'clock, the Right Hon. Dr. Ball, as President of the Department for Jurisprudence and Amendment of the Law, will open the proceedings of the section with an address, which he will deliver in Trinity College. In the same hall the presidential addresses of the other departments will be delivered at ten o'clock on each successive morning, namely—"On Education," by Sir Patrick J. Keenan, K.C.M.G., C.B.; "On Health," by Dr. Cameron, M.P.; "On Economy and Trade," by Mr. Goldwin Smith; and "On Art," by Lord Powerscourt. The meetings of the sections will take place simultaneously each day in the New Buildings, Trinity College. On Saturday, the 8th, the united meeting of the Council will be held, and the place of meeting for next year fixed. During the week, garden parties and *conversazioni* will be given by some of the leading citizens and learned societies. The Statistical and Social Inquiry Society of Ireland will hold a *conversazione* in the Royal College of Surgeons, and the Lord Mayor will give a similar entertainment in the Mansion House.

During the month of July last there were registered in the eight principal towns of Scotland the births of 3588 children; of these, 3246 were legitimate and 342 illegitimate, the latter constituting 9·5 per cent. of the whole number. During the same period, the deaths of 1900 persons were registered in these eight towns; this is the smallest number recorded in the month of July for the last ten years, and it is 518 under the average, due allowance being made for increase of population. A comparison of the deaths registered in the eight towns shows that during the month under notice the mortality was at the annual rate of 16 deaths per 1000 persons in Edinburgh, in Dundee, and in Aberdeen, 18 in Greenock and in Leith, 21 in Glasgow and in Perth, and 23 in Paisley. The Registrar-General for Scotland further shows that during July the miasmatic order of the zymotic class of diseases proved fatal to 269 persons, and constituted 14·2 per cent. of the whole mortality. This rate, however, was much exceeded in Perth, where 9 deaths, or 17·3 per cent. of the mortality, were caused by whooping-cough. Fever caused 29 deaths; of these, 12 were tabulated as typhus, 16 as enteric, and 1 as simple continued fever. Whooping-cough caused 54 deaths, measles 52, diarrhœa 49, scarlet fever 31, diphtheria 19, and small-pox 2. The deaths from inflammatory affections of the respiratory organs (not including consumption, whooping-cough, or croup) amounted to 340, or 17·9 per cent.; those from consumption alone numbering 282, or 14·8 per cent.

A movement has been set on foot at Portsmouth for the establishment of a local Sanitary Protection Association, which it is intended shall undertake the supervision of the drainage arrangements of private houses, so as to insure their proper sanitary condition. A meeting in furtherance of these views was recently held under the presidency of Mr. Alderman Cudlipp, the ex-Mayor. The Association proposes, as a supplementary object, to enable its members to procure practical advice on moderate terms, so as to obtain the best means of remedying defects in houses of the poorer classes.

The Town Council of Evesham has recently decided to adopt a scheme for supplying the borough with water by gravitation from springs in the Broadway Hills, six miles distant. The owner of the springs, Mr. Edgar Flower, of Stratford-on-Avon, has dealt liberally with the Corporation, and the whole scheme, inclusive of the necessary pipes, hydrants, etc., is estimated to cost £10,250. The matter, although only recently concluded, has been under consideration for nearly ten years.

A scheme has been suggested by some of the leading engineers in America to utilise the vast water-supply of the extreme north of that country. By closing the northerly outlet of the valley of the Mackenzie River at the line of 68°, and thus storing up the water of 1,260,000 square miles, to which could be added the water of other large areas, a lake would be formed of about 2000 miles in length by 200 of average width, which would cover with one continuous surface the labyrinth of streams and valleys which now occupy the Mackenzie valley. It would prove a never-failing feeder for the Mississippi, and would connect with Hudson Bay and the great lakes, and also with the interior of Alaska through the Yukon and its affluents. The connexion of the Upper Mississippi with Lake Mackenzie would be a comparatively easy matter, and a vast amount of navigable waterway would be added to this river. The formation of Lake Mackenzie would also contribute to the proposed ship canal from Cairo (Illinois) to the Gulf St. Lawrence by the almost straight line which cuts the Wabash Valley, the Lakes Erie and Ontario, and the Lower St. Lawrence.

At a recent meeting of the Bristol Sanitary Committee the Medical Officer reported sixty cases of typhoid fever in one of the houses of Müller's Orphan Asylum. The outbreak was, up to that time, confined to one of the houses in which little girls were placed, and some of the cases were reported to be serious. The water-supply is from wells within the Asylum grounds, and this is undergoing a careful analysis. Every precaution has been taken to prevent the spread of the outbreak, and latest accounts assert that it has not extended to any other inmates of this extensive institution; but as there are no less than five houses filled to their utmost capacity with children, much anxiety prevails, and the resources of the managers have been taxed to the uttermost.

A statement recently appeared in some of the morning journals, to the effect that the Camp Hospital at Darenth,

established by the Metropolitan Asylums Board for convalescent small-pox patients, would shortly be closed, and that no patients would be admitted after the first of the present month. A letter from the Clerk to the Managers has, however, been published, stating that, as the policy of the Managers respecting the future of this camp-hospital must, in a measure, depend upon the course the epidemic may take during the approaching autumn, the adoption of any decided steps would, for the present, be premature. Consequently, we may assume that this very useful and efficient method of dealing with convalescent small-pox patients will not be abandoned for the present.

The Local Board of Brentford, acting on the advice of Captain Galton, to whom the sixteen plans lately submitted in competition for the drainage of the town were referred, have awarded the first prize to Messrs. Gotto and Beesley, of Westminster. The selected scheme deals with the sewage by chemical precipitation in tanks, to be constructed on land adjoining the Ealing Sewage Works, the sewage being pumped up from a pumping station at the riverside, close by the soap works. The estimated cost of the undertaking is £18,000.

THE NECESSITY FOR AN AMENDED BUILDING ACT.

IN his report on the sanitary condition of the Whitechapel district for the quarter ended January 1 last, Mr. John Liddle, the Medical Officer of Health, remarks that there can be no doubt that a new Building Act is imperatively demanded, seeing that the existing Act is extremely defective. Since the public at large cannot be expected to insist upon the proper sanitary points being observed in the building of houses, the officers of local boards of health should be required to carefully examine houses in course of erection, to see that all things requisite for health are duly attended to; and should be empowered to insist upon their suggestions being thoroughly carried out. The apathy of the public in matters of health is, Mr. Liddle thinks, truly lamentable; the dangers which arise from the imperfect construction of foundations, drains, water-closets, and walls are well known, and such dangers might be prevented, if during the building of houses all the sanitary arrangements were frequently inspected by the surveyor and health officers of local boards, and no dwelling were allowed to be occupied until the local board had certified, on examination, that it was in every respect fit for habitation. He adds that unless more stringent regulations are made and acted on in the construction of houses, the health of the people must necessarily suffer. At the present time the only thing that appears to be considered in the construction of houses is, how cheaply they can be erected and finished off; and from an economic point of view it will certainly be found to be less expensive to prevent the building of unhealthy habitations, than to have to alter them after they are built, so as to render them fit for occupation. To our readers there will be nothing new in Mr. Liddle's remarks; but he does well to bring any defects in the machinery of sanitary administration clearly, forcibly, and frequently before the authorities and the public.

THE NEWCASTLE-ON-TYNE INFIRMARY.

THE Newcastle-on-Tyne Infirmary, which was established so far back as the year 1751, for the sick and lame poor of Northumberland and Durham, has recently published its one hundred and thirtieth annual report, for the year ended March 31 last. From this it is to be gathered that a large amount of good work has been done, though at a somewhat increased outlay. No remarkable feature has occurred in the professional work of the institution, although it is worthy of mention that six cases of ovariotomy have been recorded, with only one death; in the previous year there were eight cases, with four deaths. The Infirmary has been in a remarkably healthy state during the whole of the past year, especially when the number of inmates is taken into account, and there has been no case of pyæmia; only four cases of erysipelas had to be recorded, all of which were very mild. Anæsthesia was induced in 323 out of 351 cases —with chloroform alone in 290 instances, with ether alone in 23, and in 10 cases chloroform was used first and anæsthesia was kept up by ether; no casualty occurred in their use. There was a very remarkable increase in the number of accidents; of in-patient accidents there were admitted 425, against 337 in the preceding year, an increase of 88; and of out-patient accidents 2190, against 1702, an increase of 488. The cases of compound fracture of limbs sufficiently serious to require treatment as in-patients amounted to 70, as compared with 36 last year, and 37 in 1878.79; they included 11 of the thigh, with 2 deaths; 1 of the patella; 37 of the leg, with 3 deaths; 9 of the foot, with 1 death; and 12 of the arm and hand, with 1 death. There were 136 deaths during the year, of which number 73 were medical and 61 surgical cases. Of the 73 medical, 27 were from diseases of the respiratory organs, 10 being from consumption. The continued high death-rate in the medical department of the Infirmary is attributable to similar causes to those referred to in the previous report, viz., the greatly prolonged and intensely cold winter, together with the pressure in the in-patient department, necessitating the exclusion of all but severe cases.

DR. ALFRED HILL ON THE HEALTH OF BIRMINGHAM.

IN his report on the health of the Borough of Birmingham for the first quarter of the present year, Dr. Alfred Hill, the Medical Officer of Health for the district, remarks that the deaths registered during that period show a considerable decline in number. They amount to 2133, which gives a death-rate for the quarter of only 21·29 per 1000 of estimated population, against rates of 27·06, 26·15, and 22·36 in the winter quarters of 1878, 1879, and 1880 respectively. This diminished total death-rate of the quarter is, Dr. Hill adds, partly owing to the smaller mortality from the seven principal zymotic diseases, all of which have been less prevalent during the quarter; and partly to the diminished death-rate from phthisis, the developmental class of diseases, and from most of the local diseases, particularly those of the respiratory organs, as compared with the average of the five preceding years; and [this, he thinks, is very remarkable and noteworthy, when it is considered how intensely and exceptionally cold the weather was during a great part of the first three months of the present year. The average age at death during the quarter was thirty-one years and two months, against twenty-seven years and two months in the first quarter of 1880, a rise principally due to the smaller fatality of the diseases of infant life. The quality of the town water-supply is stated to be much improved when compared with what was supplied from the same source at the commencement of 1880. In fact, Dr. Hill concludes his report by remarking that in most particulars it may be said to be very satisfactory, as showing progressive improvement both in the general and special health of the borough.

THE LATE DR. ROBERT SMITH.

WE are very sorry to record the death of Dr. Robert Smith, Assistant-Physician to Charing-cross Hospital. This makes the third of the junior staff of that Hospital who has died during the past twelve months. We defer further notice of Dr. Smith's work and character to our next number.

THE ANTISEPTIC SYSTEM IN CALCUTTA.

OUR contemporary, the *Indian Medical Gazette*, remarks that the question of Hospitalism occupies a prominent place in the reports of the Calcutta hospitals for 1880. Special reports from the surgeons of the Medical College Hospital show that there has been a great decrease in the number of cases falling under that designation. The first surgeon reports 15 cases with 9 deaths, and the second surgeon 23 cases with 13 deaths. These were all the instances of septic blood-poisoning observed in the surgical wards. Of the 38 cases, 16 were admitted with the disease fully developed; in the remaining 22 cases the symptoms commenced in the Hospital The improvement, as compared with the past history of the Hospital, is attributed to stricter attention to hygienic measures as regards the Hospital generally, the wards, and the wounds. The antiseptic treatment is carried out as carefully as is practicable in all cases, and the importance of wound hygiene, as well as of ward and hospital hygiene, is fully admitted and acted on.

CHOLERA AND FEVER IN BENGAL IN 1880.

THE report of the Sanitary Commissioner for Bengal for the year 1880 shows a great decrease in the number of deaths from cholera, and a considerable increase in the deaths attributed to fever. The number of deaths registered as due to cholera during the year amounted to 39,043, against 136,363 in 1879. The decrease is attributed to the heavy rainfall of the year. But, on the other hand, fever prevailed very severely in some districts of Central Bengal, and this is supposed to have been caused by the heavy rains in October. In one district, that of Nuddea, the deaths from fever amounted to 25,035, against 7014 in 1879. Complaints of obstructed drainage and bad water came from all parts of the province. In Calcutta itself there was less cholera in 1880 than in any year since 1871, the registered mortality being 805. The number of cases treated in hospital was 356, of whom 183, or 514 per 1000, died; and this rate of mortality was considered an unusually favourable one.

THE SWANSEA HOSPITAL.

CERTAIN recent occurrences at the Swansea Hospital are not without interest to our profession. It appears that this Hospital was originally situated on the sea-shore, and thus was able to give its patients the benefit of sea-bathing. This advantage was prominently set forth in its report, formed part of its fundamental laws, and was drawn attention to in its appeals for funds. Some years ago its site was acquired by a railway company, and the Hospital was rebuilt some distance from the sea, no special provision for sea-bathing being made. When sea-baths were ordered, all that was done was that the porter fetched one or two tin cans of water from the sea. Notwithstanding this deficiency, the Committee continued, year after year, to largely advertise the Hospital as one which provided sea-bathing for its patients. Dr. T. D. Griffiths, of Swansea, the Ophthalmic Surgeon to the Hospital, and well known as one of the most scientific and highly respected of provincial practitioners, felt that this was wrong, and repeatedly drew the attention of the Committee to it, but without any result. In July last, a child suffering from scrofulous disease of the eyes was sent by the Cirencester Guardians, on the advice of their medical officer, to the Swansea Hospital, that it might have sea-bathing. Dr. Griffiths, under whose care the child came, felt it his duty to inform those who had sent her that the supposed facilities for sea-bathing, on account of which they subscribed to the Hospital and had sent the child there, did not exist. He mentioned that he had pointed out this anomaly to the Committee of Management, but that the majority were in favour of still "gulling the public." This led to a correspondence between the Guardians and the Hospital Committee, in which Dr. Griffiths's letter came before the latter body, who were so incensed by the term " gulling the public," that they asked Dr. Griffiths to resign. He refused to do so, and by the rules of the Hospital the Committee could not enforce their request unless their action was confirmed by a general meeting of the Governors. Such a meeting was therefore held. Dr. Griffiths explained that he had not intended by his language to reflect on the personal honour of individual members of the Committee ; but he justified it as applied to their corporate action. The result of the meeting was that the Committee's resolution, asking Dr. Griffiths to resign, was rescinded ; and that large subscriptions were promised to provide the bathing accommodation which was wanting. Dr. Griffiths has thus rendered a public service to the town of Swansea ; and we beg leave to congratulate the Swansea Hospital on possessing the services of a gentleman clear-sighted enough to see his duty, and bold and resolute enough to incur the risk of personal unpopularity and professional and pecuniary injury in doing it.

SIR JOHN KIRK, M.D., K.C.M.G.

THE Queen has been graciously pleased to give directions for the promotion of John Kirk, Esq., M.D., C.M.G., Her Majesty's Agent and Consul-General at Zanzibar, to be an Ordinary Member of the Second Class, or Knights Commanders of the Most Distinguished Order of St. Michael and St. George. Sir John Kirk, who was born in 1833, took his M.D. degree at Edinburgh in 1854. He was one of the Assistant-Physicians of the Civil Medical Staff of the British Hospital at Renkioi during the Crimean War, and afterwards Naturalist and Chief Officer in Dr. Livingstone's second exploring expedition to the Zambesi River in 1858. After six years' employment there, his health gave way, and he came home ; but returned to Africa as Acting Surgeon to the Political Agency at Zanzibar. Not long after, he was appointed Vice-Consul at that place, and, passing through the grades of Assistant-Political Agent and Agent, he was, in January last year, appointed Agent and Consul-General. Like many other English medical men, Sir John Kirk has rendered important service in the spread of civilisation. He induced the Sultan of Zanzibar to engage in the suppression of the slave trade in his dominions ; he was a friend of, and a co-worker with, Livingstone ; and he greatly aided other African explorers.

THE PARKES MUSEUM.

THIS Museum is closed until the end of September. In October it will again be opened free to the public on Tuesdays, Thursdays, and Saturdays ; and, during the winter, lectures on sanitary science will be given in the Museum. The lectures will be illustrated with the sanitary appliances deposited in the Museum, which now include many new contributions sent from the recent Medical and Sanitary Exhibition at South Kensington. We believe it is intended to distribute the awards to the exhibitors at the Exhibition at the second public annual meeting of the subscribers to the Museum in October or November.

WHY DOES LABOUR COME ON ?

DR. A. GEYL, of Dordrecht, has, in the *Archiv für Gynäkologie*, applied the Darwinian theory to answer the questions, to which so many more or less imperfect replies have been given :—Why does labour come on ? and, Why does it come on at the end of the ninth month ? Dr. Geyl's view is this : that it depends upon an inherited tendency to expel the child as soon as it has reached the stage of development most favourable to its separate existence, and yet permitting

of its passage through the pelvis. A woman with a tendency to expel the child; too soon, before it was properly viable, or to retain it too long, till it was too big to traverse the pelvis, would not of course transmit this peculiarity to any descendant. And it is obvious that the offspring of those mothers who expelled their young at precisely the most favourable time, when the greatest degree of development compatible with safe delivery had been reached, would have a better chance of surviving than those born a little too early or too late. Dr. Geyl explains the wide differences in the duration of pregnancy by supposing that peculiarities in this direction are transmitted ; i.e., given a race of women with small pelves, it would be to the advantage of that race, if with the small pelvis went a tendency to the expulsion of the child before it had got very big ; in the absence of that tendency the race would die out. If this were the only cause, it is plain that in the same woman pregnancy ought to always last nearly the same length of time. Dr. Geyl adduces some, but very incomplete, evidence in support of his theory. The theory, however, if true, is not an explanation. We have yet to know the mechanism by which such adaptation is effected.

THE HEALTH REPORT ON WORCESTER FOR THE YEAR 1880.

THE seventh annual report of Dr. William Strange, Medical Officer of Health to the Urban Sanitary Authority for the city of Worcester, for the year 1880, states that the general health of the population during the period under notice compares most favourably with the returns of any former year. The number of deaths registered was only 710, and, estimating the population by the Registrar's rule at 35,200, the death-rate will be found to have been exactly 20 per 1000 per annum. This is the lowest rate ever recorded in Worcester since the present sanitary regulations have been in force, and the lowest ever entered in the records of the city. The popular dread at present, Dr. Strange adds, is of fever or other infectious disorders, but the number of victims to the group of zymotic diseases is insignificant (thirty-nine in all) compared with the number who die from equally preventable causes. No doubt the year 1880 is below the average in this respect, since the city has been free from any epidemic for the last two or three years. It should not, however, be forgotten that it is especially against this class of disease that sanitary efforts are most effectual, and it cannot be doubted that vigilance in this respect has been rewarded by the satisfactory results which have now to be recorded. The results obtained from the erection of the Hospital for Infectious Diseases continue to justify the expense incurred in its establishment, for although there were only eight cases isolated in it during the past year, they were all cases which could not safely have been treated at home without detriment to the rest of the inmates. The mortuary and post-mortem room have also proved a great boon to the district. These few facts will, Dr. Strange thinks, justify the authority in feeling satisfied that the work of sanitary amelioration is being fairly and steadily carried out in Worcester.

THE PARIS WEEKLY RETURN.

THE number of deaths for the thirty-fifth week, terminating September 2, 1881, was 1015 (573 males and 442 females), and among these there were from typhoid fever 72, small-pox 19, measles 6, scarlatina 11, pertussis 6, diphtheria and croup 44, dysentery 1, erysipelas 9, and puerperal infections 7. There were also 48 deaths from tubercular and acute meningitis, 29 from acute bronchitis, 49 from pneumonia, 150 from infantile athrepsia (59 of the children having been wholly or partially suckled), and 29 violent deaths. The slight increase of 20 deaths would be regarded as one of the ordinary oscillations met with in the succession of weeks, but on examining into the cause of the increase we find that while deaths from athrepsia have decreased from 173 to 150 (though still too frequent during so moderate a temperature), those from typhoid fever have increased from 38 to 72; so that the deaths at ages between fifteen and thirty-five have increased to 237, while in the thirty-fourth week they were only 184; small-pox has also increased from 12 to 19 deaths. The deaths from measles have for some weeks been on the decline, those for the present week (6) being considerably under the mean; on the other hand, scarlatina, which in former years only caused three or four deaths per week, has this year caused from 10 to 15. Diphtheria, with its 44 deaths, remains well-nigh stationary. The births for the week amounted to 1129, viz., 573 males (434 legitimate and 139 illegitimate) and 556 females (410 legitimate and 146 illegitimate); 82 children (57 males and 25 females) were born dead or died within twenty-four hours.

SIR GEORGE C. M. BIRDWOOD, M.D., C.S.I.

Dr. GEORGE C. M. BIRDWOOD, C.S.I., of the India Office, upon whom the Queen has been pleased to confer the honour of knighthood, is the eldest son of General Christopher Birdwood, late of the 3rd Native Infantry, and Commissary-General, Bombay. He received his medical education at the University of Edinburgh, where he took his M.D. degree in 1854; and in the same year he became a Member of the Royal College of Surgeons of England, and entered the Medical Service of the late Honourable East India Company on their Bombay establishment. In 1855 he had medical charge of the Southern Mahratta Horse, Kalludghee; and afterwards was appointed, at different times, to the 2nd Brigade of Artillery at Sholapore, the 8th Madras Cavalry, the 3rd Bombay Native Infantry, and the Civil Station. In 1856 he went to the Persian Gulf in medical charge of the steamship Ajdaha and the detachment of Her Majesty's 64th Regiment: there he saw active service, and received the medal and clasp for the Persian War of 1856-57. In April, 1857, he was appointed Acting Professor of Anatomy and Physiology in the Grant Medical College. In the same year he was made Curator of the Government Central Museum at Bombay; and, with the aid of the late Dr. Bhawoo Dhajee and the leading native gentlemen, established the Victoria and Albert Museum and the Victoria Gardens in Bombay. In 1867 he was sent by Sir Bartle Frere, at the express desire of the leading merchants of Bombay, as Special Commissioner for the Government to the Universal Exhibition held in Paris; and on his return to India his services were acknowledged by his being appointed Sheriff of Bombay; and on the occasion of the proclamation of the Queen as Empress of India he was made a Companion of the Star of India. In 1869, Dr. Birdwood was obliged, on account of broken health, to leave India; and has since then chiefly devoted himself to writing on Indian subjects. Among other works, he wrote in 1878 "The Handbook to the Indian Court" at the Paris Exhibition of that year; and last year the handbook on "The Industrial Arts of India," published by the Science and Art Department in connexion with the Indian Museum. Two years ago (about) he was appointed Special Assistant in the Revenue, Statistics, and Commerce Department of the India Office, which appointment he still retains.

THE CENSUS OF 1881 IN VICTORIA.

THE increase in the population of this colony (the Australian Med. Journal for May states) is 70,000 short of the estimate formed from the yearly increase of births over deaths, and of immigration by sea over emigration—so that this large number must have passed overland into other colonies. The total population of Victoria in 1871 was 731,528, viz, 401,050

males and 330,478 females; and in 1881, 855,796, (448,510 males and 407,286 females)—the increase being thus 124,268, viz., 47,460 males and 76,808 females. The alteration in the population of the sexes is very striking. Thus, in 1871 there were 100 females to every 121 males, but now the proportion has risen to 100 to 110. This step towards greater equality of the sexes would be more welcome were it certain that it was not due to an efflux of males. The continued crowding towards Melbourne, too, is not a healthful sign, although the natural outcome of a policy framed for the encouragement of manufactures. The population of Melbourne was 139,916 in 1861, or 25·89 of the population of the colony; in 1871 it was 206,780, or 28·27; and in 1881 it is 280,836, or 32·81. While the population of the whole colony has increased by 17 per cent. during the last decade, Melbourne has gained 35 per cent. and the country districts only 9 per cent. There is also a great contrast between the numerical relations of the sexes in and out of Melbourne. In it and its suburbs there are 138,298 males and 142,533 females, or 97 males to 100 females; while in the country districts there are 310,212 males to 264,748 females, or 117 to, 100. The death-rate of Melbourne was only 19·23 per 1000 in 1879, while its average for the preceding eight years was 20·8.

VALUATION OF THE IMPURITIES IN POTABLE WATERS.

APART from any question as to the relative merits of the processes employed by different chemists for the estimation of the organic matters in water, it must be admitted that some uniform plan for comparing the general character of several waters, or of the same supply at different times, is much to be desired. The purpose for which an analysis is made is, in almost every instance, to obtain an opinion as to its fitness for drinking, yet, from the very various values assigned by men of equally high authority to one or other impurity, as indicative of recent or of remote contamination, it not unfrequently happens that analysts whose results are nearly identical give the most divergent opinions as to the suitability of a given supply for domestic use. To obviate these discrepancies by assigning a numerical value to certain units of each impurity, according to scale to be agreed on, and thus to be able to estimate and compare the total impurities in any number of waters, is the aim of a scheme proposed some time since by Mr. Wigner, and discussed at a recent meeting of the Society of Public Analysts. With regard to purely chemical tests, the difficulty of coming to a unanimity of opinion need not be great; but it is far less easy to apply such a method to the less determinate characters of colour, smell, and the results of microscopical examination. It is freely conceded by its author that any such scheme must for some time to come be merely tentative, but he trusts that by systematically translating into the terms of his provisional scale the results of the analyses of those waters whose sources, pollutions, and general characters are best known we shall be enabled to check and correct its inferences, to learn what particular impurities have been estimated above or below their true value, and thus at length to obtain a consensus of opinion. Even among the purely chemical impurities some difficulty will be experienced when, as in the case of chlorine, they may be of inorganic or organic origin, or of ammonia, which may be derived from peat or from sewage, and the deficiency of oxygen, which may be a negative character only. The scale provisionally suggested is as follows :—Colour, as seen in two-feet tube—blue, 0; pale yellow or green, 2; dark yellow or green, 4. Suspended matters—traces, 1; heavy traces, 2; turbidity, 4. Smell when heated to 100° Fahr.—of vegetable matter, 1; strong peaty, 2; offensive (i.e., animal), 4. Total solids, 5 gr. per gallon, 1; chlorine, ·5 gr. per gallon, 1; phosphoric acid, 2, 4, or 8, according to distinctness of traces; nitrogen in nitrates, ·1 gr. per gallon, 1; free ammonia, ·006,

1; albuminoid ammonia, ·001, 1; oxygen absorbed in fifteen minutes at 80° Fahr., ·002, 1; ditto in four hours, ·010, 1; hardness before and after boiling added together 5° (Clarke's), 1; heavy metals, slight traces 6, heavy traces 12. If any single valuation exceed 10, the excess is to be doubled and added thereto. Those waters whose chemical constituents fall short of 15 are of exceptional purity; and, allowing a maximum of 10 for physical characters, any water whose total valuation does not exceed 40 is considered as belonging to the first class: such, with occasional exceptions, are those supplied by the London water companies. The limit for a second-class water is at present put at 65. Anything beyond this is considered sufficient to condemn a supply altogether The scheme may need correction in many respects, especially as regards the relative importance of vegetable and animal impurities and deficient oxygenation, but it is certainly deserving of careful consideration by analysts dealing with waters of widely differing characters.

FROM ABROAD.

THE OBSTETRICAL AND GYNÆCOLOGICAL EMPLOYMENT OF CHLORAL HYDRATE.

AT a meeting of the Boston Gynæcological Society (Boston Med. Journal, July 7), Dr. Brown read a paper upon this subject, and observed that the property which renders this remedy so useful in obstetrical practice is the power which it possesses in so pre-eminent a degree of controlling all irregular, excessive, and abnormal muscular contraction. The power the hydrate is said to possess of preventing coagulation of the blood should also render it a prophylactic of great value in relation to cardiac thrombosis and pulmonary embolism. He summed up his statements as follows:— 1. Chloral hydrate may be safely and efficiently used in labour to relieve the pains of normal and of abnormal uterine contraction. 2. It suspends all undue reflex action and resulting pain of a tendency to retard labour. 3. Labour under its influence is of much shorter duration. 4. Its use in relieving pain is most striking and satisfactory when this is caused by abnormal and spasmodic muscular contraction. Dr. Weeks, while admitting the efficacy of chloral, thought its danger was somewhat underrated, and referred to the deaths tabulated by Dr. Kane in the New York Med. Record, in corroboration of his views. In obstetric practice we are always more or less exposed to the danger of collapse and hæmorrhage, and under such circumstances the patient would be poorly prepared for it if she had been previously for any time, and to any extent, under the influence of this powerful depressant. Dr. W. S. Brown observed, in relation to the excitant influence sometimes consequent on its continuous employment, that he thought it should be seldom so employed; and that in resorting to this drug we must use caution, as we should do with opium. There is here also the danger of forming a habit. He agreed with the writer of the paper that the hydrate is the best antispasmodic which we possess; and the presence of the excessive muscular action in parturition gives additional security in its use. If its therapeutical activity is dependent upon its conversion into chloroform in the blood, we can understand the uncertainty of its operation, for chloroform is the most treacherous drug known to the profession. Dr. Field expressed a strong feeling of surprise and disappointment at the general distrust or disapproval expressed in regard to a remedy which he had come, years since, to regard as indispensable and beneficent. He had not used it in parturition because he was perfectly satisfied with chloroform. This powerful remedy, dangerous or uncertain elsewhere, is safe here; for the researches first of Simpson and then of Campbell have failed to discover any case of death or injury to either mother or child from its use in private or hospital practice. Dr. Field believes that the hydrate is particularly safe with the young, and he has repeatedly prescribed five grains to a child under two years of age as a sleeping draught, with orders to repeat it once the end of an hour if not efficacious; and in cases de-

manding such resource, and with proper selection of cases, he feels perfectly safe in following this course. The hydrate, in toxic doses, is believed to act primarily upon the heart, and subordinately on the respiratory centre; and the heart, at least, ought to be especially strong in the young subject. But there must be no grave interference, on the part of disease, with the respiratory centre when chloral is given. He does not believe in the theory that the influence of chloral is dependent upon the extrication of chloroform, for a safe medicinal dose would not produce a quantity able to exert any influence; while the action of chloral is not anæsthetic, but soporific, and is not promptly set up and speedily over, as with chloroform, but rather slow in inception and of many hours' continuance. He always insisted that a sufficient dose of chloral should be given to produce positive physiological effects—fifteen, twenty, or thirty grains being given to an adult. To trust to five or ten is mere trifling, and the remedy had better be let alone. He had always felt great security in its use, and was not often disappointed in its effects; but had always carefully attended to the contra-indications:—First, chloral should either be avoided or given in greatly diminished doses, and with close watchfulness, in conditions indicating marked hyperalkalinity of the blood, whether this be produced by a course of alkaline medicine or be the result of disease; secondly, in decided asthenia of the heart; and thirdly (probably), in emphatic central congestion or inflammation. It is of the utmost importance that the chloral hydrate should be quite pure. Much mischief is done by administering the salt in too concentrated a state, and it must always be freely diluted—say one grain to a drachm. It is of necessity a bulky medicine, and there is no escape from the inconvenience. In some reports of deaths it is quite evident that herein lay the secret of the mishap, although the reporters were apparently unconscious of the fact. Concentrated chloral hydrate is a dangerous remedy, even within the limits of the therapeutical dose, and may kill, as a massive dose of oxalic acid sometimes does, almost instantly, as by shock and paralysis of the heart. Dr. Norris stated that in his large obstetrical practice he had never used chloroform, but of late years had largely resorted to chloral and found the progress of labour greatly expedited. He gives fifteen grains, and often repeats this every fifteen minutes, until sixty grains have been taken in all. He generally adds the bromide to the mixture in the ratio of one part to two of the chloral. Dr. Clarke remarked that his experience with the hydrate at the time of and after delivery has been very satisfactory, and unattended with any accident. It gives great relief in after-pains. The dose is from ten to fifteen grains. Of late he has often substituted croton chloral, which can be given in smaller dose and with less water, and occasions less burning of the mouth and throat.

ADMINISTRATION OF CINCHONA TO CHILDREN.

Having had several cases of intermittent fever lately in the Enfants Malades, Dr. Jules Simon addressed some observations (Gas. des Hop., August 25) to his class on the above subject. It is seldom, he observes, that powdered bark is administered to children; but still it is sometimes given, in café noir, after the age of four or five, in quantities of two or three grammes daily. For his own part, he prefers one or two grammes daily of the soft extract for children when more than two years old. Before that age it causes indigestion, as does also the vinum cinchonæ. Even the syrup can scarcely be borne while the child is still suckling. After the second year, the vinum is a very good medicine—that is, on the condition that it is prescribed properly. We may often see pale, anæmic little girls, for whom bark wine, iron, or phosphate of lime, etc., has been prescribed, and has done more harm than good. Certainly for the first few days a dessert-spoonful of cinchona wine given before a meal (as it is generally ordered) will produce a stimulus and a better appetite and tone; but the improvement is only temporary, and we soon find that the appetite is lost again, pains of the head supervening, and the child becoming nervous etc., Why is the improvement of so short a duration, and more apparent than real? Owing to a slight precaution being forgotten—the dilution of the cinchona wine with a little water. So diluted, and administered immediately before the meal, it will cause no inconvenience. Still, if, in spite of the addition of a small quantity of water, dyspepsia and headache should still supervene, or if constipation should occur, the cinchona should be suspended for a time. This addition of water to the wine is of very great importance, as is the suspension of the medicine when any great susceptibility exists; and the observation holds good also with regard to quinine wine. Syrup of cinchona is a tonic which may be given to a child after its fifteenth month, and the alcoholic tincture may be begun with after the second year —associating it advantageously with bitter preparations. The action of cinchona upon the alimentary canal is complex, giving tone, appetite, and slight constipation when properly administered, and inducing dyspepsia when given badly. It renders the pulse stronger, fuller, and more regular, and aids the development of the blood globules. It acts favourably on the nervous system when properly prescribed, but only does mischief when the precautions mentioned are not observed—producing stomachal vertigo and an irritability of disposition. Cinchona also has the property of diminishing the urinary secretion, and is contra-indicated in cases in which this is deficient.

Of the salts of quinia, the sulphate is the only one Dr. Simon employs, giving it in powder in café noir, or, when the child is old enough, in a wafer. Owing to its bitterness, it may be given in silvered pills of a centigramme each, which can be concealed in preserve. When the child refuses it thus, it may be given in solution, facilitating its tolerance and preventing griping by a little opium, which does not interfere with the effect of the quinine. It is best given immediately before meals. Quinine may also be given advantageously in an enema in rather larger doses and combined with a drop of laudanum. Used externally, in the form of an ointment made up with equal parts of lard, the quinia is only found in the urine by the third day in children above two years of age, and somewhat earlier in those who are younger.

THE INOCULABILITY OF TUBERCLE.

Dr. Whitney, Curator of the Warren Anatomical Museum, terminates an exhaustive review of recent investigations on this subject, which he read at the Suffolk Medical Society (Boston Med. Jour., July 28), with the following well drawn up conclusion:—

"The conclusion which we are obliged to draw is that there is still uncertainty in the matter, considering that all the experimenters are not agreed in the results which they have reached. It is true that almost all have obtained an eruption of miliary bodies after injections, inhalation, and feeding with what was presumably tuberculous material; but the interpretation as to what these really were has differed with the experimenters, the one side holding that they were simply inflammatory products, the other that they were true tubercles. Then, again, allowing that they are tubercles, is the tubercle the result of a specific process, or is it simply one of the expressions of inflammation that may arise as the result of various irritants?

"Taken by themselves, the latest expressions of Cohnheim, Tappeiner, and Orth, who are perhaps the more worthy of belief in that they have been able to avoid some of the errors of the earlier investigators, seem to point clearly to the fact that tuberculosis is an acute infectious disease; and Klebs has proposed for the nodules of syphilis, glanders, and tuberculosis the name of infectious tumours rather than that of granulation tumours, under which name they have been associated together by Virchow on account of their histological character; and Cohnheim has gone so far as to propose as a test for tubercle—not its histological structure, not its peculiar arrangement of cells, of varying size without vessels, and with a tendency to cheesy degeneration, but—its capability of inoculation. But, whatever may be the opinion of individuals, the mass of scientists have a right to demand more and clear proof; and it may confidently be expected, with the light thrown upon the subject already, that within the next five or ten years sufficient proof will be furnished to prove or disprove the question.

"So much for the scientific aspect of the question; and while we are waiting for this solution of the subject, there are hints thrown out in these experiments which may serve as guides in practice. It is with this in view that I have brought the experiments before you, according to the ways in which the substance has been introduced into the body; and these, as you remember, are by direct inoculation, by food, and by inhalation. The first need not detain us. As

to the second, there is little danger of directly eating tuberculous matter, it is true; but there is a disease of cattle which has only very slight anatomical differences from, and is believed by the greater part of observers to be identical with, human tuberculosis; and if the results obtained by certain experimenters are verified, it does not require a very acute mind to see the danger of infection that is run by all of us, but especially by children. Our present state of knowledge does not warrant us in getting up a popular excitement or scare on the subject; but it behoves us, as physicians, to thoroughly investigate the sources of supply when we place a patient on milk diet, and, above all, when we wish that a weakly child should have the milk of one cow, to be sure that that cow is healthy.

"The other possibility of infection lies in the atmosphere in the neighbourhood of tuberculous patients becoming charged with particles by their expectoration and coughing. And knowing how utterly powerless we are to cure the disease when once established, we should impress upon those in close proximity to the face of the sufferer, especially during the act of coughing. Also the great desirability of keeping a strong solution of carbolic acid or thymol in the vessels used for the reception of sputa, especially in hospitals, where these patients had perhaps best be kept in a separate ward."

GENERAL CORRESPONDENCE.

THE DISCUSSION ON "BATTEY'S OPERATION."

LETTER FROM MR. LAWSON TAIT.

[To the Editor of the Medical Times and Gazette.]

SIR,—There is such an evident intention of fairness on the part of your reporter of the proceedings in the Obstetric Section of the Congress, and the subject of the discussion on August 6 is so important, that I am quite sure you will allow me to make a few remarks upon some of the points raised.

It is perfectly certain that "complete cure" and "complete relief" are terms capable of different interpretations in the minds of different persons, but if those terms used upon my sheet be compared with the detailed accounts of some of the cases mentioned in it (published in a pamphlet which was reviewed some time ago in your own columns), I think there will be left no doubt as to the meaning I, at least, attach to those words. One of the cases, for instance, was that of a patient of Mr. Nason, of Nuneaton, who in the meeting corroborated my statement concerning it. For years before the operation this patient had been a helpless, bed-ridden cripple; by the operation all her sufferings were completely relieved, and she now follows the laborious occupation of a hospital sick-nurse. Such an instance as this I could multiply by a large number.

The criticism your reporter makes concerning the mistake in my having published a case as fatal when it turned out that the patient recovered and was cured, is a little ungenerous; I should have deserved what he said if the mistake had been the other way, and I think it would have been fairer if he had stated exactly what I said—that the mistake was not my own. Even if it had been, the explanation is simple. Nine years ago I had no idea that my practice in abdominal surgery would ever reach the proportions it now has, and at that time I was not in the habit of using a special note-book for each case, as all ovariotomists now do. The fact is, our critics submit us to an ordeal in the way of statistical investigation, to which they themselves cannot, will not, or dare not submit their own work. Such a mistake as this by no means involves your conclusion that my cases "cannot have been very carefully kept."

Unfortunately, I was obliged to leave the room before Dr. Duncan's speech was made, and therefore I am in possession of only second-hand information concerning it. If Dr. Duncan said that the menopause was not brought about by removal of the uterine appendages, he must have been singularly inattentive to the literature of the subject. I do not know what he may mean by ovarian neuralgia and hysteria, for these are certainly not terms which I can recognise as descriptive of any of the cases I have operated upon. For the relief of what he calls neurasthenic conditions I have operated only three times, and if this be what is called "Battey's operation," my experience of it is very limited. All of these three cases were operated upon for pronounced epilepsy, and we know that epilepsy kills hundreds of persons every year. In two of these cases life has been saved by the operation. If Dr. Duncan will either visit the Borough Asylum of this town; or will communicate with its superintendents, Dr. Green and Dr. Lyle; or better still, if he will read the account of the cases published in the *British Medical Journal* just a year ago, I think he will be satisfied of the accuracy of my statements.

Dr. Duncan's criticism of my table is singularly unfortunate. He says that I operated upon twenty-six cases of uterine fibroid. Not one of these cases answers his description. Uterine fibroids do not bleed: all of my cases were and have been described as bleeding myomata; and Dr. Duncan's own statements, as given in the book on "Diseases of Women" which he published in 1879 in conjunction with Dr. West, are quite sufficient for me as an authority upon the point that hæmorrhage from a uterine myoma is very fatal. And I have no hesitation in saying that, in twenty out of the twenty-one cases in which the operation was successful, life was saved. Should there be any scepticism in Dr. Duncan's mind upon this point, I shall be very glad to let the patients tell their own tales to him, or I will even send a few of them to him for his personal inspection. I can only say further, that it is a somewhat curious fact that Dr. Duncan should have had an opportunity of listening to a minutely detailed account of all these cases, when they were read before the Royal Medical and Chirurgical Society in London in May last, without taking advantage of it, and yet should now come forward and make such an altogether unjustifiable criticism as he has done.

Mr. Spencer Wells told the Section that he did not see cases in which he thought it necessary to extirpate the ovaries, and that perhaps they all went to Birmingham. It may be that this latter remark of his is nearer the truth than he intended it to be. When he says he does not see the cases, I can only explain his statement on the supposition that his memory has failed him. A considerable percentage of the cases in which I have operated have been under his own care, and I could easily recall to his recollection cases in which he has been consulted, in which he has interfered with the performance of the operation so that it was not done, and some of the patients have since died of the diseases for which it was proposed. I do not know any of them who have been benefited by what he substituted for the operation. I will remind him of only one at present, because it will also serve in some measure as a reply to Dr. Duncan. Some time ago, a lady was seen in consultation by Dr. Marion Sims, Mr. Spencer Wells, and myself. She suffered from a most serious nervous disease which was purely menstrual, which by several physicians had been regarded as hysterical, and which was clearly due to chronic ovaritis—at least, this was the opinion of Dr. Sims and myself. Everything had been done for her relief that ingenuity could devise, short of the removal of the uterine appendages, and the consultation I am speaking of was chiefly to discuss this point. Dr. Sims and myself were in favour of the operation, but Mr. Wells opposed the idea and pleaded for at least three months' delay, and to this Dr. Sims and myself reluctantly yielded assent. Unfortunately, however, before the three months had passed, the patient died of the disease for which the operation had been proposed.

Here, at least, is one case which Mr. Wells has seen, and one in which I feel perfectly certain, from my past experience, that a valuable life would have been saved if the operation had been performed; and of all the incidents of my experience in connexion with this operation, this one is the bitterest. Whilst I can fearlessly say that, so far, I have not had a single reason to regret performing the operation, I have already had a large number of reasons to regret its non-performance. I do not mean to say from this that all my cases so far have been successful. I fear that two or three of them, at least, may ultimately prove failures; but surely this is nothing unexampled in the history of a new operation!

Your reporter says, "It is indeed astounding that in a provincial town two surgeons should within ten years meet with more than 'a hundred cases in which this operation was absolutely necessary, while in the same time the

greatest living authority on diseases of the ovary found so few cases in which he could advise it that they could be counted on the fingers of one hand." Now, this sentence contains a series of mistakes which would occupy a great deal too much of your space to discuss, and besides, they will be, I think, fully entered into in a book now in the press. But let me here say that the astounding thing to me is, not that so many cases come to Birmingham, but that the hundreds, perhaps thousands, of women who are suffering from the diseases we are able to relieve here, should go about London from physician to physician, and from hospital to hospital, without obtaining relief.

The answer to the suggestion that Dr. Battey himself has operated so few times, and that therefore my cases must include a number of unnecessary operations, comes from Dr. Battey himself, who has visited me and has seen many of my cases. If he got my results, he told me, he would do many more cases. If I had not got the results I have had, I never could have continued the practice—that is, the primary results of the operation completely justify its performance if the secondary results are such as to lead to the relief of suffering.

Your reporter has largely mistaken the character of the cases, and the reasons for the operations. I do not blame him for this, because probably it is not in his line of business to follow out the literature of this speciality. Within the last two years I have written repeatedly upon this subject, and I have laid down the axiom, which so far has never been controverted, that when we find in the abdomen or in the pelvis such a condition as renders the patient's life a burden to her, our rule ought to be to open the abdomen and see what we can do. Acting upon my rule, I have been able to produce a list of cases of altogether new proceedings, and I should like to draw attention to the fact, which will strike any candid reader, that between March 14, 1874, and May 23, 1879, there is a blank during which not one of these operations was performed. Out of eight of the operations in the first period I had two deaths, and I did not feel myself justified in going on with such proceedings with only one-fourth the mortality the same as Mr. Wells's ovariotomy; but as soon as Dr. Keith showed me how to keep my ovariotomy mortality down to 3 or 4 per cent., I felt assured that many other efforts in abdominal surgery were justifiable. Since the second of these dates I have performed seventy-five such operations with only four deaths; and if I had my experience of these cases over again, two, or perhaps three, out of these four deaths would, I believe, be avoided. Let anyone look over the list, and he will immediately see that they are by no means all cases of the so-called "Battey's operation,"—most of them are cases in which I have acted upon the general principles of surgery, after having been able to throw aside the traditional fear of the peritoneal cavity. Take, for instance, the cases of hydrosalpinx and pyosalpinx. Nearly all of these cases had wandered about vainly seeking relief. Many of them had been treated by division of the cervix for dysmenorrhœa, amputation of the cervix for hypertrophy, dilatation in various ways had been employed, and therapeutical experiments of an infinite variety had been indulged in, without relief in a single instance; and now they are all completely and, I hope, permanently cured. In fact, they had been dealt with by a series of perfectly useless kinds of treatment, the result showing that the removal of the diseased organs was the only step which could be justified. Of course the ovary had to come away with the diseased tube, but these cases have nothing whatever in common with those in which it is proposed to bring about the change of life for some neurasthenic condition.   I am, &c.,   LAWSON TAIT.

THE RYDE ADDRESSES AND HOMŒOPATHS.

LETTER FROM DR. J. H. CLARKE.

[To the Editor of the Medical Times and Gazette.]

SIR,—One word in answer to your courteous remarks. The main point of your note on my letter I am well content to leave as it stands with your readers. When, however, you step aside to say that the instances of the homœopathic action of drugs are far too few to admit of induction, I cannot allow the assertion to pass unchallenged. Neither your assertion nor my denial of it—and I do deny it emphatically—nor any amount of à priori reasoning, will decide that question. For this nothing but a fair, candid, and complete trial will suffice. It is for this we contend, and until the profession at large grant it we must keep our isolated position. Personally we care very little about being tabooed, but so long as we are compelled to be the sole custodians of what we believe to be a great truth, so long must we assert our personal rights for our belief's sake.   I am, &c.,   JOHN H. CLARKE, M.D.

15, St. George's-terrace, Gloucester-road, S.W., Sept. 5.

DR. SHORTT AND PROFESSOR GAUTIER ON SNAKE-POISON.

[To the Editor of the Medical Times and Gazette.]

SIR,—In your number for September 3 you give an abstract of some researches of Professor Gautier on the cobra-poison, and especially on the efficacy of potash in decomposing and neutralizing this poison. The learned Professor seems not to be aware that this ground has already been worked out by Dr. Shortt, of Madras, and the results were described in some letters from Madras which I had the honour of sending you five or six years ago.

Dr. Shortt was led to believe that potash effectually decomposed the poison of the daboia, and published more than one case in support of his view. The difficulty of applying the antidote when once the patient has been bitten is obvious. One remarkable fact is, that when potash is added to a solution of snake-poison, it produces a bluish-black or indigo colour. This I have myself seen in some experiments on the daboia-poison which Dr. Shortt was good enough to make when I was at Madras in 1874, and which I described in the letters above cited.   I am, &c.,
R. D.

P.S.—Let me add that, to the best of my recollection, Dr. Shortt's experiments relate to the daboia, and not to the cobra-poison, and that his researches were published in the Madras Medical Journal at the time.

OBITUARY.

ARCHIBALD BILLING, M.D. OXON., F.R.C.P. LOND., F.R.S.

DR. ARCHIBALD BILLING, the "Father of the Profession," died at his house in Park-lane, on Friday, September 2, at the patriarchal age of ninety years. Born in Ireland, in the year 1791, Dr. Billing was educated at Trinity College, Dublin, and at Oxford, taking the degree of Doctor of Medicine at the latter University in 1818. He was elected to the Fellowship of the Royal College of Physicians of London in 1819, and was by several years the Senior of that grade in the College. He served the office of Censor in 1823, and was member of the Council in 1852, 1855, 1856, and 1857. From 1817 to 1836 he was a teacher in the medical school of the London Hospital, and from 1822 to 1845 was Physician to the Hospital. In the first year of his physicianship, in 1822, he instituted clinical lectures—the first lectures of the kind delivered in London,—and continued them till 1836, when, upon the establishment of the University of London, he was invited to become a Fellow of it, for many years filled the office of Examiner for degrees in medicine, and was a member of the Senate.

Dr. Billing was a Fellow of the Royal Society, one of the original Members of the Microscopical Society, a Fellow of the Geological Society, and a Corresponding Member of medical societies of Dresden, Florence, Brussels, and New York; and had been President of the Hunterian Society, and a Vice-President of the Royal Medical and Chirurgical Society. He was a frequent contributor to the pages of the Lancet and the Medical Gazette, writing papers "On the Sounds of the Heart," into the cause of which he was a well-known and original inquirer; on "A New Diagnosis of Aneurism by the Pulse at the Wrist," and other subjects. But the work by which he was best and most widely known is his "First Principles of Medicine," a work which passed through several editions, and has been translated and published in France and Germany, and republished in America. It gained him a high reputation as an original thinker, and a clear though terse writer; and he has been heard to say that the condensation of the work cost him more mental labour than the original text. He also published a small book entitled "Practical Observations on Diseases of the Heart and Lungs," but this was not received with so much favour as the former work, perhaps because his power of concentration in writing led him to think that auscultation could be taught with great ease. It should be added that he was one of the first to teach auscultation in London.

One of Dr. Billing's old pupils, to whom we are much indebted for some notes about his master, writes: "He was not a fluent lecturer, but his matter was always a profound record of the subject upon which he was speaking, and I never knew anyone who could convey so much original and practical information in so few words. He was literally beloved by the students, and greatly respected by his colleagues. He always invited his class after lecture to accompany him round the wards in order that he might demonstrate the facts which he had just been teaching. He was an advocate of the "one-faculty system," and on one occasion publicly declared that he "despised the man who was incapable of practising his profession from the administration of a glyster upwards." He was a man of wide culture and artistic tastes. His passion for high-class music was great, and his musical entertainments were supported by the best operatic artists of the day, whose society he delighted to cultivate"; and he was, we may add, a favourite consultant as a physician with them. He published a work on gems and precious stones which is very interesting, and shows his power of grasping subjects outside his profession.

Dr. Billing, at a time when physicians, and indeed all medical men, were expected to dress in sombre colours, used habitually to wear a blue coat, a primrose-coloured waistcoat, and trousers of "Oxford mixture." He had a great opinion of the value of riding as an exercise, and used frequently to go to the hospital and to his patients on horseback, with his groom behind him. He was a man of high honour and generous disposition, and was deservedly much beloved professionally and in private life. He had retired from practice for some time; but up to a very few years ago he might have been seen taking his favourite horse exercise, and it must be a consolation to his numerous friends to know that he was able to enjoy his old age, and that at the last he passed quietly away in his sleep.

RICHARD CLEWIN GRIFFITH, M.R.C.S., M.S.A.

WE have also to record the death, at very nearly the same great age of ninety, of a well-known "general practitioner." Mr. Richard Clewin Griffith died on the 5th inst. at his residence, 20, Gower-street, W.C., where he had lived fifty-three years. He attained the great age of ninety years less three days. He was in practice before 1815, having become a Member of the Royal College of Surgeons in 1812, and was among the first batch of "general practitioners." He took his father's practice, which had been established some twenty years in Tottenham-court-road, then a country suburb of London. After a few years he removed to Gower-street, where he carried on one of the largest general practices of the neighbourhood. He belonged to the old school of practical medicine, and despised theories. Like many other able men of his time, he bravely and successfully did his work. He was Mr. Cline's last dresser at St. Thomas's Hospital. He was the father of the Apothecaries' Society, of which Company he was the Master about twenty-six years ago. He helped to establish the Zoological and the Botanical Gardens and was a member of several learned societies. For several years the late Mr. Charles Brooke, of the Westminster Hospital, was his partner; and when they dissolved partnership, about the year 1845, he (Mr. Griffith) began to resign the practice of medicine, having realised a good competence. By direct male descent his family have followed the calling of medicine in London for nearly one hundred and fifty years. He was himself a link between the past (Act 1815 history of medicine and the present, and was a credit to our profession at a critical epoch of our history.

SOCIETY OF MEDICAL OFFICERS OF HEALTH.—At the last annual meeting the following officers were elected for the year ensuing:—President: Dr. J. W. Tripe. Vice-Presidents: Dr. T. Stevenson, Dr. Bristowe, Dr. Thursfield, Dr. Dixon. Treasurer: Mr. S. R. Lovitt. Hon. Secs.: Dr. J. N. Vinen, Mr. S. F. Murphy. Council: Dr. Buchanan, Dr. Dudfield, Dr. Bate, Dr. Brett, Dr. Baylis, Dr. Corfield, Mr. Corner, Mr. Jacob, Mr. G. Turner, Dr. J. Stevenson, Dr. C. Kelly, Dr. D. Thomas.

MEDICAL NEWS.

APOTHECARIES' HALL, LONDON.—The following gentlemen passed their examination in the Science and Practice of Medicine, and received certificates to practise, on Thursday, September 1 :—

Altman, Arthur Lyons, Kingston, Jamaica.
Baker, William Braine, Banbury, Oxon.
Rabbeth, Samuel, Putney, S.W.
Thane, Philip Thornton, 15, Montague-street, W.C.

The following gentlemen passed on September 8 :—

Farnker, John Joseph, Cheshunt, N.
Johnson, Samuel Ebenezer, Birmingham.
McCutcheon, James, Bradford.
Thomson, St. Clair, King's College Hospital.
Williams, Walter Treliving, Walthamstow.

The following gentlemen also on September 1 passed their primary professional examination :—

Aslanian, Bedros, London Hospital.
Gandy, Rastanji D., Grant Medical College.
Jones, John Hughes, St. Bartholomew's Hospital.

APPOINTMENTS.

₊ The Editor will thank gentlemen to forward to the Publishing-office, as early as possible, information as to all new Appointments that take place.

EDWARDS, F. SWINFORD, F.R.C.S.—Assistant-Surgeon to St. Peter's Hospital for Stone and Urinary Diseases, etc.
RHYS, JOSHUA, M.R.C.S. Eng., L.S.A.—Assistant-Surgeon to the City Provident Dispensary and Surgical Appliance Association, 164, Aldersgate-street, E.C.
TIDSFIELD, THOS. W., M.D., M.R.C.P. Lond.—Consulting Physician to the Leamington Provident Dispensary; and also Honorary Consulting Physician to the Leamington and Midland Counties' Home for Incurable Cases.

BIRTHS.

ANDREEW.—On September 11, at the Little Green, Richmond, Surrey, the wife of William Andersen, M.D., of a daughter.
DINGLE.—On September 5, at 61, Bunhill-row, Finsbury, E.C., the wife of W. A. Dingle, L.R.C.P., of a son.
DREW.—On September 1, at Portsmouth Dockyard, the wife of G. F. A. Drew, Fleet Surgeon, of a son.
FAIRBANK.—On September 5, at Moulsey House, Windsor, the wife of William Fairbank, M.R.C.S., of a daughter.
GARRETT.—On September 12, at Kenmare House, Walsall, the wife of Charles Frederick Garrett, M.R.C.S., L.S.A., of a daughter.
KIBBLER.—On September 11, at Mordaunt House, Hackney, the wife of W. Ambrose Kibbler, M.B., of a son.
NASH.—On September 5, at Herne Bay, the wife of Edmund Nash, M.D., of 123, Lansdowne-road, Notting-hill, of a daughter.
TODD.—On September 8, at Fyfield, Berks, the wife of Mark Stanley Todd, L.R.C.P., of a son.
WHITTAKER.—On September 9, at 31, Mount Pleasant-square, Dublin, the wife of Surgeon-Major J. H. Whittaker, Army Medical Department, of a son, stillborn.

MARRIAGES.

DAVIDSON—STAINFORTH.—On September 7, at Torquay, Patrick Moir Davidson, M.R.C.P., of Congleton, Cheshire, to Emily, daughter of the Rev. Richard Stainforth, formerly rector of Wheldrake, Yorkshire.
DYSON—RANKING.—On September 8, at Leamington, Arthur Francis Hawks Dyson, Esq., of Cowbit, Lincolnshire, to Isabella Augusta Minnie, youngest daughter of Surgeon-General J. Lancaster Ranking, late of the Madras Army.
HELLOWES—PEREGRINE.—On September 7, at Silchester, Edward Price Blackwood, youngest son of Price Blackwood Hellowes, Esq., of St. Margaret's, Canterbury, to Amelia Wilkie Minnie, fourth daughter of Thomas Peregrine, M.D., of The Cottage, Silchester.
HOLMES—ORCHARD.—On September 6, at Cheltenham, Thomas James Holmes, M.D., of Tudor House, Lyme Regis, Dorset, to Xarifa Zara, youngest daughter of the late Rev. George Randall Orchard, of Christ Church, North Bradley, Wilts.
ROUTH—ROUTH.—On September 8, at Hunstanton, Norfolk, Alfred Curtis Routh, M.R.C.S., to Annie Julia Adèle, eldest daughter of C. H. F. Routh, M.D., of Montague-square, London.
THATCHER—NELSON.—On September 8, at Sandal, Yorkshire, Charles Henry Thatcher, F.R.C.S., to Emily, elder daughter of the late F. W. Nelson, Esq., of Fall Ing, Wakefield.
WALTON—KEELAN.—On September 1, at Alverstoke, Hants, Haynes Walton, F.R.C.S., of 1, Brook-street, Grosvenor-square, to Kathleen Alexandra Mary, second daughter of Patrick Keelan, Fleet-Surgeon Royal Navy.

DEATHS.

BUTLER, J. M., M.D., at Greenway House, Honiton, on September 6, aged 60.
CARTER, R. S., M.R.C.S., late of Fitzroy-street, W., at Dartmouth-terrace, Lewisham-hill, S.E., on September 8, aged 62.

HAYNE, EVA LOUISA, youngest daughter of Frederick Greaves Hayne, M.R.C.S., at Northfleet, Kent, on September 9, aged 5.
HOLMAN, G., M.R.C.S., at Ivy House, Uckfield, Sussex, on September 5, in his 74th year.
KINGSFORD, C. D., M.D., at Upper Clapton, on September 12, aged 51.
PAYNE, W. G., L.R.C.P., at Bloemfontein, Orange Free State, South Africa, on August 2.
PEACOCK, J. B., L.R.C.P., at Darlington, Durham, on August 26, aged 43.
SYMONDS, FREDK., M.A., F.R.C.S., at Oxford, on September 11, aged 68.

VACANCIES.

In the following list the nature of the office vacant, the qualifications required in the candidate, the person to whom application should be made and the day of election (as far as known) are stated in succession.

CLINICAL HOSPITAL AND DISPENSARY FOR WOMEN AND CHILDREN, PARK-PLACE, MANCHESTER. — House-Surgeon. (For particulars see Advertisement.)
DENTAL HOSPITAL OF LONDON, LEICESTER SQUARE.—Dental Surgeon. (For particulars see Advertisement.)
ESSEX AND COLCHESTER HOSPITAL.—Physician. Candidates are requested to forward their names and qualifications, together with original testimonials, to the Secretary on or before October 5.
GENERAL HOSPITAL FOR SICK CHILDREN, PENDLEBURY, MANCHESTER.—Senior Resident Medical Officer. (For particulars see Advertisement.)
MELTON MOWBRAY UNION.—Medical Officer of Health. (For particulars see Advertisement.)
SUSSEX COUNTY HOSPITAL.—House-Surgeon. (For particulars see Advertisement.)
WEST BROMWICH DISTRICT HOSPITAL.—House-Surgeon. Candidates must be surgically qualified, registered, and unmarried. Applications, stating age, &c., to be sent, with testimonials, to the Honorary Secretary, William Bache, Esq., Churchill House, West Bromwich, on or before September 26.

UNION AND PAROCHIAL MEDICAL SERVICE.

₊ The area of each district is stated in acres. The population is computed according to the census of 1871.

RESIGNATIONS.

Newtown and Llanidloes Union.—Dr. William Parry has resigned the Llamorog District: area 57,299; population 6556; salary £75 per annum.
St. Albans Union.—Mr. John Robert Hutchinson has resigned the First District and the Workhouse: area 14,081; population 7853; salary £90 per annum; salary for Workhouse £40 per annum.
Sudbury Union.—Mr. Charles Chad Turnour has resigned the Sixth District: area 11,543; population 8399; salary £55 per annum.

APPOINTMENTS.

Axbridge Union.—Alfred J. Blades, M.R.C.S. Eng., L.S.A. Lond., to the Banwell District.
Gassock Union.—Charles T. Duce, L.R.C.P. Edin., L.R.C.S. Edin., to the Brewood District.
Okehampton Union.—George V. Burd, M.R.C.S. Eng., L.S.A., to the Second District and the Workhouse.
Shaftesbury Union.—Henry Robert Sherrard, L.Q.& K.C.P. Ire., L.R.C.S. and L.S.A. Ire., to the Fontmell District.
Tonbridge Union.—Arthur Claypon Horner, M.R.C.S. Eng. and L.R.C.P. Lond., to the Second District. William Fear, M.R.C.S. Lond., to the Sixth District. John Cunningham North, M.B. and C.M. Edin., to the Seventh District.
Wantage Union.—Charles W. Beresford, M.R.C.S. Eng., L.S.A., to the East Ilsley District.

VOMITING OF PREGNANCY.—Dr. Forwood (Louisville Med. News, August 27) adds another formula to the hundreds which already exist for the relief of vomiting in pregnancy. At all events, its simplicity renders it a safe remedy, which is more than can be said of some of its forerunners:—℞. Rad. calumb. conus, rad. zingib., āā ℥ss. fol. sennæ ℥j., aq. bull. Oj., —m. ft. infus.; a wineglassful before each meal. Dr. Forwood has treated more than 200 cases by this mixture, and regards it as a complete specific.

TINCT. FERRI PERCHLORIDI.—Dr. Reed, Professor of Materia Medica in the Montreal College of Pharmacy, observes that, notwithstanding so many new preparations of iron have been brought forward, this old tincture still holds its place in spite of the unpleasantness of its taste. There is, he says, a simple method of dealing with it which is not so widely known as it deserves, and which consists in merely adding a little alkaline citrate. For every drachm of the tincture add half a drachm of citrate of potash. The liquid is then converted into a beautiful green colour, and is quite free from the peculiar roughness of the iron. For a table-spoonful dose, containing ten minims, the prescription may be—Tinct. ferri mur. ℨij., pot. cit. ℨj., syr. limon. ℨiss., aquæ ad ℨij. Another advantage of the mixture is that astringent tinctures, as bark, gentian, etc., may be added without decomposition.—Canada Med. Journal, August.

WOUNDS OF THE INTESTINE.—In a paper in the Boston Med. Jour. (July 21), Dr. Whitney calls attention to what he thinks has not been yet sufficiently pointed out—namely, the characteristic appearance of the mucous membrane in wounds of the intestine made during life, the edges of the wound being covered by a protrusion of the mucous coat. The mucous coat is loosely connected with the muscular coats, and movable upon them to a certain extent. When all the coats are divided, the edges of the wound will gape from the retraction of the cut muscles, and the lax mucous coat is forced through the opening by the peristaltic movement as far as its attachments will permit, and curls back over the edges of the wound through the action of its elastic fibres. After a short time a slight thickening of all the coats takes place immediately in the neighbourhood of the wound from an infiltration of serum and new cells. Dr. Whitney relates two cases in which there was a possibility that the lesions found might have been produced in other ways than by violence before death.

APPOINTMENTS FOR THE WEEK.

September 17. *Saturday (this day).*

Operations at St. Bartholomew's, 1½ p.m.; King's College, 1½ p.m.; Royal Free, 2 p.m.; Royal London Ophthalmic, 11 a.m.; Royal Westminster Ophthalmic, 1½ p.m.; St. Thomas's, 1½ p.m.; London, 2 p.m.

19. *Monday.*

Operations at the Metropolitan Free, 2 p.m.; St. Mark's Hospital for Diseases of the Rectum, 2 p.m.; Royal London Ophthalmic, 11 a.m.; Royal Westminster Ophthalmic, 1½ p.m.

20. *Tuesday.*

Operations at Guy's, 1½ p.m.; Westminster, 2 p.m.; Royal London Ophthalmic, 11 a.m.; Royal Westminster Ophthalmic, 1½ p.m.; West London, 3 p.m.

21. *Wednesday.*

Operations at University College, 2 p.m.; St. Mary's, 1¼ p.m.; Middlesex, 1 p.m.; London, 2 p.m.; St. Bartholomew's, 1½ p.m.; Great Northern, 2 p.m.; Samaritan, 2½ p.m.; King's College (by Mr. Lister), 2 p.m.; Royal London Ophthalmic, 11 a.m.; Royal Westminster Ophthalmic, 1½ p.m.; St. Thomas's, 1½ p.m.; St. Peter's Hospital for Stone, 2 p.m.; National Orthopædic, Great Portland-street, 10 a.m.

22. *Thursday.*

Operations at St. George's, 1 p.m.; Central London Ophthalmic, 1 p.m.; Royal Orthopædic, 2 p.m.; University College, 2 p.m.; Royal London Ophthalmic, 11 a.m.; Royal Westminster Ophthalmic, 1½ p.m.; Hospital for Diseases of the Throat, 2 p.m.; Hospital for Women, 2 p.m.; Charing-cross, 2 p.m.; London, 2 p.m.; North-West London, 2½ p.m.

23. *Friday.*

Operations at Central London Ophthalmic, 2 p.m.; Royal London Ophthalmic, 11 a.m.; South London Ophthalmic, 2 p.m.; Royal Westminster Ophthalmic, 1½ p.m.; St. George's (ophthalmic operations), 1¼ p.m.; Guy's, 1½ p.m.; St. Thomas's (ophthalmic operations), 2 p.m.

COMMUNICATIONS have been received from—

The Registrar of the Apothecaries' Hall, London; Dr. Herman, London; Dr. Goyder, Newcastle-on-Tyne; Mr. J. B. Medland, London; The Sanitary Commissioner, Punjab; Mr. R. Reynolds, Leeds; The Secretary of the City Provident Dispensary, London; Mr. Mortimer, Plymouth; Messrs. Hyfod and Dikco, London; Dr. J. H. Clarke, London; Mr. J. Chatto, London; Mr. Mark H. Judge, London; Mr. H. A. Reeves, London; Dr. Hinds, Birmingham; The Secretary of the College of Practical Engineering, London; Surgeon-General C. R. Francis, London; Messrs. Arnold and Son, London; Mr. R. W. Parker, London; The Secretary of the Church of England Temperance Society; Messrs. Sampson, Low, and Co., London; Dr. S. C. Griffith, London; Mr. Lawson Tait, Birmingham; Dr. Druitt, London; Messrs. Burroughs, Wellcome, and Co., London; Dr. Wibel, Wiesbaden; The Honorary Secretary of the Society of Medical Officers of Health, London; Mr. W. Savile Clarke, Southwold; The Honorary Secretary of the Quekett Microscopical Club, London; Mr. C. Heath, London.

BOOKS, ETC., RECEIVED—

Report on the Health, etc., of Kensington—Sessional Proceedings of the National Association for the Promotion of Social Science—Report on the Sanitary Condition of the Whitechapel District—The Micrographic Dictionary, Parts II. and III.—Report on the Sanitary Condition of the Hackney District—Railway Transsaharien, par Ch. J. Masse—The Continued Fevers, by J. C. Wilson, M.D.—The Opium Question, by Deputy Surgeon-General W. J. Moore—The Case of Susan Nixon—Annual Report on the Sanitary Condition of West Sussex.

PERIODICALS AND NEWSPAPERS RECEIVED—

Lancet—British Medical Journal—Medical Press and Circular—Berliner Klinische Wochenschrift—Centralblatt für Chirurgie—Gazette des Hopitaux—Gazette Médicale—Le Progrès Médical—Bulletin de l'Académie de Médecine—Pharmaceutical Journal—Wiener Medizinische Wochenschrift—Centralblatt für die Medizinischen Wissenschaften—Revue Médicale—Gazette Hebdomadaire—National Board of Health Bulletin, Washington—Nature—Deutsche Medicinal-Zeitung—Boston Medical and Surgical Journal—Louisville Medical News—Oil and Drug News—Occasional Notes—L'Impartialité Médicale—Chicago Medical Review—Revista de Medicina—Students' Journal and Hospital Gazette—Philadelphia Medical Times—New York Medical Journal, etc.—Maryland Medical Journal—Boston Journal of Chemistry—Pharmaceutical Journal—Weekblad—Canadian Journal of Medical Science—The American—North Carolina Medical Journal—Veterinarian—Archives Générales de Médecine—Glasgow Medical Journal—Charity Record—Practitioner—St. Louis Clinical Record—Indian Medical Gazette—Therapeutic Gazette—Western Medical Reporter—Church of England Pulpit, etc.—La Independencia Medica—Analyst.

VITAL STATISTICS OF LONDON.

Week ending Saturday, September 10, 1881.

BIRTHS.

Births of Boys, 1281; Girls, 1232; Total, 2513.
Corrected weekly average in the 10 years 1871-80, 2335·4.

DEATHS.

	Males.	Females.	Total.
Deaths during the week	653	576	1229
Weekly average of the ten years 1871-80, corrected to increased population ...	750·3	677·8	1428·1
Deaths of people aged 80 and upwards ...	...	...	26

DEATHS IN SUB-DISTRICTS FROM EPIDEMICS.

	Enumerated Population, 1881 (unrevised).	Small-pox.	Measles.	Scarlet Fever.	Diphtheria.	Whooping-cough.	Typhus.	Enteric (or Typhoid) Fever.	Simple continued Fever.	Diarrhœa.
West	668993	2	7	1	2	3	...	1	1	2
North ...	905677	9	5	14	7	10	...	5	...	7
Central ...	281793	...	2	6	1	2	...	...	...	6
East	692530	3	6	7	...	5	...	1	...	7
South	1265578	13	7	20	4	9	2	3	1	17
Total	3814571	27	27	48	14	29	2	10	2	39

METEOROLOGY.

From Observations at the Greenwich Observatory.

Mean height of barometer ...	29·606 in.
Mean temperature ...	55·4°
Highest point of thermometer ...	67·6°
Lowest point of thermometer ...	44·2°
Mean dew-point temperature ...	52·0°
General direction of wind ...	Variable.
Whole amount of rain in the week ...	0·49 in.

BIRTHS and DEATHS Registered and METEOROLOGY during the Week ending Saturday, Sept. 10, in the following large Towns:—

Cities and boroughs (Municipal boundaries except for London.)	Estimated Population to middle of the year 1881.*	Persons to an Acre. (1881.)	Births Registered during the week ending Sept. 10.	Deaths Registered during the week ending Sept. 10.	Temperature of Air (Fahr.) Highest during the Week.	Temperature of Air (Fahr.) Lowest during the Week.	Temperature of Air (Fahr.) Weekly Mean of Daily Mean Values	Temp. of Air (Cent.) Weekly Mean of Daily Mean Values.	Rain Fall. In Inches.	Rain Fall. In Centimetres.
London	3829751	50·8	2513	1229	67·6	44·2	55·4	13·00	0·49	1·24
Brighton	107934	45·9	52	26	66·0	47·1	55·8	13·23	0·98	2·49
Portsmouth ...	128335	28·6	84	48	...	...	...	...	...	...
Norwich	88038	11·8	70	23	...	...	...	...	...	...
Plymouth	75262	54·0	40	25	64·2	43·8	53·0	11·67	1·71	4·34
Bristol	207140	46·5	137	64	66·1	44·2	53·6	12·01	0·75	1·90
Wolverhampton ...	75934	22·4	57	36	63·8	47·0	52·8	11·56	0·30	0·76
Birmingham ...	402296	47·9	255	112	...	...	...	...	...	...
Leicester	128120	38·5	66	52	64·0	41·5	53·1	11·73	0·39	0·99
Nottingham ...	188035	18·9	138	82	67·9	42·5	54·5	12·50	0·39	0·99
Liverpool	553988	106·3	362	257	60·7	45·0	53·9	12·17	0·02	0·05
Manchester ...	341269	79·5	252	153	...	...	...	...	...	...
Salford	177760	34·4	132	68	...	...	...	...	...	...
Oldham	112176	24·0	84	38	...	...	...	...	...	...
Bradford	184037	25·5	125	43	63·0	46·0	53·6	12·01	0·22	0·56
Leeds	310490	14·4	232	97	64·0	45·0	53·6	12·01	0·27	0·69
Sheffield	285621	14·5	202	96	65·0	43·0	53·2	11·78	0·20	0·51
Hull	155161	42·7	95	50	67·0	45·0	53·6	12·01	0·33	0·84
Sunderland ...	116753	42·2	86	50	68·0	48·0	54·2	12·33	0·52	1·32
Newcastle-on-Tyne	145675	27·1	86	57	...	...	...	...	...	...
Total of 20 large English Towns ...	7608775	38·0	5068	2636	68·0	41·5	53·9	12·17	0·51	1·30

* These figures are the numbers enumerated (but subject to revision) in April last, raised to the middle of 1881 by the addition of a quarter of a year's increase, calculated at the rate that prevailed between 1871 and 1881

At the Royal Observatory, Greenwich, the mean reading of the barometer last week was 29·61 in. The lowest reading was 29·37 in. on Tuesday morning, and the highest 29·84 in. at noon on Saturday.

NOTES, QUERIES, AND REPLIES.

Ye that questionest much shall learn much.—Bacon.

A First Year's Man.—Registration has been abolished at the College of Surgeons. Why not read our "Students' Number," which will give you the desired information. This applies also to "A Guardian" and "An Anxious Parent."

Arts Examinations.—Those correspondents who have addressed us on this subject should bear in mind what a large number of papers have to be read by the examiners. We are told that the result cannot be known for a fortnight.

Outdoor Medical Relief in the Metropolis.—It may not be without interest to notice the alterations in the arrangements for affording outdoor medical relief during the past ten years in connexion with Section 26 of the Metropolitan Poor Law Act, 1867. There are, at the present time, in existence in twenty-seven of the thirty unions in the metropolis forty-seven dispensaries for the outdoor poor. During the year ended Christmas, 1880, 1,061,877 prescriptions were made up at these establishments, as compared with 997,815 in 1877. The total number of orders for medical relief issued during the year was 114,737, showing an average of 740 to each district medical officer.

The Miraculous Cure Delusion, Paris.—It is said that medical men on the staffs of the Paris hospitals have been much perplexed lately by applications from patients for certificates that their complaints were incurable. These were refused, and the applicants assured that by ordinary care and attention they might be restored to health; but it has since transpired that the applicants were devout persons, who wanted the certificates that they might carry them to Lourdes, where their faith would make them whole.

Food Analysis and Unofficial Purchasers.—It appears that, excepting in a very few instances, ordinary purchasers are disinclined to incur the expense and trouble of analyses under the "Sale of Food and Drugs Act." The official purchasers are consequently about 97 per cent. of the whole. A striking exception to this rule, however, is to be found in the city of Bristol, where a large number of analyses are obtained by private individuals. The fact is officially attributed to the Town Council's arrangement with their salaried analysts, to examine each sample for a fee of 2s. 6d., instead of the usual maximum charge allowed by the Act of 10s. 6d.

The Drainage of Brentford.—The Local Board have decided on a scheme of drainage which deals with the sewage by chemical precipitation in tanks, to be constructed on land adjoining the Ealing Sewage Works; the sewage being pumped up from a pumping station at the riverside. The cost is estimated at £18,000.

Colonial Items.—New South Wales.—Small-pox still continued to make its appearance in Sydney. The determination of the Chinese population to keep secret any case that might break out amongst them had, much baffled the health officers. In every case discovered the patient suffering from the disease had been removed to the quarantine station, to which the Chinese strongly object. The newly formed Board of Health has recommended to the Government the formation of an ambulance and disinfecting staff.——New Zealand.—All Chinese ports have been declared infected. The Government have taken this step as a precaution against small-pox. The consideration of a new Licensing Bill has occupied a good deal of the legislation of the session, and the total abstainers have scored a point in getting the licensing bench in each district made elective, thus practically adopting the permissive principle.

Druggists, France.—It is stated that one of the first measures which will be brought before the newly elected French Chamber of Deputies will be an important Bill affecting druggists, which, after considerable deliberation, has finally been drafted by the Council of State. In future, no druggist shall be allowed to combine with his profession that of a doctor, or to sell or advertise any patent medicines or nostrums.

Furious Driving.—Reckless drivers are receiving their merited punishment at the Marylebone Police-court. Last week Mr. De Rutzen sent three men charged with this offence to prison, without the option of paying a fine, for fourteen days each with hard labour.

Our Metropolitan Sanitary Authorities: a Hint.—A dealer, who was convicted of selling bad meat at Liverpool, in his defence stated that he had only removed from London to Liverpool a fortnight previously, and was merely carrying on his trade in his old ways, but "he found the rules much more strict in Liverpool than in London."

Aid from the Working Classes.—A children's ward is to be erected at the West Kent General Hospital, Maidstone, to the memory of the late Mr. Jonathan Saunders, towards the expenses of which the friendly and benefit societies of the town have contributed £100, part of the proceeds of their recent *fête*. A workmen's collection in aid of the fund has also been commenced.

Medical Nostrums.—In the year ending March 31 last, the stamp duty on patent medicines amounted to £139,762 18s. 10½d.

Ernest, Surbiton.—The "House of Rest," established at Babbicombe, Devon is intended for women in business who find it necessary to seek a temporary sojourn in pure air by the seaside. Admission is by subscribers' tickets, or, for those who can afford it, by a moderate weekly payment, which "tends to make the house more self-supporting." The latter class showed a considerable increase last year, when altogether 143 visitors were received. The classes who avail themselves of the Rest are milliners, dressmakers, shopwomen, Post Office clerks, etc. The institution is a development of benevolence which deserves to be commended for its practical utility and advantages.

L. L. A., Bedfordshire.—The "political" objections to the Vaccination Act have been enumerated to be—first, that it does not rest with Parliament to say how a disease shall be treated; secondly, that medicine being a progressive art, the younger and fresher minds among physicians must be left perfectly free to deviate from the routine of their elders; thirdly, that it is blind tyranny for the law to say to a parent "you shall not keep your child in perfect health." It would be difficult to say which of the three is the most foolish.

Benevolence.—By the will of Mr. A. S. Wilkes, who lately committed suicide while suffering under mental depression, the Birmingham Hospital will, in time, benefit to the extent of £50,000. The deceased bequeaths the whole of his estate, which is valued at £100,000, to the Birmingham General Hospital and the Birmingham and Midland Institute on the death of his sisters, who are to hold it in trust during their lifetime. This munificent donation will place the Birmingham Hospital among the most richly endowed of provincial charities.——It was reported to the annual meeting of the Salisbury Infirmary, held last week, that the institution would receive £12,849 from the residuary estate of Sir George Bowles, and the Herbert Home £6334 from the same source.

Railway Casualties.—There were killed 143 passengers, or one in 20,030,000 in the course of 600,000,000 railway journeys made in the United Kingdom last year; and 1812, or three in 2,000,000, were injured. But of railway servants 546 were killed and 2080 injured in the twelve months.

The New Libel Act.—A principal feature of the Act is to the effect that, "No criminal prosecution shall be commenced against any proprietor, publisher, editor, or any person responsible for the publication of a newspaper, for any libel published therein without the written fiat or allowance of the Director of Public Prosecutions in England, or Her Majesty's Attorney-General in Ireland, being first had and obtained." The law is not to extend to Scotland.

SUBJECTS FOR DISSECTION.

TO THE EDITOR OF THE MEDICAL TIMES AND GAZETTE.

SIR,—For some years the scarcity of subjects for dissection has been a serious grievance at the medical schools. I have seen statements that many students cannot get parts to dissect till after Christmas—three months of their first session gone before they can actively commence the most important part of their first session's studies. To me the thing seems easy to arrange if some *practical* man were authorised by the inspector of anatomy and the anatomical teachers to carry it out. It is notorious that large numbers of unknown and unclaimed people die in the hospitals, workhouses, etc., of London, a large proportion of whom might be available for anatomical and surgical purposes. By an understanding with the masters of workhouses and other officials, and the judicious application of fees, the present dearth of "subjects" might be altogether lessened. A guinea fee to the master for each adult subject, and a second guinea divided among the minor officials, would soon alter the present state of things, and the schools would be amply supplied with subjects for anatomical teaching and operative surgery at moderate charges. At present the funerals of the known and the unknown, the claimed and the unclaimed, afford an outing and a holiday for certain officials and inmates, and fees for the undertaker. Now, if, as suggested above, these different people were fee'd, it would be a gain to most of them, and the undertaker would sustain no loss. Subsequent charges should be placed at the minimum, as extravagant charges for "parts" only lead to students dissecting just sufficient to get certificates. If the charges for "parts" be moderate it will lead to students dissecting the same parts several times over instead of only once, and the operative surgery classes will be much more satisfactory in their working and result.

I have simply sketched a plan of action; a *practical* man would carry out the details, or modify them as he saw fit. It is one man's work; let such a man be selected by the parties I have named, and by the commencement of the session the anatomical theatres would be well supplied, the supply kept up, and all the students at work, instead of learning their anatomy by looking on, or idling for want of opportunity of work. If one suitable man does it, it will be quietly done, without bobbery, fuss, and rumpus. What is proposed to be done is quite within the law, but the object sought will be defeated if done in a fussy way, or by some incompetent person, deficient in tact and judgment. With the increased fees at the London schools it is necessary that some corresponding advantages should be afforded, and the plan now proposed, if sufficiently carried out, would at once place the London anatomy classes in the front rank, resulting from which every school and medical class would be benefited by an increased number of students. I am, &c.,

Plymouth.   DEVONIENSIS.

THE LATE MR. HECKSTALL SMITH.—The will of this well-known surgeon, of St. Mary Cray, who died on May 3, has lately been proved, the personal estate amounting to over £62,000.

AN ADDRESS
ON
SCEPTICISM IN MEDICINE.

Written for the International Medical Congress

BY THE LATE

Dr. MAURICE RAYNAUD, of Paris.

Dr. FÉRÉOL, who read this address to the International Medical Congress, prefaced it with the following observations:—

Gentlemen,—It is not I who was to be here to-day. A deplorable misfortune—a grief for the entire medical body of France—has brought me to this place, I having no other right to occupy it than that given me by the friendship which, for more than twenty years, united me to Maurice Raynaud. You will excuse me, then, if under these painful circumstances I only find words for the expression of my deep regret.

You will allow me, before reading this last work of Maurice Raynaud—a work executed for you—to speak to you of him for a few minutes. I do not desire to enter into any of the details of his scientific life, but simply ask permission to make known to you somewhat of him who felt so pleased at having to present himself before you, and at entering into communication with so many illustrious *savants* and distinguished men assembled from all parts of the world. Raynaud was, one might say, the type of a worker. Work was for him not only the accomplishment of the first duty and highest function of a human being; it was an imperious craving of his mind and the joy of his life. It was so from his earliest youth. The son of a distinguished member of the University, he studied hard in literature, and produced a thesis for the Doctor of Letters degree—"Les Médecins au Temps de Molière," which we all know, and which will hold its place. For his degree in Medicine, his thesis, "Asphyxie Locale et la Gangrène Symétrique des Extremités," introduced into science the knowledge of a new disease, to which his name should rightly be given, as has been so justly done for Bright's, Basedow's, and Addison's disease.

Raynaud was not only a learned doctor, a consummate clinician, a physiologist, and a skilful experimenter, but also a man of letters and a philosopher. Of this you will be able to judge presently; but what, unfortunately, you will not be able to judge of is the oratorical talent of the man, who would not have read his address to you, but, according to his habit, would have repeated it from memory, leaving to the inspiration of the moment the right of making modifications. You would have had the pleasure of observing those sympathetic features and of listening to that firm and elegant diction, so well suited to the professor's chair—although, through circumstances which it would be too long and too delicate to explain, the official professoriate remained closed to him even to his death.

For a long time past Raynaud had exhibited obscure symptoms of organic disease of the heart, but he continued none the less to wear himself out with incessant labour. Accustomed to display in everything an indefatigable ardour, he expended his powers, without stint, whether in science, in clinical teaching, in private practice (where his devotion, equal to every demand upon it, procured for him the warmest friendships), in the free professoriate, and even in political and religious matters, in which he was most zealously interested. On June 29 he had returned to his country house, seemingly better than usual, and after dinner was playing cheerfully with his children, when he was suddenly seized with a violent pain in the region of the heart. This he recognised as angina pectoris, and at once made every disposition for his death. In three hours he had ceased to live, having preserved to the end, in spite of the horrible anguish of the terrible separation, a serenity and strength of mind and a gentleness truly admirable. He had scarcely attained his forty-seventh year.

I have been able to secure from oblivion his last work, the address which you are about to hear, and which he had not even completed; and if you find some imperfections in it, you will remember, gentlemen, that its author was not able to

put the finishing touch to it. I have, with all possible discretion and respect, completed what remained unfinished, and any blame must attach to the calamity of this premature death and to my insufficiency.

Gentlemen,—It is perhaps a strange design, and most surely it is a perilous one, which—on the only occasion I shall have the distinguished honour of addressing this great assembly—induces me to discourse to it on Scepticism in Medicine. Is it not to do the very opposite to what you might have expected of me, and for what the circumstance calls for? Your presence here, brethren of the two worlds, who have come from every point of the civilised universe to bring your contributions to the work of common progress, is this not itself alone a protest and a warning? Does it not affirm boldly that you have faith in your science and in your art? Nevertheless, I venture to flatter myself that if you consent, as I now invite you, to take a general view of the actual condition of medical science and practice, and examine your own thoughts, you will find with me that the subject which I have chosen is not entirely devoid of opportuneness; and that, in speaking to you of scepticism, I am not speaking of what is unknown, or perhaps not even absent, and which, if it is to be regarded as an enemy (this being precisely what we shall have to inquire), is, at all events, not an unknown one. I do not say, pray observe, gentlemen, that we believe less in medicine than our fathers believed in it; but I think that we believe in it differently. In this respect, as in so many others, an evolution has taken place in what we term, rightly or wrongly, the "modern spirit," which, it seems to me, it is not without interest to investigate.

And, first of all, let us explain what we should understand by this word, "scepticism." As you are well aware, by this word two things are designated which deserve to be distinguished; so that, on the one hand, we have a very clearly defined philosophical system, consisting in the denial of the foundations of certainty; and, on the other, of a certain intellectual tendency, a frame of the mind, depending as much upon habit and education as reasoning, and leading to more or less universal doubt. That the two things are often met with united, that they willingly choose their residence in the same minds and the same epochs, is just what might be expected, and should cause no surprise; but they are not, nevertheless, necessarily connected the one with the other. Of the philosophical system I have nothing to say, for this is not the occasion to advert to it; and I will content myself with noting, by the way, that according to its etymology, σκεπτομαι does not mean "to doubt," but "to examine," which is not the same thing. It is really only by an abuse of language that this confusion has become established, for which, I admit, the sceptics are principally responsible. To doubt is an excellent disposition of mind in which to undertake any examination. But why do we examine? Precisely in order that we may form an opinion—that is, escape from the state of doubt. If we are decided beforehand to suspend our judgment indefinitely, and not even arrest research even in face of demonstrated truth, it would surely not be worth while to commence the study of a question. Thus, we find established, in my view, a necessary distinction between what I may term good and bad scepticism, or, if you will permit me to call things by their proper names, between scepticism properly so called and philosophic doubt—the latter not only being in itself perfectly legitimate, but also to be laid down as the first condition of all science.

But if we no longer regard scepticism as a system, which as such we may leave to the disputants of the schools, but —placing ourselves in a far more interesting point of view to physicians—as a disposition and practical tendency, we shall also permit here, I believe, a no less legitimate distinction to establish between scepticism so understood and the critical spirit. The critical spirit is one of the most praiseworthy things in the world, and, for my part, I believe that it is better developed in our own time than it has ever been. It consists in being very exacting in the matter of proof, in the control of the most plausible assertions, and in regarding the best-established theories only as provisional outworks which serve for the grouping of facts, but which we must be ever ready to abandon as soon as a theory is demonstrated to be false or insufficient, without necessarily abandoning the facts which seemed to support it—on the condition, however, that these facts, constantly remitted to the test of experiment, issue victorious from the trial. I admit that the limit between the critical spirit and scepticism is very difficult to trace, the former being little else than the exaggeration of the latter, and the passage from the one to the other being very easy. Who can say where exaggeration commences? Which is the group of facts of a physiological and vital order, in which we can flatter ourselves in possessing such well-defined truth that there is no need to pursue it? Assuredly such facts do exist, and they are the foundations of our art, but how small is their number! while, on the other hand, how considerable, we may almost say infinite, is the number of those which, partially known, and insufficiently explored, remain an open field to investigation, and consequently to doubt! It is clear that here we have no concern with any question of authority—for authority, whatever may have been said about it, has never held anything but a precarious and constantly contested empire among us, even at times when it passed as reigning supreme. Medicine is a matter not of faith, but of knowledge, and its knowledge possess no other value than it is fitting for our reason to accord to them. Contrary to the saying of Royer-Collard, you perceive I am disposed to assign its part to scepticism; but I believe that I render this sufficiently large when I limit its domain to the vague territories bordering on the confines of criticism. I shall also stipulate, at least theoretically, that it shall have no right to invade its neighbour's possessions.

Having said this, you will easily understand, gentlemen, that it could not enter into my idea to present here the history of medical scepticism, and to institute under this point of view a regular parallel between the ancients and moderns, and still less to place all scepticism on the one side, and all belief on the other. That would be a pure *jeu d'esprit* as contrary to good sense as to history. There have been sceptics in all times, and probably there always will be, the truth being that scepticism is one of the sides of the human mind, just as extreme credulity is another. If we must absolutely choose between the two, it is to scepticism that preference should be given; for while it may be sterile in itself, at least it has the advantage of keeping before the world the salutary idea that science is not complete—which is the indispensable condition of its becoming so. Scepticism and credulity, do not they seem the two antipodes? and yet, strange to say, the experience of every day shows us that these two opposites are far from excluding each other, and are nowise irreconcilable. It is even the prominent feature of the scepticism of men of the world with respect to medicine. We approach here, gentlemen, a very small part of the question, on which I should blush to detain at length a meeting like this; but nevertheless I cannot pass it over in complete silence. We daily meet with persons who declare to us with a convinced air that medicine is entirely a conjectural science; and to such I always reply that if under this name they designate a science, in which conjecture plays some part, there does not exist a science (including astronomy, physics, and chemistry) to which this reproach might not be addressed. The entire question consists in knowing the degree of conjecture which prevails. Now, persons who speak in this way are not only ignorant of the first elements of the science upon which they pass so severe a judgment, but for the most part they only so condemn it because they demand of it more than it admits itself prepared to give. Hence the deceptions you are familiar with, and with the deceptions that torrent of injuries and inexhaustible pleasantries to which we have been accustomed for so long a period. I formerly had occasion to study closely those of our own Molière, and to estimate their value. But Molière in this only followed a tradition as old as comedy and as old as medicine. Aristophanes had already with great irreverence bestowed on the god Æsculapius the appellation "Scatophagos"—that is, the eater of excrement. That, you observe, does not date from yesterday; and a list of the detractors could not be drawn up, for it is legion. Were physicians of a vindictive disposition they would only have to exhibit the blind confidence of their detractors in the grossest empiricism. This has been the history of all time from the elder Cato, who, it is said, expelled the physicians from Rome and forbade his son to have recourse to their aid, and yet passed his time in physicking himself, his wife, his slaves, and his cattle; to Madame de Sevigné, who never exhausted her sarcasms on the inanity of medicine, outbidding Molière if possible, and at the same time inundating her friends with innumerable absurd remedies, their only guarantee being that they were not medical. All this is most wretched, and what renders it yet more sad is that we are not able to say that the alternations of disfavour and infatuation through which our art has passed are explicable by the intrinsic value of the men and their works. The caprices and oscillations of fashion have here played a greater part than the general progress of the prevalent ideas. The end of our eighteenth century in France is not generally regarded as an age of faith, and yet it was the epoch at which the medical profession attained its highest ascendency. The Duc de Lévis has left us in his memoirs a telling picture of the admiration without limit and of the tender and submissive confidence placed in contemporary medicine by the highest society of that time, and especially among the women. "I can only compare," says he, "the sentiments of these ladies for their doctors with those which their grandmothers exhibited for their directors at the end of the age of Louis XIV. And, in fact," he acutely adds, "the preference which in our days the body has gained over the soul sufficiently explains this displacement of affection." In compensation, we must observe that the fine ladies who listened to the advice of Tronchin as to an oracle, and crowded to hear the florid discourses of Vicq d'Azyr at the Société de Médecine, were probably the same who were afterwards met with as the not less numerous and still more impassioned followers of Mesmer. Much is said of the progress of intelligence, and I do not desire to contest it, but, to speak truly, we can scarcely perceive it in the subject which now engages our attention. If we look around, we now meet with the same ignorant infatuation, the same mingling of the most unreasoning scepticism with the most childish superstition, and the same spirit, at once jeering and futile, which believes everything because it believes nothing, and which rejects scientific medicine while it accepts, without shrinking, table-turning, spiritualism, and homœopathy—the whole without other rule than pure fancy! And this strange disposition is not observed only, and not even principally, among the common people. It is in the upper classes, in minds otherwise instructed and cultivated, and sometimes even among true *savants!* Let it be understood that I am speaking only of France; but I have heard that wise England herself is not exempt in this respect from the infirmities of human nature.

This is quite enough on this subject. To render it worth while to discuss the validity of a judgment we must be assured of the competence of the judge, but here that is absolutely wanting. Unfortunately, gentlemen, we may say it among ourselves, the physicians themselves have set the bad example, and the remark has often been made that never have philosophers, literary men, or poets said such bitter things of medicine as have physicians themselves. Where, for example, can we find a more harsh judgment on therapeutics than the following?—"An incoherent assemblage of opinions themselves incoherent, it is perhaps of all the physiological sciences the one in which are best depicted the eccentricities of the human mind. It is not a science for a methodical mind, but a crude assemblage of inexact ideas, of observations which are often puerile, of illusory procedures, and of formulæ as oddly conceived as fastidiously arranged. It is said that the practice of medicine is repulsive; but I say further that it cannot in some respects be pursued by a reasonable being when its principles are derived from most of our materia medicas." Who is it that thus expresses himself, gentlemen? Not the first chance person who presents himself, but Bichat, whom we all, more or less, claim, and with good reason, as one of the promoters of modern science. And it is by the hundred that we could borrow from the principal leaders of our schools, portraits as little flattering—without including Broussais, who declares, without circumlocution, that before his time medicine had only soothed men with chimerical hopes, and that, taking it altogether, it had been more injurious than useful to humanity. Admit after this that those outsiders who have passed judgment upon us may well be excused for having been a little severe. But, if we go back to the very source, was not the first word ever pronounced on medicine one of discouragement and doubt? "Ars longa, vita brevis, experientia fallax, judicium difficilis." It is the first of the aphorisms of Hippocrates, and Peisse asks ironically, how, after having written it, Hippocrates had the courage to write the second and the following. Doubtless this great dictum is, above all things, an admirable lesson in modesty and prudence; but it has not always been understood in this sense, and the fact is, that between scepticism and medicine there would seem to have always existed, I hardly know what kind of natural affinity. It cannot be a matter of mere chance that the list of sceptical philosophers contains so many names of physicians. Sextus Empiricus, Cornelius Agrippa, Sanches of Toulouse, Martin Martines, Leonard of Capua,(a) and yet others, among whom I am much tempted to count Rabelais, who belongs to us as a physician, and who, as a philosopher, although an irregular one, somewhat difficult to classify, certainly cannot be enrolled amongst the orthodox.

I just now cited Cornelius Agrippa, and it is well known that in his book medicine is especially ill-treated. But what is, I believe, but little known is that Montaigne, whose name it is difficult to omit when speaking on scepticism, has written a chapter of rare bitterness against medicine.(b) The darts here are pointed enough, and it must be admitted that many are well aimed, and we recognise the hand of a master. But we have here one of those contrivances often met with in Montaigne. In another of his books, under the pretext of an apology for the philosopher and physician Raimond Sebon, he forces him into the camp of scepticism, and, under cover of his hero, puts forth his most exorbitant propositions. Here he goes still farther, not hesitating to copy many a passage of Cornelius Agrippa—copy him even to plagiarism without referring to him. So much is this the case that the natural "dyspathie" to medicine which he pretends to have inherited from his father and grandfather, and which in him was proof against attacks of gravel, he has, it cannot be denied, found the means of expressing by the results of his readings. His theme, it is possible, was all ready, but in a great measure, at least, his arguments have been furnished him by the physician.

I have been recalling, gentlemen, some very old memories; but do not believe that I have been seeking in them material for allusions. If they raise in your minds some comparisons with the present, it is no fault of mine. Naturally, I have been only able to speak to you of visible, palpable, admitted scepticism, which has left its traces in written documents. As for that which conceals itself, and is only revealed by its

effects, the action of which is only the more deadly, it is obvious we can only guess it; but a little attention suffices for this, and we meet with it as a mute accompaniment in every page of our history. But I should only have performed an idle piece of work if, in this review of the past, I did not seek to clear up the causes of a fact so constant and so general that it would seem to be an evil inherent to medicine. Here, as always, a good etiology is the condition of good treatment. Of these causes of medical scepticism, there are, in the first place, those which are of all ages and all times, the discovery of which only requires a little knowledge of the human heart. Scepticism, which is a great force, has this particular about it, that it flatters alike two of the most deep-seated of our instincts, and which are not of those that do most honour to our nature—idleness and vanity: idleness, by dispensing with the search after truth, which requires an effort for its discovery; and vanity, by leading us, at any easy rate, to criticise and disdain the labour of others, and to indulge the sweet persuasion that we are soaring above common prejudices. This exists at the bottom of all scepticism; but God forbid that I should say there is only that in it. For a good number of the most conscientious and reflecting minds there is also the inevitable discouragement springing from the shock of contradictory opinions, the difficulty of arriving at a conviction, and the uncertainty of therapeutical results. How can we feel astonished, then, at meeting with so many physicians among the sceptics? Is it not in medicine, especially, that the phenomena are most complex and difficult to investigate, and present themselves under the most different aspects, while in essentials they are the same? Is it not in medicine that it is most difficult to lay down fixed and invariable laws without these being rendered inoperative through their numerous exceptions? Is it not this which has given rise to that multitude of systems rushing against, combating, and overturning each other, and the incessant crumbling away of which calls to mind Bossuet's famous apostrophe of the noise of empires as they fell crashing one after the other? In presence of this spectacle, it truly demands some strength of mind to prevent our deploring the vanity of the conceptions of the human mind, and to avoid the temptation of regarding them all with the same disdain. It is especially when we have lived much with the past, that we have disturbed the dust of libraries, and, in presence of those mountains of books and manuscripts accumulated for ages, reflect on the mediocrity of the result, on the little we know and on all that yet remains to be learned—it is then, indeed, that we feel a satiety, and even disgust, of books; and we can then understand the whimsical reply of Sydenham, when asked what was the best book to read. The English Hippocrates, as he has been termed, replied, "Read 'Don Quixote.'" And yet Sydenham was no sceptic, and had reserved for his perusal a book which he knew how to read admirably—the book of nature.

But, gentlemen, the true and most powerful cause of scepticism, that which has in all times, ancient and modern, made so many sceptics among us, is that medicine at the same time that it is a science is also a profession. We do not complain of this, which is one of its glories—the highest, perhaps; for by it is given satisfaction to all that is most generous and most elevated in the human heart, the desire to come to the aid of those who suffer. But it is an onerous glory. The profession outweighs the science; and the latter, whatever it may do, will always fall far short of the exactions of the former. Men, for the most part, care little for the progress of science, but when they are ill they wish to be cured, and that is why they come to us. Now, for every practitioner having a consciousness of the dignity of his art there is a painful feeling due to his powerlessness in the presence of so many ills. What a contrast is there between the immensity of the services which are expected of us, and those which we are really able to render! How are we to justify the excess of confidence of so many patients? We must, in spite of all, act and strive. Science is incomplete, as it always will be. No matter; we must do our best. This, we must admit, is a pernicious habitude for the scientific mind to acquire. By it we accustom ourselves to act by chance, in the dark, or we fall into illusions as to what we know and what we are ignorant of. In face of this alternative, certain absolute minds, little disposed to temporising, fall back upon doubt and inaction, consoling themselves with this argument—that if we may

---

(a) The best known of all, Sextus Empiricus, who, in his celebrated "Hypotyposes Pyrrhonienne," has left us a complete summing-up and, as it were, code of the scientific scepticism of antiquity, was one of us. I am well aware that he somewhere denies that the necessary relation between doctrinal scepticism and medical empiricism as taught in his day could be established. This relation he rather sought for between scepticism and methodism, to the great trouble of his commentators. But this is of little import. He was a physician—of that there is no doubt; and, like him, there were at least four or five other physicians whose names have come down to us among the principal adepts of ancient pyrrhonism. . . . Some reservations have to be made. If the medical studies favour the emancipation of the intellect, it must also be said, to their honour, that they are fitted to maintain it in a certain practical good sense, and to preserve it from those divarications into which the philosophers by profession more readily fall. Several of the writers to whom I have referred would seem often to have been judged of rather by the outside of their books, for in reality they are rather doubters than sceptics. Thus, the book of Sanches, "Quid nihil Scitur," in spite of its satirical and paradoxical form—liable, I admit, to give rise to misunderstanding—is really only a virulent recrimination, not against science, but against the scholastic method, still held in honour in his time. It may be compared not unjustly with Bacon's "Pars Destruens" of the Organum; and, in fact, the book was, in the idea of its author, but the first part of a work in which, after having destroyed, he intended in its turn to construct. It remained unfinished, and does not admit of a definitive judgment. As to Martines, who has written not only his "Philosophia Sceptica," but also a work on sceptical medicine, he certainly possessed an independent mind, and had not breathed the air of the eighteenth century in vain. But it is sufficient to prove him not to have been a true sceptic, at least in the ordinary acceptation of the word, that in support of his doctrine he invokes side by side the great names of Sydenham and Baglivi, the authority of Scripture and the Fathers; and in his polemic against Lopes of Araujo, he found himself supported by Hieronymus Feyjoo, professor of theology at Oviedo. His voluminous works are, in fact, but a prolonged plea in favour of the method of observation. In dialogues, after the manner of Plato, he attacks the Hippocratists, the Galenists, the Chemiatrists, and the Cartesians, refuting the one by the other, his final conclusion being that scientific certainty is in its nature not absolute, but only relative, this being in fact the condition of progress. You perceive, then, that pyrrhonism such as this only goes beyond that of which Sprengel distinctly declares himself the partisan. On these terms there are still plenty of pyrrhonists. Still, the affinity of which I spoke just now none the less exists; and what is still more worthy of attention is, that there runs through medical literature a current of scepticism bearing on medical matters, a dogmatising scepticism like that of Leonard of Capua, for example (Parere del Signor Lionardo di Capoa, divisato in Otto Ragionamenti, nei quali partitamente narrandosi l'origine e il progresso della medicina, chiaramente l'incertezza della medesima si fa manifesto. Napoli, 1865). This physician seems to have assumed the task of demonstrating ex professo that medicine has no existence. I am not aware that a similar spectacle has been presented to us in any other branch of science.

(b) "De la Ressemblance des Enfants aux Pères," chap. xxxvii., livre 18.

say with Comte that "to know is to do," it is not less just to affirm that to be ignorant is to be powerless.

Such, then, gentlemen, are the most important of the general causes which, in all times and countries, have ranged a great number of physicians under the banner of scepticism. Others there are which are more special to former times or to our own epoch, and on which I ask your permission to insist for a moment. I will first speak of the past. But what sense do we attach in medicine to this word, the past? Where do the ancients terminate and the moderns begin? It is to England that the reply belongs, for hers is the honour of having actually inaugurated the modern era in the medical sciences. In fact, as Daremberg has said, there are but two great periods in the history of medicine—that which has preceded and that which has followed your great and immortal Harvey. Before Harvey, the sick man was only regarded from without—sometimes, we admit, with astonishing and admirable sagacity—but still always from without, the symptoms. Since Harvey, he has been studied from within, by the functions. The internal microcosm, hitherto closed, was now opened to investigation. Harvey at the same time introduced into science the novel and fertile idea that there were permanent and immutable laws in physiology. Prior to then, nothing was known in physiology, but from that moment acquisitions commenced. But you are aware that chronology is far from always being in agreement with doctrines. More than half a century was required for the circulation of the blood to be admitted as beyond dispute—a half-century during which the new doctrine was met face to face by the most strange and distressing form of scepticism, that which persists in closing the eyes to all evidence and in combating only with dialectics as weapons the best established facts. What talents, science, and wit have been expended in pure loss by the adversaries of the "circulators," as they were then called! Guy Patin is a memorable example. Possessed of a singularly acute intellect, but closed to every new idea, and treating the pharmacopœia of his time, antimony, and the circulation with the same disdain, he reduced all therapeutics to bleeding—furnishing a striking proof that scepticism and routine may often march side by side. Who would venture to declare that the race of Guy Patin is entirely lost, and that the genius of Harvey is at the present time everywhere and absolutely triumphant? At all times, but certainly formerly more than at the present time, dogmatism has been the parent of medical scepticism. The narrowness and tyranny of dogma lead directly to doubt, especially when the dogma does not rest on a solid foundation. Now, when we sound the depths of the ancient genius, what do we find? A vague and incomplete notion of the permanence of the laws of nature. Amidst hypotheses on the *primum movens* that are sometimes mystical and sometimes grossly materialistic, we always encounter the idea, more or less consciously formulated, but always admitted, that life is a capricious, intangible force—that in all its manifestations the exception is almost as frequent as the rule, and that it is impossible, in regard to such fluctuating matters, to make any positive affirmation.

But are such modes of thought so distant from ourselves? Do we not sometimes hear it said around us that the words "never" and "always" should not be employed in medicine, where "everything happens"? Have we never heard "uncertain medicines," "unlucky diseases," etc., spoken of? Is it not scepticism we still meet with under these common expressions—a scepticism perhaps not admitted, and all the more dangerous? It is often said at the present time that there are no longer any systems, that their time is past, and that we now only put faith in facts, etc. This is a point on which I must demand permission to remain myself somewhat sceptical. Not to go beyond France, have we not had since the beginning of this century physiological medicine, organic medicine, and its opposite the vitalistic, numerical medicine, exact medicine, positive medicine, and (which is not exactly the same thing) positivist medicine? I could even name others if I wished. Moreover, this pretension to rigour and exactness is not peculiar to our own epoch; it has always existed. Do you suppose that our fathers imagined that they were pursuing a fantastic science? They also proclaimed the sovereignty of experience and the all-powerfulness of facts. It is, therefore, a mere commonplace. Yet I willingly admit that systems at the present day have lost much of their importance—until they recover it again; I admit that, for the

moment, warned by the example of the past, we no longer embrace all science in a single formula; and that our conceptions being now more modest, have, by that very fact, some chance of being true. You will observe that I attribute to the present time all the good qualities that can be becomingly exacted; and I only ask of it to well acknowledge the defects of its qualities. It is in these defects I still find some of the causes of modern medical scepticism. First of all, I may indicate ignorance. It would be more conformable to good fraternity, and even more just, to say, the abuse of science. At the present day the field of science is so vast that we are obliged to limit ourselves to portions, under the penalty of remaining unproductive. Hence the fact, certainly very peculiar to our epoch, that some of the *savants* of the highest eminence in their own specialty are absolutely ignorant of all beyond it: and as it is always more easy and much shorter to doubt than to study, here we have all ready for certain partial scepticisms—such as therapeutical scepticism, so much in use with men of the world. There are other modes of abuse of science which also may lead to doubt. The dominant character of our present medical science is, as I have already said, the direct intervention of physiology in the matter of pathology. But physiology is not medicine, and even their field of study is not quite identical. There are, it is true, the same tissues and the same organs; but their reactions are different according to whether the man is well or ill, and disease alone has the power of provoking certain modes of reaction, which to the present time at least we know not how to induce experimentally. Who would suspect, on looking at the brain, Hippocrates has said, that wine would disturb its functions? Would the most precise notions of the functions of the skin teach us anything whatever as to small-pox? However close, then, the ties may be which henceforth may unite physiology to medicine, the light which one throws upon the other is as yet very insufficient. Therefore we must not feel surprised that a good number of physiologists, and some of the most eminent of these, look upon medicine with absolute scepticism. Such was the case with Magendie, to whom much should be forgiven, for to him we owe Claude Bernard. Even the progress of pathological anatomy would seem, in certain cases, to encourage the tendency to doubt. Formerly, for example, the efficacy of bleeding in cerebral hæmorrhage was believed in, and a theory was founded on the "raptus sanguineus" and the derivation of blood by venesection. But the discovery of miliary aneurisms destroys the theory, and the lancet loses favour. But we may loudly declare that it is only for superficial minds that the conquests of pathological anatomy will bring discredit on the ancients, and lead to the outrageous conclusion that there is nothing to be done in therapeutics. The reply is too easy. Is it not thanks to the progress of pathological anatomy that we now have the proofs of the curability of phthisis and of the possible evolution towards cicatrisation of the tubercular follicle? Is it nothing, moreover, to be made aware that you are on the wrong road? At least we change it to the great advantage of the patient. But I should be to blame were I to spend more time in these easy refutations.

I have now, gentlemen, defined and described this disease, "scepticism," and we have sought for its principal causes. Has this malady a remedy? But first, I hear the objection, Is scepticism an evil? Is it an enemy whom we can combat? Is it not rather one of those sides of human nature with which we had better come to terms, as we are powerless to triumph over it? In answering such a question, before all things we should be sincere. I once had an old master, himself somewhat of a sceptic, who was one day bemoaning before me on the impotence of our art, and added, "I should not say this before young persons, for it would discourage them and they will find it out soon enough for themselves." For my part, I never could understand this mode of procedure. We should tell to all, both young and old, what we believe to be the truth. If the result of so much human labour, so much watching, and so many sacrifices counts for nothing, our duty is still to say so. Wilful error when kept to ourselves may still be decorated by the title of an illusion; but taught to others, there is but one name for it—a lie. But who will venture to maintain that we have arrived at this point? Are you not now before me a living and illustrious negation of a system which leads to ignorance in pathology and to inaction in therapeutics? Let us, then, search for the means of resisting this tendency and of strengthening our belief. The remedy for scepticism is before all things to be found in science itself—in science each day better pursued and better understood, whose incessant progress will apply the appropriate correctives to its own errors, and furnish the expected solutions to its postulates. Each theoretical progress leads sooner or later to a practical improvement, which often proceeds from a quarter where it was least expected. It does not suffice to proclaim the merits of exact science, for in every science we have both the certain and uncertain. Nor does it suffice to blame the spirit of system, as the most famous systematisers have always been the most ardent in decrying the systems of others. Neither will it even suffice to construct the edifice on the supposed solid foundation of pathological anatomy. Long, long before our illustrious master Bouillaud had taken for his epigraph the saying of Bichat, " What can observation serve when we know not where is the disease ? " Celsus had asked, " How are we to treat a diseased organ of which we have formed no idea ? "

What is wanted, first of all, is the passage into practice and into the daily habit of the mind the truth which flows from these two axioms: first, the absolute constancy of the laws which govern life; and next, the rigorous subordination of the phenomena to certain conditions which have to be determined. It is this latter law which Claude Bernard has called " determinism "—a somewhat barbarous word, perhaps, and all the more disputable since it may easily be shown that its author himself has not always employed it in the same sense. But if the term is questionable, the thing itself is not. It is no longer a system, but the very essence of the scientific spirit. I have not here to exhibit to you the applications which Claude Bernard has made of it to physiology, and it would be too long to detail those which may be made to pathology. Allow me merely to quote a few examples; first taking locomotor ataxy. Several years since this disease remained confounded in the vague group of the paraplegias. We were entirely ignorant about it, its nature, or its cause. Its treatment was a matter of chance, and some patients were cured who certainly were not the subjects of ataxy. This was the first stage in the history of the disease—the period of ignorance. Then comes the second stage, the anatomo-pathological. The lesion is discovered and recognised as incurable. This is the period of discouragement. Finally, in the third stage, it was shown that a good number (I do not say all) of these cases originated in syphilis; and if we cannot cure them radically, we are able at least, by means of specific treatment, to arrest their development. Virulent and infectious diseases furnish us with a still more striking example. When in recent times the study of spontaneous generation led to the discovery of that world of infinitely minute beings which seemed to lay siege to us in all parts, it might well be asked how the human species, how animal life itself, was able to resist these myriads of invisible enemies ever ready to profit by any defect in the organism, and effect a penetration. But, seizing hold of this very circumstance itself, a great surgeon, who is also a thinker—Lister—invents a new method which diminishes or suppresses the chances of infection consecutive to great operations, enlarges the limits of art, and insures almost infallible success of daring procedures, before which, but a short time since, all would have recoiled.

Again, we have a man of genius whose name I pronounce with pride,—my illustrious friend Pasteur, who, taking up and systematising the work of your great Jenner, has succeeded, by the methodical attenuation of viruses, in originating a prophylaxis of virulent diseases, and opening up to us new and indefinite horizons. In face of such results as these, gentlemen, where is the place for scepticism ? It would much rather be from an excess of enthusiasm that we should have to stand on our guard, were not our admiration amply justified by the importance of the discoveries already acquired. It is thus that we can reply most usefully to the sceptics. The movement has not to be demonstrated—it shows itself. Let us, nevertheless, not forget an axiom of the medicine of antiquity, which has outlived all dogmatic revolutions, and which Hippocrates defined as " medicatrix nature." It has at times been somewhat derided; but for my part, I believe in it as something as certain as the most incontestable experimental facts. The interpretations that have been given of it may indeed be disputable; but if so many explanations have been advanced, some of them faulty enough, this arises from the commanding position of the fact itself.

Recently, in a communication by Pasteur to the Academy of Medicine, I remarked that my eminent countryman, endeavouring to fix the progressive attenuation of his viruses, had taken as a criterion the resistance offered by the organism of the sheep. Such a virus kills one sheep in fifty, another one in one hundred, and another fifty in one hundred, and so on. Now, what does this imply ? This condition of " receptivity," which M. Pasteur, great observer as he is, appeals to, what is it in its nature if not that power of resistance which, existing in every living being, and differing according to species, and even according to individuals, is yet at bottom the same thing as the *vis medicatrix* ? Whatever may be said of it, here is still one of the dominant facts of medicine. This power of vital resistance, this greater or less receptivity of disease, will always be an indispensable auxiliary of the physician; and, for my own part, I would renounce the practice of my art did I not feel myself sustained by such an ally. What constitutes the incomparable difficulty of our art is the necessity of assigning a just share to this element in the cure of disease, and of reconciling it, in the interpretation of morbid phenomena, with the two fundamental axioms which I have admitted. The task is an arduous one, but, difficult as it may appear, rest assured that an agreement will be established. However this may be, taking into account this great power of vital resistance, and illumined by the light of etiology, pathological anatomy becomes no longer a mere meditation on death, but the science of indications—a profound saying bequeathed us by ancient medicine, and which will always respond to the most actual realities of our art.

When, gentlemen, certainty has been attained on these three points, our science will be well-nigh complete; and even when it is not so, we are still not entirely disarmed, for we have then the right to make appeal to empiricism and tradition; and who of us would dispense with this ? They furnish us, in the absence of a better, with a kind of certainty which is not without its value, and which does not impede our pursuit of a higher certainty. The patrimony which each medical generation bequeaths to that which follows it consists of two kinds of things—some of an absolute value, and others of only a relative value, but which are not to be disdained. In this way we have received from our predecessors opium, cinchona, and nearly all our best medicines, which have rendered us immense services, and will yet render us more before we have been enabled to definitively determine their mode of action. So we, in our turn, shall leave to our successors chloroform, chloral, carbolic acid, the salicylates, pilocarpin, and many other substances, the appreciation of which, and the explanation of their various forms of usefulness, it will fall to the future to furnish. In this way are constituted what Cabanis has so well termed the " practical certainties " of medicine; and in this way we attain the certainty proper to the clinician, which in many respects consists of moral certainty, and, although not equal to scientific certainty, yet has place and rank at its side.

The limits assigned to me do not allow of my prolonging this address; and in order to close it worthily, allow me, gentlemen, to cite to you a passage which may serve as a summing-up and conclusion, and which I borrow from Claude Bernard. I cannot do better than leave you under the impression of these simple and powerful words. " The sceptic," says our great physiologist, in his " Introduction à la Médecine Expérimentale," " is he who does not believe in science, but believes in himself. He believes sufficiently in himself to dare to deny science, and to affirm that it is not submitted to fixed and determined laws. The doubter is the true *savant*. He only doubts himself and his own interpretations; but he has faith in science, and admits, even in the experimental sciences, a criterion or an absolute scientific principle."

NOCTURNAL ENURESIS OF CHILDREN.—Prof. Gross advises the following :—Strychniæ gr. j., pulv. cantharid. gr. ij., morph. sulph. gr. iss., ferri pulv. ʒij.—to be made into forty pills or powders, and one given three times a day to a child ten years old. They will speedily relieve the irritation of the bladder, especially if conjoined with such measures as a cold bath daily, the avoidance of irritant food and late suppers, the patient lying on the side or belly, not drinking for a few hours prior to sleep, and emptying the bladder on going to bed.—*Louisville Med. News*, August 20.

ORIGINAL COMMUNICATIONS.

REMARKS ON CERTAIN ASSIGNED CAUSES OF FEVER.

By SURGEON-GENERAL C. A. GORDON,
M.D., C.B., Q.H.P., etc.

Insanitary Conditions.—Enteric or typhoid fever is designated "a filth disease";(a) so also is cholera. From this point of view an extensive series of observations has for several years been conducted, and with the following results, namely —(a) that under particular circumstances typhoid fever has arisen from contamination of air, earth, or water by the products of animal decomposition ; (b) but it is only one of several forms of disease due to similar causes ; (c) nor does the presence of the conditions named always or necessarily produce it.

In 1800 the epidemic of yellow fever, by which Cadiz was then devastated, made its first appearance in the narrow, crowded, and offensive streets and lanes of the Barrio de Santa Maria, where also the inhabitants are dirty in their persons, and crowded together in filthy rooms. The supposed introduction of the disease into that city by means of shipping could not be traced. In 1803 a similar circumstance was recorded with regard to the epidemic in Malaga ; and in 1821 the epidemic by which Spain was again visited affected the most filthy towns, while the cleanly escaped.

Dr. Mason wrote with reference to yellow fever :—" The epidemics of this kind accompanied with most mortality are those which arise from a decomposition of human effluvium in the midst of filth, poverty, or famine, great heat and moisture, crowded multitudes, and a stagnant atmosphere." He enumerates after this manner the origin and laws of febrile action, namely—1. The decomposition of dead organised matter under the influence of certain agents produces a miasm that proves a common cause of fever. 2. The whole of the agents had not in his day been explored, but they seemed to be the common auxiliaries of putrefaction—as warmth, moisture, air at rest, or stagnation. 3. The nature of the fever depends partly upon the state of the body at the time of attack, but chiefly upon some modifications in the qualities or power of the febrile miasm. 4. The decomposition of the effluvium transmitted from the human body produces a miasm similar to that generated by the decomposition of dead organised matter, and capable of becoming a cause of fever. Fevers generated in gaols and other confined or crowded scenes contaminate the atmosphere to a less distance than those from swamps, but act with greater depression on the living fibre.

On the remote causes of disease, Dr. Alison, writing in 1832, remarked that they include—(a) imperfect nourishment ; (b) deficiency of pure air and of muscular exercise ; (c) excessive exertion, mental or bodily, and deficient sleep ; (d) long-continued heat ; (e) long-continued cold ; (f) intemperance ; (g) excessive and repeated evacuations ; (h) depressing passions of mind ; and (i) previous debilitating disease. He thus continues—"Some of the causes above enumerated peculiarly affect particular organs—as heat, the liver and mucous membrane of the bowels; excessive mental exertion, the brain ; violent mental emotion, the heart, etc." And he adds, "Continued fever differs from the exanthemata in that it is never absent from any large community in Britain, whereas the exanthemata are so." He goes on to observe (" Outlines of Pathology," page 185) that "the putrefaction of animal and vegetable matter is naturally a very frequent concomitant of the process by which the poison (of fever?) is thus developed ; but the facts stated by Chisholm and Fergusson seem sufficient to show that it is not an essential part of the process. Perhaps we may assert that long-continued mental depression and anxiety, above youth especially, has been assigned with more probability than any other cause for the *spontaneous* generation of continued fever " (page 192). These remarks, although made with special reference to fever as met with in Britain, have a very important bearing upon the disease as it occurs in India and other tropical climates.

(a) New Series of Reports by the Medical Officer to the Privy Council, No. 5 for 1875, page 9.

In India at the present time, when fever occurs at a particular station, the tendency of the day is to search for its origin in local insanitary conditions, to the relative neglect of all others. The appearance of fever at a station in the Punjaub in 1880 is made the occasion for the following remarks :—" Typhoid [why so called in this instance does not appear] fever can be traced to a cause almost with as much certainty as typhus can, and in both diseases some neglect of, or deficiency in, sanitary arrangements is supposed to be the primary danger. That danger has been lurking for a long time in Lahore, and, it would seem, still remains." And so on with regard to other localities.

Dr. Hughes Bennett quotes the opinion of Dr. Murchison that typhus and relapsing fever are caused by general insanitary conditions, including overcrowding, deficient ventilation, and destitution ; *typhoid*, by emanations from decaying organic matter, or by both these causes combined. With reference to these, however, he states that the facts which came under his notice in the Edinburgh epidemic of 1846-47 cannot, he thinks, be explained by any such supposition.

In 1832, Dr. Elliotson observed that many persons are employed in the most offensive occupations with putrid animal matter, and yet fever never breaks out among them. Orfila mentioned the healthiness of knackeries, where there is immense putrefaction in summer, and the soil has been saturated for years. It is remarked, however, that although such causes do not generate fever, yet they operate strongly when other causes of disease come into play. Dr. Alfred Carpenter states that the excreta of nearly 1200 cases of typhoid fever, with all the excreta from other cases which occurred in the Croydon district, in 1875 distributed over the fields upon which the sewage of that town is utilised. In a large number of instances these excreta were not disinfected. The number of hands employed upon the farm then averaged from forty to sixty per week ; a large number of persons were also employed in removing produce from the farm. No instance was brought to his knowledge of typhoid fever, or of any other zymotic disease, arising among the people on the farm, although he studiously sought for cases of those diseases ; there was all but complete immunity from these affections among the several thousands who live within a mile of the borders of the farm. Dr. Netten Radcliffe relates a case in which exposure to air from a dead-house was the cause of erysipelas in a succession of patients suffering from surgical injuries. No case of *enteric* fever among them was mentioned.

The doubts expressed with regard to the efficiency under all circumstances of pythogenic causes to produce specific enteric fever, appear to gain force from evidence as it accumulates, and from observations on the subject by medical men. Some of the grounds upon which such doubts are based are the following :—According to the *British Medical Journal* of July 5, 1879, " At Lymington not only is the general sanitary administration lax, but the system of excremental disposal (garden privies) is both offensive and dangerous, the sewerage is defective and leaky, and the water-supply, derived from wells in porous gravel, is obviously exposed to pollution. Yet zymotic diseases have, for the last eight years, been conspicuous by their absence, and the general death-rate is only 17·5 per 1000. It was a nut to crack for the supporters of the pythogenic hypothesis, how, notwithstanding these manifold noxious influences, Lymington has managed, during all this time, to escape a visitation of infectious disease."

According to the pythogenic theory of causation, it is observed, with reference to prophylactic measures to meet the prevalence of fatal enteric fever in Paris, that such measures are as yet little known ; that, in fact, such as are adopted on that theory are without result.

Dr. Andrew Fergus, in his address on State Medicine, delivered at the meeting of the British Medical Association in 1879, observed that improved house accommodation and the supervision of medical officers of health have of late years tended in a marked manner to reduce the prevalence of *typhus* fever in the home population ; *typhoid*, he says, does not show so well, but simple continued fever shows nearly as favourable results as typhus.

According to Dr. Baldwin Latham, no sanitary evils have followed the system of sewage irrigation adopted at Croydon, nor have any persons living in the neighbourhood of that irrigation been affected with any particular disorder. The system of this kind of irrigation was first fully adopted there in 1856, the sewage farm being situated partly in the parish of Beddington and partly in the hamlet of Wallington. According to statistics during the ten years before the introduction of that farm, the death-rate there was by fever 0·95, diarrhœa 0·74; in Croydon the fever death-rate was 1·27. From 1861 to 1878—namely, after the sewage irrigation had been introduced—the fever death-rate was 0·32, diarrhœa death-rate 0·86; the fever death-rate in Croydon 0·67. Thus, taking into account the increase of population, it is shown that no evil or injury to health has arisen. In 1862, when fever was prevalent in Croydon, no deaths by it occurred either in the district of Beddington or Wallington. In the epidemic of fever at Croydon in 1865 and 1866, two deaths occurred, but at places situated at a considerable distance from the sewage farm. In 1875 and 1876, when fever was again epidemic in Croydon, one death occurred in Wallington in 1875, and none in 1876. This establishes the fact that the exposure the sewage meets with in treatment by irrigation entirely destroys whatever noxious properties it may have, so that it becomes incapable of transmitting disease. Statistics follow the remarks by Dr. Latham, the result of which is that labourers on sewage farms, and their families, are particularly healthy, and do not suffer in an especial manner from fever.

In February, 1879, a correspondent of the Madras Mail, writing from New York, thus expressed himself with regard to neglected sanitation in connexion with yellow fever:— "There is, to start with, no division of opinion as to the expediency of entirely excluding yellow fever from our country; but differences exist as to the means necessary, or those likely to be effectual. . . . . The shackles of professional routine seem to be the main cause of this. Still, some addition to the store of facts is made, for which we should be thankful; but very little has been added since 1853. The great difficulty about it—after remembering the professional ruts above alluded to—is the fact that different localities report different results. All this, however, only goes to show us that we are probably all wrong in theory, somehow or other. In New Orleans, on the one hand, the yellow fever prevailed most, began earliest, and proved most fatal in localities situated highest and in the best sanitary condition generally; and prevailed slightly, late, and mildly in the lowest and worst policed places. In Memphis, on the other hand, it was just the reverse of that—the fever following the malarial, and exposed and dirty regions in the city. This evidence seems to prove that exhaustion from malarial influences renders the subject less able to resist the attack of the imported disease; but why would not the same thing take place in New Orleans? Taking the Crescent City alone, intelligent observation, both professional and non-professional, seems to have established these three propositions:—First, prophylactics, such as quinine, carbolic acid, bitters, and the like, are useless—that is to say, the prophylactic for yellow fever has not yet been discovered. Secondly, the uselessness of disinfectants now in use—mainly carbolic acid—in arresting the progress of the fever; that acid having been tried indoors, in the gutters, and everywhere, with next to no effect, if any. Thirdly, the independence of the fever to malarial influences directly and locally. It is agreed all round that New Orleans was not in a worse hygienic—that is, more dirty—condition in 1878 than it was in 1877, 1876, or 1875; and, unless the cumulative theory be brought in, the local origin theory of the fever must be abandoned. Indeed, it seems as if, had the whole city been in a more unsanitary condition, the fever would have made less headway; and this because it made least headway where the neglect was greatest. In Memphis the condition as to sanitation seems to be almost equally bad in all parts; at least, deplorably bad in all places."

As regards India—" So far have been the measures of conservancy and scavenging hitherto applied to stations from reducing the fatality of fevers returned synonymously enteric or typhoid, and looked upon as results of filth, that, as already observed, of late years the proportionate fever mortality has increased to a very serious extent." Nor has the introduction of the dry earth system of conservancy in gaols resulted in the abolition of contagious fevers among prisoners.

From these particulars the conclusion appears natural, that although insanitary conditions are in themselves most objectionable, and tend to concentrate and intensify epidemics of disease when these occur, they are not alone sufficient to originate or produce specific fever, such as that form designated enteric or typhoid is by many writers and observers considered to be.

What, then, is the actual state of matters in regard to general sanitation? That poverty, wretchedness, and disease prevail together is a fact as definitely acknowledged by the writers of sacred history as by the most advanced "sanitarians" of the present day. That something quite beyond the mere removal of "insanitary" conditions is necessary in order to increase the health-standard of the masses is necessary, has been thus publicly declared by one of the highest authorities of our day. In the sectional meeting of the British Medical Association, 1880, Professor De Chaumont was "afraid that in our modern sanitary science we had done little more than remove the supernatural from our list of causes. Sanitary science could only advance as medical science advanced. In diagnosis and pathology modern progress had been extremely rapid and satisfactory, but of etiology or determination of the causes of disease he could not speak with such confidence, though no doubt some advance had been made. It was upon this branch, however, that the advance of sanitation towards the dignity of an exact science depended. Until we knew more of the causation of disease it was impossible to lay down rules for its prevention; but because progress was slow were we to despair? Certainly not. But the only way to effect progress was by the careful observation and recording of facts, having full faith that the day would assuredly come when those facts would range themselves in proper order, and reveal the hitherto unknown law that bound them together. But each fact must be the truth, so far as we could make it so, and its bearing must be measured and its value weighed. Medicine and the science of measurement had been long divorced. It was the province of our age to bring about a reunion of the two"—a consummation most devoutly to be wished, but, by the nature of things, unlikely to be attained.

Nor does it by any means follow that because particular circumstances and conditions in England conduce to illness, similar circumstances and conditions similarly affect peoples of other nationalities in other countries. As an illustration in point, Sir D. Wedderburn, writing in the Nineteenth Century for August, 1880, says with regard to the people of Iceland, that "altogether it is clear that crowded unwholesome dwellings, with a somewhat free indulgence in stimulants, and a severe climate, do not prevent the hardy Icelanders from attaining a good old age. The discomfort of living in such a hovel amidst damp, darkness, and evil smells can hardly be surpassed." The influence of race also has an important relation to health and to disease. Thus the native of the temperate zone does not bear tropical heat and climates as do the natives of such countries; nor do the natives of the latter bear the climate of the temperate or frigid zone as do the indigenes of these respectively. Persons of different temperaments manifest susceptibility or tendency to different diseases; so also with regard to idiosyncrasy, habits whether hereditary or acquired, constitution, and so on. Natives of Africa, India, China, and Japan live and thrive under conditions which, according to Western ideas, are most "insanitary."

With regard to the connexion between outbreaks of typhoid fever and the state of sewers and drains in the locality, the result of investigations has been that while in certain cases an apparent connexion of this kind has been traced, others have been recorded in which exposure to defective drains has neither produced typhoid fever nor any other illness; also that, when apparently traceable to this cause, it is only one or several diseases which have been similarly traced to it. Certain writers go so far as to assert that the origin of enteric fever dates from the introduction of water-closets into dwelling-houses—an improvement for which England is indebted to Sir Hugh Harrington, in the reign of Queen Elizabeth. At Gibraltar in former years, and at Malta more recently, the occurrence of that form of fever has on some occasions been traced to defective drainage.

Dr. Barker, writing in 1863, gives various examples of direct causation of what he calls enteric fever by continuous exposure to sewer-gas. But he also gives other examples of the production of typhus, scarlatina, and erysipelas from the same cause; he, moreover, notices the circumstance that, whereas the conditions related by him had existed for years without the occurrence of those diseases, so their outbreak was only temporary, although the emanations still continued to exist. He looks upon *sulphide of ammonium* in sewer-gas as the actual producing cause of typhoid fever. But, he remarks, authors have never yet informed us why *malaria*, as a result of decomposing animal and vegetable matters, produces intermittent fever in one case, typhus fever, yellow fever, plague, cholera, and dysentery in others.

In 1866, the theory of causation in this manner was opposed by Dr. Collis. He observes, with regard to the outbreak in Liverpool-road in that year, that if the drain theory proves anything as to the etiology of enteric fever, it would prove that it arose from cholera stools, and that therefore it was not specific.

In 1874, and again in 1879, Dr. Ballard traced outbreaks of enteric fever at Tolcairne, in Cornwall, to the circumstance of water becoming contaminated by sewage matters as a result of defects in sewers, thus causing neighbouring wells to become polluted. Many similar occurrences are also related.

In 1880 the remark occurs that in Calcutta enteric fever has become more frequent coincidently with the extension of the great system of underground sewerage of that city. With regard to the assigned cause of an outbreak of the disease at Millbrook, in Cornwall, the following particulars occur, namely :—" It appears that Millbrook has recently been sewered, but that the sewers have been most inefficiently and inadequately ventilated. Moreover, as they discharge into a tidal stream, the air in them is pushed back when the tide rises, and escapes at all weak and defective places. Early in the year, the air in the sewers became infected with the contagium of enteric fever, and undoubtedly spread the disease to certain other places, especially to one particular well, the overflow of which communicated with the sewer into which the infected discharges passed. The sewers have no adequate means of flushing, only one flushing-tank having been provided; and are, doubtless, therefore, sewers of deposit. Again, but one of the wells in Millbrook was found to be safe for drinking purposes. All are sunk in fissured rocks in the immediate neighbourhood of the houses; the water is, therefore, subject to pollution by soakage from the surface, from privies, leaky drains, and the like. Dr. Ballard had no doubt that the fever had been spread through the medium of these well-waters. Another source of danger was the milk-supply. There was a dairy adjoining a slaughter-house, into which entered, from a stinking untrapped gully communicating with the sewer first infected, sewer air, which had no doubt been absorbed by the milk. Of the eight regular customers of the milk-seller, six families had been attacked with fever. One family was away at the time, and only one escaped. Persons who were occasionally supplied had also had fever."

Many other illustrative examples of reports might be quoted, but these suffice for our present purpose. Here, however, is one of a different kind. The Russian diphtheria of 1880 is described as in some respects like the form of croup or bronchitis which prevailed in London during the previous winter. In Russia it prevailed during the cold weather, in the country rather than in towns, in low-lying undrained localities. As in England, diphtheria is considered a disease of childhood, spread by communication, chiefly in schools. It does not seem to have any necessary connexion with bad drainage, though often bad drainage and diphtheria go together. A similar view is expressed by Mr. Wynter Blyth. According to him, while admitting that bad drainage, nuisances, and filth might greatly aid the extension of the disease when introduced into a family, he expressed the opinion that the general sanitary condition of houses had nothing whatever to do with the selection of the spot of attack. These remarks apply also to the form of fever called typhoid or enteric.

A recent reviewer writes as follows in reference to the view of typhoid fever, that the disease in all cases can be traced to the drinking of polluted water, the inhaling of sewer-gas, or air tainted with infectious bowel-discharges: —" This view is, no doubt, sufficiently in accord with the opinions of a large number of trustworthy authorities to justify its being maintained; but we feel sure that those who entertain it will be found, as a rule, to have derived their experience chiefly in urban districts, and that observers who have been enabled to study this disease, as it so frequently occurs in isolated and otherwise healthy conditions in rural spots, will not feel so ready to accept it as an

exhaustive solution of the problem of the genesis of a disease which shades off so insensibly into uncomplicated low fever on the one hand, and into simple diarrhœa on the other."(b)

Water.—The older medical officers in India and elsewhere made frequent allusion to the effect of bad water in producing disease; but that disease was diarrhœa, dysentery, or intermittent fever. An epidemic diarrhœa occurring among a native regiment at Hyderabad, in Scinde, from the use of stagnant water, was reported on by Dr. McLennan. The state of conservancy at some of our Indian hill-stations, more especially at Simla, was described as being bad, the ravines full of dead animals. To the use of such water was attributed the affection known as hill-diarrhœa; but, although the disease often proved most persistent, it was unattended by fever. At Darjeeling the prevalence of round worms is attributed to impure drinking-water, but nothing is said regarding the occurrence of a specific form of fever from the same cause. Water taken from ravines which at the same time may be, and are, used as latrines easily accounts for their wide distribution.

Dr. Mason Good (1829) quotes from an article by Dr. Cheyne in the *Dublin Hospital Reports* (vol. iii., page 11), in which the dependence of dysentery upon the use of impure water is clearly indicated. Of this he says:—" A striking example occurred not many years ago at Cork. While the disease was raging with great violence, it was observed by Mr. Bell, the temporary surgeon, that the troops were supplied with water contaminated by an influx from the public sewers, and rendered brackish by an intermixture with the tide. He immediately changed the beverage, and had the barracks supplied by water-casks from a spring called the Lady's Well, when the disease almost immediately ceased."

In 1869 an outbreak of *typhoid* fever occurred at Wicken Bovant. Dr. Robinson, who attended all the cases, observes that " with one or two exceptions the cases have not had the characters of the fever well marked." " Diarrhœa occurred, in some cases, but was by no means a constant symptom." He records the presence of *rose* spots in one case. The number of cases was forty-five, of deaths four. With regard to the endeavour made to connect that outbreak with the use of water from a brook believed to be contaminated with fæcal matter, the statement occurs that Clark, the first or second person attacked, denies that he drank water from it at all. The supposition that he got his illness from using contaminated water from the parish well "involves the supposition that typhoid matter could travel 250 yards through gravel without thereby being rendered harmless." The conclusion arrived at, therefore, is that Clark's fever, and that which is believed to have spread from him, " was somehow or another caused by fever imported from London."(c)

At the meeting of the British Medical Association at Cork in 1879, a discussion took place on the influence of drinking-water in originating or propagating enteric fever, diarrhœa, diphtheria, and scarlatina, from which the following extracts are taken:—Dr. Fergus stated that Glasgow was, in 1866, supplied with pure water, and since then imported cases of cholera did not take any hold on the city; summer diarrhœa and diphtheria had decreased. He instanced a family, several members of which had *typhoid* fever on their return from a watering-place, where, on examination, twenty-eight of the wells were found polluted with organic matter. He considered that Nesler's solution should be used to test water before it was made use of. Dr. A. Carpenter pointed out that there are generally two causes at work in the establishment of an epidemic of enteric fever: the first, that the houses of the sufferers are exposed to the results of sewage change; the second, that the water service is in immediate connexion with the sewers. He showed that there are conditions which tend to purify underground streams, as well as the atmospheric air; also that, if a given water-supply be not super-saturated with bicarbonate of lime, the germs of enteric fever cannot increase and multiply in that water. He considered that in all cases of typhoid epidemic there was required a fitting soil as well as an " enteric germ," and that the fitting soil was generally defective sewage arrangements; that an enteric germ finding its way into otherwise pure water cannot multiply, and will not retain its vitality for

(b) *Sanitary Record*, December 15, 1880, page 235.
(c) Report of Medical Officer, Privy Council, 1869, pages 74 to 77.

any period; that if it find its way into a healthy person who has not been exposed to miasm from decomposing animal matter, it will not set up an attack of true enteric fever. He was opposed to Pettenkofer's idea that the enteric poison multiplies in the soil without reference to the bodies of patients.

Dr. Notter observed that chemical analysis could not specify the causes of enteric fever,—they could only indicate the presence of nitrogenous compounds; and where such are present, care must be taken lest the specific germ be present also. Chemical analysis was limited in its power, and might in fact mislead. The elimination of disease germs would baffle chemistry. Microscopic examination should accompany the chemical.

Dr. E. Ballard described an outbreak of enteric fever in the village of Nunney, near Frome, the outbreak being due to the use of water from a foul brook, which water, however, did not produce the fever until a case of the disease imported from a distance occurred on the summit of a gorge through which the stream flowed above the village. A similar occurrence happened in the village of Hawkesbury Upton, in Gloucestershire, from wells sunk side by side in oolite rock to privy cesspools, and thus habitually contaminated; but in that instance also after the occurrence of an imported case. Other examples were mentioned by him, including one near Birmingham, where the disease spread from washing soiled linen; another in Mosley, where it did so by infected milk; as also similar ones to the latter at Ascot, and in Marylebone in 1873.

Dr. N. Kerr instanced a case of a family among the members of which diarrhœa, scarlatina, and diphtheritic sore-throat were never absent. Their drinking water was obtained from a well into which a drain from a pigstye and cow-house opened. The drain was improved, the same well continued to be used, and these diseases ceased. From these and other instances related he considered that the same contaminated drinking-water might, without the presence of specific germs, give rise to different ailments, the poison manifesting itself as erysipelas, scarlatina, diphtheria, diarrhœa, or enteric fever.

Surgeon-General Crawford stated, as the result of his experience in India, that various forms of fever occurred in that country which could not possibly be traced to water-supply. He instanced a cavalry regiment in which three such attacks of typhoid fever took place—one at Mhow, a second at Meerut, and a third at Umballa.

(*To be continued.*)

THE DOCTRINE OF SATURNINE GOUT.
By ROBERT SAUNDBY, M.D. Edin.,
Member of the Royal College of Physicians, and Assistant-Physician to the General Hospital, Birmingham.

THE relation of lead-poisoning to gout has met with but little attention in medical literature. Though Dr. Garrod's views on this subject were received with some scepticism by certain contemporary reviewers, I know of no attempt to examine the evidence upon which they are based, or of any definite contradiction of them. Most of our standard authors content themselves with quoting Dr. Garrod; others omit the fact altogether; while the amount of information on the subject in our periodical literature for the last twenty-five years is so exceedingly small that it is easily recapitulated.

In 1854, Dr. Garrod read a paper on Gout and Rheumatism before the Royal Medico-Chirurgical Society,(a) and mentioned that out of thirty-three cases of gout in which the occupation had been noted, eight, or nearly 25 per cent., of the patients used lead in their work, and had been affected with lead-disease.

In his well-known work on gout,(b) published in 1859, and again in Reynolds' "System of Medicine," Dr. Garrod insisted very strongly on the frequency with which he had observed gout in lead-workers, without hereditary predisposition to the disease, and mentioned that Dr. Burrows told him that his own experience at St. Bartholomew's Hospital quite confirmed this view.

Dr. Garrod gives notes of the three following cases in which this association existed:—

Case 1.—Lead-Poisoning—Gout—Not Intemperate—Not Hereditary.

J. S., aged forty-four, an organ-pipe maker, uses lead in his work. Drinks beer, but not to excess. Had gout in great toe first four years ago, and since then has had five or six similar attacks. No hereditary predisposition. Had drop-wrist two years ago; never had lead-colic. Has well-marked blue line on gums.

Case 2.—Lead-Poisoning—Gout—No Note as to Habits or Family History.

R. T., aged thirty-four, house-painter, has had gout in great toe for two years, and has had two or three attacks of lead-colic. Well-marked blue line on gums. Serum contains abundance of uric acid.

Case 3.—Lead-Poisoning—Gout—Temperate—No Note as to Family History.

J. B., aged forty-one, artist, first suffered from lead-colic ten years ago. Has always lived temperately. At present has entire loss of power in both wrists. Distinct blue line on gums. Blood contains abundance of uric acid. While under observation had a decided attack of gout.

Dr. Garrod's investigations into the state of the blood and urine showed that in cases of lead-poisoning—not only in those who had previously suffered from gout, but also in those who had shown no symptoms of the latter disease—uric acid was present in the blood, but that its presence was not quite constant. The urine showed a diminution of the quantity of uric acid excreted.

Sir Robert Christison, in answer to a question from Dr. Garrod,(c) wrote that neither gout nor lead-poisoning were common among the house-painters of Edinburgh. He had known only two cases of gout in his hospital practice, both in over-fed butlers. Dr. Williamson, of Aberdeen, informed Dr. Garrod that gout was rare among lead-workers in that city.

Dr. Warburton Begbie,(d) in 1862, in some observations on "Lead-impregnation and its Connexion with Gout and Rheumatism," says he cannot confirm Sir Robert Christison's statement that poisoning from protracted exposure to lead is a very rare occurrence in Edinburgh, or that gout occurs very rarely in his hospital practice, and he gives particulars of two cases of gout in house-painters, the subjects of lead-poisoning; but in both these cases the patients, contrary to the ordinary rule in Scotland, had indulged in fermented drinks, and were intemperate men. The amount of uric acid excreted was estimated in both cases, and found to be very much diminished.

The following are abstracts of the notes of these cases:—

Case 4.—Lead-Poisoning—Gout—Intemperate—No Note of Family History.

W. B., aged thirty, a house-painter, has been intemperate, consuming ale and porter freely. Had lead-colic first four years ago, and recently has acquired drop-wrist. Distinct blue line on gums. While under observation had an attack of regular gout.

Case 5.—Lead-Poisoning—Gout—Intemperate—No Note as to Family History.

J. H., aged thirty-seven, has worked as a house-painter for nineteen years, and has often had pains in his belly. Has had three distinct attacks of regular gout in last nine years. Has a distinct blue line on gums. Has drunk freely of whisky and malt liquors.

M. Gubler, in a discussion at the Société des Hôpitaux in 1868,(e) related the case of a patient suffering from lead-poisoning, in whom there arose an articular swelling of the great toe, with redness, heat, and severe pain, giving it much the appearance of gout; but he regarded it as simple arthritis, and thought the cases observed by Garrod were merely coincidences. MM. Bucquoy and Potain had both seen gout occurring in house-painters who had no hereditary

(a) "On Gout and Rheumatism : the Differential Diagnosis and the Nature of the so-called Rheumatic Gout" (*Medico-Chirurgical Transactions*, vol. xxxvii).
(b) "The Nature and Treatment of Gout," page 292 *et seq.* London, 1859.
(c) *Op. cit.*, page 262-4.
(d) "Observations in Clinical Medicine" (*Edinburgh Medical Journal* 1862, page 129).
(e) *Medical Times and Gazette*, vol. i. 1868, page 581.

predisposition, and they declined to see simply coincidences in these cases.

In 1868, Dr. Murchison(f) published a series of cases of lead-poisoning, of which the two following illustrated its association with gout :—

Case 6.—Lead-Poisoning—Gout(?)—No Note as to Habits or Family History.

C. C., aged thirty, a japanner, who uses lead in his business, was admitted for colic. There was a distinct blue line on his gums. While in hospital, pain, swelling, and redness of the left knee supervened—symptoms which were readily relieved by colchicum and alkalies.

Case 7.—Lead-Poisoning—Gout(?)—No Note as to Habits or Family History.

J. B., aged forty-two, a house-painter, with distinct blue line on gums, complained of pains in all his limbs, and pain, weakness, and swelling in the left knee.

Dr. Wilks, in *Guy's Hospital Reports* for 1869,(g) remarked that the association not only of the major phenomenon, but of those tissue degenerations resulting from gout (notably in the arteries and kidneys), with lead-poisoning, gives it a wide pathological significance, and suggests that, if gout be mainly hereditary, lead must be supposed to exert its deleterious influence only on predisposed individuals; while if, on the other hand, gout may be set up by mal-assimilation, then lead may act like malt liquors and want of exercise, and give rise to excess of uric acid in the blood; we may then account for the gout, diseased kidney, and other conditions, for the effect of lead is not the same in those cases in which gout has intervened. These remarks were à propos of the following three cases of gout and lead-poisoning :—

Case 8.—Lead-Poisoning—Temperate—No Note of Family History.

Edward C., aged forty-four, colour-grinder, has often suffered from lead-colic, and once had what he believed was rheumatic fever. Two years ago had lead-palsy. Temperate in habits. Distinct blue line on gums. Ascites. Great muscular atrophy. Gouty deposit of urate of soda was found post-mortem in both great-toe joints.

Case 9.—Lead-Poisoning—Gout—Temperate—No Note of Family History.

William M., aged forty-four, worker in lead, had gout nine years ago. Distinct blue line on gums. Temperate habits. Urethritis; pericarditis. Post-mortem examination showed granular kidneys and hypertrophied heart.

Case 10.—Lead-Poisoning(?)—Gout—Temperate—No Hereditary Predisposition.

John W., aged forty-eight, engineer, worker in lead. A temperate man. No hereditary tendency to gout. Gouty deposit in right elbow, left knee-joint, right ear; and gouty ulcer on metacarpo-phalangeal joint of index finger.

Dr. Garrod published(h) a clinical lecture in 1870 on a case of lead-poisoning in an organ-pipe maker, who had had several attacks of acute gout.

(*To be continued.*)

ANECDOTE OF MALGAIGNE.—Dr. Diday, in one of his *spirituel* papers in the *Lyon Méd.*, August 14, referring to an analogous circumstance that occurred to himself, relates the following anecdote of Malgaigne :—" I was present at an operation for the radical cure of hydrocele performed by Malgaigne at a *maison de santé*. The puncture was well executed, and the citrin liquid having issued without any difficulty, the warm wine was in its turn injected. But it was found that this stage of the operation went on less regularly. The canula was displaced, and the liquid instead of entering the sac had been forced into the cellular tissue of the scrotum. Disconcerted for an instant, Malgaigne quickly resumed an air of assurance, and, perceiving the patient anxious, said dogmatically, 'It is nothing at all : it is one of the proper stages of the operation.' But, fatal contrariety ! never shall I forget the pallor that invaded the visage of our master, when the patient, in reply to his consolatory statement, simply said, 'Sir, I am a medical student, and I know what has happened ; pray make the scarifications necessary to prevent gangrene.' "

(f) *Lancet*, vol. ii. 1868, page 215.
(g) *Guy's Hospital Reports*, vol. xv., page 41.
(h) *Lancet*, vol. ii. 1870, page 781.

REPORTS OF HOSPITAL PRACTICE
IN
MEDICINE AND SURGERY.

MIDDLESEX HOSPITAL.

CASE OF PLEURAL EFFUSION—PARACENTESIS.

(Under the care of Dr. FINLAY.)

WILLIAM B., aged seven, was admitted on August 11, 1880. His family history was not very good, the father having suffered from pleurisy and bronchitis, and the mother's family being consumptive; four brothers and sisters, however, were quite healthy. The patient himself had previously enjoyed the best of health, his mother stating that the present was the only illness he had ever complained of. On August 1 his mother noticed that he was very "feverish," and kept him in bed for a day, when the feverishness seemed to pass off ; and it was not till three days before admission (August 8) that he complained of shortness of breath, with a short, dry cough. The shortness of breath increased since then, and he sweated a good deal at night.

On admission, he is described as a rather puny, delicate-looking child, complaining of shortness of breath, and pain which is referred to the epigastrium. He has scarcely any cough; his tongue is moist, and very thinly coated ; temperature 100°, pulse 126, respirations 48. There is obvious bulging and deficient expansion of the right side of the chest, with dulness on percussion, the only exception to this being a small area just beneath the clavicle. The vocal vibration is abolished, and no breath-sounds are audible except towards the apex, where they are markedly tubular in character. Over the left side of the chest the breath-sounds are exaggerated, but otherwise normal. The heart's maximum impulse is found outside the nipple, the sounds, which are normal, being heard very distinctly in the axilla. The urine has a specific gravity of 1033, is acid, and does not contain albumen.

On the day after admission (August 12), paracentesis thoracis was performed, the result being seventeen ounces of clear serous fluid. After this the respirations sank to 40, the dulness was markedly diminished, and breath-sounds could be heard over the upper half of the lung. The evening temperature was 100·2°.

On the 14th the temperature was 99·2°; pulse 114; respirations 38. The resonance was good as low as the nipple level, and a few sibilant sounds were heard over the upper part of the lung posteriorly.

On the following day the improvement was still more marked, there being fair resonance to within two inches of the base posteriorly, the breath-sounds being heard quite to base. The temperature was 98°, pulse 90, respirations 26, and the child's general aspect had much improved.

On the 17th and 18th some friction sounds were heard below the right nipple, but no pain was complained of.

He continued steadily to improve, and was discharged on August 27, sixteen days after admission, with no physical sign of disease remaining, beyond slightly impaired resonance at the extreme base posteriorly, the lung having apparently expanded well.

The treatment, other than the removal of the fluid, consisted of cod-liver oil and iron, with two ounces of port wine daily.

Remarks.—There is little to remark about the case except its unsatisfactory result, which may be reasonably attributed in great measure to the early performance of paracentesis. However likely small serous effusions are to be absorbed without the necessity of having recourse to operative interference, it does not seem worth while to temporise in cases where the fluid is in such considerable quantity as to greatly compress the lung and cause a risk of permanent collapse. The performance of the operation of paracentesis has been hedged round with conditions, especially as to temperature, by different authorities ; but most, if not all, of these conditions may be safely disregarded in the presence of a large effusion, which has dangers, both immediate and remote, in comparison with which any supposed risk attending the operation is of but little importance. Probably the safest guide in all cases, except those complicated by pneumonia, is the quantity of the effusion.

VICTORIA HOSPITAL FOR CHILDREN, CHELSEA.

CASE OF ULCERATIVE ENTERITIS (PROBABLY TYPHOIDAL) WITHOUT PYREXIA—PERFORATIVE PERITONITIS—DEATH—AUTOPSY.

(Under the care of Dr. W. C. GRIGG.)

[Reported by Dr. DAWSON WILLIAMS, Registrar.]

ROSINA C., aged two years and eight months, attended Dr. Grigg's out-patient department, April 20, 1881. The mother said that she had been a very healthy child until about a fortnight earlier, when she began to complain of aching in chest, belly, and head, and vomited frequently. She had been feverish at night since, and there had been some tendency to diarrhœa. The child, when first seen, appeared a little dull and heavy; the venous radicles on the face were unusually evident; and the tongue was slightly furred on the dorsum, but moist. The temperature was 99°, the pulse about 90. There was no bronchitis. The abdomen was a little tumid and tender; but no gurgling could be obtained, and the spleen could not be felt. There was no account of any injury, and the family history was good.

The patient was admitted into the hospital under the impression that the case was one of typhoid fever. The temperature records, however, during the following twelve days did not show the presence of any pyrexia; and a firm, sausage-shaped tumour, about four inches long, was indistinctly to be felt in the left hypochondrium. There was no diarrhœa, but the stools passed were light in colour and fluid. The child did not appear to be very ill; she talked and played with the children who were near her bed, slept well at night, cried for food and to be allowed to get up.

On April 28 the circumferential measurement of the abdomen was twenty inches; on the following day it was twenty-one. She had vomited twice, and the tumour was more evident. Still the temperature did not rise much, the highest point recorded being 99·4°. (The observations were made every four hours.)

On May 1 she had a slight amount of diarrhœa. On the following day she vomited twice; and the temperature reached 100° for the first time during the thirteen days she had been under observation. The abdomen was tumid, but resonant everywhere except in the lower flanks and the hypogastric region, where there was some dulness. The patient preferred to be propped up at an angle of 45°, but could lie down without distress. The left thorax below the spine of the scapula was dull; the abdomen was not markedly tender; and the tumour above referred to could not always be distinctly felt.

On the next day, May 3, the temperature fell in the morning to 97°, but rose towards midday to 100·2°. There was more tenderness and distension of the abdomen, on the surface of which the veins were now very plainly to be seen. The pulse was about 120, small and regular. On the following morning the general condition was worse: she was a little blue about the face; the abdomen was more tender, and she had some headache. The temperature rose that night to 101·2°, and after a remission about midnight again touched 101° on the morning of May 5.

On May 6 the temperature was 101·6° at 6 a.m., and a purulent discharge occurred from the left ear. The abdomen was distended and tender, and about the umbilicus there was a large ecchymosis, where a fomentation had been applied. The face had grown pinched and blue, the tongue dry, and a few sordes had collected on the lips; there was a little vomiting; the pulse at the wrist was imperceptible. During the day she grew more restless, finally, towards the evening, unconscious. Death ensued about 9.30 p.m., the temperature having reached 103° a few hours earlier. No rash was at any time seen, though carefully looked for. The patient came under observation at about the end of the second week of her illness, and died in the fifth week.

Autopsy.—The brain was remarkably wet, and the superficial vessels were full of dark fluid blood. The left pleural cavity contained about ten or twelve ounces of sero-purulent fluid, and the lung was partially collapsed. The right lung was unaffected. On opening the abdomen about one pint of a yellowish fluid, which contained scraps of curdy material, and had a fæculent odour, escaped. The intestines and their mesentery were glued together along their opposed surfaces, and both the parietal and visceral layers of the peritoneum were covered with a layer of yellowish lymph. In the left hypochondriac region one of the coils of the small intestine at the surface showed a perforation about a quarter of an inch in diameter, almost circular in outline, with clean-cut edges. A few nodules of bile-stained curdy material lay close by, and fluid fæces welled up through the opening. The lower margin of the large intestine and the appendices epiploicæ in this region were much thickened, constituting the tumour felt during life. The position of this thickening in relation to the disposition of some lymph about the perforation in the intestine suggested an effort at encapsulation, and a subsequent microscopical examination of the thickened appendices showed that the enlargement was due to an infiltration of the connective tissue with small round cells, sufficiently great to obscure the natural structure of the part in places. After removing the intestine, two other similar apertures were found in the ileum, but these may have been produced in the removal. Only two other small ulcers were found, also in the ileum. Peyer's patches were not easily recognised, and appeared as delicate sieve-like patches on the surface of the mucous membrane. The perforation through which the extravasation had occurred was situated at one extremity of a Peyer's patch. The large intestine presented nothing distinctly unusual. The spleen was dark-coloured and soft, but not enlarged. The mesenteric glands were enlarged, soft, and of a purplish-pink colour. The other abdominal organs presented nothing unusual.

Remarks.—There can be little reasonable doubt that the ulceration was typhoidal: the duration of the illness, the site of the ulceration (in the ileum), the site of the perforation (at the apex of a Peyer's patch), and the absence of any thickening about the ulcers, must be taken as conclusive. That typhoid fever may run its course without manifesting any of its ordinary symptoms, and that this is especially apt to occur in children, is well known. The entire absence of eruption, of diarrhœa, and of any marked asthenia, need not therefore excite any surprise, but the point of special interest about the case seemed to be the failure of the temperature observations to give any indication of the necrotic and ulcerative processes which were in progress in the intestines. Further, the question as to when the perforation occurred must arise; ten days before the presence of pyrexia could be noted, and sixteen days before death, a sausage-shaped tumour was felt in the left hypochondrium. The post-mortem showed that this tumour was an inflammatory thickening of the tissues along the lower edge of the transverse colon—a thickening so disposed as to overlie and partially to occlude the perforation. Perforation has been known to occur as early as the eighth day, and it is therefore possible that it had occurred thus early in this case; otherwise it seems difficult to account for the local inflammation in the neighbourhood of the perforation, which there is every reason to suppose was already in existence when the patient was first seen. The difficulties surrounding the diagnosis of enteric fever in children are in many cases extreme, and this case illustrates well the insidious nature of the ulcerative processes which may attend apparent convalescence: for it must never be forgotten that the reparation does not commence until the fourth week of the disease; that this reparation begins in the lower parts of the small intestine, and only affects the ulcers in the upper part of the ileum at a later period; and that each ulcer takes, even under favourable conditions, a fortnight to heal.

IT may be interesting to note a plague of caterpillars which visited Swatow during the months of June, July, and August, literally covering the fir trees (on which they lived exclusively) and leaving them perfectly denuded of leaves. The hill-sides in many places looked as if a fire had passed over the trees and scorched them. The Chinese were very much afraid to handle them, as they declared them to be exceedingly poisonous—and they are right so far, as I know of two foreigners who were injured by these insects. When crushed they exude a glutinous fluid of a light green colour, which is very irritating to the skin, producing an erysipelatous rash, which causes much inconvenience for ten days or a fortnight.—*Dr. E. I. Scott, in the "Medical Reports of the Imperial Maritime Customs of China."*

TERMS OF SUBSCRIPTION.
(Free by post.)

British Islands	Twelve Months	.	£1	8	0
„ „	Six „	.	0	14	0
The Colonies and the United } Twelve „	.	1	10	0
States of America . . . }					
„ „ „	Six „	.	0	15	0
India	Twelve „	.	1	10	0
„ (vià Brindisi)	„	.	1	15	0
„	Six „	.	0	15	0
„ (vià Brindisi)	„	.	0	17	6

*Foreign Subscribers are requested to inform the Publishers of
any remittance made through the agency of the Post-office.*

*Single Copies of the Journal can be obtained of all Booksellers
and Newsmen, price Sixpence.*

Cheques or Post-office Orders should be made payable to Mr.
JAMES LUCAS, 11, New Burlington-street, W.

TERMS FOR ADVERTISEMENTS.

Seven lines (70 words)	.	.£0	4	6
Each additional line (10 words)	.	. 0	0	6
Half-column, or quarter-page .	.	. 1	5	0
Whole column, or half-page .	.	. 2	10	0
Whole page	.	. 5	0	0

Births, Marriages, and Deaths are inserted Free of Charge.

THE MEDICAL TIMES AND GAZETTE *is published on Friday
morning: Advertisements must therefore reach the Publishing Office not later than One o'clock on Thursday.*

Medical Times and Gazette.

SATURDAY, SEPTEMBER 24, 1881.

SANITARY GAINS.

IT is not seldom asserted by those who are too little taught
to know, or too ill-educated to be able to comprehend, the
meaning and reality of "preventive medicine," and by
persons smarting under the cost of enforced sanitary measures, that we can show very little, if any, real gain to the
public health from all our sanitary legislation and all the
costly sanitary proceedings enforced by our complicated and
expensive Local Government Board. There is a great shout
of triumph, these hostile critics say, if, after an expenditure
of thousands or tens or hundreds of thousands of pounds on
a new drainage scheme, the death-rate of a town or city is
for a few months one or two per thousand below what it
had been during the previous five or ten years, but we have
no certain information that this improvement continues.
More, we know that sometimes it does not, and that at the
best it fluctuates; we hear as much as ever of, and suffer as
much from, "outbreaks" of epidemics; and the Registrar-
General's Reports seem year after year to tell as nearly as
possible the same story: let sanitary reformers, boards of
health, sanitary authorities, and medical officers of health
show the contrary if they would justify the faith they would
have us put in them. This kind of complaint is by no means
without excuse. It cannot reasonably be expected either
that the public in general should understand how little,
comparatively, has yet been done in carrying out only the
coarsest requirements of sanitary science, or that a considerable time must elapse before even widely spread sanitary improvements can affect the general death-rate of a
country; or that the inhabitants of a city, town, or district, in which the newest and most approved sewerage
schemes and other health-measures have been carried out,
can always comprehend that they must continue to be liable
to outbreaks of zymotic diseases so long as neighbouring
districts, towns, and cities remain without similar improvements. They need frequent and public teaching on these
points; and the Local Government Board seem to have been
—none too soon—awakened to a sense of this. In their last
Report, just published, they give a statement of the progress
of sanitary work in England, and of the results that have
arisen from the services of the local health officers, though
these have been acting, as yet, with very imperfect
"attributions and functions."

The Report states:—"Before concluding the part of our
Report which relates to sanitary administration, it may be
useful to draw attention to the annual death-rate for some
years past as indicating the effect which recent sanitary
measures would appear to have had upon the public health;"
and a table is given, showing that the annual death-rate
per thousand, from all causes, for England and Wales was
for the decennial period 1841-50, 22·4; for that of 1851-60,
22·2; for that of 1861-70, 22·5; and for that of 1871-80,
21·5; while that from seven zymotic diseases was, for the
last three decennial periods, 4·11, 4·14, and 3·36 per 1000;
and that from "fever," in the same three periods, 0·91,
0·88, and 0·49 per 1000. It appears from these figures that
while from 1840 to 1870 the death-rate of the country
remained practically stationary, in the period 1871-80 it
fell from the 22·5 of the immediately previous decade, to
21·5. To bring the significance of this lowering of the death-
rate home to the average mind, the Report states that the
interpretation of it is that, "roughly estimated, about a
quarter of a million of persons were saved from death in the
ten years 1871-80, who would have died if the death-rate had
been the same as in the previous thirty years." Further,
if twelve cases of serious but non-fatal illness be reckoned
for every death—a fair estimate,—then it would follow that
"about three million persons, or more than one-ninth of the
whole population, have been saved from a sick-bed by some
influences at work in the past decade which had not been in
operation previously." The Local Government Board are
not content, however, with demonstrating and enforcing
the triumphs of preventive medicine that are writ on the
surface of the death-rate for the period in question. The case
is really, the Report says, still stronger than has been made
out thus far. "The death-rate of rural districts is habitually
lower than that of urban districts; and as the population is
steadily concentrating itself more and more into the towns,
the death-rate of the whole country would tend to increase
if the other circumstances that affect it remained the same."
This is rather deep digging into vital statistics in order to
magnify an improved death-rate for so short a period as ten
years. Leaving out of account, however, this tendency of
the whole death-rate to constantly increase, by reason of the
constant tendency of the population to concentrate in towns,
there remains a positive and direct reduction of the mor-
tality-rate in the ten years 1871-80, equivalent to nearly
4½ per cent. Was this gain distributed generally over the
field of mortality, or chiefly wrested from any particular
class or classes of disease? and is it possible, by a close
examination of the figures given above, to discover where
any especial gain has been, and to trace any of the causes
to which it may fairly be attributed? These are questions
of great interest and importance; and the Report before us
answers them. "Comparing, then," it says, "1861-70 with
1871-80, it will be seen from the foregoing figures that,
of the entire reduction of 1·0 in the death-rate, more than
three-quarters (4·14 − 3·36 = 0·78) comes under the head of
'The Seven Zymotic Diseases'; of the diseases, that is, which
are most influenced by sanitary improvements, and most
amenable to control by the action of the sanitary authorities.
And of this three-quarters, just half (0·88 − 0·49 = 0·39), or
three-eighths of the entire reduction, is in 'Fever,' the
disease which, more than any other, shows itself in connexion
with such faults of drainage, of water-supply, and of filth-

accumulation as it is within the province of good sanitary administration to remove." It is further pointed out that the fever death-rate has fallen pretty steadily year by year from 0·80 per 1000 in 1870 to 0·32 in 1880; in the first five years of the decade 1871-80 it was 0·61, while in the last five (1876-80) it was 0·38.

The triumph thus claimed for sanitary measures may be fairly and honestly claimed, though the period showing the improved general death-rate is a short one; and the triumph is a very real one. The Board have therefore done well in providing such a short and clear statement of the facts as will be convenient for use by medical officers of health and all sanitary reformers in their battles with ignorant and obstinate opposition and obstruction, whether passive or active. It is to be hoped, moreover, that the Board will, from a contemplation of the facts thus set forth, take courage to do their work a little more boldly; so that we may never again have to lament over such a collapse of administrative energy as they have exhibited during the last two years, in dealing with one of the worst of the seven zymotic diseases, to wit, with small-pox.

THE ARMY MEDICAL REPORT FOR 1879.

THE study of Blue-books year after year is apt to be tedious and not a little depressing; and the medical history of the British Army of two years ago is not altogether an exception, for short service itself is in a state of transition, and the conditions are not the same in 1881 as they were in 1879. The alteration made in the length of service "with the colours," involving as it does prolonged residence in unhealthy climates, must affect the proportions of deaths and of invaliding, and perhaps in future years exercise a great influence over the numbers and quality of recruits. But the Blue-book for 1879 has a peculiar interest, inasmuch as it deals with the history of two campaigns, and tells us how our boy-soldiers stand fatigue and resist disease. It tells us what short service had done for the Army in 1879. It had not made the Army popular. The prospects held out to the adventurous youth of Britain, tempted indeed 42,668 lads to offer themselves for enlistment; but although the spirit was evidently good, the flesh appears to have been unmistakably weak, and 15,477 were rejected by the doctors as unfit for service. Of course this indicates nothing as to the physical qualities of the young men of England generally, but it certainly does indicate that the class of young men who volunteered to uphold the ancient glory of England, to carry her banners victorious round the world, to die for Queen and country, were at any rate a peculiar class. Were we not much in the habit of "never expressing ourselves quite as we feel," we might be tempted to say, that at least a large proportion of the candidates for military glory probably cared nothing for Queen or country, glory or banner, but took the Queen's shilling because they had "no hope" at all. The recruits seem to have been the failures of civil life, and if we turn to the causes of rejection we can see why. Out of 42,688 lads, 4454 were rejected for muscular tenuity and debility, 1953 for defective vision, 821 for disease of the heart, 573 for varicocele, and 466 for malformation of the chest and spine. These afflicted young men, at all events, could hardly be accepted as worthy volunteers for glory. They were of the class who cannot dig, and who either are ashamed to beg, or find begging unprofitable. If we look at the previous occupation of the recruits we shall be confirmed in this opinion, for no less than 25,354 had been "labourers" and husbandmen, out of the grand total of 42,688. Who can help recollecting the grand flourish of trumpets with which the idea of short service was originally introduced? Who does not remember the appeals to the

intelligent youth of England—how they were bidden to reflect on the advantages of foreign travel, the influence of culture, and the knowledge to be acquired by contact with other races, which would enable the young soldier to return to civil life a better man, a more experienced butcher, a wiser carpenter, a more skilful artisan, than the ignoble Jack, Tom, and Harry, who had stuck to their looms or counters in their little native towns, or to the tilling of the "wonted glebe"?

It is sad to note how all these expectations have been disappointed. It would appear that in 1879 the acuter intellects rather avoided the recruiting-sergeant, and we are told that out of 36,297 recruits, 5066 were unable to read, and 3592 who could read were not able to write.

Well, England hating conscription, and detesting a long pension-list, chooses to trust her honour to the recruits, in whom she does not really believe, and so on that point there is no more to be said.

Let us see how our soldiers die. At home mortality augments in proportion to length of service, rather than to increase of age. The average of the death-rate up to thirty years of age is in favour of the military man, as compared with the civilian; but between the ages of thirty and thirty-five the scale has turned, and the civilian dies at a slower rate than the soldier—that is to say, the Service has taken it out of the man. But if this be the case at home, what must it be in India, where the average expectation of life diminishes in a far higher ratio? There cannot but be great reason to fear that short service, as lately modified, will return, year after year, ever increasing numbers of unhealthy men into the ranks of the civil population of England, and it may almost be questioned whether the saving in the pension-list of the present will not be balanced by the increase in the poor-rates of the future. We said that the greater length of service with the colours in India might in the future affect recruiting. It is possible that the diseased non-pensioned soldier, when he returns to his village, will be much more inclined to "weep o'er his ailments" than to "shoulder his crutch and show how fields were won." In 1879 the death-rate of the soldier, which was only 7·55 per 1000 in England, was 21·20 in Cyprus, 99·33 at the Cape, and 25·88 in India. There was war at the Cape and war in India, and the death-rate at both places was exceptional. Isandula swelled the total and confused the statistics, and if they were less affected in India it is because Madras and Bombay were healthy, while Bengal was exceptionally diseased. In different localities the death-rate was enormous. We read of 116·67 per 1000 at "Kooldunna," and 73·15 per 1000 at Peshawur. Cyprus, although the death-rate was high, contrasted favourably with former years, and the good result must be attributed to the greater care taken of the troops, and to better arrangements, both as to diet and exposure to malaria. We hope our readers will procure for themselves the Blue-book of 1879, for the "Medical History of the War in Zululand," by Surgeon-General J. A. Woolfryes, and the "Diary of the March of the Field Force of General Roberts from Cabul to Kandahar," by Surgeon-General Hanbury, are as interesting as they are well written and instructive. We will not attempt to review them here, but we cannot help noticing how a neglect of details may affect a masterly movement. We read of the Indian Force that "Probably a worse shod army never took the field. The ammunition boot, made of raw material, and of very indifferent workmanship, loses shape and turns over at the heel after a few days' hard marching, and simply impedes progress. The native shoe, with its wide, open mouth and narrow, pointed toes, seems ingeniously contrived to cripple and blister. The little Goorkha, who is very fond of the British soldier, invariably adopts the ammunition boot, but as his foot occupies about half the boot, I do not think he is a gainer by the transaction." We quite agree that the subject of boots deserves serious attention. We notice with pleasure the Sanitary Report for Madras, because it exhibits a triumph of common sense over old prejudice.

Surgeon-General Sir A. D. Home says, with regard to amusements, "At certain stations, special recreations are permitted, such as boating and shooting, and at many stations, the men having no duty, are allowed to leave barracks at any hour they please, instead of being restricted to certain hours; the sense of freedom in this respect is probably of the greatest advantage; the medical officers generally remark that no harm has followed the permission for the men to go about in the heat of the day." And even if a little harm did follow, much would be gained by the destruction of the Demon Ennui, who reigns supreme over barracks where men are confined all day, eating out their hearts in idleness. There is a remarkable paper in the Blue-book by Surgeon-General T. Crawford, M.D., on Enteric Fever. We notice, first, his appeal for consideration for apparent mistakes in the diagnosis of this disease. He says:—"I may remark, *en passant*, that the army medical officer is, by the regulations and practice of the Service, to which he must conform, placed at a manifest disadvantage in regard to the diagnosis of disease. In order to furnish his returns promptly he has to classify a fever before the necessary time has elapsed for him to distinguish its nature. In Army life accuracy of diagnosis is sacrificed to promptitude in classification, and a most undeserved reflection is apt to be cast upon the medical officer for unavoidable errors on his part by his being compelled to do that which in a disease like enteric fever in this country is often most difficult, and sometimes impossible, in the absence of pathognomonic symptoms." That is *a doctor's* difficulty. Let us next extract from the same paper a *patient's* difficulty in India. He says: "A soldier, little more than a recruit, arrives in the country, ignorant, of course, of its language, ways, and customs; he contracts enteric fever, and goes to hospital; it is probably the first time in his life that he has been seriously ill; he finds himself among strangers and new experiences, depressed and solicitous only for perfect quietude. As he gets worse his headache is replaced by delirium, especially at night; when his febrile state is exacerbated, and he wants to get out of his bed and wander about the ward. At such time, and in the intervals of his being seen by the medical officer or medical subordinate, he has to depend for his nursing and the supply of his wants on a ward-coolie, *probably asleep in the verandah*, supplemented, perhaps, by an equally ignorant soldier-nurse, temporarily obtained from the ranks, who certainly has this advantage over the coolie—that he and his patients do speak the same language!" We are fully of opinion that the sooner a trained Army Hospital Native Corps is organised, so much the better for the chances of recovery of a sick soldier in India. It might also be as well to allow more time for the classification of disease; for sickness which can neither be diagnosed nor nursed is most unsatisfactory.

There are numerous topics on which we should like to touch, did time and space permit. The statistics of syphilis and its modification by police regulations are worthy of notice; and the mortality among children of men serving abroad calls for remark. The dual system in the Indian campaign, and the employment of civilian doctors at the Cape, are also suggestive, but we must refrain; and we conclude by complimenting the Director-General on the preparation of a Blue-book on the whole above the average in interest.

THE LATE PRESIDENT GARFIELD.

EVERY member of the profession felt deeply grieved, when on Tuesday morning the tidings came that President Garfield's long, gallant struggle for life had ended in the peace and calm of death. But no medical man can have been in the least surprised by the sad news. During all these eleven weeks, while the whole profession throughout the civilised world have been watching for and eagerly interpreting the bulletins from the President's bedside, we have refrained from offering to our readers any speculations as to the course the fatal bullet took, the meanings of the various and varying symptoms, or the probabilities or possibilities of recovery; and from all criticism of the treatment adopted. The latter would have been an impertinence towards the able and well-known surgeons in attendance; while the former would have been an idle and presumptuous display; or, at most, would only have offered once a week the interpretations and inferences that every surgeon made daily for himself. And the prognosis of medical men must for many days past have been an almost entirely hopeless one. It was abundantly clear to the professional reader of the numerous daily bulletins and reports that the President was suffering from blood-poisoning long before a word about it was allowed to appear officially; and the signs and symptoms of this grew, almost without intermission, in number and gravity. The end came at last with unexpected suddenness, and was very naturally attributed to clot in the heart and great vessels; but the post-mortem shows this was not the case.

The details of the autopsy as already furnished are highly instructive and interesting, and we give them at once, though no doubt a more exact and minutely detailed report will shortly be available. The physicians and surgeons who made the examination, report as follows:—
"The ball, after fracturing the eleventh rib on the right side, had passed through the spinal column in front of the spinal canal, fracturing the body of the first lumbar vertebra, driving a number of small fragments of bone into the adjacent soft parts, and lodging below the pancreas, about two inches and a half to the left of the spine and behind the peritoneum, where it became completely encysted. The immediate cause of death was secondary haemorrhage from one of the mesenteric arteries adjoining the track of the ball, the blood rupturing the peritoneum, and nearly a pint escaping into the abdominal cavity. This haemorrhage is believed to have been the cause of the severe pain in the lower part of the chest which the President complained of just before his death. An abscess-cavity, six inches by four inches in dimensions, was found in the vicinity of the gall-bladder, between the liver and the transverse colon, which were strongly adherent. It did not involve the substance of the liver, and no communication was found between it and the wound. A long suppurating channel extended from the external wound between the loin muscles and the right kidney, almost to the right groin. This channel is now known to have been due to the burrowing of pus from the wound, and was supposed, during the life of the President, to have been the track of the ball. On examination of the organs of the chest, evidences of severe bronchitis were found on both sides, with broncho-pneumonia of the lower portions of the right lung and also of the left lung, though to a much less extent. The lungs contained no abscesses and the heart no clots of blood. The liver was enlarged and fatty, but free from abscesses, nor were any found in any other organ, except the left kidney, which contained, near its surface, a small abscess about one-third of an inch in diameter."

THE WEEK.

TOPICS OF THE DAY.

At the recent weekly meeting of the Hackney Guardians, Mr. Wentzell, the Hackney representative at the Metropolitan Asylums Board, reported that a check had occurred to the numerical improvement of the past few weeks as to the small-pox patients, of whom there were 581 in the various hospitals under the management of the Board, against 579 reported on the 29th ult. There were on board ship 129 patients, at the Homerton Hospital 79, at Stockwell 39, at Fulham 110, at Deptford 137, and at Darenth (not now under canvas) 87. The Finance Committee having brought up a report expressing the opinion that in the estimates of the Asylums Board the item of £40,437, the estimated balance at the end of the next half-year, might have been considerably lessened by the Managers, Mr. Wentzell explained that the Managers had felt it absolutely incumbent on them to make a very great demand upon the unions and parishes, because the requirements showed a great excess; and as epidemics came suddenly, injunctions were uncertain; and as there was no telling what might be required in case of a great visitation of disease, the Managers thought it would be very unfortunate if they were left without a sufficient balance for any possible emergency. In reply to a question whether the Asylums Board had decided on steps in reference to and consequent upon the Fulham injunction, Mr. Wentzell said the Board felt themselves fettered, whatever action they took. They had done their best to meet the emergency of the epidemic; still fault was found with them. If guardians felt they had a grievance it was competent for them to take the matter into their own hands by establishing hospitals for their respective districts; but, if they meant to do this, where could sites be found for the purpose in densely populated parishes like Whitechapel or Clerkenwell? But, even then, those parishes would still have to contribute to the Asylums Board. The matter was undoubtedly one which the Legislature would have to take into practical consideration.

A medical gentleman practising in the metropolis applied lately to the magistrate of the Southwark Police-court for his advice under the following circumstances. A lady connected with the medical profession had taken premises at Stamford-street, Blackfriars-road, which she called a Ladies' Medical College; and she had issued a prospectus in which he was announced as president, without his authority. Several other names were printed as members of the council, but, in fact, these gentlemen had never been consulted in the matter. There was no council in existence, and he and those whose names had been printed wished to repudiate any connexion with the institution or its management, for which they were in no way responsible. The magistrate said the only advice he could give to the applicant was to write to the Press disclaiming any connexion with the institution.

A Sanitary Congress has recently been opened in Vienna, uniting the Austrian and German Societies for the Protection of the Public Health. The inaugural address was delivered by the Bavarian Duke Charles Theodor, who not long ago took his degree as Doctor of Medicine. He pointed out that the protection of the public health was a question that had only lately occupied attention, yet, though sanitary societies had not been in existence ten years, their efforts had already been crowned with success. The reforms advocated by them had been introduced both into public and private life, and the result was to be found in the public thoroughfares and buildings, in schools, factories, and ships —in fact, everywhere. They should not direct their endeavours to the benefit of a certain number, but to an improvement in the physical existence of the million. It was officially announced on behalf of the Government that the resolutions of the Congress would not only be carefully considered, but practically carried out. The chief subjects of the papers and discussions are epidemic diseases and their treatment; disinfection; the management of, and attendance at, funerals; water-supply; school hygiene; and sanitary improvements in cemeteries.

A long discussion recently took place at a special meeting of the Oxford Local Board to consider the action of the University delegates with reference to the sanitary condition of the lodging-houses of that city. A few months since, the University appointed an inspector to visit such premises, and to direct such alterations to be made as he might deem necessary. In the event of his recommendations not being carried out, it was clearly intimated that the renewal of the licence would not be granted. It is now alleged that in many cases the proposed improvements are quite unnecessary, and one speaker pointed out that if they were all acted upon they would cost no less than £12,000, while in many instances the lodging-house keepers could not afford to do the required work. From facts adduced it is evident that Oxford is, at the present time, in a healthy condition, whilst the main drainage works are among the most perfect in England. Ultimately it was arranged that a conference should take place between the University and city authorities with a view of carefully investigating the matter. It was stated at the meeting that there had been only eleven cases of small-pox in Oxford during the last nine years.

Our contemporary, the *Globe*, well asks the question whether it is to be wondered at that small-pox defies all efforts to stamp it out in this country, when cases such as the following are of almost daily occurrence. An outbreak of small-pox in the Leicester Industrial School at Desford has been traced to infection communicated by a boy who came from London, this boy having caught the disease through being put to sleep in a bed next to a small-pox patient in a London workhouse. As it is said that the Leicester School Board are about to institute proceedings to recover the expense they have been put to from the London guardians under whose jurisdiction this worse than negligence occurred, it is to be hoped that in a roundabout way the guilty parties may be in a measure punished; but it is lamentable to hear of such criminal carelessness on the part of those who should be bound by their position to take every precaution for preventing the spread of contagious disease.

In connexion with the subject of the fish supply for the metropolis, now under consideration, it is authoritatively announced that the question of sites is now occupying the attention of the Special Committee of the Corporation, and that instructions have been given that any suggestion as to a site forwarded to the City Architect, Guildhall, on or before the 29th inst., will be duly considered.

As a result of the recent Royal visit to the Edinburgh Infirmary, the Lord Provost, Sir Thomas J. Boyd, at a meeting of the managers held lately, laid on the table a number of proof engravings which had been sent to him by Sir Henry Ponsonby as a gift to the institution from Her Majesty. The prints are portraits of Her Majesty and the late Prince Consort, Prince Arthur, and the Princess Beatrice. The Lord Provost was requested by the managers to convey, through Sir Henry Ponsonby, their most sincere thanks to the Queen, and to express the high estimation in which they hold the gift. It was then remitted to the House Committee to hang some of the engravings in the two wards named by Her Majesty the Victoria and Albert Wards on the occasion of her recent visit, and the others in such prominent places of the institution as they may think most suitable.

A public meeting has been held in Dublin, under the presidency of the Bishop of Meath, for the purpose of promoting more permanent and efficient arrangements for the care and nursing of the Protestant sick poor in the South Dublin Union, and to consider the practicability of extending the system to other similar institutions. It was proposed, and unanimously carried—" That every effort to provide the Protestant poor in workhouse infirmaries with well-trained nurses, calls for the warm sympathy of the meeting, and of the Protestants of Ireland at large." The mover of this resolution, Mr. A. Shackleton, J.P., said it was not generally known that the infirmaries of the North and of the South Dublin Unions were the largest hospitals in that city. The usual number of patients in the former varied from 200 to 250, and the latter accommodated about 750 inmates. These hospitals received no share of the Hospital Sunday Fund. It might be observed, however, that there were a great number of ladies who visited the hospitals in the South Dublin Union, and their visits did a great deal of good, and were a source of comfort to the inmates. Before separating, an influential committee was appointed for the purpose of furthering the objects specified in the various resolutions put to and carried by the meeting.

The magistrate at the Worship-street Police-court has delivered his decision in the case which was brought before him by the sanitary authorities of the Poplar District Board of Works, in which a manufacturer of German sausages, residing in Old Ford, was charged with having on his premises a quantity of horseflesh for the purpose of preparing it for human food, the same being unwholesome. Mr. Mayne Talbot, Medical Officer of Health for the northern division of the Poplar district, in examination deposed that he examined the meat submitted to him by the inspector, but was unable to say whether it was or was not horseflesh, while to him it appeared to be fit for food. Mr. Bushby, in giving judgment, said that the contention whether horseflesh was or was not fit for human food he had not considered an important element in the case, but in the face of the evidence tendered it was impossible for him to put the law in motion; the summons would therefore be dismissed, but without costs.

The want of a public park for the recreation of the people has long been experienced in Salisbury, and recently a letter was read at the monthly meeting of the Town Council, from the solicitor to the Rev. Dr. Bourne, offering to hand over to the city his lease, and also his freehold interests in a portion of Green Croft, a large piece of land which could be used as a park, the Council to undertake to fence it and plant it with trees. The Corporation expressed their appreciation of the gift, and the matter was ordered to be referred to a committee.

An Act to amend the Metropolitan Open Spaces Act, 1874, has lately been printed. In thirteen clauses (after a long interpretation provision) power is given to trustees and others to transfer open spaces to local authorities. The Metropolitan Board, and vestry or district, may carry out the Act jointly. The statute is to apply to the City of London. Among the enactments is one to transfer disused burial-grounds to local authorities, who may improve and lay out the same for the public benefit.

SERIOUS ILLNESS OF DR. A. H. M'CLINTOCK, OF DUBLIN.

THE many friends of this highly esteemed gentleman will learn with regret of his dangerous illness. On Friday three weeks he had a stroke of paralysis, which left him speechless and hemiplegic. We understand that of late he has been making slow progress towards recovery, but his condition is still such as to give rise to the liveliest apprehensions among those who know and love him well.

THE INTERNATIONAL MEDICAL AND SANITARY EXHIBITION

IT is highly unsatisfactory to learn that the decisions of some of the judges at the recent International Medical and Sanitary Exhibition have given rise to great discontent in some quarters; and we must admit that, so far as we can judge, the complaints made (especially as to the decisions and awards in the class of drugs, medical dietetic articles, etc.) appear to be fully justified. The errors charged are of both commission and omission; all very serious, but the former the most grave and inexplicable. It is stated that an award has been given to two nostrums that ought never to have been admitted to the Exhibition—viz., an "Oriental balsam" and an infallible "worm-cure," both secret preparations, puffed in the most outrageous style. This is, of itself, bad enough, but the matter becomes worse, if it is true—and this also is alleged —that the London agent for these Eastern articles was one of the judges in the class to which they had so mistakenly been admitted. This is a matter demanding explanation and correction. As to the sins of omission, they are very numerous, and very strangely appear to relate principally, if not entirely, to articles of American manufacture, or exhibited by an American firm—a fact that certainly does not lessen the appearance of unfairness. No award has been made to the pills of McKesson and Robbins—pills of exceptional merit for originality of form and for excellence of manufacture. The compressed tablets, and the other preparations of Wyeth Brothers, have all been passed over without any kind or degree of commendation. No mention has been made of Kepler's extract of malt, perhaps the one most widely known and most largely used in this country; while all other malt extracts exhibited have been commended. And no notice has been taken of Fellows' hypophosphites; of Burrough's and Wellcome's beef and iron wine; of Bishop's granular effervescing citrate of caffeine, and other granular effervescent salts, though he was the original inventor of this most acceptable method of administering drugs; or of many other articles that might be mentioned. All these are matters that call loudly, we submit, for explanation and correction; and these will, we trust, for the sake of all the parties concerned, be given without delay

PRESENTATION TO DR. RICHARD BUDD.

ON Saturday, the 10th inst., the Mayor of Barnstaple, and a large company of ladies and gentlemen, assembled in the Town Hall of Barnstaple, for the purpose of presenting Dr. Richard Budd, of that town, with a portrait of himself and a purse of £400. Dr. Budd, who is one of the distinguished medical family of Budds of Devonshire, has recently resigned the post of Physician to the North Devon Infirmary, after having been connected professionally with it for close upon forty years; and his fellow-townsmen and friends seized the opportunity of expressing their recognition of his long and eminent services. The presentation was made, in the name of the numerous subscribers, by the Earl of Fortescue, the President of the Infirmary; and among those present at the gratifying ceremony was Dr. George Budd, who was for many years Professor of Medicine in King's College, London, and is another of the quiver-ful of brothers who have made the name of Budd famous in the profession of medicine. The portrait of Dr. Richard Budd, which was painted by Mr. Edgar Williams, a well-known Devonshire artist, is said to be an excellent likeness; and a replica of it, by the same artist, has been presented to the Infirmary by Mr. W. F. Rock, of Barnstaple. Dr. Budd, in returning thanks for the honour done him, expressed his intention of giving the money part of the testimonial as his contribution towards the erection of a detached building for the out-patients department of the Infirmary. He said that a great number of those patients are crowded together for hours at a time, two or three times a week, in the basement storey of the institution, where there is no kind of ventilation, and the contaminated air from which must ascend the wards occupied by the in-patients. We trust the friends of the Infirmary will recognise his generosity by quickly providing the additional funds for carrying out an improvement that he has so greatly at heart.

THE REPORT ON THE SANITARY CONDITION OF CAMBRIDGE FOR 1880.

In his annual report on the sanitary condition of the Cambridge Improvement Act District for the year 1880, Dr. Bushell Anningson, M.A., the Medical Officer of Health, has included the results of some observations he has made on the causation of summer diarrhœa, the inquiry having been undertaken at the instance of the Local Government Board. The space at our command will not permit us to give the whole of Dr. Anningson's remarks, but it may be stated that the conclusion at which he arrives (unwillingly, he admits, because if he is right the remedy is difficult of application) is that the area of his district in which diarrhœa is most prevalent lies along the line of sewers of low rate of inclination in poor neighbourhoods, where less heed is paid to traps. So slight, indeed, is the inclination of the sewers, that the sewage in them is practically stagnant, and ferments, producing gases which press with great force, as Dr. Anningson ascertained by direct experiment, upon the traps in some of the scullery sinks. The evil, Dr. Anningson thinks, would be palliated by ventilation of the sewer all along its line; there would even then be foul gas in the streets, but in a less concentrated state. The death-toll for the year 1880 might, if the gross sum alone were regarded, the report adds, be reckoned as light, for the total number of persons belonging to the district who have died during the period is the smallest recorded during the five years 1876-80, and is equal to a death-rate of 16·4 per 1000 living per annum. But while the aggregate extinction of life may, from its smallness, be cause for satisfaction, the sundry items are, for the largeness and qualities of one or two of them, cause for serious consideration. Compared, however, with the health-returns of other towns in the kingdom, Dr. Anningson may be congratulated on the result of his labours to improve the sanitary condition of the district entrusted to his care.

TOTAL EXTIRPATION OF THE UTERUS FOR CANCER.

This operation may be said at present to be on its trial; for surgeons are not yet agreed as to whether the prospect of benefit outweighs the risk. The statistical accounts that have as yet been published are incomplete, and therefore not quite in agreement. We want figures to show us, first, in what number of cases the operation itself proves fatal, and then, in how many of those who recover from the operation the disease returns. The statistics are not in agreement; first, because improvements are being made in the *technique* of the operation, and in estimating the probable future mortality of an operation, we must reject cases in which the operation was not done in the way which better knowledge has shown to be the safest, and also because some cases, published as cures, have afterwards relapsed. Bearing in mind these errors, the following statistics will be interesting :—Mikulicz (*Wiener Medizinische Wochenschrift*, 1880, No. 47) quotes from Ahlfeld a table of 66 cases, out of which 49 proved fatal, in 4 the operation could not be completed, and of the 13 who recovered, in 6 relapses occurred; of the remaining 7, in some the period since the operation, at the time the figures were compiled, was too short to allow the occurrence of relapse to be considered improbable. Some later statistics are more favourable. Kleinwachter, writing at the beginning of the present year, collected 94 cases of operation, with 24 recoveries; but Kaltenbach, writing about the same time, out of 88 cases enumerates 30 as successful. These figures evidently want sifting. They all relate to cases in which the uterus has been extirpated by abdominal section. Olshausen has collected (*Berliner Klinische Wochenschrift*, No. 35, 1881) 41 cases in which the uterus was removed by the vaginal method; of these 29 recovered and 12 died. To these he adds 6 performed by himself, all of whom, so far as the operation was concerned, were successful.

MEMORIAL HOSPITAL TO CANON MILLER AT GREENWICH.

Some time since we recorded the particulars of a meeting held to consider the details for erecting a hospital as a memorial to the late Canon Miller, in recognition of his services in promoting Hospital Sunday in the metropolis. The Committee then appointed have arranged all preliminaries, and a meeting was recently held at the Royal Kent Dispensary, Greenwich, when it was finally decided to raise £10,000, and to build a hospital in the rear of the Dispensary, with the view of providing accommodation for the large and densely populated district comprising Greenwich, Deptford, Woolwich, Blackheath, Lee, Lewisham, Charlton, Plumstead, and contiguous parts of South-east London. A memorial in favour of this scheme, signed by fifty-eight local medical men, was read. It was pointed out that a population of nearly one million and a half on the Surrey side of the Thames has to rely on Guy's with 700 beds, and St. Thomas's with 400 available beds, both of which, though largely endowed, are situated miles away from that portion of the district for the wants of which the new hospital would in future provide. Already upwards of £1200 has been received in private subscriptions from a few of the residents in the district who recognise the necessity of providing this new hospital. The Canon Miller Memorial Fund Committee have agreed to co-operate with the Executive Committee of the Royal Kent Dispensary in raising the necessary funds; and it has been arranged that one of the wards shall be called the Miller Memorial Ward as a recognition of the valuable services rendered to the hospitals and dispensaries throughout the country by the late Rev. Canon Miller, D.D., as the promoter of Hospital Sunday, and as a mark of esteem and affection to his memory. It was resolved to make a vigorous effort to raise the necessary funds, and to erect and open the hospital for the reception of patients on the centenary of the Royal Kent Dispensary in 1883. It was further resolved to try and carry out a plan which has proved very popular in America, by which congregations attending churches and chapels in the neighbourhood, and the workmen of the larger firms, will be encouraged to establish and endow a bed or beds in the new hospital. It is thought possible that some of those friends of the late Canon Miller who reside in distant parts of the country may desire to send contributions towards the expense of the Miller Memorial Ward.

THE PARIS WEEKLY RETURN.

The number of deaths for the thirty-sixth week, terminating September 9, 1881, was 938 (477 males and 461 females), and among these there were from typhoid fever 41, small-pox 11, measles 13, scarlatina 7, pertussis 3, croup and diphtheria 36, erysipelas 6, and puerperal infections 6. There were also 43 deaths from tubercular and acute meningitis, 15 from acute bronchitis, 40 from pneumonia, 105 from infantile athrepsia (32 of the children having been wholly or partially suckled), and 57 violent deaths. In this week's return there is observable a general diminution of mortality, in which almost every disease concurs, the only category which is aggravated being that of violent deaths. But in reality these are not deaths which belong to Paris, eighteen of them being victims of the terrible railway accident at Charenton, but registered on the list of the arrondissement in which the Morgue is situated. The true return for the week is therefore not even 938, but 920 deaths, which may be reckoned at 23 per 1000, which is that of entire France. The rise in epidemic diseases which occurred last week has subsided during the present. The births for the week amounted to 1128, viz., 608 males (443 legitimate and 165 illegitimate) and 520 females (388 legitimate and 132 illegitimate); 89 children (57 males and 32 females) were born dead or died within twenty-four hours.

A LOCAL GOVERNMENT BOARD DIFFICULTY IN IRELAND.

THE Medical Officer of the Carrigtuohill Dispensary in the Middleton Union, co. Cork, was recently dismissed under sealed order by the Local Government Board for Ireland. We are not informed what was the cause of the dismissal of Dr. Richard Ryan, the Medical Officer in question, but it is said that he was a member of the local branch of the Land League. After the dismissal by sealed order a new election was ordered. The election was held, and Dr. Ryan, being one of the candidates, was re-elected by a large majority. The Local Government Board refused to recognise the appointment, and ordered a new election. The second election took place on Friday, September 16, and again Dr. Ryan was placed at the head of the poll by a large majority. The people a few nights ago broke in the dispensary house door to show their feeling of dissatisfaction at the appointment, *pro tem.*, of a new officer.

THE HEALTH REPORT ON THE PARISH OF ST. MARY, ISLINGTON, FOR 1879.

DR. MEYMOTT TIDY's report on the sanitary condition of the parish of St. Mary, Islington, during 1879, draws attention to a marked peculiarity in the death-rate for that year, namely, its extreme irregularity. Thus, during the winter months, the severe weather and the intensity of the London fogs proved exceptionally trying to the very young and very old; but so accurately was this unusual death-rate balanced by the exceptionally low death-rates at certain other periods of the year, that, in taking the average of the whole, the annual mortality was equalised. In speaking of the various causes of death, the report notes that mortality from diseases of the respiratory organs (more especially bronchitis) is far above the average, whilst the fatal cases of diarrhœa are as far below the average—the latter due, no doubt, to the unusually low summer temperature of 1879, and to the excessive rainfalls, which kept the sewers constantly and efficiently flushed. Another point to which attention is specially directed is the unprecedented fatality from measles during the year under notice ; no less than 219 deaths have to be recorded as having resulted from this cause. All the cases, except nine, occurred in children under five years of age, and it is somewhat remarkable that nearly the whole of the 219 deaths took place between April and August. These are the months, Dr. Tidy adds, when, perhaps, least attention is paid to draughts, and to keeping the patients sufficiently warm, and probably it is to these causes, amongst others, the particularly fatal character of the outbreak is to be traced. Although it is true the deaths from small-pox recorded in the district for 1879 are few, Dr. Tidy points out that it is nevertheless important to bear in mind that the prevalence of small-pox in any given district cannot be accurately gauged by the mortality alone, seeing that it is *the one* disease which induces the sufferers of the poorer

and even middle classes to consent to removal to hospital. Thus a parish may apparently be, so far as death-returns indicate, actually free from the disease, whilst all the time patients are being removed to the various hospitals fitted for their reception.

THE LATE ARTHUR JERMYN LANDON.

WE gladly aid in making known the suggestion that a memorial brass shall be placed in the hospital church of St. Bartholomew-the-Less, to Arthur Jermyn Landon, a student of the Hospital, who fell in the discharge of his duty on Majuba Hill, in the Transvaal, on Sunday, February 27 of this year. The circumstances of Mr. Landon's death are told in the proposed inscription on the brass, which runs as follows :—"His former medical contemporaries at St. Bartholomew's Hospital have set up this tablet to keep in memory the bright example of Arthur Jermyn Landon, who, while continuing to dress the wounded amid a shower of balls in the action on Majuba Hill, was in turn mortally wounded by a bullet, and calling out to his assistants, 'I am dying ; do what you can for the wounded,' only desired for himself that his friends might be told that 'he fell doing his duty.' His habitual life was expressed in the simple grandeur of his death." Subscriptions (which need not exceed half a guinea) and names may be sent to any of the following :—C. E. Harrison, M.B., Surgeon Grenadier Guards Club, 70, Pall-mall, S.W.; Mr. Joseph Mills, or Dr. Norman Moore, the College, St. Bartholomew's Hospital, E.C.; W. E. Steavenson, M.B., the Hospital for Sick Children, Great Ormond-street, W.C.

FRENCH MILITARY REQUISITIONS TO CIVIL PRACTITIONERS.

THE serious state of things in Africa may be judged of by the fact that the French authorities have issued a circular to civil practitioners, requesting to know whether they felt disposed to lend their services to the Army Administration for attending on the troops who, in consequence of the large number of army surgeons despatched to Africa, are quite insufficiently supplied with medical attendance. Nothing like this has occurred since the Crimean War ; and painful surprise has been felt that such a step should have become necessary at the very commencement of a campaign hitherto regarded as little else than a military promenade. The circular has given dissatisfaction by the vagueness of its statements, while the pay offered is said to be contemptible; and it is proposed, instead of employing the medical volunteers in the military hospitals, to send them, at least as far as Paris is concerned, to perform duty in the detached forts which surround the capital. This, it is observed, is as much a military as a medical duty, and can only be effectually performed by those possessing military knowledge and authority. Scarcely anyone in Paris has as yet consented to sign the agreement; and the *Gazette Hebdomadaire* strongly advises civil practitioners not to undertake this laborious and ill-paid duty, in which they will have heavy responsibilities unaccompanied by authority.

THE SANITARY ORGANISATION OF DUBLIN.

LAST Monday a very important step was taken by the Corporation of Dublin in connexion with the Public Health Department of the city. This was the appointment of Dr. Charles A. Cameron as Superintendent Medical Officer of Health and Executive Sanitary Officer at a salary of £1000 a year ; and the promotion of Mr. J. G. Bolger to the position of Secretary to the Public Health Committee and Assistant Executive Sanitary Officer, at a salary of £200 a year. Dr. Cameron hereby undertakes the entire control of and responsibility for the working of the Public Health Department under the Public Health Committee of the Corporation, including attendance at the office of that Committee when not engaged in the duties of his appointment through the city, attendance at the meetings of the Committee, and the discharge of his present duties as City Analyst. He undertakes to abandon all other professional emoluments with the exception of the fees paid to him as analyst to many counties in Ireland; but he is permitted to retain his Chair of Chemistry in the School of Surgery of the Royal College of Surgeons of Ireland. It is to be hoped that these appointments will infuse new life into the sanitary organisation of Dublin. There is too eager a disposition to attribute the low deathrate which has of late held in that city to the exertions of the sanitary authorities. The improved state of the public health is much more likely due to the cool, damp summer—the temperature not having been low enough to cause the pulmonary complaints of winter and spring, while the coolness and abundant rainfall have checked the prevalence of the diarrhœal diseases of summer and autumn. Viewed from this point, Dublin has merely benefited in common with all the other large towns of the United Kingdom, from the exceptional character of the season; and Dr. Cameron's laurels have yet to be won in his capacity as Chief Medical Officer of Health for the Irish capital.

REPORTS TO THE
LOCAL GOVERNMENT BOARD ON VARIOUS
OUTBREAKS OF ENTERIC FEVER.

Melton Mowbray.—In November, 1880, the Registrar-General having informed the Local Government Board of the occurrence of three deaths from enteric fever in Melton Mowbray, and on the 13th of the same month several cases of the same disease having been reported in the town, Dr. Blaxall was instructed to institute an inquiry into the circumstances of the outbreak in relation to the sanitary condition of the town. This latter he reports to be eminently unsatisfactory, specially with reference to the means of excrement removal and disposal, the water-supply, and the drainage. With the assistance of the acting Medical Officer of Health, Dr. Blaxall instituted a thorough investigation into the causes of the outbreak then prevalent; and considers that the unsanitary condition of the town furnished all the conditions favourable to the development and spread of enteric fever, and the introductory cases of the epidemic in question were traced back so far as the previous April, resulting in forty-one families being attacked (exclusive of the initial cases), with sixty-six cases and eight deaths, besides two fatal cases reported to have been contracted in the town and to have died elsewhere. The salient points of this epidemic, the report says, may be summed up as follows : 1. The fever was confined to a particular portion of the town traversed by one line of sewers, the contents of which had become specifically infected with the contagium of enteric fever. 2. The families invaded were exposed to the escape of the infected sewer-air through the medium of untrapped or imperfectly trapped drain-inlets in the immediate vicinity of their dwellings. 3. The peculiarities in the incidence and succession of attacks arose from flooding of imperfectly ventilated sewers at the lower parts of the town forcing infected air through unguarded drain-openings at higher levels. 4. Other parts of the town beyond the immediate influence of the infected sewers were exempt from fever. The whole teaching of the inquiry, Dr. Blaxall adds, points unmistakably to the epidemic having been due to defects in conditions over which the sanitary authority can exercise control, and he warns them that the contagium of enteric fever has become so widely diffused that there is every probability that the town will be subjected to the occurrence of isolated cases, with occasional outbreaks of an extended character, unless early and efficient action be taken to improve the sanitary defects which he has enumerated.

Uckfield.—In April of the present year, Mr. W. H. Power was despatched by the Local Government Board to report on the prevalence of enteric fever in the Uckfield Urban Sanitary District. The outbreak began in September, 1880; and lasted until the following March, during which time there were thirty-eight attacks, five of them fatal. Except in certain special cases the history of one of these outbreaks in small country places would appear to be the history of the whole. Defective sewerage arrangements and a polluted water-supply, through the fouling of wells, is a tale which never varies, and Mr. Power remarks that whatever may have caused the first series of fever cases in the town, it seems quite clear that the subsequent ones, more especially those constituting the outbreak in January and February last, were due to dissemination of infection that had become, so to speak, rooted in the place. This, he adds, is not surprising, seeing that all the fever cases were treated at their homes in a town possessing in its water-supply and sewerage arrangements unusual facilities for the spread of the disease material of enteric fever ; but how far these unwholesome conditions have severally conduced to the outbreak cannot well be judged of, since the possible influence of one cannot be estimated apart from that of the other. One noticeable point elicited by the inquiry was the fact that until 1879 Uckfield had remained for some years singularly free from enteric fever. On three separate occasions during 1877 and 1878 isolated cases occurred in the town, but these, whether imported or of home production, never assumed epidemic proportions under conditions apparently singularly favourable for the reproduction of the disease. Also, there is a history of *autumnal* enteric fever, infertile at first, under circumstances seemingly conducive to its fertility, but suddenly in a particular season developing reproductive powers, to be in a subsequent season fully maintained with widely increased range. Suggestions of this sort concerning the natural history of enteric fever, are, Mr. Power observes, of no little interest, though perhaps not of immediate practical value. The recommendations attached to the report principally refer to the water-supply and sewerage.

Bridlington.—Dr. H. Franklin Parsons was instructed to report on the prevalence of enteric fever in the Bridlington Urban Sanitary District, in consequence of the Registrar-General's returns for the fourth quarter of 1880 showing thirty deaths from "fever." From tables compiled by him it would appear that although deaths from fever, described almost exclusively as enteric or typhoid, occur in the Bridlington Urban District almost every year, the mortality from that disease has not been a prominent feature until the present outbreak, during which, as far as could be ascertained, eighty-seven households were attacked, with 160 cases, and thirty-four deaths. In the present instance it was observed that the great majority of the households in which fever had broken out obtained their milk from one particular dealer, and a sample of water from a well upon his premises was pronounced by the public analyst to be "a very bad water, evidently largely contaminated with sewage." For the following reasons Dr. Parsons is of opinion that this particular outbreak of fever was connected with the milk-supply upon which suspicion had fallen :— 1. The sudden and widespread character of the outbreak. 2. The apparent absence in some cases of other circumstances which might account for the disease. 3. The especial incidence of the fever upon the households supplied with milk from the suspected dairy. 4. The undoubted pollution of the water used for dairy purposes, and the possibility of its being contaminated by the specific typhoid infection. 5. The speedy decline of the epidemic after its cause had been ascertained and measures of prevention adopted. Dr. Parsons quotes an instance of remarkable fatality connected with this outbreak, which leads him to conjecture that exposure to sewage effluvia, together with the reception of specific infection through the medium of milk, combine to develope an exceptionally severe form of the disease. Towards the end of September two neighbours jointly cleansed the ditch which formed the boundary between their respective gardens. One was a young man, a fellmonger, the other an old man with chronic heart disease ; the daughter of the latter (aged thirty-four) assisted in carrying the buckets of stuff removed. The ditch received the sewage from a row of houses, but, so far as could be ascertained, no cases of typhoid fever had at that time occurred in any of the houses drained into it. All three persons used milk from the suspected dairy. The woman and younger man were taken ill on October 1, the former dying on the 15th and the latter on the 21st; the old man was taken ill on October 4, and died on the 23rd. A married daughter, living in another quarter, who had nursed her father and sister, was taken ill five days after her return home, and died on November 24. There were many instances in which relatives and others in attendance on the sick contracted the disease. The recommendations particularly refer to an early completion of the sewerage scheme already sanctioned for the district, and to the provision of a hospital for infectious diseases.

FROM ABROAD.

Is Alcohol a Food?

At a meeting of the Philadelphia County Medical Society (*Phil. Med. Times*, July 16), held for the discussion of the various points relating to the use of alcohol, among the papers read was one by Prof. H. C. Wood, bearing the title "Is Alcohol a Food? When should Malt Liquors be preferred to Wines and Spirits in the Treatment of Disease?" He first defines what should be meant by the term "food," and protests against its restriction to those substances which, either in their entirety or in a more or less altered condition, are capable of being formed into the bodily structure. Of the substances taken into the stomach only a portion becomes an integral part of the economy, as is shown by the enormous increase in the formation of urea which follows a heavy meal of meat. The longing for and extraordinary consumption of a fatty diet by persons exposed to an arctic temperature show that the system requires an extra supply of such food, which does not induce fattening of the recipients, but acts as fuel and is burned up in maintaining the bodily heat — that is, yielding force to maintain the molecular movements of the organism. It is plain that, under many circumstances, that which is eaten is used not for reconstruction, but for force-production. If the term "food" be employed in its narrower sense, it must be acknowledged that there is no proof that alcohol is a food; but when it is in its wider and more correct sense, the question must receive quite a different answer. From this point of view, any substance which is destroyed in the system, and during its destruction yields force, is a food. The evidence that alcohol fulfils both these conditions is most positive. The questions whether alcohol is an economic food, whether it is practically useful as a food, are entirely distinct from the above.

"Looking at the matter practically, and not as to theoretic economy, it is evident that, as alcohol is usually taken and as food is usually eaten, no claim can be rightly made as to the superior cheapness of the beverage. Again, it is notorious that in America almost everyone in reasonable health consumes much more food than the system needs, so that any alcohol taken is added to that which is already in excess. In Europe it is different—a large part of the population is underfed, and a modicum of alcohol is a decided food-gain. It must be remembered, also, that as a food alcohol is superior even to lean beef, in that it requires no force to digest it. The coarse food of a European peasant is often worked up by the stomach only by the expenditure of much force; it is also repulsive to the palate. The draught of *landwein* or the schooner of beer washes down very well the morsel of black bread. Not only by stimulating the stomach does it aid in digestion, but also by readily yielding force to the system it assists in the elaboration of some refractory substances. Although I hold that the habitual use of alcohol to well-fed persons not only unnecessary, but positively harmful, it seems to me that in many cases of illness, and in those periods of life when, by reason of age, the body waxes weak, alcohol is possessed of great value. Under sixty years of age, the daily employment of wine may for most persons be very well discountenanced; but after this period has been reached, I believe the moderate employment of stimulants is very useful. The progressive failure of bodily powers points to the use of a substance which shall aid in digestion and readily supply force. In the later years of life, even the narcotic influence of alcohol is of value, easing the restlessness, the slight discomforts, the suffering of nerve-failure, incident to failing vitality.

"The question whether alcohol has food-value in disease is one not easily answered by positive evidence, because the narcotic properties of the substance are so marked as often to mask its influence as a food, and because we rarely dare to employ alcohol except with an abundance of other food. The principles already outlined are, however, as applicable in disease as in health. Recent researches in fever(a) have determined that the excessive heat-production is dependent upon excessive changes in the stored materials of the body; and it is improbable, though not impossible, that alcohol is capable of taking the place of these, and, by being, as it were, vicariously burnt, saving the tissues. The value of alcohol in low fevers, therefore, probably depends upon other qualities than its usefulness as a food, although our knowledge of fever processes is yet so imperfect that it is necessary to speak with great reserve. In chronic wasting diseases, I believe that alcohol has an actual food-value, besides being a most powerful aid to the digestion of other food."

In regard to the best mode of administering alcohol when used for sustaining the powers, Prof. Wood observes that probably all will assent to two rules—first, that it should be given in a diluted form; and, next, along with other food,—and, provided these rules be observed, he does not consider that it matters much in what form it is given. In chronic diseases, malt liquors have both advantages and inconveniences: they represent food and drink, are less likely to be abused than stronger liquids, and derive some tonic properties from their bitterness; but they sometimes disagree with the stomach. As they contain some nutritive material, there may be too much tendency to give them apart from food. The amount of solid constituents in a pint of malt liquor varies from over two ounces and a half in the strongest English ales to three-quarters of an ounce in the weakest ales and beers. "The nature of much of this solid matter is not known, but albumen, bitter and resinous principles from the hop, earthy salts, grape sugar, glycerine, and a number of complex acids, have been recognised in it. The tendency to grossness seen in beer-drinkers undoubtedly largely depends upon the solid constituents of the beer, and seems to one to indicate the proper medical use of malt liquors —namely, that they are especially to be employed in wasting diseases; i.e., where there is a tendency to the loss of the bodily fat. In regard to the choice of malt liquors, I do not think that there is any other than what we may call personal grounds for selection. That which suits the palate best usually also suits the stomach best. The choice should always settle upon the ale, porter, or beer which can be used with least inconvenience to the stomach; and when all malt liquors produce 'biliousness' (i.e., gastro-intestinal derangement) wine or diluted spirits should be substituted. As malt liquors contain nutritive material, it is less necessary to give food with them than it is with whisky or wine. Nevertheless, it is preferable in most cases that food should be taken with the ale or beer."

The Etiology of Rheumatism.

At a recent clinical lecture at the Hôpital Cochin (*Gaz. des Hôp.*, September 6), Dr. Bucquoy made the following remarks on the etiology of rheumatism:—

From an early part of this year we have had in my wards a number of persons, the subjects of acute rheumatism, as a consequence of a more or less prolonged residence in damp habitations. That does not mean that this disease is peculiar to cold seasons, for, like many other affections, it is the consequence of variations of temperature and of damp cold. But then, in order that it should become developed, certain predispositions, dependent upon age, sex, constitution, and heredity, must also exist. Age is a very important element in the history of acute articular rheumatism; and the best articles which have been written on this disease do not indicate this point very clearly. The figures furnished by statistics show us that the affection is very rare before the fifth year, that it is tolerably frequent between ten and fifteen, and that it especially makes its appearance between the years of fifteen and forty, and principally between thirty and forty. After this latter age it is rare. But from these facts the true conclusion has not been drawn, for if we are

(a) See a valuable essay upon this subject, contributed by Prof. Wood to the last volume of the *Contributions* of the Smithsonian Institution just published.

seeking for the date of the first attack we shall find that in general the disease begins prior to the thirtieth year; as, if a great number of persons attacked after that age, we shall also find these generally are suffering at that time from their second or third attack of the disease. In my opinion, then, acute articular rheumatism commences at an earlier period than that indicated by statistics, and is a disease especially of young subjects and adolescents. This fact is of importance, for the disease disappearing for the most part after the fortieth year, we may conclude from this that a case which we may have to do with after this age is not an acute articular rheumatism, but a chronic or constitutional, and not an accidental rheumatism. The question of sex is of less interest than that of age, for little difference in regard to the disease exists between males and females, as any predominance that appears to exist in men is exclusively due to their mode of life and occupations exposing them more to the variations of temperature than is the case with women. On the other hand, the question of sex is important in chronic rheumatism, which is especially the appanage of women, being exactly the contrary to what is the case in gout. With respect to the constitution most favourable to rheumatism, we find that individuals most predisposed to the disease are young persons with delicate and pale skin, fair hair, and an animated complexion. These are said to be the attributes of the lymphatic temperament, but rheumatism is not a disease confined to lymphatic individuals, as a considerable number of scrofulous persons become rheumatic at adult age. As to the part played by heredity in the etiology of rheumatism, the examination of antecedents is often difficult. Still, rheumatism oftenest occurs in those whose father or mother or grandparents are or have been the subjects of acute articular rheumatism. But the investigation should not be confined to rheumatism in the antecedents, but should be extended to arthritism in all its forms, gout, chronic rheumatism, etc., which may produce the rheumatic diathesis. Here the age and constitution play a certain part; for if the diathesis manifest itself at an early period, we find acute articular rheumatism occurring, while if such manifestations are more delayed, it is chronic rheumatism or gout which appears. Hereditary influence is not absolutely necessary for the appearance of acute articular rheumatism, and accidental external circumstances may suffice for its production. Gout belongs especially to the upper classes of society, and is not a *morbus servorum*, if we may use the expression. But the individual who contracts accidentally an acute articular rheumatism becomes an "arthritic," but not a "true arthritic." I understand by that he may have hereafter new attacks of the acute rheumatism, and that he may transmit a predisposition to the same disease, but not to manifestations of gout, nor to hæmorrhoidal or emphysematous accidents. It is not therefore a true "arthritism," for it will produce in the children only rheumatism, they not becoming true "arthritics," but remaining mere "rheumatics." So that it seems to me that we are not at present justified in confounding under one and the same condition the rheumatic diathesis and arthritism.

MEMBRANOUS DYSMENORRHŒA IN RELATION TO NORMAL MENSTRUATION.—In a paper read at the Académie de Médecine, Dr. Sinéty stated that it resulted from the observations which he had made on a great number of women, that, in the physiological condition, the uterine mucous membrane is not, as is generally taught, eliminated in menstruation; but, under certain pathological conditions, the mucous membrane of the body of the uterus exfoliates, and is expelled at the catamenial period. This phenomenon, designated as "membranous dysmenorrhœa," is usually accompanied by severe pain and loss of blood. It does not constitute a special disease or morbid entity, and is observed under very variable conditions, with or without metritis. The exfoliation is the result of an exaggeration of the normal menstrual process, inducing a too great infiltration of the deeper layers of the mucous membrane and compression of the vessels of this region, and leading to elimination of the tissues situated above this layer. It will be thus understood that anything which prevents the blood issuing, as in the normal state, by the superficial vascular network of the mucous membrane, may be a cause of membranous dysmenorrhœa.—*Union Méd.*, September 13.

REVIEWS.

Photographic Illustrations of Skin Diseases. By GEORGE HENRY FOX, A.M., M.D., Clinical Lecturer on Diseases of the Skin, College of Physicians and Surgeons, New York; Surgeon to the New York Dispensary, Department of Skin and Venereal Diseases; Fellow of the American Academy of Medicine, etc. New York: E. B. Treat, 757, Broadway. London: J. and A. Churchill, New Burlington-street. 4to. 1881.

WE have before us Parts 5 to 12 of this excellent work, the first four parts of which we noticed at the beginning of last year; and we now congratulate Dr. Fox on having brought out all the parts and completed the work in such a thoroughly satisfactory manner. We may remind our readers that each part contains four illustrations, each of which is the result of a careful selection both of the case of the disease illustrated, and of the photograph of it; and that the photographs are coloured to the desirable extent and degree by a skilled artist, who was formerly a physician, and studied diseases of the skin under Hebra in the General Hospital, Vienna. The illustrations contained in the parts now under notice are—Eczema, in its various varieties and stages; Varicose Ulcer, Psoriasis, Lupus; Epithelioma; Trichophytosis, Lichen; Kerion, Lepra Maculosa, Molluscum, Erythema; Phthieriasis, Scabies, Porrigo; Herpes Facialis, Hydroa, Erythema Circinatum and Exfoliatum, Purpura Simplex; Cornua Cutanea, Alopecia Areata, Morphœa, Scleroderma, and Sarcoma Pigmentosum. It will be seen from this list that some of the most rare forms of skin disease are illustrated, as well as those commonly met with; and this fact adds not a little to the value of the work for practitioners at a distance from the societies and hospitals. The great majority of the illustrations are unusually good, and not a few are of rare excellence; all testify to the care and skill employed in selecting and producing them. The text accompanying each plate is concise, clear, and very good, giving, in a style worthy of Dr. Fox's reputation as an accomplished dermatologist, brief notes of the case or cases illustrated, the diagnostic characters of the disease, and practical directions as to treatment. The work may be confidently recommended to practitioners as a very useful and valuable one.

A Guide to the Use of the Laryngoscope in General Practice. By GORDON HOLMES, L.R.C.P. Edin. London: J. and A. Churchill. 1881. Pp. 62.

THE author believes that the laryngoscope is still but little used in the ordinary routine of medical practice; this he attributes to the fact that a belief prevails among practitioners that tedious practice and long application are needed in order to acquire facility in the use of the instrument.

We are sure that those who may wish to undeceive themselves need only consult the book before us. It is a short but clear account, wherein will be found all that is necessary to become a good and practical worker in laryngoscopy.

It will be obvious to everyone that remedies can be more safely and more surely applied to diseased parts when the exact situation of the disease has first been ascertained, than when the remedies are used guesswise; while it is equally well known that, in general practice, "sore throat" in some shape or other is a very common complaint.

The author speaks with some authority, and his little book may be consulted with confidence by anyone wishing to learn the rudiments of this subject.

It issues from a well-known firm, and bears the finished impress which characterises all their publications.

A Sketch of the Discovery of Vaccination, and of the Evidences of its Power. By JAMES W. MILLER, M.D., Consulting Physician, Dundee Royal Infirmary, and Examiner in Medicine, University of Aberdeen. Edinburgh: George Waterston and Sons. 1881.

THIS little pamphlet, as its author announces, is not addressed to the medical profession, since nothing has been introduced into its pages which is not already well known to medical men; but Dr. Miller thinks—and we entirely agree with him —that there is among the general public a great want of information on the subject of vaccination. In lay circles it is generally considered sufficient to be acquainted with the fact that the good effects of vaccination were discovered by Jenner and, although it will scarcely be credited, among the present generation there are not a few who confuse that individual with the Sir William Jenner of our own day. The present sketch formed the subject-matter of a lecture delivered by Dr. Miller to the Naturalists' Society of Dundee in March last, and since its delivery various considerations have occurred to the author which appear to him to render its publication not only desirable, but opportune. Especially, considering the persistent, though misguided, energy with which the fallacious opinions of the anti-vaccinationists are propagated, it becomes a duty incumbent on those who really know the facts of the case to diffuse sound information on the subject for the welfare of the community, and Dr. Miller has compiled a history of small-pox and its antidote, which will be found by the non-medical portion of the public to be interesting as well as instructive reading.

GENERAL CORRESPONDENCE.

HOSPITAL OUT-PATIENTS.
LETTER FROM THE HON. REGINALD CAPEL.

[To the Editor of the Medical Times and Gazette.]

SIR,—The controversy which existed some years ago with respect to the abuse of our hospital out-patients system has in a measure subsided, but there have been letters lately upon the subject, and there are many who think that some reform is urgently needed.

I have long held the opinion that a large majority of those who attend as out-patients, do so, not so much because they get advice gratis, but rather because they secure the services of highly qualified and often first-rate men, and I believe most of them would pay if it became a rule they should do so. Cases of gross imposition are, I am sure, very rare, and a great deal too much has been made of them. In the hospital with which I am connected we had an officer whose sole duty was to register all cases, and to investigate by personal visits a large proportion of them. The result was, that not more than 5 per cent. were found to be, what we considered, ineligible. These we referred to a neighbouring provident dispensary; those in receipt of outdoor relief were referred to the relieving officer. I believe that 90 per cent. of hospital out-patients are "poor," dependent upon wages varying from 10s. to 50s. per week, but still often able and willing to pay something.

In my opinion, the class whom we wish to help would willingly become members of a provident institution *in connexion with and under the hospital roof, provided they were prescribed for by the hospital staff.* There is a strong bias amongst the poor in favour of advice from the hospital; and so long as they can obtain such advice, provident dispensaries outside the hospital will not flourish to the desired extent.

† By adopting such a course as I have suggested, the funds of the hospital would be materially benefited, and the Management would be in a position to make some pecuniary return to the medical staff for the services they now render gratuitously. Doubtless many objections will be raised to my suggestion, and it is with a view of eliciting opinions that I would ask you to insert this.

I am, &c., R. CAPEL,
September 21. Hon. Sec. Great Northern Hospital.

HOMŒOPATHY, HAHNEMANN, AND HOMŒOPATHS.
LETTER FROM DR. J. H. CLARKE.

[To the Editor of the Medical Times and Gazette.]

SIR,—You have compelled me, however reluctant, to address you yet again. For your evident desire to treat this question on its merits, and your willingness to hear both sides of the case, I thank you. Your opinions and conclusions you have a perfect right to express, and your readers to endorse if they choose. To these I take no exception. But when you state imaginary facts as the grounds of your conclusions, it is a different matter. Facts are too important to be trifled with ; and as I am sure you would be the last knowingly to distort them, I will now point out to you some of the graver errors into which you have fallen.

1. You state that, "according to the homœopathic

doctrine, the efficacy of a remedy increases more and more from the *simile* to the *similius*, and even to the *simillimum*, but the moment the last becomes, instead of like, identical, it only intensifies the mischief."

This same statement was made in your article of April 30, and corrected in my letter published a fortnight later, to which I must refer you. There is no such homœopathic doctrine. Arsenic will cure the identical supra-orbital neuralgia it has often produced—provided, of course, it be not itself the cause in this particular instance. The symptoms may be identical ; if the cause is different, a cure will take place. With this one of your chief arguments falls to the ground.

2. You say, "There is not a single remedy—except among those which act locally, as by irritating the skin or the bowels—which produces the same effect as does disease, and at best the resemblance between the effects of the two is of the most superficial and remote description."

This is astounding. One would suppose you had never heard of lead or mercurial palsy ; the nephritis and strangury of cantharis and terebinth ; the delirium, dry-mouth, and sore-throat of belladonna ; or the constipation of opium ; with a host of other equally well-known phenomena.

3. You say, "The vast majority of our professional brethren say that the law of similars has failed in their hands when fully and duly tried in that bright light which beats around the bedside of a fully equipped and active medical school, where no work can escape acute and jealous criticism."

This is no less astonishing. It is simply impossible that the vast majority of medical men should have thus tried the law of similars. During their clerkship in hospital they have had no opportunity of trying medicines for themselves ; and even if the opportunity had been theirs, they could not have had the knowledge requisite for making such use of it. And it will not be contended that the vast majority of medical men are hospital physicians and surgeons.

4. You say that Hahnemann had a very poor medical training, and that he only took to real medicine late in life.

Hahnemann was born April 10, 1755 ; commenced to study medicine at Leipsic, 1775 ; studied at Leipsic, Vienna, and Erlangen, where he took his degree August 10, 1779, in his twenty-fifth year. He commenced practice at once, and continued in practice the rest of his long life, with the intermission of one or two years, during which he supported himself, as you say, by literary work, and among other, by translating Cullen's Materia Medica into German. He soon resumed practice, and to such good purpose that Hufeland, writing in 1801, called him "one of the most distinguished of German physicians," and "a practised physician of matured experience and reflection."(a)

As for his medical training being very poor, the statement is very misleading. Judged by the scientific standard of to-day, he had, no doubt, a very poor medical training ; but then it was infinitely superior to the training Harvey had, or any of the heroes before him, for they in their college days were not taught the circulation of the blood. It would be just as fair to discredit Harvey on the same grounds. Harvey wrote concerning the blood, as Professor Huxley has lately told us, that it maintains and fashions all parts of the body: "idque summâ cum providentia et intellectu, in finem certum agens, quasi ratiocinio quodam uteretur." Hahnemann never wrote anything more absurd than this. And yet no one thinks of denying Harvey's greatness, or of grudging him his monument, because he knew nothing of protoplasm. In Harvey's day, and for some time after him, there was a despised medical sect called "Circulators" because they believed in the circulation of the blood. After a time the medical world came to admit that the sun did shine, and that the reason they had failed to see it was that they had resolutely kept their eyes shut. Then all believed in the circulation of the blood, and the sect of the Circulators ceased to exist. So it is with homœopathy now. Its adherents are at present a despised sect. The time is coming when the sect of the Homœopathists will become extinct as did that of the Circulators of old.

5. Hahnemann's peculiar dosage was not the result of persecution, but one of the causes of it. Apothecaries could not, or would not, make up his prescriptions—they were paid according to the number and quantity of the ingredients—

(a) *Hufeland's Journal*, vol. v., part ii., page 52, note.

and prosecuted him when he made up his own, even when he gave his medicines away. His taking to small doses was a mere matter of practical experience, and not the fruit of preconceived theories. That there is such a thing as *potentising* a medicine by *attenuating* it, the superior efficacy of hydrarg. cum cretâ over the crude metal is sufficient evidence to show, if there were no more, as there is plenty.

Homœopathists, as a rule, do not bind themselves down to every utterance or every practice of their master. They hold themselves entirely free to use their own judgment. At the same time they are very jealous for the honour of him to whom they owe so much, and resent every attempt to discredit him or his discovery. There are homœopathists who are not ashamed to drag his name in the dirt, or pass him by in silence, whilst they trade on the fruits of his labours, thinking to compound for their heterodoxy in the eyes of the orthodox by damning him from whom they have learned all that is best in their practice. But the bulk of the homœopathists are not of this sort; they would rather be tabooed with Hahnemann than recognised with such as these.

There are other points in your article which I might notice, but it would require too much space. I am unaware of the experiments made on healthy young men that you mention, and should esteem it a favour if you would supply the references. Again thanking you for your courtesy,

I am, &c.,   JOHN H. CLARKE, M.D.
15, St. George's-terrace, Gloucester-road, S.W.,
September 19.

OBITUARY.

ROBERT SMITH, M.A., M.D., C.M. ABER., M.R.C.P. LOND.

IT is once more our painful duty to record the early death of a young and promising member of the profession. Dr. Robert Smith, Assistant-Physician and Pathologist to the Charing-cross Hospital, whose name was becoming known even in the great world of the profession in the metropolis, dies of phthisis at Laurencekirk, N.B., on September 9, at the age of thirty-two. Born at Kincardine O'Neil, he received his education in Arts in the University of Aberdeen, where he graduated M.A. in 1872, after a distinguished career as a student. Immediately afterwards he commenced his medical curriculum in the same institution, and so speedily and certainly were his abilities recognised by his teachers that he was appointed assistant to more than one of the professors—the most important post, which he held for twelve months, being that of Demonstrator of Anatomy under Professor Struthers. Dr. Smith had fixed on the metropolis as the field of his life-work, but before coming up to town he was, for about a year, Resident Medical Officer of the Leeds Infirmary. In 1877 he was appointed Medical Registrar to Charing-cross Hospital; and, in the course of time, was elected to the posts of Demonstrator of Practical Physiology, Medical Pathologist, and, finally, of Assistant-Physician. Meanwhile, he had been elected an Examiner in Medicine in the University of Aberdeen. The most important and arduous of these offices had been held by him for only a few months, when his friends were alarmed to mark in him the symptoms of serious illness. He continued, however, to discharge the duties, which must have sorely tried his strength, until April last, when weakness compelled him to seek relief in rest and change of air. The progress of the fatal disease was never, however, in any degree arrested, and on the date mentioned above he died, after a very short confinement to bed, of what appears to have been an attack of pneumothorax.

Robert Smith was one of the most accomplished and promising of the younger generation of our hospital physicians; and Charing-cross may truly mourn the loss of such a man within twelve months of the deaths of Pearson Irvine, Sparks, and Amphlett. There can be no doubt that Dr. Robert Smith's death was the direct result of his laborious habits, which had grown out of a natural love of work in itself, a thirst for accurate knowledge, and an amount of conscientiousness which utterly disregarded personal health, rest, or relaxation. He was always a student in the strictest sense of the term, from the time when he carried off the first prizes in the Arts classes of his University, and graduated in medicine and surgery with Highest Academical Honours,

till the very hour almost of his death. After a day spent in the wards, in the out-patient room, in the physiological laboratory, or in the post-mortem room, he would devote the evening and part of the night to reading, writing, and work in every form. Never, to all appearance, a strong man, he broke down under the strain of constant application, and the anxiety that must have accompanied his struggle for position and distinction. His abilities were very good, and his knowledge remarkable for its variety, its exactness, and the readiness with which it could be commanded on occasion. Nothing that he had ever learned appeared to have been lost or forgotten; and thus the classics and the exact sciences were as familiar to him as the many departments of his own profession. In addition to these intellectual abilities, Robert Smith was endowed with a most amiable and considerate character, which expressed itself in acts of calm, quiet, gentle kindliness, and an only too disinterested regard for others. Such qualities of mind and heart rendered him one of the most successful and popular of teachers, and both in the University of Aberdeen and in Charing-cross Hospital he will long be remembered with gratitude and respect by many students. His literary work was almost entirely anonymous. For some time he had been one of the most regular contributors to our columns, and the reports of the Pathological Society have for several sessions been from his pen. He was the last man to bring forth unripe fruit, and his name is not publicly associated therefore with any literary work; but few can form any just conception of the amount of valuable writing of a routine kind which he produced. His friendship and good-comradeship will be missed and mourned by his many friends.

JAMES ROSE-INNES, M.B., C.M. ABER.

WE regret having to record the death, at the early age of twenty-six years, of Mr. J. Rose-Innes, M.B., who was Surgeon on board the *Teuton* when that vessel foundered. He was educated for the medical profession at Marischal College, Aberdeen, and the London Hospital, at the former of which he graduated M.B. and C.M. in 1880.

Shortly after taking his degrees, Mr. Rose-Innes obtained an appointment as Surgeon to the steamship *Utopia* of the Anchor Line, trading between London and New York, and whilst on his first voyage in November last year that vessel was overtaken by a heavy storm. The funnel of the *Utopia* was washed away, and the ship almost lost. On that occasion Mr. Rose-Innes behaved with conspicuous coolness and gallantry in taking charge of the passengers and emigrants. The vessel had to put back to Plymouth to refit, and she then proceeded to New York, on his arrival at which place Mr. Rose-Innes was presented with a testimonial, signed by the captain of the vessel and passengers, in recognition of his conduct. The next appointment which he obtained was that of Surgeon to the Union Royal Mail steamship *Durban*, trading between Southampton and South Africa. On his arrival at Cape Town he was transferred to the *Danube* for intercolonial service. Being required in England on some private business, he was again transferred—this time at the request of his friends—to a homeward-bound steamer. Thus he came to join the ill-fated *Teuton*, only a few hours before she met with her terrible disaster off Quoin Point. It appears, from the account of the survivors, that Mr. Rose-Innes took charge of and kept order among the passengers—some 200 in number—during the last few moments, again behaving with admirable coolness and judgment. He was well known in Aberdeen, and while his untimely loss will be deplored by his family, his friends, and college associates, they cannot fail to find some consolation in the thought that in the hour of trial he was found at his post, and died while nobly doing his duty.

RARITY OF FLIES AND WASPS.—Dr. Latour calls attention in the *Union Médicale* (September 10) to the fact that in Paris this year, notwithstanding the torrid heat of July, flies have been exceedingly rare, and wasps, the torment of the amateur fruit garden, well-nigh absent. Many of our readers will be able to confirm the observation as relates to this country. He suggests that the extreme heat of July in many instances burned up the ova and larvæ of these insects.

VITAL STATISTICS OF LONDON.

Week ending Saturday, September 17, 1881.

BIRTHS.

Births of Boys, 1245; Girls, 1248; Total, 2493.
Corrected weekly average in the 10 years 1871-80, 2513·2.

DEATHS.

	Males.	Females.	Total.
Deaths during the week	580	571	1151
Weekly average of the ten years 1871-80, corrected to increased population ...	721·6	680·7	1402·3
Deaths of people aged 80 and upwards	...	...	43

DEATHS IN SUB-DISTRICTS FROM EPIDEMICS.

	Enumerated Population, 1881 (unrevised).	Small-pox.	Measles.	Scarlet Fever.	Diphtheria.	Whooping-cough.	Typhus.	Enteric (or Typhoid) Fever.	Simple continued Fever.	Diarrhœa.
West ...	668998	2	1	6	...	1	...	3	...	8
North ...	905677	6	3	12	2	8	1	3	...	4
Central ...	261793	1	1	3	...	1	...	3	...	6
East ...	692530	2	5	9	1	4	...	3	1	8
South ...	1265678	15	5	21	3	8	...	9	1	14
Total ...	3814571	26	15	51	6	22	1	21	2	40

METEOROLOGY.

From Observations at the Greenwich Observatory.

Mean height of barometer ...	...	...	...	...	29·997 in.
Mean temperature ...	...	...	...	...	55·0°
Highest point of thermometer	...	...	...	...	66·4°
Lowest point of thermometer	...	...	...	...	40·0°
Mean dew-point temperature	...	...	...	...	51·9°
General direction of wind ...	...	...	...	...	Variable.
Whole amount of rain in the week	...	...	...	...	0·14 in.

BIRTHS and DEATHS Registered and METEOROLOGY during the Week ending Saturday, Sept. 17, in the following large Towns :—

Cities and boroughs (Municipal boundaries except for London.)	Estimated Population to middle of the year 1881.*	Persons to an Acre (1881).	Births Registered during the week ending Sept. 17.	Deaths Registered during the week ending Sept. 17	Temperature of Air (Fahr.)				Temp. of Air (Cent.)	Rain Fall.	
					Highest during the Week.	Lowest during the Week.	Weekly Mean of Daily Mean Values.			In Inches.	In Centimetres.
London ...	3899751	50·8	2493	1151	66·4	40·0	55·0		12·78	0·14	0·36
Brighton ...	107934	45·9	64	34	66·1	47·8	55·7		13·17	0·16	0·41
Portsmouth ...	128335	28·8	101	48	...	...	...		...	...	...
Norwich ...	88035	11·8	49	31	...	...	...		...	...	...
Plymouth ...	75282	54·0	55	25	66·0	42·5	53·0		12·01	0·00	0·00
Bristol ...	207140	46·5	147	59	65·0	42·2	53·3		11·84	0·00	0·00
Wolverhampton ...	75934	22·4	55	21	62·5	42·5	51·1		10·62	0·20	0·51
Birmingham ...	402296	47·9	276	124	...	...	...		...	...	...
Leicester ...	123120	39·5	92	63	63·5	39·5	52·3		11·28	0·19	0·48
Nottingham ...	186235	18·9	122	73	64·8	37·5	51·9		11·05	0·15	0·38
Liverpool ...	553998	106·3	435	299	62·2	45·3	53·1		11·73	0·16	0·41
Manchester ...	341289	79·5	239	100	...	...	...		...	...	...
Salford ...	177760	34·4	133	54	...	...	...		...	...	...
Oldham ...	112176	24·0	76	26	...	...	...		...	...	...
Bradford ...	181037	25·5	103	53	62·0	43·2	51·7		10·95	0·39	0·99
Leeds ...	310490	14·4	211	82	61·0	44·0	52·1		11·17	0·14	0·36
Sheffield ...	285621	14·5	197	90	64·0	39·9	51·5		10·84	0·21	0·53
Hull ...	161161	42·7	102	91	64·0	37·0	52·2		11·22	0·46	1·17
Sunderland ...	116753	42·2	75	38	...	...	...		...	...	...
Newcastle-on-Tyne	145675	27·1	117	50	...	...	...		...	...	...
Total of 20 large English Towns ...	7608775	38·0	5142	2521	66·4	37·0	52·8		11·55	0·18	0·46

* These figures are the numbers enumerated (but subject to revision) in April last, raised to the middle of 1881 by the addition of a quarter of a year's increase, calculated at the rate that prevailed between 1871 and 1881.

At the Royal Observatory, Greenwich, the mean reading of the barometer last week was 29·90 in. The highest reading was 30·05 in. on Friday morning, and the lowest 29·69 in. at the end of the week.

MEDICAL NEWS.

APOTHECARIES' HALL, LONDON.—The following gentleman passed his examination in the Science and Practice of Medicine, and received a certificate to practise, on Thursday, September 15 :—

Taylor, Thomas, Gloucester-street, Regent's-park.

The following gentlemen also on the same day passed their primary professional examination :—

Dabbs, Charles John, the London Hospital.
Davies, E. Cluneglas, the London Hospital.

At the Preliminary Examination in Arts, held at the Hall on September 16 and 17, 152 candidates presented themselves, of whom ninety-five were rejected, and the following fifty-seven passed and received certificates of proficiency in general education :—

In the First Class, in order of merit—

1. Evelyn Oliver Ashe and William Henry Hillyer. 3. Edward William Mulligan. 4. Charles Stancourt Ware.

In the Second Class, in alphabetical order—

H. G. L. Allford, J. E. Appleton, D. E. Ashbee, P. T. B. Beale, L. T. F. Bryett, W. J. Calvert, J. E. A. G. Becker, Wm. Robt. Cargill, I. W. Clegg, E. H. Corder, Guy Cory, Arthur Crapp, H. N. Edwards, C. Ewart, W. G. R. Farquharson, H. J. Fitzgerald, John Fitzgerald, Jas. R. Gaylard, W. H. Gatrell, R. C. Ginson, E. S. Gooddy, A. J. Gregory, C. J. Habbijam, L. Hamel-Smith, W. J. Harris, H. P. Helsham, J. P. Hocken, Frank Hues, T. W. Kelly, C. B. T. Langton, Cyprus Legg, Alfred Lloyd, A. Meyrick-Jones, F. J. Morgan, H. Nelson, S. W. Owen, C. J. Parson, C. T. Peach, J. Petherbridge, J. Rausch, J. G. Rusher, G. H. Seagrave, F. M. Sealy, G. Shillcock, J. H. Smyth, W. P. Southby, F. T. Troughton, Tamiz Uddin, Louis Vallee, John Verco, William Wilson, Bernard D. Z. Wright, and Percy Phillips Wright.

NAVAL, MILITARY, ETC., APPOINTMENTS.

ADMIRALTY.—Surgeon Arthur Vereker Smyth has been promoted to the rank of Staff Surgeon in Her Majesty's Fleet, with seniority of August 17, 1881.

BIRTHS.

ADCOCK.—On September 13, at Great Yarmouth, the wife of John Adcock, M.D., A.M.D., of a daughter.

CROWFOOT.—On September 14, at Beccles, Suffolk, the wife of W. M. Crowfoot, M.B., of a son.

HOFFMEISTER.—On September 15, at 8, Cambridge-road, Brighton, the wife of J. B. Hoffmeister, L.R.C.P., of a son.

O'CONNELL.—On September 17, at Thornfield, Hastings, the wife of Surgeon-Major E. O'Connell, A.M.D., of a daughter.

SMITH.—On September 15, at 32, Argyle-square, W.C., the wife of Sydney Lloyd Smith, L.R.C.P., of a son.

STARTIN.—On September 12, at The Highams, Surbiton-hill, the wife of James Startin, M.B., M.R.C.S., of Savkville-street, Piccadilly, of a daughter.

WHITEHEAD.—On September 15, at Belgrave House, Ventnor, the wife of John Livesay Whitehead, M.D., of a daughter.

MARRIAGES.

DAVIES—MORRIS.—On September 16, at Hebburn-on-Tyne, Hugh Walter Davies, M.R.C.S., L.R.C.P., to Mary Jane, only daughter of David Morris, Esq., of Pelaw Main, Newcastle-upon-Tyne.

FINLAY—EBDEN.—On August 17, at Rondebosch, Cape of Good Hope, Arthur W. Finlay, Esq., of 80A, Fenchurch-street, London, to Augusta, daughter of Henry Ebden, M.D.

JOHNSON—JOHNSON.—On September 8, at Sussex-gardens, Walter Johnson, M.R.C.S., to Amy Charlotte, third daughter of the late Henry Johnson, Esq., of Lincoln's-inn.

JOHNSTON—PERCEVAL.—On August 31, at Kilbell, Percy Herbert Johnston, M.D., A.M.D., eldest son of J. W. Johnston, M.D., of Park View, Cork, to Agnes Maude, eldest daughter of General J. Maxwell Perceval, C.B., Colonel 97th Regiment.

MACROBIN—JONES.—On September 14, at Clontarf, Surgeon-Major Macrobin, A.M.D., to Annabella, widow of the late Charles Gray Jones, Captain R.N., and daughter of Henry A. Dillon, Esq., Malahide, co. Dublin.

MANN—BEATTY.—On September 13, at Seaham Harbour, William Dalla Mann, Esq., of Sunderland, solicitor, to Elizabeth, youngest daughter of Thomas Carlyle Beatty, M.R.C.S., L.S.A., of Seaham Harbour.

SHAND—STUART.—On September 14, at Montrose, James W. F. Smith-Shand, M.D. Aber., to Anna, youngest daughter of the late William Stuart, Esq., of Inverugie, Morayshire.

SMITH—WHITWILL.—On September 13, at Bristol, William Alexander Smith, M.A., M.D., M.R.C.S., F.C.S., of Newport, Essex, to Mary Catherine, eldest daughter of Mark Whitwill, J.P., of Redland House, Bristol.

DEATHS.

BARRY, JOHN MILNER, M.D., F.R.C.P., at Tunbridge Wells, on September 15, aged 66.

INNES, LILIAN, younger daughter of Surgeon-General J. H. Ker Innes, F.R.C.S., C.B., Honorary Surgeon to Her Majesty, at Baveno, Lago Maggiore, on September 14, aged 13.

KNAGGS, LOUISA COLEMAN, wife of Sydney Henry Knaggs, M.R.C.S., at Stratford Lodge, Folkestone, on September 14, in her 41st year.

ROSS, WILLIAM HERBERT, fourth son of Henry Cooper Ross, M.D., at Hampstead, on September 21, aged 18.

VACANCIES.

In the following list the nature of the office vacant, the qualifications required in the candidate, the person to whom application should be made and the day of election (as far as known) are stated in succession.

CLINICAL HOSPITAL AND DISPENSARY FOR WOMEN AND CHILDREN, PARK-PLACE, MANCHESTER. — House-Surgeon. (For particulars see Advertisement.)

ESSEX AND COLCHESTER HOSPITAL.—Physician. Candidates are requested to forward their names and qualifications, together with original testimonials, to the Secretary on or before October 5.

NORTH-EASTERN HOSPITAL FOR CHILDREN, HACKNEY-ROAD, E.—Surgeon. Candidates must be Fellows or Members of the Royal College of Surgeons of England. Applications, accompanied by testimonials, to be sent to Alfred Nixon, Secretary, 27, Clement's-lane, E.C., from whom further particulars can be obtained.

QUEEN'S HOSPITAL, BIRMINGHAM.—Casualty Surgeon. Candidates must be Fellows or Members of the Royal College of Surgeons of England, Edinburgh, or Dublin. Applications and testimonials, with certificates of registration, to be sent to the Secretary at the Hospital, from whom all further information may be obtained, on or before October 5.

ST. COLUMB MAJOR UNION, CORNWALL.—District Medical Officer. (For particulars see Advertisement.)

THE NEW DOCTOR DEPUTIES.—The Chambre des Deputés elected in 1877 contained thirty-seven doctors, and the new one just elected will contain fifty-two. There are also three pharmacians in it.—Lyon Med., September 11.

THE examinations in Sanitary Science by the University of Cambridge, open to all whose names are on the Medical Register of the United Kingdom, will begin on October 4. The names of candidates must be sent to Professor Liveing, Cambridge, on or before the 28th inst.

A WINTER SANATORIUM IN THE NORTH SEA.—Geh.-Med. Rath Prof. Dr. Beneke will during September and October take up his residence at the island of Norderney, in the North Sea, and is willing to take certain suitable patients under his protection. If at the end of October he finds that there is a sufficient number of them who are desirous of wintering on the island, he will be willing to remain there with them during the entire winter; but intimations of such desire must be delivered to him not later than October 1. The provision of dwelling-places, care of the sick, the means of maintenance, communications with the Continent, etc., are now so far secured that Prof. Beneke feels that everything is ready for making this first trial of the effects of a residence here during the ensuing winter. The patients, who, from former trials, are deemed especially suitable by Prof. Beneke for a winter's residence at Norderney, are young subjects with commencing phthisis, the bad forms of scrofula (ulcerated lymphatic glands, osteo-myelitis, and obstinate affections of the mucous membranes of the respiratory organs, the ear, eye, etc.), and lastly, individuals suffering from general constitutional debility, which renders a much longer duration of life improbable, and exhibits itself in feeble development of the bony and muscular systems, anæmic decolouration, abnormal irritability of the nervous system, etc. Prof. Beneke has made every provision, and especially with regard to comfortable homes, and we earnestly hope that every success will attend his plan, dictated as it is by the warmest humanity and the most active scientific interest. He will supervise and treat the patients gratuitously, and is willing to take every responsibility as to the safe return of any patient in whom unfavourable circumstances may appear. Easy communication also renders a temporary residence on the island convenient.—Deutsche Med. Woch., August 27.

Two deaths from cholera in Shanghai, during the half-year ended September 30, 1880, are reported, but there was no epidemic of cholera or of choleraic affections, although, as usual at the approach and during the continuance of hot weather, a large mortality among native residents was announced. The cause of this yearly recurring mortality is only vaguely described, but the symptoms enumerated point to excessive consumption of more or less unripe or decayed fruit and vegetables, exposure to the direct rays of the sun, and the absorption of malarious and other poisonous exhalations from the soil, which are condensed in the dark, filthy, crowded, and unventilated ground-floor rooms in which multitudes of Chinese habitually sleep. When one considers the miscellaneous but always filthy food consumed by pigs in China, and the large extent to which pork enters into the diet of natives; when we consider, also, the fact that not only ordinary cooking, but smoking, pickling, and even saturation with chloride-of-zinc solution, are inoperative to destroy the larvæ of Trichina spiralis when encapsuled in muscle, it is not unreasonable to suppose that many of the cases of rapid death, with symptoms of collapse following on pain of a rheumatismal character, and accompanied by sweating, ascites, diarrhœa, and vomiting, which are every summer reported as occurring among the natives, are due to trichinosis. A case of this kind was brought into the Gutzlaff Hospital last August, and died a few hours after admission. By no amount of persuasion could I prevail on the relatives to allow me to take a specimen of the muscles, and therefore the diagnosis must rest doubtful. Two other members of the patient's family had died a few days before with the same symptoms, which had extended in one case over three weeks, and in the other over four. The man brought to hospital was reported to have been ailing for about a month, and his illness, it was said, began with violent pain and swelling of the abdomen.—Dr. A. Jamieson, in the "Medical Reports of the Imperial Maritime Customs of China."

NOTES, QUERIES, AND REPLIES.

Je that questioneth much shall learn much.—Bacon.

An Anxious Student.—The results of the Preliminary or Arts Examination of the Royal College of Surgeons of England—the last to be conducted by the authority of that body—will be published in our columns next week.

B. F.—The surgeon whom you mention died some years ago. Apply to any known hospital surgeon.

Cutting off the Water-Supply.—The County Court Judge of Hastings has decided that the Urban Sanitary Authority has no right to cut off the water-supply of any cistern, unless it was proved that such cistern was leaky, and thus caused a waste of water, or was open to sewage or other contamination.

Medico-Historical Houses.—The house in which Dr. Denman (the father of Lord Denman) lived is in Denman-street, formerly Queen-street. Smellie practised as an apothecary in Pall-mall. William Hunter's house in Great Windmill-street is now a French hotel; the little Windmill-street School; a carman's; and Brookes' School in Blenheim-street, a lead warehouse.

Dr. Williams.—The Museum and Library of the Royal College of Surgeons will be re-opened on Monday, October 3.

A Third-Year Student.—On and after January next all students will have to undergo the new examination, unless holding a recognised licence including medicine and midwifery.

Recreation in Army Station-Hospitals.—The Army Medical Department has at length succeeded, after urgent representations, in inducing the War Office to authorise the issue of games to all station-hospitals, in proportion to the average number of patients. It has hitherto been thought undesirable to increase the attractiveness of a stay in hospital to the not a few malingerers who sought thereby to avoid duty. But upon convalescents the beneficial influence of such recreation is so obvious, that all opposition has been overcome.

A Sanitary Improvement.—A faculty has been obtained for the conversion into a public garden of the churchyard attached to the church at the junction of Clapham- and Brixton-roads.

A Counterblast against Tea.—According to Cobbett, the drink-corrosive, gnawing, poisonous, which destroys health, enfeebles the frame, engenders laziness, debauches youth, makes old age miserable—the drink that had done a great deal to bring this nation into the state of misery in which he found it—is tea.

Private Medical Practice.—In "Cousin William," Theodore Hook calls the aunt and uncle "bold Buchaneers," from their fondness for rash domestic medical practice, and doctoring themselves from Buchan. In describing the original of this aunt at the Garrick, one morning, he declared that the old lady was so delighted with everything pertaining to physic, that she drank wine every six hours out of dose glasses, and filled her gold-fish globes with leeches, the evolutions of which she watched by the hour.

Wit at York.—A gentleman was telling, at the recent meeting of the British Association, that he was eighty-one years of age, and had never been an abstainer, when he was greeted by the exclamation (which brought down the house)—"You would have been a hundred by this time if you had."

*** Mr. Clarke has been good enough to send us the following, thinking that as the subject is so seldom dealt with in verse, it may be deemed worthy of quotation in our columns:—

WITH THE SCALPEL.

"Ubi sedes vitæ?"

(By H. Savile Clarke, in *The Burlington*.)

Here's our "subject"—tall and strong,
  With vermilion well injected
Where the blood once coursed along—
  Ready now to be dissected.
Some one never claimed, it seems,
  Friendless amid London's Babel:
Did he ever in his dreams
    See this table?

Here's a hand that once held fast
  All things pleasant to its liking;
Now its active days are past,
  Or for friendship or for striking.
Nothing colder here could lie,
  Yet on some one's palm there lingers
Sense of its warm touch,—while I
    Strip the fingers.

How the dead eyes strangely stare
  When I lift the lids above them!
Yet some woman lives, I swear,
  Who too well had learnt to love them;
Some one since their final sleep
  Holds their smiles in recollection,—
While I put them by to keep
    For dissection.

Then the heart. I take it out,
  Handling it with no compunction:
Once it wildly pulsed, no doubt,
  Well performed each wondrous function—
Sped the life-blood on its race
  In miraculous gyration;
Felt, responsive to one face,
    Palpitation.

Where was Life then? Was it hid
  In each curious convolution,
Packed beneath the cranium lid
  With such ordered distribution?
Can we touch one spot and say—
  Here all thought and feeling entered,
Here—'twas but the other day—
    Life was centred?

No! that puzzle still remains
  One unsolved supreme attraction:
Here are muscles, nerves, and veins,
  Where was that which gave them action?
Though the scalpel's edge be keen,
  Comes no answer from the tissues,
Telling us where life has been—
    Whence it issues.

We can bid the heart be still,
  Stop the life-blood's circulation;
Paralyse the sovereign will
  Through the centres of sensation.
When the clay lies at your feet,
  We can light no life within it,
Cannot make the dead heart beat
    For one minute.

Yet this thought remains with him—
  Dead he is to outward seeming,
Still the eyes so glazed and dim,
  See what lies beyond our dreaming;
Know the secrets of the spheres,
  Truth of doom or bliss supernal,
Read the riddle of the years—
    Life eternal!

So we'll leave him—ready now
  For to-morrow morning's lecture.
Little recks that placid brow
  Of our wayward wild conjecture.
It may be our fate to die
  All unwept and missed by no men:
As he lies there, we may lie,
    Absit omen!

St. George's.—There is a portrait by the celebrated Hogarth of Sir Cæsar Hawkins in the Council-room of the Royal College of Surgeons. Hogarth was a man most susceptible of flattery. Being at dinner with the celebrated Cheselden, he was told that Mr. Freke, surgeon to St. Bartholomew's Hospital, had asserted that Greene was as eminent in musical composition as Handel, to which Hogarth replied, "That fellow Freke is always shooting his bolt absurdly in one way or the other. Handel is a giant in music, Greene only a light Florimel kind of a composer." "Aye," said the artist's informant, "but at the same time Freke declared that you were as good a portrait-painter as Vandyke." Hogarth at once exclaimed, "There he was right,—and so, by God, I am! give me my time, and let me choose my subject."

Anatomist.—Yes. Galen is supposed to have only dissected apes, and judged of mankind by analogy; and though there may be reason to doubt whether this was altogether the case, it is certain that he had very little practice in human dissection.

Iago, New Cross.—The Metropolitan Hospital Saturday Fund was started seven years ago. In the first year the street collection amounted to only £258. The annual collections have steadily risen since, and last year were considerably over £1800. The total amount last year from both the street and workshop collections was about £7000.

Unlawful Sale of Intoxicants.—There is no doubt that workmen's clubs are often used for the illicit sale of intoxicating liquors, and that they require a somewhat strict police supervision. Several persons were lately charged at the Clerkenwell Police-court with having sold intoxicating liquors without a licence. The defendants were members of the Clarendon Working Men's Club, High-street, Islington, and it was in connexion with the proceedings at the club that the charges were preferred. One summons was dismissed, three were withdrawn, and the other defendant was fined £5.

A Beer-drinker.—According to the Inland Revenue Commissioners the result of their experience is, that "there is reason to believe ingredients deleterious to health are now seldom, if ever, added to beer."

COMMUNICATIONS have been received from—

Mr. Joseph Harper, Barnstaple; Dr. C. H. Leonards, Providence, U.S.A.; The President, Treasurer, and Medical Officers of Guy's Hospital, London; The President and Treasurer of St. Thomas's Hospital, London; Mr. John Blake, London; Dr. Norman Moore, London; Dr. J. W. Moore, London; The President of the Local Government Board, London; The Secretary of State for the Colonies, London; Mr. J. Chatto, London; Mr. Stone, London; The Registrar-General, Queensland; The Registrar-General, Scotland; The Dean of the Medical Faculty, King's College, London; Dr. J. H. Clarke, London; Mr. J. T. W. Bacot, Seaton, Devon; Dr. J. Anderson, London; Dr. Anningson, Cambridge; The Registrar of the Apothecaries' Hall, London.

BOOKS, ETC., RECEIVED—

Convulsions, by Edward T. Reichert, M.D.—Ethylene Bichloride, by Edward T. Reichert, M.D.—Localised Cerebral Lesions, by E. C. Seguin, M.D.—Epilepsy, by E. C. Seguin, M.D.—Dr. George Henry Fox's Photographic Illustrations of Skin Diseases, parts 5 to 12—Transactions of the College of Physicians of Philadelphia, vol. v.—General Index to the Cyclopædia of the Practice of Medicine, by Dr. H. von Ziemssen—Bigelow's Operation, by R. Harrison, M.R.C.S.—Medical Communications of the Massachusetts Medical Society—Vaccination, by P. A. Taylor, M.P.—Health-Resorts for Tropical Invalids, by W. J. Moore.

PERIODICALS AND NEWSPAPERS RECEIVED—

Lancet—British Medical Journal—Medical Press and Circular—Berliner Klinische Wochenschrift—Centralblatt für Chirurgie—Gazette des Hopitaux—Gazette Médicale—Le Progrès Médical—Bulletin de l'Académie de Médecine—Pharmaceutical Journal—Wiener Medizinische Wochenschrift—Centralblatt für die Medizinischen Wissenschaften—Revue Médicale—Gazette Hebdomadaire—National Board of Health Bulletin, Washington—Nature—Deutsche Medicinal-Zeitung—Boston Medical and Surgical Journal—Louisville Medical News—The American—Occasional Notes—Oil and Drug News—North Devon Journal, Sept. 15—Sydney Morning Herald, July 12—Journal of the British Dental Association—Liverpool Medico-Chirurgical Journal—Revue de Médecine—Detroit Lancet—Giornale Internazionale delle Scienze Mediche—Revue d'Hygiène—Hackney and Kingsland Gazette, September 17—Physician and Surgeon—Canada Lancet.

APPOINTMENTS FOR THE WEEK.

September 24. Saturday (this day).

Operations at St. Bartholomew's, 1½ p.m.; King's College, 1½ p.m.; Royal Free, 2 p.m.; Royal London Ophthalmic, 11 a.m.; Royal Westminster Ophthalmic, 1½ p.m.; St. Thomas's, 1½ p.m.; London, 2 p.m.

26. *Monday.*

Operations at the Metropolitan Free, 2 p.m.; St. Mark's Hospital for Diseases of the Rectum, 2 p.m.; Royal London Ophthalmic, 11 a.m.; Royal Westminster Ophthalmic, 1½ p.m.

27. *Tuesday.*

Operations at Guy's, 1½ p.m.; Westminster, 2 p.m.; Royal London Ophthalmic, 11 a.m.; Royal Westminster Ophthalmic, 1½ p.m.; West London, 3 p.m.

28. *Wednesday.*

Operations at University College, 2 p.m.; St. Mary's, 1¼ p.m.; Middlesex, 1 p.m.; London, 2 p.m.; St. Bartholomew's, 1½ p.m.; Great Northern, 2 p.m.; Samaritan, 2½ p.m.; King's College (by Mr. Lister), 2 p.m.; Royal London Ophthalmic, 11 a.m.; Royal Westminster Ophthalmic, 1½ p.m.; St. Thomas's, 1½ p.m.; St. Peter's Hospital for Stone, 2 p.m.; National Orthopædic, Great Portland-street, 10 a.m.

29. *Thursday.*

Operations at St. George's, 1 p.m.; Central London Ophthalmic, 1 p.m.; Royal Orthopædic, 2 p.m.; University College, 2 p.m.; Royal London Ophthalmic, 11 a.m.; Royal Westminster Ophthalmic, 1½ p.m.; Hospital for Diseases of the Throat, 2 p.m.; Hospital for Women, 2 p.m.; Charing-cross, 2 p.m.; London, 2 p.m.; North-West London, 2½ p.m.

30. *Friday.*

Operations at Central London Ophthalmic, 2 p.m.; Royal London Ophthalmic, 11 a.m.; South London Ophthalmic, 2 p.m.; Royal Westminster Ophthalmic, 1½ p.m.; St. George's (ophthalmic operations), 1¼ p.m.; Guy's, 1½ p.m.; St. Thomas's (ophthalmic operations), 2 p.m.

ORIGINAL LECTURES.

—◆—

ON ATAXIA AND THE PRE-ATAXIC STAGE OF LOCOMOTOR ATAXIA.

Delivered at the Hospital for Epilepsy and Paralysis, Regent's-park, March 28.

By THOMAS STRETCH DOWSE, M.D., F.R.C.P. Edin.

——

GENTLEMEN,—There can be no doubt, unless we have contrary proof of the most absolute and positive kind, that irregularity of movements and disturbances of volition, either in the creation of ideas or in the performance of coördinate muscular acts, are, in a very large majority of cases, due essentially to some syphilitic affection of the nervous centres, either hereditary or acquired. With this fact the physician is becoming every day of his life more familiar, and it is a misfortune of the most serious nature to the patient when these symptoms and signs of incoördination of movement are treated as mere trifles, and thought to be due merely to fatigue, or to stomach or liver derangement. I have no hesitation in saying that every case of locomotor ataxia is curable, provided it be treated sufficiently early and in the most energetic manner. This observation, which is of great import, will cause physicians both of the past as well as of the present day to shake their heads and reject a statement which hitherto has been considered untenable. So persistently has it been held that locomotor ataxia is an incurable disease that we can scarcely refer to a text-book on medicine(a) where we do not find this to be stated without any qualification. I hope that I shall, in the following pages, prove that this doctrine is erroneous, and that the conclusions upon which it is based are false, illogical, and unworthy of the present advanced stage of scientific medical research.

The disease which we know by the name of locomotor ataxia, and which we shall again refer to, is not of rapid progress until it arrives at a more advanced stage, and many cases of inveterate and incurable ataxy have come under my observation during the past three years which have existed in the pre-ataxic or curable stage for ten, fifteen, and even more than twenty years. Every case of locomotor ataxy (with very few exceptions) can be traced to a syphilitic origin, if due care be taken to inquire fully into the patient's history.

It is surprising to note for how long a time some men will suffer from attacks of unsteadiness of gait, incoördination of movement, abnormal sensations, and acute flying pains, before they think in any way seriously of the grave nature of the disease with which they are afflicted; and then, alas! when too late for any remedies to be of absolute avail, they seek advice on all sides in the most impatient and irresolute manner, deploring the helplessness of doctors to do them any good. This is unquestionably a most distressing state of things for the patient, who looks to the physician as one skilled in the art of healing, and in whose powers of discrimination and judgment in scientific detail he not only hopes, but expects, to find some remedy for his afflictions; and it is a blot upon our skill in diagnosis, no less than upon our skill in treatment, that so many cases of nervous disease are permitted to run an unchecked course, and are not unfrequently relegated to diseases caused by mere derangement of function on the part of the liver or on the part of the digestive apparatus. It is true that physicians, either from want of skill or from a too superficial examination of the patient, do frequently permit an incipient locomotor ataxy to pass from a curable to an incurable stage before taking active measures to prevent such a condition ensuing. I have had many patients to consult me for flying (so-called rheumatic) pains about the body, associated with want of sleep,

and stomach and liver derangements, who were quite ignorant that they were suffering from locomotor ataxy, and the fact that they were walking with their legs wide apart, and wearing down the heels of their boots in a manner which they had not done before, and with their eyes watching the movements of their feet, was, in their opinion, more a habit than a sign of commencing and serious mischief of the spinal cord.

In all diseases of the nervous system it is especially necessary that a careful and early diagnosis should be made, and if this were done we should see far less of the many incurable cases which are constantly presenting themselves to our notice. In this article I shall confine my remarks more particularly to ataxy of the lower limbs, and give my experience in reference to its curative treatment and its differential diagnosis in reference to some other diseases of the brain and nervous system. A physician accustomed to the treatment of the varying forms of nervous disease has generally, comparatively speaking, very little difficulty in arriving at a correct and approximate estimate of the seriousness or otherwise of the symptoms and signs which are presented by his patient, although it may be a matter of grave doubt in some cases as to the extent, nature, and position of the lesion in the brain and spinal cord, which may be the cause of those signs and symptoms. It is far too common a practice, even amongst professional men, to treat with indifference many of the incipient signs of the most serious and grave degenerations of the brain and spinal cord, and to transfer such cases to the class of " nervousness," " mimicry," and " hysteria." The man of experience is invariably more careful in making a diagnosis and in giving a prognosis concerning any lesion of the nervous system than is the man whose knowledge of such cases is less profound and of a more superficial nature. I am compelled to admit that I have in several important instances seen cases of unquestionable organic disease of the brain which were merely looked upon as due to exhaustion or functional derangement, and which required, so it was thought, only time and change of air to effect their cure. Now this, in my opinion, and even in my practice, has demonstrated to me the existence of errors of judgment in diagnosis which most certainly ought not to have had the shadow of an existence, and much less the reality of one. To believe that a patient is feigning disease because the medical man fails at once to recognise its true nature, and is unable to trace it to its origin, shows an ignorance and even culpability which is deserving of the most severe censure and reprobation. Yet so little do we know even now of the nervous system, and the marvellous power which it possesses in controlling our every thought, word, and deed, that we ought to be more careful—and, in fact, we cannot be too careful—in bringing together and training our ideas to unravel the as yet inexplicable network of fallacies which at present entangle this field for laborious study. I am quite willing to admit, however, that the diagnosis of a tumour of the brain or a tumour of the spinal cord, let it be syphilitic or otherwise, is in its early stage not unfrequently a question of great difficulty, and so also is the diagnosis of many of those slight and chronic inflammatory changes which give rise to what we now term a sclerosis, and which lead to many protracted and incurable forms of paralysis. In making the diagnosis of a progressive locomotor ataxia in that stage when our remedies shall be found of avail to bring about a cure, we have certain points presented to us for our consideration which serve as landmarks to guide us to a satisfactory issue, but these vary so greatly that it is almost an impossibility to lay down any hard and fast laws for our guidance with that degree of certainty which is at all times so desirable for teaching purposes.

Dr. Seguin, of New York, has given to the profession a clinical lecture on locomotor ataxy, which, in my opinion, is a very valuable contribution to the literature of this subject,(b) and I shall take the liberty of copying his classification, because in almost every particular I can quite endorse the soundness of his doctrine and the truth of his assertions.

For the sake of clearness and definition we divide the course of locomotor ataxy into three stages; and, as Dr. Seguin points out, "The first stage of the disease may well be designated the stage of fulgurating pains, and in

(a) Sir Thomas Watson says ("Lectures on the Principles and Practice of Physic," vol. i., page 700): "The treatment of this disorder must in the main be that which is indicated in all disorders that are incurable."

(b) A series of American clinical lectures edited by E. C. Seguin, M.D. "The Diagnosis of Progressive Locomotor Ataxia," 1873.

association with these pains we find the following signs and symptoms :—

Localised hyperæsthesia.
Diplopia from strabismus.
Ptosis from palsy of third nerve.
Small pupils.
Unequal pupils.
Numbness and slight anæsthesia of feet.
Sexual excitement.
Seminal emission.

Paresis of the bladder.
Diminished tendon reflex.
Impaired sight from atrophy of optic nerves.
Slight joint affections.
Localised anæsthesia.
Absence of paralysis or ataxia in the limbs.
General health excellent.

"The beginning of the second stage is characterised by the ataxic movements, and may be called the ataxic stage. The chief symptoms are, in order of importance :—

Ataxic movements.
Fulgurating pains.
Localised hyperæsthesia.
Ocular paralyses.
Numbness and other dysæsthesia.
Anæsthesia.
Staggering with closed eyes.
Failure of sexual power.
Absence of tendon reflex.
Rectal and vesical pareses.
Gastric crises.

Laryngeal crises.
Vesical crises.
Severe arthropathies.
Amaurosis.
Complicating common transverse myelitis.
Spinal congestion.
Paralytic dementia.
Vesical catarrh.
Preservation of mere muscular force.

"The third stage may be said to begin when the anæsthesia and ataxia are so great as to render the patient perfectly unable to stand or to use his legs. This might aptly be called the pseudo-paralytic stage. In this terminal period we may have either of the following symptoms in various groupings, or even all of them :—|

Fulgurating pains.
Ataxic movements.
Absolute anæsthesia.
Loss of sexual power.
Rectal and vesical pareses.
Paralysis of ocular muscles.
Amaurosis.
Deafness.

Various crises.
Severe arthropathies.
Disorganisation of large joints without pain.
Seeming paralysis of the extremities from anæsthesia. (and loss of muscular sense).
Dementia."

I think this classification of so much usefulness that I have not hesitated to adopt it here, because I feel sure that it is as perfect as such a differential classification can be, and it would be impossible to classify the signs and symptoms of this disease from a limited number of cases with anything approaching accuracy of detail ; also I have no doubt there are many observers who would disagree with the main order of frequency and relationship of many of the symptoms and signs which are here laid down. Of course, in going over these lists, one would have really little or no difficulty in bringing forward individual cases which would upset these methodised results of Dr. Seguin's careful and observant industry, but this would by no means invalidate the general conclusions.

Now, in progressive locomotor ataxia, or tabes dorsalis, we have a sclerosed condition of the posterior root-zones of the spinal cord, and I quite agree with Dr. Hammond(c) that the terms just mentioned to designate this disease are inappropriate—quite as much so, in fact, as calling a disease after the name of the man who first chronicled it. The term ataxy (from a priv., and τακτὸς, ordered) means a want of order, disturbance, irregularity ; but irregularity in locomotion is due to disease of the brain or cerebellum, as well as to disease of the spinal cord, so that we have to consider the especial kind of muscular incoördination which is peculiarly pathognomonic of the disease we are considering. It will be found that the legs in walking are invariably kept extended, the forepart of the foot is thrown well forward into the air, and the heel is brought down to the ground with a thud, so that the foot comes into contact with the ground by two distinct movements, and the more the patient tries to co-ordinate his movements, the less co-ordinate they become. A patient that I now have under my care, who suffers from the first stage of syphilitic ataxy, can walk with comparative comfort upon a thick Turkey carpet, but when he tries to walk upon a tiled floor his movements are so inco-

(c) "Diseases of the Nervous System," New York, 1876.

ordinate that he runs the risk of turning over, and he has to balance himself with his arms to keep himself from falling, and when the eyes are closed or when he attempts to walk in the dark he fails utterly to do so, in the most signal manner. Again, when a patient with syphilitic ataxy is in the recumbent posture, with the eyes closed, he is still unable to co-ordinate the movements of the legs, just in the same way as he is when trying to walk ; if, for instance, he is told to place one leg over the other, the leg is usually raised high in the air with an oscillating action, and falls with considerable force and without due co-ordinating power. It is by this means that we can readily distinguish an ataxy of this kind from an ataxy due to disease of the cerebellum, where the movements of the lower limbs are quite co-ordinate when the patient is lying down.(d)

It is an interesting question to consider what relationship exists between the electric-like pains and the ataxic gait in reference to precedence of origin (but this part of the question we shall enter into more fully when considering the signs and symptoms of the pre-ataxic stage of locomotor ataxy), and also whether these subjective and objective signs can in any way, according to their relationship, lead us to the conclusion that the disease is of a syphilitic nature. I am greatly inclined to believe that if we follow up our researches in this direction we shall arrive at a satisfactory result ; and although I feel sure that nearly every case of locomotor ataxy is due to syphilis, either hereditary or acquired—so much so, in fact, that it may well be called syphilitic ataxy,—still I can scarcely see that we are justified in maintaining that a locomotor ataxy is syphilitic because there is some indistinct history of the existence of a sore of many years before the ataxy made its appearance. If my own experience serves me, I should say that a prolonged first stage in locomotor ataxy is rather against, than in favour of, its being of syphilitic origin, and I base my statement upon comparative, rather than upon direct, evidence ; and for this reason, that out of twenty-three cases of this disease which I have recorded, seven have existed almost stationary in the first stage with ataxy for a series of years varying from eight to fourteen, whereas in the remaining sixteen cases, where there has been a clear history of syphilis, the troubles of the second stage, and even of the third stage, with ocular paralysis and vesical and gastric crises, have come on in from two to five years. I am not, as a rule, at all ready to admit that because a disease yields to anti-syphilitic remedies it should on this account be considered absolute that such disease was of a syphilitic character ; but in reference to disease of the posterior columns of the cord, I am bound to make the statement that whenever this condition does yield to mercury or to iodide of potassium, it is as sure a test as we can possibly have that it must have been of a syphilitic nature. With regard to the pains of locomotor ataxia, they are, I venture to think, of so peculiar and special a kind, that it would be impossible for them to be confounded with the pains of rheumatism, or with the pains of neuralgia. They certainly simulate a trifacial neuralgia with regard to their intensity, but they very rarely, if ever, take the course of a nerve, so that it would be impossible to map them out in the same manner that one frequently does a neuralgia, which invariably follows the course and distribution of the nerve affected. These pains are extremely sudden in developing themselves ; for instance, a patient of mine will complain sometimes of a peculiar feeling at the back of the thigh, which will continue perhaps for an hour or more, when he cries out, " Here it comes !" and in a second, like a lightning-shock, he is convulsed in agony. Sometimes these pains are stabbing, cutting, and tearing, whilst at other times they are burning and gnawing in their character ; and what I think makes them still more peculiar, is the way in which they sometimes yield to the most simple remedies, whilst they resist anything like heroic treatment.

A gentleman who consulted me not long ago, told me that at times the pains disappeared upon the application of aromatic spirit of ammonia to the part ; but in very severe attacks, neither morphia injections nor the internal admi-

(d) Ataxy of locomotion is made manifest by a feeling of weakness whilst standing upright and in walking, which is associated at the same time with the troubles of motor co-ordination and equilibration, and which contrasts with the integrity of healthy individual movements ; by loss of sensibility, varying in different degrees, of the skin and parts beneath it —that is to say, of the muscles, nerves, osseous and articular surfaces; by functional troubles of the genital organs (impotence or satyriasis) ; and, difficult micturition or defæcation.

nistration of chloral helped to mitigate the pain. I am quite convinced that chloral is of little use in relieving the severe pains of locomotor ataxia, and unfortunately it seems to lose its power under these conditions to induce sleep even in large doses. One of my patients suffering from locomotor ataxia, who had never previously taken chloral, thought that during one of his attacks of pain he would give it a trial, and in the course of four hours he took upwards of two drachms of this drug without any relief from the pain, and without even a tendency to sleep having been induced.

The use of morphia, on the other hand, has certainly many advantages, and if its internal use is not promptly followed by relief, I blister the skin rapidly with a strong ammoniated solution of cantharides, and apply to the blistered surface two grains of morphia rubbed up with vaseline. These pains are so vagrant, and present such an infinite variety of symptoms, that it would be almost impossible to describe them accurately. A gentleman who was a patient of mine, and of the highest intelligence, said that he utterly failed when he tried to give a succinct account of the horrible pains from which he suffered.

In the case of another gentleman, who consulted me some few months ago, I found a specific for the relief of his pains in the injection of half a grain of morphia sent well down to the sciatic nerve at the hip; and following this, I thoroughly anæsthetised him by causing him to inhale the bichloride of methylene. He usually slept after this for two hours, and he then awoke quite free from pain.

I have never seen severe measures of much use in the relief of these pains. I shall not readily forget the condition of the limb of a patient whom I was called hurriedly to see; he had rubbed the leg so vigorously with a strong hair-brush, that it was literally raw, without any good effect having been produced. The application of extreme heat and extreme cold has in some of my cases produced a relief from the pain when other remedies have failed. Within the past six months the following plan has been adopted, both upon the Continent and likewise in this country, but with very partial success, for the removal of these distressing pains. The plan has been to make a free incision right down upon the sciatic nerve, and to raise the nerve from its bearings with the surrounding parts so as to stretch it to the extent of some inches. I cannot recommend this mode of procedure, for in those cases where I have known this operation to have been performed, very little if any permanent good has been the result.

We sometimes find that when the first stage of an ataxy is prolonged the pains will leave the patient for years, and then return again in the most unaccountable manner; and again, I have found that in some old-standing cases of ataxy the patients never suffer from pain otherwise than during an electrical state of the atmosphere. It is an important fact, and one which ought not to be forgotten, that in nearly every case of locomotor ataxia the ataxic gait is preceded by these fulgurant pains; and I would here draw a marked distinction between those severe pains of a deep-seated character which are associated with the ataxic gait, and those slighter pains which are so evanescent and resemble a sharp needle or lancet thrust into the skin, and which do not infrequently resemble a neuralgia in their nature, and may exist for years before any ataxy becomes evident by objective signs; and, so far as I have seen from the writings and experience of others concerning this disease, this symptom has not been sufficiently thought of, and I would maintain, in contradiction to many observers (and Dr. Seguin amongst the number), that the pre-ataxic stage of a true locomotor ataxia can be diagnosed, and, if diagnosed, the advance of a "fasciculated sclerosis" of the posterior nerve-roots can be stopped, and an incurable locomotor ataxia prevented. I am as sure of this as I am of anything in medicine; and the following signs and symptoms are, in my practice and experience, diagnostic of what I now call the pre-ataxic stage of a locomotor ataxia:—

Pre-ataxic Signs of Locomotor Ataxy.

Inequality of pupils.	Variable patella tendon reflex, rarely absent.
Small pupils.	Spinal irritability.
Paresis of left third nerve.	Dyssesthesia. ⎫
Cutaneous fulgurating pains.	Anæsthesia. ⎬ Very
Sexual excitement.	Hyperæsthesia. ⎭ transitory.
Transitory incoördination of lower limbs.	Visual colour-changes.

Gastric and intestinal crises.	Mental depression.
Temperament variable.	Insomnia.
Retinal changes.	

I believe that I am quite right in making the statement that within the past few years our ideas concerning the signs and symptoms of a locomotor ataxy have undergone a very material change. It is not so long ago that physicians were disinclined to recognise any form of disease as locomotor ataxy provided there were no ataxic movements; but now a sclerosal atrophy of the optic disc, if associated with lightning pains and an absence of knee reflex, would be quite sufficient to lead most men to the conclusion that a sclerosal change was going on in the sensory side of the nervous system, and that incoördination of movement would invariably follow. I am now going to describe, seriatim and very briefly, the symptoms and signs of what I venture to think I am the first to note as the pre-ataxic symptoms proper of locomotor ataxy; and when I say that I am firmly persuaded that if these signs and symptoms be fairly diagnosed and properly treated, an incurable disease can be prevented, then I repeat that I think our knowledge will prove a great boon to many unfortunate sufferers. I am not at all clear in my own mind—and the conclusions arrived at by the investigations of numerous continental and home authorities appear to be not more explicit than my own—upon one point, which is this, namely:—Of all the pre-ataxic signs of locomotor ataxy, can we place most reliance upon those which affect the eye, or upon those which affect the skin? I have seen many cases during the past few years where the eyes have been affected, and there have been as well the lightning-like pains of the skin and muscles for over twenty years before there were any of the objective difficulties associated with incoördinate movements either of the speech or the upper or the lower limbs; and, speaking more particularly from my own experience, which has been considerable, I must say that, of the two most important signs of locomotor ataxy—namely, what we call the eye symptoms and the electric-like pains—I am fully inclined to believe that no case of locomotor ataxy ever existed which was not preceded by these pains, and, moreover, that these pains were the first subjective phenomena which bore upon them the initial stamp of what would inevitably follow in months, or perhaps years, and many years, to come.

Character of Pains.—Now, these pre-ataxic pains differ very greatly from the particular and special pains of a confirmed locomotor ataxy, which are commonly spoken of as fulgurant or electric-like pains. In the first place, although they come on suddenly and disappear suddenly, they are much less intense and of much shorter duration, and they vary greatly in character and intensity. This variability in character and intensity would confound one very much concerning their real nature were it not for the fact that they vary in their periodicity which is so common a condition in neuralgia and migraine. Yet, although it is not a difficult matter to diagnose a purely neuralgic pain, even when associated with locomotor ataxy, from those pains which may be considered as intimately bound up with the symptoms of locomotor ataxy, still it is much more difficult—and in our present state of knowledge I have no hesitation in saying that it is almost impossible—to diagnose pre-ataxic pains from other pains which are essentially neuralgic, unless we exercise great care and judgment, and endeavour, if possible, to find out some other initiatory and associated sign; and this is the more difficult for the reason that the pre-ataxic stage of locomotor ataxy is invariably associated with spinal irritability, and well-marked tender spinal spots can be readily elicited, which appear to be more or less connected with the pains by nervous contiguity and influence. These pains, however, have this special peculiarity, and in this respect they certainly resemble their congeners in well-marked locomotor ataxy, and that is (a point, by the way, which I have previously referred to), that they are electric-like in their arrival and departure, and almost of momentary duration. They may affect, like neuralgia and migraine, the head, eyes, face, ears, jaws, and neck; and this is due, as Mons. Pierret(a) has pointed out, to the sensory divisions of the roots of the fifth and occipital nerves becoming implicated by a commencing degenerative change in the medulla oblongata and upper

(a) "Essai sur les Symptomes Céphaliques du Tabes Dorsalis," par le Dr. A. Pierret. 1876.

cervical posterior root-zone. And they may also affect the chest, the abdomen, the genital organs, the rectum, the anus, and the lower limbs—the inner side of the calf, the inner and back of the thigh, and the outer side of the foot.

A man twenty-three years of age consulted me at the North London Hospital for Consumption, for a hard, dry cough; but what he mostly complained of, and what seemed to give him very serious anxiety, was the onset of pains of the most violent and sudden character which invaded principally his chest, but would sometimes attack the heart, the head, and even the lower limbs. I treated them in the first instance as neuralgic, but upon his second visit I found that there were an imperfect knee reflex and fairly well-marked pupillary symptoms, and, in fact, other signs indicative of a commencing ataxy. I discontinued treating him for his chest, and blistered his spine freely, and gave him large doses of bromide of potassium and ergot, and he rapidly improved.

All writers on locomotor ataxy appear to be agreed that it is ofttimes a very difficult matter to obtain a true statement from patients concerning the pains which we are now considering, and which, in fact, play so important a part in that phase of the disease which we have under our immediate observation. It is a most common thing to hear patients speak of these pains as "rheumatic" or "gouty." They say that they are very sharp while they last, but are soon over. Whenever a patient thus speaks of recurrent pains precisely similar in their action, do not let them pass without considering their exact nature with the most painful care and discrimination, and examine every spinal process with exactitude and precision. These abnormalities of sensation which we have hitherto been designating pain must now be considered rather in the light of a perversion of normal sensibility. For instance, we will first take the sensations of heat and cold. C. complains of feeling as though a hot iron were being applied to the left side over the eighth, ninth, and tenth ribs. S. will complain of a feeling at the back of the left thigh, as though a star had fallen upon it and radiated its heat to surrounding parts. D. complains of a feeling as though innumerable very fine needles were being driven into the skin of the calf of the leg, extending over a surface about the size of a crown-piece. E. will complain of a general shooting pain passing through the temples, as though a knife had been driven through. F. will complain of a creeping sensation over the left nostril, as though a number of ants were crawling over the skin. G. complains of a sense of coldness over the left shoulder, as though a lump of ice had been placed upon it. I. complains of the *left* foot becoming cold and numb, whilst the right foot is burning. B. complains of a feeling as though a rod of cold iron were being placed upon the inner part of the thigh; which, however, alternates in feeling, being sometimes cold and sometimes hot. E. will say that her back feels as though it were being scalded by boiling water; whilst R. will say that as though cold water were being poured down it. I. will complain (and this is not uncommon) that the teeth feel spongy, and as though they were made of india-rubber. P. complains of a feeling as though a tight band of variable roughness was being tied around the head. W. as though a sharp, fine knife were being driven into the peritoneum, or it may be into the rectum.

In this stage of the disease which we are now considering there is unquestionably an exaltation of sensation and sensibility. This, however, is not only extremely variable, but it may be of very short duration.

In reference to undue subjective sensibility on the physical side of the nervous system, it is demonstrated in many ways; as, for instance, a man in the pre-ataxic stage will not be able at times to sit cross-legged for more than a few minutes without experiencing a feeling of numbness (and pins and needles) and, it may be, a shooting pain running up the sciatic nerve at the back of the thigh; or if he catches his foot in walking, it jars upon the nerves, going up the leg in a manner which is quite unknown in the healthy state. Now the same condition is referable to the upper limbs. A patient of mine who suffers from initial ataxy is constantly experiencing these jarrings upon his nerves, and, although he is not an anatomist, he can map out the course of the larger nerves with the greatest accuracy, simply from the fact that he *feels his nerves*, as he very graphically expresses it.

In reference to undue sensibility on the psychical side of the nervous system in the pre-ataxic stage of locomotor ataxy, I think there can be no question of doubt, but it is often a very difficult matter to elicit this point. Men do not like to admit that they are fearful, impressionable, irascible, excitable, emotional, and so on; but the practised eye can readily detect an inward trepidation and instability, which the patient endeavours to mask by an assumed air of cool *nonchalance*, which is in truth nothing more or less than pure assumption.

I had a patient under my care a few months since who spoke of these pains as resembling the sting of a horse-fly. I have seen a patient in the greatest distress and discomfort from these pains, and they succeed each other with the greatest rapidity; they occur for the most part singly, and the patient has scarcely time to rub one part of the body before his attention is called to another part. Now, these pains may be preceded and succeeded by intense itching over a limited and circumscribed area, and this state of itching will be as rapidly migratory as were the pains just described. And if we test the sensibility of the skin of the feet and lower limbs we shall find patches which are decidedly anæsthetic; but this is more particularly marked over the plantar and dorsal surfaces of the feet and inner part of the legs. A patient of mine, who is now the subject of a confirmed ataxy, told me that the first symptom which in way alarmed him was that upon one occasion when mounting his horse he could not recognise that he had his foot in the stirrup.

There can be no question that the resistance of the cord to the reception of impressions is greatly increased in this stage—probably not enough, however, for the patient to recognise it until his attention is drawn to it; and I maintain that this increased power of resistance on the part of the cord is due in most cases to an actual congestion of its vascular supply; in fact, a vaso-motor paralysis which leads on to defective nutrition, and ultimately to degenerative change.

Thus the two symptoms which I have just described—namely, fulgurating cutaneous pains, and plantar and dorsal limited anæsthesia—are infallible signs of the pre-ataxic stage of a locomotor ataxia. If any of the other signs exist, the diagnosis is made more confirmatory; but when investigating the history of these cases (I mean of disease of the posterior columns of the cord), one frequently finds that patients will date the commencement of their illness from the time when they first became ataxic, and when they are asked concerning other subjective symptoms, such as pain, perversion of sensibility, attacks of indigestion, rapidly appearing and as suddenly disappearing sexual excitement, seminal emissions, and so on, they seem somewhat astonished that such apparent trifles and ordinary derangements of health should have ever been the important and diagnostic precursors of such a serious nervous infirmity as that from which they are suffering.

Eye Symptoms.—It is indeed highly probable, but the statement requires time and further observation for its complete verification, that special eye symptoms may exist in the initial stage of locomotor ataxy for twenty or twenty-five years. For the moment I pass over what may be actual changes in the retina, and consider those more delicate reflex processes which we find to exist in connexion with the pupil of the eye, and which have been referred to for some years by Echeverria, Voisin, Clymer, Argyll Robertson, Grainger Stewart, and others. Of all recent writers upon this subject, Professor Erbe has, I think, treated this question in the most philosophic and scientific manner, although very much remains to be done in this interesting field of observation. In the pre-ataxic stage of locomotor ataxy we often find extreme contraction of the pupil (spinal myosis), with inexcitability to light, and with preserved accommodative movements, which we also so frequently see in well-marked locomotor ataxy, general paralysis of the insane, lead-poisoning, and in other diseases of the nervous system due to syphilis. Yet, on the other hand, it may be set down as a well-ascertained fact that, although the pupil may not be, and frequently is not, contracted (for, on the contrary, it may be even abnormally dilated), it will also be found that there is an absence of reflex pupillary mobility to light; whilst, under accommodative impulses and convergence of the visual axes, they react with perfectly normal promptness. Erbs ("American Archives of Medicine," 1880) says that in 84 recent cases of tabes he found absolute reflex pupillary immobility to occur 59 times ; very weak, slow, and inexpansive action to light, 12 times : hence a total of 71 cases with diminished reaction, against 13 with normal reaction. *Out of the 71 cases, 43 belonged to the initial stage—that is, they exhibited no signs of ataxia, or only the slightest trace of it.* It is obvious, then, according to this most distinguished neurologist, that we have in this pupillary non-excitability a sign in reference to the pre-ataxic stage of locomotor ataxy which is not only remarkable, but of the utmost diagnostic importance. The absolute value of this sign may, if necessary, be further confirmed by the fact that this diminished pupillary reaction rarely ever exists in healthy individuals, but, as we have before stated, it does exist in persons suffering from various forms of nervous disease. Erb, in the article before alluded to, says that it does sometimes exist in persons not affected with tabes ; but that these patients will not develope tabes sooner or later, who will dare say ? In my own practice during many years I have given considerable attention to the so-called eye symptoms in the pre-ataxic stage of loco-motor ataxy, and I am perfectly convinced of their diagnostic value.

There is another point of importance for consideration, and it is this : In confirmed tabes we find almost invariably absence of reflex pupillary contraction, and not unfrequently an absence of reflex dilatation ; and there is this marked difference to be noted between the excitability of the pupil in the stage of pre-ataxy and in the stage of confirmed ataxy, namely, that in the pre-ataxic stage an ordinarily unexcit-able pupil can readily be excited by sympathetic or reflex irritation, both with and without the aid of electricity. For instance, if a patient in the pre-ataxic stage of locomotor ataxy (where the pupils do not contract to light in the ordinary way) is made to shut one eye, and if the lid of the closed eye be lubricated with the tip of the forefinger, exercising at the same time some amount of pressure, the pupil of the opposite eye will dilate to a degree which is really remarkable; and the same effect can be produced, but not in so marked a degree, when the faradaic brush is applied to the skin of the temples, or the mastoid process of the temporal bone, or the cervical plexuses of the sympathetic in the neck. Now, such an excitability of the pupil does not follow, under similar conditions, in a well-pronounced case of locomotor ataxy. I do not mean to say that such excitability of the pupil cannot be produced in myosis associated with lead-poisoning and general para-lysis, because I have long been acquainted with the fact that it can be, and I have frequently used this means to aid me in making a differential diagnosis. Nevertheless, in this sign, when considered with other signs, we have a most im-portant aid in diagnosis which ought not to be forgotten; neither must we fail to remember the great help which the ophthalmoscope affords us ; but I am inclined to think that in the pre-ataxic stage of locomotor ataxy the non-excitability of the pupil to light (by this I mean the sluggish pupil) is of far more value than the intraocular changes which may be met with by ophthalmoscopical examination. By way of example, I will refer to three cases of confirmed locomotor ataxy which are under my care at the present time, and two of these cases were sent to me by my friend, Mr. Mackinlay, to whom they applied for defective vision, and in whose eyes he found a rapidly ad-vancing grey sclerosis and atrophy; but, upon going into the history of these men, I found that they had been suffer-ing from the initial signs of locomotor ataxy for years before their vision became affected (this does not, I am well aware, negative the fact that a neuritis may exists, and yet vision of a kind remain unimpaired)—so long, in fact, that I feel sure that the other signs did exist prior to the changes in the optic disc. My friend, Dr. Williams, of Canonbury, brought a patient to consult me who had been under the care of one of our most eminent oculists, who said that he either was ataxic or would become so. There was complete scleroseal atrophy of one eye, with loss of vision ; but, as far as I can remember, there were no other signs of ataxy, and the man's condition was stationary, so that I am inclined to hold to the opinion just expressed, that we must look to the pupil of the eye rather than to the changes in the optic disc for a definite pre-ataxic sign; still, neither must be neglected. If we look at the physiological side of this question, I think we shall be more than ever con-

vinced that this opinion has some foundation in fact, even although Stilling of Strasburg has very recently endea-voured to prove that the optic nerve has a spinal or medullary root.(f) It is now generally admitted by ophthal-mic physiologists that certain nuclei exist in the floor of the aqueduct of Sylvius, which govern the muscles of the eyeball, the action of the pupil, and the accommodation of the eye; hence we find those objective signs through the medium of the pupil, which predicate with an almost un-erring accuracy changes in the sensory tracts of the brain and spinal cord.

Lastly, before leaving the eye symptoms, I would draw attention to the fact that inequality of the pupils is not infrequently an initial sign of locomotor ataxy. One pupil, for instance, will be widely dilated whilst the other is con-tracted, and neither pupil will react to light, but the con-tracted pupil will act under accommodation more readily than the pupil which is abnormally dilated.(g)

From examinations of the retinæ, made by myself and others, there has invariably been found a more or less degenerative change going on in the vessels and in the disc ; the former are more or less tortuous and blurred on the out-line, and the latter have a dull greyish appearance, but in many cases no changes in the disc are seen. Colour-blind-ness is a not uncommon accompaniment of ocular defects in the pre-ataxic stage. For instance, red and green are fre-quently said to be dirty yellow and brown, but blue and yellow are invariably perceived correctly. Other ocular troubles and palsy of ocular muscles are not uncommon in the pre-ataxic stage.

Patellar Tendon Reflex, "Knee Reflex," "Westphal's Symp-tom."—We now come to the consideration of a very valuable sign which is usually supposed to be a diagnostic of organic disease of the spinal cord, and, until I questioned the fact, it seems that no other observer took exception to what has generally been received by the profession as a rule to which no exception can be taken—I refer to the "knee reflex," or what is more commonly called the "patellar tendon re-flex." There is no one who knows the practical value of this sign more than myself, and it was a lucky hit of Westphal when he first found the absence of a knee reflex in disease of the spinal cord, and set to work to draw the valuable de-ductions with which we are now familiar. I admit that I am sceptical concerning too great value and importance being attached to this condition, and not only so, but also to the condition itself, and I have very good reasons in support of my statement.

In the summer of this year a gentleman from Australia was brought to consult me by my friend Mr. Brain, with many symptoms and signs of a locomotor ataxia in the pre-ataxic stage. After eliciting from him all the information I could, I tried the knee reflex in every way without any re-sponse attending my various tappings, and it certainly looked as though I had an incurable case to deal with. However, with my previous experience to guide me, I then passed the continuous current freely through the spinal cord, and the knee reflex, which before was entirely absent, now became evident in the most unmistakable and satisfactory manner. I have records of other cases, and shall refer to them again when speaking of treatment.

The question naturally arises as to what was the difference in the cord before the galvanism and after the galvanism, for it was perfectly clear to my mind that this gentleman was suffering from the pre-ataxic stage of locomotor ataxia, and that the posterior root-zones and column of the cord were in a state of inhibition or congestion, or at all events, to put it in less theoretical and less figurative language, there was some molecular condition of the cord which increased its power of resistance beyond the normal, and which was removed by the influence and stimulus of the galvanic current.

Erb has arrived at the conclusion that absence of knee reflex exists in about 95 per cent. of cases of locomotor

(f) *Lancet*, November 27, 1880.

(g) These eye phenomena have, according to Erb, the following phy-siological significance. He says:—" Between the retina and sphincter pupillæ innervated by the oculo-motorius, exists a reflex track which goes through the optic nerve to the brain, within the brain to the oculo-motorius, and in this centrifugally to the iris ; and in explanation of the reflex immobility we can only maintain that that portion of the reflex tract is affected which lies between the optic and oculo-motor centres. For the myosis we must refer to changes in the dilator pupillæ, whose centre is said to be in the medulla oblongata, and sends the principal part of its mass into the cervical cord, down to the cilio-spinal centre."

ataxia, and I am thoroughly convinced that Erb is quite right; yet I feel sure that functional absence of knee reflex will be found to exist in the pre-ataxic stage. But it must be remembered that it is by no means uncommon to find all the reflexes exaggerated in the pre-ataxic stage of locomotor ataxy as well as in the imitatory stages of the general paralysis of the insane, and I think that this may be accounted for by the possible probability that the changes in the posterior root-zones are extremely peripheral, and invade more or less the adjacent matter of the lateral columns, and so give rise to motor sensorial disturbances and to an exaggeration of automatic and other reflexes; and if future experience should prove the truth of my assertion, I think that there are few practitioners of medicine who will deny that such a condition, if it be found correct, must be an invaluable guide to a definite and curable course of treatment of a disease which is thought at the present time to be incurable. I have upon more than one occasion astonished my patient, who sought my advice on account of what he considered to be nervous dyspepsia, by tapping his knees and then proposing to him that he should have his spine dry-cupped and the actual cautery applied; and in cases of so-called nervous dyspepsia and biliousness with incoordinate movements, I must say that it is the special duty of the doctor to make sure whether the knee reflex is absent or not, and should it be absent, then to make sure whether it is due to a functional or organic arrest of the normal reflex tonus of the spinal cord; and under any circumstances, if the knee reflex is absent, to treat the assumed dyspeptic symptoms in a manner very different from what they would be treated provided the knee reflex were quite normal. I am very well aware that in ninety-nine cases out of one hundred of dyspepsia no approach even to a locomotor ataxia does exist, yet it does exist, nevertheless, in many cases where it is not even suspected; and every experienced observer must be aware that locomotor ataxy is frequently marked by functional troubles, with which, however, it may nevertheless be associated; and I repeat, with emphasis, that it is only in the initial stage of a chronic inflammatory change in the spinal cord, whether it be of the posterior root-zones and posterior columns, or whether it be of the anterior horns and anterior columns, that our treatment can be of any avail in the cure of this class of nervous disease; and after all is said and done, it avails our patient but little if we devote too much attention to the possible cause of certain phenomena, while we fail to recognise the exact moment when it is in the power of the physician to retard the onward progress of a disease which otherwise can have but a fatal termination. Above all things the physician has to be extremely careful that he does not relegate an initial locomotor ataxy to the class of nervous functional diseases which are known by the names of neurasthenia, "nervous debility," "nervous exhaustion," "hypochondriasis," and so on. Several such unfortunate cases have come under my notice during the past three months, and they have been in the hands of men who would never have failed in making the correct diagnosis if they had noted with care the pupillary phenomena which have been described.

In the month of last June I was consulted by a gentleman, about thirty-four years of age, for what he considered to be nervous depression associated with acute dyspepsia, and for this latter complaint he had sought the advice of many leading physicians, both at home and at the leading European spas, whose remedies, however, did him no good; his intellect became confused, and his legs and arms felt strange, and their movements were incoordinate; he suffered from seminal emissions and sexual excitement. The bowels acted very irregularly—sometimes he would suffer from attacks of diarrhœa, and at other times the bowels would be obstinately confined; but after an evacuation, the feeling of exhaustion was so extreme that for an hour or so he felt good for nothing, and at times he suffered great distress from the fulgurating cutaneous pains which were darting about his body. But what I want to demonstrate in this case is that the knee reflex was absolutely lost, but the continuous current applied to the spine and to the feet completely restored the reflex power of the cord, and he got quite well under the influence of bromide of potassium, solution of ergot, and bichloride of mercury. The spine was dry-cupped every third day for a month, and as no marked improvement became apparent, I applied the actual cautery to the extent of three inches every other day, first rendering the skin

insensible by means of ether spray. Now, it is an interesting and important fact that after the second application of the cautery, patellar tendon reflex was permanently regained.

In the latter part of July, S., a South American, consulted me concerning some obscure nervous symptoms from which he suffered, and which one physician attributed to nervous exhaustion, and another to anæmia of the spinal cord; normal patellar tendon reflex was greatly subdued, but rapidly renovated after the continuous current was applied to the spine. From the other symptoms I came to the conclusion that the posterior columns of the cord were congested, and that he was in the pre-ataxic stage of locomotor ataxy. I at first gave him strychnine with bichloride of mercury, but he suffered so much from sexual excitement and insomnia that the strychnine had to be discontinued. I then gave him bromide of potassium and solution of ergot, and his servant used to dry-cup the spine every day. He improved greatly under this treatment, but I lost sight of him, as he had to return home.

A gentleman, who was in the Indian Civil Service, consulted me in the fall of the year for what he considered to be neurasthenia. He was a man of excellent physique, fair and robust-looking, and of about thirty-three years of age. He contracted syphilis at the age of twenty-five. When he sat down in the chair he quietly remarked that he was all to pieces, but he certainly looked just the reverse of this, and after he had given me a somewhat extensive history of the errors of his youth, the first thing that I asked him was to cross his legs, and I must say that I was rather astonished to find a complete absence of tendon reflex. I then found out that he had suffered from neuralgias and from rheumatic pains (fulgurating pains). The pupils did not contract to light, but contracted fairly well during accommodation. There was a marked absence of the ataxic gait, but he reeled when standing erect with the eyes closed. I considered this to be a case of locomotor ataxy in the pre-ataxic stage, but no galvanic stimulation of the spine gave me any knee reflex. I told him what was my opinion of the case, and the remedies which I wished to be employed. He rather hesitated, and then remarked that as everything had hitherto failed to do him any good, he placed himself entirely in my hands. I produced slight ptyalism by mercurial inunction of the oleate of mercury, and applied the actual cautery to the spine (previously anæsthetised) every other day, and I was no less surprised than delighted to find in about ten days a most marked improvement. The reflex at the knees was returning, and the fulgurating pains had disappeared. The treatment, however, was persisted in for a month, and when discontinued ten grains of the iodide of potassium were taken three times a day. He recovered most completely.

Now, I need scarcely say that I have had many persons suffering from advanced forms of locomotor ataxia when all my remedies have been of no avail whatever, but I will never concede to the opinion expressed by many, and taught by most, that a locomotor ataxia is an incurable disease, for there is a stage of this disease, which I now call the pre-ataxic stage of a locomotor ataxia, when by prompt and energetic treatment we may safely hope for good and successful results.

LISTERISM AT MONTPELLIER.—In a clinical lecture delivered by Prof. Dubreuil at the St. Eloi Hospital, Montpellier, on a case of amputation (*Gaz. Méd.*, September 17), he observed: "Here we are working with bad surroundings, for we have to complain alike of the faulty construction of our wards, of the unsuitable manner in which they are kept, and of the defective services of the subaltern attendants, who are insufficiently looked after. So that, prior to the adoption of Lister's method, the results of our operations were detestable; but thanks be to God and to Lister, all this is now changed, and death after amputation has now become a rare exception, while formerly it was the rule. You observe that I rigorously follow out the precepts of the antiseptic method, for I really cannot understand that mania of some surgeons, who will persist in modifying the precepts of the master, even at the risk of compromising the results. As for me, I follow them out literally, and I declare to you that, in my eyes, the surgeon who at the present time does not adopt the antiseptic method commits an act of criminal folly and odious inhumanity."

ORIGINAL COMMUNICATIONS.

REMARKS ON CERTAIN ASSIGNED CAUSES OF FEVER.

By SURGEON-GENERAL C. A. GORDON,
M.D., C.B., Q.H.P., etc.

(Concluded from page 385.)

In 1879 an outbreak of typhoid fever in Bristol was traced to the circumstance that a mill-stream, the water of which was made use of by the affected, was rendered foul by fæcal percolation, and by the presence in the stream of "two hind quarters of a calf dead of 'quarter-ill'—a very contagious disease supposed to be identical with anthrax in man,—and besides these, the entrails of a bullock." On this subject the remark is made (*British Medical Journal*, May 22, 1880, page 792) that this water had been used for some time previously, and without like results. In reference to this and similar instances, the remark occurs that the oxidising effect upon animal decomposing matter produced by water is extensively acknowledged by authorities. The circumstance also is important that, in London, typhoid fever may be said not to exist, notwithstanding that the waters of the Thames are impregnated with fæcal matters coming into them above Teddington, and necessarily containing *specific* typhoid poison. This result, it is added, may arise from the oxidising power of running streams being greater than that of still waters, as of wells. Further, the remark has been made with regard to the outbreaks of typhoid during the same year at Caterham and Reigate, that contamination of water by fæcal matter, to which that outbreak was said to have been due, was but very slight indeed. Dr. Davis also acknowledges that his endeavours to trace the parentage of cases returned as fever have sometimes been baffled—that is, he has failed in all instances to detect a specific cause of a specific disease.

As examples of the very indefinite grounds upon which, in some instances, the occurrence of "enteric" or typhoid fever has been positively assigned to polluted water, the following extracts from statements on this subject are given, and their number might be extended were it considered desirable thus to lengthen them. It will, perhaps, be sufficient if we italicise the words to which these remarks more particularly refer. Thus, regarding Haverfordwest, "it is *stated* that upwards of a hundred cases have occurred, at least ten of which have already proved fatal. It is *believed* that the pollution of one of the reservoirs supplying the town with water—this reservoir being in close proximity to the cesspools of certain cottages—has been the cause of the outbreak." At Pontardawe, Glamorganshire, "the infection *seems* to have been mainly spread by the soaking into the water-sources of sewage from the privies into which the excreta were cast. . . . . One group of cases especially was traced to the use of water from a cistern which had *apparently* become infected by percolation from a cesspit, into which the excreta of a patient brought from Swansea had been thrown. The *suspected* cistern was closed on September 26; and after October 10 the outbreak ceased, so far as regards its especial *incidence* upon the houses supplied with water from this source." That is, because after a certain percentage of persons had been attacked by an epidemic disease, that epidemic itself ceased, the cause of this cessation was assigned to the fact of water from a particular well having been tainted, and to that only. At Rosewell, near Bonnyrigg, "an outbreak of typhoid fever visited *nearly every* house in the village, and proved fatal in several cases. The *water*-supply is *at present* blamed for it." That is, attention is concentrated upon one set of circumstances, rather than the general conditions under which disease occurs. On the other hand, Dr. Blyth says that to his knowledge water contaminated with the sewage of healthy persons has been drunk for a long period with impunity. Ample evidence that this is the case is furnished by what occurs in all the large cities and towns in China.

From the particulars thus given, the following conclusions are drawn, namely:—

1. That contaminated water produces diarrhœa and dysentery in those who make use of it, has been long acknowledged to be a fact.

2. The occurrence of intestinal worms has also been assigned to this cause.

3. That with the introduction of a pure water-supply certain epidemic diseases ceased to prevail.

4. That although instances are on record where persons have without evil result used water most offensively contaminated, others are also given in which communities thus making use of such water were never free from diarrhœa, scarlatina, and diphtheria.

5. That a specific fever, when prevailing as an epidemic, is capable of transmission by means of water, is reasonably established as a fact; but that contaminated water, will, of itself and by itself, give rise to specific fever, is not by any means confirmed or even rendered probable.

Food.—There are authors who believe that specific typhoid fever may be communicated by means of meat of affected animals, even when that meat has undergone the process of cooking. The following are illustrative examples of cases upon which this belief is based, namely:—

In July, 1879, at Andelfingen, in the canton of Zurich, 513 persons of all ages sat down to a cold collation of veal and ham, both of inferior quality. Of that number, 421 were subsequently seized with an acute febrile disease which was at the time looked upon as typhoid. Thirty-four other persons who had obtained meat from the same butcher were also attacked with similar symptoms; and subsequently, a further number of eleven out of fifteen who had also been supplied by the same butcher. These cases appear to have ushered in an epidemic of what was described as typhoid fever. The symptoms were those of severe gastro-intestinal irritation, with high fever, delirium, stupor, congestion of the lungs, and great prostration. No rose rash was observed, but in some cases there were petechiæ. The mortality was slight, but post-mortem examination in some cases disclosed infiltration and ulceration in "the lower part of the ileum." In others, however, "these changes were not observed." With reference to this epidemic, the significant remark occurs —"But great doubts have been expressed as to whether it was really typhoid fever, or a form of poisoning resembling sausage-poisoning."(a)

In 1845 a similar epidemic, but on a much smaller scale, occurred at Thalweil; in it "eight or ten persons were attacked with what was believed to be typhoid fever after eating bad veal."

In September, 1879, an outbreak of what was at the time considered to be enteric fever occurred on board the training-ship *Cornwall*; on that occasion forty cases took place, one of which was fatal. The cases were of various degrees of severity, but all presented the phenomena of enteric fever. They could not, however, be traced to any of the recognised causes of that disease, although Mr. Power was able to his own satisfaction to assign the disease to the use by the boys of trichinised pork; from which circumstance the prevailing affection, although in all respects similar in its phenomena to *enteric* fever, "might not have been that disease at all, but *trichinosis.*"

From these particulars the conclusion seems fair that it was questioned if the disease which arose in the instances related was really specific enteric fever, notwithstanding that its phenomena were similar to those of that disease. In the work on "Hygiene and Surgery of the Franco-Prussian War," page 225, several examples are given in which the meat of diseased cattle, both when handled in the raw state and when eaten cooked, failed to produce illness; and it is even stated that "past experience has demonstrated that the flesh of animals suffering from typhus is most unfit for food." It therefore seems to follow that this part of our subject requires further consideration. In India, tainted meat (particularly pork), fish, and shell-fish induce cholera, but cases of fever from them are unrecorded. In that country, as in others, there are people who habitually eat the flesh of animals dead by various kinds of disease, and who themselves continue to enjoy good health. Therefore the fact of a specific form of fever being thus produced has yet to be established.

The most illustrative case was described by Dr. Huguenin, of Zurich. It occurred in 1878. The food consisted of a ragout of veal, roast veal, and veal sausages. Nothing was observed with the ragout, but the cold roast veal was in part decomposed, and the sausages were manifestly bad

(a) Dr. Cayley, *British Medical Journal*, March 20, 1880, page 430.

Out of 690 persons who sat down to the collation, 290 were attacked, and all 668 persons who were infected who had partaken of the meat, besides 49 who were secondarily affected by contagion(?) without having eaten of the meat. In this instance the meat was considered to have had two injurious qualities :—(1) It was putrid ; (2) it was affected with specific typhoid poison.

Milk.—The first occasion in which the occurrence of enteric or typhoid fever as a specific disease was considered to have been connected with milk happened in 1853. In that year the *Devonport Independent* contained a record of an outbreak of that disease at Stoke as having been traced to this source. In 1871 an epidemic of the same nature at Islington was similarly traced to contaminated milk by Dr. Ballard. In 1878 Dr. Davis reported an illustrative occurrence at Bristol. Many other instances of the same kind have been more or less fully detailed in the pages of medical journals and in special reports of individual outbreaks.

It is believed, however, that, in some instances at least, the actual results to be drawn from investigations, records of which have appeared, are not of a nature to support the theory in accordance with which those investigations were undertaken and conducted ; in fact, that in addition to, and altogether beyond, contaminated milk, the operation of some other cause or set of causes has been required in order to give rise to the specific form above named, even as it occurs in England ; also, that if that form of fever really be so propagated, certain others are so also.

For the sake of more readily indicating the value attached to certain expressions in the following remarks they are italicised, as were some already given in this article.

At page 475 of the *British Medical Journal*, dated September 20, 1879, there occurs a report on what is called *milk* typhoid at Chichester, from which the following extracts are made :—As regards drainage, the city is in the same state that it was in 1865 ; it is full of wells and full of cesspools ; filth from the cesspools percolates into the wells, and much of the *water* is unusable. The rate of mortality is 20·7 per 1000. In February, March, and April, fifty persons were attacked (six fatally) in thirty houses. Many of the cases of the fever were of an uncertain type ; there was considerable *difference of opinion* as to *the real nature* of the disease ; there were some cases of undoubted *scarlatina*, some that were certainly enteric ; not a few of a *mixed* character, having at first the characters of scarlatina, subsequently putting on a *typhoid* appearance ; many had an *abortive* appearance, starting suddenly with high temperature and rapid pulse, as if to be severe, then subsiding in five or six days : this variety was known as *Chichester fever.* The cases personally examined by the Inspector *appeared* to be of a *typhoid* character, though *by no means* well marked ; only a few had any spots, and in those the spots were hardly more than points ; diarrhœa was not constantly present ; no instance of hæmorrhage from the bowels could be heard of ; the persons attacked were for the most part in *delicate health* previously.

Of fifty-nine families supplied from a particular dairy, twenty-six, or 43 per cent., had in the course of the epidemic *more or less* distinct cases of typhoid, whilst forty families in the same locality supplied by other dairymen had *complete immunity* from the disease. As to the method, however, in which the milk became affected the inspector is *much less clear.* He *believes* the cause to be that the *udders* and *teats* of the cows are washed with water obtained from the Lavant, a small exposed stream in the adjoining meadows. Surely here is an example of seeking for a particular cause of a disease, the exact nature of which is matter of question, to the relative neglect of general causes of an evidently inconstant kind.

With reference to the above report several points present themselves, namely :—1. The conditions related had not changed from 1865 ; during the interim no outbreak of typhoid is recorded as having occurred. 2. Many of the cases of fever are described as of a *somewhat uncertain type,* nor do the grounds appear on which, being so, they were decla'ed to be *typhoid*, or in what sense the term was applied. 3. Some were cases of *undoubted scarlatina*; then why enumerate them otherwise? 4. Some were of a *mixed* character, at first resembling scarlatina, afterwards putting on a *typhoid appearance.* Where did scarlatina end and typhoid begin ; or was the *typhoid appearance* a condition

of scarlatina, and how far were such cases *specific* in their nature? 5. Among diagnostics, spots and diarrhœa were by no means constantly present, and no case of intestinal hæmorrhage was noticed. Thus in the absence of diagnostics it is not stated on what grounds *diagnosis* was made. 6. As all the cases occurred in persons of delicate health, nothing is stated against these being themselves of adynamic type, such as usually occur in such persons. 7. The cause of attack is said to have been polluted milk ; but as to the precise manner in which the pollution occurred or acted, we have nothing more definite than that the inspector's "suggestion is certainly an ingenious one"—no facts are related in support of it.

Dr. Airy, who inquired into the occurrence of the above outbreak, observed that the quantity of infected water introduced into the milk must have been very small, but that no other source of infection was discovered. He further admits that the evidence against the milk was *very questionable*, but observes that the outbreak could not be explained on the hypothesis that, as a whole, it was due to sewer-gas *or any other cause than infected milk.* In other words, this investigation was directed to the discovery of specific and pythogenic causation of an epidemic fever, and to them only.

From a large number of instances illustrating the kind of evidence on which is based the conclusion that specific typhoid fever is due alone to infected milk, the following are selected :—It is stated that at Southport an outbreak of this disease was due to infected milk ; that the milk was brought from a rural district ; that thirty-two cases of the disease in all occurred ; that immediately it was discovered the disease was becoming prevalent in the town, the cause was sought for, and it was soon found to originate from some infected *milk-farms* several miles away. The sale of this milk was stopped, and the disease fully stamped out. Thus an epidemic having ceased after having attacked thirty-two persons, and its cessation contemporaneous with the interdiction of a particular milk-supply, therefore the prevalence of that epidemic was the result of contamination of that milk. Surely the circumstances as related are insufficient to bear out that conclusion.

Regarding the occurrence of "milk typhoid" at Southport, the following particulars appear, namely :—Twenty-eight cases of that affection were reported as having occurred in that town. The houses *invaded*, and their surroundings, were subjected to careful examination ; but in only *two* cases were any *sanitary defects* discovered, and these were exceedingly slight, and altogether *insufficient* to account for the outbreak. Every case, however, had been served with *milk* from a particular dairy some miles out of the borough ; and inquiry by the Southport officials revealed a well on the dairy premises *greatly polluted* by privy soakage. Chemical analysis of the water showed that, in the words of the chairman, it was "nothing but liquid sewage, and *calculated* to spread disease wherever its influence extended." When the milk-supply was stopped, the epidemic ceased at once ; but, unfortunately, not before two deaths—one of a young man twenty-one years old, and the other of a young woman aged twenty-two—had occurred. With reference to this and other similar outbreaks at the same place, it is added, in the abstract from which we quote, that "these oft-recurring epidemics, *caused* by infected milk, cannot be regarded with equanimity. In the Southport, as in the Paddington, Glasgow, and innumerable other outbreaks, the *poison* of the disease has been brought from a rural district outside the jurisdiction of the local authority who have control of the outbreak when it occurs." But, as a matter of fact, nothing appears in the record as it stands of a nature to identify the outbreak of the fever related with the particular milk-supply indicated. It is true that a well on the dairy premises is said to have been polluted with liquid sewage, but there the evidence ends.

Of a recent outbreak of fever at Bridlington we read thus : "Considerable anxiety and alarm have been occasioned at Bridlington, a seaside resort in Yorkshire, by the recent prevalence of typhoid fever in the district, and once more the outbreak *appears* to be due to the neglect of sanitary precautions in a private dairy. During the month ended October 22, 1880, no fewer than eight deaths occurred there from this disease, and in the previous month a fatal case was also recorded. *Suspicion* having rested upon a particular milk-supply, it was found, on examination, that the water used in the operations of the implicated dairy was drawn from a well *eighteen* feet deep, sunk through a *gravelly* soil in a low-lying, and in wet weather swampy, under-drained field, where a downward percolation would readily take place. In the lane where the dairy is situated, the sewage of several houses flows into an open ditch at the bottom of the adjacent gardens, which ditch is full of stagnant dirty water and mud. At one of these houses there was *recently* a case of enteric fever : an occurrence which, taken in connexion with the subsequent outbreak, raises *the suspicion* that the poison from this case *somehow* got into the water used at the dairy. The eighty-three households supplied by the particular dealer were visited, with the result of finding that, *exclusive of seven doubtful cases*, forty-eight persons in those households were suffering from undoubted enteric fever. This large incidence of the disease upon the *dairy-customers* must be held to point *very* strongly to *milk* as the cause of the outbreak ; and this is the view adopted by the medical officer of health. *It is true* that there have *been* ' *other cases* of fever' (the number is not stated) where the particular milk *was not supplied* ; but this hardly affects the main argument. From the descriptions given of it, Bridlington *seems* to be a *likely* place for epidemics of typhoid fever, from *whatever cause arising*, to occur. The health officer tells his authority that ' *other influences* have doubtless *contributed* to produce this epidemic, and, as such, I have repeatedly invoked your interposition respecting drainage, neglected ashpits and cesspools, and kindred elements for the propagation of disease.' "

Here, then, we find in the first instance the statement made that *suspicion* rested upon a particular milk-supply. Then the circumstance is assumed that *somehow* the (assumed) *poison* got into the water used in the dairy ; that *doubtful* cases occurred ; that there have been other cases where the particular milk was not supplied ; also that other influences have doubtless contributed to produce this epidemic. All this being the case, surely the grounds produced are of themselves insufficient to justify the conclusion arrived at, that the epidemic in question was due to contaminated milk, and to it alone ?

One other case need be adverted to, namely, that of Rochdale. In a brief allusion to the outbreak of *typhoid* fever at that place, " it is stated that the typhoid fever epidemic in Rochdale is increasing, the milk-supply having in all cases been *the same*. An examination has been made, and in a small cottage on the farm was found a family of nine persons, with two lodgers, suffering from severe typhoid fever. All kinds of *refuse* had been thrown upon the ground, and the water which the cattle drank had thus become poisoned." Subsequently this outbreak came under the cognisance of the county coroner, and of the results of his investigation we read as follows in an evening paper at the time, namely : " The coroner's inquiry into the causes of the typhoid fever epidemic at Rochdale was resumed yesterday. Eleven deaths from fever and fifty two cases of infection are reported to have occurred in the borough during the past two months, and in a considerable number of these cases it was shown that the milk taken by the deceased had been supplied from a particular farm. The jury were of opinion that the evidence adduced was not sufficient to prove from what particular cause the fever arose, but they considered it to have arisen either from infected milk or defective sewers." That is, the conclusion arrived at professionally has not withstood the test of investigation to which, in accordance with rules of evidence, it was thus subjected. A similar result would have doubtless followed had other instances been similarly investigated.

The *specific poison* and *de novo* theories *of causation*. The question as to whether " enteric " fever is necessarily due to the action of a specific cause, or may arise *de novo* and in the absence of such specific cause, has been much debated. In reports on fever among British troops in India some of the views on each side of that question are enumerated as follows, namely, that a form of fever may owe its cause to the combined effects of fatigue and exposure. Dr. Aitkin writes of a *specific poison generated* in the body alone. Dr. Budd, that " the living body is the soil in which the *specific poison* breeds and multiplies." He is of opinion that the specific poison of typhoid fever is as distinct as that of small-pox, measles, or scarlatina. Dr. Roberts considers that the specific poison of enteric fever is quite distinct from that of typhus. According to Klein,(b) the specific poison

(b) Sixth Report, Medical Department, Privy Council.

of enteric fever ranks with the poison of those infective diseases which are of a contagio-miasmatic character. The *de novo* origin is supported by Drs. Thin, Moore, Mr. Bowen, and others. Dr. McArthur cannot trace it to any specific poison. According to Dr. Strange, in ninety-nine cases out of every hundred, enteric fever is not from any germ or contagium derived from the intestines. According to Dr. Mackintosh, medical men are not yet agreed as to the nature of the cause. Dr. Barclay describes the causation as little understood (First Report, page 15). Pettenkofer discusses the development of enteric fever " poison " deep in the ground (Second Report, page 73). Dr. Bryden considers that the aspect under which " typhoid " fever in India shows itself is sufficient to refute all arguments based on the assumed localisation of a specific typhoid poison (page 74). Dr. Cuningham considers that in India it is not dependent for its propagation on poisoning of a specific fœcal character. According to Dr. Tuckwell, " under special and peculiar conditions, enteric fever may become instituted in the system without any external agencies " of a specific or special nature (*ibid.*). Dr. Copland believed that specific causes are not in all cases required in order to produce an attack of fever—that changes may take place spontaneously in one or more of the functions, and proceed to give rise to the worst forms of fever (page 75). Dr. Wardell also believes " that, under special and peculiar conditions, enteric fever can become instituted in the system without any external agencies other than such common causes as give rise to " lowered tone of vitality (page 153).

With regard to the " poison " which is by a large class of writers looked upon as the cause of enteric fever, Dr. Cayley writes after this manner :—"The actual nature of the poison, whether it be, according to the hypothesis most generally accepted, some kind of fungus or microzyme or protoplasm, in a word, a *contagium vivum* ; or whether, as maintained by others, it is some deviation of albumen, capable of exercising a catalytic action on other albumen," is rather more of a theoretical than a practical question. As an argument on the side of the *de novo* theory, he states that enteric fever " has often broken out in isolated situations—farmhouses far removed from, and holding no communication with, places where the disease exists,—and many such instances are given by Dr. Murchison. On the other hand, it has been proved incontestably by many instances, both in this country and on the Continent, that all the conditions supposed to be required for its generation may be present for an indefinite time, as percolation of sewage into wells supplying drinking-water ; and yet the disease does not show itself till the *poison* is introduced by the arrival of an infected person, when an outbreak at once takes place."

Professor Corfield, in his lecture on Sanitary Fallacies, enumerates among those fallacies the following opinions regarding *enteric* fever, they being, as he acknowledges, held by a considerable number of persons, namely, that like typhus, diphtheria, and cholera, it originates spontaneously —that is, *de novo* ; that it is not contagious ; that in the great majority of instances it originates from decomposing filth ; that intestinal discharges of its subjects do not contain the poison of the disease.

According to reports regarding enteric fever in England during the autumn of 1880, an unusual number of outbreaks of that disease occurred in various parts of the country ; these took place in localities where there existed no history of any previous case until the outbreak appeared, and of them it has been said that, unless they are to be accounted for on the *pythogenic theory*, " *which does not receive general acceptation*," the reason for these outbursts must be looked for in the presence of *old germs* of the disease lying latent in the soil. The statement is made that it seems important to insist upon the vitality of disease germs, and to warn investigators that they are not to readily accept the *de novo* theory because no recent previous case can be discovered to account for the appearance of the disease.

Professor Klebs of Prague believes that he has discovered the micro-organism which constitutes the specific agent of typhoid fever. He writes that he has been able to find, at the necropsy of twenty-four persons carried off by dothinenteritis, microbes in various organs : in the intestinal mucous membrane, in the thickness of the cartilages of the larynx, in the pia mater, in the foci of lobular pneumonia, in the mesenteric ganglia, in the parenchymata of the liver, and generally diffused in the organs which showed the most decided lesions. These micro-organisms showed themselves in the form of rods, about eighty micrometers in length and 0·5 to 0·6 micrometers in thickness. They have been constantly observed in the bodies of dothinenteric patients since the attention of Professor Klebs was drawn to the subject, and they are always absent from the organs, and specially the intestines, of subjects who have died from any other disease than typhoid.

On the non-specific side of the question, Dr. Davidson, of the Chester County Asylum, is of opinion that the specific germ of typhoid fever, supposed to be generated in the intestinal canal, has never yet been discovered by means of the microscope nor detected in the laboratory; and he ventures to think it is not unlikely sooner or later to be found, like some other now exploded theories in medicine, that the specific germ, so much talked about, only exists in the cinereous matter of the brains of a few theorists. These are bold opinions; but they indicate with unequivocal clearness that serious doubts are entertained, by some at least, regarding the absolute correctness of the specific poison theory of typhoid fever. Dr. Davidson believes in the pythogenic causation of typhoid fever, and in its origin from noxious gases. With reference to the organic poisonous organisms considered to have been discovered by Klein, and by him believed capable of producing enteric fever, Dr. Creighton considers that he has disproved the existence of any such organisms.

The above particulars seem to indicate the following conclusions, namely:—

1. That enteric fever may arise in the absence of specific poison.

2. That variety of opinion exists with regard to the actual cause of fever.

3. That the history of "enteric fever" in India refutes arguments based upon localisation of a specific typhoid poison.

4. That fevers of the worst forms may arise spontaneously as a result of changes taking place in the functions of the body.

5. That the existence of a specific poison capable of producing enteric fever is based upon an assumption; that the question of its existence is more of a theoretical than practical nature.

6. That the existence of a specific micro-organism capable of producing enteric fever rests at present upon the dictum of one very eminent authority.

7. But that, even should further examination confirm the statement that particular microbes are found in the organs named, the circumstance remains that their presence is no more than a result of ultimate causes upon which the morbid action, in the course of which they are developed, itself depends.

IMPURE ICE.—In an article on this subject, the Louisville Med. News (August 6) observes that many persons, alarmed at the danger of employing the drinking-water of cities, drink only melted ice during the unhealthy season; but it is a popular fallacy to suppose that freezing of water will purify it if it is contaminated, and an alarming epidemic was recently traced to ice derived from a pond. Pure ice-supply is therefore of scarcely less importance than pure water-supply. As long as ice is obtained bonâ fide from the American northern lakes, all requirements seem to be met; but, according to the writer, much of the so-called northern-lake ice is cut from small rivers and streams accessible to the surface-drainage of the surrounding country. He also states that close to the Des Plaines River, whence ice is derived for Chicago and southern consumption, is a canal so foul from the sewage of that town that no fish can live in its waters, in the vicinity of which diphtheria and other diseases are constantly prevailing. Although there may be no direct surface communication between the canal and the great river, there may be many subterraneous sources of contact; and, at all events, the exhalations from this open sewer would be readily absorbed. "If the foregoing deductions are sound, what is the remedy? We answer, Artificial ice. It is now possible to manufacture this article so rapidly and at so low an expenditure of capital that it can successfully command the market with the natural ice, no matter how ample may be the facilities of the natural-ice companies for gathering and transporting their commodity."

THE DOCTRINE OF SATURNINE GOUT.

By ROBERT SAUNDBY, M.D. Edin.,

Member of the Royal College of Physicians, and Assistant-Physician to the General Hospital, Birmingham.

(Concluded from page 395.)

Case 11.—Lead-Poisoning—Gout—Intemperate—Not Hereditary.

A man, aged fifty-nine, organ-pipe maker, was intemperate in his use of beer and gin in early life. In the four years preceding 1858 he had several attacks of regular gout. In 1858 he had lead-palsy. In 1863 he had gout again, and seven months later he had his last attack. In 1867 he had lead-palsy again. Having lost all his teeth, no blue line was observable. The urine contained a trace of albumen. There was no hereditary predisposition.

This is apparently a further account of Case 1, and so far modifies the former statement that he had always been temperate, by admitting a free use of beer and gin in early life.

In another clinical lecture, published in 1872,(a) Dr. Garrod promised his hearers a full inquiry into the relations of lead-poisoning and gout, but apparently only a part of the lecture was published, and though styled Lecture I., I can find no Lecture II., or any other of the series.

Dr. Wilks reported the following case in the British Medical Journal for 1875(b):—

Case 12.—Lead-Poisoning—Gout—No Note of Habits or Family History.

——, aged twenty-nine, has worked in lead since he was a lad, and has had colic twice. Had a well-marked blue line on gums, and painful swelling of the ball of the great toe exactly resembling gout. The urine contained a little albumen.

Dr. Wilks asks the pertinent question, in what way lead-poisoning affects the digestive and assimilative processes so as to favour the production of uric acid?

The following case occurred recently in my own practice:—

Case 13.—Gout—Lead-Poisoning—Absence of Hereditary Predisposition—Intemperate.

Matthew H., thirty-nine, married, file-cutter, was admitted as an out-patient to the General Hospital on April 21, 1881, complaining of pain and swelling of fingers and toes.

His illness began eight years ago with pain in the left foot, and he has since had repeated attacks of regular gout in his feet. His hands have been affected for six years. He has been a worker in lead for twenty-five years, and has suffered repeatedly from lead-colic, but has never had lead-palsy. He admits having often drunk too much beer on a Saturday.

His father worked at the same trade, but died of consumption at thirty-nine; he never had gout. His mother also died of consumption at forty-four. One sister died in the General Hospital of bronchitis(?) at twenty-five. No one in the family has had gout except father and a brother who works at the same trade. Patient has had nine children, of whom seven are living and healthy.

The patient presented the following condition:—Left hand: The distal joint of the middle finger and the middle joint of the little finger were much enlarged, reddened, and very painful. Right hand: The distal joint of the ring-finger was swollen, almost globular in shape, reddened, ulcerated, discharging urates and pus, and very painful. The metacarpo-phalangeal joint of the thumb and the wrist-joint were also swollen and very painful. The feet presented no deformity or swelling except two small nodules over the left external malleolus. No other joints were affected. There were no nodules in the ears. The incisor teeth had lost their enamel, and there was a distinct blue line on the gums. The aortic second sound was accentuated; pulse 84. Lungs, liver, and spleen normal. Urine 1016, clear, yellow, acid, containing a trace of albumen. Patient is in the habit of getting up two or three times at night to make water.

It was certainly a surprise to me to find that a doctrine so very generally received rested on no better evidence than these very inconclusive cases.

(a) Lancet, vol. i., 1872, page 1.
(b) British Medical Journal, vol. i. 1875, page 9.

There can be little doubt that Case 11 is a further account of Case 1, so that these should count as only one case, and as the first note of temperate habits is modified by the confession of early over-indulgence in beer and spirits in the later account, Case 1 must be rejected altogether.

If we proceed to examine these cases a little more critically, we find still further objections to them. Thus, if we look at the facts adduced as evidence of lead-poisoning, in Case 10 there is merely the statement that the patient used lead in his work.

The following table will bring out more clearly the results of such an examination of these cases and their defects:—

No. of case.	Name of reporter.	Evidence of lead-poisoning.	Evidence of gout.	Habits.	Family history.
1	Garrod	Good	Good	Temperate	Free from gout.
2	,,	,,	,,	No note	No note.
3	,,	,,	,,	Temperate	,,
4	Begbie	,,	,,	Intemperate	,,
5	,,	,,	,,	,,	,,
6	Murchison	,,	Doubtful	No note	,,
7	,,	,,	,,	,,	,,
8	Wilks	,,	,,	Temperate	,,
9	,,	,,	Good	,,	,,
10	,,	None	,,	,,	Free from gout.
11	Garrod	Good	,,	Intemperate	,,
12	Wilks	,,	,,	No note	No note.
13	Saundby	,,	,,	Intemperate	Free from gout.

The evidence of gout is marked as doubtful in three cases: in Cases 6 and 7 the only gouty phenomenon was irregular swelling of the knee-joint, and in Case 8 the theory of gout rested on the post-mortem discovery of urate of soda in the great-toe joint. The history of an attack of regular gout was present in all the others (except Case 10), and is to my mind the only satisfactory evidence.

As these cases were all published to illustrate this peculiar causation of gout, we should reasonably expect the reporters to have noted the habits of the patients and their family histories, so that we might be able to exclude the influences of alcoholic and fermented beverages and hereditary predisposition. But reference to the table will show that most of the notes are defective in one or other of these particulars. In four there is no note under either heading, and there is information on both points in four only—Cases 1, 10, 11, and 13—and, as the former two have been already rejected for other reasons, only two (11 and 13) out of the whole number remain to support the doctrine of saturnine gout. But even these, when looked at closely, do not turn out to be very effective props, for both were intemperate persons, and consequently their gout may be as justly regarded as the product of beer as of lead. It therefore appears that the doctrine of saturnine gout rests rather on authority than on demonstration.

When we turn to the writings of Dr. Garrod himself, we find that he expresses himself very cautiously as to the relations of lead-poisoning to gout, admitting that the fact that women who work in white lead manufactories, and who often suffer from lead-colic, but are not affected with gout in like ratio with men, indicates "that lead alone does not very powerfully predispose to gout."

But Wilks and Murchison, especially the former, appear to have accepted and taught, without qualification, that lead-poisoning produces gout, although, as we have seen, they have not brought forward any evidence which can be regarded as justifying this advance from Garrod's position; and doubtless the authority of these eminent names has sufficed to obtain admission for the doctrine into our text-books.

"To give a general currency," says the learned Dr. Paris, "to a hypothetical opinion, or medicinal reputation to an inert substance, nothing more is required than the talismanic aid of a few great names. The laconic sentiment of the Roman satirist is ever opposed to our remonstrance— 'Marcus dixit? Ita est.'"

No doubt our great men are very often right, but as they are not so always, and we have no means of discriminating truth from error, except by asking for proof, it is to be regretted that scientific methods should still have gained so little acceptance among those upon whom the progress of medicine mainly depends.

So long as authority takes the place of evidence, and dogmatic assertion is welcomed rather than logical reasoning, so long will medicine remain stationary or oscillate between opposite extremes of opinion.

But, admitting the unsatisfactory nature of the cases adduced, it may be argued that the doctrine is strongly supported by Dr. Garrod's discoveries that the blood in cases of lead-poisoning is loaded with urates, and that lead administered internally checks the elimination of uric acid by the kidneys.

But the assumption here made is that gout is identical with uric acid in the blood—a point which I cannot concede. Dr. Garrod does not seem to have taken the necessary precaution of examining the blood of a sufficient number of persons unaffected with either gout or lead-poisoning, or he would not have attached so much importance to his discovery. Dr. Austin Meldon states(c) that, although gout is one of the rarest affections in hospital practice in Ireland, he has repeatedly found the blood loaded with urates in otherwise healthy men lying in the accident wards.

Moreover, very many physicians recognise a pathological lithæmia not associated with gout. If we are to regard a regular attack of gout in the toe as the only conclusive evidence of the disease, then we can only express surprise that so few persons affected with lead-poisoning are also affected with gout—a difficulty which Dr. Garrod himself does not attempt to get over.

Modern research has not contributed anything further to the physiological side of the question. Rutherford has shown that lead administered internally diminishes the biliary secretion of the dog, and we may infer that lead is a general hepatic depressant; and those who regard the liver as the organ mainly concerned in the production of gout would, if saturnine gout were an established fact, find strong confirmation of their views. But in the present state of our knowledge we are warranted in no such conclusions.

THE NIGHT MEDICAL SERVICE IN NEW YORK.—The night medical service is now a year old. It seems to have been, on the whole, fairly successful, though there is much absurd talk in the daily papers about its incalculable blessings. There have been, we are told, nearly 500 calls during the past twelve months. It is proposed now, by some enthusiasts, to establish a day medical service, paying a dollar fee to the physician called on.—New York Med. Record, August 20.

QUEBRACHO IN DYSPNŒA.—Dr. Andrew Smith, in a report read at the New York Medical Society (New York Med. Journal, September) upon the use of quebracho (first employed by Dr. Penzoldt, of Erlangen, in 1879) in dyspnœa, states that it refers to thirty-two cases. Eleven of these were spasmodic asthma, with or without emphysema and bronchitis, and in nine notable relief was obtained; and taking the whole thirty-two cases of different diseases in which dyspnœa was a prominent feature, this symptom was relieved to a greater or less extent in twenty-one, not relieved in ten, and aggravated in one. "The fact that dyspnœa, depending upon such a variety of causes, may be relieved by quebracho, points to the respiratory centre as the seat of its action. Apparently it blunts the sense of want of air, and thus mitigates the suffering from a deficient supply. But this action is not necessarily only palliative. Exaggerated respiratory efforts are often in themselves an evil, not only on account of the muscular effort expended, but from the aspiration of blood into the thoracic viscera which results, especially when the dyspnœa is caused by the narrowing of the air-passages rather than by solidification or compression of the lung. Hence in many cases an agent which will moderate the violence of the respiratory movements will not only lessen the distress of the sufferer, but will increase the chances of his recovery. That quebracho will very promptly fulfil this indication there seems to be no room to doubt, while as yet there is no evidence that it is liable to produce unfavourable after-affects. The extremely disagreeable taste of the medicine, and its tendency to produce nausea, are, however, serious drawbacks to its use."

(c) British Medical Journal, vol. i. 1881, page 446.

REPORTS OF HOSPITAL PRACTICE
IN
MEDICINE AND SURGERY.

UNIVERSITY COLLEGE HOSPITAL.

THREE CASES OF REMOVAL OF THE BREAST.
(Under the care of Mr. CHRISTOPHER HEATH.)

MR. HEATH removes the entire breast, as a rule, in cases of scirrhus, and is very particular to remove at the same time any axillary glands which may be enlarged. In operating, he uses the knife but little after the first incisions, which are planned so as to include any infiltrated or doubtful skin, and strips back the skin mainly with the finger, except in very thin patients, where cautious dissection is necessary. It is more easy to distinguish breast-substance with the finger than with the eye, and thus to make sure of removing the thin margin of an atrophied breast. Should the breast be adherent to the pectoral, Mr. Heath removes some of the fibres and even large portions of the muscle, and has not found the haemorrhage severe. In dealing with the glands in the axilla, Mr. Heath employs the forefinger very freely to enucleate all the glands within reach, the deeper ones lying in close proximity to the axillary vessels. The haemorrhage accompanying even an extensive operation thus performed is found to be very slight, two or three ligatures being used on the average, and occasionally none at all.

Although employing the Listerian system, as a rule, in hospital cases, Mr. Heath finds that in private he obtains very excellent results with the employment of a solution of chloride of zinc, a drainage-tube, and a dressing of absorbent cotton. The gauze dressing is often complained of as being hot, and by shutting in the arm on the affected side it often leads to troublesome stiffness of the elbow.

For the following cases we are indebted to Mr. Stanley Boyd, Surgical Registrar:—

Case 1.—Scirrhus—Amputation of Breast—Antiseptics.

A. B., aged thirty-nine, a governess, single, began to suffer from slight pricking pain in the left breast about three months before admission, and found that using the left arm was unpleasant. The date at which she first noticed a tumour is not known. She remembered no injury to the breast. Menstruation had always been regular. As regards family history—mother died just after the birth of patient; eldest sister died of cancer uteri; father died of heart disease.

The left breast, with the exception of the lower and inner portion, was occupied by a hard new growth, which rendered the organ distinctly larger than its fellow. It was freely movable over the great pectoral. Some axillary glands were much enlarged. The patient was thin, but showed no signs of secondary deposits.

Mr. Heath removed the breast by incisions above and below the nipple; the outer end of the wound was then extended into the axilla, and three or four glands turned out. There was very little bleeding. A drainage-tube was brought out in the axilla, the wound closed by wire sutures, and a carbolic gauze dressing applied—the spray having been used. The patient slept well on the night after the operation. The wound healed rapidly. The temperature was 100·2° on the second night, and 100° to 100·6° on the third day; but after this 100° was only once registered.

On the eighteenth day she was discharged with the wound almost closed.

Patient has since completely recovered, and resumed her employment.

Case 2.—Scirrhus—Amputation—Antiseptics—Recurrence and Abdominal Affection.

M. C., aged sixty, married, noticed a small swelling in the left breast five months before admission, which caused no pain, but grew steadily. The patient's father died at sixty, three, and mother at eighty-five, but neither had any tumour. Of nine brothers and sisters, six died of phthisis and one sister of cancer. Of three children, two died of phthisis. In the left breast, immediately above the nipple, was a scirrhous growth, about two inches across, not involving either skin or muscle. There were two much enlarged glands behind the

tendon of the pectoral, and the left supra-clavicular fossa was distinctly fuller than the right. Just outside the sternomastoid a small, firm gland could be felt, which was not tender. The patient was thin, but there were no signs of secondary growths in internal organs.

The breast was removed in the usual way; the incision lengthened into the axilla, and a carbolised hemp ligature having been placed round the pedicle of the enlarged glands, they were removed. The axillary vein was exposed. No spray was used, but the parts were thoroughly carbolised after the operation, and a carbolic gauze dressing applied. The wound was closed with wire sutures, and drained from the axillary end.

The patient did not recover well from the operation. For forty-eight hours she could not pass her urine, and vomiting was frequent for five days. On the evening of the fourth day venous oozing occurred from the wound, and was stopped by pressure. On the following day the discharge was free, bloody, and offensive. The temperature till now had varied from 100° to 101·2°; the pulse from 100 to 128, rather small and compressible. After this the patient mended slowly. Granulations in the wound were large, pale, and showed very little tendency to grow together, in spite of strapping and careful bandaging. The hemp ligature with a large slough separated on the tenth day.

For a month the morning temperature was 99° to 100,° and the evening 100° to 101°, and the patient slowly lost flesh. On the thirty-fourth day a tender, firm swelling was felt in front of the lower lumbar vertebrae. On the thirty-eighth day many purpuric spots appeared, and the evening temperature was 103°. The spots had done by the forty-seventh day, and the patient left the hospital on the fifty-second day, the wound being still unhealed.

She was readmitted a few days later, improved in strength and appearance; wound unhealed, flaps firm; axilla indurated; left hand and forearm oedematous; no sign of recurrence in lungs; both legs oedematous; abdomen full and tympanitic, but a tender resistant mass could be felt just to right of umbilicus, apparently moving with respiration; liver dulness ceased just below ribs; tenderness over spleen, which was not felt.

The patient was discharged in much the same condition three week later.

Case 3.—Scirrhus—Partial Amputation of Breast—Carbolic Oil and Salicylic Wool.

E. B., aged sixty-five, a laundress, single, noticed a small, very movable swelling in left breast six months ago. There was a pricking and shooting pain in it; and she had lost a good deal of flesh since its appearance. There was no family history of tumour, the patient's mother and father having each died at eighty.

On admission there was a firm mass in the upper and outer part of left breast, freely movable over the great pectoral. It sent a short process upwards, along the anterior axillary fold, and just here the skin was involved for about one inch square. There was tenderness, but no enlarged gland, in the axilla. Above the clavicle a small movable gland could be felt, but it was not tender. The patient looked healthy, but her skin hung loosely.

Considering the patient's age, Mr. Heath decided to remove only the new growth; and this he did by semi-lunar incisions parallel to the anterior axillary fold. The wound was washed out with chloride of zinc (forty grains to the ounce), drained by a tube brought out in the axilla, and the edges were approximated by stout wire sutures. Lint steeped in carbolic oil was placed next the wound, and a thick pad of salicylic wool was secured over this by a bandage.

Free discharge rendered it necessary to change the dressings the same evening, and again on the following morning. The patient felt well, and her morning temperature remained normal till the fifth day, when it rose to 100°, pulse to 120; at the same time, patient felt ill, and a patch of cutaneous inflammation spread from wound some distance down the back. Next morning the temperature was normal, and in four days the blush had disappeared.

On the seventh evening sharp haemorrhage occurred, and was arrested by douching with iced water and pressure over a sponge. The temperature two hours later was found to be 102·8°, but on the following morning it was again normal. On the tenth day slight haemorrhage into the dressings was found, but on the eleventh day such free bleeding occurred that it was necessary to open up the wound and turn out a mass of clot. A small artery was then seen spouting, but it stopped before a pair of forceps was obtained. There was no union at this time, and the surface of the wound became very sloughy. By the eighteenth day it was granulating well; but healing was very slow, and when she was discharged on the fiftieth day a small granulating patch remained. The temperature at the period when hæmorrhage occurred was often subnormal—95° to 97°,—but after this it was only twice 100°.

The patient remains well, and there is no recurrence.

General Results.—Of 20 cases of amputation of the whole breast, often with removal of glands and muscle, 9 were treated antiseptically throughout; all were discharged healed, or almost so, in periods varying from eight to thirty-five days—twenty-two on the average. Eight were treated antiseptically—some with, some without the spray—but the dressings became septic within the first week. Of these 3 died—1 of erysipelas and pyæmia; 1 (a stout woman of fifty) apparently from cardiac syncope; 1 from asthenia, due to erysipelas and secondary deposits in liver; 1 never healed, from recurrence, and the others were slow in doing so; but two were very fat women. The average temperature was much higher than in first series. Two were dressed with salicylic wool—1 died of acute septicæmia, the other recovered well; 1 was dressed with cotton-wool, and died of septicæmia.

TERMS OF SUBSCRIPTION.
(Free by post.)

				£	s.	d.
British Islands	. . . .	Twelve Months	.	1	8	0
" "	. . . .	Six "	.	0	14	0
The Colonies and the United States of America	. . .	Twelve "	.	1	10	0
" " "	. . .	Six "	.	0	15	0
India	. . . .	Twelve "	.	1	10	0
" (viâ Brindisi)	. . .	" "	.	1	15	0
" "	. . .	Six "	.	0	15	0
" (viâ Brindisi)	. . .	" "	.	0	17	6

Foreign Subscribers are requested to inform the Publishers of any remittance made through the agency of the Post-office.

Single Copies of the Journal can be obtained of all Booksellers and Newsmen, price Sixpence.

Cheques or Post-office Orders should be made payable to Mr. JAMES LUCAS, 11, *New Burlington-street, W.*

TERMS FOR ADVERTISEMENTS.

			£	s.	d.
Seven lines (70 words)	.	.	0	4	6
Each additional line (10 words)	.	.	0	0	6
Half-column, or quarter-page	.	.	1	5	0
Whole column, or half-page	.	.	2	10	0
Whole page	.	.	5	0	0

Births, Marriages, and Deaths are inserted Free of Charge.

THE MEDICAL TIMES AND GAZETTE *is published on Friday morning: Advertisements must therefore reach the Publishing Office not later than One o'clock on Thursday.*

Medical Times and Gazette.

SATURDAY, OCTOBER 1, 1881.

INTRA-PERITONEAL WOUNDS OF THE BLADDER.

Cui persecta vesica fuerit . . . . lethale est. Such was the dictum of Hippocrates (translated into Latin), and such may be said to be the result of intra-peritoneal wounds to-day, unless the surgeon rapidly and scientifically steps in. Under any circumstances, however, the prognosis in such cases is very serious; for out of ninety-seven hitherto recorded cases, ninety-six proved fatal. The only case that recovered is that of a patient who was treated by Walter of Pittsburg (1862), by opening the abdomen and removing the extravasated urine. The mortality of extra-peritoneal rupture of the bladder is not nearly so high; for out of seventy-

six cases there were twenty-nine recoveries—that is, a mortality of 65 per cent. But to judge from the most recent utterances on the subject, everything is about to be changed now, and wounds of the bladder, when recognised early, are about to be rescued from the great mortality which in the past has attended them.

An interesting and instructive memoir will be found in the *Revue de Chirurgie* for June and July of this year, by M. Vincent of Lyons. In it he recapitulates, (I.) the historical literature of the operative treatment of vesical perforation, and then (II.) gives an account of some experiments undertaken with the object of studying the repair of incised, punctured, contused, lacerated, and gunshot wounds of that part of the bladder which is covered by the peritoneum.

I.—HISTORICAL RECAPITULATION.

What methods of treatment were adopted, previous to the era of antiseptic surgery, in perforating intra-peritoneal wounds of the bladder? The methods may be categorised as follows:—1. Simple urethral catheterism, or catheterism of the bladder, and thence, through the wound, into the cavity containing the extravasated urine, as recommended and practised by Thorp of Dublin. Thorp's case was that of a man, aged thirty, who while drunk fell off his horse. Four hours later he was suffering from an urgent desire to micturate, but was quite unable to do so. Burning pain at the hypogastrium and tension of the abdominal muscles were present, but there was neither contusion, nor vomiting, nor rigor. A catheter was passed into the bladder without difficulty, but at first no urine came. The instrument was then passed in somewhat further, and on rotating it slightly on its axis, a few ounces of blood-stained urine were drawn off. On making the patient assume various positions, some more urine was drawn off. Warm water was then injected, with a view to wash out the peritoneal cavity; and a catheter just reaching to the neck of the bladder was left in situ. This treatment, together with leeches, hot fomentations to the abdomen, and the internal use of calomel and opium, resulted in cure at the end of fourteen days. The absence in this case of all inflammatory symptoms, however, favours the supposition that the rupture was outside the peritoneum. 2. The urethra has been opened in the perinæum. Bartels, in his *Mémoire* in *Langenbeck's Archiv*, reports four cases in which this mode was adopted; but it would appear only justifiable in cases where the penile urethra was, from some cause, impassable. 3. The peritoneal cul-de-sac in front of the rectum has been punctured. This operation was inspired by an idea that all the extravasated urine would gravitate to this part of the peritoneal cavity. But Wegner has shown that the peritoneum absorbs the fluid with great rapidity during the first few moments after the extravasation, and, moreover, that irritating fluids cause peristaltic movements of the intestines, which diffuse the liquid in all directions. It is only after inflammation has set in, when the absorbent power of the peritoneum becomes exhausted, that fluids may possibly gravitate towards the lowest part of the cavity. 4. The abdomen has been punctured—(a) above the pubis; (b) in the flank on a level with the umbilicus; (c) puncture and aspiration. The indication, of course, would be collections of fluid in front of the bladder. 5. The bladder has been opened in the perinæum. Employed six times, this procedure has given two cures. It would only seem suitable for extra-peritoneal injuries. Bartels and others, nevertheless, have recommended it in intra-peritoneal cases. 6. The abdominal cavity has been opened by an incision along the median line, and the extravasated liquid removed by means of sponges. This being done, authors have agreed to sew up the abdominal wound; but as regards sewing up the hole in the bladder there has been less unanimity. Some think it unnecessary to suture the bladder, contenting themselves by leaving a catheter *in situ;* they believe that the edges of the vesical wound will approximate themselves by reason of the contractility of the organ, and that there is no need to use any mechanical agents, which must necessarily remain in the peritoneal cavity as foreign bodies, and may there prove sources of danger. It was thus that Dr. Walter of Pittsburg treated his now celebrated case, which was published in 1862. We may briefly remind our readers of the details of this case:—A young man, aged twenty-two years, received a blow in the lower abdomen during a fight. He immediately felt a severe pain, and felt a great desire to urinate without being able to do so. After some hours, the abdomen began to swell, his pulse became small and frequent, and his respiration was hurried; nausea and vomiting set in. The catheter drew off a small quantity of blood-stained urine. A diagnosis of intra-peritoneal rupture of the bladder was arrived at, and, as all the symptoms were aggravating themselves, Walter decided on laparotomy *ten hours* after the accident. The abdomen was opened by an incision six inches long in the median line; the distended intestines at once protruded. After having removed about one pint of urine and blood by means of sponges, a rupture two inches long was discovered in the fundus of the bladder. A catheter was placed *in situ,* and the patient was kept well under the influence of opium. The abdominal wall was closed, but nothing was done to the bladder-wound itself. At the end of three weeks the patient was well.

In this case, a most important point to observe is that the operation was undertaken in ten hours, and it is not unlikely that the success was due to its promptitude.

As long ago as 1716, Jacob Woyt hinted at laparotomy, with subsequent suture of the injured bladder. In his "Leçons" he says—"It is considerably more serious when the walls of the bladder are affected, for then neither suture nor art can avail anything, as the urine can so easily escape into the belly, and cannot get out through the external opening. It is true that by making a free incision into the lower belly, and drawing the bladder out through it for the purpose of sewing together the edges of the wound, one might cure the rupture, provided the inflammation did not interfere with it." Benjamin Bell has generally been credited with the idea of sewing up the wound in the bladder, but he did not write for many years subsequent to Woyt. Messrs. Willett and Heath in this country have each added some valuable experience on this subject, to which we would refer our readers for details.

We shall reserve an account of M. Vincent's experiments for a later issue.

THE ARMY MEDICAL REPORT FOR 1879.

[Second Notice.]

We return to the Army Medical Report, to see if we can learn anything by comparing the statistics of 1879 with those of previous years, and to look for the chances of improvement consequent on the suggestions and recommendations scattered through the pages of the volume. We have said all that we need say about "short service." Everyone will recollect, when that system was introduced, the appeals made in Parliament to the patriotism of the colonels, who were implored to hold their peace until the new scheme had been put on its trial. It has been put in the dock, and already the judge has summed up apparently against it, and the jury some day or another may be called upon for a verdict. Not just yet, of course; for short service, like a phoenix, is to arise again, converted into something

neither short nor long; and no doubt patriots will again be bidden not to embarrass the War Minister. But there are some points touched on in the Medical Report which are not tabooed, and people may venture to express an opinion on them without offence. Is there, for instance, any lesson to be learned from the medical history of the Zulu War? We believe it teaches us, for one thing, that the Army Medical Department should be kept up to its full strength. When the war broke out the members of that Department were discontented, and its numbers were reduced. It was necessary to employ civilians to serve with the troops. This is an objectionable step, and the regulations for the Medical Department decidedly condemn it. They permit militia surgeons, indeed, to serve with the regiments *in the field,* but all other surgeons volunteering as hospital helpers have to do duty in stationary hospitals. There is reason in this rule, and a paragraph in the Report of the Zulu War illustrates it. We read there of the frequent complaints made by civil surgeons that the medicines *they required* were not in the "field companions," and we are also told of their unwillingness to substitute one medicine for another. It is evident that on a campaign the Army-trained doctor is the right man in the right place. He has been educated, so to speak, to run on one leg, and to fight with one arm tied behind his back; he has learned by experience all he may hope to find in a Departmental medicine-chest, and he undertakes his rough and ready work without wasting time in searching for the tools which cannot be supplied. For our own part, we should be glad to see all the medical men who serve with Volunteers put through a course of Netley drill, convinced as we are that a knowledge of these apparent trifles is a matter of extreme importance, and makes all the difference between success and failure. We notice the same complaint made with regard to Medical Transport. The Report says that "the regulations were not carried out by attaching men of the Army Service Corps to the Medical Transport,—civilian conductors, Hottentot drivers, and native leaders being employed,—the result of which was that the transport arrangements were not so satisfactory as could have been wished." The civilian doctor may be the more learned, and the Hottentot driver the better whip; but where patients must be treated and bullocks driven according to *pattern,* the "Department" comes out triumphantly.

Something might be learned from the Appendix to the African Report with regard to the influence of age on disease during the Zulu campaign; but the ages of the men serving are not given, although the ages of those invalided and of those who died appear in contrasted columns. All we can note is that twenty-two lads under nineteen were invalided, and five died. It is sad to observe that such boys were serving in a campaign!

There is a curious note at the conclusion of the African Report with regard to the Black Irregular Troops. The Surgeon-General says that there was a smaller proportion among them both of admissions and deaths, and "this is accounted for by the Black Irregulars for the most part when sick returning to their homes to be treated by their witch doctors." We confess to a curiosity as to the success of the treatment by these most irregular practitioners Turning next to the Indian march of General Roberts' field force, we notice with pleasure that the men were *men.* Surgeon-General Hanbury says: "The strength of the column was in round numbers 10,000 fighting men and 8000 followers. All troops and followers composing it were carefully weeded out previous to marching from Cabul. It was, therefore, a picked force, and probably the finest that has ever taken the field in this or any other country." The force marched from Cabul on August 9, and on the 24th the Surgeon-General reports: "The Native troops, followers, and baggage-animals are much fagged and exhausted from want of sleep and regular meals; *the Europeans stand the privations and hard work much better.*"

We have already remarked on the complaint made, that probably a worse shod army never took the field! Here is again an instance of what some might deem a trifle, but bad boots were able to place hundreds of fighting men on the daily sick list! We may observe that Surgeon-General Hanbury is of opinion that the *wide-soled ammunition boot* is best adapted for both European and Native troops, but the material and workmanship must be improved, and decided attention to fitting is demanded. With regard to the length of the daily march, we learn "that about fourteen or fifteen miles were accomplished with comparative ease, but that every yard over that distance told with undoubted force." It is curious to observe how the fighting little Goorkhas were outpaced. On August 27, we are told, "the pace was so fast that it distressed the Goorkhas greatly. On this day the 24th Punjab Native Infantry led the way, and of course gave the time."

The Surgeon-General's opinion of preserved meats is worthy of attention. He says, "All the preserved meats that have hitherto come under my observation for issue to the troops are well adapted for short expeditions of two or three days. If continued longer, indigestion, dyspepsia in all its phases, diarrhœa, invariably result."

There is unhappily one thing especially to be said with regard to suggestions and observations recorded in medical Blue-books, and that is, no one ever knows whether they will be attended to. India is a long way off even now; appointments are rapidly vacated, and the new office-holders have their own special troubles, and cannot be bothered with the complaints of their predecessors. Who can tell how much longer bad boots will continue to be the rule, or that the sick soldier will still be left for long, weary nights to the mercy of Indian coolies? And if some grievances are remedied, it does not follow that people who wade through Blue-books are made acquainted with the improvement. Let us turn to the Medical Report for 1871. A few grievances are recorded there which somewhat startled us at the time. For instance, Surgeon-General Beatson made the following remarks upon bedding in India:—"The system which makes the bedding the property of the individual soldier is an inconvenient and imperfect one. The Indian system is attended with this great defect, that the amount of bedding which is sufficient for the warmer parts of India is quite inadequate for the hills or in the Punjab during the winter." We have not been able to learn, from the study of Blue-books, that any alteration has been made with regard to bedding. Again, in 1870, Inspector-General Currie remarked at Madras, "All executive officers recommend that *pillows* should be issued to soldiers in barracks, as they are to sick in hospital. I quite endorse this recommendation." Who would not? But Blue-books do not tell us whether soldiers in India had pillows in their barrack-rooms in 1879. Worse still: in 1871, Deputy Surgeon-General O'Flaherty reported, "Complaints are very general at some stations regarding the inadequacy of the lighting provided by Government, which consists of cocoanut oil lamps, affording a very insufficient amount of light"; but if the Bombay Report for the previous year be procured, it will there be found that Inspector-General Mouat stated, "It is universally admitted that the men cannot read in their barrack-rooms in the evenings unless they provide themselves with some light in addition to that provided by Government." He says *universally admitted*. Yet the lights of 1871 were no better than the lights of 1870! Are they better

now? and if not, why not? Some may call these trifles, but they are anything but that. Want of healthy occupation in India prepares the mind for intemperance and immorality; and surely the wasted hours in the dim barrack-room can bear no wholesome fruit, and drunkenness and incontinence must be expected to increase. We notice in the Blue-book for 1879 that some new regulations for governing canteens were in force in Madras and Bombay— "No restriction is placed on the amount of beer a soldier may be served with, except that he must pay for it at once, and be sober at the time. Most of the medical officers have seen no harm from this extension; some think it has acted well, others that it has increased drunkenness. The medical officers of the depôts at Poonamallee and Wellington concur in condemning the new regulation as unsuitable for such places, where the men have much time on their hands. The medical officers pretty generally condemn the issue (optional) of a dram of rum or arrack; they think it hurtful in initiating the habit of drinking in young soldiers." We also are strongly inclined to think so; and feel quite sure that confinement to barracks, want of lights, and uncomfortable bedding must tend to develope the habit which may be initiated by the dram of rum.

FATTY HEART: ITS DIAGNOSIS, PATHOLOGY, AND TREATMENT.

OUR knowledge of the disease termed fatty heart cannot be said, more especially as to its diagnosis and treatment, to be of a very definite or satisfactory character. Hence as a basis for farther advance we are disposed to welcome the *resumé* of its diagnosis, pathology, and treatment given by Professor Stoffella, of Vienna, in a lecture recently published (*Wien. Med. Wochenschrift*, 1881, Nos. 26-28).

After distinguishing between fatty infiltration—which Dr. Walshe calls "local obesity" of the heart—and fatty degeneration, or the precipitation of fat within the primitive fibres, which latter alone he means when he speaks of "fatty heart," Professor Stoffella goes on to say that the diagnosis of the disease, except in its immediate beginnings, is by no means specially difficult. He lays especial emphasis on the weak and usually toneless character of the heart-sounds, combined with the presence of the usual causes of fatty degeneration of the heart. He also notes the weak or imperceptible heart's impulse, the weak compressible pulse, usually intermittent, irregular, and slow. Dyspnœa, permanent or spasmodic, and frequent syncope, with the absence of valvular or pulmonic disease, also assist in the diagnosis. He fails to comment on the relative pulse and respiration rate, which Dr. Walshe has found in some cases 2 : 1; nor does he mention the valuable, while not, as was at first thought, diagnostic, symptom of the "Cheyne-Stokes' respiration." We fear, however, that, notwithstanding all known aids, the diagnosis of this disease will in many cases be unmade, or, if made, will partake more of the character of a probable guess than a scientific conclusion. One of the grounds on which, as we have seen, Professor Stoffella bases his diagnosis, is the presence of the usual causes of fatty degeneration. But while, as we shall see, there is a certain amount of sure etiological ground, outside that lies a residue of cases in which, beyond the hypothesis of a hereditary tendency, we must acknowledge ourselves ignorant of the cause of fatty metamorphosis of the heart-fibres.

In discussing the pathology of fatty heart, Professor Stoffella commences with some account of the physiological deposition of fat. Twenty years ago, Voit and Pettenkofer showed that the direct source of the fat in the body is not the carbo-hydrates, starch, sugar, etc., but albumen. The overplus of albumen left circulating in the blood or other fluids of the body, after deduction of that used in tissue-formation, is broken up into water, carbonic acid, and fat, while, so far as it is perfectly oxidised, it leaves the body as urea and uric acid. The amount of fat deposited will therefore depend on (1) the amount of the "circulating albumen" and (2) the small relative supply of oxygen. As to other sources of fat, it is at least doubtful if gelatine forms fat, and of ingested fat only stearin, palmitin, and olein—the varieties naturally present in the body—go towards the production of fat. While, however, albumen is without doubt the direct source of fat, it is a manifest fact that gelatine, fat, and the carbohydrates help the production of fat in the body. This they do by oxidising and splitting up more readily than albumen, thus using up the available oxygen, so that albumen is oxidised simply to fat, in place of to water and carbonic acid. By their oxidation, also, the carbo-hydrates spare the fat of the body, while, according to Voit, gelatine saves the blood and tissue albumen.

Parenchymatous fatty degeneration is fundamentally the same process as the physiological formation of fat—that is, the albuminous contents of cells imperfectly oxidised deposit fat granules as a part of the process of destruction, morbid or natural.

Fatty heart is thus, Professor Stoffella says, the expression of a disturbance of nutrition, either purely local, as in disease of the coronary arteries or advanced fatty infiltration of the heart, or general, as in anæmia and chlorosis, in alcoholism, Bright's disease, the acute exanthemata, and all marasmic diseases. How comes this about? Two sets of experiments help us here. First, Dr. Litten has shown that the muscles of guinea-pigs kept for a lengthened period in a high temperature undergo fatty degeneration—first the heart, then the respiratory muscles, and lastly the body muscles, accompanied by changes in the blood corresponding to those in typhoid fever. Again, various Continental observers have shown that if dogs and other animals are subjected to successive blood-lettings, fatty degeneration of the heart supervenes. The result is the same in both sets of experiments, therefore, and the common point between them is the poverty of the blood in red corpuscles. But the red corpuscles are the oxygen-carriers of the body, therefore a deficiency of oxygen follows, resulting in an imperfect oxidation of the organic albumen in cells and tissues. The difference between the physiological and the pathological process is, that in the first the "circulating or store albumen" becomes fat, in the second the "organic or tissue albumen."

The treatment of fatty heart recommended by Professor Stoffella follows as a natural corollary from what has just been said. Deficiency in the oxygen-carrying red corpuscles being the cause of the disease, our object is to stimulate the blood-forming function. Our most valuable agent for this is iron, and this must be used with perseverance on the part both of doctor and patient. Should the digestion be unweakened, the best preparation, according to Professor Stoffella, is the sulphate of iron in the form of Blaud's pills. Niemeyer's formula for these is—R. Ferri sulph. pulv., potass. carb. pur. â ℥ss., mucil. tragacanth. q. s. ft. mass. et div. in pil. xcvi. Of these Professor Stoffella gives three thrice daily, immediately after meals, to prevent cardialgia. Should constipation be present, add jalapin or extr. aloes aquos. Where digestion is weak, Professor Stoffella recommends the milder pyrophosph. ferri et sodæ solutum. The iron treatment must be continued for several months, combined with quinine or extr. quebracho should the dyspnœa and chest-oppression be troublesome. When the degeneration occurs as a consequence of valvular disease he would also give digitalis or quinine. The alkaline

mineral waters, mildly purgative and containing iron, usually benefit much. The diet ought to consist principally of lean meat, with green vegetables, bread, eggs, milk, rice, and a fair allowance of wine. All fats, potatoes, beer, brandy, etc., are to be excluded. The carbo-hydrates, fat, and gelatine must, however, be allowed in restricted amount, as otherwise, from the difficulty of oxidising albumen, muscular reparation and animal warmth suffer. Also, nausea and disturbance of digestion result very soon from an exclusively flesh diet, as seen in the Banting cure.

THE WEEK.

TOPICS OF THE DAY.

THE Hackney Board of Guardians appear to be determined to question the financial arrangements of the Metropolitan Asylums Board. At their last week's meeting, Dr. Millar, of Clapton, drew special attention to the items in the accounts of the Asylums Board, just issued, which, he said, called for some explicit explanation from the Managers, who, he found, were spending the ratepayers' money at the rate of half a million sterling per annum. The items for the Atlas hospital-ship, which had only 120 beds for small-pox patients, included the extraordinary sum of £2991 2s. 3d. for blankets and bedding, £3000 for furniture and fittings, £685 8s. 3d. for bedsteads, £1652 for stores and ironmongery, and £293 5s. 6d. for boots and shoes. The bedsteads thus cost £5 14s. each, while the same item for the Hackney Union Infirmary Pavilion had only cost nine shillings, so that in bedsteads alone there was a remarkable excess. The other articles showed a similar extravagant excess in price. Horse-hire for the London-fields ambulances cost £611 17s., and the uniforms for the ambulance drivers, of whom there were only four or five, came to £54 14s. 6d., the cloth being, he was told, superior, and the uniform altogether luxuriously elegant, when reasonable people might suggest that a commoner material would do for those who had to remove small-pox pauper patients. The fish and poultry bill for the Deptford Hospital reached £840 5s. 11d. for the year. He had to complain that this huge expenditure was incurred (referring particularly to the establishment of the Atlas hospital, and the ambulance station) when there were actually 200 vacant beds in the metropolitan hospitals. Mr. Martin (chairman of the Hackney Sanitary Committee) thought that the ratepayers would certainly demand at the hands of the guardians that some inquiry should be made into all this expenditure, especially as the new precept from the Asylums Board required the ratepayers to pay a precept of £9000, as against the precept of £4500 for the corresponding half-year of 1880-81. Ultimately the matter was referred to the Finance Committee for immediate investigation; and as it appeared that patients were being removed to the Atlas ship although there was room in the Homerton Hospital, instructions were given to the relieving officers to use their own ambulance for that purpose for Hackney patients.

Referring to the reported outbreak of cholera at Aden, a letter dated August 30 from that place states:—"There is a disease now prevalent here which is causing considerable alarm—entirely confined to Mussulmans—which the doctors pronounce to be sporadic cholera, being sometimes fatal in two hours. I do not believe it is anything of the kind, but is, I think, entirely due to Ramadan—the Mohammedan month of fasting, now just over. The deaths have been very numerous; the symptoms being griping pains and vomiting. The last returns show a sudden decrease of mortality. It is only reasonable to suppose that men who work all day without food, and eat a heavy meal at night, and keep that on for a month, would suffer very seriously, especially in this climate." Subsequent news, under date 20th ult., reports that during the previous week fifty cases of cholera, out of a total of seventy-eight, proved fatal.

Archdeacon Denison is a great controversialist, but he is as great and more effective as a benefactor and teacher. He has lately circulated amongst his villagers at Brent Knoll a paper setting forth the extent to which he has, after unceasing efforts during the last quarter of a century, supplied the district with water. Finding that epidemic disease prevailed for want of water, he dug for wells, and has now ten reservoirs, four springs, and eight dams, with fountains, filtering-beds, tanks, and pumps. The drinking-water is supplied through galvanised pipes direct from the springs. The six lower reservoirs are fish-pools, pools for swans and ducks, and drinking-places for cattle. The Archdeacon has spent £1500 on these works, and he now calls upon the people to take up the matter, and continue what he has so successfully commenced.

An important prosecution was recently instituted at the Chester Police-court against a druggist of that town, by the Assistant-Secretary of the Chemists' and Druggists' Association, Birmingham, for selling poison without placing a poison-label upon the bottle. Mr. Temple, representing the Society, went to defendant's premises, and requested the assistant to make up a prescription containing arsenic, and another containing two ounces of laudanum. The defendant was not qualified to retail poisons, as he was not a registered chemist and druggist. When the assistant handed prosecutor the poison he omitted to label the bottle "poison," as he should have done. Mr. Templeman admitted that the bottle bore the poison-label of another chemist when he handed it to the assistant, but the Act specified that the vendor was to give his own name and address. It was urged in defence that the defendant had frequently cautioned his assistant not to retail poisons, and that, after all, only a technical offence had been committed. The Bench, being of opinion that the defendant was not aware of his assistant's act, thought a small penalty would meet the justice of the case, and fined him 10s. without costs.

Mr. Newton, the Marlborough-street magistrate, has given his decision in the case of the summons taken out by Messrs. Jay, of Regent-street, against the Grand Junction Waterworks Company for non-supply of water to their premises in July last. The defendants argued that, as Messrs. Jay had made a special contract with them for a water-supply, they had contracted themselves out of the Waterworks Clauses Act, on which their case depended, and that therefore they had no remedy in such an emergency as that which had happened in July last, their remedy being an action for breach of contract by the Company. Mr. Newton was, however, of opinion that, although under a contract, the Company was liable to the penalties imposed by the Act of 1847, and he inflicted a fine of £10, with £6 6s. costs. The defendants gave notice of appeal. In his recent report on the general condition of the works of the Grand Junction Waterworks Company, Lieutenant Colonel Bolton, the official Water Examiner, gives an explanation of the causes which led to the failure of the supply in July last. He says: "There is no doubt whatever that the Company failed to meet the requirements of a part of their district between July 14 and 24, and that the cause of this failure is attributable to a deficiency in pumping power at Hampton, which power is limited to fourteen and a half million gallons per diem, when they actually required pumping power equal to twenty million gallons. This deficiency of pumping power would not have existed if the Company had carried out in its

entirely the project of the new works at Hampton decided upon some two years ago, but the directors were checked in their progress by the anticipated acquisition of their works by the Government in 1880, whereas the result shows that the project should have been carried out on the assumption that no such acquisition would be made, and thus a full year's time would have been saved, and the present short supply would not have occurred. By the end of the year, however, the new engines will be at work, and the pumping power of the Company will then be augmented to over twenty millions of gallons daily."

Dr. Tirard, one of the Physicians to the Evelina Hospital for Sick Children, has sent letters to the local boards and to the Charity Organisation Society, asking for aid in circumstances that cause sore trouble and vexation to hospital and dispensary physicians. He says: "I am constantly seeing cases of so-called wasting that appear to me to be often due simply to an insufficiency of proper food. The mothers, or far more often the people having the care of children, receive instructions as to the mode of feeding infants; they perhaps attend the hospital for two or three weeks, and then one day apply for a certificate of death. From an insufficient knowledge of what goes on in the homes we are rarely in a position to refuse to give a certificate; we have no direct evidence to take before a coroner, and thus I cannot but feel that our certificates of 'marasmus' (which we are obliged to give) very often cover wilful neglect. Of course, it would be easy to give information in such cases to lead to investigation after the death of a child, but my object in writing is to ascertain whether any steps cannot be taken to prevent the death. Punishment is all very well, but it seems to me that prevention would be better, if possible." Referring to the case of a child he had just seen, Dr. Tirard adds: "The mother states that she gives the child a pint of milk daily, and can afford to give more if the child would take it. We can at present find no sign of disease to account for the extreme emaciation; but we see the child whining in a low tone and constantly sucking its hands—two symptoms which are almost sure indications of insufficient food. If, by any inquiries you could make, neglect could be proved, we should have sufficient evidence to hold in terrorem over the mother, and induce her to treat her child properly." The St. Saviour's Board of Guardians have instructed a relieving officer to inquire into one of the cases mentioned.

A Blue-book consisting of more than five hundred pages has been recently issued, containing the evidence taken by the Select Committee of the House of Commons appointed to inquire into the Contagious Diseases Acts, 1866-69, their administration, operation, and effect. The Committee were instructed that they had power to receive evidence which might be tendered concerning similar systems in British colonies, or in other countries, and were to report whether the said Acts should, in their opinion, be maintained, amended, or repealed. The report states—"Your Committee have partly considered the subject referred to them, but have not been able to complete the inquiry. They have resolved to report the evidence already taken, and to recommend the reappointment of the Committee in the next session of Parliament."

On the complaint of Lord Ebury and Mr. Cook, a gentleman residing at Rickmansworth, the Rural Sanitary Authority of the Watford Union have taken proceedings against Mr. Colin Taylor, a local wharfinger, for infringing the Public Health Act by allowing offensive manure to be deposited on his wharf at Batchworth, and keeping it there longer than necessary. The case was defended on behalf of farmers in the district, who had been in the habit of landing manure at the wharf; but the Bench made an order for the abatement of the nuisance, and for the prevention of its recurrence, and directed the defendant to pay all costs.

We regret to learn that Professor William Warren Greene, of Portland, Maine, who recently attended the International Medical Congress in London, died while proceeding to New York in the Cunard steamer *Parthia*, and was buried at sea.

The arrangements necessary for the conversion of St. Margaret's Churchyard, adjoining Westminster Abbey, into a garden, for which a faculty has already been obtained, have been completed.

THE LONDON WATER-SUPPLY FOR THE MONTH OF AUGUST LAST.

THE official Water Examiner, in his report for the month of August last, remarks that the state of the water in the river Thames at Hampton, Molesey, and Sunbury, where the intakes of several of the London companies are situated, was good in quality during the whole of the month under notice. The water in the river Lea was also good during the whole of the month. These remarks, of course, refer to the condition of the water previous to filtration. The same good account is, however, confirmed by after examination; thus, Messrs. Crookes, Odling, and Tidy, in their report to the President of the Local Government Board, conclude as follows :—" Our daily examinations of the water delivered to London during the past month (August) satisfy us of its excellent quality, and of its suitability in every way for the supply of the metropolis. Further, our results, which are in accordance with those of all chemists who have examined and reported on the subject, show that the water of the Thames in its flow of some one hundred and thirty miles as a definite stream, does not acquire any increased proportion of organic matter, the amounts of organic carbon and of organic nitrogen existing in the water supplied by the companies not exceeding the amounts existing in the river water at Lechdale, where the main stream of the Thames is formed." Dr. Frankland also reports that the Thames water sent out by the Chelsea, West Middlesex, Southwark, Grand Junction, and Lambeth Companies was about the same in quality as during the last and two preceding months, being very much above the average of the water derived from this source. In every case the water was efficiently filtered before delivery. The Lea water supplied by the New River and East London Companies was also efficiently filtered, and of much better quality than usual; the New River Company's supply being indeed, as regards chemical purity, second only to the best of the deep-well waters, whilst that of the East London Company ranked with the better classes of Thames water.

DOMESTIC SCAVENGING IN DUBLIN.

AN inquiry was held on Tuesday last, at the City Hall, Dublin, by Dr. M'Cabe and Mr. Cotton, C.E., in connexion with the loan of £34,725, proposed to be raised by the Corporation of the city of Dublin for the sanitary improvement of the city. The City Accountant showed that, even with this loan, there would still be a margin within the sum Parliament allowed the Corporation to raise for sanitary improvements; and Mr. Young proved the need of the loan, and stated how it would be allotted. Dr. Charles Cameron then gave evidence as to the desirability of the Corporation taking upon itself the domestic scavenging works of the city, and stated that unless the proposed loan was obtained for the purposes set forth the work could not be carried on. The Corporation were bound to carry on the work, which was of the most vital importance as regarded the health of Dublin. He also urged the necessity of the loan being sanctioned, as affecting the condition of the tenement-dwellings of the City.

THE PARIS WEEKLY RETURN.

THE number of deaths for the thirty-seventh week, terminating September 16, was 935 (483 males and 452 females), and among these there were from typhoid fever 45, small-pox 18, measles 8, scarlatina 10, pertussis 7, diphtheria and croup 42, dysentery 1, erysipelas 4, and puerperal infections 5. There were also 42 deaths from tubercular and acute meningitis, 16 from acute bronchitis, 47 from pneumonia, 95 from infantile athrepsia (30 of the children having been wholly or partially suckled), and 24 violent deaths. The mortality continues very low, although it is 15 higher than that of the preceding week (920), the increase being chiefly due to typhoid fever, a disease which for six weeks past has been on the increase. This may be judged of by the weekly returns of cases treated at the Paris hospitals since July 30, which are as follow :—166, 175, 204, 248, 265, 317, 310, 309. With the exception of diphtheria, which maintains its terrible mean of about 40 deaths weekly, the other epidemics have declined. The efforts of the vaccinators have reduced the mortality from variola considerably. Together with the increase of the typhoid fever epidemic there has been an augmentation of deaths from diseases of the digestive organs, and it is possible that this arises from errors of diagnosis, the typhoid basis of some of the abnormal forms of some of these affections being overlooked. The affections of the digestive organs in early infancy (athrepsia), on the contrary, have undergone a great diminution, the deaths having descended from 254 at the end of July to 95 in the present week. The births for the week amounted to 1136, viz., 608 males '(443 legitimate and 160 illegitimate) and 523 females (378 legitimate and 145 illegitimate); 50 children were born dead or died within twenty-four hours.

THE LATE MR. A. B. STIRLING.

MANY an old Edinburgh student will hear with regret of the death of Mr. A. B. Stirling, a man well known to, and much esteemed by, many generations of students at the University of Edinburgh. Mr. A. B. Stirling, who was born in 1811, at Milngavie, Stirlingshire, was the son of a shoemaker, a man of great energy and vigour of character; and the son much resembled his father in force and independence of character. He was a born naturalist; as a lad, studied the habits of animals, prepared skeletons, stuffed birds, and was a keen fisher. He for many years followed his father's trade; then was a policeman, an inspector of police, and a gamekeeper. All this time he continued his study of natural history, and this brought him to the notice of the late Professor John Reid and Dr. Adamson, who employed him in arranging the University Museum of St. Andrews. Dr. Adamson recommended him to the late Professor Goodsir, who in 1856 appointed him Assistant-Conservator of the Anatomical Museum in the University of Edinburgh. In this position Mr. Stirling was able to follow fully the bent of his natural gifts; and he rapidly gained an excellent knowledge of both human and comparative anatomy, and became distinguished for his taste and dexterity in the preservation and display of anatomical preparations. He also devised new methods, was an accomplished microscopist, and invented a very useful and valuable microtome; and his microscopic preparations and injections became widely known. His knowledge of the habits and structure of fish also led him to take a keen interest in the " fungus disease " which so seriously affected salmon; and he communicated to the Royal Society of Edinburgh a series of memoirs on this disease, which contain the fullest and most exact information on its pathology that has yet been published. Our contemporary, the *Scotsman*, to which we are indebted for these notes of

Mr. Stirling, says of him : " He discharged his official duties in an ungrudging spirit. He spared no time or trouble when work was required of him. He had a kind word for all with whom he came in contact, and was ever ready to share his great store of knowledge and experience. He earned the confidence and esteem of the professors, and other medical and scientific men whose pursuits brought them into personal relation with him. He was encouraged and rewarded by the sympathy shown to him in his work ; and, unlike the naturalists of Banff and Thurso, whose careers have been recorded in so interesting a manner by Dr. Smiles, he was not left to struggle and strive in an uncongenial occupation, but found in the University a position which enabled him to cultivate science, and to promote, by his advice, ingenuity, and experience, the study of biology in this country."

REPORT ON THE HEALTH OF WATFORD FOR THE YEAR 1880.

IN presenting his annual report for the year 1880 to the Watford Local Board of Health, Dr. Alfred Brett, the Medical Officer of Health, remarks that the general sanitary condition of the district has been good. Diphtheria, mostly of a mild type, has been more frequent than it should be in a town that has the advantages of air, of soil, and of water that Watford has. In most of these cases, poisoning by sewer-gas appeared probable; in one case the water-closet, and in another the sewer, ventilated into the kitchen. Whooping-cough was also very fatal, partly caused by the coldness of the weather,—if it had not been for this, the zymotic death-rate would have been very low ; and there was not a single case of small-pox reported. The number of deaths registered in the district during the past year was 218, which gives a death-rate of 29·2 per 1000 on the actual population of 7461 at the census of 1871; but as eighty houses have been built in the district during 1880, if five people are allowed to each house, the population is probably 10,400. Assuming this latter estimate to be correct, the death-rate per 1000 will be reduced to 20·9. Again, of the 218 deaths, 39 occurred in the Union House Infirmary, and from this number 27 may fairly be deducted as the deaths of those who did not belong to the district, but came from other parishes; the total number of deaths will, therefore, be 191, equal to 18·3 per 1000. In concluding his report, Dr. Brett suggests to the Board that they should obtain more land for irrigation purposes, as it will be necessary to increase the present sewage works to meet the corresponding increase of population ; also that they should adopt the constant water-supply system, and build a home for the treatment of infectious diseases.

VACCINATION IN CHINA.

A RECENT speech of Sir John Pope Hennessy, Governor of Hong-kong, contains an interesting account of the spread of vaccination among the Chinese, not only of the colony, but of the empire. No port is more liable to the introduction of small-pox, yet it never spreads there. The health officer of the colony was also astonished to find that nearly all the young Chinese emigrants had vaccination or inoculation marks on their arms. That inoculation has been practised in China, as in other Eastern countries, from time immemorial, was already known, but the adoption of vaccination is quite recent, and he was surprised to find it so generally and perfectly performed. On inquiry he learnt that the native doctors of the Tung-wa Hospital—a charitable institution supported by the voluntary contributions of Chinese merchants and others—not only vaccinated their countrymen in the colony itself, but actually sent travelling vaccinators over the adjoining provinces of China. In this way

thousands of persons have been vaccinated during the past four years. The lymph is supplied to them by the Governor, who gets it by every mail in his dispatch-bag from Downing-street.

THE BOURTON-ON-THE-WATER COTTAGE HOSPITAL.

THE twentieth annual report of the Committee of Management of the Bourton-on-the-Water Cottage Hospital shows that this useful little local institution continues to do its work efficiently and well. During the year 1880, to which the report refers, 44 in-patients were under treatment, of whom 5 remained from the preceding year ; and of this number 37 were discharged cured or relieved, and 7 were still in hospital on January 1 of the present year. The average daily number of beds occupied was four, and the average time each patient remained in hospital was about thirty-six days, while it is satisfactory to note that there were no deaths. The number of out-patients was 487 during the year, 157 of these being new cases. The Honorary Secretary, Dr. W. C. Coles, who also fills the post of Honorary Physician to the Hospital, calls attention to the fact that some increase of donations or subscriptions is urgently required, as, although the new building admirably answers its intended purpose, yet some details still require to be carried out, and the sanitary arrangements are not entirely satisfactory, so that the balance at present in hand will not be sufficient to meet this extra expenditure. It may, however, be fairly assumed that the local gentry, who have so benevolently combined to establish this much-needed and excellently conducted charity, will not allow its usefulness to be impaired for the want of additional funds. There are still many districts in England, remote from any large centre, where the example afforded by the Bourton Cottage Hospital might with great advantage be followed.

THE DUBLIN ARTISANS' DWELLINGS COMPANY (LIMITED).

ON Monday, September 19, at the half-yearly meeting of the directors and shareholders of the Dublin Artisans' Dwellings Company, the report recommended payment of a dividend at the rate of 4 per cent. per annum for the half-year, the allocation of £196 8s. 7d. to pay off the balance of the preliminary expenses, and the carrying forward to the next account of £96 9s. 1d. The Chairman said that during the half-year they had received £1642 in rents, which was £102 more than was received during the previous half-year. Their expenses, however, were somewhat larger also, but this was partly accounted for by the severe frost of the winter, which did some damage to cisterns and pipes. The net balance of profit to be disposed of was £1103. Fifty-six new houses built in Kirwan-street had entirely answered the expectations of the directors ; and the contractor for the houses in the Coombe area was now pushing on their construction most vigorously. The sanitary condition of their property continued to be most satisfactory. On June 30 last they had 1428 inhabitants in their houses, as compared with 1304 on December 31 last. The mortality had been at the rate of 15 per 1000, while the death-rate of the city at large during the same period was 38 per 1000. He believed there was no doubt that the best way to reduce the death-rate in the city was to provide wholesome and comfortable houses for the working-classes, and he thought that nothing was more conducive to an improved morale of the people. They all had a deep interest in elevating and improving the condition of the working-classes; and as that Company had proved that they could build comfortable houses for the working-classes, and at the same time give a good return for the capital invested, he hoped that the public would come forward and take up more of the shares, and thus enable the directors to extend their operations.

FROM ABROAD.

UNIVERSITY COLLEGE MEDICAL SOCIETY.

WE understand that the annual address to the Medical Society of University College will be delivered on Wednesday, October 12, by Dr. J. Russell Reynolds, F.R.S., who takes for his subject "Specialism in Medicine." The Society will meet in the Botanical Theatre of University College; and the President, Mr. Dawson Williams, M.B., will take the chair at 8 p.m.

CALENDAR OF THE ROYAL COLLEGE OF SURGEONS OF ENGLAND.

THIS useful publication for the collegiate year 1881-82 has just been published, from which it appears that the not small army of 18,825 qualified practitioners are now inscribed in the College roll, viz.—1910 Fellows (of whom 573 obtained the distinction by examination), 16,140 Members, 978 Licentiates in Midwifery, and 497 Licentiates in Dental Surgery.

The Board of Examiners in Anatomy and Physiology conducts the primary examinations in these subjects for the diplomas of Fellow and Member, and during the past year held seven meetings for the former and thirty-nine for the latter, with the following results:—Of the 120 candidates for the Fellowship, 51 passed and 69 were referred for six months; and for the Membership there were 942 candidates, of whom 589 passed, 318 were referred for three months, and 35 for six months.

The Court of Examiners conducts the pass examinations in surgery and surgical anatomy, of candidates for the diplomas of Fellow and Member of the College. During the past collegiate year the Court has held two meetings for examinations for the former, and thirty-three for the latter. For the pass Fellowship there were 52 candidates, 30 of whom passed, and 22 were referred for one year. For the pass Membership there were 649 candidates examined, with the following results:—367 passed, 39 were approved in surgery but were required to qualify in medicine, 37 were approved in surgery and afterwards qualified in medicine, 243 were referred for six months, and 404 diplomas were granted.

The Board of Examiners in Dental Surgery held two meetings, and examined 22 candidates, 19 of whom were successful. During the past collegiate year there have been ten meetings of the Council.

With regard to the finances of the College, it appears that the income amounted to £16,848 17s. 6d., derived principally from fees paid by students on examinations, which realised £13,872 8s.; rents from chambers adjoining the College amounted to £1478; dividends on stock, £1075 9s. 5d.; fees paid by members of the Council, Court of Examiners, and Fellows on election amounted to £158 10s. The expenditure during the collegiate year amounted to £16,380 13s., the principal item being in fees paid to members of Council, and courts and boards of examiners, which amounted to £6761 13s.; salaries and wages for the officers and servants in the three departments—museum, library, and office—amounted to £4076 1s. 2d.; taxes, rates, and diploma stamps, £1395 14s. 2d.; the Barnard Davis collection of skulls, £500; the Hunterian Festival and Oration, in addition to receipts from fund, £112 15s. 2d.—leaving a balance at the bankers of £852 19s. 1d.

In looking down the list of prize essayists we see the members of the Council and Examiners represented by Mr. J. Birkett in 1848; Mr. J. W. Hulke, F.R.S., in 1859; Mr. John Wood, F.R.S., in 1861; and Mr. Christopher Heath in 1867.

On the Council we find the following gentlemen who have filled the high office of President of the College, viz.:—Sir James Paget, Bart., F.R.S.; Messrs. Prescott Hewett, John Birkett, Luther Holden, John E. Erichsen, F.R.S., and Erasmus Wilson, F.R.S.

Amongst Hunterian Orators still living are Arnott, South, Hawkins, Gulliver, Quain, Le Gros Clark, Paget, Humphry, and Holden. The recipients of the honorary medal of the College still living are Mr. George Bennett, F.R.C.S., of Sydney; Mr. W. L. Crowther, F.R.C.S., of Hobart Town; and Dr. T. B. Peacock, of Finsbury-circus.

There are some remarkable illustrations of longevity observable in the list of Fellows, several being nonagenarians. The oldest appears to be Mr. James Muscroft, of Pontefract, admitted a Member of the College in May, 1805; and presuming him then to have been of the required age of twenty-two, he must now be in his ninety-ninth year. Extreme old age is more observable amongst the Members:—Mr. Edward Ashton passed his examination so long ago as 1801, so that he is something more than one hundred years old. Nonagenarians are common amongst the Members.

FROM ABROAD.

THE PARIS HOSPITAL MORTALITY RETURNS.

DR. ERNEST BERNIER, in his report for the second quarter of 1881, states that the temperature of Paris (13·1° C.) was notably inferior to the mean of the corresponding period, which is 13·8° C.; and that the quantity of rain that fell, which during the first quarter was above the mean, sank below it in this second quarter. The general hospital mortality, as compared with that of the same quarter in 1880, underwent a great diminution, although it still remains (3624) superior to the mean of the same quarter (3338) of the nine preceding years. Still, the excess is so slight (286), that the mortality of the quarter may be considered as about normal.

1. Affections of the Respiratory Organs.—Pulmonary phthisis excepted (1589 cases, with 879 deaths), the mortality from which is regularly and progressively increasing from year to year, the affections of the respiratory organs have not exceeded the mean figure at the corresponding seasonary period, and their mortuary co-efficient is not raised above that which is proper to a hospital population, which, however, is always higher than the general mean. There were 809 cases of pneumonia, with 263 deaths (32 per cent.), 1450 cases of bronchitis with 77 deaths (5 per cent.), and 455 cases of pleurisy with 43 deaths (9 per cent.).

2. Diphtheria.—The epidemic of diphtheria remains still intense, although the number of deaths for the second quarter of 1881 is not larger than that of the same quarter of 1880. This second quarter is the normal epoch of the annual diphtheritic paroxysm, and an attenuation may be looked for in the third quarter. The total number of deaths from diphtheria in Paris for the first quarter in 1881 was 543, and of the second quarter 553; and the total number of cases of diphtheria and croup admitted into the hospitals during this second quarter was 343, with 212 deaths (61 per cent.):—viz., 150 cases of diphtheria with 70 (46 per cent.) deaths, and 193 cases of croup, with 142 (73 per cent.) deaths. On consulting the table, however, which Dr. Besnier gives of the sex and ages of the subjects of these diseases we find a discrepancy in the number of cases and deaths; and as this last table furnishes the details it must be the correct one. According to this, there were 150 cases of diphtheria admitted, with 80 deaths, viz., 18 adults (10 male and 8 female) with 7 deaths, and 132 children with 73 deaths (71 boys with 46 deaths, and 61 girls with 27 deaths)—i. e., a total of 80 instead of 70 deaths. Of cases of croup there were 2 in adults (both fatal), and 201 in children (203 altogether, instead of 193), of which number 102 occurred in boys with 73 deaths, and 99 in girls with 67 deaths. On the occasion of the death of Dr. Clozel de Boyer, one of the most promising internes of Prof. Parrot at the Hopital des Enfants, of diphtheria, Dr. Besnier renews a protest he has made before against allowing these frequent deaths of the young men engaged in the children's hospitals to go on without any attempt being made to prevent them. While, for the most trifling operations, disinfection by carbolic acid and other means is put into force, no precautions are taken with regard to those who have to perform autopsies or tracheotomies; and he suggests that these should be rendered compulsory, so that prevention of a disease that is so often incurable may be attempted. In the meantime, he proposes that the Medical Society of Hospitals should appoint a committee of those of its members who are connected with children's hospitals to consider and report upon the subject.

3. The Eruptive Fevers.—As has repeatedly been demonstrated in these reports, the eruptive fevers have a regular seasonary evolution, according to which small-pox undergoes a

decline in this quarter, while measles, scarlatina, and erysipelas increase. With respect to *scarlatina*, it is to be observed that not only is there this seasonary evolution, but its annual increase has for some time been observable. After remaining for many years extremely rare in Paris, and especially in the hospitals, it has now attacked individuals in all classes of society, and has made numerous victims at every age. "Here we have an epidemiological fact of great importance under all points of view. There would seem to be present a period of activity in the scarlatina germ which would be very favourable for an investigation instituted on the same plan as those which at the present time are pursued so actively in the pathology of animals. When shall we see human diseases submitted to the same investigations and benefited by the same progress?" During the second quarter there were admitted into the Paris hospitals 694 cases of small-pox, with 144 deaths; 195 cases of measles, with 36 deaths; 214 cases of scarlatina, with 20 deaths; and 349 cases of erysipelas, with 32 deaths.

4. *Small-pox.*—This disease exhibits a decrease not only in its proper seasonary evolution, but also in its "multi-annual" movement. Thus, while in all Paris there were registered 642 deaths from small-pox during the second quarter of 1880, there were only 296 registered during the second quarter of 1881; and from the first to the second quarter of 1881 the deaths descended from 356 to 296, and according to the seasonary law of the evolution of the disease they will descend still lower during the third or summer quarter. During the first quarter of 1881 there were received into the Paris hospitals 723 cases, of which 173 proved fatal; and during this second quarter there were 694 cases, with 164 deaths.

5. *Typhoid Fever.*—This disease underwent an exacerbation during the first quarter of this year, as it did also in the first quarter of 1880. In the first quarter of 1881 the deaths for all Paris amounted to 740, but following the seasonary law of its normal and regular decline in the spring quarter, it has sunk to 373 deaths during this second quarter—this mortality being still more than a third higher than the mean of the preceding ten years. During this second quarter of 1881 there were received into the Paris hospitals 865 cases, of which 176 (20 per cent.) proved fatal. Of the 861 cases, 480 were men, with 89 deaths; 301 women, with 65 deaths; 37 boys, with 8 deaths; and 47 girls, with 11 deaths.

MEDICAL ULTRAISMS.

Something more than amusement may be obtained from the following extracts, taken from an address delivered a while ago by Dr. Maughs, President of the Medical Association of the State of Missouri. The warnings they convey against exaggerations and perversions of specialism may not be needed so much in this country as in America, but that they are necessary will scarcely be denied.

"Within the last thirty years departments of the healing art that were embraced within the narrowest limits have widened into vast fields that engage the labours of the most intelligent and industrious to comprehend them. This has been accomplished by the division of labour whereby men of talent by devoting themselves to a single branch of medicine have been enabled to develope it to an extent otherwise impossible. But, while by this division of labour an infinite amount of good has been accomplished, which would have been impossible had all been general practitioners, there is now danger lest, all being specialists, none shall be general practitioners. Indeed, in some of our large cities, specialism is now carried to such an extreme, and the human body is so nicely mapped out and divided, that there is only left to the general practitioner or family physician the *umbilicus*. In country districts, where from necessity the physician has to treat all diseases, and consequently where specialism is an impossibility, the family doctor still holds his own; but in all our large cities and densely populated districts specialism revels in tropical luxuriance.

"Has a patient sore-throat, not the family physician who alone is acquainted with his constitutional peculiarities, but a nose and throat specialist is consulted, who, acting well his part, attacks the throat, without, it may be, any regard to the fellow who owns it. Has a feeble and delicate daughter just blushing into womanhood chorea, not again the general practitioner is consulted, but the neuro-pathologist, who, dominated by an idea, grapples with reflex spinal action and vaso-motor influences with a grip that knows no mercy to an enfeebled constitution. Has the wife a vaginal discharge, the gynæcologist is called in, who attacks the uterus with an earnestness that disregards the fact that there may possibly be a woman behind it. Has a man phthisis, not again the family physician, but the professor of physical diagnosis and diseases of the chest is called in, and here, again disregarding the man, the lungs are made accountable for the sins, it may be, of ten generations of ancestors. Has the father enlargement of the prostate, or diabetes, not the surgeon or the general practitioner, but the specialist in genito-urinary diseases is consulted. Has the grandmother cataract, not the surgeon, but the oculist is supposed to know enough of the case. Has the child some defect in hearing, not the family physician, or a nurse, but the aurist is alone supposed to be competent to wash out the ears. Has a member of the family epilepsy, an 'insane doctor' is sent for. I have seen the wife for some uterine complaint, the same day and perhaps at the same time another physician has seen the child for measles, another doctor the father for sore-throat, another the son for gonorrhœa, and the general practitioner or family physician the servant-girl for pain at the umbilicus—colic.

"Medicine has its fashions, and it is surprising to see how much good may be accomplished by simple means when fashionable. Some twelve or fifteen years ago, after the publication of Marion Sims' 'Uterine Surgery,' and the introduction of the euphonious duck-bill speculum with the left lateral semi-prone position, and the bilateral operation, it was discovered that, so potent were these, all the ills of womankind were at once met by them. In St. Louis, washerwomen, sewing-girls, and *nymphes du pavé* were chased down, rolled over in the left lateral semi-prone position, and the duck-bill being applied, were bilateralised with results truly magical. The most unpromising cases were by this simple process renovated, rejuvenated, fecundated, and delivered with wonderful certainty. One operator in St. Louis boasted of having thus blessed several hundred women within a short time. In 1868, in a paper read before this Association, I pointed out the errors of this, and showed that, instead of being the harmless operation it was said to be, several women had been allured to the bilateral Mecca, bilateralised, and then their bodies kindly returned to their friends.

"But, while the uterus has run the gauntlet, and is now permitted to rest from the importunities of the bilateralist, let no one suppose the gynæcologist less active in his philanthropic endeavours; he has only changed his point of attack from the uterus to the ovaries. Heretofore the modest, retiring ovaries, hidden away in the remotest recesses of the female economy, have been venerated as the Isis behind an impenetrable veil, being supposed in some way to be concerned in lending to lovely woman the charm of her womanhood, and to possess some importance in perpetuating the species; they are now, however, found to answer a more useful purpose, as they furnish the gynæcologist with a wide field for experiment, and that gynæcologist is an exception who has not killed half a dozen women in demonstrating the ease with which these pestiferous organs can be removed. One blessing supposed to result from such removal is that the woman becomes apathetic if not absolutely wanting in amenities towards the other sex, as well as utterly indifferent to the progress of semen, but there is no authority for this. What does the gynæcologist know about women? How many has he killed?

"In the ancient city of Cairo, in Egypt, on account of race, climate, and habitat, the nymphæ of many women are unduly developed, hypertrophied, requiring or justifying an operation for their removal; consequently the voice of the female circumcisor, as the voice of the vendor of oranges, may be heard crying through the streets, 'What woman wants to be cut?' There is a prospect, if this warfare and rivalry against the ovaries continues, that soon a like cry may be heard through the streets of St. Louis and New York, 'What woman wants to be spayed?' Normal ovariotomy (Battey's operation, as we call it—a placebo for many of the ills of womankind, it is true) often kills the woman, but this is of little consequence; it is the disease we are after, and this it cures radically: moreover, if it does kill the woman, this is not supposed to be the fault of the operation or of the operator, but must be attributed to a female weakness, and, like Sangrado's practice of blood-letting and warm water, should not be given up merely because patients are so obstinate as to die rather than to confirm the wisdom of the theory. Now, without entirely ostracising this operation—for there are extreme cases where it gives the only promise of preserving life, as in the case reported by Dr. Richmond, of St. Joseph, where, from an incurable *atresia vaginæ*, there was no possibility of giving exit to the menstrual blood, and in other conditions where life is alike endangered, or in rare and unfortunate incurable cases where the mind is secondarily affected, it affords a last hope and should be resorted to,—we venture the prediction that in ten years it will be as rare to find a gynæcologist who is willing to perform normal ovariotomy merely for convenience or notoriety, as it is now to find one who is not thirsting to do so for either or both of these reasons."

FOREIGN AND COLONIAL CORRESPONDENCE.

CASE OF INTUSSUSCEPTION IN AN INFANT.

"Ne quid nimis."

A NOTICE "On the Diagnosis of Intestinal Intussusception," which appeared in your issue of June 18 last, induces me to send you the following case, which, although of no practical value, is nevertheless not without interest to the profession; I would ask, therefore, for its insertion in your valuable columns:—

On March 30 last, at 10 a.m., I was called to see an infant seven months old. He was of fair complexion and well nourished. Up to the day before, he had enjoyed good health; and his bowels had acted regularly. But about 3 p.m. that day he vomited twice. A few hours afterwards his mother gave him two teaspoonfuls of rhubarb syrup. He had passed a not restless night; but his bowels had not been moved till next morning early, when he had two motions. At the same time he was seized with frequent vomiting. I found him lying in his nurse's arms. There were no urgent symptoms; vomiting had ceased about an hour before my arrival, the countenance was not anxious, the tongue was moist and clean, the abdomen slightly distended, and on examining it I did not detect anything noteworthy, with the exception of some tenderness on pressure. The pulse was not feeble, and was scarcely above the natural rate. There was neither fever nor lowering of the normal temperature; the pupils were not dilated. I was shown the two motions passed that morning; they were rather copious and natural. I ordered—R. Calomel. gr. iiss., pulv. jalap. gr. iss., sacch. gr. ij., to be divided into two powders, the second to be given half an hour after the first; and R. Subnitratis bismuthi gr. xxx., looch. albi 3 viij., syrupi diacodj. 3 iiss.; one teaspoonful to be given every hour, commencing an hour after the administration of the above powders.

At three o'clock in the afternoon I was sent for. On my arrival, the mother stated that soon after my departure the child began to be sick and to vomit everything he took. Accordingly, the drugs had been not long retained, and that about an hour previously he had two fæcal motions, after which he continued to pass blood. He had since continued to be sick, vomiting everything, and to pass blood and blood-stained mucus, with tenesmus. The pulse was quicker than in the morning, but there was no fever. On examining the abdomen, which was then more distended than before, I found in the left hypochondriac region, at the end of the transverse and the descending colon, a sausage-shaped tumour, about an inch and a half in length, very distinctly felt. Nothing could be made out on rectal examination.

Seeing the gravity of the illness, I requested a consultation. Meanwhile, I proceeded to inject air gently by means of an enema syringe. On account of the lump remaining unchanged, I injected cold water. As the water was injected I continued to examine the tumour. At first the water returned directly without effect, but after little more than a pint and a half had been thus injected, the tumour had entirely disappeared.

The physician called in consultation arrived just after the disappearance of the tumour. Having heard the history of the case, and after examination of the patient, he arrived at an altogether different and unexpected diagnosis: that "the case was one of intestinal irritation, and not one of intussusception."

Two hours afterwards another consultation was held with the above-mentioned and a third physician. The infant was then almost constantly sick, vomited frequently, and passed blood and mucus with straining; there was no fever; abdomen more distended, and a tumour about two inches in length and thick as a man's middle-sized finger was felt in the left iliac fossa. Passed urine as usual. The third physician was agreed with me as to the diagnosis and treatment, but the other persisted in his diagnosis.

March 31, 10 a.m.—The child had passed a bad night; sickness and vomiting continued, as also the passage of slimy mucus with blood and tenesmus. The abdomen was tympanitic; the tumour in the left iliac fossa much larger. The temperature of the skin was elevated, but the thermometer showed no fever. The respiration was not much quickened. The infant occasionally cried; waking alternated at times with coma, from which he was soon roused by the nausea. Our *confrère* persisted in his cherished diagnosis, and in supporting it observed that "in order to rightly judge we should make a good appreciation of the facts," —that is to say, he appealed to logic.(a)

At 6 p.m. we saw the child with a fourth *confrère*, who agreed with me as to diagnosis and treatment. Vomiting became less frequent. The mother stated that he had vomited some bilious-like stuff. From twelve o'clock till half-past two nothing had been passed from the anus, and thence till six o'clock (the time of consultation) he had only two motions, consisting of a very small quantity of mucus with blood, which we did not see. The abdomen was decidedly tympanitic, the general state worse. The physician last called in felt with the finger the intussuscepted bowel. Before this consultation the dissident *confrère* began to speak about an operation, which otherwise the father of the child opposed.

The child growing worse, his strength failed, and he died next day.

1881.　　　　　　　　　　　　　　D. EUSTRATIADES.

GENERAL CORRESPONDENCE.

THE HYPODERMIC EMPLOYMENT OF QUININE.
LETTER FROM DEP. SURG.-GEN. MOORE.

[To the Editor of the Medical Times and Gazette.]

SIR,—The origination of the method of using quinine by subcutaneous injection has, I observe, been attributed to several gentlemen. I therefore beg your permission to state that I first used quinine in this manner, when Assistant-Surgeon to the European General Hospital in Bombay, in 1862. The method was brought before the Bombay Medical and Physical Society in March, 1863, and in August of the same year an article of mine was published in the *Lancet*, detailing my manner of procedure in what I then designated "this novel mode of using quinine."

I am, &c.,　　　W. J. MOORE,
Deputy Surgeon-General H.M. Forces, Bombay.
Bombay, September 6.

ENTERIC FEVER IN QUETTAH.—It is reported that several cases of enteric (typhoid) fever have lately, during the summer, occurred amongst the British troops at Quettah. There has been no doubt as to the diagnosis, as it has been verified by the existence of the usual lesions at post-mortem examinations. It is stated also that a few cases have occurred among native troops there. Most of the cases among the British troops were in young men, of short service and recently out.

(a) No doubt every man, be he whom he may, not only has a right, but is compelled, unknown to him, to make use of logic; for, as a competent writer rightly says, "Even to demonstrate that we must not philosophise, it is necessary to philosophise." Unfortunately, however, for the human kind, this natural logic is far short from enabling us to judge rightly. Even the science of logic points out many dangerous sources of errors, with which even the soundest thinkers are beset, and into which we ignorant and poor in spirit so easily and so frequently fall. For which reason we ought always to bear in mind that—
"Melius est aliter ere gradum quam progredi per tenebras."

MEDICAL NEWS.

THE ROYAL COLLEGE OF SURGEONS OF ENGLAND.—
The half-yearly preliminary examinations in Arts, etc., for
the diplomas of the College have just been brought to a close,
and out of the 649 candidates examined, the following were
successful :—

Messrs. A. J. Adkins, E. D. Agnew, W. E. Allard, O. W. Andrews,
G. D. Atkinson, A. M. Atkinson, C. J. Ayres, R. G. Bagley, A. E. Baker,
T. R. Baker, William Barrett, C. A. Barstow, Charles Batchelor, R. F.
Bate, A. H. Beardmore, R. H. Beardsley, Sydney Beauchamp, E. E.
Belcher, J. C. Bell, F. H. Bence, W. L. Bentley, Alfred Berrill, W. H.
Best, W. J. Best, B. W. Bickle, A. F. Bilderbeck, J. H. Blakeney, J. H.
Blamey, J. T. Blancard, F. W. Bloomer, A. H. Blunt, J. W. Boden, R. B.
Booth, F. H. Boyer, Harry Boyle, A. F. Bradbury, Frank Bradshaw,
Horace Brenchley, A. J. Briant, F. S. Bright, S. C. Bright, Norman
Brodie, J. T. Brierley, E. E. Brook, F. J. Brown, F. R. W. Brown,
W. J. M. Brühling, F. W. A. Bryden, C. R. H. Buckby, A. E.
Bullock, Herbert Burland, F. C. Bury, L. C. E. Calthrop, Robert
Capes, F. C. Carden, T. G. Carr, F. F. Chambers, R. H. Chapman,
G. L. Cheatle, Brown Clark, J. T. Clarke, R. W. Clayton, C. H. Coffin,
O. C. Coker, W. H. Carter, A. L. Chignall, E. Colman, J. A. Coleclough,
T. Coleman, H. J. Collins, C. T. T. Comber, F. W. Cooper, W. F.
Cooper, J. G. D. Cort, J. K. Couch, E. J. Courtenay, W. R. Cox, J. D.
Cree, F. A. Cribb, A. J. Cross, H. P. Cuthbert, C. P. Curtis, J. F. Dawson,
A. G. E. de Vallancey, D. N. P. Datta, W. M. Davidson, H. Davis, Ernest
Dawson, E. I. Day, J. G. Desborough, C. E. Dew, Herbert Diemer, G. W.
Dowling, P. H. Dunn, H. de B. Dwyer, C. G. Dwyer, T. J. Dyall, S. P.
Eastick, A. D. Ellis, W. C. Ellis, Charles Ellisson, Joseph Ellison, J. F.
Farrar, R. H. Faulkner, John Fawcett, E. D. Fawkes, A. C. Fenn, D. G.
Firth, W. F. Fisher, G. E. FitzGerald, F. J. Fletcher, G. S. Flux, W. P.
Fordham, Frank Fowler, F. G. T. Fox, S. C. G. Fox, H. S. Fremlin, John
Fullard, A. N. Gamble, F. G. Gardner, B. Garrett, John Garth, George
Gautby, A. J. Gedge, C. T. Getting, Mark Glanville, James Godding,
J. H. Godwin, N. J. Goodchild, C. H. Goodman, R. F. Gordon, C.
Goullet, J. W. F. Graham, Arthur Greenhalgh, Arthur Greenwood,
T. R. E. Griffiths, M. S. W. Gunning, G. A. Gunton, W. G. Gyton,
E. S. Haddy, Edmund Hall, Rowland Hall, John Hancocks, A. E.
Hardy, C. C. Harris, D. H. Harris, S. H. Harrison, Llewellyn
Harris, D'Arcy Harvey, J. A. S. Harvey, J. M. Hay, M. H. Hay,
E. M. Hearnden, C. P. K. Hemming, Eugene Henry, H. B. Hether-
ington, F. W. Hildyard, J. H. Hill, C. P. Hird, B. B. Hoggan, J. C.
Holderness, P. K. Holman, Joshua Holt, T. E. Honey, S. P. Hosegood,
F. M. House, A. B. M. Howard, T. M. Hawkins, C. T. Hudson, P. H.
Hudson, H. Hudson, F. H. Hurcombe, A. H. W. Hunt, C. W. Jackson,
G. T. James, J. L. Jeaffreson, G. R. Jenkins, T. E. Johnson, R. L.
Johnston, A. E. Jones, G. M. Jones, R. Jones, S. Jones, O. F. Joynson,
Frank Jubb, W. E. Kelbe, H. T. Kelsall, P. J. Kitson, W. R. Laidlay,
E. J. Lang, H. Lawson, C. M. Leakey, J. W. Leech, Cyrus Legg, F. R.
Le Queene, C. S. D. Leslie, B. A. Lewis, Frederick Lewis, F. H. Lewis,
L. O. Lindridge, P. A. Linnell, T. W. M. Longmore, Ernest Loveday, W.
H. Lyon, John Maberly, P. B. Mackay, G. I. Mackfunn, F. R. Mallard,
H. E. Mansell, Richard Markland, C. L. Martin, H. F. C. Marvin,
J. F. McClean, F. H. A. McCormick, E. E. McCrea, Henry McVeagh,
N. W. W. Meadows, P. H. S. Mellish, Charles Mitzgar, A. D. Miller,
A. S. Milner, H. R. Mitchell, J. MacS. Mitchell, F. P. Moles, J. E.
Molson, J. C. Morgan, W. V. Morgan, A. O. F. L. Morrell, John Muriel,
Robert Nairn, Ben Naylor, Arthur Nicholson, B. S. G. Nightingall, R. N.
Norgate, Albert Norman, John Norton, J. F. Norton, H. B. Osburn, Peter
Paget, C. E. R. Falk, C. A. Parker, T. F. Parkinson, C. O'G. Parsons,
F. G. Parsons, J. S. Part, Frank Pearce, G. E. Pearson, R. S. Peeke, E. V.
Pegge, R. H. Perkins, A. E. D. R. Peters, W. B. Pettitt, A. J. Pickthorn,
C. H. Pilliner, L. J. Pisani, J. E. Platt, T. A. B. Plowman, W. H. H. Plow-
man, H. J. Pocock, A. B. Price, C. F. W. Price, H. T. Preston, E. A. Quicke,
Richard Ray, F. B. Reed, L. St. J. Reilly, W. V. Reynolds, W. L. Rhys, R. C.
Richards, W. H. Richardson, A. W. Riddell, J. W. Rigby, A. E. G. Roberts,
F. H. Roberts, H. B. Roberts, J. W. Roberts, Reginald Roberts, G. H.
Robinson, V. H. Rocher, S. J. Roderick, H. D. Rolleston, F. J. W.
Rogers, William Routh, O. T. Samman, J. E. Sargent, J. G. V. Sapp, T. W.
Sargent, E. P. Satchell, F. L. Seale, P. G. Selby, E. W. Sharman, Giles
Shaw, W. C. Sheard, W. F. M. Shells, J. L. B. Sherlock, A. D. Skinner,
S. C. Skipton, W. B. Slyman, B. G. D. Speedy, W. J. Spoor,
W. J. Staddon, C. T. Standing, C. J. Stanley, W. H. C. Staveley,
D. R. P. Stephens, H. W. Stephens, H. S. Stockton, H. J. Stoner, G. W.
Stringfield, B. Sumner, H. E. T. Symons, C. H. Tattershall, F. B.
Taylor, J. B. Thickins, A. W. Thompson, J. H. Thompson, F. G. Twigg,
Louis Vallée, A. E. Vidler, A. W. Wainwright, E. T. Walker, H. A.
Walker, M. E. A. Wallis, John Walton, W. P. Warburton, A. V. R.
Warde, C. L. Warke, Sydney Warren, Edwin Webster, John Webb,
Charles Welch, W. B. Welch, W. W. Welch, R. H. Wellington, L. S.
Wells, C. E. H. West, H. J. Wheeler, G. H. Whitaker, F. H. Whitehead,
R. H. W. Wilbe, G. H. Wilkinson, E. L. Williams, G. H. Williams, G. R.
Williams, T. H. Williams, A. Winterbottom, A. S. Wood, A. V. Wood,
H. de C. Woodcock, S. Woodhams, J. D. Woodhouse, J. T. Woodhouse,
J. F. Woodyatt, W. L. Woollcombe, George Wordsworth, Henry Worsley,
Alfred Wright, B. J. E. Wright, G. H. L. Wright, P. Wright, E. W. P.
Wright, W. L. Wyatt, W. H. Yeld, Stanley Yeoman, George Ley, W. A.
Mercer, F. W. Turtle, C. E. Thomas.

The preliminary examinations of the College having now
come to an end, all inquiries with respect to the recognised preliminary examinations should be addressed to the
Registrar of the General Medical Council.

APOTHECARIES' HALL, LONDON.—The following gentle-
man passed his examination in the Science and Practice of
Medicine, and received a certificate to practise, on Thursday,
September 22 :—

Wigan, Charles Arthur, Portishead, Somerset.

The following gentlemen also on the same day passed their
primary professional examination :—

Forrest, James Rocheid, St. Bartholomew's Hospital.
Vivian, George Ernest, St. Thomas's Hospital.
Whitten, Samuel, Mercer's Hospital, Dublin.

APPOINTMENTS.

*** The Editor will thank gentlemen to forward to the
Publishing-office, as early as possible, information as to
all new Appointments that take place.

LANE, J. ERNEST, M.R.C.S.—Demonstrator of Anatomy at St. Mary's
Hospital Medical School.
ORR, W. Y., M.B. Edin., M.R.C.S.—Assistant House-Surgeon to the
Northern Hospital, Liverpool, vice W. R. Parker, B.A., M.B. Cantab.,
M.R.C.S., resigned.
PARKER, WILLIAM RUSHTON, B.A., M.B. Cantab., M.R.C.S.—House-
Physician to the Northern Hospital, Liverpool, vice C. H. R. Shears,
M.R.C.S., L.R.C.P., resigned.
PHILLIPS, SIDNEY, M.D.—Demonstrator of Anatomy at St. Mary's
Hospital Medical School.

NAVAL, MILITARY, Etc., APPOINTMENTS.

ADMIRALTY.—Staff Surgeon John Sampson Levis, M.D., has been promoted to the rank of Fleet Surgeon in Her Majesty's Fleet, with
seniority of August 19, 1881.—Staff Surgeon Edward Mulcahy has
been promoted to the rank of Fleet Surgeon in Her Majesty's Fleet,
with seniority of September 17, 1881.

BIRTHS.

ADAMS.—On September 21, at 184, Aldersgate-street, E.C., the wife of
John Adams, L.R.C.P., of a daughter.
BARNES.—On September 23, at Dorset House, Ewell, Surrey, the wife of
G. R. Barnes, M.D., of a son.
BRANDER.—On August 19, at Ranchee, Bengal, the wife of Surgeon E. S.
Brander, M.B., of a son.
CLOTHIER.—On September 25, at 1, North-road, Highgate, London, the
wife of Henry Clothier, M.D., of a son.
GRIFFIN.—On September 26, at 12, Royal-terrace, Weymouth, the wife of
F. C. G. Griffin, M.A., M.B., of a son.
GROSS.—On September 24, at Westmoreland-road, Walworth, the wife of
Charles Gross, L.R.C.P., of a daughter (stillborn).
MUMBY.—On September 18, at Iver, Bucks, the wife of B. H. Mumby,
M.D., of twin sons.
PARKER.—On September 15, at Haverigg House, Gosforth, Cumberland,
the wife of Charles A. Parker, M.D., of a son.
TURTLE.—On September 19, at 35, High-street, Homerton, the wife of
James H. Turtle, M.D., of a son.

MARRIAGES.

AITKEN—BOUCH.—On September 21, at Hanover-square, Lauchlan Aitken,
M.D., of Rome, to Fanny, elder daughter of the late Sir Thomas
Bouch, C.E.
CHAVASSE—MAUDE.—On September 27, at Overton, Flintshire, Francis
James Chavasse, M.A., Rector of St. Peter-le-Bailey, Oxford, fifth son
of Thomas Chavasse, F.R.C.S., to Edith Jane, younger daughter of the
late Rev. Canon Maude, Vicar of Chirk, Denbighshire.
MARSHALL—SMYTHIES.—On September 24, at Hathern Church, Leicester-
shire, Lewis Walter Marshall, M.D., of Nottingham, to Frances
Elizabeth Ethel, youngest daughter of the Rev. E. Smythies, Rector of
Hathern, etc.

DEATHS.

BATTYE, RICHARD FAWCETT, M.R.C.P., at 123, St. George's-road, S.W.,
on September 23, in his 61st year.
BOULTON, GEORGIANA CAROLINE, wife of Albert E. Boulton, M.R.C.S., at
Horncastle, on September 21.
POLLARD, JAMES, M.R.C.S. Eng., on September 26, aged 50.
RAWBONE, GEORGE, F.R.C.S., at Athole House, Tooting, Graveney, Surrey,
on September 19, in his 83rd year.
ROGERS, EMMA WATSON, wife of Henry C. Rogers, M.R.C.S., Newport-
Pagnell, on September 26.
WINN, EMELYNE BELLE, wife of J. M. Winn, M.D., of 51, Harley-street,
Cavendish-square, on September 23.

VACANCIES.

In the following list the nature of the office vacant, the qualifications required in the candidate, the person to whom application should be made
and the day of election (as far as known) are stated in succession.

BOSCOMBE PROVIDENT INFIRMARY, BOURNEMOUTH. — Resident House-
Surgeon. (For particulars see Advertisement.)
CLINICAL HOSPITAL AND DISPENSARY FOR WOMEN AND CHILDREN, PARK-
PLACE, MANCHESTER. — House-Surgeon. (For particulars see Adver-
tisement.)
ESSEX AND COLCHESTER HOSPITAL.—Physician. Candidates are requested
to forward their names and qualifications, together with original testi-
monials, to the Secretary on or before October 5.
METROPOLITAN ASYLUMS BOARD.—Assistant Medical Officer for the
Leavesden Asylum for Imbeciles, near Watford. (For particulars see
Advertisement.)
QUEEN'S HOSPITAL, BIRMINGHAM.—Casualty Surgeon. Candidates must
be Fellows or Members of the Royal College of Surgeons of England,
Edinburgh, or Dublin. Applications and testimonials, with certificate
of registration, to be sent to the Secretary at the Hospital, from whom
all further information may be obtained, on or before October 5.

INFIRMARY OF THE CITY OF LONDON UNION.—Assistant Medical Officer. (*For particulars see Advertisement.*)

SUSSEX COUNTY HOSPITAL, BRIGHTON.—Assistant House-Surgeon. (*For particulars see Advertisement.*)

WESTERN OPHTHALMIC HOSPITAL, 155, MARYLEBONE-ROAD.—Surgeon. Candidates must be fellows or members of the Royal College of Surgeons, and have attended ophthalmic practice for twelve months. Applications to be made to the Secretary at the Hospital.

UNION AND PAROCHIAL MEDICAL SERVICE.

*** The area of each district is stated in acres. The population in computed according to the census of 1871.

RESIGNATIONS.

Bellingham Union.—Dr. James Mitchell Monteith has resigned the Fourth District: area 12,625; population 1128; salary £12 per annum.

Birmingham Parish.—The office of Assistant Medical Officer at the Workhouse is vacant by the resignation of Dr. A. C. Suffern. Salary £130 per annum.

Kington Union.—Mr. G. Foote has resigned the Kington District and the Workhouse: area 16,784; population 1740; salary £55 per annum. Salary for Workhouse £25 per annum.

Knaresborough Union.—The offices of Medical Officer for the Scriven District and the Workhouse are vacant by the resignation of Mr. W. Bulmer: area 4989; population 1945; salary £30 per annum. Salary for the Workhouse £50 per annum.

Newark Union.—The Bennington, Claypole, and Foston Districts are vacant by the death of Mr. William Bell Irving. Bennington District: area 12,770; population 2068; salary £24. Claypole District: area 3943; population 952; salary £10. Foston District: area 7868; population 1191; salary £14.

Peterborough Union.—The Stilton District is vacant by the death of Mr. Thomas Gregory Wright: area 18,420; population 3514; salary per case.

Spalding Union.—Mr. Robert E. Hunt has resigned the Pinchbeck District. Area 15,468; population 3846; salary £51 per annum.

Totnes Union.—The Totnes and Berry Pomeroy Districts are vacant by the death of Mr. A. J. Wallis. Totnes District: area 4080; population 4120; salary £82 per annum. Berry Pomeroy District: area 8181; population 2001; salary £35 per annum.

Wakefield Union.—The First District is vacant by the death of Mr. F. C. Jennings: area 732; population 21,066; salary £100 per annum.

APPOINTMENTS.

Ashbourne Union.—Arthur E. Broster, M.R.C.S. Eng., L.R.C.P. Edin., to the Brassington District.

Barnet Union.—Thomas William Thompson, L.R.C.S. Eng., L.R.C.P. Edin., and L.S.A. Lond., to the Second District.

Barton-upon-Irwell Union.—Thomas Fiddes, B.M. and M.C. Aber., to the Urmston and Flixton District.

Battle Union.—Charles Hoar, B.M., M.C. Aberd., to the Fifth District.

Blaby Union.—Edward H. Snoad, M.R.C.S. Eng., L.S.A., to the Aylestone District.

Derby.—Otto Hehner, F.C.S., as Analyst for the county, *vice* Denis Coyle, resigned.

Dover Union.—John Ormsby, L.R.C.P. Edin., L.R.C.S. Edin., to the St. Mary's District.

Hertford.—Charles Heisch, F.C.S., appointed Analyst for the County. Remuneration by fees.

Kington Union.—Arthur George Rawson Harris, L.R.C.P. Lond. and M.R.C.S. Eng., to the Eardisley District.

Reeth Union.—Francis J. Turner, L.R.C.P. Edin., L.F.P.& S. Glasg., to the Muker District.

Reigate Union.—Thomas C. Lawson, M.R.C.S. Eng., L.S.A., to the Fourth District.

St. Leonard (Shoreditch) Parish.—David Lloyd, L.R.C.P. Edin., L.R.C.S. Edin., as Assistant Medical Officer to the Infirmary and the Workhouse.

West Derby Union.—Ralph Worrall, M.D., M.Ch. Ire., as Assistant Medical Officer to the Walton Workhouse.

FORMULÆ.—1. *Hæmostatic Pills:* Dr. Huchard often employs the following formula in various kinds of hæmorrhage, as metrorrhagia, hæmoptysis, epistaxis, etc.:—Ergotine, sulph. quinine, āā two grammes, powder of digitalis, extract of henbane, āā twenty centigrammes, in twenty pills; from five to ten to be taken daily. 2. *Constipation:* Four pills daily may be given to an individual the subject of constipation, each pill consisting of powdered sulphate of iron ten centigrammes, socotrine aloes five centigrammes, and extract of belladonna one centigramme. If there be ataxy of the intestines, for the belladonna we may substitute extract of nux vomica in the dose of from five milligrammes to one centigramme.—*Gaz. des Hop.*, September 17.

DIPHTHERIA IN RUSSIA.—According to an extract from the *Journal de St. Pétersbourg*, in the *Progrès Méd.*, September 17, the fearful ravages of diphtheria during the last ten years or so have exceeded those caused by the plague or by cholera, almost all the children of some localities having been carried off. The epidemic is still spreading, and even the two capitals have begun to suffer from it. In distinction to former epidemics the present one has been called the "great epidemic of diphtheria," and it is stated to have originated in Bessarabia in 1872, whence it spread during the eight following years into many "governments." The centre of this great epidemic was therefore in the south of the empire, whence it spread to the east and north-west, following the direction of the winds of the southern region of Russia in Europe. The last governments which have become infected are those of Tamboff, Saratoff, and Samara; but the exact returns from these are not yet known. In Bessarabia, from 1872 to 1879, in 35,538 cases there were 19,949 deaths; in the government of Poltava, the worst stricken of all, of 45,543 cases, of which 18,765 died; and in that of Karkof there were 17,048 deaths in 28,750 cases. There is every reason to believe that these numbers are below the reality; and it is certain that the mortality increases in proportion to the number of cases.

ALLEGED PRECOCIOUS MENSTRUATION.—Dr. Zeller, of Beamsville, Ohio, reports the following facts of a case of precocious menstruation:—"The child is now five months old, and began menstruating at the end of two months. It has now menstruated three times at regular intervals of four weeks, the menses lasting for three or four days. The parents came to me for advice, but as the child is very healthy there is nothing to be done. Bedford relates a case where the child was as young as twelve months, but does not seem to have placed much faith in it."—*New York Med. Record*, September 3.

RECREATION GROUNDS FOR LONDON.—The inhabitants of the district of Tottenham-court-road intend to petition the trustees of the place of worship known as Whitefield's Tabernacle, with a view to converting the adjacent graveyard into a garden for the use of the public. The ground known as St. John's Burial-ground, in Horseferry-road, Westminster, will, it is understood, be brought under the notice of the Court of Arches, in order that it may be converted into a recreation-ground for the inhabitants.

GRISCOM'S FAST.—At the beginning of the fast the experimenter weighed $197\frac{3}{4}$ lbs. At the end of the seventh day he had lost $18\frac{3}{4}$ lbs.; by the thirteenth day, $19\frac{1}{2}$ lbs.; by the twenty-first day, $29\frac{1}{2}$ lbs.; by the thirty-first day, $34\frac{3}{4}$ lbs.; and by the fortieth day (when he weighed $151\frac{1}{2}$ lbs.), $46\frac{1}{4}$ lbs. His abdomen, thigh, calf, arm, and forearm were measured on the first day and on the forty-second day, when the measurements were found to have diminished as follows:—Abdomen, $43\frac{3}{4}$ to 30; thigh, 21 to $17\frac{1}{2}$; calf, 16 to $12\frac{3}{4}$; arm, $12\frac{1}{4}$ to $10\frac{1}{2}$; and forearm, $11\frac{1}{2}$ to $9\frac{3}{4}$. No marked changes are given regarding the pulse, respiration, and temperature. He drank from twenty-four to forty-eight ounces of water daily. His strength continued to the end, and he often walked considerable distances during the last part of the fast. He is said to have been watched by several respectable physicians.—*New York Med. Record*, August 13.

APPOINTMENTS FOR THE WEEK.

October 1. *Saturday (this day).*

Operations at St. Bartholomew's, $1\frac{1}{2}$ p.m.; King's College, $1\frac{1}{2}$ p.m.; Royal Free, 2 p.m.; Royal London Ophthalmic, 11 a.m.; Royal Westminster Ophthalmic, $1\frac{1}{2}$ p.m.; St. Thomas's, $1\frac{1}{2}$ p.m.; London, 2 p.m.

3. *Monday.*

Operations at the Metropolitan Free, 2 p.m.; St. Mark's Hospital for Diseases of the Rectum, 2 p.m.; Royal London Ophthalmic, 11 a.m.; Royal Westminster Ophthalmic, $1\frac{1}{2}$ p.m.

4. *Tuesday.*

Operations at Guy's, $1\frac{1}{2}$ p.m.; Westminster, 2 p.m.; Royal London Ophthalmic, 11 a.m.; Royal Westminster Ophthalmic, $1\frac{1}{2}$ p.m.; West London, 3 p.m.

5. *Wednesday.*

Operations at University College, 2 p.m.; St. Mary's, $1\frac{1}{4}$ p.m.; Middlesex, 1 p.m.; London, 2 p.m.; St. Bartholomew's, $1\frac{1}{2}$ p.m.; Great Northern, 2 p.m.; Samaritan, $2\frac{1}{2}$ p.m.; King's College (by Mr. Lister), 2 p.m.; Royal London Ophthalmic, 11 a.m.; Royal Westminster Ophthalmic, $1\frac{1}{2}$ p.m.; St. Thomas's, $1\frac{1}{2}$ p.m.; St. Peter's Hospital for Stone, 2 p.m.; National Orthopædic, Great Portland-street, 10 a.m.

OBSTETRICAL SOCIETY, 8 p.m. Specimens will be shown. Dr. Ernest Herman, "On the Relation of Anteflexion of the Uterus to Dysmenorrhœa."

6. *Thursday.*

Operations at St. George's, 1 p.m.; Central London Ophthalmic, 1 p.m.; Royal Orthopædic, 2 p.m.; University College, 2 p.m.; Royal London Ophthalmic, 11 a.m.; Royal Westminster Ophthalmic, $1\frac{1}{2}$ p.m.; Hospital for Diseases of the Throat, 2 p.m.; Hospital for Women, 2 p.m.; Charing-cross, 2 p.m.; London, 2 p.m.; North-West London, $2\frac{1}{2}$ p.m.

7. *Friday.*

Operations at Central London Ophthalmic, 2 p.m.; Royal London Ophthalmic, 11 a.m.; South London Ophthalmic, 2 p.m.; Royal Westminster Ophthalmic, $1\frac{1}{2}$ p.m.; St. George's (ophthalmic operations), $1\frac{1}{4}$ p.m.; Guy's, $1\frac{1}{2}$ p.m.; St. Thomas's (ophthalmic operations), 2 p.m.

VITAL STATISTICS OF LONDON.

Week ending Saturday, September 24, 1881.

BIRTHS.

Births of Boys, 1900; Girls, 1130; Total, 2830.
Corrected weekly average in the 10 years 1871–80, 2535·0.

DEATHS.

	Males.	Females.	Total.
Deaths during the week ...	662	617	1279
Weekly average of the ten years 1871–80, corrected to increased population ...	711·5	675·4	1386·9
Deaths of people aged 90 and upwards ...	...	...	37

DEATHS IN SUB-DISTRICTS FROM EPIDEMICS.

	Enumerated Population, 1881 (unrevised).	Small-pox.	Measles.	Scarlet Fever.	Diphtheria.	Whooping-cough.	Typhus.	Enteric (or Typhoid) Fever.	Simple continued Fever.	Diarrhœa.
West ...	666998	3	4	3	4	2	...	3	...	4
North ...	905677	8	3	17	4	8	2	10	1	11
Central ...	981795	...	...	3	1	4	...	4	1	6
East ...	692580	1	2	8	3	3	1	14	...	6
South ...	1265678	14	8	20	5	14	...	10	...	6
Total ...	8314571	26	17	48	14	31	3	40	2	33

METEOROLOGY.

From Observations at the Greenwich Observatory.

Mean height of barometer ...	...	29·930 in.
Mean temperature ...	...	56·2°
Highest point of thermometer ...	...	72·9°
Lowest point of thermometer ...	...	43·0°
Mean dew-point temperature ...	...	55·0°
General direction of wind ...	...	Variable.
Whole amount of rain in the week ...	...	1·19 in.

BIRTHS and DEATHS Registered and METEOROLOGY during the Week ending Saturday, Sept. 24, in the following large Towns :—

Cities and boroughs (Municipal boundaries except for London.)	Estimated Population to middle of the year 1881.*	Persons to an Acre. (1881.)	Births Registered during the week ending Sept. 24.	Deaths Registered during the week ending Sept. 24.	Highest during the Week.	Lowest during the Week.	Temperature of Air (Fahr.) Weekly Mean of Daily Mean Values.	Temp. of Air (Cent.) Weekly Mean of Daily Mean Values.	Rain Fall. In Inches.	Rain Fall. In Centimetres.
London ...	3829751	50·2	2330	1279	72·9	49·0	58·2	14·55	1·19	3·02
Brighton ...	107934	45·9	62	32	69·3	49·6	58·0	14·44	1·37	3·48
Portsmouth ...	128335	28·6	76	40	...	...	...	...	...	...
Norwich ...	88038	11·3	54	36	...	...	...	...	...	...
Plymouth ...	76262	54·0	45	25	66·6	43·2	57·0	13·89	0·16	0·41
Bristol ...	207140	46·5	135	61	70·0	42·4	56·7	13·72	0·33	0·84
Wolverhampton ..	75934	22·4	48	38	67·8	44·5	55·1	12·84	1·10	2·79
Birmingham ...	402296	47·9	271	117	...	...	...	...	...	...
Leicester ...	123120	38·5	81	49	...	...	...	...	...	...
Nottingham ...	188235	18·9	116	74	73·2	41·6	55·9	13·28	0·71	1·80
Liverpool ...	553938	106·3	462	246	...	...	...	...	...	...
Manchester ...	341289	79·3	221	165	...	...	...	...	...	...
Salford ...	177760	34·4	124	53	...	...	...	...	...	...
Oldham ...	112176	24·0	88	39	...	...	...	...	...	...
Bradford ...	184037	25·5	108	53	67·1	43·0	55·1	12·84	2·02	5·13
Leeds ...	310490	14·4	194	90	68·0	48·0	55·6	13·12	1·36	3·45
Sheffield ...	286621	14·5	202	94	70·2	45·5	54·4	12·44	1·39	3·53
Hull ...	155161	42·7	96	73	71·0	43·0	56·4	13·55	2·26	5·74
Sunderland ...	116755	42·2	71	35	72·0	43·0	53·7	12·05	2·49	6·32
Newcastle-on-Tyne	145675	27·1	94	62	...	...	...	...	...	...
Total of 20 large English Towns...	7608775	38·0	4811	2855	73·2	41·6	56·0	13·33	1·31	3·33

* These figures are the numbers enumerated (but subject to revision) in April last, raised to the middle of 1881 by the addition of a quarter of a year's increase, calculated at the rate that prevailed between 1871 and 1881.

At the Royal Observatory, Greenwich, the mean reading of the barometer last week was 29·62 in. The lowest reading was 29·28 in. on Wednesday morning, and the highest 30·02 in. on Saturday morning.

J. R., Doncaster.—Mr. Liebreich is not now at 16, Albemarle-street, and we believe he is abroad; but write to him at the old address, inquiring when he can be consulted.

"*First Aid.*"—It is announced that the Home Secretary expects that all who hereafter join the Metropolitan Police Force will, after three years' standing in the force, obtain a certificate from the St. John Ambulance Association.

Colonial Items.—At Victoria the foundation-stone of a new hospital for incurables has been laid by His Excellency the Governor. The total receipts for the purpose, when the mail left, were £7700, of which Mrs. Austin had given £6000; this munificent donation had been supplemented by Mr. Landsell with £1000.——New South Wales: Mr. Thomas Walker, of Concord, has given £5000 to the Sydney University for a bursary endowment. A portion of the bursaries will be made applicable to female students.——New Zealand: The publicans were exclaiming loudly against the new Licensing Bill. A licensee will not be permitted, under any pretence whatever, to leave his premises for more than fourteen days at a time. The police, under the new Act, may demand admittance to the premises at any hour of the night without giving any reason for their conduct.

Army Medical Officers, West Indies.—The serious outbreak of yellow fever at Barbadoes has led to the despatch of an extra staff of army medical officers for service in the West Indies. When the mail left, Surgeon-Major Ward had died of the fever, and Surgeon Maddam had been struck down within a few weeks of his arrival from England. It had been found necessary to place the troops in medical charge of a civil surgeon, no officers of the Army Medical Department being available for the purpose. Surgeon-Major Ward, who died at Barbadoes, had served through the Ashantee and Zulu campaigns, and was mentioned in despatches for his services when in medical charge of the troops which were wrecked in the *Lord Clyde* transport.

Vivisection.—Last week, at the annual meeting of the North Wales Medical Association, held at Colwyn Bay, near Conway, a resolution was unanimously carried in favour of allowing vivisection for scientific purposes under proper restrictions.

A Domestic Sanitary Exhibition, Brighton.—At a large and influential meeting held in this town it was decided that a domestic sanitary and scientific exhibition shall be held in the borough the week before Christmas. An executive committee, with power to appoint sectional committees, was formed, and to immediately further the work 130 season tickets were at once taken.

THE "EATON FUND."

The following subscriptions have been received :—

	£	s.	d.
Messrs. Henry Thompson and Son ...Grantham..	25	0	0
Mr. Councillor Fox	5	0	0
——— Hannett	2	2	0
——— Codling	1	1	0
——— Brown	1	1	0
Messrs. Shipman and Wilson, surgeons ...	5	0	0
J. W. Jeans, Esq., J.P., M.R.C.S. ...	2	2	0
W. H. Paterson, Esq., M.D. ...	1	1	0
H. B. Bailey, Esq., M.R.C.S. ...	1	1	0
J. F. Burdidge, Esq., J.P. ...	5	0	0
Messrs. Wyles and Burrows ...	5	0	0
T. Hopkinson, Esq., J.P. ...	5	0	0
Mr. William Thompson... ...	2	0	0
Mr. William Bedford	1	1	0
Mr. Thomas Bastow	1	0	0
Mr. Henry Yates...	1	0	0
Mr. J. W. Atkin, Gipple, near... ...	2	2	0
Miss Collins	1	0	0
F. D. Fisher, Esq., J.P.... ...	1	1	0
A Friend	1	1	0
Donations under £1 in	8	7	6
Osborne Johnson, Esq., M.R.C.S. ...	1	1	0
Lionel Beale, Esq., F.R.C.P., F.R.S...	1	1	0
T. Lauder Brunton, Esq., M.D., F.R.S. ...	1	1	0
Sir George Burrows, Bart., M.D., F.R.S. ...	1	1	0
Andrew Clark, Esq., M.D., F.R.C.P. ...	5	0	0
W. F. Walshe, Esq., M.D., F.R.C.P. ...	1	1	0
G. T. Willan, Esq., M.R.C.S.... ...	1	1	0
Francis Vacher, Esq., L.R.C.P. and S. ...	1	1	0
Edwin Saunders, Esq., F.R.C.S. ...	2	2	0
J. R. Burton, Esq., M.R.C.S. ...	1	1	0
Christopher Johnson, Esq., F.R.C.S. ...	1	1	0
Edward Lund, Esq., F.R.C.S.... ...	2	2	0
R. L. Bowles, Esq., M.D., M.R.C.P. ...	1	1	0
Henry Lewis, Esq., M.D., M.R.C.P. ...	1	1	0
Thomas Jervis, Esq., M.D., M.R.C.S. ...	2	2	0
James Bishopp, Esq., M.R.C.S. ...	1	1	0
William Cholmeley, Esq., M.D., F.R.C.P. ...	1	1	0

Additional subscriptions will be gladly received and duly acknowledged by Mr. J. Fox, 53, High-street, Grantham.

Assistants in Shops.—The protection given under the Factory and Workshops Acts to factory workmen requires to be extended and amended so as to include other classes of the employed. The law allows a draper, for instance, to keep his assistants at work in his shop until midnight, or even later, while it regulates the hours of the workshop, and a penalty is incurred for excess beyond the legal limit. Lord Stanhope's Bill, introduced last session, proposed to rectify this special anomaly; but legislation should deal with the hours of labour in other shops than those of drapers, if it meddles at all. Grocers' assistants appear to be kept at work for inordinate hours, in many districts often till past midnight. Statutable protection should include shop *employés* generally, if the well-being of these persons is to be properly secured.

Brompton Hospital.—There will be a vacancy at this Hospital during the ensuing autumn for the post of Lady Superintendent.

"Non-Intoxicating Drinks."—It seems that the Inland Revenue Board have determined that in every case in which liquor flavoured with hops, or containing more than 2 per cent. of spirit generated by fermentation, is brought before the public under any of the names usually applied to beer, such liquor is liable to be taxed as beer, according to its gravity when brewed. It is not intended to interfere with ginger-beer, treacle-beer, and innocuous decoctions, although these contain a small quantity of alcohol.

A New Eye, Ear, and Throat Hospital for Shropshire.—At Shrewsbury, last week, the Countess of Bradford opened this institution, which is intended for Shropshire and North Wales. At the same time a fancy bazaar, in aid of the building fund, was inaugurated by her ladyship, the net profit of which is about £600.

Anti-Vaccination, Bedford.—This town maintains its reputation as one of the favourite quarters of the anti-vaccinationists. No less than forty-four persons were summoned last week (the largest number ever charged at one time there) for neglecting to have their children vaccinated. The usual objections were urged by the defendants, but the magistrates imposed fines and costs in each case. The former, which had on previous occasions been 6d., was raised to 1s.—an increase which seemed to surprise the defendants.

Historical Medical Houses.—The home of the Charlotte-street School of Medicine—a school conducted for about a quarter of a century by the late Dr. G. D. Dermott, and where the late Dr. Tyler Smith delivered his first lecture, is now known as 16, Bloomsbury-street, W.C. The house was required through the necessity of taking down the next house for the formation of the new part of Oxford-street, W.C. Ever since the formation of the street the house has been occupied by a medical bookseller. The Charlotte-street School of Medicine was afterwards conducted in 27, Bedford-square, and until Dr. Dermott departed this life on September 12, 1847. Dr. Dermott may be considered the last of the great anatomical teachers—Hunter, Brookes, Carpue,—although the school was conducted as the Hunterian School of Medicine in Bedford-square, W.C., until about 1853.—E. N.

Perplexed.—You should consult the "Students' Number" of this journal. The following notice is now being sent out by the College of Surgeons to all enquirers on the subject, viz. :—"The preliminary examinations of the College having now come to an end, all inquiries with respect to recognised preliminary examinations should be addressed to the Registrar of the General Medical Council, 315, Oxford-street, W."

Illegal Death Certificates.—At an inquest held at Hammersmith by Dr. Diplock, on the body of an infant nine months old, it appeared that the child was suddenly seized with convulsions. A surgeon was sent for, but he was not at home; his assistant, however, attended, and prescribed for the deceased. The child died two hours afterwards. The assistant gave a certificate of death, but the registrar refused to accept it, and referred the matter to the coroner. The surgeon in question stated that the cause of death was hydrocephalus; his assistant was an experienced man, but not legally qualified. The coroner remarked that an unqualified assistant, however great his medical experience might be, could not give a legal certificate of death. The law only recognised medical men whose qualifications were registered. A verdict in accordance with the medical evidence was returned.

Local Sanitary Acts, Liverpool.—Amongst the private Bill applications to be made in the next session of Parliament is one by the Liverpool Corporation for powers to amend the Local Building and Sanitary Acts. The amendments proposed to be made in the existing Acts include powers to have infectious disease compulsorily registered, and that the Council may buy insanitary property by agreement if they can, instead of compulsorily.

Matthew F.—Mr. Lowe's (now Lord Sherbrooke) answer to the deputation of the Scottish Meteorological Society, in search of a grant in aid, was to the effect that he entirely disapproved of official interference in aid of scientific exertion, and of expending public money for anything which could be accomplished without it. It seemed to him improper that voluntary societies should incur a certain amount of labour and expense, and that, unable or unwilling to extend their sacrifices of time and money, they should at last apply to the Government for assistance in the accomplishment of their objects.

Dr. Young, Hong-kong, China.—Letter and enclosure received.

A New Magistrate.—Mr. Richard Axford, surgeon, has been appointed a magistrate for the Borough of Bridgwater.

Hospital Saturday Fund.—The Victoria-park Committee of the Victoria park Band [has handed to the Fund £70 from the Band's performance receipts. The total of the street collection this year is £2115, against £1896 in 1880. The workshop collection also shows a proportionate increase. On December 31 last the total collected was £6524; at the present time it is estimated that there is already £2900 in hand. Many large firms have yet to send in their collecting-sheets.

WITH THE SCALPEL.

"*Ubi sedes vitæ?*" :

A FRIENDLY REJOINDER.

All you say, my friend, is true,—
    No one could have made it clearer,
That a disappointing view
    Meets us as we search him nearer;
That the "subject," stiff and stark,
    Whom we waited many a week for,
Cannot rescue from the dark
    What we seek for.

But then all your fancied sketch
    May be wrong and quite mistaken:
He, perhaps, was but a wretch,
    And deservedly forsaken;
May have used his hands and eyes,
    Not in loving grasp and yearnings,
But to make illegal prize
    Of our earnings!

Why should you assume that he,
    Disembodied and a vapour,
Should have knowledge such as we
    Find it hard to put on paper;
Should already know the cause
    Of the works of the All-seeing,
And the everlasting laws
    Of their being?

Whether we renew our life
    After passing through death's portals,
Ever was a cause of strife
    In the creeds of puzzled mortals;
And so needs *mori* or
    Of the careless, heathen poet,
Though from true religion far,
    Serves to show it.

Let us hope that in some way
    (Never mind the 'why and wherefore')
We may still prolong our day
    To give help to those we care for.
This will surely far transcend
    Knowledge about constellations;
"Make us useful without end
    To the nations"!

September 26.   J. D.

COMMUNICATIONS have been received from—

Dr. SHEPHERD, London; Dr. LUCAS, Bombay; Mr. J. T. W. BACOT, Seaton, Devon; Dr. W. J. MOORE, Bombay; Dr. J. ANDERSON, London; Mr. BECHER, London; Mr. CHINE, Edinburgh; THE REGISTRAR-GENERAL, Scotland; THE SANITARY COMMISSIONER, Punjab; Dr. E. G. DAUVY, Campinas, Brazil; THE REGISTRAR OF THE APOTHECARIES' HALL, London; THE SECRETARY OF ST. MARY'S HOSPITAL MEDICAL SCHOOL, London; Messrs. S. and B. NOCK, Bloomsbury; Mr. J. RIGBY, Doncaster; THE SECRETARY OF THE OBSTETRICAL SOCIETY, London; Mr. J. DIXON, Dorking; THE STAFF OF CHARING-CROSS HOSPITAL AND SCHOOL, London; THE SECRETARY OF THE DEVONSHIRE HOSPITAL AND BUXTON BATH CHARITY; THE SECRETARY OF THE UNIVERSITY COLLEGE MEDICAL SOCIETY, London; Mr. J. CHATTO, London; Mr. T. M. STONE, London; Mr. R. W. PARKER, London; Dr. DOUGLAS POWELL, London.

BOOKS, ETC., RECEIVED—

Annual Congress of the National Association for the Promotion of Social Science—Annual Report on the Sanitary Condition of the Borough of Southampton—Modern Midwifery, by Rodney Glisan, M.D.—Sanitary Report of the Parish of Paddington for 1880—Epilepsy, by W. R. Gowers, M.D., F.R.C.P.—Female Diseases, by R. J. Minn, M.D.—Zur Nervendehnung bei Tabes Dorsalis, von Dr. O. Berger—Diseases of Women, by Arthur W. Edis, M.D.—Suicide, by Henry Morselli, M.D.—Orthopædic Surgery, by J. W. Haward, F.R.C.S.—Médecine Vitale et Médecine Nouvelle, par le Dr. Mariano Semmola—Girl's Own Annual—Boy's Own Annual—Health Lectures—Typhus Exanthématique, par le Docteur S. Robinski.

PERIODICALS AND NEWSPAPERS RECEIVED—

Lancet—British Medical Journal—Medical Press and Circular—Berliner Klinische Wochenschrift—Centralblatt für Chirurgie—Gazette des Hopitaux—Gazette Médicale—Le Progrès Médical—Bulletin de l'Académie de Médecine—Pharmaceutical Journal—Wiener Medizinische Wochenschrift—Centralblatt für die Medizinischen Wissenschaften—Revue Médicale—Gazette Hebdomadaire—National Board of Health Bulletin, Washington—Nature—Occasional Notes—Deutsche Medicinal-Zeitung—Boston Medical and Surgical Journal—Louisville Medical News—Funny Folks—Aberdeen Herald and Weekly Free Press—Oil and Drug News—Therapeutic Gazette—Dublin Journal of Medical Science—Night and Day—The Colonies and India, September 24—Philadelphia Medical Times—Leisure Hour—Sunday at Home—Boy's Own Paper—Friendly Greetings—Girl's Own Paper—Union Médico-Students' Journal and Hospital Gazette.

INTRODUCTORY ADDRESS

DELIVERED AT THE OPENING OF THE

MIDDLESEX HOSPITAL MEDICAL SCHOOL.

By R. DOUGLAS POWELL, M.D., F.R.C.P.,

Physician to the Hospital.

GENTLEMEN,—The first part of my duty to-day is an easy and a pleasing one—to give you all a hearty welcome on the part of my colleagues and myself, and to express the hope that we all meet with renewed health and enthusiasm, eager for the work that lies before and around us.

Happily, one has little temptation at this time of year to wander from the special purpose of an address introductory to the work of the coming session, for in the past autumn all topics of general interest have been exhausted: the harvest of science has been gathered, the harvest festivals have been held, the fruits are garnered, and seed-time has again commenced.

The duties of the student of medicine at every stage of his career were so fully and ably pointed out by Dr. Coupland in his address two years ago—an address that must be still fresh in the memories of most of you—that I am free to select a few points for my remarks to-day. One cannot have been a student, more or less, up to middle life without having gained experience from past errors and a bitter consciousness of present deficiencies that might well prompt an eloquent and instructive address to others ; and if beside any words of counsel and encouragement you detect anything in my remarks that savours of admonition, I will ask you to believe that I am talking more than half to myself.

I take it that all whom I now address have accepted the great profession of medicine as their calling ; and you have done well. In its study it is the most interesting, and in its practice it is the most beneficent, of callings. Of all sciences, Medicine embraces a wider and a freer range of thought, and gathers up the teachings of allied sciences more immediately to one end and purpose—the well-being and improvement of our kind. The pursuit of truth justifies medicine as a science ; the alleviation of suffering, and the constant endeavour—how often futile it matters not—to preserve the integrity of human life to the maximum period allotted, are the reason and justification of the practice of medicine as an art. That which is true as a science and justified as an art must in practice be a worthy means of livelihood. Fortunately for her stability in this age of tottering dynasties and threatened institutions, the aims of Medicine are aside from politics ; her growth must be with the growth of civilisation, her teachings and purpose take an ever-deepening root in the selfishness, if not in the philanthropy, of mankind.

The driest of the elementary studies of medicine would be profoundly interesting if we could but inherit or acquire the spirit of wisdom to see beforehand their full bearing and application. What drier than the bones, with their interminable prominences, depressions, rough surfaces, foramina, epiphyses, apophyses, and developments ? The tendons, ligaments and muscles, their attachments and relations ? But observe a few cases of dislocation or fracture, how, only by placing the limb in a position dictated by these very dry anatomical facts, the dislocation can be reduced, the strained muscles relaxed, the fractured bones adjusted in exact application for ready and perfect union. Observe a hundred other points of practice, based entirely upon anatomical principles, in the medical and surgical departments of this Hospital in your spare hours—and the first and second years' students, whilst awaiting opportunities for dissection, and in the interim of lectures, have many such hours,—and the light of scientific purpose will clothe the tedious dry bones with a new and living interest. In later professional life we have repeatedly to revert to early studies, looking up points we perhaps never before saw the full meaning of—facts in regional anatomy and physiology. At what I will call the

VOL. II. 1881. No. 1632.

anatomical period of your career let me, then, advise you to regard practical matters of medicine and surgery—which are aside from or beyond the special work of your time—rather from the anatomical and physiological points of view. Listen to the healthy heart and breath sounds, and take notice of such things as alterations of body-temperature, modified secretions, characters of pulse. Consider these as matters of mechanism, of chemistry, of tissue-change, which are quite within your ken. At this early time, too, take every opportunity of training the eye quickly to notice alterations in shape and outline. You will thus gain invaluable experience and reflected interest in the anatomical and physiological work proper to this period of your career. Except for the degree and kind of interest I have just alluded to in Medicine and Surgery, I think the student will do well to refrain from all clinical work until he has accomplished his primary examinations.

It has recently been well said, that to separate physiology from pathology is like attempting to divide meteorology into sciences of good and bad weather.(a) Hence I would say to those of you who are more advanced, still pursue your studies on anatomical and physiological lines, proceeding from healthy anatomy and physiology, with which you are now familiar, to consider those alterations of structure and perversions of function and nutrition which constitute disease. You must now no longer look upon disease merely as spectators interested in vital mechanism, but take part individually in the investigation of cases in the wards, and observe their course to recovery, to restored equilibrium, or to death. As the healthy structure of the body should be the study of the first period of your career, so the natural history of Disease should be the subject of your inquiries during the second period—aye, and ever onwards through your professional life. Train to the utmost by constant practice your eye, ear, and hand to see, hear, and to feel and appreciate physical signs of disease. If I might be allowed, on the part of myself and my colleagues, to give you a hint, I would say, Question more, and you will learn much more. It is impossible to know where your difficulties are unless you ask questions. Do not always expect complete or satisfactory answers—all at the bedside are learners, although some must presume to teach. Conversation is a valuable medium for clinical instruction. Strive to obtain posts of practical work—clerkships, dresserships, physician-assistantships (in-patient and out-patient), house-surgeonships, and all the other 'ships that are open to you. They are invaluable steps to future comfort and success in practice. Do not be deterred from going in for any such appointment because you think So-and-so may be better up than you are. Modesty is an excellent quality, but this form of modesty is but shirking that generous rivalry to fear which is to court failure in life. One is often astonished to see a house-surgeoncy or a physician-assistantship, for instance—appointments worth £500 to any man—with only one candidate applying for them. No one can teach you what you may in these offices learn for yourselves ; no teacher can succeed like responsibility. Practical experience of disease multiplies in value with geometrical progression, as case after case comes before us, and nothing in any walk of life is equivalent to it for strengthening and training the mind and concentrating purpose in action. I would not wearisomely extend my string of proverbs. But how shall I emphasise to you your duty and interest in this matter of ward attendance ? The "gifts of healing" are not in these days for those who have not worked hard and practically to gain them. The best of us who pass out into practice do so with an immense weight of responsibility upon us. All must feel this ; the sense of it must, indeed, at times be crushing to those who have not made the very most of their opportunities to gain at least some counterpoise of experience. There are here, gentlemen, within the walls of this great Hospital, more than three hundred disease-problems in all stages of natural and artificial solution, from which to cull your day-by-day experience. And I venture to say that a man who has taken full advantage of his opportunities in the practical way I have been speaking of, at this or any other large hospital,—such a man, I say, goes out into the world with an accumulated experience greater than he can gain, perhaps, in all the years of private practice that remain to him. It will be difficult for him to make serious mistakes, the work of his life will gather

(a) Prof. Michael Foster: Address to British Medical Association, 1880.

interest with years, and he is sure of that success and reputation which ever await honest work.

Whoever investigates the natural history of Disease in the manner I have glanced at, pursuing the lines of anatomy, physiology, and pathology, has proceeded far and on a sound basis to a true knowledge of his profession; but he has yet more to learn in the same direction. We see in the post-mortem room the last results of disease; they are very instructive and interesting to witness, and teach us some bitter but wholesome lessons in humility. But let us not neglect the study of that happier solution which the majority of the disease-problems that come before us undergo. To do so is to miss the brighter side of pathology, and to tend to fatalism in prognosis and to vacillation in practice. The processes of *repair* and *convalescence* are too often passed by in silence in our text-books, and these naturally are not sufficiently observed by the clinical student. We may, it is true, often get instructive glimpses of the processes of repair in various stages of completion in the bodies of those who have fallen victims to some intercurrent malady whilst their original disease was in course of healing, but we must supplement these casual glimpses by steady clinical research into the phenomena of returning health. And in these days of comparative precision in physical diagnosis, at least much may be done in this line of clinical pathology in advancing our knowledge of the natural history of disease. The surgeon is familiar, in the suppurating gland and in the necrotising bone, with the two processes of disintegration and healing going on side by side. In phthisis a careful examination may often tell us of the same two processes going on together—of necrotic-tissue softening and being removed, whilst a surrounding area of scar-formation limits the destruction, and is already preparing to heal up the lesions.(b) In the absence of a knowledge of the frequent association of these two processes, the physician would be guided by the signs of softening and excavation to an erroneous view and treatment of the case. Again, the phenomena attendant upon the recedence of acute inflammatory consolidations of the lung or infiltrations into the cellular tissue (*e.g.*, pelvic cellulitis) are well worthy of closer attention. Not only do we see in our day-by-day observation of the rapidity with which the products are melting away, a remarkable instance of the power of Nature to remove the results of disease, but in the course of convalescence, certain other phenomena occasionally present themselves—phenomena of slight blood-poisoning, secondary fever, chills, sweatings, and the like—presumably the result of an undue rapidity of the reparative absorption, by which an overdose, so to speak, of effete material is taken up. With due care, these cases clear up perfectly; but undoubtedly one sees in these interesting phenomena a sufficient reason for the occurrence, under less favourable conditions, of those secondary diseases—abscess, local or general tuberculosis, pyæmia—which we know to arise from neglected inflammations. Here we see, too, how closely pathological and physiological processes are connected. My object in bringing forward these examples is not to anticipate any of the teaching of the coming session, but to endeavour to excite your curiosity and interest, and to induce you to watch the vicissitudes of repair and convalescence, and thus to gain a little insight into the working of that *vis medicatrix naturæ* which was recognised by Hippocrates, extolled by Cullen, and which seems to have dazzled the result in almost complete adoration some more modern authors.

Equally with repair, we must look to *compensation* as a great principle in the natural history of disease. Compensatory function is the *modus vivendi* in chronic disease. The sources and methods and paths of compensatory function will afford you a rich field for interesting and original research. It is a subject upon which, again, our text-books are curiously silent. All the knowledge you will gain of it will be gathered in the wards and the out-patient room. Here, for instance, you will see a man walking about the ward or attending the out-patient room with apparently but little the matter with him; he is very well on level ground, but is short-breathed on exertion. There is another patient propped up in bed gasping for breath, with dropsical limbs and engorged viscera. Yet these two people have precisely the same form of valvular heart-disease, but in the one case the heart-muscle has gained power to maintain the circula-

(b) Laennec was well aware of this when he observed that phthisis was only curable in the third stage.

tion, notwithstanding its disabled valve; in the other case this compensatory power has not yet been established. In another case, again, it perhaps never will be established. This is but one illustration of compensation in chronic disease. You may observe the same principle at work in case after case, and in every region and system of the body. The *vicarious* principle by which one set of organs will temporarily bear the burdens of another is well recognised in Medicine; you will see frequent illustrations of it in the wards. I do not wish you to study these phenomena merely for the satisfaction they will afford you, nor as intellectual exercises or matters of purely scientific interest, but because of their direct practical bearings upon the treatment of disease. They are the essential conditions of life to thousands of people, and to start, to stimulate, and to maintain them in chronic illnesses are the grand objects of our art, in attaining which some of the most brilliant triumphs of therapeutics are achieved. Nor can an accurate opinion as to the future of any chronic illness be formed without taking into account what may be effected by reparative or compensatory processes or by vicarious function in restoring a working equilibrium. These constitute our wealth of vitality. Two men may stand side by side with the same disease, yet the one is bankrupt of resource, while the other has a heavy constitutional balance in his favour.

A full recognition of the *vis medicatrix naturæ* does not warrant, as it has been held to do, an expectant or hand-folded treatment of disease. Let us keenly scan the ways and means of Nature as they are manifested to us in healthy and diseased processes, and we cannot fail to find abundant room for the resources of art to aid, to direct, and to control her doings; and it is pardonable in us at least to conceive that the science of Medicine has been instituted, in the Divine order of things, thus to assist and to control Nature. There is little fear that those who have well studied the natural history of Disease will be meddlesome in therapeutics; they will understand and leave much to the *vis medicatrix naturæ*, but they cannot fail to have observed that this same *vis medicatrix* plays sad havoc with us sometimes. People would not infrequently be choked or starved by Nature's attempts at repair were it not for timely surgical interference. Well-nigh all the graver forms of valvular heart-disease are due not so much to the original lesion as to the after-attempts (Nature's attempts) at repair by cicatricial processes. The surgeon frequently suffers the greatest embarrassment from Nature's determined efforts to heal in the wrong place. Modern research has discovered that we are beset on all sides by pernicious agents, against whose insidious attacks Nature unaided is often powerless; but Art steps in, and our Pharmacopœia has of late years bristled with antiseptics and germicides. In short, you will find in practice but few cases in medicine or surgery in which you can with a clear conscience stand aside and say there is nothing to be done. You may sometimes cure those that without your aid would die; you may always relieve suffering when present, and in hopeless cases you may prolong life and strip death of some of its terrors.

What I have now said will, I trust, serve to show that Medicine has the great and fundamental interest of a growing science, in which there is room for all to work and to add their gifts from experience or research; it owns no finality within our reach, nor can its practice ever prove monotonous. And if I have not quite exhausted your patience, there are a few words I would still say to those about to pass on into practice, whether in the public services, in towns, or in country or colonial districts.

But first let me here remind you that your future success depends upon good health as well as upon good training, and hence in your eager pursuit of the *vis medicatrix naturæ* through the tangled paths I have indicated, and amidst the morasses and pitfalls of studentship, do not forget your own health; at every stage of your career your fortunes will largely depend upon the care you take of it in early days.

It is, I think, hardly enough recognised by us how large a part of our professional work is of an educational kind, and how much good we may do in this direction. I suppose it would be difficult, for instance, to calculate the educational value in the aggregate of the few brief words of advice and direction given by out-patient physicians and surgeons in our large cities in matters of hygiene, cleanliness, temperance in all things, care of children, diet, and the like. Our large and well-administered hospitals and convalescent institutions are again, in a way, schools whose inmates cannot fail to learn healthy and cleanly habits. It is refreshing to see, for example, the transformation in a gutter child who has passed through a few weeks of convalescence at some "Home"; he can scarcely fail to take back with him a very practical lesson. In each town or village throughout Great Britain and the colonies every family is brought into more or less frequent communication with a member of our body, who is generally a man of culture, of liberal views, and of wide experience in life. He cannot help in some degree literally teaching from door to door the laws of healthy living; he might do much more in this way did he think of it; and who knows better than he that these laws are in the greatest part identical with the purest morality? Many a friendly hint or word of warning may be given by the doctor to those, some of whom are perhaps beyond the reach of, or as yet insensible to, any higher teaching, and many a family may thus be saved from ruin or unhappiness.

It has been said, and the saying is, I believe, attributed to Sydney Smith, "that everyone around the sick man's couch sees the approach of Death save himself." The doctor has shaken his head, the nurse has packed her box, the friends have arranged the funeral preliminaries, even the meats are baking, whilst he with Death's grasp about him is arranging convalescent tours or counting the anxieties of the morrow. Our duty in this matter is as plain as it is often difficult and painful. We must see that our patient is made aware, directly, or indirectly through others, of his condition. A great responsibility rests upon us: first, to the patient himself, and then to his family. It is neither kind nor justifiable to deceive a man, nor even to let him remain in ignorance at such a time, and yet the greatest delicacy and care are required in conveying the needful information.

To those of you who go into the country or the colonies, let me advise a good equipment at starting. Be especially supplied with remedies for ready use. Be not content to carry about with you what may be called your side arms — thermometer and stethoscope — weapons of precision no doubt, but in diagnosis only. Even a pocket-pistol in the form of a morphia syringe is not enough! A small bag or case, containing a well-planned selection of medicines for immediate use, should be your constant companion.(c) A man can hardly be held to have any serious belief in therapeutics who is satisfied to carry about with him only the implements of diagnosis, leaving many hours behind the means of treatment. In these days, too, the doctor, on returning with remedies he should have had at hand, may find to his confusion that the squire's daughter, or some other smart young ambulance lady, has looked in, and with a pardonable disregard for professional etiquette, has cured his patient—or has at least administered such active remedies as have entirely altered the character of the symptoms he came back prepared to treat! I would commend the Army to those of you who have a taste for travel and any enthusiasm for natural history, or for investigating the effects of climate—provided also you have a good constitution and no commanding home ties. Some of the most interesting and important questions in medicine have been, and are to be, worked out by military surgeons. In the Army, however, the doctors above all things, soldiers only in discipline, courage, and patriotism. The surgeon holds a high place in a regiment, none higher if he have a love for his profession, and be a companionable fellow at the same time. He must not be tempted by nor strive for the rewards of gallantry in the field; the clarion sound suggests not to him the "crowded hour of glorious life," but equally in the din of battle, amidst the raging pestilence, or in the monotony of barrack life, his unexcited mind and ready hand are for the sick and suffering.

In conclusion, I have only further to remark, that as I have endeavoured to show that the chief labour of early studentship consists in the foundation studies of anatomy and physiology, and that the later period of studentship is

(c) Messrs. Savory and Moore exhibited at the International Congress Museum some miniature portable dispensaries suitable for military field work. Something on a similar plan might be devised for country practice. Messrs. Kirby and Sons have an admirable series of "miniature dispensaries" for ready use. Mr. Martindale has fitted a bag—" the antidote bag"—containing all the remedies and apparatus used as antidotes, as suggested in Dr. Murrell's valuable little book.

concerned with the natural history of disease in its pronounced phases, course, termination in death or recovery, and treatment, so I would add, that in the still more advanced stage of studentship upon which some of you are now entering, and from which I trust you as earnest practitioners will never emerge, we have much to find out of the beginnings of diseases—in individuals, in families, in communities. Here is worthy labour for many lifetimes.

I have now said, gentlemen, at only too much length, what it has occurred to me might be useful to old friends and new, and I am happy to make way for the more interesting business of the day, but not before I have expressed to you and to my colleagues and friends my true appreciation of the courtesy and patience with which you have listened to me.

INTRODUCTORY ADDRESS

DELIVERED AT THE OPENING OF

ST. GEORGE'S HOSPITAL MEDICAL SCHOOL.

By WARRINGTON HAWARD, F.R.C.S. Eng.,
Surgeon to the Hospital.

IT is my pleasant duty to express for my colleagues and myself our welcome to those of you who to-day have joined our school, and to those also who, after I hope a pleasant holiday, have returned to their studies amongst us—a welcome which, I assure you, we are prepared to extend to you all, not only in word but in deed. It is our hope that you have come among us for your welfare, and it will be our endeavour to help you, as far as we have power, to utilise to the best purpose the opportunities which are here afforded you of acquiring a sound knowledge of the profession which you have chosen. As an earnest of this our desire, it is the custom for one of us, at the commencement of the winter session, to address to you some words of encouragement and advice, to aid, if it may be, in starting you in the right direction at the outset of your career.

Now, in availing myself of this privilege, I do not think I need say anything to you of the advantages or disadvantages of the medical profession. You will have considered these before your entrance here, and have probably come to the conclusion that the path you have chosen is, like most others, neither all smooth nor all rough—that it has its special difficulties as well as its special attractions, its grave responsibilities as well as its grateful rewards, its opportunities of good and its possibilities of evil. Neither do I think it would be at all profitable to attempt to advise you as to the method in which you should pursue each particular study in which you are about to engage: that will be told you far better than I can, by the teacher of each special subject. What I should like to speak to you about, in the short time that is to-day at my disposal, is the spirit or tone of mind in which, as it seems to me, you may best enter upon your studies as a whole.

I am not forgetful that the liberal education which you have undergone, and the university training which many of you have enjoyed, must already have led most of you to certain habits and methods of thought which are securely fixed on well-considered bases, and which, it may be, are not usefully to be altered. Yet it is not unprofitable sometimes to review our mental condition, and it is possible that some of you may think it worth while to make this, your entry upon a new class of studies, the opportunity for taking a new departure along routes and by means not hitherto attempted by you.

I suppose the first thing that strikes the student at the outset of his medical education is the number and complexity of the subjects which he is expected to study. It soon becomes obvious that it is impossible for anyone of ordinary capacity to become equally well versed in them all. The question, then, at once occurs to him, What is the relative importance and value of these different subjects? And this involves the wider and more difficult question, how far he is to act upon his own judgment or bias, and how far upon the advice of his teachers in deciding this, as well as the other difficulties which he has to face.

As the student advances in his studies, this question will frequently recur in other shapes. For our knowledge of disease and its treatment is, to a large extent, composed of the accumulated experience of the past, while at the same time that experience, and the interpretation thereof, is every day being corrected, confirmed, and enlarged.

How far, then, you will continually be obliged to determine, are you to trust to the dictation of your teacher, and how far to depend upon your own judgment or investigation? for you cannot wholly depend upon either the one or the other. We should indeed be poor, both in knowledge and resources, if we were deprived of the great inheritance of observation and doctrine which has descended to us from our forefathers, or if we accepted nothing from the past of which we had not ourselves tested the accuracy and the value; but, on the other hand, unless we duly exercise our judgment, it will become enfeebled by disuse, and, like the weakened muscles of disease, liable to irregular and errant action, and easily turned aside by the smallest obstacle.

The knowledge of to-day is built, not with fragments from the ruins of the past, but with new material added to the solid structure which has stood the test of time. We must perforce avail ourselves of the basis furnished by the labour of those who have gone before. But we must know well the foundation, see that it is firmly established, and that the superstructure stands erect, and beware of the bias of prejudice or passion, remembering that every such deflection from uprightness introduces an element of instability into the edifice, so that the more it is added to the more dangerous it becomes, and the nearer it is to its inevitable downfall.

He therefore who, in arrogance or self-conceit, despises the teaching of his predecessors, and believes only in himself, is equally in error with him who, either from feebleness or idleness, yields his independence of thought to, and takes his opinions from, another.

How, then, are you to steer between these two dangers? How, while imbued with the lessons of the past, and yet receptive of the influences of the present, can you best use them both for your secure progress in your studies, and the attainment of the knowledge that will best help you in the exercise of your profession?

A question not easy to answer, for it involves the right balance of liberty and authority; yet a question of such radical importance that I should be glad if I could give you some aid towards its solution.

Now it may I suppose be safely said that, given the same amount of technical knowledge, his judgment will be truest whose general culture is the highest. For whatever enlarges and ennobles the mind increases the power of appreciating and discriminating the truth, and of recognising and avoiding error, so that you will learn the most—of this I am very sure—not from the man who knows best one part of our art, but from him whose comprehensive knowledge is applied by a well-trained and highly cultivated mind.

That which you have to learn from your teachers is chiefly the knowledge that has been arrived at by the observation, investigation, and reasoning of the master-minds of medicine. But it is quite useless to tell you of this unless your minds are prepared to receive, appreciate, and reason upon it, and the practical application of such knowledge you can only teach yourselves. A first essential then, for profitable reception of the teaching of others, is that we approach our studies in the student frame of mind—that is, with the consciousness that there are others who know more about the subject than ourselves.

I do not think you would take it as a compliment if I told you that you are all such wonderfully clever fellows, and have had the good fortune of being born into such an advanced and knowing age, that you may safely despise the teaching of the benighted beings who have preceded you; that you are not to believe anything that you have not yourselves proved; and that the proper and philosophical state of mind for you is one of profound scepticism of every-one and everything except yourselves.

Rather let me advise you to remember at the outset of your studies, what we in the progressive studies of our lives discern more clearly every day, that "there are more things in heaven and earth than are dreamt of in our philosophy"; that even within the limits of our own special studies there are many more things than can by us be known, at least at present, and many others which are as yet but dimly seen;

and that concerning all the Hippocratic maxim still holds good that "true judgment is difficult."

This consciousness of the imperfection and deficiency of our knowledge should engender in us modesty, toleration, and caution—mental qualities which are no less becoming than profitable to cultivate,—while the sense of the vast extent of the unknown which invites our investigation should add the stimulus of enthusiasm. These four mental qualities, then, I commend to your cultivation—modesty, toleration, caution, enthusiasm,—of which, if you will consider them for a moment, you will, I think, see the importance. First, Modesty—a, due sense of the proportion which we bear to the rest of the world: that is the true meaning of the word,—modestus, from modus, a measure, or due proportion,—a condition of mind therefore usually developed in proportion to the amount of real knowledge attained; for, as our horizon widens, we see how much more others know than ourselves, how much we have still to learn, how much there remains yet beyond our ken. Everyone knows the memorable saying of Sir Isaac Newton, that he was but as a child gathering a few shells upon the sea-shore, while the vast unfathomed ocean lay beyond. That was an example of true scientific modesty.

Then the second quality of which I spoke was Toleration. This naturally follows upon modesty; the recollection that we are fallible; so that not only ought we to tolerate an honest difference of opinion upon doubtful points, but even upon matters of which we ourselves feel very sure. Remember the difficulties of attaining absolute certitude, and, lest you think that I am exaggerating them, let me recall to you the weighty words of Mr. John Stuart Mill, who says: " On any matter not self-evident there are ninety-nine persons totally incapable of judging of it for one who is capable; and the capacity of the hundredth person is only comparative; for the majority of the eminent men of every past generation held many opinions now known to be erroneous, and did or approved numerous things which no one will now justify." "Unfortunately for the good sense of mankind, the fact of their fallibility is far from carrying the weight in their practical judgment, which is always allowed to it in theory; for while everyone well knows himself to be fallible, few think it necessary to take any precautions against their own fallibility, or admit the supposition that any opinion, of which they feel very certain, may be one of the examples of the error to which they acknowledge themselves to be liable."

To give an example of this from our own profession. I have myself lived to see an operation which was denounced as an unjustifiable barbarity, come to be looked upon as one of the greatest triumphs of modern surgery.

And if we need any further argument in favour of toleration I would remind you that intolerance has always been associated with ignorance, and has ever prevailed most with regard to those subjects which present the greatest difficulties.

The third mental quality which I commended to you was Caution. The best guarantee for real advancement in learning is that each step shall be secure—a care which is especially requisite in an age like the present, when the very rapidity of our progress and the facilities at our command, make a due circumspection the more needful for maintaining our balance. Moreover, the multiplicity of aids to investigation which we now possess tends rather to a levity and haste of judgment which is a characteristic fault of the present day, and against which we should be on our guard.

One evil of the increasing pressure and hurry under which most people now live is a want of accuracy both of observation and speech. The ancient physicians, who had but few instruments to help them in the investigation of disease, used their unassisted senses with a skill and sagacity which we may well envy, and recorded their observations in language the clearness and accuracy of which we might usefully imitate.

Some of Hippocrates' "cases" might be set forth as examples to clinical clerks. Let me give you one specimen : it may perhaps tempt you to look at the Hippocratic Treatises, which are not fashionable among the students' manuals of the day. Here is Case VIII. from the Third Book of the " Epidemics ":—

"In Abdera, Anaxion, who was lodged near the Thracian Gate, was seized with an acute fever; continued pain of the right side; dry cough without expectoration during the first days, thirst, insomnolency; urine well-coloured, copious, and thin. On the sixth day delirious. No relief from warm applications. On the seventh, in a painful state, for the fever increased, while the pains did not abate, and the cough was troublesome and attended with dyspnœa. On the eighth I opened a vein at the elbow, and much blood of a proper character flowed. The pains were abated, but the dry cough continued. On the eleventh the fever diminished; slight sweats about the head; cough with more liquid sputa; he was relieved. On the twentieth, sweat, apyrexia; but after the crisis he was thirsty, and the expectorations were not good. On the twenty-seventh the fever relapsed. He coughed and brought up much concocted sputa; sediment in the urine, copious and white. He became free of thirst, and the respiration was good. On the thirty-fourth, sweated all over; apyrexia; general crisis."

Surely a clear enough description of a case of pleuropneumonia—vivid, exact, and without needless circumlocution,—giving the gist of the matter in a few words, and without any theorising. It is always an easier thing to speculate about a case than to carefully observe and record it.

> "Our nimble souls
> Can spin an unsubstantial universe
> Suiting our mood, and call it possible,
> Sooner than see one grain with eye exact,
> And give strict record of it."

The difficulty of such accuracy is increased by what I cannot forbear protesting against, the current pollution of our language with all sorts of slang and vile metaphor, which has reached such a degree that I observe the advertisement of a "slang dictionary." This is a custom of which we have become much too tolerant, and against which the members of a scientific profession may, without any suspicion of pedantry, protest both by precept and example.

Now the habit of caution of which I have spoken will help to preserve us, not only from flippancy of language, but also from inaccuracy of thought; we shall be less likely to be led into the too ready acceptance of doubtful and ill-considered conclusions, if we are in the habit of requiring an exact statement of the premises from which they have been deduced. It will often lead us to suspend our judgment, to wait for further investigation; to weigh carefully, not only the degree, but the kind of evidence before us; and to abstain from enforcing our conclusions upon others, until we have, with due pains, tested their accuracy ourselves.

Do not suppose that this kind of caution is in the least degree opposed to real progress; quite the contrary, for it is a marked characteristic of the most actively progressive minds. In proof of which, let me give you three notable examples.

You will remember how the illustrious author of the "Advancement of Learning" insists upon this caution with regard to what you learn from books, of which he says, "Read, not to contradict and confute, nor to believe and take for granted, nor to find talk and discourse, but to weigh and consider."

Take, for a second example of far-reaching sagacity and progressive thought, John Hunter, of whom Sir James Paget says—"It was a sign of this wise caution that he always hesitated to publish his knowledge. He worked for eighteen years before he published anything in his own name. He was forty-three when he published his first book, that on the teeth. He began to collect the materials for his great work on the blood and inflammation while he was a student; some of the experiments recorded in it were made while he was House-Surgeon at St. George's Hospital. He worked at it for forty years, and began to print it only just before he died."

And for a third example of this combination of scientific caution and progress, let me remind you of the illustrious naturalist happily still amongst us, whose name is well worthy to be placed beside that of Hunter—Mr. Darwin,—who spent more than twenty years in patiently accumulating and reflecting upon facts, before publishing the conclusions upon the origin of species, with which his name will for ever be associated.

And this becoming modesty, this needful toleration, and this wise caution should be accompanied by the healthy stimulus and inspiring influence of Enthusiasm. A very necessary aid you will often find this of enthusiasm, for without it you would be deterred by the difficulties, discouraged

by the failures, or overcome by the opponents you will meet with on your road. It comes chiefly from a belief in the nobleness and rectitude of your aim, and produces a sublime indifference to obstacles, just as in pursuing a difficult journey the certain knowledge that you are on the right path helps you to disregard the roughness or steepness of the way.

Having said thus much, then, gentlemen, of the frame of mind in which I would advise you to approach your studies, let me proceed to place before you a few suggestions concerning the second part of my subject—the influence of Authority therein.

In considering the influence of Authority in medicine, three questions naturally arise :—1. What facts and doctrines are there so certainly known and established that they may be taken for granted and used as a basis of action ? 2. What authorities are we to trust, and what are to be the limits of our assent? 3. Wherein are we bound to investigate for ourselves, and to claim full liberty of action ?

1. What facts and doctrines are there so certainly known and established that they may be taken for granted and used as a basis of action ?

The answer to this question is intimately connected with the next upon the criteria and limits of authority, for a large proportion of the accepted doctrines of medicine remain unquestioned because they have the sanction of authority.

There are, of course, certain self-evident axioms in medicine, as in other sciences, to which the mind cannot but assent. But besides these there are many facts and deductions which we may safely take for granted, because established by credible witnesses, received by competent judges, and confirmed by sufficient experience. The accurate observations recorded by Hippocrates two thousand years ago are as true now as they were then, and the deductions which he made therefrom have not lost their force, but have acquired the additional sanction of antiquity, which, within certain limits, is not to be despised.

For opinions that have long prevailed have this primâ facie claim to our assent—that they have stood the test of time; and, provided always that they have been open to use and question, the presumption is that, had they been unfounded, they would have been proved to be so in the lapse of time, either by logical questioning or experimental inquiry. As Mr. Mill says, "The beliefs which we have most warrant for have no safeguard to rest on, but a standing invitation to the whole world to prove them unfounded." Now, if you investigate the origin of the beliefs in medicine which we are daily acting upon, you will find many of them to be the dogmata of the ancients sanctioned by time. You would be perhaps surprised to find how many such are derived from the Father of Medicine—Hippocrates. For instance, it is well known to all of us that erysipelas is apt to prevail during the cold east winds of the spring an observation that has, I think, been attributed to Sir Benjamin Brodie; but you will find the fact quite definitely set down in the Third Book of the "Epidemics" of Hippocrates. Hear one or two more of his aphorisms, and observe how familiar they are; for instance : "When sleep puts an end to delirium it is a good symptom." "Persons who have had frequent and severe attacks of swooning without any manifest cause die suddenly." "Persons who are naturally very fat are apt to die earlier than those who are slender." "In dropsical persons ulcers forming upon the body are not easily healed." "At the approach of dentition children are attacked with pruritus of the gums, fever, convulsions, diarrhœa, especially when cutting the canine teeth, and in those who are particularly fat and have constipated bowels." Sydenham well said that "things which have their foundation in the fancy, and not in the nature of things, will be forgot in time' whereas those axioms which are drawn from real facts will last as long as Nature itself."

The great principles upon which our art is founded remain unchanged; details must, of course, be modified in accordance with particular indications, but the general laws remain the same; just as we see in history that the laws of nations must be founded upon the unchanging principles of justice, though the application of these will be regulated to suit the varying condition of the people.

But then comes the second question, What authorities are we to trust, and what are to be the limits of our assent ?

Now there is one thing, gentlemen, which, whatever may

be your culture, you *cannot* yourselves at present possess; one thing which no genius, however brilliant—no industry, however patient—no sagacity, however penetrating—no learning, however profound—can supply the place of: I mean, Experience, which is, indeed, the great teacher of us all. I think, therefore, one criterion of authority should be the possession of experience. You remember what Aristotle says on this point: "We are bound to give heed to the undemonstrated sayings and opinions of the experienced and aged, not less than to demonstrations, because, from their having the eye of experience, they behold the principles of things."

Then, again, we may allow the authority of a person because he is exceptionally competent upon the subject he treats of. For example, on board ship we are content to prepare for bad weather because the Captain predicts it, even though we may see no sign of it ourselves. This is a kind of authority which, as Dr. Newman has pointed out, requires a certain amount of intelligence and knowledge of a corresponding kind (though not, of course, of the same degree) to appreciate the force of. It is an authority, I may remark, of which everyone is occasionally obliged to avail himself.

Another kind of authority which differs from either of the preceding is that of men of genius. I shall not attempt to define genius—it is known chiefly by its effects—but it is a kind of intellectual supremacy which we cannot afford to despise; which, indeed, we shall do well to take heed to and rejoice in. It is a light which enables its possessor to see into the heart of things—to distinguish the accidents from the essentials, to perceive clearly what others only dimly dream of.

But here let me guard myself against your supposing that I would advise you to follow blindly even these guides. "Experience" is sometimes "fallacious"; the most competent may err, the highest genius is occasionally at fault. Let it be understood, then, that although it is often right and necessary to listen to the voice of authority without stopping to question it, yet whenever possible its dicta should be submitted to the criticism of reason; and that no kind of penalty should attach to not accepting it. Authority may point out the way, but it must not compel any to walk therein.

This brings us to the third question of which I spoke, namely, Wherein are we bound to investigate for ourselves, and to claim full liberty of action?

First of all, I should say, whenever we advance towards the unknown, we are bound to use all available means of inquiry, and to claim full liberty of judgment. Here, too, is the place for the scientific use of the imagination, and for the free play of the speculative as well as of the critical faculties.

So, also, whenever it becomes your duty to form an opinion upon any new problem, you must investigate it for yourselves, and take nothing for granted. Every case of disease which comes before you for diagnosis is such a problem, and must be so examined. Here you must take nothing for granted, but see for yourselves; and having by due scientific inquiry elicited all possible facts about your case, then bring your best judgment to the estimation of their value and meaning. To rightly understand a case of disease, therefore, two processes are needful—observation and reasoning—and both require cultivation for their efficient use. There is no greater mistake than to suppose that people see a thing because it is before them; on the contrary, it needs much practice either to see what is before you, or to understand what you see.

I would beg you to observe, therefore, that although I have endeavoured to point out to you somewhat of the use and value of authority, I am equally anxious to impress upon you the absolute necessity of independent inquiry, and of exercising to the utmost your powers in that direction. No discovery, no progress, is otherwise possible; for authority is not creative—it only adds its sanction to, or explains the meaning of, what already exists. Doubtless inquiry is the better means of arriving at truth, but it is not always available; and if I have seemed to lay any undue stress upon the value of authority, it is because it has seemed to me that the tendency of the present time is wrongly to despise it, and in the pride of a fancied liberty to treat with unmerited scorn its venerable aid.

But all this has been much better said long ago in the wise words which Aristotle quotes from Hesiod:—"Best of all is ho," says that poet, "who is wise by his own wit; next best he who is wise by the wit of others; but whoso is

neither able to see nor willing to hear, he is a good-for-nothing fellow."

Having thus far, then, gentlemen, endeavoured to suggest to you something of the spirit and method in which I would advise you to pursue your studies, let me now speak very briefly of the right use of the knowledge which I will presume you, by those studies, to have gained.

And first let me remind you that we are bound by our profession to make our knowledge subservient above all things to the alleviation of suffering, and to the welfare of those who seek our aid. That our duty is not merely to know but to practise our art; that indeed, as Sydenham has well said, "our art is only to be rightly learned by its use and practice."

All the arts have two sides from which they may be investigated—the contemplative and the active, the theoretical and the practical,—and he only is the complete artist who has the mastery of both of these.

It is not enough that the painter should be familiar with the method of mixing pigments and with the analysis or synthesis of colours, nor even that he should also have contemplated with all care every detail of his subject; he must be able to use his brush—in fact, to paint.

The musician must not only be versed in the theory of harmony and the relation of sounds, but must have the power of placing these sounds in that combination and sequence which alone will produce true music.

The art of medicine is no exception to this rule. You must not be merely contemplative physicians or surgeons. It is insufficient that you have the most exact knowledge of the nature and pathology of the disease which has attacked your patient, and of the methods which may be used for its treatment. You must, besides this, have the power of applying your knowledge and of practising your art—in fact, of doing battle with the enemy with which you are confronted.

There is, perhaps, just now somewhat too great a tendency to cultivate the contemplative side of our art; to look upon our patients as "cases" which may furnish this or that interesting pathological specimen; and, it may be, sometimes to forget that *disease* can only be seen, studied, and treated in the *living*, that our specimens only show us the *results* of disease, and that when we have our pathological specimens the disease and the patient are usually beyond our treatment.

Yet do not imagine that I would depreciate scientific pathology—we cannot too highly value it; nor that I think it is always desirable or possible to treat our patients—sometimes the best we can do for them is to leave them alone: but I wish you to remember that our business is the prevention, the alleviation, and, when possible, the cure of disease and injury; that our art is an *active* one, and that we must have such knowledge of it, and be so versed in its practice, that we may always be ready at the right moment to do what is needful to be done.

I said our business is the prevention, the alleviation, and, when possible, the cure of disease. We are sometimes, perhaps, prone to think too exclusively of the last, and to forget the importance of the first two of these functions. Yet there is no more true adage than that "Prevention is better than cure"; and there is no more valuable work done in our profession than that which aids in the prevention of disease. Here, at least, I hope you will range yourselves on the side of authority, and assist in the maintenance of all possible restrictions to the liberty of spreading or originating disease.

It seems to me a curious comment on our boasted liberty, that we still allow the air we breathe to be poisoned with noxious vapours, and the water we drink to be supplied to us by trading companies, who care not what impurities it contains, so long as its sale produces a profitable dividend. I have often thought what an irony it is to preach to the poor the duty and advantage of cleanliness, when it is impossible to obtain in their miserable homes either a breath of fresh air or a drop of pure water! It is still, I am sorry to say, permissible and profitable to men to make money by the letting to poor people of wretched tenements, the air of which is poisoned with the foulness of the sewer, and the water of which has to be carried to all parts of the house from one insufficient and impure supply. Surely here is a fertile enough source of disease, and a sufficiently obvious need for a central authority, with power to regulate matters so deeply affecting the health of the people, and to protect those who are least able to help themselves. Now, by using your influence and authority to aid in remedying these and similar evils, you may do much for the prevention and diminution of some of the ills which flesh is still unfortunately heir to.

Another curious instance of the lack of the protective authority of the State is the fact that the health of the people of this country is committed to the care of medical practitioners, the only guarantee of whose fitness for the responsibility is the possession of a licence to practise, which may imply either a great abundance, or an almost complete absence, of the requisite qualifications.

I may, however, perhaps be allowed to express the hope that the Council of Medical Education may before long be so constituted and so empowered that it may be able at least to enforce a uniform standard of knowledge as the *minimum* qualification for admission to the responsibilities and privileges of a registered medical practitioner.

Just consider, also, the harm that is constantly wrought by ignorance or disregard of the commonest laws of health. How many children, for instance, annually die from improper food? How many more are sacrificed to unwise clothing? How many cases of rickets, with all its attendant deformities, do we daily see which have a similar origin? Well, by diffusing a better knowledge of these things you are as surely helping the health of the community as by the most elaborate display of therapeutic skill.

So, again, the alleviation of the misery of disease, when we cannot prevent or cure it, is a function in nowise to be despised. Unfortunately there are still many ills that we know not how to prevent or cure. Do not suppose that you have nought to do with these, for by your care and knowledge you may often greatly mitigate suffering, and render tolerable and useful lives which would otherwise be gladly resigned.

Then not forget the cure of disease. Do not forget that many diseases tend naturally to recovery, and that in such cases you will best aid your patient by taking care that his environment is as favourable as possible, and by guarding him against any impediments to the natural process of repair.

Let me remind you, also, that in the investigation of disease in the human subject you have to deal with very inconstant factors.

Here it is not like the diagnosis taught you in your botany lectures, where the plant to be examined is quite passive, gives no false evidence, originates and developes always in the same manner, and can be pulled to pieces to ascertain any doubtful point. In medicine you are dealing with that exceedingly complex and changeful subject, the human being, who often resists and embarrasses your investigations, often consciously or unconsciously throws difficulties in your way, even willingly deceives you by giving false answers to your questions, and in other ways; and *cannot*, like the plant, be pulled to pieces to see the condition of the inside.

Therefore I would advise you to cultivate your imagination, that you may be able to make allowance for the abnormal condition of your patient, for the errors of nervousness, the exaggeration of disturbed sensibility, the reticence of shame; and remember that what may seem a very small thing to you, may appear a very important one to the sufferer.

And this cultivation of the imagination will help to give you patience with the sick; you will be able to place yourselves in imagination somewhat in their position, and to be the more tolerant of their irritability or their fears. But this does not mean that you are to yield to the prejudices of your patients. That is a thing you must *never* do. One of the difficulties you will have to contend with in practice is that people are constantly endeavouring to obtain your sanction to their own follies.

Let them understand at once that this is not possible; that in this matter you are uncompromising; that no wish to please or to make things smooth will induce you to sanction that of which you do not approve. Some will ask you to let them try the rubbish of quackery, and will accuse you of intolerance because you will not assent; some will be discontented because you will not order them physic which they do not need; while others will take offence at your pointing out the errors upon which their ailments depend. Well, you can't help people being fools, but there is no need to facilitate their folly. What you have to do is to be strictly upright. As Marcus Aurelius says, " Whatever anyone does

or says, I must be good, just as if the gold, or the emerald, or the purple were always saying this—Whatever anyone does or says, I must be the emerald and keep my colour." Be careful, then, to take no part in what our great novelist has called " debasing the moral currency," by countenancing any departure from that perfect simplicity and openness of conduct, and that absolute integrity of aim, which are characteristics of the true gentleman. Do not be ashamed to say " I do not know." Have " no contrefeted termes to semen wise," and if you cannot do good to your patient, at least follow the Hippocratic maxim, and " do no harm." For if you consider how greatly you are trusted, how complete must often be the dependence of your patients upon you, and that their lives and happiness are often in your hands, it must become a point of honour to merit the trust reposed in you.

You see then, gentlemen, that the practice of your profession involves grave responsibilities, and sometimes anxious cares; and that the conditions of your work are such as to make it needful for you to cultivate habitually calmness of mind, to which end I should advise you to alternate your labours with the rest of reasonable recreation.

Probably nothing is so conducive to this desirable equanimity, or so refreshing or recreating to the mind, as the study of natural beauty and of the art which has striven to represent it.

> " For Nature never did betray
> The heart that loved her ; 'tis her privilege
> Through all the years of this our life, to lead
> From joy to joy ; for she can so inform
> The mind that is within us, so impress
> With quietness and beauty, and so feed
> With lofty thoughts, that neither evil tongues,
> Rash judgments, nor the sneers of selfish men,
> Nor greetings where no kindness is, nor all
> The dreary intercourse of daily life,
> Shall e'er prevail against us, or disturb
> Our cheerful faith that all which we behold
> Is full of blessings."

And he will not be the less intelligent a student of natural science who also appreciates the beauty of the nature he is studying; who, with whatever of anatomical interest he may study the human body, fails not to note its beauty of outline and its grace of form; who, while with scientific ardour he classifies an insect, stops to admire the brilliance of the beetle's wing; who, in the exercise of his botanical analysis, still loves the sweetness of the summer flowers; who not only knows how the prism would divide the sunbeam, but also recognises the majestic splendour of the setting sun.

Herein too you may see again the ever present influence of Authority—Nature in all its variety and complexity still subject to law; its ever expanding and progressing energy still under inexorable control, and reminding us that we ourselves are under the same Supreme Authority.

And again, when you try to face the wonderful problem of Life—its origin, its orderly development, the subtlety and precision of its processes, the multiplicity and yet the unity of its phenomena,—you will see, you *must* see, that all is under the guidance of law and authority; that disease is, as we even call it, a *disorder*, an endeavour to escape from authority; and Death—the great mystery of Death—what shall I say of it? Well, I cannot understand death. It would *seem* the triumph of disorder over the order of life —a dissolution of the bonds which hold the elements of the body in co-operative union, a release from a beneficent authority into a baneful and destructive liberty. I say it would *seem* so, but that we know there is an Authority even over death; and, knowing *that*, we come to see that the shadows that gather round us as we enter on—

> " The undiscovered country from whose bourne
> No traveller returns "

are but the shadows of evening, tinctured it may be with somewhat of its sadness as well as its calm, but still the shadows of evening, coming in the orderly progression of the day, and deepening, not into an impenetrable darkness, but into the restful night through which we all must pass to enter on the everlasting day; that even *here*, completest Liberty is only attained by deference to Authority, for the Authority is of Him " whose service is perfect freedom."

OPHTHALMOLOGICAL SOCIETY.—The first meeting of this Society for the current session will be held on the 13th inst. A list of communications promised will be given in our columns as soon as possible.

INTRODUCTORY ADDRESS
DELIVERED AT THE OPENING OF THE
ST. THOMAS'S HOSPITAL MEDICAL AND SURGICAL COLLEGE.
By Dr. ALBERT J. BERNAYS.

GENTLEMEN,—It has been the custom for many years, on occasions like the present, to address to the new students, through the medium of an introductory lecture, some observations with reference to the studies in which they are about to engage, to set before them their utility and importance, and to urge upon them such diligence in acquiring knowledge as will enable them hereafter to practise the art of medicine with credit to themselves and with benefit to their fellow-creatures. To me has been deputed the privilege of addressing you on the present occasion; and, although fully sensible of the honour conferred upon me by my colleagues, yet I confess I complied with it, not from any sense of my ability to do justice to the subject, but from my desire to co-operate with them for the general welfare.

To you, Mr. Alderman Stone, we are indebted for an unintermitted attention to the welfare of this Hospital and of the Medical and Surgical College connected with it. As Treasurer, we have always found you ready to espouse our cause and to give us most essential aid when required. Your interest, too, in the College still leads you to offer the well-known and highly esteemed prize—the Treasurer's Medal,—and we trust that you may be spared many years to present it.

We are cheered by the presence of many members of the Grand Committee and other friends of this Hospital, and to them also, in the name of my colleagues and myself, I offer our sincere thanks. I would also desire to state how much we have been gratified by the honour done to one of our colleagues. The title, so richly deserved, and so promptly carried out, conferred by Her Most Gracious Majesty upon him, assures us of the interest taken by Royalty in the noble profession of medicine, and of the fact that it has been ably sustained by Sir William Mac Cormac.

In the re-arrangement of the lectures you will observe the removal from the prospectus of a name much honoured and much lamented. In bidding his colleagues farewell, Mr. Wagstaffe reminds me that he was a first year's student in the year in which I had the honour of being appointed to St. Thomas's. I cannot fully express my feelings as to the loss of a man from whom so much might have been expected; but it is a warning to young men of the insecurity of health.

And now let me give a hearty welcome to you who have entered, or are about to enter, upon your career at this College. I presume that you have not joined us without some degree of thought, and that many of you have adopted from genuine choice the profession to which you are about to devote yourselves.

One piece of advice I would venture upon as of the greatest importance to the first year's man. It is to cultivate self-control as a habit. Without it you cannot have any individuality; you will merely go with the stream, and you will become in sentiment and in character just whatever the men you associate with happen to be. A result of self-control is a resolute will. The man who has considered his duty will carry his convictions into action. But there are sore temptations to do otherwise. The path of duty is by no means always agreeable. Yet, in the affairs of life, how great an advantage is a habit of decisive action following on a prompt and sound judgment. Without it, indeed, there is no real manhood; but to acquire it a student must be independent of mere impressions. He must learn to conquer varying moods of mind, and do the things he feels he ought to do, in spite, it may be, of strong distaste—in spite of obstacles, with no slavish regard to the world's opinions, and at times even against the judgment of those to whom he would willingly defer.

You, gentlemen of the first year, will find resoluteness of will necessary to insure application to your medical studies. You are your own masters to a very great extent, in danger of neglecting the thing you ought to do, and taking to the thing you like to do. You want novelty in work as well as in mental excitement. It *is* hard to be engaged upon a hateful task, but it is through hardship that all that is valuable in character is acquired. Habits of application are thus induced before we are in a condition to choose our own work; and it is wonderful how habit reconciles us to disagreeable tasks. Habit is indeed a noble auxiliary in good, but a terrible tyrant in evil. Every case of neglected duty is a step in moral retrogression, is a loss of moral power, is a link added to the chain which binds us to evil, and which will soon acquire the very strength of despair.

What you must do, therefore—not what people think about it—*is all that concerns you.*

May I also be allowed to recommend to you to be wary in accepting many of the opinions which are afloat with reference to your own being, and to that of your Creator? Whilst, for myself, I humbly believe that God *has* revealed Himself to us, and has not left us in total darkness, as is said by some, I would warn you against the error of supposing that by any scientific research you can find Him. Nay, "for the very forest you will not see the trees." Bacon warns us against identifying God with nature,—the Architect with his work. Darwinism only introduces confusion into nature when it removes God from the scene. And this is by no means implied in the theory.

When I was young, the denial of the literal interpretation of the Mosaic cosmogony was considered a mark of the infidel; whilst now a man is not even considered a fool when he suggests that the beginning of all life upon our globe may be accounted for by the fall of a meteorite, or a shooting star, from some other orb! To none more do we owe our present liberty of thought than to the late Dean Stanley, who only three years since delivered the address at our prize distribution, and was rightly hailed by Mr. Simon as the liberator of the conscience of mankind.

Whilst men dispute, do you act in the light of the Psalmist's teaching—

"Lord, who shall abide in thy tabernacle !
Who shall dwell in thy holy hill !
He that walketh uprightly, and worketh righteousness,
And speaketh the truth in his heart.
He that backbiteth not with his tongue, nor doeth evil to his neighbour,
Nor taketh up a reproach against his neighbour.
He that sweareth to his own hurt, and changeth not."

" If any man will do the will of God, he shall know of the doctrine."
" That the soul be without knowledge is not good."

Now, the bodily health has much to do with the power of acquiring information, and it becomes a solemn duty to promote it by all available means. Within reasonable bounds you should go in for athletic exercise, as the proper oxygenation of the blood will do away with the necessity which impels so many to the use of stimulants or sedatives. Dr. Andrew Clark defines health as " that state of body in which all the functions of it go on without notice or observation, and in which existence is felt to be a pleasure, in which it is a kind of joy to see, to hear, to touch, to live." Were it not for alcohol, few indeed would ask the silly question, " Is life worth living ? " Nor have I any hesitation in saying that very few young men require any alcoholic drinks; and, if it be true, as Dr. Clark further asserts, that 70 per cent. of the patients in the London Hospital owe their sickness to alcohol, what an opportunity does your youth offer to try the effects of more or less total abstinence ! "Wherefore should I stand in the plague of custom ? " says Shakespeare. Many will be gratified to hear that as much milk is consumed in the Students' Club of our Medical College as beer. This opportunity will make it easy to abstain altogether, and to carry out the rule never to partake of any alcoholic drink during the day's work. It is a fact that alcohol disables the quiet brain for work, and the only possible explanation of the large amount of drink which so many can carry, is, that so many have no brains, and are therefore out of court as witnesses. May I, then, advise you with all earnestness to give abstinence, or the greatest moderation, a fair trial, and not to give up the attempt until, by six months of patient trial, you have proved your inability to carry it out.

Gentlemen, students of the second and third year, to you I commit the care of the students of the first year. Be you their guides ! Help them in the dissecting-room ; keep them employed; and you yourselves will be abundantly benefited thereby. Respect their ignorance, remembering that you also were once in the same condition. Let them distinctly understand that the first year well spent will almost insure a successful career. You, gentlemen of the second year, can remind them how well our system of compulsory examinations is bearing fruit; and we can speak with hearty congratulation of the effects. In the lists recording the results of these examinations we find the names of Carpenter, Lawson, Sims, Smith, Frohwein, and Bidwell, in the first class, and no fewer than twenty-one names of other students in the second class of the first year. This is eminently satisfactory, and I seize the occasion to make prominent mention of the system, as it gives parents and guardians some guarantee of the progress, or otherwise, of our charges.

Alas! that I should have to record the death, by drowning, on September 15, of young A. B. Holberton. He was well known to me, both by his own work in the laboratory, and as the brother of one of our House-Physicians. His name stands high in the second class, and you, second year's men, will naturally miss him in your classes and in your sports. His very manliness led him into danger, and was the occasion of his death. May the warning—"In the midst of life we are in death"—not be lost upon any of us.

With reference to your studies, you have not to incur the responsibility of choice. But, just as the body is not to be a mere receiver of food, so must the mind be instructed, not crammed. You must study anatomy and physiology in the dissecting-room, in the museums, and in the laboratory, aided by the careful and diligent perusal of books, and the guidance of your teachers. As a rule, read but few books: select them well, and master them thoroughly; you will then have more knowledge than those who run through a library. In hastily running over a mass of reading, the power of attention is dissipated; the mind becomes unable to fix itself upon the subject; time is not afforded for thinking upon what you have read, and making it your own; and but for the passing pleasure you may have had while reading, your labour has been useless. The minds of many readers have thus been spoiled in youth. They have no accurate knowledge—none that is ready, that is at command. They cannot remember where to find anything they have read, and if they want to know the subject correctly, they have to go over the ground again. Persons whose power of attention has thus been injured, have adopted a plan of reading which is of great service in retaining the substance of what they read. It is to have a note-book at hand, and to stop and condense in their own words what they think worth retaining. Whether, then, the mind is engaged in perceiving, reflecting, recollecting, abstracting, or reasoning, let it be with close attention. It is only thus that minds can truly acquire, arrange, and trace the relation of facts. I say then again, read but few books, and accept with perfect confidence the statements of your teachers until you are convinced of their untrustworthiness. You will be saved much waste of time and labour, which the self-taught generally incur from want of knowing what books to use and how to use them. But beyond this clearing away of some difficulties at the commencement, and applying a forcing stimulus to make a pupil exert himself to overcome others, teachers cannot assist a student. Everyone must teach himself all but the groundwork of all branches of knowledge; and if he does not continue the activity of application, into which he was first stimulated by his instructors, after he has passed from their hands, he is in danger of falling quickly behind a self-taught person, who has by the necessity of resolute application, from the first, brought himself into habits of industrious study. It is indeed the law of all valuable, of all available, knowledge, that it must be pondered, questioned, and proved by the learner himself.

As the profession of medicine is dependent upon the qualifications and capacities of those who pursue it, you must avail yourselves of all the varied and increasing knowledge which is within your reach, if you desire to extend the knowledge of the healing art. Mystery, except to quacks, no longer offers a shelter for ignorance; and even were you inaccessible to any higher motives, subsistence would be precarious if you were not prepared to meet the criticisms of an inquiring age.

Without experiment nothing can be known. A good illustration we have in the employment of anæsthetics, against the use of which there was at one time as much ignorant opposition as there is now against vivisection.

Sir James Simpson was able to satisfy some of his opponents by recording the fact that in the creation of Eve, Adam was made to fall into a deep sleep. Students of medicine should be the last people to suggest "Cui bono?" in the application of new remedies. Well do I remember one of our former students, who was preparing for the First M.B. of the University of London: he had been much exercised by the various actions of chlorine upon alcohol, and had found no satisfaction in the production of chloral. What is the use of it? The day following he informed me of the discovery by Professor Liebreich of the application of chloral hydrate, and brought me a specimen which still graces our museum, promising also that he would never again ask what was the use of knowledge.

Consider, again, the antiseptic treatment, and the benefit which has already accrued to mankind from its employment. We owe all our present knowledge to experiment, and from what we already know of the germ theory, our hopes are great in favour of the preventive treatment in medicine and in surgery.

Who shall say that inhalation has been sufficiently studied, or that the action of many disinfectants is at all understood? Who will deny that much of the disinfection carried out in the administration of the law is not only useless, but often leads to the spread of contagion by the incomplete methods with which it is performed? Much of this can only be matter for experiment, and might be undertaken by students in their fourth and fifth years. And this leads me to a reflection which I published some time ago, and which lies buried in our Transactions. There are at every medical school a number of able young men who would delight in spending another year or more in attending the hospitals if they could find the means, and there is no doubt that the public would benefit immensely by the clinical experience thus gained. Now, according to modern notions, no gentleman can be considered educated who is without some knowledge of physiology; and I do not think he could obtain it anywhere with greater advantage than at a medical school. Teachers also of the upper classes of board and other schools might, by arrangement with the Committee of the School Board of London, obtain the means of acquiring sufficient knowledge to be enabled to impart instruction at their respective schools. Now, the medical schools being distributed over London, would furnish convenient centres for large districts, and, during the medical session of nine months, it would be easy, of an evening, to find both the men and the time to teach physiology and chemistry, both practically and theoretically. There would be no necessity for building laboratories, either for the study of physiology or of chemistry; all the appliances for practical work are at hand. Instead of a system of centralisation, which threatens to overthrow our most essentially English ideas, we should have colleges sufficiently widely apart to be convenient to the respective inhabitants of the neighbourhood; we should have unity of plan with diversity of management.

South Kensington, with reference to greater London, reminds me of a scene in "Nicholas Nickleby." Mr. Squeers is boasting of the fatness of his son, as proving the quality of the feeding at Dotheboys Hall, whereupon the gentleman to whom he appeals declares that the boy has got the whole of it. Everything is starved for the sake of South Kensington; and, at the least, it does seem a waste of means, that the museums, lecture-rooms, and laboratories should be so little employed compared with their possibilities.

Stated, then, in few words, what a spur to further study it would prove, if the able students, at the end of their fourth year, might look with certainty for the means to enable them to walk the hospital, and to study their profession practically, whilst they gave a portion of their time to observation and teaching in the laboratories! At the outside, only a small percentage of students could thus employ themselves, and I should recommend the system of payment by results as applicable to the present proposition. I assume that the authorities would give their permission, and that the scheme should be carried out with the consent, or under the guidance, of the respective professors.

It is only in the laboratory that an examination of the various nostrums which are so confidently offered to a credulous public can take place. As the late lamented Dr. Maurice Raynaud says, "People talk a great deal of the progress of knowledge, and I will not contest it; but strictly speaking, we cannot perceive much of it in the subject which occupies us (scepticism in medicine). If we look around, we shall find the same ignorant infatuation, the same mixture of the most unreasonable scepticism with the most infantile superstition, the same sneering, jesting spirit which believes nothing because it believes everything, which refuses scientific evidence, and accepts without suspicion table-turning, spiritualism, and homœopathy, all without any other reason than pure imagination. And this strange disposition is not seen only, or even principally, among the common people; it is in the upper classes, in minds otherwise intelligent and cultivated, sometimes even in learned men." And again, "In all ages, dogmatism has been the father of medical scepticism. The narrowness and tyranny of dogma lead directly to doubt, above all when it does not rest on very firm foundations. Now, when we wish to investigate the old spirit, what do we find? A vague and incomplete notion of the permanence of the laws of Nature! In the midst of hypotheses, sometimes mystic, sometimes grossly materialistic, on the *primum movens*, we always meet with this idea, more or less formulated, but everywhere admitted, that life is a capricious, indiscernible force; that in all its manifestations the exception is nearly as frequent as the rule; and that it is impossible, in these changing matters, to affirm anything positively." Dr. Raynaud spoke of France; but are not his remarks quite as applicable to ourselves? During the last year our Government received £140,000 as stamp-duty upon patent medicines, and this represents but a fraction of the medicines sold!

Of all people, amongst ourselves, the most credulous are the supporters of the so-called religious press, and of certain hobbies; you have only to read the advertisements, and leading articles even, to be convinced of the truth of my statement. In a leading article in such a journal of September 23, I find that the intelligence of a new beverage broke upon the ears of men like the morning light after a long night of heavy, thick darkness. The fearful character of mineral medicines, and the superior quality of herbs of various kinds, are the subjects most generally treated. Of the credulity of people I myself remember an apt illustration. A vendor of herbs was wont, each returning market-day, which happened to be on a Friday, to set out a long table, made of planks standing upon trestles, and among heaps of herbs to place tall bottles containing specimens of tape and other worms. After a lecture, always delivered under the very windows of a regular practitioner, in which the injurious character of calomel, tartar emetic, white arsenic, and other mineral poisons, was plainly set forth, he used to clench the argument with a quotation from Holy Writ: "And what saith the Scripture?" said he, as he thumped the table and made the worms dance. Then there was all attention on the part of his increasing audience. "And what saith the Scripture?" he repeated, again thumping the table and making the worms wriggle: "'Is there no balm in Gilead? Is there no physician there? Why then is the health of the daughter of my people not recovered?' Why? Because they used mineral medicines!" At this telling reply the herbs sold like wildfire, and the table was often cleared within half an hour.

Besides the medicines there are the drinks—mineral waters of a different composition to that vaunted in the published analyses; effervescing drinks of more benefit to the maker than the consumer, clogged with chemicals requiring as much skill in their administration as does the treatment of disease! It is for you, gentlemen, to assert your proper place in society; and to be able to speak with authority, because with knowledge: and this knowledge you can only obtain by possessing some practical acquaintance with chemistry.

Surely your own observations during the last three months must have taught you how great is the interest which the public takes in matters connected with the body. We have all been watching at the sick-bed of the late President Garfield, and have read the account of the treatment pursued with an amount of attention which we rarely give to such a subject. And do you think it unimportant to lead public opinion in these and other matters?

Another good reason why you should cultivate a deeper acquaintance with the laboratory is that you may have a better knowledge of apparatus. Very little can be done in the way of research without expensive apparatus, and very much of the hopes of the future, as to knowledge, depends

upon it. Comte stated in 1842 that it was useless and hopeless to expect to determine the composition of the heavenly bodies; nevertheless, the spectroscope has to a great extent revealed the wondrous harmony of Creation. It used to be supposed that the sun was dark, and its atmosphere luminous, but it is now seen that the body of the sun is luminous, and that the solar atmosphere is made up of comparatively cool gases, which occasion the dark lines in the spectrum, and of a chromosphere consisting principally of hydrogen, jets of which are said sometimes to reach to a distance of 100,000 miles. As might have been expected from a knowledge of the composition of our own earth, the material of the planets is not uniform, depending for their difference much upon their antiquity; but no element has yet been discovered in any meteorite which is not also found upon the earth, although some of the minerals contained in them must have been formed under different conditions. The spectroscope may yet solve for us the question as to the number of the elements. Prout suggested that hydrogen must be the primordial substance; and Lockyer considers that he has proved that certain bodies are not elements. The question is not yet answered, and at present there is no sense in dogmatising as though our knowledge were complete. Not very long since the idea that electricity could compete with gas as an illuminating power was scouted as the dream of an enthusiast; now it is much more probable that gas will be vastly extended in its use for heating rather than for lighting. Surely in the better times before us smoke will no longer be permitted to defile the air, nor will volumes of sulphurous acid be allowed to escape from our chimneys! And yet the greater portion of this nuisance could be prevented by the removal of our open fireplaces, and by the introduction of Messrs. Doulton's stoves; yet more by the employment of purified gas, from which much of the lighting property has been removed through the application of a greater heat in its manufacture.

The remainder of the address was devoted to an exposition of the recent advances in constructive or synthetic chemistry, illustrated by diagrams of formulæ.

ABSTRACT OF

INTRODUCTORY ADDRESS

DELIVERED AT THE OPENING OF

ST. MARY'S HOSPITAL MEDICAL SCHOOL.

By G. P. FIELD, M.R.C.S. Eng.,

Aural Surgeon to the Hospital.

AFTER some remarks on the history of St. Mary's Hospital, and recent changes in its staff; upon the importance of physical and mental recreation, Mr. Field said:

And now, gentlemen, may I, without presumption, venture to offer you a few words of salutary counsel, derived mainly from personal observation?

To begin with our own profession. At the head of it I see men of the highest culture, an honour to our craft and to science. We live in bright days when we can look up to such leaders as a Watson, a Paget, or a Jenner. Surely such men as these merit a life peerage! "They order this matter better in France." Would they offer a President of their College of Physicians a knighthood, and make a respectable contractor or alderman a baronet? I have always felt that these lights of our profession should take higher fees. If our leaders took five or ten guineas, it would do good in every way. They would not be obliged to work so hard themselves, the juniors would get more practice, the profession would be better thought of, and the public better served. Alluding to fees, I may relate a characteristic anecdote of the late Sir William Fergusson, who, after a successful operation on a Manchester millionaire, was asked by the patient to name the fee. "Two hundred guineas," was the reply. "Two hundred guineas!" exclaimed the patient. "Yes," said Sir William; "you forget the life-long experience required to give the proper skill, the time and toil of the journey, and the loss of practice in London." "But you have only been ten minutes about it," said old Dives. "Oh! if that's your objection," said Sir William, in his broad

Scotch, "the next time I come I'll keep ye an 'oor under the knife!" Are there not hundreds of cases in which younger physicians can give as good an opinion as the most eminent practitioners? What would junior counsel think of the Attorney-General taking the same fees as themselves? Fancy calling a Bishop, or Lord Chancellor, out of bed at three in the morning! and yet the heads of our profession run this risk. If any rich numskull has feasted too liberally at the Mansion House, he immediately sends for what he considers the first opinion, naturally thinking he will get the best for his money; but if the fee were a hundred guineas the heads of our profession would sleep peacefully, and their slumbers would not often be disturbed.

But the great difficulty seems to me to be with those who are on the border-line, such as past Presidents of the Colleges of Physicians and Surgeons. What are they to do? They are all men of eminence, but have not perhaps succeeded in becoming the fashionable doctors of the day; at the same time, they could hardly take smaller fees than others holding the same position.

As was well said here by Dr. Farquharson, "The trading mind has lately been much exercised by the unheard of, and insolent, if not illegal, attempt of some grasping practitioners to demand two guineas on a first visit! It is surely time to show the general public that if they wish the luxury of a fashionable opinion they must pay for it."

Is there any body of men who work as hard as we do, and often for nothing, being scarcely thanked, for what is termed charitable work? But charity begins at home; we have to maintain a position, we have to educate our children to a high standard, if we wish them to keep pace with the rest of the world. I think our hospital authorities ought to offer their medical officers some remuneration, instead, as is frequently the case, of making the staff pay even to become governors of the institution. Again, the Poor-law medical appointments, involving wear and tear of body and mind, by night and day, do they not demand, instead of a wretched pittance of £10 or £20 a year to gentlemen of culture and position, a requital fifty-fold as much? The public must be taught what is obviously its duty.

The Hospital Saturday we may look upon as the offering of the working-classes, amounting only to about £5000 a year. Now, if 3,000,000 out of every 4,000,000 in London subscribed but 1s. per annum each, the contribution would be £150,000. It is therefore obvious that the working-people of London subscribe less than a halfpenny a year each to the support of their hospitals. Poverty cannot be pleaded, as a recent statistical investigation has shown that, in a single square mile in London, £400,000 is spent in drink in one year!

The death of a great statesman this year has given rise to an almost endless correspondence on Homœopathy, with reference, more especially, to the propriety of meeting in consultation those who practise it, the expediency of compromise, and endeavouring to heal the breach in our ranks. The followers of Hahnemann of the present day have partly come over to us; they prescribe strong tinctures, containing drugs as powerful as any preparations to be found in our Pharmacopœia; but as long as they do this, and still believe in the efficacy of infinitesimal doses, with all due deference to Bristowe and Hutchinson, we cannot co-operate with them or be of one accord.

With regard to the Contagious Diseases Acts, the repeal of these Acts would be a public calamity. Contrasting the state of things existing before with that which now prevails after the passing of the Bill, we cannot but be struck by the difference. Ever since that change, where the Acts are in force, immorality has decreased, and therefore there is less disease. Do those who clamour for the repeal of these Acts comprehend what a dreadful scourge this disease is? Have they any conception of the horrors of a case of this kind allowed to run its course? I remember, a few years ago, every breakfast-table was inundated with appeals from these people—a majority maiden ladies, perfectly innocent in both senses of that word, with the best intentions, blessed with great energy and a wonderful amount of crass ignorance. The cry was, Is it right that women should be subjected to such degrading investigations? If Jeremy Bentham is correct, happiness results from doing the greatest good to the greatest number, and in this case the end must justify the means. A minor wrong may possibly be done to individuals, in order to confer unspeakable benefit on our race; although I firmly maintain that instances of respectable women being annoyed by the police are hardly known. The objectors declare that if men sin, they deserve to be punished. This we fully admit, but it is not the whole truth; there is such a thing as hereditary disease. Total deafness and loss of sight I know to be far from uncommon from this cause. My old teacher, Hinton, found that one-twentieth of the aural patients at Guy's Hospital suffered from hereditary syphilis. "No other cause, except perhaps fever, brings on deafness so rapid and so complete." There are few worse cases than these. And knowing all this, and having a remedy at hand, are we not to make use of it? If all the idiots, the wretched, puny, diseased mortals, who have to drag out a life of misery through no fault of their own, could rise up in judgment, they would cry shame on these sickly sentimentalists, who are working hard for the repeal of the very Acts which people of intelligence and information know to be the only way of stamping out this dreadful pestilence. I should like such persons to have witnessed in the hospitals a few cases of disease before 1866—human beings, whose condition can be described by no other term than rottenness: except perhaps in the terribly graphic words of the Psalmist, "My wounds stink and are corrupt, through my foolishness." Compare such cases with the milder type of disease that is now seen at the Lock hospitals, as the rule, and not the exception. Let them picture to themselves the offspring of such parents, who surely are visited with the sins of their ancestors for many generations. It is our duty as medical men to improve the condition of the human race, and this is best done by stamping out disease, and so preventing, in a great measure, misery and crime from riding rampant; and we shall then hand down to future times, not a feeble and sickly, but a virtuous and vigorous race.

But how are we to stamp out this disease, and what is being done to further this object?

The Contagious Diseases Act is still on its trial, on its original limited scale, at the larger naval and military stations. It has been the case now for many years, again lately shown by Surgeon-General Lawson, before the Select Committee of the House of Commons this session, that the amount of primary venereal disease is considerably less than half at the stations under the Acts, as compared with those not so protected. But, in addition to this, and what is of still more importance, the number of admissions for secondary disease has been shown to be during recent years as much as 40 per cent. less at the protected places than at the others, where it has remained as nearly as possible stationary. It would be of incalculable advantage to the public if these Acts could be extended to all the large centres of population. Seaport towns, such as Liverpool and Hull, are known to be hotbeds of venereal disease of all kinds. It is impossible, however, in the face of the fanatical and unreasoning opposition which is still being carried on, to hope that much can yet be done in this direction. The Anti-Contagious Diseases Acts Association, as shown before the Committee of the House of Commons, collects £3000 a year to carry on the agitation.

The opposition is similar in character to that which prevails against vivisection and vaccination, and is almost confined to places far away from the working of the Acts, where there is an almost complete ignorance as to their operation and effects. The testimony given this session from places where these measures are in operation is overwhelming, not only as regards the diminution of disease, but the improved condition of the towns, in the suppression of street solicitation, riotous demeanour, etc. Clergy of all denominations have given most striking evidence to this effect, as well as to the facilities afforded for the reformation of fallen women and the suppression of juvenile prostitution, which they find now to be almost a thing of the past. It would be well if the profession generally would make themselves more familiar than they are with these facts, so as to be able when opportunity offers to guide public opinion in the right direction. There is one point which is well worthy of mention, and which has been brought out by the labours of Surgeon-General Lawson. He has ascertained from the Registrar-General's Returns the proportion of deaths from syphilis in the different parts of England and Wales, taking three quinquennial periods from 1865 to 1879, and he has found that in the counties south of the Thames and the Bristol Channel, in which are situate all the stations under the Acts, except Colchester, there has been a decline in the deaths from syphilis, comparing the first with the third period. of 14 per cent. In all the other groups of counties, Midland, North Midland, and Northern, there has been an advance of 14, 37, and 15 per cent. respectively. The death-rate varies in the different groups of counties; but the only place north of the Thames where there has been a decrease, is London, where the rate is very high, but has fallen 9 per cent. These are most remarkable statistics, and being given chiefly on the authority of Mr. James Lane, cannot be doubted; they are of especial interest when it is considered that three-fourths of the recorded deaths from syphilis are of children under one year of age. Further investigation in this direction is much to be desired, for if it can be shown that legislation of this kind can make a really serious impression on hereditary syphilis, the benefit which would accrue to the community could hardly be over-estimated.

As to the Anti-vivisectionists, let them turn their attention to Hurlingham, where the bleeding bird wantonly killed sometimes drops into the very lap of the fashionable lady; to pastimes and sports, which are not altogether free from the charge of cruelty, and see what a cloud of hornets will buzz about their ears! Public opinion would be far more outraged at the bare idea of stopping man's amusement of this kind, than it is even moved at present by the attempt of some to smother scientific research which is for the public weal. Talking now of selfish motives, some of the special hospitals, who advertise in the *Times*, generally in the season, are worthy of notice. First, we have the president, perchance a great and good man, but a child in the ways of the world, and who cannot see that some of these so-called special hospitals seem to be established for the advantage (direct or indirect) of the medical officers, who probably obtain a payment out of every patient; and next, the secretary, not unfrequently a retired but not retiring military gentleman, who, it is not uncharitable to suppose, receives a percentage out of every subscription. A lady said to me the other day, "Do you know anything of such and such a hospital? I have had six circulars from it during the last four months. It seems to be a capital way of advertising the senior medical officers, at the expense of the institution!" I think it is a crying evil that general hospitals in this great and fabulously rich city should be obliged to close their wards for want of funds, while other places of little worth are springing up daily from the importunity of clever promoters, who set to work in the same way as they would to float a company.

Mr. Field also referred to the growth of specialism, the International Medical Congress, medical evidence in courts of law, and to recent advances in general and in medical science, and concluded in the following words:—

I have ventured to counsel you as to the mode of beginning and continuing your medical life. I have pointed out some of the abuses of our time, regarding which it is our duty, as medical men, to speak plainly, "for if the trumpet give an uncertain sound, who shall prepare himself to the battle." It will be for you to carry on these reforms, and "to pass the torch of truth from hand to hand." I have just told you what has been effected by great men of late years, and have especially dwelt on the achievements of our own profession. As much as has been done, can be done, and more. We cannot all secure distinguished success, but we can all gain an honourable position in society, our chief reward being the knowledge of benefits rendered to mankind.

Permit me, gentlemen, as one deeply interested in your welfare, to entreat you to refrain from grasping at the fleeting and deceitful shadows of life. Cling earnestly and firmly to everything that is honest and true. Let a strong sense of duty pervade every thought, word, and deed. Then, and then only, can you reasonably expect to ride calmly, through the storms of this troublesome world, into the haven of perfect peace. You will then be able to look back with feelings of satisfaction upon an honourable career, in which it has been your privilege to mitigate the sufferings of that being, of whom our great dramatist has said, "What a piece of work is man! How noble in reason! how infinite in faculties! in form and moving how express and admirable; in action, how like an angel; in apprehension, how like a god!"

ORIGINAL COMMUNICATIONS.

ON PROLAPSE OF THE OVARIES.(a)

By G. ERNEST HERMAN, M.B. Lond.,

Assistant Obstetric Physician to the London Hospital; Physician to the Royal Maternity Charity; Honorary Librarian to the Obstetrical Society of London.

I OFFER some remarks on the subject of prolapse of the ovary, because, taking together all cases in which it occurs, it is a very common condition; it gives rise to definite symptoms; and, when existing alone, it can generally be successfully treated. It is sometimes the only morbid condition present; but far more commonly it is found accompanying other diseases of the internal genitals. It is briefly mentioned in most of the text-books on diseases of women, and it has recently been made the subject of an able monograph by Dr. Paul F. Mundé, of New York.(b) That which seems to me yet to be desired in the descriptions of this condition in the systematic works, and even in Dr. Mundé's paper, is a closer adherence to the principle of studying *the simplest cases only*. A case in which several morbid conditions occur together, seldom can teach us much as to the natural history of any one of them. But if we are familiar with the signs and symptoms which any morbid condition causes when occurring alone, it is then easy to recognise the part it plays in modifying the clinical phenomena due to any other maladies with which it may co-exist.

Taking together all the cases in which prolapse of the ovary is met with, they may be divided clinically into three groups, which are the following:—First, those associated with diseases of the other pelvic organs; more particularly with perimetritis, and with the backward displacements of the uterus. I mention this group first, because I have little to say about such cases. In them the symptoms are of course complex, and not those of ovarian displacement simply; and the treatment has to be modified in each case in accordance with the sum of the conditions present. In studying the symptoms and natural history of prolapse of the ovary, such cases do not help us. I therefore pass from them.

The second group is of cases in which prolapse of the ovary coexists with well-marked oöphoritis. In these cases it has been made a subject of argument whether it is the swelling of the ovary from inflammation that leads to the displacement, or the prolapsus which causes the oöphoritis. There is no doubt that the former statement is true of some cases—I think, with Mundé, of the majority. It is possible that the latter may also hold good of some; but I am not convinced that it is the rule. It is to be regretted that many authors have put this class of cases together with that next to be mentioned.

The third class is, cases in which ovaries apparently otherwise normal are prolapsed. Dr. Mundé, in the paper that I have referred to, although he recognises this class of cases as different from the preceding one, yet does not make the distinction clear. He says:—"Displacement of the ovary is a very common and, by itself, highly distressing affection, worthy of a separate place in the text-books, and requiring, and capable of, efficient treatment independently of the congestion and enlargement of the organ which may or may not accompany it." Again—"It must be admitted, however, that cases are not infrequently met with in which the prolapsed ovary excites no local symptoms whatever except that of pain during coition." These quotations show that Dr. Mundé is familiar with ovarian prolapse independently of inflammatory conditions of the organ; and I think it is unfortunate that in the descriptions he elsewhere gives of the symptoms, he should not have separated the two classes of cases. He enumerates, for instance, as symptoms of ovarian prolapse, "a dragging sensation in each groin and down the thighs, some bearing-down and weight in the pelvis, sacralgia, pain in either hip, slight radiating neuralgic pains in the groins and thighs"; and in another place, speaking of the symptoms, he says, "The majority of them are met with in almost every aggravated form of uterine disorder, and that none of them are distinctive of ovarian disease." This latter statement seems to me only correct from Dr.

(a) Read before the Hunterian Society.
(b) American *Gynæcological Transactions*, vol. iv., 1879, page 184.

Mundé's point of view; because he reasons from complicated cases, in which the symptoms caused by other diseases accompany those produced by the ovarian prolapse. *Simple cases alone* can tell us what these latter symptoms are. There is another point upon which greater precision is to be wished; that is, a clearer distinction between *direct* and *indirect* symptoms. He says:— "As constitutional symptoms may be mentioned—a feeling of lassitude, of distaste for mental and physical exertion; an excitable, irritable disposition, alternating with melancholy and hallucinations; various hysterical and nervous symptoms, occasionally hemichorea, and neuralgic pains in the leg of the affected side." Now most of these, it is well known, are met with in nervous exhaustion from any cause. Anything, in the ovary or elsewhere, productive of long-continued suffering and anxiety, may lead to most of the symptoms here set down. They have no special connexion with prolapse of the ovary, or even with the ovary at all. They are not symptoms of prolapse of the ovary, but spring from a state of the nervous centres which it, as well as many other causes, may produce. The most that can be said of the connexion is, that they are indirect consequences which sometimes follow prolapse of the ovary.

The late Dr. Rigby, who, I believe, was the first to call attention to the symptoms caused by the displacement now under consideration, did so by describing at length a case which some might think was one of prolapse of the ovary with oöphoritis : for his patient, who was a single woman, had pain not only during defæcation, but also coming on when she could hardly tell the exciting cause of the attack. His account is followed, in the references which they make to the subject, by West, Barnes, and Schroeder, each of whom mention sudden paroxysmal pain as well as pain during certain functions. Other authors who mention the occurrence of this displacement, among whom I may mention Mackintosh, Denman, Tilt, Scanzoni, Hodge, Emmett, refer to it only in connexion with other morbid states of the organ, such as cystic disease and oöphoritis, of which the displacement is an occasional complication.

I will now submit to your consideration notes of some cases of prolapse of the ovary, and then offer some remarks on the clinical facts which they teach.

The first case which I have, although it is not quite so simple, nor are my notes so full, as I could wish, yet the patient's statements were quite definite enough to make it very instructive.

Mrs. R., aged twenty-three, was sent to me in November, 1877, by Dr. Talbot King, of Hackney. She had had one child in June, and had been ill since, suffering chiefly from hæmorrhage. She had a retroflexion of the uterus, for which a Hodge's pessary was adjusted, which was worn with comfort until February, when it was removed. On July 29, 1878, she again consulted me. Her chief complaints now were of pain in defæcation and in sexual intercourse, the pain on each occasion lasting two or three hours, and being accompanied with nausea. Other symptoms, which did not trouble her so much, were pain in micturition, and frequent desire to pass water, pain in the sacral region, in the nape of the neck, and in both iliac regions. She should have menstruated on the 12th, but had not done so, and her breasts were slightly painful.

On examination, I found the uterus in the axis of the pelvic inlet, and slightly enlarged ; being, as was afterwards shown, about six weeks pregnant. Low down behind the uterus was a movable, tender, oval swelling, of about the shape and size of a normal ovary. Pressure upon this body produced pain which the patient identified as being like that which she suffered on the occasions mentioned. Her appetite was good, but the bowels were confined. She had rested much, hoping that thereby the pain would be relieved, but without improvement.

She was advised to take three times daily a mixture composed of one drachm of sulphate of magnesia in an ounce of peppermint-water, and a thick elastic ring pessary was put into the vagina.

On August 12 I again saw her. The pain on intercourse had been quite absent. After this date I saw no more of the patient till November 12, 1880. She then told me that the instrument had been removed about a month after I had seen her, and that then the dyspareunia had returned, but had got better towards the end of pregnancy.

The points in this case to which I ask attention are

these :—1. That before the prolapse of the ovary she had a retroflexion. The causal conditions of backward displacement of the uterus and of prolapse of the ovary are in the main identical, both being alike results of slight yielding of the pelvic floor, into which the uterus is implanted, and upon which the ovary rests. 2. The symptoms of which the patient chiefly complained. These were, pain in defæcation (the bowels being constipated) and in sexual intercourse—symptoms arising out of the altered position of the ovary, in a manner obvious enough. The character of the pain is noteworthy ; it was a pain of considerable duration, lasting two or three hours, and accompanied with nausea. 3. The effect of treatment. A thick elastic ring (watch-spring covered with india-rubber) was put into the vagina. The result was that the pain in intercourse went away. After a month the ring was withdrawn, and the dyspareunia returned. As pregnancy advanced, and the enlarging uterus lifted the ovaries out of the pelvis, this symptom spontaneously got better. I regret that I can throw little light on the other symptoms in this case. The prescription first given for the pain in defæcation was not efficacious ; and I did not have the opportunity of modifying the treatment. Other cases will illustrate what I have to say on this symptom. The other pains, the irritability of bladder, etc., may have been due to oöphoritis, or they may have been reflex only, and a result of the pregnancy. I was inclined to think the latter, but did not see enough of the patient to make me sure about it. I adduce the case on account of the three points I have drawn attention to, which it illustrates.

F. E. C., aged twenty-six, stonemason's wife, came to the obstetric out-patient department of the London Hospital on December 15, 1877. Before her marriage she had been a nurse in the London Hospital, and, probably from the experience so gained, she was unusually clear and precise in her description of the troubles from which she suffered.

Her statement was, that she had been married three years and a half ; had had one child, two years ago, but no other pregnancy. Until this confinement she had been quite well. The labour was a bad one, instruments being used ; she had "a slight touch of inflammation" afterwards ; hæmorrhage continued for three weeks, and she lost blood on and off more frequently and more copiously than she had been accustomed to at her menstrual periods, for nine months subsequently. Five months after her confinement she began to have a yellow discharge : this came on gradually, and latterly had been copious. During the last six months the catamenia had been regular, but scanty, only lasting two days, and not accompanied with any pain. Her great complaint—that which had brought her to the hospital—was of dyspareunia. This had been present ever since the confinement, and was very severe. She could not hold her water very long. These troubles—dyspareunia, discharge, and irritability of bladder—were the only ones from which she now suffered. She had no pain of any kind except the one mentioned, nor had she ever had since the confinement. The bowels were regular.

She was a fairly well-nourished and healthy-looking woman. The uterus was rather low down, but was not altered in shape. The vagina was rather lax, but there was nothing else abnormal about it, nor about the vulva. There was no tenderness about the vaginal orifice or its neighbourhood. There was a slight erosion round the os uteri. The uterine cavity measured two inches and three-quarters in length. Low down, behind and to the right of the uterus, was felt a movable body of the shape and size of an ovary. When this was pressed upon, the patient at once complained of pain, and said that the pain so caused was like that for the relief of which she had come to the hospital. A metal Hodge's pessary was put in ; and she was also given an astringent injection to be used twice daily.

She attended rather irregularly, the next note I have being on May 4, 1878. She had used the injection, and had found out for herself how to take out and replace the pessary. She found that she could not wear it more than twenty-four or thirty-six hours, because if she did she suffered pain in the coccygeal region and the genitals swelled. But after she had worn the instrument she found that the dyspareunia was much better. The discharge had now ceased. As the Hodge's pessary caused pain, it was removed, and a thick elastic ring put in its place.

The next important note is on July 16. She then said

that the dyspareunia was better, but that she had much discharge. She had found that when she was without the ring the discharge ceased, but the dyspareunia returned. With the ring the discharge was abundant, but the pain became slight.

I did not see her again till March 11, 1879. She then said that since her former attendance she had had some illness which had obliged her to call in a medical man in her neighbourhood. She was now so far well that she did not think it necessary to attend at the hospital.

I next saw her on February 3, 1880. Since her last attendance she had been treated several times for "ulcera. tion of the womb" by cauterisation; each time marital ab. stinence had been enjoined during treatment, and after the ulceration was pronounced well she had gone to the country for a week or two. On her return she found the pain gone. The "ulceration" was accompanied with discharge, which stopped after the cauterisation. For the last three months the pain on intercourse had been returning. It was referred to the left ovarian region, and each occasion was followed by discharge lasting about two days. There was a very slight erosion round the os. The tender ovary-like body was felt to the right of and behind the uterus as before. On account of the discharge caused by the india-rubber ring, the patient preferred an instrument of different material; a Hodge's pessary was therefore put in.

February 13.—She said that intercourse had taken place without any pain.

January 19, 1881.—I heard from another nurse that this patient had again been under the care of a medical man in her neighbourhood. He had tried various pessaries, and had at length fitted her with a thick elastic ring which exactly suited her. She now thought herself quite well.

This case also is not so complete as I should wish, but it shows some important points. First, the etiological condi. tions. There were frequent hæmorrhages persisting for nine months after delivery, probably due to defective in. volution of the uterus. There was a lax and capacious vagina, a condition due partly to defective involution after labour, and partly to the chronic vaginitis which was present, and had doubtless led, as all inflammations do, to softening and consequent relaxation of the part affected. The uterus was low in the pelvis, and there was irritability of the bladder, a symptom frequently associated with yielding of the pelvic floor. The conditions enumerated are all such as are the forerunners and accompaniments of descent of the uterus. Second, dyspareunia was the only symptom which was so troublesome as to make her seek advice. Not a pain was felt, or had been felt, except when the ovary was touched. She had no pain on defæcation; but, unlike the other cases, the bowels were quite regular. Lastly, the relief which fol. lowed the application of an instrument which gave support. Unfortunately, the patient attended so irregularly, and took her treatment to so large an extent into her own hands, that the demonstration of the effect of treatment is not here so clear as I should have liked it to be.

(*To be continued.*)

REMOVAL OF THE UTERUS FOR CANCER.—The *Presse Médicale Belge* of September 18 has an article strongly de. precatory of the present mania for the performance of this operation leading to its being undertaken when the diagnosis is uncertain and the probability of ultimate cure hopeless. The writer furnishes references to eighty-one cases, with their results, which have been performed since Freund's typical operation in 1878. Of these cases, fifty-eight are recorded as fatal, to say nothing of unfinished operations and relapses. "In the presence of such results, is not our opposition to so grave an operation for uterine cancer amply justified? Two objections will be taken. It will be said, 'But there are some cures.' If we accept as definitive cures temporary recoveries, this may be so; but, even here, who will answer for it that it was really cancer for which the operation was performed? If we require more than mere affirmation, we can only accept with doubt this word 'cure' with its numerous reticences. Secondly, it may be affirmed that in many cases the patients have not died from the con. sequences of the operation. We reply that diseases co-existing with cancer of the uterus were evidently a contra-indication to the operation, and a reason the more for not resorting to it."

ON AGARICUS IN THE TREATMENT OF NIGHT-SWEATING.

By R. NORRIS WOLFENDEN, B.A., M.B. Cantab.,
Lecturer on Practical Physiology at the Charing-cross Hospital School.

I REGARD every new drug that can be pressed into the service of checking the debilitating night-sweats of phthisis as invaluable. Having made extensive trial of those com-monly in vogue, I have found many sadly wanting, and only one, viz., atropia, that yielded really excellent results. Given in one-seventieth of a grain doses, it rarely fails. But atropia is a drug of great power, and capable of producing great physiological effects, and though accidents are very rare, such an accident as an overdose might easily occur; and dispensing is not always faultless. If, therefore, any preparation could be found, possessing the advantages of atropia without its toxic properties, I should prefer to use it.

It is now about eighteen months since I first made trial of a preparation which had previously been used in France, viz., agaricus. The complete success of this preparation has led me to consider it of value equal to atropia, and the superior of atropia from the fact that it is quite innocuous. Ten grains, too much or too little, produce no toxic effects. Equally powerful with atropia, then, in its action, it has the advantage of being harmless. It is a light, bulky, brown powder, of very bitter taste, and is best administered made into a confection with a little jam. Twenty grains are usually quite sufficient, given at bedtime, though thirty grains may be necessary to quite check the sweating, the only inconvenience attending the administration of large doses being the great quantity of the powder. However, patients make no objection to the bitter taste, etc., when they find how much they benefit by it.

I have administered it in nearly forty cases of night-sweating, with complete success. A few cases from my note-book, taken just as they come, are as follow :—

1. A female, subject of chronic tubercular phthisis, sweated copiously at nights. Agaricus gr. xxx. given, at first every night. From the first dose the sweats ceased entirely. After-wards she had some diarrhœa, and the dose was reduced to twenty grains, sweating still being checked. When she left off the powder, sweating returned.

2. A male, the subject of tubercular phthisis, whose night temperature was generally 108°, and who sweated profusely, wetting the bedclothes, was ordered agaricus gr. xx. The first dose stopped the sweating, and it never recurred while agaricus was administered.

3. A male, with advanced pneumonic phthisis, sweated copiously. Agaricus gr. xx. checked the sweating. As he also had chronic diarrhœa, it was combined with gr. ij. of Dover's power.

4. A male, with tubercular phthisis, sweated regularly and profusely at night. Agaricus gr. xx. at first diminished the sweats, and after three nights stopped them altogether. When he left off the agaricus, sweating recurred.

5. A male, with fibroid phthisis, also sweated very profusely every night. Pulv. agaricus gr. xx. checked the sweats con-siderably; twenty-five grains stopped them altogether, and he never sweated again.

6. A girl, who had complicated cardiac disease and con-gested lungs. She used to sweat much every night. Pulv. agaricus gr. x. om. nocte stopped the sweats entirely.

These cases could be multiplied, were it not taking up too much space. They are in no way picked, but merely the first half-dozen in my note-book. I am convinced that in agaricus we have a most useful and powerful, and at the same time harmless, drug. The only ill effects of a large dose that I have seen are—first, sickness, which stops on diminution of the dose; or diarrhœa, which can be averted by combination with one or two grains of Dover's powder. The cases that I have experimented on have all been phthisical, except one, and therefore I cannot speak of its effect on sweating other than phthisical. I believe it to be a preparation worthy of extensive trial, and of such equal efficacy with atropia that it may supplant it.

REPORTS OF HOSPITAL PRACTICE

IN

MEDICINE AND SURGERY.

CHARING-CROSS HOSPITAL.

PULSATILE AORTA—ANÆMIA—DEATH—AUTOPSY.

(Under the care of Dr. POLLOCK.)

[For these notes we are indebted to Mr. ALBERT LEAHY.]

JANET F., aged fifty-three, married, was admitted into the hospital under the care of Dr. Pollock on June 9, 1881, with the following history. She had experienced a "curious throbbing sensation" in the abdomen for the last five or six months, and for many years past she had suffered from dyspepsia, with pain and sickness after her food. She has never had any blow or other violence on the abdomen. Her bowels have always been very constipated. She has suffered from rheumatism. During her present illness she has lost flesh very considerably, her weight having come down from thirteen stone to nine stone in the last six months. She had an erythematous rash on her a few days ago: it appeared first on the forearms, and then on her face. Her father died, aged seventy-eight, of senile decay; her mother is still alive and well; but she has lost a sister and a brother from phthisis.

The "present condition" on admission was noted as follows: —She complains of considerable pain, of an aching and continuous character, whenever she is in a sitting posture, but which is much relieved by lying down. She feels "a curious throbbing sensation" in her abdomen, which is most plainly felt in the lumbar and inguinal regions on the right side, and which she compares to the ticking of a watch. She says that, after sitting up for some time, her legs begin to swell. Her throat is very sore. Tongue is raw-looking and glazed from loss of its epithelium; it is very foul and coated in the early mornings; there is also considerable stomatitis. She is very thirsty; appetite quite gone. During the day she suffers from delirium and is very strange in her manner. There is no headache. She has a double femoral hernia. Pulse 124; temperature 99°.

On examining the abdomen, a well-marked pulsation, synchronous with the heart's beat, was found in the middle line and immediately over the aorta. This pulsation did not extend laterally, and was not so distinctly expansile as in the sac of an aneurism. It was, moreover, diffused lengthwise, and could be felt more or less over the whole length of the aorta. It was thought, on making deep pressure on the left side of the median line, that a hard prominence could be felt coming forwards from the spine, and distinctly behind the pulsation. Over the pulsating area a loud systolic bruit was audible, which was increased on pressure and was loudest in the epigastric region. There was a tympanitic note over the aorta, which was due to the intestines in front of it; but over the hard prominence on the left side the percussion-note was distinctly dull. Her throat, when more carefully examined, was found to be much inflamed, with several small ulcerated spots on the posterior wall of the pharynx, as well as something very like false membrane. The uvula was elongated and œdematous.

Treatment.—An effervescing medicine was ordered.

June 11.—She passed a very restless night, suffering from muttering delirium; complained of headache, and difficulty in swallowing. Tongue very hard and dry; thirst excessive. She vomited once. Temperature 102°; pulse 120.

14th.—She was suddenly seized with difficulty in breathing and died.

Post-mortem Examination.—Heart: Tissue anæmic and fatty; otherwise normal. Lungs: They were both emphysematous, and the left at its base was œdematous. Liver small and fatty. Kidneys pale and anæmic; capsules adherent. Spleen small and soft. Stomach and intestines appeared healthy. Brain congested; tissue soft; there was some turbid fluid in both lateral ventricles. The aorta was pushed forward and to the left by a scattered osteophytic new-growth, involving the bodies of all the lumbar vertebræ, especially the adjoining portions of the fourth and fifth. The nature of the growth was not very apparent.

TERMS OF SUBSCRIPTION.

(Free by post.)

				£	s.	d.
British Islands	. . . .	Twelve Months	.	£1	8	0
,, ,,	. . . .	Six ,,	.	0	14	0
The Colonies and the United } States of America . . . }	Twelve ,,	.	1	10	0
,, ,, ,,	. . . .	Six ,,	.	0	15	0
India ,, ,,	. . . .	Twelve ,,	.	1	10	0
,, (viâ Brindisi)	. . . .	,, ,,	.	1	15	0
,, ,, ,,	. . . .	Six ,,	.	0	15	0
,, (viâ Brindisi)	. . . .	,, ,,	.	0	17	6

Foreign Subscribers are requested to inform the Publishers of any remittance made through the agency of the Post-office.

Single Copies of the Journal can be obtained of all Booksellers and Newsmen, price Sixpence.

Cheques or Post-office Orders should be made payable to Mr JAMES LUCAS, 11, New Burlington-street, W.

TERMS FOR ADVERTISEMENTS.

			£	s.	d.
Seven lines (70 words)	. . .	.	.0	4	6
Each additional line (10 words)	. .	.	0	0	6
Half-column, or quarter-page	. .	.	1	5	0
Whole column, or half-page	. .	.	2	10	0
Whole page	. . . . .	.	5	0	0

Births, Marriages, and Deaths are inserted Free of Charge.

THE MEDICAL TIMES AND GAZETTE is published on Friday morning: Advertisements must therefore reach the Publishing Office not later than One o'clock on Thursday.

Medical Times and Gazette.

SATURDAY, OCTOBER 8, 1881.

THE OPENING OF THE MEDICAL SCHOOLS.

THE summer is over and gone; the vacation is past, and with it the holiday weather; chill October—very chilly, so far—is again upon us; and the voice of the lecturer is once more heard in our medical schools. As the 1st of October, the normal date for the commencement of the great winter session in England and Ireland, fell this year on Saturday, the opening of the great majority of the schools was put off till Monday this week; but at St. Thomas's Hospital the Introductory Address, by Dr. Albert Bernays, was delivered on Saturday last. The old custom of commencing the session by only an "introductory" address by one of the staff was observed at but three of the schools—namely, St. Thomas's, St. Mary's, and St. George's. At the Middlesex and Westminster Hospitals the distribution of the prizes for the past year, and at University College and Charing-cross Hospital a conversazione, followed the address; while at King's College, Sir John Lubbock opened the session. At St. Bartholomew's, Guy's, and the London Hospitals no address of any kind was given.

At St. Thomas's Hospital, Dr. Bernays gave the students some hints to guide them in their work, advising them strongly to cultivate the habit of self-control, and touched, among other things, on the freedom—or liberality, so called —of thought as regards religious matters in the present day, recommending them to be wary in accepting many of the opinions afloat with reference to their own being, and to their Creator. He spoke of the high value of scientific research: we owe, he observed, all our present knowledge to experience, which is but the result of experiment: and he dwelt at length on the immense advantages that would arise to general education, to medical science, and to individual medical men, could our medical schools be employed as centres for teaching physiology and chemistry, practically and theoretically. Our museums, lecture-rooms, and laboratories are now but little used as compared with their capabilities; while it would give a great spur to educational and scientific work could the more able of our students look forward to continuing, after the completion of the ordinary curriculum, their hospital and clinical studies, while they gave a portion of their time to teaching in the laboratories under the guidance of the professors. Work of great and direct value to the public, and which can only be properly and fully done in well-appointed laboratories, could then be fully done in examining the nature and character of the nostrums offered to the public, in the analysis of mineral waters, natural and artificial, and in other work of like kind.

Dr. Douglas Powell, in the admirably thoughtful and instructive introductory address which he delivered to the students at the Middlesex Hospital, and which we have the satisfaction of being enabled to publish to-day in full, pointed out how the driest of the elementary studies of medicine would become profoundly interesting could we but see beforehand their full bearing and application; and he urged the students in "the anatomical period of their career"—that is, during the first and second years of their studies—to use their spare hours in the interim of lectures, and while awaiting opportunities for dissection, to observe practical matters of medicine and surgery from the anatomical and physiological points of view. Let them train the ear in listening to the healthy heart- and breath-sounds; the touch in recognising characters of the pulse; the eye in noticing quickly alterations in shape and outline; and so on : but beyond this kind of training, to refrain from all clinical work. The more advanced students should still work on anatomical and physiological lines, proceeding from healthy anatomy and physiology to those changes and perversions of structure, formation, and nutrition that constitute disease. Now also, and always, the student must train to the utmost, by practice, eye, ear, and hand, to see, hear, feel, and appreciate all physical signs of disease. Dr. Powell advised the students to be eager questioners. "Question more, and you will learn much more. It is impossible for teachers to know where your difficulties are, unless you ask questions; but do not always expect complete and satisfactory answers—all at the bedside are learners, although some must presume to teach." He insisted, not a whit too strongly, on the immense value of all posts of practical work—clerkships, dresserships, house-surgeonships, etc.; every post that gives practical experience and responsibility. It is simple truth that "no one can teach students what in these offices they may learn for themselves—no teacher can succeed like responsibility"; and Dr. Powell gave very valuable advice when he added here, "Do not be deterred from going in for any such appointment because you think So-and-so may be better up than you are. Modesty is an excellent quality, but this form of modesty is but skirking that generous rivalry, to fear which is to court failure in life." We commend also especially to our readers Dr. Powell's remarks on the high value of a careful and close study of the processes of repair and convalescence, and the pregnant illustrations he gives of its teaching; and his observations on *compensation* as a great principle in the natural history of disease. "Compensatory function," he said, "is the *modus vivendi* in chronic disease. The sources and methods and paths of compensatory function will afford a rich field for interesting and original research. It is a subject upon which our text-books are curiously silent. All the knowledge you will gain of it will be gathered in the wards and the out-patient room." He also spoke well and wisely on not trusting blindly and too much to the *vis medicatrix naturæ*. "That power ofttimes plays sad havoc with us; and you will find in practice but few cases in medicine or surgery in which you can with a clear conscience stand aside and say 'here is nothing to be done.'" He dwelt at some length

on the educational duties of the medical practitioner; referring to the value of his opportunities of giving words of advice in matters of hygiene, cleanliness, temperance in all things, care of children, diet, and the like. And he gave some good and useful hints as to the equipment with which the practitioner in the country or the colonies should be provided on his daily rounds. The whole address should command careful and thoughtful study.

Mr. Warrington Haward, in his excellent address at St. George's Hospital, which also we have the pleasure of giving at length, took for his subject "Liberty and Authority in Medicine." He pointed out to the students the spirit or tone of mind in which they should enter on their studies as a whole. They would be continually obliged to determine as to how far they were to trust to the dictation of their teachers, and how far to depend upon their own judgment and investigation, for they could not wholly depend upon either the one or the other. We should all be poor indeed, both in knowledge and resources, if deprived of the great inheritance of observation and doctrine that has come to us from our forefathers, or if we accepted nothing from the past of which the accuracy and value have not been tested by ourselves. But, on the other hand, our reason and judgment must be duly exercised, or, enfeebled by disuse, they, like muscles weakened by disease, will be easily turned aside by the slightest obstacle, and be liable to irregular and errant action. The question was how to steer well and safely between the danger of despising the teachings of our predecessors, and that of yielding our independence of thought to and taking our opinions from others; and Mr. Haward addressed himself to the task of giving his hearers some aid towards its solution. He pointed out that consciousness of the imperfection and deficiency of knowledge should engender in them, and lead them to cultivate, modesty, toleration, and caution, while the sense of the vast extent of the unknown that awaits and invites investigation should add the stimulus of enthusiasm. Modesty is the due sense of the proportion which we bear to the rest of the world, and it is, therefore, usually developed in proportion to the amount of real knowledge attained. This sense naturally leads to toleration—the expression of our recognition of our own fallibility. Caution—the best guarantee for real advancement in knowledge—is especially requisite in the pressure and hurry of the present day. On this Mr. Haward enlarged, pointing out how neglect of a wise caution leads to inaccuracy of thought, observation, and speech. To these virtues—this becoming modesty, needful toleration, and wise caution—should be added, if possible, the healthy stimulus and inspiring influence of enthusiasm; which comes, Mr. Haward told the students, "chiefly from a belief in the nobleness and rectitude of your aim, and produces a sublime indifference to obstacles, just as, in pursuing a difficult journey, the certain knowledge that you are on the right path helps you to disregard the roughness or steepness of the way." Mr. Haward then discussed these questions :—1. What facts and doctrines are so certainly known and established that they may be taken for granted and used as a basis of action? 2. What authorities are we to trust, and what are to be the limits of our assent? 3. Wherein are we bound to investigate for ourselves, and to claim full liberty of action? We cannot here note, in even the most cursory manner, Mr. Haward's scholarly and learned handling of these questions. Our readers have the address, and they will reap a full harvest of profit and pleasure in studying it. We will only add that, with regard to the first question, Mr. Haward shows that the doctrines to be received must be established by credible witnesses, received by competent judges, and confirmed by sufficient experience; and that many of the beliefs in medicine upon which we are daily acting are the *dogmata* of the ancients, sanctioned by time. Under the second question, the limits and *criteria* of authority are considered, and it is contended that its *dicta* should, when possible, be submitted to the criticism of reason, and that no penalty should attach to not accepting them. In answer to the third question, he said that whenever we advance towards the unknown we are bound to use all available means of inquiry and to claim full liberty of judgment. This was the place for the scientific use of the imagination, and for the full play of the speculative as well as of the critical faculties.

Dr. Vivian Poore, who delivered the introductory address at University College, discussed the *locus standi*, the advantages and disadvantages, of medicine as a profession and as a science, insisted on the necessity of an acquaintance with the principles of the collateral sciences, and pointed out how the continued and inevitable growth of medicine and its allied sciences makes it more and more difficult to confine medical education within reasonable, or what seem reasonable, limits as to time and expense; and then addressed himself to discuss and criticise *Medical Language*. This, he said, is certainly a branch of medical knowledge which " does but encumber whom it seems to enrich," and it is an encumbrance entirely of our own creating, which has brought and still brings ridicule upon us, and is a heavy burden and impediment to ourselves. Everyone, almost, will sympathise in Dr. Poore's desire for a purified and international medical nomenclature, and his scorn and wrath at our hybrid jargon and barbarous technicalities. To compare, he says, the feeling caused by the language we—not seldom, alas ! —meet with in medical writing with that produced by reading masterpieces of pure English composition, as Gray's Elegy, " would be like comparing the pleasurable movement of a first-rate carriage on our wooden pavements with the rumbling joltings of a springless waggon over a corduroy road." It may be objected that it is hardly fair to compare professional writing with Gray's Elegy, or with any poetry (except Browning's), but the illustration is graphic and telling; and Sir Thomas Watson and some other medical authors have shown us how lucid, simple, and flowing medical writing may be. Of course we must have technical terms, and numbers of old terms must be retained, however much our professional nomenclature may be purged. But surely men need not continue, as they do, to invent horrible, barbarous, and clumsy polyglot terms; and men might learn to use, even in professional writing and speaking, to a much greater extent than they do, the language " understanded of the people,"—though that cannot be used on all occasions.

Time and space prevent our saying more now of the Introductories of this year; but we have certainly shown that they at least equal in excellence and fitness those of any former occasion. To certain, here unnoticed, we must return again.

AN OLD TALE RETOLD.

In the course of the present year there has appeared in Paris a book which has acquired some notoriety even there for the filth it contains, and the barefaced audacity with which its contents are narrated. It is entitled " Memoires de Mr. Claude, Chef de la Police de Sureté sous le Second Empire," and, as is now the almost universal fashion in France, describes the Second Empire not only as a sink of iniquity, but also as the origin of all the evils which have come upon France since the days of what was supposed to be its greatest glory and happiness. We cannot see our way to praise the condition of things in that whited sepulchre, but this much may be said —that the French themselves seemed to enjoy it mightily while it lasted; and we are safe in saying that whilst the Empire lasted no such pestiferous books as those of Zola, for instance, would have been tolerated, and such a one as that to which we now refer would have been impossible. But great is Republican virtue—it is a cloak which nowadays covers a very great multitude of sins. All this may seem out of our ordinary route, and in a certain sense it is so, but in turning over these so-called Memoirs we happened upon a tale now nearly forgotten—in this country, at least—which is narrated in the book with perhaps more than its ordinary effrontery, but which will bear relating again. The story is that of La Pommerais, who was executed for poisoning his mistress by the use of digitalin. The case was fully investigated at the time by Tardieu and Roussin, and is largely narrated in their book on poisoning. The medico-legal evidence was not very strong, but the circumstantial details left no room for doubt.

According to Claude, La Pommerais was a very good-looking man, but with a certain forbidding expression, and the " eye of a vulture." The first time the two met was in the Bois de Boulogne, where a cab, in which were La Pommerais and one of his mistresses, came in collision with that in which was M. Claude, driven by a gentleman equally distinguished with La Pommerais himself, for he too lost his head subsequently for a double murder. When next the policeman and the doctor came in contact, La Pommerais had assumed the title of Count, was practising as a homœopathic physician, but had become connected with a band of sharpers or worse. One of these bore the assumed title of Marquis, and the Marchioness was the lady formerly seen with La Pommerais. Although respectably connected, La Pommerais never seems to have been very well off. Whatever he had was very soon wasted, and, not being overburdened with scruples, he would seem to have helped himself wherever he could. Moreover, he pushed himself everywhere, and in some fashion or other became acquainted with a Madame Dubizy and her daughter, to the latter of whom he became attached, but the mother was unwilling for a marriage, the position of the lover being anything but satisfactory. However, by hook or by crook— according to Claude, by the exhibition of borrowed securities, —he at last obtained the consent of the friends, was engaged to, and subsequently married, the young girl. Money matters were not, however, quite so satisfactory as he would have liked, for the old lady persisted in retaining the management of them in her own hands. This undoubtedly led to her death.

Meanwhile, however, we find an interesting episode in Claude's Memoirs. One day, calling on the " Marchioness," he noticed the cast of a hand, which he was told was that of La Pommerais. Interested in the science of reading character by means of the hand, the policeman asked leave to examine it. Probably no better instance could be given of the character of the author himself than what he has written about this hand. Roughly translated, the passage runs as follows : —" The cast of this hand was remarkable for the development of the palm on the side of the little finger and the length of the thumb. This exaggerated development of the palm, called at this spot the ' *hill of Mars*,' indicated a nature perverse and the instincts of an assassin. The length of the thumb announced an inflexible will. The '*line of life*,' turning round the base of the thumb, was large and shallow —that signified murder. Finally, under the ' *hill of Saturn*,' situated at the base of the first finger, the '*head line*,' separated into two portions, indicated death by beheading. On these revelations, which I held for certain, since I had examined the hands of so many criminals, my countenance expressed astonishment, stupor, and alarm," etc. With such nonsense does the worthy Claude entertain his readers.

One morning some time after this scientific investigation,

Madame Dubizy called upon Claude to ask for protection against her son-in-law, who, she said, wished to get rid of her, as she would not part with her own fortune as well as that of her daughter; but as she would lay no formal complaint against La Pommerais, nothing could be done. Some time after this she died, as was supposed at the time and said, by a sudden attack of cholera, but in reality poisoned, and La Pommerais entered into full possession of his wife's fortune. "After this," says M. Claude, "I made myself his friend the better to look after him." But the worthy homœopath was now in funds, and could launch out, which apparently he did with good effect. Claude tells us that in the record (dossier) kept by the police against him it is noted that such men as Andral, Nélaton and Conneau were to be seen in his house. Nevertheless, he lived beyond his income, was crippled by debts, and, besides the expenses, already great enough, of his own private dwelling, "kept several mistresses." All this time, says M. Claude, he loved his wife dearly, and was equally beloved by her. Among these mistresses, unfortunately for her own sake, was a Madame Pauw, the widow of a painter, who had died leaving her and her children very badly off. After his marriage, La Pommerais for a time abandoned the widow, but when his mother-in-law died, thinking apparently that she was well-nigh friendless, he renewed the acquaintance on the old footing, but with the most sinister objects in view. He persuaded the widow, after the manner of our countryman Palmer, to insure her life, he taking all responsibility. This he managed by means of a friendly and unscrupulous insurance agent, to the extent of over half a million of francs. His story to the widow was this: The insurance was to be effected, but once effected, she was to be taken ill, when the various companies would be only too glad to compromise the matter by compounding for an annuity, which they would not suppose would go over a long period. This business being settled, she was to recover her health, and so find herself provided for during her lifetime. The shammed illness having duly begun, the insurance companies became alarmed, and sent their medical agents to examine Madame Pauw, but they could find nothing to account for the "illness." Presently, however, the sham became a reality, and, after a night passed with La Pommerais, the unfortunate woman speedily died.

Meanwhile this worthy M. Claude had provided himself with a warrant for the arrest of his friend La Pommerais—for had he not read La Pommerais' fate in the model of his hand which he had given to the Marchioness d'Arnesano, already referred to? However, a few days after Madame Pauw's death, her sister, a Madame Gouchon, brought a complaint at the Police Office against La Pommerais. This complaint was limited, however, to a suggestion that the death of Madame Pauw was due to poisoning by an individual who was interested in her life insurances. "This charge, though vague enough, was quite clear to me, who had watched La Pommerais since the death of his mother-in-law." However, the body of Madame Pauw was examined, and that of Madame Dubizy was disinterred and likewise examined, the whole being entrusted to Tardieu, who, as we have said, was assisted in the chemical part of the work by Roussin. Matters taken from Madame Pauw's stomach, and matters which she had vomited, were extracted, and the extract given to dogs, in some instances proving fatal with the signs of poisoning by digitalis. We hardly think that the test applied in this way would give every satisfaction at the present day. Nevertheless, the accompanying evidence—especially the purchase and disappearance of a large quantity of digitalin—was so strong that La Pommerais was condemned, and, what seems to strike M. Claude with some surprise, without extenuating

circumstances (so dear to the minds of a French jury), though the worthy gentleman, who had evidently studied his poisons well, defended himself with skill and "audacity." Sentence of death was pronounced, but every effort was made to save him, though in vain. But he could not meet his fate without something of that theatrical display so dear to Frenchmen. Claude says:—"La Pommerais, before mounting the scaffold, had a look of his hair cut off, and gave it to the priest. It was brought to his lips, and he gave it a final kiss—last and pitiful mark of the affection which Madame La Pommerais could claim from her criminal spouse." In many respects the career of La Pommerais reminds us of that of Palmer, but salved over by a fulsome sentimentality covering a vile immorality to which the English criminal was a stranger.

THE WEEK.

TOPICS OF THE DAY.

A MEETING has been held to form an association with the object of rescuing the poor from the hands of unqualified experimenters. The meeting took place at the residence of Dr. Hewitt, Lancaster-gate, Hyde-park, and was attended by many medical practitioners and others, the object being the formation of an association for the total suppression of medical practice other than that sanctioned by the law of the State. Dr. Hewitt was requested to preside, and as a preliminary it was announced that letters had been received from Mr. W. J. Payne, the City Coroner; Mr. S. F. Langham, Deputy Coroner for Westminster; and other gentlemen, expressing their keen sense of the necessity which existed for the course which the Association intended to take. The Chairman then explained that the poorer neighbourhoods of London and other large cities were infested with unqualified medical practitioners—men practising without a diploma, and doing an incalculable amount of harm to their patients. This fact had been prominently brought forward at numerous inquests. Many of these quacks practised in so-called dispensaries, and took the small fees of the poor people, while they were simply permitting their diseases to gain a deadly hold upon them. The law had given the profession ample remedy against these persons, and it was the general belief of all the doctors he had conversed with that the time had arrived when the law should be strictly and remorselessly enforced. He therefore moved that a committee be formed for the purpose of establishing a British Medical Defence Association, on a basis so strong that it shall invite the co-operation of all registered medical practitioners, and gain all information possible regarding the class of persons against whom it will be expedient to proceed. After some discussion the motion was carried unanimously. It does not appear to have been stated to the meeting that two associations for the suppression of unqualified practitioners already exist, and have done good work—viz., the Medical Defence and the Medical Alliance Associations.

Once more the Hackney Board of Guardians have felt it their duty to take exception to the course pursued by the Metropolitan Asylums Board in dealing with the present small-pox epidemic. At their last meeting the removal of the bodies of dead small-pox patients from the Atlas hospital-ship for interment was the subject of discussion. Dr. G. C. Millar mentioned the case of a youth belonging to Hackney, who, instead of being admitted into the hospital at Homerton, was removed under the regulations of the Metropolitan Asylums Board to the ship, where he died eight days afterwards. The body was then removed back to Homerton Hospital, awaiting interment at Ilford. Dr. Millar complained that all the patients dying on board the Atlas were removed to Homerton for burial—a procedure which he thought was bad, considering that Hackney had already a large small-pox hospital and an ambulance station in its midst. Mr. Wentzell, the Hackney member of the Asylums Board, in explanation, said that the hospital was full when the youth in question was sent to the *Atlas*. He could not help thinking that if there had not been so much clamour by the people of the metropolis about Fulham and Hampstead, no hospital-ship would have been needed at all. If a number of parishes were allocated to the ship, of course it was natural that their patients should be sent thither. The deceased were covered with charcoal, and the coffins were filled with it, so as to reduce the possibility of infection. It should be borne in mind that the system of dealing with the patients was entirely under the direction of the medical superintendents, who had absolute control. It was, however, moved— "That this Board has heard with great alarm that it is the practice of the Metropolitan Asylums Board to remove the dead bodies from the ship *Atlas*, for all the parishes and unions allocated to that vessel, to the Homerton Small-pox Hospital previous to burial." This was duly seconded, and carried by twenty votes to one, and it was agreed to forward a copy of the motion to the Metropolitan Asylums Board.

At a recent inquest held by Mr. George Collier, in Bethnal-green, as to the deaths of two children, twins, the son and daughter of a carman, evidence was given, showing that the mother was delivered by a midwife, who stated that the children were prematurely born and would not live. Two days after the boy died, and the girl the day following, the midwife giving certificates. An undertaker took the bodies away, but the coroner's officer, hearing of the matter, made search for them, and succeeded, after the lapse of forty-eight hours, in tracing them to the house of a widow in Brick-lane. These facts having been proved, Dr. Matthew Corner, of Mile-end, was sworn, and gave evidence to the effect that had the children been attended by a medical man at birth, their lives, in all probability, would have been saved. Death had resulted from inanition. The Coroner, in summing up, appealed to the Press to make the case known. He regretted to say that such cases were of common occurrence, and their continuance was a source of vast danger to the community. He did not say that any foul play was apparent in this case, but the illegal practices of midwives in giving certificates in cases where children were not stillborn, and the burying of children's bodies by undertakers in a surreptitious manner, were calculated to make murder easy in the extreme: it was a monstrous evil. The jury agreed with the views of the Coroner, and returned a verdict in accordance with the facts. Mr. Collier told the midwife that she had acted illegally in giving the certificates, and he warned her that if she repeated the offence she would be punished.

The City Sewers Commission resumed their sittings after the recess, and Dr. Sedgwick Saunders, the Medical Officer of Health, reported that during the previous week 266 houses in the City had been inspected, of which 17 required sanitary improvement; that 13 tons 9 cwt. of diseased meat (including nearly two tons of Australian meat) had been seized at the markets, and that six cases of scarlet fever had been registered. The deaths in the week had been 24, or at the rate of 24·32 per 1000 of the population, and the births 17·22 per 1000. Dr. Saunders, replying to Mr. Deputy Rudkin, said his attention had been called to the state of Fireball-court, City, the houses in which were in a very dilapidated condition. Recently there had been some structural alteration going on, but the sooner the place was entirely swept off the face of the earth the better. This matter was ultimately referred to the Streets Committee for consideration.

Some important business was transacted by the Metropolitan Asylums Board at their first meeting after the recent recess. The complaints of various local authorities in the metropolis against the expenditure of the Managers were taken into consideration, and Mr. Proudfoot moved that the facts should be sent in the form of the following letter to the various complaining boards:—"That the estimates for the half-year ending Michaelmas, 1881, were prepared by the Committee of Finance so far back as February last, when the extent of the provision which had to be made to meet satisfactorily the exigencies of the recent epidemic of small-pox was not, and could not have been, contemplated. That at the time the said estimates were in course of preparation the total number of beds at the disposal of the Managers for the treatment of small-pox cases amounted to 669 only, and the Finance Committee made their calculations upon the basis that all those beds might be occupied during the whole of the ensuing half-year, but they did not anticipate the large number of extra beds that were subsequently required. That on June 25 last, when the epidemic was at its height, no less than 1568 beds, or nearly 1000 more than could reasonably have been estimated for, were occupied by small-pox cases; and, to meet the increased demand for hospital accommodation, it was found necessary to erect temporary huts at the Deptford and Fulham hospitals, to establish a camp for convalescent patients at Darenth, and eventually to fit up and furnish the hospital-ships *Atlas* and *Endymion*. That the total cost of this additional accommodation amounted to over £40,000, exclusive of, and beyond, the extra administrative expenses incurred and the cost of the daily maintenance of the patients. That the number of small-pox patients treated in the hospitals of the Managers during the three months ending on June 30 last was 3983, as against 3794 cases treated the whole of the preceding twelve months. That if the balance which it is estimated the Managers will be credited with at the end of the next half-year (£40,487) is exceptionally heavy, it should be observed that no amount has been estimated for such contingencies as the establishment of a convalescent hospital or hospitals, the interest on additional loans, or the expense attending the adapting and cleansing one or more of the small-pox hospitals for the treatment of fever cases, the latter of which expedients it is expected may, unfortunately, have to be resorted to during the approaching autumn or winter." The letter concludes by stating that, greatly as the Managers regret that the additional amount will have to be met by rates levied during the winter months, the fact that the epidemic prevailed during the past spring and summer left them no option in the matter. Mr. Galsworthy, the vice-chairman, seconded the motion for the adoption of the letter as an answer to the allegations of undue expenditure on the part of the Board, and it was finally agreed that the Clerk should be ordered to send copies to all the local authorities.

The Earl and Countess Fitzwilliam recently opened the first coffee-palace established at Peterborough—a limited liability company, of which the Dean of Peterborough is President, having been started for the promotion of the undertaking. Earl Fitzwilliam expressed the great pleasure he and the Countess experienced in being present to inaugurate the new building. Many movements of all descriptions, he said, had sprung up of late years, but none were more important than this, which had for its object the endeavour to make people, women as well as men, temperate and sober in their habits. The members for the borough, the Hon. J. W. Fitzwilliam and Mr. Whalley, and the Dean of Peterborough and the Mayor of that town, also took part in the proceedings, and so far the experiment has been launched under the very best auspices.

At the Henley Police-court, last week, the Thames Conservators summoned the Rural Sanitary Authority for polluting the river Thames by allowing the drainage of Caversham to enter the stream. The case excited much interest, and the defence set up was that the Authority had done their utmost to prevent the pollution. The analyst to the Conservators proved that the sample of water taken at the drain was concentrated sewage, and caused by old sewage-matter being allowed to run into the river. Ultimately the Bench inflicted a penalty of 40s. Notice of appeal was given.

At a recent inquest held at Bristol touching the death of a woman who had succumbed to puerperal fever, the evidence showed that four other females, attended by the same mid-wife, had died from this cause, and that the Medical Officer of Health had remonstrated with the woman, declaring that she was a centre of infection. The midwife, despite this caution, attended deceased, who died two days afterwards. The inquiry was ultimately adjourned.

It seems almost incredible, and certainly ought not to be possible, that with the present sanitary organisation in the metropolis such a state of things could exist as was recently described at an inquest held by Dr. Danford Thomas at the Coroner's Court, St. Pancras. A child, aged eight months, whose parents resided in Eden-street, Hampstead-road, had died suddenly, not having been medically treated. Dr. Gibson, of Fitzroy-square, deposed that he was sent for to the above address, where the man and woman and four children lived in a room at the top of the house. He found the child very emaciated, with hardly a particle of fat on the body. On making a post-mortem examination he ascertained that death had resulted from effusion of serum on the brain and chronic inflammation of the bowels, and this condition, he said, had been caused by the horribly un-sanitary state of the house. The stench arising from the basement was quite unbearable; a pigsty would not have smelt so bad. No doubt if the child had had proper nourish-ment and air its life would have been saved. Eliza Camp, another lodger in the same house, stated that there had been a stoppage in the closet for more than a month past, and the sewage matter overflowed into the area. She had lived in the house for about fourteen weeks, and had not been able to drink the water from the cistern all that time, as it was full of refuse and of a dirty green colour; about a fortnight ago a dead cat was taken out of it. The sanitary inspector of St. Pancras said his attention had been called to the house in question, which was one of the worst in the district. He had to threaten the agent to the owner, Mr. Smith, of George-street, who had some repairs done to the pipes, though they had now become as bad as ever. He could not get at the owner, and believed the house was in Chancery. The Coroner intimated to the officer the expediency of shutting the house up if such a state of affairs could not be remedied. After some further evidence, the jury returned a verdict in accordance with the medical testimony, and cen-suring the parents for negligence. Might they not rather have censured the St. Pancras sanitary authorities; or, at least, have strongly called their attention to the house?

It is difficult to understand why the metropolitan magis-trates do not always endeavour to strengthen the hands of the various sanitary authorities in their efforts to prevent the spread of small-pox. This was especially apparent in a case which recently came before Mr. Marsham, at the Green-wich Police-court, for decision. A bootseller, of Southwark-park-road, was summoned, at the instance of the Rotherhithe Vestry, for neglecting to carry out the disinfection of his house in a proper manner after notice had been served on him. The defendant was an anti-vaccinationist, and threw

every possible obstacle in the way of the officials in reference to small-pox. Eight cases of this disease had occurred in his house. A young child was first attacked, and was nursed by his wife; it recovered, but the wife took the disease and died, and two other children also succumbed. The defendant borrowed a suit of clothes from a young man in an oil-shop opposite to attend the funerals, and, after he had returned them, the young man was attacked with small-pox, and died. Four other children of the defendant were stricken, three of whom were taken to the Deptford Small-pox Hospital on a compulsory order of the magistrate, defendant obstinately refusing to permit their removal before. In the houses sur-rounding the defendant's, sixteen other cases subsequently occurred. Defendant had been applied to respecting the disinfection of his premises, and said it had been carried out, but he failed to produce a certificate from a medical prac-titioner, as required by the Sanitary Act of 1866. The Vestry did not dispute the fact that some sort of disinfection had been attempted, but they contended that it was necessary that the process should be conducted under the superintend-ence of a medical man, and they ventured to express a hope that the magistrate would take their view of the case, and thus strengthen the hands of the Sanitary Authority. Mr. Marsham, however, seemed to think that there was some amount of feeling in the matter, and he eventually dismissed the summons, stating that he failed to see that the defen-dant had shown negligence in disinfecting his premises. As we before remarked, the tendency of decisions such as this is decidedly mischievous, and Mr. Marsham seems to have ignored the fact that, even if a certain amount of disinfec-tion had been carried out, the necessary certificate prescribed by the law had not been produced.

ARMY MEDICAL SCHOOL.

THE winter session of the Army Medical School commenced at Netley, on Monday, the 3rd inst., with an opening address by Professor De Chaumont, F.R.S. Twenty-four surgeons on probation for the Army Medical Service, and ten for the Indian Medical Service, had joined on the previous Saturday. In addition to the thirty-four gentlemen already named, Colonial Surgeon Dr. Rowland, of the Gold Coast Colony, has arrived to go through the courses of practical instruction at the School.

THE VITAL STATISTICS OF SCOTLAND FOR THE JUNE QUARTER OF 1881.

THE Registrar-General of Scotland's report for the second quarter of the present year, ending June 30 last, shows that during that period there were registered in the different registries under his control the births of 33,351 infants and the deaths of 17,389 persons; it would appear, therefore, that the birth-rate for Scotland has been 0·129 per cent. below the average of the corresponding quarter of the ten years immediately preceding, and the death-rate has been 0·292 per cent. below the average of former years. Of the eight principal towns, Paisley had the highest and Edinburgh the lowest birth-rate. For every 10,000 in-habitants, the births were at the annual rate of 420 in Paisley, 406 in Greenock, 405 in Glasgow, 397 in Leith, 365 in Dundee, 355 in Perth, 353 in Aberdeen, and 331 in Edinburgh. Of the 33,351 births, 2625 (or 7·9 per cent.) were illegitimate; the rate of illegitimacy was highest in the mainland rural, and lowest in the insular rural districts. In eight counties the illegitimate births were at least 11 per cent. of the whole; in Sutherland, on the other hand, they were only 3·7 per cent. The deaths regis-tered during this quarter constituted an annual proportion of 191 deaths to every 10,000 of estimated population—a rate which is considerably lower than that for the corresponding quarter of the ten years immediately preceding. The annual death-rate did not, in fact, exceed 18·6 per 1000 of the population estimated for the middle of this year from the numbers enumerated in April last. This rate is the lowest recorded in the second quarter of any year since the establishment of civil registration in 1837. In Dundee the annual death-rate per 10,000 of estimated population was 188; in Aberdeen, 197; in Leith, 201; in Perth, 202; in Greenock, 204; in Edinburgh, 212; in Paisley, 231; and in Glasgow, 250. The natural increase of population during the quarter, without regard to emigration or immigration, was 15,462. During the quarter under notice zymotic diseases caused 971 deaths, of which number only 2 were due to small-pox. The meteorological remarks for the second quarter of 1881 show that the characteristics for the month of April were a high barometric pressure, small range thereof, low mean temperature, dry air, little rainfall, and much wind from the north and east. The mean temperature for May, unlike all the preceding months of this year, was somewhat above the average, the daily range of temperature was large, and the rainfall somewhat greater than the average. June was nearly an average month, except as to mean temperature, which was 2·0° lower than usual; the rainfall was but slightly in excess, as also the number of days on which it fell. The prevailing direction of the wind over the country was west-south-west.

THE YELLOW FEVER IN SENEGAL.

GREAT excitement (*Progrès Méd.*, October 1) prevailed on the rumour being spread that the yellow fever had been imported into Dunkirk by the *Emma Treckmann*, which had arrived from Bathurst and was inadvertently admitted without undergoing quarantine. Bathurst is separated from Senegal by the river Gambier, and is only about forty leagues distant from Gorée, where the yellow fever has either prevailed or been imminent. Four of the crew of the *Emma Treckmann* were taken to the hospital next day, but on minute examination being made, the medical authorities pronounced the disease to be Senegal fever, and not yellow fever. A letter from St. Louis (Senegal) states that the disease has not ceased its ravages, and that sixty-four out of seventy-four cases that were admitted during the fortnight ending September 7 died. The greatest consternation prevails in the colony, all the shops and workshops being closed.

THE LOCAL GOVERNMENT BOARD.

AT the last meeting of the Metropolitan Asylums Board a letter was read from the Local Government Board, in answer to a communication requesting advice with reference to the proceedings taken by residents in Fulham to prevent the Fulham Small-pox Hospital from being used for small-pox patients of the metropolis generally. As usual, the Asylums Managers obtained no help whatever from the Local Government Board, and even but little advice. That Board stated that it was impossible that assent could be given to the wishes of the residents of Fulham in restricting the Asylum in that district to cases arising within the area under that local authority, as the adoption of the like principle in other parts of the metropolis would leave large districts wholly without accommodation for small-pox and fever patients, to the great danger of the public generally. With regard to the interim injunction obtained against the general use for the metropolis of the Fulham Hospital, the Board felt unable to advise the Managers in regard to a proposed appeal against the continuance of the injunction, and after an expression of inability to understand upon what principle the complaint could be supported against the use of the Hospital for patients coming more than a mile distant, while

it was to be left free for the use of those within that distance, the Board advised reference to counsel's opinion on some of the points raised. After considerable discussion, the Managers decided that the legal advisers of the Asylums Board should be instructed to take the steps necessary in the case.

THE ORIGIN OF THE LIQUOR AMNII.

DR. WIENER, of Breslau, has experimentally investigated upon dogs and rabbits the above subject, with especial reference to the part played by the fœtal kidneys in the production of the amniotic fluid. His results are communicated to the *Archiv für Gynäkologie*. The amnion is of course a fœtal membrane, and therefore it might be supposed that, at least in the early months of pregnancy, the fluid within it was in some way furnished by the fœtus. From the fact that the liquor amnii contains urea, some have supposed that the fœtus passed urine into it. But some experiments which have been made by Zuntz, and confirmed by the author, show that when a solution of an indigo salt is injected into the maternal blood, the liquor amnii becomes coloured by the pigment, although none of it enters the fœtal circulation or stains the fœtal tissues. And according to Fehling and Ahlfeld, the secretion of urine by the fœtus during intra-uterine life is very scanty and slow. If these facts be correct, it would seem that the liquor amnii in the later months of pregnancy is mainly furnished by the mother, and that fœtal urine does not, as a rule, form a part of it. To determine both whether the kidneys act, and whether their secretion does add to the amount of the liquor amnii, Dr. Wiener injected the indigo solution, with a hypodermic syringe, directly into the fœtus. This he says is not difficult to do. He found that when introduced thus into the fœtal circulation it was excreted by the kidneys, and tinged the liquor amnii. He concludes, therefore, that the kidneys do actively act in intra-uterine life, that the urine is passed into the amniotic sac, and that the liquor amnii largely consists of fœtal urine. His experiments give a little additional support to what might have been inferred from the facts, that, as mentioned, the liquor amnii commonly contains urea, and that in cases of malformation and occlusion of the fœtal urethra, the bladder and kidneys are found distended with urine.

DUST AND GERMS.

WHEN some years ago Professor Tyndall published his observations on the constituents of the dust which during the summer months covers the walls and the furniture of our houses, our food, and our persons, and presumably enters our alimentary and respiratory passages, the matter was taken up eagerly by the daily press, and created a sort of scare in the popular mind. The study of bacteria and disease germs was then, however, in its infancy, and scientific men, believing that the organic particles detected by that observer were, for the most part, composed of mere dead and inert matter, the excitement to which it had given rise speedily subsided. As long back as 1864, Mr. Samuelson had indeed demonstrated that infusoria, algæ, and various spores were more abundant in the dust collected in dry than in wet weather; but the whole question has been recently investigated with great care by M. Miquel, who, at the Observatory of Montsouris, has for some time devoted his whole attention to the examination of atmospheric dust. He finds that the spores it contains may be resolved into two classes:—1. Protorganisms of a vegetable nature, algæ, and moulds, averaging 30,000 to 40,000 in a cubic metre of air, though varying in number with the weather, but shown experimentally to be for the most part quite harmless; and 2. Bacteria, including micrococci, bacilli, and vibrios averaging only 100 in the cubic meter, but some of which are capable of producing grave disturbance to health, if not actual specific disease. Both classes multiply under the influence of warmth and moisture, but their relative abundance in the dust varies remarkably, and inversely with the degree of humidity of the air. The former during rain may reach the extraordinary number of 200,000 in the cubic metre, and sink during drought to 4000 or 5000. On the other hand, the bacteria almost disappear during rain (thirty to fifty per cubic metre), but mount to 200 when dry weather has been maintained for many days or weeks. For these differences M. Miquel has advanced an ingenious and a satisfactory explanation. The spores of the lower fungi are, for the most part, developed at the extremity of filaments arising from their mycelium, and are easily detached by the wind, while the moisture which favours their proliferation is no obstacle to their dispersion. On the contrary, the minute particles which compose the joints of bacteria adhere closely to moist earth, and are only raised by the wind when long drought has reduced the soil to the state of drifting dust. Hitherto M. Miquel has found the oscillations indicating the number of bacteria in the air to preserve an inverse relation to the rainfall with the utmost constancy; and he and M. Bertillon have, they believe, observed a direct relation to subsist between the number of bacteria and the prevalence of eruptive fevers, though they admit that the period during which their observations have been conducted is too short to exclude the fallacy of mere coincidence. In the country, especially where a large extent of grass checks the desiccation of the soil, analyses of the air reveal an extremely small number of bacteria, and it does not seem unreasonable to refer, in part at least, to their paucity the rapidity with which surgical cases recover under such circumstances, and their freedom from erysipelas and septicæmic complications.

THE PARIS WEEKLY RETURN.

THE number of deaths for the thirty-eighth week, terminating September 23, was 947 (514 males and 433 females), and among these there were from typhoid fever 29, small-pox 15, measles 8, scarlatina 2, pertussis 5, diphtheria and croup 33, erysipelas 8, and puerperal infections 7. There were also 42 deaths from tubercular and acute meningitis, 22 from acute bronchitis, 56 from pneumonia, 93 from infantile athrepsia (40 of the children having been wholly or partially suckled), and 38 violent deaths. In spite of the small increase of 12 deaths this week, an examination of the prevalent causes of death shows that there has been rather an amelioration in the public health—the violent deaths and organic diseases accounting for any increase. The typhoid epidemic, judging from the smaller number of deaths and of admissions into the hospitals, is fast decreasing—the deaths this week having sunk from 45 to 29, and the admissions from 98 to 81. Scarlatina, also, has only caused 2 deaths in place of 10, and diphtheria 33 instead of 42. On the other hand, small-pox is a little on the increase (15 instead of 10); but the proportion of deaths to cases need not give rise to any uneasiness. The births for the week amounted to 1165, viz., 578 males (429 legitimate and 149 illegitimate) and 587 females (431 legitimate and 156 illegitimate); 56 children were born dead or died within twenty-four hours.

THE VACANT CHAIR IN OXFORD.

WE understand that Professor Morrison Watson, of the Owens College, Manchester, is a candidate for the chair of Human and Comparative Anatomy at the University of Oxford.

PROFESSOR PASTEUR AND THE YELLOW FEVER.

OF Professor Pasteur's journey in quest of yellow fever germs, M. Latour (Union Méd., September 24) writes as follows:— "This journey to Pauillac is a courageous act. In spite of his immortal works and in spite of his genius, an ineffaceable blot tarnishes the name of Galen, and posterity has never forgiven him his cowardly abandonment of Rome when a prey to an epidemic of plague. Professor Pasteur, who is not in early life, for he was born in 1822, and whose health has suffered from a serious accident, has, in the midst of his brilliant career, and all the celebrity which his admirable discoveries have bestowed on his name, and when he ought to be enjoying some of that repose so legitimately acquired, given up his holidays, and the vivifying air of his Jura mountains, to go—where? To shut himself in a lazaretto in company with some unfortunate beings who have brought with them the fearful yellow fever from Senegal, in order to search in their dejections, at the peril of his life, for the microbe that may perhaps be the cause of this terrible affection, and in the hope of being able, by his skilful and patient 'culture,' to find the 'vaccinator' for the black vomit, as he has found it for anthrax and chicken-cholera. Whatever may be the result of his expedition, it will do none the less honour to Professor Pasteur. Even if his generous hopes are not realised, he will, at all events, have given proof of his great courage in having undertaken these perilous experiments on a disease which, by infection or contagion, prostrates the most robust."

STATISTICS OF THE RECENT SMALL-POX EPIDEMIC IN THE METROPOLIS.

THE returns presented at the last meeting of the Metropolitan Asylums Board from the various small-pox hospitals, showed that during the previous four weeks there had been admitted 332 patients—namely, 63 to Homerton Asylum, 65 to the ship Atlas, 24 to Stockwell Asylum, 57 to the Fulham Asylum, and 123 to Deptford Asylum. In the whole, 56 had died, 311 had been discharged, and 440 remained under treatment in the hospitals and ship, and 38 in camp at Darenth—in all 478, being a decrease, as against the numbers a month ago, of 81. In the previous four weeks, 408 were admitted, 80 died, 479 were discharged, and 559 remained under treatment. The fever returns were less satisfactory. During the previous four weeks 244 fever patients were received at the Stockwell and Homerton Asylums, as against 147 in the four weeks immediately preceding; 27 died and 129 were discharged, leaving 335 under treatment, as compared with 254 at the date of the previous return. An interesting return was also presented, showing the numbers of small-pox patients sent into the Asylums Board's small-pox hospitals by each district of the metropolis for the first two quarters of the year. In the first quarter the City of London Union sent 50, and in the second 23; the Fulham District sent 102 in the first quarter, and 132 in the second; Greenwich, 263 and 469; Hackney, 530 and 308; Holborn Union of parishes, 123 and 190; Lewisham, 41 and 24; Mile-end Hamlet, 97 and 98; the Poplar Union of parishes, 66 and 49; St. George's, Hanover-square, Union of parishes, 66 and 49; St. George's-in-the-East, 107 and 52; St. Giles's, Bloomsbury, Union of parishes, 14 and 31; St. Giles's, Camberwell, 285 and 245; St. John's, Hampstead, 3 and 12; Shoreditch, 196 and 451; Chelsea, 64 and 66; Paddington, 20 and 41; St. Marylebone, 34 and 102; Lambeth, 254 and 202; Islington, 169 and 217; Kensington, 100 and 133; Bethnal-green, 355 and 203; St. Pancras, 72 and 85; St. Olave's Union of parishes, 111 and 274; St. Saviour's, Southwark, 190 and 190; the Strand Union, 14 and 30; Stepney Union of parishes, 122 and 47; Wandsworth and Clapham Union of parishes, 143 and 133; Whitechapel, 125 and 53; Woolwich, 49 and 53; Westminster Union of parishes, 12 and 17; and the Port of London, 2 in the first quarter only. The total shows that 3794 patients were received in the first quarter and 3983 in the second.

EXFOLIATIVE VAGINITIS AND MEMBRANOUS DYSMENORRHŒA.

IT has been a common reproach to gynæcologists that they are too fond of assuming that disorders of the general system, more particularly hysteria and allied nervous symptoms, when met with along with uterine disease, are its result. Dr. Cohnstein, in a paper on the subject of membranous dysmenorrhœa and exfoliative vaginitis, published in a recent number of the *Archiv für Gynäkologie*, goes to the other extreme, and, reasoning from a number of cases which he has collected (which collection makes his paper very valuable for purposes of reference), concludes that membranous dysmenorrhœa is not the cause, but the result, of hysteria, or of disorder of the general health. He points out that in nearly all the cases of his collection the general health was much deteriorated; that we know of no local treatment which will cure membranous dysmenorrhœa; that membranes are sometimes passed at the menstrual period without pain; that in many cases impairment of the general health preceded the painful menstruation. It is very difficult to see in what way hysteria should so modify the functions of the uterus as to make it excrete a membrane each month; and hysteria itself is a thing so difficult to define that it seems hardly possible that proof should be forthcoming of Dr. Cohnstein's theory. But, without going as far as he does, we think he has done good service in calling attention to the facts that nervous and hysterical symptoms going with uterine disease are not of necessity caused by it, and that menstrual pain is modified by the state of the general health n this way—that an amount of pain which a strong, healthy woman would think too trifling to mention, will put a feeble, neurotic individual quite *hors de combat*. In the latter case treatment of the general health may, without modifying the local condition, so improve the patient's power of bearing pain as to remove her from the condition of invalidism.

DEFECTIVE PROVISION FOR THE INSANE IN THE UNITED STATES.—Dr. Folsom, Lecturer on Mental Diseases at Harvard Medical School, in an address to the American Medical Association on the "Relations of the State to the Insane" has the following passage:—"In Massachusetts, with a census population of 1,783,812 in 1880, there were 4600 insane officially known; 3124 were in public or corporate asylums at the end of the year, or 175·13 to every 100,000 people. This ratio had increased from 9·55 in 1820, 11·34 in 1830, 61·99 in 1840, 84·97 in 1850, 110·55 in 1860, 130·44 in 1870. Two new hospitals just finished in that State are already crowded to accommodate 1200 patients. From all parts of our Union a similar story might be told, except that too often the over-filled asylums would be found wretchedly inadequate to care for a half or a quarter of those fairly needing their shelter. In Massachusetts, 1 in 350 of the population is insane; and there cannot be, I think, less than 100,000 in the whole United States, of whom hardly a third are even receiving asylum care, unsatisfactory as that is in some places, while the utter wretchedness of those in gaols, poorhouses, and often private dwellings, is almost beyond belief. Of the total number, probably between 10 and 20 per cent. are by our present methods permanently curable, and not far from 70 per cent. should be wards of the State." Dr. Folsom, while strongly impressed with the necessity of instituting some means of official supervision, states that although a "lunacy commission, with the power given to such boards in Great Britain, would be out of the question for obvious reasons," yet the appointment of a United States Commissioner of Insanity, with chiefly advisory duties, is very desirable. State boards and commissions would be too much under the influence of local politics.—*Boston Med. Jour.*, August 4.

THE SOCIAL SCIENCE CONGRESS, 1881.

ON Monday evening, October 3, the opening meeting of the twenty-fifth annual Congress of the National Association for the Promotion of Social Science was held in the Bijou Theatre of the Exhibition Palace, Earlsfoot-terrace, Dublin. There was a large attendance of Members and Associates. The President, the Right Hon. Lord O'Hagan, Lord Chancellor of Ireland, delivered the inaugural address, choosing for his subject a review of the principal legislative enactments affecting Ireland since 1861, when the Social Science Congress met in Dublin for the first time. Lord O'Hagan spoke of reforms which had been effected in the Judicial System, in the Lunacy Laws, in the Jury System; in Primary, Intermediate, and University Education (including the education of women, the modification of reformatories, and the establishment of industrial schools). He alluded to the Sunday Closing Act, the Irish Church Act, and Land Reforms, and, in conclusion, touched on the topics of Irish manufactures and the fine arts. The portion of his address, however, which possesses most interest for the medical profession is that in which he sketched the sanitary reforms of the past twenty years. In the year 1861, Ireland had, as its chief sanitary authorities, expiring parish vestries, clothed with antiquated powers, which had been vested in them so far back as the year 1818. There were some other bodies acting for similar purposes, under statutes which had once had equal application to England and Ireland, but had continued in action there after they were repealed in England. Five years after the meeting of the Congress, in 1866, the vestries were finally abolished, and the guardians of the poor were entrusted with sanitary powers identical with those existing in England and Wales. The change was great and wholesome, and was pushed to better issue when the Local Government Board was created in 1872. It was armed with large authority, and acted with energy and success. An Act of 1874 developed the sanitary system and brought it into full operation throughout the country. Under that Act the whole of Ireland is divided into sanitary districts, called urban sanitary districts and rural sanitary districts. The urban districts consist of towns having a population exceeding 6000. The governing body of the town is made the sanitary authority. The rural districts consist of the Poor-law unions, and the boards of guardians are the sanitary authorities. There are fifty-six urban sanitary districts, and 163 rural sanitary districts; and in each of those districts a complete sanitary staff has been organised under the orders of the Local Government Board.

The medical officer of the dispensary district is, in all cases, the sanitary officer or medical officer of health. The principal duty of the sanitary authorities and their officers consists in the inspection of their districts, and in taking all necessary steps to compel the removal or abatement of nuisances, provide a proper supply of water, and (construct, or cause to be constructed, where it may be necessary, proper sewers and drains. The Public Health Act of 1878 repealed all previous Sanitary Acts, re-enacting, amending, and consolidating their provisions, so as to comprise in one statute the entire sanitary law as it at present exists in Ireland. The principal subjects dealt with in the Act are—Sewerage and Drainage, Scavenging and Cleansing, Water-Supply, Abatement and Removal of Nuisances, Lodging-houses, Markets and Slaughter-houses, and Infectious Diseases. Thus the scope of the statute is comprehensive, as the machinery for effectuating its purposes is complete. He rejoiced to say that its worth has been widely recognised. The increasing activity of the local authorities was demonstrated by the amount of their expenditure for the last six years, as it appears in the audited accounts of the Board, and still more strikingly by the amount of the loans obtained from the Board of Works, in those successive years, on the recommendation of the Local Government Board, "for objects," in the words of the Public Health Act, "which may be deemed sanitary improvements." The sums had steadily increased from £37,584 in 1875-76 to £365,179 in 1879-80. In 1880-81 it had fallen a little below £200,000.

It was not easy to over-estimate the importance to Ireland

of the sanitary work which is thus proved to have been done. It had been of double advantage, by relieving the poor at seasons of sore distress, and securing the permanent improvement of the health of the community. In a department so deeply affecting the comfort and the happiness of a people, Ireland need not be ashamed of the progress she is making and has made. And for her that progress was especially important. Health and social morals run closely together. Cleanliness and godliness are in alliance; and wholesome and commodious dwellings are important instruments of civilisation. The squalidness of his home drives the artisan for light and solace to the public-house. The mud cabin, with its single room and crowded foulness, is not very compatible with the formation of ordered industry; and, save in a country still marvellously pure, its inmates would be subjected to many dangers. It is of great consequence, for reasons like these, which might be largely multiplied—that our sanitary work should extend not merely to lodging-houses, but, as far as may be, to the dwellings generally of the humbler classes; and that the English effort in that direction, which has been successfully prosecuted under the benevolent guidance of Lord Shaftesbury, should have wide and cordial imitation here.

Many will think that the President's description of the existing sanitary organisation in Ireland partook too much of the *couleur de rose*, but this is perhaps allowable on a festive occasion.

At the conclusion of the address, a vote of thanks to the President, proposed by the Lord Mayor of Dublin, seconded by Professor Bonamy Price, and supported by the Hon. Dudley Field, of New York, was carried by acclamation.

On Tuesday and the following days the departments of the Congress met in their respective rooms in Trinity College.

FROM ABROAD.

The Holding of Patents by Doctors.

In the prospect of alterations being made in the code of medical ethics, which has now long been adopted by the American Medical Association, the editor of the *New York Medical Journal* for August calls attention to the desirability of abrogating that portion of it which declares it to be "derogatory to professional character for a physician to hold a patent for any surgical instrument or medicine." He believes that such a prohibition would never have been inserted or suffered so long to remain had it not been coupled in the same sentence with the statement that it is also derogatory to "dispense a secret nostrum."

"Whether," he says, "this grouping of the two acts for common denunciation was an ingenious device on the part of those who abhorred the idea of a physician holding a patent, and who chose this way to spread their abhorrence, we are unable to say; but it is certain that the idea of dispensing secret nostrums is revolting to high-minded men, and when they find this practice classed in the same category with the possession of a patent, it is no wonder that, without giving the matter much thought, they gradually come to look upon the latter as a hideous offence. Very little reflection is needed, however, to show how diverse the two are, and how monstrous it is to class them together. The code' has no denunciation for the holder of a copyright; and yet there is no essential difference between a copyright and a patent. A copyright covers a publication, and every one acknowledges that about this there can be no secrecy—hence to couple the holding of a copyright with the dispensing of a secret nostrum would carry its own refutation.

"But a patent is also a publication, and nothing of secret composition or secret mechanism can be patented. Analogy shows us, then, that there is nothing in the nature of things to justify the assertion that it is derogatory to professional character for a physician to hold a patent. As a matter of fact, we find that some physicians do hold patents, and that they are not looked upon by their professional brethren as having debased themselves by so doing. We understand that Paquelin's cautery is patented. Whether the patent is held by the inventor or by the maker matters little, for now held by any other person than M. Paquelin, it must

have been held by him originally. Who has whispered that M. Paquelin has degraded himself? Is an act right in France, but wrong in America? What then shall be said of Dr. Dawson, who patented a cautery-battery of his invention? We have not heard that he has lost caste; and, for our part, we admire the independence he showed in acquiring and holding the patent-right as much as we admire the ingenuity displayed in the construction of the battery. By declining to throw obloquy upon these gentlemen the profession has shown that it does not regard the possession of a patent as derogatory. That declaration in the code that so sets it down is therefore a dead letter, and ought to be expunged."

Therapeutical Action of Digitalis on the Heart.

Prof. H. C. Wood, on introducing this subject to the notice of the Philadelphia Medical Society (*Phil. Med. Times*, July 2), having referred to the current opinions in regard to the action of digitalis upon the nervous apparatus of the heart, claimed for it a peculiar effect on the heart-muscle. This influence, which has been amply shown both by experiment and clinical observation, renders digitalis particularly serviceable in the condition of heart-disease in which the increased work required of the heart is greater than the increase of the power—without regard to the particular valve that may be affected. It improves the nutrition of the heart by regulating its contractions and lengthening the diastolic interval, doing away with the rapid, imperfect contractions which interfere with the blood-supply of the cardiac muscle. In such cases the nutrition of the heart suffers, because it is necessary to have lateral distension of the aorta in order to fill the arteries in the muscular tissue. A little digitalis steadies the heart, and therefore improves its condition and retards degeneration. In chronic valve-trouble of the heart, digitalis is serviceable, and sometimes must be given in large doses. A half-drachm dose of the tincture apparently saved from impending death two cases of advanced heart-trouble, which afterwards got well enough to attend to their business. It enables the heart to gather up its strength, and keeps it going until the last. By the surgeon, digitalis is often used improperly. Thus, it is not rarely given in aneurism, where the great danger is from increased lateral pressure, not want of forward pressure. In acute diseases, with failing heart, digitalis may be employed. Such a condition may occur in asthenic or in the advanced stages of sthenic pneumonia. In the early stage of sthenic pneumonia it is improper to give it. When the lung is consolidated throughout a large extent, the heart is overworked; by-and-by it begins to fail, the pulse getting rapid and feeble; and now digitalis comes into play. It will save life in such a condition, when without it the patient must die. In a case of alcoholic pneumonia, ten minims of the tincture given every two hours, day and night, reduced the pulse from 150 or 160 to 60.

"Two points in conclusion—(1) in regard to the cumulative action, and (2) in regard to the cause of the slow action of digitalis. The remedy acts slowly in producing its full effect, and its effects are very permanent when they do appear. Digitalis acts slowly and cumulatively, not only because of its special influence upon the heart, but because it only comes very slowly in contact with the heart-structure, since it osmoses slowly into and out from the body. The practical point is this: watch the kidneys when giving large doses of digitalis; if water is not passed freely, then cumulative action will be apt to occur. . . . The longer the digitalis is in acting, the more likely it is to have a lasting effect. After abdominal tapping, the digitalis often shows itself in reducing the heart's action. Either it has been lying in the intestines unabsorbed, or in the cellular tissue; probably all the fluids are saturated with the drug. Digitalis is a very useful remedy in cases of syncope and collapse. Formerly, alcohol alone was used. One of the advances of modern therapeutics has been to teach the danger of giving large doses of alcohol in cases of surgical shock. Belladonna and digitalis are proper remedies, given by hypodermic injection. The pulse begins to fill up in twenty minutes or half an hour. No irritation is produced at the point of puncture. Throw in twenty minims at once, and expect to find the result in half an hour. He did not wish his remarks to be understood as declaring that digitalis was entirely without danger, but he had used it in hundreds of cases, and had seen men apparently dying revive under its effects. It is important to stop it as soon as evidence appears in the pulse that it is beginning to be absorbed. Used in this way, he did not believe that there would ever be any serious cases of poisoning with it."

After a short discussion, Prof. Wood said that he would touch upon two or three practical points that had been raised. First, as to the choice of preparation: the infusion seemed to be generally preferred; but probably the only reason for this being considered more efficacious was that it was given in relatively larger doses than the tincture. He believed that either preparation obtained from an unknown druggist is not infrequently unreliable. He believed that gastric disturbance (of which, however, he has seen very few cases) is less likely to occur with the tincture than with the infusion. He had not made much use of digitalin, which in fact is not the alkaloid, but merely a purified extract: it is uncertain in its composition and in its results; and as the dose of digitalis is so small, there is no need for resorting to so uncertain a substance. Dr. Wood wished to be distinctly understood as discountenancing the employment of large doses until the smaller had failed. In conclusion, he made a few remarks on the experimental investigation of the subject.

"The action of digitalis on the frog's heart is that it is rarely arrested in diastole, more frequently in systole. As regards the question of its effect upon the pneumogastric nerve, in some cases the effect is to destroy life in this manner. In such cases we can restore the action of the heart by cutting the pneumogastric nerve. As a rule, however, the effect is greater upon the heart than it is upon the nerve, and the animal dies of cardiac spasm. It has the same effect upon the pulse of mammals; the full effect produces a weak pulse, sometimes dicrotic. This he had seen beautifully illustrated in man. It means that there are two antagonistic effects upon the heart—upon the heart-muscle, and on the brake action. This is undoubtedly the explanation of the dicrotic pulse and of the double wave written upon the manometer. Later the arterial pressure is found to be falling. Looking at the heart, the dilatation becomes less, the diastole becomes imperfect, only a small amount of blood now enters its cavities on account of the cramp of the muscular tissue, just as in the tetanic spasm of the muscles in strychnia-poisoning; and then come cramp of the muscles of respiration and death. The pulse becomes frequent in digitalis-poisoning, because the heart is so constricted that the blood is dammed back and cannot get into the aorta."

OBITUARY.

JOSEPH BROWN, M.B., C.M., F.R.C.P. Edin.

The announcement of the untimely death of Dr. Joseph J. Brown, Medical Superintendent of the Fife and Kinross Asylum, will occasion sincere sorrow amongst a large circle of friends and acquaintances. After graduating in the University of Edinburgh with honours in 1871, he acted as House-Physician in the clinical wards of the Royal Infirmary, a post secured after a severe open competition. After quitting the Medical School, he devoted himself to the study and treatment of insanity, and acted as Assistant Medical Officer, first at Saughton Hall Asylum, and subsequently at Morningside. A vacancy having occurred in the superintendentship of the Fife and Kinross Asylum, through the promotion of Dr. Fraser to the post of Deputy-Commissioner in Lunacy, Dr. Brown was the successful candidate. By the painful death of Dr. Brown the department of medicine which has to deal with lunacy has lost one who had achieved much, and who needed only the progress of time to permit of his name being enrolled amongst those of the eminent men whose humanity, soundness of judgment, and personal benignity have lightened the darkness of insanity in this country, and have converted English, and especially Scotch, asylums into institutions which are more easily admired than imitated in other lands.

SIMPLE REMEDY FOR CHAFES (Prof. H. C. Wood).— Bathe the parts well in tepid water, dry well with soft cloths, and apply, by means of a soft sponge or cloth, the following: —℞. Zinci acet. gr. xv., morphiæ acet. gr. ij., glycerin., aq. rosær., āā ℥ij.; m. Apply to chafed parts twice or three times a day.—*Louisville Med. News*, September 10.

VITAL STATISTICS OF LONDON.

Week ending Saturday, October 1, 1881.

BIRTHS.

Births of Boys, 1312; Girls, 1206; Total, 2518.
Corrected weekly average in the 10 years 1871–80, 2491·3.

DEATHS.

	Males.	Females.	Total.
Deaths during the week	635	582	1217
Weekly average of the ten years 1871–80, corrected to increased population ...	716·0	677·0	1393·0
Deaths of people aged 80 and upwards ...	...	...	81

DEATHS IN SUB-DISTRICTS FROM EPIDEMICS.

	Enumerated Population, 1881 (unverified).	Small-pox.	Measles.	Scarlet Fever.	Diphtheria.	Whooping-cough.	Typhus.	Enteric (or Typhoid) Fever.	Simple continued Fever.	Diarrhœa.
West ...	668968	1	2	8	...	2	1	3	1	7
North ...	905677	4	5	15	6	7	2	15	...	8
Central ...	281788	...	2	5	2	2	...	11	...	5
East ...	692830	2	4	10	3	8	...	10	...	5
South ...	1265678	8	4	17	1	8	1	9	...	9
Total ...	3814571	15	17	55	12	27	4	48	1	34

METEOROLOGY.

From Observations at the Greenwich Observatory.

Mean height of barometer	30·067 in.
Mean temperature	53·2°
Highest point of thermometer	70·4°
Lowest point of thermometer	38·3°
Mean dew-point temperature	50·3°
General direction of wind	S.W. & N.E.
Whole amount of rain in the week	0·36 in.

BIRTHS and DEATHS Registered and METEOROLOGY during the Week ending Saturday, Oct. 1, in the following large Towns:—

Cities and boroughs (Municipal boundaries except for London.)	Estimated Population to middle of the year 1881.[*]	Persons to an Acre (1881.)	Births Registered during the week ending Oct. 1.	Deaths Registered during the week ending Oct. 1.	Highest during the Week.	Lowest during the Week.	Weekly Mean of Daily Mean Values.	Temp. of Air (Cent.) Weekly Mean of Daily Mean Values.	Rain Fall. In Inches.	In Centimetres.
London ...	3829751	50·2	2518	1217	73·4	38·3	53·2	11·78	0·36	0·91
Brighton ...	107934	43·9	68	33	66·0	45·3	54·2	12·33	0·03	0·08
Portsmouth ...	128335	28·6	83	39	...	...	...	...	...	...
Norwich ...	88038	11·8	61	31	...	...	...	...	...	...
Plymouth ...	74262	54·0	47	19	64·0	43·7	54·3	12·39	0·81	2·06
Bristol ...	207140	46·5	160	75	...	...	...	...	...	...
Wolverhampton ...	75034	22·4	36	24	62·9	38·5	51·6	10·90	0·15	0·38
Birmingham ...	402296	47·9	274	132	...	...	...	...	...	...
Leicester ...	123129	38·5	92	48	...	...	...	...	...	...
Nottingham ...	188235	18·9	125	68	65·6	37·2	52·2	11·22	0·51	1·50
Liverpool ...	553988	106·3	424	241	...	...	...	...	...	...
Manchester ...	341269	79·5	250	147	...	...	...	...	...	...
Salford ...	177760	34·4	141	73	...	...	...	...	...	...
Oldham ...	112176	24·0	66	41	...	...	...	...	...	...
Bradford ...	184037	25·5	125	77	65·0	43·2	53·6	12·01	0·20	0·51
Leeds ...	310490	14·4	211	97	64·0	41·0	53·0	11·67	0·55	1·40
Sheffield ...	285621	14·5	240	87	64·0	39·0	52·7	11·50	0·63	1·61
Hull ...	165164	42·7	95	72	64·0	38·0	51·9	11·08	0·28	0·71
Sunderland ...	116755	42·2	102	37	72·0	46·0	56·5	13·61	0·88	1·47
Newcastle-on-Tyne	145675	27·1	105	48	...	...	...	...	...	...
Total of 20 large English Towns...	7608775	38·0	5223	2307	73·0	37·2	53·3	11·84	0·42	1·07

* These figures are the numbers enumerated (but subject to revision) in April last, raised to the middle of 1881 by the addition of a quarter of a year's increase, calculated at the rate that prevailed between 1871 and 1881.

At the Royal Observatory, Greenwich, the mean reading of the barometer last week was 30·07 in. The lowest reading was 29·87 in. on Sunday at mid-day, and the highest 30·24 in. on Thursday morning.

NEW INVENTIONS AND IMPROVEMENTS.

PAGE'S PATENT VAPORISER AND CRESOLENE.

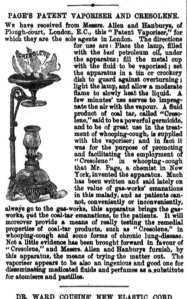

WE have received from Messrs. Allen and Hanburys, of Plough-court, London, E.C., this "Patent Vaporiser," for which they are the sole agents in London. The directions for use are: Place the lamp, filled with the *best* petroleum oil, under the apparatus; fill the metal cup with the fluid to be vaporised; set the apparatus in a tin or crockery dish to guard against overturning; light the lamp, and allow a moderate flame to slowly heat the liquid. A few minutes' use serves to impregnate the air with the vapour. A fluid product of coal tar, called "Cresolene," said to be a powerful germicide, and to be of great use in the treatment of whooping-cough, is supplied with the vaporiser; and in fact it was for the purpose of promoting and facilitating the employment of "Cresolene" in whooping-cough that Mr. Page, a chemist in New York, invented the apparatus. Much has been written and said lately on the value of gas-works' emanations in this malady, and as patients cannot, conveniently or inconveniently, always go to the gas-works, this apparatus brings the gas-works, *quâ* the coal-tar emanations, to the patients. It will moreover provide a means of really testing the remedial properties of coal-tar products, such as "Cresolene," in whooping-cough and some forms of chronic lung-disease. Not a little evidence has been brought forward in favour of "Cresolene," and Messrs. Allen and Hanburys furnish, by this apparatus, the means of trying the matter out. The vaporiser appears to be also an ingenious and good one for disseminating medicated fluids and perfumes as a substitute for atomisers and pastilles.

DR. WARD COUSINS' NEW ELASTIC CORD TOURNIQUET.

MESSRS. ARNOLD AND SONS have sent us a specimen of a "new elastic cord tourniquet" invented by Dr. Ward Cousins, which is a powerful and efficient instrument. It

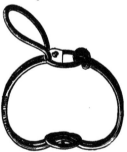

consists of three parts—1. An endless elastic cord; 2. A metal clamp by which the cord can be instantly tightened or loosened; 3. A metal ring fitted with a crossbar for the purpose of connecting the cord, in any position, with an elastic pad. It can be very speedily and easily adjusted on a limb so as to completely control the circulation; and it is adopted for all surgical operations in which such an instrument is needed. The comparative ease with which it can be applied is indicated by the fact that it admits of self-application to any limb with one hand. We must add that this "new elastic cord tourniquet" appears to us to be a revised edition of the "spring tourniquet" invented by Dr. Ward Cousins, and brought out by Messrs. Wright, of Bond-street, which we noticed last year; and it is a prettier and more "finished" instrument.

MEDICAL NEWS.

APPOINTMENTS.

*** The Editor will thank gentlemen to forward to the Publishing-office, as early as possible, information as to all new Appointments that take place.

BULTEEL, MARCUS H., M.R.C.S., L.R.C.P.—Surgeon to the Provident Dispensary of the Royal Albert Hospital and Eye Infirmary, Devonport.

NAVAL, MILITARY, ETC., APPOINTMENTS.

ADMIRALTY.—Surgeon Edward Elphinstone Mahon (for gallant conduct at the action of Majuba Mountain) to be Staff-Surgeon in Her Majesty's Fleet, with seniority of July 18, 1881. Staff-Surgeon James Trimble to be Fleet-Surgeon in Her Majesty's Fleet, with seniority of September 20, 1881.

BIRTHS.

ARNOTT.—On September 29, at The Vicarage, Bussage, near Stroud, Gloucester, the wife of the Rev. Henry Arnott, F.R.C.S., of a daughter.

HARVEY.—On September 30, at 26, Rue Wissocy, Boulogne-sur-Mer, the wife of J. S. Harvey, M.R.C.S., of a daughter.

LUCEY.—On September 28, at The Elms, Bush Hill-park, Enfield, the wife of William C. Lucey, M.D., of a daughter.

STEWART.—On September 29, at 19, Charlotte-square, Edinburgh, the wife of Professor Grainger Stewart, M.D., of a son.

MARRIAGES.

BABER—LEWIS.—On September 13, at Brompton, J. J. Y. Baber, Esq., second son of John Baber, M.D., of Thurloe-square, South Kensington, to Edie Elizabeth, elder daughter of the Rev. L. W. Lewis, Vicar of Meopham, Kent.

BYRCH—BREMNER.—On September 27, at Chatham, Captain Edward Berry Byrch, Royal Marine Light Infantry, to Jessie Florence, second daughter of John T. U. Bremner, M.D., Deputy Inspector-General of Hospitals and Fleets, Royal Navy, of Melville Hospital, Chatham.

CONOLLY—ROUCH.—On September 29, at Greenwich, Beaumont Rowley Conolly, M.D., to Helen Rouch, of Madeira.

DRURY—D'ARCY.—On September 26, at Kensington, Richard Drury, M.D., to Isabel Jane, youngest daughter of the late Rev. John D'Arcy, Rector of Galway.

SIMPSON—WHEELER.—On October 3, at Bow, Philip John Simpson, M.R.C.S., L.S.A., of the Royal Hospital, Chelsea, to Rhoda, eldest daughter of George Wheeler, Esq., of Bow.

SNOW—NORTON.—On September 17, at Weston-super-Mare, Herbert Lumley Snow, M.D., to Florence Charlotte Amelia, eldest daughter of S. Norton, Esq., of Weston-super-Mare.

DEATHS.

ADDISON, W., F.R.C.P., F.R.S., at 10, Albert-road, Brighton, on September 26, in his 80th year.

BOISRAGON, T. S. G., M.D., at Denbigh-street, Pimlico, on September 20, in his 72nd year.

HITCH, SAMUEL, M.R.C.P., at Eastbourne, on September 29, in his 81st year.

MURPHY, ROBERT, Surgeon-Major A.M.D., at Fort Lahore, India, on September 1.

PLAYFAIR, GEORGE RANKIN, M.D., late Inspector-General of Hospitals, Her Majesty's Indian Army, at 26, Longridge-road, S.W., on October 4.

TURNBULL, EDGAR LICHFIELD, son of G. H. Turnbull, M.D., at Kelso, N.B., on October 2.

VACANCIES.

In the following list the nature of the office vacant, the qualifications required in the candidate, the person to whom application should be made and the day of election (as far as known) are stated in succession.

GATESHEAD DISPENSARY.—Assistant-Surgeon. (*For particulars see Advertisement.*)

HOSPITAL FOR EPILEPSY AND PARALYSIS, ETC., PORTLAND-TERRACE, REGENT'S-PARK.—Physician. Applications and testimonials to be sent to the Secretary, at the Hospital, from whom all particulars can be obtained, on or before October 12.

HULME DISPENSARY, MANCHESTER.—House-Surgeon. Applications to be sent to Dr. Wahltuch, Honorary Secretary, Medical Staff, by October 20.

INFIRMARY OF THE CITY OF LONDON UNION.—Assistant Medical Officer. (*For particulars see Advertisement.*)

KINGSTON RURAL SANITARY AUTHORITY.—Medical Officer of Health. Candidates must be legally qualified medical practitioners. Applications, stating what diplomas they hold, age, residence, with recent testimonials as to character, to be sent to Anthony Temple, Clerk to the Rural Sanitary Authority, on or before October 10.

KINGSTON UNION.—Medical Officer. Applications to be sent to Anthony Temple, Clerk to the Guardians, on or before October 10.

LEEDS PUBLIC DISPENSARY.—Resident Medical Officer. Applications to be sent to Dr. E. H. Jacob, 12, Park-street, Leeds, before October 15.

UNION AND PAROCHIAL MEDICAL SERVICE.

. The area of each district is stated in acres. The population in computed according to the census of 1871.

RESIGNATIONS.

City of London Union.—Mr. G. E. Miles has resigned the office of Assistant Medical Officer and Dispenser at the Bow Infirmary. Salary £100 per annum, and board and lodging.

Malling Union.—Dr. F. A. Smith has resigned the Second District: area 12,043; population 6547; salary £100 per annum.

South Molton Union.—Mr. Timothy Daley has resigned the Eighth District: area 10,552; population 1496; salary £30 per annum.

Warminster Union.—Mr. Thomas Flower has resigned the Warminster and Corsley Districts. Warminster District: area 7108; population 6039; salary £117 10s. per annum. Corsley District: area 5085; population 1252; £52 10s. per annum.

APPOINTMENTS.

Newport (Salop) Union.—John Davies, L.R.C.P.E., L.F.P.&S. Glasg., L.S.A. Lond., to the Second District.

Tisbury Union.—Samuel R. Holdsworth, L.R.C.P. Edin., L.R.C.S. Edin., L.S.A. Lond., to the Hindon District.

A NEW SMALL-POX HOSPITAL AT PARIS.—The Paris Assistance Publique is about to erect a new special hospital for small-pox patients in the commune of Alfort, twelve kilometres from Paris. At present these patients are isolated in special pavilions attached to the St. Louis and St. Antoine hospitals; but it is found that the disease is propagated from these hospitals to the surrounding districts, and it is for this reason that it has been determined to found a small-pox hospital in the open country.—*Gaz. Méd.,* October 1.

ANTISEPTIC TREATMENT OF ABSCESS.—Dr. Lucas-Championnière recommends the following procedure :—Before opening an abscess, in whatever region it may be placed, we should carefully wash the skin, especially if it has been covered by a poultice, with a strong carbolic acid solution (crystals 50 parts, glycerine 50 to 75 parts, and water 1000 parts). The bistoury should also be dipped in the solution. The contents of the abscess are to be discharged, and some of the above solution injected, care being taken that the injected liquid has a free issue. The end of a caoutchouc tube is introduced into the wound, having a thread attached to it to facilitate its removal, and it is then covered by a thick layer of charpie, impregnated with a solution of carbolic acid 25 parts, glycerine 25 parts, and water 1000 parts. Finally, over all is laid a layer of gummed silk. At the end of twenty-four hours the tube is removed in order that it may be cleansed and shortened, when it is again covered with the charpie moistened with the weaker solution. Under this treatment the amount of suppuration is diminished, the redness of the wound becomes insignificant, and the cicatrices which result are much less apparent. Dr. Lucas recommends this procedure especially in abscess of the breast.—*Union Médicale,* September 15.

IMPROVEMENTS IN HYPODERMIC INJECTION.—Dr. Mason recommends the following as the best way of dealing with the piston of the hypodermic syringe when its packing gets worn and loose, so that it does not work readily. Remove the small nut at the end of the piston and take half of the packing off (it is usually in two parts), and place between them a piece of chamois skin. Cut it round, leaving it somewhat larger than the packing. It will absorb water, swell, and completely fill the barrel. A trial of this will convince the most sceptical of its value over all other devices to do away with the most annoying feature connected with the use of the syringe. With regard to the solution of morphia to be used, he thinks, to obviate the sediment which usually forms, it is better to make it as it is wanted at the bedside, which, after a little practice, may be done very quickly. "After determining the quantity of morphia, plunge the syringe (*minus* the needle) into water, and draw up as many minims of water as it has been determined to give minims of Magendie's solution. Place these in a teaspoon and add sulphate of morphia until it will take up no more. After the solution is completed, put, say, five additional minims of water to it, stir, and be positive that all is dissolved. The air which is apt to collect in the syringe is readily expelled by holding the syringe perpendicular, with the needle upwards. The liquid will gravitate to the bottom, and the air will be expelled by simply pushing the piston upwards until the fluid is seen to pass from the point of the needle. The number of abscesses which follow the hypodermic use of morphia will, I think, diminish if this method is used."—*New York Med. Record,* September 3.

NOTES, QUERIES, AND REPLIES.

Ye that questioneth much shall learn much.—Bacon.

M.A. Oxon.—The list of successful candidates was published in this journal last week. Out of the 610 candidates examined, no less than 293 were rejected. Write to the Registrar of the General Medical Council.

Re-organisation of the Indian Medical Service.—The Bombay *Gazette* states that the Government of India have sent home an important despatch relating to the re-organisation of the Indian Medical Service, in which it is proposed that the Medical Department of India should be amalgamated with the British Army Medical Department, on a plan similar to that followed when the Indian Corps of Engineers were incorporated with the Royal Engineers.

M.A. Cantab.—The gentleman named by you holds the same degree as yourself, and is moreover a *Fellow* of the College. He sends you the following enigma :—

> "To be called by my name you would highly disdain,
> Though with titles of honour I rank in the list.
> By law and by custom I single remain,
> Though unless I am double I cannot exist."

Answer—*A Fellow.*

Disputed Jurisdiction.—Some time ago it was mentioned in these columns that the new Coroner for Middlesex—Dr. Danford Thomas—immediately on his election claimed to have jurisdiction in Holloway Prison; Mr. W. J. Payne disputed this, and appealed to the Court of Aldermen on the matter. Mr. Payne subsequently addressed a letter on the question to the Home Secretary, who, in his reply, states that after having consulted the law officers of the Crown, as to whether the Coroner for the City of London or the Coroner for the Central Division of Middlesex was entitled to exercise jurisdiction in Holloway Prison, he is advised by them that the thirtieth section of the Prisons Act of 1877 preserved the jurisdiction of the Coroner for the City of London in all prisons in which he had jurisdiction at the time of the passing of the Act.

Cremation.—In Germany, cremation seems to be gaining public favour. The furnace at Gotha has now been used fifty-seven times since its erection in December, 1878. Twenty-three of these cases occurred this year.

The Penalties of Milk Adulteration.—At West Hartlepool two heavy penalties have been inflicted by the county magistrates for milk adulteration. In the first case a farmer, charged for the third time with the offence, was fined £30 and costs, or three months' imprisonment. In the second the fine was £10 and costs, or six weeks' imprisonment. If magistrates would more generally treat persons convicted of milk adulteration with similar justifiable severity, the dishonest practice would probably not continue to so great an extent as it does.

Goats.—A prominent feature in the Exhibition at the Agricultural Hall, Islington, was the collection of goats. The object of the British Goat Society is to improve the breed of these animals, and to utilise their adaptability as a milk-supply. On the Continent and in Ireland the goat is regarded as the poor man's cow.

Unqualified Medical Assistants.—The evidence of a medical assistant, given at an inquest held by the Deputy Coroner for the city of Manchester, on the body of a woman aged fifty-two years, should not escape observation. He said he had prescribed for the deceased. He was an unqualified assistant to a surgeon at the latter's dispensary, 129, Collyhurst-street. His employer did not live there, but at Stockport, and had five dispensaries, at each of which there was an assistant. Witness had no medical qualification of any kind. He had been in his present service thirteen months; had previously been employed in a druggist's shop, by a firm of manufacturing chemists, and as apprentice to a grocer and chemist. He attended the deceased in the absence of his employer, and prescribed medicine for her. He did not send for his employer, and when he called the next morning he found that the woman was dead. He charged sixpence for the medicine and sixpence for the visit. The jury returned a verdict of "Death from natural causes," and both the Coroner and the jury commented strongly on the evidence. But the verdict was absurd; and what was said about, or is to be done as to, the conduct of the principal !

Hygienist.—Kensal-green Cemetery was the first in London—opened in 1832. Acts respecting burials passed 1850, &c.

The Working-Class Tenements, Birmingham.—On the holding of two inquests in Birmingham, last week, the Borough Coroner had occasion to comment upon the wretchedness of deceased's dwellings, which he characterised as shockingly appalling. In other towns, he said, such groups of wretched tenements had been removed under the Artisans' Dwellings Act, in order that the working-classes might have built for them proper and sanitary dwellings.

Compensation for Damage by Sewerage Works.—Sir W. Hart-Dyke, Bart., M.P., has recovered £7960 compensation from the Darenth Valley Main Sewerage Board for damage done to his estate, Lullingstone Castle, by the sewer laid through it. He claimed £30,000.

WITH THE SCALPEL.

"Ubi sedes vitæ?"

ANOTHER REJOINDER.

Here's our subject. Young and strong,
With sentiment not *too* infected.
We own life short if art be long,
And common sense must be respected.
Not ours to seek the soul departed,
Not ours to ask who gave it birth;
From other will than ours it started—
We too are earth.

Why should we ask if *this* were hero,
Or martyr dying for his creed?
He might be Paul or might be Nero;
His carcase serves us in our need.
His soul? Ah! that we cannot tell;
But wise men say the angels bright,
Who asked what they did know full well,
Lost all their light!

We know that time in future years
May bring poor suppliants to our feet,
To crave for help, with prayer and tears—
God grant we may not *curses* meet.
We shall deserve them if we waste
The chances gone without recall,
While shaping to our separate taste
The Lord of all!

And duty done—though age may moan,
It need not ask for further light;
Bolder he puts his armour on
Than he who doffs it after fight.
Contented with the daily bread,
Meekly accepting God's decree,
The workers, *hoping*, downward tread,—
And so will we!

A MEDICAL STUDENT.

Benevolence.—Sir Richard Wallace, M.P., has presented to the East Suffolk and Ipswich Hospital £200 to assist in liquidating a debt on that institution, with the intimation that, if necessary, he will consider the desirability of increasing his yearly subscription.

Cardinal Manning on Liquor Legislation.—The Cardinal, addressing the Catholic Total Abstainers at Liverpool, said a Sunday Closing Act was as certain for England as that summer would return next year. He believed that the last Parliament would be the last friendly to the liquor traffic, for in the House of Commons at the present moment there were 240 members prepared to vote in favour of local option.

Novel Condition of a Licence.—A publican applying for a licence to the Birmingham Bench, pleaded, as a reason why a licence should be granted, that he intended "to serve no women, good, bad, or indifferent"; and the magistrates in granting the licence did so only on the condition that women were not to be admitted on the premises at all.

Paterfamilias.—In consequence of the outbreak of cholera at Mecca, the Sanitary Board at Constantinople have resolved to enforce ten days' quarantine against vessels from the Red Sea. Ships from Egyptian ports will be inspected by medical inspectors, and such as have passed through the Suez Canal, after undergoing quarantine in Egyptian ports, will be subject to forty-eight hours' observation.

Non-Registration of Milk Shops.—Two purveyors of milk in Glasgow have been fined £4 and £2 respectively for neglecting to register their shops. It is satisfactory to observe that these traders are receiving proper supervision by the authorities.

Urban and Rural Sanitary Works.—The Sheffield Town Council have appointed a committee of inquiry to consider the advisability of purchasing the waterworks supplying the town.——A commodious and completely arranged new dispensary has been opened in Union-street, Hereford. The cost of the building, exclusive of site, has been £1000.——A new cemetery, situated on the Evesham-road, Stratford-on-Avon, comprising an area of six acres, has been opened, the cost of which is about £1880.——The new sewerage works of Canterbury are, after much delay, perfected and in full working order. The total cost has been £8300. The sewage farm covers twenty-two acres and a half of land.——The Galashiels Town Council have accepted the offer of Mr. Scott, of Gala, of the cricket-ground as a public park, the Corporation having undertaken to keep it in order.——New sick wards are being added to the workhouse at Newport, Isle of Wight.——The Town Council of Ashton-under-Lyme have agreed to accept the offer of Stamford Park, estimated to be worth £40,000, to be kept up at the joint cost of the Local Authorities of Ashton, Stalybridge, and Hurst as a public park.——The Town Council of Leamington are about to make improvements and additions to the waterworks.——The sewering of Kenilworth is rapidly progressing towards completion.——The Local Board of Richmond, Surrey, have adopted the recommendation of their water engineer that the artesian well should be deepened from 400 to 1200 feet by a central bore.——The Local Authority of Kirkintilloch have decided on plans for the formation of a water reservoir at an estimated cost of £6000.——The Mexborough Local Board are about to carry out works for the disposal of sewage.——The Burnley Corporation have resolved to go to Parliament with a view of obtaining increased powers to construct new reservoirs and other sanitary improvements.

Anti-Quack.—Will the epigram written by Garrick when he quarrelled with Sir John Hill do for you, as he was a great quack?—

"For physic and farces, his rival there scarce is—
His farces are physic—his physic a farce is."

COMMUNICATIONS have been received from—

Mr. G. P. FIELD, London; Mr. WHARTON BARKER, Philadelphia; Messrs. W. and A. GILBEY, London; Dr. VIVIAN POORE, London; Dr. HERMAN, London; Dr. BERNAYS, London; THE SECRETARY OF THE CLINICAL SOCIETY, London; Dr. ALFRED POPE; Dr. NORMAN KERR, London; THE SECRETARY OF THE HUNTERIAN SOCIETY, London; Dr. LEONARD, Rhode Island, U.S.; THE SECRETARY OF GUY'S HOSPITAL, London; Dr. J. MURPHY, Sunderland; THE CHAIRMAN OF THE NATIVE GUANO COMPANY, Aylesbury; Surgeon-Major F. R. HOGG, Netley; Mr. J. CHATTO, London; Mr. R. W. PARKER, London; Mr. T. M. STONE, London.

BOOKS, ETC., RECEIVED—

Atlas of Skin Diseases, by Louis A. Duhring, M.D., part ix.—Outbreaks of Small-pox in Maidstone, by M. A. Adams, F.R.C.S.—Historisch-Geographischen Pathologie, von Dr. August Hirsch—Gerichtsärztliche Praxis, von Dr. H. Friedberg—Annual Report of the Board of Works for the St. Giles District—The Young Doctor's Future, by E. Diver, M.D.—On Epidemics of Dengue Fever, by J. Christie, A.M., M.D.—Transactions of the American Gynecological Society for 1880—University College Hospital, Report of Surgical Registrar for 1880—Male Sexual Organs, by S. W. Gross, A.M., M.D.—Assainissement de Paris—Medical Electricity, by Roberts Bartholow, A.M., M.D., LL.D.—Report of the Board of Works for the Poplar District, 1880-81.

PERIODICALS AND NEWSPAPERS RECEIVED—

Lancet—British Medical Journal—Medical Press and Circular—Berliner Klinische Wochenschrift—Centralblatt für Chirurgie—Gazette des Hopitaux—Gazette Médicale—Le Progrès Médical—Bulletin de l'Académie de Médecine—Pharmaceutical Journal—Wiener Medizinische Wochenschrift—Centralblatt für die Medizinischen Wissenschaften—Revue Médicale—Gazette Hebdomadaire—National Board of Health Bulletin, Washington—Nature—Occasional Notes—Deutsche Medicinal-Zeitung—Boston Medical and Surgical Journal—Louisville Medical News—Oil and Drug News—Monthly Index—Archives Générales de Médecine—Veterinarian—Glasgow Medical Journal—Centralblatt für Gynäkologie—The American—Border Advertiser—Weekblad—Monthly Homœopathic Review—Maryland Medical Journal—Indian Medical Gazette—Medical Temperance Journal—Reporter—Edinburgh Medical Journal—Liverpool Daily Post, October 4.

APPOINTMENTS FOR THE WEEK.

October 8. *Saturday (this day).*

Operations at St. Bartholomew's, $1\frac{1}{2}$ p.m.; King's College, $1\frac{1}{2}$ p.m.; Royal Free, 2 p.m.; Royal London Ophthalmic, 11 a.m.; Royal Westminster Ophthalmic, $1\frac{1}{2}$ p.m.; St. Thomas's, $1\frac{1}{2}$ p.m.; London, 2 p.m.

10. *Monday.*

Operations at the Metropolitan Free, 2 p.m.; St. Mark's Hospital for Diseases of the Rectum, 2 p.m.; Royal London Ophthalmic, 11 a.m.; Royal Westminster Ophthalmic, $1\frac{1}{2}$ p.m.

11. *Tuesday.*

Operations at Guy's, $1\frac{1}{2}$ p.m.; Westminster, 2 p.m.; Royal London Ophthalmic, 11 a.m.; Royal Westminster Ophthalmic, $1\frac{1}{2}$ p.m.; West London, 3 p.m.

12. *Wednesday.*

Operations at University College, 2 p.m.; St. Mary's, $1\frac{1}{4}$ p.m.; Middlesex, 1 p.m.; London, 2 p.m.; St. Bartholomew's, $1\frac{1}{2}$ p.m.; Great Northern, 2 p.m.; Samaritan, $2\frac{1}{2}$ p.m.; King's College (by Mr. Lister), 2 p.m.; Royal London Ophthalmic, 11 a.m.; Royal Westminster Ophthalmic, $1\frac{1}{2}$ p.m.; St. Thomas's, $1\frac{1}{2}$ p.m.; St. Peter's Hospital for Stone, 2 p.m.; National Orthopædic, Great Portland-street, 10 a.m.

HUNTERIAN SOCIETY (London Institution) (Council Meeting, $7\frac{1}{2}$), 8 p.m. First General Meeting: Introductory Remarks by the President. Mr. J. Hutchinson, "On Second Attacks of Syphilis."

ROYAL MICROSCOPICAL SOCIETY, 8 p.m. Mr. B. Wills Richardson, "On Multiple Staining of Animal and Vegetable Tissues."

13. *Thursday.*

Operations at St. George's, 1 p.m.; Central London Ophthalmic, 1 p.m.; Royal Orthopædic, 2 p.m.; University College, 2 p.m.; Royal London Ophthalmic, 11 a.m.; Royal Westminster Ophthalmic, $1\frac{1}{2}$ p.m.; Hospital for Diseases of the Throat, 2 p.m.; Hospital for Women, 2 p.m.; Charing-cross, 2 p.m.; London, 2 p.m.; North-West London, $2\frac{1}{2}$ p.m.

OPHTHALMOLOGICAL SOCIETY, $8\frac{1}{2}$ p.m. Mr. J. E. Adams, "On Uniocular Diplopia." Dr. W. M. Ord, "On Cases of Uniocular Diplopia." Mr. J. E. Adams, "On Cases of Suppurating Ophthalmitis from Septic Embolism." Dr. Brailey, "On a Case of Tuberculosis of Eye." Dr. Walter Edmunds—1. Tubercle of Choroid; 2. Perineuritis Optica twenty-four hours after Fracture of Skull—(microscopical specimens). Living specimens at 8 o'clock.

14. *Friday.*

Operations at Central London Ophthalmic, 2 p.m.; Royal London Ophthalmic, 11 a.m.; South London Ophthalmic, 2 p.m.; Royal Westminster Ophthalmic, $1\frac{1}{2}$ p.m.; St. George's (ophthalmic operations), $1\frac{1}{4}$ p.m.; Guy's, $1\frac{1}{2}$ p.m.; St. Thomas's (ophthalmic operations), 2 p.m.

CLINICAL SOCIETY, $8\frac{1}{2}$ p.m. Dr. Wiltshire, "On a Case of Ruptured Ovarian Cyst." Mr. Christopher Heath, "On a Case in which a Large Odontome was Successfully Removed." Mr. C. B. Keetley, "On a Case of Charcot's Joint Disease" (living specimen). Mr. C. T. Dent, "On a Case of Strangulated Hernia" (Littré's).

ABSTRACT OF

INTRODUCTORY ADDRESS

DELIVERED AT THE OPENING OF

UNIVERSITY COLLEGE MEDICAL SCHOOL.

By G. V. POORE, M.D., F.R.C.P.,

Professor of Medical Jurisprudence, University College, Assistant
Physician to University College Hospital, etc.

AFTER some observations on the advantages and disadvantages of the medical profession, and on the importance of an acquaintance with the principles of the collateral sciences, Dr. Poore said:

There is one branch of medical knowledge which most certainly "does but encumber whom it seems to enrich," and which I think we should strive as much as possible to be rid of altogether. It is a branch of knowledge, if indeed it can be spoken of as such, which is entirely of our own creating, which has, in times past, brought much deserved ridicule upon medicine, and which, albeit that it seems to me to savour more of pedantry and quackery than of wisdom, has, I fear, become with most of us a vicious and incorrigible habit. I allude to *medical language.*

The unwieldy proportions which this cumbersome branch of knowledge has assumed may be judged of by the "Dictionary of Medical and Scientific Terms" which is now in course of publication by that useful body, "The New Sydenham Society." This dictionary, a work which reflects the greatest credit upon its learned compilers, was commenced more than two years ago. It already consists of 800 closely printed large octavo pages, and the compilers have as yet only reached the third letter of the alphabet. If the present proportions be maintained, the dictionary will extend to some 8000 pages, and will contain more than 300,000 terms, which the already over-weighted student will be expected to master; and if the present rate of word-making is maintained by medical and scientific professors, the appendix, which will be necessary when the work is completed at the beginning of the next century, will be bigger, possibly, than the parent book. Why is it that doctors and men of science seem entirely to forget the use of their mother-tongues? What excuse have we, who inherit the most expressive language in the world (the language of Shakespeare and Milton, of the Translators of the Bible, of Huxley, Herbert Spencer, and Sir Thomas Watson), to offer for this huge collection, mostly of Pedantic Jargon, which never formed a part of the language of communication of any nation which ever lived upon the earth? I fear that we are as deserving of ridicule in this matter now, as we were in the days of Molière and Fielding; and as I firmly believe that this fatal love of long words has contributed not a little in the past to check the advance of medical science, I trust I may be excused for dwelling upon the subject for a few minutes.

In making use of language to express our thoughts, we ought to be sure—(1) that the words used really express the idea which it is wished to convey; (2) that they are the shortest; and (3) that they are the most familiar words which are available. Words must be as objective as possible, i.e., they should bring the subject with the utmost vividness before the mind's eye: and therefore those words to which the eye, and the ear, and the mind have been accustomed for the longest time (vernacular terms used from infancy) are the best; and as it is equally obvious that a word of two syllables requires twice the mental attention that is necessary for the comprehension of a word of one syllable, it is clear also that, other things being equal, the shortest words are the best. We need not be, as almost seems the case, under any superstition that scientific facts, if they be facts, differ from common facts and require other than common words for their expression. Neither need we fear that by the use of short vernacular terms our literary style will be otherwise than improved. Let us rather take comfort from such a masterpiece of English composition as Gray's Elegy, in which the words of more than two syllables, other than present participles, may almost be counted upon the toes and fingers. To compare the feeling produced by reading a stanza

VOL. II. 1881. No. 1633.

of this exquisite poem, with that evoked by the perusal of a paragraph of what passes for English in some medical writings, would be like comparing the pleasurable movement of a first-rate carriage on our wooden pavements with the lumbering joltings of a springless waggon over a corduroy road.

If the advantages of expressing ourselves simply are so obvious, why, it will be asked, do we continue to use the polysyllabic gibberish which passes current as the language of science, but which proves, I think, that we have not yet come to a right comprehension of the scientific use of language? The only justification which can be given for it is the desire, which we all must share, that there should be a common language to serve for the interchange of thought between scientific men of all nations; and the fact that these specially coined words are possibly comprehensible to a select clique of some few nations is supposed to compensate for the fact that they are not only perfectly incomprehensible, but absolutely repellent, to the millions of all nations. Do not let us suppose that the terms we use are "classical"; far from it. Hippocrates and Celsus, were they to revisit the earth, would be as little able to understand them as are the classical scholars of the present day. We owe only a very small minority of them to the fathers of medicine. Those great men, be it remembered, wrote their great works in their own vernacular, well knowing that if a man wishes to express himself with clearness, and without ambiguity or fear of being misunderstood, he must use the language with which he is most familiar, and which conveys the most definite ideas to his own mind. By using a language "not understood of the people" for the expressing of scientific facts, we undoubtedly seriously curtail the area from which we draw our scientific recruits; and I take it that one explanation of the scientific fervour which pervades the whole of Germany is to be found in the fact that scientific terms are in that country very largely derived from the German vernacular, and that he who only knows the German language is not necessarily confronted in a German scientific book with words which compel him to close the volume almost as soon as opened with a sigh of helplessness and hopelessness. There may be those who still think that it would be an advantage to science if Latin were still its common language, as it was two centuries ago, but it is hardly conceivable that science would have advanced by leaps and bounds as it has done if its professors had continued to express their ideas in a language which could never become, like their vernacular, really a part of themselves and the active machinery of their thoughts. It must be admitted that our long words have not hitherto been of much use as a means of international communication. The scientific work of the French and Germans is still a sealed book to us, unless we have learned the French and German languages; and those who listened to the polyglot discussions which lately took place at Burlington House must have been impressed with the fact that, however desirable a common language for science may be, we never were farther from its attainment than at present.

Now, the only branches of knowledge which have anything like a common international language are *Mathematics, Chemistry,* and *Music,* and in these international communication is only possible as long as professors rigidly adhere to the use of the symbols which have come to represent the elements of their respective sciences, and as soon as they attempt to write or talk about the facts which these symbols represent, all mutual interchange of thought is at an end. Now, in order to have anything like an international language for medicine, the first step must be to definitely settle upon a set of names or a code of symbols to represent the elements of Anatomy and Histology. This we have already got to a certain extent, but there is not yet a perfect international agreement as to the names to be applied to some of our best-known anatomical elements. As a sample of this I may allude to the fact that the nerve which we call *musculo-spiral* is universally called *radial* on the Continent; and that several muscles of the hand and arm have one name on the Continent, and another name in this country. I will not weary you by giving other instances, but I would suggest to the promulgators of international congresses the desirability of appointing a committee to settle once and for all the names by which the anatomical and histological elements of the human body are henceforth to be known. I do not, of course, mean to suggest that existing names should be altered. Utterly bad as many of them are, we have become accustomed to them by use, and the very antiquity of many of them, and the fact that some are derived from the names of the older anatomists, serve to give an historic interest to dry facts, and to remind us how laboriously and slowly our knowledge has been pieced together by the great men who have preceded us.

Although we are, I think, bound to accept and continue to use existing names, it is, nevertheless, interesting and instructive to compare the Saxon anatomical and physiological terms, so wonderful in their simplicity and striking individuality, which originally came to us by the light of nature, with those which have since been added by the light of science. We cannot conceive simpler words, or words less liable to misconception, either by the eye or ear, than *head, neck, eye, nose, skin, back, mouth, tooth, leg, arm, gut, touch, pain, ache, taste, smell, right, sound, sweat*, and many other most expressive monosyllables, some of which we happily still continue to use, while others have been cast aside as " vulgar " (whatever that may mean).

Although we still use the simpler words, we seem half ashamed of them, for whenever we get a chance we make use of our hybrid jargon, and give our pure-bred Saxon the cut direct. The chances are, that, if a medical writer wishes to speak of the *mouth*, he calls it the *oral orifice ;* the *nose* becomes the *olfactory organ ;* the skin of the back is the *dorsal integument ;* touch is *tactile sensibility ;* pain is an *algesic phenomenon ;* a fit of the *stomach-ache* is a *gastralgic crisis ;* *tears* become *lachrymation ;* and *sweating*, a *diaphoresis*. In compound words this tendency is more marked, and it is strange how completely we have cast aside the pure Saxon *lore* in favour of *logy*, an Anglo-Greek mongrel. The man who talks of *ophthalmology* or *odontology* would certainly not consent to use such expressions as *eye-lore* or *tooth-lore ;* and the professor of *anthropology* would certainly tell us that he had nothing to do with *folk-lore*. Now, I believe that, even in scientific anatomy, each nation would do well to adhere, as far as possible, to its own vernacular monosyllables, for since anything like a common medical language is not to be dreamt of, and since it is necessary to learn French and German in order to understand French and German medical writings, these terms, which are always amongst the simplest and oldest in the language, are never a source of difficulty. The Greek and Latin terms given by the older anatomists, cumbersome and singularly inexpressive as many of them are, must be retained ; but if they be retained, they must be retained *in their original form*. If these original terms be translated into the vernacular, we get a worse confusion than ever. Let me illustrate this by an example. Some three hundred years before Christ, Herophilus, a Greek anatomist of the Alexandrian school, described that C-like bend of the gut which is just beyond the stomach. This bend being about as long as twelve fingers are wide, he called *the dodekadactyl*, and this term was ultimately translated by the Latin writers into *duodenum*, the word which is now in common use. Although the word itself is neither short nor expressive, it should be retained and used in its Latin (the commonest) form. The Germans, however, are not content to receive the old word merely as a symbol, but, looking back to its original form, they have had regard to its original meaning, and have perversely *translated* it into their own vernacular, and thus *the dodekadactyl* of Herophilus has become the *Zwölf-fingerdarm*, or twelve-finger-gut of modern Germany. Now, although an anatomist may know all about the *duodenum*, it does not, I regret to say, necessarily follow that he knows how the name arose or what is its meaning ; and although he might be well enough acquainted with German to translate the three words, *Zwölf, Finger*, and *Darm*, he might be sorely puzzled to know what was alluded to. I could give you many other instances in which the Germans have thus disguised landmarks which would otherwise be easily recognisable by all. Our barbarous technicalities are merely symbols, and, if literally translated, they are often misleading, as the meaning we attach to them is usually arbitrary and purely conventional. Thus the man who was under the impression that " Bacillus anthracis " (which, according to the Latin and Greek dictionaries, means the *little rod of the coal*) was a new name for a patent poker, was sadly mistaken. When dealing with anatomical elements, anything like variety of expression is not to be thought of. To speak, for example, of the "latissimus dorsi" in one sentence, and of " the broad muscle of the back " in the next, is only likely to puzzle the

reader and throw him off the scent. In like manner, the way in which the French speak of the " teres major " as the " grand rond," and of the " serratus magnus " as the " grand dentelé," is merely misleading.

I believe that the establishment of an absolute international agreement as to the names to be given to the few hundred elements with which we have to deal, is a matter really worth striving after, and a fit subject for the consideration of an international committee. Perhaps such a committee might have some power given to it of altering names, for the unwieldiness of some is out of all proportion to their utility, and it would almost seem as if some names were meant to bear an inverse proportion to the size and importance of the thing designated. We must be very far off from even so much community of expression as is enjoyed by chemistry, when one of our most insignificant anatomical elements rejoices in the name of " levator labii superioris alæque nasi." Possibly we might be allowed to speak familiarly of this little muscle as the " sneerer," just as men and women whose names occupy many lines in the parish register are habitually known to their familiars as Jack or Gill, as the case may be.

If we had one common name only (instead of an indefinite number, as is now the case) for the elementary factors of our frames and tissues, and if diseases were named solely with reference to their anatomical seat and the process producing them, we should have attained, I believe, as far as it is possible to attain, a code of expressions capable of international use. As international communication is the only conceivable reason for employing other than vernacular words, so is it also a reason for adhering to our vernacular terms outside the restricted province which I have defined For international communication we must make ourselves familiar with each other's languages. That is certain. And it is manifestly of importance that each nation should try to keep its language pure, in order that it may be the more easily learnt. The practice of concubinage with the dead languages merely has the effect of producing a mongrel language (as unproductive as are all other mules), of huge bulk and monstrous form, which has to be learnt as an additional study.

I may here mention incidentally that the universal adoption of the metric system of measurement would do more for the facilitating of international communication than the coining of any number of words.

It seems to be the pitiable ambition of some writers to seize upon a trifling fact, and to give it the longest name they can invent with the aid of a lexicon ; and if such a practice be not vigorously discouraged, medicine may become again what it once was—" a rhapsody of words." Some, possibly, are under the impression that their dictionary-made expressions may gain for them a reputation for classical learning. They cannot afford, as did John Hunter, to rely for their reputation upon the facts which they discover, and who, when he was twitted with his want of knowledge of Greek and Latin, wrote thus characteristically to a friend —" Jesse Foot accuses me of not understanding the dead languages ; but I could teach him that on the dead body which he never knew in any language, dead or living." The defence has lately been put forward for scientific jargon that every trade or profession *must* have its own technical terms. I confess I cannot see the *necessity*. The tailor, so far as I know, derives no advantage from calling his smoothing-iron a " goose " ; and seamanship is not advanced because a sailor's " companion " is one thing at sea and another thing on shore. It seems to me that technical terms ought, as far as possible, to be discouraged, because the coining of new words when they are not wanted, and the giving of strange and conventional meanings to common words, must increase the difficulty of acquiring any art or handicraft. Many technical terms are maintained for selfish and trades-union purposes, and with the object of covering a simple matter with a veil of secrecy. Let Medicine take care that she be not suspected of similar unworthy objects.

Many of our long words exercise a most unwholesome fascination upon the student, and I have known some who appeared to think that a parrot-like use of words was the main object of medicine, and who have talked, for example, of " sclerosis," as if the word itself had some magic power of explaining every symptom of disease, and defined at once the process at work and its situation. I may be wrong in supposing that our English equivalent " hardening " would be more likely to make the student think, not only of the *hardness*, but also of the "why?" and the "where?"

Words (which are but the shadows of facts) are, unlike natural shadows, very often not true. It has been most unfortunate that such a word as "vivisection" should ever have been applied to so mild a process as that of pricking an animal with the point of a lancet. The word is so vivid in itself, and so calculated to raise in the mind all the horrors of the Inquisition and the writhings of witnesses under cross-examination, that we cannot be surprised at a cardinal and a judge combining together to suppress the practice utterly. Sometimes the shadow will remain, although we are unable to find the substance. Such a shadow is the word "homœopathy." If the term "*like-cure*" had been used, just as "*water-cure*" is used for hydropathy, the proper limits of its application would long ago have been determined, and the word would never have been worshipped to the same extent as a fetish by the faithful among the public.

Among unworthy motives which have induced us to have long words, must be reckoned the desire to appear more learned than we are, and there was a time, perhaps, when there was very little true knowledge behind the verbiage which was the chief stock-in-trade of the profession. Now, however, times are changed. Pathology, or the study of disease, has become a true science, and we are no longer content merely to translate the symptoms of which the patient complains into Greek or Latin, as the case may be, and call it a diagnosis. We now recognise when a patient comes to us complaining, for example, that he has lost power on one side of his body, that by calling his trouble "hemiplegia" we make no forward step. It is merely telling him in Greek what he had confided to us in English. It is rather a step back, for it throws what has been called "the decent obscurity of a dead language" over a matter which is self-evident. Our duty now is to discover the *cause* of his symptoms, to form a *judgment* or *diagnosis* on the disease process at work and its exact situation, and to make a *forecast* or *prognosis* as to his chances of recovery and the best means of bringing it about.

There is in human nature a tendency which is expressed by the words "Omne ignotum pro magnifico,"—a tendency to put an undue value upon the unknown. It was this natural tendency which led the hero of Warren's famous novel, "£10,000 a Year," to make the fatal experiment of applying to his hair the pomade called "Cyanochaitanthropopoion," and it is the same tendency which leads the public to buy anything, no matter how common or how worthless, to which the vendor has given a name that is utterly incomprehensible to them. By pandering to this tendency I doubt not that medical terms have been in reality an unspeakable, though delusive, comfort to the public; and that the lady who was told by the physician "that there was still in her husband's lung a perceptible amount of '*whispering pectoriloquy*,' although the '*ægophony*' had happily completely disappeared," derived from the information the same kind of consolation as did the old woman who, listening to a deep and learned sermon by her rector, found solace in "that blessed word Mesopotamia."

The advantage of using plain language is nowhere more manifest than in courts of law, where the life or reputation of a fellow-creature may depend upon your making yourselves perfectly understood by the twelve plain men who constitute the jury. If, however, you do not cultivate the habit of using simple terms at all times, you will find that they are not forthcoming when you want them; and if you cannot tell a plain unvarnished tale, you will lay yourselves open to the imputation that you cannot speak plainly because you do not understand the question. You must always bear in mind that not only the jury but the counsel and judge also are probably completely ignorant of terms which to you have become a second nature. Reporters for the press are also equally ignorant, and unless you are very careful you will probably be mortified by finding that, owing to a non-comprehension of your language by these gentlemen, your evidence, when it appears in print, will seem to you and your professional brethren a mass of rubbish.

I trust that what I have said will lead you to think seriously on this important matter of medical language, and I would finally impress upon those who are beginning their studies how necessary it is to be sure and understand every technical phrase they come across. To those who are soon to be adding to our sum of knowledge I would say, Be merciful

to posterity; do not coin new words if you can possibly help doing so, and remember the simple lines of good George Herbert:—

  "Let forrain nations of their language boast
    What fine variety each tongue affords;
  I like our language as our men and coast—
    Who cannot dress it well, want wits, not words."

INTRODUCTORY ADDRESS

DELIVERED AT THE OPENING OF

KING'S COLLEGE HOSPITAL MEDICAL SCHOOL.

By SIR JOHN LUBBOCK, M.P., F.R.S.

THE opening address at King's College was delivered by Sir John Lubbock, M.P., F.R.S. It was an obvious and most pleasant privilege, he said, to congratulate those present, especially, of course, Dr. Barry and the staff, on the prosperity, efficiency, and progress of the College. The history of King's College had, indeed, been one of constant progress and success, and he was the more glad to be able to attend on the present occasion because it might be said to be the jubilee year of the College. There were now no fewer than seven distinct departments at work, with more than 1500 regular students, to say nothing of about 800 more attending the subsidiary courses. He might add that, as regards the future, the Council were establishing a new department for women's education, to be carried on, indeed, in a separate locality, but as an integral part of the College, and under the same government. King's College set a good example in giving some share of encouragement to all the great subjects of human knowledge. It was, indeed, well worth considering whether the time had not arrived when the University of London might initiate a system under which the students at King's College and other educational institutions of the metropolis might have the advantage of a course of lectures on subjects, perhaps, too special for any single college or school to undertake. Nor was this the only way in which education might be promoted by such combined action. The question, however, was one of much difficulty, and perhaps hardly suitable for discussion on such an occasion as that. Sir John Lubbock proceeded:—You are, most of you, destined for one of the noblest of our professions—that of ministering to the health of your fellow-creatures. But, gentlemen, there is one person of whose health you are bound to be especially careful—I mean your own. As medical men, you will not, I am sure, suppose that I intend to imply that you should think much about it; to be over-anxious about one's health is the very way to make one's self ill. On the other hand, it is most desirable to lay down a well-considered course of life, and, if warning symptoms appear, to consider what is the cause to which they are due. I would also impress on you to economise your time, and to arrange your work so as never, if you can help it, to waste a moment. But when I say this I by no means intend to recommend any of you to be constantly at work. Quite the reverse. A certain amount of amusement is most desirable; regular exercise is absolutely necessary to all ordinary constitutions. But a great many people, so far, at least, as my experience goes, for want of a little forethought, lose a great deal of time in what is neither work, exercise, nor amusement. This is the waste of time which I deprecate, and against which I would caution you. But once again let me say that, far from deprecating holidays, I would strongly recommend them. The late Sir H. Holland made it, I believe, a rule to allow himself three months every year. That is, no doubt, more than most could spare. Still, if you can, by all means give yourself good long holidays and the rough change, then your work during the rest of the year will be worth all the more. One way in which much time may be obtained is by utilising small opportunities. Frequently we have ostensibly five minutes to spare before the arrival of some train or an appointment with a friend. It seems hardly worth while to begin on anything for so short a time. Never mind, your friend will often be late, and you will in this way gain many a valuable hour. In reading, again, I am often astounded at the reckless way in which time is squandered. It happened to me, if I may be pardoned a personal reference, many years ago, to be taken by some friends to Scotland for a holiday. I trusted to them for books,—they trusted to me. We were in the far North, miles away from any railway, and before I could get a fresh supply of books I had read " Cœlebs in Search of a Wife " through three or four times. I shall never forget it; but it was a most valuable lesson, and I never go anywhere now without carefully selecting plenty of books. Indeed, I am often astonished at the want of care with which many persons select their reading. Few, indeed, have more than a very little time to devote to it, and one would, therefore, have supposed that the utmost care would be given to select the very best. Yet, how often do we see our friends take up the first book that comes to hand. They go to bed early, perhaps, in the evening at a country house, and, carelessly remarking that they must have a book, they take up any one that happens to be on the table, just as if a book was a book, and one book was as good as another. I need not say there are many books which are deadly poison, which contain the bacteria of mental disease, as certain in their operation as any of the infusions of the physiologist. I doubt whether anyone ever read a trial for murder without being distinctly the worse for it. But, without condescending to the literature of the police-courts, it is surely very sad that so much valuable time should be wasted over mere padding. The fact that we have so little time for reading renders it all the more desirable to make the most of what we have; and if care be taken, I think you would be surprised how many of the great standard books of the world you will be able to read, even during a very busy life, if you husband your time, and do not throw it away upon rubbish. You will often hear a remark made with surprise, that the busiest people have the most leisure. And there is much truth in it. For those who economise, who really make the wisest use of their time, not only can do more than others, but even, if I may so say, have time over. We all know how often large subscriptions are raised by small individual contributions. We are constantly asked to give a guinea, or perhaps even only a shilling, towards some important object. I am not, of course, going to ask you to-day for any pecuniary contribution, however infinitesimal. What I would, however, beg is that you will each of you make some small contribution to the great edifice of human knowledge, that you will record some one fact or observation; and if you once make a beginning I do not doubt that you will continue. Depend upon it, you will have the opportunity of doing so. You may even, without any great effort of your own, be in a position, if you cultivate the habit of observation, to have opportunity which the most learned and able would envy. I do not ask you to take my word for this. Dr. Billings, in his interesting address on Medical Literature delivered before the International Congress, justly observed that " Chance may present to the most obscure practitioner an opportunity for observation which the greatest master may never meet." I do not, of course, mean for a moment to imply that any of you will be among the " most obscure practitioners "; but if such opportunities are open to them, how much more to you with your great advantages! I would also venture to impress upon you very strongly the importance of cultivating habits of business. One of the most eminent of your profession assured me not long ago that, when he thought over the many cases he had known of men even of good ability and high character who had been unsuccessful in life, by far the most frequent cause of failure was that they were dilatory, unpunctual, unable to work cordially with others, obstinate in small things, and, in fact, what we call unbusiness-like. And when you have done your best do not be anxious. Sir James Paget has given some interesting statistics, which show that out of 1000 medical students whose career he followed, rather more than 300 left the profession or died early, more than 600 attained fair, some of them considerable, success. Out of the whole number only fifty-six entirely failed. Of these fifty-six, fifteen never passed the examinations, ten failed through ill-health or accident, and ten through intemperance or dissipation—happily a small proportion, to which we must add, however, about twenty of those who left the profession. These figures seem to show that out of the whole 1000 less than fifty entirely failed, except through gross misbehaviour on their own part. You have, therefore, no reason to fear but that with diligence and prudence you will have a happy

career before you, though it is no doubt true, as stated in an excellent article in a recent number of the *Lancet*, that no one should think of entering the medical profession who is not prepared to throw himself into it heart and soul. In the case of companions—I will not call them friends—again, it is surprising how little care is exercised. Many people seem to trust almost to the chapter of accidents: they make friends with a man because they travel by the same train, belong to the same club, or are thrown in with him by some other accident. By all means be friendly with everyone who has done nothing to render his companionship undesirable, but for real friends try to secure the very best; you will naturally select those who have congenial tastes, but above all, endeavour to win those from whose stores of knowledge you may gain instruction, who may advise you wisely in cases of difficulty, and raise you by the stimulus of a noble example and the spectacle of a well-spent life.

ORIGINAL COMMUNICATIONS.

ON PROLAPSE OF THE OVARIES.

By G. ERNEST HERMAN, M.B. Lond.,
Assistant Obstetric Physician to the London Hospital; Physician to the Royal Maternity Charity; Honorary Librarian to the Obstetrical Society of London.

(*Continued from page* 442.)

H. R., a aged twenty-six, labourer's wife, came to the obstetric out-patient department of the London Hospital on March 8, 1879. She stated that she had begun to menstruate at fifteen, and had from the beginning been regular, the flow lasting about a week, but varying in quantity. Since about the age of twenty, menstruation had been accompanied with much pain, which was accustomed to come on the day after the flow began, and to last a day or two. It was referred to the situation of the ovaries, the left being the worse. It would come on suddenly, and last about two hours. It was relieved by lying down. She was married when aged twenty-four. Since then the pain at her menstrual period had been getting worse; but in other respects the menstrual function had not altered. There had never been any sign of pregnancy. She had suffered from dyspareunia ever since her marriage: it varied in severity, but was on the whole steadily getting worse. She also complained of a feeling of " bearing-down," of too frequent desire to micturate, and inability to retain the urine when the desire to pass it was felt; of pain during defæcation; of leucorrhœa, and heat of the vulva. All these had been coming on since her marriage. The bowels were regular. She was a healthy-looking woman, who presented no sign of disease in any part of her body except the pelvic organs. The vagina was capacious; the uterus in the normal position (in, or nearly in, the axis of the pelvic inlet), of natural size and shape. Behind and rather to the left of the uterus a body was felt, of the shape and size of the ovary, and tender. She was given mag. sulph. ʒj., aq. menth. pip. ʒj., ter die.

March 18.—Her last menstruation ceased on the 17th, after lasting a week. The amount was not so much as usual, and there was no pain to speak of. This, she says, is the first time for six years that she has menstruated without pain. The bowels have been freely open, and the pain in defæcation is less. The dyspareunia is no better. This she now lays especial stress upon; she says it is, and always has been, her chief complaint. On local examination the state of things found is the same as when the last note was made. When the ovary-like body behind and to the left of the uterus was pressed upon, she said that the pain produced was like that felt during coitus. A thick elastic ring was put into the vagina.

At each following visit she reported her symptoms as being better.

On April 5 she said she now had no pain of any kind. The dyspareunia had ceased, and so had the dyschezia.

On April 19, having just finished menstruating, she stated that the period had passed over without pain. She thought herself quite well. She was advised to continue wearing the instrument, and to come in three months.

She accordingly came on July 26. She said she had continued to take aperient medicine until May 3. On leaving

It off the pain on defæcation returned, she began again to suffer from leucorrhœa, the bowels became confined, and she was troubled with nausea and flatulence, with colicky pains in the abdomen. There was no dyspareunia. The catamenia had been regular and painless. The ring was removed, and the patient was advised to take aperient medicine, so as to insure regular action of the bowels.

August 16.—Since the last note the bowels have been regular. She has no dyschezia, no dyspareunia. Has a slight feeling of weight in the pelvis on exertion. No discharge; can retain urine longer than formerly. Has no pain at any time, and thinks herself well.

January 21, 1881.—She again attended at the hospital, and stated that her symptoms had returned a month or two after the date of the last note. The only symptoms she has are those formerly mentioned—dyspareunia and dyschezia; the bowels are confined.

28th.—A thick elastic ring put in.

May 1, 1881.—Since the last note, has taken an aperient mixture. Bowels open regularly; no pain in defæcation. No dyspareunia. Catamenia regular, flow lasting eight days; pain very slight. Some days has an aching in the back and numbness in the feet; other days feels quite well.

I would ask attention in this case, as in the last—first, to the conditions accompanying the ovarian displacement. There were signs and symptoms such as go with slight prolapse—a loose and capacious vagina, with leucorrhœa from vaginal catarrh; and a feeling of "bearing-down" with irritability of the bladder. Next, to the two chief symptoms, which were, pain on sexual intercourse, and (the bowels being habitually constipated) pain on defæcation. Third, to the effect of treatment. Aperients removed the pain in defæcation, but not the dyspareunia. The latter symptom disappeared when a thick elastic ring was worn. The pain in defæcation returned when the bowels were allowed to get confined, and again went away when they were kept freely open. I may also call attention to the fact, upon which I shall not make further comment, that the patient suffered from dysmenorrhœa, and that this ceased after aperients had been given. I have seen other cases in which menstrual pain has been completely removed by aperients; but not a sufficient number to enable me to state in what their peculiarities consist.(a) That leucorrhœa is aggravated by constipation will be familiar to all; therefore I need not dwell on the exemplification of that fact by this case,—nor need I enlarge upon the fact that flatulent dyspepsia is a not infrequent result of constipation.

A. L., aged twenty-seven, a gardener's wife, came to the Obstetric Out-patient Department of the London Hospital on October 15, 1879. She had had two children, the younger being nine months old: it had been weaned a fortnight. She had not menstruated since her confinement. The complaints she mentioned were abdominal pain, pain in micturition, inability to retain her urine long, and pain in defæcation. On examination, the uterus was found in its natural position, not enlarged, the cervix small and healthy. Behind and to the left of the uterus an ovary-like body was felt, which was not particularly tender. Nothing else wrong was detected.

I unfortunately have no note of her treatment, nor any further note of her condition, until July 21, 1880, when her medical attendant, Mr. Culpin, of Stoke Newington, brought her again to me; and he explained, what she herself had not liked to state at the hospital, that her chief trouble was dyspareunia. This had been present ever since her confinement, and had been worse the last three months. There was also pain on defæcation, which resembled that caused by intercourse. Behind and to the left of the uterus an ovary-like body was to be felt as before, which was very tender. A thick elastic ring was put in, and an aperient mixture was prescribed.

September 4, 1880, is the date of my next note, which is, that there is no longer any pain, either on defæcation or on intercourse.

January 16, 1881.—In answer to an inquiry from me, Mr. Culpin tells me that about two months ago, he removed the pessary for a few days, but the pain returned, and he replaced it, with relief to the pain. She still wears it.

This case is simpler, and therefore more instructive, than either of the former ones. The patient, from modesty, did not mention her chief symptom when she first came, and her statements then were vague; therefore I need not occupy time with remarks upon her condition when first seen. When she came with her medical man the account of her symptoms, given through him, was clear and definite. Her only troubles were dyspareunia and dyschezia, both these pains being identical in kind. A thick elastic ring relieved the former, and aperients the latter. When the ring was removed the pain in intercourse returned, and was again relieved when the instrument was replaced.

[Reported by Mr. W. H. Price.]

C. G., aged twenty-seven, porter's wife, was sent to me by Dr. Wheeler Brown, of Stoke Newington, on March 18, 1880.

Her complaints were of dyspareunia, dyschezia, irritability of bladder, with pain in micturition, leucorrhœa, also of flatulence, and headache.

She said she had always lived well, and had never had any serious illness. She began to menstruate at the age of fourteen, and had been regular every month since, except during pregnancy. Before marriage the flow was very scanty, only lasting one day, and was accompanied with much pain, sometimes enough to lay her up. Since marriage the flow had been more copious, lasting three days, and the ago, pain had been far less acute, never laying her up. She married when between nineteen and twenty. Her first child was born about three years after marriage; the labour was natural, but after it she was ill for four months with "bad breast." Her second child was born four years ago, prematurely, in the eighth month of pregnancy; there was slight flooding before the child was born. After the delivery she had no bad symptoms of any kind; she lay in bed a fortnight. Ever since the confinement she had suffered from a feeling of "bearing-down," and also from dyspareunia, which had been especially severe during the last twelve months, this pain being accompanied with nausea and with faintness, and lasting for nearly an hour. For two years she had suffered from leucorrhœa, and occasional pruritus of the vulva. For twelve months she had not been able to hold her urine so long as formerly, and had occasionally had pain in passing it. For the last three months her bowels had been confined, and she had had pain in defæcation, the pain thus occasioned resembling that caused by intercourse. For the same time, but never before, she had been a good deal troubled with headaches; her stomach had often swelled, making her uncomfortable, a condition which she attributed to wind.

On examination, she was not anæmic, and was well nourished; the abdominal walls were lax, and no tumour was to be felt. There was slight tenderness in the left ovarian region. Per vaginam, the uterus was found in the normal position, and quite movable; its shape was natural, and its cavity measured two inches and a half long: the cervix was healthy, with the exception of slight redness of its posterior lip. A movable body, of the shape and size of the ovary, and tender, was felt low down, and to the left of the uterus. She was given mag. sulph. ʒss., acid. sulph. dil. ♏ v., dec. cinch. ʒj., three times daily; and a thick elastic ring was put into the vagina.

April 6.—She can hold her urine better; the bowels are regular, and there is now no dyschezia. The dyspareunia is now "nothing to speak of."

April 21.—No dyspareunia; no dyschezia. Menstruated two weeks ago: pain same as usual. Told to come in two months.

June 16.—Complains of occasional pain in left ovarian region; is otherwise quite well. Ovary-like body still to be felt.

September 22.—Pain in left side better; dyspareunia "nothing to speak of."

As in the former cases, I would ask attention here first to the etiological conditions. The patient had a long illness—abcess of the breast—following confinement; and quickly after this she became pregnant again: a course of events obviously likely to debilitate the patient. From this second confinement she dated the symptoms for which she came to the hospital. Besides the symptoms characteristic of prolapsus ovarii, she had those which commonly go with yielding of the pelvic floor: a feeling of "bearing-down" and irritability of the bladder. There was chronic vaginal catarrh, by which relaxation and yielding of the walls of that canal was favoured. Her main symptoms were, as in the other cases, pain in intercourse and in defæcation, both pains

(a) In his work on Dysmenorrhœa, published since this paper was written, I find that Dr. Heywood Smith states that constipation is "a fruitful source of dysmenorrhœa" (page 111).

being said to resemble one another, and being described as lasting nearly an hour, and being accompanied with nausea and faintness. There was, as is usual when dyschezia is a prominent symptom, constipation; and to the loaded state of the large bowel are to be attributed the flatulence and the headache of which the patient complained. The relief afforded by treatment was in this case, as in the others, practically complete: the dyschezia was removed by freely opening the bowels; and when the support of a thick elastic ring was given to the tender part, the dyspareunia became "nothing to speak of."

(To be continued.)

RARE ACCIDENTS.

Reported by Mr. CHARLES McIVHOR GOYDER,
Senior House-Surgeon to the Newcastle-on-Tyne Infirmary.

I SHOULD be unwilling to publish these few isolated cases of curious injury if by so doing no useful purpose would be served. I think, however, that if a rare accident is recorded in such a manner as to show its mode of production, the appearances after the injury, and the result of treatment, the case may usefully and instructively add to the number of recorded instances of such injury.

Compound Comminuted Fracture of the Astragalus without Fracture of Malleoli—Recovery with Movable Joint.

James A., aged forty, master of a tug-boat, a man weighing upwards of fifteen stones, was admitted into the Newcastle-on-Tyne Infirmary, under Mr. Russel's care, February 5, 1877, suffering from injury to right foot.

Two hours before admission the patient attempted to step from the rail of his boat to the deck below, a distance of two feet. Having placed his right foot upon the link of a cable chain lying on the deck, he threw the whole weight of his body on to the right leg, when the foot suddenly slipped from the chain to the deck, producing the injury. The patient was a healthy man, and had never suffered from syphilis or rheumatism, but had taken large quantities of whisky daily.

Upon examination, the foot appeared inverted, the external malleolus projected about an inch through a transverse wound over the outer ankle. There was no fracture of the malleoli, but the lower end of the fibula was cleanly divested of all the structures attached to its tip. Upon introducing a finger into the wound, two small chips of bone came away, cancellous in structure and covered in part by a compact layer; a great many smaller fragments were removed from the ankle-joint, when the astragalus was found to be almost completely broken up into comminuted fragments. There was no bleeding, and the foot in other respects was quite natural in appearance. The case was treated antiseptically and placed upon a back-splint with foot-piece, and two side splints.

The patient did well up to April 5, when he got an attack of phlegmonous erysipelas. An abscess formed, which travelled up the sheath of the peronei muscles, and was opened; after which the wound quickly healed, and the patient became an out-patient on May 17, his leg and foot being placed in an immovable bandage. He was discharged cured on June 30, 1877.

Condition Four and a Half Years after.—I saw this patient to-day (August 24). He follows his employment, and walks without any aid. The right leg is shorter than the left, but not sufficiently so to make him halt in his walk. There is good movement at the ankle-joint, and the scar of the wound over the external malleolus, together with that of the opening made into the abscess, are the only remaining marks of the injury. He cannot bear his whole weight on the fore part of the foot, and in walking plants the whole surface of his foot on the ground at once. A ground plan of his feet shows that the right foot is one-fourth of an inch shorter than the left—a fact which he tells me his shoemaker has found out since the injury; the breadth of the sole also is markedly less on the right side, owing to atrophy of the plantar muscles.

Remarks.—This accident results from the application of a crushing force to the upper surface of the astragalus. The inversion of the foot was apparent, and resulted from the projection of the external malleolus through the wound.

The strange part of the case is the fact that there was no fracture of the malleoli whatever, and that the patient recovered with a movable ankle-joint. Mr. Bryant ("Practice of Surgery," second edition, vol. ii., page 416) mentions an exactly similar case, "in which the bone was crushed into fragments, and extruded from below the external malleolus," and in which a good recovery was made. Sir Astley Cooper ("Dislocations and Fractures into Joints," page 331) describes a case under Mr. Liston's care, which died of pyæmia. Mr. Erichsen ("Science and Art of Surgery") does not mention compound fracture of this bone specially. Gross ("System of Surgery"), Hancock ("Surgery of Foot and Ankle-Joint"), Holmes ("System of Surgery"), and Miller ("System of Surgery") do not mention the accident.

Depressed Fracture of the Malar Bone without External Wound—Recovery.

W. N., aged twenty-three, admitted September 29, 1879, under Dr. Luke Armstrong, complaining of an injury to the face. He states that, whilst intoxicated, he fell flat upon the kerbstone, striking the right cheek.

Upon examination, there was a large blood-tumour over the right malar region, the skin covering it being deep red in colour, contused, abraded, and ecchymosed. There was, however, no external wound. The right eyeball was very prominent and the eyelids œdematous; there was no concussion of the brain. When, by the aid of ice and cold lotions, the blood-tumour was dispersed and the eyelids were of their normal size, the true nature of the injury was apparent. There was marked flattening over the right malar bone—the finger, travelling down the external angular process of the frontal, reached a hollow where naturally the prominent malar bone should be. From this hollow, by a gentle slope, the finger reached the zygoma behind and the upper jaw below. The malar bone could be felt firmly fixed in its new position, pushing the contents of the orbit forwards and from the outer wall. The sight was good; the pupils equal, susceptible to light; the fundus oculi showed no injury or venous engorgement; the muscles of the right eyeball were acting.

Three weeks after, when the man was discharged, the exophthalmos persisted, and the depression in the right cheek gave a peculiar appearance to the man's face.

Condition Twenty-three Months after Accident.—I saw this man to-day (August 23). The right eyeball is not now at all prominent, and although it is easy to find that the malar bone is somewhat depressed, yet there is very little deformity remaining. Patient is in good health and follows his employment. I am indebted to Drs. Wicks and Wear (the latter of whom sent the case in after the accident) for the opportunity of seeing the patient again.

Remarks.—It seems remarkable that a force sufficient to depress and impact the malar bone—one of the buttresses of the skull—can be exerted directly, without the skin covering it being broken; and it appears essential that the surface producing the injury should be smooth. This accident is described by Miller ("System of Surgery," vol. ii., page 764) under the head of "fracture of the malar bone and zygoma." Gross ("System of Surgery," vol. i., page 948) says this fracture is very uncommon, always produced by direct violence, and invariably attended with severe contusion. Mr. Erichsen ("Science and Art of Surgery," seventh edition, vol. i., page 396) states that a fracture of the malar bone is usually accompanied by external wound. The accident is not described by Holmes ("System of Surgery"), except as a complication of fractured jaw. I regret that I have not access just now to the works of Hamilton or R. W. Smith.

Dislocation Upwards of the Scaphoid Bone of the Tarsus.

Patrick C., aged thirty-one, labourer, was admitted into the Percy ward, under Dr. Luke Armstrong's care, on December 20, 1880, having injured his right foot.

He stated that whilst walking across an inn-yard in the darkness he mistook his way, and fell down the open trap of a beer cellar, a distance of seven or eight feet, alighting on his toes and the forepart of his right foot. He felt something give way at this moment, and could not place his foot on the ground without extreme pain afterwards. The patient was a strong, healthy man, well developed, and free from rickets. The right foot was partially extended at the ankle-joint, and its inner border was somewhat short. Upon the dorsum, in a situation corresponding to the scaphoid bone, was a marked prominence, wider from side to side than from before backwards, with edges well defined, but covered by upraised tendons, etc., its anterior margin being on a line laterally with the proximal end of the fifth metatarsal bone on the outer side, and with the proximal end of the internal cuneiform on the inner side. There was a very noticeable arching of the sole of the foot, and flexion at the ankle-joint caused great pain.

Under chloroform, the foot was extended and abducted, the toes being bent down, when the displaced bone slipped into its normal position with a jerk.

There was very little inflammation following the accident; no difficulty was experienced in retaining the bone in its position, and he was discharged cured five weeks after the accident.

Remarks.—The case is of interest from its rarity. Mr. Erichsen ("Science and Art of Surgery," seventh edition, vol. i., page 517) mentions the accident. Mr. Bryant ("Practice of Surgery," second edition, vol. ii., page 355) describes a case of dislocation inwards under Mr. Cock's care. Hancock ("Surgery of Foot and Ankle-Joint," 1873, pages 435 and 436) makes no mention of simple dislocation of the scaphoid alone, although he relates a case of compound dislocation which recovered under Mr. Wheelhouse, of Leeds, and two cases of dislocation of the scaphoid and cuneiform together. Gross ("System of Surgery," edition 1872, vol. ii., page 80) relates a case of dislocation of scaphoid and cuboid from astragalus and os calcis, but no case of scaphoid alone. Holmes ("System of Surgery") does not mention the accident.

P.S.—I wish to express my thanks to Mr. Russel and to Dr. Luke Armstrong for their kind permission to publish the above cases.

GUY'S HOSPITAL: PRIZE LIST.—The medallists and prizemen for the session 1880-81 are as follow:—Treasurer's Gold Medal for Surgery—Lockhart Edward Walker Stephens, Emsworth. Gurney Hoare Prize—Edwin A. Starling. Beaney Prize—Edwin A. Starling, St. Leonards-on-Sea. Michael Harris Prize—Albert Martin, Wellington, New Zealand. Third Year's Students—Thomas Carr, Brixton, first prize, £35; William Thomas Frederick Davies, Swansea, second prize, £20; Walter Thomas Harris, Ipplepen, Devon, certificate; John Oscroft Littlewood, Ashfield, certificate; John Henry Booth, Chesterfield, certificate. Second Year's Students—Albert Martin, Wellington, New Zealand, first prize, £25; Arthur Ernest Larking, London, second prize, £10; Francis Heatherley, London, certificate; John Herbert Hawkins Manley, West Bromwich, certificate; Thomas Hugh Miller, Virginia, certificate; Allan Glaisyer Minns, Thetford, Norfolk, certificate. First Year's Students—George Elliott Caldwell Anderson, Cape Town, first prize, £50; Reginald Maurice Henry Randall, Sydenham, second prize, £25; Alfred Herbert Tubby, Kennington, certificate; Ernest Willmer Phillips, Brighton, certificate; William Henry Bowes, Herne Bay, certificate. Open Scholarships in Arts—1880, Richard Moody Ward, Ashburton; 1881, Albert Edward White, Swansea. Open Scholarships in Science—1880, Henry Walter Pigeon, Clifton, Bristol; 1881, John Wychenford Washbourn, Gloucester.

A NEW FEBRIFUGE PREPARATION.—At the Government Cinchona Factory in British Sikkim, a new product, which claims to be an improvement on the cinchona febrifuge, is a "crystalline febrifuge." The peculiarity of this preparation is that it consists of the mixed sulphates of the crystallisable alkaloids only. By rejecting those that are not crystallisable it is expected that the nausea which sometimes follows the taking of the febrifuge will also be eliminated.

IMPURITY OF THE AIR OF PARIS.—According to M. Miquel, in the *Annuaire de l'Observatoire de Paris pour 1881*, a cubic metre of the external air contains upon the average 30,000 spores. This figure may be increased during the prevalence of the moist heats of summer to 200,000, and may be as low in winter as 1000 when the atmosphere is cold and calm and has been recently traversed by snow or rain. In the park of Montsouris the air is found to be five or six times as pure as in the centre of Paris, and the atmosphere of the wards of the best kept hospitals is five or six times more impure than the humid atmosphere of the sewers!—*Lyon Méd.*, September 18.

REPORTS OF HOSPITAL PRACTICE

IN

MEDICINE AND SURGERY.

EAST LONDON HOSPITAL FOR CHILDREN.

TWO CASES OF TRACHEOTOMY IN YOUNG CHILDREN.

(Under the care of Dr. HORATIO DONKIN.)

[For these notes we are indebted to Mr. J. SCOTT BATTAMS, Resident Medical Officer.]

Case 1.—Gastro-intestinal Catarrh—Membranous Laryngitis —Tracheotomy—Death—Autopsy.

THOMAS P., aged ten months, was admitted into Princess Mary ward on July 18, 1881, under the care of Dr. Donkin, for gastro-intestinal catarrh.

Previous History.—Mother healthy; its father is delicate—he suffers from cough. It is one of ten children, eight of which are living. One died of "wasting and water on the brain," the other of "paralysis on one side and blindness." The mother has had one miscarriage; no history of syphilis. The child was healthy and plump when born. It was fed on condensed milk and bread. It has not been thriving for two months, during which time it has suffered on and off with diarrhœa and offensive stools: "all its food has seemed to run through it." It had cried a good deal, and has drawn up its legs as if in pain. For the past fortnight its mouth has been sore and ulcerated, and it has vomited its food.

Present Condition.—Child very much wasted; it seems too weak to cry, and only moans. It coughs a little. It has four teeth. Its skin is inelastic and hangs in folds. On examining the chest, some high-pitched resonance is found in the upper half of the right lung; no other physical signs.

July 28.—The child has improved somewhat on suitable food and treatment.

29th.—About 9 a.m. the child's breathing was noticed to be very hurried, although it was reported to have taken its breakfast apparently well a short time previously. The alæ nasi were dilating; respirations 60; temperature 103°, as against 99·4° Fahr. on the preceding evening. There was sinking-in of the epigastrium and lateral parts of the chest with each inspiration. There was no dulness on percussion; on auscultation no air could be heard entering the lungs. The child has had a cough more or less throughout, but this morning it was decidedly "croupy" in character. With a view to relieve any spasm which might exist, a mustard bath was ordered, and four grains each of chloral and bromide of potassium were given. No improvement having resulted in the next hour or so, an emetic of sulphate of zinc was administered, after which the child vomited, but was not relieved. There was no struggling for breath, as in cases of so-called croup coming on suddenly, for the breathing was hurried rather than laboured. There was a general suffusion of the face, with fulness of the veins at the root of the neck. Early in the afternoon, Dr. Donkin saw the child, and after another emetic, which failed to bring about any relief, he requested Mr. Parker to see the child with a view to tracheotomy.

The operation was performed accordingly, after which the respirations fell from 60 to 38 per minute. One small bit of membrane was got up by means of the feather, together with a quantity of thick tenacious mucus. The trachea was found to be remarkably small, hardly admitting the smallest canula. The child seemed relieved; but its temperature remained high, and the respirations soon again increased in frequency.

30th.—The temperature remained high (103°). At 10 a.m., pulse 160; respirations 52 to 60 per minute. The tube was taken out and changed. The tube found blackened in one or two places; feathers were passed down, and the trachea cleansed with a weak solution of potash. No membrane was got up. Bowels had acted four times in the twenty-four hours. Milk diet and beef-tea, with a little brandy, were ordered as diet. Temperature 103·2° at 6 p.m.

31st.—The child seemed worse. Temperature 103·8° at

11 a.m. There was very little secretion from the trachea; the wound looked dry and unwholesome; the tube on removal was found blackened. The child's condition now being very bad, one-sixteenth of a grain of pilocarpine was injected subcutaneously. This did not produce much salivation, but the child sweated rather freely.

August 1.—Died at 2 a.m.; shortly before which he was convulsed. The cyanosis was never very marked.

Autopsy.—Larynx, trachea, and lungs removed *en masse.* The mucous membrane of the larynx and trachea was much injected throughout; there was no membrane. In the primary subdivisions of the left bronchus there was a tough false membrane, almost occluding them. The lower lobe of the left lung was livid red, in places almost black, dense as liver-substance, quite airless, and sinking at once in water. On squeezing it, black blood issued from the vessels, and thread-like pieces of membrane from all the air-tubes. The lower lobe of the right lung and lower part of the middle lobe were airless, sinking at once in water. They were full of frothy fluid, not the tenacious secretion as in the left lung. There was no membrane in the right main bronchi. There was recent pleurisy on the left side ; about three ounces of blood-stained serum were found in the pleural cavity. To a less extent also there was pleurisy on the right side. The diaphragm was adherent to both lungs by recent lymph. The other organs presented no special points of interest.

Case 2.—Apparently Sudden Onset of Dyspnœa—Tracheotomy —Expulsion of Membrane—Death—Autopsy.

Elizabeth G., aged eleven months, admitted into Enfield ward, under the care of Dr. Donkin, September 30, 1881, at 10 p.m. It had just been seen by a doctor, who advised it to be brought at once, "as it might require an operation."

Previous History.—The mother (from whom it was very difficult to get any exact information) stated that the child had had a cough for a week or more, which had been worse for the past two days. It had seemed pretty well until one o'clock of this day, at which hour its breathing was noticed to be "very noisy and frequent." Its cough now had a "barking" character about it. The child was a well-developed girl, well nourished, and seemed to have been well cared for ; her limbs were large and firm.

Condition on Admission.—The child appeared exceedingly well-nourished and large for its age. Its face was flushed. Temperature 101° Fahr.; pulse 140 ; respirations 40, stridulous, chiefly noticeable during inspiration. The lower ribs sank in with each inspiration, and there was great recession of the epigastric region, as also of the supra-sternal notch. The child cried with a hoarse, whispering voice. On examining the pharynx, it was found to be congested and swollen, as were the tonsils. No membrane could be seen anywhere. There were some enlarged glands at the angles of the jaws. The lungs, on percussion, appeared normal, but on auscultation, dry sibilant rhonchi were heard over the lower and back portions. A mustard bath was ordered at once, and an emetic of ipecacuanha ; the child vomited some mucus and some curdled milk. On being put to bed in the usual steam tent she seemed better, and slept for some time.

October 1.—5.30 a.m.: Mr. Battams was called up to see the child, and found the dyspnœa much worse. Expiration as well as inspiration was laboured and prolonged ; face pale; lips bluish. Temperature 100° Fahr.; pulse very small, it seemed to be arrested by each inspiratory effort. The recession of the soft parts of the chest even more marked. There was some convulsive jerking of the arms and body, and every now and then she tried to raise herself, as if for breath. Tracheotomy was therefore at once performed. Before the tube was inserted the trachea was wiped out with feathers and a solution of potash, and a large piece of tough white membrane, an inch and a half long, was withdrawn, and some smaller pieces were coughed up. At 8 a.m., respirations 54; pulse 140; temperature 99° Fahr. 12 noon: Child seemed comfortable. It had taken its food well. The skin was dry and burning hot. 11.30 p.m.: Several pieces of membrane had been expectorated, or brought up with the feather. The breathing generally seemed easier and moist.

2nd.—Child looks well, is cheerful and plays, takes food well. Some dryish tenacious mucus has been expectorated. Temperature 101·6° Fahr. at 11 p.m.

3rd.—Breathing easy and quiet. A good deal of mucus was expectorated from the trachea ; wound rather inflamed and infiltrated. Was seen by Mr. Parker, who removed the tube and cleared out the trachea with sponge and a feather. The tube was found to be blackened. Temperature at 10 a.m. 99·4°, evening 101·6° Fahr.

5th.—The child's general condition was hardly so favourable, although it was difficult to specify why or how. It took food, seemed cheerful and played, but was extremely pale. Bowels acted twice. Temperature at 6 p.m. 102°. There was a resonant percussion-note all over the chest.

6th.—Towards 2 p.m. the breathing became more hurried, respirations 60, pulse 120, temperature 99·8°. There was no secretion from the trachea. For a day or two the amount of secretion had diminished, although steam had been kept up, and a solution of potash had been sprayed over the trachea from time to time. The exterior wound was unhealthy, and the soft tissues of the neck were swollen and rather infiltrated. The tube when removed was found much blackened. The symptoms all became aggravated towards night.

7th.—At 4 a.m. the child died, evidently from lung-collapse.

Autopsy, twelve hours after Death.—There was a good layer of adipose tissue all over the body. The tongue, larynx and pharynx, trachea, and lungs were removed together. The mucous membrane of the larynx and trachea was greatly inflamed and swollen. There were large patches of membrane in both main bronchi, which extended far down into the lungs, preserving its firm membraniform character. The thymus was very large : it reached quite up to the isthmus of the thyroid, and must have been seen in the tracheotomy wound. The lungs themselves, except on their surfaces and along their margins, were inflamed and airless ; the greater part of them when cut in pieces sank in water. There was no pleurisy. The heart extended over to the right of the mid-sternal line ; the right side was distended with blood, so that the right ventricle contributed to form the apex ; the left side was firmly contracted and empty. The liver weighed fourteen ounces ; it extended below the ribs for at least three fingers' breadth; its substance was fatty. Spleen, kidneys, and other abdominal viscera quite normal. Bladder empty. Head not opened. There were a few spots of membrane on the under surface of the epiglottis, but none in the pharynx elsewhere.

Remarks (by Mr. Parker).—These two cases presented remarkable contrasts as regards the children—the one was poor, thin, and weakly ; the other was apparently strong and robust ; and the former lived two days, the latter five days. In the first case there had been gastro-intestinal catarrh for some time before the laryngitis became manifest ; while, in the second, the child appears to have been running about until within a few hours of the onset of the disease. In neither of the cases, however, was there any cyanosis, or that struggling for breath which characterises disease commencing primarily in the larynx ; yet we never detected any pharyngeal mischief in either. On the contrary, in both cases, the respiration throughout was characterised by its frequency and shallowness rather than by any increased effort. In the first case the frequency of the respiration (which always betokens lung-complication) led me to hesitate as to the desirability of tracheotomising the child. After the operation, however, some temporary relief was obtained. The trachea proved to be exceedingly small, not much larger than a good-sized goose-quill, and we were obliged to dispense with the double tube and only use the inner and small one of our smallest size. The whole track of the mucous membrane of the larynx was in a catarrhal condition, and this, owing to the small size of the tube, doubtless greatly increased the difficulty of breathing. But it cannot be doubted that the lungs were almost *hors de combat* at the time of the operation, for within two or three hours the respirations varied from 52 to 60 per minute. The lungs in both cases were solid in their interior, while on their surfaces and along their margins they were highly emphysematous. This emphysematous condition accounts for the resonance on percussion—a point which is apt to mislead ; while auscultation, owing to the conduction of loud tracheal gurgling from the tracheotomy-tube, renders it difficult to rightly gauge the lung-condition within the chest. In the former of the two cases, pilocarpin was tried, but not very thoroughly ; the post-mortem conditions, however, do not justify any hope that it could have had any beneficial effect.

TERMS OF SUBSCRIPTION.
(Free by post.)

British Islands	Twelve Months	.	£1 8 0
,, ,, ...	Six ,,	.	0 14 0
The Colonies and the United } States of America . . . }	Twelve ,,	.	1 10 0
,, ,, ,, . .	Six ,,	.	0 15 0
India ,, ...	Twelve ,,	.	1 10 0
,, (viâ Brindisi)	,, ,,	.	1 15 0
,, ,, ...	Six ,,	.	0 15 0
,, (viâ Brindisi)	,, ,,	.	0 17 6

Foreign Subscribers are requested to inform the Publishers of any remittance made through the agency of the Post-office.

Single Copies of the Journal can be obtained of all Booksellers and Newsmen, price Sixpence.

Cheques or Post-office Orders should be made payable to Mr. JAMES LUCAS, 11, New Burlington-street, W.

TERMS FOR ADVERTISEMENTS.

Seven lines (70 words) . .	.	£0	4 6
Each additional line (10 words)	.	. 0	0 6
Half-column, or quarter-page .	.	. 1	5 0
Whole column, or half-page .	.	. 2	10 0
Whole page	.	. 5	0 0

Births, Marriages, and Deaths are inserted Free of Charge.

THE MEDICAL TIMES AND GAZETTE *is published on Friday morning: Advertisements must therefore reach the Publishing Office not later than One o'clock on Thursday.*

Medical Times and Gazette.

SATURDAY, OCTOBER 15, 1881.

SOMETHING MORE ON THE INTRODUCTORIES.

AMONG the Introductories not referred to last week were two of some interest, as coming from laymen. One of these was perhaps, in the strict sense, no Introductory at all, coming as it did after the regular address; but the position of the speaker, Lord Derby, was such as to give his words a weight which could not fail in a very great measure to overshadow what had been said before. With regard to Lord Derby's remarks, they are, like most others made by him, all very true, but contain nothing very new. Their real value lies in the kindliness which they carry with them, and the appreciation of the work of medical men on the part of such a prominent man as Lord Derby. He dwelt, as will be seen by the report given elsewhere, on the peculiar advantages which accrue from the study and practice of medicine to the student himself. For he endeavoured to show that the satisfaction derived from the study of our profession was greater than that to be got from pure science or from classical knowledge, inasmuch as we have always a clear end in view, and that end cannot be other than good.

"Your privilege," he said, "the privilege of your chosen employment, is—and a high and enviable one I call it—that you can largely satisfy the intellectual impulse to know and to discover on the one hand, while on the other you can equally, in the ordinary routine of your duty, do useful service to your fellow-men. The ultimate mystery of existence can never be solved, but on the conditions of existence every successive generation of inquirers throws clearer and clearer light; and in that line of research, never exhausted nor capable of being exhausted, there is space enough for the highest ambition, and interest enough to compensate for much of mere drudgery and dulness. But there is another and perhaps a more practical aspect in which the profession of which we speak may be regarded. Medical science applies itself more directly than any other to the promotion of human well-being and the prevention of human suffering."

Of this kind of beneficial labour there are, he said, two varieties—the one public and the other private; the one concerning the health of the community at large, the other that of the unit, the individual, or the family. As regards the former, Lord Derby pointed out that on it depended the welfare and supremacy of the race, but he was also careful to show that here the medical man had a difficult position to maintain— "when money is on one side and health on the other, and when plain speech may give serious offence in quarters where offence is dangerous." Perhaps he would not have been wrong here to give a word of warning which would apply better to the public officer than it does to the practitioner. This advice was to avoid needless pugnacity and antagonism; for more harm has been done by these troublesome characteristics to the cause of sanitary science than by all the rest of the opposing forces put together. Nor should these other words be neglected: "For the great office, as I most seriously call it, of a trusted medical adviser there is wanting more than fine science, though that must necessarily be the basis; he must have tact, judgment, firmness in opinion, courtesy and gentleness in expression."

But, alas for many of us, he has to add that in all departments of life much gratuitous work is done. "But I assert," he said, "with some confidence that the absolutely gratuitous assistance given by the medical profession to those who are unable to pay for it far exceeds that which is bestowed or demanded in any other line of life; and it is not less creditable to those who give it because custom has in great measure caused it to be expected as a matter of course. Whether it is equally creditable to the public that it should be expected to the extent it is, is a different question, into which I need not now enter."

So much for Lord Derby. Let us turn now to what Sir John Lubbock had to say at King's College. One idea he dwelt on in the earlier part of his discourse has been raised over and over again, but as now brought forward by one powerful to aid it, might seem to have a chance of being realised. This was the institution of special courses of lectures for students by the University of London. Three chief difficulties have always stood in the way of any such scheme—one is the intense mutual jealousy of the various teaching and examining bodies in London; another, the great distances which separate nearly all from any central point; and thirdly, and not least important, the inertia of the student, and his unwillingness to take up anything which will not pay when examination time comes round. One has only to look at the mode in which the various lectures at the Colleges, and even at the University, are regarded, to have these truths thrust in upon them. Moreover, it is not to be denied that the scanty time allowed to the student to gather up the fragments of such an enormous variety of subjects as he is now expected to be familiar with, give him but little time to attend to anything which is not absolutely needful. Yet we can easily conceive a course of lectures which would do more to widen the breadth of the student's view and strengthen the grasp of his mind, than any amount of the grinding and cramming so much in vogue.

Of the rest of Sir John Lubbock's address, little need be said. It speaks for itself; though were he as familiar with students' ways as we are, he would hardly have thought it necessary to warn them against over-work or advise them to take plenty of holidays. At all events, Mr. Bond, at Westminster, took care to speak against that over-indulgence in athletic sports—one form of holiday-making which is far too much thought of at the present time.

Something was said of Dr. Poore's lecture at University College last week, and this week we publish its most important portion, with regard to which we would venture on a few additional observations, partly because we believe in the importance of the subject-matter, partly because, whilst in certain respects holding with Dr. Poore, we are also bound in some degree to dissent from him.

Dr. Poore's remarks on medical language may, in one way, be said to be founded on the Dictionary now issuing by the New Sydenham Society, with its cumbersome form, and what must be its unwieldy bulk, chokeful of the vilest hybrid terms that could well be imagined. And it is not uninteresting to notice that a very great number of these terms have been elaborated by men who know little Latin and less Greek. They can be compared to nothing save to those fearful names invented by tradesmen to stupefy their customers or to entice them into purchasing a very ordinary article concealed under a very uncommon name.

Dr. Poore is very strong on the subject of using our mother-tongue in medicine, as in every-day life; and whilst in this we heartily concur, good and appropriate scientific terms have their value, provided they are not used to conceal a want of knowledge which outwardly they seem to carry with them. For one thing, they often enable us to avoid long and roundabout descriptions by indicating with a single word the thing described. Dr. Poore cites the example of Germany in compounding all scientific terms from the vernacular, but we should say that this is an example which ought to deter rather than to encourage our use of English expressions. There is, indeed, no greater drawback to the study of German than this cumbrous mode of framing scientific terms. They repel the student, and, though easy enough to one who has mastered scientific German, they are quite as much a mystery to the commonalty as are those expressive terms, "Cryptoconchoid siphonostomata," or another, which used to be the terror of our earlier days, "methyl-ethylamylophenylammonium." These are words actually in use, and not invented for the occasion, as that one of Dr. Warren's, which Dr. Poore cites—which, by the way, was a dye, and not a pomade, to which the term would be inapplicable. Nevertheless, we say that the German system is equally objectionable, and that it constitutes a real barrier to the study of German which is not to be found in any other language with which most people are acquainted. There is an example which Dr. Poore unconsciously gives of the proper use of scientific terms. A patient comes, complaining "that he has lost power on one side of his body." We say he has "hemiplegia." True, this is no additional knowledge—it is only expressing the same thing, with perhaps something more, in Greek; but it is at least shorter to write and less roundabout to pronounce than is the other mode of expression. The mischief lies when either form of words is taken as real knowledge, and not as a symbol only.

Elsewhere Dr. Poore complains that certain common words are "considered 'vulgar,' whatever that may mean." Now here again we must join issue with Dr. Poore. Certainly there are plenty of good English words to which there can be no possible objection, but there are others which, from whatever cause—perhaps their very commonness, i.e., vulgarity—do produce a feeling of repugnance to their use on the part of the speaker or writer, as well as on the part of the listener. The common names of many parts of the body belong to this category, especially, let us say, those relating to the organs of generation and their diseases. A good example we saw the other day in a volume of hospital reports, where, in all the cases of stricture, it was noted whether the patient had had "clap." The word is expressive enough, but its use would be resented by many. And we must remember that nowadays, in the wards of most hospitals, our teaching must be carried on in the presence of ladies, to whom certain forms of expression could not fail to be distressing. Still further, if there is a lesson to be inculcated in the minds of students

at the bedside, it is that of gentleness and consideration for the feelings of others, whether sick or well.

Thus, whilst strongly upholding and daily practising the use of plain and simple language, we must maintain that good scientific terms have their uses, though they may be readily abused; and that there are limits beyond which plain English cannot be carried with advantage either to oneself or to others with whom we have to do.

THE GERM THEORY AT THE SOCIAL SCIENCE CONGRESS.

THERE is nothing upon which the mind dwells with more real satisfaction than the spectacle of some hard-won discovery, the fruit of much uncheered thought and much unpaid labour, taking its place decisively among the familiar truths and household doctrines of mankind. It is only the very highest achievements of the mind, the very masterstrokes of genius, that are destined to enjoy that wide currency. There is no more grateful acknowledgment of their merits than that they are taken up and understood by the world at large; and if we were to name in one word the quality which enables them to pass into the common and every-day understanding of men, we should say that it is their simplicity. The grandest discoveries are those that can be stated in the simplest terms; and they are, for that reason, those that most readily find currency in men's minds. This wise world of ours is mainly right; and the popular, though not always speedy, adoption of a new truth is at once the most valuable, as it is the most grateful, tribute that the philosopher receives. But the public taste for an uncomplicated formula is so strong that it is sometimes misled by appearances. While the best discoveries of science are the simplest, there are other doctrines which are simple only because they are superficial. Nothing can be simpler, in medical theory, than that the ailments of the body are well-defined and clean-cut entities, for each of which there is an appointed and appropriate specific remedy. It cannot be doubted that the homœopathic medicine-chest and the homœopathic theory are things that, if we may use a vulgarism, have "fetched" the public not a little, more especially in those new countries where the sentiment of equality tends to level the differences in technical knowledge between the doctor and his patient. Those of us who know something of the complex diseased states which the deadhouse reveals are apt to smile when we see the symptomatologist (or the homœopath) resorting to his remedies with a light heart. The homœopathic theory is too simple by half. Another theory which has entered readily and deeply into the public mind is based on the view that certain diseases are due to the lodgment in the body of specific micro-organisms. Far be it from us even to suggest that the specific-germ theory is to pathology what the homœopathic theory is to practice. It is vouched for by too many respectable and honoured names to be made the subject of so compromising a comparison. But our friends, the germ-theorists, will forgive us if we take this opportunity of pointing out that the public is being immensely fetched (to use the word again) by the simple and attractive notion of numerous common diseases being caused by aërial swarms of organisms which have, as it were, declared war against mankind. The members of the Social Science Congress who listened to Dr. Cameron, M.P., at Dublin the other day, probably know little or nothing of the complexities of morbid anatomy and pathology. The explanation of disease held up to them had the signal merit of simplicity, and they may be pardoned if they do not inquire too closely whether the simplicity is of the right sort. No one would wish to say that the specific-germ theory of disease is a pathological nostrum. But it is only too evident, from the prelude and tone of Dr. Cameron's address, that it may be made to strut and swagger in the garb of that objectionable thing.

Dr. Cameron, speaking from the chair of the Public Health Section of the Congress, began with the following general observations, which we take leave here and there to italicise. "There never has been," he said, "a period since the days of Æsculapius, during which so much has been accomplished to entitle medicine to take a place among the exact sciences as within *the last ten or fifteen years.* Up to that period we knew diseases *only as groups of effects.* Of their causes we had no certain knowledge. As the methods of research adopted became *stricter and more systematic,* a mass of information was accumulated, pointing generally in one direction, and enabling more accurate hypotheses to be framed "—the germ theory, of course, the grand solution of all our difficulties, the last word in the theory and therapeutic indications of disease. Dr. Cameron is understood to have for a good many years ceased to observe the concrete occurrences of disease, and he has presumably failed to keep pace with the advances in abstract theory. On the other hand, if report speaks truly, he has had, as a journalist, the opportunity of knowing the responsibility that attaches to public writing and to public speaking. We have to express our regret that Dr. Cameron should have thought fit, before a lay audience, to read so unhesitatingly the lesson of certain experiments, which certainly have their significance, although the wisest heads in the profession are for the time at a loss to say what precisely that significance is.

The seven years' keeping, which Horace recommended for poetry, is perhaps not too long a term of probation for startling discoveries in pathology. The specific germ of hydrophobia has enjoyed a scientific reputation of only two or three months; and another minute organism, on which Dr. Cameron lays much stress, and which has the peculiar property of resisting a very high temperature, the specific germ of tubercle, has been known (in France at least) for only a few weeks. Time will try the specific-germ theory, as it tries all things; and that theory will receive an honoured place in the body of pathological doctrine if it is found to deserve it. But at the present moment it is only right that we should keep in mind the past achievements of pathology. The "last ten or fifteen years" may or may not stand out boldly in the history of medicine as the golden time when the specific germs of disease were sought for and found; but, at any rate, pathology has a past, and a present, and a future altogether independent of that or any other single theory. In the house of disease, if one may so say, there are many mansions. If the truth were known, the "stricter and more systematic methods of research," which Dr. Cameron claimed for the germ-theorists, are not by any means their exclusive prerogative. Up to ten or fifteen years ago, it seems, we knew diseases only as groups of effects; of their causes we had no certain knowledge. Dr. Cameron is unconsciously a dualist of the deepest dye. He will separate the cause from the effect, and, like a true man of business, he will go straight for the cause. There are circumstances, however, in which the tortoise outruns the hare. Pathology has steadily advanced on the lines laid down by Morgagni more than a century ago; it is still *de sedibus* and *de causis morborum* that the question arises, and not more about the causes of disease than about its seats. Those who are patiently working at the problems of disease in the old morphological and in the newer physiological directions need not be discouraged if their work is temporarily thrown into the shade by the more glittering achievements of the "last ten or

fifteen years." The desire on the part of the public to isolate the very causes of disease, and to stamp them out, does credit to its goodness of heart. But it is based upon an intellectual conception of disease which is curiously inadequate to the complexities of the case.

THE WEEK.

TOPICS OF THE DAY.

BETWEEN unqualified medical practitioners and uncertificated midwives the lower classes of the community would appear to be in bad case. We last week alluded to an inquest at the East-end of London which terminated with a warning from the coroner addressed to the midwife who appeared before him as a witness. We have now to record a somewhat similar case. Mr. George Collier opened an inquiry in Banner-street, St. Luke's, touching the death of an infant who only lived fourteen hours. The father deposed that his wife was attended in her confinement by a midwife whom he believed to be certificated; a nurse was also engaged, and he gave authority for calling in a medical man should the services of one be required. The nurse, in evidence, stated that after the child was born the midwife told her it could not possibly live, and recommended that she should go and consult a doctor about it. Witness went to Dr. Yarrow's surgery, and explained to that gentleman the condition of the child, but did not ask him to come and see it. Dr. Yarrow offered some suggestions as to its treatment, which were adopted, but it ultimately died, and she then went to his house to ask him to give a certificate as to the cause of death, and this he, of course, declined to do. Dr. G. E. Yarrow, of Old-street, St. Luke's, said that he saw the child after it was dead, when he refused to give a certificate: he had since examined the body, and found the cause of death to have been convulsions; moreover, the lungs did not appear to have been properly inflated. Had a medical man been called in when the child was born, in all probability it would have lived; and he considered there was great neglect on the part of the midwife in not sending for medical assistance. The Coroner remarked that it had not been proved to his satisfaction that the midwife was properly certificated, but, whether or not, she had been guilty of most reprehensible conduct in taking upon herself to say the child would not live, since the medical evidence had proved that if a doctor had been called in to see the child after it was born it would in all probability have been alive then. He was sorry to say the present case was not the only one which had been brought under his notice lately, and they were continually occurring; therefore the sooner a stop was put to the employment of these incompetent midwives, the better it would be for society. As the woman was not present in court, the inquiry was adjourned, in order to give her an opportunity of attending and offering an explanation of her conduct; and as in the end it was proved that she had strongly recommended the husband to send for a medical man, the blame was accordingly shifted to him.

Some heavy, but by no means too severe, sentences have recently been passed for the disgusting practice of exposing bad meat for sale. At Salford two butchers were charged with this offence. The borough meat inspector visited their premises, and in both shops found horseflesh dressed for sale, and beef which was so congested as to be unfit for human food. The animals had evidently died a natural death, and had not been slaughtered in a proper manner. Both these defendants were sent to prison for two months, without the option of a fine. A pork-pie manufacturer of Leicester was brought before the borough magistrates, charged with having on his premises no less than two tons and a half of hams, bacon, and beef which were unfit for the food of man. Dr. Johnstone, Medical Officer of Health for Leicester, and Dr. Malvey gave evidence as to the shocking condition of the meat, which, when chopped up for conversion into pies, was highly seasoned to conceal its condition. Dr. Johnstone further remarked that no human being would eat meat in such a condition as that examined by him, if he knew what he was about at the time. The defendant persisted that he had no wrong intention in the matter, but the Bench sentenced him to two months' imprisonment without hard labour, an appeal to the quarter sessions being allowed.

The owner of Nos. 2 and 4, Charles-street, Lisson-grove, was recently summoned by the Marylebone Vestry for allowing nuisances to exist on those premises to the danger of health. Mr. W. E. Greenwell, solicitor to the Marylebone Vestry, prosecuted, and stated that fourteen cases of typhus fever had already occurred in the street named. The houses were constantly under the notice of the Vestry, and proceedings were being taken under Torrens's Act. The surveyor had examined No. 4, and found under the flooring of one of the rooms of the basement sewage matter to the depth of five feet, and under the floor of the basement of No. 2 liquid sewage matter to the extent of two feet, due to defective sewerage. Though the two houses were reported by the Medical Officer of Health for the parish as unfit for habitation, they had several families in them, and persons were even living in the room adjoining that under which the sewage was found. Further evidence having been given, Mr. Cooke made an order that the two houses be cleared of the occupants at once, and that the offensive matter be removed within a week.

The Sanitary Commission of the Porte, with the consent of the Imperial Government, has wisely decided that, in consequence of the outbreak of cholera at Mecca, ships having on board pilgrims for the Mohammedan holy places shall not be cleared for the Red Sea ports. A Russian steamer from Odessa, arriving recently in the Golden Horn, was obliged to land a number of pilgrims before proceeding on her voyage. They will be sent back to Russia by another steamer. The Porte would seem to be ready to take all reasonable measures which the medical authorities may suggest to prevent the spread of the epidemic.

An extraordinary and important meeting of the Vestry of St. Marylebone has been held for the purpose of considering communications which had been addressed to them, with a view to secure co-operation in a determination to obtain a more adequate and cheaper fish-supply than is at present provided for the metropolis. Communications were read from Westminster, the Strand district, and other West-end and Northern local bodies, and also from Newington, Wandsworth, and other places on the southern side of the metropolis. The whole of them expressed an opinion that the monopoly of the fish and other markets should be at once taken away from the Corporation of London, and placed under the control of the Metropolitan Board of Works, or some representative body; and some suggested that, inasmuch as the large proportion of fish brought to London was by the railways, the London market should be as near the termini of the great railways as possible, and the space near King's Cross, which had been cleared by the Midland Railway Company for a potato market, was the most appropriate. The following resolution was eventually agreed to : "That the Vestry of St. Marylebone is of opinion that the Metropolitan Board of Works should be empowered by Act of Parliament to create or erect markets in such convenient positions as would offer to the inhabitants of the metropolis generally the best means of expeditiously obtaining an adequate supply

of fish." Meanwhile, the Special Committee of the Corporation of the City of London, to whom it was referred to select and report as to the sites suitable for a new fish market, the cost of erecting the necessary buildings thereon, and also as to the probable outlay involved in improving Billingsgate and its approaches, have received 100 plans and suggestions upon the subject of the reference. They have selected thirty plans from the number, and have commenced visiting the sites indicated in them. No time will be lost in prosecuting the matter, as the Corporation will have to arrive at some decision before Lord Mayor's-day if they intend to promote a Bill upon the subject of the fish-supply of the metropolis in the coming Parliamentary session.

A dangerous practice, which is perhaps only due to thoughtlessness, was exposed at a recent inquest held by Dr. Danford Thomas on the body of a little girl aged three years. The mother of the deceased, who resides in Clerkenwell, deposed that her daughter became very ill on Monday, the 26th ult., after eating some sweets, and she died on the following Wednesday. It was explained that in the description of sweets eaten by the deceased, certain packets were advertised to contain a farthing as an inducement to the children to buy them, and one of these had unfortunately come into the possession of the child, who had swallowed it. Dr. Smythe, of Colebrooke-row, Islington, who attended the child prior to her death, was of opinion that the sulphate of copper from a coin—probably a farthing—concealed in one of the sweets which the deceased ate, produced peritonitis or inflammation of the bowels, from which she died. During twelve months he had attended a dozen cases arising in a similar way, one of which nearly proved fatal. The Coroner thought the vendor of these dangerous mixtures should be cautioned not to sell any more of them. The jury returned a verdict in accordance with the medical evidence.

At the last meeting of the Bethnal-green Vestry the Clerk called attention to the deficiency of the water-supply in different parts of the parish. He instanced that for four days he had been unable to wash his hands at the Vestry offices, and said that the state of things was much worse in the houses of the poor. Several vestrymen testified to the non-supply of water in the different parts of the parish, and the Vestry Clerk further complained that letters which he had written to the water company on the subject had been disregarded. The Vestry finally instructed the Sanitary Committee to take immediate steps in the matter.

In accordance with the scheme propounded by Lady Strangford, classes for the instruction of soldiers' wives in elementary nursing are in course of formation at Eastney Barracks, Portsmouth, at Newport, at Sandhurst, at Taunton, and at Woolwich. The instructor is to be Mr. Crookshank, M.R.C.S.

CHANGE OF ADDRESS OF THE MEDICAL COUNCIL OFFICE.

It may not be out of place to call the attention of our numerous readers to the circumstance that, owing to the re-numbering of Oxford-street, the offices of the General Medical Council are now numbered 299, instead of 315, as formerly. With every wish to bow to the decision of constituted authorities, we cannot help thinking that the re-numbering of such an important thoroughfare as Oxford-street must have been productive of many hardships, and—what is more important—of great inconvenience to the public, who do not seem to realise the fact that it is better, in addressing a letter, to put no number at all than to insert a wrong one. In the former case the postman is bound to find the office or owner, provided always he lives in the street ; in the latter case he has only to leave it absolutely as directed.

THE VICTORIA CROSS.

THE Queen has been graciously pleased to signify her intention to confer the decoration of the Victoria Cross upon the undermentioned officer, whose claim has been submitted for Her Majesty's approval, for his conspicuous gallantry during the recent operations in South Africa (Basutoland):—Surgeon-Major Edmund Baron Hartley, Cape Mounted Riflemen, for conspicuous gallantry displayed by him in attending the wounded under fire at the unsuccessful attack on Moirosi's Mountain, in Basutoland, on June 5, 1879; and for having proceeded into the open ground under a heavy fire, and carried in his arms, from an exposed position, Corporal A. Jones, of the Cape Mounted Riflemen, who was wounded. While conducting him to a place of safety the corporal was again wounded. The Surgeon-Major then returned under the severe fire of the enemy in order to dress the wounds of other men of the storming party. It is not often that the medical profession is thus honoured. Dr. Hartley is a Devonshire man, and the eldest son of Dr. Hartley, of Warwick-square, S.W. After leaving St. George's Hospital in 1874, he proceeded to South Africa, with the idea of entering on private practice, but war soon broke out, and he was appointed Surgeon to the Cape Mounted Rifles. Subsequently he was made Principal Medical Officer of the Colonial Forces.

NAVAL MEDICAL SUPPLEMENTAL FUND.

AT the quarterly meeting of the directors of the Naval Medical Supplemental Fund, Dr. H. J. Domville, C.B., Inspector-General, in the chair, the sum of £75 was distributed among the several applicants.

LIVERPOOL MEDICAL INSTITUTION: OPENING OF THE SESSION.

THE present session of the Liverpool Medical Institution was opened on August 6, when over a hundred members attended the opening meeting. The introductory address was delivered by the President, Mr. Reginald Harrison, who, after the usual obituaries and references to current events, took for his subject the prevention of disease by ambulances. He showed how deficient all English cities were in having suitable conveyances for fractures, etc., and pointed out the evils that had arisen to the injured in consequence. He compared the state of affairs in Liverpool in this respect with what obtains in New York, and finally proposed the maintenance of similar ambulances in connexion with all the Liverpool hospitals to what he saw at the City of New York Hospital. This want was considered to be a very pressing and obvious one by the large audience, and Drs. Turnbull and Waters, in proposing and seconding a vote of thanks to Mr. Harrison, both expressed a hope that all those present would join in an endeavour to bring the subject to a practical issue. The rooms of the Medical Institute were tastefully decorated with flowers, and a very interesting collection of photographs of disease, surgical appliances, hardened brains, etc., the contributions of the members, was exhibited. The President exhibited several specimens of micro-photography sent to him by Dr. Woodward, of America.

MIDLAND MEDICAL SOCIETY.

AT the annual meeting of this Society, on October 5, the following gentlemen were elected to the offices of the Society:—*President*: Mr. John Manley. *Treasurer*: Mr. J. Farmar. *Secretaries*: Messrs. H. Eales and T. F. Chavasse. *Members of the Council*: Mr. J. F. West, Dr. Welch, Dr. Sawyer, and Mr. Garner. The inaugural address this year will be delivered on October 19, by T. Clifford Allbutt, M.A., M.D., F.R.S.

DR. NEALE'S "MEDICAL DIGEST."

ELSEWHERE, in our advertising columns, will be found a notice referring to a new edition of Dr. Neale's "Medical Digest." The former edition was published by the New Sydenham Society, but the forthcoming one he desires to bring out by means of a private publisher. With that end in view, Dr. Neale seeks subscribers, with no view to profit, but simply to cover expenses, which must be very great, altogether independent of the enormous amount of work Dr. Neale has bestowed on this labour of love. We need not say how cordially we recommend Dr. Neale's scheme to the consideration of all our readers; the book itself is well worthy of every word of praise we can give it. The price at which it is to be published is exceedingly moderate, and ought to put it within the reach of all.

THE NEW SAVOY THEATRE.

THIS new theatre is situated between the Strand and the Victoria Embankment, close to the Savoy Chapel and the "Precinct of the Savoy." It stands on historical ground, near where once stood the old Savoy Palace, and is of interest, inasmuch as some provision has been made for the health of the public. In the first place, the electric light is to be universally used both in the auditorium and on the stage. Swan's system of incandescent lights has been adopted; and though, unfortunately, the arrangements were not quite completed, we could fully appreciate the vast importance, from the health and comfort point of view, of thus lighting a public building by lamps which add neither heat nor the products of combustion to the air. The principal carriage entrance, too, deserves attention. The approach is on the Embankment by a private road, and there is a covered pavement of upwards of seventy feet, which allows six or seven carriages to take up at the same time. The difficulty of getting one's carriage at the close of a crowded house is well known, and it is a fruitful source of lung-mischief in this cold, damp, uncertain climate of ours. Mr. D'Oyly Carte may be congratulated on being one of the first managers who has successfully grappled with both difficulties.

DR. M'CLINTOCK, OF DUBLIN.

WE are happy to learn that this esteemed gentleman, whose dangerous illness we announced some time ago, is making most satisfactory progress towards recovery. The paralysis is gradually disappearing, and Dr. M'Clintock was able to come down to his study last Monday. He hopes to leave town shortly, with a view of seeking complete rest and change of air.

DEATH OF PROFESSOR SCHUTZENBERGER.

THE greatest medical celebrity of French Strasburg has just died in consequence of an attack of pneumonia. Born in 1809, and appointed Professor of Clinical Medicine in 1845, Dr. Schutzenberger, although the subject of a painful disease, performed all the duties of his chair during thirty-five years, and became the centre of all medical activity at Strasburg, promoting every modern investigation, and raising the clinic of that Faculty into the first place in France. After the German occupation he struggled for a long time in the endeavour to still maintain a French medical school in the city with which he had been so long identified.

TRAINING IN SANITARY SCIENCE.

OF the successful candidates at the recent examination for the certificate in Sanitary Science at Cambridge University, five—viz., Drs. Burgess, Fraser, Mukhopadhyá, and Whitelegge, and Mr. Walford—were pupils at the Hygienic Laboratory of University College, London.

PROFESSOR PASTEUR AND THE YELLOW FEVER.

PROF. PASTEUR, the *Gazette Hebdomadaire* observes, has had all his trouble and expense for nothing. When he reached Pauillac on September 14 all the dead from yellow fever had been buried, and the sick were convalescent. He awaited fresh transports for a fortnight, but none of the ships brought others than convalescents, although one of the ships had eight, and the other six, patients die on board during the passage. Prof. Pasteur therefore returned to Paris, but the researches which he intended to undertake will be pursued in the very focus of the epidemic, as Dr. Talmy, a naval medical officer, has volunteered for this perilous mission, and has just left for Senegal, furnished with all necessary instructions. It is said also that Dr. Monard, a physician attached to one of the thermal establishments, is also about to set off on the same errand.

ENTRANCE SCHOLARSHIPS.

THE competition for the two Entrance Scholarships in Natural Science at St. Thomas's Hospital Medical School, of £100 and £60, resulted in a tie between Mr. J. S. Hutton and Mr. H. Sydney Jones, and the value has therefore been divided equally between them, viz., £80 each.

At St. Mary's, Mr. A. R. S. Anderson has obtained the Scholarship in Natural Science, tenable for three years—£75 the first year, £50 the second, and £25 the third. Mr. W. Williams has obtained the second—£60 the first year, £25 the second, and £15 the third.

SERIOUS ILLNESS OF DR. THOMAS HAYDEN, OF DUBLIN.

ON Saturday week, Dr. Hayden, while attending a meeting of the Senate of the Royal University of Ireland, had a severe rigor, and very shortly afterwards unmistakable signs of a rapidly extending consolidation of the lungs made their appearance. Within forty-eight hours from the first seizure his life was in imminent peril, and for several days it hung in the balance. The unremitting care of his colleagues, Dr. C. J. Nixon and Dr. F. R. Cruise, aided by the advice of his friends, Dr. Banks and Dr. Lyons, M.P., has, under Providence, so far been rewarded by a gradual rally from the very prostrate and dangerous condition in which Dr. Hayden lay at the end of last week.

MEDICO-CHIRURGICAL SOCIETY OF GLASGOW.

AT the meeting of this Society in the Faculty Hall, on Friday, October 7, the following were elected office-bearers for the session 1881-82 :—*President :* Dr. George Buchanan. *Vice-Presidents :* Dr. J. B. Russell and Dr. Peter Stewart. *Council :* Dr. Bruce Goff (Bothwell), Dr. George Willis (Baillieston), Dr. George Mather, Dr. H. C. Cameron, Dr. Robert Forrest, Dr. Lapraik, Dr. D. Maclean, Dr. J. C. Woodburn. *Secretaries :* Dr. Joseph Coats, Dr. W. L. Reid. *Treasurer :* Dr. Hugh Thomson. The President then gave an introductory address, in which he adduced a number of interesting facts regarding the changes in the medical profession and schools of Glasgow during recent times. The subject of vivisection being introduced by the President, the following resolution was put from the chair and carried unanimously :—"That it is the opinion of this Society that experiments on animals are necessary for the advance of medicine, and that no obstacles should be thrown in the way of competent men performing such experiments. Further, that this Society strongly deprecates the infliction of unnecessary pain, and would support any law which would check this without obstructing competent observers, as the present law does." Afterwards a committee was appointed to carry the resolution into effect in co-operation with similar committees from the Faculty and other bodies.

LONDON HOSPITAL BIENNIAL FESTIVAL.

THE biennial festival of the London Hospital Medical College was held on Monday, October 3, under the presidency of Dr. Robert Barnes. A good number of the staff, old students, and friends of the institution, including Mr. J. H. Buxton, the Chairman of the Hospital, gathered round the chairman on this occasion. Dr. Barnes expressed in warm terms the pleasure with which he looked back on his connexion with the London Hospital, and the harmony which had always prevailed between himself and his former colleagues there ; and Mr. Buxton spoke of the interest which the Committee felt in the welfare of the School, and their sense of its importance to the Hospital.

THE ORIGIN OF TUBO-OVARIAN CYSTS.

DR. HENRI BURNIER contributes to the *Zeitschrift für Geburtshülfe und Gynäkologie* a case of the above rare kind, which occurred in the practice of Professor Schroeder. The patient gave a history clearly indicating antecedent peritonitis. When the cyst was removed, it was found that the Fallopian tube, much dilated, opened directly into it, the opening being as big as a shilling (*Marktstückgrosse*). Ray-like processes of mucous membrane, continuous with and resembling that of the tube, spread out from the opening over the inner wall of the cyst, some of them meeting at the opposite pole of the cavity. This mucous membrane was everywhere covered with cylindrical epithelium. On examination of the cyst-wall, Graafian follicles could be found, more or less abundantly, in every part of it, except where the tube entered it. The mode in which Dr. Burnier supposes this tumour to have arisen is the following :—First, an attack of peritonitis causing adhesion of the peritoneal surface of the fimbria of the tube to the ovary. Then, a Graafian vesicle ripening and coming to the surface at the site of this adhesion. Owing to the greater resistance caused by the inflammatory thickening, this follicle cannot burst, but becomes distended into a cyst (hydrops folliculi). At the same time, the secretion of the Fallopian tube, being retained, dilates the tube (hydrosalpinx). We thus have two collections of fluid, separated by a septum consisting of the wall of the follicle and the fimbria of the Fallopian tube. This septum becomes absorbed, and a tubo-ovarian cyst is the result. The adhesion between the tube and the ovary at the site of the dropsical follicle prevents this from projecting from the surface of the ovary, as such follicles are wont to do, and therefore it can only grow by stretching out the healthy tissue of the ovary round it. Hence the presence of Graafian vesicles at every part of its circumference. Dr. Burnier examines the recorded cases of tubo-ovarian cyst. Three of them, he finds, support this theory, and the others contain nothing against it. The theory of Veit, which assumes the coincidence of catarrh of the tube and hydrops folliculi, Dr. Burnier regards as quite compatible with his own view. Richard's theory, that the fimbria of the tube embrace the ovary at the time of bursting of the follicle, and that the tubo-ovarian tumour results from the bursting of a dropsical follicle, and effusion of its fluid into the tube, Dr. Burnier regards as untenable—first, because there is not enough evidence that the fimbria do embrace the ovary when the follicles break ; and, secondly, because it does not account for the presence of cylinder epithelium within the tumour.

NEWCASTLE COLLEGE OF MEDICINE.

THE introductory lecture at the Newcastle College of Medicine, which is in connexion with the University of Durham, was delivered by Dr. James Murphy, of Sunderland, the Lecturer and Examiner in Botany at that school. The subjects dealt with, however, need hardly detain us.

THE PARIS WEEKLY RETURN.

The number of deaths for the thirty-ninth week, terminating September 30, was 832 (433 males and 399 females), and among these there were from typhoid fever 21, small-pox 4, measles 12, scarlatina 5, pertussis 12, diphtheria and croup 37, dysentery 3, erysipelas 10, and puerperal infections 5. There were also 37 deaths from tubercular and acute meningitis, 14 from acute bronchitis, 34 from pneumonia, 88 from infantile athrepsia (47 of the children having been wholly or partially suckled), and 26 violent deaths. The diminution of deaths has been very considerable, but must not be entirely attributed to the decrease of disease. It arises in some measure from the great *villégiature* which takes place in Paris at this time of the year, and which especially embraces school-children and their relatives. Still, the condition of things is very favourable, as in former years there have been normally from 880 to 890 deaths per week at the same epoch. Small-pox and typhoid fever have diminished—the one from 15 to 4, and the other from 29 to 21; but diphtheria still causes 32 deaths. The births for the week amounted to 1249—viz., 638 males (456 legitimate and 182 illegitimate) and 611 females (434 legitimate and 177 illegitimate; 36 were born dead or died within twenty-four hours.

STATISTICAL SOCIETY.

The usual annual competition for the "Howard Medal" (1882) will take place as formerly. The Council have again decided to grant the sum of £20 to the writer who may gain the "Howard Medal" in November, 1882. The essays to be sent in on or before June 30, 1882. The subject is—"On the State of the Prisons of England and Wales in the Eighteenth Century, and its influence on the Severity and Spread of Small-pox among the English population at that period.' The essays also to present a comparison of the mortality by small-pox among the prison population of England and Wales during the eighteenth century, with the mortality from the same cause during the last twenty years. Further particulars or explanations may be obtained from the Assistant-Secretary, at the office of the Society, King's College entrance, Strand, W.C.

COMPULSORY NOTIFICATION OF INFECTIOUS DISEASES IN BOLTON.

In order to conform with the instructions of the Local Government Board, that annual health-returns are to be made up to the end of December in each year, Mr. Edward Sergeant, the Medical Officer of Health for the town of Bolton, in issuing his seventh annual report, for the year 1880, has included the statistics and transactions of the previous fifteen months. The report remarks that zymotic diseases were very prevalent in the locality during this period, and gave rise to 692 deaths, equal to 24·4 per cent. of the entire mortality, and 4·5 per 1000 of the population. As compared with the previous year the zymotic death-rate was more than doubled, and showed an average higher than any recorded for the preceding ten years. This increase of infectious disease was, in Mr. Sergeant's opinion, exceptional, and entirely due to the great prevalence of measles and scarlet fever, and the extreme fatality from diarrhœa. Small-pox was more or less prevalent from March to August, and was traced to have originated in one of the large cotton-mills of the neighbourhood, presumably introduced by raw cotton, since the first six patients attacked were employed at this mill, and took part in the earlier process of cotton manipulation. Mr. Sergeant affirms that the compulsory notification of infectious disease has, during the past fifteen months, given every satisfaction, and proved of immense value in limiting the spread of contagion. The

number of cases reported amounted to no less than 1646, and, as a rule, considerable care was exercised by the medical men in promptly making returns, there being every reason to believe that the reported infectious disease fairly represented the total amount. The advantages, in fact, of this compulsory notification of infectious disease are so manifest that Mr. Sergeant expresses his opinion that before long the matter will have to be dealt with by a general Act of Parliament; and in the meantime, large towns like Liverpool, Manchester, Salford, and others are seeking powers for the introduction of the system.

DELIQUESCENT SALTS IN STREET-WATERING.

The observations of M. Miquel on the constant presence of bacteria—septic, if not pathogenic at all times—in the dust of towns, have recalled attention to the question of the expediency of adding deliquescent salts (if also germicidal, so much the better) to the water used for laying the dust in streets. The idea is not new, the experiment having been made at different times in Glasgow, Paris, and elsewhere, but abandoned for reasons with which we are unacquainted. M. Houseau, from four years' experience at Rouen, finds that the addition of calcic chloride actually reduces the cost of watering by one-third; for while, under the old system, the operation had to be repeated four times a day, a single watering now sufficed for not less than five or six. The solution employed was the waste liquor from the manufactories of pyroligneous acid, containing, besides calcium chloride, notable quantities of iron and volatile tarry matters also of value as antiseptics. The only reason for its abandonment at Rouen was that improvements in the manufacture of the acid so reduced the strength of the residual liquor that it could no longer be used with advantage commercially. But if the sanitary benefit as well as the comfort of preventing the dispersion of dust were fully realised, no doubt other sources of calcium chloride with the accompanying tar products—as, for example, the manufacture of ammonia from gas liquor—could be found, which would not materially, if at all, increase the cost of street-watering.

SMALL-POX IN SENEGAL.

The last accounts from St. Louis announce that to the epidemic of yellow fever there is now added one of small-pox, which has especially attacked the native inhabitants of Senegal. The disease is the more alarming as most of the blacks are unvaccinated, and the authorities find their efforts crippled by the almost complete absence of vaccine virus in the colony. A supply has been immediately forwarded by the Minister of Marine.

BAD MEAT PROSECUTION AT BIRKENHEAD: IMPORTANT VARIANCE IN THE SCIENTIFIC EVIDENCE.

A cargo of American cattle was brought from America in the steamship *Istria*. During the passage some of the animals suffered from splenic fever and were destroyed. The others were placed in the Woodside lairage. A Mr. Smith bought one animal, and an inspector who saw it just after it was killed condemned it as unfit for food. Whilst getting an order to destroy the carcase, the defendant removed it, and although "no menagerie-keeper would feed his animals upon it," yet it was sold and eaten by the inhabitants of Scotland-road, Liverpool. The evidence of the inspector as to the unfitness of the animal for food was supported by Dr. Vacher, Medical Officer of Health for Birkenhead, and Mr. Moore, the Inspector of Cattle for the Privy Council, and others. On the other hand, Mr. Luge, Chief Inspector of Meat in Liverpool, not only had passed the carcase as fit for food, but he and his family had eaten of it without any other than the usual effects of eating meat. Another inspector and several others gave evidence to the same effect, and Dr. Vacher explained its innocuousness by its being well cooked. In spite, however, of the apparently conclusive proofs that the animal was not unfit for food, the defendant was fined £5 and costs.

THE EPIDEMIC OF YELLOW FEVER IN THE WEST INDIES.

THE accounts of the progress and continuance of this epidemic are very distressing. Dr. Manning, a civil practitioner of forty-two years' experience in the island of Barbadoes, states that he has never witnessed an epidemic of more virulent type. Since early in June last, cases of yellow fever had been occurring among the civil population of Barbadoes, and remittent fever with considerable mortality had been prevalent among the troops, among whom, on July 29, the first undoubted case of yellow fever occurred, although probably many of the previous fatal cases were of the same nature. The men of the Royal Artillery have been the greatest sufferers, and among those of the 1st Battalion Royal Lancaster Regiment the disease has been very prevalent and fatal. The cases among the troops up to latest date had been fifty-one, and ,the deaths thirty-seven. Among the victims were the daughter of the American Consul (one of the earliest cases) ; the wife and child of Lieutenant-Colonel Nicolls, commanding the Royal Artillery ; Surgeon-Major Ward and his wife ; and Surgeon J. Ronayne, a very promising young officer. The Chaplain, an officer of the Army Hospital Corps, and another medical officer, also suffered from the disease. No form of treatment appears to have given satisfactory results. The cases had become less frequent among the troops since their having been placed under canvas on Gun Hill, but a fresh outbreak has since taken place. It has been stated that, notwithstanding the extreme urgency of the situation, the Local Board of Health of Barbadoes declined to sanction the landing on ;the island of three officers of the Army Medical Department specially despatched from this country, the assigned reason being that a slight case of small-pox had occurred, the patient having become completely convalescent, on board the ship in which they had arrived. Blundering bumbledom and common sense continue at variance all the world over.

WE greatly regret that Dr. Russell Reynolds' address on Specialism at University College reached us too late for insertion this week.

DISCHARGE OF A SWALLOWED BODY FROM THE CHEST.

—In the New York Med. Record for September 10, Dr. White relates a remarkable case. A young man was treated by him from March 9 for acute pleurisy, from which he soon recovered as regarded the acute symptoms ; but his convalescence was tedious and accompanied by fever, night-sweats, and great debility, so that he was not considered as cured until the end of April. Two or three weeks afterwards he complained of a dull pain at the seat of the old pleuritis, where was also a large, flat swelling, about fifteen inches in circumference. His general health was very feeble, and fever was present. An abscess was found to be present at the side of the chest, and was opened, and owing to the tediousness of its course and its not healing, dead bone was supposed to be present. What seemed like small spicula of bone protruded from the upper part of the opening, but on introducing a probe no bone could be felt. On another examination, June 21, what was supposed to be bone was found to be loose, and was removed by the fingers. It proved to be a head of rye with half an inch of its straw attached to it, and was perfect as on the day when the patient swallowed it, while threshing, on March 5—i.e., 109 days before.

REMARKS MADE AT THE OPENING OF THE NEW UNIVERSITY COLLEGE AT LIVERPOOL.

By the EARL OF DERBY.

THE Liverpool School of Medicine, now fused with the new University College, was opened by an address from Professor Lodge. At the close of the prize distribution in the medical department, however, Lord Derby, who is President of the College, said :—

You students have selected, from among the various occupations open to you, one of which the interest and importance can scarcely be exaggerated. The services of the soldier or the sailor, invaluable as they are, are not always—happily, in our day they are not often—in requisition ; but the war against disease is constant and never-ending. The lawyer, bound by his instructions and by the customary requirements of his profession, cannot always feel that his success, however honourable and deserved, is the triumph of justice ; but the saving of life is work which no man can regret, however slight the apparent value may be of the individual's life so rescued. The ecclesiastic and the politician live in an atmosphere of controversy, and are daily compelled to affirm and to act upon convictions which, nevertheless, fall far short of certainty. The art of the physician may err also, but if it does, nature has a very speedy and effectual way of pointing out his mistake. The student of abstract science gratifies in the fullest measure the intellectual requirements of his nature, and he may be sustained by a perfectly just conviction of the ultimate utility of his work ; but the stimulus of a direct and visible result is most frequently wanting to his exertions. Your privilege, the privilege of your chosen employment, is—and a high and enviable one I call it—that you can largely satisfy the intellectual impulse to know and to discover on the one hand, while on the other you can equally, in the ordinary routine of your duty, do useful service to your fellow-men. Intellectually considered, the subject of your study is that which most deeply concerns us all. It has grown into a proverb that the proper study of mankind is man ; and in this age, when the intimate connexion of body and mind is recognised—when we know that no thought, no feeling, no emotion, can pass over the human frame without leaving traces of its passage—the enormous importance of studying the physical organisation of our race is less than ever likely to be disregarded. The ultimate mystery of existence can never be solved, but on the conditions of existence every successive generation of inquirers throws clearer and clearer light ; and in that line of research, never exhausted nor capable of being exhausted, there is space enough for the highest ambition, and interest enough to compensate for much of mere drudgery and dulness. But there is another and perhaps a more practical aspect in which the profession of which we speak may be regarded. Medical science applies itself more directly than any other to the promotion of human well-being and the prevention of human suffering. And it does more than that. Those who practise it are the guardians, so to speak, of the national health, and I need not tell what is implied in that practice. The struggle for existence between races, as between individuals, is incessant. The strongest must win in the end ; and the very first condition of a strong race is that it shall be physically healthy. In no age of the world have sanitary matters attracted so much attention as in ours, and in the extension of life and the diminution of disease we are reaping the fruit of what has been done during the last twenty or thirty years. I need not point out, in connexion with that subject, how great is the power and the influence of the medical adviser on distress ; nor need I dwell on what is obvious enough—the demand made upon him for courage and honesty to speak the whole truth where scientific matters are in question, where money is on one side and health on the other, and when plain speech may give serious offence in quarters where offence is dangerous. But it is not in such questions alone that the moral as well as the intellectual qualities of the physician are constantly called into play. He has to deal, not with dead matter, but with men and women ; he has to witness and experience their caprices, their passions, their weaknesses, and of these last at least he sees more than the members of any other profession, and that is no light burden to bear. He must be firm, under penalty of being useless. He must be sympathetic, or the experience of his daily life will force him into cynicism. He must avoid needless pugnacity and antagonism, yet without yielding in any essential point to the quackery and empiricism in which a half-educated public delights. But, on the other hand, he probably enjoys more of the confidence of those with whom he has to do than any other adviser. We do not in these days confess ourselves to priests, but we do confess ourselves— generally with great sincerity—to our lawyers and our physicians. For the great office, as I most seriously call it, of a trusted medical adviser there is wanting more than fine science, though that must necessarily be the basis; he must have tact, judgment, firmness in opinion, courtesy and gentleness in expression. One thing more I will add—there is happily in all departments of life much unpaid service freely and ungrudgingly rendered, often by men who might be excused if they thought first of their own scantily provided families. But I assert with some confidence that the absolutely gratuitous assistance given by the medical profession to those who are unable to pay for it far exceeds that which is bestowed or demanded in any other line of life; and it is not less creditable to those who give it because custom has in great measure caused it to be expected as a matter of course. Whether it is equally creditable to the public that it should be expected to the extent it is, is a different question, into which I need not now enter. What I here say to you medical students may be summed up in one word—Respect your profession and respect yourselves. You have great examples before you, you have noble traditions to follow, you have exceptional opportunities of leading a life not only blameless but intellectual and publicly useful. Remember that each one of you, young as he may be, can do something to honour or, so willing, to discredit his profession. I have no doubt which your choice will be; and I hope many of you may look back from a respected and honoured professional position on these early days of discipline and training, when you stand on this platform as prizemen in our new University College.

THE HEALTH OF TROOPS AT QUETTAH.

(From a Correspondent.)

WE regret that the health of our troops still across the frontier is unsatisfactory; the general appearance of the men being anæmic, worn-out, and of poor physique. The sick-list is high, the prevailing diseases being diarrhœa, dysentery, hepatitis, fever, and some cases of enteric fever. It is questionable, even after the intended withdrawal of the troops from the Peshin, that Quettah, from a hygienic standpoint, would be a desirable station—permanent, or even temporary. Before the Government finally resolve or commit themselves to the permanent retention of Quettah, and before much more money is expended on additions in the shape of barracks, etc., on contaminated and condemnable sites, we venture to urge the paramount and absolute necessity of a thoroughly searching and impartial inquiry on the hygienic suitability of the place for garrisoning troops, who would not, within short spaces of time, need being relieved in consequence of being rendered hors de combat by disease, thus frustrating the raison d'être of the defensive intent for which they are placed there. Such an inquiry would reveal many weak and unfavourable points as regards the station. For the inquiry to be searching it should, as a sine quâ non, be made by experts of special knowledge. To be impartial, it should be conducted by gentlemen of independent character and opinion, who would have nothing to lose or gain by the results.

RUSSIAN VISITORS TO THE CONGRESS.—The total number of Russian physicians who took part in the International Medical Congress was 31, viz., 17 from St. Petersburg, 5 from Warsaw, 3 from Moscow, 2 from Kasan, 2 from Wilna, and one each from Dorpat and Charkow.—St. Petersburg Med. Woch., September 24.

THE NEW MEDICAL SCHOOL BUILDINGS AT CHARING-CROSS HOSPITAL.

THE Charing-cross Hospital and School of Medicine entered upon a new era in its history at the beginning of the present winter session. On Monday, October 3, the governors, officers, and old and present students connected with the institution, celebrated in an informal manner, by a conversazione, the opening of the new Medical School, and the consequent extension of the Hospital proper. The event deserves record, not only as a sign of advance in one of the most promising of the smaller metropolitan schools, but also as an evidence of the recognition in these days of the importance of the practical departments of medical education, to which a considerable portion of the building is devoted.

From the foundation of Charing-cross Hospital, some fifty years ago, the School has continued to be situated within the Hospital buildings. The two departments, however, have, within the last few years, more than once outgrown each other, and for this reason, as well as from hygienic considerations, it was determined to separate the scientific and clinical departments from each other, and to locate the former in a special building. A site was therefore secured upon it after the designs of Mr. J. J. Thomson; and the two buildings were connected by means of a subway under the street.

The building meets the eye on looking along Agar-street from the Strand, the front being in red brick in a free-classic style, with something of the so-called Queen Anne element in it. Entering a decorative porch, one finds oneself in a wide vestibule and hall, from which the administrative rooms, the library, and the museum open, and from which the staircase rises communicating with the upper floors. The museum is a spacious apartment, forty-one feet by twenty-four feet, lighted by large windows at either end. The whole of the wall space is fitted with cases for anatomical and pathological specimens, the upper shelves being reached by means of a gallery running round the room; and the woodwork consists entirely of pitch-pine. A curator's room and a special room for toxicological specimens are connected with the museum. The library measures twenty-seven feet by twenty-four feet, and is specially fitted and furnished for a reading-room as well. On the first floor are located the chemical and physiological departments, with a lecture theatre. The physiological laboratory measures thirty-three feet by twenty-one feet, and is remarkably well lighted, and fitted with every requisite for chemical and microscopical work. The chemical department consists of a suite of three rooms for lectures and practical classes, and for the more strictly scientific work of the lecturer. On the upper floor the chief features are the dissecting room, the post-mortem room, and an anatomical lecture theatre. These three rooms have the comparatively novel feature in common, that they occupy the upper part of the building, and are open-roofed. The light is thus entirely derived from the top, and the windows are fitted with patent opening and closing apparatus, so that thorough ventilation can be constantly carried on. The dissecting-room is especially handsome, measuring forty-one feet by twenty-four feet, and accommodating twenty dissecting-tables. The walls are of cement, with a dado of slate for diagrams; the floor is of red and black tiles; and there are provisions for flushing the entire place with water, when desired. The post-mortem room is provided with raised platforms for the students during the necropsies. The basement remains to be described. Here we find, first, a large students' room fitted with lavatories, etc., injecting room, porters' rooms, and the central heating apparatus. On the basement we also find the entrance of the subway to the Hospital, and the lower end of the lift, which is carried to the top of the building, with an opening at each floor, and which is chiefly intended for the conveyance of bodies to the pathological and anatomical departments.

It is hardly necessary to enter into the more purely

architectural details of the building. The warming is effected chiefly by warm-water pipes, but most of the rooms also contain open fireplaces. These and the walls and fittings are designed in the style of the exterior; and the furniture has been specially selected to harmonise with the whole. The cost of the building is said to be about £11,000.

At the *conversazione*, on October 3, the various departments were thrown open to inspection, and in every room some objects of interest—scientific or artistic—were displayed. In the lower theatre a quartette band under the direction of Dr. Wolfenden discoursed excellent music, which appeared to be highly appreciated.

As we have already said, advantage has been taken of the removal of the Medical School from the Hospital buildings, to greatly extend the out-patient department, which has been completely rearranged. At the same time, extra accommodation has been provided for the resident staff. Altogether Charing-cross Hospital has reason to be heartily congratulated upon the remarkable improvements which have been made upon it within the last few years, both in the wards, in the out-patient department, and in the School.

GUNSHOT WOUNDS AMONG MEN
OF THE
ARMY HOSPITAL CORPS AT MAJUBA HILL.

ELSEWHERE will be seen a letter from Surgeon-General Longmore with regard to a small fund which has been got together for two men in the Army Hospital Corps who singularly distinguished themselves at Majuba Hill. Both were so seriously wounded as to incapacitate them for further service, and to one of them the Victoria Cross has been awarded. The following details of the nature of their wounds will doubtless interest many. Unfortunately, the only member of the Army Medical Department hurt was mortally wounded, and died almost on the spot.

Case of Corporal Farmar, A.H.C.—This man was attending to the wounded on Majuba Hill, under the directions of Surgeon Landon, when the Boers, having gained the summit, directed a fire upon the troops who were retreating past the spot where some of the wounded had been collected. Surgeon Landon, who, with his assistants, remained with these disabled men, was shot, as well as some of the wounded men themselves. Corporal Farmar then held up in his right hand a bayonet with a triangular bandage fastened to it, as a signal to the Boers, who are believed to have been about fifty yards off, that they were not combatants. He was immediately struck by a bullet in the forearm. He next, saying that he had still another arm, held up the *extempore* flag of truce with his left hand, but this arm was also directly hit. In the first of the two wounds, the bullet struck and partially fractured the right ulna on its inner aspect, just above the styloid process, injured the ulnar nerve, and tore its way out by the base of the metacarpal bone of the little finger. Sensation in the parts supplied by the palmar branches of the nerve still continues very dull and imperfect. The cicatrix of the wound adheres to the bone and is tender on pressure. In the second wound, that in the left arm, the bullet entered in front, just above the bend of the elbow-joint, partially fractured the humerus near its inner border, and escaped just behind the prominence of the inner condyle. The ulnar nerve on this side was completely severed, and he has never since had any sensation in the parts supplied by the nerve below the wound. When the bullet passed through the limb he felt as if he had received the shock of a strong galvanic battery, and the hand and arm remained quivering and very painful afterwards. The hand and forearm are now much wasted; the little finger is strongly contracted, and, in addition to total loss of sensation in the little finger and ulnar side of the ring finger, there is marked diminution of temperature in these situations. Owing to alteration of shape in the lower part of the humerus, the result of the gunshot fracture, the elbow is permanently contracted. The forearm can be flexed on the arm fully, but cannot be extended beyond an angle of forty-five degrees. The injuries disable him from ordinary manual labour.

Case of Private Sealey, A.H.C.—Private Sealey was half kneeling, dressing a wounded man of the 92nd Regiment, when a bullet struck and passed through him near the left shoulder. The wound of entrance was two inches and a quarter above the top of the anterior fold of the axilla, an inch and a half below the coracoid process; that of exit was nearly directly opposite, about two inches above the posterior axillary fold. The axillary nerves appear to have escaped entirely. He merely felt a blow locally, and, not realising the fact that he had been shot, went on bandaging the patient. The missile must have been a rifle-bullet of narrow diameter, and traversing with very high velocity, for the cicatrix of the exit opening is exactly similar in size to that of the entrance-wound, viz., three-eighths of an inch in diameter. Within a minute or two after receiving this wound, and while still dressing the patient, he was struck by another bullet in nearly a corresponding place on the right side. This bullet entered just below the acromio-clavicular articulation, between it and the coracoid process, nearly four inches above the top of the anterior axillary fold, passed downwards and backwards, and escaped at the inferior margin of the scapula, about two inches and a half above its inferior angle. A small gap remains in the border of the scapula, whence a piece of bone appears to have been punched out. During the healing process some small fragments of bone escaped by both openings. The instant he was hit on this side the man felt pain through the whole limb, and the arm dropped useless, so that the nerves were evidently injured by the passing projectile. They have since recovered their function, but, owing to deep cicatricial contractions, the arm remains seriously disabled. He cannot extend it above an angle of forty-five degrees from his side, and all the movements of the shoulder are impaired. The left arm is also weak, and any attempt to elevate it above the level of the shoulder causes much pain. The injuries just described were aggravated by the colonial ambulance waggon, in which Sealey and several other wounded men were brought down from Mount Prospect Hospital, being overturned by the way. Private Sealey was much bruised about the chest at the time of this accident. It is remarkable that in each of the two wounds, close as they were to the articulation, the joint itself should have escaped being opened. From both wounds being so nearly on the same level, so close to each other, and following in such quick succession, it was probably the same Boer who fired both shots. It is not unlikely that Corporal Farmar's two wounds were also inflicted by one man.

I am tempted to add the following anecdote, which has not hitherto been made public, regarding Surgeon Landon, of the Army Medical Department, who was mortally wounded on the same occasion. It not only illustrates the immense value of the subcutaneous injection of morphia in certain cases in field practice, but affords additional testimony to that which has already been published regarding the cool and thoughtful character of that much-regretted young officer. Surgeon Landon was kneeling attending to a wounded man, when a bullet wounded him in the loin, and he at once fell forward. The lower half of his body became at the same time completely paralysed. Dr. Landon at once recognised the nature of his injury, and told Corporal Farmar he must die. After the firing had ceased, some Boers came down among the wounded, and with them a man who said he was a doctor. At this time, Corporal Farmar, who, as before mentioned, had had both ulnar nerves injured, was suffering excessive pain in the two arms, and Dr. Landon, who had brought in a field case, which he had carried slung from his shoulder, some morphia solution and syringes, advised some of the solution to be injected for its relief. The Boer doctor attempted the operation in one arm, but, from the bungling way in which he set about it, it was evident the proceeding was not familiar to him. Dr. Landon then caused the upper part of his body to be propped up against a boulder of rock, and in that position administered the injection in both Farmar's arms in succession. The result was, the corporal obtained such relief from the pain that he shortly afterwards, in spite of the rain and general discomfort, fell asleep, and remained so for several hours. When all the circumstances of the occasion are remembered, it is difficult to imagine a more perfect example of professional heroism than was afforded by the conduct of Surgeon Landon, from the time when the Majuba fight commenced, to that when death put an end to his own suffering. T. L.

SOCIAL SCIENCE CONGRESS IN DUBLIN.

HEALTH DEPARTMENT.

ON Tuesday, October 4, the Health Department, under the presidency of Dr. Charles Cameron, M.P. for Glasgow, was engaged in discussing the first of the three special questions set down for consideration at the Congress—namely, " Is it desirable that hospitals should be placed under State supervision ? " The question was introduced in a paper by Mr. Henry C. Burdett, F.S.S., which was read by Dr. J. W. Moore, in the unavoidable absence of the author. The consideration of the question was continued in a paper by Dr. Prospere De Pietra Santa, of Paris, on " Hospital Administration in Paris and London." A discussion followed, and Dr. Charles A. Cameron, Superintendent Medical Officer of Health for Dublin, moved a resolution to the effect that the Council of the Social Science Association be recommended to take measures to promote an inquiry, with a view of securing an independent supervision over the administration of all public hospitals. Dr. Darby, of Bray, seconded the resolution, which was unanimously agreed to.

In the afternoon a paper by Major F. Duncan, LL.D., on " First Aid to Injured Persons " was read for the author by Mr. F. R. Davies, President of the Dublin Centre of the St. John Ambulance Association. The paper referred to the introduction into England by the Order of St. John of improved vehicles for the transport of injured persons. From this had sprung the existing St. John Ambulance Association, branches of which existed in Great Britain, Ireland, and the colonies, and which has already instructed over 30,000 pupils of both sexes and all classes in the first treatment of injured persons.

After a brief discussion, the chair was taken by Dr. Chaplin, of Kildare, the President of the Royal College of Surgeons in Ireland, and Dr. Cameron, M.P., President of the department, read a paper on " Animal Vaccination." He accounted for the falling off in our results by a deterioration of the vaccine virus cultivated (as regards ordinary vaccination) for generations on what Chauveau's researches had proved to be an unnatural soil. As illustrating this falling off, he exhibited a table giving an analysis of over 10,000 cases recorded in London in 1852-67, and over 4000 recorded there in each of the periods 1871-73 and 1877-79. In cases exhibiting marks of cicatrices the mortality had in the first period been 7·6, in the second 8·15, and in the third 8·45. In cases classified as bearing good cicatrices the figures were respectively 1·8, 3·32, and 4·70 ; in the best class—those recorded as showing four good cicatrices —0·87, 1·5, and 3·33 ; and so on, the falling off manifested being most alarming in the best vaccinated class of cases, while the percentage classified as good in each successive period also showed a marked falling off. These facts, Dr. Cameron maintained, were themselves sufficient to call for a change in our system. The motive which had originally given rise to the cultivation of lymph on calves was a desire to avoid all possibility of the inoculation of a loathsome human disease which had been frequently communicated through the ordinary virus. Such mishaps were in this country very rare, but the fact that they might occur, in the writer's opinion, rendered it the duty of the State, which enforced vaccination, to provide against all avoidable accidents. As to the possible dangers which anti-vaccinators had suggested might attend on animal vaccination, the answer was that when it was practised, as in Belgium, Holland, and the United States, no such accident ever had occurred, and, assuming their theory to be correct, the danger attendant on the operation was no greater than that which lay in every cup of milk or mouthful of meat consumed. No danger from inflammation attended the use of the cultivated animal virus—in fact, there was much less trouble from that than under the ordinary practice. For purposes of revaccination animal lymph presented a three-fold advantage. It " took " in a greater percentage of cases ; universal experience showed that much larger numbers of persons got themselves revaccinated when it was available than when it was not, and when required it could be produced in unlimited quantities. This was not the case with humanised lymph, which was always difficult to obtain when the presence of an epidemic rendered an abundant supply most urgent.

A discussion followed, after which the Section adjourned.

On Wednesday, October 5, the Section took up the second special question, namely, " Is it desirable that there should be a system of Compulsory Notification of Infectious Diseases ? and if so, what is the best method of carrying such a system into effect ? and what is the best mode of enforcing the isolation of cases of infectious diseases ? "

Mr. Collins, the secretary of the department, read a paper by Mr. W. H. Michael, Q.C., on the subject. The author thought that some general measure rather than private legislation was desirable ; but he did not think the time had yet arrived for passing a compulsory measure for the isolation of persons who were suffering from infectious diseases.

A paper was read by Dr. J. W. Moore, M.D. Univ. Dub., F.K.Q.C.P., Physician to the Meath Hospital and to Cork-street (Fever) Hospital, Dublin, on the question. The author pointed out that " notification " and " registration " should not be used as synonymous terms. Two things would seem to be necessary in the case of outbreaks of epidemic infectious diseases—first, the immediate compulsory notification of such outbreaks to the sanitary authorities ; secondly, the early registration of all cases of these affections, and the publication of the tabulated results at frequent intervals by the general registration offices of each division of the United Kingdom. Whatever system of notification is finally adopted should apply uniformly to the whole country, for local and piecemeal legislation is most mischievous in this case. Four methods have been suggested or adopted, viz. :—1. Direct notification by the medical attendant. 2. Indirect notification by the medical attendant. 3. Notification by the head of the sick person's family, or by the occupier of the infected house. 4. Dual notification by both the medical attendant and the head of the family or the occupier. Dr. Moore described each system in detail, and discussed its merits and demerits. He expressed himself in favour of a modified system of indirect notification by the medical attendant, in accordance with which it should be incumbent on the sanitary authority to acknowledge at once to the medical attendant the receipt of the information from the head of the family, the medical attendant to send a duplicate certificate to the sanitary authority should their acknowledgment not reach him within a short specified time. In conclusion, the author advocated the payment of an adequate fee to the medical practitioner for every certificate given by him in accordance with the provisions of the proposed Act of Parliament.

Dr. Stewart Woodhouse, M.A., read a paper on " A Proposal obviating the Difficulties connected with the Compulsory Notification of Infectious Disease." The writer, while recognising the desirability of reporting to the sanitary authority every case of infectious disease, believes that the measure introduced to the House of Commons last session for this purpose would meet with the strenuous opposition of the medical profession, who should be the chief machinery in executing it—on the ground that it would violate the secrecy due to their patients.

A prolonged and very interesting discussion ensued. Dr. Jacob regretted that he had to assume a position of uncompromising antagonism to the system of compulsory notification which had been proposed. He did not hesitate to admit fully that the greatest advantage was to be gained by the notification of infectious diseases. His quarrel was with the way in which the papers proposed to carry notification into effect. The subsequent speakers were Mr. Hastings, M.P., who made an eloquent appeal to the members of the medical profession not to take up an isolated and selfish position on this question, but, casting aside all other considerations, to regulate their conduct solely by a desire to fulfil a high and holy purpose of their profession, namely, the prevention of the spread of disease ; Mr. Edmund Dwyer Gray, M.P.; Dr. Cameron, Medical Officer of Health for Dublin ; Mr. Dalgleish, Town Clerk of Jarrow ; Dr. Grimshaw, the Registrar-General for Ireland, who strongly supported the views of Dr. Moore and Mr. Michael ; Dr. Chaplin, the President of the Royal College of Surgeons in Ireland ; Miss Downing, a delegate from the Vigilance Association for the Defence of Personal Rights, of London, who declared herself strongly opposed to the Bills of both

Mr. Hastings and Mr. Gray; Mr. H. M. Collins, the secretary of the department; Dr. Norwood; the Rev. Mr. Kerr; and Mr. Thompson, of Manchester. The President, in closing the discussion, remarked that the State had a right to expect duties from medical men in return for the monopolies it gave them.

We must postpone until next week an account of the proceedings in the Health Department on Thursday and Friday.

FROM ABROAD.

THE SYSTEMATIC WEIGHING OF INFANTS.

UNDER this title, Dr. Haven recently read a paper before the Boston Society for Medical Observation (*Boston Med. Jour.*, September 8), observing that this procedure substitutes scientific data for mere personal opinion. First advised by Prof. Guillot, in 1852, it did not come into any general use until later. In 1866, MM. Blache and Odier strongly urged the practice of regular and frequent weighing, and since that time it has been gradually introduced in France and Germany, Prof. Parrot having done much to popularise it. Dr. Haven states that although practised by a few persons interested in the study of pediatrics in the United States, it has seldom been employed there by the general practitioner, or in many of the institutions devoted to the care of children; and the same statement may be repeated as regards our own country.

"A balance responding to two or three grammes (almost any in ordinary household use will do this), and a set of weights, preferably metric, are the necessary instruments. The child should be weighed as soon after birth as practicable, being dried and wrapped in a piece of warm flannel. The weight of this should be previously ascertained, or if always used may be disregarded, being a constant factor, and not affecting the results, except in the slight original addition. During the first eight or ten days the weighing should be daily. The existence, persistence, and termination of the so-called physiological loss are thus determined. The original weight should be regained from the fifth to the eighth day. After this, weekly weighings for the first five months, and later fortnightly, will suffice. The best time is the morning, when the child's toilet is made. The daily gain should be about 25 grammes for the first five months, at which time the weight at birth should have become doubled; after this its gain gradually decreases to about 10 grammes at the end of the fifteenth month, when the initial figures should be quadrupled. These numbers are the mean of a very large number of French observations, and have the demerit of being too exact. In general, however, the average daily gain in the first few months should not be below 20 grammes. If it is, the child is badly nourished, is sick or going to be so. There are exceptions to this rule, the gain being sometimes less, sometimes greater. It is, however, always in direct proportion to the original weight. If this is very small the gain may be correspondingly small. The technical difficulties in carrying out this method are slight—certainly in any institution they would be so; and any mother or nurse of ordinary intelligence can be trusted to secure accurate results.

"Its advantages are, that it affords absolute knowledge on several points. Is the food affording sufficient and proper nourishment to the babe? Is it getting a fair start in life? This question is often the most important, and at the same time the most difficult, to solve. The scales give us information far more reliable than the intelligence of the mother, the education of the training-school graduate, the experience of the monthly nurse, or even than the experience, intelligence, and education presumably combined in the physician himself. Again, in the treatment of disease, are the desired results being attained? This we can tell with certainty: exactly what food—usually the most important of all treatment—is best suited for the child. We can tell in the wasting diseases of children, when the struggle for life is often severe, if we are gaining or losing ground. There are many other advantages I will not go into here. The effect on the mothers of the better class is not, I think, to be despised. It inculcates the habit of systematic observation of their children, and correct deductions therefrom. It enforces the all-important connexion between the diet and the health of the child—a truism, an axiom to the physician; unfortunately, not so to many of the most intelligent mothers. In dispensary practice, who that has suffered from the maddening prolixity, or the sullen ignorance, of the majority of mothers of that class would not be rejoiced to get, as he can by this method, in a moment's time, some satisfactory and reliable evidence as to the condition of the child, the success of his treatment, and how far his dietetic instructions have been followed?"

Dr. Haven prints some "weight-charts" which show the many points concerning which the balance gives accurate information. At the discussion which followed the paper, Dr. Draper observed that each observation made in this way furnishes new and valuable information. The normal weight of the new-born child is important also in a medico-legal aspect. About 3500 grammes is the normal weight. In answer to a question whether there is any difference in the weight of children of primipare and multipare, Dr. Haven states that not only is the initial weight of the first-born child under the average, but its daily increase is also less. Observations taken in France show that the children of primipare increase less rapidly in weight, the milk of the mother being not only less nourishing, but also less abundant. Dr. Minot believed it of importance to note other things at the same time as the variations in weight, such as the age and health of the parents. Another interesting point would be a comparison of the weights of children fed upon different foods. The comparative value of the different forms of infants' food could in this way be ascertained better than in any other. Dr. Minot had seen, this winter, a curious condition of things in a child. It was thirteen months old and unable to use its legs. The reflex function of the legs was lost. The child looked intelligent and could speak a little. It was found that it had been fed on condensed milk. It was first put on cow's milk and then upon Mellin's Food. Improvement was immediate. It was soon able to move its legs, and before long could do so very well indeed, till it was able to stand and walk by pushing a chair before it. No medicine was used. The case looked very like one of infantile paralysis.

VACCINATION OF ERECTILE TUMOURS.

On exhibiting before the Académie de Médecine (*Bulletin*, September 20) a case of erectile tumour which he had treated by vaccination, Dr. Constantin Paul observed that while this mode of treatment was no novelty, yet as long as we had at our disposal only the limited amount of vaccine virus derivable from the vaccination of children, it could only be applied to tumours of small dimensions. Moreover, the procedure adopted has been faulty, and often failed. Punctures were made at a certain distance from each other, but if one or more of these failed, intervals existed in the resulting cicatrices, and the operation was more or less unsuccessful. Now that we may obtain any amount of heifervirus we are able to resort to more effective procedures, and the one which Dr. Paul employs is, first to cover the tumour with a layer of this virus, and then, by means of a cutting needle, to practise beneath it superficial incisions. These have to be made with extreme lightness, and as superficially as possible, as the skin over these tumours is reduced to a very thin membrane; and if this be pierced through its whole substance, a troublesome hæmorrhage, which might frustrate the operation, would be produced. The issuing of some "sanguinolent serosity" shows that the vessels are open, and that absorption has become possible; and as the opening takes place immediately under the vaccine virus, the contact with this liquid becomes certain and immediate.

This is, in fact, the procedure which Dr. Paul adopts for ordinary vaccination. A drop of vaccine virus is deposited on the skin, and a superficial incision is made with a cutting needle beneath the liquid, so that this cannot escape from immediate contact with the vessels. In this way vaccination never fails, although calf virus is less fluid than human virus. The usual procedure has two inconveniences: sometimes the lancet gets wiped in penetrating, and the virus remains outside; or in some cases, when the needle is used, this penetrates into the subcutaneous cellular tissue, and gives rise to erysipelatous phlegmon. During the eight years that he has employed this plan, Dr. Paul has had occasion to treat four cases of erectile tumour with a more or less considerable surface, and in all the results have been satisfactory.

Dr. Blot, commenting upon the paper, observed that Dr. Paul's paper was couched in words somewhat too vague, not sufficiently distinguishing the different kinds of erectile tumours. But this distinction, made long since by all surgeons, is of the greatest importance, as the treatment varies according to whether we have to do with one or the other kind; while for some even abstention should be the rule, for the simple reason that they are cured spontaneously. Of those which require treatment some are more or less superficial, while others are dense and more or less deep-seated. They are distinguished as cutaneous and sub-cutaneous. The superficial or cutaneous ones, which Dr. Blot terms *taches sanguines*, to avoid confounding them with the others, are alone curable by vaccination, and even all of them are not so. But when the thickness of the tumour is more or less considerable, from a millimetre to a centimetre or more, we should not think of treating it by vaccination, which has the double inconvenience of not being able to cure the disease, and, what is of greater consequence, of giving it time to increase. We know, in fact, with what rapidity erectile tumours of this second category may increase in all directions. The size of a lentil at the time of birth, they may in the course of two or three months attain the extent of the palm of the hand. Vaccination applied to such as these may produce a superficial cicatricial tissue, which changes the colour of the tumour, rendering it whitish instead of violaceous; but it does not cure it. "This is, in fact, precisely what has taken place in the case exhibited to us by Dr. Paul, so that we must guard against illusions as to the results obtained. I feel the more authorised to dwell upon these distinctions, as, being the director of the vaccination service of the Academy, I have frequently young infants sent to me by my *confrères* with the request that I would apply the virus to tumours which, by their volume, density, and depth, are not suitable for this treatment. As to the operative procedure in cases in which vaccination may be applied with a chance of success, I prefer that which I employ to the one Dr. Paul has described. Instead of applying the virus to the intact skin, and scarifying only as the second stage of the operation, I perform the two stages on the inverse order—that is to say, I commence by *practising* over the whole diseased surface a series of superficial scratches (*éraillures*) resembling in their disposition those lines which in drawing are termed hatchings. I allow any blood that may issue to *almost* completely cease flowing, and then, while all these minute furrows are still *moist and raw*, I perform the second stage by applying an abundant quantity of the liquid virus. In a few minutes all is perfectly dry; and in this way I avoid the washing away of the virus by the blood. But I must repeat, in conclusion, that it should be well known that, under a great number of circumstances, vaccination is insufficient, and that we should, in order to obtain a complete cure, have recourse to other means. On this occasion I do not intend to pass these in review, and will only say that the actual cautery has been of great service to me. Prof. Gosselin, in corroboration of what Dr. Blot had stated, observed that since 1844, thanks to the labours of Auguste Bérard, the distinction has been well established between cutaneous and subcutaneous erectile venous tumours. Vaccination, in his opinion, is of no efficacy except for the cutaneous tumours, which are the most rare. As to the child exhibited at the Academy, vaccination has not cured the tumours of which it is the subject, and in Prof. Gosselin's opinion they can only be cured by the actual cautery. Dr. Blot repeated that the question was one of great importance, in view of the absolute ignorance which the majority of practitioners exhibit in this matter. Quite recently one of them sent for vaccination an infant having the entire cellular tissue of the cheek invaded by an erectile tumour. Dr. Paul, in reply, observed that by vaccination a cutaneous lesion, and never a subcutaneous lesion, is produced, the thin vascular dermis, all ready for hæmorrhage, being transformed into a whitish non-vascular cicatrix, which forms a barrier against hæmorrhage. If the subcutaneous veins are also too developed, nothing prevents the operation being completed by the actual cautery. As to the procedure recommended by Dr. Blot, he has often tried it, and condemns it as giving

rise to much too large and irregular pustules. M. Jules Guérin stated that since 1840 he has performed subcutaneous section for this disease with frequent success.

CHOLERA IN CANDAHAR IN 1879.

THAT the occupation of Candahar and Southern Afghanistan generally has been not without its baneful results on the health of our troops cannot be gainsaid. The following illustration of the *importation of cholera* into Afghanistan, which is gathered from an official report, is interesting. The disease was prevailing at Sukkur, in Sind, in the early part of the summer of 1879; from there the traffic and the march of the troops (prior to the completion of the railway to Sibi) were by the rough road across a sandy plain, and cholera ran up this line to Quettah and to Candahar. It is noteworthy, however, though in accord with accepted views, that such troops as marched by a new route from Candahar to Peshin avoided the disease, the ravages of which were concentrated on the trunk road and its immediate vicinity; but every regiment that marched along the trunk road took up cholera as a certainty.

The 3rd Goorkhas suffered terribly in this epidemic. Surgeon-Major J. W. Johnston, the medical officer of the regiment, states that his men were "exceedingly prostrated by fever; from June 21 to July 5, 254 cases passed through hospital"; and he is of opinion "that the exposure and harassing duties incidental to service in Afghanistan, and the want of accustomed stimulants, tended to conduce to a special form of fever such as sometimes prefaces a cholera epidemic. The bulk of those who suffered were weaklings convalescing from fever. No less than 31 out of 36 deaths from cholera that ensued at headquarters were fever cases. The sum of these factors gives us a known determining condition, which, aggravated by the loitering sequelæ of fever, created a luxuriant but local individualised malific condition, well adapted to receive and fructify any epidemic aura." Cholera first appeared in a detachment of this regiment quartered at Abdul Rahman, which is two stages on the Quettah side of Candahar. This was on July 4. It then spread to the headquarters of the regiment at Candahar. The total number of cases in this regiment was 78; 49 died and 24 recovered. On July 8 the first case occurred in the 25th Regiment of Punjaub Native Infantry, under the medical charge of Surgeon Murphy. In this corps cases continued to occur, "in spite of evacuation of barracks and moving men short distances round the square in tents. On August 5 there was an increase, five men being admitted on that date. Next morning half the regiment was moved out into camp, about one mile away on the plain north-west of the city. Amongst those left behind in the square, two cases occurred on August 6, one on the 7th, and one on the 9th. The companies that had been moved out remained free until the night of the 9th, between which and the 11th there were nine admissions. On the 11th the whole regiment was moved into Mir Dil Khan's garden, about a mile and a half." Dr. Johnston notes the curious circumstance that, out of an establishment of 140 dooly-bearers, only four men were attacked, and these four were employed in carrying cholera patients from the old to the new encampment.

CHANGES OF DOCTORS IN AMERICA.—There are in the United States 110 medical schools, having an annual attendance of 12,000 students, 3000 of whom are graduated every year, and go forth to battle with life and competing M.D.'s. This, associated with the historico-statistical fact that there are only about 600 persons to each physician now in the United States, makes appropriate the question—What are we to do? Taking into consideration the fact that some of the more fortunate of the profession have more than their *pro ratâ* of patrons, others must have proportionately less; and while this is well enough for the former, it is, to say the least, quite sufficient to produce a lack of patients to the latter: and patients are just as requisite to the doctor in the battle of life, as is patience to any other class of mankind.—*New York Med. Record*, September 10.

REVIEWS.

Lectures upon Diseases of the Rectum, and the Surgery of the Lower Bowel. By W. H. VAN BUREN, M.D. London: H. K. Lewis. 1881. Pp. 412.

WE learn from the preface that this is a second edition, largely re-written, and containing much new experience, both personal and that derived from other works on the subject. The contents are arranged as lectures, which were delivered at the Bellevue Hospital Medical College, at which establishment the author is Professor of Surgery.

The author enters straightway *in medias res*, giving in the first lecture an account of pruritus, erythema, herpes, eczema as seen about the anus, together with the varieties and causes of haemorrhoids. Here the reader will find much useful information on subjects which are difficult to treat unless the real cause of the disorder is well made out. We miss a chapter, which, in diseases of the lower bowel especially, is one of great importance. Our own best-known authority on the subject—Mr. Curling—commences his work on Diseases of the Rectum with an introductory chapter, full of useful hints as to the class of persons subject to these diseases, mode of examining rectum, the use of anæsthetics, and some general remarks on operations on the rectum. This chapter concludes with a sentence which we cannot forbear to transcribe:—"It may seem superfluous to remark that no operation, even of a trivial character, should be performed on the anus or rectum without due inquiry into the state of the patient's general health. I have heard of diffuse inflammation of a fatal character arising after the removal of a small excrescence from the anus, and after the division of a fistula; and of pyæmia occurring after the removal of hæmorrhoids; and although all operations are more or less liable to ill consequences, they very rarely happen after operations on the anus and rectum, except where the precaution alluded to is neglected." Doubtless, in the course of the work now before us, very much of the above quotation will be found; but the advice, especially in lectures delivered before students, is of such importance that its repetition can never harm.

Van Buren's lecture on internal hæmorrhoids is very practical; it places the subject before us in a clear, forcible manner. In contrasting internal with external piles, our author says—"We have seen the external form of the disease characterised mainly by inflammation and pain, and these features are temporary. *Internal piles*, on the contrary, form more slowly, attain greater development, and are less frequently the seat of acute pain and swelling; they are more chronic in their nature, invariably complicate themselves with more or less prolapse of the mucous membrane of the rectum, and, as their name implies, are a constantly existing source of loss of blood." In discussing prolapse of the rectum, the student's attention is drawn to the fact that it is not simply the thickened, infiltrated mucous membrane of the rectum which "comes down," but that all the coats of the rectum are included. In the former condition, which is called partial prolapse, the tumour never attains a large size, and the folds *radiate*, as against being *transverse* in cases of complete prolapse; but in the latter the tumour may assume almost any proportions. Another point of importance in the complete cases is insisted on, viz., that it always contains more or less peritoneum. In treating of intussusception, it is needless to say that laparotomy is advised in suitable cases, after other measures have failed. "I cannot discuss, here and now, the considerations which influenced Brinton in 1867, and Ashhurst in 1871, and others who had carefully studied the history of this subject, to conclusions against abdominal section, or gastrotomy as it was then called, in intussusception; but the reasons justifying interference given by Hutchinson, Marsh, and Sands—above all, their success—seem to me to make it our duty, in the presence of so hopeless a condition as prolapse with invagination of this kind, to stand ready to imitate them."

We cannot pretend to follow our author through all his chapters. They will well repay careful study. The last lecture is somewhat mixed up, treating, as it does, of congenital malformations, fæcal impactions, foreign bodies, neuralgia, and sundry other points. The hygiene of the rectum, too, comes last, while, as we think, it ought to have been discussed first. As regards congenital malformation, our author might with advantage have written more fully, and that because, to use his own words, "cases of this kind may happen to any medical man who takes charge of women in childbirth; and where the aid of a surgical expert is not within reach, a human life may depend upon the promptness and capacity for intelligent action of the accoucheur."

Dr. Van Buren only gives four forms of defect in development, and these are based on the visible condition of or about the anus. His first form, in which the natural position of the anus is "skinned over" simply, hardly seems worthy the term "congenital malformation." The corresponding cloaking of the vagina is well known; and both cases only require the introduction of an oiled finger-tip to restore the parts to their natural condition. Further explanations, however, amplify this somewhat scanty arrangement, while a foot-note refers "to other and rarer varieties besides those indicated in the text." A further shortcoming is the manner of treating those cases in which the rectum opens into the vagina—the commonest form of the malformation, we believe, in female children. Rizzoli's method of detaching the rectum from the vagina, and then of attaching its extremities to the incision through the incised sphincter, might at least have been mentioned. It appears to us that this is one of the class of cases most easy to operate on, and most likely to prove successful afterwards. Speaking of the general treatment of such cases, some useful hints will be found, especially concerning the danger of cicatricial stricture of "the usual obstinate character." Whenever there is a deficiency in the rectum itself, mere incision through the "imperforation" will not suffice. If mucous membrane cannot be brought down to the external orifice, contraction of the new opening will take place, whatever be done. We are not, therefore, to content ourselves with an opening through which meconium can pass, though for a time it may seem to answer. "The proper course to pursue, after failure to find the rectum from the perineum, is to open the sigmoid flexure of the colon in the left groin with the view of establishing an artificial anus in this locality." Few surgeons of to-day will be disposed to differ from this advice. This surgical proceeding "was first suggested by Littré, of Paris, in 1710, after examining the dead body of an infant that had died on the sixth day after birth with malformation of its rectum." There was a perfect anus and *cul-de-sac* below, and a blind rectal pouch above, with an interval of fibrous material between them. In the hope of saving life in a similar case, the eminent anatomist proposed to open the belly of the child, and bring the intestine to the wound, "which should thenceforward be prevented from closing, that it might perform the function of an anus." But it was not till 1783 that this operation was performed.

We have said enough to show the kind of lectures which we have before us. They are all interesting and suggestive, and both student and practitioner will find them a reliable guide in this department of practice.

LIST OF PRIZEMEN AT THE LIVERPOOL SCHOOL OF MEDICINE.—*Lyon Jones Scholarships*: Mr. F. C. Larkin and Mr. A. H. Wilson. *Winter Session*: Third Year Subjects—Medicine, Surgery, and Pathology: Mr. J. F. Joseph, Silver Medal; and Mr. E. Williams, Silver Medal—*equal*. Second Year Subjects—Advanced Anatomy and Physiology: Mr. W. O. Travis, Torr Gold Medal; Mr. F. C. Larkin, Bronze Medal; Mr. A. W. Dawson, Hon. Certificate, and Mr. H. A. Bredin, Hon. Certificate—*equal*. First Year Subjects—Elementary Anatomy and Physiology and Chemistry: Mr. E. P. P. Macloghlin, Bligh Gold Medal; Mr. C. J. Lewis, Bronze Medal; Mr. A. W. Collins, 1st Hon. Certificate; and Mr. G. S. Wild, 2nd Hon. Certificate. Histological Prizes: Mr. W. O. Travis, Mr. F. C. Larkin, and Mr. H. Robinson. *Summer Session*: Medical Jurisprudence and Toxicology: Mr. E. P. P. Macloghlin, Silver Medal; Mr. G. Abbott, Hon. Certificate, and Mr. J. W. M'Vitie, Hon. Certificate—*equal*. Materia Medica: Mr. W. T. Thomas, Silver Medal; and Mr. W. O. Travis, Hon. Certificate. Botany: Mr. E. C. Larkin, Silver Medal. Practical Chemistry: Mr. H. Clare, Silver Medal, and Mr. F. C. Larkin, Silver Medal—*equal*; and Mr. W. O. Travis, Hon. Certificate. Comparative Anatomy: Mr. F. C. Larkin, Prize; Mr. P. O'Brien, Hon. Certificate; and Mr. T. D. C. Barry, Hon. Certificate. Students' Debating Society's Prizes: 1st Essay, Mr. E. P. P. Macloghlin; 2nd Essay, Mr. F. A. Saunders. Reports of Medical Cases, Mr. T. P. Lowe; Reports of Surgical Cases, Mr. W. H. Wright.

GENERAL CORRESPONDENCE.

FARMAR AND SEALEY FUND.
LETTER FROM SURGEON-GENERAL T. LONGMORE.

[To the Editor of the Medical Times and Gazette.]

SIR,—It will be remembered that when the reports of the disaster at Majuba Hill, on the Transvaal border, reached this country, public attention was called to the admirable manner in which certain medical officers and men of the Army Hospital Corps had distinguished themselves by their efforts to assist and protect the wounded under the peculiarly trying circumstances of that sad occasion. The gallant conduct of Corporal Farmar, A.H.C., was particularly brought to notice in the official despatches, and this non-commissioned officer has since had the special honour of receiving the Victoria Cross at the hands of Her Majesty the Queen at Osborne. When Corporal Farmar and another man of the Army Hospital Corps, Private Sealey, who had also made himself conspicuous by his attention to the wounded, and who, like Corporal Farmar, had been severely wounded himself while dressing them, reached Netley, it was found that both men had become incapacitated by the effects of their wounds for active manual exertion in the future. With the permission of the Director-General of the Department, a subscription was started by some of the medical officers, and officers, non-commissioned officers, and men of the Army Hospital Corps, with a view to supplement the Government pension which the two disabled men would receive in regular course on their discharge from the service; and my object in now writing is to state that this fund, which at present amounts to £278, must shortly be closed. In the meantime, any additional subscriptions to the fund may either be sent to the address of Surgeon-General Shelton, head of the Medical Branch, 6, Whitehall-yard, who has kindly taken the trouble to collect subscriptions, or to myself; and I shall, with your permission, report hereafter the total amount of the fund, and the manner in which it has been distributed.

I am, &c.,   THOS. LONGMORE, Surg.-Gen. H.P.,
Netley, October 5.   Prof. of Military Surgery.

P.S.—As the wounds of both Corporal Farmar and Private Sealey present some features of surgical interest, I send a short report of them.

A NINE MONTHS' CRUISE.

[To the Editor of the Medical Times and Gazette.

SIR,—It is within the experience of most medical men to have a patient suffering from some slight affection of the lung, larynx, etc., who requires the bracing air of the sea, and occupation for the mind; and the difficulty of finding such a combination is only too well known. That has now been achieved by the proposed cruise of the Ceylon round the world. This yacht, of over 2000 tons, formerly a P. and O. steamer, is fitted up not only with home comforts, but with all the luxuries of a ladies' and gentlemen's club. It has its boudoir, smoking-, reading-, and dining-rooms ; a cuisine where the various delicacies obtained during the voyage will be cooked à la Francatelli, so that the passenger will have the " bird's-nest soup," " the turtle steak," " a slice of buffalo," and " a canvas-back duck " brought to his own table. There will be no worry of hotels or shore-boats, as a steam launch will run to and from the ship whenever wished for, thus freeing the passenger from nuisance and expense. Starting, as the Ceylon does, on October 20, the traveller will find in the Mediterranean sunny skies that will be with him to the Bosphorus, through the Suez Canal to India, China, and Japan, whilst the heat will make him enjoy the shady groves of King Kalakua's home, and the fogs and winter snows of London will be but visions in the mind of the now invigorated and healthy patient. The Ceylon carries two surgeons, so that the health as well as the comfort of the voyagers is well looked after, and any special treatment recommended would be carried out to the best of the ability of the medical men on board. I enclose my card, and shall be glad to answer any letter sent to you.

I am, &c.,
SENIOR SURGEON TO THE "CEYLON."

THE HYPODERMIC EMPLOYMENT OF QUININE.
LETTER FROM DR. R. NEALE.

[To the Editor of the Medical Times and Gazette.]

SIR,—At page 424 of your journal, as well as in other medical periodicals of same date, Mr. J. W. Moore, writing from Bombay, claims to have been the first to introduce this method of administering quinine. A reference to the "Medical Digest," section 402.4, will, at a glance, show that Dr. James McCraith, of Smyrna, anticipated Mr. Moore's report. Dr. McCraith, in two admirable papers, published in the Medical Times and Gazette, August, 1862, pages 120, 307, claims "the discovery of what is tantamount thereto" for his friend and confrère Dr. Chasteaud.

I am, &c.,   RICHARD NEALE, M.D.
60, Boundary-road, South Hampstead, N.W., Oct. 8.

MEDICAL NEWS.

UNIVERSITY OF CAMBRIDGE.—SANITARY SCIENCE EXAMINATION.—The following gentlemen have satisfied the Examiners in both parts of the examination :—

Adams, G. E. D'Arcy, M.D.	Oram, A. M., M.D.
Bruce, R., M.R.C.S.	Potter, H. Percy, F.R.C.S.
Burgess, P., M.B.	Smith, W. R., M.D.
Fraser, W., M.B.	Stevenson, R. D., C.M.
Hill, A. Bostock, L.R.C.P.E.	Sykes, W. J., M.D.
Moodie, R., M.D.	Walford, E., M.R.C.S.
Mukhopadhya, S. C., M.B.	Whitelegge, B. A., M.R.C.S.
	Willoughby, E. F., M.B.

APOTHECARIES' HALL, LONDON.—The following gentlemen passed their examination in the Science and Practice of Medicine, and received certificates to practise, on Thursday, October 6 :—

Beatley, William Crump, 42, Bloomsbury-square.
Brewster, William, St. Bartholomew's Hospital.
Miller, James, Brunel-street, S.E.
Simons, Charles Nathaniel, Leton, Beds.
Rogers, Harry Cornelius Edwin, 114, Stanhope-street.

The following gentleman also on the same day passed the primary professional examination :—

Culhane, Francis J. F., University College.

APPOINTMENTS.

. The Editor will thank gentlemen to forward to the Publishing-office, as early as possible, information as to all new Appointments that take place.

WOOLLEY, GEORGE TALBOT, M.R.C.S. Eng.—House-Surgeon to St. Peter's Hospital for Stone and Urinary Diseases, etc., vice Mr. W. R. Williams, F.R.C.S., resigned.

BIRTHS.

BERNAYS.—On October 6, at Old Charlton, S.E., the wife of Herbert L. Bernays, M.R.C.S., of a daughter.

DANIELL.—On October 10, at Strood, Kent, the wife of Herbert E. Daniell, M.B., of a daughter.

FARMER.—On October 9, at Hexham, Northumberland, the wife of Farmer, L.R.C.P., of a daughter.

HARRIS.—On October 10, at 57, Darnley-road, Hackney, the wife of Robert Harris, M.B., of a son.

KIRKMAN.—On October 5, at The Briars, Silverhill Park, St. Leonards-on-Sea, the wife of W. P. Kirkman, M.D., of a daughter.

LYON.—On October 7, at Houghton-le-Springs, Durham, the wife of Walter Lyon, M.A., M.D., of a son.

SCOTT.—On October 4, at Musselburgh, N.B., the wife of Thomas R. Scott, M.B., of a son.

THOMPSON.—On October 9, at 9, Cranley-place, South Kensington, the wife of Reginald E. Thompson, M.D., of a son.

MARRIAGES.

APPLEBE—COWPER.—On October 5, at Boddington, Edward Alexander Applebe, L.R.C.P., of Hay, Brecon, to Alice Whateff, youngest daughter of J. W. Cowper, Esq., of Lower Boddington, Northampton.

BROWN—KELSON.—On October 5, at Hackney, J. Alexander Brown, M.R.C.S., of Coombe Lodge, Peckham, S.E., to Kate, daughter of the late Thomas Kelson, Esq., merchant, of Archangel.

FLORENCE—BARNES.—On October 4, at St. Marylebone, Ernest Badinius Florence, Esq., barrister-at-law, of 14, Emperor's-gate, South Kensington, to Ada Constance Sedley Carr Jackson, youngest daughter of Robert Barnes, M.D., of Harley-street, Cavendish-square.

HEAD—BREW.—On October 5, at Pant&c, Mon., Harold Ellershaw, son of Alfred J. Head, Esq., of Theydon Bois, Essex, to Rachel Eveline, daughter of Charles A. Brew, M.R.C.S., of Fonrhydyrun, Mon.

JAKINS—VOSPER.—On October 4, at South Petherwin, Percy S. Jakins, M.R.C.S., of 9, Omaburgh-street, Regent's-park, to Emily, daughter of the late William G. Vosper, Esq., of Brock Hill, South Petherwin, Launceston, Cornwall.

McCheane—Langmore.—On October 5, at Norfolk-square, W., Alfred Cobbett, son of the late John McCheane, Esq., J.P., of Portsmouth, to Ada Caroline, daughter of J. C. Langmore, M.B., F.R.C.S., of 20, Oxford-terrace, Hyde-park, W.

Moir—Gibson.—On October 5, at Maybole. N.B., William Brown Moir, M.D., of Fort William, N.B., to Jane Hutchison, eldest daughter of the late John Gibson, Esq., of Melton Abbey, Dorset.

McCullagh—Cockburn.—On September 19, at Rangoon. British Burmah, Captain James Robert McCullagh, Royal Engineers, Survey of India, to Jessie, daughter of J. Balfour Cockburn, M.D., A.M.D.

Ralfe—Davies.—On October 11, at North Benfleet, Charles Henry Ralfe, M.A., M.D., F.R.C.P., to Elizabeth, daughter of David Davies, Esq., late of Tyllwyd, Llanwrda.

Russell—Walton.—On October 7, at Hanover-square, Rowland Harrison Russell, Esq., to Bessie, daughter of Haynes Walton, F.R.C.S., of 1, Brook-street, Grosvenor-square, W.

Wade—Ambler.—On October 5, at St. Leonards-on-Sea, Arthur Law Wade, M.D., to Louisa Jane, second daughter of the late Thomas Benjamin Ambler, Esq., of Hornsey Rise, London.

DEATHS.

Curtis, William, M.R.C.S., at Alton, Hants, on October 7, in his 79th year.

Lidbetter, Walter Reginald, son of T. G. Lidbetter, M.R.C.S., at Quadrant Villa, Canonbury, on October 10.

Mahaffy, Surgeon-General E, M.D., C.B., late of Her Majesty's Bombay Medical Service, at Castle Hill, Maidenhead, on October 3.

Merrett, William Gwillim, M.R.C.S., at Dalton House, Beckford, Gloucestershire, on October 2, aged 82.

Thompson, W. J., M.D., M.R.C.S., at Dublin, on October 3, aged 75.

VACANCIES.

In the following list the nature of the office vacant, the qualifications required in the candidate, the person to whom application should be made and the day of election (as far as known) are stated in succession.

Birmingham General Dispensary.—Resident Surgeon. Candidates must be registered, and possess both a medical and surgical qualification. Applications, together with original testimonials and certificates of registration, to be sent to Alex. Forrest, Secretary, on or before November 18.

Bristol General Hospital.—House-Surgeon. Candidates must be members of the College of Surgeons of London, Edinburgh, Glasgow, or Dublin, and also Licentiates of the Apothecaries' Company of London or Dublin, or possess some other recognised medical qualification. Applications, enclosing testimonials of good moral character and ability, with certificate of registration, to be sent to the Secretary, on or before November 5.

Dispensary of the General Hospital for Sick Children, Gartside-street, Manchester.—Medical Officer. (For particulars see Advertisement.)

Hospital for Sick Children, Great Ormond-street, W.C.—Assistant-Physician. (For particulars see Advertisement.)

Hulme Dispensary, Manchester.—House-Surgeon. Applications to be sent to Dr. Wahltuch, Honorary Secretary, Medical Staff, by October 20.

Inverness District Asylum.—Assistant Medical Officer. Candidates must be duly qualified and registered. Applications and testimonials to be forwarded to Dr. Aitken, Medical Superintendent (from whom all further particulars can be obtained), not later than October 20.

Leeds Public Dispensary.—Resident Medical Officer. Applications to be sent to Dr. E. H. Jacob, 12, Park-street, Leeds, before October 15.

Richmond Hospital.—House-Surgeon. (For particulars see Advertisement.)

St. Thomas's Hospital, S.E.—Assistant-Physician. (For particulars see Advertisement.)

UNION AND PAROCHIAL MEDICAL SERVICE.

*** The area of each district is stated in acres. The population is computed according to the census of 1871.

RESIGNATIONS.

Chester Union.—The City and North-Eastern Districts and the Workhouse are vacant by the death of Mr. Thomas Brittain. City District: area 2768; population 33,340; salary £100 per annum. North-Eastern District: area 12,415; population 7418; salary £50 per annum. Salary for Workhouse £100 per annum.

Thetford Union.—Mr. C. V. Willett has resigned the Brandon District: area 18,034; population 2690; salary £45 11s. per annum.

APPOINTMENTS.

Aston Union.—Henry James Kelly, M.D. St. And., M.R.C.S. and L.M. Eng., and L.S.A. Lond., to the Castle Bromwich District.

Saffron Walden Union.—William Alexander Smith, M.B. Oxon., M.R.C.S. Eng., to the Third and Fifth Districts.

Stroud Union.—Benjamin Walker Cawthorne, M.B. and C.M. Edin., to the Fifth District.

Ticehurst Union.—Charles Hoar, B.M., M.C. Aber., to the Robertsbridge District.

Wakefield Union.—William H. Haley, L.R.C.P. Edin., L.R.C.S. Edin., to the Wakefield District.

ANALYSTS.

Tiverton.—Mr. John P. McNeill, M.D., reappointed Analyst for the Borough for one year.

Wakefield.—Alfred Henry Allen, F.C.S., appointed Analyst for the Borough for one year. Remuneration by fees.

The Cholera.—The Governor-General of Algeria has come to the decision that the Mecca pilgrimage shall be interdicted to the Algerians this year. The decision has been founded on the advice given by the Hygiene Committee on being consulted by the Minister of Agriculture and Commerce as to the measures which shall be adopted in consequence of the appearance of the cholera at Aden. In issuing this interdiction, the Governor-General explains in a note that the measure, founded on the precedents of 1874 and 1875, is rendered necessary by the interests of the public health. The most rigorous enforcement of the regulations relating to quarantine is also ordered.—Union Méd., October 4.

Queen's College, Birmingham; Prize List, 1881.—Medicine—Medal and First Certificate, F. Leslie Phillips; Second Certificate, Arthur T. Holdsworth. Surgery—Medal and First Certificate, Henry Leonard Swinson; Second Certificate not awarded. Pathology—Medal and First Certificate, Arthur Thomas Holdsworth; Second Certificate, not awarded. Anatomy—Senior Division: Medal and First Certificate, Charles Edwin Purslow; Second Certificate, Edward Dennis Vinrace. Junior Division: Medal and First Certificate, Charles Edwin Purslow; Second Certificates, George Hyde Melson and Arthur Frederick Mossiter, equal. Practical Anatomy—Senior Division: Medal and First Certificate, Charles John Evers; Second Certificate, John Dudley Price. Junior Division: Medal and First Certificate, Charles Edwin Purslow; Second Certificate, Arthur Frederick Mossiter. Physiology—Medals and First Certificates, Charles John Evers, and John Dudley Price, equal; Second Certificate, Arthur William Scott. Practical Physiology—Medal and First Certificate, John Dudley Price; Second Certificate, Arthur William Scott. Chemistry—Medals and First Certificates, Charles Edwin Purslow and George Hyde Melson, equal; Second Certificate, James Bernard Wall. Botany—Medals and First Certificates, Charles Edwin Purslow and George Hyde Melson, equal. Materia Medica—Medal and First Certificate, William Aston; Second Certificate, George Hyde Melson. Forensic Medicine—Medal and First Certificate, Frank Leslie Phillips; Second Certificate, Charles John Evers. Midwifery—Medal and First Certificate, Frank Leslie Phillips; Second Certificate, John Dudley Price. Practical Chemistry—Medals and First Certificates, William Aston, and Thomas Young, equal; Second Certificates, John Woodward Crowther and — Richards, equal. Sands-Cox Prize—Arthur Thomas Holdsworth. Ingleby Scholarship—Frank Leslie Phillips.

Professor Marey's New Physiological Station.—At the request of Prof. Marey, of the Collège de France, there is about to be established a physiological station in the Parc des Princes, in the Bois de Boulogne. Prof. Marey has been enabled to pursue his numerous investigations into the physiology of the muscles and nerves at his laboratory at the Collège; but in consequence of the want of space he has been surrounded by difficulties when studying the functional movements of various animals. The new physiological station in the Bois de Boulogne, comprising grounds which are 3500 metres in extent, will allow him to pursue his experiments with ease.—Revue Méd., September 10.

Sinuses Treated by Tents.—Dr. Edward Williams calls attention to the frequency with which the knife may be dispensed with by the employment of tents in the treatment of simple sinuses. A narrow slip of sticking-plaster is rolled up lengthwise, just as a piece of paper is rolled in order to light a lamp or cigar, and, having been pushed to the bottom of the sinus, may be left there for three or four days until it excites a healthy suppuration. The tent is then removed, and the sinus allowed to heal up from the bottom like a fresh wound, bringing its walls together, if necessary, by a bandage or strips of adhesive plaster. This plan will not take the place of the knife in all cases, but it certainly may in many; and fistulæ in ano have often been cured in this way, or by the seton, which acts in the same way. Two other applications of the same principle are mentioned by Dr. Williams. One of these is the keeping an ordinary urethral bougie for five or ten minutes within the uterus in cases of chronic endometritis, this forming a good substitute for cauterising and curetting the surface of the organ. The other is keeping this same bougie à demeure in the male urethra for a time in gleet and seminal emission. These conditions are kept up by a kind of chronic prostatic urethritis, with probably a granular condition of the mucous membrane. The prostatic portion is supersensitive, and sometimes bleeds a little on the passage of an instrument.—Boston Med. Jour., August 3.

VITAL STATISTICS OF LONDON.

Week ending Saturday, October 8, 1881.

BIRTHS.

Births of Boys, 1238; Girls, 1230; Total, 2468.
Corrected weekly average in the 10 years 1871–80, 2541·9.

DEATHS.

	Males.	Females.	Total.
Deaths during the week	679	683	1362
Weekly average of the ten years 1871–80, corrected to increased population ...	744·6	692·4	1435·0
Deaths of people aged 80 and upwards	...	...	39

DEATHS IN SUB-DISTRICTS FROM EPIDEMICS.

	Enumerated Population, 1881 (unrevised).	Small-pox.	Measles.	Scarlet Fever.	Diphtheria.	Whooping-cough.	Typhus.	Enteric (or Typhoid) Fever.	Simple continued Fever.	Diarrhœa.
West	668993	1	2	10	2	5	...	4	...	7
North ...	905677	5	4	16	1	8	...	13	...	4
Central ...	281793	...	...	5	4	2	...	7	2	5
East ...	692530	1	4	7	2	4	...	11	...	13
South ...	1265578	6	11	17	3	5	...	11	2	9
Total	3814571	13	21	55	12	24	...	46	4	38

METEOROLOGY.

From Observations at the Greenwich Observatory.

Mean height of barometer	30·037 in.
Mean temperature	47·1°
Highest point of thermometer	61·6°
Lowest point of thermometer	35·2°
Mean dew-point temperature	43·2°
General direction of wind	N.E.
Whole amount of rain in the week	0·69 in.

BIRTHS and DEATHS Registered and METEOROLOGY during the Week ending Saturday, Oct. 8, in the following large Towns :—

Cities and boroughs (Municipal boundaries except for London.)	Estimated Population to middle of the year 1881.*	Persons to an Acre. (1881.)	Births Registered during the week ending Oct. 8.	Deaths Registered during the week ending Oct. 8.	Temperature of Air (Fahr.) Highest during the Week.	Temperature of Air (Fahr.) Lowest during the Week.	Temperature of Air (Fahr.) Weekly Mean of the Highest and Lowest Daily Values.	Temp. of Air (Cent.) Weekly Mean of Daily Mean Values.	Rain Fall. In Inches.	Rain Fall. In Centimetres.
London	3529751	50·8	2468	1362	61·6	35·2	47·1	8·39	0·69	1·75
Brighton ...	107934	45·9	59	34	57·2	35·0	46·0	7·78	0·34	0·86
Portsmouth ...	128335	29·6	74	44	...	...	...	...	...	...
Norwich ...	88038	11·8	45	22	...	...	...	...	...	...
Plymouth ...	73262	54·0	47	24	59·9	35·2	48·6	9·23	0·22	0·56
Bristol ...	207140	48·5	143	49	61·0	32·5	46·2	7·89	0·37	0·94
Wolverhampton	75034	22·4	44	29	59·4	34·0	46·4	8·00	0·38	0·97
Birmingham ...	402296	47·9	284	133	...	...	...	...	...	...
Leicester ...	123120	38·5	96	41	...	...	...	...	...	...
Nottingham ...	188035	18·9	99	68	60·2	36·0	49·1	9·50	0·47	1·19
Liverpool ...	553988	106·3	412	243	59·7	39·2	49·1	9·50	0·31	0·79
Manchester ...	341289	79·5	250	143	...	...	...	...	...	...
Salford ...	177760	34·4	138	69	...	...	...	...	...	...
Oldham ...	112178	24·0	68	35	...	...	...	...	...	...
Bradford ...	184037	25·5	101	63	61·0	41·9	49·1	9·50	0·33	0·84
Leeds ...	310400	14·4	189	112	61·0	42·0	50·0	10·00	0·35	0·89
Sheffield ...	285621	14·5	210	100	59·0	41·0	48·2	9·00	0·40	1·02
Hull ...	155161	42·7	93	65	59·0	39·0	48·2	9·00	0·40	1·02
Sunderland ...	116755	42·2	92	39	...	...	...	...	0·40	1·02
Newcastle-on-Tyne	145675	27·1	116	69	...	...	...	...	...	...
Total of 20 large English Towns ...	7605775	38·0	5036	2739	61·6	32·5	43·0	8·69	0·39	0·99

* These figures are the numbers enumerated (but subject to revision) in April last, raised to the middle of 1881 by the addition of a quarter of a year's increase, calculated at the rate that prevailed between 1871 and 1881.

At the Royal Observatory, Greenwich, the mean reading of the barometer last week was 30·04 in. The highest reading was 30·32 in. on Friday morning, and the lowest 29·70 in. by the end of the week.

NOTES, QUERIES, AND REPLIES.

Be that questioneth much shall learn much.—Bacon.

A. P. T.—Apply to Sir W. Mac Cormac, Harley-street.

Archæologist asks for some information respecting the curious and remarkable seal recently found on Wash Common, the scene of the first Battle of Newbury, September 20, 1643, near the spot where the Falkland Memorial is erected. The seal, which is circular, is made of brass, measuring one inch and eight-tenths in diameter. It bears the device of a skeleton, with the surgeon's knife in the dexter hand, and an hour-glass on the sinister side. The legend with which it is inscribed is as follows :—"The . Sosciety . and . Loyalty . of . Chyrurgeons . Hall . London." It is supposed to have been used by the Serjeant-Surgeons, who always attended the king in person.

Banting.—Dr. Cheyne weighed in 1715 more than thirty stone, but afterwards, by changing his habits and living on milk and vegetables, reduced himself to less than half that weight.

Food Adulteration, Paris.—The report of the newly established Analytica Laboratory in Paris shows that out of 455 samples of wine purchased by the inspectors in the month of June, 318 were found to be adulterated. Out of 72 of cider, 16; of 180 of milk and cream, 123; of 19 of butter, 10—Not fewer than 48 of the 54 samples of spices analysed were condemned ; and the samples of chocolate and sweetmeats were scarcely more favourable.

Mr. Manning.—The celebrated Dr. Radcliffe left to St. Bartholomew's the yearly sum of £500 for ever towards "mending the patient's diet, and the further yearly sum of £100 for buying of linen."

Mad Dog.—No definite period has yet been fixed for the poison of hydrophobia to lie dormant in the system. The Council of the College of Physicians made it the subject for the Jacksonian Prize in 1810, when Mr. Boden, of Bath, carried it off ; and a special honorarium on the subject was awarded at the same time to Mr. Gillman, of Highgate. Mr. Chatto, the Librarian of the College, will no doubt show you the essay. Again in 1857 it formed the subject for the prize, but there was no award.

A Fellow.—When Wat Tyler was slain by Sir William Walworth his body was carried into St. Bartholomew's Hospital, and laid in the Master's Chamber.

Magisterial Leniency.—The Report of the Commissioners of Lunacy, just issued, discloses the leniency with which magistrates deal with cruelty to lunatics on the part of their keepers. The cases cited are, first, that of an attendant who had struck a patient on the head with his wand key with such violence as to inflict a wound "dividing the temporal artery and reaching the bone." For this offence he was simply fined by the Maidstone borough magistrates 40s. and costs. In another case, an attendant was convicted of having "grossly assaulted a patient," and fined 20s. and costs. No comment on these judicial sentences is made by the Commissioners.

Trees in Public Thoroughfares.—Dr. Vinen, Medical Officer of Health, has suggested to the St. Olave's Board of Works the desirability of planting trees in the widest part of Tooley-street, and of continuing them, as the new street is formed, through the district. They would not only be ornamental, but beneficial from a sanitary point of view. The matter was referred to a committee.

Vigilans.—The intention of the Committee of the Hulme Dispensary, Manchester, to establish a hospital for indoor patients as an adjunct to the dispensary, for which purpose they had secured premises in Moss-side, has not met with the success they hoped. The hospital scheme, however, is in suspense, and not abandoned.

J. Jenner N.—The total amount received by the bequest to Owens College, Manchester, of the late Mr. C. F. Bryer, of Gorton, who died in June, 1876, was £114,899 8s. 7d., thus—from the residuary estate £98,519 9s. 3d. in respect of capital, and £16,379 19s. 4d. in respect of income which had accrued since the death of the testator.

A Utopia.—A temperance colonisation society has been organised at Toronto, Canada, with the object of colonising a tract of land of about two millions of acres in the North-West Territory of the Dominion, with the proviso that no intoxicating liquors shall be introduced into the settlement.

Violating the Factory Acts.—At Sittingbourne Petty Sessions, Mr. J. A. Redgrave, sub-inspector under the Factory Acts, appeared in support of eight different complaints against a brickmaker for offences against the provisions of these Acts. The infringements were—neglecting to exhibit an abstract of the Acts, and to obtain certificates of fitness of children before employing them ; and employing children full time instead of half a day. Fined £5 3s. 3d.

A Memorial Rejected.—A memorial, signed by upwards of six thousand persons, in favour of re-acquiring Kingsland-green, has been presented by a deputation to the Hackney District Board of Works, but after some discussion that body declined to further entertain the matter, having already given it consideration.

New Baths, etc., Margate.—The Margate magistrates have granted a provisional licence for new buildings for baths, winter gardens, etc., being erected on the site of the old rink, at an estimated cost of £30,000.

The Welsh Sunday Closing Act.—Two conflicting decisions have been given with respect to this Act. At Hawarden the magistrates decided that the Act was in force, and accordingly fined the defendants; while the Swansea Bench ruled that the Act did not come into operation till the licensing meeting next year. But the latter case will probably rule the future decisions, as it appeared that the stipendiary magistrate had communicated with the Home Secretary, and through him had got counsel's opinion. That opinion was to the effect that the Act not having passed till August 27, it would not come into operation until the licensing-day of 1882.

Sanatorium, Torquay.—The Local Government Board has sanctioned a loan of £3000 for the purpose of erecting a sanatorium at Torquay.

Diphtheria, Russia.—A report issued by the local doctors states that 77 per cent. of the cases in the epidemic now raging in the province of Orel prove fatal.

Cheap Meat.—It is a noteworthy fact, that notwithstanding all the outcry that was raised concerning the failure of the Australian frozen meat imports, three weeks ago, the meat itself was sold by the ton, and purchased by the consumers. There were some wholesale dealers who were candid enough to admit that the quality of the cargo was superior to that of the average American meat. The chief difficulties in the way of making the abundant herds of Australia serve for food in this country would appear to be in a fair way of being overcome, and the cost of Australian beef will have an appreciable effect upon the present prices of English and American meat.

Health at Hampstead.—Dr. Gwynn, Medical Officer of Health to the Hampstead Vestry, in his annual report states that the death-rate of 1880 was 13·8 per 1000; that of London being 22·2.

Workhouse Infirmary Nurses.—There can be little doubt reform is needed in the nursing arrangements at many of the workhouse infirmaries. This subject came before the notice of the Woolwich Board of Guardians last week, on the appointment of a girl of twenty years of age as a nurse at the infirmary. One guardian protested against appointing such young persons to nurse the aged and sick poor. Another observed, " that the Woolwich Union Infirmary had become so notorious that no nurse would stop there. Week after week it was reported to the Board that 'Nurse So-and-so' had resigned, and they were really compelled to get whom they could."

Mortality, New York.—During the hot season the deaths in New York were almost unprecedented—nearly five thousand in excess, during the nine months of this year, of those in the same period last year; and the great majority ascribable to the excessive heat.

Proposed Association of Local Authorities.—A meeting of representatives of local boards has been held in Manchester for the purpose of considering the desirableness of forming an association of local boards. The objects of the proposed society were to meet at certain periods to consider matters affecting local boards generally, and to consider, if necessary, any Bills that may be brought before Parliament affecting local authorities. A resolution was carried—"That it is desirable to form an association of local boards, rural sanitary authorities, and improvement commissioners, within an area to be hereafter decided upon." A Committee was appointed to draw up a circular, embodying the results of the meeting, and to draft rules, etc., for the guidance of the association.

London Smoke.—It is computed that above ten millions of tons of coal are burned in London every year. Fifteen years ago the consumption was only six millions.

Electricity is Life?—Is the hobby ridden too hard? At the rate of the enclosed paragraph we may expect our medical schools to be closed in some future time, and our present race of medical students will become simply students of electricity and natural science. Anatomy, pathology, etc., will be relegated to the same limbo as alchemy and astrology in " the good time coming." Shall we, any of us, live to see it? Deranged, decaying, sluggish, or over-active vital processes may be duly regulated, and there is health and no physic. It is to be hoped our present race of doctors will by that time be independent of the change of fashion or treatment, or it may go badly for them :—

" We have been treated to a great deal of speculation as to the future uses to which electricity is to be put when we only know a little more about it and are a little better acquainted with its vagaries than we are at present. It appears, however, that none are to benefit so much by it as the agriculturists. No more artificial manures; no more carting of stuff on to the land: no horses required on a farm,—for electricity is to supply the place of everything. Every farmer has but to supply himself with a given number of reservoirs of electricity, according to the size of his farm and his special requirements, to have all he can want. Electricity will manure his fields; it will propel his carts, his ploughs, his harrows, and his market trap; it will drive his machinery for thrashing, grinding, pulping, chaffing, etc.; and when he desires to have two crops in the place of one, he has but to turn on his electric light at night and have two days instead of one. At least, so Professor Siemens told his audience at the last meeting of the British Association. Is there anything electricity cannot be made to perform? for a noted aëronaut said the other day electricity would enable man to fly."

APPOINTMENTS FOR THE WEEK.

October 15. Saturday (this day).

Operations at St. Bartholomew's, 1½ p.m.; King's College, 1½ p.m.; Royal Free, 2 p.m.; Royal London Ophthalmic, 11 a.m.; Royal Westminster Ophthalmic, 1½ p.m.; St. Thomas's, 1½ p.m.; London, 2 p.m.

17. Monday.

Operations at the Metropolitan Free, 2 p.m.; St. Mark's Hospital for Diseases of the Rectum, 2 p.m.; Royal London Ophthalmic, 11 a.m.; Royal Westminster Ophthalmic, 1½ p.m.

Medical Society of London, 8½ p.m. Address by the President (Dr. Broadbent). Mr. Thomas Bryant, "On a Case of Amputation for Knee-Joint Disease in a Man with Phthisis." Mr. Jonathan Hutchinson, "On Ulcers of the Tongue."

18. Tuesday.

Operations at Guy's, 1½ p.m.; Westminster, 2 p.m.; Royal London Ophthalmic, 11 a.m.; Royal Westminster Ophthalmic, 1½ p.m.; West London, 3 p.m.

Pathological Society, 8½ p.m. Specimens: Dr. R. E. Carrington—Fracture of the Base of the Skull and Cervical Spine. Dr. Stephen Mackenzie—Hæmato-Chilionia (living specimens); Filaria Sanguinis Hominis shown in Freshly-drawn Blood. Mr. Gay—Mammary Tumours, Recurrence. Dr. Fowler—1. Primary Cancer of Liver (card specimens); 2. Aneurism and Rupture of the Aorta; 3. Membranous Band in Left Auricle. Mr. Bryant—Cyst containing Oil removed from the Parotid Region of a Girl.

19. Wednesday.

Operations at University College, 2 p.m.; St. Mary's, 1½ p.m.; Middlesex, 1 p.m.; London, 2 p.m.; St. Bartholomew's, 1½ p.m.; Great Northern, 2 p.m.; Samaritan, 2½ p.m.; King's College (by Mr. Lister), 2 p.m.; Royal London Ophthalmic, 11 a.m.; Royal Westminster Ophthalmic, 1½ p.m.; St. Thomas's, 1½ p.m.; St. Peter's Hospital for Stone, 2 p.m.; National Orthopædic, Great Portland-street, 10 a.m.

20. Thursday.

Operations at St. George's, 1 p.m.; Central London Ophthalmic, 1 p.m.; Royal Orthopædic, 2 p.m.; University College, 2 p.m.; Royal London Ophthalmic, 11 a.m.; Royal Westminster Ophthalmic, 1½ p.m.; Hospital for Diseases of the Throat, 2 p.m.; Hospital for Women, 2 p.m.; Charing-cross, 2 p.m.; London, 2 p.m.; North-West, 2 p.m.

Harveian Society, 8½ p.m. Dr. Fothergill, "On Emulsionising of Fats."

21. Friday.

Operations at Central London Ophthalmic, 2 p.m.; Royal London Ophthalmic, 11 a.m.; South London Ophthalmic, 2 p.m.; Royal Westminster Ophthalmic, 1½ p.m.; St. George's (ophthalmic operations), 1½ p.m.; Guy's, 1½ p.m.; St. Thomas's (ophthalmic operations), 2 p.m.

AN ADDRESS
ON
SPECIALISM IN MEDICINE.

*Delivered before the Medical Society of University
College, London.*

By J. RUSSELL REYNOLDS, M.D., F.R.S.,
Consulting Physician to University College Hospital, etc.

THERE was a time when every man was his own doctor, priest, and lawyer; and, with a due or undue regard to himself and his immediate relatives, may have exercised the functions of those three professions to the entire satisfaction of himself and of those about him. But the age of perfect capacity to do everything has long since passed—if a man would pay due regard to anyone but himself; and yet it is not so very long since that I have seen persons who thought themselves able, not only to do all these things, but to command the Channel Fleet, or to correct telephonic apparatus with its last and newest improvements, if such delicate operations were only confided to their charge. But are such persons competent and sane? or are they self-important people, who are ignorant and crazy?

When knowledge was very small, people who thought that they possessed it were very great; when information is very great, and the means for acquiring it are also vast, the want of wisdom and the power to use it may make men very small.

Some departure from the primal condition of man soon became necessary; and yet, not many centuries ago, the "wise man," the "seer," the "priest," was the person to whom those about him would go if there was anything wrong in their mind, body, or estate; and it was mainly to the priest that such appeal was made. He was the man who could give help in the rough times; and he often did so well—giving counsel to those suffering with morbid thoughts, and medicines to those with upset bodies, and advice to those who did not know how to arrange about their neighbour's landmark; and also comforting those whose hearts were tired about the meaning of it all, and the ending of it all in some other world than this. He was the only man who knew anything outside his own daily routine of work; and so he was not only the parson or priest, but the doctor and the lawyer.

But what have we now? There are so many professions, and so many subdivisions of the work of each of them, that time would fail me to say anything of any other than our own. The priest, the doctor, and the lawyer, have been distinctly separated in the general nature and character of their several lines of work; and yet often they follow their respective callings hand in hand, and with mutual help. And it is with no disrespect to either profession that I say it is not outside the experience of some that the priest feels the pulse, and occasionally asks questions which he might have left unasked; and sometimes gives drugs, often of harmless "homœopathic" sort; but sometimes does things, and more often says them, which may be mischievous; and that the doctor goes outside his vocation in the matter of prayers and tracts; and that the lawyer does not always see the distinction that the clergyman sees in ritual or doctrine, or that the physician holds to be of importance in regard to public or domestic health. We know that it is so; but we might do well, perhaps, to regard these acts in the light of spasmodic activity of the organs left in a rudimentary state, in either one or the other, by the processes of differentiation, evolution, and specialism, that have brought us to the positions we now occupy. I draw a sharp and broad line between those three words and their outcome in modern present life. "Differentiation" means "division of labour"; "evolution" means its upward growth in utility to all; and "specialism" means its abuse.

With the expansion of human life, and the increasing complication of its requirements, division of labour becomes a necessity. The "simple cell," with its simple elements, may, as it does in some "low forms of organisation," as we

term them, do all that the cell needs to do. But some cells, looking equally simple, have within them powers that necessitate, for their real use, a differentiation of those powers; and so, out of a "primordial cell," with some appropriate materials and conditions, muscles, nerves, and the like are grown and rendered useful. And so it is with human life, and all its complex social arrangements. Some of the differentiated elements must do one thing, and some another; and so the "corporate body" (as it is sometimes called) of humanity requires this aid.

There would be simply waste of time if I were to say anything more about the entire necessity for division of labour. It would be waste of words for me to tell you, members of this "Medical Society"—for you must all know it quite well—that you cannot, every one of you, attain to the proficiency, in all of the several branches of your calling, to which others have attained by special work. You must be content, first of all, to master what is common to all, i.e., the knowledge that will fit you to undertake all the work that will come before you in after life—the common knowledge of facts and of principles, without which you can have no good ground from which to start in any "special" work that you may wish to do.

Next let me say a few words about "evolution." Your able Assistant Clinical Professor, Dr. Poore, said, in this theatre, a few days ago, in the admirable and wise address which I had the great pleasure of hearing, many weighty things, well worthy of your consideration, as to the meaning and use of words. Let me urge upon you to realise that which he said, and to see carefully to it that such words as "evolution" and "survival of the fittest" do not, in themselves, convey the whole of biologic or social science. Evolution does not involve in its primary meaning all the disturbing elements that may derange its processes, when these have been brought into it from outside by perverse activities of surrounding forces; nor does the phrase "survival of the fittest" distinctly convey to every mind an answer to the question: "Fittest" for what? When I used these words, a few moments ago, it was my intention to convey to your minds that which, in the progress of time, has to be observed and valued in our profession, viz., the progress from the lower to the higher ranges, from the simple to the complex; and, so far as individual work may make it so, the giving of the results which special labour could, or can, alone obtain, to those whose circumstances were such that they could not obtain this information for themselves. The results of their toil have often been given by these special workers to those who have no time nor opportunity for such direction of their industry; and they are of vast advantage to those who can use them well. By such mutual help all may derive advantage, and medical science may be carried, as it has been, to a higher stage of usefulness than that which it could otherwise have attained. But by the expression "survival of the fittest," it seems to me sometimes questionable whether or no that expression, unqualified, will express exactly what we mean by "professional progress" in any other sense than "progress of the individual." The response to the earnest feeling expressed in the words "Il faut vivre" may be perhaps answered now, as it was years ago, by "Je n'en vois pas la nécessité." In many instances, this division of work and this process of evolution have resolved themselves into "specialism"; and it is to that I wish now to direct your attention. It is, in my view, the wrong side of two right things and processes : the abuse of divided labour, and evolution of knowledge.

At the outset, let me remind you that there are thousands of members of our profession, practising in town and country life, who are absolutely free from the vice of "specialism"; but as absolutely dependent, if they do their work well, on the labours of the "specialists." All honour to them; their life is hard, and in the country beset with difficulties and risk to which the London or town practitioner is not exposed. The one has to undertake anything and everything, at a moment's notice; to treat apoplexy or pneumonia; to set a broken limb; encounter a case of placenta prævia; treat croup and diphtheria, cholera and chicken-pox; and to do this single-handed; and in the vast majority of instances he is equal to the occasion. In all sudden or acute maladies, he must do something before any outside help can come, and he must often do this promptly, and do it well. The practitioner in a town is equally liable to sudden calls and immediate responsibilities; but within ten minutes he can generally summon to his aid a professional brother to share his responsibility, or advise him from special knowledge as to what he should do, and so much mitigate his sense of care.

But if the country practitioner be thus well informed, and able to do his work, and to do it well, let me ask, In what way was he fitted for this work? And to this I answer, without hesitation, to the work of specialists, who have taught him, in the wards of hospitals, and in systematic lectures, and by their writings, what their special work has enabled them to teach, and which they could not, by any but the rarest gifts or the rarer accidents, have obtained in any other way. Other men have sown, and they have reaped or entered into their labours.

It is not possible that the courses of instruction that are given in this College and Hospital could have been made of any use to the general practitioner unless the teachers had already been taught by their own "special" devotion, or by that of others, to separate branches of inquiry, so numerous that life is by far too short for any one man, by his own industry, to acquire even a superficial knowledge of them all, or of a hundredth part of them. The results of years of labour are summed up by your teachers, and these fit you to undertake the work of life. These, in physiology, in medicine, and in surgery, are the outcome of special work, digested, sorted, and put forth into shape the most usable for those who have to learn.

But, when I speak of "specialism," the word carries us into a region quite other than that of helpful work—into that of miserable retrogression, instead of "evolution"—into that of the "survival," not of "the fittest," but of the charlatan and the quack. You may not know all or even much of this; and I hope that you never may, because there is a belief in my mind that specialism may die out. I may not live to see it; but you, many of you, will; for, foolish as people are, they are beginning to see through much of it, if not all.

But let me make one word of distinction between specialism and the adoration of great names. For the former, our profession is to blame; for the latter, the public. I have known distinguished surgeons go down into the country to say whether or no a patient with rheumatic fever had endo- or peri-carditis, when neither of them would know which end of the stethoscope to use. I have known physicians treating onychia or stone, and doing minor operations in surgery, for which, as the results proved, they were quite incompetent; but also men in both major branches of the profession who have declined to accept such responsibilities, and who referred the applicants for relief to those who could help them wisely and well. Great names will often override specialism; but, as I have said, this is due to the fault or ignorance of the public, and has its reward.

If you ask me what I mean by specialism, I should say: "It is a morbid condition of the mind—of physician or surgeon, as the case may be—which shows itself in his regarding every patient who comes under his care as a sufferer from the particular disease which he has studied; of seeing the symptoms only from the point of view which he has assumed, and made quite clear—to himself—and of treating it in a manner which no one like himself understands; and of treating it to the utmost degree of attention, frequency, and speciality of treatment that his patient's patience will endure."

It is well to classify "specialities" and their commonly attendant "specialisms," and this which is now proposed is a somewhat "natural order." First of all, the distinction between those who deal with men, women, and children; then, secondly, those who treat either of those groups of patients as sane, or insane; thirdly, those who divide certain parts of the human being upon a somewhat regional anatomico-physiological basis, and take as their fields for cultivation, nervous system, respiratory system, digestive system, and the like; fourthly, those who make particular diseased conditions, such as gout, fever, their line of study; fifthly, those who take special lines of work, such as medico-legal practice in courts of law.

1. *Men, Women, and Children.*—To what does specialism often lead? There are many surgeons in large cities who never, except by caprice, accident, mistake, or good nature, find a lady in their consulting-rooms. They have to treat what they find in the so-called "sterner sex," and their practice becomes somewhat closely confined to a particular class of maladies that most frequently arise from

irregular modes of life, of which many of them are ashamed. There are those who have chosen this speciality, and done what they have to do, with good to their patients, credit to their profession, and honour to themselves. But this cannot be said of all. Are there not some who prey upon the sense of shame, and extort money for needless operations and worthless drugs, holding in terror over their victims the knowledge of facts that have been confided to them, and using that knowledge, which is power, to benefit, not their patients, but themselves? Are there not undergraduates and others who dare not "call in the family doctor"? and are there not "potent, grave, and reverend seniors," who are just as anxious as their sons may be that nothing of their malady should be known at home?

The consulting-room—as sacred as the confessional—is degraded to the lowest depths of degradation when it is used, or abused, as the engine of terror and extortion. But yet debts are incurred, and bills are drawn, and Jews are sought for, aye, and Christians too, in order to meet the so-called "obligations" of these sufferers. The surgeon has the power in his hand, and he knows it, and wields it often with a cruelty that no words of mine can utter, or efficiently contemn.

The surgeon who resorts to no such baseness as this might, I think, in another way, be helped if, occasionally, he had some other things to do, and were, every now and then, consulted by some few of what is called the "softer sex," of pure life, and exalted character; some one of virgin soul, or matron dignity, who might break in upon the routine of daily practice, and teach, by their bearing and their anxiety, a higher lesson than that which is learned mainly in the chatter of the clubs. The surgeon becomes rough-and-ready, and there are hundreds to speak well of his skill; but often his roughness has risen to such point that men will say, "I cannot again see So-and-so, he is so outrageously rude and overbearing."

We know that there are a very large number of physicians, and a very small number of surgeons, who devote their lives to the treatment of women, and who do their work well; never shunting a duty, never over-stating a case, never condescending to anything in their practice that they would object to inspection by the *élite* of their professional brethren. They have studied, have learned, and have taught; and their lives are as valuable as they could wish them to be.

But we know that there are others of whom this cannot be said. Physicians have coined names for trifling maladies—if they have not invented them—and have "set fashions" of disease. They have treated, or maltreated, their patients by endless examinations, speculations, applications, and the like; and this sometimes for months, sometimes for years; and then, when by some so-called accident the patient has been removed from their care, she has become quite well, and then there has been no more need for caustic, speculum, or pessary.

The profession is not altogether to blame for this. Such is the want of education on physiological matters, that women do think and feel a great deal more about any "irregularities" of a certain kind than there is reason for them to think or feel. They attach an amount of importance to dysmenorrhœa entirely out of proportion to that which they render to dyspepsia; and tight-lacing and ball-dressing, and all that they involve, are disregarded, so long as these special functions are not disturbed. But when anything goes wrong in such way that the "lunar periods" are put out, then the specialist is consulted; and happy is it for them if the doctor himself does not suffer from specialism. If he does not, he treats the patient as she ought to be treated. If he does, too often he "makes a case" of it; and then follows the whole ritual of what I need not describe.

Some years ago *ulcerative uteri* was the fashion, and applications of various sorts were made two and three times a week in order to cure a malady which some eminent men, in special practice too, said did not exist. Lately I have rarely heard of this complaint; the disease has died a natural death, or has met with a violent end. But now, according to some authorities, there is scarcely any woman living whose uterus is where it ought to be. It is anteflexed, or retroflexed, or verted this way or that way, so that all kinds of contrivances have to be adjusted or readjusted in order to cure backache, vesical irritation, albuminuria, hysteria, and I know not what besides. Now, when this is all done by some one who knows with what he is dealing, and honestly deals with it, as many do, much good may be accomplished. But when imitators of the good workers take such cases in their hands, nothing but harm can follow. There is meddling and muddling of the most disreputable sort, and the patients after a time grow sick of it and give it all up, and get well; or they go on from bad to worse, and become chronic invalids, and a great trouble to themselves, their relations, and their friends.

There are the consulting-rooms of some doctors that are as they ought to be; there are others soothed by "a dim (can I say?) religious light," into which the patients are ushered, and in the dim silence of which all this kind of "treatment" goes on. And not only so, but in their own homes, patients are sometimes treated by—or shall I say to? —a vaginal injection of warm water, which the physician himself must administer.

This kind of thing is "specialism," and in one of its worst forms. It is the taking advantage of a natural solicitude on the part of women, and of their undue anxiety; and, instead of correcting it by steady purpose and common honesty—of pandering to the weakness of human nature, petting their patients into a feeble condition of dependence, and rendering them unfit for life in all its personal and domestic relations.

If some surgeons may be at fault in seeing life only as they read it in the clubs, surely some specialistic physicians are also to blame in looking at life only as they see it through a speculum; and it would be of advantage to them if they could occasionally have men for their patients, and so lose a little of that tendency to soft words and compliments in the use of which they are such conspicuous adepts.

There is not much that need be said about specialism with regard to children. They are virtually unsexed, and so do not fall into the hands of either of the classes of practitioners that I have mentioned. But it is quite possible for the man who deals solely, or even mainly, with children's diseases to take an exaggerated view of their differences from those with which adults may be afflicted, and so construct a pathology and a therapeutics which may be of disadvantage to the profession and of no real use to the child. Specialism can scarcely be said to exist here, unless it be in the physician sometimes taking upon himself the functions of the nurse, and seeing almost all things from a nursery point of view.

2. *Sane and Insane.*—The speciality of the physician who directs his attention mainly, or, it may be, even exclusively, to the charge of the insane, is a most direct advantage to the profession and the public; and this is demonstrated by the fact of its general recognition. This is true, however, only when the physician is at the same time competent to treat the other bodily ailments that may ramp themselves around the brain-disease with which he has primarily to deal.

The fault of "specialism," however, in this department is, that the so-called "mad-doctor" fails, sometimes, to see anything from a sane point of view. The *mens sana* is a myth to him, and he cannot bring himself to believe in its existence. He may think that it exists *in corpore sano* of his own possession, and in other *corpora* of his friends; but, beyond that narrow range, the sane mind is not to be found in those who are suffering from anything which may perturb the current of their thoughts. He may be right in regarding all people as somewhat mad, but he may be wrong in thinking that all men are so far mad as to require restraint.

There can be no doubt as to the fact that men and women have been in the past, and sometimes—but much more rarely—in the present, dealt with as insane, when they were simply incompetent, vacillating, eccentric, extravagant, or perverse. But, the mode in which "specialism" becomes mischievous in these physicians is this: that they have but one idea; and that is, that the patient must be secluded, or sent to an asylum to be treated; and the upshot of such advice often is that the patient is not "treated" in any other sense than that he or she is delivered over to the care of attendants, who are not always of the best-informed, the wisest, or the kindest sort.

The physician who is affected with "specialism," in regard to the insane, seems to take his stand upon the threshold of an asylum—half in, half out,—and, holding that to be the stand point for the observation of human life and human history, bases his creed with regard to both of them upon

the facts that lie behind him, and does not look, face-forward, into the world beyond.

3. *Regional Physiology.*—There are "specialisms" in regard of nervous system, of lung and heart systems, of digestive systems, and the like; and, with regard to them, I have but this to say: that the faults lie in the incompetency which many who have devoted themselves to one line of study often exhibit in their analysis and diagnosis of cases, into the complicated conditions of which their speciality of study has prevented them from entering.

Thus, I have known learned and distinguished "head doctors" speak of grievous palpitation of the heart as a merely nervous phenomenon, when the patient had dilated heart, with obvious valvular disease; of dyspnœa of very trying sort as a "nervous condition," when there were, in addition to dyspnœa, cough, expectoration, and the physical signs of emphysema, chronic bronchitis, dilated bronchi, and enfeebled heart; of short breathing described as "hysterical," when one-half of the chest was filled with fluid.

On the other hand, "heart and lung doctors" have failed to trace that anything was the matter, because the stethoscope could tell them nothing, when it was obvious that disease of the spinal marrow in some cases, and disease of the kidneys in others, was the cause of altered breathing.

Again, it has often been my lot to see "digestion doctors" worrying their patients with blue pill and elaterium, and bringing them to the verge of extinction from not having been able to discern that a diseased heart was the *fons et origo* of their sufferings.

4. *Special Diseases.*—With regard to these, "specialism" is sometimes more interesting and amusing than directly mischievous. There are consumption doctors, cancer doctors, gout doctors, and the like. If the former send their patients to the Riviera, or the uttermost parts of the earth, when it was unnecessary for them to make such pilgrimages, they, at least, have had the benefit of seeing new scenes, and sometimes of acquiring the knowledge of a foreign tongue. If "cancer doctors" have given, with grave looks and graver forebodings, a diagnosis and prognosis that may have been most distressing, yet sometimes tears have been turned into joy when the tumour has disappeared, and the cancer of the liver has turned out to be a gall-stone. If "gout doctors" have given their patients very wise instruction as to life and diet, they have been often rewarded by the extermination of "the fear of the evil" that the patient suffered from, and have found favour in their sight.

5. *Lines of Practice.*—The one illustration that I will give now is that of the "specialism" which affects many members of our profession when they are in the frequent habit of giving evidence in courts of law; and I will take for example that which happens in the case of railway accidents. It is pretty well known who, among the physicians and surgeons of the day, will be called upon for the plaintiffs, the injured, and who for the defendants, the company. So familiar in legal circles has this knowledge become, that the phrase, "So-and-so is a very rising witness" has been used, and not unfrequently. What does this mean but that members of our profession, whose only object should be truth and justice, "take sides"? Many years ago much of this came under my notice, and I alluded to it in some lectures which I had the honour to deliver before the College of Physicians; but for many years I have declined to take any part in such proceedings, owing to the manner in which evidence was given by what I must call "party witnesses."

It seems to me quite unpardonable that six or eight members of our profession should meet together, and go through the farce of a so-called "consultation," when neither one of the physicians or surgeons, on either side, would interchange a single word with one another. I have tried to break through this absurdity more than once, and sometimes have succeeded in my attempt. But more frequently I have failed, and have given it up; and this because I have heard said in courts of law such things as were so utterly unscientific, ignorant, or perverse, that it was simply impossible to deal with them. One instance will suffice. After rather understating a case of hemiplegia, the result of accident, it was urged, "on the other side," by an eminent surgeon, that the man was shamming because, forsooth, he did not exhibit ptosis, strabismus, and dilated pupil, and that he had never seen a case of hemiplegia in which those three things did not co-exist.

There are some members of our profession who have

become specialists in this direction, who seem to think that everything that a man tells them of his subjective symptoms are matters of fact and of great importance; and, on the other hand, there are those who regard every plaintiff as either a knave or a fool, and most probably a combination of the two, but who never believe that any man is injured in a railway accident unless he has broken his neck or has a compound fracture of his thigh.

It is time that this specialism should come to an end; and we of our profession can bring it to an end, if we will but insist upon it that the meeting together of the doctors is a consultation, and not a farce.

There are many other points upon which I should have liked to speak to you, of the specialisms that have so limited an area that it is quite impossible for any man who is restricted to any one of them to make a large income, unless he does so by inducing his patients to pay him needless visits; such, for example, as to touch his throat with something every day, to turn the screw on his "instrument for the back" two or three times a week, or to do something to the Eustachian tube with equal frequency. But what I have said is enough to guard you, I hope, from falling into these mistakes, these "worse than crimes, these blunders."

In conclusion, let me revert to an illustration used at the outset, with regard to what "differentiation" means—viz., the springing into being of varied structures, with their varied uses, and of their development into the being of a perfect whole—a living thing, with complex powers—all its parts subservient to the ends for which they were intended, and for which they are so ordained as to conduce to the "survival of the fittest." But let me carry the illustration yet farther, and say that all these different members are members one of another, and that when any member suffers all the other members suffer with it; and that, when any physician or surgeon does that which is ignoble, he not only does injury to himself, but to the whole of the noble profession to which he belongs.

MEDICAL WOMEN IN BOSTON.—At a meeting of the Suffolk Medical Society, where Dr. Bowditch proposed resolutions censuring Harvard University for refusing to furnish medical instruction to women, and the Massachusetts Medical Society for refusing to admit them as members, it was stated that there were now more than a hundred women engaged in the practice of medicine in the city of Boston alone, this being more than one-eighth of the entire number of all the various professors of medicine. " At present," said one of the speakers, " we are practically driving every woman who would be a physician into quackery. A large number of the students of the Boston (Homœopathic) University are women, not because they desire to be homœopaths, but because it is the one place where woman is welcome to a free rivalry in medical study." The resolutions proposed by Dr. Bowditch were negatived.—*Boston Med. Jour.*

SUDDEN DEATH AFTER FRACTURE OF THE LEG.—In one of his clinical lectures (*Gaz. Hop.*, No. 86), Prof. Verneuil referred to the case of a man sixty years of age, strong, robust, and tall, who had been in hospital for two months and a half for the fracture of both bones of the leg. He was treated as usual, had exhibited no bad symptoms whatever, and in fact was just about to be sent to a convalescent hospital prior to dismissal, when (the only thing that had excited attention having been some alteration in his features) he suddenly died, his face having a violaceous aspect. Prof. Verneuil believed that this must have occurred from embolism, which is not very rare after fracture. It is produced by thrombosis of some of the veins in the vicinity of the fractured bone, which is the cause of the œdema that so commonly accompanies fracture of the leg. Through a sudden movement or muscular effort, one of the clots which have thus formed in the inferior vein, and which are usually not very adherent, may become detached, and, entering the femoral and iliac veins, and eventually reaching and obstructing one of the branches or the bifurcation of the pulmonary artery, give rise to sudden death, as in asphyxia. However, in this case the diagnosis was erroneous, for the most careful examination of all the veins and the pulmonary arteries failed to show the existence of any clot. The heart was absolutely empty, and the brain, minutely examined, exhibited no disease.

ORIGINAL COMMUNICATIONS.

A CASE OF POISONING BY RESORCIN.

By WILLIAM MURRELL, M.D., M.R.C.P.,

Lecturer on Materia Medica and Therapeutics at the Westminster Hospital; Senior-Assistant Physician at the Royal Hospital for Diseases of the Chest.

ATTENTION has of late been directed to this new drug by the publication of papers on its physiological action by Dr. Julius Andeer of Würzburg, Professor Lichtheim of Berne, Dr. Dujardin-Beaumetz of Paris, Dr. Callais, and others.

Resorcin, resorcenal, or metadioxylbenzene ($C^6H^4H^2O$) is a compound isomeric with hydrochinon, a substance recently introduced by Brieger as an antipyretic. It was discovered in 1864 by Hlasewetz and Barth,(a) who obtained it by fusing galbanum resin with potash. They named it resorcin(b) partly because it was procured from a resin, and partly from its analogy to orcin, which had been extracted in 1829, by Robiquet, from lichens. It is also formed by the action of potash on assafœtida, ammoniacum, sagapenum, and acaroid resins. Umbelliforine and brazilin also yield it when similarly treated. Körner(c) has prepared it synthetically, and it is frequently obtained as an intermediate product in the manufacture of eosine.

Commercial resorcin is red in colour, and has a strong smell resembling carbolic acid. Pure resorcin, which alone should be used for medicinal purposes, is met with in beautiful white feathery crystals, having very little odour, but a sweet pungent taste. It is freely soluble in alcohol, ether, glycerine, and vaseline, but is insoluble in chloroform and bi-sulphide of carbon. It has a neutral reaction, and burns with a bright flame. Its solutions give with perchloride of iron a deep violet colour, and with fuming sulphuric acid a yellowish orange tint. It forms a white precipitate in albuminous fluids, the precipitate being probably an albuminate of resorcin.

The observations of Andeer(d) and Brieger, and more especially the experiments of Dujardin-Beaumetz and Callais,(e) have shown that it arrests almost all forms of fermentation, and that it is a powerful antiseptic. For surgical purposes it presents many advantages over carbolic acid; it is probably less poisonous, less irritating; is almost odourless, and is very soluble in water.

In rabbits, dogs, and other animals it exerts a powerful action on the nervous centres, producing epileptiform convulsions. The respiratory movements become superficial and very rapid, and usually the heart continues beating for some time after breathing has ceased. Dujardin-Beaumetz and Callais frequently noticed a considerable elevation of temperature in rabbits which had received a toxic dose.

Its action on man has as yet been but little studied. The ordinary dose is said to be from one-half to three grammes, but more may be given. Lichtheim(f) found that after the administration of a full dose there occurred giddiness and buzzing in the ears, the face became flushed, the eyes brighter than before, the breathing quickened, the pulse more frequent by several beats and generally somewhat irregular. In from ten to fifteen minutes after the dose had been taken, the skin became moist, and a few moments later the whole body would be bathed in perspiration. He found that it reduced the temperature in fever-free patients by five or six degrees Fahr., and from this he was induced to employ it as an antipyretic. When given in large doses it often induces symptoms of intoxication, with illusions and moaning respiration, but—and he especially refers to the fact—no symptoms of collapse were ever noticed, either during or after its administration. Andeer, on one occasion, took ten grammes of resorcin in 250 grammes of water. In fifteen minutes he lost consciousness, and was seized with epileptiform convulsions. He recovered in five hours.

(a) " Annal. Chem. und Phar.," pages 130, 354.
(b) Flückiger and Hanbury, "Pharmacographia," 1879, page 318.
(c) *Comptes-Rendus*, pages 63, 564.
(d) " Einleitende Studien über das Resorcin zur Einführung in die praktische Medicin," von Dr. Justus Andeer, Würzburg, 1880.
(e) *Bulletin-Général de Thérapeutique*, Bulletins des 15 et 30 Juillet.
(f) *Correspondenzblatt für Schweizer Aerzte*, July 15, 1880.

Therapeutically, resorcin has been employed in the treatment of acute rheumatism, ague, and typhoid fever, and for the reduction of the temperature of phthisis. In the form of spray or powder it has been used in diphtheria, and is said to be a good dressing for syphilitic and other sores.

My own experience of resorcin is very limited, but the symptoms produced in one case by an overdose were so marked, that I think it only right to publish it. From a consideration of its physiological action I was in hopes that the drug might do good in asthma, and, having an obstinate case under treatment, I determined to give it a trial. The patient, a young woman of nineteen, had suffered from spasmodic asthma for two years, and had been under treatment for eighteen months. Her attacks usually came on once or twice a week, but sometimes oftener. They lasted sometimes only five or six hours, but not uncommonly a couple of days. In the intervals she was perfectly well and had no cough. On physical examination of the chest a little emphysema was detected, but nothing more. She was not febrile, her temperature for three weeks varying from 97·6° to 99·4°. She had received a great deal of treatment, including arsenic, belladonna, ipecacuanha, lobelia, iodide of potassium, citrate of caffeine, stramonium and datura tatula, jaborandi and pilocarpine, Jamaica dogwood, quebracho and its alkaloid, nitrite of amyl, nitro-glycerine, iodide of ethyl, pure terebene, hypodermic injections of morphia and atropia, nitre papers and tablets, cubebs cigarettes, Himrod's and the Green Mountain powder and sprays, and inhalations of all kinds. In addition, she had been carefully dieted, and change of air had been tried. Nothing seemed to do her much good, with the exception of a particular American preparation of *Grindelia robusta*, which, although it succeeded admirably for a time, ultimately lost its effect. At last it was determined to try resorcin. Accordingly, after a few preliminary observations with smaller doses, she was given during a severe paroxysm half a drachm in a little milk. She experienced no difficulty in taking it; her breathing became easier almost at once; and in half an hour she fell asleep, sleeping comfortably for three hours, when she awoke free from shortness of breath. The urine passed on the following day was of an olive-green colour, as if carbolic acid had been taken. The same dose was given on two other occasions during a paroxysm, but failed to give relief. The dose was then increased to a drachm. Immediately on taking the powder, which was given in a little milk, she experienced a decided sensation of giddiness; this was followed almost immediately by heaviness over the eyes and drowsiness, the dyspnœa was relieved, and in a quarter of an hour she was fast asleep. This was tried on four different occasions, and always with the same result. The pupils were not affected, there was no diplopia and no tinnitus aurium. The action on the urine was more marked with the larger dose. She generally perspired freely during her attacks, but still the resorcin seemed to act as a diaphoretic. She was satisfied that the powder eased the breath, but she postponed taking them as long as possible on account of the giddiness they produced.

The dose was now increased to a drachm and a half without the production of symptoms other than those already mentioned.

On the morning of Sunday, December 5, at about half-past five, she was found to be suffering from one of her usual asthmatic attacks. At seven she was given two drachms of resorcin in a little milk. Almost immediately, as she subsequently told us, it flew to her head, and she felt giddy and had "pins and needles" all over. In a few minutes she became insensible, and was found lying on her side with closed eyes and clenched hands, faintly moaning. She had not been sick, but was bathed in profuse perspiration and was very cold. Dr. Jessop was at once sent for, and at 7.10 found her in the following condition:—"Insensible; in a profuse perspiration from head to foot; groaning; pallid, lips blanched; tongue dry; no foaming at the mouth or smell in the breath; pupils equal, normal; conjunctive insensible to touch; teeth clenched; skin cold and clammy, and temperature evidently low. No facial paralysis; no paralysis of mouth or œsophagus; pulse imperceptible at the radials; chest-walls almost motionless. On stethoscopic examination, very little air was found to be entering the lungs; no rhonchus; heart-sounds very faint, and heard with difficulty—no distinction between first and second sounds. Abdomen not distended; walls flaccid. No

than legs; total absence of reflex action on tickling foot; no patellar reflex; no tetanus; no spasm, either tonic or clonic." Dr. Jessop, realising the urgency of the case, forced open her mouth, and poured down about two ounces of olive oil. He then applied the stomach-pump, and in a few minutes the stomach was emptied and thoroughly washed out with tepid water. He next injected a scruple of sulphate of zinc and a drachm of mustard, and the patient vomited slightly. She was flicked with a wet towel, and an endeavour was made to get her to walk, but she was found to be absolutely powerless. The pulse at the radials was now weak and thready, and the temperature in the axilla was only 94°. In a few minutes the breathing improved, and the conjunctive were found to be slightly sensitive. The extremities were still cold and sweating. From half-past seven to eight, patient was gradually coming round, and could answer in monosyllables, although she seemed hardly to understand what was said to her. The axillary temperature was now 95°. At eight the feet were warmer, consciousness was returning, and the pulse under the influence of brandy became stronger. At half-past eight she was given an inhalation of nitrite of amyl; the temperature was 96°, and it gradually rose to the normal. At a quarter to nine she was conscious, and we were satisfied that she was out of danger. At 11 a.m. the temperature was 99°; at 3 p.m., 102·2°; at 6 p.m., 100·4°. On the following and subsequent days it was normal. There was never, at any time, ptosis, strabismus, or salivation. The first urine passed presented the usual olive-green colour, but this disappeared in about twenty-four hours. There was no action of the bowels.

At first I was somewhat puzzled to account for the severity of the symptoms, but the explanation is simple. Until the administration of the last dose we had been using an impure resorcin. The two-drachm dose was given from a fresh specimen which was much purer than that at first used. The first sample was dark in colour, stained the paper in which it was kept, lost about two-thirds of its weight on exposure to the air, and was undoubtedly contaminated with carbolic acid. The second specimen was lighter in colour, was quite dry, and almost free from carbolic acid smell. It was understood that it was prepared by the action of sulphuric acid on benzine vapour. It was not absolutely pure, but probably contained not more than 2 or 3 per cent. of impurity.

The symptoms developed in this case present several points of interest. The general resemblance to poisoning by carbolic acid is very apparent. The cold sweats, stupor deepening rapidly into collapse, with complete abolition of sensory and reflex movement, are noteworthy. The fall of temperature is very remarkable. The condition of the urine is also noticeable. It is difficult, without further experiments on the lower animals, to say exactly how resorcin acts, but it is undoubtedly a cardiac depressant, and probably exerts, in addition, a direct action on all the organs involved. Respecting the treatment adopted by Dr. Jessop, it may be said that it was the best that could possibly have been employed. The olive oil probably prevented further absorption until the stomach was emptied by the stomach-pump. In poisoning by carbolic acid, the exhibition of alkalies in solution and in large excess has been recommended, and Baumann and Sonnenburg have suggested the use of sulphate of sodium as an antidote. Should the condition of collapse continue, it would be advisable to administer a hypodermic injection of atropia. Dr. Andeer considers that albuminate of iron and red wine are the best antidotes in resorcin-poisoning. What is the largest dose of pure resorcin that may be given with safety, I am not prepared to say, but I have often given forty grains every four hours without the production of any unpleasant symptom.

LEUCORRHŒA OF CHILDREN.—Dr. Bouchut treats this first by frequent washings with bran water, Goulard water, or walnut-leaves water, and then by touching the mucous membrane of the vagina with a solution composed either of 10 centigrammes of corrosive sublimate to 300 grammes of water, or of 20 centigrammes of nitrate of silver to 30 grammes of water. Charpie, imbibed with antiseptic substances, is placed between the labia, and tonics and anti-diathesic

ON PROLAPSE OF THE OVARIES.

By G. ERNEST HERMAN, M.B. Lond.,

Assistant Obstetric Physician to the London Hospital ; Physician
to the Royal Maternity Charity ; Honorary Librarian
to the Obstetrical Society of London.

(Concluded from page 462.)

I WILL now offer some remarks on the points which these cases suggest. First, as to the *causes* of prolapse of the healthy ovary. It seems to me, in most cases, a gradual process, brought about, like most displacements of the uterus, by conditions which favour yielding of the pelvic floor. These conditions are of two kinds—those which weaken the pelvic floor (such as child-bearing and long-standing vaginal catarrh), and those which increase the pressure upon it (such as the frequent and prolonged straining at stool consequent upon constipation. Dr. Goodell, in the discussion of Dr. Mundé's paper, is reported to have said, " I have observed that in a majority of cases this dislocation occurs in lean persons, persons with lax fibre, and with the retentive power of the abdomen much weakened by the loss of fat." My own experience is quite in accord with Dr. Goodell's statement. Although my patients are all stated to have been well nourished, yet none of them were fat ; and I think that, had I inquired minutely into the point, I should have found that each of them considered herself thinner than she had been. It is said that sudden concussions of the body, as in falls, etc., may produce this displacement of the ovary. This is possible, but cases so produced are rare. I have seen one case in which urgent symptoms were supposed to have been the result of a sudden dislocation of the ovary, but they had all passed off when my attention was called to the patient, and the case had not been at all closely investigated. It is also stated that the ovary may be pushed down by tumours—uterine fibroids, fæcal accumulations, etc. This must be very rare. Dr. Mundé, however, narrates a case in which the ovary was, in his opinion, pushed down by a tumour of the kidney.

Next, the *symptoms*. All these cases had in common two symptoms, which were very pronounced, and for the treatment of which they presented themselves. These were, pain on defæcation and on sexual intercourse. The mode in which these symptoms are produced will be too obvious to need elucidation. The pain in defæcation was always associated with constipation. The two kinds of pain were said to resemble one another. The pain was of considerable duration, lasting some time after the cause which occasioned it—according to one patient nearly an hour, according to another two or three hours ; and it was by some said to be accompanied with nausea and faintness. Some of the patients had other symptoms, but these were comparatively trifling, and were such as are commonly found along with slight degrees of prolapse—"bearing-down," irritability of bladder, etc. But except these minor troubles, these patients had nothing whatever to complain of, and felt perfectly well in the intervals between the events which occasioned pain. It is in this that the important distinction appears to me to lie between prolapse of a normal ovary, and similar displacement associated with oöphoritis. With the latter condition the pain is more or less constant ; the patient is scarcely ever free from pain, and her suffering is aggravated by the menstrual period, as well as by the functions referred to. The distinction between these two kinds of cases is important, not merely for the ascertaining what is the effect of displacement, but for prognosis.

I have spoken of these cases as being instances of prolapse of healthy ovaries. It may be asserted, in objection to this, that healthy ovaries are not tender ; that tenderness is proof of disease ; and that my cases are specimens of ovaritis with descent. This objection I see no way of completely disproving. It is impossible to say that there may not be many women whose ovaries are prolapsed, but are not tender, and cause no symptoms ; for such patients would not seek advice, and the condition of the female pelvic organs cannot be explored in the routine way that the lungs or eyes can be examined. Again, the disease not being fatal, it is only accidentally, so to speak, that we can expect the opportunity of examining the condition of the organ anatomically, and ascertaining whether there is evidence of inflammation or not. If tenderness be proof of inflammation, then there is ovaritis in these cases. Without entering here upon a discussion of the clinical phenomena which indicate ovaritis, I may simply say that I do not regard tenderness alone as enough to prove its existence ; and I think that the *onus probandi* of showing that in cases such as these inflammation is present lies upon those who affirm it. I do not say that it is certain that inflammation was in these cases absent, but merely that there is not sufficient evidence of its presence.

I think it unnecessary to discuss the point, because it is not here of practical importance. We have here a group of cases in which the symptoms are such as entirely depend upon an altered position of the ovary—i.e., that were this body in its usual place, out of the way of contact, there would be no symptoms. Further, they can be relieved by treatment of a definite and simple kind. Whatever name we choose to give to the changes present, I think it desirable to separate these cases from those in which the symptoms are not so evidently dependent upon the change in position, and are not so easily relieved by treatment. The cases I have described are *the simplest cases in which prolapse of the ovary calls for treatment,* and as such they deserve recognition and separation.

The physical signs are easily made out. The patient complains of dyspareunia and dyschezia. There is no tenderness, nor anything abnormal, about either anus or vaginal orifice. Per vaginam, the uterus is movable, and natural as to size, shape, and position. But behind, and a little to the side of the uterus, a movable body is felt, of about the size and shape of an almond, which is very tender. When the finger presses this body the patient at once complains, and when questioned says that the pain produced by such pressure is like the pain from which she suffers. Any doubt which may exist will be cleared up by an examination per rectum, by which the same body will be felt, but of course in front of the bowel. If the abdominal walls are very thin and loose, and the examiner expert at examining the pelvic organs bimanually, he may be able to feel the ligament of the ovary, and the Fallopian tube as a cord running from the corresponding corner of the fundus uteri to this little tumour. But even without this, the diagnosis will be pretty certain.

The *treatment* is simple. The pain in defæcation is due to the pressure of descending scybala upon the ovary. The treatment is therefore to prevent the formation of scybala, by at least keeping the bowels regular, or still better, by making them slightly loose. When this is done, the pain in defæcation is either no longer felt, or at least greatly lessened. By getting the bowels to act regularly we not only thus get rid of a cause of pain, but remove a powerful agent in the production and maintenance of the prolapse ; for the straining to empty the rectum, and the passage of the fæcal masses downwards, must tend to force the ovaries lower down each time the patient goes to stool. For regulating the bowels in these cases, saline aperients are best, because they produce soft or fluid evacuations. None of these are better than sulphate of magnesia. To prevent the discomfort caused by its violent action, and yet to get a sufficient effect, the best way is to give it in small doses, frequently repeated—*e.g.*, 5ss.–3j. three times a day. The dyspareunia was relieved in all these cases of mine by the use of a thick elastic ring made of watch-spring covered with india-rubber. This produces benefit, I think, in two ways ; partly by pushing up and supporting the prolapsed ovary, and partly by occupying the vagina, and so protecting the tender part from contact. There are two inconveniences which these rings are apt to cause : First, all india-rubber instruments form with the vaginal secretions an exceedingly ill-smelling compound, which may be so irritating as to lead to a slight degree of vaginitis. This happened in the second case. It is to be avoided by cleanliness. The patient who is wearing any india-rubber instrument should frequently syringe the vagina with cold or tepid water. The second is, that not having, like a Hodge's pessary, a posterior curve upwards, the part of the pessary which lies behind projects slightly into the rectum, and if the motions should be large and hard, there may arise pain and difficulty in defæcation, and the ring may even be forced out during the efforts at expulsion of the fæces. This inconvenience will not arise if the bowels be kept regular and the motions soft.

The measures described may, however, be disparaged on the ground that they are only palliative, and that the object to be aimed at in treatment is not merely to relieve symptoms, but to put the ovaries in their proper position and keep them there. Can this be done? For if it can, it is proper to do it. It has, I am told, been recommended to push up the ovary every day with the finger—a manipulation which is perfectly useless, and therefore objectionable. Dr. Mundé recommends putting the patient in the knee-elbow position and then letting the vagina become distended with air, for, when this is done, the anterior wall of the vagina, with the uterus and ovaries, will fall forwards. Often, Dr. Mundé says, the displacement will not return, and, if it should do so, it may again be redressed by the same manœuvre. In a case in which the prolapse is recent, and the result of some transitory cause, I can quite imagine that simple reposition in this manner may effect a complete and permanent cure. But where (as in the majority of cases) the displacement depends upon a general yielding of the parts by which the ovary is naturally supported, I have found it to return when the patient reassumed a more usual position. Dr. Mundé has given much attention to the construction of pessaries for keeping up the ovary, and therefore it is evident that he has met with many cases in which simple replacement of the ovary was not enough. Dr. Mundé's pessaries are modifications of Hodge's. This pessary, by raising and anteverting the uterus, may lift the ovaries upwards by means of their attachment to that organ. But if this is not accomplished, the pressure of the hard rigid bar of the Hodge's pessary will make the patient worse. Dr. Mundé's modifications, which consist in skilfully shaping the posterior end of the instrument so as to avoid pressure on the ovary, may be adequate to prevent this. But it is difficult and troublesome so to fit a pessary, and it is possible that the patient may get tired of experiments in this direction before the proper shape has been hit upon; and when the result attained at last is no better than is secured by a simple elastic ring, the trouble seems to me scarcely worth taking. The measures I have recommended are equally suitable if the ovary be inflamed; other treatment may be required in addition; but laxatives, and the support of a thick elastic ring, will not do harm, but the reverse. An ill-fitting Hodge's pessary may, on the contrary, do mischief.

The only part of the subject that remains to be spoken of is the prognosis. This has to be considered in respect of two alternative conditions: first, what will happen if the patient be let alone; and second, what will be the result of treatment. As to the course of these cases, if they are left without treatment, I cannot speak with the certainty to be derived from watching a number of cases. But, judging from the length of time these patients had been ill before they came to me, and from the fact that those who were at first treated in ignorance of the cause of their symptoms did not get well until measures were directed to the relief of the local suffering, I do not think that this disease tends, as a rule, to spontaneous recovery. Next, as to the effect of treatment, which is usually satisfactory. In this, as in every disease, we cannot predict the effect of remedial measures unless the diagnosis has been accurately made. If the case be simply one of prolapse of the normal ovaries, then the treatment described will be followed by relief to the symptoms. But before promising such benefit, it is needful to be sure that oöphoritis is not present. If the patient be in pain at all times, and not simply when the causes which have been mentioned come into operation, or if she have great suffering at the menstrual period, then the prognosis should be guarded. Although relief may be given in these, it will not be so complete, nor will the treatment be so simple.

There are many questions arising out of this subject to which I have not referred, some of them being the subjects of controversy, and others being unimportant. I have endeavoured simply to trace the broad outlines of the subject—the characteristic symptoms, and the important points in treatment; and I think that anyone who may meet with a case of the kind, and will apply what I have said, will find that his experience will confirm my statements.

NITRITE OF AMYL IN CHORDEE.—This will be found a very effectual remedy in chordee and painful priapism. Three to five drops by inhalation is the proper dose.—New York Med. Record, September 24.

REPORTS OF HOSPITAL PRACTICE
IN
MEDICINE AND SURGERY.
—
UNIVERSITY COLLEGE HOSPITAL.

LARGE LABIAL (INGUINAL) HERNIA—RADICAL CURE.
(Under the care of Mr. RICKMAN GODLEE.)

SUSAN L., aged fifty-seven, was admitted into University College Hospital, under the care of Mr. Godlee, on March 26, 1881. About thirty-three years ago she found a small protrusion at the external abdominal ring, which remained quite stationary for some five years. It then began to increase in size until two years ago, when it suddenly came down into the labium as a very large swelling. It was reduced with some difficulty by the medical attendant who was called in. There was great pain while it remained down. She has attended at several other hospitals, but has not succeeded in keeping the hernia up at all.

State on Admission.—There is, on the left side, an inguinal hernia, occupying the labium majus, as large as a child's head; there is direct impulse on coughing; and the hernia is easily reducible. There was a slight inguinal hernia upon the opposite side. The patient was thin, and old for her age.

March 30.—The patient being under ether, Mr. Godlee, after having reduced the hernia, which was retained within the abdomen by the hand of an assistant, made an incision, three inches long, over the external ring, by transfixing the pinched-up skin; he then dissected down on to the sac, and separated it from the surrounding structures. The sac was then dragged out of the labium, and was opened; the finger was passed into the inguinal canal, to make sure that all intestine had been reduced, after which the sac was sewn across, just external to the external abdominal ring, by several overlapping but disconnected sutures of fine catgut; the portion of the sac beyond the line of sutures was next cut off. The pillars of the external ring were then approximated with six stout catgut sutures, the two upper of which passed through the stump of the sac. A drainage-tube was next inserted, which reached to the bottom of the labium, and the wound was stitched up. The strictest antiseptic precautions were used throughout.

31st.—Re-dressed. There was very little discharge; it consisted of blood and serum. The labium contained some blood. Patient has vomited several times. At 2 a.m. an enema of starch and opium was given to check some diarrhœa, the result of treatment before operation, but this was not retained. A dose of opium was given by the mouth. She complained of pain in the abdomen; it was confined to the neighbourhood of the wound. Tongue moist and fairly clean. Pulse 54, intermittent; temperature 100°. A soft catheter was ordered to be passed every six hours. Temperature in the evening 101·6°.

April 1.—She passed a good night. The vomiting has ceased; her bowels have not acted. Tongue clean. Temperature 101·8°; pulse 80, very intermitting. On re-dressing the wound, the labium appeared as if distended with blood. The discharge from the wound was odourless, but blood-stained; drainage-tube taken out, cleaned, and cut shorter. There was slight fulness and some tenderness in the left iliac fossa, but none elsewhere.

6th.—Patient has gone on well since last note. The wound has been dressed antiseptically as usual. Temperature has fallen almost to the normal; and the general condition has been good. To-day there was a good deal of bloody discharge from the labium; it was quite free from odour, and, on examination of the fluid, stained with aniline violet, it was ascertained that no bacteria were present. The labium was aspirated, and about four ounces of a treacly, port-wine-like fluid were withdrawn. There was a puffy swelling above the iliac crest, due to effused blood.

7th.—Labium as full as ever.

9th.—Mr. Godlee incised the labium, and let out the effused blood.

15th.—The labium is now like a loose bag of skin, except at its lowest part, where there is a firm mass (? a clot). Temperature normal.

29th.—Some sloughing has been taking place in the wound during the last few days, and the patient's general condition is less satisfactory. Temperature 103°; pulse 104. She has not taken her food so well, and has complained of a feeling of chilliness. This high temperature came on suddenly, and only lasted two days. It did not appear to be due to the condition of the wound.

May 6.—The slough is separating, and the wound looks healthier. It is to be syringed out with equal parts of carbolic lotion (one to twenty) and solution of copper sulphate (gr. viij. to 3j.).

29th.—The wound has almost healed; it is to be dressed with boracic lint.

June 11.—Patient was discharged.

Remarks (by Mr. Godlee).—I consider that in this case the operation was indicated by the fact that the hernia was of great size, and also because, after repeated and careful attempts, it was found quite impossible to retain it by any truss that we could devise; the condition of things, moreover, was not only a source of great inconvenience to the patient, but of considerable pain, so that she was disabled from following her usual occupation. I also thought I was justified in doing it, as I considered that by the strict adoption of antiseptic measures any question of danger to life might be eliminated. A serious cause of inconvenience afterwards was the accumulation of blood in the labium, and it seems probable that the constant leakage through the wound had a good deal to do with the slowness of healing. I avoided making a puncture at the lower part of the labium, which would, no doubt, have prevented this inconvenience, as an opening so low down might have endangered the antiseptic element of the case. That no putrefaction did occur was proved by the microscopic examination of the blood which was removed by the aspirator. The slowness of healing previously referred to was a noteworthy feature of the case. Some sloughing, probably of part of the aponeurosis of the external oblique, occurred, and the separation of the sloughs was very tedious; but even after these had been completely removed the wound remained in a most indolent condition. At last, however, complete cicatrisation took place, and the patient was allowed to go about with a double truss, it being considered unwise to try experimentally at present whether or no a sufficiently good cure had been obtained to enable her to dispense with all artificial support. It is hardly to be expected, indeed, that it will ever be thought wise to give it up; but as it is, the relief obtained is, I think, more than sufficient to justify the operation.

CONGENITAL DISLOCATION OF THE FEMUR.—Dr. Pravas, the Director of the Lyons Orthopædic Institution, in a communication to the Lyons Société des Sciences Médicales (Lyon Méd., July 31), states that between 1863 and 1878 he had under his care 125 cases of congenital dislocation of the femur, and in 107 of these cases he has noted the facts of whether the dislocation was double or single, and the sex of the patient, viz.:—

	Double.	Right.	Left.	Total.
Males . . .	7	1	3	11
Females . .	44	28	24	96
	51	29	27	107

From these statistics it results that the dislocations occur in an enormous proportion in females (90 per cent.) compared to males, that the single dislocations are almost as frequent on the one side as on the other, and that the double dislocations are nearly equal in number to the unilateral. After discussing the four principal hypotheses of the etiology of the affection—(1) the action of external forces, whether by reason of the position of the fœtus or the manœuvres during delivery; (2) the action, whether by excess or deficiency, of the muscular powers; (3) intra-uterine diseases of the hip-joint; (4) an original vicious conformation, due to primary alteration of the germ, or arrest of development—Dr. Pravas observes, "It appears to me legitimate to conclude that, if these dislocations may result from multiple causes, the most general one is to be sought for in an anomaly of the organisation, this hypothesis admitting, in the great majority of cases, the greatest amount of probability." As one explanation of the greater frequency of the affection in females, he observes that, notwithstanding the greater development of the pelvis in the female, the cotyloid cavities are less deep than in males, varying in the former from 20 to 25 centimetres, and in the latter from 25 to 35.

TERMS OF SUBSCRIPTION.
(Free by post.)

British Islands	Twelve Months	.	£1	8	0
,, ,, ...	Six ,,	.	0	14	0
The Colonies and the United States of America . . .	} Twelve ,,	.	1	10	0
,, ,, ...	Six ,,	.	0	15	0
India	Twelve ,,	.	1	10	0
,, (vid Brindisi)	,, ,,	.	1	15	0
,, ,, ...	Six ,,	.	0	15	0
,, (vid Brindisi)	,, ,,	.	0	17	6

Foreign Subscribers are requested to inform the Publishers of any remittances made through the agency of the Post-office.

Single Copies of the Journal can be obtained of all Booksellers and Newsmen, price Sixpence.

Cheques or Post-office Orders should be made payable to Mr. JAMES LUCAS, 11, New Burlington-street, W.

TERMS FOR ADVERTISEMENTS.

Seven lines (70 words) . . .	.	£0	4	6
Each additional line (10 words)	.	0	0	6
Half-column, or quarter-page .	.	1	5	0
Whole column, or half-page .	.	2	10	0
Whole page	.	5	0	0

Births, Marriages, and Deaths are inserted Free of Charge.

THE MEDICAL TIMES AND GAZETTE is published on Friday morning: Advertisements must therefore reach the Publishing Office not later than One o'clock on Thursday.

Medical Times and Gazette.

SATURDAY, OCTOBER 22, 1881.

DR. RUSSELL REYNOLDS ON SPECIALISM IN MEDICINE.

THE address of Dr. Russell Reynolds on Specialism in Medicine, which was delivered before the Medical Society of University College, and which we publish this week, is one which we are sure will afford both pleasure and profit to our readers, for it is both wise and witty. Such a combination is unfortunately too rare in professional speeches or writings; consequently, when we do come across anything of the kind we are ready to enjoy it all the more thoroughly.

As regards specialism, Dr. Reynolds goes to the root of the matter, for he begins with the earliest days, when each head of a family was prophet, priest, and king; but it was long, long after this that the doctor made his appearance—n fact, the existence of such an individual, as contradistinguished from the magician or medicine-man, indicates a relatively high growth of civilisation. But the idea of this composite function is the fundamental one in the earlier part of Dr. Reynolds' address, his purpose being to show how, as time goes on, a "differentiation"—or, to make use of the term employed in social life, a "division of labour"—becomes absolutely necessary. Of this Dr. Reynolds says, "In many instances this division of work and this process of evolution have resolved themselves into 'specialism.'" This "is, in my view, the wrong side of two right things and processes—the abuse of divided labour and evolution of knowledge." But, as the speaker took care to point out, there is a good and there is a bad form of specialism. There is that kind of specialism, let us say, seen in the time and trouble many hospital physicians and surgeons take to thoroughly master everything known about their cases for the purpose of giving it out again to their pupils. And there are few men who, having once devoted themselves specially to any one case or set of cases—who have sought by every means in their power to master the whole subject, the better to enable them to teach—who are not better able than most others to speak with authority on all that relates to it. In this sense, these men are specialists; but it is in a good sense.

The word is, however, commonly employed in a totally different fashion. Thus, Dr. Reynolds says, "When I speak of 'specialism,' the word carries us into a region quite other than that of helpful work—into that of retrogression, instead of evolution; into that of the survival, not of the fittest, but of the charlatan and the quack." And further on he thus humorously defines specialism—"If you ask me what I mean by specialism, I should say: 'It is a morbid condition of the mind—of physician or surgeon, as the case may be—which shows itself in his regarding every patient who comes under his care as a sufferer from the particular disease which he has studied; of seeing the symptoms only from the point of view which he has assumed, and made quite clear—to himself—and of treating it in a manner which no one like himself understands; and of treating it to the utmost degree of attention, frequency, and speciality of treatment that his patient's patience will endure.'"

But he is careful to distinguish between specialism and the adoration of great names. The latter makes many people run to him who is best known to fame—often a medical case to a surgeon; much more rarely *vice versâ*. And, as Dr. Reynolds says, it is notorious that many surgeons of the highest standing will, and do, treat medical cases, though they never had the slightest medical training. A notable instance of this was that of a surgeon now deceased, who whilst alive, occupied the highest position in his walk of the profession. But there is another tendency on the part of the public which it is well to bear in mind. Often it has occurred to us, as doubtless it has occurred to many others, for a patient to make his or her appearance, with the inquiry, if it has not already been made at the door, Are you the doctor—who is famous for this, that, or the other thing?—in each case the maladies differing *toto cælo*; but clearly the patient was ready to bolt if he or she could not be assured that we were really the famous one. In the case of the true specialist, as defined above, there never is such a difficulty, for, as Dr. Reynolds says, he promptly concludes that if a patient comes to him it can be for one thing, and one thing only. All kinds of absurd stories are abroad, illustrating this kind of "morbid condition"; one of these relates to the time to which Dr. Reynolds alludes, when *ulceratio uteri* was the fashionable disease. As the story goes, a lady made her appearance before a well-known practitioner, affected with this particular form of mania. Promptly, and without any time being allowed for explanation, the disease was discovered, and, equally promptly, the appropriate remedy applied. And with the injunction of "Not a word now, madam," the patient was dismissed. Again and again, so goes the story, the same farce was enacted, until the lady was declared cured, when at last she [was allowed to speak, only to say, "But, dear me, doctor, I came to consult you about my eyes!" As in most other] legends of the same kind, the satire implied is at least *ben trovato*. It must, moreover, be said that, in the hands of an unscrupulous individual, there is no form of specialism so dangerous as this. There are, indeed, men in this line of practice of the highest honour, alike esteemed by the public and their professional brethren; but opportunities for the abuse of the influence over the patient acquired in it are only too plentiful, and unfortunately they are too often taken advantage of in more than one way. There is an uneasy feeling abroad that women are not the same after a course of this kind of special treatment; and it is hardly to be wondered at, if, as we have heard, such a thing as an arrangement of mirrors, by which a patient may see the process of cure in her own case, is even to be found among us.

With regard to the different forms of specialism enumerated and discussed so ably and so well by Dr. Reynolds, we would only allude to one more—that is, to the railway witness. Fortunately, the race of hard swearers seems dying out: the most eminent members of our profession will no longer have anything to say to such business; and some of those who formerly swore the hardest are now a little more cautious. Unfortunately, this caution is not always duly appreciated either by judge or jury, who prefer clear and definite statements to those of one who tries to state his belief in all honesty; and this seldom can be done in the blunt, sledge-hammer fashion in favour with those who are paid to make up their minds on behalf of one side, and one side only. But we have already said more than enough as regards this address. It gives us real pleasure to read it; it is both healthful and pleasant, and we are sure that those who take the trouble to peruse it will think with us.

INTRA-PERITONEAL WOUNDS OF THE BLADDER.
II.—EXPERIMENTAL INVESTIGATIONS.

FOR the purpose of these experiments a medium-sized dog was used. On distending the bladder with water, it was found pyriform in shape, with its anterior wall in contact with the abdominal parietes, from which it is separated by the omentum. The bladder in the dog is covered in all directions by peritoneum, from which fact it follows that all wounds of this viscus are intra-peritoneal. The organ may be reached by making an incision just above the symphysis pubis, and drawing out the bladder.

As regards the form of suture, Dr. Vincent recommends two, which he calls sero-muscular and sero-serous, and which sufficiently explain themselves. The latter is the better, as the peritoneal surfaces are those from which the most plastic material is exuded. But a combination of the two may be even better still. For the purpose of testing whether the sutures have been placed sufficiently near each other, he recommends that the bladder should be injected with some coloured fluid, such as milk, before the abdominal wound is closed, using sufficient force to distend the bladder moderately. If the milk escape through the sutured bladder, more stitches must be applied at that point. Our author thinks the stitches ought not to be distant more than two millimetres from each other. In dogs he never found this kind of suture give way, and he has seen them void considerable quantities of urine a few hours after the experiment. But in man it would be advisable to keep in a catheter, and moreover to wash out the bladder every few hours with some antiseptic solution, in order to get rid both of the urine and of any other product which might be secreted. The material used for the sutures in the experiments was ordinary linen thread. Catgut is too rapidly absorbed. Metallic wire is also good. In answer to the question whether the edges of the wound shall be revivified, Dr. Vincent says that this can only be necessary some hours after the accident, or after gunshot wounds with marginal burning. He had not practised it in any of his experiments; it was especially unnecessary with the sero-serous suture. Nevertheless, in man it might be necessary in some cases, if the edges of the wound were much damaged, or gangrenous, or likely to become gangrenous. As regards antiseptic dressings, in dogs it was impossible to think of any dressings at all, beyond, every now and then, irrigating the external wound with carbolised water.

The experiments themselves would take up too much space were we to attempt anything like a detailed account. We may just state, however, that the bladder was punctured, and that small portions of its walls were removed, and after urine had extravasated it was then immediately sutured; that gunshot wounds were produced, as also wounds by tearing with the fingers, and that after urine had extravasated and been in the abdomen a certain number of hours, the sutures were applied. In both series of cases the peritoneum was carefully cleansed before sewing up the abdominal wound.

The results may be summed up as follows:—Immediate union has been obtained in all kinds of wound of the bladder when the suture has been *immediate*. Treatment (opening the belly, suture of the bladder, removal of urine and extravasated blood from the abdominal cavity, with subsequent suture of the abdominal wall) has been successful, even after six and a half and eight and a half hours after intra-peritoneal extravasation. On the other hand, the operation has constantly proved useless when practised twenty-four and a half, twenty-five, or twenty-five and a half hours after extravasation, the animals having succumbed to urinary intoxication rather than to the violence of the peritonitis. A vigorous dog may survive an extensive wound of the bladder with intra-peritoneal extravasation of urine about forty-eight hours when left alone. But it is well to bear in mind that in dogs, as in human beings, the susceptibility of the peritoneum differs widely; but even this would not materially affect the final issue.

On the whole, therefore, one may venture to assert that success will belong to the surgeon who operates early; laparotomy must be undertaken early if it is to save the patient. On the other hand, the presence of peritonitis, unless severe, or of uræmic symptoms, does not necessarily render it inadmissible. In civil practice this is not difficult, provided the patient applies early enough, and that the surgeon arrives promptly at a correct diagnosis; and it may be said that an error in diagnosis, leading to a laparotomy in a case where the bladder turned out not to be injured, would be less serious than the want of recognition of an extravasation which had taken place. In the former case, the surgeon would at least be able to discover the causes of the symptoms which he believed were due to rupture of the bladder, while, due precautions being taken, the danger to life would be quite insignificant.

Dr. Vincent thinks that our present antiseptic dressings warrant operations which formerly would have savoured of almost unpardonable temerity. "*Autre temps—autre chirurgie.*"

GEOLOGICAL DISTRIBUTION OF GOÎTRE.

THAT goître is in some way connected with drinking-water is a belief deeply rooted in the popular mind in every part of the world where the disease prevails endemically. The notion which has found favour in some quarters, that it is caused by the use of snow-water, is completely exploded by the fact that it is absent from the region of "Greenland's icy mountains," and is met with where snow is never seen, as in Sumatra. The almost universal prevalence of goître in limestone districts, and especially where dolomite or magnesian limestone is present, seems to indicate a close relation between it and these formations; indeed, such a mass of positive evidence has been accumulated as to place the question, in the opinion of many judicious observers, beyond the reach of doubt: while, on the other hand, the immunity enjoyed by the inhabitants of neighbouring districts, differing only in not lying on these formations, appears to lend strong support to this view. Again, in the valley of the Saskatchawan, those individuals who are by circumstances compelled to use in their expeditions snow-water, surface-water, or the streams which in summer traverse the plains, escape, while those who remain at home and are restricted to the water of the river itself suffer severely. Further

confirmatory evidence has been collected by Drs. Aitken and Parkes from various sources to such an extent that it would seem idle to reopen the question; but in 1867 Dr. de St. Lager, of Lyons, minutely investigated the distribution of goître in France,[a] and Professor Lebour, of Newcastle-upon-Tyne, has more recently attempted the same for England. In the former country the importance of goître, as a disqualification for military service, gives a practical value to the inquiry which is wanting here, but unfortunately the French statistics refer only to males, whereas females are everywhere more liable to the disease. The statistics are therefore so far imperfect, though the most complete of any we have at present. The first thing which strikes one on glancing down the list of formations on which goître is endemic, and on which it is not, is what one would have expected, viz., the general preference for calcareous strata shown by the disease in question; but on closer inspection one sees that several of these are free from endemic goître, while it prevails extensively on geological formations where lime in any form is absent, as the Kimmeridge and Oxford clays, and the Cambrian. But the point in which the goîtrous and non-goîtrous limestones differ, and in which the former agree with the few non-calcareous but goîtrous formations, seems to be the presence in all places where goître is seen of pyrites, and its absence from all those where it is not. This is especially well-marked in the Eocene and in the coal-measures. In England, again, goître is absent from the alluvial and tertiary formations generally, and nearly so from the oolites and lias, rare on the chalk, but present, as in France, on the gault and greensand, as well as the Wealden, in all of which much pyrites is found. On the new red sandstone it is endemic in several places, as Crediton in Devonshire, and especially at Wombourne, near Wolverhampton, where the soil is highly ferruginous. Its headquarters, however, may be said to be the vast beds of grits, shales, and limestones forming the carboniferous rocks in Cumberland, Derbyshire, and Yoredale, in Yorkshire, but to this there are some remarkable exceptions. At South Shields and Sunderland, where the water companies draw their supply from wells sunk deep into the magnesian limestone, goître is as unknown as in London; and when we remember that it occurs in the Weald of Kent, and the lignitiferous beds of the Paris basin, but not in the neighbouring gypseous marls or *calcaire grossier*, the conclusion seems irresistible that it is not in limestone *per se*, but in certain combinations of ferruginous and earthy salts, most frequently found in such formations, though not absolutely limited to them, that we must seek for the real cause of goître. The results of Professor Lebour's inquiries, which he has pursued during the past ten years, with the assistance of medical men and geologists in various parts of the country, were, early in the present summer, laid before the Northumberland and Durham Medical Society in a paper which has since been reprinted separately, though for private circulation only.

THE WEEK.
TOPICS OF THE DAY.

THE Devonshire Hospital at Buxton, which has for so many months been undergoing the process of enlargement, was recently formally reopened by the Duke of Devonshire. The increased accommodation, as will doubtless be remembered, has been provided through a grant of £34,000 obtained from the Convalescent Fund of the Lancashire Cotton Districts, the Duke of Devonshire giving more ground for the buildings on merely nominal terms. By dint of good manage-

(a) Dr. de St. Lager, "Études sur les Causes du Crétinisme et du Goître Endémique," Paris, 1867.

ment on the part of all concerned, the charity has not been entirely closed during any time that the extension works have been in progress, so that the reopening of the Hospital is not to be taken literally. The Duke of Devonshire was accompanied upon the occasion by Lord Edward Cavendish, Mr. Hugh Mason, M.P., Mr. Cheetham, M.P., Mr. T. W. Evans, M.P., and many of the gentry of North Derbyshire. After the religious ceremony, performed by the Vicar of Buxton, the Duke said that they had at first entertained hopes that possibly the extension might have been opened under the auspices of the Prince of Wales, but, unfortunately, owing to the many demands upon His Royal Highness's time, those hopes had to be abandoned. In reviewing the past history of the Hospital, his Grace remarked that it now entered upon a new stage of existence, with great additions to its advantages, and on a greatly enlarged scale, and he thought it would be gratifying to the Governors of the Cotton Districts Fund to find that their munificent grant would be the means of admitting annually to the benefits of the institution not many fewer than 1500 patients, in addition to those hitherto received. The Hospital was then declared open for the reception of patients, and the company were entertained at luncheon. The Earl of Derby, who was expected to attend to represent the Governors of the Cotton Districts Fund, was unable to be present on the occasion.

Once more we have to report a meeting of the Lower Thames Valley Main Sewerage Board, which took place at Kingston, and was presided over by Sir Thomas Nelson. In the course of the proceedings, a letter was read from the Local Government Board, acknowledging the receipt of a copy of a resolution passed by the joint Board with regard to the terms upon which the West Kent Main Sewerage Board were willing to arrange for the discharge into their sewers of sewage from the Lower Thames Valley district, and stating that the Board much regretted to learn that the last proposals of the West Kent Board were such that the joint Board had felt themselves unable to agree to them. At the same time, the Board could not but consider that, under the circumstances surrounding the case, the difficulties would best be met by an arrangement which would admit of the discharge of the sewage of the district into the West Kent system, and they asked whether steps might not be taken to bring about a conference between the two authorities, with the view of reverting to the original proposal. The Board would afford every assistance in their power towards promoting such a conference, and they would be prepared to instruct one of their inspectors to attend it if his presence should be deemed desirable. In the long discussion which followed, it was explained that the Board had already adopted a separate scheme of Mr. Hawksley's, and it was ultimately resolved, by a large majority, "That the West Kent scheme not being at present an assured success, and this Board having no knowledge of, and being incapable of foreseeing, the possible and probable results that may accrue from the construction thereof, are of opinion that it is not desirable to further consider the matter, having no guarantee that such a combination will prove either economical, efficient, or final." It was stated by the Chairman that the time was very shortly coming when they would have set there four years, and the only result they had to show for it was an unfortunate expenditure of a very large sum of money, which had absolutely resulted in nothing.

At a recent meeting of the Hackney District Board of Works, a member asked if Dr. J. W. Tripe, the Medical Officer of Health for the Hackney District had any report to present on the subject of the evil smells of Hackney,

about which so much has lately been written. Dr. Tripe remarked that all he had at that time to explain was that a summons had been taken out, at the instance of the Metropolitan Board of Works, against an offending firm, but the hearing had been postponed. Mr. John Runts, the Hackney member at the Metropolitan Board of Works, said the summons had been adjourned in order to enable the defendants to make certain alterations which would, it was hoped, remedy the nuisance complained of. Another member remarked that it was exceedingly desirable that action should not any longer be delayed, for the reports which had appeared in the newspapers were proving very disastrous to the parish of Hackney—people who were coming to reside in Hackney were writing letters to ask the real sanitary condition of the parish; and the quickest way to disabuse their minds would be to bring about a speedy remedy of the evil where it existed. Dr. Tripe said it was a matter really not under the control of the District Board, but he would promise the Board that now the matter had been taken in hand it would be promptly dealt with.

The Governor-General of India has been pleased to make the following appointments to his personal staff:—To be Honorary Surgeons: Surgeons-General W. R. Cornish, C.I.E., and A. J. Payne; Deputy Surgeon-General W. J. Moore, Brigade-Surgeon J. A. Marston, Surgeons-Major G. Farrell, T. E. Charles, M.D., R. W. Cunningham, M.D., and C. A. Atkins, and Surgeon A. H. Rowe—all of the Army or of the Indian Medical Service. These appointments are similar to those of Honorary Surgeon to Her Majesty the Queen in this country.

The City Commission of Sewers at its last meeting considered a report of their engineer, Colonel Hayward, on the subject of the disposal and destruction of refuse from the streets of the City, which was eventually ordered to be printed for further discussion. Many complaints have recently been made as to the inadequate manner in which the streets of the City are cleansed; the street-orderly boys with their brushes and shovels perform their duty in a very slipshod manner, and generally contrive to leave a fine layer of malodorous material spread thinly over the surface of the roadway. The constant traffic pulverises this thin deposit, and the atmosphere becomes charged with unwholesome particles which are inhaled by the crowds of passers-by. It is to be hoped, therefore, that Colonel Haywood's scheme deals with the proper collection of street refuse as well as with its disposal and destruction. A letter was also read from the Vestry of St. Botolph, Bishopsgate, calling attention to the present filthy condition of several houses in Windsor street and Widegate-street, which is seriously prejudicial to the health of the inhabitants, and it was referred to the Sanitary Committee, in conjunction with the police, to stop the overcrowding which was reported to be practised there, some families sleeping in these wretched premises from six in the evening until two o'clock the next morning, and then including young children and women) being turned out to make room for other lodgers for the rest of the night. It was stated incidentally that these premises belonged to one of the officers of the Commission. Surely if this be true there should be little difficulty in bringing about an amended state of affairs!

An inquiry was recently held in Whitechapel by Mr. Collier, Deputy Coroner for East Middlesex, relative to the death of a child aged nine months. It appeared that the deceased had been ailing for the last four months. During the latter part of the time he had been under the treatment of a herbalist, who had the effrontery to give the mother the following certificate of death:—"This is to certify that I saw George Thomas Croney, aged nine months, on Friday morning last, October 7, and gave him a little mixture for consumption of the bowels and bronchitis, from which he was suffering, but he died on Tuesday morning, October 11, 1881, at a quarter to six o'clock.—C. M. Wilson, 364, Cable-street, Shadwell, October 10, 1881." When the mother took this document to the registrar of births and deaths for the district, he very properly refused to accept it. Dr. Joseph Loane was called to prove that the cause of death was from convulsions. The Coroner, in summing up, said that the herbalist had been guilty of gross misconduct in giving the mother of the deceased a certificate of death, and might have brought himself within the reach of the criminal law. The jury ultimately returned a verdict in accordance with the medical testimony, and added, as a rider, that they considered the conduct of the herbalist who attended the deceased, and gave a certificate of the cause of death, deserving of great blame.

The governing body at Gonville and Caius College, Cambridge, have recently issued an order as to the Thurston Speech, which up to the present time has been delivered annually on May 11, the day of the commemoration of Dr. Caius, the orator being chosen from the medical graduates of the College in rotation. The subject of the speech was, "The Progress of Medicine from the time of Dr. Caius," the speaker receiving the sum of £18. In lieu of this annual speech, the governing body have decided that in future there shall be given triennially about £54 in money, or in any other form that may be thought best, to that member of the College who has published in the course of the preceding three years the best original investigation in physiology (including physiological chemistry), pathology, or practical medicine—the person to whom the prize is awarded being required to give an account of his investiga-tion in the form of a lecture (or otherwise, as the governing body may think best) in the College. If within the specified period no investigation of sufficient merit shall have been made, the money shall be carried forward to augment future prizes. This scheme is to come into operation immediately, and the prize will be first awarded in 1884.

A circular has been issued by the Council of the Hospital Saturday Fund, urging foremen, employers, and others to send in the result of their collections by the end of the present month, about which time, it is hoped, the accounts of the Fund may be closed. The Council announces that the amount already received (viz., £8000) considerably exceeds any former total at the close of the Fund. Of the 37,000 sheets issued, about 20,000 have up to the present time been returned.

The Medical Acts Commission met this week for the first time after the recess, at 2, Victoria-street, Westminster.

THE ARMY LIST.

An inconsistency of arrangement of the departments of the Army may be observed in the recently revised monthly and quarterly Army Lists. In the official list of the War Office in the quarterly Army List for October the heads of departments are arranged in what may be considered to be the natural and suitable order of precedence—namely, the Chaplain-General, the Director-General of the Army Medical Department, the Commissary and Assistant Commissary-General at Headquarters, and the Principal Veterinary Surgeon; but in the body of the book the arrangement is as follows:—The Chaplain's Department, the Commissariat and Transport Staff, Medical Department, Ordnance Store Department, Army Pay Department, and Veterinary De-partment. One would think that the relative positions of the departments as given in the official list of the War Office should be observed throughout the work, instead of interposing the Medical Department between the Com-missariat and the Ordnance Store Department, the analogy between the two last-named branches of supply being borne in mind. That an attempt has been made to re-arrange the departments on some fixed system is evident from the Chaplain's Department, which in the Army List for Sep-tember is last in the series, having in the October issue been placed first. No special reference has, however, been made to any scriptural authority for this alteration in relative precedence.

ROYAL COLLEGE OF SURGEONS.

At a quarterly meeting of the Council on the 20th inst., Mr. John Croft, Surgeon to St. Thomas's Hospital, was elected a member of the Court of Examiners in the vacancy occasioned by the resignation of Mr. John Marshall, F.R.S., Vice-President of the College.

THE FUTURE PLANS OF THE METROPOLITAN ASYLUMS BOARD.

At the last meeting of the Metropolitan Asylums Board, Sir E. H. Currie brought up the report of a special com-mittee appointed to consider the action which should be taken to provide increased accommodation for fever patients without materially limiting the restricted accommodation for small-pox patients at present possessed by the Board. The Committee recommended that, with the consent of the Local Government Board, the Homerton Small-pox Hospital should be closed against small-pox patients, forty reserved beds being, however, retained for very severe small-pox cases arising in the district allocated to Homerton Hos-pital, and that all the small-pox cases arising in the Homerton Hospital District should be sent to the Atlas ship, to which Dr. Gayton and his assistants were to be transferred. The Hospital, thus closed, could be pre-pared for fever patients, and, moreover, the Deptford Committee could provide a hundred beds for the same class of patients. The Committee further recommended that the ambulance arrangements carried out at Hackney for small-pox patients should be extended to the conveyance of fever patients by vehicles, nurses and drivers being ob-tained for the exclusive purpose of conveying fever patients. The Committee recommended also that the ambulance station at Hackney should be under the Homerton Com-mittee, and that a special committee should be appointed to manage the Atlas, the duties having hitherto been carried out by the Darenth Committee. In moving the adoption of the report, Sir E. Currie stated that it was necessary there should be ample provision on the south side of London for small-pox patients, since the disease was still very rife on that side. With regard to the Managers making their own arrangements for ambulance service, he related that in one district he found it had been the custom to send a hearse-like vehicle, with the usual long-tailed horse, to collect patients. On one occasion it took three patients from different places, each patient taking a friend. Anything more disgust-ing and dangerous, he thought, it was impossible to conceive ; and he laid upon the manner in which the ambulance service had been carried out a great deal of the out-cry which had been raised against the Board's work. The Local Government Board, he said, had given its entire concurrence to the Managers organising the ambulance system. Mr. Hodges remarked that he had had much ex-perience on the Homerton and Deptford Hospital Com-mittees, and could attest that nothing could be worse than the ambulance arrangements of the parishes for the convey-ance of the sick poor to the hospitals. Mr. E. Galsworthy said the proposals submitted by Sir E. Currie in regard to the ambulances would, if carried out, put an end to evils which could scarcely be mentioned. In answer to questions, Sir E. Currie stated that the small-pox patients now at Darenth were not in camp—that having been broken up—but in wards in one of the new buildings. He added that the stores of the camp, blankets and beds, valued at about £8000, might be distributed to the other small-pox hospitals of the Managers, as he did not think it was possible the Board would be able to form another camp there. The locality objected to a camp of metropolitan small-pox patients, and he hoped the necessity for a camp would not arise, for there would be difficulties in the way of forming one at Darenth. Mr. Galsworthy gave notice that at the next meeting he would move that the Local Government Board should have its attention specially drawn to the injunctions which had been obtained in courts of law against the Managers' action (action sanctioned and approved by the Local Government Board), to the threats of other like proceedings, and that the Local Government Board should be requested to state whether the Government was prepared to take any steps for the protection of the Managers in the discharge of their onerous duties under the Act of 1867.

THE YELLOW FEVER AT BARBADOES.

THE latest reports describe the health condition of the island as not satisfactory. Sickness still prevails among both the civil inhabitants and the troops, and cases of yellow fever with fatal results continue to occur among all classes, but with rather less frequency among the troops. The rains have set in pretty generally throughout the island, with frequent thunder and lightning, from the occurrence of which a salutary change is hoped for.

LONDON SANITARY PROTECTION ASSOCIATION.

WE have received the prospectus of this Association—of which Professor Huxley is Chairman, and Sir William Gull, Dr. Acland, Dr. Bristowe, Dr. Andrew Clark, Dr. Burdon-Sanderson, Mr. Holmes, and others, members of Council, —with an intimation that their first general meeting is to be held in the Society of Arts Room, Adelphi, next Tuesday evening at eight o'clock, Professor Huxley in the chair. All members of the medical profession will be admitted on presenting their cards at the door. This Association has not been established for purposes of profit, but has, we believe, been doing much good work quietly for the last nine months in giving skilled advice as to the sanitary condition of houses, both those in course of construction and those already building, and would, if it grows into a large institution—as we trust it will,—effect a great improvement in the health of private houses. It is at present only young, and still struggling for life. Medical support is very necessary for its growth, and of this we trust it will receive an ample share. An account of the work already carried out will be given at the meeting by Professor Fleeming Jenkin.

THE PARIS WEEKLY RETURN.

THE number of deaths for the fortieth week, terminating October 7, was 881 (457 males and 424 females), and among these there were from typhoid fever 27, small-pox 14, measles 14, scarlatina 3, pertussis 5, diphtheria and croup 31, dysentery 2, erysipelas 4, and puerperal infections 8. There were also 40 deaths from tubercular and acute meningitis, 15 from acute bronchitis, 36 from pneumonia, 95 from infantile athrepsia (35 of the children having been wholly or partially suckled), and 27 violent deaths. The sanitary condition thus continues good, and, in fact, 19 of the deaths ought to have been registered last week instead of this. The only cause of death which offers sensible

augmentation is that from puerperal infections, which contributes 8 deaths in from 1100 to 1200 parturient women. The births for the week amounted to 1448—viz., 573 males (404 legitimate and 169 illegitimate) and 575 females (408 legitimate and 167 illegitimate) ; 102 infants (56 males and 46 females) were born dead or died within twenty-four hours.

THE ROYAL UNITED HOSPITAL, BATH.

THE mode in which the staff of this institution is appointed has recently been the subject of some discussion in the local papers. It is alleged that this Hospital is managed in an exclusive spirit ; that, excepting the three physicians and three surgeons, the profession in Bath is shut out from it, it being practically impossible for any medical man not on its staff to set foot within its walls. This is attributed to the vicious method by which the staff is appointed—viz., by popular vote—a mode of choice in which family influence and personal popularity go for much more than professional ability. The lady friends of the candidates, a newspaper correspondent says, press the claims of the rival doctors in a most offensive and pertinacious way upon men of business. A reform which some think desirable is that assistant-surgeons and assistant-physicians should be appointed, so that when vacancies occur in the senior staff a junior should be ready to go up. Besides this, the patients, it is thought, would be better attended to if there were members of the permanent staff who could take the place of the seniors during their absence, or otherwise assist them if necessary. The younger members of the profession, it is pointed out, are generally better acquainted with the theoretical part of their work than their elders, although they may be lacking in experience; and it is a strength to the staff of a provincial hospital to be reinforced by young men fresh from the schools. The above statements as to the present management of the Bath Hospital are taken from ex parte accounts ; we give no opinion as to their correctness: but we have no doubt of the weight of the considerations urged by those who wish for reform. Elections to a hospital staff ought to be made by those who are competent to judge of the merits of the candidates, not by the popular voice or the efforts of female canvassers. It is a gain to a hospital to enlist in its service the zeal and more modern knowledge of the younger members of the profession. A large hospital in a provincial town ought to be a centre of union for the whole profession in that town, useful to all, and not merely an appendage to the private practice of a few.

THE QUEEN'S UNIVERSITY IN IRELAND.

WHAT was probably the last—certainly the penultimate—meeting to confer degrees of the Senate of the moribund Queen's University in Ireland was held in St. Patrick's Hall, Dublin Castle, on Thursday afternoon, the 13th inst. The attendance of graduates, as well as of the general public, was unusually large. His Grace the Duke of Leinster, Chancellor of the University, presided. The Chancellor, in his opening address, observed that this day closed the thirty-second academic year of the University, and that during it upwards of one thousand students had been under instruction by the University in its colleges (the Queen's Colleges) at Belfast, Cork, and Galway. In the Faculty of Medicine there are two Previous University Examinations in addition to the Degree Examination. At these examinations 532 students of the University had presented themselves, and 2 extern candidates. Of these, 72 had passed for the degree of Doctor in Medicine, 53 for the degree of Master in Surgery, 34 for the diploma in Midwifery, and 286 at one or other of the two Previous Examinations. Seven of the candidates for the degree of Doctor in Medicine, and 15 of the candidates at the Previous Examinations, had been awarded high University distinctions. Among the recipients of honorary degrees were John Cleland, M.D., F.R.S., on whom was conferred the degree of Doctor of Science, *honoris causâ*; and William Thomson, B.A., M.D., M.Ch., who received the degree of Master of Arts, *honoris causâ*. The "Peel Prize for English Composition," open to the competition of undergraduates in Medicine, was awarded to William S. McKee, of Queen's College, Galway, for his essay on the selected subject, "Insanity." The "Peel Exhibitions," awarded at the First University Examination in Medicine, were adjudicated as follows:—First, Robert Crawford, Belfast, £20 a year for two years; second, Frederick James Burns, Galway, £15 a year for two years.

THE STRANGE FATE OF A QUOTATION.

IN Dr. Russell Reynolds' address is to be found a quotation, which we had supposed to be tolerably well known even in this country, and certainly we had given our worthy contemporaries, the *Lancet* and the *British Medical Journal*, the credit of knowing something of the French language. Nevertheless, the said quotation appears in the columns of these journals in two different versions—it is true, not both equally bad, for that in the *Lancet* is absurd beyond the wildest imagination, but both such as would justly earn for a schoolboy a hearty caning, if such things be still permitted in an enlightened age. Thus the *Lancet* puts the former portion of the saying, "*Il faut que vivra*," which the *British Medical Journal* makes "*Il faut que vivre*"; whilst, as regards the second part, the *Lancet* says, "*Je ne vois par la necessité.*" The *British Medical Journal* had scholarship enough to substitute an *s* for an *r* in *pas*, and to insert a necessary accent, but left the quotation as inexact as ever.

SOCIETY FOR RELIEF OF WIDOWS AND ORPHANS OF MEDICAL MEN.

THE Quarterly Court of Directors was held on Wednesday, October 12, at 5 p.m., in the rooms of the Royal Medical and Chirurgical Society. The chair was taken punctually at 5 p.m. by the President, Sir Geo. Burrows, Bart. The Court was unusually well attended. The deaths of two of the oldest members of the Society, Dr. Billing, V.P., and Mr. R. C. Griffiths, were announced. Two new members were elected. The deaths of two widows were reported; one had been in receipt of grants since 1833, receiving for herself and children the large sum of £2272, the husband having been a member for only nine years, paying but eighteen guineas. Applications were read from sixty widows, nine children, and three recipients from the Copeland Fund, and a sum of £1250 10s. was recommended to be paid them at the next Court. The expenses of the quarter were £37 15s. The Treasurer reporting favourably of the state of the funds, the Directors resolved to give the same present this Christmas as last to the widows and orphans receiving grants. An application was approved of from one widow, and a grant of £30 was given to an orphan towards his self-maintenance.

EXTIRPATION OF THE KIDNEY.

THIS operation, being one which has only recently been at all frequently performed, but which will doubtless take its place among the recognised resources of surgery, has yet to have its risks, results, and the best method of performing it settled by comparison of a large number of cases. The most complete account of it which the English reader has at his disposal is that communicated by Mr. A. E. Barker, of University College Hospital, to the Royal Medical and Chirurgical Society. A later summary of experience, comprising a larger number of cases, is given by Kroner, in a paper published in a recent number of the *Archiv für Gynäkologie*; this will therefore, doubtless, be read with interest. At the time Dr. Kroner wrote, the operation had been performed forty-one times, or rather, forty-one cases of its performance had been published. The following were the diseases for which it was done:—In 8 cases, for hydronephrosis; in 1, for cystic disease of doubtful origin; in 10, for malignant tumours of the kidney; in 2, cases of movable, but otherwise healthy, kidneys; in 1, the organ was removed along with a retro-peritoneal fibroma; in 1, on account of a fistulous communication between the ureter and the abdominal wall; in 1, for ureto-uterine fistula; in 1, for ureto-vaginal fistula; in 4, for renal calculus; in 2, because the presence of a stone in the kidney was suspected; in 4, for pyo-nephrosis; in 4, because of damage the result of injury; in 1, for disease, the nature of which is not clearly explained; in 1, part of the kidney was removed along with a hydatid cyst. In 21 of the cases the operation was performed by the abdominal incision, with 14 deaths; and in 20 by the lumbar incision, with 5 deaths; but in 3 other of these the result is not stated. Dr. Kroner does not think the higher mortality of the operation by abdominal incision is from any greater danger attending it, but because these cases included those in which the diagnosis was uncertain, and the abdomen was opened tentatively. As Dr. Kroner gives his authority for each case that he quotes, his paper is of much value for the purpose of reference. He also discusses the treatment of hydronephrosis by incision and drainage. He can only find five cases on record, three of which died. He comes to the conclusion that it is impossible to secure obliteration of a hydronephrotic sac. If there be any bit of secreting tissue left, this will, when the pressure of the retained fluid is removed, go on secreting urine. Injection of the sac with iodine is fruitless. To find the orifice of the ureter and restore its patency, is so difficult as to be practically impossible.

SIR PATRICK DUN'S HOSPITAL, DUBLIN.

DR. MACALISTER, Professor of Anatomy and Chirurgery in the School of Physic in Ireland, has requested of the Board of Trinity College to be relieved of his duties as Clinical Surgeon to Sir Patrick Dun's Hospital, in order to devote all his time to his professorship. Dr. Macalister's request was granted on Saturday last, and Dr. Charles B. Ball was appointed Clinical Surgeon, *locum tenens*.

DR. AIRY'S REPORT ON AN OUTBREAK OF SMALL-POX AT BOURNE BRIDGE, ONGAR.

IN the early part of the present year, Dr. Airy was despatched by the Local Government Board to inquire into an outbreak of small-pox which had occurred in February last in a house at Bourne Bridge, in the Ongar (Essex) Union. The inhabitants of the house, numbering eleven persons, belonged to the working class, and were all of one family; and Dr. Airy calls attention to the fact that the four youngest children, who had all been well or fairly well vaccinated, escaped the disease altogether, while those who caught it suffered more or less severely according as their vaccination marks were less or more satisfactory and recent. Two deaths resulted from this outbreak in the house in question. In the first case, that of the father, no marks of vaccination could be seen, although it was stated that he had been vaccinated in childhood. The doctor, provided by the parish, is of opinion that his death was greatly due to the cold of the room in which he lay; the eruption was wholly suppressed, and the skin discoloured. The second fatal case was that of a neighbour who was called in to nurse the family; in her case, also, no marks of vaccination were seen, and the disease was confluent. The doctor in attendance—Mr. Sanders—had offered to vaccinate her in the first instance, but she objected, saying that she had no fear of small-pox. The origin of the outbreak seems involved in some mystery. The first case occurred in the person of one of the sons, a labourer, aged nineteen, and, according to all the evidence procurable, he would appear to have contracted the infection of small-pox about January 28 or 29, while he was staying at home out of work on account of the severity of the weather. No case of small-pox existed at that time in the locality; no one appears to have visited the house; and no second-hand clothes or other suspicious articles had been brought to it. The eruption appeared on February 11, and one of his brothers was taken ill on the 15th, and the father on the 17th of that month. If small-pox, Dr. Airy remarks, could be contracted from a person in whom the disease was still in the incubation stage, we might take it for certain that the second son and his father had caught the infection from this first case; but if this cannot be admitted we must suppose that they all owed their infection to some common cause which was operative over a space of at least nine days. For example, it is possible that the clothes of some member of the family may have become infected by unnoticed contact with some person who had small-pox, and may so have become a standing source of infection at home. But there was no trace or recollection of any such occurrence. Still, Dr. Airy adds, we must look to some such unnoticed contact for the origin of the outbreak, or else to some wholly unsuspected channel of infection. A suggestion was made of the disease being caused by some diseased sheep kept in close contiguity to the house, but all Dr. Airy's inquiries failed to trace the origin of the outbreak to this cause. In concluding his report on this peculiar outbreak, Dr. Airy relates that on a subsequent visit to the district, on April 14, he learnt that another case of small-pox had recently occurred at another house in the same hamlet, but 200 yards away from the first house affected. Not the slightest intercourse had taken place between the two families, but it was elicited that when the bedding and clothes of the first persons who had died were burnt in the open air, the wind carried the smoke in the direction of the second cottage; and Dr. Airy was convinced that there remained no mode or medium of infection in this second case, upon which suspicion could be fastened, except conveyance, by the wind, over a distance of 200 yards, of infectious matter derived possibly from the ventilated sick-room, possibly from the clothes or bedding as they were brought out to be burnt, or as they were burning, or possibly from the dead body of the last of the two fatal cases in the act of removal.

AN EXPOSURE OF QUACK REMEDIES.

THE President of the Sanitary Board of Carlsruhe, Herr Karl Schnetzler, and Dr. F. Neumann, have recently issued a curious and useful tract, addressed to the thousands of persons of the lower orders who buy the numerous quack medicines so freely advertised. The pamphlet has a biographical and a chemical section : the former, compiled from the records of the police administration, gives the real names and the personal history of some of the most noted and successful of the advertising quacks. Not one of these "doctors" has ever undergone the slightest medical training; most of them are uneducated men; not a few have been condemned in the police-courts; but nearly all of them, in spite of frequent fines, have become prosperous traders, while some are enormously wealthy. The people are reminded that in all cases this wealth has been built up on the stupidity and blind confidence of their thousands of dupes, who never take the pains to test the authenticity of the marvellous wares which are advertised. The second section gives a chemical analysis of the most popular and successful of the advertised medicines, and shows what mischief the worst among them may effect upon the patient, and how cheaply and easily the less hurtful are produced. We fear, however, that, in spite of the efforts of these gentlemen, the trade in quack medicines will continue to flourish in Baden, as it does in places which might even boast of a more enlightened community.

KING AND QUEEN'S COLLEGE OF PHYSICIANS IN IRELAND.

AT the annual stated meeting of the College, held on St. Luke's Day, Tuesday, October 18, the following officers were elected for the ensuing year :—*President :* George Johnston, M.D. *Censors :* John William Moore, M.D., (*Vice-President*); Christopher J. Nixon, M.D.; Reuben Joshua Harvey, M.D. ; Arthur Vernon Macan, M.D. *Additional Examiners :* George Frederick Duffey, M.D.; Arthur Wynne Foot, M.D.; Walter George Smith, M.D.; John Mallet Purser, M.D. *Examiners in Midwifery :* Fleetwood Churchill, F.C.P.; and John Rutherford Kirkpatrick, M.B. *Registrar :* John Magee Finny, M.D. *Treasurer :* Aquilla Smith, M.D. *Professor of Medical Jurisprudence :* Robert Travers, M.A., M.B. *Representative on the General Medical Council :* Aquilla Smith, M.D. *Agent to the Trust Estates :* Charles Uniacke Townsend, Esq. *Law Agents :* Messrs. Stephen Gordon and Sons. At this meeting also Dr. Walter George Smith was elected King's Professor of Materia Medica and Pharmacy, and Sir Edward B. Sinclair, M.D., Knt., was elected King's Professor of Midwifery and Diseases of Women for a further term of seven years. Professor Helmholtz, of Berlin University, was elected by acclamation to the Honorary Fellowship of the College.

THE AUTOPSY OF PRESIDENT GARFIELD.

ALL the American medical papers which have just reached us are full of details of the illness, death, and post-mortem examination of President Garfield. In most of them the report of the autopsy, signed by the various medical attendants, is given at full length. One of them—Dr. Hayes' quarterly (the *American Journal of the Medical Sciences*)—is illustrated by some very striking woodcuts of the parts injured, which may be interesting to some of our readers. It is stated that for forty-two days' attendance on President Garfield, Drs. Bliss, Barnes, Woodward, and Reyburn, the four surgeons, each charged the Government $4200, or $100 each per day. Dr. Agnew's bill for the same number of days for " consultations, operations, and visits " was $32,600 ; and Dr. Hamilton for " visits and consultations " rendered a bill for a similar amount. These charges altogether amounted to $82,000, or a trifling sum of between £16,000 and £17,000.

REPORT ON THE URBAN AND RURAL SANITARY DISTRICTS OF TAUNTON, 1880.

IN his eighth annual report on the health of the borough of Taunton for the year 1880, Dr. Henry J. Alford, the Medical Officer of Health for the district, remarks that not only is the number of deaths below the average of the preceding decade, but, what is of greater importance from a sanitary point of view, the number of deaths from preventable diseases is considerably below the average, especially from those diseases which are either due to " filth " in the widest acceptation of the term or to the absence of those sanitary requirements which are essential if infectious diseases are to be checked. During the past year a great improvement has been effected in the water-supply of the town, and the public supply has been largely substituted for well-water, which in nearly every case has exhibited traces of sewage-pollution. The sewerage of the district has also been considerably extended, and great attention has been paid to the ventilation of the sewers. A marked improvement has also to be recorded in the dwellings of the artisan class, and Dr. Alford expresses a confident opinion that the death-rate will greatly diminish when the working-classes have exchanged their overcrowded and often dirty courts and alleys for the fresh air and better-built houses which are now being erected in the neighbourhood. The statistics of the Rural Sanitary District of Taunton, which is also under the supervision of Dr. Alford, exhibit a like satisfactory result : there is an improvement in the district generally, and people are more alive than formerly to the necessity of cleanliness; although constant supervision is still necessary. Several cases of small-pox were traced to infection from rag-sorting in a large paper factory in the neighbourhood; but prompt isolation and disinfection were successful in preventing the disease from becoming epidemic. The report points out that mortuaries in some of the larger villages would be a great boon, as the living and the dead are often huddled together in a shocking manner; and the health of the district would benefit proportionally.

INTERNATIONAL MEDICAL CONGRESS MEDAL.

WE are requested to state that a few copies of this medal remain, which it is wished to dispose of before closing the account. Copies will be forwarded by the Hon. Secretary-General, 13, Harley-street, on receipt of post-office order. The cost to members is 10s. 6d., or 11s. to cover postage. Cost of extra medals, or to non-members, 21s., or 21s. 6d. to cover postage.

THE HEALTH OF THE METROPOLITAN POLICE FORCE IN THE YEAR 1880.

IN issuing the annual report on the health of the Metropolitan Police Force during the year 1880, Mr. Holmes, the Chief Surgeon, remarks that the return of sickness for the past year is so nearly identical with those issued for the few preceding years—calling for no special comment—that only the ordinary particulars are given in their proper sequence. In the first place, when the nature of the duty is taken into consideration, with all its exposure to different phases of weather, it is somewhat surprising to find that only 4895 members of the Force were placed upon the sick-list during 1880, the total for the preceding year having been 5099; throughout the year under notice the average daily number of men on the sick-list was 285·9, and the average daily loss on the whole Force by sickness was 3 per cent., which is, as nearly as possible, the same as in preceding years. Rheumatism (" chronic " and " muscular "), coryza, bronchitis, and tonsillitis were the chief diseases resulting from exposure, claiming altogether a total of 2685 cases, against 3033 in the preceding year. One fact deserves to be specially recorded, namely, that, thanks to the protection accorded by revaccination, though small-pox was more or less epidemic in London during the whole of the past year, no case occurred throughout the whole of the Force. The number of deaths in the Town and Woolwich Divisions during the year was 66, and of these no less than 23 were attributed to consumption and disease of the lungs, 6 to pneumonia and pleurisy, 5 to bronchitis, and 11 to disease of the heart. The causes of invaliding during the year may be noted, beginning with the most frequent : From age, long service, and debility, 57 ; rheumatism, rheumatic gout, and sciatica, 56 ; consumption and "diseases of the lungs," 28; direct results of injuries incurred on duty, 15; disease of the heart, 15; defective vision, 13; bronchitis, 10; gout, 8; insanity and mental afflictions, 8; varicose veins and ulcer, 5; deafness and vertigo, 4 each ; fistula in ano, epilepsy, disease of the liver,

and disease of the brain, 3 each ; diseases of joints, amputation of the leg, pneumonia, pleurisy, erysipelas (sequelæ of), and tender feet, 2 each.

RUPTURE OF THE UTERUS SUCCESSFULLY TREATED BY DRAINAGE.

Two cases in which this usually fatal accident was successfully treated by drainage, are reported in a recent number of the Centralblatt für Gynäkologie (1880, No. 26). One is reported by Dr. Morsbach. The patient was aged thirty-five, and had had four children, the last five years previously. Labour came on at full term. When vigorous pains had lasted five hours, the midwife ruptured the membranes. After this, the patient, who had till then been standing, felt herself obliged to lie down; and the pains ceased. Three powders, obtained from a chemist, were given to bring on pains, without effect. Ten hours after the rupture of the membranes, Dr. Morsbach saw the patient. The os uteri was about eight centimetres in diameter, and the feet could be felt presenting, but high up. A dose of ergot was given, without effect. The patient was then narcotised, and it was discovered that there was a rupture of the vagina and cervix uteri, and that the child was in the abdominal cavity, except one foot, which was within the uterus. The foot was seized, and the rent carefully enlarged by numerous small incisions with scissors, till it would allow the child to be extracted. The hand was then inserted, and the placenta, which was in the peritoneal cavity, was removed. Two thick caoutchouc drainage-tubes were put into the rent, and a pad of salicyl wool between the thighs. Slight pyrexia followed, lasting a little more than a week, with abdominal tenderness and tympanites. One drainage-tube was removed the next day, and the other on the fourth day. The patient got up on the fourteenth day. Fourteen weeks afterwards she thought herself quite well. There was then a deep fissure in the cervix posteriorly, the bottom of which could not be reached by the finger, and a cicatrix in the posterior vaginal wall. Dr. Morsbach thought it possible that the midwife may have ruptured the uterus when she thought she was only rupturing the membranes, for she admitted that she had found great difficulty in doing what she did. The other case occurred in Berlin, and is reported by Dr. M. Graefe. The patient was in labour with her thirteenth child. The pains continued for six hours, and then suddenly ceased. An hour afterwards she was found in a state of collapse, the face presenting, an arm down in front, and a foot behind. Incomplete rupture of the uterus was diagnosed, and the patient was removed to the hospital. When she got there it was plain that the child was in the abdominal cavity, the contracted uterus being felt in front and to the left of it. The hand was introduced, a foot seized, and the child extracted ; then the placenta was removed. The uterus was found ruptured transversely, only about three fingers' breadth of its wall remaining entire. The peritoneal cavity contained much clotted blood and meconium. It was washed out with a 2½ per cent. carbolic acid solution, and then a thick drainage-tube, thirty centimetres long, put into the abdominal cavity, and secured by a silk suture to the posterior commissure. A bandage was put round the abdomen, and on it an ice-bladder. During the first two days the pulse was hardly perceptible. Hiccough and vomiting were troublesome during the first five days. The temperature did not rise till after the sixth day, when she began to have evening exacerbations of fever, which continued until the beginning of the fourth week, after which the temperature remained normal. After the sixth day the parts were irrigated from one to three times daily, through the tube, with a 2½ per cent. solution of carbolic acid. The tube was removed on the thirtieth day. The patient left the hospital, well and strong, on the thirty-fifth day. Dr. Graefe remarks, that whatever be the position this treatment will ultimately take, as compared with laparotomy, in these cases, there can be no doubt of its advantages in country practice, where the necessary assistants, instruments, etc., for laparotomy often cannot be had in time to be of service. These authors were led to adopt this mode of treatment by a paper by Dr. Richard Frommel, which will be found in the *Zeitschrift für Geburtshülfe und Gynäkologie*, Bd. V., Heft II. This author there reports eight cases, seven treated by laparotomy, all of them fatal; one by drainage, which recovered.

THE COMBINED SANITARY DISTRICT OF WEST SUSSEX.

THE seventh annual report on the condition of the Combined Sanitary District of West Sussex for the year 1880 affords ample proof of the largeness of the task imposed upon the Medical Officer of Health in thoroughly supervising all the healthy and unhealthy portions of the large area entrusted to his care. Dr. Charles Kelly possesses, however, as Professor of Hygiene in King's College, special qualifications for the duties he is called upon to perform, and this may be considered fortunate when it is stated that no less than ten sub-districts go to make up the Combined Sanitary District of West Sussex. Although the annual sanitary history of each of these is given in the report under notice, want of space precludes our noticing each separately. Dr. Kelly's summary shows that in the Combined District the birth-rate for the year 1880 was 30·3, and the death-rate 14·9 per 1000 persons living. The excess of births over deaths for the past six years was equal to 7345, but the population has increased from 81,872 in 1875 to 86,146 in 1880, or an increase of 4274, so that 3071 persons must have left the district during this period, over and above the results of immigration and emigration. The low birth-rate in West Sussex is stated to be chiefly due to the distribution of the population at various ages; the emigration of young people to large towns bringing about an excessive proportion of old people in rural districts. On the other hand, the low death-rate—conspicuous amongst the rates for the south-eastern division (including Kent, Surrey, Sussex, Hampshire, and Berkshire), which has always a lower mortality than the other registration divisions—may, Dr. Kelly thinks, be fairly placed to the credit of the improved sanitary measures which have of late years been introduced and enforced, not in West Sussex only, but all over the kingdom.

CLINICAL THERMOMETERS.—Some time ago we noticed the serious errors that had been detected in the clinical thermometers in use in the United States, and the circular which was issued from Yale College respecting them. Since then, thermometers have been accurately tested and re-tested at Kew Observatory, and from these a number have been constructed for comparison. The result has been very satisfactory, for, according to the *Louisville Med. News* (September 8), during a twelvemonth 1667 certificates have been issued with thermometers for clinical and physiological researches. And so much have the instruments made by the American makers improved, that while in 1880 four-fifths of all the thermometers received from seven makers for examination were in error over a third of a degree, and 2 per cent. had errors exceeding a whole degree; in 1881, four-fifths of all the thermometers sent in had errors of less than three-tenths of a degree. "A significant fact in connexion with this work is that about fifty physicians' thermometers, taken from actual practice, had errors exceeding a degree and a half. This may explain the many reports of affections presenting a marvellously high temperature with recovery, where authorised clinical records of the same, based upon correct thermometrical readings, would call for a prognosis of death."

SOCIAL SCIENCE CONGRESS IN DUBLIN.

HEALTH DEPARTMENT.

ON the morning of Thursday, October 6, an address was delivered before the Congress at large by Dr. Charles Cameron, M.P. for Glasgow, the President of the Health Department, in the Front Hall of Trinity College. The Right Hon. Lord O'Hagan, President of the Congress, occupied the chair, and there was a very large attendance, which included the Presidents of all the Sections.

Dr. Cameron selected for his theme the light cast by recent discoveries upon the nature of virulent and infectious maladies, the practical account to which those discoveries have already been turned, and one or two lessons which they suggest in connexion with the preservation of the public health. We have already dealt with this address, but we may be excused for quoting its concluding portion:—" In the first place, all this teaches in every line the necessity, from the standpoint of public health, of regarding every person suffering from an epidemic or contagious malady as a hot-bed swarming with living organisms which cause and spread the disease. It should be the duty of the public sanitary authorities to provide convalescent homes for patients recovering from serious infectious diseases, where they might be taken care of until all danger of the propagation of infection by them had ceased. Were this duty attended to, the recent discoveries as to the nature and causation of disease leave not the smallest doubt that we might be spared many epidemics, and that one disease especially—scarlatina—might be made to show a very different death-tale in our tables of mortality. In the second place, the whole history of the chain of discoveries which have furnished the topic of this address seems to teach the enormous importance of the study of comparative medicine and pathology—of medicine and pathology, not in their connexion with human diseases alone, but as branches of a science affecting the whole animal and vegetable world. Unless greater prominence be given to such studies, this country can hardly hope to hold her own against her neighbours in the cultivation of medical science. And no greater misfortune could befall the nation. But we must beware, while crying out for fresh enactments and extended powers, not to overlook the fact that throughout the kingdom those powers which the law already provides for the preservation of public health are but half enforced."

At the conclusion of the address, Dr. Grimshaw, the Registrar-General for Ireland, moved a vote of thanks to Dr. Cameron for his able and learned address. This resolution was seconded by Mr. William Johnston, Fishery Commissioner, and carried by acclamation.

The Health Department met subsequently to discuss the third and last special question—"Is any further Legislation desirable in order to more effectually prevent the Overcrowding of Dwelling-houses?" The discussion was opened with a general paper by the Hon. the Recorder of Dublin, on "The Overcrowding of Dwelling-houses from a Dublin Standpoint."

This was followed by a paper on the "Amelioration in the Condition of the Lowest Class of Dwellings," by Dr. Charles A. Cameron, S.Sc.C., Cambridge, Fellow and Professor of Hygiene, R.C.S.I., Medical Officer of Health for Dublin.

The next paper was one by Mr. Edward Spencer, Secretary of the Dublin Artisans' Dwellings Company. The author divided his paper into two parts: the first giving an account of the operation of the Dublin Artisans' Dwellings Company (Limited) since its formation in 1876; while the second part was devoted to a consideration of some of the difficulties which surround the provision of accommodation for the working-classes in Dublin, and the best means of surmounting those difficulties.

In the discussion which followed the reading of the three foregoing papers, the speakers were Mr. Henry Wigham, Mr. E. Dwyer Gray, M.P., Mr. Edmundson, the Right Hon. the Lord Mayor, Mr. Robert O'Brien Furlong, B.L., Secretary of the late Royal Sanitary Commission, Mr. T. W. Russell, Mr. Rawson Carroll, Alderman Harris, and Mr. Haughton.

Mr. Collins, Secretary to the Department, submitted the following resolution, which was carried, viz.—"That it is the opinion of this Section that it is desirable that the Corporation of Dublin should seriously consider the propriety of providing proper dwellings for the labouring classes under the provisions of the various Acts of Parliament relating thereto, and requests the Council to submit to the Corporation this expression of its opinion."

A paper by Mr. Edwin Chadwick, C.B., on "The Progress of Sanitation: Preventive as compared with Curative Science," was taken as read, and the Section adjourned.

THE FRENCH MEDICAL SERVICE IN TUNIS.

A WEEK or two since, Dr. Lereboullet, a retired medical officer of the French army, and now one of the sub-editors of the Gazette Hebdomadaire, published in that journal extracts from numerous letters of medical officers engaged in the Tunisian war. These displayed a startling condition of things, exhibiting the effects of the predominance of the commissariat (intendance) department over the combative and medical departments, which had done so much mischief in the Crimean, the Italian, and the Franco-German Wars. Deficiencies in food, in hospital accommodation, and an absence of almost rudimentary organisation, abounded, while large sums had been expended to prevent the recurrence of errors that had so often before proved so disastrous; but although long Parliamentary discussions had laid bare the errors that had to be corrected, nothing seems to have been done. These statements in the Gazette obtained a wide circulation throughout Europe in the columns of the lay press, including those of the Times; and general indignation, and something like consternation, have been produced at the fact revealed, that after so many years and such expenditure nothing has been done. In the number of the Gazette for October 14, Dr. Lereboullet returns to the subject, stating that he has received numerous confirmatory letters, and exposing the shortcomings of the explanations which the Government has published. After passing these in review, he terminates his article with the following observations:—

"Everyone must remember the obstinate resistance offered by General Farre to all those who endeavoured to get the Bill carried for the reform of the administration of the army. Those who read this journal at that time will not forget what we then predicted. Rejecting the autonomy of the medical body, and delaying by every kind of reticence and subterfuge the vote on the Bill, the urgent necessity of which was patent to all, General Farre, at the outset of an expedition so difficult to conduct, has allowed a state of things to persist which the experience of our former wars had condemned. He imagined that the undisputed zeal, devotion, and intelligence of the officers of the Intendance would supply their complete ignorance of the most serious medical questions; and he took no pains to ascertain which would be the diseases that in the months of June and July would be likely to seize hold of troops consisting of unacclimatised young soldiers, unaccustomed to African warfare, and, above all, predisposed to typhoid fever. He took them from everywhere—from the north and east of France, and even from garrisons where typhoid fever had prevailed. On receiving, if he has received them, the medical reports, he has never thought of immediately advising the disinfection of camps and barracks where typhoid patients had sojourned, and preventing other troops occupying them."

The Progrès Médical, commenting on the revelations brought to light, observes—"Nothing can be more sad, but still it must be said, that all the efforts, all the sacrifices made by the country in order to reconstruct its army have been a pure loss. Let a war break out to-morrow, and, as in 1870, we shall find our army without matériel, without provisions, and without medicines; and whatever may be the merits of the general in command, we shall witness the same disasters. We are persuaded that this expedition to Tunis will render us a great and immense service. It demonstrates that the position given by our military laws to the Intendance should be reversed, if our armies are ever to acquire any solidity. Superior, at the present time, to the combative and the medical services of the army, it should be made subordinate to them, being created for the satisfaction of their needs, and not to judge those needs."

FROM ABROAD.

CHANGE OF COLOUR OF THE HAIR FROM PILOCARPIN.

DR. PRENTIS, Professor of Therapeutics at the Washington Medical College, relates, in the Philadelphia Med. Times (July 2), a very complicated case of pyelitis, with anuria, in which change of the hair of the head from light blond to nearly black, seemed to be a consequence of the hypodermic use of pilocarpin, the hair being also thicker and coarser than before, and its growth more vigorous. Examined microscopically, the colour was found to be due, not to a dye, but to an increase of normal pigment. There was also a corresponding change of colour in the hairs of other parts of the body, but in a less degree. The pilocarpin was commenced on December 16, and the hair was first noted as beginning to change on the 28th. Although a similar case to this has not been recorded, it is well established that jaborandi increases the nutrition of the hair, stimulates its growth, and renders it thicker. In terminating the narration of this remarkable case, Prof. Prentis recapitulates the chief points of interest:—1. The prolonged period of total suppression of urine, this extending once over a period of eleven days, while for twenty-one days it might be considered as total, the daily average being less than a teaspoonful. 2. The value of pilocarpin in eliminating urea from the system and averting the consequence of uræmic poisoning. The usefulness of this drug in uræmia and in the various forms of dropsy is becoming well known, but it seldom happens that its beneficial effects are so strongly marked as in this case. The uræmia was extreme, and the case at one time so apparently hopeless that it became a serious question whether so distressing a course of treatment was justifiable. 3. The amount of fluid eliminated during "a sweat." "I have hesitated to state the amount eliminated—fourteen pints (by vomiting and saliva seven pints, saturated blanket five pints, and body-clothes two pints), which is about a seventh of the patient's weight—because it seems almost incredible; but a careful reconsideration satisfies me that the statement is not exaggerated. I think it possible that the amount was increased by the hot-bottle pack." 4. The effects produced in this case by the pilocarpin upon the stomach and bowels would seem to indicate that it excites a watery discharge from their mucous membrane, as well as from the skin and salivary glands. 5. The hypodermic use of pilocarpin is the preferable mode of employment. The hydrochlorate is perfectly soluble, and its use is unattended with pain or irritation. Its action is more prompt and the effects are sooner over than when administered by the stomach. 6. "There was no dropsy in this case. In two other cases of pyelonephritis occurring in my practice, which resulted fatally, there was no dropsy. Uræmia, or rather anuria, is not sufficient to cause dropsy, but when combined with a drain of albumen (albuminuria), dropsy soon results."

THE PARIS FACULTY OF MEDICINE.

The following are the lectures which are to be delivered at the Paris Faculty during the winter session of 1881-82:—1. Medical Physics—Prof. Gavarret will lecture once a week on Biological Physics and the Mechanical Phenomena of Vision; and Prof. Gariel three times a week on General Physics, the General Properties of Bodies, Heat, and Electricity. 2. Medical Pathology—Prof. Jaccoud, on Diseases of the Liver and Kidneys. 3. Anatomy—Prof. Sappey, on the Figurated Elements of the Blood and Lymph, the Lymphatic Vascular System in Man and Animals, the Sanguineous Vascular System, the Organs of the Senses, and the Apparatus of Innervation. 4. General Pathology and Therapeutics—Prof. Bouchard, Nervous Excisions in Disease. 5. Medical Chemistry —M. Hanriot (as a substitute for Prof. Wurtz), Inorganic Chemistry (Metalloids and Metals) in its Applications to Medicine and Toxicology. 6. Surgical Pathology—Prof. Duplay, Surgical Affections of the Cranium and Spinal Column, Diseases of the Nose and Nasal Fossæ, and Diseases of the Ear. 7. Operations and Apparatus—Prof. Léon le Fort, Therapeutics of Surgical Affections of the Joints, the Arteries and Veins, of the Head and Neck. 8. Histology—Prof. Robin, Tissues and Anatomical Systems, and their Accidental Modifications. 9. *History of Medicine and Surgery*—Prof. Laboulbène, History of the Popular Diseases of France, and Medical Biography. 10. *Medical Clinics*—Prof. Sée, at the Hôtel-Dieu ; Prof.Lasègue, at the Pitié ; Prof. Hardy, at the Charité ; and Prof. Potain, at the Necker. 11. *Clinic of Mental Pathology and Diseases of the Encephalon* — Prof. Ball, at the Asile Ste. Anne. 12. *Clinic of Diseases of Children*—Prof. Parrot, at the Enfants Assistés. 13. *Clinic of Syphilitic and Cutaneous Diseases*—Prof. Fournier, at the St. Louis. 14. *Surgical Clinics*—Prof. Gosselin, at the Charité; Prof. Bichet, at the Hôtel-Dieu ; Prof. Verneuil, at the Pitié ; and Prof. Trélat, at the Necker. 15. *Ophthalmological Clinic*—Prof. Panas, at the Hôtel-Dieu. 16. *Midwifery Clinic*—Prof. Depaul, at the Clinique d'Accouchement et Gynécologie.

The clinical professors lecture daily, and the others three times a week. In addition to the above, Prof. Brouardel gives a practical conference on Legal Medicine at the Morgue once a week, M. Farabœuf gives a course of Practical Anatomy, and M. Gay conferences on Physics. There are also *auxiliary courses*—on Medical Chemistry, by M. Henninger ; on Medical Natural History, by M. Lanceson ; on Internal Pathology, by M. Legroux ; on External Pathology, by M. Marchand ; on Midwifery, by M. Budin ; on Physiology, by M. Rémy ; and on Pathological Anatomy, by M. Straus.

INFLUENCE OF MALARIA IN MODIFYING ACUTE DISEASE.

The following interesting extract(a) is from the pen of Dr. Alexander Jamieson, Shanghai :—

The multiform modifications imposed by acute or chronic malarial saturation on the natural course of specific diseases deserve careful study, as also do various independent typhoidal conditions hitherto undescribed, which occasionally end in death, and which are in all probability manifestations of acute malarial poisoning. To include them, the application of the term "malaria" may require to be widened, so as to include the vehicles of poisons other than that or those productive of the group of affections now classed as malarial. There can be little doubt that we are already within sight of a new and scientific general pathology, whose foundations will have been laid in those investigations into the history of blood-parasites and of aërial and soil germs which are being ardently pursued all over the world, and in China notably by Manson, of Amoy. Those investigations will doubtless bring to light the causes of such cases as I refer to below, in which a non-traumatic septicæmia of unknown origin was accompanied by the gastro-enteritis described by Bergmann as existing in artificial septic poisoning. Hitherto I have observed these typhoidal conditions only in young male adults newly or lately arrived, but I have heard of other instances which prove that neither sex, nor age, nor duration of residence, is a necessary factor.

Two cases have recently been under my care, one of which I saw shortly before death, while the other I had an opportunity of watching from the beginning. The symptoms were those of profound blood-poisoning—depression, rapid exhaustion, variable but never high temperature, profuse sweating, yellow staining of the skin, night delirium (sometimes tranquil, at other times wild) ; transudation of altered blood through all the mucous membranes except that of the mouth ; profuse stools, discharged without pain or straining, and consisting of broken-down blood without any tendency to coagulation, but containing here and there a small black or crimson clot ; scanty bloody urine, laden with urates, expelled with difficulty ; persistent vomiting, occasionally tinged with blood ; epistaxis ; and frequent expectoration of blood-stained mucus, without, however, any true hæmoptysis. In neither of these cases was there distension of the abdomen or gurgling or pain in the cæcal region. In neither was there any exanthem until, in one case three, and in the other two, days before death, when a mottling of petechiæ, resembling the typhus rather than the typhoid rash, appeared on the abdomen. There were no sordes on the mouth, nor was there swelling of the gums. In neither were there any chest symptoms other

(a) From the *Medical Reports of the Imperial Maritime Customs of China.*

than those of congestion of the lungs. In neither was there any sensible enlargement of the liver, and in one only was there a slight increase (to the extent of about an inch below the costal border) of the splenic dulness. These cases were treated with hot cataplasms to the abdomen kept on night and day, and internally quinine, ergot, wine, lemon and orange juice, and occasional small doses of salines, with concentrated nourishment, but in neither did any benefit result from the treatment adopted.

REVIEWS.

The Principles and Practice of Surgery : being a Treatise on Surgical Diseases and Injuries. By D. HAYES AGNEW, M.D., LL.D., Professor of Surgery in the Medical Department of the University of Pennsylvania. Profusely illustrated. Vol. II. Philadelphia : J. B. Lippincott and Co. London : 16, Southampton-street, Covent-garden. 1881.

In the *Medical Times and Gazette* of January 3, 1880, will be found the review of the first volume of this colossal treatise. We have now before us the second volume, consisting of 1666 pages, and illustrated by 788 figures. In his preface to this volume the author tells us that the third, which when published will complete the work, "is in progress of rapid preparation."

It has been a cause of regret that three years have elapsed between the issue of the first and second volumes, and it is to be hoped, for the sake of those who have purchased both and intend to make them their text-book on surgery, that an equally long interval will not separate the third from the second volume. It cannot, however, be a matter of surprise that so long a time passes before one part follows the next, if we consider what an enormous task the author has set himself to accomplish. The period must needs be a very busy one to the writer.

The amount of labour performed by some of the older physicians and surgeons, of which their writings are the proof, has often excited admiration. It was only the other day that an American surgeon, wishing to ascertain all that could be discovered about Sir Charles Bell and his life's work, advertised in one of the British medical papers for information, and was at once supplied by an enterprising London bookseller with a catalogue of no less than seventy-three books, articles, and pamphlets ; and this catalogue was shortly followed by an intimation that he (the bookseller) had just discovered ten others also from the pen of Charles Bell. It may, however, be fairly questioned whether the labour of producing a book of moderate dimensions was, formerly, equal to that requisite for a well-executed article on any given subject of medical or surgical practice nowadays. The quantity of literature—books, journals, and contributions to societies—which must be consulted in order to produce an article thoroughly up to the present time is of itself enormous, and the task can only be roughly judged, not even approximately measured, by the result.

Bearing this in mind as we read over the pages of Dr. Agnew's work, we are satisfied that there are amongst us in these days men comparable in industry to their most energetic predecessors. Moreover, we repeatedly found in Dr. Agnew's work proofs of what we have often remarked in studying the admirable and exhaustive articles which appear from time to time in the *American Journal of Medical Sciences*—namely, extensive research, minute and careful examination of the work of others, shrewd criticism, and well-balanced conclusions.

The second volume of Dr. Agnew's treatise does not, however, equal the first. There is no chapter in it which at all comes up to the exhaustive chapter in vol. i., on Injuries of the Osseous System, nor even to that on Injuries of the Chest and Abdomen. There are, too, evidences of hurry, and of the carelessness which arises out of hurry, scattered everywhere throughout the text, and occurring even in places where it might have been supposed that extreme attention would have been given to accuracy. Take, for instance, the tabular lists on pages 102 and 103 ; the references to the very first case are wrong, and the "characteristic phenomena" of other cases are inaccurately quoted. Even the names of distinguished surgeons and authors are misspelt—in some instances spelt so as to make it difficult to ascertain who is really meant. "Stanly," for Stanley ; "Jessup," for Jessop, though uncomplimentary inaccuracies, do not give rise to doubt in the reader's mind; but when "Cline" takes the place of Cline, "Southam" for Southam, and "Laird" for Lund of Manchester; and when the surname of another surgeon, whose invention is recommended, is left to the imagination of the reader, and a drawing of an instrument stands in the Christian name of its inventor, much more confusion is caused and a greater injustice is done.

It might have been thought, too, that sufficient interest in operations on the kidneys had been excited during the last two or three years, and that sufficient care had been taken to distinguish the different operations from one another by appropriate names, to have prevented the author of the most recent text-book from describing nephrotomy as an operation which "is performed either through the lumbar region or through the anterior parietes of the abdomen"; and from enumerating all the conditions under which nephrectomy is suitable and justifiable as cases adapted for "nephrotomy."

We should have supposed, also, that the intention and action of Davy's "rectal lever" had become by this time pretty well known to surgeons; or if not, that, at least, a surgical author before referring to it would have ascertained that it was devised for the purpose of compressing the common iliac artery, not the abdominal aorta; that it has been found to answer its purpose admirably in now quite a large number of cases: and that to give it countenance by quoting a single successful case in which it was employed is doing but scant justice to an established and deservedly well-established method of preventing hæmorrhage during amputations at the hip-joint, and top of the thigh.

In the chapter on Dislocations there are several defects. There may be good reason for describing "dislocations of the acromial extremity of the clavicle" as "dislocations of the scapula," but there is more reason to put the student or practitioner on his guard against the possible errors in diagnosis of dislocation of the inferior angle of the scapula; yet this is not done. In dislocations of the shoulder it is undesirable to lead the student to seek for "a loss of from one to two inches in the vertical circumference of the shoulder-joint of the affected side," instead of an increase to that extent. Also it is useless to be still burdening the memory or encumbering descriptions with all the details of the mode of employing the pulleys for hip-joint dislocations, and to be copying diagrams from Astley Cooper in which the partial outline of the acetabulum is made to look like a deformed trochanter minor. Even in Cooper's large and original plates reference to the letterpress is almost necessary to enlighten one on this point; but in the copies, in this as in numerous other works, which have been made of these plates, it is quite impossible for the uninitiated to divine what these peculiar dotted curves are intended to represent. So experienced a surgeon and so industrious an author as Dr. Agnew might, too, have been expected to make himself acquainted with other views besides those of Bigelow on the mode of production of dislocations of the hip. The writings of Fabbri, Tillaux, and Morris are not alluded to, though it may justly be said that the paper by the latter in the sixtieth volume of the *Medico-Chirurgical Transactions* has had the effect of simplifying what was confused in our views of the nature of these accidents, and of pointing out how the character of the lesions explains the *modus operandi* of the method of reduction by manipulation.

In the treatment of carbuncle the value of solid carbolic acid in hastening the separation of the sloughs and checking the spread of the inflammation is not mentioned; indeed, cauterisation is only alluded to to be dismissed as a "barbarism"; and heat and moisture, or blistering, are the remedies preferred.

The symptoms of tuberculous disease of the bladder are said to be "by no means characteristic, differing very little from those common to morbid growths in the bladder." If the author had said that the difficulty lay in distinguishing the exact locality of the disease along the genito-urinary tract, we should have agreed with him; but surely, when the general health and constitution of the patient are considered, and instrumental and digital examination give no evidence of stone or growth in the bladder, the symptoms of tubercle are usually characteristic enough to enable the surgeon to form a positive diagnosis.

The section on Ovariotomy is most unsatisfactory. The remarks on the mode of securing the pedicle convey no definite instruction or advice to the reader. He would certainly not gather from it that at the present time the ligature, and the intra-peritoneal method of applying it, is the most approved. Spencer Wells is said to be still the champion of the clamp, Keith of the cautery; and when a ligature is applied, the practice of "bringing the threads out at the lower part of the wound, as advised by Clay, or through the vagina, the plan of Greene," would appear, from the author's account, to be as good and as much to be recommended as any other. The method described of closing the wound is extremely clumsy and tedious, and the advice given with regard to diet is calculated to increase the mortality of the operation if very rigidly followed.

In the chapter on Diseases of the Mouth there is a paragraph on carbuncle on the lips; the frequency with which this disease leads to phlebitis and thrombosis of the cerebral sinuses is not noticed, and the author contents himself by saying that a suggestion has been thrown out "that the tendency to constitutional symptoms may be due to the readiness with which the facial veins receive morbid materials."

Two methods are described and illustrated for removing portions of the tongue affected with epithelioma, by strangulation with ligatures. The objections to this proceeding are surely overwhelming, and it can hardly be supposed that any surgeon would resort to such practice. The distinctive characters of epitheliomatous and syphilitic ulcerations would require revision before being accepted as commonly correct.

Next as to the illustrations, with which this volume, like its predecessor, abounds: there are two which are so bad as regards the information they are intended to convey that it is not conceivable the author would have allowed them place in his book if he had taken time to consider them. One is on page 312, showing the disposition of surgeon and assistants in performing amputation of the leg: whilst an assistant is engaged exclusively in handing a saw to the surgeon before the flaps have been commenced, no one is appointed to look after the artery. The other illustration to which we refer is on page 671, and is intended to show the position of patient, operator, and assistants in the operation of lateral lithotomy. Nothing can possibly convey a worse or more erroneous impression. Surely, if instruction is to be given in this way, care ought to be shown in the construction of the sketches. It may further be remarked of the illustrations that a large number are quite superfluous; whole pages are given up to drawings of instruments, which would be becoming enough in the illustrated catalogue of a surgical instrument maker, but are quite out of place in a modern work on surgery. There are no less than six drawings, showing as many "positions" in which the knife ought to be held by the operator; and two or three pages are devoted to verbal instruction on this head; though, in spite of them all, each surgeon will doubtless continue, as Sir William Fergusson long ago recommended, to employ the position which is most convenient and suitable to himself.

A very large number of the illustrations seem to be familiar to us, or to be so nearly the same as, that it is hard to distinguish them from, those we are accustomed to in certain well-known works. We may be wrong in this, and we prefer to think we are, as there is no acknowledgment of the source of many of them, either in the list of illustrations or elsewhere.

The size of the work might have been kept down, had the author not introduced matters which are more fittingly dealt with in other works than text-books on surgery. Overflowing as the field of surgical practice is with so many large and different subjects, and voluminous as a treatise on them all necessarily must be, there is no excuse for trespassing on the domain of the physician-accoucheur, by entering in detail into questions of the symptoms and treatment of uterine malpositions, uterine flexions, inversion of the uterus, dysmenorrhœa, and malignant disease of the uterus.

On the whole, however, if it has been felt by any that another text-book on surgery was needed, Dr. Agnew is succeeding in meeting the want very well, in spite of the several shortcomings, to some of which we have alluded; and in spite of the fact that this second volume cannot be said to be brought well up in all respects to the latest period.

GENERAL CORRESPONDENCE.

INTRA-PERITONEAL WOUNDS OF THE BLADDER.

LETTER FROM DR. R. NEALE.

[To the Editor of the Medical Times and Gazette.]

SIR,—In your editorial article upon Intra-peritoneal Wounds of the Bladder (October 1, page 415), it is stated that, out of 97 reported cases, 96 have proved fatal, the exception being a case under the care of Dr. Walter, in 1862. A reference to the "Medical Digest," section 1053-3, will prove that this is not absolutely correct.

Mr. Chaldecot (Lancet, July, 1846, page 112) reports a case in which the bladder was ruptured by a fall, severe peritonitis following, which was healed by large doses of opium. In twenty-two hours water flowed through the catheter, and all the symptoms abated. Six days subsequently, wishing to avoid the catheter, the patient strained violently, and all the symptoms of peritonitis reappeared, and again yielded to appropriate remedies. Mr. Skey, who saw the case, agreed that the symptoms were due to rupture of the bladder. The patient, although never subject to gout, had a severe attack three days after the accident, due to the absorption of the effused urine, a relapse following the strain on the sixth day.

M. Perrin relates a case in which a man fell on the leg of a chair, which pierced the bladder through the anus. A gush of urine followed the extraction of the foreign body, and the wound healed on the twenty-fifth day. Fifteen days later, retention came on, due to a piece of trouser cloth blocking the urethra.

The Medical Times and Gazette (November, 1879, page 608) contains an exhaustive clinical lecture upon a case of recovery from ruptured bladder, due to violence, delivered by Henry Morris, M.A., M.B., at the Middlesex Hospital.

I am, &c.,　　　　RICHARD NEALE, M.D. Lond.

P.S.—The above is a good illustration of one of the many advantages to be derived from a free use of the "Medical Digest."

60, Boundary-road, South Hampstead, N.W., October 6.

DOCTORS TO PILGRIM SHIPS.

LETTER FROM MR. T. COMFIELD.

[To the Editor of the Medical Times and Gazette.]

SIR,—As doctors will soon be in request for steamers intended to call at Yembo and Jeddah, ports in the Red Sea, for pilgrims returning home after performing their hadj at Mecca, I think it would be well if attention were drawn, from time to time during the next few weeks, to the fact that cholera has this year broken out among those pilgrims, and also to the fact that quarantine is therefore now enforced against all ships carrying them home.

Medical men intending to go out as doctors to pilgrim ships would also do well to remember—

1. That a steamer carrying pilgrims to or from a port under British rule would only be allowed to take about two-thirds of the pilgrims she could, and almost surely would, take to any other port. Pilgrim ships are so crowded with pilgrims, and encumbered with their bulky belongings, that this is a very important point to be remembered.

2. That, unless the steamer is taking pilgrims to or from a port under British rule, no place is set apart for the sick; and the law does not require (or, at all events, did not last season) any drugs, medical comforts, or surgical instruments or appliances to be carried for the pilgrims. On this point I would remark that I was told on all sides, even up to Jeddah itself, and without a dissenting voice, that the pilgrims would take no medicine, but I found, with but few exceptions, that it was quite the reverse.

3. That as cargo steamers only are employed in the pilgrim trade, doctors will find the living, as a rule, very rough, and probably no congenial society on board.

Previous to last season, only those pilgrim ships which went to or from British India ports had to carry doctors, but now all carrying over a hundred pilgrims have to carry a doctor of some sort or another.

The most repulsive feature in a pilgrim ship, to my mind, is the almost universal lousiness—I refer to pediculi corporis, not capitis—of the pilgrims. I could never look round at

any time of the day, during any period of the voyage, without seeing a considerable number of them overhauling their garments, searching for their tormentors.

I am, &c.,　　　　THOS. COMFIELD, L.R.C.P., etc.

14, Caistor-villas, Stoke Newington, N., October 15.

NEW ELASTIC CORD TOURNIQUET.

LETTER FROM DR. J. W. COUSINS.

[To the Editor of the Medical Times and Gazette.]

SIR,—If you will kindly re-examine the two spring tourniquets, I think you will be convinced that the new instrument made for me by Messrs. Arnold and Sons is really more than a "revised edition" of the old tubular spring tourniquet.

First. The old form of clamp is discarded for a strong metal ring, fitted with a toothless plate, which opens only upwards. This arrangement has the special advantage that it does not cut the rubber.

Secondly. The pad is done away with altogether, and pressure upon the artery is obtained by quite a novel contrivance. The cord is simply passed through a strong ring with a cross-bar, and in this way the elastic cord is converted in any position into an elastic pad.

Thirdly. The new tourniquet consists of three separate pieces. The cord is an endless ring, which can be attached to the metal ring and released again in a moment. This arrangement has the advantage that the instrument can be conveniently cleaned, and also that no portion of the rubber is constantly on the strain in the same position.

I am, &c.,　　　　J. WARD COUSINS,

Surgeon to Royal Portsmouth Hospital.

Southsea, October 18.

OBITUARY.

GIOVANNI CABIADIS.

It is with extreme regret that we announce the untimely death of Dr. Giovanni Cabiadis, the intelligent, zealous, and indefatigable Sanitary Officer in the service of the Ottoman Health Department. Dr. Cabiadis was a native of Mytilene, and graduated at the University of Pisa in 1867. He died at Bushire, in the Persian Gulf, on September 26, from suppurative inflammation of the liver, the consequence of repeated attacks of the Yemen malarial fever, caught in the discharge of his duties. While still suffering from the effects of this fever, he went, at the desire of the Board of Health, to Mesopotamia to superintend the sanitary measures that were to be carried out there in order to stamp out the plague, and in so doing he aggravated the malady from which he was suffering, and thus accelerated his untimely end. By his death the Ottoman Health Department has lost the best man it had, and those who knew him have lost an intelligent, active, warm-hearted friend.

A DISPENSING QUESTION IN FRANCE.—Dr. B., called to a child suffering from croup, gave the father a prescription to get made up. The pharmacien, on the pretext that the emetic ordered would endanger the child's life, refused to dispense it. The prescription was shown to another physician, who concurred with the pharmacien as to its dangerous character. Dr. B. was not called to the child again, who died. The father on several occasions commented upon the conduct of Dr. B., attributing his child's death, to some extent, to his unskilful procedure. Hereupon Dr. B. brought an action for 5000 fr. against the father and the pharmacien, the former for his libellous statements, and the latter for having refused to dispense the prescription. He lost the case, and had to pay the costs, the judge determining that a pharmacien had no right to alter a prescription even when he believed it dangerous, his duty being to immediately refer to the prescriber for explanation. But, on the other hand, if he dispenses a dangerous prescription, he is criminally liable for the consequences. He is under no obligation to dispense it at all, providing his refusal is not founded on a desire to injure the prescriber. The confirmation by another physician of the view of the dose taken by the pharmacien was held to exonerate him from any suspicion of that kind.—Revue Méd., October 1.

REPORTS OF SOCIETIES.

THE CLINICAL SOCIETY OF LONDON.

FRIDAY, OCTOBER 14.

JOSEPH LISTER, D.C.L., F.R.C.S., F.R.S., President,
in the Chair.

NEW HONORARY MEMBERS.

THE PRESIDENT announced that the Council had decided
to recommend to the Society the election of Sir James Paget
as a British Honorary Member, and of nine distinguished
gentlemen, who lately attended the International Medical
Congress from abroad, as Foreign Honorary Members of the
Clinical Society. The announcement was received with
applause.

CASE OF RUPTURED OVARIAN CYST.

Dr. WILTSHIRE read notes of this case. A lady, aged
twenty-eight, just convalescent from typhoid fever, fell,
while in a hansom cab, struck her abdomen, and burst an
ovarian cyst which she had had about three years. Severe
shock and collapse ensued, but under opium and restoratives
she slowly recovered, and, two years after the accident, remained quite well and free of her tumour, with the exception of a small mass, supposed to be the remains of the
collapsed cyst and pedicle. Though an expectant plan of
treatment was elected, in the belief that no hæmorrhage
was going on, yet the propriety of immediate operative
interference was discussed, chiefly in relation to the question
of rapid death from internal hæmorrhage, and its arrest-
ment by means of abdominal section, accompanied, of
course, by removal of the ovary. Operation in connexion
with ruptured dermoid purulent, infective, or strangulated
(twisted) cysts, and peritonitis was also referred to, and
allusion was made to the treatment of dangerous intra-
peritoneal hæmorrhages from ruptured ectopic gestation,
varices of the broad ligament, ruptured uterus, etc. The
prognosis in rupture of infective ovarian growths was adverted to, and the views of pathologists and surgeons thereon
respectfully sought.

The PRESIDENT remarked that the case was one of great
anxiety, as a decision respecting the treatment, whether that
should be expectant or active, must be at once arrived at.
Was the cyst single or multilocular? If multilocular, it
would be well, perhaps, to rid the patient of the fluid lying
within the peritoneal cavity, and of the other cysts, by one
operation at once. Whereas, if the cyst were single, the
expectant treatment might with propriety be pursued. But
the treatment would probably depend on the condition of the
patient at the time of the surgeon's visit. The solid mass
detected before the rupture afterwards dwindled away. Was
not that a remarkable circumstance?

Dr. WILTSHIRE, in reply, stated that he had not seen the
patient before the accident; but Dr. Oldham, who had previously been consulted, had thought she had a multilocular
cyst. He (Dr. Wiltshire) wished to learn what was the
prognosis of such cases, and had recorded the case in order
to elicit opinions respecting the course of treatment to be
pursued.

ODONTOMA OF THE LOWER JAW.

Mr. CHRISTOPHER HEATH contributed particulars of this
case, in which he had removed a large odontome. It was one
of the rare tumours described by Broca as odontomes odonto-
plastiques, and consisted of a mass of dentine studded with
nodules of enamel. The mass weighed 815 grains, and
measured an inch and a half by an inch and a quarter. The
patient was a young lady aged eighteen, who had never been
able to close the teeth properly, but otherwise was supposed
to have gone through the first and second dentitions naturally. Last Christmas she had some pain and uneasiness
about the right angle of the lower jaw; and in April her
father, a dental surgeon, extracted the second bicuspid
tooth, there being no molars then present. A dentist, who
was subsequently consulted, thought he detected an encysted
tooth, and tried to extract it with the elevator. The result
was an acute attack of periostitis. Profuse suppuration
ensued; and, on firm pressure near the angle, pus could
be forced up from the interior of the bone. Under treat-

ment, the inflammation subsided, and the patient went to
the seaside; and on her return there was apparently some exposed bone, with greatly hypertrophied mucous membrane on
each side. A month later, after imprudent bathing, sudden
increase of pain and swelling took place; and she consulted
Mr. Heath, who found great enlargement of the bone, with a
fungus-like growth in the mouth, and apparently bare bone,
the appearances closely resembling those ordinarily found in
a case of sarcoma of the jaw. An operation involving removal
of a portion of the jaw was declined, and the swelling slowly
diminished again. In September, Mr. Heath undertook an
operation for removal of the supposed sequestrum of bone,
and, after considerable trouble, succeeded in elevating the
mass described from its bed, since which the jaw had slowly
contracted to its proper shape.

Mr. VASEY learnt, upon inquiry, that there was no history
of a blow to the jaw.

The PRESIDENT considered the case to be one of great
interest practically, because a tumour of the lower jaw was
got rid of by a process of simple extraction; pathologically,
because of its rarity. Surgeons should be on their guard
lest they might remove a portion of the lower jaw instead of
extracting the tumour.

CASE OF CHARCOT'S JOINT-DISEASE.

Mr. C. B. KEATLEY read particulars respecting this case,
and exhibited the patient. He was a shopkeeper, aged
thirty-four, married ten years, having three healthy children.
Up to October, 1880, no other symptoms than the following
had been noticed:—(1) slight "weakness on the legs," of
twelve years' duration, and attributed by the patient to the
lameness occasionally produced by a "corn" beneath the
right great toe; (2) pains in the muscles, described as rheumatic; (3) attacks of diarrhœa, occurring fortnightly for
long periods at a time. But, in October, 1880, the "corn"
ulcerated, and the corresponding great toe became greatly
swollen. About a week afterwards the hip, groin, and thigh
of the same side (the right) swelled enormously, but were
pale and comparatively free from pain, i.e., such pain as did
exist was not synchronous with the occurrence of the great
swelling. A deep fluctuating point being opened towards
the lower part of the front of the thigh, several ounces of
synovia, or a synovial-like fluid, escaped. In two months the
patient was able to stand again, and move the joint freely,
but there was then discovered an inch and a half of shortening, a tendency to eversion, and a peculiar "scrunching"
or crepitus on manipulating the hip in a certain manner.
The joint was also somewhat loose. Apparently, the head of
the femur had disappeared. From this time, for nine months,
the limb steadily increased in usefulness; the power of spontaneously rotating it both inwards and outwards seemed to
also return. But then the left hip was attacked exactly like
the right, but not so acutely. This attack came on whilst
the patient was being severely purged by two pills and two
black draughts, prescribed by a chemist on the theory
that the patient looked "bilious." While the swelling of
the left hip was subsiding, after the manner of that on the
right side a year before, severe pains attacked the front and
inner side of the left thigh, and the left knee also, but passed
away after some hours. At present the patient had only
occasional slight pains in the left thigh, but great numbness on the front aspect above the knee. He could
already get about on crutches, and even stand without
them. There was now evidence of the left hip having undergone anatomical changes like those of the right. The right
great toe joints had been also deformed since the swelling
thereof twelve months ago. The corn was represented by a
thin red scab. There were various symptoms of tabes dorsalis
besides those above-mentioned. These were loss of patellar
tendon-reflex, of iris reflex, of the power of standing with the
heels together and the eyes shut, partial loss of sensation in
the outer sides of both feet, perverted sensation in the right
foot, slight deafness of the left ear, and (?) an ataxic gout
disguised by the joint-affections. And, though there were
no gastric crises, there were what might be termed "intestinal
crises," viz., the above-mentioned periodical attacks of diarrhœa. In the case of each hip, the subsidence of the general
swelling left a marked enlargement of the inguinal glands,
which persisted some time. The internal treatment had
been iodide of potassium with salicylate of soda, five grains
of each three times a day. Was it justifiable to try nerve-
stretching in this case? There were some grounds for enter-

taining such an idea? In most of the cases, now not few in number, in which nerve-stretching had been done for the lightning pains, general as well as local benefit had accrued, not only by way of lessening the pain, but also by diminishing, or even removing, the incoördination. And the same general improvement as regarded the whole neurosis had been observed in leprosy, when the pains of that disease had been treated by nerve-stretching. Done antiseptically it was by no means a very serious proceeding. Moreover, to do nothing in such a case as this did not secure for the patient a very good prognosis. If the speaker had any evidence to show that nerve-stretching had checked the visible changes in the skin in leprosy, he would be still more inclined to try it. Could any of his hearers speak as to that point?

Dr. DYCE DUCKWORTH thought the cases of this disease must be much more common in France than in this country. Sir James Paget, at the recent International Medical Congress, stated that he had not seen such a specimen from any such case in any museum, nor any living example of the affection; and he was invited to ask Professor Charcot to describe the cases in question. Dr. Benjamin Ball first described the ulceration of the feet. As regarded the question of nerve-stretching as a mode of treatment, some good observers were opposed to it.

Dr. BUZZARD remarked that a similar ulceration of the toe had occurred in a case reported to the Society by Dr. Greenhow ten or eleven years ago. The ulceration was due to a trophic change connected with disease of the nervous system. The diarrhœa in this case, consisting of three or four liquid motions a day for two or three days, had for years come on every fortnight or so. He also had heartburn, but there was no vomiting. He (Dr. Buzzard) had suggested an association of tabetic arthropathy, with the "gastric crises" mentioned by Charcot; he had seen the latter six times in nine cases of the former in his own practice. He thought the gastric crises were due to sclerosis of the posterior cornua of the spinal cord, continued up to the medulla oblongata, there influencing the vagus, and that possibly in that part of the nervous system was a centre which presided over joints. Such a centre would explain the relationship of acute rheumatism and heart disease. The muscles in the neighbourhood of the affected joints exhibited only normal excitability. In this patient the periodical diarrhœa and heartburn might be taken as an equivalent of the gastric crises.

Dr. ALTHAUS considered the case a very rare one. The œdema present here from the commencement of the joint-affection was not usual. The early joint-swelling was generally hard, not œdematous. As regarded the union of gastric crises and joint-affections, the former he declared frequent, but the latter very rare; so that he did not think there was much connexion between the two. As to the centre in the medulla oblongata supposed to preside over the joints, it was an ingenious supposition, but could not at present be proved. The pathology of the disease was mysterious, and it was difficult to see how the joint-affection came about. It had been suggested by professor Volkmann that the joint-disease was due to injury received by ataxic patients. But he (Dr. Althaus) did not consider this correct, as it often occurred in the early stages of tabes, even when the ocular symptoms were the only ones that could be recognised. This patient had had no injury to his joint. As regarded the operation of nerve-stretching, it might perhaps be done advantageously in certain defined cases.

Mr. H. PAGE said that until quite lately the Museum of the Royal College of Surgeons had contained no specimen of the joint-disease in tabes. But at the International Medical Congress Mr. Macnamara had exhibited two specimens of hip-disease in ataxia; and a patient in St. Mary's Hospital was walking along when he had suddenly felt his hip "give way," so that the limb suddenly became three or four inches shorter than the other. He was subsequently discovered to have ataxia. Mr. Page had exhibited at the Congress a patient having enlarged joints of the foot, the bones of which moved freely on one another, and the movement gave no pain. He had sores on the feet such as were found in these other cases, and he had called them "gathered corns." They were not very painful. He was examined, and found to have well-marked tabes dorsalis. Whilst under observation, the other foot had become enlarged at the tarsal and ankle joints, and the bones were freely movable upon one another, as if the foot

were a bag containing loose bones. He (Mr. Page) had kept that second foot at rest, as the first had been so treated and had been cured. The patient had left the hospital with the foot in plaster-of-paris bandage, and was much improved. He had never had pain in the parts affected, but had gastric and intestinal crises, and profuse hæmaturia, for which no surgical cause could be discovered. Physicians and surgeons must have their eyes open to look out for these patients. The patients often had, when first seen, no ataxic symptoms; they could still walk with their eyes shut.

The PRESIDENT remarked on the rarity of the affection. He had seen one case of the kind under one of the surgeons at King's College Hospital. Perhaps it was the very rarity and abnormality of the cases which kept them out of the museums.

Mr. KEATLEY, in reply, stated that a patient might have ocular and other symptoms for years before he became ataxic. This patient had not his knees affected. The joint-disease was liable to be bilaterally symmetrical. The disease was not likely to be mistaken for any other disorder. This man's hip and thigh were much more swollen after being affected for one week, without there being any pain, than were any other hip or thigh he had ever seen affected with any other disease; and yet in two months the swelling was nearly all gone, the limb was shortened,—and all this had occurred with scarcely any pain. The disease certainly had most distinct features, and was easily recognisable.

THE PATHOLOGICAL SOCIETY OF LONDON.

TUESDAY, OCTOBER 18.

SAMUEL WILKS, M.D., President, in the Chair.

FRACTURE OF A CERVICAL VERTEBRA.

DR. CARRINGTON showed a specimen of this disease which had been taken from a man who had fallen into a ship's hold a distance of ten feet. There were no special symptoms for the first few days to indicate the nature of the accident, and he was treated as an out-patient for two or three days. The man got up after his fall. He spat up some clotted blood, and had some difficulty in swallowing. He was admitted into Guy's Hospital under Dr. Wilks, the nature of his injury not being apparent even yet. His symptoms pointed to the pharynx and larynx, which were examined with the laryngoscope; a sloughy ulcer was observed at the root of the tongue. The temperature was raised; but there was no paralysis of any kind. The ulcer was diagnosed as possibly diphtheritic in nature. The man died, delirium tremens having supervened. At the post-mortem examination an abscess-cavity was found between the bodies of the vertebræ and the soft structures of the cervical region. This contained fœtid pus. There was a fracture across the body of the sixth cervical vertebra, but without any displacement, for the posterior common ligament was normal, and there was no pressure of any kind on the cord, which also appeared normal. The spinal canal contained a little pus; the putrid inflammation had spread up to the meninges of the base of the brain. Some blood was found extravasated about the root of the tongue.

Dr. CARRINGTON showed also, as a card specimen, a similar preparation from the Guy's Museum. The prævertebral abscess had opened into the œsophagus. The exact nature of the case was not at first very evident. The man had lived twenty-four days.

CHYLURIA—FILARIA SANGUINIS HOMINIS.

Dr. STEPHEN MACKENZIE showed a well-marked example of this condition. The man (who was present) was aged twenty-six years. He was born in Madras, of European parents; was in the Artillery, and during his stay in India had always enjoyed good health. He felt the change of climate considerably on his arrival in England. He first noticed that his urine was increased in quantity, and then that it was slimy, and subsequently milky in appearance. One day he experienced great pain in the back, then had a severe attack of hæmaturia, which lasted some eight or ten days. He was admitted into hospital for this. The chylous urine was faintly alkaline; he passed on one occasion as much as fifteen pints, at other periods from four to eight pints during the twenty-four hours. The milkiness, when examined with the microscope, was found to be due to minute granules: there were no casts; no sugar. The character of the day and of the night urine varied—that passed by day contained more blood and more filariæ, that passed by night was more milky in appearance. The blood was found to contain numbers of filariæ. The maximum number was found about midnight, while at 9 a.m. the blood was almost quite free from them, and remained so until about 9 p.m., when the filariæ again began to show themselves. On postponing the meals for an hour or two during the day, no difference in the migration of the filariæ was observed; but if the man was kept up all night, and allowed to sleep all day, then their periodicity was exactly reversed. Reference was made to the fact that the mosquito was found to be the intermediary host, and specimens from these creatures from Australia and China were shown and described.

Dr. COBBOLD, in answer to a request from the President, remarked on the early history of the filaria, describing five epochs:—The first described by Wücherer in the urine; second, Lewis's discovery of them in chyluria, and in the blood and other tissues of these patients; third, Bancroft's notice of them in lymphatic abscess of the arm; fourth, Manson's discovery of the intermediary host (the mosquito); fifth, Manson's further discovery of filarial periodicity. He thought the pathological importance of these creatures could hardly be exaggerated.

Dr. GEORGE HARLEY said the germ theory of disease was becoming every day more important. Filariæ were known to attack horses and other animals. All germ diseases were periodical—scarlet fever, ague, etc. He had recently heard that rice-fermentation had its period, which was doubtless analogous. The question, what became of the filariæ in the intervals, was one to be solved.

Dr. VANDYKE CARTER regarded the periodicity as an accident; the parent worm was lodged somewhere in the lymphatics of the urinary tract, which discharge itself at certain times. Many of these cases have periods of intermission. Perhaps the flow of lymph carries the young filariæ into the blood after taking food. This would account for the inverted migration in Dr. Mackenzie's case, where the man was kept up at night and made to sleep during the day. Filariæ existed in the blood of many persons without producing any derangement whatever.

Mr. WALTER PYE confirmed the identity of this filaria with that described by Dr. Patrick Manson.

RECURRENT FIBROMA OF BREAST.

Mr. GAY showed a specimen of this disease, which he had removed for the seventh time quite recently. The first removal took place in 1865, the woman being then sixteen years of age. The tumour was situated, not in the gland itself, but among the outlying fat. There was no glandular infection, and the scars always remained healthy, but there had been local recurrence seven times. The present tumour was identical with the preceding ones, and consisted of spindle cells in a homogeneous matrix of a soft colloid nature.

ANEURISM OF DESCENDING AORTA, AND IN TWO OTHER PLACES LOWER DOWN.

Dr. FOWLER showed an unusual form of aneurism of the descending aorta, which was adherent to the apex of the lung, into the substance of which it had burst. The aorta also presented two other aneurisms further down, one of which was dissecting. The man had been seized with pain, and then began to cough and expectorate blood. He had six recurrences. He died, two hours after his admission to the Middlesex Hospital, of hæmoptysis. The aorta was highly atheromatous.

MEMBRANOUS BAND IN LEFT AURICLE.

Dr. FOWLER also showed this specimen, which was probably a congenital peculiarity. It appeared to be connected with the valve of the foramen ovale at one point, and to the wall of the auricle at the other extremity, and had been so directed (probably) by the blood-current in early life. The patient was also the subject of primary cancer of the liver, but this was not reported on this occasion.

CYST, CONTAINING OIL, OVER PAROTID REGION.

Mr. BRYANT stated that he had removed the cyst from near the parotid region of a young woman, aged nineteen. It

had existed at birth, and slowly but steadily increased in size. The cyst was translucent, and before removal was thought to contain serum. After removal this fluid was found to resemble oil, which, however, became solid. The girl was well in all other respects.

Mr. DORAN inquired as to the structure of the epithelium of the cyst-wall.

Dr. COUPLAND suggested whether it had any connexion with the branchial clefts.

Mr. DAVIES-COLLEY had once removed a similar cyst from an out-patient.

Mr. BRYANT promised that the wall of the cyst should be examined.

Mr. HUTCHINSON showed a man with a large patch of Lupus Lymphaticus on the left shoulder.

Mr. MORRIS showed drawings of an unusual form of Fracture of the Femur.

MEDICAL NEWS.

UNIVERSITY OF DURHAM.—FACULTY OF MEDICINE. —FIRST M.B. EXAMINATION, October, 1881.—The following candidates have satisfied the Examiners :—

Abbot, Frederick Ernest.	Johnston, George David.
Blair, Charles S.	Keatinge, E. P.
Bredin, Howard Albert.	Parsons, John Inglis.
Buxton, William Maberly.	Pridew, Septimus T.
Charpentier, Ambrose Edward.	Rodman, George Hook.
Dawson, Arthur William.	Thurston, Daniel.
Hill, H. Gardiner, M.R.C.S.	Travis, William Owen.
	Watson, Robert W.

Thirty-four candidates entered. One failed in Chemistry and one in Botany. Each of these is admissible for re-examination in the subject alone in which he failed.

UNIVERSITY OF EDINBURGH.—Appended is a list of candidates who received respectively the degrees of Doctor of Medicine, Bachelor of Medicine, and Master in Surgery, in the University of Edinburgh, on Monday, August 1 :—

The Degree of Doctor of Medicine (with the Titles of the Theses).—John Adam (M.A. Edin.), Scotland, M.B. and C.M., 1877—Typhoid Fever. Reginald Gervas Alexander (M.A. Cantab.), England, M.B. and C.M., 1871—Description of a Portable Clinical Urine Case. Henry Joy Clarke, England, M.B. and C.M., 1878—Cases in Clinical Surgery. Charles Stuart Clouston, Orkney, M.B. and C.M. (with Second Class Honours), 1885—Acute Rheumatism, and its Treatment by Salicylates. David Collie, Scotland, M.B. and C.M., 1878—The Treatment of some Varieties of Insanity. Alexander Robert Coldstream, Scotland, M.B. and C.M., 1874—The Therapeutics of Pilocarpine. Joshua John Cox, Ireland, M.B., 1876—Upon Endocarditis, especially its Ulcerative Form. James Thomas Richard Davison, Argentine Republic, M.B. and C.M., 1878—The Physiological Action and some of the Therapeutic Uses of Strong Doses of Digitalis. Henry George Deverell, India, M.B. and C.M., 1877—Angina Pectoris. Charles Edward Douglas, India, M.B. and C.M., 1877—Spinal Irritation. George Alexander Gibson (D.Sc. Edin.), Scotland, M.B. and C.M., 1876—The Physiological Action of Duboisia on the Circulation. Matthew Hay, Scotland, M.B. and C.M. (with First Class Honours and Ettles Prizeman), 1879—The Action of Saline Cathartics. William Lamb, Scotland, M.B. and C.M., 1876—A Contribution to the Physiology of the Splanchnic Area. Robert Lawson, Scotland, M.B. and C.M., 1871—The Physiological Action of Extractive Hyoscyamine, and its Employment in the Treatment of Insanity. Alexander Bruce Low, Scotland, M.B. and C.M., 1878—Penetrating Wounds of Joints. Peter M'Bride, Hamburg, M.B. and C.M., 1876—Certain Nervous Symptoms and their Origin. William Alexander Macnaughton (M.A. Edin.), Scotland, M.B. and C.M., 1875—Puerperal Eclampsia. Duncan M'Donald (B.Sc. Edin.), Scotland, M.B. and C.M., 1872—Treatment of Malarious Fevers. Roger M'Neill, Scotland, M.B. and C.M., 1877—The Diagnostic and Prognostic Value of the Initial Rashes of Small-pox. William Birkmyre Miller (M.A. St. And.), Scotland, M.B. and C.M., 1872—Syphilis. Robert Moodie, Scotland, M.B. and C.M., 1869—Scurvy; with an Outbreak of Scurvy at Thrill in the Kuram Valley. James Murray (M.A. Edin.), Scotland, M.B. and C.M., 1876—A Clinical Study of Pityriasis Rubra. Arthur Murray Oram, Australia, M.B. and C.M., 1878—Rickets. Henry Robert Oswald, India, M.B. and C.M., 1875—An Epidemic of Enteric Fever. William Edward Pountney, England, M.B. and C.M., 1874—Hæmorrhage during Pregnancy, Labour, and after Delivery. Oliver Cromwell Shaw, England, M.B. and C.M., 1877—Hystero-Epilepsy, with Special Reference to Metalloscopy. Thomas Sanctuary, England, M.B., 1875—Dilatation of the Stomach: its Causes, Symptoms, and Pathological Changes. Andrew Smith, Scotland, M.B. (with Second Class Honours), 1876—The Infectiveness of Phthisis. David George Thomson, Scotland, M.B. and C.M., 1878—The Prognosis in Insanity. Leslie Batten Trotter, England, M.B. and C.M., 1874—Goitre in the Forest of Dean. William Turner (M.A. Aberd.), Scotland, M.B. and C.M., 1879—Version versus Forceps as a Method of Delivery in Cases of Deformity of the Pelvic Brim. William Henry Williams, England, M.B. and C.M., 1874—Medical Supervision of Schools. Robert Lamley Williamson, England, M.B. and C.M., 1877—The Operation of Skin Grafting. John Wilson, Scotland, M.B. and C.M., 1878—Medical and Surgical Cases. German Sims Woodhead, England, M.B. and C.M., 1878—Medulla Oblongata.

The Degree of Bachelor of Medicine and Master in Surgery.—James Hepburn Aitken, Scotland; Francis Joseph Baildon, England; John

Hutton Balfour, Scotland; William Burney Bannerman, Scotland; Barclay Josiah Baron, England; John Francis Bateson, England; Richard Charles Bennett, Trinidad; William George Birrell, Scotland (received the degrees on November 27, 1880); John Lyell Black, Scotland; Robert Henry Blaikie, Scotland; Thomas Borthwick, Scotland; Robert Bowes, Scotland; William Edward Bradley, England; William Haig Brodie, Scotland; Thomas Brown, Scotland; David Bruce, Australia; Robert Cathcart Bruce, India (received the degrees on November 27, 1880); John Greig Buchan, Orkney; James Arthur Lawrence Calder, Jamaica; Henry Martyn Clark, India; Francis Richard Sandford Corser, England; James Wharton Cox, Sydney; Dixon Grey Crawford, India; William Robert Dalzell (M.A. Edin.), India; Camille Victor Delepine, France; William Doig, Scotland; William Jones Doule, Scotland; Arthur Conan Doyle, Scotland; James Dunlop Dunlop, Scotland; Robert Pearns, Scotland; James Mitchell Ferguson, Scotland; Manley Montague Fitzpatrick, England; Frank Fraser, England; John Ilceock Fraser, Scotland; William Walter Baldock Fry, England; John Lockhart Gibson, Australia; Alexander Grant (M.A. Edin.), Scotland; Leonard Grant, Scotland; Ogilvie Grant, Scotland; David Rogerson Hamilton, Scotland (received the degrees on January 29, 1881); William Harding, England; Alfred Hartley, England; Septimus Harwood, England; Sydney Walter Haynes, England; Joseph Heath, Ireland; David Hepburn, Scotland; Christian Lawrence Herman, Cape Town; James Heweteon, England; Josias Matthiam Hoffman, Africa; William Hosegood, England; James Gilpin Houseman, England; Louis Ralston Huxtable, Tasmania; Francis Wm. Innes, Rangoon; Frederick Adolphus Jelly, England; Robert M'Kenzie Johnston, Scotland; Charles Kennedy, Scotland; William Watt Kerr (M.A. Edin.), Scotland; Herbert Dove King (M.A., B.Sc. Edin.), England; Roger Kirkpatrick, India; Robert Laidlaw, Scotland; Robert Laurie, England; Robert James Lawson, Scotland; George Leslie, Scotland; Charles Low, Australia; James Macdonald (M.A. Edin.), Scotland; Roderick John Johnstone Macdonald, England; George Hugh Mackay, Scotland; Samuel Mackew, England; Norman Maclean, Scotland; Archibald Lyle Macleish (M.A. Edin.), Scotland; William Aitken Macleod, Scotland; Alfred Macpherson, England (received degrees on November 27, 1880); John Farquhar Macrae, Scotland; John David Malcolm, Scotland; Walter Mercer, Scotland; James Mill, Scotland; William Morrison, Scotland; George Harold Mounsey, England; Henry Ferguson Mudie (M.A. St. And.), Scotland; Walter Galbraith Murray, Ireland; Robert Hector Munro, Scotland; Thomas Patrick Mylne, Scotland; Charles Edward Nichol, England; Brooke Owen Norfor, India; Walter Stewart Ogilvy, Scotland; James Orr, Ireland; Augustus Alexander Pechell, England; George Chapman Steele Perkins, England; Henry Whitby Phillips, England; George Proudfoot, Scotland; George James Renwick, (B.A. Sydney), Australia; Thomas Ridgley, England; David William Leone Ritchie, Scotland; John Robert Stevenson Robertson, England; George Virgile Rohan, Mauritius; James Maxwell Ross (M.A. Edin.), Scotland; Ernest Daniel Rowland, England; Alexander Fraser Russell (M.A. Edin.), Scotland; Johannes Sauer, Africa; William Christiaan Scholtz, Cape of Good Hope; Robert Scot Skirving, Scotland (received the degrees on April 20, 1881); Alfred Hynam Sevier, Russia; Robert Smith Sibbit, England; Robert Fraser Sinclair, Scotland; Wm. James Sinclair, Orkney; John Smith (M.A. Edin.), Scotland; Simon Woronzow Smith, America; James Greig Soutar, Scotland; John Sorley, Australia; Alex. Mitchell Stalker (M.A. Edin.), Scotland; Daniel Stalker (M.A. Edin.), Scotland; John Prince Stallard, England; Peter Standen, England; Gavin Stiell, Scotland; Charles Stuart, Scotland; Robert Thomas Sutherland, Natal; Adolphe Harrison Thomas, England; John Thomson, Scotland; Matthew Barclay Thomson, Australia; John Batty Tuke, New Zealand; John Patrick Tulloch (M.A. Edin.), Scotland; John Valentine, Scotland; Anthony (?)abert Viljoen, Cape of Good Hope; Edward Brooking Cornish Walker, England; Alfred Ward, England; James Smith Watson, Scotland; John Waugh (M.A. Edin.), Scotland; Arthur Poulett Lethbridge Wells, England; David Welsh, Scotland; Robert Crosbie Welsh, Scotland; John Humphry Williams, Wales; Richard Fredk. Williamson, England; George Wilson, Scotland; Henry John Wolseley, Demerara.

The Degree of Bachelor of Medicine.—Henry Hyslop Aitchison, England; Frederick John William Cox, Scotland; John Horn, England; William Young Orr, Scotland; Robert Wilkie Smith, Scotland (received the degree on April 20, 1881).

The Degree of Master in Surgery.—Robert Wilkie Smith, M.B., Scotland.

The Ettles Prize for 1881 has been awarded to Barclay Josiah Baron, M.B., C.M. The Beaney Prize has been awarded to David Hepburn, M.B., C.M. The Goodsir Prize has been awarded to Matthew Hay, M.D. The Wightman Prize has been awarded to Francis William Grant. The Buchanan Scholarship has been awarded to James Heweteon, M.B., C.M.

QUEEN'S UNIVERSITY IN IRELAND.—At a meeting of the Senate of the University, held in St. Patrick's Hall, Dublin Castle, on Thursday, October 13, the following Degrees in Medicine and Surgery and Diplomas in Midwifery were conferred by the Chancellor His Grace the Duke of Leinster :—

The Degree of Doctor in Medicine (M.D.).—First Honour Class: Havelock Henry R. Charles, Cork; Thomas Sinclair, Belfast; George Luck Galpin, Cork; William Henry Lendrum, Belfast; Francis M'Laughlin, Galway; James Pinkerton, Belfast; David Semple, Belfast. Upper Pass Division: Warwick Long Child, Belfast; Timothy Dilworth, Cork; William Walter Gibson, Galway; Patrick F. Graham, Cork; James W. B. Hodson, Belfast; John Kennedy, Belfast; William J. R. Knight, Galway and Belfast; John S. Logan, Belfast; Robert W. S. Lyons, Belfast; Samuel Macaulay, Belfast; William Odilo Maher, Lower Edward J. Parry, Galway. Lower Pass Division: Robert Anderson, Belfast; William G. K. Barnes, Cork; John G. Black, Galway; John Blair, Cork; Samuel Connor, Belfast; James Craig, Belfast; Charles Daly, Cork; John Dodd, Belfast; Chas. Dundee, Belfast; Alexander John Fleming, Belfast; David Forsyth, Belfast; Robert Henry, Belfast; John L. Jaquet, Cork; Samuel W. Johnson, Galway and Belfast; Edward M'Connell, Belfast and Galway; Thomas S. M'Connell, Belfast and Galway; Robert James M'Cormack, Belfast; Beattie M'Farland, Belfast; Wahab M'Murray, Belfast; John R. M'Neil, Belfast; William N.(?) M'William, Belfast ;(?) William Arthur Moynan,

Galway; William Nelson, Belfast; David Valentine O'Connell, Galway; Arthur O'Keeffe, Cork; Richard M. Ralph, Belfast; Robert Stewart, Belfast; Jeremiah Sugrue, Cork; Edward James Holmes Sullivan, Cork; George M. Thompson, Belfast; Felix C. Vinrace, Galway; Chas. Wiseman, Cork; Henry Harper, Galway; Michael Jennings, Galway; Walter C. Johnson, Cork; Samuel F. Loughead, Cork; Daniel Lynch, Cork; Joseph R. M'Donnell, Galway; Jeremiah M'Kenna, Cork; James Minnie, Belfast; Gerald Mitchell, Cork; David T. Montsith, Belfast; David J. O'Malley, Galway; George H. Powell, Galway and Cork; John Redmond, Belfast; Archibald O. Robinson, Belfast; Robert L. Rutherford, Galway; David M. Saunders, Cork; William D. Sexton, Cork; James Simpson, Belfast; Henry Sinclair, Cork; John M. Trimble, Belfast; Charles H. Wheeler, Belfast.

The Degree of Master of Surgery (M.Ch.).—David Taylor Monteath, M.D., Belfast; David J. O'Malley, M.D., Galway; William Smyth, M.D., Belfast; William G. K. Barnes, Cork; John Blair, Cork; Havelock H. R. Charles, Cork; Timothy Dilworth, Cork; John Dodd, Belfast; Alex. John Fleming, Belfast; George Luck Galpin, Cork; Patrick F. Graham, Cork; Robert Henry, Belfast; James W. B. Hoddson, Belfast; John Kennedy, Belfast; William Henry Lendrum, Belfast; J. Smythe Logan, Belfast; R. W. Steele Lyons, Belfast; Saml. Macaulay, Belfast; Robert J. M'Cormack, Belfast; Wahab M'Murray, Belfast; John Robinson M'Neill, Galway; W. Odilo Maher, Cork; William A. Moynan, Galway; William Nelson, Belfast; Arthur O'Keeffe, Cork; James Pinkerton, Belfast; David Semple, Belfast; Thomas Sinclair, Belfast; Robert Stewart, Belfast; Jeremiah Sugrue, Cork; Ed. J. Holmes Sullivan, Cork; George Matthew Thompson, Belfast; Felix Coulson Vinrace, Galway; Robert Alexander, M.D., Belfast; Richard Campbell, M.D., Belfast; W. Naunton Davies, M.D., Belfast and Galway; James Geraghty, M.D., Cork; James Mullin, M.D., Galway; John F. L. Mullin, M.D., Galw[a?]y; James A. Oakshott, M.D., Cork; James B. White, M.D., Belfast; James F. White, M.D., Galway; Edward Horan, M.D., Cork; Joseph Anderson, M.D., Belfast; Daniel Lynch, Cork; Jeremiah M'Kenna, Cork; James Minniece, Belfast; John Mitchell, Cork; George H. Powell, Galway and Cork; David M. Saunders, Cork; Henry Sinclair, Cork; John M. Trimble, Belfast; Charles H. Wheeler, Belfast.

Diploma in Midwifery.—James Minniece, M.D., Belfast; James Mullin, M.D., Galway; James F. White, M.D., Galway; David Taylor, M.D., Belfast; J. Greer Black, Galway; John Blair, Cork; Havelock H. R. Charles, Cork; Warwick L. Child, Belfast; Samuel Connor, Belfast; Charles Daly, Cork; Timothy Dilworth, Cork; Patrick F. Graham, Cork; John Kennedy, Belfast; William H. Lendrum, Belfast; J. Smythe Logan, Belfast; Robert J. M'Cormack, Belfast; William Odilo Maher, Cork; David V. O'Connell, Galway; Arthur O'Keeffe, Cork; James Pinkerton, Belfast; Richard M. Ralph, Belfast; David Semple, Belfast; Thomas Sinclair, Belfast; Edward J. Holmes Sullivan, Cork; George Matthew Thompson, Belfast; W. Naunton Davies, M.D., Belfast; James A. Oakabott, M.D., Cork; James B. White, M.D., Belfast; Daniel Lynch, Cork; Jeremiah M'Kenna, Cork; George H. Powell, Galway and Cork; John Redmond, Belfast; David M. Saunders, Cork; Henry Sinclair, Cork.

KING AND QUEEN'S COLLEGE OF PHYSICIANS IN IRELAND.—At the usual monthly examinations for the Licences of the College, held on Monday, Tuesday, Wednesday, and Thursday, October 10, 11, 12, and 13, the following candidates were successful :—

For the First Professional Examination—

Andrew, Letitia Harvey. | McCabe, Alfred Alex. Donald.

For the Licence to practise Medicine—

Abbott, George.	McFarland, Francis Edward.
Bonynge, Francis George.	Magrane, Vincent John.
Brennan, Mark Andrew.	Nolan, Lyster Andrew.
Dempsey, Patrick Joseph.	O'Connor, Daniel Michael.
Jones, Walter William Stockton.	Parsons, Charles.
Lumley, Charles Louis.	Penny, John Alexander Cairns.

Tuthill, John.

For the Licence to practise Midwifery—

Abbott, George.	Magrane, Vincent John.
Bonynge, Francis George.	Nolan, Lyster Andrew.
Hall, Nicholas.	Parsons, Charles.
Jones, Walter William Stockton.	Penny, John Alexander Cairns.
Lumley, Charles Louis.	Tuthill, John.

The following Licentiates in Medicine of the College having complied with the by-laws under the Supplemental Charter of December 12, 1878, have been duly admitted to the Membership :—

Cheasure, George Cochet, 1866, Surgeon-Major, Indian Army.
Cooper, John Nield, 1874, London.
Westby, George, 1877, Liverpool.
Smith, Richard Baker, 1877, London.
Russell, Thomas O'Dwyer, 1877, Limerick.
Cameron, James Cheasure, 1878, Montreal.

The numerals placed after the names indicate the year in which the Licence to practise Medicine of the College was obtained.

APOTHECARIES' HALL, LONDON.—The following gentlemen passed their examination in the Science and Practice of Medicine, and received certificates to practise, on Thursday, October 13 :—

Deane, Herbert Edward, Sutherland-gardens, St. Peter's-park.
Donald, James, St. Leonard's-place, Kingston.

At the recent examination for the prizes in Materia Medica and Pharmaceutical Chemistry, given annually to medical students by the Society of Apothecaries, the following were the successful candidates—viz., First, Joseph

Walker, of the Liverpool School of Medicine, a Gold Medal; Second, Herbert Tanner, of St. Mary's Hospital, a Silver Medal and Books.

APPOINTMENTS.

. The Editor will thank gentlemen to forward to the Publishing-office, as early as possible, information as to all new Appointments that take place.

Murphy, James, B.A., M.D.—Consulting Surgeon to the Monkwearmouth and Southwick Dispensary.

NAVAL, MILITARY, Etc., APPOINTMENTS.

Admiralty.—Staff-Surgeon George Mair, M.A., M.D., has been promoted to the rank of Fleet-Surgeon in Her Majesty's Fleet, with seniority of September 30, 1881. Fleet-Surgeon Edward Beumton Brooster has been placed on the retired list of his rank from October 7, 1881.

BIRTHS.

Cassidy.—On October 15, at 22, Guilford-street, Russell-square, the wife of Joseph Lamont Cassidy, M.D., of a son.

Graves.—On September 12, at Meerut, North-West Province, India, the wife of Surgeon-Major W. Graves, A.M.D., of a son.

McDonagh.—On October 17, at Mornington Villa, 211, Hampstead-road, N.W., the wife of James McDonagh, jun., M.R.C.S., of a son.

Richards.—On October 12, at the County Asylum, Hanwell, the wife of J. Peeke Richards, M.R.C.S., of a daughter.

Shaw.—On October 15, at St. James's Lodge, Enfield Highway, Middlesex, the wife of George Shaw, M.R.C.S., of a son.

MARRIAGES.

Boissier—Harington.—On October 11, at Bath, Arthur Henry Boissier, L.R.C.P., M.R.C.S., of Pocklington, Yorks, to Octavia Georgiana, youngest daughter of the late Colonel T. L. Harington, 5th Regiment Bengal Light Cavalry.

Mowan—Garraway.—On October 18, at Ospringe, Kent, the Rev. Richard Turnill Mowan, of Charlton, Dover, to Ada, daughter of Edward Garraway, M.R.C.S., of Faversham.

Rice—Cook.—On October 13, at Plumstead Common, George Rice, M.B., C.M., to Florence Mary, eldest daughter of John Cook, Esq., Merton Villa, Plumstead Common.

DEATHS.

Gwillim, William, M.R.C.S., at Burton-on-Trent, on October 14, aged 86.

Rawson, Thomas James, M.D., at Barrowville, Carlow, Ireland, on October 12, in his 73rd year.

Sexton, Septimus, M.D., Staff Surgeon Royal Navy, H.M.S. Magpie, at Hong-kong, China, on October 11.

Simpson, George Alexander, M.D., of Highgate, London, at Banchory-terrace, Kincardineshire, N.B., on October 15, aged 96.

Sparrow, Ethel Gordon, only daughter of G. Gordon Sparrow, L.R.C.P., at Hazlemere, East Southsea, on October 11, aged 6 months.

Whiting, John, M.R.C.S., of St. Bartholomew's Hospital, late Surgeon of British India ss. Chyebassa, in London, on October 8, in his 26th year.

VACANCIES.

Birmingham General Dispensary.—Resident Surgeon. Candidates must be registered, and possess both a medical and surgical qualification. Applications, together with original testimonials and certificate of registration, to be sent to Alex. Forrest, Secretary, on or before November 19.

Bradford Infirmary and Dispensary.—Dispensary and Visiting Surgeon. Candidates must be registered as legally qualified medical and surgical practitioners. Applications, stating age, with copies of recent testimonials as to moral character and professional ability, to be sent to William Maw, Secretary, on or before October 25.

Bristol General Hospital.—House-Surgeon. Candidates must be members of the College of Surgeons of London, Edinburgh, Glasgow, or Dublin, and also Licentiates of the Apothecaries' Company of London or Dublin, or possess some other recognised medical qualification. Applications, enclosing testimonials of good moral character and ability, with certificate of registration, to be sent to the Secretary, on or before November 5.

Dental Hospital of London, Leicester-square.—Assistant Dental Surgeon. (For particulars see Advertisement.)

Dispensary of the General Hospital for Sick Children, Gartside-street, Manchester.—Medical Officer. (For particulars see Advertisement.)

Eastern Dispensary, Bath.—Resident Medical Officer. (For particulars see Advertisement.)

French Hospital and Dispensary, 10, Leicester-place, Leicester-square.—Resident Medical Officer. Candidates must be fully qualified and able to speak French. Applications, with particulars of professional qualifications and testimonials, to be sent to F. Borel, Assistant-Secretary.

Hospital for Sick Children, Great Ormond-street, W.C.—Assistant-Physician. (For particulars see Advertisement.)

Jersey General Dispensary.—Resident Visiting and Dispensing Medical Officer. Candidates must possess the double qualification, and be unmarried. Applications to be made to the Hon. Secretary, Jersey General Dispensary, 11, Elizabeth-place, Parade, Jersey.

Richmond Hospital.—House-Surgeon. (For particulars see Advertisement.)

St. Mary, Islington, Workhouse and Infirmary.—Resident Assistant Medical Officer. (For particulars see Advertisement.)

Wigan Infirmary.—Junior House-Surgeon. Applications to be made to the Secretary, not later than October 27.

South Devon and East Cornwall Hospital, Plymouth.—House-Surgeon. Candidates must be duly qualified. Applications, with testimonials, to be sent to J. Walter Wilson, Hon. Sec., on or before Nov. 7.

UNION AND PAROCHIAL MEDICAL SERVICE.

. The area of each district is stated in acres. The population is computed according to the census of 1871.

RESIGNATIONS.

Stething Union.—Mr. J. J. Lay has resigned the Fourth District: area 13,167; population 2231; salary £72 per annum.

Halifax Union.—The Skircoat District is vacant by the death of Dr. W. Elliott: area 3756; population 11,573; salary £35 per annum.

Monmouth Union.—M. T. G. Prosser has resigned the Monmouth District: area 14,424; population 7526; salary £40 per annum.

APPOINTMENTS.

Chertsey Union.—John Macdonald, M.D. Edin., to the Walton District.

Newhaven Union.—John Pollington Grover, M.R.C.S. Eng., L.R.C.P. Edin., L.S.A. Lond., to the Second Division of the Third District.

Newton Abbot Union.—William Harvey, M.R.C.S. Eng., L.S.A., to the Teignmouth District.

Poplar and Stepney Sick Asylum District.—Philip Thornton, L.R.C.P. Edin., M.R.C.S. Eng., L.S.A., as Assistant Medical Officer at the Asylum.

Ruthin Union.—Thomas Griffith Jenkins, L.R.C.P. and L.M. Edin., M.R.C.S. Eng., L.S.A. Lond., to the Workhouse.

Stokesley Union.—Anthony Snowdon, L.R.C.P. Edin., L.R.C.S. Edin., to the Hutton District.

Totnes Union.—John Raby, M.R.C.S. Eng., L.R.C.S. and L.R.C.P. Edin., to the Totnes District. Alfred G. Chitty, M.R.C.S. Eng., L.R.C.P. Edin., to the Berry Pomeroy District.

Union-upon-Severn Union.—John W. George, M.R.C.S. Eng., L.S.A., to the Fifth District.

Examinations for Trichinæ in France.—The Journal Officiel announces that laboratories for the microscopical examination of salt pork of foreign origin are about to be established at all points of the coast and frontier where salted provisions arrive. They will be under the direction of experts in microscopy appointed by the Minister of Commerce. Any of these who may not be deemed sufficiently instructed in the matter will have the opportunity afforded them of attending gratuitously a course of twelve lectures on microscopy and helminthology under the direction of M. Joannes Chatin. There is every sign of the Government having the intention to speedily repeal the prohibition of the importation of salted meats from America, and to replace it by a permanent system of inspection of all foreign bacon and pork whencesoever it may arrive. The prohibition has caused great agitation, as this important article, it is said, at the port of Havre alone amounts to 40,000,000 kilogrammes per annum, and the working-classes are thus deprived of a substantial and cheap food. It has been supposed that salting kills the trichina, but this is a complete error, more complete cooking being, in fact, required to effect this end than for fresh pork. This micrographic service is the first attempt at a central organisation of the various services relating to public health, and it is to be hoped that it will not stop here, as wine, milk, etc., are liable to various pernicious adulterations which would be advantageously dealt with by experts under the control of a central administration.—Union Méd., October 6.

Medical Women in the United States.—At the meeting of the American Social Science Association at Saratoga, Dr. Emily Pope presented some statistics concerning the practice of medicine by women, which were evidently gathered with much care. According to these, there are in the United States 470 women physicians, of whom 390 are engaged in active practice. Of those heard from, 75 per cent. were single when they began to study, 19 per cent. were married, and 6 per cent. were widows; 341 practise regular medicine, and 13 homœopathy; 77 report that they have supported themselves from the beginning of their practice, 34 in less than one year, 57 after the first year, 34 in two years, 14 in three years, and 10 in various periods over three years; 289 are in general practice, 45 make a speciality of female diseases, and 4 of ophthalmology. These statistics show that a larger percentage of women engage in general practice than is usually supposed. Other investigations have led to the conclusion that nearly one-half follow some speciality, generally that of gynecology, obstetrics, or the diseases of children. As regards health, it was stated that, of 130 who have practised less than five years, 76 report health good, 51 health improved, and 3 health not good. On the whole, the figures show that the practice of medicine has been successfully followed by these four hundred American women. It has furnished them a livelihood, and has neither impaired their health nor interfered markedly with their social relations.—New York Med. Record, September 17.

VITAL STATISTICS OF LONDON.

Week ending Saturday, October 15, 1881.

BIRTHS.

Births of Boys, 1256; Girls, 1194; Total, 2550.
Corrected weekly average in the 10 years 1871-80, 2577·2.

DEATHS.

	Males.	Females.	Total.
Deaths during the week	741	719	1460
Weekly average of the ten years 1871-80, corrected to increased population ...	738·3	710·9	1449·2
Deaths of people aged 90 and upwards ...	...	...	51

DEATHS IN SUB-DISTRICTS FROM EPIDEMICS.

	Enumerated Population, 1881 (unrevised).	Small-pox.	Measles.	Scarlet Fever.	Diphtheria.	Whooping-cough.	Typhus.	Enteric (or Typhoid) Fever.	Simple-continued Fever.	Diarrhœa.
West ...	669908	1	5	6	3	5	...	4	1	8
North ...	905677	3	6	17	3	5	...	10	1	2
Central ...	261796	...	3	3	2	4	...	4	...	6
East ...	692530	...	3	11	3	8	...	6	1	7
South ...	1965578	19	18	29	2	9	...	9	...	8
Total ...	3814571	23	35	66	13	32	...	33	3	26

METEOROLOGY.

From Observations at the Greenwich Observatory.

Mean height of barometer	29·602 in.
Mean temperature	49·0°
Highest point of thermometer	62·4°
Lowest point of thermometer	37·2°
Mean dew-point temperature	44·3°
General direction of wind	W.S.W.
Whole amount of rain in the week	0·51 in.

BIRTHS and DEATHS Registered and METEOROLOGY during the Week ending Saturday, Oct. 15, in the following large Towns:—

Cities and boroughs (Municipal boundaries except for London.)	Estimated Population to middle of the year 1881.*	Persons to an Acre. (1881.)	Births Registered during the week ending Oct. 15.	Deaths Registered during the week ending Oct. 15.	Temperature of Air (Fahr.) Highest during the Week.	Temperature of Air (Fahr.) Lowest during the Week.	Temperature of Air (Fahr.) Weekly Mean of Daily Values.	Temp. of Air (Cent.) Weekly Mean of Daily Mean Values.	Rain Fall. In Inches.	Rain Fall. In Centimetres.
London ...	3829751	50·2	2550	1460	62·4	37·2	49·0	9·44	0·51	1·30
Brighton ...	107934	45·9	60	44	60·5	38·5	48·9	9·39	0·22	0·56
Portsmouth ...	128835	28·6	79	40	...	...	...	...	...	...
Norwich ...	88038	11·8	58	28	...	...	...	...	...	...
Plymouth ...	76293	54·0	53	24	61·8	38·8	50·1	10·06	0·40	1·02
Bristol ...	207140	46·5	112	60	61·5	41·2	49·7	9·83	0·96	2·44
Wolverhampton ...	75934	22·4	51	31	57·8	31·5	46·1	7·54	1·22	3·10
Birmingham ...	402296	47·9	287	174	...	...	...	...	...	...
Leicester ...	123120	38·5	87	33	61·0	35·3	46·8	8·23	1·13	2·87
Nottingham ...	189235	18·9	152	92	60·0	33·7	47·5	8·61	1·19	1·84
Liverpool ...	553098	106·3	374	296	59·0	37·4	48·1	8·95	1·61	4·09
Manchester ...	341269	79·5	203	143	...	...	...	...	...	...
Salford ...	177760	34·5	108	67	...	...	...	...	...	...
Oldham ...	112176	24·0	75	43	...	...	...	...	...	...
Bradford ...	184037	25·5	124	74	57·1	35·0	47·3	8·50	2·05	5·21
Leeds ...	310490	14·4	191	102	59·0	37·0	48·1	8·95	1·15	2·92
Sheffield ...	285621	14·5	182	94	58·0	35·0	47·3	8·50	2·01	5·11
Hull ...	155161	42·7	108	79	60·0	34·0	44·9	7·17	1·10	2·79
Sunderland ...	116758	42·2	100	45	66·0	35·0	49·2	9·55	0·94	2·39
Newcastle-on-Tyne	145675	27·1	90	54	...	...	...	...	...	...
Total of 20 large English Towns ...	7605772	38·0	5049	2953	66·0	31·3	47·9	8·83	11·11	2·69

* These figures are the numbers enumerated (but subject to revision) in April last, raised to the middle of 1881 by the addition of a quarter of a year's increase, calculated at the rate that prevailed between 1871 and 1881.

At the Royal Observatory, Greenwich, the mean reading of the barometer last week was 29·60 in. The lowest reading was 28·87 in. on Friday morning, and the highest 29·95 in. by the end of the week.

NOTES, QUERIES, AND REPLIES.

Je that questioneth much shall learn much.—Bacon.

A Provincial Demonstrator.—Mr. Charles Hawkins, a late Member of the Council of the College of Surgeons, is the Government Inspector of Anatomy for the Metropolitan Schools; and it is a fact worthy of notice, that in the year ending September 30 last a larger number of subjects have been supplied for dissection than in any year since the passing of the Anatomy Act in 1832.

Vesalius.—Formerly the bodies of all murderers hanged at the Old Bailey were claimed by the College of Surgeons, and distributed by that institution amongst the metropolitan schools for dissection. The last so claimed was that of Smithers, executed for setting fire to his house in Oxford-street, and thereby causing the death of two young ladies lodging in his house. The statement in *Notes and Queries*, that "dissection of murderers' bodies was made *optional* in 1832, and abolished in 1880," is not correct; the notice was subsequently corrected in that journal on the 1st inst. by a correspondent ("Lex") evidently acquainted with the true case. The skeletons of Jonathan Wild, John Thurtell, and the skull of Eugene Aram, are in the Museum of the College of Surgeons.

Thomas Guy.—A great increase in the cost of treating hospital patients has taken place in the last dozen years. In 1867, in St. George's Hospital, each patient cost £4 17s. 9d., increased last year (1880) to £6 17s. 3d.

Sorting Rags and Small-pox.—The recent outbreak of small-pox in Maidstone (striking for the large number of seizures within a few days) is traced to its origin by apparently conclusive evidence in the report of Dr. M. Algernon Adams, Medical Officer of Health for the borough. With two exceptions, for which other incidental causes are alleged, there appears no doubt that every case was due to infection disseminated in the sorting of rags at a paper-mill. The testimony to the efficacy of vaccination which the outbreak affords is forcibly shown.

Inquirer.—The premises in Chatham-street, Piccadilly, Manchester, formerly occupied by the Chatham-street School of Medicine, to be opened in that city in May next.

Liquor-drinking, Russia.—The Congress of Experts at St. Petersburg, charged with the inquiry into the evils caused by excessive drinking in Russia, have resolved to advise a diminution in the number of licensed liquor houses, and also the vesting in the communal authorities the right of opening liquor shops under regulations to be decided by a sub-committee for that purpose, which has been appointed.

Colonial Items.—Victoria: Small-pox has not yet appeared in this colony, and recent returns show that 39 per cent. of the children has been vaccinated. Several wealthy colonists have lately made large donations to the various charities. One gentleman has given £1000 to the Bendigo Charity and £1000 to the Hospital for Incurables. Another gentleman has made a similar donation for the past four years on the occasion of his birthday. New South Wales: Small-pox is still spreading in Sydney and suburbs, notwithstanding the efforts of the authorities. Great complaints were made of the incompetency of the Board of Health. Ou-Chong and Co., Chinese merchants, of Lower George-street, had sent in a claim for £3000 to the Colonial Treasurer. They assert that their premises had been quarantined unnecessarily, and that their loss had exceeded the sum mentioned; whilst they deny that any person on their premises had at any time been affected with small-pox. South Australia: The census returns show that the male adult population of the colony is increasing rapidly. Queensland: A mining town called Mount Perry, about two hundred miles north-west of Brisbane, has been attacked with a deadly epidemic, somewhat resembling inflammation of the lungs.

Army Medical Officer, Bayswater.—The Minister of War, Paris, has ordered an inquiry to be made into the alleged insufficiency of medical service in North Africa.

Sanitary Legislation, United States.—The sanitary part of house-plumbing has been placed, in New York and Brooklyn, under the control of legislation. From a New York scientific journal—the *Sanitary Engineer*—we learn that a law has been passed, coming into operation in March next, and applying to that city and Brooklyn, which requires all plumbers to be registered, and places their work, as well as that of drainage, under official supervision. The registration is intended to secure that only duly qualified men shall be entrusted with such responsible work. Under the Health Act, local authorities in this country have superintendence over the construction of drains and fittings, but there is nothing to restrain the selection of poor materials and the bad or defective workmanship so often complained of.

P. N. P., Hants.—It is forty-three years since the Poor-law Board, at the instance of Mr. Chadwick, who was then their Secretary, obtained the famous report from the late Dr. Southwood Smith, which was the foundation of sanitary work and legislation in England. In 1848 the first Public Health Act and the Epidemic Diseases' Prevention Act were passed.

Praiseworthy.—A cheque for £30, the amount realised by a cricket *fête* held at Upton Shrubbery, West Ham, between members of the H Division of Police and the Burton Brewery Cricket Club, has been handed by Inspector Smith, H Division, to the Secretary of the East London Hospital for Children, Ratcliff Cross.

Fides, Hove.—Very soon after the discovery of vaccination most of the governments of Europe made provision for affording its benefits to their respective populations. As early as 1803 an ordinance on the subject was promulgated in Sweden; Denmark and many of the German States speedily following the example. The first Austrian regulations date from 1808. By the time Jenner died (1823), there was hardly a government in Europe, except Great Britain, in which the practice was not directly or indirectly rendered compulsory. The first law regarding vaccination in England was enacted in 1840. From that year began the system of public vaccination free of charge. By Lord Lyttelton's Bill of 1853 the operation was rendered compulsory, under penalty of 20s., upon parents and guardians.

Bad Eyesight of London School-Children.—Attention is directed by Mr. Baily, Inspector of Schools in the Hackney district, to the prevalence of bad eyesight among the children, which he attributed partly to the vitiated atmosphere which London school children breathe, and to their possessing fewer opportunities for healthy recreation than children in the country.

A Parent, Kensington.—With the view of securing healthy lodgings for University men, the University authorities of Oxford have appointed a qualified sanitary engineer to ascertain the sanitary condition of all houses licensed to receive University men, and they have announced that unless by the close of the year such alterations as may be deemed necessary shall have been made, a licence to receive University men as lodgers will be withdrawn. Some 650 houses in the town have been inspected and reported on, and such alterations as are required to render them healthy residences have been ordered, on pain of losing the licence to let.

C. Randall N., Brompton.—In the United Kingdom, it is estimated, there are over 52,000 blind people. The census of France for 1876 showed that there were then actually 31,631 persons deprived of vision in that country. Of this number 5978, or nearly a sixth, set down as blind from birth, have in reality been so afflicted only from infancy.

Legally, or not Legally, entitled to Fees: Important Case.—The adjourned hearing of the case of Dr. Simpson and the Board of Guardians of Dover was before the County Court judge last week, and decided. It appeared that Dr. Simpson formally brought an action against the Guardians for £38 18s. for 137 cases of successful vaccination performed by him in a period of fourteen months, during which he acted as the house-surgeon to the workhouse. The Guardians did not dispute the claim, but they were disinclined to discharge it in consequence of an objection raised by the Local Government Board on the grounds that the appointment of medical officer had not been confirmed by them. The Judge gave a verdict for the plaintiff for the full amount, and said he had hoped that in the interim which had elapsed the Local Government Board would have allowed the claim.

The Advantage of Official Pressure.—The Barton-upon-Irwell Rural Sanitary Authority has resolved to seek power to borrow £600 for a cottage hospital for infectious diseases for the use of the inhabitants of Worsley and Swinton. The Local Government Board had pressed the Local Authority to make provision for cases of infectious disease by the erection of a joint hospital for the whole of the union, and the proposed hospital is simply an experiment: if it be found to answer, other similar hospitals will be erected by the Authority.

Deficient Water-Supply.—The annual report of the Inspector of Nuisances to the Rural Sanitary Authority, Lichfield, states, *inter alia*, that nothing had been done with regard to the water-supply of Brereton, where there were about forty houses without any good water-supply. The inspector understood that the South Staffordshire Waterworks Company had the power to oppose any company supplying Brereton with water for several years. He did not know whether any steps had been taken to arrange with the Company to supply Brereton. Hagleslade was still without an adequate supply of water, there being only one pump to the whole of the dwellings, and that at a long distance from the houses.

COMMUNICATIONS have been received from—

Mr. Henry Gant, London; Dr. Stephen Mackenzie, London; Dr. Radcliffe Crocker, London; Dr. Richard Neale, London; Sir William Mac Cormac, London; Mr. J. Ward Cousins, Southsea; Dr. E. Sargeant, Bolton; Dr. Comfield, London; Mr. J. Hamilton Craigie, London; The Secretary of the Society of Medical Officers of Health; Mr. R. Clement Lucas, London; Mr. Camillo de Figuiredo, Manchester; Mr. Lawson Tait, Birmingham; The Secretary of the Royal Medical and Chirurgical Society; Dr. Moore, Dublin; Messrs. Arnold and Sons, London; Dr. William Murrell, London; Mr. R. W. Parker, London; Mr. J. Onatto, London; The Honorary Secretary of the Medical Society of London; The Secretary of the Society for the Relief of Widows and Orphans of Medical Men, London; Mr. D. J. Fox, Stepney; Mr. Bartlett, Birmingham; Professor Bentley, London; Dr. E. F. Willoughby, London; Professor Paget, Cambridge; Mr. G. Cowell, London; Mr. A. De Watteville, London; Dr. F. T. Roberts, London; The Registrar of Apothecaries' Hall, London; Dr. U. Pritchard, London; Mr. Stone, London; Dr. Semple, London; Dr. N. Chevers, London; Dr. De Castro, London; Dr. Gillespie, London; The Secretary of the Quekett Microscopical Club, London; Dr. Sangster, London; Dr. Francis, Clapham; The Secretary of the College of Medicine, Newcastle-on-Tyne; Mr. W. Haward, Clinical Society, London; Mr. F. Mason, London; Mr. T. Holmes, London; Dr. Kidd, London.

BOOKS, ETC., RECEIVED—

The Students' Handbook of Chemistry, by H. L. Greville, F.I.C., F.C.S. —Imperial Maritime Customs, China, Report on Opium—A Report on the Fevers of Cyprus, Malta, and Gibraltar, by Henry Veale, M.D.—Transactions of the American Otological Society—The Perfect Way in Diet, by Anna Kingsford, M.D.

PERIODICALS AND NEWSPAPERS RECEIVED—

Lancet—British Medical Journal—Medical Press and Circular—Berliner Klinische Wochenschrift—Centralblatt für Chirurgie—Gazette des Hopitaux—Gazette Médicale—Le Progrès Médical—Bulletin de l'Académie de Médecine—Pharmaceutical Journal—Wiener Medizinische Wochenschrift—Centralblatt für die Medizinischen Wissenschaften—Revue Médicale—Gazette Hebdomadaire—National Board of Health Bulletin, Washington—Nature—Occasional Notes—Deutsche Medicinal-Zeitung—Boston Medical and Surgical Journal—Louisville Medical News—Oil and Drug News—Westminster Review—Chemist and Druggist—Philadelphia Medical News—Lincolnshire Chronicle, October 14—Weekblad—Revue de Médecine—Revue de Chirurgie—Bath Herald, October 15—Church of England Pulpit, etc.—Journal of the British Dental Association—Canadian Journal of Medical Science—Centralblatt für Gynäkologie—Revue des Sciences Médicales—Manchester Examiner and Times, October 15—Birkenhead News, October 15—Boston Journal of Chemistry—Supplement of the New York Journal and Obstetrical Review—La Independencia Médica—New York Medical Journal—American Journal of the Medical Sciences—Boston Medical and Surgical Journal—Anales del Circulo Medico Argentino—The Colonies and India—Archives of Medicine—Martin's Chemists' and Druggists' Bulletin—Essex Telegraph, October 15—Western Medical Reporter.

APPOINTMENTS FOR THE WEEK.

October 22. Saturday (this day).

Operations at St. Bartholomew's, 1½ p.m.; King's College, 1½ p.m.; Royal Free, 2 p.m.; Royal London Ophthalmic, 11 a.m.; Royal Westminster Ophthalmic, 1½ p.m.; St. Thomas's, 1½ p.m.; London, 2 p.m.

24. *Monday.*

Operations at the Metropolitan Free, 2 p.m.; St. Mark's Hospital for Diseases of the Rectum, 2 p.m.; Royal London Ophthalmic, 11 a.m.; Royal Westminster Ophthalmic, 1½ p.m.

Medical Society of London, 8½ p.m. Mr. Thomas Bryant, "On a Case of Amputation of the Thigh for Knee-joint Disease in a Man the subject of Phthisis." Dr. Radcliffe Crocker, "On a Case of Congenital Syphilis with Enlarged Spleen and Thickening of the Cranial Bones."

25. *Tuesday.*

Operations at Guy's, 1½ p.m.; Westminster, 2 p.m.; Royal London Ophthalmic, 11 a.m.; Royal Westminster Ophthalmic, 1½ p.m.; West London, 3 p.m.

Royal Medical and Chirurgical Society, 8½ p.m. Mr. Jonathan Hutchinson, "On Gangrenous Eruptions in connexion with Chicken-pox and Vaccination." Mr. Clement Lucas, "On a Case of a Healthy Child suckled by a Mother inoculated with Syphilis subsequent to its Birth."

26. *Wednesday.*

Operations at University College, 2 p.m.; St. Mary's, 1¼ p.m.; Middlesex, 1 p.m.; London, 2 p.m.; St. Bartholomew's, 1½ p.m.; Great Northern, 2 p.m.; Samaritan, 2½ p.m.; King's College (by Mr. Lister), 2 p.m.; Royal London Ophthalmic, 11 a.m.; Royal Westminster Ophthalmic, 1½ p.m.; St. Thomas's, 1½ p.m.; St. Peter's Hospital for Stone, 2 p.m.; National Orthopædic, Great Portland-street, 10 a.m.

Hunterian Society (London Institution), 8 p.m. Mr. Stevens will show a Tumour of the Brain. Mr. J. E. Adams, "On Injuries to the Arteries of the Lower Extremities."

27. *Thursday.*

Operations at St. George's, 1 p.m.; Central London Ophthalmic, 1 p.m.; Royal Orthopædic, 2 p.m.; University College, 2 p.m.; Royal London Ophthalmic, 11 a.m.; Royal Westminster Ophthalmic, 1½ p.m.; Hospital for Diseases of the Throat, 2 p.m.; Hospital for Women, 2 p.m.; Charing-cross, 2 p.m.; London, 2 p.m.; North-West London, 2½ p.m.

28. *Friday.*

Operations at Central London Ophthalmic, 2 p.m.; Royal London Ophthalmic, 11 a.m.; South London Ophthalmic, 2 p.m.; Royal Westminster Ophthalmic, 1½ p.m.; St. George's (ophthalmic operations), 1¼ p.m.; Guy's, 1½ p.m.; St. Thomas's (ophthalmic operations), 2 p.m.

Quekett Microscopical Club (University College), 8 p.m. Ordinary Meeting.

Clinical Society, 8½ p.m. Mr. C. T. Dent, "On a Case of Strangulated Hernia (Littré's) or Partial Enterocele." Dr. Churton (Leeds), "On a Case of Cholesterin-containing Fluid in the Pleura." Mr. Reeves, "On a Case of Stricture of the Pharynx and Œsophagus, with special reference to Gastrotomy and Œsophagotomy." Dr. Stephen Mackenzie, "On a Case of Excessively High Temperature."

PATHOLOGY, PAST AND PRESENT.

AN INAUGURAL ADDRESS

Delivered in the University of Edinburgh, October 26, 1881.

By J. W. S. GREENFIELD, M.D., F.R.C.P. Lond.,

Professor of General Pathology, University of Edinburgh.

GENTLEMEN,—Coming before you to-day for the first time as the formal occupant of the Chair of Pathology in this University, it is fitting that I should, in accordance with precedent, address to you some statement of the past history of the chair, and of the present relations of my subject to the study of medicine.

Just fifty years ago the first separate course of General Pathology in this University was commenced. Previously, indeed, it had formed a part of the course of the Institutes of Medicine, in its three branches of Physiology, Pathology, and Therapeutics, just as there was but one chair of Anatomy and Surgery. The growing importance and extended knowledge of Physiology would soon have rendered such a separation inevitable, had not the prerogative of the Crown somewhat rudely and forcibly intervened, and without consultation with any of the Medical Faculty, or indeed with anyone, appointed Dr. John Thomson Professor of General Pathology, and made attendance upon his lectures imperative upon all candidates for graduation.(a) No wonder that the Medical Faculty viewed such a course with disfavour, and that such eminent pathologists as Alison, Syme, and Christison were strongly opposed to the foundation of the chair in such a manner. It is not worth while to follow the course of the disputes and difficulties which ensued, or to revive long-buried controversies. The founders of the chair have at least the credit of foresight in seeing what must in a few years have come to pass, and profiting by it; and Professor Thomson was, as his "Lectures on Inflammation"(b) show, no mean pathologist in his earlier days. During his tenure of the Professorship, pathology did not suffer in the school, but it was by the labours of his colleagues rather than his own that it was enriched. On his death in 1841 he was succeeded by Dr. Henderson, who retained the chair till 1869. I know not what influence may have been exerted by it during his long tenure of office, but it cannot have been marked in the hands of one who, whatever his genius and accomplishments, was in the strange position of professing a subject whose methods are practical and whose principles are the basis of scientific medicine, whilst he practised a system of therapeutics(c) originating in groundless theories, and uncontrolled by scientific observation. Thus for thirty-eight years after its foundation the chair, instead of advancing on the lines of observation and research which should have made it a distinguished aid to science, remained practically useless for that purpose.

It would ill become me to attempt any worthy record of my distinguished predecessor, Dr. Sanders. What he was as a man, as a physician, and as a pathologist, you already know full well. His character and life-work are fresh in the memories of all; and we this day mourn his loss. This only will I say with regard to what he did for this chair : recognising the great importance of pathology as a branch of practical medical education, convinced that to be of real value it must be grounded on observation rather than theory, and that morbid anatomy in its fullest development must be one of its main supports, he set himself to work to build up, step by step, a full and thorough teaching of pathology in all its branches. And he thus accomplished, not merely a complete course of systematic teaching, but he so organised and arranged the means and appliances for practical study as to be prepared for any future developements of the science. What he has done in this respect will yet, I trust, bear fruit

(a) The Chair of General Pathology in the University of Paris was founded by Louis Philippe, after the Revolution in 1830, in a somewhat similar way, and Broussais appointed first Professor.
(b) Published in 1813.
(c) Dr. Henderson became a homœopathist.

v. II. 1881. No. 1635.

for many future years, though he did not live to see and enjoy its full fruition. Let us remember that it is to him we owe the establishment of laboratories for the practical study and teaching of pathological anatomy, histology, and chemistry, and that whatever future researches may be carried out in the new laboratories will be in a measure due to his influence.

But it is time that I should define to you the scope of the subject taught from this chair.

Pathology has been defined as the Science of Disease, as distinguished from Physiology, the Science of Health, bearing a similar relation to the morbid structure and functions of the body which physiology does to its healthy conditions. The name "General Pathology," as given to this chair, was, I believe, intended to distinguish the subject from that special pathology which is to be learnt in the study of surgery and medicine, and to include all those general facts and laws relating to disease which can be advantageously studied apart from the special diseases of which they form an element.

So long as disease was regarded as a sort of morbid entity, as the working of a spirit or evil humour which entered into the body and settled down upon and deranged the action of various organs, so long only could pathology be studied apart from morbid anatomy. We have gradually come to see that the derangement of function which we call disease is inseparably connected with an altered physical or chemical condition, which in many cases becomes obvious as a structural change, and that if we would understand the nature and course of disease, we must investigate the conditions of structure which underlie the outward phenomena.

It is in this way that morbid anatomy, in its widest sense, has come to be inseparably linked with general pathology.

Pathology, then, includes in its scope—

Morbid or *Pathological Anatomy*, i.e., the study of all the altered conditions of diseased organs, in their characters physical and chemical, and their relations to one another, whether revealed by the naked eye, the microscope, or in other ways. It investigates, too, the conditions of their occurrence, and seeks to elucidate the mode in which the visible changes have been brought about.

Grouping together those changes which are alike in the several organs or tissues, and eliminating that which is peculiar to the individual organs, it establishes certain groups or orders of morbid changes which form the subject of *General Morbid Anatomy*.

But it goes yet further, and by investigating the mode in which the altered constitution of the organ affects its function, and gives rise to symptoms, it forms a great part of the basis of the subjects of *Pathogenesis* and *Pathological Physiology*.

But pathology, as including the science of disease, is not content with registering its effects; it traces them back to their origin, and, under *General Ætiology*, it endeavours to study the general causes of disease, whether external to the body or within it, and to investigate their mode of action.

And, lastly, finding that there are processes of deranged action, morbid modes of motion, so to speak, which, grouped in various ways, enter into a multitude of diverse diseases, but which have fixed laws that govern their course, we group these together for study under the heading of what is more strictly defined as *General Pathology*.

I have emphasised this connexion between general pathology and morbid anatomy, or, to put it in a wider form, between disease and its physical basis, because in the history of medicine we find that, in proportion as this connexion has been recognised, has been the advance in its exact knowledge. Yet we must ever bear in mind that the study of the forms and reactions of *dead* matter can only guide us to a certain point; that it is *living* matter with which we have to do, and that it is by the exact study of the phenomena of life that we must bridge over the chasm between dead morbid anatomy and living pathology. If we start with the study of phenomena without the guide afforded by the knowledge of their physical conditions, we shall never reach solid ground, but wander in the quagmires of speculation; whilst if we omit to recognise the properties of life we shall equally fail. It is thus that physiology, biology, and experimental pathology, together with clinical medicine, are the inseparable adjuncts of morbid anatomy in working out scientific pathology. It is thus that the study of living matter in all its forms, and of the influences which act upon it, are of vital importance to the pathologist.

I would now ask you to look back at the history of morbid anatomy, in order to realise how it has grown and acquired its present position as the groundwork of pathology. For, until morbid anatomy had successfully asserted this position, pathology had no scientific existence, and the theories and doctrines evolved by a combined observation of symptoms and a use of the imagination have passed into the region of historical curiosities.

Morbid anatomy was studied at a very early period of the history of medicine. Hippocrates (460 B.C.) is usually spoken of as the earliest to pay attention to it; but there can be little doubt that in India, long before Hippocrates, there was some knowledge and use of it. Erasistratus and Herophilus are said by Pliny to have studied it. Aretæus(d) seems far to have excelled his predecessors in his acquaintance with it. But Celsus, who probably lived in the time of Tiberius, and whose work, " De Re Medica," is still in use as a subject of examination by some medical bodies, appears to have attached no importance to it as a part of the study of disease. Galen,(e) in the second century, studied morbid anatomy both practically and historically, and recognised more fully than his predecessors how often structural change was associated with functional derangement.

But just as the Mohammedan conquest of India was to destroy Indian medicine, so did the overthrow of the Roman Empire arrest all progress in science in Europe; and medical science, during the Middle Ages, became obscured, and lost, instead of gaining, knowledge. The history of morbid anatomy is practically a blank until the seventeenth century, although here and there isolated observations were recorded by anatomists and surgeons. With the revival of science came the revival of medicine.

Nearly fifteen hundred years elapsed before the next work of value on morbid anatomy, when the " Sepulchretum "(f) of Bonetus appeared, a work in which some systematic attempt was made to connect the appearances in the dead body with disease in the living.

Eighty years later the first great systematic work on morbid anatomy—that of Morgagni(g)—was published. Morgagni was a pupil of the illustrious Valsalva at Bologna, and was Professor of Anatomy at Padua from 1715 to 1771. In this work he brings together an enormous amount of accurate observation upon morbid anatomy, both from his own personal work and from other sources, and attempts to show how the changes found were related to the production of symptoms.

Morgagni, therefore, took the first step towards the establishment of a scientific pathology by attempting to localise disease. But it needed the discoveries of structure and function to complete the connexion between morbid anatomy and pathology.

The next work of importance(h) was that of Matthew Baillie,(i) who, in 1799, began to publish the first illustrated

(d) Aretæus of Cappadocia, who lived in the time of Vespasian, goes even so far as to mention the production of hemiplegia of one side in disease of the opposite cerebral hemisphere, and of paralysis of the same side in disease of the spinal cord. He describes, too, intestinal ulcers, and speaks of jaundice as caused by obstruction of the bile-ducts by scirrhus or by inflammation.

(e) Galen (130-200 A.D.) left on record a large amount of pathological lore, but how much originated with himself is doubtful. It is to him that we owe the introduction of pathological experiments upon living animals.

(f) " Boneti Sepulchretum," published 1679. There is an attempt to trace disease to their anatomical seats, but much that is fabulous, and too little personal observation.

(g) J. B. Morgagni, born in 1682, studied under Valsalva at Bologna, became Professor of Anatomy in Padua University in 1715, and held that post till his death in 1771. He was a great friend of Santorini. His great work, " De Causis et Sedibus Morborum per Anatomen Indagatis," was arranged mainly on the basis of symptoms and order of symptoms, cases being taken in which like symptoms were observed, and the symptoms discussed in the light of post-mortem examination. This method was the only one possible in his day, when the seats of various functions had been but very imperfectly determined; and it was in accordance with the semeiological system of medicine of his day. It was a first step to the localisation of disease to localise the cause of the most prominent symptoms. The aphorisms of Hippocrates had still a remarkably strong hold even upon so independent an observer as Morgagni, and he hardly ventured to question them in the face of the strongest evidence.

(h) Those of Lieutaud in 1767, and Ludwig in 1785, may also be mentioned.

(i) " On the Morbid Anatomy of some of the most important parts of the Human Body," illustrated by engravings, London, 1799. Nearly half of the drawings are from " specimens in Mr. Baillie's collection," and many others " from Mr. Heaviside's collection," which was given thirty

work on morbid anatomy. But it was to John Hunter that Baillie was indebted, both for inspiration and for the material from which most of his drawings were made, and it is, I believe, to the influence of John Hunter, renowned alike as anatomist, physiologist, and pathologist, that we may in a great measure trace the revival of pathology which followed.

With the beginning of the present century began the real and thorough study of morbid anatomy. It seems strange that so simple and obvious a method of studying disease should have been little practised for so many hundred years, and that within the lifetime of some here to-day it has grown to its present vast proportions.

We owe to great anatomists, who in most cases were also surgeons, the commencement of this movement of revival. They had most to do with the dissection of dead bodies, and the deeper and more attentive study of anatomy was a guide to altered as well as to healthy structure. The systematic application of these studies to medicine was yet to come, and it was in France that the first great movements took place.(k) The names of Bichat, Laennec, Andral, and Cruveilhier are pre-eminent amongst the many active workers. Of Bichat I shall have to speak later. Laennec,(l) during his earlier years, devoted himself ardently to pathological research, but his labours, after his discovery of mediate auscultation, were mainly directed to that subject, although his influence greatly assisted in the work.

In the earlier years of this century the French medical world was under the domination of the ideas of Broussais, who, in 1816,(m) promulgated his doctrine of so-called " physiological medicine," in which the stomach became the centre and source of all diseases, and varying degrees of inflammation of the stomach and intestines the starting-point of all pathological changes. Against such theories, the school of pathological anatomy of Bayle and Laennec, Cruveilhier and Andral, asserted itself, and gradually made good the cause of the " medicine of observation," grounded on clinical study joined to morbid anatomy.

Cruveilhier, the great anatomist, supported the cause by his extensive observations,(n) subsequently embodied in his great work on morbid anatomy.

But to Andral(o) must be given the credit of fighting, step by step, the detail of the battle against the almost overwhelming opposition of Broussais and his followers, who included a great part of the medical world. In 1823 he published the first volume of his " Clinique Médicale," in which were arrayed, in opposition to Broussais, a great series of clinical and post-mortem observations, which demonstrated the falsity of the speculations of Broussais. It was the first great move in the conflict of scientific pathology founded on observation, against mere speculation, which ended in the complete overthrow of Broussais' system, so that when Andral succeeded Broussais in the chair of General Pathology in 1839, Broussais' system had already become extinct. That Andral was a diligent morbid anatomist, as well as a brilliant physician and pathologist, is shown by a fact which he casually mentions, that he had examined the thoracic duct and principal lymphatic vessels in more than six hundred subjects.(p) It was Andral's especial merit

years later to the Hunterian Museum. We must remember that John Hunter's museum was practically the first museum containing specimens of pathological anatomy. Other museums were founded at Amsterdam in 1789, at Leyden in 1795, Berlin in 1796, and later those of Vienna, Florence, and Paris did much to aid in fixing observations.

(k) Text-books of pathological anatomy began to appear towards the early part of the century—that of Conradi in 1796, Voigtel in 1804, Meckel in 1811, Otto in 1814, all of German origin.

(l) Laennec was born in 1781, came to Paris in 1800, and studied under Corvisart and Bichat. His work on pathological anatomy was mainly done between 1804 and 1812. For three years he lectured on morbid anatomy as successor to Bichat. In 1815 he discovered mediate auscultation, and his subsequent labours, till his death from phthisis in 1826, were almost entirely on this subject.

(m) " Examen de la Doctrine Médicale généralement adoptée."

(n) Cruveilhier published his first paper on Pathological Anatomy in 1816 (" Essai sur l'Anatomie Pathologique"). In 1825 he was appointed Professor of Anatomy in the University of Paris, and in 1829 commenced the publication of his great illustrated work on Pathological Anatomy (" Anatomie Pathologique du Corps Humain," vol. i.). In 1835 he was transferred to the chair of Pathological Anatomy.

(o) Andral lectured on Pathological Anatomy in Paris before 1825, in the extra-mural school (Enseignement libre). In 1828 he was appointed Professor of Hygiene in the University of Paris, and in 1830 transferred to the chair of Internal Pathology. His " Précis d'Anatomie Pathologique," the complement of his " Clinique Médicale," was published in 1829. He died in 1876, at the age of seventy-nine. He was the pupil of Laennec and Lærminier. To the latter he owed his opportunities for acquiring material for his " Clinique Médicale."

(p) " Précis d'Anatomie Pathologique."

that he was not content merely to record morbid appearances, but in every case sought to trace their causes,(q) and to discover how they were related to each other, their order of causation and succession, and the part they played in the production of disease. From this time morbid anatomy has become not merely an observing and recording, but an interpreting science.

Nor must I omit the names of Louis, Bouillaud, Gendrin, Reynaud, and Chomel, who in more special ways advanced pathological anatomy and clinical medicine together.

In England, during the same period, partly from the same causes, and partly through the direct influence of the French school, great attention was being paid to morbid anatomy, especially in relation to diseases of particular organs, and the results were becoming apparent about the time when this chair was founded.

In London, three men, all of whom were students and graduates of this University—Hope, Carswell, and Bright—were especially pre-eminent in this direction.

Hope, who had studied under Laennec and Andral, was, I believe, one of the first to introduce and teach the method of auscultation in this country. To him we owe the first correct explanation of the mode of production and localisation of cardiac murmurs,(r) and his first work in this direction was done when he was Resident Physician and Surgeon in the Royal Infirmary of Edinburgh in 1824 and 1825. In 1833 he published a valuable Atlas of Morbid Anatomy.(s) But his work was eclipsed by that of Robert Carswell, which appeared in 1838. Carswell's immense industry and artistic ability enabled him to produce a very large number of admirable drawings in addition to those published in his work on pathological anatomy, many of which, purchased and presented to this University by his friend Professor Thomson, we have still in daily use for purposes of illustration.(t)

But of the three men who at the time of the foundation of this chair were conferring the greatest services on morbid anatomy and medicine, Richard Bright must take by far the highest rank. He was then Lecturer on the Practice of Medicine at Guy's Hospital, and had just completed the publication of those "Reports of Medical Cases" (1827 to 1831), by which his name will be handed down to all succeeding generations; for they contain in the foremost place those observations on kidney-disease with which his name is indissolubly connected, and they show that the same method by which he arrived at his great discovery—acute and careful clinical observation, combined with exactly recorded and delineated post-mortem examination, and the whole informed by careful inductive reasoning—was applied to every part of his work. In the same work is contained an accurate description of a series of cases of enteric fever, and drawings and descriptions of the condition of the intestines, which have not, I think, been since surpassed; indeed, he may be said to have worked out the clinical history and pathology of the disease as far as was then possible.

We have thus reached the period of the foundation of

(q) How far Andral was in advance even of some of the distinguished pathologists of his day may be judged from these words of Bayle.—"The end of morbid anatomy is to bring new light to nosology; its utility is limited to supplying a new means of comparing those organic diseases which are of the same nature, and distinguishing those which, in spite of similarity of symptoms, are of entirely different nature, and belong to another order of disease." And he adds—"One would have a very false idea of pathological anatomy if one imagined that it could throw any light upon the essence of organic diseases, on their immediate cause, or on the mechanism of their production. Pathological anatomy only gives us the knowledge of organic lesions."

(r) His fully detailed evidence, confirmed by numerous experiments on animals, was published in his work on "Diseases of the Heart" in 1832, when he was Physician to St. George's Hospital.

(s) Hope grouped together the diseases of each organ in his illustrations, but in the text followed Andral's classification of the various morbid changes into lesions of (1) circulation, (2) nutrition, (3) secretion, (4) the blood, and (5) innervation. Hope's great ability and faithfulness as an artist, and his mastery of clinical medicine, as shown in his work on "Diseases of the Heart," make his Atlas of especial value. I ought also to mention in this connexion Robert Hooper, who for nearly thirty years was engaged in collecting materials for an Atlas of morbid anatomy, to illustrate the diseases of all the principal internal organs. Only two parts of his work—those on the Brain, in 1828, and on the Uterus, in 1832—ever saw the light, but I have had the good fortune to obtain possession of more than 200 water-colour drawings, made for this purpose, dating from 1797 to 1834, many of which were made by such men as Howship, Hope, and others equally capable.

(t) Carswell's published work cannot be said to have done justice to his powers, and the arrangement which he adopted for illustrating the various processes of inflammation, analogous tissues, atrophy, hypertrophy, and, so on, by examples of each in various organs, though valuable at the time has produced much confusion, for he was often in error as to the nature of the process.

this chair, and it is interesting to consider who were then the active leaders in pathological advance. The period was one of the epochs of great activity and of rapid strides in the advance of science. It was in the same year that the British Association for the Advancement of Science was founded, and amongst its earliest members were many of the leaders in medical science of the day. And it was a period of great pathological revival and creation, whether we regard the men who were foremost in the medical world, the discoveries which were made, the works which were published, or the increased foundation of chairs for teaching the subject. In France, Cruveilhier and Andral at Paris, and Lobstein at Strasburg, were the recognised leaders. Louis, who had published his great work on Phthisis in 1825, his "Anatomo-pathological Researches" in 1826, and that on "Gastro-enteritis" in 1829, was living and active; and Rayer, known by his work on "Diseases of the Skin" (1827), was preparing for his more important work on "Renal Disease," published in 1839.

In Germany there was less obvious activity, but Gläge and Fick were doubtless working at those micro-pathological problems which were brought out in 1838; Rokitansky was amassing those stores of knowledge which, ten years later (1841-46), he gave to the world; and Johannes Müller was making those researches on the structure of tumours which were to supplement his physiological studies.

In London, too, besides the men I have named, there were others who greatly contributed to the advance of pathology. Addison had just published his first work,(u) and Hodgkin, who had begun to lecture on morbid anatomy in 1827 (published in 1836-41), had just completed a Catalogue of the Museum of Guy's Hospital (1830).

In Edinburgh there were great men and great pathologists. Alison published the outlines of his lectures on physiology and pathology in 1831, and the pathology separately in 1833. Christison, who had for nine years been a professor in the University, and was already distinguished both in toxicology and pathology, had published his great work on "Poisons" (1829) two years before, and in the same year his first paper on "Dropsy in relation to Diseased Kidney," a subject in which he afterwards did such valuable work.(v) Abercrombie, Monro, and Gregory were still in active practice.

I have thus briefly traced the outward history of morbid anatomy to the time of the foundation of this chair, when it had successfully asserted its position as an essential basis of pathology. Everywhere attention was being devoted to it, and no case was considered complete in which the morbid appearances were not noted. But naked-eye morbid anatomy had its limits as an interpreter. The functions even of some important organs were but little understood, and the way in which visible changes were brought about, or how they were related to disease, could not, owing to imperfect means of research, be fully appreciated. We are apt to smile at the notion entertained by Laennec, that the yellow masses in cirrhosis of the liver, from which he gave it its present name, were a morbid deposit, and the belief that the morbid "granules" described by Bright in diseased kidneys were some material whose nature could be solved by chemical analysis. But it was only by the use of the microscope, and the discoveries of physiology on the structure and functions of organs, that more enlightened views became possible. This was to be the next step in advance.

The dawn of the new era may be traced to the beginning of the present century, and may be said to have begun with new ideas of structural anatomy preceding the fuller knowledge of function. For until the primary analysis of the structure of the body had been made, until the minuter elements had been grouped into classes, and their individual functions and powers determined, it was impossible to reduce to any general expression the derangements to which they were subject. The first step to this was the rearrangement and classification of the tissues, due partly to Haller, but mainly to the genius of Bichat, who must be regarded as the founder of general morbid anatomy, as well as of general anatomy. He not only classified the tissues and organic systems, but he entered into their pathology, and asserted that "each tissue has its own diseases." Apart from his own work in this direction, he rendered

(u) "On the Disorders of Females connected with Uterine Irritation," 1830.

(v) "On Granular Degeneration of the Kidneys." Edinburgh. 1829.

possible the subsequent advances in the study of diseases of systems and tissues, in which Laennec and Gendrin were the pioneers.

The general application of the microscope to vegetable and animal histology was the means of the next great advance. It is true that so early as the middle of the seventeenth century, the microscope had been employed in histological and pathological research, by Hooke, Leeuwenhoeck, and Malphigi (1686), and that early in the present century many discoveries had been made in normal histology; but it is none the less true, that until after 1830 it had not been possible to apply it systematically to pathological histology. Nor was it till 1847 that the work of Schleiden on "Vegetable Histology," and later of Schwann on the "Comparison of the Cellular Structure of Vegetables and Animals," laid the foundation of our modern histology. Johannes Müller was the first to systematise pathological histology as applied to tumours, and was followed by Henle, Glüge, and Vogel. Nor must we omit the names of Kölliker, Bowman, Goodsir, and Sharpey, who did such good work in normal histology.

It is unquestionably to Virchow that we owe the great advance by which histology came to take a first rank as an aid to pathology, and from the date of his great work on "Cellular Pathology" (1858) we may reckon the era of modern pathology. His work, dedicated to Professor Goodsir "as one of the earliest and most acute observers of cell-life, both physiological and pathological," put a new life into pathology. Starting from the discoveries of Schleiden and Schwann on the cellular structure of vegetable and animal tissues, he showed how in the cell is the vital unit of all organised structures, how intimately its changes are associated with all the processes of organic life, both in health and disease, with the development and maintenance of the tissues, and in all their functional reactions, whether normal or abnormal. He showed, moreover, how cell-changes are concerned in all morbid growths, and in a vast number of diseases, and how in cell-systems and cell-territories disease processes may often be localised. It would be impossible for me to do justice to the many side-lights which he threw upon disease. I do not think that all Virchow's most absolute dicta can be accepted at the present day, or that we can reduce all pathology to the simplicity of cell-reaction. But apart from this, and its great value as a study in histology and physiology, Virchow's work did incalculable service to pathology in sweeping away old fallacies, in compelling attention to the most minute changes which lie at the root of disease, and in showing how in these minute changes are to be sought both the evidence and the explanation of functional disorder. Nor must we overlook the great value of his cellular pathology as a system, taking the place, to a large extent, of the humoral, solidistic, and other pathological systems which had preceded him.

Had we lived in the days of Brown and Broussais we should better appreciate the revolution which Virchow's doctrines effected, and what solid ground was substituted for previous speculation.

What the atomic theory has been to chemistry, and the wave theory to physics, that the cell theory has been to pathology.

And I would especially notice that it is not in any mere knowledge of cellular structure and arrangement, or in the relations of cells to development, that the value of Virchow's system consists. Nothing could have been farther from the central idea of his teaching than the mere mechanical application of cellular structure to the elucidation of the phenomena of life and of disease. It is the living cell, endowed with vitality and with function, governed by laws of existence, capable of self-multiplication and propagation, and arranged in organic systems, which he studies. It is the cell as the living active agent in the production of disease, and the arrest or perversion of its action by disease-producing causes, which have the highest place in his thoughts. It is by this link that the study of histology is connected with pathology, and that in turn this is joined to evolution and development—the link by which all other biological studies come to have an intimate bearing on pathology. However far we may transcend cellular pathology, we cannot neglect it in any future study.

We have thus reached a point at which the era of modern pathology may be said to begin. In the first thirty years of the century we have the awakening, the new impulse to the study of morbid anatomy both in its relations to normal anatomy and to clinical medicine, and side by side with this, though as yet separate, the renewed study of general anatomy. In the next thirty years we have the more general application of morbid anatomy to clinical medicine as an expounder of the phenomena of disease, and at the same time the fuller knowledge of structure and function of the several organs, and the working out of detailed normal and pathological histology rendered possible by the improvement of the microscope. We may reckon the end of the thirty years, 1860, when Virchow's work had had time to be known, as the culminating point of this period, and the entrance of our present epoch.

During the twenty years which have passed since Virchow's great work, pathology has made immense progress. Morbid anatomy has discovered lesions and diseases before unknown, and has connected them with the symptoms and functional derangements with which they are associated. New processes of disease have been discovered, and old ones explained. Such discoveries as those of Cohnheim on inflammation, and the work done on the subject of microscopic parasites, have revolutionised whole fields of pathology. Our knowledge of minute structural changes has become encyclopædic. Look which way we will, the array of facts and discoveries seems almost overwhelming, and every day new ones are added to the store.

But, gentlemen, this is not the time for me to speak to you in detail of modern pathology. This it will be my duty to unfold to you in due course. I would rather try to impress upon you the spirit in which the subject of pathology is to be approached, and how it stands related to your past and future studies.

(To be continued.)

UNIVERSITY OF CAMBRIDGE.—EXAMINATIONS FOR THE DEGREES OF M.B. AND M.C.—The above examinations will begin on Tuesday, December 13. Candidates for the degree of M.B. are requested to send their names to the Prælectors of their several Colleges on or before November 26. The certificates of candidates for the degree of M.B. are to be sent to the Secretary; and the names and certificates of candidates for the degree of M.C. to the Regius Professor of Physic, Dr. Paget, Cambridge, on or before December 3.

STREET-NAMING AT LYONS.—In the new street-naming which has been undertaken at Lyons, the Municipal Commission has determined that every street shall be named after a celebrated man; and for the medical quarter in which the new Faculty is established the names of doctors are to be employed. But the number of streets, quays, and squares requiring to be thus baptised is so numerous that the difficulty in finding indigenous medical celebrities to furnish the names must have been considerable, especially as there is not a single doctor on the Commission. The consequence is that no one, not even a doctor, can explain the reason why some of these names have been chosen; and this lavishing of honours on unknown or questionable persons naturally indisposes persons of legitimate ambition desiring to find themselves in such company. Moreover, what is to be done with regard to future celebrities, whose places will all be taken by others, and who it will be difficult to displace in their favour?—Lyon Méd., September 29.

THE CENTRE OF POPULATION OF THE UNITED STATES.—"Westward the star of empire takes its way." The Popular Science Monthly says that the centre of population of the United States appears now to have reached a point in latitude 39° 03', about five miles west of Covington, Kentucky, ten miles east of the boundary line between Indiana and Ohio, and fifty-one miles west and a few miles south of the point it reached in 1870. It has moved west about 450 miles since 1790. It is interesting to note that this westward march of the empire is at an average rate of about five miles a year, and that this snail-like pace has not been much quickened by free railroad communication, and the consequent settling up of vast regions of western territory. At this rate, Louisville, or its meridian, will hardly be reached in eleven years; while St. Louis will have to wait about sixty-one years before she can claim the coveted honour of being in every sense of the word the central city of the Republic.—Louisville Med. News, September 10.

CLINICAL LECTURES
ON DISEASES OF THE ABDOMEN.

By FREDERICK T. ROBERTS, M.D., B.Sc., F.R.C.P.,
Professor of Materia Medica and Therapeutics at University College,
Physician to University Hospital, and Professor of
Clinical Medicine, etc.

LECTURE III.

A CLINICAL CLASSIFICATION OF ABDOMINAL
DISEASES.

THE diseases of the abdomen being so numerous and varied, a mere acquaintance with the nature and clinical characters of the several affections of each organ or structure is far from being sufficient for diagnostic purposes, and often leaves the practitioner in great doubt and uncertainty as to the nature of a case. I therefore am now going to attempt a classification of these diseases from a more comprehensive point of view, which I hope may be of some practical use to you, founded upon the groups of cases which, according to my experience, come under one's observation in actual practice. In this classification I shall exclude, except where it is absolutely necessary to allude to them, diseases of the female generative organs, which demand special study; and also purely surgical affections, although there are some conditions which must be noticed, which are on the confines between medicine and surgery, or which, originally belonging to the class of medical cases, subsequently became surgical in their nature.

In the first place, cases of abdominal disease must be recognised as divisible into three main groups, according to their mode of onset and severity, namely:—I. Sudden, or Hyper-acute; II. Acute, or Sub-acute; III. Chronic.

I.—SUDDEN OR HYPER-ACUTE.

As these terms imply, cases belonging to this group are characterised by suddenness or marked rapidity of onset; with intensity and urgency, or even extreme danger, in the symptoms or morbid conditions and their effects. They may prove immediately or speedily fatal; or be attended with evident grave symptoms, either local, general, or both; or be merely of a painful character, without any particular danger. In some instances belonging to this class, paroxysmal attacks of a severe type constitute a special feature in their clinical history. Cases of sudden or hyper-acute lesions or symptoms connected with the abdomen may be arranged in the following way:—

1. Conditions resulting from External Injury.—These, of course, belong to the domain of surgery, but it is important to recognise a class of cases in which rupture of some internal organ, such as the liver or stomach, or of a tube, such as the ureter, has occurred from some indirect or comparatively slight injury, which has scarcely attracted attention, or has not caused any external signs of injury in connexion with the abdominal walls. Such cases might come under the notice of the practitioner as if belonging to the medical group, especially if there were no history of injury, and under such circumstances they would be very puzzling, or, indeed, incomprehensible.

2. Poisoning by Corrosives or Irritants.—This is an important group of cases in which abdominal organs are implicated, and the symptoms are more or less urgent and grave. They include not only those due to the effects of the recognised irritant and corrosive poisons, but also those in which the irritation depends upon articles taken as food or drink, such as decomposed animal or vegetable foods, fish or shell-fish in certain individuals, special articles of diet, bad water, etc. Moreover, it must be remembered that the poisons may not only be taken by, or administered to, the patient, either designedly or accidentally; but may enter the system by inhalation, being suspended in the atmosphere in the form of a fine powder, as happens in the case of arsenic derived from arsenical wall-papers, and consequently serious symptoms might rapidly supervene, for which no apparent cause could be found.

3. Affections attended with Spasm or Cramp.—These are of common occurrence in practice; and the spasm may affect the muscles of the abdominal walls, the stomach (generally called "cramp"), the intestines ("colic"), or the diaphragm. The prominent feature of these cases is pain having certain characters, often very intense, and not uncommonly accompanied with other alarming symptoms; but as a rule they are not really dangerous, and recovery usually takes place.

4. The Passage, or attempted Passage, of Calculi, or rarely of other Objects (Clots, Worms, etc.) along certain Tubes.—Practically we have to deal in this group with calculi, the others being extremely rare, and it includes mainly two classes of cases, namely—(a) those in which a biliary calculus or gall-stone passes along the bile-duct to the intestine; (b) those in which a renal calculus passes along the ureter to the bladder. It may possibly happen that a calculus escaping from the pancreas gives rise to symptoms. Cases belonging to this class are often remarkably sudden in their onset, and attended with urgent and dangerous symptoms or effects.

5. Ruptures and Perforations within the Abdominal Cavity.—This group is intended to include those cases in which a rupture or perforation within the abdomen occurs independently of any external injury, and in many instances without any immediate obvious cause. They are of great consequence, and are necessarily attended, as a rule, with grave danger to life.

6. Certain forms of Intestinal Obstruction.—Some cases of intestinal obstruction are extremely acute in their onset and symptoms, and in this connexion the different forms of strangulated hernia must not be forgotten.

7. Special Diseases.—These include chiefly cholera, choleraic diarrhœa, yellow fever, and dysentery in some instances.

8. Special Symptoms.—Of symptoms connected with the abdomen which may become suddenly or rapidly urgent in themselves, and thus demand particular attention, may be mentioned vomiting, hæmorrhage from different parts, and retention of urine. The condition last mentioned may occur not only in recognised surgical cases, but also in those which come within the scope of medical practice.

II.—ACUTE OR SUB-ACUTE.

This division scarcely needs definition, but it includes conditions presenting various degrees of acuteness in their onset and symptoms, merging on the one hand into the group already considered, and on the other into cases of a sub-acute character.

1. Acute Affections of the Abdominal Walls.—These are of three kinds, namely:—(a.) Painful affections, without any obvious morbid changes, including muscular rheumatism, and severe neuralgia or hyperæsthesia, especially met with in some hysterical subjects. (b.) Localised inflammation, often ending in suppuration—a class of cases which may be exemplified by "bubo" in the groin, but the inflammation may involve any part or structure of the abdominal walls. (c.) Subcutaneous accumulations, either of fluid (œdema), or of gas (emphysema). These conditions are seldom limited to the abdomen, the œdema being usually a part of acute general dropsy, and the collection of gas a part of more or less extensive subcutaneous emphysema.

2. Acute Congestion of Abdominal Organs.—Many cases are referred to this category in ordinary practice which really do not belong to it, but unquestionably clinical phenomena, more or less obvious and important, do arise from acute congestion of certain abdominal viscera, more especially the liver, kidneys, and spleen.

3. Acute Disorders of the Digestive Organs.—Under this head I would include certain derangements of the digestive apparatus, evidenced by prominent symptoms, but not really of a serious character, and due to a variety of causes. The most familiar are those cases recognised under the terms acute dyspepsia, biliousness, and sick-headache. Many cases of ordinary diarrhœa may also be included. Not only may the stomach or intestines be affected, but also the liver or its duct, and the pancreas. The condition is often one of catarrh of the mucous surfaces; but it may depend upon some mere functional disorder, due to injurious articles taken into the alimentary canal, or to some centric nervous disturbance, as in sick-headache.

4. Acute Inflammation of Structures within the Abdomen.—This constitutes a numerous and somewhat complicated group, inasmuch as any structure or organ within the abdomen may be implicated, and even two or more at the same time; while the inflammation varies considerably in its

intensity, extent, and pathological consequences and effects. Nevertheless, it is possible for practical purposes to bring the majority of cases under certain subdivisions, and I submit for your consideration the following arrangement :—

a. Peritonitis, including all cases in which the peritoneum is acutely inflamed ; and these, although presenting much diversity, and not uncommonly being associated with inflammation of other structures, are sufficiently well-defined as a group.

b. Inflammation affecting the Alimentary Canal.—The less severe cases of mucous catarrh have already been referred to, but there are others in which the inflammation is more serious, and may become extremely grave, involving the mucous membrane more or less extensively, or it may be all the coats at some limited portion of the alimentary tube. The signs of these different conditions are usually tolerably definite. In this connexion the effects of irritant poisons must be again noticed, as these not uncommonly set up acute inflammation.

c. Inflammation around Organs.—This may involve the capsule of an organ (as in the case of peri-hepatitis); or the cellular tissue which surrounds it, which is well exemplified by peri-typhlitis (inflammation around the cæcum), perinephritis (inflammation around the kidney), and many cases of pelvic abscess. The cases differ in severity, and when the cellular tissue is affected the inflammation tends to terminate in suppuration.

d. Special Inflammations connected with the Urinary Organs.—These cases fall into two groups, namely : (i.) Cases of acute desquamative nephritis or Bright's disease, characterised by very definite and striking symptoms ; (ii.) Cases in which the urinary mucous membrane is inflamed in some part of the tract, in medical practice divisible into those in which the pelvis of the kidney is implicated (pyelitis), and those in which the bladder is involved (cystitis). Here the inflammation often terminates in the formation and discharge of more or less purulent material.

e. Inflammation ending in Abscess.—It has seemed to me most expedient for practical purposes to bring cases thus characterised under one head, but they may be further classified thus :—(i.) Those in which the abscess forms in the substance of an organ. It very rarely happens that an abscess forms in the walls of a hollow viscus, but in actual practice such an event may be put out of consideration. The organs within the abdomen to be specially borne in mind, as liable to become the seat of abscess, are the liver and kidney. Very exceptionally the spleen, pancreas, suprarenal capsules, or absorbent glands may be thus affected. (ii.) Cases in which pus, usually mixed with other fluids, accumulates within a hollow viscus or space, usually as the result of some obstruction to its escape. This may happen especially in connexion with the gall-bladder or renal pelvis. (iii.) Cases of inflammation beginning in the cellular tissue, and ending in the formation of abscess. These have been already alluded to, where the inflammation begins around organs ; but a similar condition may originate from diseased bone, injury, and other causes. (iv.) Cases of localised inflammation of the peritoneum, ending in limited suppuration, owing to the presence of adhesions.

5. *Acute Atrophy.*—This is a peculiar and very rare class of cases, in which certain organs become the seat of rapid fatty degeneration with atrophy, these morbid changes being attended with striking and grave symptoms, and the termination quickly fatal. The liver and kidneys are the abdominal organs in connexion with which clinical phenomena are specially noticed, and particularly the liver.

6. *Acute Tuberculosis.*—Structures within the abdomen are frequently involved in acute tuberculosis, but it rarely happens that this can be positively made out during life by any definite symptoms.

7. *Embolism.*—Emboli are liable to lodge in certain organs in the abdomen, especially the spleen and kidneys, and may possibly give rise to acute symptoms referred to these organs. Subsequent changes may also be set up, of an inflammatory nature.

8. *Special Diseases.*—Typhoid fever and dysentery belong to this group, these diseases being attended with prominent lesions and symptoms connected with abdominal structures.

9. *Trichinosis.*—This is an acute affection at the outset, due to the entrance of trichinæ into the alimentary canal, and they usually originate very severe abdominal symptoms.

(*To be continued.*)

ORIGINAL COMMUNICATIONS.

A NOTING ON SOME PECULIARITIES OF CONTAGIOUS OPHTHALMIA, AND ON THE USE OF BICARBONATE OF SODA.

By BRINSLEY NICHOLSON, M.D.

ABOUT 1855-57, when an assistant-surgeon stationed in King William's Town, British Caffraria, we had an outbreak, in our regiment, of contagious ophthalmia. The contagiousness, besides being shown in individual cases, was also shown by its attacking at first one, and then two, and finally four companies, the remainder remaining untouched, while the two first attacked suffered most. The instance of the fourth company was most instructive. During the outbreak, it and another had, according to Army instructions from home, been added to the regiment, and they were of course formed out of the other companies. Among the men thus told off were two chronic cases (but then doing duty) from an affected company, and the first case that occurred in this new company came from the hut occupied by these two.

The outbreak began, first, so far as circumstances could prove, from a case of chronic granular lids, then doing duty, but who, at some previous time, had had two attacks—one, at least, in Dublin ; and both, if I remember rightly, in Ireland—of ophthalmia. There was too a report among the men that he had also gonorrhœa at the time of the outbreak, but this was never proved, nor do I think it likely, for we had no gonorrhœa cases just then, and in what might be called a military village, otherwise so slightly populated, the soldiery forming its chief population, had there been one case, there would have been several others at the very least. Our men's quarters were very fair wattle and daub huts, of rather large size, thatched, and floored with hard daub that took a polish. But after-inquiry showed the cause of the spread of the disease. While the officers of the store department liked to have in store, say within the Cape Colony, a goodly show of numerous and brightly shining articles of barrack equipment ready to send anywhere, and on any emergency, the soldiers beyond the colony were only furnished with one hand-basin for every three or four men. The river was some little distance off, and hence the number using one basin usually made use of the same water for their morning ablutions. Hence the spread of the disease. When afterwards convalescent cases, i.e., cases for which there was no room at headquarters, and thought likely to be benefited by rest, greater absence from temptations, and change of air—when such were sent to either of the two isolated outposts that we occupied, and kept without the walls, and furnished with separate equipment, there was at these posts —about seven and twelve miles out in different directions— no occurrence of the disease. Neither were the men of any other corps in King William's Town at all affected.

I first took charge of fresh cases late in the attack, and will thus succinctly describe them. A man came in, saying that, well on the previous day, his eye (generally one eye) during the night had become as he then showed it. Enlarged and tortuous vessels ran across the eyeball ; the conjunctiva of it and of the lids was greatly chemosed, inflamed, and granular, the outer lids were swollen and much bulged, purulent matter ran freely from the eyes, and there was photophobia and great pain. Any local treatment – astringents, sedatives, etc.—was of little avail: a forty-grain solution of nitrate of silver brushed lightly across seemed in three or four instances to bring some amelioration, but its reapplication, even after three or four days, was resented. General treatment—lowering medicines, sedatives, sudorifics, mercury, etc.—seemed of equally small service. But gradually, under time and care, the cases improved and become chronic, the result being granular lids which I never cured nor saw cured. There also, of course, remained such differences as to congestion, chemosis, watering, and photophobia as depended on the different states and constitution of the patients. Some had ulcerations of the cornea, with opaque spots and sometimes protrusion of the iris. There were also what I should call an unusual number, chiefly during the more chronic stage, of a somewhat chronic form of iritis, readily reduced by small doses of the iodide of mercury. Some were distinctly due to a syphilitic taint, but in others I could neither detect nor elicit that origin.

Two points of interest, however, I noted as regards the commencement of the disease. On closer inquiry it turned out that the men had felt their eyes weaker and more watery three or four days previous to what they had called "the attack." Again, a man was admitted with the usual symptoms in his left eye. Within the first week I one day noticed that his right looked weakish and watery, and immediately everted the upper lid. On it I found *three islands of red granulations*, the rest of the conjunctiva looking perhaps a little reddish, but otherwise normal. Nor was I a day too soon; the next day that eye was as the other. Subsequently I saw one, if not two, other similar cases. Hence it became clear that the disease I am describing *commenced with granulation*, differing in this from the ordinary cases where granulation is a secondary result.

I now come to the period when, during the first part of the outbreak, I had to attend only to the chronic cases, such as best bore being sent out of our small hospital. These had been, I believe, treated latterly chiefly with the sulphate of copper applied in substance to the granular conjunctiva. They came out with paler and less mountainous, more undulating and smaller, granulations; but trifling wateriness of the eye, or even none; and the conjunctiva of the eyeball clear and healthy-looking. But under barrack—or, rather, barrack-hut—life, and the temptations which assail men who have long been confined to hospital with a merely local disease, and who, when outside it, had little or nothing to do, their eyes readily degenerated. The granulations became redder and more prominent, the eyeballs both more congested and watery-looking, and there was more or less discharge of water, blinking, and photophobia. Lotions of acetate of lead (my favourite lotion), or of sulphate of zinc, etc., with or without sedatives, were all tried; till at last I had all but come to the determination of commencing at one end of the medicine-chest, and going through it, in search of a remedy. Luckily, before I gave myself up to this despair, I hit upon the bicarbonate of soda in impalpable powder, introduced once a day between the lids, or placed on the everted lid, which was at once reverted. This only caused a short stinging pain, which the men bore readily, for they said "it dried their eyes"—that is, the granulations resumed their ordinary colour and appearance, the eye lost its bloodshot and watery look, the tears ceased, and so did the photophobia. There was not more than one case in which the granules seemed to disappear, but the following will illustrate the benefits of the treatment:—Two patients in hospital were each affected in both eyes, and habitually passed their time sitting on their beds. Their lids were greatly swollen and chemosed, as well as the sclerotic conjunctiva. Their eyes almost streamed with water, requiring constant mopping, and there was great photophobia. Not thin, but flabby and pale, they were excellent specimens of the ophthalmic cachexy. Each sat on his bed, as I have said, because it was too troublesome to walk about blinded. When they did go out, they felt for guidance by the ward dining-table, stopping some twenty times to wipe away the water and to allow them to blink a little before advancing any farther. Under the soda treatment, their eyes so improved in every respect that they forsook their bed-sittings and moved about in comparative comfort, and their general health improved also. So, in after years, whenever I had chronic cases which became worse under exposure or other causes, and where I thought it advisable to have recourse to the nitrate of silver or sulphate of copper, I found it very useful to first reduce the irritation and congestion by this means, especially where, as on board ship, there is seldom a fit hospital or means of keeping the patients from draughts or other exposures. The plan of treatment I almost always found the most useful was—on two mornings, the bicarbonate of soda; on the third, oxide of zinc; on the fourth, a rest from treatment; and then a recurrence in the same order. The oxide of zinc, however, was omitted during the first few days when the eye seemed too irritated and congested. Sufficiently satisfied with the bicarbonate of soda, I did not give so great a trial to the bicarbonate of potash as I wish I had; but from such trials as I made, the latter, like the carbonate of soda, was more irritant, and therefore less efficacious.

A similar treatment has, I believe, been adopted by others

in granular lids, but it is only much later that I became aware of this. Nor am I now aware whether my adoption of it was later than, or prior to, that of others. On this point I am indifferent. But I would say that having, since my retirement from the Army, thought over means for better getting rid of that opprobrium to surgery, granular lids—though not improbably my imagination is too sanguine—I would be greatly obliged to the ophthalmic surgeon of a hospital, or to any other medical man, who would send me such a chronic case. The means that I would use are, I may as well add, officinal, and in no way dangerous.

306, Goldhawk-road, Shepherd's-bush, W.

CONCEPTION WITH IMPERFORATE HYMEN.

By Surgeon-General C. R. FRANCIS, M.B. Lond.

Mrs. A., the wife of an officer in India, consulted me on account of persistent "morning sickness." She was tall, well formed, of dark complexion, thirty years of age, and had been married rather more than four months. The mammæ were tumid, with prominent nipples, and an indistinct areola. In the absence of any other probable cause for the morning sickness (which, however, the patient herself confidently believed to exist), and in the presence of symptoms which, added to it, are supposed to be almost diagnostic of pregnancy, I ventured to suggest that Mrs. A. was as "ladies wished to be," etc. The husband told me that his wife considered this very unlikely; indeed, he added, "She says it is *impossible*."

Ruminating upon this decided declaration on the part of an inexperienced married woman, I came at length to the conclusion that the sexual act had not been consummated. And yet the husband was, in the full flower of his youth and, apparently, vigorous enough. Being well aware that conception was quite possible, even though the hymen should not be perforated, I marked the page in "Gooch's Diseases of Women," where the story is told of John Hunter demonstrating the fact to a sceptical student, and sent the book to Captain A., with a note, in which I asked him if "that" (an unperforated hymen) was what his wife meant. He replied, in returning the book, that it was.

Another month or two passed away; the morning sickness continued unabated. The lady—still unconvinced, though wavering—became increasingly languid, and, as the hot season was setting in, it was thought desirable that she should pass it in the cooler climate of the Hills. Mrs. A. was sent, therefore, to a well-known sanatorium in the Himalayas. Time wore on, and in due course the pains of labour were felt. Until quite latterly Mrs. A. had discredited the idea of her being in the family-way. The "quickening" had not been distinct enough to make any impression, and it was only when the progressive abdominal enlargement became conspicuous that she admitted the possibility, and supposed it must be so. The medical officer who attended Mrs. A. in her confinement, wrote to me subsequently that the final exodus of the head of the child had been impeded by a toughish membrane, which was stretched tensely across the vagina. This membrane was, obviously, the imperforate hymen, which must have been of unusual density thus to offer a barrier to so large a body as the forcibly propelled head of a fully developed fœtus. It was, however, naturally ruptured, and the birth was satisfactorily completed. A few days afterwards, poor Mrs. A., who had suffered much, and complained latterly of palpitation of the heart, died somewhat suddenly. There was no post-mortem, but, from all I could gather, the immediate cause of death was embolism.

Clapham-common, S.W.

PRIZE QUESTION.—The Prize Committee of the American Medical Association have selected the following question—"What are the special modes of action or therapeutic effects upon the human system of water, quinia, and salicylic acid when used as antipyretics in the treatment of disease?" The essays must be founded on original experimental and clinical observation, and must be forwarded to the Chairman of the Committee of Award by January 1, 1883.—*Louisville Med. News*, October 1.

REPORTS OF HOSPITAL PRACTICE
IN
MEDICINE AND SURGERY.

THE ROYAL FREE HOSPITAL.

CASE OF MALIGNANT DISEASE OF LUNG.
(Under the care of Dr. COCKLE.)
[From notes taken by Mr. R. BROOKES, House-Physician.]

ANN L., aged forty-four, a cook, was admitted into the Boys Ward, June 23, 1881, with dyspnœa and hæmoptysis. There was a strong consumptive family history, her father and two sisters having died therefrom. Two months previously, caught cold, had a severe cough, with pain in left side, sharp and stabbing in character. Brought up, by coughing, a "teacupful" of blood about a week after, and the sputa for the next few days were streaked with it. Has suffered from severe night-sweating. Six months ago weighed (so she said) 15 st. ; on admission weighed 12 st. 3 lbs.

The patient is a fairly healthy-looking woman; good colour; slightly anxious, careworn expression of countenance; muscles soft and flabby. Measurement of chest—left, eighteen inches ; right, eighteen inches and a half. Absolute dulness over the whole of the left side of the chest, back and front, extending in front one inch to the right of the sternum. Complete absence of vocal fremitus, vocal vibrations, and breath-sounds. The heart is displaced downwards and to the right. Apex-beat felt most distinctly to right of the ensiform cartilage. No bulging of intercostal spaces. Left decubitus ; any movement from this position caused a violent fit of coughing. Extreme restlessness, attacks of dyspnœa causing her to sit up in bed and hold on to something for support. Temperature ranged from 98° to 100° throughout ; on one occasion only (July 24) it reached 103°, from no apparent cause. Respirations from 30 to 50.

On July 20, had an attack of diarrhœa, which defied all ordinary astringents, lasting three weeks, and stopped finally by means of solid opium in pill—one grain every four hours.

The chest symptoms remained unaltered throughout. About a week before death she began to improve; her appetite came back, and she began to gain flesh rapidly, weighing 12 st. 6 lbs.

August 17.—Whilst sitting on the night-stool became suddenly unconscious, and after slight convulsions, lasting five minutes, she died.

Autopsy, thirty-six hours after Death.—Well nourished ; no post-mortem lividity; rigor mortis absent. Level of diaphragm—left side, eighth rib; right side, fifth rib. On removing the sternum a soft mass was cut into, as it was closely adherent to the costal cartilages on the left side. The mass occupied the position of the lung, portions of which could be seen through the thinned pleura. The heart was displaced downwards, and to the right the pericardium was filled with dark fluid blood. The left pleura (parietal layer) was very thick except at the anterior part, which was adherent to the tumour and sternum. On opening it a quantity of sanguineous serum escaped. The upper part of the pleural cavity was filled by the mass described, and the lung ; the lower part was filled with œdematous lymph and blood-clots. The visceral layer of the pleura which enclosed the lung and the tumour was thickened in some places and thinned in others, showing protruding masses of the tumour. Thick bands of adhesions stretched across from parietal to visceral layer. Two or three rounded processes projecting from the lung were apparently caused by formation of adhesions and subsequent rupture. A section of the mass from behind to the root of the lung showed the tumour to be growing from the root of the lung along the bronchi (both outside and in). The peripheral part of the lung was dotted over with light brown spots and patches, composed of disintegrated lung-tissue and pus, which could be easily washed away by a stream of water, leaving small circular depressions and cavities. The larger bronchi were filled with a gelatinous material, composed entirely of new growth. The new growth obliterated the left pulmonary vein, and was growing into its interior. It also extended along the pulmonary artery through the pericardium close up to the heart. The aorta was unaffected—only adherent by its under surface to the mass under the arch. Valves healthy, except two or three small warty growths on the mitral. There was no apparent cause for the hæmorrhage into the pericardium beyond a patch of redness on the left side of the pericardium in close connexion with the growth. There was a large mass of tumour in the abdominal cavity situated in front of the left kidney, growing apparently from the lumbar glands. The growth was firmly adherent to the capsule, compressing but not infiltrating the kidney-structure. The descending colon was adherent to the mass, and on opening it three or four circular ulcers were seen on the posterior surface about the size of a "sixpence." Some nodules two or three inches higher were prominent under the mucous membrane. No constriction. No growths in other organs. The microscope showed the tumour to be a small round-celled sarcoma.

Remarks, by Dr. Cockle.—This case offers much of clinical interest. Its several particulars, principally those subjoined, left little doubt in my mind as to the existence of malignant disease of the left chest : (1) the very peculiar physiognomy so expressive of intense anxiety and pain ; (2) the marked and rapidly progressive emaciation ; (3) the constant and excessive pain in the left chest ; (4) the absolute, complete, and unchanging dulness, under percussion, of the entire left chest, extending above the clavicle, and to the left sterno-clavicular angle. It may be, though not certain, considering the extent and seemingly more indurated state of the abdominal mass, that the affection commenced in the lumbar glands ; if so, the perfect latency of all abdominal symptoms, not alone before those of the chest were developed, but also to the very close of the case, was, to say the least, remarkable. The suffering was always exclusively referred to the left side of the chest. Death was evidently the direct result of sudden hæmorrhage into the pericardium. I cannot call to mind any similar occurrence in my experience of malignant disease of the chest.

SLOW PULSE.—M. Laure brought a man, twenty-six years of age, to be exhibited at the Lyons Medical Society, with a very slow pulse. He had latterly suffered from attacks of syncope, a sense of oppression, and palpitation. A careful examination of his heart revealed absolutely nothing abnormal, and the sphygmographic tracing denoted a feeble amount of tension, and slightly resembled the tracing derived from aortic insufficiency. The pulse varied from twenty-six to forty in a minute, digitalis and bromide of potassium exerting no sensible influence on it, while the rate is always reducible to twenty-six or twenty-four if the patient stands up for a few minutes.—Lyon Méd., No. 32.

PEABODY'S BUILDINGS.—Mr. Peabody's original gift, of half a million sterling, for the erection of model lodging-houses, has now become £720,000. This large increase on the capital of the trustees is stated by the trustees' surveyor to be due to the income from the buildings, the occupants of which include all grades of the working-classes. The entire expenses of the management of the trust are, according to the same authority, under £300 per annum. The mortality in these dwellings—calculated upon sixteen years' experience—has been at the rate of only 16·7 per 1000 per annum, while the general death-rate for the whole metropolis during the same period has been 23·4. According to the surveyor's evidence before the Select Committee on Artisans' Dwellings, the death-rate in crowded districts surrounding the buildings may be taken at thirty or forty to the thousand. Why should this fund so accumulate, when poor people are perishing for want of house-accommodation?

BLACK RAIN.—A curious phenomenon has been observed during September in different localities of the Department of the Seine-Inférieure. The housewives were astonished at finding that the pots and pans which they put out were filled with a black liquid, instead of the limpid water they were accustomed to. Whatever precaution was taken as regards cleanliness of vessels or of the roofs on which the water fell, the water collected continued black. This phenomenon has been observed more than once before in the same part of France. It has always taken place in September, so that it may be supposed to be due to some circumstance peculiar to this season. May this not be an excessive abundance of the emission of cryptogamic sporules? It is an interesting problem for investigation.—Union Méd., October 20.

TERMS OF SUBSCRIPTION.

(Free by post.)

British Islands	. . . . .	Twelve Months	.	£1 8	0
,,	. . . . .	Six	,,	. 0 14	0
The Colonies and the United States of America	. . . }	Twelve	,,	. 1 10	0
,, ,, ,,	. .	Six	,,	. 0 15	0
India	. . .	Twelve	,,	. 1 10	0
,, (viâ Brindisi)	. . .	,,	,,	. 1 15	0
,,	. . .	Six	,,	. 0 15	0
,, (viâ Brindisi)	. . .	,,	,,	. 0 17	6

Foreign Subscribers are requested to inform the Publishers of any remittance made through the agency of the Post-office.

Single Copies of the Journal can be obtained of all Booksellers and Newsmen, price Sixpence.

Cheques or Post-office Orders should be made payable to Mr. James Lucas, 11, New Burlington-street, W.

TERMS FOR ADVERTISEMENTS.

Seven lines (70 words)	. . .	.£0 4	6
Each additional line (10 words)	. .	. 0 0	6
Half-column, or quarter-page	. .	. 1 5	0
Whole column, or half-page	. .	. 2 10	0
Whole page	. . . . .	. 5 0	0

Births, Marriages, and Deaths are inserted Free of Charge.

The MEDICAL TIMES AND GAZETTE *is published on Friday morning: Advertisements must therefore reach the Publishing Office not later than One o'clock on Thursday.*

Medical Times and Gazette.

SATURDAY, OCTOBER 29, 1881.

A FORGOTTEN CHAPTER IN THE HISTORY OF PATHOLOGY.

A SHORT time ago there passed away one whose name might well have been famous had not the reputation of Dr. Thomas Addison, of Guy's Hospital, to a great extent overshadowed the less brilliant, but not less eminent, Dr. William Addison. Moreover, Dr. William Addison was before his time, and the discoveries he made lay neglected until rediscovered long years after. There are few now alive who could give us any information as to the early years of Dr. William Addison, for he was eighty when he died, and we are left very much to his published works. Many years ago he retired to Brighton, and ill-health compelled him at a comparatively early age to give up practice. Nevertheless, as we have seen, he attained an age considerably beyond the ordinary span of life—another illustration of the fact that the weakliest do not always perish first.

It is rather, however, of certain portions of his work that we here desire to speak, the more especially as much of its earlier portions was published in the columns of the old *Medical Gazette*, our immediate predecessor. The first of these communications, as far as we know, and that with which we have now to deal, appeared in that journal in 1840-41. The papers were entitled "On the Blood," but really far exceeded the scope this implied. Many facts therein recorded have been noticed in that mine of information, Dr. Druitt's article on Inflammation, unfortunately buried in "Cooper's Surgical Dictionary," to which, or rather to the original, we would refer inquirers into this curious part of historical pathology. It will be remembered that in the year 1867 a great stir was made in the medical world, owing to the discovery by Cohnheim that in inflammation, the blood, and the bloodvessels, took a most active part. Up to that time Virchow's notion had been generally accepted that the connective tissue or fixed corpuscles were the chief agents concerned in multiplying, under irritation, and with a due supply of nutritive material, so as to create heaps of pus corpuscles or other new formations, and that the bloodvessels simply served as a means for conveying an increased quantity of nutrient elements to the part. Cohnheim showed that the white blood corpuscles inside the bloodvessels were likewise active, gathering together on the inner walls of the vessels, and then worming their way through to the tissues beyond. Indeed, he maintained that this was the sole way in which new cells were, in the first instance, at least, heaped together in any given spot, as in the formation of an abscess. Dr. W. Addison had forestalled this view in every particular, and when it is borne in mind what difficulties attended microscopic research in those days, it seems something wonderful that such a result could have been attained. The microscopes were bad and unwieldy, apparatus and reagents were alike unknown. Yet William Addison, and later Augustus Waller, succeeded in demonstrating what was at the time of Cohnheim almost completely forgotten—what was, even at the date we have mentioned (1867), supposed to be the outcome of a marvellous ingenuity and care, and only attainable by the quieting influence of curare upon the frog, the usual subject of experiment. Well do we remember the first demonstration of this kind given at the Pathological Society, and the feeling of wonder which it inspired, even though the experiment was not quite successful.

In 1841, then, Dr. Addison had recorded the increase of white corpuscles in the blood of a part the subject of inflammation; Dr. C. J. B. Williams had observed, about the same time, their tendency to adhere to the walls of vessels; and both had seen them outside the vessel itself. In 1843, in the *Provincial Transactions*, Addison enunciated his views more clearly, and especially he maintained that "the central part of a white corpuscle is alive, and that by virtue of its vitality it exercises certain movements by which a division into parts ensues." But it was not until 1846, after Waller's experiments had been made public (*Philosophical Magazine*, 1846), that Dr. Addison, in a new work on Healthy and Diseased Structure, was able to formulate his doctrines clearly and precisely. What he said then is, however, very striking—"During inflammation, using the word in the general sense, there is a more or less marked increase of colourless elements and plasma in the parts affected. At first—in the first stage—these elements adhere but slightly along the inner margin or boundary of the nutrient vessels, and are therefore still within the influence of the circulating current—belonging at this period as much, or rather more, to the blood than to the fixed solids. Secondly—in the second stage—they are more firmly fixed in the walls of the vessels, and are therefore now without the influence of the circulating current. Thirdly—in the third stage—the new elements appear at the outer border of the vessels, where they add to the texture, form a new product, or are liberated as an excretion." Surely it would be hard to find a more accurate description than this of what are popularly supposed to be Cohnheim's original discoveries. Original, no doubt, in a sense, they were, for we have no reason to believe that Cohnheim was acquainted with the work of either Addison or Waller. Thus we see how fatal it is sometimes to live before one's time, and how still more fatal it is that the name of a discoverer should be overshadowed by the name of another whose fame is worldwide. Very many men—those, too, who know something of both writers—are apt to confound the one with the other, even at the present day.

THE INFLAMMATORY ORIGIN OF TUMOURS.[a]

MOST people who hear inflammation alleged as a cause of tumours will naturally think that the word is used in some special and restricted sense. It is inflammation without the *rubor* and the *calor*, with *dolor* only occasional, and with nothing but the *tumor* for certain. If, however, that which all the world understands as inflammation be for the moment put on one side, it may be admitted that there are certain morbid processes which are connected with inflammation on the one hand, and with tumour-formation on the other. The repairing of the breach in the tissues made by an inflammation follows much the same lines as tumours sometimes take when they arise in the tissues without any inflammatory commotion : the thickening of a mucous membrane from chronic catarrh sometimes takes unaccountably the polypoid form; the filling-up of a repeatedly inflamed bursa patellæ by connective-tissue growth often results in a round mass as large as an orange, which may well pass for a tumour, and may be removed as such. In considering the pathology of tumours, it is always profitable to go back upon those points which are in contact with the inflammatory process, whether in the interest of common sense or of philosophical analysis. The inflammatory origin of tumours, which is the subject of the paper referred to below, fails, of course, in universal applicability, just as the fashionable German hypothesis of persistent embryonic rudiments is only half the truth, or something less than half. But if there ever is to be a comprehensive hypothesis for tumours, it can only be arrived at by an appreciative consideration of the various points that have been somewhat exclusively dwelt upon by various minds. Out of the diversity will come forth unity, and the grand generalisation of the future will probably take something from each of the narrow generalisations of to-day. In any case, let us not altogether undervalue work which is animated by the presence of an idea, insufficient though the idea may be; human nature, even in Germany, begins to assert itself against the intolerable dulness of the purely "objective" method, and we have lately had the refreshing spectacle of professors of high repute taking some recreation in the way of hypothesis-making of the old sort. *Gens humana ruit per vetitum nefas,* and we are to be headed by no less respectable a pathologist than Professor Cohnheim. The reaction is perhaps extreme, but the incubus of un-idea'd pedantry is worth getting rid of even at some cost. It is in this spirit that we welcome the present observations on inflammation as a cause of tumours.

Nothing stands out more clearly from the facts put together by Dr. Formad, than that the excitations which ordinarily lead to inflammation sometimes lead to tumour-formation, more especially if they continue in action over a long time. But the real issue that is raised thereby is, if we may venture to say so, for the most part disregarded by this author. Under what circumstances is it that excitations of the ordinary kind lead to persistent and even malignant tumours, and not to transient inflammations? For example, we are properly reminded that cases of enchondroma and osseous tumours in young persons have been clearly traced to blows, fractures, and other injuries. But is not the significant thing here that the injury happened during the growing period, in a part where the process of growth is special, and in individuals so constituted that the process of growth in them might be easily diverted from the physiological track? Again, many epitheliomas of the lip, tongue, and other places are

traced to long-continued irritation from a tobacco-pipe, ragged tooth, or the like; but Professor Thiersch has shown us that it requires an almost senile condition of the connective tissue, a certain disturbance of the "histogenetic equilibrium" between the epithelial and the sub-epithelial layers, before the characteristic encroachments of an epithelioma, in preference to an inflammatory reaction, can take place. Once more, "Lücke and Virchow found that whenever an autopsy revealed cancer, or any tumour of stomach or œsophagus, the clinical history nearly always revealed 'drunkard.'" Even if this were a general truth (which it is far from being), those victims were only a small fraction of all that come under that melancholy designation; they are merely the unfortunates upon whom the tower of Siloam fell. So also, it may well be (as Dr. Formad inclines to think) that gall-stones have been the excitant in every case where cancer has been set up in the gall-bladder; but cancer of the gall-bladder is one of the rarest of maladies, and gall-stones not one of the least common. We inevitably come to predisposing causes after we have gone through all possible views of the exciting cause, and we shall probably find it hard to avoid such halfway resting-places as "dyscrasia" or "taint." Dr. Formad admits a predisposition of a particular kind—a predisposition acquired, and acquired through external influences. The inflammatory process, he thinks, creates conditions in the tissues, which directly, and more than any other cause, predispose to tumour-formation. Cicatricial tissue is certainly a direct product of the inflammatory process, and cicatricial tissue is sometimes a kind of halfway house to cancer. But that is about the only instance of tissue-predisposition that can be traced back to inflammation; and the predisposition of the tissue of a scar is probably not so much due to its being the termination of a long-past inflammatory process, but rather to its inherent embryonic character. The notion that the inflammatory process predisposes the tissues to tumour-formation, reveals to us the sense—the somewhat lax sense—in which inflammation is used throughout the article referred to. It is well known that certain tumours (of the sarcomatous kind) are made up of cells of the embryonic type, and that is the slender basis of observation upon which the tumour-hypothesis of Cohnheim has been reared to its giddy height. Dr. Formad properly remarks that the embryonic cells do not need to be pre-existing (as Cohnheim will have them) in order to form a tumour; "they can be, and always are, created by inflammation." But it is really departing altogether from the meaning of words to describe that beautiful and orderly return of cells to their embryonic character which one may sometimes see in the beginning of a sarcoma and in the extension of a cancer, as an inflammation. It is just the difference between a tumour-process and an inflammatory process—a difference which is not obliterated by discovering analogies or parallelisms between them. Or, to take another instance, the infiltration of sub-epithelial tissue, which is apt to occur in long-standing catarrh, has doubtless a great significance for the origin of cancer in those organs (stomach and os uteri) which are exceedingly liable to catarrh. But is it always reasonable or conducive to a just view to claim that catarrhal process for inflammation? Observations have shown that there may be wandering and infiltration of cells into the stroma of a glandular organ, while neither is the excitant of an inflammatory kind, nor are the cells white blood-corpuscles. Here is a physiological analogy suggesting that there may be even catarrhs which hardly belong to inflammation. A remarkable instance of a long-continued catarrhal process in a mucous membrane, leading to tumour-formation, is found in the case of the glans penis in the horse, in the enormous dendriform masses

(a) "The Inflammatory Origin of Tumours." Paper read before the Pathological Society of Philadelphia, by H. F. Formad, M.D., Lecturer on Experimental Pathology in the University of Pennsylvania. (Seguin, *Archives of Medicine*, October, 1881.)

of warty growths which are apt to form when the sheath remains continuously unretracted, and the natural desquamation of the epithelium tends to accumulate. But no good purpose is served by insisting upon the inflammatory nature of such a catarrh as that, or by claiming the resulting growths as a product or as one of the terminations of inflammation. It is again the difference between the tumour process and the inflammatory process that we have to face.

The strictly original observations in the essay which has given us occasion for these reflections and criticisms relate to three cases of fibroma—two of them were from the uterus and broad ligament respectively, and one was from the finger. No one will be surprised that Dr. Formad should have failed to find in these tumours "perfect endothelial sheaths surrounding the bundles of fibres, such as were so beautifully seen in a preparation of tendon made for comparison simultaneous with the fibroma specimens." It is also credible that the cell-plates so well seen in tendon are not discernible in the fibrillar tissue of cirrhosis. But do those facts, and practically those facts alone, constitute a sufficient reason why "fibromata should be classed as a product, or rather as one of the terminations of inflammation?" This observer will doubtless find, when he has examined more fibromata, that there are among them those, especially in early life, which have nothing of the structure of cicatricial fibrous tissue, but the most perfect physiological type of interlacing bundles of wavy fibres, of uniform breadth and orderly arrangement, and possibly with cell-plates all complete. Dr. Formad's paper cannot be said to have effectually bridged over the gulf between tumours and the products of inflammation, but it serves the useful purpose of recalling those of us who have our pet theories of tumour to certain aspects of the tumour-process that ought not to be left out of sight.

THE WEEK.

TOPICS OF THE DAY.

In his capacity as President of the Manchester Infirmary, Lord Derby presided recently at a meeting held in the Town Hall, in aid of the funds of the institution. He explained the financial position of the Infirmary as follows:—It had been found necessary since 1877 to make alterations and improvements in the Hospital, at a cost of £23,000, while the Hospitals at Cheadle and at Monsall had cost £11,000 more. It was absolutely necessary to put up a building for the use of the nursing staff, and that would involve an additional outlay of £5000. Further, the ordinary business of the Infirmary had been carried on during the last five years at a loss on the whole of more than £21,000. The capital fund of the charity had lessened by some £30,000. In addition to this loss, there had been a falling off of income owing to the bad times, and the net result was that, whereas the receipts from all sources stood in 1877 at £28,000, these were now below £21,000. It was calculated that the cost at which the Infirmary could be maintained on its present footing was £27,000 yearly, which gave a deficit of about £6000 per annum. His Lordship said that unfortunately nothing was more costly than effective sanitary work, and nothing was more important: the very first condition of sanitary improvement was fresh air and plenty of it; and fresh air in hospitals meant increased space, and this again meant increased outlay in buildings, and not only that, but a larger outlay to keep up the buildings. Those present were well aware that nothing had been spent on the Infirmary in the shape of architectural ornament. In making his appeal to the public for assistance he would add one suggestion on his own responsibility. He would recommend an effort for increased subscriptions, rather than to replace the capital. The times

were not favourable for large donations; people were more willing to subscribe a moderate sum yearly than a large sum down; and when it was known that an institution had come into large capitalised means the effect invariably operated to lessen the annual subscriptions. During the meeting subscriptions of several thousand pounds were announced, some of them by instalments spreading over five years.

Recently, at the Thames Police-court, Joseph James Sewell, a medical practitioner of Pimlico-road, was summoned, at the instance of the Medical Alliance Association, for unlawfully making a false certificate or declaration concerning the death of Anne Harvey, of St. Leonard's-road, Bromley, contrary to the Births and Deaths Registration Act, 1874. It appeared that in August last Mrs. Harvey was *enceinte*, and on the 1st of that month she was very ill, and her husband sent for a doctor. A person named Knight, in the service of a Dr. Ford, attended her, and between eight and nine o'clock the same night the child expired. Nobody but Knight looked after her until the child died, and Mrs. Harvey subsequently died on the 17th of the month. Her husband was not aware that Knight was an uncertificated medical man, or he would not have allowed him to attend his wife. A boy in Mr. Harvey's service was sent to Dr. Ford's shop, and asked the defendant for a certificate of the child's death, and he immediately wrote one out, setting forth that the child had died of debility, although he had never attended it. The certificate was sent in the usual way to the registrar of births and deaths for the district, and he entered it in the register. The magistrate said it was the policy of the law that the best possible information should be given to the registrar of births and deaths, and a true answer or declaration rendered to him. It was quite clear that there was no sort of duty on the defendant to give a certificate as to the cause of this child's death, and he had wilfully given a false certificate under the Act. It was not a matter which ought to be treated lightly, and he should fine the defendant £10 and 2s. costs.

M. de Lacerda has lately discovered a fact of considerable scientific and practical importance, which he has communicated in a note to the Paris Academy, namely, that permanganate of potash counteracts very effectively the poison of snakes. In a first series of experiments, a water solution of the poison was injected into the cellular tissue of dogs, under the legs, and its usual effects were large swellings, with abscesses, loss of substance, and destruction of tissues. But when an equal quantity of filtered (1 per cent.) solution of permanganate of potash was injected one or two minutes after the poison, those local injuries were quite obviated; there was merely a slight swelling where the syringe had entered. Next, introduction into the veins was tried, and the permanganate again succeeded admirably. In only two cases out of more than thirty was there failure, and this is attributed to the animals experimented on being very young and weak, and badly fed; also to the antidote being administered at too long an interval after the poison, when the heart was already tending to stop. In one series of cases the permanganate solution was introduced half a minute after the solution of venom, and the animal operated on showed no derangement beyond a very transient agitation, and acceleration of the heart's action for a few minutes. In another series, the characteristic troubles caused by the poison were allowed to manifest themselves (dilatation of the pupil, quick breathing and heart action, contractions, etc.) before the antidote was applied. In two or three minutes, sometimes five, the troubles disappeared; a slight general prostration followed for fifteen to twenty-five minutes; after which the animal would walk, and even run about, and resume its normal aspect. Other dogs poisoned similarly, but not receiving the antidote, died more or less quickly.

At a recent meeting of the members of the North-Western Association of Medical Officers of Health, held at Manchester, Mr. Francis Vacher, Medical Officer for Birkenhead, read a paper on "Milk-Inspection and the Control of the Milk-Supply." After summing up the regulations which obtained in respect to the sale of milk, and the powers vested in local authorities for insuring a pure supply, Mr. Vacher proceeded to point out some of the causes which tended to make the control of the Authority less efficient and thorough than it should be. Amongst other reasons were the facts that properly qualified inspectors were not appointed; that the responsible duties of deciding on the fitness or otherwise of dairy premises were handed over to irresponsible sub-committees; and that the regular storing and selling of milk was allowed in all sorts of general shops, samples being rarely taken for analysis, except owing to specific complaints. It appeared to him that additional powers were wanted to enable a local authority to veto the sale of milk by vendors coming from without such authority's district, to require all licensed milk-sellers to notify cases of infectious disease appearing in their premises, with ability to close such premises till the removal of the infected animal and disinfection of the premises. He might also add, that were the supervision of the important work of milk-inspection committed to one responsible officer under the Local Government Board, local authorities would be encouraged to do their utmost to give effect to the Privy Council's regulations, and any other powers possessed by them in this respect, and any amendment of the law which might be necessary would be pointed out and brought under the attention of those able to undertake it.

It is reported from America that the Mayor of New York has issued a proclamation to the inhabitants, calling their attention to the perilous state of things arising from the deficiency in the water-supply, caused by the long drought. The inhabitants are therefore exhorted to practise economy in using water, as, unless copious rains set in shortly, the entire reserve supply will be exhausted about the 8th prox., at the present rate of consumption, and New York will then be dependent on the natural flow of the Croton River, which at the present time supplies 10,000,000 gallons daily, or about a ninth part of the quantity of water now used in the city. The Mayor further points out that, in such a case, it would be impossible to check any conflagrations that might break out.

As many invalids who have been recommended to seek winter quarters at Algiers are hesitating to proceed thither for fear of finding themselves endangered by the Arab insurrection, the resident English chaplain there has sent a communication to the London press, in which he says:—"It should be understood that the insurrection of Bou Amema (of which, latterly, we have heard next to nothing) when at its height did not come within 150 miles of Algiers itself; while the more serious war, which is in Tunisia—not in Algeria at all,—must be, at least, 400 miles distant. So little fear is felt of an Arab rising in Algiers itself, that building in the suburbs has been going on even more than usual."

The second series of lectures on Domestic Sanitation, delivered by Dr. B. W. Richardson, F.R.S., to the Ladies' Sanitary Association, has commenced. In the course of these lectures it is announced that the structure and functions of the nervous system will be presented, and in this division the physical and mental training of the young will be considered.

The terrible epidemic of yellow fever in the West Indies has shown that the effects of the disease are most severely felt by the resident Portuguese and by native-born Englishmen, who have not lived long enough in the colony to become acclimatised.

The Local Government Board has declined to assent to the proposal of the Eastbourne Board of Guardians to pay Mr. Nicholls, the vaccination officer, 1s. 4d. for each case of successful vaccination. We agree with the remark of one of the local justices at the last meeting of the Guardians, when the question was under discussion, that it is absurd to make any fee to the officer depend on the result of the operation. Moreover, in Eastbourne there exists an organised opposition to the Act, and it appeared it frequently happened that the vaccination officer had to call half a dozen times before he could induce the parents to comply with the Act. The general feeling of the meeting was that some concession should be made in the officer's favour, and ultimately it was unanimously agreed that permission be obtained to make the fee 1s. in all cases.

At an inquest held by Mr. Collier, Deputy Coroner for the Eastern Division of Middlesex, a juryman refused to take the oath because "he did not believe in life or death," whereupon he was asked to affirm; but he replied he was of no religion, he did not believe in anything, he should not consider an oath or affirmation binding on his conscience. The Coroner remarked, after that statement, he could not allow him to go on the jury; he was sorry for him if what he stated was correct. Why he said that was, that he had found many persons made the same observations as this juror in order to be exempt from serving. In this case, however, the juror would have to wait until the inquiry was finished.

ARMY MEDICAL DEPARTMENT.

IT has, we believe, been arranged that Surgeon-General Shelton, whose retirement from the service on having attained the full limit of age dates from October 28, is to retain his position at the War Office as head of the medical branch of the office of the Director-General of the Army Medical Department. He will thus be a supernumerary in the establishment until the assumption by Dr. Crawford, in April next, of the duties of Director-General. This arrangement, while enabling Dr. Crawford to nominate for selection the medical officer whose services he may prefer in such an important position, will not interfere with the ordinary progress of departmental promotion. It is also, we understand, intended that Deputy Surgeon-General Irvine, who in December next will have completed the usual period of five years' tenure as head of the sanitary branch of the Director-General's office, shall continue to perform those duties for a further period of two years. This arrangement has been made in consideration of his having, since November last, on the amalgamation of the sanitary and statistical branches which took place after the death of Deputy Surgeon-General Lydd (head of the statistical branch), carried on the work of the combined branches. As, according to the Warrant of November, 1879, the Deputy Surgeon-General at headquarters receives a rate of pay considerably below that to which he would be entitled if in charge of a home-district, it is probable that many medical officers of that rank would prefer general administrative duty to the official work for which a peculiar aptitude and experience are so necessary.

KING AND QUEEN'S COLLEGE OF PHYSICIANS IN IRELAND.

ON St. Luke's Day, the following Fellows of the College were appointed examiners, in addition to those mentioned last week:—Dr. Hawtrey Benson, additional Examiner in Medicine; Dr. Fleetwood Churchill, additional Examiner in Midwifery; Dr. Christopher J. Nixon, additional Examiner in Anatomy.

AN UNSANITARY VILLAGE.

At a recent meeting of the Lincoln Board of Guardians, Dr. Harrison, the Medical Officer, submitted the following report to the Rural Sanitary Authority :—" Several children have been suffering from scarlet fever in the parish of Hykeham. The attention of the inspector of nuisances has been called to several nuisances from defective drainage, etc. Three houses in this village are overcrowded, having only one sleeping room for man, wife, and four children. Complaint having been made of a nuisance arising from a certain trade carried on at Hykeham, I visited the premises, and found the business complained of was the manufacture of sausage-skins and catgut. Sheep's intestines are received fresh from the various slaughter-houses, and subjected to certain processes, portions of the intestines being prepared and salted, to be used for sausages, while other portions are made into catgut and sent to Saxony for manufacture into strings for musical instruments. Bone-boiling is also part of the business. Butcher's bones are subjected to prolonged boiling; the fat rising is taken off and sold as dripping. Inside the shed where the business is carried on the smell was very offensive, but I failed to detect any nuisance off the premises. A few days after my visit, I received a letter asking permission to build a shed further removed from the high-road, for the purpose of carrying on this business. I advised that a rural sanitary authority had no power to sanction the use of premises for any noxious trade, and had no power to prevent it, but that any business carried on must be conducted in such a manner as to give rise to no offensive effluvia, or steps would at once be taken for the abatement of the nuisance."

AMPUTATION OF THE GRAVID UTERUS WITH CANCEROUS CERVIX.

REMOVAL of a gravid uterus with cancerous cervix has been completed, for the first time in this country, by Mr. Spencer Wells. The procedure combines the advantages of Porro's operation—i.e., the removal of the body of the uterus so as to prevent a further pregnancy—and Freund's excision of the entire uterus when affected with cancer. The operation was done, after consultation with Drs. Playfair and Graily Hewitt, last Friday (October 21). On the sixth day after operation the patient was going on very satisfactorily. The uterus is now in the Museum of the College of Surgeons, and the report of the case will, in all probability, lead to an important discussion at the Royal Medical and Chirurgical Society on November 23. At the International Medical Congress the feeling appeared to be strongly against Freund's operation, and Porro's was not seriously considered. Both operations are of great interest to surgeons and obstetricians, and we trust that some of the leaders in each branch will do what they can towards the formation of sound professional opinion on a new subject.

THE PATHOLOGICAL ANATOMY CHAIR AT THE VIENNA FACULTY.

THIS chair, one of the great glories of the Vienna University, is in a singular state of abeyance. Since the death of Prof. Heschl, who for a short time held it as successor to his great master Rokitansky, the electoral body, consisting of the professors, have been debating month after month as to who should be its new occupant, and, after numerous and prolonged deliberations, have successively proposed Profs. Eppinger, Kundrat, and Arnold—men who, though they have shown themselves able teachers in their respective more limited spheres, were not generally deemed in professional circles as fitting occupants for so famous a chair; and as the Minister of Public Instruction possesses a veto, this has probably been exercised, for no appointment has yet been announced as final. At first sight, the prophecy would seem to be about to be realised, that the political liberties now possessed in Germany would soon draft off from the professoriate some of the ablest minds who heretofore found within its shelter the only possibility of exerting their influence. This is not the case, however, in this instance, for two men of the highest calibre—Prof. Cohnheim of Leipzig, and Prof. Klebs of Prague—have been announced as candidates, and none more distinguished in the ranks of progressive medicine could probably be found. Prof. Cohnheim, we believe, has no desire to hold the post; but Prof. Klebs' candidature has received the approbation of some of the highest celebrities. Some strong objections (arising, according to some, from the germ-fiend which is said to have taken possession of Prof. Klebs, rendering him, in the opinion of some of the older electors, too exclusive a personage to fill such a chair advantageously) to complying with this recommendation evidently influence the professorial body, so that they keep falling back upon insufficient substitutes, and things remain, months after the post should have been filled up, *in statu quo*.

THE HEALTH OF BOURNEMOUTH DURING THE YEAR 1880.

THE annual report of the Medical Officer of Health for Bournemouth (Mr. Philip W. G. Nunn), for the year 1880, shows that that period has, from a public health point of view, been a very satisfactory one; the small amount of infectious disease, considering the rapid increase of population, being a matter for congratulation. Mr. Nunn rightly calls attention to the serious diminution of late years in the number of pine-trees in the district; and points out that trees of this class are of special benefit to the locality, which largely owes its celebrity as a health-resort to them, and without them would lack one of its greatest attractions. We agree with him in holding that the matter should at once be taken up by the ground landlords, as well as by all house-owners. The great increase of building operations in the neighbourhood, with other causes, is gradually ruining this English Arcachon, and when it is too late the authorities will become cognizant of the fact. We are glad to learn, on the testimony of Mr. Nunn, that the majority of the hotels in Bournemouth now fulfil the conditions of the model by laws of the Local Government Board, so far as they relate to drainage, etc. As the hotel-keepers have so readily followed his suggestions, he trusts that the lodging-house keepers of the town will also see the necessity of following so good an example.

A NEW CLINICAL TELEPHONE.

PROF. SABATUCCI has contrived a medical hydro-telephone from which he predicts great results in clinical medicine. It is constructed as follows:—Two leaden cylinders (five centimetres in diameter and half a centimetre thick) are each closed with two very fine iron laminæ. To the anterio part of each is fitted a wooden mouthpiece, like that of a Bell telephone, connected to a caoutchouc tube, through which one may hear at a distance. The posterior part has a very sensitive electro-magnet communicating with a microphone and battery. One tube is applied to each ear. Words or sounds produced before the microphone and heard but faintly, are rendered intense and distinct by introducing liquid into the cylinders. The less dense the liquid the better. Two sounds may be compared, and their intensity exactly measured, by varying the quantity of the liquids and noting the effects through the tubes.

THE PARIS WEEKLY RETURN.

THE number of deaths for the forty-first week, terminating October 14, was 1001 (537 males and 464 females), and among these there were from typhoid fever 30, small-pox 7, measles 14, scarlatina 5, pertussis 5, diphtheria and croup 35, erysipelas 4, and puerperal infections 3. There were also 42 deaths from acute and tubercular meningitis, 26 from acute bronchitis, 40 from pneumonia, 88 from infantile athrepsia (32 of the infants having been wholly or partially suckled), and 23 violent deaths. The general sanitary condition continues good, in spite of an increase of 120 deaths upon the former week, for epidemic diseases take no part in this augmentation. This results almost exclusively from the fatal termination of old chronic affections, which will not bear the first diminution of temperature. Thus phthisis alone contributes 67 deaths. So also the increase especially presses on individuals above sixty years of age; while all the epidemic diseases, which are the diseases of the young, have generally declined. The births for the week amounted to 1158, viz., 551 males (393 legitimate and 158 illegitimate) and 607 females (440 legitimate and 167 illegitimate); 105 infants (62 males and 43 females) were born dead or died within twenty-four hours.

THE COLLECTIVE INVESTIGATION COMMITTEE OF THE BRITISH MEDICAL ASSOCIATION.

THE Collective Investigation Committee of the British Medical Association are about to appoint a secretary, whose salary is to be £200 per annum, with addition for travelling and other expenses. They ask members of the profession who may desire the appointment to make application to F. Fowke, Esq., Secretary to the Association, 161A, Strand, before November 20.

LONDON SANITARY PROTECTION.

AT the first general meeting of the London Sanitary Protec. tion Association, after an account of certain financial details had been given by the Treasurer (Mr. Holmes), Prof. Fleeming Jenkin said that the cost was small, the importance great, and already many similar institutions had been established all over the country. Inspections had been made of 108 houses, and of these seven were found to be entirely with. out drainage, the drains having become completely choked. In several instances no suspicion existed of this state of things, for the sewage was making its way into the soil under the houses. In thirty-three houses the drains were found not to be gas-tight, and allowed the sewage-gas to go into the houses. This was discovered in a very simple way, namely, by pouring a little oil of peppermint into the sewer, from which the smell rose into the house. In twenty-seven cases the overflow-pipes from cisterns were connected with the drains. Prof. Huxley said that when they came to congregate three or four millions of people on a surface of fifty square miles, if care were not taken they would be decimated, not as in the old days, by the black death, but by other diseases which were readily disseminated by the system of water drainage if it were imperfect. The old cesspool was, he thought, far less dangerous than an imperfect system of water drainage, which was a perfect machinery for dissemi. nating disease, while the water drainage if in perfect order was the best that could be. Therefore the question was, how were we to see that this water sewage system was main. tained in a reasonably perfect condition. A government inspection, he did not think would be tolerated by house. holders, and it would be most expensive. The best mode was that of a regular sanitary inspection by our own engineers, and this was what the Association offered at a cheap rate. He hoped it would become extensive and useful. The offices of the Association, where members are enrolled and arrange. ments for house inspection can be made, are at Adelphi Chambers, John-street, Adelphi, directly opposite the Society of Arts.

DEATH OF M. HOUEL.

THOSE of our readers who have frequented the Musée Dupuytren, Paris, for the purpose of study will regret to learn that the able and obliging Conservator has just died suddenly. He had recently completed a catalogue of the contents of the Museum, accompanied by an atlas, and was always at the service of his colleagues in making known to them the riches of the Museum, with which he was so inti. mately acquainted. He had served as President of the Société de Chirurgie, and at the time of his death belonged to numerous scientific societies. He was also a *professeur agrégé* at the Faculty, and Chevalier of the Legion of Honour.

MIDLAND MEDICAL SOCIETY.

ONE hundred and sixty members and visitors of the Society assembled at the Grand Hotel, Birmingham, on the 19th inst., to hear the inaugural address, "On the Surgical Aids to Medicine," given by Dr. Clifford Allbutt, F.R.S.; John Manley, Esq., President, in the chair. After acknowledging the distinction conferred upon him by the invitation of the Midland Medical Society, the speaker proceeded to discuss some of those subjects which occupy the borderland between medicine and surgery. The main division into medicine, surgery, and midwifery was good, owing to the limits of human capacity, so that it had never been possible for one man to attain distinction in both medicine and surgery together. But while recognising these necessary divisions of work, we must avoid the dangers of isolation. There was a tendency for physicians and surgeons to work too little together, and cases were frequently only given up with a confession of failure. The speaker repudiated any by-laws which might forbid him to fully use any needful instrument, though, on the other hand, the better he knew his cases the more loyally and intelligently would he seek the aid of a surgeon where surgery was concerned. Reference was made to the ophthalmic and aural surgeon in the treat. ment of head-affections, and the manifestations of scrofula were often curable by surgical interference. In diseases of the thorax the early application of surgical means was often of signal service. Laparotomy, Dr. Allbutt spoke of as one of the greatest surgical triumphs. Its application to hepatic abscesses, to gall-stones, various diseases of the kidney, were not yet fully appreciated; but sooner or later it might be possible for the physician to reach and promptly cure ulcers of the stomach. Reference was also made to nerve-stretch. ing and the treatment of painful and stiffened joints; and the physician was urged to be unsparing in the use of his forefingers, as many pelvic diseases might thereby be de. tected and relieved. In the course of the evening many interesting experiments in chemistry, physics, and physi. ology were demonstrated by Drs. Tilden, Poynting, and Haycraft, Professors of the Mason College. There was also a display of instruments and drugs.

ENGLISH REGISTRAR-GENERAL'S RETURN, JUNE QUARTER.

THE following are some of the particulars gathered from the Return of the Registrar-General for England for the second quarter of the present year, ending June 30 last. The births registered during that period numbered 225,467, or 7089 less than the number in the corresponding quarter of last year. The annual birth-rate was equal to 34·7 per 1000 of the estimated population, was 1·4 below the average rate in the corresponding quarter of the ten years 1871-80, and was lower than in the second quarter of any year since 1869, when it did not exceed 34·1. The birth-rate during this quarter was but 23·0 in Herefordshire, 29·2 in Cornwall, 29·6 in Dorsetshire, and 29·9 in Devonshire, but it ranged upwards in the other counties—to 37·6 in Nottinghamshire, 39·8 in Staffordshire, and 42·4 in Durham. In twenty of the largest English towns the birth-rate for the quarter under notice averaged 35·3 per 1000, against 38·0 and 37·6 in the corresponding periods of 1879 and 1880. During this quarter the deaths of 120,825 persons were registered in England and Wales, showing a considerable further decline from the numbers returned in recent corresponding quarters. The annual death-rate did not exceed 18·6 per 1000 of the population, estimated for the middle of this year from the numbers enumerated in April last, and was 2·3 below the average rate in the ten preceding corresponding quarters, whilst it was the lowest recorded in the second quarter of any year since the establishment of civil registration in 1837. The nearest approach to it occurred last year, when the rate in the June quarter was 19·5. The average rate in the second or spring quarters of the forty-three years 1838-80 was equal to 21·8 per 1000, and 3·2 higher than the rate recorded in the quarter under notice. The excess of mortality in the urban, compared with the rural population, was considerably below the average: in equal numbers living, the deaths in the urban were as 111 to 100 in the rural population; the relative proportion in the second quarters of the ten years 1871-80 having been 114 to 100. In twenty of the largest English towns, including London, and having an estimated population of about seven millions and a half of persons, the death-rate averaged only 20·5 per 1000, corresponding with that which prevailed in the second quarter of last year; in the corresponding periods of 1878 and 1879 the death-rate in these towns averaged 22·7 and 22·3. The total number of deaths attributed to zymotic diseases was 12,167, and the death-rate from them was 1·87, being the lowest yet recorded in the Quarterly Returns; the only occasion on which the rate was nearly as low was the immediately preceding quarter, when it was 1·89. There has been, therefore, for the first two quarters of the present year a remarkable immunity from zymotic disease in this country. Whooping-cough is responsible for the greatest number of deaths (2617), and the mortality from small-pox, which in the three preceding quarters had been successively 69, 208, and 730, rose still further to 1213, furnishing the highest record since the second quarter of 1877. The report, however, remarks that the experience of past years gives rational grounds for anticipating with much confidence that the mortality from this disease will be found to have been considerably reduced in the third quarter of the present year. Of the 1018 fatal cases of small-pox that were registered in London itself, 420, or 41·2 per cent, were certified to have been unvaccinated; 207, or 20·3 per cent, to have been vaccinated; while concerning the remaining 391 no information on this point was given.

AN ERROR.

WITH much regret we find that an error crept into a quotation of a quotation from the columns of our contemporary the *Lancet* in our last week's number. It is very far from our desire that anything of the kind should ever occur, for we have no wish to live in enmity with our brethren, still less to misrepresent them. Under the circumstances it would be ungracious on our part to enter into any discussion of the form in which the quotation actually appeared in the *Lancet*, though that by itself is quite enough to show how apt all of us are to err.

THE GERMAN ASSOCIATION OF NATURALISTS AND PHYSICIANS.

THE opinion recently expressed in different quarters, that the British Association for the Advancement of Science had almost outlived its time, and that it would be a judicious act for it to consent to its dissolution, has been shown by the energetic proceedings and great success of the meeting at York to have been somewhat premature. It probably might be more accurately addressed to her elder sister the Versammlung deutscher Naturforscher und Aerste, which, at its fifty-fourth meeting, held in September at Salzburg, exhibited a great falling off, both in the numbers and the position of its members. When Prof. Pettenköfer's address at the first general meeting, was occupied with his well-worn subject on the Soil in its relations to Public Health, and this is described as having been received with great enthusiasm, it is evident that the recent advances of science do not form the leading objects of attention with this body. The second general discourse was delivered by Prof. Weismann of Freiburg, on the Duration of Life; and the third came from the Astronomer of the Vienna Observatory, Dr. Oppolzer, on the question, Does Newton's Law of Attraction suffice for the explanation of the Motions of the Heavenly Bodies, or is there reason to regard it only as approximate?" At this meeting, also, Obermedizinalrath Kerschensteiner, of Munich, delivered an address on the occasion of the 340th anniversary of the death of Theophrastus Bombastes Paracelsus. It seems that the numbers of the visitors to these congresses are diminishing, for while 1000 were present at Baden-Baden, and 800 at Danzig, there were not many more than 600 at Salzburg. Several of these only came for a day or two, others turned up for the festivities, while the ladies and many other persons could not be said to represent the scientific element. The medical portion of the congress is too much split up into minute sections, so that some of these, as that of ophthalmology, could not be formed at all. The numbers of special congresses which are now held of course sap the strength of the parent body, especially when this is too much subdivided. There was also a remarkable absence of eminent persons, so that on several questions no discussions were maintained. The belief seems to have been pretty prevalent that this in some degree arose from the disinclination of Germans to come to a congress held on Austrian soil, but this surely can scarcely be credible!

THE HEALTH OF BRISTOL DURING THE YEAR 1880.

MR. DAVID DAVIES, the Medical Officer of Health for the city and county of Bristol, in presenting his summary for the year 1880, remarks that the sanitary condition of the district, as indicated by the returns of mortality, has, on the whole, not been unsatisfactory, either in comparison with the returns of former years, or with those of other large centres of population. During the year under notice 4276 deaths were registered, giving a rate of mortality of 20·0 per 1000. The previous year's returns showed a rate of 21·4 per 1000. The deaths from zymotic diseases were, however, less during 1879 than in the past year, the rate in the former year having been 2·2 against 3·3 in 1880. Only one death was recorded from small-pox, the infection being clearly traceable to a neighbouring city. Although several cases followed upon this one, by dint of prompt isolation and continuous watching of the houses infected the disease was eventually stamped out. Scarlet fever, Mr. Davies records as the most unmanageable of all the zymotic diseases, and during the past year was accountable for 244 lives. The families mostly affected are those who visit and are visited unceremoniously by their neighbours; day-schools of various kinds are also the frequent means of disseminating it, chiefly through the almost criminal recklessness of parents in sending their children to school from infected houses, without communicating the fact to the governors of these establishments. In his last quarterly report, Mr. Davies has suggested some additions which should be made to the powers of medical officers of health in this matter, and one of these is, that in the event of a refusal to allow of the removal of a case of scarlet fever, a caution should be prominently affixed to the house where the patient lies, and all ingress and egress should be regulated by the sanitary authority. He admits that the public are not yet prepared to accept such an innovation on personal liberty, but he contends that this disease can never be successfully combated in crowded cities except by some compulsory law of the kind indicated.

THE MOBILITY OF THE PELVIC ARTICULATIONS.

DR. KORSCH, of St. Petersburg, contributes to a recent number of the *Zeitschrift für Geburtshülfe und Gynäkologie* an account of an experimental investigation of the above subject. He had dilators so constructed that two opposite parts of the instrument could be separated, and both the extent of their separation, and the force required to effect it, measured. This instrument he applied to different parts of the pelvic cavity, and measured the extent to which its diameters could be altered, and the force required to do it. His experiments were made on the bodies of recently delivered women, of pregnant women, of non-pregnant women, and of men. The following are the conclusions he comes to:—1. Both during pregnancy and in patients suffering from large uterine or ovarian tumours, there is not only yielding of the pelvic articulations, but widening of the pelvic diameters. 2. At the pelvic inlet, the greater widening is of the transverse diameter; at the outlet, of the antero-posterior diameter. 3. To enlarge the pelvic inlet requires nearly double the force needed to widen the outlet. 4. Widening of the transverse diameter of the pelvic inlet is accompanied with shortening of the antero-posterior diameter; but widening of the latter does not alter the former. 5. When the transverse diameter of the brim has been enlarged to the maximum extent, the conjugate may still be slightly lengthened; but when the maximum increase in length of the conjugate has been attained, the transverse diameter cannot be widened. 6. When the transverse and antero-posterior diameters of the inlet are simultaneously expanded by pressure, the amount of increase in each is not so much as when each is separately expanded. 7. Widening of the pelvic outlet diminishes slightly the conjugate, but leaves unaltered or slightly increases the transverse diameter of the brim. 8. The converse takes place when the inlet is widened. 9. In the majority of the cases the greatest amount of mobility was in the sacro-iliac synchondrosis. 10. In those joints of which the mobility was increased, the quantity of synovial fluid was usually somewhat greater. 11. Lengthening of the antero-posterior diameters depends upon the movement of the sacrum; that of the transverse diameters upon yielding of the symphysis pubis. 12. Increase in size of the synovial cavity of the pubic articulation leads to a greater mobility of the joint. 13. The number of deliveries has, apparently, no influence on the mobility of the pelvic articulations.

MORTALITY IN HUNGARY.

A CORRESPONDENT of *La France Médicale*, writing from Buda-Pesth, gives some curious details as to the mortality in Hungary. According to Dr. Szalardi, the population of the country, numbering at the last census 11,000,000, had only increased by 11,000 in the last ten years; and yet the birth-rate is enormous, not less than 50 per annum for every 1000 living, while in the most prosperous of other European countries it does not exceed 36 to 40. M. Szalardi attributes this high mortality to the frequency of irregular unions, the neglect of the children among the poor, and to the prevalence of malaria in the lowlands contiguous to the great rivers. From other sources we learn that for the whole of the Austrian Empire in the years 1853-74 the mean death-rate was 32·2, birth-rate 39·9, and marriages 17·2; those of England being 22·2, 34·9, and 16·8. If these statements of Szalardi be correct, there must be an urgent need for reform in the social, moral, and sanitary condition of a country which has but two towns with more than 50,000 inhabitants. We cannot but think that there is a mistake somewhere, especially as the Magyars, who were estimated by Chovanetz in 1850 at 4,800,000, are at present returned as 6,700,000. The suppression of the military frontier as a separate government renders comparison between different censuses difficult, but, so far as we can make out, the aggregate population of Hungary, the Banat, Croatia, Slavonia, and the frontier has increased in twenty years from 11,800,000 to 13,400,000. A comparison of the increase or decrease of the several nationalities, of which Hungary contains nearly as many as Europe itself, and of the most diverse races and habits, would be very instructive. Which of these are the greatest sinners M. Szalardi does not inform us, but we know that the Croats have been stationary since Safarik wrote in 1835.

VITAL STATISTICS OF SCOTLAND.

THE monthly report of the Registrar-General for Scotland for August last shows that the births of 3638 children were registered during the period in the eight principal towns, together with the deaths of 2033 persons; this latter number is 284 under the average for the month of August during the last ten years. A comparison of the deaths registered shows that this mortality was at the annual rate of 16 deaths per 1000 persons in Dundee and in Leith, 18 in Edinburgh and in Perth, 19 in Aberdeen, 20 in Greenock, 23 in Glasgow, and 27 in Paisley. Of the 2033 deaths, 828, or 41 per cent. were those of children under five years of age. The zymotic class of diseases caused 351 deaths, or 17·3 per cent. of the whole mortality. This rate was, however, considerably exceeded in Paisley, where measles, whooping-cough, and diarrhœa prevailed. The deaths from inflammatory affections of the respiratory organs (not including consumption, whooping-cough, or croup) amounted to 322, or 15·8 per cent. Those from consumption alone numbered 238, or 11·7 per cent. One male and six females were aged ninety years and upwards, the eldest of whom was a widow ninety-nine years of age.

ANOMALIES OF THE CORONER'S COURT.—At the conclusion of an inquest held in St. Luke's, a few days since, the Foreman said : I am supported by my brother jurymen. Mr. Coroner, in asking whether you can allow us a small fee. The Coroner said he was sorry he had not the power, or he would willingly do so. The Foreman observed : Fees are payable in some districts. The Coroner replied : They are payable in Surrey and in the City, which is a liberty in itself ; but otherwise they are not allowable in Middlesex. A juryman remembered that on one occasion he received a fee at the Middlesex Hospital—nine years ago or so. The coroner rejoined that it must have been under some special circumstances, as the Middlesex magistrates had long done away with fees in the county. The foreman thought it very unfair to have them in one part and not in another. The coroner admitted it was so, but he could not help it ; they must apply to the magistrates if they thought it an injustice, but the magistrates were scarcely likely to help them, on economical grounds. The jury then withdrew.

ABSTRACT OF

INTRODUCTORY ADDRESS

DELIVERED AT THE OPENING OF

THE UNIVERSITY OF GLASGOW MEDICAL SCHOOL.

By MATTHEW CHARTERIS, M.D.,

Professor of Therapeutics and Materia Medica.

THE address to the medical students at the opening of the winter session of the University of Glasgow, on Tuesday, October 25, was delivered by Dr. Matthew Charteris, Professor of Therapeutics and Materia Medica.

After alluding to the International Medical Congress, and more particularly to Professor Pasteur's address, Dr. Charteris said :—

The wide range of speculation and inquiry opened up in these and kindred subjects, the obvious deductions that could be drawn, naturally made men pause and consider other and more pertinent questions, through which we, as a profession, are called before the bar of public opinion . Whether we wish it or not, we are judged by those whose servants we are, and from whom we obtain the means of our livelihood. Our motives are scrutinised, our inner life laid bare, and our systems and our inherent morals keenly inspected. Our deeds are now enveloped in no mystery, nor are our actions read in an unknown tongue. We cannot screen ourselves behind our ancient and noble lineage, nor can we expect sympathy only because of the antiquity of our art. We cannot hope that those of the far distant past will be our protectors. Their learned treatises, their weighty arguments, their subtle nosologies, their ingenious plans for coping with disease, are judged by the clear and cutting logic of the nineteenth century, and the mere records which they have left us will avail us little, unless they can be used in the living present as true to all time. The age in which we live is peculiar and characteristic. It abjures sentiment. It is intensely realistic. It is distinctly practical and somewhat sceptical, and before the judgment of this sceptical, unsentimental, utilitarian, and prosaic age we are called and asked for our position and our watchword in the face of the discoveries which science is revealing. The question is put by the public to the profession as a whole—"Have you utilised recent investigations in treating the diseases of every-day life ? "

Dr. Charteris then considered modern resources of therapeutics as applied to (1) acute zymotic diseases ; (2) general diseases and diseases of individual organs. With regard to the latter he said :—

We are called in, for the instinct is strong in man, and has been so in all times, to try something in disease, no matter how fatal or how hopeless it may seem. The physician then represents the high and holy union which rendered the persons of our predecessors divine. He is the vague embodiment of superior knowledge, which awakened superstitious dread. He is the master of the situation, and as such is recognised in lands the most savage and countries the most civilised. His lightest wish is law. Like Pallida Mors, in whose shadow he walks, his knock is heard at the peasant's hut and at the palace of the king.

If to this yearning appeal the oracle is dumb—if he stands there, the faithless exponent of the healing art, and suggests nothing and knows nothing, then his visit is one of evil omen. . . . To the sick man this conduct is death. To the friends and to the public it is cool and heartless cynicism, and an open confession, either of incapacity, or of lack of care, if not of both. To the impartial critic it means "medical suicide," for he sees that if the policy of expectancy is carried to its legitimate conclusion there is a sapping of the foundations of therapeutic faith. There is a lowering of the public interest in scientific inquiry. There is no use in "having doctors at all."

The position assumed is no imaginary one. It is openly advocated by some. It is attempted to be justified by others, because it is better to leave well alone in our efforts to deal with disease, lest by stumbling strokes of medical aid we do more harm than good. We may stab (they say) the salutary recuperative efforts of nature, instead of inflicting any injury on the malady. We thus adopt the Fabian policy of delay.

Such a doctrine is properly fatal to our position in the eyes of the public, and it is necessarily false to the best interests of the profession (and besides, it is not in accordance with present facts). The acquaintance with pharmacology is based on intelligent premises. We endeavour to test the actions of medicines by the method of research inaugurated by Morgagni, and followed up by his successors in the present day. . . .

Therapeutics takes up a position which is critical but not antagonistic to its ally. It acknowledges that physiology is not medicine, and that we cannot trust to it alone ; for we must recollect that the most significant testing-ground for medical agents is the hospital ward and actual practice. It states that the action of a medicine may be accurately described so far as it affects a healthy human being or animal. . . . But disease cannot be imitated, and a man in health and the same man in disease are two dissimilar entities, so far as the action of the medicine or particular drug is concerned. We take it up, therefore, with no preconceived theory as to its efficacy. We try it at the sick-bed, and if it succeeds we hail it with gratitude. If it does not succeed, or only imperfectly so, we say that it has not answered its purpose, or probably that it is inferior to some better-known and more trusted friend.

Looking at what has already been accomplished by the cordial working of these two methods, I can truly say that I know of no disease, unless pronounced hopeless by its nature, which cannot be benefited by medical aid. I mean by this not the nurse's attention, but the physician's skill. In some things we may have conflicting statements. We may have different roads proposed, strangely opposite methods recommended, and it may be puzzling to the young beginner to know which to accept. Time will solve these perplexities as it has solved many a harder problem. If a remedy is found good only in one man's hands, and not in any other's, it will not long occupy a prominent place in the therapeutic roll-call. It soon sinks to merited oblivion. On the other hand, ours is an open creed, and if merit there be, time will place it in the proper niche.

Dr. Charteris concluded his address as follows :—

Future graduates of medicine, carry the hope of progress with you into the work of your after life, and you will feel yourselves loyal sons of men whose names are dear to every student's heart. Deal gently with the weaknesses of the old masters as revealed in their writings, and with no scornful hand lay bare their errors in judgment and discrepancies in treatment. They failed in much, but they achieved much ; and in the dim and shadowy past in which they lived, remember that their lights were feeble as compared with yours. Seek not to destroy the belief in the ars medicandi which they helped to rear with great labour and which they cherished with faithful care.

"The proper study of mankind is man," and man sends for you to study him, not in the glow of his physical strength and pride of intellectual might, but in his day of danger and hour of bodily weakness. He does so in the hope that you may do him good, and not that you may regard him simply as an instructive and interesting case of physical or mental decay. Remember this in the time of your pupilage, and when you have passed from the threshold of this University into the busy pursuits of your after life, and so reflecting and so acting, your student days will be true and earnest, and your future career sustained by the rich reward of merited success.

Place before you no other standard, however seductive the prospect, than the desire to diminish the suffering and extend the term of the troubled years of those who have trusted themselves or theirs to your honour and your skill. The mission you have chosen is noble ; see that you walk worthily and warily in the attempt to fulfil the work of your choice.

PROPORTION OF DOCTORS.—According to the Medicinal Zeitung there are in every 10,000 inhabitants in Italy 6·10 doctors, in France 2·91, in Germany 3·21, in Austria 3·41, in Hungary 6·10, in Switzerland 7·06, in England 6·00, and in North America 16·24.—Wien. Med. Woch., September 24.

ALKALI WORKS' REGULATION ACT, 1881.
(44 AND 45 VIC., C. 37.)

AN important circular letter has just been issued by the Local Government Board, calling upon the sanitary authorities in England and Wales to furnish certain information, with the view of giving effect to the provisions of this Act. The Board ask for a return from each district, showing the description of all the different works which will be affected by the Act, the parishes in which the works are situated, and the names and addresses of the proprietors or managers. It is stated in the circular letter, that in addition to alkali works, the following works will, by operation of the Act, be brought under skilled inspection from and after January 1 next, viz.:—Sulphuric acid works, chemical manure works, gas-liquor works, nitric acid works, sulphate of ammonia and muriate of ammonia works, chlorine works, or works in which bleaching-powder or bleaching-liquor is made; works in which the extraction of salt from brine is carried on, and cement works, or works in which aluminous deposits are treated for making cement. It is explained that, in order that all works of this description may be brought under inspection (with the view of preventing the escape of noxious and offensive gases from the works, or rendering them harmless or inoffensive), the Act requires that every work shall be registered in the manner prescribed by the Board, and, after April 1, 1882, shall not be carried on unless certified to be so registered. The information asked for in the return is to enable the Board to determine what arrangements shall be made for the inspection of all works and for the issue of instructions to the proprietors, pointing out to them the steps to be taken to obtain the requisite certificates of registration. The Board state that they entertain no doubt that, with the assistance of the medical officer of health and inspector of nuisances, there will be no difficulty in supplying the information required. In conclusion, the Board direct attention to Sections 19 and 28 of the Act, which they think of considerable importance. The former provides that if any sanitary authority applies for an additional inspector, and undertakes to pay a moiety of the salary, the Local Government Board may appoint such an officer, who is to reside within a convenient distance of the works he is required to inspect. The latter section provides that any person injured by a nuisance from any noxious or offensive gas, wholly or partially caused by the acts of several persons, may proceed against and recover damages from any one person in proportion to his contribution to the nuisance, although the act of such person will not separately have caused a nuisance. It is also pointed out that complaint may be made to the central authority by any sanitary authority on the representation of any of their officers or of any ten of the inhabitants of the district.

FROM ABROAD.

PROFESSOR BALL ON THE PATHOLOGICAL ANATOMY OF GENERAL PARALYSIS.

PROF. BALL, in a lecture delivered on this subject at the Ste. Anne Asylum (*Revue Méd.*, 1881, No. 34), observed that when in an autopsy of a subject of this paralysis we remove the brain, the lesion which strikes us at first sight exists in the form and appearance of the encephalic mass—a lesion characterised by a general atrophy affecting the whole of the organ, its weight and volume, and also characterised by localised atrophy. Above all, we find an enfeeblement and an atrophy of the frontal region, and then a general collapse, the brain no longer holding itself in position, but sinking down on the table and losing its volume, its amplitude, and its consistence. Its circumference is no longer ovoid, but irregular, and presents projections analogous to those which are observed on a soil that has undergone convulsions. The scales show us the diminution of weight and volume, all the more remarkable as the brain at this period of life is in its full development. A man attacked with general paralysis usually dies between the thirty-fifth and forty-fifth year of his age—that is, when the functional conditions are in the highest vigour. If after making this general survey of the mass of the brain we proceed to the details, we meet with a primordial lesion characterised by the thickening of the arachnoid. This membrane, in fact, is opaque, whitish, or lactescent at certain points of predilection—that is to say, at the temporal lobes, and especially the anterior lobes, the frontal lobes, and the convexity of the encephalon; while the occipital or posterior lobes possess an absolute immunity. Thus we have a great preponderance of meningeal lesions in front, which is the general rule. If we examine the arachnoid with some attention, not only do we recognise the white, opaque patches, but also certain tracts running parallel with the vessels, the sinuosities of which they trace out; and also the almost constant existence of whitish filaments uniting the arachnoid to the dura mater and the pia mater. The pia mater is also notably thickened, tenacious, and resisting, and is torn with more difficulty than in the normal brain. On its surface also are to be observed vascular islets, true capillary networks, contrasting with the paleness of the surrounding parts, some of which are due to an obvious hyperæmia, and others to a serous infiltration, which is also found beneath the pia mater, filling in any lacunæ which may exist there. These lesions of the pia mater correspond exactly, as regards seat, with those of the arachnoid—the whitish, opaque, lactescent patches,—there being also the same predilection for the frontal lobes and the convexity of the brain, and the same exemption of the posterior lobes.

But the examination of the brain would be incomplete if the arteries of the base were neglected. We do not meet with in these the atheromatous lesions so frequent in the different diseases of the brain, as the arteries are never found in this condition at the ages at which these cases occur. The vessels are, in fact, dilated and increased in calibre. If by the aid of these facts we take a general survey of the brain, we find an atrophy of the convolutions, especially in the region of predilection; and in the majority of cases a diagnosis of general paralysis may be made after the first glance at the brain as a whole. When we try to raise the meninges, we find more or less numerous adhesions uniting the surface of the convolutions to the enveloping membrane, so much so that with the pia mater we tear off a portion of the grey substance. The adherent points may be very circumscribed or very extensive, few or numerous, but they are always confined to the upper surface of the convolutions, and never descend or penetrate into their furrows or anfractuosities. The losses of substance through detachment of the pia mater are sinuous, anfractuous, and irregularly disseminated, resembling the face of a subject upon whom small-pox has impressed indelible traces. The localisation of these adhesions is the same as that of the meningeal lesions, that is, always at the front and the convexity, the posterior region remaining absolutely free. There is, then, in progressive paralysis a general law that all the lesions are absolutely localised in the more noble parts of the brain, the occipital lobes being constantly exempted.

These adhesions of the pia mater, although very frequent, are not constant; and, if we are to believe the English authors who have occupied themselves with this question, they are absent in a fifth of the cases. This is principally the case when the disease is characterised by a rapid evolution and a speedy death—a kind of urticaria of the brain, if we may so speak, which leaves no traces of its passage. It is also the same sometimes in general paralysis with the most chronic evolution, in which the convolutions have become so atrophied as to preserve no traces of meningo-cephalic lesions.

Although, in the majority of cases, very apparent, we must know how to search for these lesions with care, and all the more so because it is difficult to strip the convexity of the brain thoroughly of its envelopes, and there is thus danger of the lesions escaping notice. Thus it is generally a wise precaution to harden the brain by allowing it to macerate for several weeks in a solution of nitric acid, one-tenth strong. It results that, the pia mater destroyed, we can observe on the brain with great facility the lesions hollowed out in it, the vestiges of the destroyed adhesions.

Continuing the examination by a section of the brain, we find atrophy of the cortical substance, to such a degree that it is sometimes reduced to a millimetre in thickness. The white substance has also undergone change. It is indurated as if sclerosed, yellowish, and easily separable from the grey substance. As to the bony walls, we find in many cases thickening of the vault of the cranium, or at least an increased vascularisation, a vascularisation of the diploë, a congestion of the osseous tissue, with a more or less rusty tinge. Sometimes there is *ramollissement* of the bones of the cranium as well as of the adhesions of the dura mater to the osseous tissue, the bones being not solid, as in the aged insane, but soft and easy of detachment. The internal surface of the dura mater also has a rusty appearance. The sinuses of the encephalon are gorged with blood, and sometimes there are true lesions, as hæmorrhagic pachymeningitis, and blood-cysts. Finally, the cavities of the ventricles are pretty often dilated and filled with a certain quantity of serosity.

All the lesions enumerated would not, if met with separately, be of any serious importance for the anatomopathological study of general paralysis, while taken conjointly, as a characteristic whole, they are of true value, it being by progressive atrophy that we are able to explain the symptoms of the continuous decline of the patient.

REVIEWS.

Selections from the Works of Abraham Colles. Edited, with Annotations, by ROBERT McDONNELL, M.D., F.R.S. London : The New Sydenham Society. 1881. Pp. 481.

THESE Selections consist chiefly of Colles' observations on the venereal disease, and on its treatment by small doses of mercury. There are some minor selections, among the best known of which is that " On the Fracture of the Carpal Extremity of the Radius."

The value attaching to this work is historical rather than practical; for now much of the doctrine which Colles taught, and which required all the weight of his authority to make accepted, is known to most students who apply for their diplomas, while the use of mercury " in small doses " —small even as compared with what Colles ordered—is the all but universal treatment of syphilis at the present time.

To rightly understand the great merit of Colles' teaching, one must be fully posted in what were considered as the authoritative doctrines of syphilis and its treatment, not less than the teachings and the science of surgery generally about the year 1800, when Mr. Colles became a member of the Royal College of Surgeons in Ireland. We of to-day, with unparalleled advantages in education, with an inexhaustible supply of literature within reach, bringing us into contact with the views and teachings of almost every school in Europe, shall find it difficult—not to say impossible —to carry ourselves back to the time when Hunter's often erroneous and always dogmatic teaching was still paramount; and without this it will be hardly possible to gauge aright Mr. Colles' new teachings. That they should have become established doctrine is the natural result of increased experience and of persistent teaching.

And yet when we bear in mind that Colles lived in an age antecedent to the introduction of iodide of potassium, we are brought face to face with a fact which our present knowledge of its essential value in syphilis makes it difficult to bridge over.

Next in interest and importance to the use of mercury in small and long-continued doses, which Mr. Colles first introduced, are his teachings on hereditary syphilis. It seems to have been generally taught that when an infant showed symptoms of syphilis it was supposed to have been infected in its passage through the genitals of its mother, or that its parents, one or both, were affected with primary or secondary symptoms at the time of its conception. It was Colles who first clearly established that an infant might be born of apparently healthy parents, and yet show unmistakable and severe signs of syphilis; and it was he, too, who first drew attention to repeated abortion as a sign of still active syphilis in parents who might not themselves show any active or outward manifestation of the syphilitic taint, and that small doses of mercury were the remedy for this condition. Such observations may not appear of great value to-day, when the

doctrine is so generally known and acted upon; but it is easy to be wise after the event—easy to follow when a way has been cleared.

That which has since been called Colles' Law is as follows :—" I have never," says Mr. Colles, " seen or heard of a single instance in which a syphilitic infant (although its mouth be ulcerated) suckled by its own mother had produced ulceration of her breast; whereas very few instances have occurred where a syphilitic infant had not infected a strange hired wet-nurse, and who had been previously in good health." The further outcome of this doctrine necessarily teaches that a woman may become syphilised by giving birth to a syphilitic child, and that without herself showing any of the ordinary signs by which syphilis is usually recognised.

This is, of course, an important point, and it opens up, in view of the protective action of vaccination against variola, and of M. Pasteur's new observations of vaccination against anthrax, etc., the possibility of our one day being able to protect against syphilis by introducing designedly into the system some modified virus, which shall be as efficacious and as little harmful, against the disgusting malady syphilis, as vaccination is against variola. When we bear in mind the terrible secondary consequences of syphilis on every part of the system, we must admit that this consummation is devoutly to be wished for.

The editor has given us a memoir of Mr. Colles, which will be read with interest. We wish he had given us a detailed list of all Mr. Colles' writings. Many notes are interspersed through the text by the editor, which add considerably to the value of the book.

Atlas of Pathological Anatomy. By Dr. LANCEREAUX, Professeur Agrégé à la Faculté de Médecine de Paris, Médecin de l'Hôpital de la Pitié; and M. LUCKERBAUER, Artist. Translated by W. S. GREENFIELD, M.D., with additional Plates drawn by Mr. W. HURST. London : J. and A. Churchill. Plates LXX.

THE medical public are without doubt deeply indebted to the Messrs. Churchill for the zeal and enterprise they have manifested in placing before them such admirably illustrated works as Bentley and Trimen's " Medicinal Plants," and Godlee's Anatomical Plates; but if we are not greatly mistaken, their debt of gratitude is still more justly due for the volume whose title heads this notice. The name of Lancereaux has long been recognised in this country as that of an excellent and careful writer. And of Dr. Greenfield's qualifications we need not speak. An excellent French scholar, Dr. Greenfield is also one of the best pathologists of the day, as is evidenced by his translation to the Chair of Pathology in Edinburgh, vacant through the lamented death of Dr. Sanders. It is, however, much to be regretted that the translator did not see his way to publish the text which accompanies the plates in the original French edition; but, as he says that this would have necessitated a complete remodelling of the work, it had to be abandoned after much labour had been expended on it. Undoubtedly this is a great loss, but we must perforce be content with the somewhat copious descriptions given of the various figures in each plate, though we greatly miss the history which attaches to each individual illustration, whilst it renders the work of criticism doubly difficult.

The first five plates are devoted to diseases of the stomach and intestines. One form of disease with which we are not very familiar in this country is largely illustrated—that is, alcoholic inflammation of the stomach. Unfortunately that is common enough, but here it is represented as going on to ulceration of the most marked kind. On the other hand, the only form of malignant disease figured is a papillary epithelioma; not a sign of carcinoma, either here or in connexion with the intestine. Two other forms of local mischief are figured which are seldom seen among us : these are uræmic gastritis and enteritis, both of the ulcerative—the latter, perhaps, rather of the sloughing—kind. Three forms of enteritis are very well figured, viz., those connected with acute and chronic dysentery, and simple ulcerative enteritis; which, by the way, is not unlike what we speak of as tubercular. In Pl. III. there are some very good examples of pigmentation from obstructed circulation, and an excellent drawing of that peculiar form of malignant disease found in the rectum (the author calls it epithelioma), characterised by the great multiplication of tubules with columnar cells. In Pl. V. a curious illustration occurs of hæmorrhages in the intestinæ during scarlatina, together with enlarged mesenteric glands, the so-called scarlatinal buboes. Pl. VI. is devoted to the peritoneum and the pancreas. Pls. VII. to XIII.—a very valuable series—illustrate diseases of the liver. Pl. VII. is largely occupied by very good illustrations of advanced cirrhosis (the earlier changes are not represented) ; whilst Pl. VIII. contains drawings of gummatous changes (showing, by the way, a very well defined boundary wall), abscess, yellow atrophy (here also called exudative hepatitis), and cancer of the ordinary kind, and said to be primary. In Pl. IX. three forms of disease are represented, namely, tubercle, that form of cylindrical epithelioma already spoken of as being frequently found in the rectum, and melanotic sarcoma ; whilst Pl. X. is chiefly notable for illustrations of the changes dependent on the so-called hepatic adenoma. Degenerations follow, especially the so-called amyloid, and the fatty ; of these the illustrations are both good and instructive, particularly those of different kinds of fatty liver ; whilst Pl. XIII. is chiefly devoted to pigmentations and cysts. Pl. XIV. is excellent ; it deals entirely with splenic mischief, but one or two points in the description deserve notice. Thus, the Malpighian bodies are in one place so described, in another they are spoken of as splenic glomeruli ; whilst splenic infarcts are also spoken of as splenic embolisms, which might lead one to think they too were totally different. Pl. XVI. is in brief occupied with representations of glandular sclerosis and glandular leukæmia ; whilst in Pl. XVII. we have some very interesting illustrations of leukæmia, melanæmia, and certain vascular maladies, mainly inflammatory, embolic, and thrombotic ; and so, too, of Pls. XVIII. and XIX., and to a certain extent Pl. XX. The microscopic sections of these emboli are especially interesting. Pl. XX. is of a mixed kind, partly referring to embolism, partly to changes in the valves of the heart. One embolism of a branch of the Sylvian artery shows well how a fibrinous or white plug grows at its distal extremity by accretion of coagulated blood. Pl. XXI. is mainly devoted to peri- and endo-carditis, illustrating what is here called villous—what most frequently we term vegetative or warty—change, as well as the ulcerative forms. Pl. XXII. is largely microscopic ; it still deals with heart-changes, as does Pl. XXIII. Some of the drawings refer to endocardial and some to myocardial change. One drawing in Pl. XXII. represents what is called a growth, the result of villous endocarditis, but it is mainly composed of spindle-shaped cells, many with double nuclei, such as we commonly associate in this country with a more malignant form of disease ; whilst Pl. XXIII. is chiefly notable for various forms of fatty degeneration. Pls. XXIV., XXV., and XXVI. deal with diseases of arteries. Endarteritis is here represented in at least three forms—the nodose, the warty, and the form where the deposit is in plates—all of which we are apt to group as atheroma. One drawing in Pl. XXV. is very interesting from a practical point of view. It is taken from a patient the subject of angina pectoris, and in it the nerves are seen in close contact with the inflamed aorta, whilst a microscopical drawing shows the nerve-fibres granular, and the interfibrillar material filled with young cells. In Pl. XXVI. the most interesting drawing is one of multiple cerebral aneurisms of small size, so often associated with cerebral hæmorrhages.

Pl. XXVII. introduces the diseases of the respiratory organs ; nothing, however, is here very striking, except that the author figures the diphtheritic membrane as purely corpuscular, with a certain proportion of leucocytes ; no other formed structures are to be seen. Pls. XXVIII., XXIX., XXX., and XXXI. are devoted to the lung, especially illustrating pneumonia and phthisis. The drawings of caseous and sclerous pneumonia are, to our mind, exceptionally good and exceedingly instructive. There is also a single representation of miliary tuberculosis. Pl. XXX. is devoted almost entirely to pigmentary changes ; whilst XXXI. deals rather with the diseases of the pulmonary appendages.

Pls. XXXII., XXXIII., XXXIV., and XXXV. are, inasmuch as the author is a recognised authority on renal diseases, of far more than usual interest, dealing, as they do, almost entirely with renal maladies. The most important of these are the two forms of inflammation—the acute and chronic, or yet again what might be called the catarrhal and

the sclerous ; and the various forms of degeneration—the fatty, the lardaceous, the cystic, and (which has special reference to the ureters) the tubercular. Nevertheless, in Pl. XXXII., Fig. 1 is not correctly described. The cortical substance is spoken of as being figured brownish-yellow ; in reality, it is uncoloured. On the whole, we are inclined to reckon more highly the unenlarged than the microscopic drawings in this series ; the interstitial tissue seeming in almost every microscopical drawing to be over-abundant, whilst, in certain others, glomerular and tubular epithelial increase is left unnoted. Probably the explanation of this imperfection is in great measure due to the absence of the accompanying text. Then, again, several illustrations are devoted to renal infarcts—not one to show the origin and connexion of the renal cysts with which we are so well acquainted. On the other hand, the appearance of the true cystic kidney is exceedingly well given.

Pl. XXXVII. is occupied with illustrations of disease of the testis ; in several places the references cannot be made out, and the description of Fig. 6 is entirely omitted. Moreover, there is no illustration of any form of malignant disease. Pls. XXXVIII. and XXXIX. are mainly occupied with uterine changes ; and here we must give a just meed of praise to the microscopical sections, which are beautifully executed and highly instructive.

To many the plates XL. to XLVI. inclusive will be among the most useful and the most valued in the whole publication. They deal exclusively with the nervous system, and afford excellent representations of morbid conditions with which many of us are not well acquainted, whilst in XLIX. we have also various figures of the retina as seen by the ophthalmoscope in different forms of disease. The figures of the diseases of muscles and bones need hardly detain us, though they are among the best in the book. One or two plates of skin diseases are added, and a kind of supernumerary plate, mainly in connexion with diseases of the heart, brings Lancereaux's share of the volume to a close.

The first thing that strikes one with regard to Dr. Greenfield's additions to the foreign plates is the great difference in colouration, these being much brighter and more abundant in carmine than are the French. They come, moreover, in no very distinct order. Thus, Pl. LXI. contains five figures, four of which represent caseous tubercle in various parts ; LXII., LXIII., and LXIV. relate almost entirely to phthisis ; LXV. and LXVI. also to lung ; LXVII. mainly to lymphadenoma ; whilst LXVIII. and LXIX. are devoted to illustrations of intestinal ulceration ; and LXX. is of a mixed kind. But Dr. Greenfield's share of the work is not thus lightly appreciated ; for, above all things, he has had the difficulty not only of supplementing the work where he thought it deficient, but of rendering the descriptions both clear and, at the same time, in idiomatic English.

And now what do we think of it all ? There is no great difficulty in expressing an opinion. We have gone over the whole carefully—and this has cost us days of labour,—plate by plate and figure by figure ; for it must be understood that a plate does not represent one subject, and one subject only. Each is crammed full of separate illustrations, often in such a way as to lead to some little trouble in disentangling them, for each figure is in turn mapped out by letters, which had to be followed up separately from the accompanying description.

Founding our opinion on such a basis, we may safely say that there is not such another book available to the English-reading public. We do not pretend that it is perfect in every respect. To give an illustration of each form of morbid process known in every part of the body would be a superhuman task. But what the Atlas pretends to do it does. We have in it an excellent epitome of pathological knowledge demonstrated before our eyes, so that we may see what elsewhere we may read of, or verify what we have found in a post-mortem research. And it is especially in the naked-eye appearances that the strength of this volume lies. As regards microscopic structures, no staining material seems, as a rule, to have been used, so that certain of the differentiations of structure are thus left less apparent. But it must be remembered that the class for whom such a volume as this has a special value is precisely that for which anatomical, rather than microscopical, lesions have their chief value. But on every ground we would most heartily recommend this Atlas to our readers and their friends as worthy of all honest commendation.

REPORTS OF SOCIETIES.

THE OBSTETRICAL SOCIETY OF LONDON.
WEDNESDAY, OCTOBER 5.

Dr. MATTHEWS DUNCAN, President, in the Chair.

MR. F. WALLACE showed an Anencephalous Fœtus with Spina Bifida.

Dr. HERMAN showed a translucent Sac, one inch and three-eighths by three-quarters of an inch, which had been passed by a woman who supposed herself three months and a half pregnant, and was followed after some hours by a placenta with a rudimentary cord. Within it, attached to its wall, was a solid body as big as a pin's head. He re-garded the specimen as the dropsical membranes of a blighted embryo.

Dr. EDIS exhibited two Polypi Uteri. The first was the size of a walnut, and intra-uterine. It was removed by torsion with ovum forceps from a woman aged forty-six, who had suffered from severe periodical hæmorrhages for twelve months. The second was a fibroid polypus, as large as a goose's egg, and was removed from the vagina by écraseur.

Dr. WILTSHIRE exhibited two pendulous Cysts from the labia minora. They were removed from different patients and contained translucent fluid. Such cases were extremely rare, and were mentioned by no author except by Schröder.

Dr. BRUNTON showed plaster casts of a Fœtal Head which he had delivered for a neighbouring practitioner. Forceps above the brim, and version, had been tried in vain. He applied his modification of Assalini's forceps, then failing with them, retained them upon the head, amputated the body to gain room, and perforated between the blades.

Dr. GALABIN showed microscopic sections of a Membrane which was periodically discharged in the middle of the intermenstrual interval in a case of cervical endometritis. It consisted of an exudation made up of fibrin and cells, some of which showed a tendency to grow into processes. At the edge was a border of inverted cervical epithelium, which had been brought away with the exudation.

Dr. WILTSHIRE thought the fortnightly exacerbations explicable on the hypothesis of hebdomadal periodicity which pervaded the menstrual function. He knew many cases of fortnightly menorrhagia. Did the specimen show any tendency towards the commencement of epithelial cancer?

ON THE RELATION OF ANTEFLEXION OF THE UTERUS TO DYSMENORRHŒA.

Dr. HERMAN read this paper, the object of which was to inquire as to the correctness of the widely accepted theory that anteflexion causes dysmenorrhœa by leading to nar-rowing or temporary occlusion of the uterine canal at the point of bending. The evidence required to prove this was of two kinds, anatomical and clinical. The anatomical was first considered. First, it had to be shown that in anteflexion the canal was bent at an angle, and that, as figured dia-grammatically in many works, a spur of tissue projected in-wards and blocked up the canal. But in four specimens of anteflexions in London museums the curve was quite gradual; there was no angle, nor dilatation of the uterine cavity. Next, the author had searched in vain for any case of reten-tion of the menstrual blood and dilatation of the uterine cavity, for which no other cause than an anteflexion existed, or of a pelvic hæmatocele, dependent upon stenosis of the uterine canal from anteflexion. The clinical evidence was then discussed. The arguments in favour of the theory fell into four groups :—1. That drawn from the patient's sensa-tions. 2. That drawn from the apparent hindrance to the passage of the uterine sound. The author gave reasons for thinking these arguments inconclusive. 3. That drawn from the frequent association of anteflexion with dysmenorrhœa. The author pointed out that, before concluding from this asso-ciation that the anteflexion is the cause of the dysmenorrhœa, it was necessary to know how often anteflexion occurs without functional disorder of the uterus. He quoted summarised statistics from various other observers, which showed that out of 431 women, anteflexion was present in 185, and the uterus was straight and in the axis of the pelvis only in

153. He had himself examined 102 women, who applied for treatment, not for functional disorders of the uterus, but for local contagious disorders, and in 40 of these he found the uterus markedly anteflexed. Of the 53 in whom the uterus was slightly or not at all bent, in 38 there was little or no pain at the menstrual period, and in 15 severe pain ; but of the 49 in whom there was pronounced anteflexion, in 33 there was little or no pain at the men-strual period, and in 16 severe pain. So slight a difference, the author thought, was practically none. As to the effect of treatment, the author pointed out that dysmenorrhœa with anteflexion was often curable by rest, by vaginal pessaries, by depletion, by incision, or by dilatation of the cervix—remedies which do not straighten the uterus. Benefit following the use of intra-uterine stems might be due to their effect in dilating the canal, in stimulating the uterus, or to the preparatory treatment. In cases in which the first-mentioned kinds of treatment had failed, there was no evidence that intra-uterine stems succeeded. The purport of the paper was summarised in the following propositions : —1. That there is no anatomical evidence that anteflexion causes any hindrance to the escape of menstrual fluid. 2. That there is reason to think that well-marked anteflexion is present in nearly half of all women who have not borne children. 3. That, therefore, it is to be expected that anteflexion and dysmenorrhœa would frequently coincide. 4. That dysmenorrhœa is practically as common when the uterus is straight as when it is anteflexed. 5. That painless menstruation is practically as common when the uterus is anteflexed as when it is not. 6. That when dys-menorrhœa and flexion go together, the severity of the pain bears no relation to the degree of the bending. 7. That dysmenorrhœa associated with anteflexion is frequently cured without straightening the uterus. 8. That there is no evidence that straightening the uterus invariably or even frequently removes dysmenorrhœa which is associated with anteflexion, and in which other methods of cure have been ineffectual. 9. That these facts show that the relation between anteflexion and dysmenorrhœa is not that of cause and effect, but merely that of coincidence.

Dr. GERVIS, after expressing his admiration of the care and ability shown in Dr. Herman's paper, ventured to doubt whether his deductions were valid, even if his facts remained unchallenged. He believed it to be quite possible for even a flexion of the uterus to exist, and yet no obstruction to be produced, provided the calibre of the cervical canal was not intruded upon by the bend. In one of the specimens cited there was no obstruction in the canal, though a very marked curvature was present. It was a question whether it would not be well to recognise a class of cases of antecurvature, as distinct from sharp flexion ; and Dr. Herman's cases of anteflexion without symptoms would mostly belong to these. He still believed that, if there were obstruction to the cervical canal, there would be the symptoms characterising obstructive dysmenorrhœa.

Dr. AVELING asked Dr. Herman what method he had adopted in discovering the amount of displacement, and in distinguishing between anteflexion and anteversion. Also whether the condition of the bladder had been considered in each case ? Dr. Aveling thought anteflexion was the cause of obstruction, resulting not only in dysmenorrhœa, but in sterility.

Dr. HERMAN explained that he estimated the anteflexion by bimanual examination.

Dr. GALABIN thought great credit was due to Dr. Herman for his scientific paper. But, unfortunately, statistical in-quiries always came out in support of the previous opinions of the authors. Dr. Graily Hewitt's recent statistics on the causation of hysteria would, if free from any influence of unconscious bias, demonstrate the extreme importance of anteflexion as completely as Dr. Herman's would, on a similar hypothesis, now demonstrate the contrary. Again, Dr. Emmet had published statistics of many hundreds of cases, from which he inferred that flexion of the body of the uterus was *invariably* associated with pain during the menstrual flow. Dr. Herman had made no distinction between the symptoms of congestive and obstructive dysmenorrhœa. If it were true, as held by Schultze, that permanent straightness of the nulliparous uterus is itself a proof of induration from chronic metritis, Dr. Herman's figures would be quite con-sistent with obstructive dysmenorrhœa being commoner among anteflexed uteri, for congestive dysmenorrhœa might be commoner among the straight. It was contrary to all physiological analogy to expect permanent distension of the uterus from partial obstruction of the canal, for in stricture of the urethra we found not a distended bladder, but a contracted bladder with hypertrophied walls. It was a drawback that the statistics were taken from prostitutes, amongst whom congestive dysmenorrhœa might well so preponderate over obstructive, that all trace of the causation of the latter would be lost when no distinction was made between the symptoms. He thought the four preserved uteri cited, which might be cases of congenital anteflexion, insufficient to prove that anteflexion never caused obstruction. This should be decided by the fresh uterus. If it were suspended in a bottle by the fundus, gravity would diminish the flexion a little, and obliterate any flattening of the canal, even if it existed. It was contrary to his own experience that strongly marked anteflexion existed in nearly 50 per cent. of nulliparous women, but, as Dr. Herman examined only by the bimanual method, his statistics perhaps applied rather to uteri which could be brought into anteflexion by pressure from above.

Dr. HEYWOOD SMITH thought that Dr. Herman had rather exaggerated the description of the uterine canal in anteflexion in saying that there existed a spur of tissue projecting backwards into the canal. The antecurve of the fœtal uterus was shown in a section of the pelvis in the museum of the Hospital for Women. Marion Sims' operation was not intended to straighten the uterus, but to cut a new and straight canal. His explanation of sterility with anteflexion was that the os was tilted forwards, and lifted above the pond of semen that gravitated into the posterior cul-de-sac. In many cases, frequent reposition of the uterus and the passing of a thick sound relieved the dysmenorrhœa. Patients with anteflexion described the pain as preceding the flow, and being of a forcing character, and felt in the hypogastrium.

The PRESIDENT complimented Dr. Herman on the excellence of the method which he had pursued in the study of this subject. It was a great point in his demonstration that the dilated uterus and the spur-like obstruction at the internal os, so frequently depicted, were never seen. No such specimen was described except from imagination, and none was found in museums. Specimens well described showed no dilatation of the uterine cavity and no spur, and he believed there was no obstruction. By statistics, and by a mass of other evidence, Dr. Herman had brought his opinions far nearer to proof than those had done who held other views. Much had been made of the condition of supposed obstruction. Now, a specimen of anteflexion, with complete atresia or closure of the cervical canal, was shown lately to the Society, and in it there was no spur and no dilatation of the uterine cavity. If there was only a small or very contracted passage, there was still room enough for blood to pass freely, not only the few ounces in a few days of a menstrual period, but so much as to let the woman bleed to death in a short time. Along with Dr. Gamgee, he had, some years ago, published a paper in the Journal of Anatomy and Physiology, showing the facility of the passage of blood through capillary canals; and there was much clinical evidence to the same effect.

Dr. HERMAN, in reply, said that he had not disputed the existence of obstructive dysmenorrhœa; but it did not follow that the obstruction was due to flexion. He had stated in his paper the precautions he had taken to prevent any bias due to preconceived opinion in his own mind from affecting the result. Dr. Hewitt's paper only showed that a number of invalids got well under the influence of rest and good diet. Dr. Emmet's statistics did not bear on the question, because he only examined patients who consulted him for some uterine trouble. It was possible that some of those he had himself examined might have dysmenorrhœa induced by their mode of life. Still, if anteflexion caused dysmenorrhœa, there ought to have been a decided preponderance in the frequency of dysmenorrhœa among those whose uteri were anteflexed. In saying that stenosis of the canal should lead to dilatation of the uterine cavity, he had only quoted what was stated and shown diagrammatically in many books; and the words "spur" or "promontory" were not his own, but were used in works of high repute. Theoretically, fluid would flow a little more readily along a straight tube than a curved one, but in the case of the uterus the difference would be infinitesimal. It was

very rarely possible to distinguish congenital from acquired anteflexion. He did not know any way of diagnosing anteflexion so certain as bimanual examination. He did not think that in his cases anteflexion had been produced by the method of examination; if it were so, it was remarkable that his figures agreed so nearly with those of other observers.

OBITUARY.

ALFRED H. McCLINTOCK, M.D. GLASG., LL.D. EDIN., FELLOW AND EX-PRES. R.C.S.I.

OUR readers will have learnt with sad surprise that on Friday, October 21, Dr. McClintock breathed his last. But a few days previously his state was so satisfactory that he was able to be moved from his city residence in Merrion-square, to the seaside at Ballybrack, co. Dublin, and his many friends began to hope that, although complete recovery could not be expected, yet life might be spared, so that for some years to come the beloved father might rest by his fireside, and the amiable and faithful friend might enjoy the pleasures of social life. But God willed it otherwise, and the call went forth—"Well done, good and faithful servant, enter thou into the joy of thy Lord."

Alfred Henry McClintock was the second son of the late Henry McClintock, Esq., of Dundalk. He was born on October 21, 1821, so that he died on the sixtieth anniversary of his birth. At an early age he selected the profession of medicine as his calling in life, and in 1842, when only just of age, he became a Licentiate in Surgery and Midwifery of the Royal College of Surgeons in Ireland. Two years later he graduated as Doctor of Medicine in the University of Glasgow. Not long afterwards he was appointed Assistant-Master in that great school of obstetrics and gynæcology, the Rotunda Lying-in Hospital, Dublin. He was not slow to turn to good account the vast experience gained in the wards of the Hospital, and in 1848 he appeared as the joint author with the late Dr. Samuel Hardy, of Dublin, of "Practical Observations on Midwifery and the Diseases incidental to the Puerperal State." In 1851, when he was Vice-President of the Dublin Obstetrical Society, McClintock contributed to the pages of the Dublin Quarterly Journal of Medical Science a remarkable paper on "Secondary Hæmorrhage after Parturition," which was only one of a brilliant series of valuable contributions to the pages of the same journal.

Three years later he became Master of the Rotunda Hospital, at the exceptionally early age of three-and-thirty. The first few months of his residence in the Hospital were overshadowed by an outbreak of puerperal fever in December, 1854, which lasted until the middle of the following February. This epidemic McClintock described in the nineteenth volume of the Dublin Quarterly Journal, page 454. Of 182 lying-in women admitted between the commencement of December, 1854, and the middle of February, 1855, 38 (that is, 1 in every 5) were unequivocally affected with the symptoms of the disease; while out of these 38 so affected, 17 recovered and 21 died. It is worthy of note that the epidemic subsided coincidently with the rigorous frost of the winter of 1855. One paragraph in this report of the epidemic is specially worth quoting, for it bears testimony to McClintock's character for honest observation and prudent inference. He writes:—"With this impression strong upon my mind I entered upon the task of collecting and arranging the materials which form the substance of this paper, endeavouring to the best of my humble ability to observe closely, to record faithfully, and to infer cautiously."

Professional advancement and honours early awaited the writer of these words. As the years went by he was chosen in succession President of the Dublin Obstetrical Society, President of the Pathological Society of Dublin, and President of the Royal College of Surgeons in Ireland, of which he had become a Fellow in 1844. He was elected an Honorary Fellow of the Obstetrical Society of London, the American Gynæcological Society, the Edinburgh Obstetrical Society, and the North of England Obstetrical Society; and an Honorary Member of the Gynæcological Society of Boston, United States of America. The University of Edinburgh conferred upon him the degree of Doctor of Laws, LL.D., on the occasion of the visit of the British

Medical Association to that city in 1875, and the University of Dublin gave him the Degree of Master in Obstetric Science (Magister in Arte Obstetriciâ), honoris causâ, in 1877.

In this latter year he contributed to the *British Medical Journal* a highly important paper on "Fœtal Therapeutics." At this time he was also engaged in editing, for the New Sydenham Society, an edition of "Smellie's Midwifery," Mr. Jonathan Hutchinson, the able Secretary of the Society, having written to him in May, 1875, a very courteous letter, asking him, on the part of the Council, to undertake the task. If we may be allowed here to express an opinion of the work, we would say that it owes its chief value, from a modern point of view, to the editor's careful annotations, whether critical, explanatory, or historical.

But hard work was now beginning to tell on the trusted and busy practitioner. For many years an affection of the heart was known to exist, and the symptoms became aggravated in the beginning of 1880, so that Dr. McClintock had to give up work. He went to Canada, where he remained for several months, at last returning home much better, but not well. On the first Monday in June, in the present year, he signalised his vacation of the Presidential Chair of the Royal College of Surgeons by entertaining at a *recherché* breakfast the President, Council, and members of the Irish Medical Association. His last public act was to preside over the Section of Midwifery at the recent International Medical Congress in London. How well he fulfilled the duties of that arduous post, and with what laurels he was crowned!

On Friday, September 2, Dr. McClintock left his house in Merrion-square, as usual, to visit his patients. While actually paying a visit, he noticed himself that he had lost the power of speech. He returned to his carriage, and drove home. Shortly afterwards, a more decided stroke of paralysis left him speechless and partly hemiplegic. There is a touching pathos in an incident which occurred some days afterwards. His medical attendants, visiting him, expressed their gratification at some marked symptoms of improvement in his state. He shook his head, and, asking by signs for writing materials, with his left hand he traced the word "*Death*" upon the page. Alas, that his prognosis should have been so soon verified! The improvement, it is true, went on for a few weeks; but then came suppression of urine, and, after a few days of suffering, rest in death.

　　　　　　　　　　　　　　　　J. W. M.

HEMERALOPIA IN DISEASES OF THE LIVER.—In an article on this curious affection, in the *Archives Générales de Médecine*, Dr. Parinaud comes to these conclusions:—Hemeralopia in affections of the liver exhibits itself ordinarily by crises of variable duration, under the influence of accessory determining causes. It is special to chronic diseases, and particularly to cirrhosis. It becomes developed after the disease of the liver has continued for some time. It does not seem to be produced by icterus, but by a special change in the blood resulting from disturbance of the hepatic function. It is of serious signification. It is probable that in the hemeralopia termed essential, the ocular disturbance depends, as in affections of the liver, upon change in the blood, which is not that of common anemia, and that this change acts on the organ of sight by modifying the secretion of the visual purple.—*Gaz. des Hôp.*, October 8.

ARSENIATE OF SODA IN PSORIASIS.—Dr. Guibout prescribes 1 centigramme of the arseniate with 1 gramme 60 centigrammes of the extract of gentian, dividing into ten pills, of which from two to three are given at each of the three meals; or, instead of the pills, from 1 to 2 tablespoonfuls of the arseniate, 10 centigrammes in 500 grammes of distilled water, may be taken at each meal. The arseniate is to be continued in some forms of the disease for from six to twelve months after the disappearance of the eruption. Repeated purgatives must be given, and if the patient is robust, alkaline preparations, while if he is weak and anemic, tonics and preparations of iron must be resorted to. As an external application, 10 to 15 parts of pyrogallic acid to 100 of lard may be employed, soapy baths being used every two or three days for cleansing the skin. Juniper oil (*l'huile de cade*) used in frictions twice a day may be substituted for the baths. The treatment should be completed with alkaline baths.—*Union Méd.*, October 20.

VITAL STATISTICS OF LONDON.

Week ending Saturday, October 22, 1881.

BIRTHS.

Births of Boys, 1353; Girls, 1228; Total, 2581.
Corrected weekly average in the 10 years 1871-80, 2539·8.

DEATHS.

	Males.	Females.	Total.
Deaths during the week	842	744	1554
Weekly average of the ten years 1871-80, corrected to increased population ...	781·7	721·0	1504·7
Deaths of people aged 90 and upwards ...	...	...	53

DEATHS IN SUB-DISTRICTS FROM EPIDEMICS.

	Enumerated Population, 1881 (unrevised).	Small-pox.	Measles.	Scarlet Fever.	Diphtheria.	Whooping-cough.	Typhus.	Enteric (or Typhoid) Fever.	Simple continued Fever.	Diarrhœa.
West ...	668993	1	5	8	2	6	1	7	3	2
North ...	905677	4	13	12	8	8	1	13	1	2
Central ...	281793	...	1	5	3	2	...	11	...	1
East ...	692530	2	1	8	3	13	1	7	1	4
South ...	1265579	7	10	15	5	10	2	15	4	8
Total ...	3814571	14	30	48	21	39	5	53	9	18

METEOROLOGY.

From Observations at the Greenwich Observatory.

Mean height of barometer	29·811 in.
Mean temperature	48·7°
Highest point of thermometer	54·5°
Lowest point of thermometer	38·1°
Mean dew-point temperature	39·8°
General direction of wind	E.
Whole amount of rain in the week	0·32 in.

BIRTHS and DEATHS Registered and METEOROLOGY during the Week ending Saturday, Oct. 22, in the following large Towns:—

Cities and boroughs (Municipal boundaries except for London.)	Estimated Population to middle of the year 1881.*	Persons to an Acre.	Births Registered during the week ending Oct. 22.	Deaths Registered during the week ending Oct. 22.	Highest during the Week.	Lowest during the Week.	Weekly Mean of Daily Mean Values.	Weekly Mean of Daily Mean Values. (Cent.)	In Inches.	In Centimetres.
London ...	3829751	50·2	2681	1586	54·5	38·2	43·7	6·50	0·52	1·31
Brighton ...	107984	45·9	81	43	53·5	33·0	45·4	6·43	0·92	2·34
Portsmouth ...	128335	28·6	106	53	...	...	...	...	...	...
Norwich ...	88633	11·8	77	27	...	...	...	...	...	...
Plymouth ...	75282	54·0	38	24	57·8	33·9	47·3	8·50	0·71	1·80
Bristol ...	207140	48·5	151	62	54·0	30·1	42·5	5·84	0·21	0·53
Wolverhampton ...	75084	22·4	64	25	50·4	28·3	39·9	4·39	0·83	2·12
Birmingham ...	402296	47·9	288	175	...	...	...	...	...	...
Leicester ...	123120	88·3	98	50	50·2	27·5	41·4	5·22	0·96	2·44
Nottingham ...	189035	18·9	119	64	52·8	27·2	42·1	5·82	0·62	1·57
Liverpool ...	553988	106·3	435	307	...	...	...	...	...	...
Manchester ...	341289	79·5	282	135	...	...	...	...	...	...
Salford ...	177760	34·4	149	84	...	...	...	...	...	...
Oldham ...	112176	24·0	76	54	...	...	...	...	...	...
Bradford ...	194037	25·5	111	63	50·8	29·4	41·6	5·34	1·40	3·56
Leeds ...	310490	14·4	189	99	53·0	29·0	43·2	6·72	0·92	0·66
Sheffield ...	288621	14·5	231	110	53·0	29·0	42·8	5·91	1·81	3·34
Hull ...	155181	42·7	134	89	48·0	29·0	41·0	5·00	0·51	1·30
Sunderland ...	120788	42·2	103	45	60·0	35·0	46·5	8·06	0·54	1·37
Newcastle-on-Tyne ...	145675	27·1	97	50	...	...	...	...	...	...
Total of 20 large English Towns ...	7656775	38·0	4518	2047	60·0	26·2	44·9	6·26	0·73	1·85

* These figures are the numbers enumerated (but subject to revision) in April last, raised to the middle of 1881 by the addition of a quarter of a year's increase, calculated at the rate that prevailed between 1871 and 1881.

At the Royal Observatory, Greenwich, the mean reading of the barometer last week was 29·81 in. The highest reading was 30·24 in. on Monday morning, and the lowest 29·13 in. by the end of the week.

NEW INVENTIONS AND IMPROVEMENTS.

TAPPING AND A NEW ANTISEPTIC TROCAR.

*(By John Ward Cousins, M.D. Lond., F.R.C.S., Surgeon to
the Royal Plymouth Hospital.)*

It was an old-established rule in surgery, long before the
introduction of antiseptic treatment, that every precaution
ought to be taken in all tapping and exploring operations to
prevent atmospheric contact with the interior of the cyst or
cavity. The old-fashioned trocar is not well adapted for
this purpose. Some years ago I used a flexible tube attached
to the canula, and through its side I introduced the trocar,
so that on its withdrawal the perforation was closed by the
elasticity of the tube. This, however, was a very clumsy
proceeding.

The syphon trocar invented by Mr. Charles R. Thompson,
of Westerham, has been very generally employed of late
years, and a modification of it has been introduced by Mr.
Spencer Wells for the purposes of ovariotomy. The protection against the admission of air depends wholly upon the
action of the piston, which must fit the canula accurately and
also be well greased so that its action may be easy and secure.

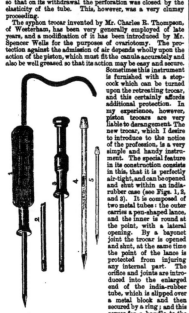

Sometimes this instrument
is furnished with a stop-
cock which can be turned
upon the retreating trocar,
and this certainly affords
additional protection. In
my experience, however,
piston trocars are very
liable to derangement. The
new trocar, which I desire
to introduce to the notice
of the profession, is a very
simple and handy instru-
ment. The special feature
in its construction consists
in this, that it is perfectly
air-tight, and can be opened
and shut within an india-
rubber case (see Figs. 1, 2,
and 3). It is composed of
two metal tubes : the outer
carries a pen-shaped lance,
and the inner is round at
the point, with a lateral
opening. By a bayonet
joint the trocar is opened
and shut, at the same time
the point of the lance is
protected from injuring
any internal part. The
orifice and joints are introduced into the enlarged
end of the india-rubber
tube, which is slipped over
a metal block and then
secured by a ring ; and this
serves for a handle to the
instrument. It is adapted for all kinds of tapping ; it
can be used also for exploring or injecting purposes ; or
it can be very readily attached to the exhausting apparatus of the aspirator. The trocar is manufactured by
Messrs. Arnold and Sons, of West Smithfield, in three convenient sizes. I have now employed it in every variety of
operation, and with special advantage in cases of paracentesis
thoracis. The opening and closing action within the india-
rubber case is very readily accomplished, and the necessary
movement can be easily performed by anyone after a little
attention to the construction of the instrument.

Fig. 4 represents a simple form of exploring tube to which
an india-rubber bag can be adjusted. The capillary drainage-
tube, Fig. 5, is intended for the treatment of anasarca ; it
can be left in the subcutaneous tissue without any risk of
injury to the deeper parts, and its position can be altered
without another puncture of the skin.

THE Würzburg University will next year celebrate
its 400th anniversary.

MEDICAL NEWS.

APOTHECARIES' HALL, LONDON.—The following gentle-
men passed their examination in the Science and Practice of
Medicine, and received certificates to practise, on Thursday,
October 20 :—

Cheyne, Robert, Nottingham-place, W.
Coles, William James, George-street, Croydon.
Marshall, John Gissell, Wallingford, Berks.
Neligan, James Charles, Ballina, co. Mayo, Ireland.

The following gentlemen also on the same day passed their
primary professional examination :—

Greenway, John Henry, Guy's Hospital.
Pryce, Thomas Davies, St. Bartholomew's Hospital.
Sarzana, Ettore, St. Bartholomew's Hospital.

APPOINTMENTS.

** The Editor will thank gentlemen to forward to the
Publishing-office, as early as possible, information as to
all new Appointments that take place.

BIRD, ASHLEY, M.R.C.S., L.S.A. Lond.—Assistant Medical Officer to the
City of London Infirmary, Bow-road, E.

BIRTHS.

CASSAN.—On October 25, at Gainsborough, the wife of Theodore Cassan,
L.R.C.P., M.R.C.S., of a daughter.

CORFIELD.—On October 19, at 10, Bolton-row, Mayfair, the wife of Professor Corfield, M.D., of a daughter.

CRIGHTON.—On October 22, at 3, Cambridge-villas, Twickenham, the wife
of George C. Crichton, M.B., L.R.C.S., of a son.

DAVIDSON.—On October 14, at Coventry, the wife of Charles Davidson,
M.D., of a daughter.

GROSS.—On October 15, at Melksham, Wilts, the wife of S. Gross, M.D.,
F.R.C.S., Staff Surgeon R.N. (retired), of a son.

MANDERS.—On October 17, at Agincourt House, Yorktown, Surrey, the
wife of Horace Manders, F.R.C.S., of a son.

SCOTT.—On October 25, at Shirley Lodge, Shirley, Hants, the wife of E.
R. Scott, Surgeon-Major A.M.D., of a daughter.

SEXTON.—On October 22, at 6, Almorah-crescent, St. Helier's, Jersey, the
wife of Edward James Sexton, M.D., Bombay Medical Establishment,
of a daughter, stillborn.

MARRIAGES.

HALFORD—SEQUEIRA.—On October 19, in London, Henry John Alford,
Esq., to Amelia Louisa, only daughter of H. L. Sequeira, M.R.C.S., of
Jewry-street, Aldgate, and Waltham Lodge, Tulse-hill.

DEATHS.

BARNARDO, ISABELLE FLORENCE, wife of F. A. Ernest Barnardo,
L.K.&Q.C.P., at Birkdale Park, Southport, on October 17, aged 36.

BROTHER, EDWARD BRERETON, Fleet-Surgeon Royal Navy, at the Naval
Hospital, Haslar, on October 20.

DAVIDSON, ELLEN DRANE, wife of Charles Davidson, M.D., at Coventry,
on October 25, in her 30th year.

GILCHRIST, MARY, wife of James Gilchrist, M.D., at Linwood, Dumfries,
on October 17, in her 86th year.

GREENHOW, T. M., M.D., F.R.C.S., at Newton Hall, Potternewton, Leeds,
on October 25, in his 90th year.

HARDING, ROBERT, L.R.C.P., L.R.C.S.I., late Assistant-Surgeon Royal
Navy, at Wellington, New Zealand, on July 3, aged 44.

LYDALL, HAROLD WYKEHAM, son of Wykeham H. Lydall, M.D., at
19, Mecklenburg-square, on October 24, aged 3 months.

VACANCIES.

BIRMINGHAM GENERAL DISPENSARY.—Resident Surgeon. Candidates must
be registered, and possess both a medical and surgical qualification.
Applications, together with original testimonials and certificates of
registration, to be sent to Alex. Forrest, Secretary, on or before
November 14.

BRISTOL GENERAL HOSPITAL.—House-Surgeon. Candidates must be
members of the College of Surgeons of London, Edinburgh, Glasgow,
or Dublin, and also Licentiates of the Apothecaries' Company of London
or Dublin, or possess some other recognised medical qualification. Applications, enclosing testimonials of good moral character and ability, with
certificate of registration, to be sent to the Secretary, on or before
November 5.

EAST SUSSEX, HASTINGS, AND ST. LEONARDS INFIRMARY, HASTINGS.—
Assistant-Surgeon. Candidates must be fellows or members of the
Royal College of Surgeons of London, Dublin, or Edinburgh. Applications, with testimonials, to be sent to William J. Gant, Secretary, not
later than November 14.

EVELINA HOSPITAL FOR SICK CHILDREN, SOUTHWARK-BRIDGE-ROAD, S.E.—
Physician. *(For particulars see Advertisement.)*

ROYAL PIMLICO DISPENSARY, 104, BUCKINGHAM PALACE-ROAD, W.—Medical
Officer. Candidates must reside in the district. Applications and testimonials to be sent to W. C. Meates, Secretary, at the Dispensary, on or
before November 7.

SOUTH DEVON AND EAST CORNWALL HOSPITAL, PLYMOUTH.—House-
Surgeon. Candidates must be duly qualified. Applications, with testimonials, to be sent to J. Walter Wilson, Hon. Sec., on or before Nov. 7.

UNION AND PAROCHIAL MEDICAL SERVICE.

APPOINTMENTS.

Barrow-upon-Soar Union.—John William Sellers, L.R.C.S.&P. Edin., to the Barrow-upon-Soar District.

Liverpool Parish.—St. David G. Walters, L.R.C.P., L.R.C.S. Edin., as Assistant Medical Officer at the Brownlow-hill Workhouse.

Nantwich Union.—Edward Potts, M.R.C.S. Eng., L.S.A., to the Tarporley District.

Newtown and Llanidloes Union.— Daniel Ferguson, L.R.C.S. Edin., L.R.C.P. Edin., to the Llanwnog District.

Warminster Union.—Frederick J. Flower, M.R.C.S. Eng., L.S.A., to the Warminster and Corsley Districts.

CONVALESCENCE OF CONTINUED FEVER.—Dr. Braive, in his dissertation on this subject, comes to these conclusions: —1. The pulse and the temperature approach the normal; but still, the pulse sometimes remains frequent, and that for a long time. 2. The weight of the body is constantly on the increase; and wherever we find it diminishing or remaining stationary we have reason to fear some accident, and must search out for its cause and nature. 3. The muscular force increases daily in a constant and regular manner. 4. Urea is excreted in a large quantity during confirmed convalescence, so that it may sometimes be double the weight of that excreted in the normal conditions. When convalescence is nearly completed the quantity diminishes, more and more approaching the physiological condition.—*Gaz. des Hop.*

EPIDEMIOLOGICAL SOCIETY OF LONDON.—The following is a list of the officers and other members of Council for the session 1881-82:—*President:* George Buchanan, M.D., F.R.C.P. *Honorary Vice-Presidents:* The Earl of Shaftesbury, K.G.; Right Hon. Lord Mount-Temple; Edwin Chadwick, Esq., C.B. *Vice-Presidents:* Gavin Milroy, M.D., F.R.C.P.; Sir William Jenner, Bart., K.C.B., M.D., D.C.L., F.R.S., Physician-in-Ordinary to Her Majesty the Queen; Henry W. Acland, M.D., F.R.S., Regius Professor of Medicine in the University of Oxford; J. W. Reid, M.D., Director-General Navy Medical Department; William Farr, M.D., D.C.L., F.R.S.; Sir William Muir, K.C.B., M.D., Director-General Army Medical Department; John Simon, Esq., C.B., D.C.L., F.R.S.; Sir Thomas Watson, Bart., M.D., F.R.S.; Benjamin W. Richardson, M.D., F.R.S.; Robert Lawson, Esq., Inspector-General of Hospitals, Royal Army (retired); Sir William R. E. Smart, K.C.B., K.I.H., M.D., R.N., Inspector-General of Fleets and Hospitals (retired); J. Netten Radcliffe, Esq.; John Murray, M.D., Surgeon-General (retired); Sir Joseph Fayrer, K.C.S.I., M.D., LL.D., F.R.S., Q.H.P. *Treasurer:* R. Thorne Thorne, M.B., F.R.C.P., 45, Inverness-terrace, W. *General Secretaries:* Shirley F. Murphy, 158, Camden-road, N.W.; G. C. Henderson, M.D., 121, Gower-street, W.C. *Secretary for Navy:* Walter Dickson, M.D., R.N., Medical Officer to the Hon. Board of Customs, 14, Trinity-square, Tower-hill, E.C. *Secretary for Army:* Robert Lawson, Esq., Inspector-General of Hospitals (retired). *Foreign and Colonial Secretaries:* Germany and Russia, Dr. Collie; Sweden, Norway, and Denmark; Dr. Charles Fredk. Moore; Portugal and the Brazils, Dr. Donnett, R.N.; East Indies, Dr. John Murray; West Indies and South America, Dr. G. C. Henderson; China and Australia, Dr. Squire; Indian Ocean and East Africa, Dr. J. Christie; North America, Dr. Joseph Ewart. *Other Members of Council:* Robert Cory, M.D.; W. H. Corfield, M.D.; Edwin Haward, M.D.; Sir A. D. Home, K.C.B., V.C., M.D.; Norman Chevers, M.D.; J. Burdon Sanderson, M.D., F.R.S.; Hermann Weber, M.D.; Surgeon-General C. A. Gordon, C.B., M.D., Q.H.P.

FRACTURES IN HEMIPLEGIA.—In a communication to the Paris Hospital Society, Dr. Debove observed that in his practice at the Bicêtre he had frequent occasion to see fractures in the subjects of hemiplegia, these fractures always occurring on the hemiplegic side, there being every reason to believe that changes took place in such cases in the osseous tissue, rendering it more fragile. In one case of chronic hemiplegia, he found that not only the fractured bone itself, but all the bones on the same side, had undergone such change. They were less heavy than on the sound side, the medullary canal was larger, and the substance of the diaphysis was less compact. Examined histologically, the Haversian canals were found much dilated and the bone porous. Chemical examination also shows that the diaphysis contains a larger quantity of fat. These fractures usually consolidate rapidly, the callus being somewhat more voluminous.—*Gaz. des Hop.*, October 20.

NOTES, QUERIES, AND REPLIES.

He that questioneth much shall learn much.—Bacon.

An Old F.R.C.S.—According to the last published calendar there appear to be 1210 Fellows, of whom 573 obtained the distinction by examination. The annual election takes place the first Thursday in July.

A Governor of the Hospital.—You will find a very interesting letter in the *Daily News* of about the middle of June last from Mr. Charles Hawkins, in which he states that the cost of treating hospital patients, which in 1867 amounted to £4 17s. 9d., increased last year (1880) to £6 17s. 3d.

Medical Acts Commission.—We hope shortly to give you the desired information.

A Teacher.—Perhaps you refer to the observation of Charles Dickens, that—"we hear sometimes of an action for damages against the unqualified medical practitioner who has deformed a broken limb in pretending to heal it; but what of the hundreds of thousands of minds that have been deformed for ever by the incapable pettifoggers who have pretended to form them!" Many teachers, as well as yourself, agree with Mr. Holden.

Dr. McD.—Mr. John Marshall, F.R.S., Vice-President of the College of Surgeons, succeeded the late Mr. Richard Partridge as Professor of Anatomy in the Royal Academy. The Professorships of the Academy are held for a period of five years, subject to reappointment.

Extraordinary Longevity.—The obituary of the *Times*, of the 24th instant, contained some remarkable illustrations of prolonged existence in nine persons, viz., six ladies and three gentlemen whose united ages amounted to 784 years, giving an average of 87 years and more than one month to each. As usual, the fair sex took the lead, the oldest having arrived at the great age of 98 years, the youngest of the same sex being 80. Of the gentlemen the oldest was 91 and the youngest 84 years of age. The following were the respective ages, viz., 80, 83, 84, 85, two at 85, two at 91, and one at 98. The same obituary recorded the deaths of eight nonagenarians, averaging 74 years and rather more than four months. On the 18th inst. was interred, in the churchyard of Hockham, Norfolk, a well-known and respectable man known as "Tinker Joe, the costermonger," who had arrived at the patriarchal age of 112 years. He was followed to his grave by a large number of his sons, daughters, grandchildren, and great-grandchildren, and friends from all parts of the county. The coffin-plate bore the following inscription:—"Joseph Ashton, died October 8, 1881, aged 112 years." He was never known to have a day's illness, and to the end was in the full use of his mental powers. On leaving the grave, the rector, the Rev. J. Spurgin, said: "Peace be to thee, memorable old friend."

J. G. G., M.D.—The Swiney Lectureship in Geology is tenable for five years, and is restricted to Doctors of Medicine of the University of Edinburgh.

Dr. Williams.—The late Mr. George Langstaff's collection has been for many years in the Museum of the College of Surgeons. The Council gave Mr. Bransby Cooper £1500 for the museum of his uncle, the well-known Sir Astley Cooper.

The Sea Shell Mission.—This Mission continues unostentatiously to prosecute its endeavours to brighten the hours of many a poor sick child in the metropolis: 1600 boxes of shells have now been sent to as many poor sick children. In addition 900 scrap-books have been prepared by the friends of the Mission, and sent to amuse as many weary children.

T. T. N., Bloomsbury.—Hospital nursing reform has been actively going on in England over twenty years, in Scotland about eleven, and in Ireland during the past five or six years. There are about four hundred appointments open, in the United Kingdom, in connexion with the medical charities alone, for nurses, varying in value from £35 to £150 per annum, exclusive of residence, board, etc. The authorities of the Nightingale fund find that about 80 per cent. of their probationers ultimately continue as trained nurses.

Medical Adventurers, America.—A lady at Long Branch, says the *Boston Courier*, died recently from the effects of eighteen bottles of anti-fat medicine which she had taken in ten months. This is one case that has been brought to light; probably hundreds of others have committed suicide in a similar manner; and there are thousands to-day who are shortening their lives by taking similar compounds. The people who make these mixtures and put them upon the market ought to be reached by the law in some way. We forbid druggists to sell poison without a physician's recipe, and yet allow adventurers and quacks of all descriptions to offer "anti-fat" and "anti-lean" preparations which poison the blood, and bring in most cases death to their customers!

The Remaining Wing of Old St. Thomas's Hospital.—It is proposed to convert these premises into baths and washhouses for the parish of St. George the Martyr, Southwark. Negotiations are now going forward which are likely to result in the purchase of the buildings by the Vestry, and their immediate adaptation for public baths and washhouses.

A Sea-Water Supply at Newcastle-on-Tyne.—The Town Council have decided to apply for Parliamentary powers to bring salt water into the borough from the sea at Whitby for sanitary and other purposes. The estimated cost is £50,000.

The West of Scotland Convalescent Seaside Homes, Dunoon.—By the twelfth annual report these Homes for the past year had been unprecedentedly prosperous. They had been in active operation since August, 1869, and had from the first been a great success. The total cost of the new wing was £7985 16s. 9d. Of that sum £4048 11s. 6d. remained a debt. The ordinary revenue had been £4217 8s. 5d., showing a marked increase on any previous year. The total expenditure for the same period was £3613 17s. 11d. The industrial classes had subscribed £1452 15s. 2d. It is expected that the proceeds of the contemplated bazaar, to be held in St. Andrew's Halls in March next on behalf of these Homes, will entirely wipe away the debt of £4040 11s. 6d.

Suicides, France.—Recently published statistics show an increase of suicides of not less than 78 per cent. From 1851 to 1856 the annual average was 3639, or one suicide for 9823 inhabitants, while in the latest return the annual number is 6496, or one suicide for 5161 inhabitants.

Cremation Abroad.—At Copenhagen, at the last meeting of the Society for Cremation, the Secretary-General announced that the Society numbered 1400 members, among whom were eighty-three distinguished physicians and many well-known Protestant ministers. The system adopted does not cost more than from 5s. to 7s. each burial. In Italy, as the result of a series of lectures in various capitals of Europe by Dr. Pimi, new societies have been formed, which now number nine in all Italy, and new crematories have been constructed in Rome, Varese, Pavia, Cremona, and Leghorn. In Hungary also measures have been taken to establish societies for cremation.

Quis.—We imagine you refer to Sir Philip Perrin's address to his critics—

"Think, not, O man, who dost this book review,
I fancy all within is good and new;
Much it contains has been already said,
And may perchance be elsewhere better read."

Dax.—1. The expenditure of the country upon imported dairy produce during 1879 has been estimated at no less than £11,000,000. 2. The powers given to inspectors of markets and police-constables, acting under the authority of the municipal authorities and justices of the peace, to inspect milk *in transitu* between the purveyor and purchaser are under the provisions of the Contagious Diseases (Animals) Act, 1878. 3. Butterine and oleo-margarine, we believe, are synonymous terms. Many convictions have already taken place for selling oleo-margarine as butter under the Sale of Food and Drugs Act.

In Memoriam.—A new window to the memory of Dr. W. Hall Ryott has just been placed in Thirsk Church, at the foot of which is the following inscription:—This window is erected by numerous friends to perpetuate the memory of William Hall Ryott, for many years a most able and beloved medical practitioner in this town."

Voluntary Sanitary Aid.—The freedom of the town of Hastings from infectious diseases for the past eleven years is noteworthy. This immunity, it is stated, is largely due to the efforts of the Sanitary Aid Association—a voluntary organisation of which Sir Thomas Brassey, M.P., is President. In connexion with this Society, a meeting was held in the town last week, at which Mrs. Johnstone—who was the originator of the Association—read a paper on the subject. Sir Thomas Brassey, who occupied the chair, in course of some highly commendatory observations on the good work Mrs. Johnstone had done in the borough by promoting sanitary economies in the secluded houses of the poor, and the self-sacrifice it had imposed upon her, spoke of the importance to a town like Hastings of maintaining a reputation for its sanitary condition.

Elephant's Milk.—According to Dr. Charles Doremus (America), the milk of the elephant is the richest that he has ever examined. It contains less water and more butter and sugar than any other, and has a very agreeable taste and odour.

Contravening the Licensing Act.—A manager of a local club has been fined by the Hampstead magistrates £20, with the alternative of a month's imprisonment, for having consented to the sale of intoxicating liquors on unlicensed premises after two previous convictions under the Licensing Act. Similar convictions for contravening the Act of Parliament on the part of "club" *employés* demonstrate that these offences are increasing.

PERIODICALS AND NEWSPAPERS RECEIVED—

Lancet—British Medical Journal—Medical Press and Circular—Berliner Klinische Wochenschrift—Centralblatt für Chirurgie—Gazette des Hopitaux—Gazette Médicale—Le Progrès Médical—Bulletin de l'Académie de Médecine—Pharmaceutical Journal—Wiener Medizinische Wochenschrift—Centralblatt für die Medizinischen Wissenschaften—Revue Médicale—Gazette Hebdomadaire—National Board of Health Bulletin, Washington—Nature—Occasional Notes—Deutsche Medicinal-Zeitung—Boston Medical and Surgical Journal—Louisville Medical News—Oil and Drug News—Arrowsmith's Christmas Annual, 1881—Revue D'Hygiène—Brain—Australian Medical Journal—União Medica—Journal of Anatomy and Physiology—Christian Commonwealth.

BOOKS, ETC., RECEIVED—

The Sanitary Chronicles of the Parish of St. Marylebone—A Contribution to the History of Hygrometers, by G. J. Symons, F.R.S.—Annual Report of the West Cheshire Provident Dispensary, Birkenhead—Histology, by Thomas E. Satterthwaite, M.D.—Diseases of the Chest, etc., by E. Fletcher Ingals, A.M., M.D.—Scheme for a Central Fish Market for London, by J. J. Cayley, J. Boyes, and H. H. Bridgman, A.R.I.B.A.—Études de Thérapeutique, par le Docteur A. Luton—Report on the Health, etc., of Kensington, September 11 to October 8, 1881—The Use of the Ambulance in Civil Practice, by Reginald Harrison, F.R.C.S.

COMMUNICATIONS have been received from—

Dr. M. Charteris, Glasgow; Mr. Lawson Tait, Birmingham; Dr. Lucas, Quettah; Mr. Morgan, London; The Registrar of the Apothecaries' Hall, London; Dr. McCall Anderson, Glasgow; Dr. Warner, London; Mr. Pridgin Teale, Leeds; Mr. Arthur Durham, London; Dr. Henry Ashby, Manchester; The Secretary of the Anthropological Institute, London; Dr. Thomas Oliver, Newcastle; Mr. R. J. Godlee, London; Dr. W. S. Greenfield, Edinburgh; Dr. Herman, London; Dr. Goodhart, London; Dr. Creighton, London; Mr. J. Hutchinson, London; The Sub-Librarian of the Obstetrical Society of London; Mr. J. Chatto, London; The Honorary Secretary of the Medical Society of London; The Honorary Secretary of the Pathological Society of London; Dr. F. Churchill, London; Dr. Mickle, Bow; The Secretary of the Obstetrical Society of London; Mr. Brookes, London; Dr. G. Johnson, London; The Sanitary Commissioner, Punjaub, India; Mr. Morris, London; The Secretary of the Midland Medical Society; Dr. Harley, London; Dr. Guye, Amsterdam; Mr. Stone, London; Dr. Anningson, Cambridge; Mr. W. R. Thomas, Sheffield; Dr. Anderson, London; The Secretary of the London Sanitary Protection Association; Dr. Ross, Manchester; Mr. Gardiner Brown, London; The Secretary of the Harveian Society, London; Mr. T. Chavasse, Birmingham; Dr. Druitt, London; Messrs. Walsh and Co., London; Dr. Duncanson, Edinburgh; The Secretary of the Local Government Board, London; The Secretary of the Sanitary Assurance Association, London; Dr. G. Buchanan, Glasgow; Mr. W. Whitehead, Manchester.

APPOINTMENTS FOR THE WEEK.

October 29. Saturday (this day).

Operations at St. Bartholomew's, 1½ p.m.; King's College, 1½ p.m.; Royal Free, 2 p.m.; Royal London Ophthalmic, 11 a.m.; Royal Westminster Ophthalmic, 1½ p.m.; St. Thomas's, 1½ p.m.; London, 2 p.m.

31. *Monday.*

Operations at the Metropolitan Free, 2 p.m.; St. Mark's Hospital for Diseases of the Rectum, 2 p.m.; Royal London Ophthalmic, 11 a.m.; Royal Westminster Ophthalmic, 1½ p.m.

Medical Society of London, 8½ p.m. The President (Dr. Broadbent) will exhibit a Case of Paralysis of the Seventh, Eighth, and Ninth Nerves, with Atrophy of the Muscles affected. Dr. Churton (of Leeds), 1. "On Two Cases of Aneurism of the Left Ventricle"; 2. "Notes of a Case of Primary Dilatation of Tricuspid Orifice"; 3. "On a Case of Shedding of the Epidermis of the Sole of the Foot following a Quinine Roseola occurring Three Times."

November 1. Tuesday.

Operations at Guy's, 1½ p.m.; Westminster, 2 p.m.; Royal London Ophthalmic, 11 a.m.; Royal Westminster Ophthalmic, 1½ p.m.; West London, 3 p.m.

Pathological Society, 8½ p.m. Specimens: The President—1. Ear of Corn discharged through the Chest; 2. Drawing of Muscæ Volitantes. Mr. Hutchinson—Lupus Lymphaticus. Mr. Eve—Cases of Striped Muscle Tumours connected with the Kidney. Mr. Morris—Longitudinal Fracture of Shaft of Femur. Dr. Dawson Williams—Tumour of Kidney chiefly composed of Muscular Fibre. Dr. Isambard Owen—Necrosis of Skull-cap after a Burn. Mr. Pearce Gould—1. Absence of One Half of Cerebellum; 2. Abscess in Head of Tibia. Dr. Norman Moore—Malignant Disease of Kidney following Renal Calculus. Dr. Broadbent—Remarkable Thickening of Pericardium. Dr. Samuel West—Extra-Uterine Fœtation.

2. *Wednesday.*

Operations at University College, 2 p.m.; St. Mary's, 1¼ p.m.; Middlesex, 1 p.m.; London, 2 p.m.; St. Bartholomew's, 1½ p.m.; Great Northern, 2 p.m.; Samaritan, 2½ p.m.; King's College (by Mr. Lister), 2 p.m.; Royal London Ophthalmic, 11 a.m.; Royal Westminster Ophthalmic, 1½ p.m.; St. Thomas's, 1½ p.m.; St. Peter's Hospital for Stone, 2 p.m.; National Orthopædic, Great Portland-street, 10 a.m.

Epidemiological Society, 8 p.m. Inaugural Address by the President (Dr. Buchanan), "On Aids to Epidemiological Knowledge." Dr. G. C. Henderson, "On the Progress of Zymotic Micro-pathology."

Obstetrical Society, 8 p.m. Dr. J. Matthews Duncan, "On Shortness of the Cord as a Cause of Obstruction to the Natural Progress of Labour." N. W. Jastreban (St. Petersburg), "On the Normal and Pathological Anatomy of the Ganglion Cervicale Uteri."

3. *Thursday.*

Operations at St. George's, 1 p.m.; Central London Ophthalmic, 1 p.m.; Royal Orthopædic, 2 p.m.; University College, 2 p.m.; Royal London Ophthalmic, 11 a.m.; Royal Westminster Ophthalmic, 1½ p.m.; Hospital for Diseases of the Throat, 2 p.m.; Hospital for Women, 2 p.m.; Charing-cross, 2 p.m.; London, 2 p.m.; North-West London, 2½ p.m.

Harveian Society, 8½ p.m. Mr. Edmund Owen, "On the Treatment of Joint-Affections in Childhood."

4. *Friday.*

Operations at Central London Ophthalmic, 2 p.m.; Royal London Ophthalmic, 11 a.m.; South London Ophthalmic, 2 p.m.; Royal Westminster Ophthalmic, 1½ p.m.; St. George's (ophthalmic operations), 1¼ p.m.; Guy's, 1½ p.m.; St. Thomas's (ophthalmic operations), 2 p.m.

PATHOLOGY, PAST AND PRESENT.

AN INAUGURAL ADDRESS

Delivered in the University of Edinburgh, October 26, 1881.

By J. W. S. GREENFIELD, M.D., F.R.C.P. Lond.,

Professor of General Pathology, University of Edinburgh.

(Concluded from page 514.)

GOING back to the standpoint, that pathology is the investigation of deranged *life*, of abnormal *living* processes, it will be obvious to you that morbid anatomy alone, even combined with histology and chemistry, cannot be our guide beyond a certain point, that knowledge limited to structure cannot serve to show us fully how function and living action are affected. In some cases, indeed, our present morbid anatomy fails us entirely, as in the case of epilepsy or of typhus fever ; though we hope with better methods to discover their organic cause. But even in the simplest cases, where our induction seems to be a direct one from anatomical changes, we find that we are in reality presupposing a knowledge of function. Take, for example, the simple case of impaction of a calculus in the ureter. By simple mechanical pressure of the pent-up urine, the pelvis and calyces dilate, the kidney substance gives way, and gradually atrophies, and at last remains as a sort of shell of tissue, which for all intents and purposes of kidney-function is effete. Surely, you will say, morbid anatomy shows us all this at a glance. But you have assumed a knowledge of the function of the kidney in secreting urine, and the possibility of its partially continuing its functions for a time, even when the outflow of urine is checked. And if you go more deeply, and inquire what are the subsequent intimate changes in the structure of the organ, and what the effects upon the system, you will find that you are involved in a multitude of complicated pathological problems. And if you would trace back the disease to its source you must determine what constitutional causes led to the formation of the calculus, by what physical or chemical processes it came to be formed, and why and how it found its present lodgment.

Thus it is that to make morbid anatomy and histology worthy of the name of *pathological* anatomy, we require the knowledge of function and its mechanism. We must know where and how altered structure is connected with perverted function, whether as cause or effect ; and this we owe to physiology and to comparative and experimental pathology. There has been too great a tendency to overlook this vital fact, and to regard the investigation of structure as the be-all and end-all of pathology. It has unfortunately by many been thought enough that we should know the naked-eye and microscopic appearances of diseased organs, without any intelligent idea of how they are brought about, or in what relation they stand to the phenomena of disease. We have sought rather to find in structure the characteristics of disease, than to make it a guide to the understanding of disease. We have been passing through what we may call the slough of histology. For example, the tubercle corpuscle of Lebert, the cancer cell, the giant cell, the micro-cyte, all have had their day as absolute criteria of particular diseases. But I will go further, and say that in a great part of our microscopical work on diseased organs we have been too apt merely to observe visible changes, without paying attention to the more important processes which underlie them. Yet surely this should not be. We must and ought to study structure and chemical composition as thoroughly and deeply as possible, by all the means in our power, but we must not rest there. It is the great merit of Virchow's great work, that, passing by the mere study of structure for structure's sake, he sought to show how the morbid change had been developed, what was its bearing upon living action, and in what way it stood related to normal processes of evolution, growth, and function.

I have said that in great measure we owe this further connecting link between morbid anatomy and pathology

to physiology, comparative pathology, and experimental pathology.

Physiology is the first great guide. Normal development and normal life in all its departments have their imitations in abnormal growth and abnormal life, whether excessive, perverted, or deficient. Transfer some morbid growths to the embryo, and what is disease becomes healthy development. Magnify and transfer the normal secretion of milk, and you shall have, under different conditions, a fatty degeneration. Even inflammation—that great bone of contention—seems to be ranging itself by degrees as a greatly exaggerated physiological process. Indeed, it is by our knowledge of the normal structure, composition, and function of every minutest part that we gain our knowledge of what is disease, and in part of how it is brought about.

Hence it is that every physiological discovery, however minute, becomes of vital importance for the advance of pathology. Many discoveries, which seem of small importance in their physiological aspects, become of great value in the field of pathology.

Pathology, in its turn, enlightens and advances physiology. The subtle processes of disease often reveal normal structure far more fully than the most skilful manipulations of the histologist upon healthy tissues, and follow out the track of dissections 'which no scalpel could trace. Waxy degeneration of the liver, and the course of secondary degenerations in the spinal cord, afford striking examples. So, too, the reactions of disease, aided by simple micro-chemical reagents, serve to distinguish varieties of chemical composition too minute for analysis. Pathology, too, often corrects physiological theory as regards function. It has been well said, that the value of an hypothesis consists, not in explaining the instances which have preceded it, but in standing the test of subsequent instances. Pathological observation has thus often served to demolish hypotheses which had stood the test of instances specially designed to try their strength.

If I were asked what is the present standpoint of pathology, I should unhesitatingly say that it is the physiological, or, if you will, the biological standpoint. In other words, pathology is governed by no theory, and limited by no methods, other than those which equally govern and limit physiology. If a cellular physiology could suffice to explain all the phenomena of healthy life, a cellular pathology might equally serve for disease life. And whatever method or instrument of research is requisite for the full investigations of the phenomena of healthy life in all its manifestations, is equally or still more requisite for studying the phenomena of disease life.

It is from this point of view that the study of clinical medicine and pathological experiment are, in my opinion, the inseparable adjuncts of pathological study. That would be a strange physiology which should conduct its study on dead animals alone, and no less strange a pathology studied only on dead subjects.

The history and course of each particular case, the hereditary antecedents, the physiognomy and conformation, the symptoms and their order and mode of death-production or recovery, are so many phenomena of disease life which we must minutely study in order truly to understand the pathology of each particular case, and rightly to connect structure with function. If we could, after opening the body case, set the body machine going again like a watch, and observe how the wheels interlock, or where the obstruction is, or, separating one part, set that in action, and so piece by piece discover where and how its stoppage came about, we might rest content with morbid anatomy. But the human machine, once run down or stopped, can only be set in action again by the hand of the Creator. We can and must imitate the action by study upon inferior machines ; but precious as such results are, they will not and cannot fulfil all the conditions of the diseased human body.

I have shown how physiology and pathology must go hand in hand, and that the discoveries of physiology are essential to pathology, and this leads me to say a word on the subject of experiments on animals, both physiological and pathological. No one who knows anything of the history of physiology can for a moment question that it is by this means that a large part of our most important knowledge has been gained, and could have been gained in no other way. And no one can study or teach pathology, without constantly referring to and making use of the knowledge thus gained.

He is worse than a coward, who, knowing this, and making use of his knowledge, would claim for himself, whether directly or by implication, any higher moral ground, because he is not personally engaged in such investigations. We cannot, if we would, do without the knowledge acquired for us in this way by physiologists. If we could pull out all that has been built upon this knowledge, our fabric of pathological science would totter and fall, just as would the whole of modern medical science if it could eliminate all that physiologists and surgeons and pharmacologists have gained for the benefit of humanity by experiments on animals.

But pathological experiment has its own proper work. In this country, for the time, it is so seriously hampered that research by its means has become almost impossible. Science does not walk easily in fetters, even if adjusted with the sanction and co-operation of its votaries. It has indeed been objected that we cannot induce in animals the natural processes of disease, and that the results of experiments on animals are fallacious when applied to man. In a certain sense this is true; for, of course, as in all other experiments, we require the use of judgment and discretion. But the statement is very largely grounded on a sort of belief that as man is mentally so far superior to the lower animals he must likewise be widely removed from them in general organisation and structure.

It is by the study of Comparative Pathology that we have come to learn how intimately the processes of disease in the lower animals may resemble those in man, and it is by experiments upon the diseases which they have in common with man that we have come to appreciate those differences in constitution and in reaction to disease which enable us in a great measure to control the results of experiments.

Comparative pathology—that is, the study of the diseases of the several classes of animals, and the study of the same disease in its reactions upon different classes of animals—is to a very large extent a growth of late years. Just as I have remarked that the growth of human morbid anatomy followed in the wake of the progress of normal anatomy, so has the study of comparative pathology followed the development of comparative anatomy, comparative physiology, and comparative embryology.

It is true that a study of diseases of animals has been, to some extent, conjoined with the study of comparative anatomy and physiology, and that Harvey, Hunter, and Jenner were well aware of the valuable information to be derived from a comparison of human with animal pathology. It was well known that some of the lower animals were subject to certain morbid growths and parasites analogous to those which afflict man, such as warts, cancers, and hydatids; and that some animal diseases, such as hydrophobia, could be communicated by inoculation to man. And long before Edward Jenner discovered that cow-pox could be transferred to man, it was suspected that small-pox was primarily an animal disease.

But we have only recently come to understand the full bearing of those endemics and pestilences which have in all ages desolated the animal world, and to see that we stand on common ground with the brute creation in being subject to the same or to analogous plagues, and that by the study of these, under their simpler conditions, we may hope to throw light upon the forms affecting man. It is in this branch of comparative pathology—that relating to infectious and contagious diseases—that we see best the value and importance of experimental pathology, in the direct benefits which it confers on the whole brute creation, as well as upon man. And it is in this field that have been gained some of the most remarkable triumphs of modern pathology, which bid fair to revolutionise the science and treatment of infectious disease.

Gentlemen, I have no idea of giving you now any description, however summary, of the past and present state of what has recently been called "Bacterial Pathology." But as it is to myself a subject of intense interest, and one upon which attention and expectation are now largely centred, I may venture in a few words to indicate its importance to you as a subject of study, and to point out its bearings on the pathology of the future.

We find the germs of the discoveries on this subject in three different sets of observations. Common observation of epidemic and malarial diseases had brought the convic-

tion that the *materies morbi*, the contagium or seed of these diseases, must be something infinitely small, light, and portable, capable of floating in the air, of remaining long dormant, and, on finding a suitable soil in the human body, of producing a certain definite series of symptoms, occurring often with great regularity in the time of appearance and order of development. In the case of some of these diseases, the virus, whatever its nature, was not exhausted in the body, but multiplied ten thousand fold, and, as in the case of small-pox, one might inoculate a certain definite minute quantity and produce a local disease, which, by contagion (a) to other healthy persons, might cause hundreds of cases, in each of which the poison was reproduced. Clearly, then, it was also capable of indefinite self-multiplication under suitable conditions, and must be something more than a mere chemical poison.

This, then, was the starting-point of the germ theory as applied both to zymotic diseases, such as measles and scarlet fever, and to certain wound infections, such as erysipelas. But microscopic research failed to detect these germs, and though the theory was discussed and maintained, it could not yet assume a definite scientific form.

Then came the great discoveries of Pasteur (b) on fermentation, and the recognition of bacteria as the accompaniments and apparent agents of putrefaction. The idea that each infectious disease might be a sort of fermentation produced by a fungus, now grew into a more definite shape, and the germ theory received expansion upon this basis. You may some day read the history of the many germs and fungi which were discovered and lost again, and I will not detain you with the many marvels which were seen, or believed to be seen, under the microscope. But all the time the true was being worked out with the false, though the erroneous observations of some, and their contradiction by others, have tended to make many scientific men disbelieve both true and false.

The first accurate light upon the question came in the investigations upon anthrax or splenic fever, and, out of the multitude of results of research on this and other contagious diseases, I shall venture to select, by way of illustration, one in which I am especially interested. In 1850 the presence of a minute foreign organism of a rod shape in the blood of animals dying of this disease was discovered (c) by Rayer and Davaine. Davaine gave to these bodies, which he showed to be of vegetable nature, the name of *bacteridia*, (d) to distinguish them from *bacterium termo*, which they resembled except in being devoid of movement. Then came the discovery that they could be cultivated artificially in fluids outside the body, and the demonstration by Koch that they formed seed spores which could remain a long time dormant, but under suitable conditions grow and multiply. With this also came the perfecting of the proof, afforded mainly by experiment with the artificially grown fungus, that the fungus or bacillus was the essential virus of the disease.

Here, then, was one instance—but a solitary one—in which a disease, having many characters of a contagious disease, was proved to be due to a fungus, which, when inoculated, gave rise to the disease, and was reproduced in the blood. But long before this proof had become complete, the researches of Klebs, Panum, Bergmann, Sanderson, and many others, had shown that the bacteria of decomposition were apparently the active agents in what we know as blood-poisonings following wounds, and that similar organisms were to be found in some of the allied diseases, such as diphtheria and erysipelas. Now, so far as we are acquainted with the history of these diseases, they have this sharp distinction from the zymotic diseases : that they do not give any protection from a future attack, and that they are essentially allied to putrefaction, both in their causes and phenomena. The admirable scientific and practical experiments which Lister worked out when a professor in this University, and the investigations of Koch on wound-infections, have established with certainty the fact that these blood-poisonings are effected through the agency of bacteria. Might it not then be that splenic fever was merely one of

(a) This, I need hardly say, was the reason why inoculation of small-pox was made penal.
(b) Published 1857 to 1861.
(c) The discovery is usually attributed to Pollender, but his independent discovery was not made till 1855.
(d) The name *Bacillus anthracis*, given by Cohn the botanist, is that by which this organism is now usually known.

these common blood-poisonings, and that its study could throw no light on the zymotic diseases? In animals it appeared to be communicable by ordinary ways of infection or contagion, but to man only by inoculation, and it was seriously questioned whether even in the lower animals it could be produced except by inoculation.

The question was in this state until about three years ago, when it was discovered by Dr. Sanderson and Mr. Duguid that a cow might be inoculated with splenic fever from a guinea-pig, and, though suffering severely, not die of the disease. In continuing these experiments, I found that a cow once so inoculated resisted the results of further inoculation to a very remarkable degree; in other words, that practically it could thus be rendered insusceptible to future attack of the disease. This fact at once showed that splenic fever followed the same rule with regard to protection as the ordinary zymotic diseases, and did away with one of the barriers to the acceptance of the bacterial germ theory.

In making a series of experiments with a view of obtaining, in a suitable form for inoculation, this virus modified by transmission through the guinea-pig, I found that if one cultivated the bacillus under particular conditions it gradually lost its activity, and at last became practically inert. It at once occurred to me that, by making use of this fact, I might obtain a virus so far modified as to be sufficient when inoculated to insure protection, and yet not to endanger the life or safety of the animal inoculated. And this I found could be done with success.(e)

M. Pasteur has recently published the results of a very large series of experiments(f) made by a precisely similar method, and with results fully confirming those which I published more than a year ago. And, although I venture to claim for England whatever merit may be due to priority of the discovery, I none the less rejoice that the facts should have been so fully established in France. My experiments were made with a small and inadequate sum of money furnished by the generosity of a private society, and in the face of all the difficulties interposed by law; whilst M. Pasteur is encouraged and abundantly supplied with means by the liberality of the French Government.

But I must not now dwell upon the many points of interest opened up by recent discoveries on bacterial contagion. What I wish to emphasise is the immense field of research which is opened by these discoveries, and the hopeful anticipation of the possible prevention and remedy of a multitude of the most deadly scourges of our race. And all this—indeed, all the certain progress in this field of research, which, bear in mind, promises as much for the animal world as for man—has been the outcome of experiments on animals. Every step in these inquiries is necessarily made by inoculation of living animals, and every result must be checked by the same means. If experiments on animals were stopped, or even if, in other countries, they were subjected to the same restrictions as in England, I can honestly say, speaking from experience, that I believe these inquiries, which may save hundreds of thousands of lives of both cattle and men, would be practically arrested, or would at least take many years for their development. And it is not only in this more direct manner that such discoveries are of interest, for they promise, I need hardly tell you, to throw great light upon the whole question of contagion. Much has yet to be learnt, much to be made certain, many conflicting testimonies to be reconciled, before we can fully accept the bacterial hypothesis of zymotic infection; but we may yet look hopefully forward to its establishment.

I have thus briefly referred to some of the main branches of pathological investigation; and I have incidentally referred to the relations of physiology to pathology. But there is one subject which must not pass unnoticed, viz., What is the relation of pathology to therapeutics? I think it is true to say that it is by the intimate study of pathology that we must hope for advance in the scientific application of remedies. Up to the present time pharmacology is mainly chemical and physiological, whilst treatment is

(e) *Journal of the Royal Agricultural Society*, vol. xvi., part 1, April, 1880, and vol. xvii., part 1; *Proc. Roy. Soc.*, June 17, 1880; *Lancet*, December 18, 1880, and January 1, 1881; *British Medical Journal*, December and January, 1880-81.
(f) Communicated to the International Medical Congress, London, 1881; and published as a Parliamentary paper, August 24, 1881. Vide *Times*, August 17 and 24, 1881.

mainly empirical; in other words, most of our acquaintance with the mode of action of drugs is based on experiment on healthy animals, whilst most of our actual use of them in disease is based on experience or on theory. That there are notable instances in which knowledge of physiological action has led to correct application in disease, everyone knows; such, for example, as the use of nitrite of amyl, of digitalis, of jaborandi, and of salicylic acid. But these triumphs have been based either on a knowledge of the intimate nature of the morbid process, or on a happy combination of knowledge of physiological action with a speculation on the pathology of the disease, which turned out to be correct. In the latter case the experiment has solved the pathology of the disease as well as its remedy, just as we may open a box and solve the structure of its lock by trying, out of a number of keys, one which we think looks about the right size and shape.

But how shall we hope for scientific advance in therapeutics? Pathological experiment is exceptionally possible. The pharmacologist does his best in discovering all he can of the physiological properties of drugs; the therapeutist exerts his knowledge, ingenuity, and experience in practical application; but he who can say, Here lies the centre and source of the disease, and this is its precise mode of development and the way in which function is affected; this is the point which you must touch, and in such a way must you touch it,—it is only he who can say this who bridges the gulf which separates empirical from rational therapeutics.

And lastly, I come to inquire what is the present position of pathology in relation to medical education and practice?

I have shown that the separation of pathology from physiology became essential, partly in consequence of the growth of both subjects, and partly from a divergence of their methods. The "Institutes of Medicine" arrived at a practical exclusion of pathology and therapeutics by the mere force of growth of its primary subject, physiology, and the requirements of its teaching. But other causes were at work. So long as pathology was regarded as a subject to be studied mainly on the basis of physiology, normal and experimental, aided by instances drawn from bedside experience, and speculations upon them, so long only could they conveniently be studied together. But with the growth of the study of morbid anatomy and histology as the basis of rational pathology, showing, as they did, conditions inexplicable by, and unknown to, any physiological law, a temporary separation became inevitable, and pathology, following its own path through the dead-house and laboratory, has but recently emerged upon the same open plain to which the more direct path of physiology had already led; and the two again walk side by side, mutually supporting and assisting each other, and in their turn aided by and aiding all the other branches of biology.

In a somewhat similar way the teaching of pathology has become separated from that of systematic medicine. Not that it can be or should be excluded from it, but that its complete study requires a more extensive treatment. In most cases the study of pathological anatomy was the first to receive special separate attention, and it is still so in many foreign and most English schools. In proportion to the increased attention to morbid anatomy as a subject worthy of special scientific study, apart from its obvious utility as a corrective to diagnosis and a guide to the course of individual cases, so did the difficulty of fully treating it in lectures on the symptoms and history of special diseases increase. Morbid anatomy in its turn threw light upon medicine, and by its means, diseases formerly regarded as identical came to be separated, and their symptoms and course had to be discussed in greater detail and with increased care, and so the possibility of considering even all common diseases in one course of lectures became much diminished. The special training and methods of study increased the need of separation, and the development of pathological histology has made the necessity for division still more remediless.

In many English schools the subject of General Pathology is not specially treated, but retains its place as a part of systematic medicine and surgery. The separation and union with other branches of pathology is, I believe, more scientific and more beneficial. That this is so I make bold to maintain on these grounds:—First, that what we understand by general pathology is very largely based upon the study of pathological anatomy in its widest sense. Some have gone so far as to make the term general pathology almost synonymous with general pathological anatomy—an undoubted error. But beyond question the foundation of pathology must be largely laid in pathological anatomy, from which, moreover, it draws many of its illustrations.

In its study, too, general pathology has methods which are widely different from those of systematic medicine and surgery. It aims at the establishment of general as distinguished from special laws; it studies processes underlying widely divergent maladies; it seeks its proofs in all regions of life, whether in human physiology, in experimental and comparative pathology, in the processes of growth and degeneration in plants, and in the rare and costly experiments by which nature sometimes solves pathological problems at the expense of human suffering and life.

And if I may add a practical and utilitarian reason, a separate course of general pathology saves the double teaching of its subjects in special medicine and surgery. General pathology, like actual life, knows no distinction into the corresponding external and internal pathology. Its illustrations are equally drawn from both, and it teaches the changes and processes which are common to the whole system and to its several structures. Hypertrophy and atrophy, degeneration and repair, inflammation and morbid growths, know no separation into external and internal. General pathology is thus the common meeting-ground of medicine and surgery, uniting the isolated discoveries of each into one harmonious whole. And it does more, for, introducing those arguments and discoveries afforded by general biology and by comparative pathology, it elucidates that which could not be explained by study on man alone.

Of the importance of Morbid Anatomy as a branch of medical education, I need not say more than I have already said. The history of pathology, and the immediate benefits to be gained from its study, as well as the requirements of examining bodies, have made it one of the ordinary branches of medical education. But whilst in England gross naked-eye morbid anatomy has been well worked at, especially in relation to clinical medicine and surgery, we have somewhat fallen behind in pathological histology and pathological chemistry. Perhaps the notion that we excel in clinical discovery, fostered by the great results attained by Bright, Addison, W. Jenner, Hughes Bennett, Murchison, Wilks, and many others, has led to some disregard of those improved methods of research afforded to us by science. And it must be added that these means have but recently arrived at such perfection as to enable teaching to be carried on with facility on a large scale. But certain it is that both in France and Germany the general knowledge of microscopic pathology has hitherto been far in advance, and the teaching much more thorough than in England. That this has been so is not to be attributed to any want of encouragement by example of the great discoverers of former or recent times. Going over the names of those in England who have been eminent as clinical surgeons and physicians of late years, I find very few who have not in their earlier and less occupied years been largely addicted to microscopic pathology, unless engaged in some other more special branch of scientific investigation of disease. Jenner, Paget, Bowman, Gull, Lister, Wilks, Hutchinson, Bristowe, Quain, Hughes Bennett, Sanders, Grainger Stewart, and a host of others, might be adduced as instances. These men, following the example of Bright and others, have used the best and most recent means to study thoroughly and record completely all the phenomena of disease falling under their observation, and have proved in the warfare of practice that disease may be overcome by science better than by rude assault.

Nor has it been due to any want of enthusiasm on the part of students or of the younger generation of medical men, as is abundantly proved by the work done for pathological societies, and by the large number who for this very purpose have sought foreign schools to complete their studies. It is, I believe, entirely due to the neglect of teaching and examining bodies. This University, which is unique in having a Professorship of Pathology, also stands, I believe, almost, if not quite, alone in requiring any special examination in pathology, including morbid histology, for a medical degree. And this fact has reacted upon the teaching, which, many schools, has been allowed to remain incomplete and inefficient. Attendance upon lectures on pathological

anatomy is now required by many examining bodies, but I say with some confidence that, with one or two exceptions, there has scarcely existed, if there does now exist, in the London Medical Schools, any course in which pathological histology is systematically taught so as to comprehend a practical study of the principal changes in all the important organs.

I speak thus distinctly upon the subject, because I am convinced of its importance, and desire to draw attention to it. It is to the honour of this University that pathology occupies so important a place in its curriculum.

We have thus glanced at the condition of teaching in relation to general pathology, morbid anatomy, and histology. There is, however, one subject upon which I must say a word, viz., Pathological Chemistry.

Much has been expected of pathological chemistry, yet hitherto it has made but small advances. It was expected that mere ultimate analysis would solve many pathological problems. When Bright gave the account of granular disease of the kidneys, it was thought that chemical analysis would decide what was the nature of the morbid granules, and thus settle the pathology of the disease. So, too, at a later period, it was thought that the discovery of some particular chemical product was distinctive of a particular disease, e.g., leucine and tyrosine in the urine as pathognomonic of acute yellow atrophy of the liver. Pathological chemistry has thus passed through the same phases of faith as pathological histology. It is becoming gradually recognised that pathological chemistry must stand on similar ground with morbid histology in its relation to physiology, that it must be by comparison with the normal chemical processes and chemical reactions in the body that the chemistry of disease must be investigated, rather than by means of ultimate analysis or of discovery of organic compounds peculiar to disease. Both of the latter have, of course, their own proper value.

Pathological chemistry thus waits for the advance of physiological chemistry, and the great difficulty and complexity of this subject make advance necessarily slow.

But perhaps you will ask what influence the study of pathology has upon the actual practice of surgery and medicine.

Not uncommonly it is alleged that the special study of pathology is a waste of time, nay, positively injurious to the development of acquaintance with practical work. There is, in truth, a limit of time and energy both to students and practitioners, and in the case of both, time and energy may be ill-apportioned for the practical object in view—the treatment of disease—especially when so many subjects must be crowded into so short a time.

But the rare facilities offered for the study of pathology during the student career, and the far greater difficulty in acquiring opportunities in after life than is the case with many other subjects, render its thorough study at this time especially important, if it is worth studying at all.

No one, I suppose, questions the importance of carrying the studies of the bedside in fatal cases to the test of the post-mortem room, or the advantage of gaining that acquaintance with the different appearances presented by diseased organs which will enable them to be recognised in after life. These, and the supposed power of stating at a glance whether a microscopic scraping of a tumour is malignant or non-malignant, have been gravely asserted to me by a hospital surgeon as being "all that a student wants to know of pathology."

If there were no science of pathological anatomy, if all its multitudinous incidents were connected by no general laws, if there were no intimate connexion between symptoms and structure, and no possibility of tracing the processes of disease and connecting them with the changes in the organs, we might perhaps allow this. And if it were possible without any practical demonstration to teach what we know of the alterations of minute structure in disease, their origin and course, and the way in which these affect function, the study of pathological histology by students might be to a large extent given up. But since we have eyes to see and hands to work, and the microscope enables us to apply both to the ready investigation and recognition of these processes, we prefer the practical method of study, as both easier and more effective, as well as more interesting, and of daily increasing value in after life.

And will not that man who is acquainted with what has

hitherto been learnt of the causes and processes of disease in its more widely distributed forms, of the laws which condition its occurrence, and the general course which it takes, be far more likely to take a rational view of the symptoms, and of the effect of remedies? Will he not see in each case, however trivial, the application of general laws, and, conversely, will he not often be able, in some exceptional occurrence, to extend those laws by fresh observation?

Thus, knowing the gross forms and results of disease, intimately acquainted with the conditions which give rise to them, the interactions of the several organs, the changes of minute structure which lead to impairment of function, guided by general pathology, his views corrected and enlarged by knowledge of the results of experimental and comparative pathology, the surgeon or physician will, in his every-day round of work, take rank as a scientific observer: no case, no symptom, will be trivial to him; each, unimportant though it may appear in itself, will serve as a guide to some more general or deeper seated cause; and whilst he will be delivered from the tedium of routine, he will also be saved from its dangers.

Gentlemen, I have endeavoured to trace out to you something of the history of the chair during the fifty years of its existence, and to show you in brief outline how the subject of pathology has come to assume its present condition as a great and all-important branch of medical science. I have endeavoured to impress upon you the fact that it has intimate relations with all the other branches of your medical studies, between which, indeed, it forms the connecting link. The exact studies of anatomy, physiology, chemistry, and biology have prepared you to enter upon this study; and in proportion to the extent and practical accuracy of your knowledge of these subjects will be the possibility of your advance in pathology. I have given you some faint idea of the importance of this study in its bearings on your future work, when you will have to do with the immediate study and treatment of disease.

Enter then upon your work with the conviction that what you now learn is to form the groundwork of a study which will last you a lifetime, and lay the foundations as deeply and broadly as possible. Make it your object to advance the science of pathology by diligent and careful observation, in which everyone may assist, and avoid as far as you may all barren theoretical discussions.

If, in what I have said, I have in any way awakened an interest and quickened your curiosity by what may now seem in a measure obscure, no effort on my part shall be wanting to make clear to you, step by step, the science of pathology in all its branches.

Carry with you into your work, whether at the bedside, in the post-mortem room, the laboratory, or the lecture theatre, the belief that pathology is a living, not a dead study: let this belief make the routine of its drier bones instinct with life and action, and you shall find that the reality of its interest and its value immeasurably transcend what I have endeavoured faintly to depict.

THE GRASP OF A MADMAN.—After several attacks of delirious fever, a *restaurateur* of Vincennes had been sent to Bicêtre, and having been treated during eleven months, was dismissed in an apparently satisfactory state. Next day, having been drinking with all his customers, he again showed signs of insanity, and his wife sent for M. Coste, their doctor, who ordered him a strict diet and abstinence from drink. On hearing this, the madman was seized with an attack of furious delirium, and rushing upon the doctor, drew him to the window, which he threw open, and seizing M. Coste by the neck, held him suspended in the open air. More dead than alive, the doctor dared make no struggle, while his dangerous patient howled like one possessed, and threatened to let him drop. The neighbours, finding how things stood, obtained a ladder, and one of them mounting it, got hold of the unfortunate doctor. He was, however, not yet saved, for the lunatic refused to relax his hold, and, in fact, did not abandon his prey until a blacksmith had burned his hands with a hot iron. The madman was taken back to Bicêtre.—*Lyon Méd.*, Oct. 23.

THE foundation-stone of a new infirmary in the Mayday-road, Croydon, close to the Workhouse, was laid last week. It will provide accommodation for 400 beds, and is estimated to cost £100,000.

ORIGINAL COMMUNICATIONS.

A CASE OF

EXCESSIVELY HIGH TEMPERATURES,

BELIEVED TO BE FICTITIOUS.[a]

By STEPHEN MACKENZIE, M.D., F.R.C.P.,
Physician to, and Lecturer on Medicine at, the London Hospital.

THE patient was re-admitted, under the care of Mr. Rivington, on October 21, 1879, complaining of pain in the stomach and back. After remaining in the surgical wards until December 31, 1879, she was transferred to my care.

It was then elicited that an injury to her leg—a knock when going upstairs—thirteen years before was the cause of an ulcer of the leg for which the limb had been removed, and that she had been under treatment for it several times previously; Mr. Hutchinson having, several years prior, removed a piece of necrosed bone, advising at that time removal of the limb. She is stated to have had typhoid fever six years ago, and following this a cough, with, on many occasions, spitting of blood—half a teacupful at a time. Since then she has always had a cough in the winter, and spits blood, she states, occasionally. Two years ago, she states that she was laid up with typhus fever for thirteen or fourteen weeks. Soon after the original accident which caused the ulcer on her leg she took opium to relieve pain, and she has continued the habit ever since. The largest quantity she has taken in the twenty-four hours has been one drachm and a half of solid opium. This quantity she has been in the habit of taking for the last six years.

The patient is a short, dark-complexioned woman, with apparently fair intelligence. She is of a somewhat complaining nature, and has given a good deal of trouble to the authorities in this way; so much so that further admission has been prohibited. She was admitted on the present occasion for pain and swelling of the stomach. The abdomen was much distended, and stated to be tender on pressure. It was everywhere resonant on percussion. The bowels were irregular, the tongue clean. The stump was slightly erythematous and tender on pressure; a sinus existed, from which oozed a little nearly clear fluid. Urine 1010, acid, no albumen, urea 0·5 per cent.; pulse, 78, full; heart and lungs normal; respirations 30; temperature on several occasions normal.

No important peculiarity was noticed as regards temperature, etc., until January 13, 1880. It is then stated that the patient "had a slight rigor this morning at about 8.30." Temperature at 11.15 a.m. was 109·2°; pulse 72; respirations 24.

January 14.—Patient had a bad night; complains of pain in head. Has vomited several times during the night. This morning tongue clean, bowels confined. Temperature at 11 a.m. 106·4°; pulse 76; respirations 26.

15th.—Patient had a bad night; slept very little. Vomiting and pain in head continue. Tongue coated with white fur. The highest temperature occurred between 1 p.m. yesterday and 4 a.m. this morning, when on several occasions it was 113°. As the thermometer did not register higher, the temperature may probably have exceeded this. At 10 a.m., temperature 107·2°; pulse 108; respirations 30. No special pain in stump, which is not discharging more than usual.

16th.—Patient passed another very bad night. Vomiting still continues. The highest temperature registered was 114° at 4 p.m. yesterday. At noon to-day, temperature 107°; pulse 90; respirations 28. Urine contains more urea, 1·4 per cent.

17th.—Patient passed a better night; the temperature, therefore, was not taken during the night. Has had one slight rigor this morning. Pain in head less; has vomited once. Temperature at 11 a.m. 99·4°; pulse 68; respirations 20.

19th.—Patient had a very bad night. Pain in head severe; vomiting has ceased. Has had some slight rigors. Temperature at 11 a.m. 106·4°; pulse 90; respirations 26. The highest temperature since last note was at 6 p.m. yesterday, when it was 112°. Patient has lost four pounds and a half in weight.

20th.—Pain in head still severe; vomited again this

(a) Read before the Clinical Society, October 28, 1881.

morning; complains of giddiness, everything appearing to revolve from right to left. Temperature at 11 a.m. 110°; pulse 76; respirations 26.

22nd.—Highest temperature at 4 a.m. this morning, when a new thermometer marked to 130°, procured for the purpose, registered 120·8°. Pain and vomiting continue. Temperature at 12 midday 102·2°; pulse 74; respirations 28.

23rd.—Head still bad; vomiting has ceased. Highest temperature at 4 a.m. 116·8°; temperature taken at 12·45 p.m.—in axilla 105°, in rectum 99°, in mouth 98·8°; pulse 78; respirations 24.

26th.—Slept a good deal in the night; pain in head not so severe; no vomiting. Highest temperature at 4 a.m. 113·6°; at 11 a.m. 99° in both axillæ; pulse 72; respirations 20.

27th.—The temperature at 4 p.m. yesterday was 116·8°, at 3 a.m. to-day 114·8°, at 6 p.m. 110·8°. No extraordinary temperatures were recorded from this date until April 5. During this period the temperature was irregular, and occasionally reached 102° or 103°. Her general condition remained stationary. There was erythema of the stump; the abdomen was distended.

The following is a record of the daily thermometric observations:—

January 13.—11.15 a.m., 109·2°.

14th.—1 p.m., 108°; 2 p.m., 108·2°; 4 p.m., 107·4°; 5 p.m., 108·5°; 7 p.m., 109·6°; 8 p.m., 106·8°; 9 p.m., 102·6°; 11 p.m., 106·4°; 12 p.m., 113°.

15th.—3 a.m., 113°; 4 a.m., 113°; 5 a.m., 111°; 10 a.m., 107·2°; 12 noon, 111·6°; 2 p.m., 112·2°; 4 p.m., 114°; 6 p.m., 109·2°; 8 p.m., 110·2°; 10 p.m., 113·3°.

16th.—2 a.m., 107·4°; 5 a.m., 113°; 7 a.m., 107·8°; 9 a.m., 108·7°; 12 noon, 107°; 2 p.m., 114·2°; 4 p.m., 111°; 9 p.m., 111·8°; 12 p.m., 98·6°.

17th.—4 a.m., 100°; 10 a.m., 103°; 12 noon, 99·2°; 2 p.m., 98·8°; 4 p.m., 99·2°; 6 p.m., 101·8°; 8 p.m., 104·6°; 10 p.m., 1 5·8°.

18th.—5 a.m., 108°; 8 a.m., 107·6°; 10 a.m., 106°; 12 noon, 107·7°; 2 p.m., 106°; 4 p.m., 110·4°; 6 p.m., 112°; 8.30 p.m., 108°; 12 midnight, 103·7°.

19th.—3 a.m., 106·4°; 5 a.m., 105°; 9 a.m., 102·4°; 11 a.m., 106·6°; 2 p.m., 108·8°; 4 p.m., 101·6°; 6 p.m., 102·8°; 9 p.m., 102·2°; 10 p.m., 102·7°; 12 p.m., 106°.

20th.—6 a.m., 108°; 9 a.m., 102·4°; 11 a.m., 110°; 3 p.m., 101·7°; 6 p.m., 104·4°; 8 p.m., 105·8°; 10 p.m., 103·6°.

21st.—2 a.m., 101°; 9 a.m., 106 2°; 11 a.m., 106·1°; 9 p.m., 109·2°; 10 p.m., 104·6°.

22nd.—2 a.m., 102·6°; 4 a.m., 120·8°; 9 a.m., 110°; 12 a.m., 102·2°; 2 p.m., 101·4°; 4 p.m., 104·2°; 6 p.m., 108·2°; 8 p.m., 110·2°; 10 p.m., 107·2°.

23rd.—2 a.m., 110·4°; 4 a.m., 116·6°; 9 a.m., 107·4°; 12 a.m., 109·4°; 2 p.m., 108·4°; 4 p.m., 114·2°; 6 p.m., 104·2°; 8 p.m., 106·6°; 10 p.m., 108·7°.

24th.—2 a.m., 103·6°; 4 a.m., 105·2°; 10 a.m., 104·2°; 12 a.m., 111·2°; 2 p.m., 113·2°; 4 p.m., 109·2°; 6 p.m., 107·2°; 8 p.m., 101·6°; 10 p.m., 111·4°.

25th.—4 a.m., 105·8°; 10 a.m., 106·5°; 12 a.m., 105·4°; 2 p.m., 110·6°; 6 p.m., 102·6°; 8 p.m., 107·2°; 10 p.m., 111·2°.

26th.—4 a.m., 113·6°; 10 a.m., 99·2°; 12 a.m., 99·2°; 2 p.m., 106·6°; 4 p.m., 116·8°; 6 p.m., 110·8°; 8 p.m., 107·5°; 10 p.m., 105·2°.

27th.—3 a.m., 106·2°; 10 a.m., 114·8°; 12 a.m., 98·8°; 2 p.m., 99°; 4 p.m., 108·2°; 6 p.m., 106°; 8 p.m., 110·6°.

On April 5 the patient complained of headache, and vomited once. On placing a thermometer in the right axilla, and leaving it there for some time (ten minutes) unwatched, the thermometer registered 106·8°. The clinical clerk then placed a thermometer in each axilla, leaving them there unwatched for ten minutes. At the end of this time that in the right axilla registered 109°, that in the left axilla had the mercury driven into the bulb at the top of the thermometer—113°. The special thermometer was then placed in left axilla and left unwatched for ten minutes, when it registered 99°. A thermometer was then placed in each axilla, and allowed to remain ten minutes, the patient being watched; the temperature in each axilla was 99°.

April 10.—Temperature—unwatched 104°, watched 99°.

Various fluctuations of temperature, none exceeding 105°, followed during the next month.

On the evening of May 11 the patient had another high rise of temperature. The thermometer when first placed in the axilla registered 110°; taken five minutes afterwards by the nurse (who stood at the table the while), it was normal; taken two hours later by the House-Physician, it was still normal.

May 17.—For the last few days the patient has been complaining of pain in the stump, most severe at a certain point over the cicatrix. The temperature at various times has risen to 108° and 104°. This evening she complains of a good deal of pain. The temperature was found at first to be 105°. Taken a little while afterwards with two thermometers (shown to register alike) in the same axilla, one registered 105°, the other 104°. The patient was not watched. Within ten minutes, taken by the clerk, who held the thermometers in the axilla, it was found to be 98·8°. Pulse 88, respirations 34. It was noticed that the patient shook the bed with voluntary tremor, and that when "the respirations" were asked for the breathing became quicker.

24th.—Complains of much pain in leg, head, and back. Her temperature this morning was 109·2°, pulse 88. The temperature taken a second time was 98·6°. Two thermometers were subsequently placed in the same axilla, and registered respectively 105·9° and 106·5°. Directly afterwards the temperature was again taken, the thermometer being under direct observation, and found to be 99°.

This evening the temperature of patient has shown some strange variations. The nurse took it at 8.30, when it registered 106°. At 8.55, sister took it with two thermometers in the same axilla; one was found to be 107°, and the other 107·2°. Immediately afterwards the House-Physician placed two thermometers in the same axilla, and held them there. At the end of ten minutes both were found to be normal.

For the next week variations in temperature were the rule, but none were extremely high. The difference between two thermometers in the same axilla for the same time was from 1° to 4°.

From this time till her discharge the temperature was about normal, two thermometers being placed in the axilla and agreeing.

The stump remained painful and erythematous; the abdomen distended. She complained frequently of the latter. I convinced myself, by repeated and thorough examinations, that there was nothing the matter with it, and that the distension was quasi-voluntary. The patient's general condition seemed practically the same, whether she had an ordinary or an excessively high temperature. After leaving the hospital she went to Colchester on a visit to some friends. Whilst there the pain and vomiting returned. She was treated without benefit, and at the end of three weeks returned to London and sought readmission into the hospital on August 16, 1880.

She then complained of severe pain in epigastrium, increased by food; vomiting everything except milk and soda-water. Some blood was stated to be occasionally vomited. The abdomen was distended, presenting a bulging appearance; everywhere resonant, and fluctuation-wave absent.

A chart of her temperatures on this occasion showed similar fluctuations to those on the last occasion, and a few notes only are necessary.

Thus, on August 19, when a temperature of 110° was recorded, the thermometer had been left unwatched. When found to be so high, a fresh thermometer (the index of the former being destroyed) was placed in the axilla, and the temperature found to be normal. On September 13 the temperatures of two thermometers in the same axilla for the same time were 106·5° and 101°. On the 15th, 111° and 110° when not watched, when watched 105° and 104°. On the 17th the thermometers registered 105° and 102° respectively. On one occasion the clinical clerk noticed the patient fumbling under the clothes when she thought she was unwatched.

On no occasion when the patient was strictly watched, or the thermometers held in the axilla, were excessively high temperatures observed.

The patient was discharged on September 24, 1880.

Desirous to follow up the case, I went, in September, 1881, to the patient's address, when a friend told me she was in a Poor-law infirmary, dangerously ill, and not expected to recover. I visited her there, and found she was under treatment for an "abdominal tumour," which required a generous diet, with extras and stimulants. No excessively high temperatures had been recorded, for the simple reason that the thermometer had not been on any occasion employed. I have seen her this afternoon (October 28, 1881), and her temperature in the axilla was normal.

I have brought this case before the Society because several cases have been recorded within the last few years where extraordinarily high temperatures have been observed—notably one before the Society in 1875, by Mr. John Teale, in which the temperature was stated to be certainly 122°, and possibly 125°. Cases have been published by Dr. Greig Smith, Dr. Ormerod, Mr. Julius Cæsar, and Dr. Horatio Donkin. The latter has collected and analysed many of the published cases, including the first part of the present case. Dr. James Little, of Dublin, has had a case under his care in which (in the *Medical Times and Gazette*) the temperature is stated to have reached 130·8°.

I desire to state my unhesitating belief that in my case, whilst under my own care at least, the excessively high temperatures were fictitious. At the same time I do not wish to imply that all cases of such paradoxical tempera_tures are of the same nature. The fact that some cases, recorded by good observers, are believed to be genuine, renders it desirable, in my opinion, that a fictitious one should be exposed, to put all on their guard in investigating cases of this kind.

I base my belief that this case is fictitious on the following grounds :—

1. That the patient was a neurotic woman, and an "educated hospital patient," *i.e.*, had been in the hospital several times, and knew the importance attached to high temperatures.

2. That when, on one occasion, the temperature was simultaneously taken in the mouth, rectum, and axilla, the temperature in the mouth and rectum corresponded and were normal, whilst that in the axilla was 6° higher.

3. That when two thermometers were simultaneously placed in the same axilla there was as much as from 1° to 4·5° difference.

4. That there was no correlation between the high temperatures, the pulse, and the respirations.

5. That on no occasion when the thermometer was held in the axilla, or the patient closely watched, was an excessively high temperature observed.

The other objective symptoms—the erythema of the stump, the vomiting, and abdominal distension—were, in my opinion, self-induced.

I have attached no importance to consecutive observations, as Dr. Donkin has argued, from cases observed by himself and others, that the high temperatures may be excessively evanescent, and thus not incompatible with life. It would be an unjustifiable assumption, however, that in this case, in the hourly or bi-hourly observations, the temperatures, if genuine, should have been excessively high always when taken, and have fallen between the times of the observations. If we admit that there is no warrant for such an assumption, we have to consider the possibility of the bodily temperature being maintained for days at a height of from 106° to 113°, or 120°, not only with recovery, but without other symptoms of corresponding gravity.

It is of course *possible* that the temperatures were genuine in the first instance, and that the patient, finding the importance attached to the symptoms, kept up an interest in her case.

I have not been able to ascertain how the high thermo_metric readings were produced. I have taxed the patient with their voluntary or unconscious causation, but this is strenuously denied. That the mercury may be driven to the summit of the thermometer by gently shaking it when inverted, and that when rubbed in a fold of linen the mercury can be driven up to 105° or 110°, in a minute or less, I have experimentally ascertained. Thermometers vary much in the mobility of the index. When some of the observations were taken the patient had hot poultices to the chest or abdomen, or hot bottles. At a later period these were not allowed.

Postscript.—The patient has, since this paper was read, confessed to me that she caused the high temperatures by means of poultices, hot bottles, etc. She did it sufficiently cleverly to elude the vigilance of those taking the observa_tions. When the temperature was taken in my presence it was never abnormal.

REMARKS ON A CASE OF UNUSUAL TEMPERATURE.

By WALTER RIVINGTON, F.R.C.S.,
Surgeon to the London Hospital, etc.

NOT having seen the notes of this case prior to publication, I should like to add one or two observations by way of correction and enlargement. The patient is a widow, and has been so for the last two years. She had three children: one was stillborn, another died of croup at three years, and the third of bronchitis at six years of age. There are some scars on her right leg which she attributes to an accident whilst dancing, and the ulcer on the amputated leg arose, according to her account, from an injury to her shin twelve years ago. There is no overt history of syphilis. Her leg was at first treated for rheumatism. Afterwards an ulcer formed, and she came under the care of a surgeon at the hospital, who removed some necrosed bone, which was "like charcoal," and advised her, she says, to part with the limb eleven years ago. She went home and poulticed her leg, and it healed up, and she was able to get about again. But five years later the ulcer broke out again, and the limb gradually became useless, the muscles contracting, and extending the foot and flexing the knee. As a speculation I ordered mercury and iodide of potassium, which she took for a time with some advantage, but not sufficient to make the limb worth preserving. At the time she was laid up at home with her leg she began to eat opium, and continued the practice for many years. She took daily a drachm and a half of the gum opium, which she bought for a shilling, or rather more, for she spent nine shillings a week on the drug. When she first came under my care she brought a supply of opium with her. The amputation was performed at the lower third of the thigh by long anterior and short posterior flaps, under the carbolic spray. No case ever did better, for in a week the flaps had united, and the line of union was scarcely conspicuous on the face of the stump. I was exhibiting it as an example of the benefit of Lister's system. A few weeks passed, and I could not account for the fact that the corners of the flaps did not and would not unite. The patient complained of pain in the stump, and it continued to discharge pretty freely. I enlarged one of the openings, inserted my finger, and found a little nest of pieces of drainage-tube, four or five in number, which had been introduced by the dresser or house-surgeon, without any tangible security for their re_turn. (In passing, I may remark that this occurrence is not uncommon. About the same time, I had under my care a man who had come from another hospital with discharging openings in his scalp. Nothing would induce the sinuses to heal till the openings were enlarged, and some pieces of drainage-tube from the sister institution had been detected and removed.) After this the stump healed well, and there was only a very small opening, not leading beyond the subcutaneous tissues, when she was sent into the country to a convalescent home. When she returned, the stump was soundly healed, but there was a circumscribed blush over the upper flap, with increased heat, some swelling, and great tenderness. This condition, she told me, was due to a recent accident. Of any previous injury in the ward when she got up I know nothing. Being very reluctant to dis_turb a good stump, I kept her quiet in bed with lead lotion for weeks without benefit. The enlargement of the end of the bone could be felt as an irregular growth, and at last I consented to interfere. The end of the bone was more than a little enlarged, for it resembled a small mushroom, owing to an outgrowth from the periosteum. There was no necro_sis. Possibly the bone was sclerosed—a condition which might be overlooked in microscopic examination. All went on well after the operation, and the patient was apparently cured. She has now returned. Her symptoms were con_stant sickness, and great pain and tenderness in the stump, especially on pressing on the end of the bone, which seemed a little enlarged, whilst an aperture had formed in the centre, leading down to the bone. I have again removed a slice of bone under the thymol spray. The sickness is abating. The temperature is inclined to fall, having been down to 97°. With regard to the high tem_peratures recorded before the second operation, I may remark that I did not myself have the opportunity of seeing them; they were capricious and fugitive, and during my visits they were absent, but they were recorded by trustworthy observers. Caution was especially needed in the present case, for it has been found that the patient's statements are not separated by any clear line of demarcation from the unreliable. As an illustration of the effect of the mind on the body, it may be mentioned that for three weeks during her first stay in the hospital, water was substituted for solution of morphia as a hypodermic injection, and produced an effect as sedative as the narcotic itself. The thermometer used was the best that the institution afforded at the time.

22, Finsbury-square, November, 1879.

AN ACCOUNT OF

ONE HUNDRED AND TEN CONSECUTIVE CASES OF ABDOMINAL SECTION

PERFORMED SINCE THE 1ST OF NOVEMBER, 1880. (a)

By LAWSON TAIT, F.R.C.S.

Analysis of the Series.

	Cases.	Deaths.
Exploratory incisions	14	0
Removal of one ovary for cystoma	38	2
Removal of both ovaries for cystoma	9	0
Removal of parovarian cysts	4	0
Removal of both ovaries and tubes for { Myoma	11	1
Hydrosalpinx	5	0
Pyosalpinx	3	0
Chronic ovaritis	2	1
Opening and draining of pelvic abscess	11	0
Hepatotomy	4	0
Enterotomy for intestinal obstruction	2	0
Hysterotomy	4	2
Cæsarian section	1	1
Extra-peritoneal cysts (peritoneum not opened)	2	2
	110	9

In giving an account of the work which I have done during the last twelve months, I shall continue the practice which gives, as I believe, the only just method of showing its value, or the general progress which is being made in this department of surgery, by placing on record every case in which I have opened the abdomen, in a tabulated statement. This, as will be seen, contains columns, two of which will serve sufficiently for the identification of any particular case, should my critics require it. A third column gives the nature of the disease, and another the kind of operation performed; whilst the results are given for the primary effect of the operation in all cases, and for the secondary effect in a few, chiefly those in which malignant disease has killed the patient after recovery from the operation.

It is first of all to be noticed that the number of operations has increased nearly 45 per cent. over those performed last year, and as by far the larger number of the cases have been placed under my care by my professional brethren, I take this as a most gratifying proof that the results I have obtained are satisfactory to them.

The total mortality amounts to nine deaths, or only 8·2 per cent., a result which would be remarkable enough in itself if all the cases had been mere ovariotomies, but still more so when its details are examined. If I had confined the definition of "abdominal section" strictly to those cases in which the peritoneal cavity was opened, I should eliminate two of my deaths (Nos. 26 and 56), but none of my successful cases, and thus the total mortality would be reduced to 6·4 per cent. I include these two cases, however, the details of which will be given further on, in order that no charge may be made against me of dealing unfairly with my results.

Of the fourteen exploratory incisions, I may say that they all occurred in cases of malignant disease. In many of them I was certain that the disease was of a hopeless kind before I operated, but I offered the patients the chance of a harm-

(a) Read before the Midland Medical Society, November 2, 1881.

less opening in order that I might be sure that I had made no mistake. In a few of the cases there was doubt, and in two I was wholly mistaken, having been under the impression that I was dealing with ordinary cystoma, whilst the disease was really malignant sarcoma. Two per cent. of error is, however, not large, and I am greatly comforted by the fact that this percentage has immensely diminished during the last few years.

I now make exploratory incisions to make sure I am not wrong, whereas formerly I used to make them only to find. I was entirely mistaken. They serve the purpose of complete tappings, and, as the patients uniformly recover, they do no harm at all.

By far the most satisfactory statement I can make, both for myself and for the general advancement of abdominal surgery, is that there is not a single incomplete operation on the list. Not a single tumour which I have attacked have I not completely removed; and the reproach which has been made on the operation for the removal of small ovaries (the so-called oöphorectomy), that there was such a large proportion of incomplete operations, will, I hope, no longer be applied with justice to my practice. Increased experience, and greater boldness and manipulative dexterity thereby acquired, have enabled me to complete a large number of the operations in the list now submitted, which, two or three years ago, would have been left unfinished.

Of the operations which were formerly grouped together under the name of ovariotomy (and most improperly so), I have performed fifty-one with only two deaths, or 3·49 per cent. These were all cases of cystic tumours affecting one ovary in thirty-eight cases, both ovaries in nine cases, and the tubules of the broad ligament in four cases. The mortality obtained in this group is most satisfactory, and is an immense advance on anything hitherto obtained, save in the practice of Dr. Keith, of Edinburgh, to whose teaching and example it is very largely due—a fact which I here proclaim by no means for the first time. I have already said enough of the so-called antiseptic system of Lister to be able to say that it has been finally dismissed from this department of surgery as having done far more harm than good. I venture to predict a similar fate will meet it everywhere else; and I take to myself some credit for having burst one of the largest, best blown, and most attractive bubbles ever displayed to a surgical audience.

The main factors in the success, as I have said before, and as I have increasing reason to believe, are three—the discontinuance of the clamp treatment of the pedicle, increased personal experience, and a general improvement of the conditions under which operations are performed. There can now be no question that our former high mortality was mainly due to the clamp, and for this Mr. Spencer Wells is solely responsible. Before his day the intra-peritoneal treatment had been completely established by Mr. Baker Brown, in whose hands its mortality was reduced to 10 per cent. between 1865 and 1867. Neither Mr. Spencer Wells nor anyone else got results from the clamp, after 1867, much better than 25 per cent. mortality. Mr. Baker Brown's ruin was, therefore, a great misfortune for humanity, and Mr. Wells has never yet explained on what grounds he neglected the lesson of Baker Brown's practice, and why it was left for Dr. Keith to put ovariotomy in its legitimate position. For twelve years Mr. Wells went on with a mortality more than double that which he would have had with the cautery; and, unfortunately, he led others into the same mistake. Not only this, but the whole progress of abdominal surgery, which has been so rapid during the last four years, was retarded, for no one dared to perform operations which are now completely to be justified, so long as ovariotomy was fatal in one case in every four.

One item to be classed under the head of the general improvement is of very great importance, which is, that I get the patients now in a much earlier stage of the disease than I used to do, for my professional brethren generally send me their patients as soon as the presence of a tumour is recognised. This is proved by the fact that only two out of the fifty ovarian tumours which I have removed during the past twelve months had been tapped before they were sent to me. If ovarian tumours were never tapped I believe that 98 per cent. of recoveries would be the rule in ovariotomy. The two deaths which I speak of occurred in cases where the patients were so situated that the disease was not recognised till too late. One, sent to me by Dr. Williams, of

Dyffryn, had obstinately refused to be examined till she was at death's door from persistent vomiting. Her emaciation and exhaustion were extreme, yet the operation was performed within a few days of the recognition of the case by Dr. Williams and Dr. Roberts, of Portmadoc. She went on very well till the third day, when, during an attack of vomiting, she was suffocated by the vomited matter being drawn into the trachea. Death was quite sudden. I had left her not many minutes before, and had felt no unusual anxiety about her recovery. Had the operation been performed three months before, her recovery would have been certain.

The second death occurred in a case sent to me by Dr. Hamp, of Wolverhampton, within a few days of her being seen by him. She had been under some one else, who had failed to recognise either the nature of the case or its gravity. She was of enormous size. The operation was prolonged and serious from the adhesions. It was a case which I ought, I fear, to have drained; certainly I should do so now. And here I wish to make a recantation of what I have said about drainage. I have no doubt now that Dr. Keith is right when he says that drainage will save three or four cases in each hundred. Previous to August last I had often said that I never had drained, and that I did not think I had lost anything by abstaining from the practice. I fear I was in error, yet my splendid results without it almost justified my belief. But there comes a train of striking coincidences in every line of life, and it came to me in August last. I spent a few days with Dr. Keith in that month, and at his table we discussed drainage, and I expressed my views about it. Dr. Keith told me that I would alter my opinion; and I can only say with Solomon, that he is a fool who never does so, and he is a wise man who does so seldom. Dr. Battey accompanied me home from Edinburgh, and next morning he assisted me to remove a large ovarian tumour, at the base of which was a large malignant adhesion which I had to tear across. The hæmorrhage from it was very profuse, and I had to pack the pelvis with sponges for its arrest. Looking across the table to Dr. Battey, I said, "I think I had better change my opinion now, and use a drainage-tube." He concurred, and I fastened in a tube. The patient made an easy and uninterrupted recovery, and went home, though since then she has succumbed to the cancerous growth.

Next morning I removed, with Dr. Battey's assistance, an enormous tumour, in which the pelvic adhesions were as formidable as it is possible for them to be; again I drained, clearly with advantage; and—to make a long story short—I have done so in four other cases, all with the happiest results. These six cases were so very bad that I do not think I could reasonably have expected them all to have recovered without drainage, and I retract everything that I have hitherto said on the subject. I have also re-opened the wound in two cases which were doing badly, in the stage of acute peritonitis, have cleaned it out, and then fastened in a drainage-tube; and both cases from that moment mended and made speedy recoveries. So satisfied have I been with the results in these cases, that the next case of peritonitis to which I am called, of whatever sort it be—even puerperal,—I shall advise and perform, if allowed, abdominal section, shall cleanse out the cavity and drain it; and, if the operation be not deferred till the patients are moribund, I believe this treatment will prove eminently successful. Our views of peritonitis will, I am certain, soon undergo an immense alteration. The terms "septicæmia" and "septic peritonitis," for which Mr. Spencer Wells is mainly responsible, and which have appeared in the mortality column as the explanation of the deaths after ovariotomy, are simple nonsense, and have led us astray altogether. In future we shall treat the peritoneum on the same principles as we treat other suppurating cavities, and with quite as secure results. Upon this subject I have much more to say, but cannot find space here. It will be fully discussed in a work now in the press.

I do not find that removal of both ovaries for cystoma is in any way a more formidable operation than removing one, and the removal of parovarian cysts has been in my hands uniformly successful.

One Hundred Consecutive Cases of Abdominal Section performed since November 1, 1880, by Lawson Tait, F.R.C.S.

No.	Residence.	Medical attendant.	Age.	Married or single.	Disease.	Operation.	Date.	Hospital.	Private.	Recovered.	Died.	After result— Remarks.
							1880.					
1	Malvern	Dr. Weir	64	W	Cystoma	Left ovary removed	Nov. 1		P	R		
2	Liverpool	Dr. Parry	44	M	Malignant sarcoma	Hysterotomy	" 2	H			D	
3	Wolverhampton	Dr. Lycett	19	S	Pelvic abscess (?)	Exploratory	" 2		P	R		
4	Bradninch, Devon.	Dr. Stephenson	42	W	Myoma	Both ovaries removed	" 16	H			D	Intestinal obstruction.
5	Feckenham, Worc.	Dr. Leacroft	50	M	Cystoma	Right ovary removed	" 20		P	R		Had tetanus, and gangrene of tumour.
6	Walsall	Dr. Day	56	M	Malignant sarcoma	Exploratory	" 25		P	R		
7	Hednesford	Dr. Marsh Stiles	41	M	Parovarian cyst	Removed	Dec. 2	H		R		
8	Coventry	Dr. McVeagh	21	S	Cystoma	Left ovary removed	" 7	H		R		
9	Nuneaton	Dr. Hammond	20	S	Dermoid cyst	Opened and drained	" 10	H		R		Complete cure.
10	Birmingham	Dr. J. W. Taylor	44	S	Myoma	Both ovaries removed	" 18	H		R		
11	Knighton, Radnor	Dr. Coventon	43	M	Cancer of liver	Exploratory	" 20	H		R		
12	Stratford-on-Avon	Dr. Gill	42	S	Cystoma	Right ovary removed	" 21		F	R		Died of cancer of liver, Mar. 30, 1881.
							1881.					
13	Hembleton, Worc.		58	M	Cystoma	Right ovary removed	Jan. 4	H		R		
14	Baddesley, Warwck	Mr. S. F. Palmer	40	M	Cystoma	Right ovary removed	" 5		P	R		Complete cure.
15	Wolverhampton	Dr. Totheriek	11	S	Pelvic abscess	Opened and drained	" 7	H		R		Complete cure.
16	Coventry	Dr. Plowman	32	M	Myoma	Both ovaries removed	" 15	H		R		
17	Leamington	Dr. McFie Campbell	21	S	Chronic ovaritis	Both ovaries removed	" 26	H		R		
18	Coventry	Dr. Fenton	23	S	Suppurating kidney	Exploratory	" 28	H		R		
19	Llanbedr, Merion.	Dr. Williams	40	M	Cystoma	Right ovary removed	Feb. 2		F	R		
20	Birmingham	Mr. H. Bracey	15	S	Cystoma	Right ovary removed	" 2	H		R		Complete cure.
21	Brierley Hill	Dr. D'Arcy Ellis	41	M	Cystoma	Both ovaries removed	" 5	H		R		Complete cure.
22	Birmingham	Dr. G. P. Hadley	56	M	Cyst of liver	Hepatotomy	" 6	H		R		Complete cure.
23	Dyffryn, Merion.	Dr. O. Williams	49	S	Cystoma	Left ovary removed	" 7		P	R	D	
24	Leamington	Dr. Thompson	25	M	Hydatids of liver	Hepatotomy	" 7	H		R		Complete cure.
25	Birmingham	Dr. Kenny	43		Myoma	Both ovaries removed	" 12	H		R		
26	Shifnal	Dr. Lamb	51	M	Extra-peritoneal cyst	Removed	" 13		P	R	D	
27	Chesterfield	Dr. Booth	32	S	Cystoma	Left ovary removed	" 14		P	R		Complete cure.
28	Leamington	Dr. W. Tomkins	21	S	Hydatids of liver	Hepatotomy	" 15	H		R		
29	Birmingham	Mr. Raffles Harmar	49	M	Cystoma	Left ovary removed	" 17	H		R		
30	Loominster	Dr. Barnett	23	S	Cystoma	Left ovary removed	" 19	H		R		
31	Birmingham	Dr. J. W. Taylor	53	M	Large spleen	Exploratory	" 26	H		R		
32	Nuneaton	Mr. R. B. Nason	58	M	Cystoma	Both ovaries removed	" 27		P	R		
33	Wooton-und.-Edge	Dr. Forty	25	S	Cystoma	Both ovaries removed	March 2		P	R		
34	Leicester	Dr. Cox-Hippisley	31	M	Cystoma	Both ovaries removed	" 5	H		R		
35	Church Stretton	Dr. McLintock	87	M	Double pyosalpinx	Both ovaries removed	" 6		P	R		
36	Harbury, Warwick	Dr. Lattey	63	M	Cystoma	Both ovaries removed	" 9	H		R		
37	Lancaster	Dr. Cassidy	56	M	Cystoma	Right ovary removed	" 9		P	R		

No.	Residence.	Medical attendant.	Age.	Married or single.	Disease.	Operation.	Date.	Hospital.	Private.	Recovered.	Died.	After result—Remarks.
							1881.					
38	Peckenham	Dr. Lescroft	53	M	Fibrocyst of uterus ...	Hysterotomy	Mar. 10	H	...	R	D	
39	Solihull	Dr. Page	22	S	Cystoma	Both ovaries removed	„ 12		P	R		
40	Wolverhampton ...	Dr. Walton Hamp ...	21	S	Cystoma	Left ovary removed ..	„ 16	H	...	R	D	Obstructed intestines.
41	Rugby	Drs. Simpson & Sadd	39	M	Urinary cyst	Opened and drained	„ 19	H	...	R		Had a miscarriage, and died of it.
42	Ashby-de-la-Zouch	Dr. Betts	43	W	Cystoma	Right ovary removed	„ 16		P	R		
43	Birmingham	Mr. J. Greene	26	M	Pyosalpinx	Opened and drained	„ 28		P	R		
44	Ombersley	Dr. Hughes	61	M	Cancer of omentum...	Exploratory	April 2		P	R		Died subsequently of cancer.
45	Cannock	Dr. Moses Taylor ...	38	M	Cystoma	Right ovary removed	„ 2	H	...	R		
46	Birmingham	Dr. Bailey	30	M	Cystoma	Left ovary removed..	„ 9	H	...	R		
47	Darlaston	Dr. Sutton	33	S	Myoma	Both ovaries removed	„ 20		P	R		Complete cure; tumour has wholly disappeared.
48	Fazeley	Dr. Buxton	55	M	Malignant cystoma...	Exploratory	„ 25	H	...	R		Died subsequently of cancer.
49	Birmingham ...	Mr. H. Bracey	15	S	Malignant cystoma...	Exploratory	„ 26	H	...	R		Same patient as No. 20.
50	Birmingham	Mr. Hall Wright ...	12	S	Intestinal obstruction	Enterotomy	„ 27		P	R		
51	Coleshill	Dr. Taylor	29	S	Chronic ovaritis ...	Ovaries and tubes removed	„ 28	H	...	...	D	
52	Cradley	Dr. Standish	29	M	Cystoma	Left ovary removed	„ 29		P	R		
53	Nottingham	Dr. Huthwaite ...	47	M	Cystoma	Right ovary removed	May 7		P	R		
54	Lichfield	Dr. Bastable	36	M	Cystoma	Right ovary removed	„ 7		P	R		
55	Birmingham	Dr. Cox	57	M	Ruptured cystoma ...	Right ovary removed	„ 19	H	...	R		
56	Hanley	Dr. Craig	39	M	Extra-peritoneal cyst	Removal	„ 19		P	...	D	Complete cure.
57	Birmingham	Dr. Welch	7	S	Hydatids of liver ...	Hepatotomy	„ 20	H	...	R		
58	Darlaston	Dr. Cameron	40	M	Cystoma & hydrosalp.	Both ovaries removed	„ 21		P	R		
59	Nuneaton	Dr. Hammond	20	S	Dermoid cyst ...	Opened and drained	„ 27	H	...	R		Same patient as No. 9.
60	Dolgelly	Dr. E. Jones	29	M	Malignant sarcoma...	Exploratory	„ 31		P	R		
61	Birmingham	Dr. Drummond ...	27	W	Suppurat. haematoma	Opened and drained	June 9	H	...	R		
62	Cradley	Dr. Standish	29	M	Pyosalpinx	Tubes and ovaries removed	„ 13	H	...	R		
63	Malvern	Dr. Weir	48	M	Ruptured cystoma ...	Right ovary removed	„ 15		P	R		
64	Droitwich	Dr. Cuthbertson... ...	43	M	Myoma	Both ovaries removed	„ 16	H	...	R		Complete cure.
65	Birmingham	Mr. Hall Wright ...	47	M	Myoma	Both ovaries removed	„ 17	H	...	R		
66	Atherstone	Dr. Handford	33	M	Chronic peritonitis ...	Exploratory	„ 18	H	...	R		
67	Shustoke	Mr. O. Pomberton ...	35	M	Papilloma	Exploratory	„ 29	H	...	R		
68	Aston	Mr. Lawson Tait ...	31	M	Cystoma	Left ovary removed	July 4	H	...	R		
69	Wellington, Somer.	Dr. Edwards	22	S	Ruptured cystoma ...	Both ovaries removed	„ 5		P	R		
70	Walsall	Dr. G. Sharp	39	M	Cystoma	Left ovary removed	„ 6	H	...	R		Pregnant 4 mos.
71	Ashby-de-la-Zouch	Dr. Betts	34	M	Cystoma	Both ovaries removed	„ 7		P	R		
72	Derby	Dr. G. Copestake ...	35	W	Cystoma	Left ovary removed	„ 13		P	R		
73	Redditch	Dr. Bosworth ...	34	M	Double hydrosalpinx	Both tubes and ovaries removed	„ 14		P	R		
74	Alfreton, Derby ...	Dr. J. J. Bingham ...	45	M	Cystoma	Right ovary removed	„ 26		P	R		
75	Aston	Dr. Smith	33	M	Double pyosalpinx ...	Opened and drained	Aug. 2	H	...	R		
76	Birmingham	Dr. D. Nelson ...	38	M	Cystoma	Right ovary removed	„ 2	H	...	R		
77	Chirk	Dr. Aylmer Lewis ...	17	S	Cystoma	Left ovary removed	„ 2		P	R		
78	Durham	... ...	47	M	Myoma	Hysterotomy	„ 3	H	...	R		
79	Birmingham	Mr. Lawson Tait ...	40	M	Parovarian cyst ...	Removed	„ 8	H	...	R		Pregnant 4 mos.
80	Maentwrog, Wales	Dr. Roberts	63	M	Hydatids of liver ...	Hepatotomy	„ 15		P	R		
81	Stourbridge	Dr. Hammond Smith	27	M	Hydrosalpinx	Removed both tubes and ovaries	„ 19	H	...	R		
52	Derby	Dr. Rice	18	S	Cystoma	Right ovary removed	„ 22		P	R		
53	Sutton-in-Ashfield	Dr. J. J. Bingham ...	25	M	Cystoma	Both ovaries removed	„ 24	H	...	R		Died subsequently of cancer.
84	Ironbridge, Salop .	Dr. Law Webb ...	38	S	Myoma	Both ovaries and tubes removed	„ 25		P	R		
85	Birmingham	Dr. Kenny	43	S	Myoma	Both ovaries and tubes removed	„ 27		P	R		Complete cure.
86	Aston	Dr. Fairley	36	M	Pelvic abscess ...	Opened and drained	„ 17	H	...	R		
87	Worcester	Dr. Coombes	52	M	Cystoma	Left ovary removed	Sept. 3	H	...	R		
88	Adderbury, Oxon.	Dr. Colgrave	46	M	Cystoma	Right ovary removed	„ 5	H	...	R		
89	HorseBuckley, Wor	Dr. Woodward ...	51	M	Parovarian cyst ...	Removed	„ 12	H	...	R		
90	Bilston	Mr. Lawson Tait ...	35	M	Cystoma	Left ovary	„ 13	H	...	R		
91	Wolverhampton ...	Dr. Pope	40	M	Myoma	Both ovaries and tubes removed	„ 19		P	R		
92	Birmingham	Dr. Kenny	30	M	Cystoma	Left ovary removed	„ 20		P	R		
93	Festiniog	Dr. Evans	39	S	Malignant sarcoma...	Exploratory	„ 23		P	R		
94	Llandulas, N.W. ...	Dr. Turner	48	M	Parovarian cyst ...	Removed	„ 24	H	...	R		
95	Liverpool	Dr. McFie Campbell...	22	S	Suppurat. haematoma	Opened and drained	„ 29	H	...	R		Same as No. 17.
96	Oldhill	Dr. Ker	25	M	Hydro and pyosalpinx	Opened and drained	Oct. 3		P	R		
97	Broseley	Dr. Bartlam	51	S	Myoma	Both tubes and ovaries removed	„ 4	H	...	R		
98	Walsall	Dr. Sharp	37	M	Hydrosalpinx	Right tube removed ...	„ 7	H	...	R		
99	West Bromwich ...	Mr. Langley Brown ...	55	S	Myoma	Enterotomy (?) ...	„ 9		P	R	D	
100	Leominster	Dr. Edwards	35	S	Deformed pelvis ...	Cæsarian section ...	„ 11		P	R		
101	Birmingham	Dr. Madden... ...	47	M	Papilloma	Exploratory	„ 11		P	R		
102	Bridgnorth	Dr. Collis	23	M	Pelvic abscess ...	Opened and drained	„ 12	H	...	R		
103	Birmingham	Mr. J. R. Harmar ...	63	W	Cystoma	Right ovary removed	„ 15		P	R		
104	Birmingham	Mr. Hall Wright ...	34	M	Double hydrosalpinx	Both tubes removed	„ 19	H	...	R		
105	Wolverhampton ...	Mr. S. F. Palmer ...	57	S	Cystoma	Both ovaries removed	„ 21		P	R		
106	Dudley	Mr. Berry	31	S	Double pyosalpinx ...	Both tubes and ovaries removed	„ 21		P	R		
107	London	Dr. T. Chambers ...	29	M	Double hydrosalpinx	Both tubes and ovaries removed	„ 24	H	...	R		
108	Ombersley	Dr. Roden	63	M	Cystoma	Right ovary removed	„ 24	H	...	R		
109	Wolverhampton ...	Dr. Scott	34	M	Cystoma	Right ovary removed	„ 29		P			Pregnant 4 mos.; acute peritonitis.
110	Ludlow	Dr. Brooks	37	S	Myoma	Hysterotomy	„ 30		P	...	...	

REPORTS OF HOSPITAL PRACTICE
IN
MEDICINE AND SURGERY.

SAMARITAN FREE HOSPITAL FOR WOMEN AND CHILDREN.

SOLID OVARIAN TUMOURS.
(Under the care of Mr. KNOWSLEY THORNTON.)
(Continued from page 674 of last volume.)

Case 1.—Removal of Large Solid Dermoid Tumour.
(No. 11 in Ovariotomy Tables.)(a)

C. H., married five years, aged twenty-six, came under my care as a hospital patient in September, 1876. (The Samaritan was closed at the time, and in consequence I operated upon her in a nursing home, but include her case among my hospital patients, and therefore give it here.) She had had two children, the youngest being nearly three years old.

History.—Did not quite regain her size after last confinement, but otherwise felt well, and nursed for nine months, when, a period coming on, she weaned her child, and immediately became, as she thought, again pregnant. The single appearance of the menses occurred in August, 1874, and she had no further discharge till April, 1875, and then only a slight coloured discharge for a day and a half. It was stopped by the application of a cold wet napkin to the vulva. She assured me that during this time she had all the symptoms of pregnancy, and that she continued to feel the movements of the child for two weeks after this discharge. When I examined her, in September, 1876, there was still sufficient milk in both breasts for it to squirt out on pressure, though the breasts were evidently wasting. The increase of size had continued up to December, 1875, and since that time there had been little, if any, change.

On examination, I found the abdomen occupied by a very large solid tumour, in the centre of which there was an irregular mass very much resembling a child. Vaginal examination revealed the presence of a healthy mobile uterus of normal size, in front of which the lower part of the tumour could be felt, with an angular, bony mass in it. I found a slight fœtid serous discharge from the umbilicus, and learned that this had been going on for six months. The umbilicus was very dark in colour, and formed a tumour of the size of half a hen's egg.

The diagnosis which most commended itself to me was that of dermoid tumour of the ovary, but there was the question of encysted extra-uterine fœtation, and the possibility that the latter condition and ovarian tumour might both be present. The patient's general health was failing very rapidly, and I therefore determined to perform an exploratory operation at once. The operation was performed on September 11, 1876, and is noteworthy as being my first attempt at Listerian ovariotomy. How poor an attempt and how unsuitable a case no one now knows better than myself. The discharge from the umbilicus made it a septic case to begin with, and how I overlooked this fact at the time I cannot imagine. There were also many failures in the details of applying the method, and many things were done which I now know to be wrong.

The operation was a very formidable one—the tumour practically a solid sarcoma (though it contained some small cysts), with masses of bone, skin with hair, etc., irregularly diffused throughout. The umbilical tumour was formed of thickened and brawny skin, with small cysts in it, and from the latter the serous discharge had apparently taken place. Its under surface was adherent to the tumour and to the omentum, the latter being also extensively adherent to the tumour, and full of little sago-grain growths, which I have no doubt were the result of direct infection. The right ovary was also diseased, as is so often the case with malignant tumour. Both pedicles were secured by short silk ligatures soaked in carbolic oil. (I have since found that the silk when soaked in oil does not absorb well, and is very apt to cause abscess.) I also put in a glass drainage-tube, but hardly any serum came away, and it was removed in

thirty-six hours. The tumour weighed nineteen pounds after removal, and the incision necessary to extract it was fully eight inches long.

The patient did not do well from the first, and died on the fifth day. No post-mortem was allowed, and I am not at all sure what was the actual cause of death. Temperature and pulse suggested septicæmia, but there was no sickness, flatus passed well, the abdomen was perfectly flat, and there was no rapid decomposition of the body after death. On the fourth day, temperature and pulse both came down, and the patient seemed so much better that I confidently expected recovery; but in the afternoon she suddenly became comatose, and remained so till she died next day.

The solid parts of the tumour presented the microscopic characters of a mixed sarcoma; the dermoid portions contained perfect skin, with hairs, follicles, etc., and there were large irregular plates of bone, some of which contained teeth; the small cysts which were scattered through the mass had, when not covered with patches of skin, the usual cyst lining, through which small solid papillomata were sprouting.

Case 2.—Removal of Solid Dermoid Tumour from Left Side, and of a small one from Right Side.
(No. 143, Ovariotomy Tables.)(b)

T. P., single, aged thirty-four, came under my care at the Samaritan in October, 1879. She was a very stout, florid woman, and apparently in robust health. The lower abdomen contained a very hard, mobile tumour, with evidences of adherent intestines along its upper border. Menstruation quite regular.

History.—In November, 1878, began to suffer with pain in the abdomen, and noticed that she was getting large and that the abdomen was hard. Pain became severe and constant in June, 1879, so that she could not sit up straight, and in July increase of size became very rapid.

My diagnosis was either dermoid ovarian, or ovarian with twisted pedicle—the latter diagnosis being suggested by the paroxysmal character of the pain, and the fact that after the severe pain in June the growth of the tumour appeared to have been arrested for nearly a month.

On November 5, I performed ovariotomy, and removed a very solid nodular tumour from the left side. An attempt to tap the tumour after I had exposed it only gave exit to some dark blood and creamy fat, and after removal I found that the whole mass was a soft, brain-like sarcoma, with small plates and spicules of bone, and other dermoid structures, scattered irregularly through it. The tumour was accidentally destroyed, and I had no opportunity of examining it microscopically, but I have no doubt it was of similar nature to the tumour described above, the sarcoma being of a much softer kind. The other ovary was affected with similar disease, and was also removed. It was as large as a small cocoanut. Both pedicles were ligatured and dropped in. The patient made a rapid recovery, and left the hospital apparently quite well, on the twenty-third day after operation.

Within the year she began to suffer pain in the abdomen, and enlarged again, dying at her own home in the country on July 20, 1880. No post-mortem was made, but there can be no doubt, from the account of the case which I received, that there was very general malignant disease of the peritoneal surfaces.

Remarks.—It is worthy of special note that, in spite of the complete disorganisation of both ovaries, menstruation continued with perfect regularity up to the time of operation. So far as I could learn, there was no return of the menses afterwards. These two tumours, or rather four tumours, seem to belong to a class which has not previously been described—the whole ovarian stroma taking on not only a malignant sarcomatous growth, but also forming dermoid structures, not, as is usually the case, from small circumscribed centres, but from the cell-elements throughout, so that sarcoma and dermoid structure become jumbled together in a confused mass. The only approach to anything of the kind that I have seen, except in these two cases, was in some small solid growths in a case of double dermoid operated upon some years ago by Mr. Spencer Wells. The condition seemed in this case to be confined to these small

---

(a) Ovariotomy Tables. *Transactions of Medical Chirurgical Society,* vol. lx., pages 311-13.

(b) Ovariotomy Tables. *Transactions of Medical Chirurgical Society.* Now in the press.

solid masses, which projected into the cyst-cavity in one tumour, the remainder of this tumour and the whole of the other presenting the usual characters of a dermoid ovarian cyst, *i.e.*, partly dermoid, but mainly ordinary multilocular cysts. When last I heard of this patient, some years after the operation, she was in perfect health. The unfortunate result of the operation in the first case I have recorded seems hardly a subject for regret, when considered side by side with the second. And in the first, infection of both parietes and omentum had already occurred; while in the second there was no evidence of this condition at the time of operation, and yet fatal recurrence took place within the year. This last case is one of the six referred to in my previous remarks on page 214.(c)

(*To be continued.*)

TERMS OF SUBSCRIPTION.
(*Free by post.*)

				£ s. d.
British Islands	. . . .	*Twelve Months*	.	£1 8 0
„ „	. . . .	*Six* „	.	0 14 0
The Colonies and the United }	*Twelve* „	.	1 10 0
States of America . . . }			
„ „ „	. .	*Six* „	.	0 15 0
India	. .	*Twelve* „	.	1 10 0
„ (*viâ Brindisi*)	. . .	„ „	.	1 15 0
„ „	. . .	*Six* „	.	0 15 0
„ (*viâ Brindisi*)	. . .	„ „	.	0 17 6

Foreign Subscribers are requested to inform the Publishers of any remittance made through the agency of the Post-office.

Single Copies of the Journal can be obtained of all Booksellers and Newsmen, price Sixpence.

Cheques or Post-office Orders should be made payable to Mr. JAMES LUCAS, 11, *New Burlington-street, W.*

TERMS FOR ADVERTISEMENTS.

			£ s. d.
Seven lines (70 words)	. . . .	.	£0 4 6
Each additional line (10 words)	. . .	.	0 0 6
Half-column, or quarter-page	. . .	.	1 5 0
Whole column, or half-page	. . .	.	2 10 0
Whole page	. . . . .	.	5 0 0

Births, Marriages, and Deaths are inserted Free of Charge.

THE MEDICAL TIMES AND GAZETTE *is published on Friday morning: Advertisements must therefore reach the Publishing Office not later than One o'clock on Thursday.*

Medical Times and Gazette.

SATURDAY, NOVEMBER 5, 1881.

PROFESSOR GREENFIELD ON PATHOLOGY, PAST AND PRESENT.

THE opening day of the session in the Edinburgh Medical School furnishes the student, as he listens to lecture after lecture, with the impression that the very last lecture he has listened to is on that particular subject which is the greatest of all subjects in his medical curriculum. Professor Greenfield therefore had a twofold advantage, in that he was making a first appearance in his chair, and that his office is one which he cannot well magnify too much. Whatever amount of attention Pathology as a separate subject may receive in our schools and examination boards, we are probably all agreed in a general or abstract kind of way that it is a very important subject—indeed, the very foundation of the whole superstructure of professional skill and usefulness. But Professor Greenfield had an opportunity, which he did not neglect, of doing something more. The metropolitan University of Scotland is not only unique in having a Professorship of Pathology, but it stands almost alone in requiring a separate and special examination in pathology, including morbid anatomy, for a medical degree.

"And this fact," he adds, "has reacted upon the teaching, which has, in many schools, been allowed to remain incomplete and inefficient. Attendance upon lectures on pathological anatomy is now required by many examining bodies, but I say with some confidence that, with one or two exceptions, there has scarcely existed, if there does now exist, in the London Medical Schools any course in which pathological histology is systematically taught, so as to comprehend a practical study of the principal changes in all the important organs."

Regarding Professor Greenfield's address, and the varied subject-matter of it, let us say at once that it betokens a catholicity of mind which should prove a valuable quality to one who has daily to address a class of two or three hundred students. A professor, it has been well said, is much more than a speaking text-book; he is all that is excellent in several text-books, and in the text-books of several languages, whilst he has his own experience to fall back upon to aid and guide him in their interpretation. The incumbent of the Edinburgh Chair of Pathology cannot afford to be either limited in his knowledge of facts, or crotchety in his theories, or bigoted in his statements. He has the whole history of pathology behind him; and Professor Greenfield, in the part of his address which we published last week, has spoken of the great men of former times with the respect that is their due. He has before him in the present the various concurrent, if not always convergent, lines of work which are being followed by men of various aptitudes and tastes; and there is evidence, in that part of his address which we publish to-day, that he is no less aware of that existing variety than sensible of his own responsibility as a teacher towards it. Not morbid anatomy and histology alone, not experiment alone, not clinical observation alone, but each and all of these enter into the programme which he unfolded before the Edinburgh students. He utters a timely note of warning that it is possible to make too much of morbid histology. "We have sought rather to find in structure the characters of disease, than to make it a guide to the understanding of disease. We have been passing through what we may call the slough of histology. For example, the tubercle corpuscle of Lebert, the cancer-cell, the giant-cell, the microphyte, all have had their day as the absolute criteria of particular diseases." We are especially glad to be told that even the microphyte has ceased to be the absolute criterion of particular diseases. The text, indeed, gives "microcyte," but that new-looking word, if it has not been coined by the compositor, can hardly be, on internal evidence, other than the equivalent of the term which we have ventured to substitute for it.

This inaugural address strikes the true note when it says that the standpoint of pathology is the physiological, or, if we prefer it, the biological standpoint. It must be a gratifying circumstance to Professor Virchow, in his mature age, to find that the philosophical view of pathology which he has valiantly contended for during all the years from his early work of 1848 down to his latest deliverance in St. James's Hall, is the view that necessarily commends itself to everyone who has the grasp of mind to expound the scope of pathology at all. Professor Greenfield, indeed, has a tale of a hospital surgeon who once gravely asserted to him that the capability of telling from a scraping under the microscope whether a tumour was malignant or not was "all that a student wants to know of pathology." That accomplishment—if it were a real one—is not so small as it may look to some advanced morbid anatomists of a special school; but, at any rate, rule-of-thumb pathology is not enough. What the Edinburgh Chair gives the opportunity of teaching, and what has been and will, we are sure, be still well taught from it, is the fascinating subject of diseased processes and their relation to healthy processes. It is a living knowledge of very different value from that of purely dead matter, which the practitioner will carry with him, as Professor Greenfield says, into his every-day round of work—"and whilst he will thereby be delivered from the tedium of routine, he will also be saved from its dangers." Speaking from a Chair specially devoted to Pathology, the Professor was not at all likely to represent his subject as being what some would have it to be—only a part of physiology. Both subjects deal with the phenomena of life, but in pathology it is *vita præter naturam*. The one subject has its proper field, and so has the other, only that the greater includes the less. The methods, however, are the same. Whatever method of research, we read in this address, is requisite for the full investigation of the phenomena of healthy life in all its manifestations, is equally or still more requisite for studying the phenomena of disease life. That would be a strange physiology which should conduct its study on dead animals alone, and no less strange a pathology studied only on dead subjects. Perhaps it was not superfluous, in view of the pretensions sometimes set up for physiology, to have added that it would be an equally strange pathology that was studied only on healthy persons. But biology comes first, and we can only understand what constitutes disease when we know what is the condition of things in ordinary health. No one could think of beginning the study of physiology from a basis of morbid anatomy and diseased processes.

"NAVEL-ILL" IN CHILDREN.

It is well known to obstetric practitioners that there is met with sometimes in new-born children an affection of the navel which appears to lead to pyæmia. Some years ago Mr. Jonathan Hutchinson communicated to the Obstetrical Society of London an account of a similar disease occurring in lambs. In those which he had dissected he found purulent inflammation of the umbilical veins, with pyæmic abscesses in the liver, and in some peritonitis, pleuritis, pneumonia, and joint-affection also occurred. In the following year Dr. George Roper brought before the same Society two cases of umbilical phlebitis with pyæmia. Both the cases had occurred in the practice of the same medical man, and the mother of one of the children had died from pyæmia. His paper contained a reference to the work of Dr. Hasse (published by the Sydenham Society), in which that author had collected ten cases of a similar affection. Dr. Arthur Edis, on the same occasion, brought forward a case which he had met with, in which an identical form of disease led to the death of the child. These are almost the only accounts of the subject in our literature.

A recent paper by Dr. Max Runge, of Berlin,(a) contains an interesting account of a larger number of cases than either of the authors above referred to were able to collect. In the Strasburg Lying-in Charity, during the summer of 1876, five cases of navel affection occurred out of 120 deliveries. There were no cases of puerperal fever. In the summer of 1879 an epidemic of puerperal fever appeared, many women dying; but there was no disease among the children. From March to June, 1880, the health of the mothers was exceedingly good; but twenty-six infants suffered from navel affection, sixteen of whom died. Dr. Runge has altogether seen forty-five cases, in twenty-four of which a careful post-mortem examination was made. In every one of the cases he found inflammation of the umbilical arteries, the umbilical vein being healthy. In eight cases this was the only morbid condition present. In one there

(a) *Zeitschrift für Geburtshülfe und Gynäkologie*, Bd. VI., Heft 1.

was syphilitic disease in lungs, supra-renal capsules, and epiphysal cartilages. Twice cerebral hæmorrhages were present, in one accompanied with gangrene of the scalp from pressure with forceps, and in one with gonorrhœal ophthalmia. In fourteen cases there were morbid changes present which were undoubtedly connected with the umbilical affection. In five, pneumonia or pleurisy were the only affections which occurred; in four others they existed along with other changes; and in one (the syphilitic one above mentioned) there was peritonitis. In two there was jaundice, in two erysipelas, in three hypertrophy of the spleen, and in one infarctions of micrococci in that organ.

Dr. Runge draws the following conclusion from his cases: —Inflammation of the umbilical arteries is not in all cases a local disease tending to recovery. It may, *per se*, cause death, and it may lead to pyæmia. In the cases in which pyæmia occurred (except the one with gangrene of the scalp) there was no channel except the umbilicus through which the infective poison could have entered the circulation He believes that the process begins in the connective tissue around the arteries, and then extends to the vessel itself, producing thrombosis and the subsequent changes seen. The precise time at which the morbid process began could not be ascertained. None of the children died during the first three days, three died on the fourth day, eleven between the fifth and eighth days, and ten on or after the ninth day.

He then considers the etiology of the disease. It has been supposed that the infection was derived from disease in the mother. This is negatived in Dr. Runge's cases by the fact that, with the exception of one that died from eclampsia, one that had cystitis, and another in whom there was metritis, all the mothers were well.

The diagnosis is exceedingly obscure. In many of Dr. Runge's cases its existence was not suspected during life. That pus can be squeezed from the umbilicus has been stated to be a sign of this disease; but our author finds that this is only seldom the case with arteritis, and that it occurs in other conditions, so that it is not to be relied on. It has been said that jaundice occurs with umbilical phlebitis, but not with arteritis: this is shown by Dr. Runge's cases to be erroneous. From the uncertainty of the diagnosis it follows that the prognosis is equally obscure. The death-rate of umbilical disease in the cases observed by our author was about 45 per cent.

Assuming that the disease under consideration arises from septic infection, and that the septic infection gains access to the system through the umbilicus, the most obvious source of such infection is the dead bit of the cord between the abdominal wall and the ligature. To prevent the disease, therefore, it would seem to be first necessary to insure an aseptic condition of this structure. Dr. Runge has therefore carried out a careful experimental investigation into different methods of dealing with the remnant of the cord after its ligature. He compared the behaviour of different bits of cord, under the following conditions :—1. Simply exposed to the air; 2. Enclosed in a glass case, so that evaporation of moisture was prevented; 3. Wrapped in a rag soaked in carbolic oil; 4. Wrapped in a dry rag. He found that Nos. 1 and 4, which were simply kept dry, quickly mummified without smell; No. 2, in which evaporation was prevented, soon stank; No. 3 did not get fœtid, but did not shrivel up. From these experiments the best way of dealing with the bit of cord is obvious.

A most important point remains to be mentioned, viz., that, with the prevalence of this navel affection, there were a remarkable number of cases of purulent ophthalmia. What the connexion is—whether the eyes were infected from the umbilicus, or *vice versâ*—our author is unable to express an opinion.

Another point of interest is, that a striking number of the children who died were premature. This, in fact, seems the chief element in prognosis; for the children at term who were attacked mostly survived.

For the prevention and cure of this malady the chief points seem to be :—1. To keep the bit of cord which remains attached as dry as possible; 2. The greatest care in washing and dressing the child, so that there shall be no possibility of contact between contagious pus or the maternal discharges and the eyes or umbilicus of the child. As an application to the umbilicus, Dr. Runge recommends a powder composed of salicylic acid and starch.

WORK IN THE TREATMENT OF INSANITY.

DR. SAMUEL MITCHELL, the Medical Superintendent of the South Yorkshire Asylum, near Sheffield, reports to the Visiting Justices that in the general treatment of the lunatic patients under his care, leading prominence is given to employment. As soon after admission as the requisite degree of mental quietude and bodily strength has been acquired, it is expected that some kind of work, sufficient to keep the mental and bodily faculties in exercise, shall be engaged in, as affording the most hopeful means of cure. With this view, many patients have been kept at work on the farm, in the kitchen-garden, and in levelling and laying out the airing courts; and others have assisted in the various workshops. No difference of opinion can exist nowadays as to the value of employment as one element of treatment in certain forms of insanity. Its usefulness has been long known, and is now universally recognised. Forty years ago, Dr. Hill, of the North Riding Asylum, taught that spade-labour was a panacea in mental diseases; and since then the Commissioners in Lunacy have persistently called attention to the subject of the occupation of the inmates of the asylums under their supervision. The danger now seems to be, not that occupation may be neglected, but that its importance may be exaggerated. The simplicity of its application as a means of treatment, the official favour bestowed on heavy returns of patients usefully employed, the economical results of lunatic industry, and the magisterial and popular notion that asylums and prisons have something in common, and that what is good for convicts must be good for lunatics, all tend to encourage a rather amplified and indiscriminate resort to occupation as a remedial measure in insanity. It would be deplorable should our asylums become vast workshops instead of hospitals, and should their medical superintendents sink the physician in the task-master. That there is some danger of such a decadence, phrases found in asylum reports like that of Dr. Michell, that "work is the most hopeful means of cure" in insanity, seem to suggest. If work be the most hopeful means of cure, the wonder is that insanity should abound amongst us, and that lunatic asylums should be constantly multiplying, putting forth new wings, and throwing off new blocks. There is work enough and to spare, and occupation might be provided for those who need it, without any such credential as a certificate of unsound mind. We fear the truth is that work has an etiological as well as a curative relation to insanity. Our asylum population is not all drawn from the indolent and leisured classes, but includes many with bodies and brains exhausted or worn out in the hard struggle of bread-winning. And a majority of those pauper lunatics, at any rate, whose mental trouble springs not from wear and tear, but from other sources, such as hereditary predisposition or bodily illness, have been hard at work up till the outbreak of their insanity. In them, work, if "the most hopeful means of cure," has certainly not proved most effectual means of prevention. The first duty

of an asylum is, we take it, to provide not toil, but repose—not attrition, but reparation; its paramount duty is to bring all the resources of science and experience to bear upon the relief and resolution of nervous disease. Amongst these resources occupation takes its place —a conspicuous place too—but to exalt it above all other resources, and to claim for it all-healing powers, is to convert it into an engine of cruelty, and to bring it ultimately into contempt. Wholesale occupation in an asylum would be worse than general idleness. What is wanted is not mere occupation as such, but varied, interesting, well-chosen occupation, suited to the individual wants of patients. A man emerging from an acute attack of madness is not to be driven back at once into his habitual activities, and the monotony of his workaday life, but is to be guided rather into "fresh fields and pastures new," where he may obtain at once exercise and refreshment. A woman under similar circumstances is not to be instantly reduced again to domestic drudgery, but is rather to be taught some new pursuits that may divert her thoughts from morbid channels, engaging attention without overstraining it, imparting an additional interest to her lot, and fostering self-respect.

The selection and regulation of work for the insane require medical knowledge and sympathetic insight. Without these, work may be chosen that is unsuitable, and pushed to a degree that is oppressive. With these, it may be made a powerful and beneficent adjunct to medical treatment. Dr. Mitchell, we are glad to notice, in spite of his theory as to the precedence to be given to work over the pharmacopœia, rest, education, religious instruction, diet, hygiene, and all other means included in the modern treatment of insanity, justly estimates its utility in actual practice, and does not unduly insist on it in the institution over which he so ably presides. Only 50 per cent. of the male patients and 70 per cent. of the female patients under his care are usefully employed.

THE WEEK.

TOPICS OF THE DAY.

THE amount of agitation necessary to secure the adoption of any measure, however good, can only be realised by those who have endeavoured to bring about a radical reform, and much credit is due to the delegates from the vestries and district boards of London who meet in St. Martin's Hall from time to time, with a view of obtaining a less expensive and more satisfactory supply of water for the metropolis. These gentlemen recently held a meeting, when their chairman, Mr. E. J. Watherston, explained that they had assembled to urge the Government to take steps to deal with the water question next session, to which end it was necessary that Parliamentary notices should be given during the present month. The consequences of the inability of the Government to legislate on this subject last year, he observed, were most serious, owing to the re-assessment of the metropolis, of which the water companies had not been slow to avail themselves. Further delay was very much to be deprecated. The Grand Junction Company, and the Southwark and Vauxhall Company, failed last summer in their high service supply. Moreover, if the question were shelved any longer, either by the apathy of Parliament, or by the action of those who desired the previous unification of London government, it was difficult to see how Parliament could avoid granting extended capital and fresh powers to the water companies, all of which would add considerably to their claims for compensation when the inevitable day of purchase arrived. As it was, the revenues of the companies had increased, and were increasing at a rate even beyond all previous calculation—a circumstance attributable not only to the normal increase of houses, estimated at about 25,000 annually, but also to the fact that the companies, released from the arrangements for purchase, had, in many instances, although admittedly within their Parliamentary limits, raised their charges upon the basis of the re-assessment of metropolitan property. Some discussion took place as to the action which the conference ought to take, but ultimately it was agreed to transmit a memorial to the Prime Minister, representing the increasing charges which the ratepayers of the metropolis had to pay to the water companies, without obtaining any equivalent in the shape of a purer or more copious water-supply, and urging the Government to legislate on the subject next session on the lines of the report of the Select Committee of last year.

At the last meeting of the City Commission of Sewers, Dr. Sedgwick Saunders, the Medical Officer of Health, reported that during the week over six tons of diseased meat had been seized at the slaughter-houses and markets. Public attention having been directed to the alleged overcrowding of houses in Windsor-street, and other streets in Bishopsgate, a night inspection had been made, and, while the result did not justify the charge of overcrowding, it was impossible to exaggerate the dirty condition of the premises, owing to the filthy habits of the inmates. In Windsor-street there were 12 houses with 108 rooms, in which 359 people dwelt ; in Widegate-street, 7 houses, 48 rooms, and 88 persons ; in Sandy-row, 6 houses, 49 rooms, and 124 persons ; and in Catherine-Wheel-alley, 3 houses, 16 rooms, and 73 persons. No persons were found sleeping in the basements ; and the allegations freely made by irresponsible persons, that large numbers of persons occupied these rooms in the night alternately, had not been borne out. The structural condition of the majority of the houses would not justify any attempt to demolish them, although it must be admitted that the habits of the occupants were not conducive to health, morality, or decency. The disposal of the refuse of the City was also discussed, and it was proposed to conduct, at an expense of over £9000, experiments on a patent process for consuming it ; the subject was ultimately adjourned, in order that the Court might obtain counsel's opinion upon matters involved.

The City of London Union recently discussed the question of appointing a vaccination officer for the City. The Guardians have been in correspondence with the Local Government Board ever since June last on the subject, but the latter body objected to the appointment of a salaried officer, and insisted that the remuneration should be by fees   Dr. Stevenson attended the meeting, and in the course of his remarks said the recent epidemic of small-pox had shown that the disease in the metropolis was most prevalent in three classes of persons—viz., " emigrants " to London from the provinces (very nearly three-fourths of whom consisted of workhouse boys, who obtained their living by any means), the unvaccinated, and the badly vaccinated, which was the largest class of all.   At least 40,000 infants annually escaped without vaccination.   Only by the vaccination officers doing their duty thoroughly could they hope to get rid of small-pox.   The question of the appointment of an officer upon the terms mentioned by the Local Government Board was ultimately referred to a committee for consideration.   The Hackney representative at the Metropolitan Asylums Board reported to his Vestry that the present number of small-pox cases in the various hospitals of the Managers was 451, against 428 at the expiration of the previous fortnight.   Fever was gradually increasing, there being 445 fever patients in the hospitals, against 380 at the last fortnight's report.   The increase of fever had

been so marked that the Managers had decided to divide the Deptford Hospital, using one half for fever and the other half for small-pox ; so that when the accommodation for fever patients was fully occupied at the two existing hospitals there would be room available at Deptford.

At a general meeting of the magistrates for the county of Middlesex, held last week, the Committee for Accounts and General Purposes brought up a report showing the salaries and disbursements of the various coroners for the quarter ended September 30 last, viz.:—Sir J. Humphreys, salary £551 18s. 6d., disbursements £351 7s. 8d. ; Mr. G. Danford Thomas, salary £524 18s. 4d., disbursements £365 2s. 3d. ; Dr. Diplock, salary £162 10s., disbursements £135 7s. ; Mr. W. J. Payne, salary £13 12s. 4d., disbursements £14 8s. ; Mr. C. St. Clair Bedford, salary £118 11s. 6d., disbursements £106 18s. 6d.—showing a total of quarter's salaries and expenditure of £2344 14s. 3d.

The Commissioners appointed to inquire into the causes of accidents in mines, with a view to ascertain whether the resources of science furnish any practicable expedients that are not now in use, and are calculated to prevent the occurrence of accidents or limit their disastrous consequences, have just issued a preliminary report.   In this report, however, they confine themselves to giving a summary of the evidence already taken, without indicating any definite conclusions of their own.   They reserve the expression of any such conclusions until the completion of the experimental and other investigations upon which they are still engaged.

It is to be regretted that the magistrates generally will not combine in an effort to put down the disgusting traffic in bad and unwholesome meat which is still openly carried on in our midst ; and the only method to effect this would be to abolish fines and inflict imprisonment in every case. Recently a butcher carrying on business at Otterton, Devon, was summoned before Sir T. S. Owden, at Guildhall Police-court, by the Chief Inspector at the Central Meat and Poultry Market, for sending the carcase of a cow to that market for sale as human food, the same being diseased and unfit for the food of man.   The offence was clearly proved.   Sir T. S. Owden thought it a very bad case, and fined him £20, and £3 3s. costs, or one month's imprisonment.   The fine and costs were paid.   At Preston, also, a butcher was fined £10 and costs, or two months' imprisonment, for having in his possession a large quantity of meat unfit for human food, some of it being quite rotten. It was stated that most of this flesh was sold to shopkeepers in the town for making sausages and meat pies.

The Committee of the Indian Medical Service Defence Fund have issued a circular to the subscribers, in which they state that their attention has been called by many members of the Service to the rumours that very serious additional changes in the constitution of the Indian Medical Department are imminently impending.   It is, they say, of course of the highest importance that all proposals for such a purpose should be carefully criticised, and instant measures adopted to induce the Government to refrain from all changes calculated either to ultimately damage the public service, or inflict unnecessary or unavoidable hardships and injury on individuals.   The Committee are willing to use their best efforts in this direction, but this will involve a certain amount of expenditure in time and money : the former they willingly place at the free disposal of their late brother officers ; for the latter they regret that they must appeal to the members of the Service themselves, and the circular suggests the manner in which the additional funds might be procured.

At a recent meeting of the Smoke Abatement Committee

a letter was read from the American Minister, acknowledging the receipt of Lord Granville's note on the subject of the exhibition proposed to be held in London in the coming autumn, of apparatus of all kinds devised to prevent smoke, or to consume smokeless fuel, and promising to give publicity to the objects of the exhibition in his country, as well as to adopt any measures which may be found practicable for contributing to its interest and success. The hon. secretary of the Smoke Abatement Committee further reported that the directors of the Gas Light and Coke Company had liberally decided to give the gas required for the purposes of the exhibition gratuitously, and a vote of thanks was accorded to the Company. It was further reported that applications for space had been received very numerously from leading houses among the manufacturers of improved domestic grates and heating apparatus, as well as from the inventors and manufacturers of various novelties for the consumption or reduction of smoke.

The Medical Acts Commission met at 2, Victoria-street, Westminster, on October 18 last, and four following days. There were present the Earl of Camperdown (chairman), the Bishop of Peterborough, the Right Hon. W. H. F. Cogan, the Right Hon. G. Sclater-Booth, M.P., Mr. Simon, C.B., Professor Huxley, Dr. Robert McDonnell, Professor Turner, and the Secretary. The following witnesses were examined :—Dr. John K. Barton ; Mr. William Stokes, of Dublin ; Dr. J. Magee Finny, and Dr. J. W. Moore, Irish Medical Association ; Dr. B. W. Richardson, Medical Defence Association ; Mr. Thomas Collins, Apothecaries' Hall, Ireland ; Professor Struthers, Aberdeen University ; Professor P. Redfern, Queen's University ; Professor T. R. Fraser, Edinburgh University ; Mr. John Tomes, British Dental Association ; Mr. Thomas Edgelow, Association of Surgeons practising Dental Surgery ; Rev. Samuel Haughton, M.D., Dublin University ; Professor Young, Glasgow University ; and Dr. J. G. Greenwood, Victoria University.

A very serious epidemic of scarlet fever is reported to be raging at Hull, and the Medical Officer of Health there has reported that 128 fresh cases were discovered in the course of the week, the deaths from the disease in one fortnight having amounted to no less than sixty-eight. The fever is stated to be distributed all over the town, and the medical officer attributes its rapid spread to the carelessness of the inhabitants in mixing indiscriminately with each other while members of their families are suffering from the fever.

UNUSUAL TEMPERATURES.

In our number for November 1, 1879, there appeared the brief report of a case which had been under the care of Mr. Rivington in the London Hospital. The patient, as is usual in these cases, was a female, and about the troublesome age of forty-two. She had already been an in-patient, and her left thigh had been amputated for an intractable ulcer. The stump did not do well, and she was readmitted to have it dealt with. At this time the temperature was 99° Fahr.— that is, about February 26. On March 11 the temperature was 98·2°. Then began the curious variations. On the 14th it ranged from 107·8° to 100°; but after this having been said it will be better to leave the rest to the statements of Dr. Stephen Mackenzie, under whose care she came, and to Mr. Rivington's notes made at the time, elsewhere published in our columns.

THE METROPOLITAN WATER-SUPPLY FOR SEPTEMBER, 1881.

It is to be gathered from the report of the Water Examiners on the supplies issued by the metropolitan water companies during the month of September last, that the state of the water in the Thames at Hampton, Molesey, and Sunbury, where the intakes of several of the London companies are situated, was good in quality during the whole of the month, with the exception of two days, the 27th and 28th, when it became indifferent ; the water in the river Lea was also good during the whole of the month—remarks which, of course, refer to the condition of the water previous to filtration. The report presented to the Local Government Board by the analysts acting on behalf of the water companies says : "Altogether the water supplied by the metropolitan companies during the month of September continues to be of excellent quality, though no longer presenting that exceptional freedom from other than blue colour by which it was characterised during the summer months." Dr. Frankland's report states that of the water drawn from the Thames, by the Chelsea, West Middlesex, Southwark, Grand Junction, and Lambeth Companies, that sent out by the Lambeth Company alone maintained the quality of the last month's supply, whilst that distributed by the other companies exhibited a deterioration. With the exception of that furnished by the Chelsea Company, the water was in every case delivered in an efficiently filtered condition. Of the Lea water, that supplied by the New River Company was superior to any derived from the Thames, whilst that sent out by the East London Company was better than average Thames water. Both supplies were efficiently filtered before delivery. The deep well water furnished by the Kent and Colne Valley Companies and by the Tottenham Local Board of Health was of its usual excellent quality for drinking; and the Colne Valley Company, by softening their supply with lime, thereby rendered it also suitable for washing and all other domestic purposes.

TYPHUS FEVER IN LISSON-GROVE.

Some of our lay contemporaries have lately been occupying themselves with the unsanitary condition of certain streets opening out of Lisson-grove. We doubt not that their powerful advocacy will so draw public attention to these "fever dens," that, like others in the past, they will soon have to disappear. Such infected spots are dangers to the public health, quite apart from all local considerations ; and all efforts to stamp out infectious disease will be futile so long as such plague-spots are allowed to exist. We hear from the Medical Superintendent (Dr. Lunn) of the New Marylebone Infirmary that only two real cases were admitted, subsequently to be sent off to the Homerton Fever Hospital, where one (female) died. It is comforting to find that the amount of typhus said to exist seems to have been exaggerated ; but, bearing in mind the nature of the malady, it is to be regretted that conditions under which the fever is known to arise should have been allowed to exist so long.

THE TROUBLES OF THE METROPOLITAN ASYLUMS BOARD.

Amongst various items of business transacted at the last meeting of the Metropolitan Asylums Board a letter was read from the Local Government Board with reference to the ambulance station in London Fields. Mr. Hedges said it was essential that every provision should be made for the removal and reception of fever patients. This epidemic was fast getting ahead of them. Four of their nurses at Homerton had been seized with typhus fever, and every one of these nurses would cost the ratepayers at least £50. Sir E. H. Currie said the Local Government Board evidently wished for information as to the length of time it would take to remove Marylebone patients by the ambulances to the various hospitals. Mr. Galsworthy said he thought it was disgraceful on the part of Marylebone that the outbreak had not been discovered until three weeks after its commencement. The small-pox statistics showed that there' was an increase of sixteen cases during the past fortnight, as compared with the previous period. Sir E. H. Currie said it was a sorry state of affairs, and pointed out that, during the fortnight ended the previous day, there had been 175 cases admitted, as contrasted with 113 in the former period. For the past fortnight there had been 181 cases of fever admitted to the hospitals, being an increase of 48 in the total number remaining under treatment. Mr. Galsworthy moved—"That, having regard to the interlocutory injunction recently granted by the High Court of Justice, restraining the Managers from continuing the use of the Fulham Hospital, constructed at the expense of the ratepayers generally, for the purpose for which it was established—viz., for metropolitan pauper patients, irrespective of area,—and restricting the use of such hospital to patients within a limited area, as well as to the injunction granted by the Court of Queen's Bench against the use of the Hampstead Hospital, and to the several threats of legal proceedings, the Managers are of opinion that the time has arrived when the General Purposes Committee should seek an interview with the President of the Local Government Board, and ascertain whether he is prepared to take steps, and, if so, what steps, to enable the Managers to carry out their duties according to the spirit and intention of the Metropolitan Poor Act, under which the Metropolitan Asylums Board was constituted." Mr. Galsworthy explained that the Managers had lately had difficulties to contend with which had never been contemplated. Mr. Sedgwick seconded the motion. Sir E. H. Currie said that the Managers wanted to feel that their efforts to stamp out loathsome epidemics had the approval and support of the Government of the day. He agreed with Mr. Galsworthy that there must be some limit to their patience. The motion was then unanimously agreed to.

ARE GOVERNMENT BUILDINGS EXEMPT FROM INSPECTION BY THE LOCAL SANITARY AUTHORITY?

TOUCHING the death, from typhoid fever, of a telegraphist employed in the Exeter Post-office, the poisonous atmosphere he breathed while at his work being strongly suspected as the primary cause of the disease, the Sanitary Committee of the Corporation made an application to inspect the premises. This the Postmaster refused to allow, alleging that Government offices were exempt from the operation of the Public Health Act. Subsequently the Sanitary Inspector obtained a magistrate's order to inspect the building, when a disgraceful condition of things was discovered. The instrument-room in the telegraphic department was overcrowded, and the entire sanitary arrangements of the place so defective as to endanger the health of the employés in it. These facts were brought to the notice of the Local Government Board by the Corporation. The Board communicated with the Postmaster-General on the dangerous nuisance, and a letter has been received by the Corporation, intimating that a new post-office would be erected as soon as possible. The exemption claimed by the local Postmaster could not, of course, be legally sustained.

OPENING OF THE DUBLIN MEDICAL SCHOOLS.

THE inauguration of the present session has been overshadowed by the deaths of two most distinguished members of the profession in Dublin—men not merely of local, but of European reputation in their respective branches of medical science—we refer to Alfred Henry McClintock and Thomas Hayden. In the former the Royal College of Surgeons has lost an ex-President, whose name shed lustre on the chair he last year so ably filled. In the latter the King and Queen's College of Physicians has to deplore the loss of a Fellow who, it was hoped, was soon to fill the Presidential chair. Dr. Hayden's death has caused the postponement of the inaugural addresses at his own—the Mater Misericordiæ —hospital, and at the House of Industry Hospitals. At St. Vincent's Hospital, Dr. M. F. Cox, who was appointed Physician some months ago on the lamented death of Dr. Cryan, delivered the introductory address on Thursday, October 27. Having alluded to Dr. Cryan, and to Mr. W. H. O'Leary, M.P., who had been one of the surgeons of the Hospital, Dr. Cox briefly sketched the history of the institution. On Monday, October 31, Mr. William Stoker, who had been recently appointed a Lecturer on Surgery, opened the Ledwich School of Medicine in Peter-street with an eloquent address, in which he dealt with several important topics relating to medical education and examination. On the same day, at 1 p.m., the introductory address was given by Dr. Rawdon Macnamara before the President and Council of the Royal College of Surgeons.

THE OBSTETRICAL SOCIETY.

AT the meeting of the Obstetrical Society, on Wednesday evening, the President announced to the Fellows the death of Dr. A. H. McClintock. Dr. Barnes proposed, Dr. Priestley seconded, and Dr. Beverley Cole, of San Francisco, supported, a resolution expressing their sense of Dr. McClintock's distinguished services to obstetric science, and of the loss which the Society had sustained in his death. A paper by the President was then read and discussed, and subsequently Dr. Beverley Cole exhibited a new gas cautery, which he stated is superior to Paquelin's. Dr. Cole says it is less liable to get out of order, and more quickly and easily got ready, than Paquelin's, but that remains to be tested.

THE VIRCHOW JUBILEE IN BERLIN.

PROFESSOR VIRCHOW completed his sixtieth year of life, and at the same time the twenty-fifth of his professorate, on October 13 last. We learn from our contemporary, the Berliner Klinische Wochenschrift, that a committee has been formed for the purpose of establishing what should call an exhibition (to be styled the "Rudolph Virchow Stiftung"), for the promotion and furtherance of scientific research, bearing especially on the study of man. Many of Germany's first names are to be found on this committee. We doubt not that the outcome will be worthy of the country which claims the great student of man and mankind as her son. Many other countries will probably vie with Germany in doing honour to one whose teaching is valued and appreciated wherever medicine or anthropological science is cultivated. All subscriptions are to be sent to Herr Ritter, banker, 2, Beauthstrasse, Berlin C., before the middle of November. Elsewhere it will be seen that Dr. Bristowe has undertaken to collect subscriptions in this country.

THE FISH-SUPPLY OF THE METROPOLIS.

AT the last week's meeting of the Metropolitan Board of Works, the Works and General Purposes Committee's report was brought up, on the subject of a site for a fish market for the metropolis, recommending the Board to approve a site at Blackfriars which had been suggested by the engineer and architect, and to apply to Parliament in the next session for power to acquire the site for the purpose contemplated. Mr. Dalton, in moving the adoption of this report, said the question was one of the most important that had been before the Board for some time. Billingsgate Market was found to be inadequate to fulfil the purpose for which it had been designed, and although the City Corporation had determined to improve the approaches, yet it would not now be desirable to leave to Billingsgate the whole fish-supply of the metropolis. After explaining the action taken by the Board, the speaker went on to say that the site at Blackfriars was within a mile of Billingsgate, south of the Thames, with a frontage in the Blackfriars-road, and with a railway in the middle of the site, for the conveyance of railway-borne fish. It was not proposed to disestablish Billingsgate, or to oppose the Corporation; but if it should hereafter be considered desirable to unite the sale of railway-borne fish with that of river-borne fish, it could be easily done by building a wharf on the river-side. Mr. Thompson moved as an amendment—"That the Board do apply to Parliament for power to acquire a site at York-road, King's Cross, for the purposes of a fish market." He deprecated the intended site at Blackfriars, unless it was intended for the south of London only, and showed that the Great Eastern, Great Northern, and Midland Railways had carried 81,000 tons of fish to the metropolis last year, against 7000 tons carried by lines south of the Thames. Mr. Elt seconded the amendment, and explained that the position was not only superior, but the site could be acquired for much less money than that selected at Blackfriars. Mr. Richardson also proposed, as an addition to the recommendation of the Committee, that the Board do approve the site proposed at Shadwell. After some discussion, Mr. Thompson's amendment was put and rejected. Mr. Richardson's amendment was also defeated by a large majority. The Board next divided on the original motion, when the recommendation of the Committee was rejected by seventeen votes to sixteen. The chairman said he never remembered such a course having been pursued before, and he could only suggest that they should consult the Home Secretary. A member remarked that it was perfectly clear that the Board had determined not to ask for Parliamentary powers in the forthcoming session.

ROYAL COLLEGE OF SURGEONS IN IRELAND.

AT a meeting of the Council of the College, held on October 20, 1881, the undernamed gentlemen were elected examiners for the ensuing year to examine candidates for the diploma in Dental Surgery, viz.:—B. Wills Richardson, Edward A. Stoker, Edward S. O'Grady, Henry Gregg Sherlock, John Henry Longford, and Frederick St. Barbe Taylor, Esqs.

CERTIFICATES IN OPHTHALMIC SURGERY.

ON Saturday week, October 22, there was a meeting of the physicians and surgeons of the clinical hospitals of Dublin, to consider the vexed question of charging special fees for the certificates in ophthalmic surgery now required of candidates by the University of Dublin and the Royal College of Surgeons in Ireland. The meeting was held in one of the halls of the College of Physicians, Kildare-street, Dublin, and Dr. Gordon occupied the chair. A prolonged discussion took place, when the following resolution was adopted by a large majority:—"Resolved, that the fee for general hospital practice having been fixed in July, 1877, by unanimous consent, at twelve guineas for nine months, eight guineas for six months, and five guineas for three months, and no alteration having been made in the requirements of students in general clinical teaching, we are of opinion that no alteration should be made in this fee, and that pupils requiring a special certificate for ophthalmic surgery should pay an additional fee for it. This rule not to apply to students who, under previous regulations, have completed their hospital attendance before November, 1880." It was arranged that a copy of this resolution should be forwarded to the medical board of each clinical hospital for

approval and signature by the respective honorary secretaries. This was done, and at an adjourned meeting, held at the College of Physicians last Saturday afternoon, October 29 (Mr. Wharton in the chair), it was announced that every hospital had signed the resolution approving it. A proviso attached by two hospitals, that the rule of requiring a special fee should not apply to students who had joined the hospital class before October 1, 1881, was unanimously agreed to by the meeting, which then adjourned.

MEDICAL SOCIETY OF THE COLLEGE OF PHYSICIANS IN IRELAND.

THE annual general meeting of the Society, for the election of office-bearers, was held in the large hall of the King and Queen's College of Physicians in Ireland, Kildare-street, Dublin, on Wednesday, October 26. The chair was taken by Dr. J. W. Moore, Vice-President of the College. The following members of the Society were elected as officers for the session 1881-82, viz.:—*President:* George Johnston, M.D., President of the College of Physicians. *Vice-Presidents:* John William Moore, M.D., Vice-President of the College of Physicians; Thomas Fitzpatrick, M.D. *Council:* J. Hawtrey Benson, M.D.; Fleetwood Churchill, F.K. & Q.C.P.; John Magee Finny, M.D.; Arthur Wynne Foot, M.D.; Samuel Gordon, M.D.; Thomas Wrigley Grimshaw, M.D.; Reuben Joshua Harvey, M.D.; Thomas Hayden, F.K. & Q.C.P.; Surgeon-Major Jackson, C.B.; Henry Kennedy, M.B.; Christopher J. Nixon, M.D.; Walter George Smith, M.D. *Honorary Secretary and Treasurer:* Alexander Nixon Montgomery, M.K. & Q.C.P.

LUNACY IN THE ISLE OF MAN.

THE streak of silver sea around the Isle of Man has had a very distinct influence on the character of the mental diseases which prevail there. A pent-up population has intermarried to an extraordinary degree, and the result is that congenital mental defects abound there to an extent unknown in any other part of the kingdom. Of the patients admitted into the Isle of Man Asylum, 10·9 per cent. labour under congenital impairment of intellect, whereas, of all patients admitted into asylums in England and Wales, only 4·1 per cent. are thus afflicted. Hereditary predisposition can be clearly traced in 34 per cent. of the lunatics in the Isle of Man; but only in 18 per cent. of those in England and Wales. On the other hand, the moral causes of insanity, including domestic sorrow, anxiety, business trouble, religious excitement, fright, and nervous shock, are much more powerfully operative in England and Wales than in their adjacent island. Contrary to what might have been anticipated, intemperance causes a less proportion of insanity in the Isle of Man, which was long so celebrated for its smuggling and illicit stills, than in England and Wales. The Isle of Man Asylum, which is under the superintendence of Dr. Outterson Wood, contains now about 150 patients.

THE PARIS WEEKLY RETURN.

THE number of deaths for the forty-second week, terminating October 21, was 920 (502 males and 418 females), and among these there were from typhoid fever 28, small-pox 10 measles 11, scarlatina 5, pertussis 2, diphtheria and croup 44, dysentery 2, erysipelas 13, and puerperal infections 6. There were also 39 deaths from acute and tubercular meningitis, 16 from acute bronchitis, 41 from pneumonia, 73 from infantile athrepsia (25 of the infants having been wholly or partially suckled), and 22 violent deaths. The favourable state of the public health continues to be maintained, and even increased, since there have been 81 deaths less than during the preceding week. The fluctuation in the number of deaths from phthisis, arising in some degree from fortuitous causes, explains somewhat the lower number of deaths this week. Thus, while they amounted to 158 in the fortieth week, and suddenly to 225 in the forty-first, they have again sunk to 178 in the forty-second week. The births for the week amounted to 1161, viz., 607 males (443 legitimate and 164 illegitimate) and 554 females (409 legitimate and 145 illegitimate) ; 89 infants (50 males and 39 females) were born dead or died within twenty-four hours.

A MODEL SYLLABUS.

WE have received a copy of the Syllabus of the Combe Lectures on Physiology and the Laws of Health, which are to be given by Professor Stirling, of Aberdeen. It is certainly the best thing of the kind we have seen. The plates with which it is freely illustrated are quite good enough for all actual purposes, and are infinitely superior to some of the trash we have occasionally put before us as fitted for school boards and the like. What we would therefore counsel Dr. Stirling to do would be to extend the letterpress somewhat, modifying slightly its character, so as to render it available for school teachers generally. In this way a really trustworthy guide on animal physiology would be made available to all. The great part of the expense has been already incurred as regards the diagrams, and the modification of the letter-press would entail no great amount of labour or trouble.

COMPULSORY NOTIFICATION OF INFECTIOUS DISEASES.

AT a recent meeting of the Lancashire and Cheshire Branch of the British Medical Association, held at Bolton, Mr. Edward Sergeant, Medical Officer of Health for that borough, read a paper on " The Sanitary Measures necessary for the Suppression of Infectious Disease." The paper commenced by observing that the basis of all such sanitary work is formed undoubtedly on information obtained by the prompt notification of the cases of infection as they occur. It is of the utmost importance to get at the starting-point of an epidemic, so as to nip its progress in the bud, or, if not at first successful, to follow up the attack until the enemy is subdued. Without such information, the medical officer of health is comparatively powerless in the presence of infectious disease, and has to rely on the uncertain intelligence picked up in various ways, or remain in blind ignorance until the information of a death from the disease is received from the registrar, and by that time, in all probability, the seeds of infection have been scattered far and wide throughout the community. The seriousness of this want of knowledge is frequently exemplified in the extensive outbreaks of small-pox and typhoid fever. Mr. Sergeant went on to show that in the Public Health Act of 1875, although the local authorities are empowered to make provision against infection, they are yet entirely without means of ascertaining the first appearance of infectious disease ; hence the introduction of local Acts to remedy this defect. The rise and progress of local legislation were next described, culminating in the Bills of Mr. Gray and Mr. Hastings, which, had they not been shelved in the last session of Parliament, would have supplied a general Act for the whole country more acceptable to the public generally than the sporadic efforts of different sanitary authorities. After expressing a hope that these Bills would be re-introduced, Mr. Sergeant read a table he had compiled which strikingly exemplified the beneficial effects that had resulted from the introduction of compulsory notification into the borough of Bolton. During the last five years, he said, small-pox had been imported into his district more than a dozen times, and on each occasion the prompt information received from the medical attendant had enabled him to isolate the patient, and limit the outbreak to the first case. Medical men, as a body, Mr. Sergeant thinks, are averse to having placed on them the onus of reporting the occurrence of cases, and argue that they should only be required to give the necessary certificate to the occupier of the house, or to the custodian of the sick person, who should be made responsible for its safe delivery to the Corporation. On this principle, the compulsory clauses in operation at Nottingham and Norwich are framed. The Burton-on-Trent Act requires the occupier to give notice only when a medical man is called in, and thus has a tendency to induce delay in seeking medical advice, and perhaps lead to the employment of unregistered practitioners. The dual method of reporting, by placing the duty alike on the occupier and medical attendant, commended itself most to the lecturer's views, since it takes away from the medical man the idea that he is violating the interests or privacy of his patient, because he is simply performing a duty which the patient or his friends are equally responsible for carrying out. Mr. Sergeant next proceeded to deal with the question of the proper description of hospital accommodation to be provided for infectious patients, and he concluded a very interesting address by remarking that, in dealing with the subject under consideration, he had paid attention to it principally from a medical officer of health's point of view, as, without compulsory notification and proper hospital accommodation, these gentlemen felt themselves to be almost powerless.

DEATH OF PROFESSOR BOUILLAUD.

THE veteran physician, Professor Bouillaud, known so well to three generations of practitioners, has just died at the age of eighty-six. We shall shortly furnish an account of his life and work.

EPIDEMIOLOGICAL SOCIETY OF LONDON.

THE Epidemiological Society have appointed a special Committee, consisting of Dr. Robert Cory, Dr. John McCombie, and Mr. Shirley Murphy, to ascertain the evidence which the present state of medical knowledge supplies as to the conditions affecting the protection against small-pox afforded by vaccination. The Committee, in pursuance of this object, have issued a series of questions, to which they beg replies from all. Forms will be sent on application to Mr. Shirley Murphy, 158, Camden-road, London, N.W. The queries are as follows :—

1. What cases of small-pox have come under your observation among children under ten years of age who have been vaccinated in infancy ? and of these, which have died ?

2. What number of cases of small-pox at ages specified in Forms B and B 1 have come under your observation among those who have been vaccinated in infancy ?

3. What cases of small-pox after revaccination have come under your observation ? In answering this question, please state, as far as possible—(a) the number and character of the primary vaccination cicatrices ; (b) the age of the patient at the time of secondary vaccination, the number and character of the resulting cicatrices: if none remain, please state the fact, as well as any fact as to the maturity of the vesicles or intensity of the inflammation ; (c) the character of the attack of small-pox, and the result ; (d) the age of the patient at the time of the attack of small-pox ; (e) the sex of the patient.

4. (a.) How many persons have you known to be in personal attendance on cases of small-pox ? (b.) How many of these had previously had small-pox ? (c.) How many of these have contracted small-pox ? (d.) How many of those who did not contract small-pox were revaccinated ? (e.) How many of those who contracted small-pox were revaccinated? Of the last, state the character of, and date of, vaccination the date, character, and result of attack of small-pox.

5. How many cases of small-pox have come under your observation in which the patient had previously suffered from this disease?

6. Have you ever met with a case of insusceptibility to primary vaccination? and if so, how many?

7. Have you ever vaccinated any child whose mother suffered from small-pox during the pregnancy? and if so, with what results?

THREE WEEKS IN THE MEDITERRANEAN.

A SEA-VOYAGE, with all its attendant advantages, is apt to become a little wearisome from its monotony; and many who are fond of the sea for a time, and who derive the greatest benefit from it, are deterred on this account from spending their holiday in this way. It seems scarcely worth while, for example, to spend three weeks out of four on board ship for the sake of six or seven days in America.

The trips in the Mediterranean that are made by MacIver's steamers (the well-known Cunard Line) offer a capital opportunity for combining the advantages of a life at sea with the most varied and interesting change of scene. A few lines, therefore, describing how some weeks may be comfortably spent on board one of them will perhaps interest some of your readers whose holiday will not extend beyond a month; it will show them how they may, in a most enjoyable way, visit some of the health-resorts to which they are, perhaps, frequently sending their patients; and it will also, if they are not already acquainted with it, add another to the possible list of voyages which patients may be recommended to take.

The Cunard steamers follow two distinct lines in the Mediterranean—one called the Levant line, running to Syra, Smyrna, and Constantinople, and calling at Gibraltar and Malta; and the other, which is subject to a certain amount of variation, calling at a number of ports on the west coast of Italy and Sicily, and at various places on one side or other of the Adriatic. It is quite obvious that these expeditions cannot conveniently be made at all times of the year, as the heat would no doubt be unbearable in the middle of summer; but from the middle of September onwards the traveller is likely to meet with a certain amount of heat undoubtedly, but nothing excessive; and though he may expect to encounter winds characteristic either of the particular region or the time of year, he need not anticipate anything very dreadful in the way of storms. The steamers are intended for cargo principally, but they have excellent cabin accommodation. In the vessel in which we travelled (the Aleppo) the cabins were, with the exception of two large rooms, all on deck, and thus afforded the maximum of light and ventilation; and we believe that this arrangement is found on most of the other vessels on the Mediterranean line. They are about 2000 tons burden, and therefore, though much smaller than the huge modern American liners, are amply large enough for comfort and safety.

Starting, then, from Liverpool on September 11, we left the rain and discomfort which was the lot, at that time, of those at home, for splendid fine and calm weather across the much dreaded Bay of Biscay, the dangers of which, we begin to think, from our own experience, and from what we hear from others, have been somewhat highly coloured. The passengers were thirty-one in number, all on pleasure bent, and the traditional amusements of a sea-voyage made the five days to Gibraltar pass pleasantly enough. On the fourth day the Portuguese coast below Lisbon was in sight the whole time, but before Cape Finisterre no land was sighted at all. After rounding Cape St. Vincent, we met an uncomfortable hot moist wind, "the Levanter," which often blows here, making the sea moderately rough and keeping the deck quite moist, though the sun was blazing overhead. This, it must be confessed, was not invigorating, and as it causes a flat cloud to hang over the town of Gibraltar starting from the top of the rock, it renders the atmosphere of this place particularly close and disagreeable. At Gibraltar the stay is only a few hours—just time enough to visit the fortifications, and, if the weather is favourable, to ascend the rock.

The next three days are spent in reaching Genoa. On the first of them good views may be had of the desolate coast of Spain, and, if the weather be clear, of the Balearic Isles. It is then that the most unpleasantly hot weather of the whole voyage is likely to be met with. If the traveller is fortunate he will pass along the Riviera by daylight, and, as the course is close to the land, he will have an excellent opportunity of observing the nature of the country, the manner in which it is protected by the range of Alps behind, and the extreme beauty of the situation altogether. But if this is not sufficient, the stay at Genoa is two or three days, which will give him ample time for making expeditions by train or carriage along the Cornice road, if he prefers so doing, to investigating the palaces and churches with which the city abounds, or spending some quiet hours in the almost tropical Palavicini Gardens at Pegli, some few miles off. There is a fine old hospital at Genoa, with a quite magnificent marble staircase, and enormous wards, containing on the average about a hundred beds each, arranged in two rows along each side. We were surprised at the great air of cleanliness about the place, the absence of smells, and the excellence of the kitchen; and pleased to notice a good supply of antiseptic sprays. They are building a new hospital of enormous size on the pavilion system, which will, however, take some time to finish. After leaving Genoa, a night at sea brings you to Leghorn, and a day on land is quite sufficient to visit Pisa, and see its tower, cathedral, and baptistry. Another night and a day bring you to Naples, and the day supplies you with some of the most glorious coast scenery imaginable, concluding, perhaps, at sunset, with the entrance to the Bay of Naples—a sight not soon to be forgotten. At Naples the stay is not supposed to be longer than one day, but in our case was prolonged to two, which gave us time to visit Pompeii, to ascend Vesuvius, and to see the Museum as well; and, by the kind arrangement of the captain, we steamed out a little before sunset so that we might obtain a good view of the island of Capri. Next morning we were in front of Palermo, which is interesting in many ways. The scenery in Sicily is particularly bold, and the vegetation and colouring remarkably rich. Palermo is becoming fashionable as a winter health-resort. It is very much shut in by hills, and looks towards the north, but the temperature is said to be extremely pleasant, and not liable to that sudden fall about sunset which is so unpleasant and dangerous in some parts of the South of France.

There is great talk still about the brigands in Sicily and it is difficult to discover how far there is any danger to the casual traveller. The probability is that whatever risk there may be is greatly exaggerated; still, on the road to Monreale, where there is a fine old Moorish cathedral, rich to a degree in mosaic ornamentation of the walls, riflemen are posted at intervals, with the ostensible object of protection against these ruffians. To anyone who is content to stay in the town, or who can overcome his nervousness on this score, Palermo would indeed be a delightful place to spend the winter. The Sicilians are very free with the use of the knife in their private quarrels—another rather unpleasant feature of the inhabitants. A paper was presented to the late Medical Congress by a gentleman who had been in charge of the hospital at Palermo for ten years, and during that time more than 3000 cases of knife-wounds had been treated in this institution, which, he remarked, represented a comparatively small proportion of the actual cases occurring in the town. It is clear that the process of civilisation in this island is not yet complete.

A day each at Messina and Catania give time enough to see these places satisfactorily, as well as the Straits of Messina, and Etna from the distance; and, indeed, if anyone were desirous of ascending the mountain, he might accomplish this by leaving the steamer at Palermo and joining it again at Catania. After leaving Catania, a voyage of two days and three nights takes you up the Adriatic, during which time a considerable part of the South Italian coast is visible, and the Albanian shore and Corfu may be seen in the distance on the other side.

We hope any of our readers who are disposed to make this expedition will not be kept outside Trieste, as we were, for twenty-four hours, but they must remember that if the Boreas is blowing hard this contretemps is quite on the cards. The voyage to Trieste had occupied twenty-one days, and the end of our possible vacation looming ahead, compelled us to leave the ship at this point, and come home overland by Venice, Milan, Turin, etc.; but if it had been possible to devote two months or ten weeks to repose, the return voyage by Venice, Fiume, Patras, and perhaps some other Greek ports, would have been full of interest.

Much of the pleasure of a few weeks spent in this way depends upon the character of one's fellow-passengers, but still more perhaps upon the manner in which the captain does his part in making things agreeable on board ship and facilitating the expeditions on land. We cannot conclude without saying that, in this respect, Captain McNay, of the *Aleppo*, leaves nothing to be desired.

FROM ABROAD.

THE AUTOPSY OF PRESIDENT GARFIELD.

THE *New York Medical Record* of October 8 publishes a minute account of the case of President Garfield, furnished by Dr. Bliss, his medical attendant, and illustrated by lithographs. After praising the explicit and straightforward character of this document, the Editor of the *Record* observes—

" The mistake in diagnosis, deplorable as it may seem, was natural, if not positively unavoidable, considering all the conditions present; in fact, now that the autopsy has disclosed the precise locality of the ball, it is a matter for congratulation that its real track was not suspected before death. As proved by the autopsy, there lay directly in the course of the missile the blood-sac, an injury to which by an explorative operation must have resulted in instant death. Never before has it been so clearly demonstrated that the sin of omission in surgery (if such a term may be allowable in this connexion) was more excusable than that of commission in the shape of officious operative interference. It is comforting to think that the error in diagnosis has no possible bearing upon the ultimate result, and that, in fact, it was a means of avoiding serious mishaps in other directions. . . . . Certain it is that the autopsy proves that the missile could not have been reached from any direction and removed without sacrificing the life of the patient by the wounding of large and important vessels in the neighbourhood, inflicting irreparable injury to vital organs, and thus directly inviting death. The ball could not be in a better situation for rapid and complete encystment. The traumatic aneurism formed upon the wounded splenic artery was in such a situation as virtually to press upon the portion of the track next to the ball, and secure its prompt closure. The ball itself might have remained harmless in that position for an indefinite number of years. But, in saying thus much, it must be considered that there were other attendant conditions which made it impossible for the patient to recover. . . . . As an evidence that the dressings were properly made and the freest possible drainage given to all accessible parts of the wound, it is only necessary to refer to the fact that the original track in the external soft parts (*sic*), and that the fractured twelfth rib had firmly united by bone, which could hardly have been possible if for any considerable period it had been bathed in pus. For the same reason, the eleventh rib, which, unfortunately, was not removed at the autopsy, is said to have been in a state of healthy repair."

AMERICAN OBSTETRICS AND GYNÆCOLOGY.

Dr. Chadwick, of Boston, in his " Address on Obstetrics and Diseases of Women," delivered at the last meeting of the American Medical Association, held at Richmond, Va., furnishes (*Boston Med. Jour.*, September 15) a complete survey of the periodical medical literature upon these subjects which has appeared during the last five years in European countries and in the United States, and it will be seen from his " General Conclusions " which we here transcribe, he claims for American practitioners a most decided superiority, at all events as far as this kind of writing is a test of merit, over those of all other countries :—

" The above quantitative analysis of obstetric and gynæcological literature, with regard to nationalities, manifests the predominance of America in this branch of medicine. America contributes more journal articles than any other nation; supports by contributions, both literary and pecuniary, as many special periodicals as France, and twice as many as either England or Germany; and carries on as many special societies as all the other countries of the world together. England,

despite the labours of Wells, Keith, Thornton, Barnes, Duncan, Tait, Leishman, and Playfair, is fast losing its pre-eminence in this branch of medicine, and has recently demonstrated its inability to support even one special journal, by the discontinuance of the *Obstetrical Journal*. France is exhibiting an ' unnatural activity' under special influences already adduced (academic theses and professorial competition) ; Germany holds on the even tenor of its way; while Belgium, Italy, Spain, Denmark, and Russia are awakening to a more active participation in the advance and dissemination of obstetric and gynæcological lore.

" I have throughout these pages restricted myself to a quantitative study of this literature. I cannot close without giving in a few words an estimate of the quality of each nation's contributions. Germany unquestionably advances pure science more than any other nation. The papers in its three journals are the most profound and the most critical. France manifests a great dearth of original ideas, and a most discursive style of discussion, but considerable painstaking historical research. Its journals are prolix, and, for the most part, profitless reading, and exceed in number the legitimate demand. England exhibits a waning interest in this branch of medicine, little originality, but a notable discrimination in adopting new theories and applying them to practice. Its only special journal died a natural death last year. To America I have no hesitation in according pre-eminence in this special field. Our countrymen meet the emergencies incident to child-bearing with a quickness of perception and readiness of action rarely seen in other countries. Their ingenuity has led them to devise new operations in gynæcology, and to carry them out with brilliant results, so that to-day the practice of that branch has reached a stage here far in advance of other nations. Of course our natural aptitudes lead many of us to over-estimate the beneficial results of surgery, but, taken all in all, close observation and study in most of the countries of Europe have confirmed me in the opinion that in obstetrics and gynæcology America leads the world. The two most prominent exponents of our branch in America, the *American Journal of Obstetrics* and the *Transactions of the American Gynæcological Society*, present a more happy blending of scientific facts and practical suggestions than is found in any other special gynæcological or obstetrical periodicals in the world.'

REVIEWS.

On Epidemics of Dengue Fever, their Diffusion and Etiology By JAMES CHRISTIE, A.M., M.D., Lecturer on Public Health, Anderson's College, Glasgow. Reprinted from the *Glasgow Medical Journal* for September, 1881.

IN this interesting contribution to the history of Dengue-epidemics, which was read at the International Medical Congress in the Section of State Medicine, Dr. Christie insists upon the great importance of establishing a correct chronology of these outbreaks, as he considers that, hitherto, this very important question has not obtained the accurate attention which it demands.

Dr. Christie finds that three epidemics of dengue are reported as having occurred within the Eastern hemisphere, —the first during the years 1779 to 1784, the second from 1823 to 1829, and the third from 1870 to 1875, or, if we take into account certain recent sporadic appearances, from 1870 to 1880.

The accounts which we have of the epidemic of 1779 to 1784 are of a fragmentary nature, and Dr. Christie thinks that it is by no means certain that they really refer to an epidemic of dengue. He, however, notices that Gaberts describes an epidemic as having been prevalent in Cairo in 1779, and that Brylon refers to a similar epidemic, which was called Knockel-Koorts (bone fever), which prevailed in Batavia in the same year. Mr. Persin, an Indian missionary, mentions an epidemic of a disease resembling dengue, which was prevalent in 1780 on the Coromandel Coast, Africa, Arabia, Persia, and Thibet ; while Fernandez de Castilla and Nieto de Piña describe an outbreak of a similar disease called *la piadosa*, which occurred in Cadiz and Seville in 1784 to 1785. Dr. Christie thinks it probable that these were but " the fragments of a great, though partially " [imperfectly ?] " recorded epidemic which existed from 1779 till 1785 or

1788." As, however, the above are the whole of the historical details of this outbreak afforded by Dr. Christie, we must agree with him that he has failed to prove that an epidemic of dengue occurred in the years 1779-84.

We have abundant evidence of an outbreak of this disease in 1823-29. Dr. Christie holds that "systematic writers have sadly distorted the chronology of this epidemic, each after the other having copied the mistakes of his predecessor, representing it as having had its origin in Burmah; or in Burmah, the Bengal and Bombay Presidencies simultaneously." After this we should have presumed that Dr. Christie would have been most careful in arraying the authorities upon which he rests his belief that this epidemic originated on the East Coast of Africa. Upon this point, however, his data are very imperfect.

The facts which he cites appear to us to afford little more than a presumption of the accuracy of his confident statement that "the first appearance of the disease was in the island of Zanzibar, or somewhere on the East Coast of Africa, in 1823." He shows that, when dengue prevailed generally in Zanzibar in September, 1870, "the older inhabitants recognised the disease as one which had been epidemic about forty-eight or forty-nine years before, and they gave to it its former designation—Ki-dinga Pepo." He notes that "the term dinga or denga, used to designate the disease on the East Coast of Africa in 1823 and in 1870, is almost identical with that given to it in the island of Cuba in 1828. The disease appeared four years later, in 1827, in the Danish island of St. Thomas." Dr. Stedman, the earliest historian of the epidemic, and the only one who writes of its introduction into St. Thomas, says the contagion was supposed to have been brought by a vessel from the coast of Africa, which touched at St. Thomas; but whether this vessel was from the West or from the East Coast of Africa, Dr. Stedman does not say. Dr. Christie, however, states that, at the time of the appearance of this epidemic in St. Thomas, and long after, an extensive slave-trade was carried on between the Portuguese territories in the Mozambique Channel, Brazil, and Cuba. He considers that "the vessel from the coast of Africa which touched at St. Thomas would probably be a slave-ship from the Mozambique Channel, bound for Cuba." He adds, that when the disease was thus introduced into the island of St. Thomas in September, 1827, the English negroes there called it the Dandy Fever, and that "when the disease appeared in the Spanish island of Cuba" [where it was present in March, 1828] "it was called Dunga; but was afterwards changed to Dengue, which means fastidiousness and prudery, the name by which it has been ever since known."

We must repeat that, in our opinion, the above data, which we have gathered piecemeal from Dr. Christie's by no means very sequent historical narrative, must be regarded as suggesting, but not as demonstrating, the accuracy of his assumption that "Denga was prevalent in Zanzibar in 1823." To pursue Dr. Christie's narrative from this point. He finds that the next we hear of this epidemic is in Guzuratte, in the Bombay Presidency, a district which has the closest commercial connexion with Zanzibar, by means of native craft, during the south-west monsoon, which begins to blow in April and continues till November. Dr. Kennedy, Surgeon to the Residency at Baroda, says: "The epidemic passed through the whole province of Guzuratte during the hot months" [of 1824], "and was most severely felt at Baroda during the last week of May and the beginning of June." We next hear of the epidemic in Calcutta. Dr. Christie cites the narratives of Drs. Twining, Cavell, Mellis, and Mouat, which our readers will find in the first and second volumes of the Transactions of the Medical and Physical Society of Calcutta. Dr. Twining saw his first cases on May 23 and 24, 1824. Dr. Christie shows that, during the prevalence of the epidemic, there was a general movement of troops from all parts of British India towards Burmah, so that every facility existed for its rapid transit from the West Coast to the East Coast of India. Regarding Rangoon, Dr. Christie says we know that it was taken by storm on May 11, 1824, and that a great amount of sickness prevailed. Dr. Hamilton, of the 13th Regiment, under date July 30, writes—"The type of fever which so generally pervaded the troops during the latter part of June and the commencement of July was purely inflammatory, ushered in by more than usual articular pains." Dr. Waddell, in an article "On the Diseases which prevailed among the British

Troops at Rangoon," says—"The pyrexial epidemic which visited Calcutta in May, and spread over a great portion of India during the two succeeding months, also prevailed at Rangoon in June and July. It chiefly affected the officers of the Army, of whom but few escaped."

Dr. Christie gives an account of the outbreak of the last great epidemic of dengue at Zanzibar in July, 1870. During its prevalence there the Red Sea ports, Southern Arabia, the Persian Gulf, Cutch, the Bombay Presidency, Ceylon, and the Seychelle Islands, were all exposed to infection, as vessels sailed to these places; but, as a matter of fact, with the exception of the coast of Africa and the adjacent islands, the epidemic did not extend, except to Aden and the Red Sea ports, until the early months of 1871, when the disease had become all but extinct in Zanzibar. At this point Dr. Christie's narrative appears somewhat contradictory, as at page 5 he tells us that the epidemic ceased to excite public attention after the close of 1870, and at page 7 he says that "there is reason to suppose that Bombay was infected direct from Zanzibar in August, 1871, as cases were observed at that date by Dr. Da Cunha." It was recognised at Aden by Drs. Turner, Reade, and Welsh, about the end of June.

Dr. Christie adds—"That Aden played an important part in the dissemination of the disease is evident from the fact that Port Said was infected in September, Mattra and Calcutta in the same month, and Batavia in November."

The expression, "is evident," in the above quotation, forms the text of our chief objection to Dr. Christie's narrative. He accepts as proofs data which, as we apprehend, many of his readers will only allow to be suggestions.

Dr. Christie does not allude to the very extensive outbreak of dengue in Calcutta in the hot and rainy season of 1853, which is described in the first volume of the Indian Annals of Medical Science, by the late Dr. Edward Goodeve. He would probably argue that it was endemic; but it was certainly very prevalent, at the same time, in and about Howrah, on the opposite bank of the Hooghly. Dr. Goodeve's observation, that the disease especially affected European seamen living on board their vessels or in the town, would appear to favour the view that it was imported from seaward.

Most of Dr. Christie's arguments tend to the conclusion that the disease spread by contagion. We know that at least some of those who observed the disease in India in 1853 and 1872 considered that they had no evidence of contagion. We do not think it needful to enter into Dr. Christie's merely speculative question—"Is it not possible that the cholera-germ, or the materies morbi of cholera, may be so modified by the products of human decomposition as to give rise to a hybrid disease, such as dengue?" Having seen two great outbreaks of Dengue in India, and having practically studied the cholera of that country for many years, our mind is quite incapable of perceiving any of those points of common resemblance, the existence of which would be needful to convince us that dengue is a hybrid of cholera. If such be the case, it appears inexplicable that while, in the midst of every kind of stink and filth, cholera never dies in Calcutta, the cholera-germ should never have undergone this modification giving rise to the appearance, upon a vast scale, of the hybrid disease save in 1824 and 1872 and in two intermediate years!

THE PARIS NIGHT SERVICE.—Dr. Passant, in his report for the quarter ending September 30, states that there were 1687 visits paid, or 18·3 per night. Of these, 676 (40 per cent.) were paid to males, 837 (50 per cent.) to females, and 174 (10 per cent.) to children under three years of age. Of these visits, 149 were for croup or other laryngeal affections, 201 for various affections of the lungs and heart, 369 for gastro-intestinal affections and other diseases of the abdomen, 11 for strangulated hernia, 13 for retention of urine, 114 for metritis, metrorrhagia, and miscarriage, 117 for labour, 293 for cerebral and other affections of the nervous system, 10 for insanity, 25 for alcoholism and delirium tremens, 24 for rheumatism, 49 for eruptive affections, 25 for typhoid fever, 89 for external or internal hæmorrhage, 84 for wounds and contusions, 27 for fractures, dislocations, and sprains, 4 for burns, 13 for poisoning, 2 for asphyxia from charcoal, 4 for drowning, 4 for suicides. In 41 cases the patients were dead before the practitioners could reach them.—Gas. des Hop., October 13.

REPORTS OF SOCIETIES.

ROYAL MEDICAL AND CHIRURGICAL SOCIETY.

Tuesday, October 25.

Andrew Whyte Barclay, M.D., President, in the Chair.

On Gangrenous Eruptions in connexion with Chicken-pox and Vaccination.

Mr. Jonathan Hutchinson read a paper on gangrenous eruptions in connexion with [chicken-pox and vaccination. The paper commenced with a narration of the details of a case which had been briefly brought before the Society two years ago. A child in perfect health was vaccinated with several others from the arm of a healthy infant. None of the other children suffered. In this child nothing unusual happened to the vaccination vesicles, which ran their course naturally. On the eighth day after vaccination, however, an eruption came out on the body and limbs, which three days later was diagnosed by the vaccinator as variola. Some of the spots had at this time become dusky and threatened to slough, and afterwards gangrene attacked large numbers of them. Between the eleventh and the twenty-first day no surgeon saw the child. It died on the latter date, and, an inquest having been held, the Coroner requested Mr. Hutchinson to examine the body and to report on the nature of the disease. The body, which on a former occasion was shown to the Society, and of which drawings were again produced, was that of a well-grown, healthy child. It was covered with gangrenous sores, the sloughs being black and, in many instances, extending into the subcutaneous cellular tissue; some of them were as large as shillings. There were numerous smaller sores on which no gangrene had occurred. The sores were arranged with tolerable symmetry over the scalp, face, trunk, and limbs, but the hands and feet were exempt. A post-mortem examination by Dr. Barlow showed no disease of internal organs. The child had died from exhaustion in connexion with the extensive affection of the skin. The author stated that, so far as he knew, this was the first example of a gangrenous eruption following immediately upon vaccination, and that he was inclined to regard it as an instance of the vaccinia exanthem running, in connexion with idiosyncrasy, an unusual course. Since the case was first brought before the Society in November, 1879, another almost similar one had occurred in Dublin, and had been carefully recorded by Mr. William Stokes. By the kindness of Mr. Stokes, drawings representing the condition of his patient were presented to the meeting. In this instance the patches of gangrene, although larger, were fewer in number and more superficial, and the infant, although for a time in great danger, eventually recovered. The two cases were almost exactly parallel, excepting that in Mr. Stokes' case a much shorter interval between the vaccination and the appearance of the eruption was assigned by the mother. There were, however, great doubts as to her accuracy and truthfulness, since the medical man, whom she asserted vaccinated the baby, said that he had certainly not done it on the day that she alleged. The eruptions affected the same parts in the two children. In both the hands and feet were exempt, and in neither did the vaccination spots themselves become gangrenous. The author next proceeded to another part of the subject—the attempt to demonstrate that chicken-pox does occasionally assume a gangrenous form, and present conditions very similar to those just described in connexion with the vaccinia exanthem. He had, he said, for ten years or more, been in the habit of recognising a gangrenous form of varicella, and several patients suffering from it had come under his care at the Moorfields Hospital, with suppurated iritis. In some cases the disease had proved fatal, but in the majority the patient recovered, with deep scars, and sometimes with great damage to the eyes. In the worst cases the eruption involved the whole thickness of the skin, and left an abruptly-margined, punched-out ulcer. The author quoted from a paper published by Dr. Witley Stokes, of Dublin, in 1807, in which this malady was, he thought, clearly described. Dr. Witley Stokes said that it was well known in many parts of Ireland under the names of "the white blisters," "the eating hive," and "the burnt holes." Dr. Witley Stokes had noticed the resemblance of the disease to chicken-pox, but had attempted to diagnose between them, alleging that in chicken-pox, fever always precedes the eruption, and that the pustules always dry quickly. The author of the present paper contended that neither of these distinctions would hold good, and drew attention to the fact that Dr. Witley Stokes had, like himself, observed that the eruption usually occurred in very healthy children, at its first stage was like chicken-pox, that severe inflammation of the eyes sometimes occurred, and that the worst cases ended fatally. The final proof upon which the author relied that the eruption was no other than a modification of varicella, was that he had seen it repeatedly occur to one child in a family, whilst several others were going through varicella in its ordinary form. For two examples of this he had recently been indebted to the kindness of his friends Dr. Barlow and Dr. David Lees, of the Children's Hospital. Of one of these cases a drawing was shown. The author referred to some wax casts in the Guy's Hospital Museum, which he said well illustrated the condition he had been describing. They had been named rupia escharotica, but he could have no hesitation in believing them to be examples of gangrenous varicella. In conclusion, he urged that if the proof were accepted, that, in connexion with idiosyncrasy in perfectly healthy children, the eruption of varicella might occasionally assume a severely gangrenous type, there could be but little difficulty in admitting the same possibility as regards the vaccinia exanthem. By the term "vaccinia exanthem" he intended to designate a general eruption, sometimes of an erythematous, sometimes lichenoid, and sometimes vesicular, which, although infrequent, is admitted by all experienced vaccinators to be occasionally seen. It has been especially described by Mr. Ceely, and is referred to by Hebra and others. It is, of course, the analogue of the skin eruption in variola.

The President remarked that some years ago a case came under his notice, where an elderly physician, desiring to have his whole household revaccinated, gave the example himself. The spots became perfectly black; but after a time they dried up, and there was no further trouble.

Dr. Crocker had seen a similar case to some of those reported by Mr. Hutchinson. It occurred in a child fifteen months old. It had been vaccinated; nine days later, shotty papules, as the mother said, appeared all over the body. Nine months after this a new growth of papules appeared on the legs, and pustules formed round the hair-follicles, then spread on the legs, ultimately leaving shallow and clean ulcers; but on the feet some were sloughy. The child died in convulsions; it had been badly fed, and the surroundings were unhealthy. Another child had an eruption something similar, but not so extensive. In another case, he had seen an eruption in some respects similar, but more like pemphigus. This did well with watery applications; those of a greasy nature did not suit.

Dr. Barlow had for years been observing such cases as those narrated, and had seen altogether about fifteen. When the eruption was general and simultaneous the disease was probably varicella; but some, like those mentioned by Dr. Crocker, were purely local, and to those the term "varicella" would hardly apply. In his own cases the primary eruption was mainly vesicular, not papular. The vesicles collapsed, and the slough separated, leaving behind a sore, just as if it had been trephined out, and going right down to the bone. Not one of the children was healthy; several had lung-mischief, and all examined after death had tubercle.

Mr. Parker mentioned a case of herpes in an unhealthy child, where the parts sloughed. In a case of varicella the vesicles were blood-stained.

Dr. Hilton Fagge said he had used the term "rupia escharotica" as regards the Guy's Museum specimens simply for the sake of distinction, and with no preconceived notions of relationship. He was rather inclined to think the view that this was allied to scrofula rather than to varicella was the correct one.

Dr. Habershon remarked on Mr. Hutchinson's use of the term "idiosyncrasy." Was there in any case a previous exanthem or constitutional syphilis?

Dr. Druny mentioned a case which he had seen at the Children's Hospital. Here the affection was only local, but it might be that only certain groups of pustules took on this kind of action.

Mr. Hutchinson, in reply, said he was disappointed that no one had taken up the point as to vaccinia. Most, however, were inclined to accept the varicella idea of the origin of these sores. He had never said that all gangrenous sores in children were of varicellar origin. In all the cases he had seen he had been able to refer them to nothing except varicella. It was very likely that in varicella only certain patches would become gangrenous, especially where there was any local irritation, as about the folds of the skin.

Mr. Clement Lucas showed a Healthy Child suckled by a Syphilitic Mother. The mother had only become infected some months after the child was born.

Mr. F. Mason had seen two such cases. He alluded to a case recorded by Mr. Henry Lee, where a child, born healthy, was being suckled by its own mother. Another—a syphilitic child—was given her to nurse; this infected the mother, but her own child remained intact.

THE CLINICAL SOCIETY OF LONDON.

Friday, October 28.

Joseph Lister, D.C.L., F.R.C.S., F.R.S., President, in the Chair.

Papers were read by Mr. Dent, Dr. Churton, and Mr. Reeves; but the most important paper of the evening was undoubtedly that by Dr. Stephen Mackenzie, which unfortunately was only begun at the time the meeting ordinarily disperses. We give, however, the full details of the case (as formerly reported on November 1, 1879), after it came under Dr. Mackenzie's care, together with the very interesting additions which have been made to it. It has been announced that Dr. George Harley intends to bring the subject again under the notice of the Society; should he do so, an earlier hour for its consideration will be desirable, as it would be unfortunate that such a discussion should be again baulked by continuing a meeting when all men are tired out. The other papers we hope to publish next week. Dr. Stephen Mackenzie's and Mr. Rivington's remarks will be found on pages 541 and 543.

Mr. J. W. Teale, of Scarborough, said that great doubts had been thrown on the genuine character of his case, and that usually such temperatures occurred in highly neurotic females; but it was not so in the case he had recorded, for the patient, a young lady, was strong, healthy, and active. At the time, however, the illness occurred, high temperatures were not so very much regarded. Every care was taken to verify the state of the temperature, and undoubtedly the patient was very ill. He suggested that in such another case a committee should be appointed to watch over it. He referred to a case under the care of Dr. Little, of Dublin, where the temperature rose as high as 133·6°; this was registered by a specially prepared thermometer, made by Casella, and examined at Kew.

[With regard to Dr. Little's case, that gentleman writes as follows:—"The young woman, who was my patient, presented on admission the appearance of a person severely ill of one of the specific fevers in which (as we usually say) the head was chiefly affected. I believed the case to be one of epidemic cerebro-spinal meningitis. Subsequently it transpired that she had received an injury of the head, and had been leading a wild life. My present opinion is that she had ordinary meningitis arising under these conditions. At that time the high temperature (about 106°) was associated with corresponding symptoms, and her entire body gave to the hand the sensation of being very hot. At the time when the astonishing temperatures were reached, there was a want of correspondence between the temperature and the other symptoms, and she did not show the general heat of surface. She was not hysterical, but a thoroughly bad, unreliable girl, and was several times caught at the thermometer case. At the same time, the observations were made with the greatest care, with various instruments, and while she was surrounded by observers during the time the thermometer was in the axilla. She subsequently showed similar phenomena while under Dr. Purser's care in Sir P. Dun's Hospital. When the very high temperatures were first observed, she seemed during their continuance to have great distress in her head, but during the later weeks of her

stay such was not the case. I believe the girl had actual cerebro-spinal mischief, but I am quite at a loss to explain the temperature."]

Case of Paradoxical Temperature.

Dr. Mahomed gave some details of a case with paradoxical temperature. M. W., aged twenty-two, was admitted into Guy's Hospital, September 30, 1878. She was under the care of Dr. Moxon, but for a considerable part of the time during which she exhibited extraordinary temperatures she had fallen temporarily under Dr. Mahomed's charge; she had also been under the care of Dr. Goodhart. She died March 30, 1880, having been under observation for eighteen months. She was an excitable, vivacious, and rather hysterical woman, by occupation a nursemaid. She said that she had passed through a mild attack of scarlatina seven years ago, and that it was followed by general œdema. She had previously been under the care of Dr. Habershon, during December, 1866, suffering from anæmia and irregular menstruation. She then exhibited no unusual symptoms. She was on the present occasion admitted for phthisis, chiefly affecting the left lung. She had suffered from cough for four months. Hæmoptysis occurred for the first time five days before admission. Her symptoms were those of acute phthisis from the time she entered the hospital. She suffered much from hectic fever, night-sweats, and pain in the left chest. She frequently complained of nausea, and sometimes vomited. She was liable to headache, neuralgia, and fits of depression. Her temper varied greatly. She was very weak. Her temperature was taken regularly morning and evening from the beginning of March, 1879. During March, April, and May it varied between normal in the morning and 102° in the evening; on some occasions it reached 103°. From the first week in June it attained a higher level, only occasionally falling below 101°, and frequently rising to 103°, often to 104°, and even to 104·8°. On July 23 it first became phenomenal, the thermometer registering 106·4°; and on July 25, 107·4° at 8.45, and at ten o'clock the same evening 110·8°. On this occasion it was noticed that her respirations were hurried, but otherwise she was much as usual. During the rest of July and August no temperature was recorded lower than 102°, but only on five days did it rise above 106°. On each of these occasions several high temperatures would be recorded on the same evening, each usually higher than the preceding, the observations being often terminated by the index becoming lodged in the end of the thermometers employed. In the beginning of September the clinical clerks were changed, and she had one who was new to his work. She came under Dr. Mahomed's care soon afterwards. Her case had now excited general interest, and she appeared to give free rein to her fancy, and produced all sorts of variations in her temperature in the most reckless manner. The thermometers placed simultaneously in various parts of her body would give various readings at the same moment, and two or more successive observations on one part would give variations from normal up to 120° within a few minutes of each other. During September, Dr. Mahomed made many observations on the patient, which were recorded on the "bed letter," and were to have been copied into the report, but unfortunately the "bed letter" was lost before they had been copied. The first observation made was in the presence of Dr. Taylor and several students who were standing round the bed. Three thermometers were used at the same time—one being placed in her mouth and one in each axilla; they were not held in. On removal, on one side the thermometer registered about 102°, in the mouth 107°, and on the other side 114°. (These numbers are not exact.) The thermometers were then all changed, the highest temperature being now recorded in the opposite axilla, and that in the mouth was about 104°. They were again changed, with again fresh results. It appeared that the only check to the position of the index was the length of scale of the thermometer, it being frequently, and at this time indeed usually, lodged in the small expansion of the tube at the top. Some thermometers were now procured from Mr. Hawksley which had a scale for several hundred degrees, but these were non-registering, and by means of them only ordinary temperatures were obtained. The House-Physician, Mr. Baldwin, obtained a self-registering clinical thermometer with a scale reaching to 130°, and with this an indication of 128° was given on October 15. She appears to have felt that she had gone too far on this occasion, for comparatively few high temperatures were recorded after this—only about thirteen times during the next five months. It was especially noteworthy in this case that a high temperature was never indicated by a non-registering thermometer, though they were often used. She frequently objected to the use of these, which were of larger size than the ordinary clinical thermometer, calling them "horse-thermometers." Dr. Taylor obtained the loan of some surface thermometers, which were strapped on the chest-wall, but gave none other than ordinary results, although extravagant temperatures had been recorded immediately before. The high records could be obtained at any time in the day, and appeared entirely under the control of the patient, who would frequently state beforehand that the temperature would not be high. The high temperatures were not accompanied by any corresponding increase of pulse rate or respiration, though afterwards her breathing was sometimes noticeably hurried, as if from exertion. No high temperature was ever obtained by Dr. Mahomed when he kept his hand on the arm of the patient during the time the thermometer was in the axilla. No increase of temperature of the skin or in the axilla could be detected by the touch during or immediately after the record of an extraordinary temperature, nor was the bulb of the thermometer hot at the time of removal, as it would necessarily have been had the temperature of the body been really high. Other indications of fraudulent symptoms were obtained under the following circumstances:—During the latter part of September she professed to be unable to retain any food on her stomach and to be living entirely on lemonade and soda-water. Dr. Mahomed had her placed in a private room and strictly watched on September 30. On October 1 she only took two ounces of milk; on the 2nd it had increased to fourteen ounces; on the 5th it reached a pint, and on the 8th two pints in the twenty-four hours. Her urine had been measured, and the urea it contained estimated during the whole of September and October, but it gave no indication of a decreased or increased diet. It must, however, be stated that the recorded quantities of urine and the amounts of urea are too variable to be reliable. Although during June, July, and August her temperatures had been progressively increasing and always high, yet her body-weight, which was 115 lbs. on December 9, 1879, had only decreased to 112 lbs. on September 9, 1880, being a loss of only 3 lbs. in nine months. During the next three months she lost 10 lbs., her weight falling to 102 lbs. by November 30; but her physical signs of disease had been steadily increasing throughout this period. She was frequently charged with outwitting her doctors, and asked to explain how she did it. She generally denied any deception, but often smiled, and sometimes said, "Why don't you find it out?" Her method, however, was never discovered. On March 14, 1880, she unfortunately developed the ordinary symptoms of scarlatina, and died on March 30. The necropsy revealed nothing unusual; there was advanced disease of the left, and more recent of the right, lung. Dr. Mahomed remarked that it was easy to send the index of an ordinary clinical thermometer up to the top, in from ten to fifteen seconds, by rubbing it between the slightly moistened finger and thumb, exerting at the same time considerable pressure on the bulb. The same result can be obtained by enveloping the bulb of the thermometer in several folds of silk, and placing it in the mouth, then inspiring by the nose and expiring by the mouth. This, no doubt, is produced by the evolution of the latent heat of the watery vapour of the breath, as it is condensed on the silk.

Dr. WILLIAMS asked if any temperatures were taken during sleep.

Dr. GEORGE HARLEY referred to a case reported by Wunderlich, where before death the temperature was 112·5°, and after death 113·3°. This seemed a puzzle; but in a case of death from scarlatinal pericarditis, fifteen hours after death, there was marked heat on opening the body.

THE report of the Dwellings Committee of the Charity Organisation Society shows that about three millions sterling are now in the hands of 876 building societies in all parts of England. The influence of railway facilities in inducing artisans to obtain dwellings in the suburbs has been such, that workmen earning only ordinary wages have become, through these societies, possessors of the houses they occupied.

GENERAL CORRESPONDENCE.

PROFESSOR VIRCHOW'S TESTIMONIAL.

LETTER FROM DR. J. S. BRISTOWE.

[To the Editor of the Medical Times and Gazette.]

SIR,—Kindly allow me, through your columns, to inform the many admirers and pupils of Virchow in this country that I have undertaken to receive subscriptions towards the testimonial, which our brethren of Germany are intending to present him with, on the occasion of the completion of the twenty-fifth year of his professorship in the University of Berlin, and of his sixtieth birthday. The presentation is to take place on the 19th inst.; it is important, therefore, that subscriptions should be sent to me in sufficient time to be transmitted to Germany before that date. For the guidance of subscribers, I may mention that the subscriptions in Germany range from 20s. upwards, with an average of 50s.; and that I shall be happy to receive either cheques, crossed "Bank of England," or post-office orders, on the office in Vigo-street, London, W., made payable to myself. I am, &c.,   J. S. BRISTOWE.

11, Old Burlington-street, W., November 2.

P.S.—The following subscriptions have been received:—Sir James Paget, £5; Sir Wm. Mac Cormac, £2 10s.; Dr. Gerald Yeo, £2 2s.; Dr. Bristowe, £2 2s.; Dr. Ord, £1 1s.

OBITUARY.

THOMAS HAYDEN, F.K.Q.C.P., M.R.I.A., ETC.

ONCE more have the hopes of a wide circle of friends and professional brethren been doomed to disappointment. The improvement in Dr. Hayden's state, which we chronicled three weeks ago, proved but transitory, for with the setting-in of the searching easterly winds of the last ten or twelve days of October, a gradual failure of strength showed itself, and the tide of life ebbed slowly, until on Sunday, October 30, he passed tranquilly away.

Thomas Hayden was the son of the late John Hayden, Esq., of Parson's Hill, near Fethard, co. Tipperary. At an early age he enjoyed the pupil of his relative, the late Dr. Hayden, of Harcourt-street, Dublin, and studied in the wards of the Meath Hospital. In 1850 he obtained the licence of the Royal College of Surgeons in Ireland, and soon afterwards was appointed to the Chair of Anatomy and Physiology in the Ledwich School of Medicine, Peter-street, Dublin. Here he quickly won distinction as a 'painstaking and efficient teacher. In 1854, on the founding of the Catholic University, Dr. Newman (then the lately appointed Rector, afterwards Cardinal Newman) conferred upon Dr. Hayden the post of Professor of Anatomy and Physiology in the School of Medicine attached to the University. This professorship he held to the time of his death. In 1860, Hayden joined the King and Queen's College of Physicians as a Licentiate, and in 1867 he was elected a Fellow of the College, having previously resigned his Fellowship in the Royal College of Surgeons. In 1861 he was chosen to be Physician to the Mater Misericordiæ Hospital, where he did excellent work during the remaining twenty years of his life, as his splendid treatise on "The Diseases of the Heart and Aorta," published in 1875, amply testifies. His worth was fully recognised by the College of Physicians, for he was elected Censor of the College in 1869, 1870, 1875, and 1876. During the latter two years he was Vice-President, and, had he lived, he would, without doubt, have been the next Fellow chosen to fill the presidential chair.

Among other distinctions which he enjoyed, we may mention the Membership and Vice-Presidentship of the Royal Irish Academy, and the Corresponding Membership of the Academia Physio-Medico-Statistica of Milan. In 1879, also, he was named in the charter of the Royal University of Ireland as a member of the Senate of that new University. He likewise filled the presidential chair of the Pathological Society of Dublin.

As to his private and professional life, we can only say, with his biographer in the Dublin Freeman's Journal, that "amongst those who knew him well, Dr. Hayden was beloved and esteemed for his kindly nature and his stainless and honourable character. He truly represented the best and noblest attributes of the medical profession in Dublin."

MEDICAL NEWS.

UNIVERSITY OF EDINBURGH.—MEDICAL AND SCIENCE DEGREES.—The following candidates have passed the First Professional Examination, October, 1881:—

M. S. P. Agancor, Alfred Aikman, M. S. Altounian, J. M. Balfour, M. M. Basil, B. K. Basu, James Bell, G. L. Bonnar, Frederick Bond, J. E. Bottomley, Paul Bowes, Herbert Bramwell, D. M. Brown, T. A. Brown, J. R. Burns, C. J. Burton (Science), J. M. Cadell, Henry Cauldwell, Edward Carmichael, Thomas G. Churcher, E. W. Clarke, J. G. Cossins, A. H. Croucher, A. S. Cumming, Daniel Davies-Jones, Alexander Davidson, A. N. Davidson, D. E. Dow, Thomas Easton, Edwin Eckersley, George Fisher, J. W. Fox, A. E. Grant, Benjamin Griffiths, J. S. Haldane, P. B. Handyside, W. C. Helme, George Hewlett, W. H. Hill, Archibald Hood, T. A. F. Hood, Robert Howden, R. E. Horsley, C. W. Howatson, A. W. Hughes, B. E. Iastrzebski, David Jack (Science), R. Jackson, Hugh Jamieson, Hugh John, John Johnston, Thomas Johnstone, G. H. Kenyon, Henry Ker, Francis Kraemer, David Laing, W. S. Lang, A. W. M. Leicester, W. M. Little, H. J. Mackay, William Mackay, F. L. M'Kenzie, J. H. M'Kenzie, N. J. M'Kie, John M'Myn, Archibald Macqueen, G. D. Malan, J. W. Martin, D. J. Mason, Angus Matheson, R. T. Meadows, William Miller, Duncan Menzies, Robert Mitchell, B. M. Moorhouse, A. E. Morison, E. J. B. De Moulin, Daniel Mowat, W. J. Munro, J. H. Neale, J. H. Neethling, Sydney Partridge, Ian Paterson, M. G. Pereira, F. A. Pockley (with distinction), G. Y. Polson, H. P. Prankerd, H. H. Pridie, Joseph Priestley, J. M. S. Preston, E. E. T. Price, A. C. Purchas, Alwin Raimes, T. E. Rait, C. A. Ranny, John Ring, G. M. Robertson, John Robertson, J. S. Robertson, T. H. Robinson, Joseph Rutter, A. O. Schorn, William Shand, John Simpson, George Smith, William Sneddon, T. S. Smitwoog, Arthur Solomon, J. C. Steedman, H. F. D. Stephens, A. J. Stiles, H. J. Stiles (with distinction), J. W. Stirling, J. M. Stormonth, G. H. H. Symonds, John Sykes, T. S. Tanner, J. C. Taylor, Thos. Taylor (Science), W. Taylor, A. Thomson, D. G. P. Thomson, H. A. Thomson, J. A. Thomson (Science), T. Thyne, Alfred Turner, J. W. O. Underhill, David Wallace, David Walker, E. F. S. Walker, N. P. Walker, L. W. Watson, A. K. Watt, E. G. Westenra, G. E. C. Wood, J. E. Wolfhagen, J. C. Young.

ROYAL COLLEGE OF PHYSICIANS OF LONDON.—The following gentlemen were admitted Members on October 27:

Ranking, John Ebenezer, M.D. Oxford, Tunbridge Wells.
Salusbury, Harrington, M.D. London, 21, Huntley-street, W.C.
Springthorpe, John William, M.B. Melbourne, 49, Manor-park, S.E.
Willcocks, Frederick, M.D. London, 52, Scarsdale-villas, W.

The following gentlemen were admitted Licentiates on the same day:

Bickle, Leonard Watkins, 7, Albert-square, S.W.
Clowes, Herbert Alfred, M.B. Durham, Guy's Hospital, S.E.
Dawson, Rankine, 45, Crosier-street, S.E.
Drysdale, Alfred Edgar, 5, Stanford-road, W.
East, Frederick William, M.B. Durham, 2, Clapton-square, E.
Foley, James Leslie, M.D. Montreal, 17, Horton-road, E.
Gubbin, George Frederick, Westminster Hospital, S.W.
James, Charles Alfred, Dispensary, Stoke Newington, N.
Jennings, Charles Egerton, London Hospital, E.
Macnamara, James Thomas, 19, Paris-street, S.E.
Mark, Leonard Portal, 11, Queen Anne-street, W.
Martin, John Michael Harding, M.D. Brussels, Blackburn.
Miller, Herbert Percy, 26, Stoke Newington-road, N.
Palmer, John, Middlesex Hospital, W.
Ross, James, M.D. McGill, 45, Crosier-street, S.E.
Shearman, Percy Edward, 6, Grove, South Wimbledon.
Twynam, George Edward, 18, Blandford square, W.
Usher, John Edward, M.D. New York, 39, Argyll-square, W.C.

ROYAL COLLEGE OF SURGEONS.—The following gentlemen, having undergone the necessary examinations, were admitted Licentiates in Dentistry at a meeting of the Board of Examiners on the 28th ultimo, viz.:—

Hedley, W. Snowdon, M.R.C.S., A.M.D.
Richardson, Francis, Derby.
Turner, William A., Chichester.
Mason, C. Browne, Exeter.
Headdey, H. Parry, Oxford.

One candidate was rejected. The following were the questions on Anatomy and Physiology, and on Surgery and Pathology, submitted to the candidates, when they were required to answer at least one of the two questions in each (from two to four o'clock), viz.:—1. Describe the course and branches of the internal maxillary artery. 2. Describe the functions of the tongue and the nerves concerned in each. Surgery and Pathology—1. What do you understand by a "ranula"? Give its symptoms, pathology, and treatment. 2. Give an account of the process of healing (1) of a simple incised wound; (2) of a lacerated and contused wound. The following were the questions, on the same day, on Dental Anatomy and Physiology, and on Dental Surgery and Pathology, when the candidates were required to answer two out of the three questions in each (from five to eight o'clock), viz.:—1. State the periods of eruption of the several temporary teeth. Into what groups do they, in this respect, admit of being divided? and what pauses occur in the process? 2. Describe the structures met with in a complete vertical section through the sac of a developing tooth at the period of commencing calcification. 3. Mention the various methods of attachment of the teeth to the jaws. Give examples of each variety. Dental Surgery and Pathology—1. What are the most frequent causes of death of the pulp? By what structures are so-called dead teeth in relation with surrounding living tissue? and what morbid conditions may lead to their ultimate loss? 2. State the conditions under which you would consider the following materials the most suitable for filling teeth, viz.:—gutta-percha, zinc oxychloride, zinc phosphate, and copper amalgam. 3. Describe the morbid appearances and ordinary causes of the different conditions known by the terms gingivitis, Rigg's disease, and blue gum.

APOTHECARIES' HALL, LONDON.—The following gentlemen passed their examination in the Science and Practice of Medicine, and received certificates to practise, on Thursday, October 27:—

Kenny, Frederick Hamilton, Norwich.
Palmer, John, Middlesex Hospital.
Underwood, John Charles, Little Gaddesden, Hemel Hempstead.

The following gentlemen also on the same day passed their primary professional examination:—

Boyton, Edward T. A., St. Bartholomew's Hospital.
Case, William, University College.

APPOINTMENTS.

. The Editor will thank gentlemen to forward to the Publishing-office, as early as possible, information as to all new Appointments that take place.

STALLARD, J. PRINCE, M.B., C.M. Edin.—House-Surgeon to the Worcester General Infirmary.

NAVAL, MILITARY, ETC., APPOINTMENTS.

ADMIRALTY.—Fleet-Surgeon William Redmond has been placed on the retired list of his rank from October 26, 1881. Staff-Surgeon John Mockridge has been promoted to the rank of Fleet Surgeon in Her Majesty's Fleet, with seniority of 22nd ult.

BIRTHS.

BOURKE.—On October 26, at 40, Redcliffe-square, the wife of Surgeon-Major Isidore McWilliam Bourke, of a daughter.
CARMICHAEL.—On October 24, at 5, Berlin-place, Pollokshields, Glasgow, the wife of Dr. D. Carmichael, of a daughter, stillborn.
CROWDY.—On October 22, at Highgate, N., the wife of Frederic Hamilton Crowdy, M.B., of a daughter.
FLINT.—On October 29, at Westgate-on-Sea, the wife of Arthur Flint, L.R.C.P., M.R.C.S., of a son.
HO PKINS.—On October 31, at 88, Highbury New-park, the wife of Alfred Boyd Hopkins, M.R.C.S., of a daughter.
HUTCHINGS.—On October 26, at Southborough, Tunbridge Wells, the wife of Edward J. Hutchings, M.R.C.S., of a son.
SAUNDERS.—On September 20, at Cape Town, the wife of Henry W. Saunders, M.B., F.R.C.S., of a son.
WEBB.—On October 23, at Kingsbridge, South Devon, the wife of W. H. Webb, M.R.C.S., of a daughter.

MARRIAGES.

BERRIDGE—CAMPION.—On November 1, at Redhill, Surrey, William Alfred Berridge, M.R.C.S., of Redhill, to Beatrice, second daughter of Frederick Campion, Esq., of Frenches, Redhill.
CLIFTON—READ.—On the 29th ult., at Edgbaston, Birmingham, Arthur C. Clifton, M.R.C.S. Eng., to Emma, daughter of the late John Mabyn Read, of Helston, Cornwall. (No cards.)
FULLER—BIRKETT.—On October 25, at Ramsgate, Thomas Warburton Fuller, M.B., to Florence, eldest and only surviving daughter of the late George Birkett, M.D., of Northumberland House, Stoke Newington.
OLIVER—JENKINS.—On October 27, at Consett, Thomas Oliver, M.D., of Newcastle-on-Tyne, to Edith Rosina, eldest daughter of William Jenkins, J.P., of Consett Hall, co. Durham.
WINANS—BELCHER.—On October 27, at Brighton, Walter, eldest son of William Louis Winans, Esq., of Baltimore, U.S.A., to Caroline Rowland, second daughter of Henry Belcher, M.D., of Brighton.

DEATHS.

EDIS, FREDERICK POOLEY, F.R.C.S., Surgeon-Major in Her Majesty's Indian Army, at Santa Barbara, California, on October 10, in his 39th year.
FOULIS, DAVID, M.D., at 191, Hill-street, Glasgow, of diphtheria, on October 31, aged 35.
FOWLER, ROBERT STRANGE, M.R.C.S., at 67, Marland-place, Southampton, on October 30, aged 77.
GARNETS, WILLIAM, M.R.C.S., at Repton, on October 21, aged 49.
GROSSEGOAN, EDWARD GEORGE, M.D., Assistant Medical Officer of the Borough Lunatic Asylum, at Milton, near Portsmouth, on October 27.
GOODWIN, ELIZABETH, wife of Robert Docksey Goodwin, F.R.C.S., at Monument House, Ashbourne, on November 1.

McCLINTOCK, A. H., LL.D., M.D., late President of the Royal College of Surgeons, Dublin, at Laughlinstown, co. Dublin, on October 21.

MacDOUGALL, A., L.R.C.S., at Jordan-lane, Morningside, Edinburgh, on October 30, in his 78th year.

MACKRETICH, S., M.D., Surgeon-Major 5th Punjab Infantry, at 22, Fitzroy-square, on October 27, aged 44.

OLIVER, JOHN RICHARD, L.R.C.P., A.M.D., at Barbadoes, on October 6.

RANDALL, Surgeon-Major J. G., of Woolwich, at the residence of his father, John Randall, M.D., 25, Nottingham-place, W., on October 30, aged 36.

ROGERS, GEORGE OSBORN, M.R.C.S., at The Elms, Newport Pagnell, on November 1, in his 76th year.

VACANCIES.

BIRMINGHAM GENERAL DISPENSARY.—Resident Surgeon. Candidates must be registered, and possess both a medical and surgical qualification. Applications, together with original testimonials and certificates of registration, to be sent to Alex. Forrest, Secretary, on or before November 16.

CARMARTHEN AND JOINT COUNTIES ASYLUM.—Assistant Medical Officer. Applications, with testimonials, to be forwarded to Dr. Hearder, Medical Superintendent.

EAST SUSSEX, HASTINGS, AND ST. LEONARDS INFIRMARY, HASTINGS.—Assistant-Surgeon. Candidates must be fellows or members of the Royal Colleges of Surgeons of London, Dublin, or Edinburgh. Applications, with testimonials, to be sent to William J. Gant, Secretary, not later than November 14.

EVELINA HOSPITAL FOR SICK CHILDREN, SOUTHWARK-BRIDGE-ROAD, S.E.—Physician. (For particulars see Advertisement.)

MIDDLESEX HOSPITAL, W.—Surgical Registrar. (For particulars see Advertisement.)

ROYAL PIMLICO DISPENSARY, 104, BUCKINGHAM PALACE-ROAD, W.—Medical Officer. Candidates must reside in the district. Applications and testimonials to be sent to W. C. Meates, Secretary, at the Dispensary, on or before November 7.

SOUTH DEVON AND EAST CORNWALL HOSPITAL, PLYMOUTH.—House-Surgeon. Candidates must be duly qualified. Applications, with testimonials, to be sent to J. Walter Wilson, Hon. Sec., on or before Nov. 7.

UNION AND PAROCHIAL MEDICAL SERVICE.

. The area of each district is stated in acres. The population is computed according to the census of 1871.

RESIGNATIONS.

Nottingham Union.—Mr. J. H. Webster has resigned the Fourth District; salary £100 per annum.

Settle Union.—Mr. James Hartley has resigned the Long Preston and Kirkby Malham Districts. Long Preston: area 16,396; population 1372; salary £15 per annum. Kirby Malham: area 22,328; population 878; salary £14 per annum.

APPOINTMENTS.

Bury Union.—Archibald B. Telford, M.D. Glasg., L.R.C.S. Edin., to the Pilkington District.

Kington Union.—Richard A. Billiald, M.R.C.S. Eng., L.R.C.P. Lond. to the Kington District.

Peterborough Union.—Llewellyn Thelwall, L.R.C.P. Edin., L.R.C.S. Edin., to the Stilton District.

Sudbury Union.—Charles W. Whistler, M.R.C.S. Eng., L.S.A., to the Sixth District.

Thirsk Union.—Charles Tweedy, M.R.C.S. Eng., to the Knayton District.

Tynemouth Union.—Joseph E. Gofton. L.R.C.P. Lond., M.R.C.S. Eng., to the North Shields District. Frank Rennie, B.M. and M.C. Edin., to the Whitley District.

ALLEGED IMPROPER MEDICAL TREATMENT: EXCULPATION OF THE PRACTITIONER.—At an inquest held by Mr. Carttar, West Kent Coroner, a few days since, at Lee Green, on the body of a man aged twenty-nine years, it appeared the deceased had been ill, and was attended by Dr. Cooper, who injected the arm with morphia, using the sixth part of a grain, for the purpose of inducing sleep; the deceased, who had rheumatic fever, having complained of pains in the joints. His wife saw him alive at eleven o'clock at night, and at seven the next morning found him dead by her side. Considerable feeling had been exhibited in the neighbourhood with regard to the death; rumours circulated alleging improper medical treatment, and a local newspaper had stated it was due to an overdose of morphia. The coroner, in consequence, entrusted the post-mortem examination to an independent medical practitioner, Dr. Forsyth, of Greenwich, who was assisted by Mr. Ware, of Guy's Hospital, there being also present Dr. Goodhart of Guy's, Dr. Cooper, Mr. Hartt, Mr. Clutterden, and Mr. Kennedy, surgeons. Dr. Forsyth expressed himself satisfied with the treatment pursued by Dr. Cooper. It was an unusual and unfortunate case, but the remedies used were those he would have prescribed himself. Dr. Cooper complained of the charges made against him; but the jury expressed perfect satisfaction with the treatment adopted, and returned a verdict "That the deceased died from syncope, from the dilated state of the heart," adding a rider, that they considered Dr. Cooper had shown every attention to deceased during his lifetime, and was in no way to blame for his untimely end.

VITAL STATISTICS OF LONDON.

Week ending Saturday, October 29, 1881.

BIRTHS.

Births of Boys, 1378; Girls, 1375; Total, 2753.
Corrected weekly average in the 10 years 1871-80, 2611·0.

DEATHS.

	Males.	Females.	Total.
Deaths during the week	822	766	1568
Weekly average of the ten years 1871-80, corrected to increased population	805·1	753·6	1558·7
Deaths of people aged 90 and upwards	...	...	65

DEATHS IN SUB-DISTRICTS FROM EPIDEMICS.

	Enumerated Population, 1881 (corrected.)	Small-pox.	Measles.	Scarlet Fever.	Diphtheria.	Whooping-cough.	Typhus.	Enteric (Typhoid) Fever.	Simple continued Fever.	Diarrhœa.
West	668996	1	5	7	1	4	...	7	...	2
North	905377	7	3	14	7	4	1	12	...	5
Central	381795	...	...	7	4	4	...	5	...	1
East	692520	2	4	11	2	9	2	7	1	3
South	1265576	14	7	26	11	9	1	17	...	8
Total ...	3814571	24	19	65	25	29	4	49	1	19

METEOROLOGY.

From Observations at the Greenwich Observatory.

Mean height of barometer	29·766 in.
Mean temperature	43·5°
Highest point of thermometer	53·0°
Lowest point of thermometer	34·2°
Mean dew-point temperature	39·9°
General direction of wind	N.E. & N.
Whole amount of rain in the week	0·98 in.

BIRTHS and DEATHS Registered and METEOROLOGY during the Week ending Saturday, Oct. 29, in the following large Towns:—

Cities and boroughs (Municipal boundaries except for London.)	Estimated Population to middle of the year 1881.*	Persons to an Acre. (1881.)	Births Registered during the week ending Oct. 29.	Deaths Registered during the week ending Oct. 29.	Temperature of Air (Fahr.).			Temp. of Air (Cent.).	Rain Fall.	
					Highest during the Week.	Lowest during the Week.	Weekly Mean of Daily Mean Values.	Weekly Mean of Daily Mean Values.	In Inches.	In Centimetres.
London ...	3829751	50·2	2753	1568	52·0	34·2	43·5	6·39	0·98	2·49
Brighton ...	107984	45·9	67	45	57·0	35·6	44·1	6·73	0·24	0·61
Portsmouth ...	128335	26·2	98	50	...	...	...	...	...	...
Norwich ...	88038	11·6	57	41	...	...	...	...	...	...
Plymouth ...	75269	54·0	64	48	51·2	37·9	48·2	9·00	0·76	1·93
Bristol ...	207140	46·5	123	82	50·4	34·7	44·0	6·67	0·84	2·08
Wolverhampton	75934	22·4	59	37	48·6	30·5	41·2	5·11	0·02	0·05
Birmingham ...	402296	47·9	286	148	...	...	...	...	...	...
Leicester ...	123120	38·5	91	54	48·0	30·5	41·7	5·39	0·30	0·76
Nottingham ...	188335	15·9	151	76	48·8	33·0	42·7	5·95	0·80	2·03
Liverpool ...	553968	106·3	395	280	...	...	...	...	...	...
Manchester ...	341289	79·5	241	158	...	...	...	...	...	...
Salford ...	177760	34·4	127	71	...	...	...	...	...	...
Oldham ...	112176	24·0	84	60	...	...	...	...	...	...
Bradford ...	194037	25·6	123	74	47·4	35·2	41·9	5·50	0·47	1·19
Leeds ...	310490	16·4	263	114	49·0	35·0	42·7	5·95	0·90	2·29
Sheffield ...	285621	14·5	208	92	47·0	34·0	41·8	5·45	0·25	0·63
Hull ...	155161	42·7	125	99	48·0	32·0	41·9	5·50	0·75	1·90
Sunderland ...	116758	42·2	91	47	50·0	35·0	43·8	6·58	0·91	2·31
Newcastle-on-Tyne	145675	27·1	110	70	...	...	...	...	...	...
Total of 20 large English Towns ...	7605775	38·0	5516	3202	51·2	30·5	43·1	6·17	0·60	1·52

* These figures are the numbers enumerated (but subject to revision) in April last, raised to the middle of 1881 by the addition of a quarter of a year's increase, calculated at the rate that prevailed between 1871 and 1881.

At the Royal Observatory, Greenwich, the mean reading of the barometer last week was 29·77 in. The lowest reading was 29·13 in. at the beginning of the week, and the highest 30·07 in. on Thursday evening.

NOTES, QUERIES, AND REPLIES.

He that questioneth much shall learn much.—*Bacon.*

H. J.—You cannot refer to better sources than Virchow's address at the International Medical Association, and Professor Hermann's pamphlet on Vivisection.

Physiologist.—Professor Owen succeeded Sir Charles Bell as Professor of Anatomy and Physiology at the Royal College of Surgeons.

On Dit.—It is said that Dean Stanley's death was primarily due to the bad drainage at Westminster. The terribly defective sanitary condition of the deanery is now being thoroughly examined.

The Anti-Vaccinator's New Objection.—On the hearing of several summonses by the Brighton magistrates, last week, against persons charged with disobeying orders already made upon them to have their children vaccinated, the defendants, twelve in number, urged, with one exception, the usual defence—the cruelty and injustice of the law; but the latter took a new objection, and called upon the magistrates to refuse the administration of the oath to the vaccination officer on the ground that he was an atheist. This the latter denied, and said he had not any objection to the oath; upon which the defendant rejoined, that those who ignored the perfection of the Almighty's handiwork, as did the supporters of vaccination, were just as atheistic as those who repudiated the existence of a Supreme Being. The Bench was not at all impressed with the validity of this new line of objection, and fined each defendant 10s. and cost.

M.A. Cantab.—The gentleman is quite correct in the statement he made, as you will see by the following dates of their respective foundations—Oxford, 886; Cambridge, 1110; St. Andrews, 1412; Glasgow, 1450; Aberdeen, 1494; Edinburgh, 1582; Dublin, 1593; London, 1836; Durham, 1837; and Queen's University in Ireland, 1850.

A Staff Surgeon.—Sir Charles M'Grigor, the army agent, succeeded his father as the *second* baronet. He filled the office of Director-General of the Army Medical Department for thirty-six years.

Antiquary.—We have not yet received any reply to the query respecting the seal probably of the Serjeant-Surgeons. The celebrated ring given by Queen Elizabeth to the Earl of Essex was long in the possession of the Warner family. The last of the family who held it was Mr. Joseph Warner, a member of the Court of Assistants of the Royal College of Surgeons, in 1800. Mr. Robert Keate, of St. George's Hospital, was the last member of that Court, viz., in 18[illegible].

Dens Sap., Leicester-square.—The following gentlemen are members of the Board of Examiners in Dental Surgery of the Royal College of Surgeons, viz:—Mr. J. Birkett, chairman; Mr. L. Holden; Mr. T. Holmes; Mr. A. Coleman; Mr. A. Winterbottom; and Mr. C. S. Tomes. The list of successful candidates, and the questions submitted to them, will be found in another page.

Hospital Saturday Fund and a Seaside Convalescent Home.—At the usual monthly meeting of the Board of Delegates of this Fund and Convalescent Homes, held by permission at the Westminster Hospital a few days since, the following resolution was adopted:—"That, with a view of establishing a seaside convalescent home in connexion with the Hospital Saturday Fund, a special meeting be held by the vice-presidents, and that other gentlemen likely to be interested be invited to attend, to consider what steps should be taken to carry such a project into effect." It is not intended to take the funds of the Hospital Saturday Fund to establish the "home," but to apply to the vice-presidents and employers of labour for subscriptions in aid of the object.

Sympathiser.—The children in the foundling hospital are generally disposed of by apprenticeship—the girls at the age of sixteen to domestic service for a terms of four years, and the boys at the age of fourteen (such of them as do not volunteer into the bands of the Army or the Navy) as mechanics for a term of seven years.

Official Neglect: its Consequences.—The Derby Town Council have been considering the question of accommodation for small-pox patients. A sanatorium erected some years since has been neglected and allowed to get into a dilapidated condition. During the present small-pox outbreak the Infirmary Committee have refused to accept patients, and they have consequently had to be isolated in their homes, at the cost of the Sanitary Authority. The repairs at the sanatorium will amount to £315, and a motion to vote that sum produced a desultory and prolonged discussion by the Council. Ultimately, however, a resolution that the sanatorium should be at once put into repair was adopted.

Sanitarian.—At the forthcoming Health Congress and Sanitary Exhibition at Brighton, in December next, Dr. B. W. Richardson will deliver the inaugural address. A special feature of the Exhibition will be the erection of a number of model artisans' dwellings in the grounds of the Royal Pavilion.

COMMUNICATIONS have been received from—
Professor Spence, Edinburgh; Mr. J. Bell, Edinburgh; Dr. Mahomed, London; Mr. Parker, Bath; The Secretary of the Indian Medical Defence Fund, London; The Registrar of the Apothecaries' Hall, London; Mr. S. Snell, Sheffield; Mr. Oglesby, Leeds; Dr. Creighton, London; The Secretary of the Native Guano Company, Aylesbury; Mr. Stone, London; Dr. McCraith, Smyrna; Mr. Lawson Tait, Birmingham; Mr. John Marshall, London; Dr. Crichton Browne, London; Dr. A. de Watteville, London; Mr. Walter Rivington, London; The Honorary Secretary of the Medical Society of London; Mr. J. Chatto, London: The Registrar of the Royal College of Physicians, London; Mr. Bone; Mr. F. A. C. Hare, London; Dr. Greenfield, London; Mr. H. Jackson, Barnstaple; The Secretary of the Hunterian Society, London; The Secretary of the Clinical Society of London; The Assistant-Secretary of the Royal Microscopical Society of London; The Secretary of the University of Edinburgh; Mr. C. Puzey, Liverpool; The Secretary of the University of Durham College of Medicine; Mr. J. W. Teale, Scarborough; The Secretary of the Odontological Society of Great Britain, London; Mr. Dent, London; The Secretary of the Statistical Society, London; The Registrar-General, Scotland; Dr. E. Lancereaux, Paris; Dr. Bristowe, London; The Honorary Secretary of the Royal Medical and Chirurgical Society.

PERIODICALS AND NEWSPAPERS RECEIVED—
Lancet—British Medical Journal—Medical Press and Circular—Berliner Klinische Wochenschrift—Centralblatt für Chirurgie—Gazette des Hopitaux—Gazette Médicale—Le Progrès Médical—Bulletin de l'Académie de Médecine—Pharmaceutical Journal—Wiener Medizinische Wochenschrift—Centralblatt für die Medizinischen Wissenschaften—Revue Médicale—Gazette Hebdomadaire—National Board of Health Bulletin, Washington—Nature—Deutsche Medicinal-Zeitung—Boston Medical and Surgical Journal—Louisville Medical News—Oil and Drug News—Journal of Psychological Medicine and Mental Pathology—Weekblad—Centralblatt für Gynäkologie—Detroit Lancet—Students' Journal and Hospital Gazette—El Observador Medico—The American—Chicago Medical Review—Ophthalmic Review—St. Louis Courier of Medicine—Boy's Own Paper—Sunday at Home—Leisure Hour—Girl's Own Paper—Friendly Greetings—National Board of Health Bulletin Supplement—National Anti-Compulsory Vaccination Reporter—Indian Medical Gazette—The Veterinarian—Science—Morningside Mirror—Archives Générales de Médecine—Birkenhead and Cheshire Advertiser, October 29—Musical Education—Vaccination Inquirer—Monthly Index—Glasgow Medical Journal—Monthly Homœopathic Review—Revue Mensuelle de Laryngologie, d'Otologie, etc.

APPOINTMENTS FOR THE WEEK.

November 5. *Saturday (this day).*

Operations at St. Bartholomew's, 1½ p.m.; King's College, 1½ p.m.; Royal Free, 2 p.m.; Royal London Ophthalmic, 11 a.m.; Royal Westminster Ophthalmic, 1½ p.m.; St. Thomas's, 1½ p.m.; London, 2 p.m.

7. *Monday.*

Operations at the Metropolitan Free, 2 p.m.; St. Mark's Hospital for Diseases of the Rectum, 2 p.m.; Royal London Ophthalmic, 11 a.m.; Royal Westminster Ophthalmic, 1½ p.m.

Odontological Society, 8 p.m. Dr. Richardson, "On Caries of the Teeth in relation to Food and Feeding." Casual communications from Mr. Christopher Heath, etc.

Medical Society of London, 8½ p.m. General Meeting, after which the Ordinary Meeting will take place. The President will show a Case of Disease in the Floor of the Fourth Ventricle. Dr. Allchin will exhibit a specimen of Renal Disease showing Pyelitis with Calculi. Dr. Drysdale, "On the Origin of Vaccinia and its Bearing on Animal Vaccination."

8. *Tuesday.*

Operations at Guy's, 1½ p.m.; Westminster, 2 p.m.; Royal London Ophthalmic, 11 a.m.; Royal Westminster Ophthalmic, 1½ p.m.; West London, 3 p.m.

Anthropological Institute (Council Meeting, 4½ p.m.), 8 p.m. Ordinary Meeting.

Royal Medical and Chirurgical Society, 8½ p.m. Mr. John H. Morgan, "On Two Cases of Congenital 'Macrostoma,' accompanied by Malformation of Auricles, and the presence of Auricular Appendages." Mr. H. Langley Browne, "On Simultaneous Ligature of the Subclavian and Carotid Arteries for Innominate Aneurism."

9. *Wednesday.*

Operations at University College, 2 p.m.; St. Mary's, 1¼ p.m.; Middlesex, 1 p.m.; London, 2 p.m.; St. Bartholomew's, 1½ p.m.; Great Northern, 2 p.m.; Samaritan, 2½ p.m.; King's College (by Mr. Lister), 2 p.m.; Royal London Ophthalmic, 11 a.m.; Royal Westminster Ophthalmic, 1½ p.m.; St. Thomas's, 1½ p.m.; St. Peter's Hospital for Stone, 2 p.m.; National Orthopædic, Great Portland-street, 10 a.m.

Royal Microscopical Society, 8 p.m. Mr. B. Wills Richardson, "On Multiple Staining of Animal and Vegetable Tissues."

Hunterian Society (London Institution) (Council Meeting, 7½), 8 p.m. Dr. Robert Barnes, "On Antiseptic Midwifery, and Septicæmia in Midwifery."

10. *Thursday.*

Operations at St. George's, 1 p.m.; Central London Ophthalmic, 1 p.m.; Royal Orthopædic, 2 p.m.; University College, 2 p.m.; Royal London Ophthalmic, 11 a.m.; Royal Westminster Ophthalmic, 1½ p.m.; Hospital for Diseases of the Throat, 2 p.m.; Hospital for Women, 2 p.m.; Charing-cross, 2 p.m.; London, 2 p.m.; North-West London, 2½ p.m.

11. *Friday.*

Operations at Central London Ophthalmic, 2 p.m.; Royal London Ophthalmic, 11 a.m.; South London Ophthalmic, 2 p.m.; Royal Westminster Ophthalmic, 1½ p.m.; St. George's (ophthalmic operations), 1¼ p.m.; Guy's, 1½ p.m.; St. Thomas's (ophthalmic operations), 2 p.m.

Clinical Society, 8½ p.m. Mr. Golding Bird, "On Cases of Gastrostomy." Adjourned Discussion on Mr. Reeves' paper "On Two Cases of Malignant Stricture in which Gastrostomy was performed." Mr. Clement Lucas, "On a Case in which a Pebble was removed by Tracheotomy from the Right Bronchus." Dr. Mahomed and Mr. Cripps, "Two Cases of Direct Transfusion of Blood for Hæmorrhage in Typhoid Fever."

INAUGURAL ADDRESS
DELIVERED IN
THE DEPARTMENT OF SURGERY
IN THE NEW BUILDINGS OF
THE UNIVERSITY OF EDINBURGH,
October 25, 1881.
By JAMES SPENCE,
Professor of Surgery.

THE circumstances under which I commence my surgical course this session prevent me entering at once into my subject, as I usually do. We meet to-day in peculiar circumstances. We have left the time-honoured class-rooms where we formerly met, for new buildings more adapted to the requirements of modern teaching. I am, therefore, naturally brought to speak of the reasons which led to University extension and the advantages which the new arrangements present for facilitating thorough instruction in the different departments of medical science. On such an occasion it may also be useful to look back on the rise of the teaching of surgery in this city, for the Edinburgh School of Surgery has long possessed distinctive characters in its teaching. The causes which led to extension of the University were chiefly the increased number of subjects taught in it, the institution of new professorships, and consequently increased demand for class-rooms, together with the great inconvenience of two or three professors teaching in the same class-room. What was still more felt in teaching the medical and physical sciences was, the want of proper accommodation for the practical work which forms so marked a feature of modern instruction; and last, not least, the gradual increase of students demanded increased accommodation.

How these requirements have been fulfilled in the magnificent buildings in which we meet to-day, you can scarcely fully judge, for they are yet in an unfinished state. The very lack of accommodation in the old University buildings made us anxious to "go in and possess the land," and so it has happened that, instead of waiting for a general medical exodus and the formal inauguration, we have each taken possession so soon as our departments were ready. Yet even this seeming irregularity has its compensating advantage, inasmuch as it enables each teacher to speak as to the manner in which the requirements of his own department have been fulfilled. Last year the Anatomical Department was opened by my excellent colleague, Professor Turner, who spoke (as well he might) in glowing terms of eulogy of the accommodation provided for anatomical teaching, and of the magnificent casket of stone in which the architect had set his and the other departments, of which, as he justly said, both the University and the city may feel proud. Being of less æsthetic and poetical temperament than my colleague, I will not weaken his eulogy by any faint praise of mine. I would only, as a practical person, venture to hope that when the scaffoldings are removed, and the building seen in its beauty, a discerning and generous public will not be slow to mark that the work is not complete, nor permit that beauty to be marred from want of funds to raise the campanile and other essential features in the architect's plan.

When, in common with other Professors, I was asked to consider what accommodation would be required, I confess I felt a grave responsibility, as my term of possession was not likely to be long. From my experience in the past, and from my views as to the necessities of practical instruction, I indicated—1st. A Lecture-room and Retiring-room; 2nd. Practical-room for the bandaging classes in winter, and for operative surgery in summer; 3rd. A Museum for the Professor's private collection.

As regards the Lecture-room, the general instruction to the architect was that each subject of medical study should be provided with a distinct lecture-theatre. Only those who, like myself, have felt the great inconvenience of the lecture-room being occupied by different lecturers, can fully

appreciate the advantages we now possess. These will, I trust, be more and more evident in the facilities afforded to the student for examining the preparations, appliances, and diagrams used to illustrate the lectures. I think I may congratulate you on the theatre we now occupy. So far as I can judge from its construction and appearance, it seems in its present state all that could be wished in regard to gradual elevation of the seats, distribution of light, means of ventilation, and acoustics.

The only question that arose after its construction was well advanced was with regard to space. The amount of accommodation originally arranged for was 250 students, which at that time was considered an ample margin; but meanwhile there had been rapid increase in the number of students, and at the same time it was found that there was only accommodation for 248, whilst the class numbers of last session were 242. This led to the question of introducing a gallery, as has been done in the class-room of the Professor of Practice of Physic. It was found, however, that by some lesser changes accommodation could be made for 270. I was, I confess, very averse to a gallery if it could possibly be avoided, but at the same time I had to consider the interests of the class and of my successor in time to come, and this was met by the Building Committee undertaking that the alteration would be made whenever the increase of the class required it; so that while the interests of the class for the future have thus been secured, we in the meantime enjoy what I consider the benefits of its present construction.

The Practical-room had long been sorely wanted; in fact, in the old building I was dependent on the courtesy of some of my colleagues for the use of their class-rooms when not occupied. The practical-room now provided is amply sufficient for the practice of bandaging and surgical appliances, because these can only be properly taught to limited subdivisions of the class. In regard to operative surgery in summer, I hope that the possession of the practical room will enable me to carry out some important changes in teaching that subject, even with the present limited means at our disposal.

The third requirement I indicated was a room fitted as a Museum for the Professor's private collection. To many this might not seem so essential, as the Professor has the right to obtain specimens from the University Museum; but I thought that anyone likely to be elected Professor of Surgery in this University would certainly possess a collection of his own, far more useful to him for teaching purposes than specimens from the general museum. In my own case, I rarely use specimens from the general museum, and only such as I have myself prepared, or with the histories of which I am intimately acquainted. Thus the specimens in my own collection serve as notes of lecture, bringing to mind the peculiarities and important features in different forms of surgical disease. Hence I considered a proper museum-room a most valuable adjunct to the Department of Surgery, and I feel no little satisfaction in finding my collection at length placed in a museum-room in which the preparations can be seen and utilised. Besides these more important requirements there are smaller work-rooms, and ample storage accommodation. Altogether I think that we have every reason to be satisfied with the manner in which the architect has provided for the Department of Surgery, and it must lie with us to show that we can make good use of our new advantages.

I have said that, in our present circumstances, it may be useful to look back on the rise of surgical teaching in Edinburgh, as I think that we will find in its earliest beginning the spirit which has all along been its distinguishing character—a love of teaching for its own sake; the desire of acquiring and advancing professional knowledge, and conveying that knowledge to others.

In speaking of the Edinburgh School of Medicine, it is not unusual to date its beginning from about 1720 to 1726, when Monro and others were appointed by the Town Council to lecture in the University, when lectures on Anatomy, Institutes of Medicine, Botany, Materia Medica, and Practice of Physic were regularly delivered. That no doubt marks the formation of a regular school, but that school was only the culmination of a system of teaching which had been long in operation amongst many difficulties. Brilliant as was the school which then arose, it nevertheless had its foundations in the past. If we wish to learn its early beginning, and the spirit which then, and ever since, has actuated medical teaching in Edinburgh, we must go much further back than 1790—back for now nearly four centuries—to 1505. In that year the " Surgeon's Craft " in this city applied to the Municipal Council for a charter of incorporation, which was granted, and confirmed by Royal authority in 1506. Their application is curious and interesting in many respects, but I have always considered it specially interesting as exhibiting the true spirit—a desire to advance both themselves and others in professional knowledge on a firm basis. After asking powers to prevent anyone practising surgery who had not passed a proper examination, they ask for a special privilege: " that we may have anis in the yeir an condampnit man after he is deid to mak anotomen of, quhairthrow we may haif experience Ilk ane to instruct uthers." This was a bold demand in these early days when superstition prevailed. Late in the same century, Charles V., the Emperor of Spain, then perhaps the most powerful and civilised of European nations, called a Council of Divines to decide whether dissection of the human body was permissible, and the result was a very uncertain sound. Fortunately, our municipal authorities of that time were strong-minded men, and possessed of sound common sense—men who did not expect people to make bricks without straw : they saw the spirit of the request; they saw that if the public was to be really benefited by medical treatment they must give the surgeons the means for advancing their own knowledge and of instructing their apprentices or pupils of the craft; and so the Town Council granted their request. From this transaction, so honourable to all concerned, we may trace the institution of demonstrators or teachers of anatomy, which ultimately, in the person of Monro, led to the commencement of the Medical School of the University. Having obtained their charter, the surgeons instituted a regulation equivalent to a preliminary examination. At that time there was no medical school : all teaching was by apprenticeship to members of the incorporation : and whilst, as we have seen, the surgeons had obtained for themselves and their pupils the means of instruction in the important subject of anatomy—the basis of all medical or surgical knowledge,— they also provided against uneducated persons being admitted to the profession, by this rule: " Item—that na Maisteris of the said Craft sall tak ane prenteis or feit man in tyme cuming, to use the Surgeon's craft, without he can baith wryte and reid." This may seem to you a very slender amount of requirement for entrance to the professional studies ; but when you consider that at that time many of the nobility and gentry of the kingdom did not possess these qualifications, that many an important State document bears simply " his mark +," instead of the signature of some powerful baron, you will see it was a comparatively high standard; and the same spirit has ever since distinguished the Surgeons. Few corporate bodies or universities have done more to secure a good preliminary as well as a thorough professional education than the Royal College of Surgeons of Edinburgh. As time went on, the teaching gradually assumed a more regular character under what were termed the demonstrators. Gradually other subjects were taught at the Surgeons' theatre. On February 9, 1726, the teachers of the different subjects applied to the Town Council to have these departments taught in the " Colledge," and were at that date appointed as Professors, and so the Medical School of this University was constituted.

In what spirit do we regard these early records of our School ? Do the slender requirements of the " Surgeons' preliminary " excite a smile ; or do we plume ourselves on our advance, as we compare the state of medical science then and now ? Should we not rather admire the mental powers and indomitable perseverance of the men who, working in dark and troubled times, did so much to establish our science on a sure foundation ; and consider what we owe to these pioneers of our profession ?

Whilst we may fairly congratulate ourselves on the present state of medical science, we should remember that we have entered on their labours, and are reaping where they sowed. Nothing is easier than to sneer at old-fashioned theories and practice, and congratulate ourselves on the high position of modern medicine. Speaking of such a spirit, Lord Macaulay remarks—" It is not thus we ought to judge of the events and the men of other times. They were behind us. It could not be otherwise. But the question in respect to them 'is not where they were, but which way were they going—

were their faces set in the right or wrong direction ? " I think I may claim for these early fathers of Edinburgh surgery that their faces were set in the right direction, and that they went forward in it right manfully, so that their spirit and example have influenced our School for good ever since.

Although surgery as a distinct department was not established in this University until 1831, its importance had been long recognised, and the institution of a Chair of Surgery was pressed upon the patrons in a petition from the College of Surgeons in 1777, but was resisted by Monro as interfering with his subject. The Surgeons thereupon subsequently instituted a Professorship of Surgery for their own College, their first Professor being the late eminent Dr. John Thomson (afterwards the first Professor of General Pathology in this University). He was succeeded by John Lizars, and on his resignation, the College abolished their Professorship, as the University Chair of Surgery had meanwhile been created. But surgery has long had eminent exponents in Edinburgh. John and Charles Bell, Allan, Liston, Syme, Lizars, Fergusson, and Miller are names which must always excite admiration and be held in reverence as those who have done much to advance surgical science to its present high position.

We honour these our great predecessors for the work they did; but whilst, as I have said, we have entered on their labours, we must not be content to rest in them— that would not be to profit by their example or to emulate the spirit in which they wrought. Their aim was progress, and if we would follow them aright we must strive to advance. How then shall we best use the advantages we now possess for this great end ? At first sight, it would seem that with the complete arrangement of each department—with a theatre admirably constructed for lecturing and demonstrative teaching, a museum where you have means of seeing morbid specimens illustrative of disease, and a practical-room in which the student is taught to use surgical appliances and perform operations ; there should be no difficulty in regard to complete instruction. Nor would there be, if the student could devote his whole attention to one subject. But the teacher must keep in mind the Apostolic injunction, " Look not every man on his own things, but every man also on the things of others "; and hence the difficulty of arranging the practical classes so that they may not interfere with other subjects of study. This difficulty, I foresee, will be a growing one, and one which, after some experience, I believe can only be overcome by lengthening the period of study. Meanwhile, we must meet the difficulty as best we can, by arranging different days and hours for practical instruction. The details of these arrangements I shall announce hereafter.

The advance in physical diagnosis by the introduction of instruments which enable us to observe disease with precision, necessitates the study and habit of using them ; and the tendency to study specialities, particularly in surgery, is on the increase.

I have no intention of entering on the difficult problem of medical education, but I desire very briefly to point out what I consider as essentials in pursuing your studies. First, and all-important, let your study of anatomy be thorough. The students of the present day have great advantages, and yet in our final surgical examinations I do not find the result such as I used to expect from the advantages they possess. I begin to think that there is too much done to assist instead of leaving them to gain their knowledge for themselves—more slowly, it may be, but more thoroughly. The proverb "Lightly come, lightly go," has an application here. Special dissections, preserved so as to be seen and studied ; frozen sections, or casts from such sections ; anatomical plates and diagrams, are all most useful aids in their proper place : but nothing can take the place of the study of the bones of the human skeleton and actual careful dissection of the body, the student working for himself, and only applying to the demonstrator when at a loss.

Again, there is the mistaken idea about surgical anatomy, as if that were confined to a few regions of the body. As all parts of the body are liable to injury and disease, so all human anatomy is surgical. It will depend upon the accuracy of your knowledge gained in dissection, and your having accustomed yourselves to apply anatomical and physiological facts to surgery, whether you will become skilful in the diagnosis and treatment of surgical disease. From studying a finished dissection, however perfect, you will not gain that kind of knowledge. The recognition of the textures gained in dissection; the original relation and nature of the tissues removed to display the more important organs, can only be gained by personal, and let me add, thoughtful dissection; for it is quite possible to make a clean dissection mechanically, whilst the mind may be engaged in wandering thoughts and vain imaginations.

Another department of professional study which requires notice is pathology, or the phenomena of disease, and morbid anatomy—the changes in texture consequent on injury or disease, or the development of new formations, as tumours. Here you must be prepared to study your subject from somewhat different points of view—1. The clinical aspects and the appearances recognisable by the eye'; 2. The investigation of the minute structural changes revealed by the microscope. The former is the method we chiefly use in teaching surgery in the lecture-room and hospital. The other you will be taught in pathological lectures, and especially learn for yourselves in the pathological laboratory. Both are necessary; each comes to aid the other. I think it must be evident, however, that, for practical purposes, the clinical method is most important. It enables the student to observe the more evident symptoms and progress of disease with a view to diagnosis and treatment. The purely pathological investigation of diseased structure can only be pursued when the patient is dead, or when the morbid part has been removed from the living body. Then it is of great value in settling questions connected with the character of disease, and, in some degree, throwing light upon the origin or development of growths, and the changes in the intimate structure of diseased organs. Like most things, it has its weak points: the tendency to raise theories on insufficient bases, and the arbitrary classifications and changes of nomenclature of different investigators. It is, however, a science which will gradually become of more importance as it is more fully studied, and if kept in right relation to clinical observation. Whilst, therefore, in teaching surgery the clinical method is most essential, I should be sorry to be misunderstood in regard to the importance of pure pathological science.

In regard to practical surgical teaching—the classes for bandaging and surgical appliances—I take some credit for making that department more generally attended to. It used to be cast as an opprobrium on the Edinburgh School, that many of our graduates and licentiates did not know how to bandage a limb! When appointed to this chair, I thought the best use I could make of my University assistant was to employ him to teach and superintend the students of the class, in sections, so that all might have the opportunity of gaining practical acquaintance in this important department. I need hardly dwell on its value. The application of bandages on the lay figure and the living, an acquaintance with the different forms of splints and apparatus, and a knowledge of the instruments used in operations, and the mode of arranging them, must commend itself to all; and, as it forms an integral part of the course, every member of the class can avail himself of the instruction.

Finally, as to the study of specialities and new aids to physical diagnosis. In reference to specialities, these chiefly concern the advanced student. Your first business is to obtain a good knowledge of general principles and broad views of surgery and medicine, and then turn to specialities. In regard to new aids to physical diagnosis, refuse no aid, for we need them all; only do not throw away the methods which have been found useful in the past—use them still. Some of the new methods and instruments for diagnosis, such as the ophthalmoscope and laryngoscope, will at once commend themselves. Others may seem less likely to become of practical value; do not throw them aside—study their use, and try to improve them.

In fine, in this and new methods of treatment, proceed on the Apostolic advice, "Prove all things; hold fast that which is true."

CHILDREN'S HOSPITAL AT WARSAW.—Prof. A. Walther has published in a Warsaw journal a frightful account of the state of the Asylum for Illegitimate Children at Warsaw. Every nurse has charge of two sucklings, and the mortality rose in 1879 and in 1880 to more than 46 per cent. No supervision whatever is exercised over children put out to nurse in the country.—*St. Petersb. Med. Woch.*, October 29.

AN ADDRESS ON

THE SANITARY CONDITION AND LAWS OF MEDIÆVAL AND MODERN LONDON.

Delivered before the Society of Medical Officers of Health, October, 1881.

By JOHN W. TRIPE, M.D., M.R.C.P. Ed.,
President of the Society.

THE annual address from this chair becomes every year more difficult, both as regards the selection of the subject and the matter itself, in consequence of the able manner in which my predecessors have presented their views before you. After much consideration, I decided on selecting for my subject the Sanitary Condition and Laws of Mediæval and Modern London. Of course it is impossible in the time usually occupied by these addresses to do more than briefly sketch the salient points of my subject. Indeed, I am in some doubt if many of my hearers may not consider it beyond the bounds of our organisation; but I hold the opinion that the present can only be fairly judged by looking at the past, and the future can be predicated only by a consideration of both.

If we look carefully at the legislative measures which were in force in Mediæval London, including, of course, not only Acts of Parliament, but also the civic ordinances, we should almost wonder at the prevalence of plague, sweating sickness, and other pestilences, which more than decimated the population from time to time, as well as the large fires which so frequently devastated portions of the city. The laws and ordinances in existence at that time ought to have prevented both, but they were generally neglected, and, at the most, only spasmodically enforced, in the same way as our leet juries have neglected their work, for they had the power, and rarely used it, of condemning uninhabitable houses, and removing many of the nuisances which materially affected the comfort, if not the death-rate, of the population of England. The chief reason for this neglect appears to be that the Acts and ordinances were much in advance of the habits and ideas of the population, and, therefore, fell into disuse almost immediately after the passing of the Acts.

In the time of the early Norman kings, most of the houses of London were built in a very primitive manner, viz., of wood, or mud and clay mixed with straw, and covered with a thatch of straw or rushes, so that when a fire broke out it often became of considerable magnitude, and, as water had to be brought from the nearest streams, it was often necessary to pull down adjoining houses with large hooks to prevent the spreading of the fire. An extensive fire which occurred in London in the reign of King Stephen led to an ordinance being issued in the first year of the reign of Richard I. (1189), known as Fitz-Elwynne's Assize of Buildings. This contained many important regulations, not only as regards the structure of buildings, but their appurtenances. Thus, it was ordered that the party-walls of new houses should be made of stone three feet in thickness; that if the expense were borne equally by both, the land was to be taken equally from both; but if the neighbour of the one wishing to build were too poor or objected, the latter was to give three feet of land for the other to build on, when the wall, which was to be raised sixteen feet high, became their joint property. If they agreed to make a joint gutter to carry off the rain-water, they might do so; but, if not, each had to provide his own gutter to carry the water on to his own land or the highway. There was also a curious provision that, if a man built a stone wall on his own land, and carried the eaves over his neighbour's, the latter was required to make a gutter for carrying off the water either on to his land or the highway. Another regulation, which must often have interfered not only with the light, but the ventilation of houses, was that a person might build against the windows of his neighbour, unless there was an agreement in writing to prevent him from doing so. If, however, the new building was considered to be unjust, there was power of appeal. The "Assize" also stated that, in consequence of the fire previously mentioned, which destroyed houses from London-bridge to the Church of St. Clement Danes, many of the citizens built stone houses and covered the roof with thick tiles. It will be noticed that the regulation height of the stone wall was sixteen feet, to admit of two storeys, the upper being called the "solar," which was the chief room in the house, and was entered by means of a ladder or staircase, the latter being usually placed outside. Above the solar was erected a pent-house, overhanging the foot-way, the eaves of which were to be sufficiently high to allow a man on horseback to ride under them. The goods sold at the stall or shop were suspended under the eaves or placed on a board, whilst the stall, placed outside the house, was not allowed to be more than two feet and a half wide. At this time, comparatively few of the smaller houses had either glazed windows or chimneys, and were, therefore, cold, dark, and dirty; but early in the fourteenth century these were commonly found in all houses. In better class houses both were ordinarily met with in the reign of Richard I.

In the articles of the Wardmote made in the reign of Edward II., it was expressly provided that no chimneys be henceforth made, except of stone, tiles, or plaster, under pain of being pulled down, and that all houses within the franchise should be covered with tiles, etc. It was also provided that all who dwelt in great houses should have a ladder or two in case of fire, so that low houses were by no means universal at that time. That houses were subsequently built of wood, or wood and daubing, is very evident from the frequency with which fires occurred, and the distance to which they spread.

A very graphic description of London in 1850 is given by a contemporary anonymous writer. He states that, although there are numerous large vacant spaces within the walls, belonging to the mansions of the nobility, the halls of city companies, as well as to the monasteries and convents, yet the populated parts were intersected by narrow streets, lanes, and alleys, encumbered with houses, whose apartments, jutting out storey above storey, almost touched one another at the top, so as to make the streets dark and unwholesome. The houses were much overcrowded, and several statutes were passed to prevent, not only overcrowding, but the building of new houses. Indeed, this was carried to so great an extent by Queen Elizabeth, that it was ordained in 1580 that every newly built house should have four acres of land, and numerous houses were pulled down, and the builders and workmen were punished by fine, or imprisonment without bail, for disobeying this law. It was also ordered that two newly built houses should be thrown into one to reduce the number; and, at the time of the Plague, the "Harbinger" had power to put infected persons into these houses. This proclamation was issued "because there are such great multitudes of people brought to inhabit small rooms, whereof the greater part are seen very poor, yea, such as must live of begging, or by worse means, and they heaped up together, and, in a sort, smothered with many families of children and servants in one house or small tenement."

How these evils were to be cured by restricting the number of houses I fail to see; indeed, it seems to me, that so far from being a means of preventing, the proclamation must have led to more overcrowding. At a later date, Sir W. Davenant referred, in a letter, to the contiguity of the top storeys of houses, which were, he says, so close together that the inhabitants of houses on opposite sides of the streets could shake hands. This style of building is even now to be seen in Mercerie-lane, Canterbury, but the storeys do not overhang so much as is stated by these writers.

The interior of the smaller houses is described, up to the time even of Chaucer, in anything but flattering terms, as we learn from his "Canterbury Tales." Very many were dark, badly ventilated, and filthily dirty, not only from the want of chimneys, but from the habits of the people. In the better class houses, although there were glazed windows and chimneys, yet the floors are described as being filthy in the extreme. Even as late as the reign of Henry VIII., we learn from a letter written by Erasmus to Dr. Francis, "that the floors are commonly of clay, strewed with rushes, under which lies unmolested an ancient collection of beer, grease, fragments, bones, spittle, excrements of dogs and cats, and everything that is nasty." Of course this description refers to the ordinary living room, which was situated on the ground floor, the solar and other upper rooms, if any, having boarded floors. In the reign of Henry III., and for many years afterwards, dogs, "genteel dogs excepted," were not allowed to go at large under a penalty of 3s. 4d. to the use of the Chamber, but were kept at home, and pigs

also, except those belonging to the Hospital of St. Anthony, were to be retained on the premises or in the house. If found running about the streets, the persons seizing them were directed to kill and keep them for their own use, or to give them back at the price of fourpence for each pig. In spite of this edict, pigs were kept in pigsties in the streets, and to remedy this four men were elected and sworn in to see "to the removal of the sties, and killing of all pigs, except those of St. Anthony's Priory, that might be found at large in the streets, fosses, or suburbs of London." To prevent pigs not belonging to St. Anthony's Priory being claimed by the renter, he was sworn not to put a bell on, or to claim any which were not given to the Priory in pure alms. The references to swine in the "Liber Albus" are very numerous. As it is generally supposed that most of the excrement was cast into the streets for the rakers to remove, I will refer to a passage about "necessary chambers," from Fitz-Elwynne's Assize. Concerning these, it is ordained that, if the pit of such chamber be lined with stone, the mouth shall be two feet and a half from the land of the neighbour, but if not so lined, it must be three feet and a half away. These pits were emptied by nightmen, and taken to lay stalls at Mile-end, Dowgate or Puddle Dock, or to White-friars. At a later date the lay stalls at Mile-end are described as being intolerable nuisances, and were not removed until quite recently, as, when a boy, I received a practical evidence of their existence.

The streets both within and without the walls were narrow, and became more injurious when the houses were built higher, and especially when what were known as "middle rows" (like that lately removed in Holborn) were built in the roadways of several streets. Where permanent buildings were not erected, shops, and even smithies, were frequently placed there. Aldgate-street, Cornhill, Cheapside, Newgate-street, Ludgate-street, and many others had middle rows. These were in existence at the time of the great fire of London, and must have materially assisted in rendering the City unhealthy.

Although sewers are mentioned by Fitz Stephen as being in use at the time he wrote, which was in the reign of Richard I., yet he most probably meant merely the channels in the centre of the streets which communicated with other channels leading to the Thames. These latter are especially directed in several ordinances to be kept clean. The streets were paved with small stones without any raised footpaths, and sloped down to a channel in the centre, which carried off the rain-water and most of the slops. Fishmongers were especially ordered not to cast their slops into these channels. There was also another regulation that nothing was to be thrown out of the windows between sunrise and nine at night, under a penalty of 8s. 4d.; and that any-one who sustained damage by such an act was to be recouped by the person emptying the slops. It was especially mentioned that "urine boles and ordure boles" were to be brought down and cast into the channel. It is evident from these regulations that the streets must have been in a filthy condition even when the pavement was in good condition; but, as each person had to pave the street in front of his house, and keep the channel clean and in order, the pavement must have been often in a very bad state. That this was so, especially outside the boundaries of the City, is shown by the frequency with which ordinances were issued, or Acts of Parliament passed, for paving these thorough-fares. Thus, in the time of Henry VIII., the roadway between Temple Bar and Westminster was directed to be paved at the expense of the owners and occupiers of houses abutting on the street, and kept in order from tolls to be paid by those riding on or driving along it. This is the first notice of a toll on horses and carriages, and it is said to have answered very well. As the streets were narrow, and there was not any raised path for foot-passengers, posts were placed at a short distance from the walls of the houses to protect persons using the paths from the horses and carriages, and were said to be a great annoyance. As the pent-houses overhung the pavement, the passengers kept as close to the walls as possible. This often led to quarrels and loss of life, so that, what with pools of dirty water under foot, and deluges of rain above, the condition of a wayfarer after passing through the City on a rainy day must have been anything but conducive to good health, especially as umbrellas were not then used.

Although the citizens were required to keep the pavement

and channels clean, they were not called upon to remove any of the filth swept up, but a class of men termed rakers were appointed and paid under the articles of the wardmote for each City ward, who were ordered to place it in carts, and take it to the places ordained for its reception. These were at Mile-end and the other places previously mentioned. Frequent ordinances were also made, forbidding that the filth was to be thrown into the river Thames or any of its tributaries, the chief of which was the Fleet. There were also special articles of each wardmote, prohibiting anyone from throwing dung or other filth into the streets, and especially offal. Butchers appear to have been rather frequent offenders on this point. In the fourth book of the "Liber Albus," as well as in other books, there are enumerated many special regulations for the removal of filth; the cleansing of the hythes and fosses, lanes and streets; for the custody of the conduits and watercourses; and for the cleansing of the Fleet Ditch. There were also divers other ordinances as to pent-houses, rain-gutters, stalls, jetties, cellars, and pavements. It was the special duty of the "scavengers" to superintend the streets, as the oath taken by them on their appointment sufficiently shows. As the oath is somewhat curious, I quote it at length :—" You shall swear that you shall diligently oversee that the pavements within your ward are well and rightly repaired, and not made too high in nuisance of the neighbours; and that the ways, streets, and lanes are cleansed of dung and all manner of filth for the decency of the City; and that all chimneys, furnaces, and reredoses are of stone, and sufficiently defended against peril of fire; and if you find anything to the contrary, you shall show it to the alderman, that so the alderman may ordain for the amendment thereof. And this you shall not fail to do, so God your help and the saints." It will be seen from this that the "scavager" was a surveyor and an inspector of nuisances, whilst the rakers actually removed the filth. The provision for the removal of street-filth was not great—viz., twelve carts, with two horses each, for the whole of the City.

The regulations respecting the prevention of fouling the water-courses and the Thames, especially by butchers, appear to have been rarely enforced, as, in 1361, Edward III. sent a letter to the mayor and sheriffs, commanding, "that all bulls, oxen, hogs, and other gross creatures, to be slain for the sustentation of the said city, should not be killed at a less distance than Stratford-le-Bow on the one side, and Knightsbridge on the other, so that the air of the city might no longer be rendered corrupt and infectious by means of the putrid blood and entrails which the butchers had been accustomed to throw into the streets or cast into the Thames." The penalty was forfeiture of the carcase and imprisonment. In the twelfth year of the reign of Richard II., butchers were allowed to erect slaughter-houses on the banks of the Thames, and carry away the offal in boats, and throw it into the Thames; but this was repealed in the sixteenth year of the same reign, when butchers and others were prohibited from throwing offal, etc., into the Thames, under a penalty of £40. A similar law was enacted in the reign of Henry VII., showing that the convenience of killing beasts in the City had prevailed over the law.

The first Commissioners of Sewers were appointed by statute in the sixth year of Henry VI., which Act was almost a dead letter; but, in 1531, a commission was appointed to survey the walls, streams, ditches, banks, gutters, sewers, gotes, calcies, bridges, etc.; and by a subsequent statute, in the third James I., the powers of the Commissioners for London were extended to all places situated within two miles of London. The word "sewers" is used as well as gutters; so that, in 1531, there must have been some sewers in London, but what they were I have not been able to ascertain, as there is no mention whatever of sewers in the "Liber Albus," or in any book of this date to which I have had access. Pauli, however, when speaking of London in the time of Edward III., says, "that special care was taken by the civic authorities to secure good draining for the running off of rain-water, as well as for the arrangement of sewers."

The water-supply of London was obtained at first from the River of the Wells, i.e., the Fleet, from the Wallbrook, Langbourne, the Thames, and from numerous wells dug in the gardens adjoining the houses, and also from numerous public wells. In the reign of Henry III., twenty-first year, liberty was granted to Gilbert Sanford to convey water from

Tybourne by pipes of lead, six inches in diameter, into the City. One of these pipes supplied the Cheapside conduit, near Bow Church. Other conduits were quickly built, including one in Cornhill, called the "Tonne." One of the most celebrated was in Fleet-street, known as the St. Christopher. In 1285, the so-called Great Waterworks were opened at Westcheap, when large quantities of red and white wine flowed from the pipes. A very fine conduit was erected in 1655, in Leadenhall-street.

The earliest attempt to supply London with water by mechanical means was made by Peter Morris, who carried pipes into the houses on the Thames side of Gracechurch-street. The pressure was sufficiently strong to throw water over St. Magnus Church, and was obtained from the Thames in 1582. The City granted him two arches of London-bridge, and the right to take water from the Thames for 500 years. In 1594, other works of a similar kind were erected near Broken Wharf, for the supply of houses in Westcheap, and around St. Paul's, up to Fleet-street. The supplies being insufficient, the New River Works were commenced in 1608, and opened in 1613, with results which I need not mention.

The laws against vendors of food, who sold tainted meat, poultry, fish, etc., were very severe. Thus, in the "Liber Albus," we read of persons being put into the pillory for selling putrid meat, stinking capons, rabbits, pigeons, partridges, fish, eels, conger, pigs, and stinking boiled meat. A similar punishment was also inflicted on those who sold "false shoes," and putrid wine.

The fire of London is usually said to have led to such an alteration in the overcrowded and narrow thoroughfares as prevented subsequent outbreaks of the plague. For reasons presently to be stated, I am of opinion that this was not the case.

It is true that the sanitary condition of the new part of the City was much better than the old, as the filth in the houses and streets was destroyed by the heat, but the rebuilding was on the old lines; and, although most of the new streets were widened, yet nearly 4000 additional houses were said to have been erected, partly on the gardens of the large merchants, and partly on those belonging to the City halls and other buildings. A careful comparison of maps induces a strong belief that this statement is incorrect. The chief improvement consisted in the better class and greater uniformity of the buildings, the removal of the middle rows, which interfered so much with traffic and ventilation, and the building of most of the houses without overhanging floors. The pavements were also improved, but were made with small stones, as before. The streets were rendered of a more uniform level, by filling up the lower, and reducing the higher portions. Thus, Ludgate-hill was reduced from 10 to 20 inches at the upper part, and raised from 6 feet to 8 feet 7 inches at the lower. Thames-street and the adjoining streets and lanes were also improved in a similar manner. I lay before you two maps, one of London in 1560, and the other in 1720, showing that the old streets, many under new names, were rebuilt on the old sites.

This very brief sketch of mediæval London would be incomplete without some reference to the prevailing diseases of the period, and especially to the plague, as well as to the population of the City. It appears from the bills of mortality that most probably the deaths in the City exceeded the births. Graunt, in his essay on the subject, states that the excess of deaths was very considerable, and was made up by immigrants, about 6000 of whom he believes came to London every year. He and other writers thought, that with the exception of the period, 1640-1660, when baptism was neglected, or the entries not made, the baptisms may be taken as a near approximation to the births; but when we consider that Mr. Rickman estimated that about 2½ per cent. of the children born in 1821-30 were either baptised at home, or not baptised at all, it is not likely that the registers were more to be relied upon in 1603-67, than in 1821-30. It appears from the bills of mortality, that, during the hundred years 1601-1700, there were 1,572,635 deaths registered, of which as many as 188,571 were due to the plague; that there were only 984,499 christenings entered; but a comparison of the years before and after the twenty years 1640-60 shows that at least 50,000 must be added to the total number to bring it up to the average. This would make 1,034,499 christenings, which, with 25 per cent. added, makes up a total of 1,293,124, or an excess of deaths over baptisms amounting to 279,511. There is no doubt but that, especially in the plague years, a large number of deaths were not registered; indeed, De Foe estimates the mortality from the plague in 1665 at nearly 100,000, whilst the registers show only 68,596, and other authorities support him in his opinion. At any rate, I think we may take it for a fact that the deaths in London exceeded the births during this century. The mean annual number of deaths for each ten years in this century (1601-1700), within the bills of mortality, was 11,169 in 1601-10, 8167 in 1610-20, when but few died from the plague; 13,746 in 1621-30, 11,942 in 1631-40, 10,818 in 1641-50, 12,900 in 1651-60, and as many as 25,280 in 1661-70. During the remaining three decenniads, the numbers were respectively 19,117, 22,363, and 20,770. These latter numbers, as well as the baptisms, point to a large increase having taken place in the population of the City during these thirty years. It is somewhat singular that the number of males entered on the registers as having been buried was largely in excess of the females, for, between 1628 and 1661, there were 209,436 males entered, and only 190,474 females. The same occurred, but to a smaller extent, with the baptisms, as there were 139,782 males, against 130,866 females. This may have been caused by the greater importance, socially considered, of male than female baptisms and deaths.

The plague caused a very large number of deaths in the twelfth, thirteenth, fourteenth, fifteenth, and sixteenth centuries, as well as in the seventeenth. It is reported that about 100,000 died in London in 1852, 30,000 in 1401 and in 1499, and nearly as many in 1582 and 1587. In 1603, as many as 36,000 were entered on the registers; in 1625 they were nearly as numerous; in 1636, 10,000; in 1646, 10,415; in 1647, 10,462; in 1649, 10,499; and in 1651, 10,804 deaths were recorded. From that time, until it broke out in 1665, there was a comparative cessation of its attacks. Its final disappearance is commonly attributed to the Fire of London; but that is clearly an error, as the disease broke out, on the two last occasions, in the same street in Whitechapel, and thence spread, affecting chiefly the poor, to the City itself. Now, after 1665, although Whitechapel and the localities in the neighbourhood of the Thames, east of where the fire occurred, remained unchanged, the plague did not appear amongst the inhabitants of those places, nor amongst those of St. Martin's and St. Giles's, who are described as being "very filthy in their habits." It is quite clear, as only thirty deaths were registered from plague after 1665, that some cause must be looked for, other than the fire, to account for its cessation. During the seventy years, 1601-70, there were registered 761,608 deaths from all causes, and 188,571 from plague, so that 21 per cent. of the deaths from all causes occurred from plague. As the returns were made by the parish clerks, and as large numbers of the dead were buried in unconsecrated ground, there should be about 20 per cent. added on to the numbers just given. Mr. Rickman stated his belief, that in 1821-30, about one-sixth of the total burials were not returned by the parish clerk. As also an examination of the bills of mortality shows, that instead of a smaller number of deaths being recorded from "causes other than plague," there were almost always more when the plague prevailed; it is probable that during those years not less than 25 per cent. of the total deaths were caused by plague. In the twenty years, 1611-20, and 1631-40, which included one period during which the plague was rife, and the other when it caused only a few deaths, the percentages of deaths from various causes, plague excepted, were as follows:—From old age, 8·6 per cent.; from ague and fever, 12·9 per cent.; or with purples and spotted fever added, 13·9 per cent.; chrisoms (by which is meant deaths immediately after christening), and infants, 17·4 per cent.; from consumption and cough, 24·1 per cent.; from bloody flux, 4·2 per cent.; from dropsy, 5·2 per cent.; from small-pox, 5·7 per cent.; and from teething and worms, 7·7 per cent. There was not any death mentioned from scarlet fever. It is commonly supposed that this omission arose from the deaths from this disease being entered under the names of measles or sore-throat; but as the former is credited only with a mortality of 0·4 per cent., and the latter of 0·2 per cent., this can scarcely be the case.

I have not been able to meet with any description of scarlet fever in England at this date, whilst the malignant sore-throat which devastated the shores of the Mediterranean

about this time, and reached England about the time of the Fire of London, corresponds pretty accurately with it. At a later period, viz., 1728-57, the deaths from fevers, including malignant, scarlet, spotted, and purples, were 14·8 per cent. of the deaths from all causes; small-pox 8 per cent., convulsions 27·7, consumption 17·0, cough and whooping-cough 0·5, asthma and tissick 2·1, making 19·6 deaths per cent. from chest affections. The deaths from old age were returned at 7·8 per cent. The ages at death at this last-named period were as follow:—36·2 per cent. of all the deaths occurred under two years, and 3·7 between two and five years, making 45 per cent. under five; 3·4 between five and ten; 3·1 between ten and twenty; 7·7 between twenty and thirty; 9·6 between thirty and forty; 9·7 between forty and fifty; 8·0 between fifty and sixty; 6·3 between sixty and seventy; 4·5 between seventy and eighty; 2·3 between eighty and ninety; and 0·4 above ninety years of age. These may be summarised as 45 per cent. under five years of age; 6·5 per cent. between five and twenty years; 35 per cent. between twenty and sixty; and only 13·5 per cent. above sixty. These figures must be considered very unsatisfactory, as the mortality at five years is extremely high, and also between twenty and sixty, whilst above sixty it is very small, in consequence of the excessive number of deaths below sixty years of age. Before the Fire of London the ages at death were, doubtless, looking at them from a moral point of view, still more unsatisfactory.

(To be continued.)

ORIGINAL COMMUNICATIONS.

SOME NEW FACTS CONNECTED WITH THE ACTION OF GERMS IN THE PRODUCTION OF HUMAN DISEASES.
By Dr. GEORGE HARLEY, F.R.S.

PROLOGUE.

As the medical, like all the other professions, alas! contains its full quota of ignorant, as well as of learned, men, and the old adage which says, "Nothing beats the assurance of ignorance," was typically verified a few months ago by one of the would-be supposed etymologically learned of our brethren, with more temerity than discretion attacking me in no very gracious terms for, as he in his wisdom expressed it, daring to upset the beautiful spelling of our mother tongue by sweeping away the landmarks of its etymology. In case there exist among the subscribers to the *Medical Times and Gazette* other members of the profession who from being equally unacquainted with the principles of modern comparative philology, and the history of English orthography, should feel their nerves ruthlessly shocked by my practical exposition of how our mother tongue can, not only be simplified, and consequently beautified, but in a measure restored to its original common-sense purity of orthographical construction by omitting from every word in the language—EXCEPT PERSONAL NAMES—all redundant, and consequently useless, duplicated consonants. Which probably few of my readers are aware did not exist in early English words, and were scarcely even so much as introduced into them until the time of Queen Elizabeth. When a "duplicated consonant fabrication mania" appears to have seized upon authors. For they then began apparently to vie with each other in cramming—without either rhyme or reason—into words as many duplicated consonants as they possibly could. Not only reckless alike of the time, labor, and material they went in consequence thereof compelled to throw uselessly away, but regardless of the fact that in so doing they were destroying the original simplicity, as well as the original beauty, of early English spelling. This is easily shown by placing side by side a few of the pure, with a few of the adulterated words. Thus leg became legge; ham, hamme; son, sonne; shot, shotte, etc. Until at length, in the end of the seventeenth and beginning of the eighteenth centuries, wiser generations sprang up, who, refusing to have their time unnecessarily wasted and their personal comfort inconvenienced by being compelled, for the mere sake of fashion—there is a mere fashion in orthography, as there is in everything else—to write a great host of redundant, and consequently utterly meaningless, duplicated consonants, began gradually to omit them. A proces which received in 1711 a great stimulus from the pen of Dean Swift in a public protest against useles duplicated consonants which he embodied in a leter adresed to his friend Robert Harley, the then Prime Minister. Just as I in 1878 —exactly 167 years afterwards(a)—did to our late Prime Minister, Lord Beaconsfield, not only in nearly the same form, but almost under identical similar circumstances.

Dean Swift's leter, backed up as it was by the advocacy of some other equaly inteligent and advanced thinkers, soon began to show visible efects in the improvement which speedily took place in speling by the omision of great numbers of the obnoxious leters. An improvement which, though slowly, has been gradualy going on ever since. So that now we no longer burden ourselves by writing sinne, but, omiting two leters of the alphabet, write only sin. Nor fullfill, but fulfil; nor welloome, but welcome; nor waggon, but wagon; nor allmost and allike, but almost and alike; and so on with hundreds of other words, to the advantage not only of the time of the writer and the materials of the printer, but also to the eyes of the reader. Such being undeniably the case, I ask, " Why should we in this utilitarian age wait upon 'Father Time' to eliminate for us the ofending leters, instead of ourselves having the moral courage to act up to our inate comon-sense principles, and sweep them al away at once? When, by so doing, we know that we wil not only diminish labor and save money, but restore our language to its original simplicity and beauty. While the inovation—if inovation it can logicaly be caled—wil ofer (contrary to the ideas expressed by my unlearned assailant) no impediment to the labors of the scientific comparative etymologist." For, strange to say, the results of modern Philology have shown that the suposed clerical teachings of our school days—that English words are spelt on an etymological basis—is uterly false. Not even 5 per cent. out of the whole 50,000 words constituting modern English (beyond purely technical terms) having anything whatever to do with etymological orthography. So that the etymological argument which one sometimes hears raised by the semi-educated against improving our language and economising our time as wel as our money by the omision of mute leters, is as foolish as it is groundless.

I decline to interfere with the speling of personal names: for as a man has a right in England to cal himself by what name he wil, to him must also be conceded the right of speling his name in whatever way suits his fancy.

In the advocacy of this rational plan of reforming our national orthography, I am equaly prepared to bide my time and bear abuse. For, as the late Profesor Sharpey said, in a leter he adresed to me, and which I carefuly preserve, as it is writen, not alone entirely without duplicated consonants, but without any mute leters whatever, the plan of omiting useles duplicated consonants can only be oposed by the illiterate, for it is founded not only on the principles of comon sense, but on the natural law of linguisticsc evolution. Which is the abreviation of words. Aded to which it has the aditional advantage of not only diminishing the cost of our books, but their size—a point which is of no smal degree of importance, seeing that the shelves of both our public and private libraries are rapidly becoming insuficient for their acomodation. In fact, the only argument that I can see which can logicaly be sustained against the scheme is the very trivial one, that the apearance of the words from being new is at first ofensive to the eye. That, however, as the reader wil soon be able to judge for himself, is but a trifle. For he wil find that after he has read a few pages the inovation wil cease to atract his atention. While the imense advantages acruing from its adoption will gradualy become aparent to his mind's eye, as has been explained in my little book on " The Simplification of English Speling."(b)

CHAPTER I.

THE ETIOLOGY OF THE INCUBATION PERIOD OF INFECTIOUS, CONTAGIOUS, AND INOCULABLE DISEASES—EXPLAINED ON THE GERM THEORY.

From time imemorial it has been observed that there always exists a more or les clearly defined latent period of incubation between the reception of contagion or infection, and the

(a) My leter, entitled, "A Conservative Scheme for National Speling Reform," was afterwards published, in the shape of a sixpeny pamphlet, by Hodgson and Son, Gough-square, E.C.
(b) Trübner and Co., price 2s. 6d.

first outburst of the signs and symptoms of the comunicated disease. For example, syphilitic and glanders contagion, as wel as scarlatinal and smal-pox infection, are equaly wel known never to produce imediate results. No mater however virulent their subsequent efects may be, or however rapidly fatal they may ultimately become.

It is likewise noticed that, though subject to great individual variations, the periods of incubation are, in each particular form of disease, so uniform when regarded as a whole, as to admit of being prety wel calculated. In the inoculable clas—such as vaxinia—almost to an hour. In some of the infectious group—such for example, as measles—to within a day.

Modern research has even taken us a stage beyond this, and shown that not alone do individual forms of disease poses definite uniform periods of incubation; but that the three clases of Infectious, Contagious, and Inoculable diseases, when comunicated to diferent patients in precisely the same way— no mater whether they are comunicated by infection, contagion, or inoculation—have precisely the same periods of incubation, at least to within very narow limits of divergence. This is a clinical fact which has not hitherto been suficiently apreciated. Hence it is one to which I must cal special atention. Meanwhile I have further to remark regarding the periods of incubation in general, that they are not only, as everyone knows, liable to variations—sometimes being abnormaly shortened, at other abnormaly lengthened,—but, as I shal show, the variations in the periods of incubation are, and ocasionaly have been, so exceedingly great as to have been either entirely misinterpreted, or even been totaly overlooked. After having made this statement, I fancy it wil surprise some of my readers to find me ad that even the most startling cases of Incubation anomalies are one and al of them perfectly explicable and comprehensible when interpreted, as they shal presently be, acording to one universal and normal biological law.

I shal now proceed to substantiate each of these statements, and in order to facilitate the understanding of my views I shal begin by caling atention to the folowing usualy overlooked facts in conection with the modus operandi of the Incubation proces :—

(a.) That in al cases where Disease-germs are introduced into the human system by contagion or inoculation, they invariably give origin to a primary local lesion at the point of their introduction. In syphilis, caled a sore; in vaxinia, a vesicle.

(b.) The first blush of the primary local lesion after inoculation invariably apears—but with rare exceptions afterwards to be specialy aluded to—within the narow limits of from one to three days. And this, too, even in those cases where the constitutional disturbance and the secondary manifestations of the comunicated disease folowing upon it are exeptionaly long in making their apearance. This has been particularly noticed in cases of hydrophobic inoculation. Where, although the usual redness, heat, and sweling may have ocured at the biten parts within the normal limit of three days, the constitutional disturbance has delayed its apearance for many months—even for years.

(c.) The same law which holds good as regards the period of incubation of local primary manifestations after inoculation holds equaly good in al cases of axidentaly acquired disease by contagion—syphilis, glanders, and erysipelas, for example.

(d.) The periods of incubation in diseases comunicated by infection, and which have no primary local lesions, but first make themselves manifest by the constitutional disturbance they create—in the shape of fever and nerve symptoms— although not identical to a day, are nevertheles also prety uniform as regards the date of their first apearance.

Unfortunately there is scarcely any point in clinical medicine where the data—from defective observations—have been les definitely ascertained than that of the exact periods of incubation in infectious diseases. They are, however, on the whole, suficiently wel determined to enable me to turn them to statistical acount. If I leave out of the calculation doubtful and exeptional cases, I find that the periods of incubation most generaly given in text-books are, for—

Erysipelas	5 to 14 days.
Scarlet fever	5 ,, 15 ,,
Typhoid fever	6 ,, 12 ,,
Chicken-pox	7 ,, 12 ,,
Smal-pox	10 ,, 20 ,,

These, when taken colectively, give in round numbers a general average in the periods of incubation of from six to fourteen days. As seen, the variations are not great. For between the two earliest—5 to 10—there is only 5 days, and between the two latest—12 to 20—only a diference of 8 days. These diferences are, no doubt, due to the fact that the diferent species of pathogenic germs' egs, though probably not to the same extent as the egs of distinctly diferent species of birds, as wel as the ova of distinctly diferent species of quadrupeds, fishes, and insects, take diferent periods to hatch, develop into mature animals, and reproduce their species. And this, no doubt, is the true explanation of the fact that the atacks of the diferent kinds of infectious, contagious, and inoculable diseases normaly run their respective courses in diferent periods of time.

I shal, however, go a step further than this, and state that, from a calculation I have made of the very few wel-authenticated cases of incubation of infectious diseases, where it has been posible for the reporters to furnish perfectly reliable data, both as regards the exact time of the infection, and the first apearance of the constitutional disturbance it engendered, not the earlier, but the later number of days above given—that is to say, 14 instead of 6½—most truthfuly represents the general average period of incubation in the above tabulated group of infectious diseases.

I think that I may here mention that on one ocasion I had an exeptionaly good opportunity of ascertaining with tolerable exactitude the normal incubation period of measles. It hapened thus:—Two whole months and ten days after the last child of a family of three who were atacked—al within a week of each other—with measles, was pronounced by me to be convalescent, and al the rooms of the house on the day and night nursery floors had been completely washed and fumigated, forty children asembled at a party in the dining and drawing rooms of the house. Into neither of which rooms had the afected children even so much as entered until they had been considered perfectly wel. Now comes the interesting part of the mater. Fifteen out of the forty juvenile guests were atacked with measles. Three of whom had had it before, and on careful inquiry I found that every one of those fifteen children had sickened between the thirteenth and fifteenth day after the party. In fact, only three out of these fifteen were said to have sickened, one as early as the thirteenth, two as late as the fifteenth day. And it so hapened that from these three children having had measles before, they were the most likely to have been the least carefuly noticed, so that I unhesitatingly say fourteen days was in that instance the exact period of incubation of this epidemic atack of measles.

This general uniformity in the duration of the periods of incubation of germ diseases I explain acording to the great natural biological law that the ova of al animals, and the egs of al birds, and reptiles of analogous species, size, and habits, poses tolerably uniform definite periods of incubation—varying slightly in a few individual cases; but stil, on the whole, manifesting a marked degree of uniformity.

Having said this much on the regularities of the incubatory periods, I have next to cal atention to, and atempt the explanation of, the strange, and at first sight aparently meaningles, as wel as unaccountable, iregularities which they ocasionaly present. The two forms of human disease which are said to present the greatest anomalous exentricities in this respect are, strange to say, the most diverse from each other that can be imagined, both as regards their origin, their mode of comunication, and their pathological symptoms. The one is the infectious Eastern Plague, whose periods of incubation vary from a few hours to forty days. The other is the inoculable hydrophobia, even more erratic stil, varying in the periods of its development of constitutional symptoms from 15 to 2555 days. In the case recorded by Hassinger it was 780 (Trans. Med. Gesel. Vien.). In a case recorded by Dr. Hughes (Medical Times and Gasete of 1854) the symptoms of hydrophobia did not develop themselves until five years after the bite; while in a still more extraordinary case recorded by Mr. Hale Thompson in the first volume of the Lancet, the period of incubation extended to 2555 days—seven years. It is briefly as folows :—

A lad eighteen years of age, five years after having been severely biten by a dog on the right hip, was thrown into prison. During the time of his confinement he was noticed to be sulen, and scarcely ever spoke. After being two ful

years in prison, he was sudenly seized with "most decided" symptoms of hydrophobia and died in three days. The scar of the bite was stil visible on the hip."

Added to these there are stil others which, as a rule, poses the most definite periods of producing primary local lesions—and from their being the direct result of intentional inoculation and axidental contagion, have the least right to be guilty of iregularities in their periods of incubation—which nevertheles sometimes behave even in a stil more exentric maner than either plague or hydrophobia.

As I am not writing for mere writing's sake, but with the view of advancing, as far as in me lies, the onward progres of Rational Medicine, I shal not shrink from citing two of the most startling cases of extraordinarily prolonged latency from those very two clases—Inoculation and Contagion. Even although, by so doing, I may be placing aditional dificulties in the path of the explanation I have selected to pursue. Al I can say in extenuation of my temerity is, that I enjoy the hope that, like most other exeptional cases, those I am about to cite wil in the end only tend to strengthen the rule, and thus prove of advantage to the germ theory of disease. In any case they wil have the great advantage of interesting those of my readers who have not paid much atention to anomalous examples of exesively prolonged incubation.

The first case I shal relate is one which fel under my notice in 1858, while I was acting as Physician to the Northern Dispensary. It was the case of a vaxine pustule which my eye axidentaly fel upon while I was examining a child's chest with the stethoscope, and which the mother spoke of as merely " a big pimple." On inquiry I found, to my astonishment, that the child had not been recently vaxinated. On the contrary, it had been vaxinated in two places on the arm now afected a year before, but neither of them had taken. So the woman informed me, " the pimple could have nothing to do with that." A careful examination of the vesicle, however, showed me that it was a true vaxine pustule; and strange to say; notwithstanding the extraordinary time it had taken to apear, by subsequent watching and inquiry I found that it ran, as nearly as posible, the ordinary nine-days course, as if it had comenced its active career at the usual period.

The second case I have to relate, though perhaps les remarkable, is nevertheles equaly instructive, as it shows how the most virulent form of syphilitic poison may, after remaining for months—comparatively speaking—dormant in the system, break out with fearful violence. The case was that of an English gentleman who became inoculated in America, and from whose prepuce, one hundred days after the conection, I got Mr. Henry Lee to remove by the knife a split-pea sized hard tumor, which I diagnosed as syphilitic. There was at the moment of this litle tumour's removal no other sign or symptom of syphilitic impregnation in the patient. Yet the wound left by its removal would not heal, and within a few weeks afterwards al the usual train of symptoms folowing in the wake of a true Hunterian chancre made their apearance, and it was not until nearly seven months later that the sore, by the aid of mercury, ultimately healed.

The spindle-shaped cels found in the litle tumor, when it was examined microscopicaly, was aditional confirmation of its chancreous nature. (See page 202 of the second edition of my Histological Demonstrations, where a woodcut is given of the fusiform fibre-cel elements of hard chancre.) Dr. J. Bergmann of Baltimore, and Professor Klebs of Prague (Archiv für Experimentela Pathologie und Pharmakologie)—have examined fresh prepuces in cases of Hunterian chancre; and in hundreds of sections found colections of micrococi and fungoid germs firmly adhering to and partly filling the lumen of the lymphatic vesels; and they consider that the natural history of syphilis is explained by the existence of these bodies.

These two examples of the exeptionaly prolonged latency of incubation astonish one, not, I believe, on acount of the rarity of their ocurence, but solely on acount of the rarity of their detection and interpretation. Had the child in question not been atacked with bronchitis, and no medical man's eye falen upon the pustule, neither its true nature nor its true history would ever have been discovered. For the mother, knowing that the child had not been recently vaxinated, put the vesicle down in her mind as a mere big pimple, and would consequently never have spoken of it to a doctor. Again, as regards latent chancreous tumors. No one knows how often they ocur from the fact that, even if a patient axidentaly—as mine did, when I was examining him for liver disease—cals the atention of his physician or surgeon to a litle hard, painles lump on his prepuce, probably from neither the one nor the other having ever seen or heard of a blind chancre-tumor, he is told, "Oh, it's nothing; leave it alone and it wil go away of itself." And when in the course of time it softens and breaks, the presence of the sore is atributed to the efects of a recent conection. In this way the true nature of the case is never discovered—never even so much as dreamt of. Thus it is, perhaps, that thousands of valuable observations, thousands of valuable pathological facts, are never heard of. For not only have children eyes that do not see and brains that fail to reflect, but even men (aye, wel-educated men too) go through life without either seeing, remembering, or reflecting; and hence milions of valuable facts remain undiscovered in every department of art and sience.

I may now mention that exactly the reverse of this retardation of incubation of disease has been known to ocur. Sometimes, not only local signs, but constitutional symptoms, folow on the heels of contagion and inoculation, as wel as of infection, with startling rapidity. Cases of this kind are so comon that I need not take up time by citing any of the published ones, but only alude to one which was verbaly comunicated to me by Mr. E. Bellamy, Surgeon to the Charing-cros Hospital, where the secondary efects of syphilis—sore throat, ulcerations of the alæ of the nose, and papular eruptions—manifested themselves in a gentleman aged thirty-seven, of not over-sober habits, within the brief period of seven days after the suposed inoculation.

(*To be continued.*)

REMARKS ON

A CASE OF HIGH TEMPERATURE, WITH SCARLATINOID RASH (ROSEOLA)

OCCURRING AFTER EXCISION OF THE KNEE-JOINT.

By CHAUNCY PUZEY,
Surgeon to the Liverpool Northern Hospital.

On February 15, 1879, at the Liverpool Northern Hospital, I excised the right knee-joint of a young man, aged twenty-one. The case was one of old-standing disease, with partial anchylosis and some deformity, and in which a recent injury had started fresh mischief, rendering operative measures advisable. The operation was conducted on strict Listerian principles; and the patient was anæsthetised with ether. Vomiting lasted more or less persistently for four or five days after the operation. This, according to my observation, is a singular exception to the rule that ether does not cause prolonged nausea. I think the symptom is worth noting in this particular instance, as showing the tendency to nervous disturbance which appears throughout the case. With this exception, everything proceeded favourably for nine days; the temperature never rising over 100° until the evening of February 24, when the night temperature was marked 102·6°, the pulse 100.

Next morning the temperature was 100·4°, the pulse 100. On the 26th the temperature at 9 a.m. was 100°; at 12 noon, 104°; at 2.30, 100°; at 9 p.m., 99·4°. The wound was looking perfectly healthy; all healed, except where the two drainage-tubes were inserted.

For the next three or four days the temperature was about normal; and all went on well until March 2, the fifteenth day after operation, when, about midnight, the man, because he had not been able to make satisfactory use of the bed-pan, watched his opportunity when the night nurse was out of the ward, took off the side-splints, and was caught in the passage, hobbling along to the closet, with only the back splint on his leg.

When I changed the dressings next day (March 3) I expected to find things in a mess, but, to my relief, found everything looking perfectly well and the bones in accurate apposition; but that evening the man had a slight "chill," and his temperature rose to 102·4°.

Next morning (March 4) the temperature was 101·6°, pulse 130; there was a general scarlet blush uniformly over the whole surface of the body, the tongue covered with moist

whitish fur (it having been up to this period quite clean); he had had a bad night, vomiting frequently; there was no redness of the fauces. Quinine and bromo-hydric acid were prescribed. The wound looked well, and appeared to be aseptic. That night the temperature was 102·6°; pulse 142; the tongue more furred; the fauces slightly dusky; skin dry. The urine was examined and found free from albumen. Inquiries were made as to the possibility of any fever having been conveyed to him, the result of the inquiries being to negative such an idea.

Next morning (March 5) the eruption was very bright and punctiform. Vomiting of mucous and watery fluid tinged with bile had been frequent through the night. A dose of calomel and opium was given, and a mixture containing bicarbonate of soda and hydrocyanic acid was substituted for the quinine. The pulse this day was 130; the temperature 103·4°.

On the 6th the temperature was 102·4°, the pulse 120; the sickness had nearly ceased; the tongue was quite clean; the rash still bright, but more in patches.

On the 7th the temperature was 100·4°, the pulse 100; the vomiting had ceased.

On the 9th the rash had quite disappeared without desquamation; the tongue was clean, slightly glazed; there was a little diarrhœa; the temperature had fallen to 99·8°, and the pulse to 88.

On the night of the 10th the temperature ran up to 102°, and at 7 a.m. of the 11th was marked 109° by the nurse (this at the time was considered to be a mistake, but probably was after all correct); at 11 a.m. it was marked 103·2° by the House-Surgeon, and in the evening was down to 99·8°.

For a few days the temperature remained pretty steady between 99° and 100°, and then came some astonishing bounds, so apparently inexplicable (considering the otherwise satisfactory state of the patient) that I should have doubted the correctness of the marking had it not been made by Messrs. Jones and Neale, the House-Surgeons, who tested the correctness of the marking by two thermometers, one in the axilla and the other under the tongue. They were as follows :—March 20, at 8 p.m., 106°; at about 1 a.m., on the 21st, 105°; a few hours later, 102°; at 2 p.m., 101° in the evening, 100·6°. At this time there was no apparent constitutional disturbance; the wound was looking quite well, absolutely free from any redness or tension, but there was a little smell about the dressings—more the frowsy smell of decomposing perspiration than that of putrid pus—in fact, there was a mere trace of pus from the drainage-tubes.

After this, there was nothing particular to note about the case, except that the temperature remained abnormally high, never being below 99·2°, very frequently 101·2°, and occasionally above 102°. There seemed to be no relation between the state of the wound, or the patient's general condition, and the variations in the temperature. The antiseptic dressings were continued for five weeks in consequence of a small sinus remaining; and then iodine-and-carbolic lotion was used for the sinus, no further dressing being required. The man was kept in bed, with the leg on an iron back-splint, for twelve weeks, at the end of which period there was slight antero-posterior mobility. A plaster-of-Paris splint was then applied, and the patient was allowed to get up. After three or four weeks, some irritation was felt about the outer side of the knee, and, on removing the bandage, part of the skin near the cicatrix was found eczematous, and this condition lasted for several weeks, so that it was not until the beginning of July that it was considered prudent to allow him to leave the hospital, with a gutta-percha splint to support the leg.

Remarks.—With regard to the rash, it and the patient's general appearance so much resembled that of scarlatina, that though at first I put the case down as one of those instances of surgical roseola which have been lately under discussion; yet, on the second day, when the tongue was furred, the pulse and temperature so high, the throat somewhat affected, and the stomach so much disordered, I felt considerable doubt on the subject, and consulted with my colleagues as to the propriety of isolating the patient. The fact of the length of time which had intervened between the operation and this attack was rather against surgical roseola. However, the verdict was against scarlatina, and the result proved its correctness. But the question arises, What caused this disturbance? The first reply would probably be, of course, septic absorption, especially when the high temperatures are taken into consideration. But then again occur several inconsistencies or discrepancies which are hard to explain. Throughout the case there was a minimum of suppuration; there was primary and absolute union of all the wound except where the drainage-tubes were inserted; there was no after-exfoliation of bone; and until at least three weeks after the operation, there was entire absence of smell and of bacteria from the discharge. Then, again, the first rise of temperature took place several days before the exanthem appeared, the patient at that time being perfectly well; and further, the highest temperatures were marked a fortnight later, that is, nearly a week after the disappearance of the rash. The temperature, which certainly had been normal before the operation, never touched the normal point after, and six months after was still higher than the standard. The markings were often lower at night than in the morning, and the pulse and respiration frequently bore no relation to the temperature. I was at first incredulous; and Mr. Neale, the House-Physician, who had had some previous experience of curious temperatures at the Westminster Hospital, was sceptical, until he satisfied himself on the morning of March 20. After fully considering the case, I do not know how to explain these matters except as being due to that nervous disturbance which has been found (I think it has been pretty well established) to be the cause of remarkable variations of temperature, even of different parts of the body at the same time, in those disorders which are, for want of a better name, termed "hysterical." The subject of these remarks was of such an extremely excitable and emotional temperament that the term "hysterical" would have been perfectly applicable to him. When these high temperatures were noticed, he was invariably flushed and apparently excited; the hands and tongue tremulous; and any attempt at examining the affected limb caused loud exclamations of pain, sobbing, and shedding of tears, afterwards followed by just as unreasonable laughter. I should add that the man was carefully watched to see that no tricks were played with the thermometer, such as friction of the bulb in order to raise the temperature; and I ascertained practically myself that no elevation of the mercury could be caused by rolling the bulb in the mouth against the tongue.

The foregoing account was read before the Liverpool Medical Society some two years ago, but has not been published. At the time when the notes were taken a discussion was going on in the medical papers as to the causation of certain scarlatinoid manifestations occurring after surgical operations. And now, the subject of excessively high temperatures being prominently brought forward, I think this case is somewhat to the point, and may be of some interest.

The remarks I made at that time I leave unaltered. I have seen no reason to change my opinions regarding the case, although since then I have read carefully, and with much interest, the accounts of like cases since published, and the arguments therefrom deduced. Mr. J. E. Neale, the House-Physician, and Mr. Hughes-Jones, the senior House-Surgeon to the hospital, took the temperatures on most occasions themselves. The former of these gentlemen had avowed himself a disbeliever in these high temperatures, but was finally convinced against his will, after having, as may be imagined, taken every precaution against fallacy or any fraud on the part of the patient.

I may add that I saw the man twelve months after the operation. Anchylosis was complete and firm; the limb strong and useful; the patient himself in first-rate health, but still with a tendency to flushing of the skin and to nervous stuttering of speech when questioned about himself.

A GARFIELD MEMORIAL HOSPITAL.—The *New York Med. Record* states that the admirable project has been set on foot at Washington of erecting a hospital to perpetuate the memory of President Garfield. An important meeting of highly influential persons was held on October 5, when it was resolved to appoint a committee of twenty-five to carry out the objects of the meeting. Subscription lists will at once be prepared, and the whole country and foreign nations would be asked to place the memorial hospital on a broad national and international basis of common humanity.

REPORTS OF HOSPITAL PRACTICE
IN
MEDICINE AND SURGERY.

MIDDLESEX HOSPITAL.

MULTIPLE CEREBRAL HÆMORRHAGE FOLLOWING THROMBOSIS OF CEREBRAL SINUSES—DEATH— AUTOPSY.

(Under the care of Dr. COUPLAND.)

[From notes taken by Mr. J. H. MINCHENTON, Physician's Assistant.]

WALTER P., aged thirty-one, single, and a glass-cutter by trade, was admitted on December 28, 1880. He had for some years been subject to bronchitis and rheumatism in the winter months. His habits were "said" to be temperate. At eleven o'clock the night before, he was seen by his brother in bed, sleeping soundly, breathing heavily, and supposed to be intoxicated. He hiccoughed violently all through the night. At 4 a.m. to-day he was found wandering about undressed, apparently awake, but insensible, and as no word could be got out of him he was put back to bed, his brother thinking that he was "speechless drunk." He has not complained—in fact, has not spoken since—but has mumbled and tried to speak. As he has been kept in bed, it was not noticed till this morning that he had lost power in his arm. Neither his landlady nor his brother, who came with him, seemed to know much about him; the latter did not appear to be quite sober.

On admission the man's temperature is 98·8°; pulse 48; respirations 40. He is lying on his back in bed, with his left eye quite closed, right eye nearly so, breathing rapidly and more or less stertorously. Pulse is slow and regular, but small. He seems to understand when spoken to, and mumbles an unintelligible answer; indicates that he has no pain. He is constantly hiccoughing, and frequently yawning, and smells strongly of drink. He moves his left hand and arm readily when told to do so, and has good grasping power with the hand. His right arm he cannot move much, but raises it a little way towards his head, though he cannot grasp at all with the hand. There is apparently diminished sensation in right arm and right side of face, as he does not flinch when a pin is sharply pricked into it, and he does when the opposite sides are treated in the same way. He moves both legs freely up and down in bed. Reflex action in right leg is diminished, but not abolished. Face is not drawn to either side, and there is no difference in naso-labial sulci; if anything, there is slight drooping of the right angle of the mouth, but this is not certain. There appears to be some ptosis of left upper eyelid, but there is no strabismus. The right pupil is contracted and responds sluggishly to a stimulus of light. The left pupil is dilated and will not act at all. His tongue protrudes strongly to the right side when he attempts to put it out, but he cannot readily perform this act; it is thickly coated with a yellowish-white fur. Abundant mucous râles are heard over both fronts, but heart-sounds appear normal. His urine on being drawn off contained no albumen and no sugar.

At 9 p.m. he was lying in the same position, moaning and apparently sleeping. Pupils unaltered. Some frothy mucus exuded from his mouth. At midnight he was breathing stertorously, loud tracheal râles being audible, and he was quite insensible. Four hours after he died.

The autopsy was made by Dr. Fowler, ten hours after death. Rigidity was marked. The body was well nourished, and there were some bruises over both legs. Abdominal and omental fat were in excess; intestines contracted, and no fluid in the peritoneal cavity. At base of left lung there were some recent adhesions and lymph; at apex some fibrous adhesions; no fluid in pleura. The pericardium was normal and contained no fluid; the sub-pericardial fat over the right ventricle was in considerable excess. The heart weighed nine ounces and a quarter, and the right auricle contained a fibrinous clot extending into the right ventricle and pulmonary artery; the auricle and ventricle also contained some fluid blood. The superior and inferior venæ cavæ also contained post-mortem clot and fluid blood. Pulmonary and aortic valves normal, except some slight atheromatous degeneration of the latter. The pulmonary veins and left auricle contained some small gelatinous clot of recent formation. Left ventricle was firmly contracted; the tricuspid and mitral valves were normal. The trachea and bronchi contained a quantity of slightly frothy turbid yellow fluid; the mucous membrane of the bronchi was everywhere injected. The left lung was emphysematous on the surface; on section, deeply congested and œdematous. The cut surface of the upper lobe showed numerous capillary extravasations. The right lung was in a similar condition. Along the edge of the upper lobe there were some lobules in a condition of extreme emphysematous distension; these were surrounded by a tract of collapsed lung-tissue. Spleen weighed four ounces and three-quarters. The upper half, except the extreme apex, was of a dark purple colour, mottled by prominent Malpighian bodies. A wedge-shaped spot at the lower edge was in a similar condition. This change was probably the result of an embolus in one of the vessels, but the point could not be decided. Kidneys—right, five ounces and three-quarters; left, six ounces. The capsule peeled off easily, leaving a smooth surface. The cortex was congested, and to a less extent the medulla also. The pelves contained a considerable quantity of fat. Stomach: Around the termination of the œsophagus there were several adherent flakes of recent fibrinous exudation; the stomach contained about twelve ounces of brownish turbid fluid. The vessels of the mucous membrane along the greater curvature were minutely injected, presenting a bright red velvety appearance; this extended over a surface about as large as the palm of the hand. Intestines: The mucous membrane of the duodenum and upper part of the jejunum was also injected. Liver (forty-six ounces) was very congested. Brain: On removing the calvaria, the vessels of the dura mater were found to be somewhat distended with blood. There were no adhesions between the dura mater and the surface of the brain, except along the edges of the longitudinal sinus. The pia mater was everywhere injected. The left lateral and straight sinuses were filled with a clot, partly fibrinous and partly black post-mortem clot. The right lateral sinus contained a clot of similar nature. The right cavernous sinus and right Sylvian vein were also plugged with fibrinous clot. Around the optic commissure and tract, involving the left third nerve and corpus albicantium, and extending backwards along the left side of the pons Varolii, there was a thin layer of recently extravasated blood. Sections of the substance of the hemispheres showed numerous puncta cruenta. The vessels of the choroid plexuses and velum interpositum were full of dark blood. Over the superior vermiform process of the cerebellum and adjacent laminæ there was a very thin layer of blood. The lateral ventricles were free from fluid. The corpora striata were normal. A section of the left optic thalamus showed a patch of softening at the posterior part, in size about equal to a hazel-nut. The left crus cerebri was also softened, and marked by punctiform and linear extravasations. The corpora quadrigemina were normal, but the left cerebellar peduncle was soft from hæmorrhagic extravasations. On section through the pons, a hæmorrhage was found, involving the whole of its substance, except a thin layer along the posterior border; the hæmorrhage extended forwards into the crura on each side. The vessels were free from atheroma.

Remarks.—This case is thought worthy of record for two reasons—one pathological, the other clinical. On the former head it is open to question how far the clotting, evidently in progress in the dural sinuses, determined the wide-spread and scattered hæmorrhagic extravasations, which attained their maximum in the pons. In the absence of any previous history of cerebral disturbance it is plain that the thrombosis could not have been complete until the apoplectic seizure took place, which coincided with the rupture of vessels on the surface and in the substance of the brain. That such rupture may ensue on complete blocking of the main dural sinuses was shown by Bright long ago, and admirably depicted in his valuable *Medical Reports*, vol. ii., plates 5 and 6; and it is hard to explain the occurrence of such multiple extravasations except on the view of suddenly heightened tension in the cerebral arteries (even though non-atheromatous) produced by the completion of the venous plugging. The clots described in the sinuses were mostly only partially ante-mortem, and then not of old standing; whilst no determining cause of such clotting was obvious, the patient not being exhausted by previous cachexia, as in most cases of thrombosis in the sinuses. Clinically, the case points to the ingravescent nature of the apoplexy, for although, in addition to the almost complete destruction of the pons, there were also hæmorrhages in the arachnoid at the base of the brain, and considerable extravasations in the left crura cerebri and cerebelli, yet there was, when the patient was first seen, only incomplete right hemiplegia and hemi-anæsthesia, with contraction of the right pupil, and fixed dilatation of the left, and slight left ptosis, in addition to the apoplectic state, which deepened towards the close. The rapidly fatal issue is sufficiently explained by the extensive and important regions which were destroyed by the hæmorrhages.

TERMS OF SUBSCRIPTION.
(*Free by post.*)

				£	s.	d.
British Islands	. . . . .	*Twelve Months*	.	£1	8	0
"	. . . . .	*Six* "		. 0	14	0
The Colonies and the United }		*Twelve* "		. 1	10	0
States of America . . . }						
" " "	. . . . .	*Six* "		. 0	15	0
India " "	. . . . .	*Twelve* "		. 1	10	0
" (*viâ Brindisi*)	. . . . .	"		. 1	15	0
" "	. . . . .	*Six* "		. 0	15	0
" (*viâ Brindisi*)	. . . . .	"		. 0	17	6

Foreign Subscribers are requested to inform the Publishers of any remittance made through the agency of the Post-office.

Single Copies of the Journal can be obtained of all Booksellers and Newsmen, price Sixpence.

Cheques or Post-office Orders should be made payable to Mr. James Lucas, 11, New Burlington-street, W.

TERMS FOR ADVERTISEMENTS.

			£	s.	d.
Seven lines (70 words)	. . . .	.	.£0	4	6
Each additional line (10 words)	. .	.	. 0	0	6
Half-column, or quarter-page	. .	.	. 1	5	0
Whole column, or half-page	. .	.	. 2	10	0
Whole page	. . . . .	.	. 5	0	0

Births, Marriages, and Deaths are inserted Free of Charge.

The Medical Times and Gazette *is published on Friday morning; Advertisements must therefore reach the Publishing Office not later than One o'clock on Thursday.*

Medical Times and Gazette.

SATURDAY, NOVEMBER 12, 1881.

WAITING FOR TRIAL.

When charging the grand jury at the recent Derbyshire and Leicestershire Assizes, Mr. Justice Mathew told them that since the calendar was printed one unfortunate prisoner named in it had committed suicide. This prisoner was charged with a most serious offence—viz., the felonious wounding of his wife, with intent to murder her,—and had remained in custody since July 20, a period of upwards of three months. The case was an illustration of the importance of holding trials speedily, for it was impossible to over-estimate the sufferings which some accused persons underwent while a charge was hanging over them. They were so informed, Mr. Justice Mathew continued, by those in charge of persons in custody; and this was shown in one melancholy way in the number of cases in which prisoners made attempts on their lives. Strange to say, it was noticed that untried prisoners were most liable to this offence, and, more singular still, the attempt was most frequently made by prisoners who might anticipate an acquittal, or conviction of an offence less grave than the one charged in this instance. Bearing these things in mind, Mr. Justice Mathew seemed to think it decidedly desirable to hold not fewer than four assizes in a year, and his humane judgment on this point will commend itself to public approval, and reflect somewhat unpleasantly on the grumblings of some of his brethren on the Bench, who are never tired of deploring that the elaborate and costly machinery provided for the administration of the criminal law should be set in motion when there are only a few insignificant cases to be tried. But these cases, however insignificant they may seem to the judge, are momentous enough to the parties principally concerned in them, and it cannot be tolerated that even a single prisoner should be subjected to any unnecessary protraction of the anxiety which he experiences when waiting for trial. This anxiety is of a peculiarly wearing description, as is seen not only by the suicides to which it leads, but by the loss of body-weight which it generally involves. It is notorious that prisoners often emaciate when in suspense, while waiting for trial, and begin to put on flesh immediately after conviction and a heavy sentence, thus showing how profound is the effect of painful uncertainty on bodily nutrition. But a serious impairment of the nutritive functions sometimes entails very grave consequences, and it may well be that the seeds of consumption and other fatal maladies are occasionally sown in the constitutions of innocent persons during imprisonment while under a temporary cloud of suspicion.

And there is another reason why trials should be held with all due promptitude after the commission of offences, and that has reference to the witnesses rather than the prisoners. Evidence deteriorates with keeping, and is most trustworthy in the fresh state. Some sense-impressions are fugacious, and others tend to become permanently organised in memory, and both classes of impressions contribute to the vitiation of testimony. Fugacious impressions, as they vanish, leave gaps and rents in recollection; and organised impressions, as they root themselves, become insulated, admit of no qualification, and are insisted on with obstinate persistence. A vast majority of persons will be able, under examination and cross-examination, to recall any event, conversation, or set of circumstances, with much greater fidelity one month after their occurrence than after an interval of three, four, or six months. Thus justice suffers when trials and offences are too far separated from each other.

Our judges receive large salaries, have long holidays and handsome retiring pensions, and they must be content to work as hard as physicians and surgeons of equal eminence and age are in the habit of doing. Mr. Justice Mathew is entitled to gratitude for the sagacity and candour with which he has spoken on behalf of prisoners waiting for trial.

MEDICAL EDUCATION AND REGISTRATION IN AMERICA.

THE conditions under which men should be allowed to practise medicine—the amount and kind of knowledge which they should be obliged to show; the way in which their possession of that knowledge can best be tested; the length of the preliminary training which they ought to be required to undergo; the extent to which the details of that training should be regulated by compulsory rules or left to individual option—these are questions upon which there are wide differences of opinion in this country. Changes which some would regard as progress, others would consider retrograde. A glance at the customs with regard to these questions which prevail among the great communities of our own kin on the other side of the Atlantic, cannot but be instructive; for their regulations differ much from ours, and we can learn the probable effect of certain proposed changes here by observing the effect of similar ideas carried out into practice there.

Here in England we have nineteen licensing bodies, some of which are suspected, whether reasonably or not, of trying to undersell the others by granting their diplomas on easier terms. Such underselling as prevails, however, cannot go below a certain minimum, for if a licensing body were actually and frequently to put on the Register men grossly devoid of professional knowledge, it is possible that the Medical Council would really do something. But in America this underselling can and does go on unchecked. Any body of men can unite together and give any diploma they please, to whoever they like, and on what conditions they think fit. And any person, with or without a diploma, can practise medicine. There is therefore what may be called free trade in medicine. The provision of competent medical advisers is left, so far as the central authority is concerned, to the unhampered operation of the law of supply and demand.

The statement just made, although true on the whole, yet requires now some qualification. A few years ago it was strictly in accordance with fact. But it has not worked altogether well. Some States have come to the conclusion that it is well that there should be some means by which the public should be able to distinguish between properly trained and qualified medical men, and ignorant pretenders to skill in healing. The regulations by which they have mostly sought to do this are of two kinds—first, by verification of the diplomas by virtue of which anyone wishes to practise; and second, by examination of those who have no such diplomas. Those who have satisfied one of these two tests are then registered. Laws embodying provisions to this effect have been passed (with differences in detail) in the States of New York (in 1880), Illinois (1877), California, New Hampshire, Vermont, Pennsylvania (1875), Alabama, and Texas (1879). These laws will certainly lead to improvement in the matter in question, although it will only be a partial and limited amelioration, as we shall show.

The first method by which one who wishes to practise in one of the States named, can get permission to do so, is by producing a diploma. The law of New York runs thus:— "If he has a diploma conferring upon him the degree of Doctor of Medicine, issued by an incorporated university, medical college, or medical school, without the State, he shall exhibit the same to the faculty of some incorporated medical college or medical school of this State, with satisfactory evidence of his good moral character, and such other evidence, if any, of his qualifications as a physician or surgeon, as said faculty may require. If his diploma and qualifications are approved by them, then they shall endorse said diploma, which shall make it, for the purpose of his licence to practise medicine and surgery within this State, the same as if issued by them." In Illinois and California the law is much the same. The New Hampshire Legislature has gone a little further. "The Board shall issue licences, without examination, to all persons who furnish evidence by diploma from some medical school authorised to confer degrees in medicine and surgery, *when said Board is satisfied that the person presenting such diploma has obtained it after pursuing some prescribed course of study and upon due examination.*" The law of Vermont resembles this. In Pennsylvania it is still more explicit. "The possession of a diploma regularly issued by a medical school acting under a charter from this or other State or country shall constitute the sufficient licence for the person to whom such diploma is granted to practise singly or jointly, medicine, surgery, or obstetrics, as set forth and empowered in said diploma: *Provided, however,* that a diploma that has been, or that may hereafter be, granted for a money consideration, or other article of value alone, or that has been or may hereafter be granted to anyone who has not pursued the usual course of studies required by a legally chartered medical school, shall not be considered a sufficient qualification under this Act." These regulations are obviously fair and liberal towards the various teaching and degree-conferring bodies which exist. Their practical defect lies in the number and widely divergent character of the bodies whose diplomas are thus accepted as a sufficient stamp of professional education. Some are simply "bogus" diplomas. There is no central authority to restrain a body which does not openly sell its titles of honour from giving them on ridiculously easy terms, and prescribing only a short and insufficient curriculum. This is so real an evil that in some States no provision of the kind we have quoted exists in the law, but everyone who wants to practise in the State must undergo examination. This is the case in North Carolina, in Texas, and, we believe, in Massachusetts. A law of this kind is a hardship to a man of mature years, who may be, very likely, superior to the examiners in scientific attainments and practical skill, but yet may not have at his fingers' ends the anatomical and chemical minutiæ, a knowledge of which is rightly expected from students. We may, indeed, mention the case of Dr. Storer, a physician with high British qualifications, who, when he settled in practice in Boston, was asked to undergo an examination by men with regard to whose fitness for their position it would have been more appropriate to have asked Dr. Storer's opinion, than theirs about him. Dr. Storer refused to submit to such a test; and suffered no particular harm, in the long run, from having done so. This case points out two defects in the system. One, upon which we will not here further comment, is that it scarcely seems to us that there is care enough taken to secure the best possible examiners. In North Carolina they are elected by ballot. We do not think this a matter of great permanent importance, because if it should from experience become clear that it is defective in this way, we doubt not that the defect will be remedied. The other is, that, at least in North Carolina, there is no penalty for non-compliance with the law except the disadvantage of not being able to recover fees; so that the quack has a legitimate excuse for exacting payment in advance.

The matters upon which we have hitherto commented only concern the Americans themselves and the few Englishmen who may want to practise in that country. But the effect of this system upon medical education is a much more serious matter, and, from the place which Americans are taking in medical literature, concerns the whole civilised world. It is manifest that when one school gives a diploma cheaply, easily, and quickly, another school which exacts a longer, more thorough, and therefore more expensive, training, and the passing of a more difficult examination, is at a disadvantage. In an American journal we read the following with reference to the Bellevue Hospital Medical College, New York:—"The Faculty stated last year that for several years they had endeavoured to induce students to attend three courses of lectures (passing their examinations in the elementary departments at the close of the second session), and that those who had followed this course had shown in their examinations a grade of qualifications much higher than the standard usually attained by students under the old system. The experience of the session of 1880-81 has led the Faculty reluctantly to the conclusion that to persist in the requirement of attendance during three courses will be to incur a risk as regards the interests of the College, which they do not feel justified in assuming." The lamentable fact shown in this passage should be well considered by those who think that it would be an advantage to set the student free from regulations, to get his knowledge how and when he best can. This has been the system in America, with the result that one of the best schools has to avowedly "advance to the rear," and assimilate its programme to that of the inferior ones. But we are glad to see that Boston and Philadelphia maintain the progressive attitude.

American medical literature is very voluminous, and characterised by great originality, inventive genius, industry, and practicality; and their schools by the multiplication of specialists and special chairs. The fault which we generally have to deplore in American books is the want of exact and comprehensive knowledge of other branches of medicine besides the writer's own. This is a result which might be expected. A man becomes a specialist before he has mastered the elements of medical science.

We notice also the hindrances which the laws of most States place in the way of anatomical research. This, no doubt, is an effect as well as a cause of the imperfections of American medical education. When lay Americans become convinced, by the style of men they see in it, that medicine really is a science, and that its professors know what they are talking of, they will doubtless listen to their representations and provide what they are assured is needed. But under a state of things in which great numbers of those who call themselves doctors of medicine are quacks, devoid alike of knowledge and principle, we cannot wonder that the medical profession in America has not the weight in State Councils that ought to belong to its utterances.

SPONGE-GRAFTING ON THE HUMAN SUBJECT.

AN interesting and, it seems to us, a new and important contribution to what we know of the *surgical* healing process—if we may use such a term—comes from the pen of Dr. Hamilton, Pathologist to the Royal Infirmary, Edinburgh, and is published in the current number of the *Edinburgh Medical Journal*. He speaks of it as "Sponge Grafting"; and, although the experiments which led to its discovery were of a purely scientific character, it is not unlikely that they may prove to possess even greater interest from a clinical standpoint.

Dr. Hamilton, while engaged in the study of the "process of healing," was led to the belief that in the process of organisation of a blood-clot or a fibrinous exudation the effused material itself only plays a mechanical and passive part, and that their vascularisation is not owing to new formation of bloodvessels, "but rather to a displacement and pushing inwards of the bloodvessels of surrounding tissues." With a view to test this, after sundry trials, he selected carefully cleaned and soft sponge. We will give his own reasons for this selection:—"The reasons on which I grounded this hope were: Firstly, that it is a porous tissue, and in this respect would imitate the interstices of the fibrinous network in a blood-clot or in fibrinous lymph. In the second place, it is an animal tissue, and, like other animal tissues, such as catgut, would, if placed under favourable circumstances, become absorbed in the course of time. Thirdly, that it is a pliable texture, and can, consequently, be easily adjusted to any surface, or be cut of convenient size to be placed in a cavity. If, therefore, the blood-clot or fibrinous exudation merely acts mechanically in the process of organisation, there is no reason why sponge or any other porous texture should not similarly become vascular and organised."

It would hardly be advisable on such short acquaintance with the subject-matter of this paper to pronounce an absolute judgment. We shall think it over.

THE WEEK.

TOPICS OF THE DAY.

As a sequel to the want of sanitary supervision which has lately been exposed in Marylebone parish, a very large and important meeting of the Marylebone Vestry was recently held at the Court-house for the purpose of determining, in the capacity of Sanitary Authority, whether the property in Charles-street, Lisson-grove, described as the "fever dens" of the parish, should be subjected to reconstruction, or whether the houses should be entirely demolished under the provisions of the Artizans' and Labourers' Dwellings Act. The proceedings excited very deep interest, and amongst those present were the representatives of the owners of the condemned property; Admiral Oliver, Chairman of the Sanitary Committee; Dr. Richardson, Dr. Saunders, and others. After a lengthened discussion it was eventually resolved that the order be at once issued that the houses in question should be entirely demolished.

The annual collections in the churches and chapels of Birmingham on behalf of the medical charities of the town were made on the 30th ult. for the twenty-third time. The returns show a considerable falling-off from those of recent years, the total received being barely £3000, as compared with £4386 last year, and £6414 in the year 1878. Several returns have, it is true, still to be collected, but it is feared that these will not materially affect the total. On the other hand, the Hospital Sunday and Saturday collections in Liverpool this year produced £10,027, an increase of £306 over last year. Since the fund was instituted in Liverpool, the total amount realised has reached £92,000. The Mayor recently announced, at a meeting of the Hospital Sunday Committee, that by the death of a Miss Hamilton £16,000 had fallen into the hands of the Liverpool Corporation for distribution among the charities of the city.

A shocking example of the difficulties which interfere to prevent the stamping-out of infectious diseases in the metropolis was afforded by the particulars which transpired at a recent inquest held by Dr. Danford Thomas at the Coroner's Court, King's-road, St. Pancras, on the body of Annie Griffiths, aged twelve, of Sidney-street, in that locality. The evidence given showed that the deceased had been ailing for a short time. Her parents believing that she was "down with the fever," no particular notice was taken of the matter, the fever being prevalent in the neighbourhood. Ultimately, Dr. Thompson was called in by the parochial authorities to attend the deceased, and found her suffering from scarlet fever, of which she died. The case was of the most virulent kind, and death was inevitable from the first. The sanitary inspector for the district stated that some persons living in the same house as the deceased carried on a laundry. The Coroner said that the poor were crowded together; they slept in the same bed, and the fever of one was transmitted to another. The infected bedding was often sold, and the disease thereby propagated. The inspector explained that the sanitary officer had no power to order the removal of a case of fever to the hospital. A juror said he thought that, when a case of fever occurred in a crowded neighbourhood, where a whole family lived in one room, the officer should be authorised to remove that patient. The Coroner remarked that the poorer classes had an objection to the removal of their relatives to the parish hospital; but if they only knew how well the fever hospitals were conducted, and had the least idea how well the patients were treated, and how many comforts they obtained which they could not command at home, they would take the earliest opportunity of removing their friends to the hospitals constructed for the reception of those suffering from contagious diseases. A verdict in accordance with the evidence was returned.

The Local Board of Twickenham having applied to the Local Government Board for sanction to borrow an additional sum of £10,000 for sewerage works, Major Hector Tulloch, R.E., one of the inspectors of the latter authority, has just held a public inquiry into the subject-matter of

such application. About £70,000 has already been expended in the drainage of the town, which, it is stated, is so near completion that no further loan beyond that now asked for will be required. The precipitation and filtration scheme in progress is that of the town surveyor, Mr. H. M. Ramsay. It was understood, at the termination of the inquiry that Major Tulloch would recommend the Local Government Board to sanction the proposed loan.

A deputation from the Health Committee of the Local Board of Chester, consisting of the Mayor, Dr. Kenyon, Mr. I. Smith, Deputy Town Clerk, and Mr. Lloyd (Chester Water Company), and accompanied by the Duke of Westminster, recently had an interview with the President of the Local Government Board and Sir John Lambert, K.C.B., to urge upon that Department to put in force the Rivers' Pollution Act, or the Public Health Act, against the Llangollen Local Board for polluting the river Dee with sewage and other matters, to the great injury of the health of the inhabitants of Chester. The case put forward was that the sewage of Llangollen so contaminated the river Dee, that instead its being beautiful crystal water, it was a river of sewage, and all efforts made to induce Llangollen to divert the present corruption had wholly failed. Mr. Dodson, in replying, promised that the representations made to him should be duly and promptly considered, and the decision of the Board made known at the earliest moment.

A public meeting was recently held at the Hampstead Vestry Hall, Haverstock-hill, to further the scheme for providing a park for Paddington and North-West London. Major-General Lowry presided, in the absence of Sir T. Chambers, Q.C., M.P. After explaining the object sought to be carried out, which we have more than once placed before our readers, the following resolutions were put and carried:—"That it is of high importance for the physical and moral welfare of the population of London that every effort should be made to preserve for public use any open spaces still available for the purposes of parks or recreation grounds within the metropolitan limits." Also, "That the open space still remaining uncovered with buildings in the thickly populated neighbourhood of North Paddington, and limited by Portsdown and Shirland roads, is situated in a locality of which the density of population is already great and is rapidly increasing, and that it would be highly beneficial to public interests that this space should be secured as a park for the people." The subscriptions already promised or paid amount to over £32,000, and it is believed that if not less than £100,000 be raised by public subscription, the Metropolitan Board of Works would make up the remainder of the money (£250,000) to purchase the land.

Lord Derby, President of the University College, Liverpool, has presented the sum of £400 to the Medical Faculty of the College, to found a new annual prize for medical students.

The Local Board of Warminster has finally decided to apply to the Public Works Loan Commissioners for a loan of £5000, to carry out a system of sewerage for the town, which has been in abeyance for a considerable time.

THE VIVISECTION PROSECUTION.

At last some of those ladies and gentlemen—for the most part elderly and well-to-do—who are fond of dogs and cats have plucked up courage to attack one who certainly has done good service by examining the brain-functions in living animals. They have even gone the length of engaging Mr. Waddy, Q.C., and two other barristers to appear in a police-court. The persecuted is Dr. Ferrier: the persecutors being, we believe, to a body which holds that it is better that any number of human creatures should die rather than that one cat should perish. But the peculiarity of the whole case is this : that it should be taken up now, founded as it seems to be, according to newspaper records, on a speech by Professor Goltz at the international medical meeting held as far back as August last, and that Goltz's examples of living animals and of the results of his operations thereon should be brought forward in the public prints at least as evidence against Dr. Ferrier. We alluded to both sets of experiments at the time, and we knew then that both of Dr. Ferrier's monkeys were alive and well. The ground apparently taken by the persecution was that these monkeys should have been destroyed at once, thus totally destroying all reasonable grounds for the experiments. But, somehow, wilful cruelty to animals does not seem to make much in the way of wrong in the eyes of these people. Men may kill and slay as they like, even to the extent of the Frenchman's notion of English sport—"Let us go out and kill something!" —but when anything is done which is to benefit science, or even such low beings as mankind, they are interfered with at every step—the vilest accusations are heaped upon them—too much dirt can never be thrown at them.

MEATH HOSPITAL AND COUNTY DUBLIN INFIRMARY.

THE inaugural address of the session 1881-82 was delivered on Thursday, November 7, in the theatre of the institution, by Dr. Arthur Wynne Foot, Physician to the Hospital. There was a very large audience of visitors and students.

ROYAL MEDICAL AND CHIRURGICAL SOCIETY.

AT the ordinary meeting of this Society, on Tuesday last, Mr. Morgan exhibited two cases of a somewhat uncommon malformation—macrostoma congenitum. The cases themselves were interesting : but we can hardly agree with Mr. Morgan that one of the chief points of interest lay in the fact that the majority of cases hitherto observed has been found in girls. Virchow's case—one of the few dissections which have been made—was not referred to. Mr. Langley Browne, of Birmingham, next related a case of simultaneous ligature of the subclavian and carotid arteries for innominate aneurism. The immediate effects of the operation have been highly successful.

AN EXHIBITION OF FOOD PRODUCTS.

THERE has just been held at the Agricultural Hall, Islington, an exhibition of food stuffs, and of machinery and utensils used in the preparation of articles of food. Since the inauguration of the system in 1851, it has become the fashion to organise exhibitions of all kinds; and it must be admitted that this method of promoting healthy rivalry has resulted in great advantages to the public. Quite recently in the same building an exhibition of beverages, and the materials and machinery used in their production, was held, and it was considered that the present, or second annual, exhibition of articles of food would most appropriately follow. There are nearly twice as many exhibitors as there were at the first Food Exhibition held last year; but it would seem that the subject was scarcely as yet been sufficiently ventilated, since neither the colonies nor the United States are so fully represented as they undoubtedly should be. Several continental firms have, however, accepted the invitation to submit their products in competition with our own, and in this class must be included condensed milk, preparations of cocoa, chocolate, coffee, gelatine, dried vegetables for soups, and preserved meats of several kinds; then there are many samples of foreign cheese, Russian sardines, Norwegian anchovies, caviare, etc. Messrs. Thurber and Co., of New York, are prominent exhibitors of farinaceous foods, canned meats,

vegetables, fruits, and honey, and they not only exhibit all the products of which we on this side of the Atlantic have heard so much, such as hominy, succotash, etc., but a lady has been in attendance giving a course of lessons on cookery. It would be impossible to specify all the articles introduced into the Exhibition, but we may briefly mention food for infants—headed by the preparation of Messrs. Savory and Moore; diabetic foods; baking, egg, and custard powders; self-raising flour; veal and ham, and pork pies; ham-cured herrings; refined sugars; salt for preserving fish, curing meat, "sweetening" rank grass, etc. ; preservatives for fresh meat, fish, and butter; jams, pickles, and other condiments. The judges of the show are Dr. Danford Thomas, Dr. H. C. Bartlett, Dr. J. Milner Fothergill, and Mr. C. W. Wigner, F.C.S. During the Exhibition the Hall has been lit by electricity, thirty-two lamps on the Brush system having been used for the purpose.

THE ARMY MEDICAL WARRANT, 1881.

WE would have this week commented on the provisions of what we suppose we must call the new Army Medical Warrant, though it dates back to June 25, 1881. Unfortunately, its contents seem as ambiguous to those most nearly concerned as they do to us. We cannot tell what is meant by the statement that all holders of medical commissions are to take rank as medical officers only above the rank of Brigade-Surgeon, and by the omission of all reference to promotion to the rank of Surgeon-Major, together with certain other verbal flourishes which may mean little or may mean much. Before another week passes, being duly instructed ourselves, we hope to be able to instruct our readers. Meanwhile we, like themselves, are in the dark.

SIR ERASMUS WILSON, F.R.C.S., F.R.S.

IT has been officially announced that the Queen has been graciously pleased to confer the honour of knighthood upon Mr. Erasmus Wilson, President of the Royal College of Surgeons of England, in consideration of his munificent gifts for the support of hospitals and the encouragement of medical study. Mr. Wilson's life-work as an anatomist and dermatologist has made his name honoured wherever scientific medicine is studied and practised, in the old world and the new; and his generous activity in good works is well known to and appreciated by the profession and the public in England. The honour of knighthood cannot really add anything to the lustre of his fame; but we may cordially congratulate him on the fact that his well-known name will for the future be graced with the sign-manual of his Sovereign's approval and distinction.

THE EPIDEMIC OF YELLOW FEVER IN THE WEST INDIES.

So virulent and persistent has this epidemic now become that orders have been issued for the immediate withdrawal of all the white troops from Barbadoes to England. Consequently, the 17th and 18th Batteries, 7th Brigade, Royal Artillery, and the headquarters and four companies of the 1st Battalion Royal Lancaster Regiment, are, it may be hoped, by this time on the homeward voyage in H.M.S. Orontes, and may shortly be expected in England. Whether yellow fever be or be not of contagious nature, it is undeniable that local conditions, the unfavourable influences of which are intensified by defects of sanitation such as are known to exist in the West Indies, particularly in towns and districts occupied by the coloured population, are decidedly favourable to the extension of yellow fever, its congener cholera, as well as enteric and the eruptive fevers, so that when such a step is practicable, the entire removal of an affected population is the most speedily effective method of putting an end to the epidemic. It is not easy to determine how long it may be necessary or advisable to keep the affected island denuded of troops—probably three or four months at the least. It is, however, a fair subject of anticipation to hope that the local authorities will fully avail themselves of the interval at their disposal for the removal of all known defects in sanitation, both urban and rural. In addition to the previous victims of the epidemic, we have much regret in recording the deaths of Colonel Blake, commanding the 1st Battalion Royal Lancaster Regiment; Deputy Assistant Commissary-General Drumgoole; and of two young medical officers—Surgeons J. R. Oliver and W. Deane-Freeman, M.B., the former of whom entered the Army Medical Department in March, and the latter in July, 1880. We understand that the vessel in question is likely to touch land at Dover, and that the matter of quarantine is now under consideration. During the present temperature it would seem somewhat superfluous.

GLASGOW OPHTHALMIC INSTITUTION.

The Glasgow Ophthalmic Institution having been reconstructed, and a large addition made to its indoor accommodation, was opened on the 7th inst. by the Earl of Stair (the patron of the Hospital), the Lord Provost and some of the magistrates, Sir James Watson, Mr. White of Glasgow, the Chairman, and other leading citizens and medical practitioners. The Earl of Stair spoke in very high and affectionate terms of the usefulness of the Institution, and of the good work which it has done in Glasgow from its commencement about twelve years ago.

THE BACILLUS MALARIÆ.

The fourteenth Supplement of the *Bulletin of the American National Board of Health*, July 23, contains an elaborate report by Surgeon Sternberg, U.S.A., upon the results of an inquiry which the Board requested him to undertake. This consisted in the repetition of the experiments instituted by Klebs and Tommasi-Crudeli in the vicinity of Rome, and which resulted in the discovery of *Bacillus malaria*. These new experiments were made with swamp-mud collected near New Orleans or from the gutters of the city, and are described in considerable detail. As the result, a great number of minute algæ, including bacteria of various forms, were found, many of these being susceptible of successful cultivation in Klebs' solution of fish-gelatine, which, previously innocuous, acquires pathogenetic properties as a consequence of the presence of these organisms. Infectious disease may by their agency be induced in the living rabbit, which is capable of transmission. "Some of these organisms closely resemble, and are perhaps identical with, the *Bacillus malaria* of Klebs; but there is no satisfactory evidence that these or any other of the bacterial organisms found in such situations, when injected under the skin of the rabbit, give rise to a malarial fever, corresponding with the ordinary paludal fevers to which man is subject. . . . . While, however, the evidence upon which Klebs and Tommasi-Crudeli have based their claim to a discovery is not satisfactory, and their conclusions are shown not to have been well founded (as regards rabbits), there is nothing in my researches to indicate that the so-called *Bacillus malaria*, or some other of the minute organisms associated with it, is not the active agent in the causation of malarial fever in man. There are many circumstances in favour of the hypothesis that the etiology of these fevers is directly or indirectly connected with the presence of these organisms or their germs in the air and water of malarial localities. The truth or falsity of this hypothesis can only be settled by extended experimental investigations; and while further experiments upon animals may lead to more definite results, it seems probable that the *experimentum crucis* must be made on man himself." Dr. Sternberg terminates his report with some suggestions as to how further experiments can best be carried on.

ST. JOHN AMBULANCE ASSOCIATION: DINNER TO MAJOR DUNCAN.

The medical men who have given instruction in ambulance and nursing work to the pupils of the St. John Ambulance Association in the metropolitan district dined together on October 27 at Limmer's Hotel, Conduit-street. The object of the dinner was to express to Major Duncan, who was the guest of the evening, the cordial admiration of the lecturers for the part taken by him in organising the work of the Association. The chairman, Dr. Sieveking, in proposing Major Duncan's health, spoke very warmly of the self-sacrificing labour and of the care and good taste with which all this useful work had been conducted. In replying, Major Duncan thanked the medical profession, without whom nothing could have been done, for their hearty co-operation, and said that every day brought fresh proof of the usefulness of the instruction given. He, personally, and the Association also, owed a great deal to their chief secretary Captain Perrott, to whom much of the credit for their successful organisation was due. Captain Perrott and Sir Wm. Mac Cormac were among the guests; and the hospitals, the Army, and the general profession were well represented at the dinner. All the arrangements were most carefully made by Mr. Cantlie and Mr. Crookshanks, the honorary secretaries.

RICHMOND HOSPITAL, SURREY.

H.R.H. THE DUKE OF CAMBRIDGE has kindly consented to preside at a dinner early in the new year; and H.R.H. the Duchess of Teck has kindly promised to open the new wards in the summer.

THE PARIS WEEKLY RETURN.

The number of deaths for the forty-third week, terminating October 28, was 1084 (552 males and 482 females), and among these there were from typhoid fever 47, small-pox 10, measles 12, scarlatina 5, pertussis 7, diphtheria and croup 52, dysentery 1, erysipelas 11, and puerperal infections 7. There were also 89 deaths from tubercular and acute meningitis, 34 from acute bronchitis, 70 from pneumonia, 69 from infantile athrepsia (26 of the infants having been wholly or partially suckled), and 26 violent deaths. This week's return contains therefore an increase of 114 deaths—the first effects of the advance of the cold season. The increase chiefly arises from bronchitis and pneumonia (104 in place of 57), two important zymotic diseases having also increased their ravages, viz., typhoid fever from 28 to 47, and diphtheria from 44 to 52. "In this number we continue the publication (the seventh monthly) of the number of civil funerals. On comparing the several monthly returns, we may observe how constant is the proportion of such funerals, viz., from 20 to 21 per cent.: that is, for four funerals with some kind of religious rite, there is one which is purely civil (not counting the born-dead). This remarkable fixity shows plainly that fortuitous circumstances have nothing to do with the matter, but that we have under observation a phenomenon which is deeply rooted in the fixed ideas of an important portion of the Parisian population." The births for the week amounted to 1174, viz., 599 males (456 legitimate and 143 illegitimate) and 575 females (428 legitimate and 147 illegitimate); 107 infants (61 males and 46 females) were born dead or died within twenty-four hours.

MIDLAND MEDICAL SOCIETY.

The first meeting of the session was held on Wednesday evening, November 2, in the Medical Institute, Birmingham. In the absence of the President, Mr. Ross Jordan was voted to the chair. Forty members and visitors were present. The following gentlemen were elected members of the Society :—Mr. E. Cooke Johnston, Dr. A. Harvey, and Mr. Pugh. Mr. Lawson Tait showed a living case on which laparo-enterotomy had been performed for intestinal obstruction. The operation relieved all the symptoms, and subsequently the fæces passed per rectum, and the artificial opening gradually closed, leaving a very small fæcal fistula, through which small quantities of motion occasionally passed. Mr. Tait also exhibited a large vesical calculus. The patient was a woman who had been operated upon by another surgeon three years ago for vesico-vaginal fistula. After leaving the hospital where she had been treated all the old symptoms returned. An examination showed that a silver suture had not been removed, and that the urine dribbled through the openings made by the stitch, which also had acted as a starting-point for the formation of the stone. By enlarging the openings existing, Mr. Tait was enabled to remove the suture and the calculus. Mr. May showed the following tumours :—(1) Cystic testicle, the result of traumatism; (2) sarcoma of the mamma; (3) sarcoma of the parotid; (4) sarcoma growing from the great toe; (5) tumours of bursæ. Mr. Tait then read a paper, "On One Hundred and Ten Consecutive Cases of Abdominal Section since November, 1880" (published in the *Medical Times and Gazette*). A discussion ensued, in which the following took part—Dr. Bassett, Mr. Thomas, Mr. Chavasse, Mr. Ker, Mr. Jordan Lloyd, Mr. B. May, Dr. Simon, Dr. Robinson, Mr. Ross Jordan. Mr. Tait having replied, the meeting terminated.

ARMY MEDICAL DEPARTMENT.

Among the passengers on board the ill-fated *Clan Macduff*, lost during the recent gales in the Channel, on the voyage from Liverpool to Bombay, was Surgeon Creed C. H. Smyth, of the Army Medical Department, who, having recently exchanged with a medical officer serving in India, in addition to being a passenger, appears also to have been in the position of surgeon to the ship for the projected voyage, so sadly terminated. His body has been recently picked up at Old Head, Kinsale, and buried in the neighbouring churchyard at Templetrim. It is stated that a brother of his on board the same ship was also lost.

NERVE-STRETCHING.

The surgery of the nervous system continues to form the subject of numerous communications to medical journals both at home and abroad. In No. 38 of the *Centralblatt für Chirurgie*, we find an account by Holl of Vienna, of two methods of cutting down upon the buccal nerve and excising a portion of it, in order to relieve a neuralgia of that part of the face which it supplies. He records three cases by Michel, Schuh, and Billroth, in which the nerve was reached by an incision through the cheek along the anterior border of the masseter. The author draws attention to the fact that in this way the main trunk of the nerve cannot be reached, and that, in order to do this, it should be sought from the interior of the mouth. He gives directions for performing this operation as follows :—If the mouth be widely opened, a groove is seen running near the anterior border of the internal pterygoid muscle, from the depression behind the tuberosity of the upper jaw, which portion of bone can be felt beneath the mucous membrane, to the last lower molar tooth. An incision in the line of this groove through mucous mem-

brane and some glands leads to the nerve; it is only necessary to free it from some surrounding fat, to enable the surgeon to remove a portion of it one or two centimetres long. He adds that the feasibility, and, indeed, ease of performance, of the operation has not only been demonstrated on the dead subject, but upon the living, it having been actually performed by A. Wölfler in Billroth's clinique. Cases of neuralgia of the buccal nerve are not, we imagine, common, but if one were met with, the suggested operation seems a rational one. In the same number we find a paper by M. Benedikt, recounting three cases of stretching of the great sciatic nerve for locomotor ataxy, and one of the facial in a case of long-standing paralysis with secondary *tic spasmodique*. The ataxic cases were all remarkably improved, not only as regards the pains and other disturbances of sensation, but also in respect of the ataxy, paralysis of the bladder, and even amblyopia. It is mortifying to observe that the effect of this operation appears to vary so widely in different cases. Those which we have ourselves seen have not yielded such brilliant results as seem to be frequently obtained by our German brethren. Is it possible that we are not in the habit of doing the actual stretching vigorously enough in this country ? or is it that cases differ very much in their amenability to treatment in this way ? The facial case seems to have presented considerable difficulty from the fact of the nerve being much degenerated and embedded in cicatricial tissue. The operation was, however, successfully carried out, with relief to the tic, and also, strange to say, a rapid improvement of the paralysis. This last result is doubly remarkable, as, in all cases we have seen or read of, a very prolonged paralysis of the muscles supplied was the immediate result of the stretching. No doubt there is much still to be learned, both as to the *modus operandi* of nerve-stretching and as to the classes of cases in which it is likely to prove beneficial.

THE ÆSCULAPIAN CLUB.

Medical men engaged in busy practice in the outlying suburbs of London are scarcely less exposed than their country brethren to the danger of degenerating into mere routinists, and this tendency shows itself, we fear, in the proceedings of some of the local medical associations. Sensible of this, a number of practitioners in North London have formed themselves into a society, under the name of the Æsculapian Club, meeting fortnightly from October to May at the residence of one of the members. The papers and discussions are naturally for the most part clinical. An important aim of the club is mutual assistance in obtaining good records of post-mortem examinations—an advantage too rarely to be obtained in private practice. Few of us have, we hope, forgotten the immortal letters of Sydenham on the epidemic constitution of the year, and in practice we have good reason to fall back on what many would call antiquated notions. From a somewhat extensive knowledge of what is to be seen at the various hospitals in London, year by year, we are strongly inclined to think that Sydenham's "epidemic constitution" is too much forgotten. It must remain largely with general practitioners to give us a correct notion of the fever now prevailing in London. Here is clearly work to be done.

PATHOLOGICAL SOCIETY OF DUBLIN.

The annual general meeting of this Society, for the election of officers and transaction of other business, was held in the Anatomical Theatre of the School of Physic, Trinity College, Dublin, on the afternoon of Saturday, November 5. The chair was taken, in the first instance, by the outgoing President, Dr. Arthur Wynne Foot. After the signing of the minutes, Mr. Edward Hamilton proposed, and Dr. J. W. Moore seconded, a resolution to elect Mr. William Stokes as President of the Society for the ensuing session. The motion having been carried by acclamation, Dr. Foot vacated the chair, which was then taken by Mr. Stokes. Mr. Hamilton moved, and Dr. Nixon seconded, a vote of thanks to Dr. Foot for his dignified conduct in the chair as President during the past year. Dr. Foot acknowledged the vote of thanks. Dr. J. W. Moore moved, and Dr. Nixon seconded, the following resolution, which was adopted in silence, viz.: —"That the members of the Pathological Society of Dublin desire to accord their sense of the great loss which the Society, as well as the cause of pathological science, have sustained by the lamented death of Dr. Thomas Hayden, one of the Vice-Presidents, and some time President, of the Society." The following officers for the session 1881-82 were elected: —*President:* William Stokes, M.D. *Secretary and Treasurer:* Edward H. Bennett, M.D. *Secretary for Foreign Correspondence:* John William Moore, M.D. *Vice-Presidents:* John Thomas Banks, M.D.; Samuel Gordon, M.D.; Edward Hamilton, M.D.; George H. Kidd, M.D.; William Moore, M.D.; T. Jolliffe Tufnell, F.R.C.S.I. *Council:* John Kellock Barton, M.D.; Anthony H. Corley, M.D.; George F. Duffey, M.D.; John Magee Finny, M.D.; Arthur Wynne Foot, M.D.; Reuben Joshua Harvey, M.D.; James Little, M.D.; Thomas Evelyn Little, M.D.; Robert McDonnell, M.D.; Christopher J. Nixon, M.B.; John Mallet Purser, M.D.; John Benjamin Story, M.D. *Committee of Reference of Morbid Growths:* Phineas S. Abraham, Reuben J. Harvey, Thomas E. Little, John Mallet Purser; with the President and Secretaries *ex officio.* Resolutions were subsequently passed, authorising the Council to take steps to effect an amalgamation of the medical societies of Dublin, and to arrange for the holding of special evening meetings of the Society from time to time for the reception of reports by the Committee of Reference.

HISTOLOGICAL RESEARCHES ON FAVUS AND RINGWORM.

M. BALZER (Médecin des Hopitaux) gives the result of his researches on favus and ringworm in the *Archives Générales de Médecine* (October, 1881). Of the different parts or elements belonging to the ordinary mould-fungi, only two are found in those of favus and ringworm—(1) spores, either free, in chains, or in masses; (2) tubes or mycelial threads. The spore consists of a central, somewhat granular, nucleus enclosed in a more or less resisting covering or envelope—the epispore. The mycelial threads are of two kinds, viz., those containing a substance similar to that forming the nucleus of the spores, and corresponding to the vegetating portion of the fungus—thallus; those in which the contents are segmented with more or less regularity—the latter are the sporophores or sporiferous tubes. In the process of germination the spore elongates and forms a tube; in the interior of this the nuclear substance buds into lateral processes, thus forming branched mycelium, or it becomes segmented so as to constitute a sporiferous tube; the segmentation of the envelope itself ultimately shuts off the separate segments of nuclear substance, and thus are formed new spores, each in its turn to pass through similar stages of evolution. The fungus of favus (*Achorion*) is first developed amongst the rete cells at the mouth of the hair-follicle. The superficial layers of epidermis adhering round the hair are prevented from being raised by the growing mass of fungus, and thus is produced the cup-shaped or umbilicated crust peculiar to favus. This cup-shaped vegetation seems, however, not to be peculiar to the fungus of favus. The *Oidium albicans* is said to form cup-shaped crusts in the alimentary canal (Parrot). The achorion only attacks the hair after some time; the hair-cuticle is never involved. The hair is

invaded both directly and indirectly through its root. Unna denies the latter mode of invasion, asserting that the fungus never quits the horny tissue of the epidermis, stopping short of the young and succulent cells of the bulb and Malpighian layer. The author, however, has seen the fungus (achorion) penetrating the internal root-sheath, invading the external root-sheath, and even pushing its way between the connective-tissue bundles of the true skin. The reactive inflammation set up by its presence leads to absorption and the production of the cicatrices which are seen after the cure of favus. In ringworm, mycelial threads of the fungus (*Trichophyton*) are specially well seen amongst the epidermic scales. They are long, straight, and narrow, crossing each other in all directions; they do not branch so much as the mycelial threads of the achorion. The spores of the trichophyton are, as a rule, not so large as those of achorion, but in some cases of herpes circinatus they attain a large size. When united in a row, their opposing surfaces become flattened, and give them the appearance of barrels arranged end to end. It is a striking fact that the mycelium is found for the most part in the scales, while in the affected hairs spores abound. This may be due to the fact that the fungus has full opportunity of development when sheltered in the hair-follicle, but less chance in the epidermic scales, which are continually being shed at the surface. In a diseased, but as yet whole, hair the trichophyton is seen occupying its peripheral portion, always covered by the hair-cuticle, which is itself not attacked. The fungus first invades the sheath of the hair, then the root, where it takes the form of sporiferous tubes; later on these tubes advance into the hair, and become segmented into detached spores. In the next stage the parasite invades the whole hair, excepting the medulla. Lastly, the hair (still bounded by the cuticle) resembles an elongated sac filled with spores. These different degrees of spore-infiltration may, of course, co-exist in different parts of the same hair. In preparing specimens for examination, the hairs or fragments of epidermis are first submitted to one or more washings in ether or absolute alcohol—this is to free them from fat; the material is then placed in a solution of soda or potash (10 to 40 per cent.), to render the epithelial elements more transparent. The nuclei and tube contents may be stained with eosin or aniline blue. The foregoing is a short abstract of M. Balzer's paper.

WONFORD HOUSE HOSPITAL FOR THE INSANE.

IN the eightieth annual report on Wonford House Hospital for the Insane, near Exeter, for the year 1880, the Resident Medical Superintendent, Dr. Sutherland Rees Philipps, remarks that the health of the patients has been remarkably good during the whole of the period. Although many of the inmates are old and feeble (the average age is over fifty), and the winter was unusually severe, there was no serious illness of any kind, and not a single case of any acute chest-affection. Some patients admitted in former years with symptoms of lung-disease have improved considerably, and there is now no patient with any apparent sign of active lung-mischief. The open, airy situation, good drainage, free southern exposure, and proximity to the sea, combine to influence favourably the health of all the inmates. The dietary has been improved without any increase of expense; in point of fact, the cost of maintenance of each patient, which in 1878 was £1 18s. 9½d. per week per head, and £1 14s. 1d. in 1879, was in 1880 reduced to £1 18s. 10d. Milk was given to some of the patients instead of beer with apparent advantage, evidenced by an increase of weight in some weakly patients. No patient has been restrained or secluded, though the Hospital contains a full proportion of troublesome cases. With the introduction of cheerful colour-

and decoration into the wards, excitement and outrage have materially lessened, and there has been neither suicide nor accident of any kind. The report contains some remarks of Dr. Philipps', which we recently noticed, on the subject of providing lady-companions for the insane in place of the ordinary female attendants at present provided.

REVIEWS.

Tropical Dysentery and Chronic Diarrhœa, Liver Abscess, Malarial Cachexia, Insolation, with other forms of Tropical Disease; and on Health of European Children and others in India. By Sir JOSEPH FAYRER, K.C.S.I., LL.D., M.D., F.R.S., President of the Medical Board, India Office; Honorary Physician to the Queen and to the Prince of Wales. London: J. and A. Churchill, New Burlington-street. 1881.

IF any branch of the fraternity of physicians have ever merited the larger designation of *physici, i.e.,* professors of natural science in all its branches, that appellation has, without question, been validly earned by the members of that noble old Service—the Indian Medical Department. Formerly, before the days of the Prinseps, the Oldhams, and the Blandfords, nearly the whole of the domain of Indian science was discovered and administered by medical men. In very old times, when "interlopers,"—that is, persons who not being in the service of the East India Company, ventured out to India as adventurers—were summarily deported by Government, men who, being remarkable for science outside the realm of medicine, were wanted in India, were occasionally admitted as surgeons, but otherwise employed. It was thus with John Leyden, the poet and Oriental scholar, who died at Java in 1811. Much more recently, Wallich, the botanist; Cantor, his nephew, the naturalist; and Aloys Sprenger, the great Arabic scholar, became, in like manner, ornaments to the Indian Medical Service. Many others, who entered the Department in the regular course, have become leading authorities in general science. Among these may be mentioned Faulkner and McClelland, as geologists; Wight, Thomas Thomson, Hugh Cleghorn, Balfour, Thomas Anderson, and King, as botanists; Jerdon and Day, as naturalists. We would strongly recall to the minds of our readers the now almost forgotten facts that, early in last century, William Hamilton, a surgeon, having cured the Great Mogul of a hydrocele, obtained permission, which had been long denied, for his countrymen to settle at Calcutta, when his masters, the Company, had cashiered him for obeying the monarch's summons; that a surgeon and man of great learning, John Zephaniah Holwell, who has left us that narrative of the Black Hole, the unaffected power of which Macaulay failed to improve upon, was, by no reason except that of being the best man available, twice created Governor of Bengal; that Dr. Montgomerie, of Bengal, discovered gutta-percha; and that Sir William O'Shaughnessy Brooke, of the same presidency, introduced the use of the electric telegraph in India. As long as the Government treat their Indian surgeons well, encouraging men of the best attainments to enter their service, there will never be wanting in the East those who will gratuitously devote years of labour to the cultivation of science for its own sake. We use the word "*gratuitously*" with emphasis, it being a very remarkable fact that, although the scientific works of Indian surgeons would form a large library, the merit, as scientists, of these officers has never, save in three or four exceptional cases, received any signal recognition from their Government, until August last, when the Companionship of the Indian Empire was bestowed upon a medical officer retired from each of the three Presidencies, each of these three aged physicians having devoted the scanty leisure of a lifetime to the cultivation, in India, of medicine and its allied sciences. We trust that this small beginning affords presage of the coming of better times for the Department.

Among Indian medical men of widely comprehensive scientific erudition none stand higher than the author of the recently-published medical work, the title of which heads this notice. Every brother officer who served with Sir Joseph Fayrer in India recognises his eminence as a surgeon, a physician, a naturalist, and an administrator; and

his works on Surgery in the East, on the Thanatophidia of India, and upon many other important subjects, have obtained European reputation.

We consider that the vital interest of its topics, and the masterly ability and commanding knowledge—the result of twenty-five years' practical experience—with which he has given them to the profession, will secure an equal reputation for this his latest work, which deals with subjects of leading importance strictly within the province of the Indian physician.

Besides the subjects named in its title, this volume contains chapters of great value on the Bael Fruit, and its medicinal properties and uses—a drug in the value of which long and patient experience has given us little faith; on Bronchocele, a disease which, in some parts of India, is extensively prevalent not only in man, but in some of the lower animals; and on Dengue, of which four great outbreaks have occurred in India within the last sixty years. Sir Joseph Fayrer considers that this disease is "endemic in India," and states that cases occur sporadically every year in Calcutta. We notice that our author mentions that, when dengue became most extensively epidemic in 1824, it extended from India to Burmah. He has thus avoided the blame which Dr. James Christie, in his recently published monograph,(a) has freely bestowed upon former commentators on this subject, remarking that "systematic writers have sadly distorted the chronology of this epidemic, each after the other having copied the mistakes of his predecessor, representing it as having had its origin in Burmah; or in Burmah, the Bengal and Bombay Presidencies simultaneously." This volume also contains an excellent paper on Elephantiasis Arabum, a disease of which the author had almost unequalled practical experience during his fifteen years' service as first surgeon in the largest hospital in India, in Bengal, the very hotbed of Barbadoes legs and of gigantic scrotal tumours, from which, occasionally, the man is removed, he being lighter than his excrescence. The last chapter is on the Rainfall in India—one of the first subjects upon which the author wrote after his arrival in India, he thus becoming a pioneer in that great field of research into atmospheric phenomena, which subsequent observers have largely investigated. This monograph is quite worthy of the late President of the Asiatic Society of Bengal, embodying, as it does, a vast mass of closely packed figures and facts arrayed to the utmost practical advantage by one who has always taken a deep personal interest in the subject.

We need not recommend the chapters on Tropical Dysentery, Chronic Diarrhœa, Liver Abscess, Malarial Cachexia, and Insolation, to Indian medical officers. Their author's reputation will command the full attention of those who are still learners in India, who will find them replete with the soundest and most recent knowledge—knowledge which has, in recent times, robbed these formidable maladies of half their terrors, by making them avoidable and, in a large majority of cases, remediable. Men of large Oriental experience will, we are confident, peruse these chapters with heartily appreciative gratification, as in them they will find truly reflected, as if in a pure mirror, those diseases with which it has been their lot to contend from the day on which their foot first touched the shore of India. To practitioners in the United Kingdom and elsewhere in Europe these pages will be almost equally useful. Marsh disease, so modified as rarely to be differentiated with ease except by those who have either seen or carefully studied in books the cognate diseases of the East and West Indies, is almost universally prevalent throughout the British Isles. We declare it to be a fact that he who resides in certain districts almost immediately south of Blackfriars-bridge is almost as liable to dysentery as he who dwells in the marshes of Kent or Essex is subject to intermittent fever, asthma, and facial neuralgia. Everywhere around the coasts of our own islands, paludal influence—whatever that may be—gives virulence and deadliness to small-pox, scarlatina, measles, and pertussis. The causation of that anæmia which, in various forms, so much prevails in temperate climates, has still to be investigated by the light of tropical experience. The English pathologist must be desirous to learn, for his own guidance, why phthisis, scirrhus, rheumatic fever, cardiac disease, and stone are rare diseases in Bengal. There are days in every English summer

(a) "Epidemics of Dengue Fever," *Glasgow Med. Jour.* for September, 1881.

on which every man who walks down the sunny side of Bond-street does so at the imminent risk of being struck down by insolation. Every woman in England has been liable to bron-chocele, from Queen Anne Boleyn, in the sixteenth century, on whom it was merely a prettiness, giving roundness to her "litel" neck, down to the London charwoman of to-day, to whom it is death by suffocation. Upon these and a hundred other points, in which the maladies of the East and West either touch each other or stand widely apart, men like Sir Joseph Fayrer, who have studied disease with close applica-tion and great ability, both at home and abroad, and the scientific masters of our profession throughout Europe, should never cease to confer until they have succeeded in establishing a single and indivisible pathology for the whole world. We trust that our author may be long spared to take a leading part in this great work, and that he will speedily publish another volume as replete as this is with sound facts and safe opinions.

GENERAL CORRESPONDENCE.

THE TESTIMONIAL TO PROFESSOR VIRCHOW.
LETTER FROM DR. J. S. BRISTOWE.

[To the Editor of the Medical Times and Gazette.

SIR,—Allow me to acknowledge in your columns the follow-ing subscriptions, in addition to those previously announced, towards the above testimonial, and to request intending subscribers to communicate with me on the subject with as little delay as possible.   I am, &c.,   J. S. BRISTOWE.
11, Old Burlington-street, W., November 10.

Ernest Hart, Esq., £1 1s.; Felix Semon, M.D., £1 1s.; F. J. Mouat, M.D., F.R.S., £5 5s.; W. Aitken, Esq., M.D., F.R.S., £2 2s.; Sir William Gull, Bart., F.R.S., £2 10s.; E. Bronner, Esq., £1 1s.; Bisset Hawkins, M.D., F.R.S., £2; Saml. Wilkes, M.D., F.R.S., £1 1s.; Sidney Coupland, M.D., £1 1s.; N. Montefiore, Esq., £2 2s.; S. H. Philipson, M.D., £1 1s.; D. Drummond, M.D., £1 1s.; J. Marion Sims, M.D., £2 10s.

PROVISION FOR THE INDIGENT POPULATION OF PARIS.—According to the budget of the Assistance Publique for 1882, submitted to the Préfet de la Seine, there are 125,000 regis-tered indigent persons to be cared for, and to these have to be added 48,000 sick treated at their own homes but not regis-tered as indigent, 16,000 lying-in-women confined at their own residences, and 30,000 necessitous persons requiring only temporary aid—making a total of 219,500 individuals. If to these there be added the sick, children, and aged per-sons cared for in the various establishments of the Assistance (viz., 137,513), the children placed out in the country or assisted in their families (28,000 in number), and 180 others received into the Lambrecht Asylum, we have a population of 385,143 individuals, who, for one reason or another, are under the charge of this department. In 1881 the number of beds at the disposal of the various hospital services was 22,000; and the number of days of treatment, which in 1880 was 6,722,254, is calculated for 1881 at 7,414,560. The sum calculated to be required for 1882 amounts to more than 34,000,000 fr.—Union Méd., November 5.

THE VIVISECTION SENTIMENTALITY.—That pleasant French traveller, Henri Havard, tells us that on his first visit to Holland he used to see heavy barges dragged along the canals by a big dog and a woman, harnessed to the same rope, while the man steered. On a later voyage he missed the big dogs, and saw only the woman, or perhaps two women, tugging at the heavy boat. Informing himself as to the reason of this change in the habits of so conservative a race as the Dutch, he learned that the local Society for the Pre-vention of Cruelty to Animals had secured the passing of an Act prohibiting the harnessing of dogs: so the women had to do it all themselves! In similar style, the antivivisection-ists of England and this country are striving to prevent some very few of the lower animals from being used for the purposes of science, when the inevitable consequence of their success would be that the progress of medical know-ledge—which means the relief of pain, the restoration to health, and the preservation of life—would thereby be retarded. —Phil. Med. and Surg. Reporter.

REPORTS OF SOCIETIES.

THE CLINICAL SOCIETY OF LONDON.
FRIDAY, OCTOBER 28.

JOSEPH LISTER, D.C.L., F.R.C.S., F.R.S., President, in the Chair.

(Concluded from page 561.)

A CASE OF STRANGULATED HERNIA (LITTRÉ'S) OR PARTIAL ENTEROCELE.

MR. C. T. DENT contributed this paper. After remarking that the term "Littré's hernia" had now acquired rather a loose significance, and that several varieties had been described since M. Littré's original article, the author narrated the case of W. G., aged thirty-seven, a phthisical, emaciated man, of intemperate habits, who was admitted into St. George's Hospital in February, 1881. The patient had never noticed any rupture till the day before admission, when he observed a tender swelling in the left groin. Two days previously, he had vomited after taking food. The day after admission he vomited again after taking some milk, and the bowels acted several times. The swelling was of the size of a small Tangerine orange, and slightly tender. It gave no impulse during coughing. The tongue was dry and red. There was marked distress. The diarrhœa con-tinued, and while he was being put under ether he passed a quantity of fluid fæces. The hernial sac was greatly in-flamed and thickened, and the parts were so matted together that careful dissection was necessary. On dividing a slight constriction, the hernia was felt to go back; the sac was not opened. The tissues were so lax, that the entire sac was readily displaced beneath Poupart's ligament. The symptoms were relieved for the first two or three days, but persistent diarrhœa then set in, and proved fatal on the sixth day. Post-mortem, extensive disease of the lungs was found. The hernia proved to have consisted of a portion only of the circumference of the jejunum; a dark semi-gangrenous ring corresponding to the con-stricted part was seen on the gut. Extensive enteritis of the ileum was found, which may have accounted for the diarrhœa. The case resembled those described by M. Littré, in that there was no intestinal obstruction, fæces passing freely; and in that hiccough was absent, the vomiting not persistent or stercoraceous, whilst the abdomen was not distended. It was peculiar in the following points :—1. It occurred in a man; 2. The jejunum was involved; 3. The hernia must have existed for some time without being noticed; 4. There was no diverticulum or sacculation of the gut, which, at the post-mortem examination, was found at a considerable distance from the sac. In conclusion, the author advocated the removal of a great part of the hernial sac when, as in this case, it was thickened, inflamed, and ulcerated; and the closure of the neck of the sac by deep sutures.

The PRESIDENT remarked that it was said that here there was no constipation, as there was no complete obstruction. But constipation was often found in a purely omental hernia. He remembered a case where there was a purely fatty femoral hernia, yet all the ordinary symptoms were present. At the post-mortem examination, a mass of fat was found constricted by Gimbernat's ligament.

Mr. ROYES BELL suggested that it would have been better to open the sac. The author thought that it would not be wise to sew up the sac; he had seen this done, and the case go on remarkably well.

Mr. WARRINGTON HAWARD said that if the orifice of the sac was to be left open for the escape of inflammatory products, this was certainly an argument for opening the sac. He thought it a good plan to sew together the neck of the sac; but then the lower portion should be cut away or opened.

Mr. HOWARD MARSH thought that it was a common belief that there is no peritonitis except the contents of the sac escape.

A CASE OF DOUBLE HÆMORRHAGIC PLEURISY, WITH FORMATION OF CHOLESTERIN.

Dr. T. CHURTON (Leeds) reported the following case :—A man, aged thirty-eight, of originally good constitution always temperate, not syphilitic, had, in 1876, a wide-spreading axillary abscess, the discharge from which lasted six months, as a result of a wound on the left hand. His health was never perfect after this time, and in 1878 he became positively ailing, was short of breath, and lost flesh. He had no cough, no haemoptysis, and scarcely any pain in the chest. He gradually grew worse until 1880, when he was admitted into the Leeds Infirmary. He then complained of loss of appetite, wasting to the extent of twenty pounds in twelve months; occasional vomiting, pain in the right side and between the shoulders. Complete dulness on percussion was found in both axillary regions; respiratory sounds, fremitus, and resonance were greatly diminished or absent. The dulness was of irregular outline, but sharply defined. On exploratory puncture in the left axilla, a brown greasy fluid (exhibited) was obtained. It was composed of red blood-cells, disintegrated and frayed at their edges, and scales of cholesterin in great abundance in a highly albuminous, but not spontaneously coagulating, plasma. There appeared at this time to be only a very small quantity of fluid on this side, but on aspirating the right side in the fourth space, after failing to get anything in the fifth space, two ounces of a dark red fluid were withdrawn. This also contained cholesterin crystals in abundance; the patient's temperature was normal. There was no disease of other organs. For the next twelve months the left side gave very little trouble; it was aspirated once (August 10, 1881) during that time, one ounce of the same kind of fluid as before, but lighter in colour, being obtained. The right cyst, however, refilled again and again, and the fluid was more deeply reddened than at first. Aspirations were performed on July 4 (four ounces); August 10 (sixteen ounces); November 22 (twelve ounces); December 23 (quantity not recorded); March 3, 1881 (eighteen ounces); May 4 (quantity not recorded). Up to this date his general health had improved, he ate and digested food well, could walk about and do light work easily, especially after each operation; but now, remaining in hospital with a view to the abolition of the pleural cyst by any possible means, he became involved in a quarrel with a nurse, and while in a nervous and agitated state, drank some cold water, which caused immediately a feeling of chilliness through his whole body. He became feverish and slightly delirious. On June 29, thirty ounces of fluid, now containing pus-cells, though still glittering with cholesterin, were withdrawn from the right side. On July 2, forty ounces were removed, and on July 10, as the fluid had again accumulated, and the temperature reached 103°, an incision was made, at Dr. Churton's request, by Mr. W. H. Brown, the House-Surgeon, in the right chest, seventh space, posterior axillary line. Thirty-eight ounces of similar fluid (specimen shown) escaped; the temperature fell to 99° within three days, but again rose to 103°. Dr. Churton then discovered that there was a recent accumulation of fluid upon the left side, and twenty ounces of clear but cholesterin-bearing fluid were thereupon withdrawn. The patient did not, however, improve. Pulse 120; respirations 28; temperature 102°. He fancied poison was being given to him by various people, and left the hospital on July 19. He continued to take quinine and steel. On September 10 he had pulse 110, respirations 24, temperature 99° (evening). He was still unable to walk across the room. There was a little clear fluid on the left side (explored); no cholesterin in the pus from the right side. The wound was fistulous and valvular; there were signs of gradual expansion of the lung on both sides; a probe passed through the fistula seemed to reach the right lung at once. He went to Bridlington for a month; there he gained six pounds in weight, and otherwise improved so greatly that he could walk a mile. He returned on October 17. Unfortunately, the narrow pus-channel became blocked, and he lost ground. On October 27 the following note was made: Pulse 120, respirations 27, temperature 102°; the discharge of pus was re-established; he was walking about. The dull area in the left axilla had diminished almost to nothing; a needle passed in at the dullest spot, above the seventh rib, found nothing. This part of the chest did not in him move in respiration; for this reason, apparently, there was little respiratory murmur in the lower axilla; fremitus and resonance were found there, but were not nearly so distinct as on the front of the chest, where also the breath-sounds were, as they always

had been, intensified. The right side was resonant throughout; the respiratory sounds, though feeble, were unmistakably heard in the axilla and elsewhere; fremitus and resonance were distinctly present. Two or three ounces of inoffensive pus (without cholesterin) flowed from this side daily. There were no râles. He had some phlegm, and occasional expulsive cough. While at rest he had no subjective discomfort. He was going to Scarborough for a month. The author believed that chronic pleurisy had caused the formation of a thick false membrane over a part of the lung (on each side); that blood-cells had escaped by diapedesis into the cyst thus formed; that the false membrane had at length undergone fatty degeneration, having as one of its final products cholesterin. Dr. Méhu (Archives Générales de Médecine, September, 1881) had asserted (page 277), as the outcome of very numerous observations, that cholesterin in crystals was never met with in fluids which had not been encysted at least six months. In this case it was once found in fluid from the left pleura, which had almost certainly not been there many days; more-over, a shred of membrane, derived from the left pulmonary pleura, which blocked up the aspirating needle, was found to consist of small cells and cholesterin-crystals in almost equal quantity. Although Fräntzel had stated ("Ziemssen's Cyclopædia," vol. iv., page 670) that when pleurisy appeared simultaneously on both sides it was commonly of tubercular nature, and, moreover (page 614), that relapsing hæmorrhagic pleurisy generally stood in more or less close connexion with the eruption of tubercles, yet, having regard to the facts that the patient had continued in fair health and with a normal temperature for a whole year, while frequent aspirations were being practised; that the left chest had become almost normal; that an apparently accidental empyema on the right side had not been fatal; that the part of the right lung formerly compressed had, probably from the suppuration and disintegration of its thick false membrane, been able at length to re-expand to a great extent; and that since the empyema the patient had in every way greatly improved at the seaside once (and might therefore reasonably be expected to do so again), Dr. Churton did not despair of his ultimate recovery.

Dr. S. MACKENZIE said that he thought that bloody fluid was usually referred to a cancerous origin.

Dr. POWELL asked if the corpuscles were greatly disintegrated, and whether the cholesterin was due to changein the wall of the sac, or to disintegration of the corpuscles. He did not think blood-staining so very important.

Dr. C. T. WILLIAMS thought it curious that the two pleuræ should form and contain two different fluids. What was the condition of the liver? It was quite possible to have tubercle without any marked rise of temperature.

Dr. GREEN did not think that bloody fluid must of necessity have a cancerous origin.

Dr. COUPLAND was of the same opinion as regards the bloody fluid. The cholesterin might come from a degenerated false membrane.

Mr. PARKER suggested that the one side might have been infected by the other.

Dr. SILVER said that, as regarded the origin of the cholesterin, a figure in Lancereaux's Pathological Atlas might throw some light on it. This was a drawing of a cyst of considerable size rising from the upper surface of the diaphragm, and contained within the pleural cavity. Its contents were rich in cholesterin.

The PRESIDENT said that we frequently found cholesterin in serous collections, as in hydrocele; and here its formation was often rapid.

Dr. CHURTON said the great point in this case was the rapid formation of the strange material. Cholesterin was undoubtedly often found elsewhere. Here there was no liver-disease.

TWO CASES OF MALIGNANT STRICTURE OF THE OESOPHAGUS IN WHICH GASTROSTOMY WAS PERFORMED, WITH SPECIAL REFERENCE TO OESOPHAGOSTOMY IN NARROWING OF THE TUBE.

Mr. REEVES contributed this paper. After narrating the two cases, he pointed out how, having done gastrostomy in deference to the wishes of his colleagues, he should proceed to act in any suitable case of stricture of the oesophagus. He said that the most recent information showed that malignant obstruction was most common in the upper part of the tube, occurring in that situation in about half the cases; and, although a much larger number of observations was needed to arrive at a correct conclusion, still there was sufficient justification for the rules he wished to lay down, which were the following:—1. Because of the great mortality after gastrostomy, and also because of more frequent occurrence of malignant stricture in the upper portion of the tube, œsophagostomy was by far the preferable operation. 2. Even in cases where the stricture was situated as low down as the manubrium sterni (its depth rarely being very great), œsophagostomy was indicated as a preliminary or exploratory operation; and, if it were found that the little finger or sound could not be passed through the narrowing, gastrostomy might then be performed. 3. If it resulted that the opening in the œsophagus had been made below the stricture (as in most cases would be desired), the operation could be completed by stitching the mucous membrane to the edges of the wound, and the stricture might, if thought proper, be dilated through the opening either at the time of opening or subsequently. 4. If the diseased œsophagus were reached, and no opening into it could be made through healthy walls, then it might be carefully performed either by the finger or the thermo-cautery. 5. Œsophagostomy had been many times done, œsophagostomy several, and never had these operations caused any grave local or general symptoms, or, as operations, led to the death of the patient; where gastrostomy had proved most fatal. 6. The operation should be done on the left side of the neck, and a sound, if possible, be passed, that of Vacca-Berlinghieri being the best. The skin-incision should be rather nearer the mid-line than that for ligature of the common carotid, and should extend from half an inch above the episternal notch to the level of the upper border of the thyroid cartilage. The surgeon should stand on the left of the patient, looking obliquely down and across his or her body. A tube with a funnel-shaped end should be passed, tied in place, and nourishment administered as soon as the tendency to vomit caused by the anæsthetic had passed off. It was necessary to make the opening in the walls with a sharpish stab, to prevent the loose mucous membrane being pushed before the knife. The edges of the wound might be stitched up, and care taken that no food entered it. 7. The operation should be undertaken before the patient's strength was much exhausted, and even before obstruction was complete, because frequently attempts to swallow produced spasmodic suffocative dyspnœa, as in the first case related. 8. In severe cases of simple fibrous or syphilitic stricture in the tracheal or upper thoracic portion of the tube, œsophagostomy was indicated, as then the operation might be curative as well as palliative.

The discussion of this paper was deferred, Mr. Golding-Bird promising to open the discussion on Mr. Reeves' case by bringing before the Society a report of five similar cases operated on by him in the past year.

THE PATHOLOGICAL SOCIETY OF LONDON.

Tuesday, November 1.

Samuel Wilks, M.D., President, in the Chair.

An Ear of Corn discharged through the Chest.

The President showed an ear of corn which had been discharged from the interior of the chest through an abscess in the chest-wall. The patient was a girl aged ten years; when seen she had an abscess over the scapula, which, when punctured, let out air and pus. After a few days the ear of corn was expelled, and the abscess then healed. He had little doubt but that it had been inspired, and had then gradually worked its way through the wall of the chest. Such cases were not very uncommon. In Watson's "Practice of Physic" several such cases were mentioned; but they all died.

Dr. Goodhart remarked that he had seen two cases of gangrene of the lung due to the presence of foreign bodies in the bronchi, and in neither of which was there any history as to how these bodies had got into the lung, for at no time did there seem to have been any severe or urgent symptoms.

Dr. N. Moore thought it might be a form of grass,

the ears of which possessed a certain rotatory movement which carried them forward.

Mr. Eve said there was a specimen in St. Bartholomew's Museum of abscess in the lung due to impaction of an umbrella ferrule in the bronchus, and in which there was no evidence to show how the ferrule got there, for the patient had died of phthisis.

Drawings of Muscæ Volitantes.

The President showed these, which had been observed by himself. He believed that no drawings were to be found in English books, neither was that pathological condition of the vitreous which gave rise to them at all accurately described. He asked whether they were new formations or due to some modification of existing structures.

Mr. Hutchinson said that he had seen many drawings made by patients who suffered from them; they all resembled those shown to-night, and, although he had no morbid specimens to show, he believed they were caused by some disturbance of the normal tissues of the eye.

Myo-sarcomatous Tumour of Kidney.

Mr. Eve showed two specimens of this unusual condition. The first case was sent to him by Mr. Brickwell. It was removed from a child aged thirteen months, who, when first seen, presented a soft, semi-fluctuating tumour as large as a hen's egg in the right flank. The general health was at first good. The tumour grew rapidly, and its increase in size was attended with great loss of strength, and with interference with the digestive organs, and then with the respiration. The child died from collapse. The tumour occupied the right lumbar region, extending from the margins of the ribs to the pelvis, and internally as far as the umbilicus. It measured seven by four inches, and was about four inches thick; its consistence was uniformly firm and of a yellowish-white colour, with interlacing bundles of fibres passing in all directions. Microscopically, it was found to consist of striated muscle fibres, either scattered about or aggregated into bundles, with some intervening fibrillated tissue. Nodules of round-celled sarcoma tissue were seen scattered throughout. The individual fibres were narrow and long, and distinctly striated. Mr. Eve also described a specimen of "medullary disease of the kidney of a child" from the College Museum, which, on microscopic examination, he had found to contain muscular fibre. The tumour was round, one inch in diameter; it was attached to the hilus of the right kidney, which was otherwise healthy. A nearly identical tumour was also growing from the hilus of the left kidney. No cases were recorded in the Transactions of the Society, nor had he found any similar cases in our English literature. Eberth (Virchow's Archiv, vol. lv. had described a myo-sarcoma of the kidney in 1872, and Cohnheim had since recorded a similar case in vol. lxv. of the same Archiv. Landsberger and Marchand had also published other cases in vol. lxxiii. On contrasting all these cases, the clinical features were found to agree as well as the pathological; the patients were all children under eighteen months of age. In four out of the six cases the disease was bilateral, and in five the tumour was found to consist of striated muscle fibre. In two were found secondary growths, and one of these two contained muscular fibre. In one case a third tumour was attached loosely to one of the kidney tumours. The substance proper of the kidney was not invaded in any instance; the tumour was within the capsule on the surface of the kidney, or attached to the hilus, or it divided the kidney into two parts. The kidney was not infiltrated—a fact which showed that the tumour did not originate from the kidney proper. Cohnheim had suggested what appeared to be the true explanation of the occurrence, viz., that by a faulty segmentation of the protovertebræ some of the germinal muscle cells had got displaced and mixed up with the rudiments of the uro-genital organs, and that they subsequently developed into this pathological condition.

Tumour of Kidney—Myo-sarcoma.

Dr. Dawson Williams showed another tumour of the kidney, similar to the last described. It was removed from the body of an infant aged thirteen months, who died in the Victoria Hospital for Children. The child had been under the care of Mr. Walter Pye, but was moribund when admitted, and died of exhaustion. Post-mortem, a tumour weighing 1 lb. 13 oz. (equivalent to about one-sixth of the total body-weight) was found taking the place of the right kidney. It was completely encapsuled, and the ureter could be traced into its inner aspect. Microscopically, it was found to have a fibrillated structure. The fibres were arranged in bundles, which crossed and interlaced in every place. Some of these fibres were slightly spindle-shaped, and gave an indication of a nucleus. Others, however, were elongated, in some cases branched, and in most cases showing transverse striation, as in voluntary muscular fibres. In those fibres which were largest and best developed this striation was very definite and unmistakable. In some parts of the tumour, tracts of small round-celled growth occurred, intermingled with muscular bands, and every gradation in size and form could be traced between the well-developed muscular fibres and these round or slightly spindle-shaped cells. In all parts of the tumour, sections of the kidney tubules and globular tracts of nucleated tissue, which were believed to be altered Malpighian bodies, were encountered.

Mr. WALTER PYE said he could have no doubt that the fibres were really striated muscle fibres; and it was interesting to observe that in this last case the tumour grew from the kidney itself, and thus differed from the cases to which Mr. Eve had referred. Malpighian corpuscles and kidney tubules were seen scattered among the fibres, some of which showed colloid degeneration.

All the cases were referred to the Morbid Growths Committee.

LONGITUDINAL FRACTURE OF THE FEMUR.

Mr. MORRIS showed photographs of this condition from a specimen in the Lyons Museum. He thought them interesting, as that particular form of fracture had been denied.

FATTY DEGENERATION OF ONE LOWER LIMB.

Mr. CROSS showed the amputated limb of a man aged twenty-two, who had been suffering from caries for about ten years, first of the wrist, then of one ankle. He had had suppuration in one or other joint for years past, and during the last four had been bedridden. The lower extremities were equal in length, and the size of the bones appeared identical. The right leg, however, was œdematous, and the knee-joint anchylosed, while the left one was thin and wasted. He amputated in the middle of the thigh. After removal the limb appeared to be a mass of fat, with fibrous septa, in the centre of which were the bones: they were much altered; the tarsal bones were hardly distinguishable; the cancelli were large and filled with margarin. The bones of the opposite side did not appear to be affected in this way, though they were much atrophied.

NECROSIS OF CALVARIA AFTER A BURN.

Dr. ISAMBARD OWEN showed this specimen, which he had removed from a man, who some years before death, in an epileptic fit, had fallen into the fire and severely burnt himself. Several smaller pieces of bone had been removed in St. George's Hospital. The present piece was removed post-mortem; it was found loose, resting on granulation tissue. The dura mater was much thickened.

CONGENITAL ABSENCE OF ONE HALF OF THE CEREBELLUM.

Mr. A. P. GOULD showed the occipital bone of a man, which he had obtained from the dissecting-room of the Westminster Hospital. Unfortunately, the brain was so much decomposed that anything like an accurate description was out of the question. The man was aged eighty years at the time of his death. No head symptoms had ever been noticed. The right hemisphere of the cerebellum was completely absent. The spinal cord appeared quite normal. The cerebellar fossa was normal on the left side, while that on the right side was shallow, ill marked, and it was crossed by the superior longitudinal sinus; the groove for this sinus was absent from its usual place. He believed the malformation to be congenital.

Mr. TREVES thought it might be hypertrophy of the bone due to wasting of the cerebellum.

Mr. EVE referred to specimens in the College Museum, which Sir James Paget explained on that hypothesis.

Mr. HUTCHINSON mentioned Van der Kolk's case, which was similar.

Dr. BARLOW asked as to the condition of the cerebrum, whether it too was atrophied.

Mr. GOULD, replying, thought the presence of the groove for the lateral sinus over this part of the fossa was almost certain proof of the congenital nature of this abnormality.

ABSCESS IN THE HEAD OF TIBIA.

Mr. GOULD said this specimen was removed from a patient in the Westminster Hospital, aged twenty-seven years, who, fourteen years previously, had noticed a swelling over the inner tuberosity of the tibia, for which he was treated in the Homœopathic Hospital. A sinus had remained. In July last, the knee-joint having become inflamed and useless, the leg was amputated, the man being very hectic at the time. On examining the bones after amputation it was seen that there was an abscess-cavity, containing several small sequestra, in the head of the tibia, and that the articular surface of the tibia was eroded in two places, but the joint did not actually communicate with the cavity in the tibia. The walls of this cavity were much sclerosed.

CALCULUS IN A CARCINOMATOUS KIDNEY.

Dr. N. MOORE showed this specimen. The kidney was very much enlarged, and its pelvis was occupied by a calculus weighing about three ounces and a half. There was some calculoid material plugging the ureter, which was considerably thickened. There were no secondary deposits. Microscopically, the new growth was found to be epithelioid, originating in the kidney tubules. It was no doubt, therefore, a primary cancer of the kidney, apparently resulting from the long-continued irritation of the stone. The patient was only twenty-five years of age. Many years ago, when a child, he had fallen from a swing, and had complained of kidney pain, and had since passed blood in his urine, and also pus.

The PRESIDENT remarked on the analogy of this case with cancer of the liver produced by the irritation of gall-stones.

SARCOMATOUS (?) THICKENING OF PERICARDIUM.

Dr. BROADBENT showed a portion of pericardium which was greatly thickened. At the root of the great vessels it measured one inch and a half in thickness. It did not collapse when opened, and contained blood-stained fluid in its cavity. The heart was small. It had been removed from a man aged twenty-three, who had suffered from severe and recurring dyspnœa. Mr. Savory had tapped the pericardium, without, however, drawing fluid. He thought that the thickened pericardium had compressed the roots of the great vessels, and so given rise to the dyspnœa. He wished the specimen to be referred to the Morbid Growths Committee, as it had been suggested that the new growth was inflammatory, while he himself inclined to the idea of its being sarcomatous in its origin.

CARD SPECIMENS.

Dr. SIDNEY COUPLAND showed a specimen of Cancer of the Kidney, associated with Renal Calculi.

Mr. SHATTOCK showed a specimen of Sacculi of Small Intestine from a patient lately under Mr. Beck's care.

INTERNATIONAL MEDICAL CONGRESS.—We understand that Mr. Barraud's picture of members of the late Congress is now nearly completed, and will be published this year. It will contain about five hundred portraits of the leading English and foreign medical men, from all of whom Mr. Barraud has been fortunate enough to secure special sittings.

A NEW INSTRUMENT FOR LOCAL ANÆSTHESIA.—Mr. Thomas Taylor, of the Agricultural Department, Washington, has devised a new freezing microtome, and, after the same principle, a new method of applying a freezing mixture to the skin, to induce local anæsthesia. The apparatus, in both instances, consists of a hollow metal cylinder, through which runs a spiral tube. The latter is connected by a tube with a vessel containing a freezing mixture of ice and salt, and bears at the opposite extremity an escape-tube of smaller calibre. As the freezing-mixture enters the cylinder, the fluid which results from the melting escapes by the escape-pipe, so that while it is in use the apparatus will always be in action. According to Mr. Taylor, the tongue will cling to the apparatus and become anæsthetised in a few seconds. It seems that ether spray has had its day of usefulness.—N.Y. Med. Record, October 1.

OBITUARY.

WILLIAM BREWER, M.D.

THE death of this eminent physician and philanthropist ought not to pass without some notice, however short. If we may use a familiar mode of speech, he was eminent as a physician among politicians, and as a politician among physicians. We believe that he never aimed at a large private practice, but such of his brethren as had the privilege of meeting him in consultation found him extremely acute and able in his treatment, and quite conversant with the latest modes of doctrine and theory. He appears to have been a man of large private fortune, and thoroughly imbued with literary and artistic tastes. His reading was varied and profound, and there was hardly any subject he could not illustrate from the stores of a deep and varied erudition.

It was, however, in the field of political or State medicine that his services were most conspicuous. For very many years he was one of the vestrymen of St. George's, Hanover-square.

During a short period he was M.P. for Colchester, and later, was Chairman for the Metropolitan Asylums Board, established for the purpose of relieving the mass of sickness and pauperism, and combating the epidemic and infectious diseases, which are such a tax upon the ratepayers of London. In all these important capacities he laboured unflaggingly, and battled bravely with the difficulties which environ every attempt at improvement or reform. But anyone who wished to know more of the character of the man should have witnessed his liberal patronage of the Parochial Schools of St. George's, Hanover-square, and seen how every teacher and every scholar looked up to him with affection and gratitude.

The inhabitants of this great parish ought not to let Dr. Brewer pass away without some abiding memorial of his character and services.

Dr. Brewer died at his house in George-street, Hanover-square, on November 3.

DAVID FOULIS, M.D.,

WHOSE untimely death has left an unfilled blank among the practitioners of the West of Scotland, was born in St. Andrews, but brought up in Paisley, to which his father had removed soon after his birth.

He entered upon his medical studies in the University of Glasgow in the year 1862.

Subsequently he went to India, and engaged in mercantile pursuits for seven years. Finding the occupation not congenial and not suited to his habits and disposition, he returned to student-life in Glasgow, and graduated in the University in 1873.

He afterwards studied for twelve months on the Continent, and acquired a special interest in affections of the throat, chiefly in Vienna.

On the removal of Dr. Coats to the Western Infirmary, Dr. Foulis applied for, and secured, the vacant appointment of Pathologist to the Royal Infirmary, a position which he occupied until his death. He was also attached to the Hospital as Dispensary Surgeon, and it was expected that at the next vacancy he would have been elected Surgeon to the wards.

Dr. Foulis, as a student, was distinguished among his compeers, and showed a keen interest in scientific work. His appointment as Pathologist gave him rare opportunities of studying disease, and he has enriched the excellent hospital museum by 700 specimens during the seven years of his incumbency. His views of pathology were marked by keen common sense, and he never assumed the position with a partisan of any theory. In the recent discussion on tubercle at the Glasgow Pathological Society, his speech was noted as being imbued with caution and tempered with rare discrimination.

As a surgeon he was bold and cool, and students, as they looked at his calm, intellectual face and his skilful hands, averred that Foulis could never fail. His every movement engendered confidence, and showed such refinement of mind and decision, that older Edinburgh men often likened him to Syme. His operation of removal of the larynx in 1878 attracted great attention, and he was rapidly rising to the front rank as a consultant in throat diseases.

On Saturday, October 15, he operated on two bad cases of diphtheria in different parts of the city. On the Sunday week following, and for a day or two, he complained of shivering and general malaise. On Tuesday his throat was sore and his voice husky, but he did some professional work. On Wednesday morning the diphtheritic membrane showed itself on his palate, but the symptoms were not specially alarming till Sunday, from which time he sank rapidly. For some days there was reason to fear extension of the disease to the larynx, but no actual trouble resulted, the breathing remaining perfect to the last. On the Monday afternoon he died quietly and without pain, struck down by the virulence of the poison; and three days afterwards was buried at Sighthill Cemetery, a short distance from the Royal Infirmary, where the greater part of his daily professional life was spent.

His death, we have said, has created a great blank. To those who knew him best, his loss seems irreparable; and life seems sad and joyless since David Foulis was taken away, for his spirit was gentle and his friendship was leal, and he was loved as it is given to few men to be loved in the present day. Those who knew him only by repute feel the loss occasioned by the demise of a young and rising surgeon, in whose growing reputation they felt professional pride, and whose fame was extending far beyond the city of his adoption. These feelings, we believe, are taking practical shape in an endeavour to perpetuate his name by a lasting memorial, the exact form of which has not yet been determined.

ANTISEPTIC RULES IN BILLROTH'S CLINIC.—According to Dr. Bauer, in the St. Louis *Clinical Record*, these are, more especially in laparotomy operations, as follow :—The first rule is the observation of *scrupulous cleanliness* in the operating and sick rooms. If the slightest doubt is entertained as to their purity, the rooms are sprayed with 5 per cent. carbolic acid for several hours. This measure is intended to clear the air of bacteria and to precipitate suspended germs. The second rule applies to the *thorough disinfection* of all articles of dressing, instruments, and the hands of the surgeon and of his assistant to prevent contact-infection. The sponges should be new, and soaked for several days in a 5 per cent. carbolic acid solution. The third rule permits but *one assistant*, and he and the surgeon alone are allowed to handle intra-peritoneal parts. The fourth rule commands *carbolised ablution* of the abdominal integuments, but excludes the spray during the operation, as useless, if not directly noxious, on account of the rapid absorption of carbolic acid by the peritoneum, and the consequent danger of poisoning. The fifth rule is directed against the danger of spontaneous infection.—*New York Medical Record*, October 1.

AMERICAN STUDENTS IN VIENNA.—Most of the American students (says a correspondent of the *College and Clinical Record*) are making a specialty of the eye, ear, and throat. The clinical material here is immense. The finest of all is the touch course in the lying-in ward. It is worth a trip for that alone. In one course you have the opportunity of examining at least a hundred pregnant women, in all the different stages, and of applying the forceps and other manipulations, under the guidance of the professor. There is nothing that can bear favourable comparison to it in America. Excepting Paris, Vienna is the most expensive city in Europe. The climate is exceedingly changeable, demanding of one great discretion as regards clothing. Allow me to correct a false impression that nearly all Americans possess regarding the cheapness of student life in Europe. If a student attends all the courses he wishes, and obtains comfortable board, it is not possible to spend less than $100 per month. This is even calculating very closely, for everything is very dear.

PROF. CYON TURNED DUELLIST.—Dr. J. Cyon, formerly Professor of Physiology at the St. Petersburg Medico-Chirurgical Academy, who at present is residing in Paris as the editor of the Bonapartist newspaper *Le Gaulois*, was, in consequence of some statement in that journal, challenged to fight a duel with the editor of another newspaper. He received, according to the *Wratsch*, a wound in the wrist.—*St. Petersb. Med. Woch.*, October 29.

MEDICAL NEWS.

ROYAL COLLEGES OF PHYSICIANS AND SURGEONS, EDINBURGH. — DOUBLE QUALIFICATION. — The following gentlemen passed their First Professional Examination during the October sittings of the examiners :—

Ernest Herbert Schäfer, Middlesex; John Gormley, County Roscommon; Theodore Mailler Kendall, Sydney, N.S.W.; Thomas Sharples, Preston; Searle Monteith Haward, London; Alexander Willox McFadyen, Stirling; Francis Gurney Mason, Newark; William Stephen Johns, Norfolk; Eustace Julian d'Gruyther, India; Odoardo Tomaso Achile Villani, Van Vestrant, London; Edmund Eyre, Limerick; James Mayer, Ballina; aaloe; John Gover O'Neill, Hastings; Robert Currie, County Antrim; Edmond Walsh, County Cork; Alfred Ellison Muncaster, Manchester; John Oldershaw, Derby; Arthur Wellesley Wales, Belfast; Frederick Cyril Joseph Capes, London; William Henry Clifton, Wiltshire.

And during October and November the following gentlemen passed their Final Examination, and were admitted L.R.C.P. Edin. and L.R.C.S. Edin. :—

John Thomas Dickie, Edinburgh; Louis Fitz-Patrick, Dublin; Robert Andrew Stirling, Melbourne; Thomas Sharples, Preston; Henry Simpson Wood, Melbourne; Alexander Macdonald Westwater, Edinburgh; John Rusby Seymour, London; Edwin William Reilly, Calcutta; Robert Hall Nailer, Madras; James Callaway, Gloucestershire; James McGregor, Portsmouth; Edgar Eastricke Hanson, Cornwall; John Henry Whitham, Cambridgeshire; William Henry Pretz, Colombo, Ceylon; Malcolm L. Cameron, Canada; Dadabhoy Sorabji Shroff, Bombay; William Gunn, Canada; Maurice Frank Jones, Bombay; John Buchan Spence, Berwickshire; Theodore Mailler Kendall, Sydney, N.S.W; Howard Boxboro Elliot, Iroquois, Ontario; James Hayward Hough, Cambridge; Duncan McTavish, Canada; Thomas Cormack, Canada; William Ebenezer Berryman, Madras; Francis William Joshua, Cirencester; Ernest Offord Stuart, Woolwich; Alfred Llewellyn Perkins, Owen Amman; John Trimble Elliott, County Armagh; John Mackenzie, Sutherlandshire; Harold Athelstane Baines, Melton Mowbray; John Oliver Chisholm, Jedburgh; Robert Joseph O'Farrell, Galway; Michael Augustine Lyden, Galway; Frederick Erskine Paton, Broughty Ferry; John Norman Thompson, Madras; William MacGregor, Ceylon; William Bird, Yorkshire; James Ballantine Hogg, Edinburgh; Anthony Bailey, Yorkshire.

ROYAL COLLEGE OF SURGEONS OF ENGLAND. — The following gentlemen passed their primary examinations in Anatomy and Physiology at a meeting of the Board of Examiners on the 7th inst., and when eligible will be admitted to the pass examination, viz. :—

Barefoot, John R., student of the Madras School.
Betts, J. Howard, of the Kingston School.
Boswell, H. St. George, of the Edinburgh School.
Brown, John E., of the Edinburgh School.
Byrne, George, of the Manchester School.
Bury, Peter R., of the Edinburgh School.
Drury, Alfred E., of the Birmingham School.
Gemmel, Archibald B., of the Glasgow School.
Hall, W. Hamilton, of the University College Hospital.
Heyd, Herman E., of the Montreal School.
Kirby, Ernest D., of the Edinburgh School.
Ley, Henry J., of the Edinburgh School.
McConnel, H. Wilson, B.A. Cantab., of the Cambridge School.
Richards, George W., of the London Hospital.
Roberts, Sidney M. F., B.A. Cantab., of the Cambridge School.
Sharp, Charles J., of the Liverpool School.
Welpton, John, of the Leeds School.

Seven candidates were rejected. The following gentlemen passed on the 8th inst., viz. :—

Alexander, George F., student of the Edinburgh School.
Bourne, Alfred, of the Newcastle School.
Castaneda, T. Perez, of the Paris and Madrid Schools.
Dodd, George H., of St. Thomas's Hospital.
Gill, John McH., of the Glasgow School.
Godson, John, of the Birmingham School.
Hacking, John R., of the Manchester School.
Hunt, Bertram, of St. Bartholomew's Hospital.
Lowers, Thomas R., of the Melbourne School.
Logan, Robert, of the Edinburgh School.
McDougal, James E., of the Liverpool School.
Murray, Robert W., of Guy's Hospital.
Otway, H. Carrol, of St. Bartholomew's Hospital.
Steinthal, Walter A., of the Manchester School.
Styan, Thomas G., B.A. Cantab., of the Cambridge School.
Watson, J. Costsworth, of the Edinburgh School.

Eight candidates were rejected. The following gentlemen passed on the 9th inst., viz. :—

Abbott, Frederick E., student of the Newcastle School.
Banerjee, Mahendra N., of King's College Hospital.
Barnes, R. Wickham, of the Liverpool School.
Cardozo, S. Nunes, of the Madras School.
Cuff, Robert, of Guy's Hospital.
Dixon, Arthur H., of St. Bartholomew's Hospital.
Eakridge, Richard B., of the Manchester School.
Fletcher, W. W. Ernest, of St. Bartholomew's Hospital.
Gilbertson, James H., of St. Bartholomew's Hospital.
Marsden, Herbert H., of the Liverpool School.
Montgomery, W. A. Dawson, of the Toronto School.
Nunnerley, Philip J., of the Madras School.
Opie, Edward A., of St. Bartholomew's Hospital.
Phosira, John J., of the Charing-cross Hospital.
Volckman, Bernard, of the London Hospital.

Nine candidates were rejected.

Primary Examinations :—The following were the questions on Anatomy and Physiology submitted to the candidates at the written examination for the diploma of membership of the Royal College of Surgeons on Friday, 4th inst., when they were required to answer four, and not more than four, of the six questions, viz. :—Anatomy : 1. Describe the lower half of the radius. 2. Describe the manner in which the several bones of the pelvis are connected together. 3. Describe the popliteus muscle, its attachments and relations. 4. Describe the dissection necessary to expose the sub-occipital triangle and its contents. Describe fully the course of each of the arteries entering into the anastomoses about the scapula. Show how, by means of these anastomoses, the collateral circulation may be carried on after ligature of the third portion of the subclavian. 6. Describe the intercostal nerves—their origin, course, and distribution. Physiology : 1. Describe the structure, distribution, and functions of the glands of the skin. 2. What is meant by reflex action? Give examples of it, and, in the examples given, mention the course by which the afferent and efferent impulses are conveyed. 3. Describe the chemical constitution of the neutral fats, their relation to soaps, and their preparation for absorption in the small intestine. 4. Describe the structure of a lymph-gland. What are its functions? 5. Describe the microscopic appearance, the physical and chemical characters, and the uses of tendon. 6. What is urea? Where is it formed? and how can it be quantitatively estimated?

ROYAL COLLEGE OF SURGEONS, EDINBURGH. — The following gentlemen passed their Final Examination, and were admitted Licentiates of the College, on October 21 last :—

George Haddow, Galston; Alexander Bruce Low, Edinburgh; Alexander Stookes, Liverpool; Rudolph John Maas, Michigan, United States.

The following gentleman having likewise passed his Final Examination for the diploma in Dental Surgery, was admitted L.D.S. on October 20 last :—

Mathew Finlayson, Alloa.

APOTHECARIES' HALL, LONDON. — The following gentlemen passed their examination in the Science and Practice of Medicine, and received certificates to practise, on Thursday, November 3 :—

Buchan, William Augustus, Plymouth.
Francis, John Arthur, St. Bartholomew's Hospital.
Macmillan, Colin, Nottingham.

The following gentlemen also on the same day passed their Primary Professional Examination :—

Gravely, Frank, University College.
Sutton, Henry Martyn, St. Thomas's Hospital.

APPOINTMENTS.

⁎ The Editor will thank gentlemen to forward to the Publishing-office, as early as possible, information as to all new Appointments that take place.

COX-MOORE, R. W., L.D.S.R.C.S., F.S.S. Lond.—Honorary Dental Surgeon to the United Kingdom Benefit Society.

DRAPER, JOHN B., M.R.C.S.—House-Surgeon to the Hulme Dispensary, Manchester, vice J. Stuart, M.D., resigned.

MARX, [LEONARD P., L.R.C.P. Lond., M.R.C.S. Eng., 'L.S.A.—House-Surgeon to the Richmond Hospital, Surrey, vice Mr. Robbins, resigned.

REDMOND, JOSEPH MICHAEL, M. and L. K.Q.C.P.I., L.M., L.R.C.S.I., Senior Demonstrator of Anatomy to the Catholic University School of Medicine, Physician to the Fever Hospital, Cork-street—Physician to the Mater Misericordiae Hospital, Dublin, vice Hayden, deceased.

NAVAL, MILITARY, Etc., APPOINTMENTS.

ADMIRALTY.—Staff-Surgeon Bradley Gregory has been promoted to the rank of Fleet-Surgeon in Her Majesty's Fleet, with seniority of October 29, 1881.

BIRTHS.

COLEMAN.—On November 7, at Holly Lodge, Streatham, the wife of A. Coleman, F.R.C.S., of a daughter.

GREENFIELD.—On November 7, at 7, Heriot-row, Edinburgh, the wife of W. S. Greenfield, M.D., F.R.C.P., of a son.

LOCH.—On November 4, at 3, Porchester-place, Oxford-square, W., the wife of J. H. Loch, M.D., Bengal Medical Service, of a son.

ORTON.—On November 5, at 20, Lower Phillimore-place, Kensington, W., the wife of George Hunt Orton, F.R.C.S., M.B., of a son.

ROBATHAN.—On November 3, at 20, York-villas, Prestonville, Brighton, the wife of G. B. Robathan, M.R.C.S., of a son.

THURNAM.—On November 3, at Yardley-Hastings, Northamptonshire, the wife of F. Wyatt Thurnam, M.B., of a daughter.

MARRIAGES.

Purcell—Allen.—On November 1, at Eden-grove, N., Edward Godfrey Purcell, M.D., to Anne Dodman Reeve, niece and adopted daughter of Mrs. E. Allen, of 165, Highbury New-park, N.

Smith—Manson.—On November 8, at Aberdeen, Patrick Blaikie Smith, M.D., of Aberdeen, to Helen, third daughter of the late John Manson, Esq., of Fingask, Aberdeenshire.

Wheeler—Tasker.—On November 3, at Hanover-square, W., J. Wheeler, M.D., C.M., of Pembridge-gardens, to Jane Tasker, of Gibraltar.

DEATHS.

Barton, William, son of George Kingston Barton, M.D., late of Shanghai, at Ventnor, on November 3, aged 23.

Brewer, William, M.D., Chairman of the Metropolitan Asylums Board, at 21, George-street, Hanover-square, on November 3.

Casement, Henrietta Louisa, wife of Brabazon N. Casement, M.B., at Magherintemple, co. Antrim, on November 3, aged 21.

Figgins, Henry, F.R.C.S., late of Birmingham, at Crabtree, Sheffield, on November 4, aged 68.

McCaroghee, Joseph, M.D., at Chichester, on November 5, aged 3.

Spackman, Mary, wife of F. C. Spackman, M.R.C.S., at Faringdon, on October 29, aged 47.

Temple, Alfred Robert, M.R.C.S., at 1, Belvoir-terrace, Trumpington-road, Cambridge, on November 3, in his 71st year.

VACANCIES.

Belgrave Hospital for Children, 79, Gloucester-street, Warwick-square, S.W.—House-Surgeon. Candidates must be qualified. Applications, with testimonials, to be sent to the Hon. Sec., at the Hospital, on or before November 28.

Birmingham General Dispensary.—Resident Surgeon. Candidates must be registered, and possess both a medical and surgical qualification. Applications, together with original testimonials and certificates of registration, to be sent to Alex. Forrest, Secretary, on or before November 16.

Carmarthen and Joint Counties Asylum.—Assistant Medical Officer. Applications, with testimonials, to be forwarded to Dr. Hearder, Medical Superintendent.

Charing-cross Hospital, West Strand, W.C.—Assistant-Physician. (*For particulars see Advertisement.*)

East Sussex, Hastings, and St. Leonards Infirmary, Hastings.—Assistant-Surgeon. Candidates must be fellows or members of the Royal College of Surgeons of London, Dublin, or Edinburgh. Applications, with testimonials, to be sent to William J. Gant, Secretary, not later than November 14.

Evelina Hospital for Sick Children, Southwark-bridge-road, S.E.—Physician. (*For particulars see Advertisement.*)

General Infirmary at Gloucester, and the Gloucestershire Eye Institution.—Ophthalmic Surgeon. Applications, enclosing qualifications and testimonials, to be forwarded to the Committee, under cover to the Secretary, on or before December 7.

Rubery Hill Asylum, near Bromsgrove, Worcestershire.—Assistant Medical Officer. Candidates must be registered, duly qualified in medicine and surgery, and unmarried. Applications, stating age, with copies of testimonials, to be forwarded to the Medical Superintendent, on or before November 14.

St. Mary, Islington, Workhouse and Infirmary, Upper Holloway, N.—Resident Medical Officer. (*For particulars see Advertisement.*)

Stroud General Hospital.—House-Surgeon. Candidates must be duly registered. Applications to be made to John Libby, Esq., Hon. Sec., New Mills, Stroud.

UNION AND PAROCHIAL MEDICAL SERVICE.

⁂ The area of each district is stated in acres. The population is computed according to the census of 1871.

RESIGNATIONS.

Bingham Union.—Mr. T. P. Wright has resigned the East District and the Workhouse: area 19,122; population 4386; salary £40 per annum; salary for Workhouse, £20 per annum.

Penistone Union.—Mr. Charles Rowley has resigned the Silkstone District: area 8830 acres; population 5809; salary £26 per annum.

St. Mary (Islington) Parish.—Mr. Mickley has resigned the office of Medical Officer for the Workhouse and Infirmary: salary £200 per annum, residence and allowances. Mr. John J. Gordon has resigned the office of Assistant Medical Officer: salary £100 per annum, residence and allowances.

APPOINTMENTS.

Knaresborough Union.—Arthur O. Wiley, L.R.C.S. Ire., L.R.C.P. Edin., to the Scriven District. Martin C. Sweeting, M.R.C.S. Eng., L.R.C.P. Edin., to the Workhouse.

Liverpool Parish.—John G. Barns, L.R.C.P. Lond., M.R.C.S. Eng., as Assistant Medical Officer.

Orsett Union.—Alfred H. Mason, L.R.C.P. Edin., L.F.P.&S. Glasg., to the South Ockendon District.

Spalding Union.—John K. Brigham, M.D. and M.C. Ire., to the Pinchbeck District.

Reading Union.—Henry S. Little, M.R.C.S. Eng., L.S.A., to the First District.

At the examination for the degree of Doctor of Medicine of the University of Brussels, just concluded, W. Renner, M.R.C.S. Eng., and L.K.Q.C.P. and L.M. Ire., of Sierra Leone, and Assistant to the Professor of Clinical Ophthalmic Surgery, University College Hospital, passed with great distinction (*le grande distinction*).

Mr. C. C. Aldred, M.R.C.S., J.P., has just been elected Mayor of the borough of Yarmouth for the fourth time.

Deaths in Moscow in 1880.—There occurred during 1880, in Moscow, 20,807 deaths (11,667 males and 9140 females), the greatest mortality occurring from March to July inclusive—May, however, being an exception. The greatest number of deaths occurred under two years of age, viz., 7183—therefore more than a third of the entire number. *St. Petersb. Med. Woch.*, October 22.

Statistical Society.—The first ordinary meeting of the present session will be held on Tuesday, the 15th inst., at the Society's rooms (King's College entrance, Strand, W.C.), with the President, James Caird, Esq., C.B., F.R.S., in the chair. It is understood that the "Land Question" will be the subject of Mr. Caird's opening address. The chair will be taken at 7.45 p.m.

Prof. Pirogoff.—The state of the health of Prof. Pirogoff, according to the *Sarja*, published at Kiew, is in a very doubtful condition. In spite of this he is working unremittingly on the second volume of his book on the Sanitary Condition of the Troops in the Turkish War; and it is stated, that on the completion of this work he intends writing an autobiography.—*St. Petersb. Med. Woch.*, Oct. 22.

The Vienna Chair of Pathology.—The dead-lock in this election still continuing, the Minister of Public Instruction has directed that Privat-Docens Dr. Chiari, Prosector at the Rudolph Hospital, shall, during the present winter course, undertake the duties of the chair.

APPOINTMENTS FOR THE WEEK.

November 12. *Saturday (this day).*

Operations at St. Bartholomew's, 1½ p.m.; King's College, 1½ p.m.; Royal Free, 2 p.m.; Royal London Ophthalmic, 11 a.m.; Royal Westminster Ophthalmic, 1½ p.m.; St. Thomas's, 1½ p.m.; London, 2 p.m.

14. *Monday.*

Operations at the Metropolitan Free, 2 p.m.; St. Mark's Hospital for Diseases of the Rectum, 2 p.m.; Royal London Ophthalmic, 11 a.m.; Royal Westminster Ophthalmic, 1½ p.m.

Medical Society of London, 8½ p.m. Mr. Wordsworth will exhibit a child the subject of Congenital Absence of Both Eyeballs. Mr. Francis Mason will show the parts removed from a Case of Congenital Deformity of the Rectum after Littré's Operation. Dr. Robert Lee, "On the Cutaneous Diseases of Children." Dr. Stephen Mackenzie, "On Pityriasis Rubra and its Allies."

15. *Tuesday.*

Operations at Guy's, 1½ p.m.; Westminster, 2 p.m.; Royal London Ophthalmic, 11 a.m.; Royal Westminster Ophthalmic, 1½ p.m.; West London, 3 p.m.

Statistical Society, 7¾ p.m. It is understood that the "Land Question" will be the subject of Mr. Caird's Opening Address.

Pathological Society, 8½ p.m. Specimens: Dr. S. West—1. Case of Extra-Uterine Fœtation; 2. Pulsation of the Liver (living specimen). Mr. R. W. Parker—Thorax of an Infant with Rickety Deformity. Mr. F. S. Eve—Ossified Adenoma of Skin. Dr. Douglas Powell—Aneurism of Aorta, with Secondary Pouch. Mr. Pearce Gould—1. Two Teeth from an Infant three days old; 2. Specimen of Odontoma. Dr. Isambard Owen—Hypertrophied Toe Nails seven inches long.

16. *Wednesday.*

Operations at University College, 2 p.m.; St. Mary's, 1¼ p.m.; Middlesex, 1 p.m.; London, 2 p.m.; St. Bartholomew's, 1½ p.m.; Great Northern, 2 p.m.; Samaritan, 2½ p.m.; King's College (by Mr. Lister), 2 p.m.; Royal London Ophthalmic, 11 a.m.; Royal Westminster Ophthalmic, 1½ p.m.; St. Thomas's, 1½ p.m.; St. Peter's Hospital for Stone, 2 p.m.; National Orthopædic, Great Portland-street, 10 a.m.

Association of Surgeons Practising Dental Surgery (Council Meeting, 7¾ p.m.), 8½ p.m. Casual communications.

17. *Thursday.*

Operations at St. George's, 1 p.m.; Central London Ophthalmic, 1 p.m.; Royal Orthopædic, 2 p.m.; University College, 2 p.m.; Royal London Ophthalmic, 11 a.m.; Royal Westminster Ophthalmic, 1½ p.m.; Hospital for Diseases of the Throat, 2 p.m.; Hospital for Women, 2 p.m. Charing-cross, 2 p.m.; London, 2 p.m.; North-West London, 2½ p.m.

Harveian Society, 8½ p.m. Dr. G. O. Henderson, "On a Case of Small pox followed by Ataxy." Dr. Cavafy, "On a Case of Sciatic Nerve stretching in Locomotor Ataxia."

18. *Friday.*

Operations at Central London Ophthalmic, 2 p.m.; Royal London Ophthalmic, 11 a.m.; South London Ophthalmic, 2 p.m.; Royal Westminster Ophthalmic, 1½ p.m.; St. George's (ophthalmic operations), 1¼ p.m.; Guy's, 1½ p.m.; St. Thomas's (ophthalmic operations), 2 p.m.

VITAL STATISTICS OF LONDON.

Week ending Saturday, November 5, 1881.

BIRTHS.

Births of Boys, 1347; Girls, 1271; Total, 2618.
Corrected weekly average in the 10 years 1871–80, 2733·4.

DEATHS.

	Males.	Females.	Total.
Deaths during the week ...	849	796	1645
Weekly average of the ten years 1871–80, corrected to increased population ...	823·6	772·1	1595·7
Deaths of people aged 80 and upwards ...	...	...	50

DEATHS IN SUB-DISTRICTS FROM EPIDEMICS.

	Enumerated Population, 1881 (unrevised).	Small-pox.	Measles.	Scarlet Fever.	Diphtheria.	Whooping-cough.	Typhus.	Enteric (or Typhoid) Fever.	Simple continued Fever.	Diarrhœa.
West ...	669908	...	4	12	...	3	...	4	2	2
North ...	905677	3	8	26	5	11	3	14	1	4
Central ...	281795	...	1	4	2	...	...	5	...	1
East ...	692530	1	3	13	3	11	...	11	...	3
South ...	1265978	8	16	39	3	11	2	19	1	3
Total ...	3814871	12	39	95	13	40	5	53	4	13

METEOROLOGY.

From Observations at the Greenwich Observatory.

Mean height of barometer ...	... ...	29·797 in.
Mean temperature ...	... ...	43·1°
Highest point of thermometer ...	... ...	63·8°
Lowest point of thermometer ...	... ...	26·9°
Mean dew-point temperature ...	... ...	39·6°
General direction of wind ...	... ...	S.E. & S.W.
Whole amount of rain in the week ...	... ...	0·19 in.

BIRTHS and DEATHS Registered and METEOROLOGY during the
Week ending Saturday, Nov. 5, in the following large Towns:—

Cities and boroughs (Municipal boundaries except for London.)	Estimated Population to middle of the year 1881.*	Persons to an Acre, (1881.)	Births Registered during the week ending Nov. 5.	Deaths Registered during the week ending Nov. 5.	Temperature of Air (Fahr.) Highest during the Week.	Temperature of Air (Fahr.) Lowest during the Week.	Temperature of Air (Fahr.) Weekly Mean of Daily Mean Values.	Temp. of Air (Cent.) Weekly Mean of Daily Mean Values.	Rain Fall. In Inches.	Rain Fall. In Centimetres.
London ...	3829751	50·8	2618	1645	63·3	26·9	43·1	6·17	0·19	0·48
Brighton ...	107984	45·9	69	45	59·5	36·2	44·1	6·73	0·52	1·32
Portsmouth ...	128335	26·6	65	43	...	...	...	...	...	...
Norwich ...	88036	11·8	54	38	...	...	...	...	...	...
Plymouth ...	75262	54·0	52	35	58·0	29·1	45·5	7·50	1·45	3·66
Bristol ...	207140	46·5	145	74	60·4	25·0	42·8	6·00	0·78	1·98
Wolverhampton ...	75934	22·4	50	23	59·3	25·7	39·8	4·23	0·58	1·47
Birmingham ...	402296	47·9	281	192	...	...	...	...	...	...
Leicester ...	123120	38·5	79	53	59·6	30·5	41·0	5·00	0·90	1·53
Nottingham ...	189235	18·9	148	79	60·8	30·2	40·8	4·89	0·73	1·85
Liverpool ...	553968	106·3	411	302	...	...	...	...	...	...
Manchester ...	341289	79·5	249	150	...	...	...	...	...	...
Salford ...	177760	34·4	124	78	...	...	...	...	...	...
Oldham ...	112176	24·0	72	56	...	...	...	...	...	...
Bradford ...	184037	25·5	136	78	58·0	26·5	37·6	3·12	0·85	2·16
Leeds ...	310490	14·4	199	112	57·0	29·0	39·0	3·89	1·74	4·42
Sheffield ...	285621	14·5	215	118	60·0	29·5	39·9	4·39	0·94	2·39
Hull ...	155161	42·7	97	52	58·0	30·0	40·5	4·72	0·69	1·75
Sunderland ...	116758	42·2	85	48	57·0	30·0	41·9	5·50	0·33	0·84
Newcastle-on-Tyne	145675	27·1	95	64	...	...	...	...	...	...
Total of 20 large English Towns ...	7808775	38·0	5220	3317	63·3	25·0	41·3	5·17	0·78	1·98

* These figures are the numbers enumerated (but subject to revision) in
April last, raised to the middle of 1881 by the addition of a quarter of a
year's increase, calculated at the rate that prevailed between 1871 and 1881.

At the Royal Observatory, Greenwich, the mean reading
of the barometer last week was 29·80 in. The highest was
30·06 in. on Sunday evening, and the lowest 29·59 in. on
Thursday afternoon.

NOTES, QUERIES, AND REPLIES.

Is that questioneth much shall learn much.—Bacon.

First Prosecution under the New Malt Act.—At Halesowen, a brewer, of
Shelton, Birmingham, has been fined £20 for defrauding the Inland
Revenue by neglecting to enter in a book sixteen pounds of sugar used
in brewing. Defendant denied using the sugar, and the analytical
chemist stated that the ale possessed 1 per cent. of glucine, which, not
being entered, was a fraud under the new Act. It transpired that this
was the first case of the kind under the Act.

St. Thomas's Hospital.—It is stated that the governors have determined
to ask the Duke of Edinburgh to allow himself to be nominated for
election as President.

"State Medicine."—This study—hitherto not much encouraged—is making
progress, as the Cambridge University examinations show. At the
examination just concluded at the University for certificates in "State
Medicine," there were about fifty candidates. Surprise may be expressed
that the proper training for the public medical officer was not earlier
provided for.

The Summoning a Coroner's Jury.—At St. Bartholomew's Hospital, last
week, there was a difficulty in getting the necessary number of jurymen
to serve, and the question arose as to service of the summonses. In two
cases they had not been personally served, but left in the office letter-
boxes on the Saturday afternoon, and were not seen till the following
Monday morning.

A Grievance Removed.—A circular, just issued by the Lords of the Admiralty, removes a grievance, on the part of the Naval Medical Service,
of long standing. The obligation of doctors to transmit to the Medical
Director-General of the Navy duplicates of the Service certificates of
conduct given them by their commanding officers, is dispensed with.

A Novel Objection.—A Jew, on being summoned to serve as a juror at an
inquest held recently by Mr. Payne, the City Coroner, pleaded, as an
excuse for non-attendance, that he was "A descendant of Aaron the
high priest, and was prohibited to be in the presence of a dead body
other than that of one of the nearest kindred." These being several
other members of the Jewish persuasion on the jury, the Coroner inquired
whether it was true that the objector was prohibited from performing
this public duty as he asserted, and their unanimous reply was in the
negative. "If," remarked one Hebrew, "he were a priest and a
descendant of Aaron, he would be precluded from serving, but his name
shows that he is not."

Deaths of Infants.—Mr. S. F. Langham, Deputy-Coroner for East Surrey,
held on the 4th inst. three inquests on infants [who had been found
dead in bed by their parents.

Anglosaxe.—The disposition to disease in differences of race in countries
inhabited by mixed races is very remarkable; for example, in the United
States the English and Welsh seem more liable to be affected with
scarlet fever, diphtheria, croup, apoplexy, and paralysis, and enjoy a
comparative immunity from consumption, typhoid and typhus fevers.
Among the Irish there is a marked liability to consumption, and an
extraordinary mortality from Bright's disease. The Germans show a
comparative immunity from consumption, scrofula, and cancer, and a
decided liability to small-pox, typhoid and typhus fevers, and other
febrile affections. The Swedes, Danes, and Norwegians exhibit a greater
tendency to dysentery, diarrhœa, typhoid and other fevers, with a remarkable exemption from apoplexy, paralysis, cancer, Bright's disease,
and bronchitis.

The Order of St. John, Jerusalem.—The supply of diets granted to convalescent patients of the Charing-cross and King's College Hospitals
has now been extended by the Order to the Royal Free Hospital, Gray's-
inn-road, and the Finsbury Dispensary.

Doctors' Doorplates in America.—We take the following from a Canadian
contemporary:—
"Anent doctors' signs, the *New York Record* says:—'The brazen sign is
large; it covers the whole door-post, it stretches from window to window;
its lettering is brilliant, and it is set off with scroll-work in the corners;
the passer-by sees it, and cannot but read it; small boys shout out the
name as they go by, and adults mutter it over till they reach another block.
It is judiciously placed so that the street-lamp illumines it at night. It
affects the more public ways, and it indicates the astute and enterprising
physician. He is one who maintains a dignified composure between the
code which says, "Thou shalt not advertise," and the Bible which says,
"Let thy light so shine." In these days, when æstheticism is in the
ascendant, when every man of thorough culture lunches at least once a
week on the sight of a lily, it would be strange if a love of the beautiful
did not affect the style of that corner slab of modern civilisation—the
subject of this discourse. The æsthetic sign, in its apparent development,
consists of a black marble slab, in which the physician's name is carved
and gilded. When especially "intense," the letters are old Roman, with
golden punctuation marks, which delicately suggest to the looker-on that
he come to a full stop. Some superficial critics have already classified
these evidences of the union of the beautiful with the pilular, as "mortuary signs"—a name which is uncanny, and which stamps its user as a
Philistine.'"

Cookery Training.—An interesting special report on the position and prospects of practical cookery in our public elementary girls' schools has just been issued by the Committee of the Liverpool Training School of Cookery. The neglect into which instruction in cookery has fallen in these institutions is properly complained of, and some striking examples of successful attempts to establish efficient cookery classes without the assistance of the Boards are given. The pamphlet will well repay reading.

Good Templar.—Some complaint has lately been made that what are called temperance drinks contain a good deal of alcohol, but the percentage, although larger than is usually supposed, is insufficient to produce drunkenness. The new liquor law for Holland came into operation on the 1st inst. Its principal points are—adaptation of the number of drinking-houses to the population of every township; forbidding sale of liquor in unlicensed houses; and an increased malt-tax.

U. N. O., Essex.—The pamphlet entitled "How Baby was Saved" is intended as an antidote to a little story which the anti-vaccinators are actively circulating under the title "How Baby was Killed."

The Coffee-house Movement, Edinburgh.—By the annual report of the Edinburgh Coffee-house Company it was shown that, pecuniarily, the results of the past year had not been so great a success as anticipated, and in consequence no dividend would be declared. It is fully believed, however, that a good foundation for the future has been laid. The receipts were £609 10s. 5d., the donations £87, while the expenditure was £678 11s. 4d.

Anti-Vaccination Demonstration, Eastbourne.—In lieu of payment of fines under the Vaccination Acts the police last week seized a chest of tea and a mahogany couch, the property of Messrs. P. and S. Luck, which were submitted to public auction in the town. In the evening a procession, accompanied by a brass band, paraded the principal streets, followed by a large portion of the inhabitants. During the route the Compulsory Vaccination Acts and all who upheld them were denounced.

HORÆ SUBSECIVÆ MEDICÆ-PHYSICÆ.

"*Nec desit ponderis hilum.*"—Lucretius.

TO THE EDITOR OF THE MEDICAL TIMES AND GAZETTE.

SIR,—Visiting lately a friend, who is at the same time a zealous florist and consummate Latinist, I found him in his garden, where he called my attention to the curious fact that, of the five sepals of the rose, two have the entire margin serrated, two have smooth margin, and one has one-half of the leaf with smooth, and the other half with serrated margin; and repeated the following lines, which were new to me, and which, as they may be so also to many of the readers of the *Medical Times and Gazette*, I will here transcribe:—

"Quinque erant fratres in eodem tempore nati;
Duo erant barbati; duo sine barbâ nati;
Et alter qui manebat, solum medium barbam tenebat."

How many of our medical students and of the English Navy surgeons of to-day have read "Roderick Random"? To those who have not done so I advise the perusal. Such a state of medical education and of general society as Smollett pictures existed until a much later period than is generally supposed. I and many of us knew individuals who were traditional depositories of that order of things. There is much to be learnt from the desultory reading of old literature. The other day, in reading Fielding's "Humphry Clinker," I saw that the alcoholic treatment was employed in Scotland in the last century in small-pox. Here in San Paulo, from time immemorial the popular and successful treatment of measles has consisted in the administration of rum with canine excrement, with a severe diet for forty days, as to food and exposure to cold. The use of beef within the time named by a convalescent from measles is followed often by death from intractable diarrhœa, and always by serious chronic intestinal suffering.

From the Rio journals I learn that the Brazilian Government has communicated to that of England the experiments made in the Emperor's presence by Dr. John Baptist de Lacerda with permanganate of potash in hypodermic or venous injections as an antidote to snake-venom. He uses a 1 per cent. solution, injecting in the vicinity of the wound the contents of a Pravas syringe four times repeated.

Are English physicians in the habit of prescribing an infusion of senna prepared from follicules, previously treated by alcohol in order to extract the resin, to which, or to its oxidation, the griping quality of senna is due? The famous and unfortunate quack (broken on the wheel at Venice), the Count de St. Germain, gave his name to a preparation of senna which owes its virtues to this manipulation with alcohol, and subsequent washing and drying.

An example of the recognition of the value of the old medicine in our sceptical days is to be found in the rehabilitation of cochineal as a therapeutic agent—a cardiac sedative, and a valuable remedy in certain cases of diseased kidney. May not the virtues of this insect be derived from the juices of the cactus on which it feeds, and from which it derives its colour? The *Cactus grandiflora* is, in the form of tincture, much used here in heart-ailments as a sedative.

Will any dentist or physiologist do me the favour to say if the extraction of carious milk-teeth prejudices in any way the growth or normal formation of the second or permanent teeth? I propose the question because, having, as the family physician, directed the extraction of some painful decayed teeth in a child of five years of age, the dentist who was called to perform the operation refused, alleging that by so doing the matrix of the growing permanent teeth would be injured.

Is there any inconvenience in prescribing conjointly in an 8-oz. mixture half an ounce of cherry-laurel water and two drachms of bicarbonate of soda? I inquire, because I heard a physician-graduate, it is true, of Rostock—say that in this way a poisonous combination might be formed. I remained silent, as is my wont when I hear any proposition made which seems to me strange, and as to which I cannot quote an authoritative decision.

Is the milk of a pregnant woman considered in England to be productive of injury to the child who receives it from the breast? Here, such milk is absolutely poisonous.

I have already mentioned in this journal a substance called in Portuguese *Viegrino*, from a Dr. Vieyra, who was the chief means of its introduction to the notice of the profession. I again speak of it, recommending it strongly as a substitute for quinine in all cases except the pernicious forms of disease, in which a physician would not at present be justified in abandoning the use of quinine in massive doses. *Viegrino* is a body of the type of santonine. It is obtained from the *Cinchona ferruginea*, which is found in the virgin forests of San Paulo and Minas Geraes. The dose is that of quinine. It does not produce gastric disturbance. It is dear, being produced as yet only on a small scale.

The Brazilian Government is taking measures to promote in Brazil the culture of the quinine-yielding cinchona, with a view to the increase of articles of exportation, and so of the national wealth.

I am, &c., RICHARD GUMBLETON DAUNT, M.D. Edin.,
Brazilian Citizen.

Campinas, San Paulo, Brazil, September 1, 1881.

COMMUNICATIONS have been received from—

DR. SIMON, Birmingham; THE SECRETARY OF THE CAMBRIDGE MEDICAL SOCIETY; Dr. LEWIS KIDD, London; Messrs. STRUVE AND Co., Brighton; Mr. B. J. TUCK, Seaford; Mr. H. A. LEDIARD, Carlisle; Dr. WOLFE, Glasgow; THE SECRETARY OF THE HARVEIAN SOCIETY, London; Dr. LINDSAY STEVEN, Glasgow; Professor T. G. STEWART, Edinburgh; THE REGISTRAR OF THE APOTHECARIES' HALL, London; Dr. WILLOUGHBY, London; Mr. NUNNELEY, Leeds; THE DIRECTOR OF THE ANTHROPOLOGICAL INSTITUTE OF GREAT BRITAIN AND IRELAND; Mr. BOWES, London; Mr. H. A. ALLBUTT, Leeds; Mr. J. ROUSE, London; Professor S. SHAND, Aberdeen; Dr. HERMAN, London; Dr. J. W. ANDERSON, Glasgow; Mr. J. CHATTO, London; THE HONORARY SECRETARY OF THE MEDICAL SOCIETY OF LONDON; Mr. T. STONE, London; THE HONORARY SECRETARY OF THE PATHOLOGICAL SOCIETY OF LONDON; THE SECRETARY OF THE STATISTICAL SOCIETY, London; Messrs. STREET AND Co., London; Mr. J. PUZEY, Liverpool; Mr. BECHER, London; THE SECRETARY OF THE RICHMOND HOSPITAL, Surrey; THE SECRETARY OF THE KING AND QUEEN'S COLLEGE OF PHYSICIANS IN IRELAND; Dr. COLQUHOUN, London; Dr. CHARTERIS, Glasgow; Dr. MACNAMARA, Kensington; THE SECRETARY OF THE ROYAL INSTITUTION, London; Dr. J. W. MOORE, Dublin; THE SECRETARY OF THE ROYAL COLLEGE OF PHYSICIANS, Edinburgh; Dr. HUGHLINGS-JACKSON, London; Dr. CRICHTON BROWNE, London; Mr. CHAVASSE, Birmingham; Mr. H. CRAIGIE, London; Dr. DRUITT, London; Dr. G. HARLEY, London; Dr. W. RENNER, London; Mr. C. O. ALDRED, Yarmouth; Professor SPENCE, Edinburgh; Messrs. F. NEWBERY AND SONS, London.

BOOKS, ETC., RECEIVED—

Zoological Atlas: Anatomy of Invertebrates, by D. M'Alpine, F.C.S.—Contributions to the Study of the Toxicology of Cardiac Depressants, by Edward T. Reichert, M.D.—On the Physical Examination of the Mouth and Throat, by G. V. Poore, M.D.—Om Typhus Exanthematicus, of Dr. F. W. Warfvinge—On the Diagnosis of Abscess of the Liver, by M. C. Furnell, M.D., F.R.C.S.—Chemical Laboratories at the Owens College, Manchester, by H. E. Roscoe, B.A., F.R.S.—The Care of the Body, by W. T. Gairdner, M.D.—The Brain and its Functions, by J. Luys—Historical Sketch of the Medical Societies of Baltimore, Md., from 1730 to 1880, by G. Lane Taneyhill, A.B., M.D.—The Transactions of the Edinburgh Obstetrical Society, vol. vi.—The Influence of Barometric Changes upon the Body in Health and Disease, by Andrew H. Smith, M.D. New York—Report on the Health of the Borough of Birmingham for the Quarter ending October 1, 1881—Mittheilungen aus dem Kaiserlichen Gesundheitsamte, von Dr. Struck—Report on the Sanitary Condition and Vital Statistics of the Parish of St. Matthew, Bethnal-green, during the Year 1880-81—On Chorea, by Octavius Sturges, M.D.—An Index of Surgery, by C. B. Keetley, F.R.C.S.—Diphtheria, by Robert Bell, M.D.—Pasteur and Jenner—Galen de Temperamentis Linacre Gant, 1521, by Joseph Frank Payne, M.D., F.R.C.P.—Table of the Average Weights of the Human Body, etc., by Dr. Boyd.

PERIODICALS AND NEWSPAPERS RECEIVED—

Lancet—British Medical Journal—Medical Press and Circular—Berliner Klinische Wochenschrift—Centralblatt für Chirurgie—Gazette des Hopitaux—Gazette Médicale—Le Progrès Médical—Bulletin de l'Académie de Médecine—Pharmaceutical Journal—Wiener Medizinische Wochenschrift—Centralblatt für die Medizinischen Wissenschaften—Revue Médicale—Gazette Hebdomadaire—National Board of Health Bulletin, Washington—Nature—Deutsche Medicinal-Zeitung—Boston Medical and Surgical Journal—Louisville Medical News—Practitioner—Edinburgh Medical Journal—Literary Microcosm—Chicago Medical Review—Therapeutic Gazette—Routledge's Christmas Number—North Carolina Medical Journal—Archives de Neurologie—Student's Journal and Hospital Gazette—Philadelphia Medical Times.

ADMINISTRATION OF IODIDE OF POTASSIUM AND THE VARIOUS BROMIDES.—Dr. Seguin has found that, on mixing the iodide and water in equal parts by weight, a loss of one-fifth of volume takes place: that is to say, a drop of the solution only contains four-fifths of a grain. A patient who takes 100 drops does not get, as is commonly supposed, 100 grains of the salt, but only eighty of this solution. Dr. Seguin directs that a definite number of drops be given in a liberal quantity of Vichy water, and, when this is not obtainable, with a spoonful of Vichy effervescing salts in a glass of cold water; or, if Vichy cannot be procured, a good-sized pinch of bicarbonate of soda should be added to a glass of water. The advantages which he believes are derived from administering these substances in weak alkaline waters, surcharged with carbonic acid, are the diminution of gastro-intestinal irritation, so that very large doses fail to excite this, and the nauseous taste is greatly masked. He prefers administering these remedies thus on an empty stomach.—*New York Med. Record*, October 22.

AN ADDRESS ON
THE SANITARY CONDITION AND LAWS OF MEDIÆVAL AND MODERN LONDON.

Delivered before the Society of Medical Officers of Health, October, 1881.

By JOHN W. TRIPE, M.D., M.R.C.P. Ed.,
President of the Society.

(Concluded from page 570.)

I now approach the most doubtful part of my subject—viz., the population and death-rates of mediæval London. The bills of mortality originally embraced the ninety-seven parishes within the city walls, and the sixteen parishes without the walls, which were within the liberties of the City. The out parishes were originally nine, but were increased in 1626 by the addition of the city of Westminster, and in 1636 by the further addition of Islington, Lambeth, Stepney, Newington, Hackney, and Redriff. The calculated population within the bills was variously estimated, as Graunt in 1665 believed there were 460,000 inhabitants, Sir W. Perry estimated it at about 650,000, and others a much larger number. Graunt's calculation was based on one fact only—viz., that three persons died out of eleven families per annum in some of the City parishes. He then averaged the space built over as having fifty-four families in a hundred yards square, and thus concluded that there were 48,000 families, each consisting on an average of eight persons, including apprentices and servants. It is obvious that such a calculation as this could not afford a reliable total. Besides which, Barrington states, as the result of a census of a City parish near the end of the seventeenth century, that there were only six persons in each house, which is below the present average for all London. The inscription on the Monument states that 13,200 dwelling-houses placed on 436 acres were destroyed by fire. There were seventy-eight acres of the City left untouched, which would give about 2275 more houses, making a total of 15,475 houses. It is also stated (see Brayley) that nearly 4000 more houses were built in the vacant spaces left by the fire, which would increase the total to 19,475 houses within the walls. Now, the census of 1801 showed that there were then only 8738 houses within the walls, and a population of 63,832 persons. It is admitted by all writers of the eighteenth century that the population of London proper decreased during that century, so that we may fairly assume that in 1665 it was rather considerably (say 20,000) above that number. Sir W. Petty stated that there were 11,053 houses within the walls in 1665, but even this must have been in excess of the true number. At six to a house this would give a population of 77,000 persons, and Graunt says there were 12,000 families in the City in 1635, which at five and a half to a family would give 66,000. There was, however, a census made in 1631 of the population residing in the City wards, by which the number was returned at 130,178. This included the population in the wards of Bridge Without, Cripplegate Without, and Farringdon Without, which numbered 45,951 persons. In addition, there were those residing in Bishopsgate Without, the part of Aldersgate, and also of Portsoken without the walls, giving an estimated total of 54,396 persons to be deducted from the 130,178, leaving 75,782 persons as residing within the City walls. The mean annual number of deaths registered during the sixty-three years 1604-66, inclusive of the plague, was 3181, and, with 20 per cent. added on for deaths not registered by the parish clerk, we get an annual total of 3727 deaths. These divided by the population give an annual death-rate of 49·2 per 1000 population amongst the residents within the walls of the City. I am aware that, to a certain extent, the results are unsatisfactory but after every considerable search amongst old writers and the bills of mortality, they are the best I can give.

I now propose making a great leap and commencing my account of the sanitary condition of Modern London at the year 1834, when a Committee of the House of Commons

inquired into the administration of the sewers rate of the metropolis. It appeared from their report that other sewer authorities had recently sprung into existence in London, and obtained powers from Parliament to drain the districts which were not included in the 23rd Henry VIII., cap. 5. In carrying out their schemes, the newly appointed Commissioners did not provide separate outlets to the Thames, but in most cases connected their system of sewers with those constructed in the City for carrying off the local drainage. The Committee reported that there was a want of system or combination between different trusts which had led to much inconvenience, for where the line of communication with the Thames was not complete, the improvements in one district had proved injurious to another. Thus, the enlarged sewers in the Holborn and Finsbury division having been connected with the City sewers, the latter became inadequate to carry off their contents, and led to the inundation of numerous houses in the vicinity of the river, by forcing back the sewage of these houses, and even caused a silting up of many of the small City sewers. The City Engineer also complained that a sewer taking water from the Tower Hamlets was connected with the Irongate City sewer, compelling the City Commissioners to rebuild it at a great expense. At this time Cheapside and Leadenhall-street were not sewered, as they formed the highest ground, and had cesspools for excrementitious matters. As these cesspools were dug through the clay or loam down to the gravel, the whole of the fluids percolated into the earth, as it was said, "for the benefit of the water drinkers." One witness also stated that whilst all the inhabitants paid sewer-rates, persons were not allowed to make a connexion with a sewer except on payment of 17s. 6d.; that no one was compelled to drain his house; and when he did, he was forbidden under a penalty to connect his privy cesspool, even as an overflow, with the sewer. As an illustration of the large areas left undrained, I will quote from the evidence of Mr. James Peake to the Commissioners of Sewers. When asked if there was any sewer from Virginia Row to Shoreditch, a mile in extent, also as regards numerous courts in Whitechapel, he replied there was none. Speaking of the first-named area, he said, "I cannot speak as to the state of the inhabitants; I know it is very wretched. The whole of this land was excavated for brickmaking, and has been reduced to an unnatural level"; and as regards the latter, that it is the filthiest place imaginable, and densely populated. But he added that he did not consider it to be any part of his duty to alter or carry up a sewer with reference to the health of the inhabitants, but only as regards the necessities of the adjoining property. Is it to be wondered at that typhoid fever, diarrhœa, and similar diseases made these localities their permanent place of abode? The Commissioners of Sewers not only neglected to make sewers where they were most urgently required, but when asked to trap the inlets to those already made, they decided that the "stink should not be kept down," as the sewers must have vents somewhere, and it was better to have them in the streets than in the houses. The regulations also of the different Commissions were not the same, so that a man having property in Finsbury, Westminster, the City, or Tower Hamlets might find himself subject to a penalty for acting in the same manner in all these divisions of London. There was, however, one fortunate circumstance arising out of these divisions, viz., that Mr. Roe, the engineer to the Holborn and Finsbury Commissioners, was a scientific and practical man, who made the new sewers in his district of an egg-shape instead of a circular form, and thus proved, before the Metropolitan Board of Works began their system of drainage, that the egg-shape, or a slight modification thereof, is the best form for making sewers. He also pointed out the ease with which sewers can be cleansed by flushing with water.

Evidence was also given at the same Commission as to the condition and construction of house-drains, which, I am sorry to say, is applicable to a large number of drains at present. In answer to questions, it was stated that the builders generally put in the drains anyhow, so that sewer-gas frequently found its way into the houses; that, in his (Mr. Oldfield's) opinion, house-drains should be made entirely by the persons in charge of the sewers, or under the immediate control of officers having competent skill; and that drains should not be covered up until they had been thoroughly examined by these officers. If this were done even now, much suffering and many deaths would be prevented.

This inquiry, supplemented by the labours of Dr. Southwood Smith, Mr. Edwin Chadwick, and many others, having made manifest the evils arising out of the imperfect drainage of London, an Act was passed in 1855, entitled "The Metropolis Local Management Act," which gives power to the Metropolitan Board of Works not only to construct and maintain main sewers and the appurtenances thereto, but also to control the construction of local branch sewers to be made by the metropolitan vestries and district boards of works. In pursuance of these powers, the Metropolitan Board have expended the sum of £5,625,969 in carrying out their scheme for the main drainage of London, and also repaid the sum of £275,000 which had been borrowed by the old Commissioners of Sewers. The sewers at present constructed not having been effectual in preventing the flooding by storm-waters of many parts of London, a number of new sewers, termed "storm relief sewers," are about to be made, at an estimated cost of £708,000. These have been rendered necessary by the extension of the metropolis and consequent substitution of the impermeable surfaces of roads, roofs of houses, and paved yards, for absorbent grass land, and the additional sewage of the new houses. It can scarcely, however, be considered that the present scheme is final, as the state of the Thames even at Gravesend is anything but satisfactory, whilst near the outfalls the stench from the river this year has been exceedingly bad, so that before long a very large additional sum must be expended in providing a new outfall nearer to the sea. Some idea of the extension of London since 1856 may be formed by the rateable value of property, which was then £11,250,000, and has now increased to about £27,500,000.

In addition to these works the Metropolitan Board have constructed the Victoria, Albert, and Chelsea embankments and approaches at a cost of nearly £4,500,000; made the Northumberland Avenue at an expense of £704,000; and other street improvements, which have cost about £5,500,000. They have expended £860,000 in purchasing and pulling down injurious dwellings; have spent £417,500 on parks and open spaces; and no less than £1,443,000 in freeing metropolitan bridges from toll. All these have been done in accordance with Acts of Parliament conferring on them the necessary powers to do these things, and in addition to carry out other useful measures for improving the well-being of the inhabitants of this metropolis. Amongst these I may mention the Buildings Acts and clauses of the Metropolis Local Management Acts, by which the Metropolitan Board of Works have control over the formation of streets, and the line and height of buildings therein, and the materials to be used in their construction. By the Act of 1878 they have power over the building of theatres and music-halls, and—what especially concerns the health of future inhabitants of new houses—authority to require the covering over with concrete the whole foundation of houses built on made ground.

They have also, under the provisions of the Slaughterhouses Act, issued by-laws for the conduct of the following businesses:—viz., a slaughterer of cattle, the business of a knacker, blood boiler, bone boiler, manure manufacturer, soap boiler, tallow melter, tripe boiler, catgut maker, fat melter or extracter, and, I think, some others. They have also issued by-laws for the proper management of cowsheds, dairies, and milk-shops, and, as regards the two latter, for keeping the milk in a clean and wholesome condition, and for preventing its contamination by any person suffering from a dangerous infectious disorder. As regards slaughterhouses and cowsheds, the vestries and district boards have powers somewhat in excess of those possessed by the Metropolitan Board of Works, which have in some parishes led to a conflict between the officers of the two authorities. The Metropolitan Board have to administer 110 Acts of Parliament, ninety of which directly or indirectly have a tendency towards the improvement or preservation of the public health of this great city. I would also mention the Metropolitan Asylums Board and the Board of Guardians, the former of which, although a Poor-law authority, provides hospitals for the isolation and treatment of those suffering from dangerous infectious disorders, and the care of imbeciles; whilst the latter, by its medical and relieving officers, provide for the treatment and sustenance of the sick in their own homes. A very large amount of structural work has also been executed by the vestries and district boards of the metropolis.

In 1874, a statement was compiled and published by the Metropolitan Board of Works, from returns supplied by these local authorities, showing that during the preceding eighteen years 635 miles of new sewers had been constructed, at a cost of £1,731,474; that 7,198,607 square yards of paving had been laid down, at an outlay of £3,038,406. Also that £709,395 was expended on other street improvements, and £587,592 on other sanitary works, the total expenditure amounting £6,067,228. They had also added 17,480 new lamps to those in lighting before 1856. The length of streets and roadways under their control was 1410 miles in 1874, against 925 in 1856. During the seven years which have elapsed since the date of this return a very large additional amount of sanitary work has been carried out; and it is as well to state that several of the vestries and boards did not make a return under all the headings, so that the total sum expended in 1856.74 was in excess of that just mentioned.

The earliest modern permanent legislation for the removal of nuisances and the prevention or mitigation of epidemic, endemic, or contagious diseases dates from the passing of the Nuisances Removal and Diseases Prevention Act, 1848, which was amended in 1849. There was, however, a temporary Act passed previously, in 1845 or 1846, to which I need not further refer. These Acts were supplemented in 1860 by an Amendment Act, and in 1866 by the Public Health Act, more commonly known as the Sanitary Act, 1866, which materially altered the existing sanitary law.

The powers conferred on local authorities are so well known that I need not allude to them in detail, and will merely say that they enable local authorities, amongst other things, to require the repair of any premises which are in such a state as to be a nuisance and injurious to health, so that within a due amount of pressure on the part of medical officers of health the provisions of some of the Artisans' Dwellings Acts need not be enforced. I think it will be generally admitted that the powers of the Nuisances Removal Acts, if actively carried out, are sufficient for the removal of most nuisances, although there are certain difficulties in the mode of procedure, especially as regards trade nuisances. I have found the abatement of these to be both troublesome and expensive, as well as, in many instances, unsatisfactory. There are, however, other clauses in these Acts which appear to have almost escaped notice in some parishes, viz., the prevention of black smoke escaping from chimneys attached to furnaces used for driving steamengines, or for any trade purposes whatsoever; the provision of a mortuary, and of a room for making post-mortem examinations, and one or two others of less importance.

The passing of the Sanitary Act in 1866 constituted a new era in sanitary legislation. It is true that it was passed during a time when cholera was epidemic; as, indeed, the Amended Nuisances Removal Act was; but it is none the worse for that. The most important clauses are (a) the 20th, which says, "it shall be the duty of the nuisance authority to make from time to time an inspection of the district, with a view of ascertaining the existence of nuisances, and of enforcing their removal." It is to be noticed that the word is "shall," and not "may"; and yet I believe that this very important clause has not been carried out in its entirety any more efficiently or generally than if the usual word "may" had been employed. I know that in several metropolitan parishes and districts a regular and systematic inspection of most of the poorer houses is made, but in others it is more or less neglected. It will be noticed that the word is "district," so that no exception is made as regards the better class of houses, or any premises whatever.

Another very important set of provisions are those which empower the local sanitary authorities to disinfect the clothes, beds, bedding, and other things, that have been exposed to infection; to require the owner or occupier of a house in which there has been an infectious disease to disinfect the same, or to do it themselves; to maintain carriages for the conveyance of the infected sick; and to provide a hospital for the reception of the sick. All these duties are permissive, except that of serving the owner or occupier of a house with notice to disinfect, which is imperative. There are other well-known clauses for preventing the spread of infectious diseases, which forbid the exposure of infected persons and things.

There is another important clause, viz., the 35th, which empowers the sanitary authority, with the sanction of the

Secretary of State, to make regulations for houses let in lodgings. In many parishes and districts this has not been carried out; in some the regulations have been made, but are rarely enforced, whilst in others they have not been made at all. It is also to be regretted that the regulations differ very much, so that what is overcrowding in one district is not overcrowding in another. The providing of hospitals for the sick by the metropolitan sanitary authorities has been almost entirely ignored, except as regards a few for small-pox, as it is considered that it is better that there should be only one authority, and that a central one, for carrying out this obligation; and it is, therefore, generally left to the Metropolitan Asylums Board. I must say for myself that I think this to be the best plan.

The Metropolis Local Management Act conferred upon the local authorities the powers of the Paving and Sewers Commissioners, so far as their own districts were concerned; and I think it will be admitted by all who are acquainted with the work that these powers have been fairly used. The amount of work done, and money expended, has been enormous, as was shown by the report to which I have already referred.

There is, however, in my opinion, one unfortunate and important omission, viz., that the local authorities have not generally made regulations, which they have the power to do, for the making of drains of such level, direction, form, and manner, and of such materials and workmanship, and with such branches thereto and other connected works and apparatus, and water-supply, and water-supply apparatus, as they shall order. Also for the making of such drains under their survey and control. If the works are not done to their satisfaction or to that of their officers, they may either alter, amend, or reconstruct the same at the expense of the owner of the premises, and summon him for the penalties provided by the Acts. I have referred to these at some length, as the power to make regulations for carrying out these important works, and for their strict supervision whilst in progress, are not sufficiently used. For want of these regulations a very large proportion of the waste-pipes from kitchen sinks, baths, wash-basins, and even cisterns, are connected directly with the house-drains, and the inlets are only protected by bell-traps, or as regards the last-named are not trapped at all. Rain-water pipes having their heads near bedroom windows are frequently connected with drains without a trap. I need scarcely say that the sanitary condition of a house in which these defects exist can only be described as bad, and even as being dangerous to the health of the residents.

The law as it at present stands, as regards the isolation of persons suffering from infectious diseases, is also defective, because the words "being without sufficient lodging and accommodation" have been ruled to refer only to the patient, and not to the other occupiers of the house. This requires immediate amendment, as a medical officer of health ought to be able to obtain an order for the removal of a person so afflicted, who cannot be properly isolated from healthy people. We also want legislative measures to make the registration of infectious diseases compulsory, and to provide additional hospital accommodation for cases of dangerous infectious disease without exposing those making and conducting them to actions as at present, provided they are made and conducted in the best possible manner, and to the satisfaction of some competent central authority.

As twenty-five years have passed away since medical officers of health were appointed to the metropolitan districts, it may be useful to take a cursory glance at the progress made. The works carried out by the Metropolitan Board of Works, and by the vestries and district boards, have already been referred to; and I need scarcely remind those who were familiar with London thirty years ago that it ought to be a much more healthy place of residence now than it was then, even although its bounds have been very greatly extended, and the population increased. Not only have numerous uninhabitable dwellings been removed, and in many cases replaced by better built habitations, which are less overcrowded, but many of the streets have been widened, and new streets made through densely crowded poor neighbourhoods. A very large number of cesspools have been emptied and filled up, and replaced by water-closets connected with the sewers; the yards behind the houses of the poor have been in most instances properly paved and drained; the houses themselves frequently white-

washed; and other sanitary works performed. Overcrowding has been diminished in many localities, and the density of the population in the City of London also much diminished. To show the amount of work carried out in my district, I may state that since 1855 as many as 6965 cesspools have been abolished; 10,898 choked drains have been either cleansed and repaired or reconstructed; 2094 yards have been provided with means of drainage; and 4513 repaired or newly paved; additional means of ventilation have been supplied for 2989 houses; and a better water-supply, or improved water-supply apparatus, provided for 5119 houses. In addition, since 1866, above 6000 houses have been inspected annually, and all those requiring it have been regularly whitewashed, cleansed, and repaired.

As, doubtless, as much or more sanitary works have been done in other parishes and districts there ought to be a decided improvement in the death-rates of the metropolis. On making an examination of the returns of the deaths registered in London I find that in the decennial averages since 1840 the death-rates at all ages and from all causes taken together are lower than they were, as in 1841-50 the mean was 24·87; in 1851-60 it was 23·77; in 1861-70 it was 24·43; and in 1871-80 only 22·79 per 1000 inhabitants. Indeed, during the last decade it was lower than the number just stated, as the population of London was decidedly under-estimated. As the death-rate at all ages, and from all causes, is not considered so good a test of the sanitary condition of a locality as the proportion of deaths of infants under one year to the total mortality, and especially to each 1000 births, I have ascertained these, and with, to me, somewhat unexpected results.

In 1841-50, the proportion of deaths of infants under one year to total deaths in London was 19·97 per cent.; in 1851-60 it was 21·91 per cent., in 1861-70 it was 23·56 per cent., and in 1871-80 it was 24·87 per cent. The annual increase for 1851-60, as compared with 1841-50, was 1·94 per cent.; for the next decennial, 1·65 per cent.; and for 1871-80, 1·34 per cent.—being a diminution of about 0·32 per cent. in the rate of increase for each decennial period. If this should go on at the same rate up to 1891-1900, the proportion would be 25·51 deaths amongst infants out of each 100 deaths at all ages. The annual mortality of infants under one year to 1000 births was 157 in 1841-50, 155 in 1851-60, 162 in 1861-70, and 158 in 1871-80. There is, therefore, no improvement shown in this age-period of the population. If we turn to the zymotic death-rate of London, and compare it with that of all England, the retrospect is a little more satisfactory, as, for each decennial period, the annual numbers per 1000 population were 4·44, 4·55, 4·79, and 3·85; or for the twenty years 1841-60, 4·49; and for 1861-80, 4·32. The reduction in 1871-80 in the death-rate from these diseases was almost entirely due to a smaller number of deaths from typhoid fever. It is true that there was a diminished number from scarlet fever, but these were counterbalanced by the excess from small-pox. To show the relative number of deaths from the chief zymotic diseases, I quote the following from the last annual summary of the Registrar-General:—Weekly average, 1840-79: Deaths from small-pox, 19; measles, 29; scarlet fever, 47; diphtheria (twenty years), 9; whooping-cough, 45; fever, 40; and diarrhœa, 43;—so that diarrhœa and scarlet fever have produced the largest mortality amongst these diseases.

Although the figures I have just given show that the fear expressed by some sanitarians, that improved sanitary measures might have the effect of prolonging the lives of weakly children, and thus eventually deteriorating our race, is unfounded, yet they indicate the great necessity that exists for protecting our infants from vicissitudes of weather, of affording them plenty of warmth, and especially of avoiding the process of so-called hardening, which has led to the loss of so many lives. Whilst, however, undue exposure to cold is to be avoided, the access of fresh air to the living and sleeping rooms should not be prevented; plenty of good suitable food should be given, and the interior of the dwellings should be kept as clean and free from nuisances as possible. The comparatively small mortality amongst the infants of the professional and upper classes, about 8, during the first year of life, out of every 100 born, against about 20 amongst the poorer classes, shows the frightful and unnecessary waste of infantile life. It was too much to have expected that during the short period under review any great improvement had taken place in infantile mortality, but it is much to be regretted that the sanitary measures, which, with better food, clothing, and houses, have so decidedly improved the health of the elder children and adults of this great city, have not also exercised a decidedly favourable influence on the health and longevity of our infantile population.

Before concluding, I again desire to express my conviction that imperfect construction of house-drains, for want of proper supervision, and the numerous inlets which frequently exist for the entrance of sewer-gas into houses, cause much injury to health, and may account to a certain extent for the high death-rate of young children. By sewer-gas I do not allude only to gas from sewers, but especially to that evolved from foul or partly choked house-drains, which I believe to be far more injurious than ordinary sewer-gas. The most common way by which these gases enter houses is by the pipes from kitchen sinks or baths and wash-basins, which so frequently communicate, as well as the rainwater pipes, directly with the house-drains. These should, wherever possible, be cut off, and if not, should be properly trapped. Bell-traps should never be used, as they rarely act as traps, and are frequently used as playthings by children, especially by those of the poor. I have dwelt particularly on these defects, because I have witnessed much injury to health from their existence, and also because the number of inspectors at present employed in most parishes and districts is not sufficient to find out and abate these and other nuisances. I believe that additional legal powers for the abatement of nuisances is not so necessary at present as an increased staff in the medical officer's and surveyor's departments to effectually carry out the existing laws.

LEAD IN FOOD, ETC.—Dr. Gautier, in a paper read at the Académie de Médecine on the "Continuous Absorption of Lead in our Daily Food," calls attention especially to alimentary substances contained in metallic boxes and soldered by means of lead alloys, which must be the means of incessantly introducing a very appreciable amount of lead into the economy. The articles of food most loaded with this poisonous metal are fish preserved in oil, potable waters that have remained in leaden cisterns or pipes, seltzer waters and acid drinks and condiments, such as white wines and vinegar. Lead surrounds us on all sides, our dwellings being painted with it, and our culinary vessels, etc., contaminated with it. The danger from this source is latent and insidious, but none the less continuous and certain.—Union Méd., November 10.

TREATMENT OF OPHTHALMIA NEONATORUM.—In an article upon this subject in the Louisville Med. News (October 22), Dr. Cheatham, of the University of Louisville, observes that the first of all indications is extreme cleanliness, no material being employed for this purpose that cannot at once be thrown away. Sponges and syringes should be entirely discarded. The syringe, especially, may be the vehicle of contagion, and has often proved a dangerous instrument for the eyes of the surgeon or attendant using it; while even in careful hands its tip sometimes penetrates the cornea. Bits of absorbent cotton or soft old cloths will be found to be by far the best cleansing material. After cleansing the eye, Dr. Cheatham puts a drop or two of a five-grain solution of tannic acid into it, and allows it to remain for a minute or two, when it will be found that the matter is coagulated and can be easily removed in strings or shreds. Removing these by means of a little absorbent cotton twisted on a match, the solution is again dropped in, and the coagulum removed as before. Tannic acid does not suffice in all cases, and then a fifteen-grain solution of nitrate of silver should be used in the same manner as the tannic acid, with the precaution of washing out the eye almost immediately with a solution (a teaspoonful to the half-pint) of common salt. There is no danger of staining the eye, even with a much stronger solution, if proper precautions are taken in applying it. When œdema of the lids occurs, it may be promptly reduced by the application of iced cloths. The lids should be previously well anointed with some unctuous substance, as the delicate skin under constant moisture is liable otherwise to become excoriated. In mild cases, sulphate of zinc, alum, or borax will suffice in place of the nitrate. When ophthalmia neonatorum is seen early and promptly treated it never need result in the loss of an eye.

ORIGINAL COMMUNICATIONS.

SOME NEW FACTS CONECTED WITH THE ACTION OF GERMS IN THE PRODUCTION OF HUMAN DISEASES.

By Dr. GEORGE HARLEY, F.R.S.

CHAPTER I.—Concluded.

THE ETIOLOGY OF THE INCUBATION PERIOD OF INFECTIOUS, CONTAGIOUS, AND INOCULABLE DISEASES—EXPLAINED ON THE GERM THEORY.

IN general it is easy enough to state medical facts, but not always equaly easy satisfactorily to explain them; and as these exentricities in the periods of incubation may be considered as belonging to the not easily explainable category, I must ask a litle indulgence while atempting to make the mater plain. For, in order to avoid ambiguity, it wil be necesary for me to digres a litle, and begin by (1st) directing the reader's atention to the fact that the posesion of a period of incubation before manifesting pathological activity is by no means the special atribute of living Disease-germs. For it is a quality equaly posesed, though in a much les striking maner, by almost every form of toxic agent, no mater whether it belong to the animal, vegetable, or mineral kingdom. Thus, for example, the most rapid of al known poisons, hydrocyanic acid, takes a few seconds to produce visible results, opium as many minutes, arsenic an equal number of hours. Here, however, the similitude between the living and the dead noxious agents ends. For, although syphilitic germs develop their constitutional efects in as many hours as hydrophobic ones take days, the rapidity or tardidity of the apearance of the symptoms is not, as in the case of dead deleterious agents, in direct proportion either to the quantity introduced or to the chanel of their introduction. For, although we have it in our power to make a dead deleterious agent kil in a few seconds, or to retard its action for hours—strychnia, for example, when introduced into the jugular vein kils in thirty seconds. While the same quantity introduced along with the food into the digestive canal does not extinguish life at al. While a larger quantity takes from two or three hours to kil. With germs we have no such power. Introduce them into a bloodvesel, into the subcutaneous celular tisue, into the lungs, or into the stomach, and yet they wil take, with but litle variation, the same time to produce their constitutional (not their primary local) efects. The element of quantity seems, however, to have some slight influence; but nothing in comparison with the element of quantity as in the case of dead poisons.

2nd. Again, while not only the elements but the chanels of introduction and the quantities introduced are important factors in the periods of incubation required by dead substances to produce their toxic efects, age and constitution have almost an equal influence. Thus, while a drop of tincture of opium will kil a new-born babe in the space of an hour, its mother wil swalow a hundred of them with perfect impunity. A very diferent mater from the efects of pathogenic germs, whose efects and periods of incubation are almost identical in the aged and in the young.

One element alone, in the case of pathogenic germs, stands out in prominent grandeur. The element of predisposition. An element playing alike its part in the control of dead as wel as living deleterious agents. But with this striking diference, that while in the case of the dead it usualy plays a minor, in the case of the living it invariably plays the major, part.

From a careful consideration of the foregoing facts, it is seen that, although the modes of action in the production of the periods of latency of dead toxic agents and living animal germs are not identical, they are nevertheles aparently under the influence of the same comon law. The discovery of the nature of this comon law would no doubt be a potent lever in the elucidation of the point now under consideration; but as it involves the unearthing of a philosophic explanation of the causes of the periods of latency manifested by al kinds of dead toxic agents, its consideration is beyond the scope of this article. So I must leave it, and at once return to the special consideration of the causes giving rise to the diferent periods of incubation met with in human infectious.

and contagious diseases, and explain my ideas of the *rationale* of germ-action in this respect.

My explanation, I think, wil be easily enough understood when it is known that it is founded upon the idea that it reqires a multitude of every single given species of pathogenic germ to be able to produce human disease. One single germ not being potent enough to produce by itself a visible local or constitutional efect, any more than one single raindrop can by itself drive a water-mil-wheel. 'Tis the agregate of both which alone suffices—in the one case to produce disease, in the other to set in motion the water-mil.

Time, moreover, is an element equaly required by both in order to enable them to manifest their power. In the case of the raindrop, for example, it is not alone necesary that it should fal to the earth and be there joined by a number of others, and colect into tiny triklets, but the triklets must unite together to form litle streams, which in their turn must unite to form a watercourse of suficient volume and rapidity of movement to turn the mil-wheel.

The time elapsing between the faling of the raindrops and their seting the mil-wheel in motion is their latent period of "power incubation."

I might perhaps have even chosen a beter form of simily than raindrops—which would be this:—Suposing a boy let loose a pregnant rabit on a litle fertile iland in a lake. At first the existence of its inhabitant concealed away in the gras and bushes would escape the notice of even a careful observer. A year afterwards, however, the first liter of the solitary doe would not only have arived at maturity, but probably propagated its species four or five times over; and now the suply of the iland's provender, from being but limited, and each rabit possesing a famous apetite, would become exhausted. Consequently, not only would al the gras disapear from the iland, but the bark of the bushes would also be consumed, and, as a natural consequence, they would cease to flourish, and the once luxuriantly healthy litle iland would be transformed into a baren waste. Al that is required to make the simily complete is to look upon the luxuriant iland as a healthy human being, and the rabit as a pathogenic germ, *e.g.*, the baren waste as the diseased body, and the time occupied in the extinction of the iland's vegetable fauna as the period of incubation of disease. In the same maner, then, as it required time for the raindrops to set the mil-wheel into visible motion, and the rabits to convert the luxuriant litle iland into a baren waste, so in precisely like maner it requires the same elements of time for the inoculated germ to produce its visible efects in its human host. For it must have time given it to hatch a brood. The brood to develop into maturity. To reproduce its species, and to multiply suficiently abundantly, either localy to produce a primary local lesion, or generaly in the bloodvesels and lymphatics to induce constitutional disturbance.

The time thus required for the development of a suficient number of germs in the human body to throw its working gear out of order and give rise to visible local signs or general constitutional symptoms, is what I regard as the incubation period of disease.

Next as regards my explanation of the *rationale* of the causes of the exentric periods of incubation ocasionaly met with in cases of infection and contagion.

When I say that I believe that rational medicine is simply comon sense on a scientific basis—that there is nothing diferent in the laws regulating the healthy and the diseased actions ocuring in the human frame, from those regulating every other part of the universe and al that it contains, the reader wil not feel surprised at my propounding my explanation of the causes of incubation's exentricity in the form of the folowing three propositions :—

1. Notwithstanding the exeedingly minute size of pathogenic organisms, they belong either to the animal or vegetable kingdom, or are hybrids; and partake of a litle of both.

2. Every species of animal, be it nude or clothed, with legs or without legs, large or smal, as wel as every species of plant, from the enormous *Wellingtonia gigantica* to the almost invisible lichen on the rock, develops, arives at maturity, and propagates its kind with a speed in direct proportion to the suitability of its surroundings. When the surounding circumstances are favorable, it multiplies rapidly; when the surounding circumstances are unfavorable, slowly. So in like maner, we may supose, do disease

germs. When planted in a favorable host they develop rapidly; and in what we term a non-predisposed host, slowly.

3. As some of my readers may think that the above is scarcely a comprehensive enough explanation of the extraordinarily prolonged periods of incubation above cited, I must suplement it by reminding them that pathogenic germ-egs, like the ova of insects, the spawn of fish and mushrooms, the seeds of plants and trees, may lie inactive, when in unfavorable conditions for development, for months or even years, and yet burst into activity when the conditions of their surroundings become suited to their requirements. It is a wel-ascertained fact that comon mushroom spawn wil develop perfectly after having been kept stored up for several years. Added to which is an equaly wel-known fact that man has it within his power not only to retard or hasten the germination of the seeds of plants, but even the ova of animals. The egs of insects, for example, placed under diferently colored pieces of glas, develop with diferent degrees of rapidity, and precisely the same thing I observed ocurs with the spawn of the frog. The transformation of the chrysalis into the buterfly is hastened by heat and retarded by cold. The hatching of the spawn of the salmon folows an exactly similar law. Surely, then, we can have litle dificulty in understanding why things like germs, posesing, as I shal afterwards show, an unusual amount of latent life— an amount almost equal to what is posesed by the seeds of plants—should lie inactive when the tisues of the human body are unsuited for their wants, and yet imediately burst into activity so soon as the conditions of their suroundings become favorable for their development. I shal say nothing more on this point at present, as when I come to discus the causes of periods of quiesence existing between epidemics of diseases, the latent life of germs wil receive further elucidation.

The reader who doubts that the germ theory of disease explains the unusualy extended abnormal periods of the incubation of contagious, infectious, and inoculable diseases, wil please to do me the favor of defering judgment until after he has perused what I shal say when attempting the explanation of the long intervals of quiesence which are ocasionaly observed between the cesation of one epidemic and the reapearance of another of a similar kind in the same locality; and I shal now pas on to the consideration of the causes of exeptional brevity in the periods of incubation.

About the causes of abnormaly brief periods of incubation I think there can exist but trifling dificulty, as a satisfactory explanation of it is extractable from examples of imensely rapid germ-development, such as ocured in the case of an experiment of Pasteur's, which conclusively shows that pathogenic germs, when placed under favorable circumstances, develop, not only into hundreds and thousands, but milions, in the brief space of a few hours. This was wel and beautifully incidentaly ilustrated, in so far as the point before us is concerned, by Pasteur in his experiments with the germs which produce the disease known as chicken-cholera. It was thus :—

Pasteur found that by merely alowing the germs adhering to a finely-drawn-out end of a glas rod, which had received them by being diped in chicken broth containing chickencholeraic germs, to come in contact with perfectly clear, pure, and wholesome chicken-broth, the germs multiplied so rapidly in it that within a few hours silky cloud-waves of germs could be seen floating in it, and within twenty-four hours the whole had asumed a turbid apearance in consequence of the multitudes of germs it contained. At the same time the broth had lost its benign, and aquired fatal properties. Thus, for example : before it had been inoculated with germs, one, two, ten, even twenty cubic centimetres of it could be injected under the skin of a healthy fowl without inducing either disease or death; whereas, in twenty-four hours after its inoculation with the infinitesimaly smal quantity of minute germs, it had become so virulent by the multiplication of them in the liquid, that the injection of the mere fractional portion of a drop of it under the skin of an equaly healthy fowl would not only produce its death, but transform its blood and tisues into a focus of cholera-germ poison.

Added to this, I may cite three diferent cases in which, after the deaths of the patients, I was an eye-witness of the astounding rapidity with which germs may be generated. In one of the cases, so rapid were the efects of decomposition from germ-development that their progres was actualy visible to the eyes of the bystanders. The first case I shal refer to was one of death from a poisonous dose of cyanide of potasium—a dead toxic agent. The second was one of death from putrid blood infection—a living animal poison. The third, a case of suden death from heart-disease in a patient of a roten constitution. In al these three cases there was a most unusualy rapid development of germs, and, as a consequence, a most extraordinarily speedy putrefaction of the tisues, due partly to the agents introduced into the system, and partly owing to the state of the weather. The details of the cases are briefly as folows:—

First Case.—Notwithstanding my familiarity with the fact that in al cases of death from hydrocyanic acid, or any of its salts, decomposition of the body takes place with unwonted rapidity, I was astonished to find that the body of what had been a beautiful, healthy, blonde girl of eighteen years of age thirty-six hours before, was, when I saw her, a green, blotched, and distorted-looking corpse, such as one sees in the disecting-room six weeks or so after death.

The second case was no les remarkable. It was that of a girl aged about thirteen, if I remember right, who died, after a few hours' ilnes, in a fulsome "Blood manufactory" for sugar-refining purposes in the East-end, regarding the cause of whose death I was requested to report by Mr. (now Sir) John Humphreys, the coroner. She, too, I saw within thirty-six hours of her death, and, like the case above described, she was a green, putrefying corpse, smeling most ofensively—like a dog that died after I had injected into his veins an ounce of putrid filtered water from a disecting room macerating trough. The girl's death I atributed to infection received from one of the blood-preparing vats, which I verily believe—although the father of the girl and proprietor of the manufactory stoutly denied it—had contained diseased horse-blood, from the knacker's yard. The whole establishment, notwithstanding that it had been furbished up with lime whitewashing in anticipation of my visit, smelt so abominably that I had to inspect it with my handkerchief over my nose.

The third case is the one which apears to me, as I have no doubt it wil do to the reader, the most extraordinary of al. The cause of the rapid development of the germs seemed to be the sultry state of the weather, more than anything else, on a predisposed constitution. On this ocasion I was present along with Dr. Priestley at the autopsy of a fat, wealthy old gentleman of from sixty-six to seventy years of age, living in a fine house surounded by fine pleasure-grounds in the outskirts of London. Where the sanitary arangements, I imagine, were al that could be desired. Yet, notwithstanding al this, and that life had only fled the body within two days, the corpse of this man was one mas of coruption. A human body exposed to the air for a month even in sumar time could not have presented a more corupted apearance. The skin was of a dark yelowish-green hue, covered with a layer of slimy moisture; the abdomen enormously distended; the face bloated out of human expresion. In fact, I never in my life saw anything aproaching to it, exept on one ocasion in the Morgue at Paris, when I saw the distorted carcase of a human being which had been fished out of the Seine after decomposition had wel set in.

Now comes the most extraordinary feature in this case. The smel of the corpse, notwithstanding two windows in the room being ful open, and Condy's fluid al around, was simply diabolical. But that even nothing to the strange sight my eyes beheld in the form of human tisue decomposition made visible. As I stood by—as near as my olfactory nerves would permit, which I should think would be at about from four to six feet distance—and watched the surgeon performing his unenviable ofice, I saw globules of gas actualy forming under the cuticle of the sides of the chest and abdomen—the body being open—run together into buls, which coursed along like living things under the epidermis. Sometimes by rapid starts, sometimes slowly. Unite together into great blebs, which ultimately burst, and discharged their noxious gaseous contents! This startling fact of the visible formation of gas has an important bearing, as wil be subsequently seen, on the germ theory. For the very esence of germ growth and multiplication, as I shal afterwards demonstrate, is its asociation with the evolution of gas, coupled with the disengagement of heat.

I ought not to leave this point without puting one more important fact on record, and that is, that germ development may continue uninteruptedly, after death from germ

disease, for many hours, and keep up the bodily temperature above the normal standard. I observed this in the case of a wel-nourished, plump servant-girl of one-and-twenty, whose body, after fifteen hours' sojourn in the cold post-mortem room of University Colege Hospital, in the winter time, felt quite hot to the touch, certainly feeling to my hand at least of a temperature of 102°. Unfortunately, having no thermometer in my pocket, I neglected to send for one and take the temperature. However, I have no doubt, from being experienced in manual temperature-taking, 102° is not above the mark. On the thorax being opened it steamed with heat, and on puting my hand to the heart it felt quite hot.

Now comes the question, What was the cause of this body retaining its abnormaly high temperature for fifteen hours after the death of the patient? I believe, germ development. The girl was wel nourished, and, ful, no doubt, of germ pabulum, for she had sucumbed rapidly to a virulent atack of scarlet fever with violent cerebral symptoms; and from the pabulum in her system not being exhausted at the time of her death, the growth and multiplication of the scarlet fever germs continued just as they had done, though perhaps to a leser extent than before death.

My views of the rationale of germ action in tisue and fluid decomposition wil be more fuly given in a book I am now engaged upon, in a chapter on the modus operandi of pathogenic germs. So, having shown with what imense rapidity germs may develop under favorable circumstances in the human body, both before and after death, I may leave the subject for the present.

From the foregoing data it is seen that the germ theory satisfactorily acounts not alone for the normal, but even for the abnormal, periods of incubation in the Infectious, Contagious, and Inoculable groups of disease. It behoves me, therefore, to endeavour in the next chapter to make it yield an equaly satisfactory explanation of the Periodicity of Disease.

AN ATTEMPT TO CURE EPILEPSY BY LIGATURE OF THE CAROTID OR VERTEBRAL ARTERIES;

WITH REPORTS OF SOME CASES IN WHICH LIGATURE OF ONE OR BOTH OF THESE VESSELS WAS PERFORMED.

By WILLIAM ALEXANDER, M.D., F.R.C.S.,
Visiting Surgeon to the Liverpool Workhouse.

EPILEPSY has, from the remotest historical time until the present, been a comparatively frequent and a much dreaded disease. Up to very recent years the subjects of it were supposed to be either under Divine punishment or possessed by devils, and the cure was sought for naturally in priestcraft, witchcraft, or astrology. We do not hear much now of sidereal combinations, and ful, amulets are still worn by epileptics, and in many districts priests and holy places are still credited with power to cure this disease.

Turning from popular to scientific medicine, we find that the symptoms of epilepsy have received much attention within the past few years. The morbid anatomy of patients who have died from it has been narrowly scrutinised by the most powerful microscopes of our most clever pathologists, and much progress has been made in this direction in telling us what essential epilepsy is not. It is not the result of a tumour, for that is not always found. It is not the result of sclerosis of particular regions, but the sclerosis is probably the result of the epilepsy, etc.

What the disease is, is still a theoretical consideration. According to some, the phenomena exhibited in what is called an epileptic fit are due to a nerve-storm raging somewhere amongst the grey matter of the cerebral convolutions. This storm causes the muscular apparatus of the body to vibrate in a peculiar manner, just as an electrical storm causes the telegraph needle to vibrate spontaneously and irregularly.

According to others, the subjects of epilepsy are aflicted with a hyper-sensitive medulla. According to them, reflex phenomena produced by gastric or other iritation causes vaso-motor disturbances and consequent changes that explain the epileptic symptoms.

Many other theories have been broached, and many of them are interesting and more or less plausible, but as the curative procedure about to be described does not depend upon any of them, they need not be further referred to.

Epilepsy is an irregularly periodic disease, similar to some varieties of insanity, hysteria, and several other so-called functional diseases. A period of perfect freedom from disease is followed by a single fit or a number of fits. A semi-somnolent period succeeds the fit, characterised by lassitude and exhaustion. Then comes the period of quiescence, during which changes are taking place in the cerebro-spinal system that will bring about a recurrence of the fits sooner or later.

In the early stages of simple epilepsy an autopsy reveals nothing visual or tangible to the most elaborate investigator. Hence the theories that supply the place of facts.

It seems, however, certain that an epileptic attack is the result of some abnormal nutrition, of some part of the brain or medulla. This abnormal nutrition, not being apparently due to a vascular change or a nervous lesion, may possibly be due to an alteration of the normal relations between the vascular supply and the nervous demand of some part of the brain. In all probability the affected spot may be in any part of the brain. Hence the great differences between the prodromata, the invasion, and the character of the fits in different individuals.

The nature of the irritation may be simply hyper-nutrition of nerve-cells, by which these cells become too active, and produce a disturbing influence on surrounding structures. During the exhaustion of the fit their nutrition is impaired, and time is necessary for them to recover their hyper-excited state. A fresh fit then comes.

Or the nature of the change may be an alteration of the normal osmosis that ought to exist between nerve-tissue and the blood-stream. An excessive amount of sanguineous fluid may be effused from the vessels, and excite the nerve-tissue of a particular part, or the waste materials of the affected spot may not be carried away with sufficient rapidity, and the epileptic attacks may somehow restore the balance. On either supposition the fit is brewing during the quiescent state.

Or the affected part may be simply hyper-sensitive, and the epileptic attack reduces its sensibility for a certain period.

On all these theories the well-known effect of regulated, unirritating diet on the frequency of epileptic fits can be explained.

Bromide of potassium and belladonna are the most valuable drugs in epilepsy, and they are generally supposed to act upon the disease through their influence upon the cerebral circulation.

From these and other similar considerations it seemed to me probable that cases of simple epilepsy might be cured through more or less permanent diminution of the cerebro-spinal vascular supply.

The medulla is supplied by the vertebral arteries. These arteries do not freely communicate with any others on the medulla, and ligation of one or both would sensibly diminish for a time the vascularity of that part. Indeed, in my first operation, I feared paralysis of the lower extremities or altered cardiac action. Educated in the " sensitive medulla theory," my attention naturally turned to the vertebral arteries. But post-mortem examinations have in some cases shown me that the epilepsy was caused by a distinct lesion in the convolutions, and in the early stage of such cases ligature of the carotid on the affected side might have proved useful. True, the collateral circulation is in the brain almost instantaneously established, but it is conceivable that the force of the blood-stream, its direction and osmotic properties, are changed by the ligation; and one or all of these may be all that is necessary to cure epilepsy. Hence the following operations:—

Case 1.—Josiah R., aged seventeen years, a foundling, has been under my observation since October 17, 1879. He had no fits for the first fortnight after admission. In November he had sixteen fits, and in December he had four fits. During the year 1880 he had 183 attacks. The longest period of freedom from an attack was from the 17th till the end of December. During the first half of 1881 he had 147 fits. During the month of June he had sixty-six fits. During May and part of June he was five weeks free—the longest period of quiescence he has ever known. All this time he was taking a drachm of bromide of potassium daily in three doses, yet the record shows that the disease was getting a stronger hold upon him, and the fits were not only becoming more frequent, but more severe.

The patient had his first fits between the age of fourteen and fifteen years; they were, he supposed, brought on by a fright at school. Nothing is known of his family history.

On July 6, 1881, I tied the left vertebral artery, the patient being anæsthetised by means of chloroform. Beginning about the middle of the clavicular attachment of the left sterno-mastoid muscles, one incision was made outwards along the clavicle for about two inches, and another upwards along the external border of the sterno-mastoid for upwards of two inches. The triangular flap was turned outwards. The sterno-mastoid muscle was very wide, and a portion of the clavicular attachment was cut through, and the muscle retracted inwards. The external and internal jugular veins were also drawn towards the middle line, and the dissection carefully carried down until the outer belly of the omo-hyoid muscle came into view. This was cut across, and turned out of the way. The phrenic nerve now came into view on the outer side of the wound, and the transverse cervical artery was also seen, tied, and cut across. A large vein ran close to it; this was drawn outwards. On clearing the tissue beneath, the large vertebral artery was easily seen and tied. Before tying the vessel the patient was allowed to become sensible, and at the moment of tying, Dr. Stuart, whose hand was on the pulse, told me that it gave a bound, and then went on naturally. The wound was then closed and dressed antiseptically, and the patient put to bed. He slept during the afternoon and evening. At 6 p.m. his temperature was 100·2°. The mixture of bromide of potassium that he had been taking for the past two years was continued.

On July 9 his temperature was normal, and never had risen above 101·2°. Everything went on well till July 15. During the evening of this day his temperature rose to 104°, and next morning some secondary hæmorrhage began to ooze from the wound. The wound was freely opened, and the blood seemed to come from some small veins at the base of the triangular flap. The wound was plugged with oiled lint, and a nurse told off to watch the case specially, with directions how to act until help came. A few recurrences of hæmorrhage occurred afterwards, but these were restrained by pressure until Dr. Forbes came, and it always ceased when he opened up the wound freely. The increase of temperature gradually subsided, until by July 20 it was normal. The wound now filled up readily by granulations. On August 6 the patient was allowed out of bed, and from that until July 21 he gained in flesh and strength. On August 21 he left the hospital, against the wish of the nurse, to go to church, and the excitement of escaping brought on a fit, followed on his return to the wards by another. Next day I sent him to bed and prescribed—℞. Ammoniæ bromidæ ℨj., potassæ bromidæ ℨij., tinct. belladonnæ ℨj., aquæ ad ℨx., —m.; ℨj. qq.h. Up to August 27 the patient had several semi-hysterical and semi-epileptic attacks. He did not " work " at all in the last four or five, and in several of them he was never unconscious.

From that up to September 28 he was up daily the greater part of the time, walking about and helping the nurse. He even watched different cases for her, and had not a single fit. He believes he is quite cured, and on the above date asked leave to go to New York with a friend who promised to take him. I gave him a bottle of medicine to take with him, the prescription, and discharged him. He promised to write to me as soon as he got over, and from time to time afterwards.

I heard from him on October 27. He has been working since his discharge, and has had no fits.

Case 2.—William W., aged twenty-five, a carter, was admitted to my wards on July 6, 1881. His father was killed by a fall from a horse. His mother is living, and he has had thirteen brothers and sisters. Two of the thirteen died in infancy. No epilepsy in the family. Some years ago (probably five or six), whilst following his occupation as a sailor, he fell from aloft, and hurt his head. He was only slightly stunned. A week afterwards he had a fit, and he was then taken to the Royal Southern Hospital, where he had several. He had no fits previous to the accident on board ship. Latterly the fits have become more frequent and more severe, and when they are severe his left arm " works " and twitches very much. The nurse describes the fits as lasting from five to twenty minutes. The twitchings of the left arm are very severe, and his head is dashed violently from side to side.

On July 6 the left ulnar nerve was stretched, in the upper

part of the internal intermuscular septum, for the purpose of relieving the pain complained of there after the epileptic attacks. Bromide of potassium was prescribed. The wound healed without any trouble, and the twitchings were lessened, but the epileptic attacks continued as usual.

On August 17 I ligatured the left vertebral artery by cutting down upon its course. Between the sterno-mastoid muscle and the scaleni muscles there is a depression in the necks of all but excessively stout individuals. Along this hollow, in a direction upwards and outwards, I made an incision about four inches long. The incision began just outside and on a level with the point where the external jugular vein dips over the edge of the sterno-mastoid. The internal jugular vein soon came into view, and was drawn inwards; next a zone of glandulo-adipose tissue appeared, and on tearing through this with a probe or director, the transverse cervical arteries with one or two veins could be seen. These were retracted to the outer side. The wound was now pretty deep, and a good light and careful retraction of the lips of the wound were necessary, as excessive or rough handling might have injured the internal jugular vein on the inside, or the phrenic nerve on the outside; while at a short distance below lay the pleura surmounted by the subclavian vessels and their branches. In this case, when I reached this stage of the operation, and scratched through the fascia covering the longus colli, no vertebral artery could be seen. I then separated the fibres of that muscle, and came upon it just below its entrance into the spinal canal. The heart did not show any disturbance when the ligature was tied. The wound was washed out carefully with carbolic acid and stitched up completely, drainage-tubes being superfluous in this region, where absorption and union are so rapid that tension does not occur. The operation was almost completely bloodless.

Just after the operation the patient had a fit. During the afternoon his body twitched a good deal, but there was no unconsciousness or other symptom of epilepsy.

When I saw him in the evening he was in great distress. A nurse had put on an elastic bandage to retain the antiseptic dressings in close contact with his neck, and had drawn it so tightly that his chest was gradually compressed until costal respiration was impossible. Removal of the bandage gave him intense relief.

On the 18th and 19th he had two fits. The wound healed up readily and without any elevation of temperature.

I saw him to-day (November 1), and he had not had a single fit since August 19. He has taken the same medicine since the operation that he had taken for some time before the operation took place.

Case 3.—The third case, and the last that I will publish at the present time, was a very unfavourable one.

Cornelius M., aged nine years, an epileptic from birth, first came under my care in September, 1880. He is also idiotic to a certain degree, but would probably receive much benefit from treatment in an idiot asylum. The fits, however, incapacitated him from being received there, and it was without much hope of success that I ligatured his left vertebral artery. Before the operation he had, from his admission in September, 1880, till June, 1881, 161 fits, or, on an average, sixteen fits per month. The operation was performed on July 13, by the same incision as in Case 1. The vertebral artery was very small, and for that reason also success was not expected. The patient turned out very intractable under the dressings, and it was impossible to preserve antiseptic precautions. The temperature went up on the third evening to 103°, and on the 16th it reached 106°. This high temperature did not affect the patient very much. He was quite lively, and very restless. The wound healed readily under the open method, and by July 20 the temperature was normal.

On July 23 the patient was very much excited, and the nurse thought he was going to have some fits; but after 9 p.m. he became quiet, and went to sleep. On July 29 the patient had a fit, the first since the operation. Up to August 9 the patient had six more slight fits, and on August 10 he had several epileptiform attacks during the day. I then sent him to the epileptic ward, as I considered his case hopeless without ligature of some other vessels, and the patient was so unmanageable that I dare not venture on further operation.

I saw him to-day (November 1), and happened to casually inquire as to the number of fits he has had lately. I was surprised and gratified to find that he has not had a single fit since he came down.

In all these cases I ligatured the left vertebral arteries. I have at present in hospital three other cases whose wounds are healed, but whose cases I will not publish for some months. In one I ligatured the left vertebral; in another the left vertebral and the left common carotid simultaneously; and in a third the left vertebral and right internal carotid consecutively. It is interesting to mention here that in the first of the last three the patient became insane after the fits. In some fits he has had since the operation he has not been insane and scarcely unconscious. This patient came under my observation for the purpose of being sent to a lunatic asylum.

I have been induced to publish the first three cases thus early because the effect has been so striking in all, because many medical men have been inquiring about the matter, and because the publication of the cases will draw attention to the subject, and the rapidity with which the utility or uselessness of the procedure will be proved will be so much greater than if I were to continue to prosecute the subject alone.

It is unfortunate that the operations proposed are so formidable to the *surgeon*. They are, however, in these days of antiseptics, very safe for the patient if undertaken by practical operators. The common carotid artery is easy of access, but not so effectual as the vertebral. The latter is deeply placed, and the place of access to it is surrounded by important structures, accidental wounds of which would be fatal. It is therefore to be hoped that imperfectly performed operations will not bring discredit upon the treatment before its utility is thoroughly tested. The mode of ligature of the vertebral described in Case 2 is the best.

The points to be considered are—

1. Is the effect produced by the operation permanent or temporary?

2. In what kinds of epilepsy is the treatment likely to be most useful?

3. What vessels, if tied, are most likely to affect the disease?

4. To what extent is mental deficiency or idiocy a contra-indication to an attempt to cure epilepsy by this method?

I do not come forward as an advocate of this method, as I do not yet know whether the success may not be accidental. I have simply stated the considerations that led me to the above operations, and their results. At a future time I hope to be able to state more facts, and I am only anxious that some way should be found to successfully relieve the sad condition of the multitude of epileptics in Great Britain.

UNIVERSITY COLLEGE HOSPITAL.—A letter has been received from a branch of the "People's Contribution Fund" in aid of this Hospital, by the Committee of that Fund, signed by over three hundred workmen and their employers (Messrs. Brooks and Co., of Lyme-street, Camden Town, Cumberland Market, N.W., and Bartholomew-road, N.W.), tendering "their sincere and heartfelt gratitude to the Secretary and Resident Medical Officer, for their generous and prompt response to the call, in an urgent case of sickness, made on behalf of a workman in the firm's employ, who was suddenly stricken down by illness." Further, they have subscribed their names in thanks to those officers who were instrumental in this act of kindness, asking that *three* more collecting-boxes may be placed in their hands, in order that a voluntary collection in aid of the funds of the Hospital may be made at stated periods.

TETANUS IN BALTIMORE prevailed so extensively during July and August as to have almost presented the character of an epidemic. Twenty-six deaths from it were reported during the period June 30 and August 3. In addition there were five deaths from trismus nascentium. The source of the wound was, in most cases, toy-pistols, and the seat of injury, as a rule, the hand. The cases of tetanus during this period nearly all ended fatally. Various forms of treatment were tried, among them nerve-stretching, but not often with success. In the case wherein the nerve was stretched, the symptoms improved temporarily, but the patient eventually died. There were no unusual meteorological conditions to account for the prevalence and malignity of the disease.—*New York Med. Record*, October 8.

REPORTS OF HOSPITAL PRACTICE
IN
MEDICINE AND SURGERY.

GENERAL HOSPITAL FOR SICK CHILDREN, PENDLEBURY, MANCHESTER.

ACUTE BRONCHITIS AND COLLAPSE OF LUNG— DEATH.

(Under the care of Dr. ASHBY.)

C. D., aged three years, was admitted to hospital, March 16. He had had a cough for a week, but on the 13th, three days before admission, became suddenly blue, screamed, worked his arms about, and had much difficulty in getting his breath. This attack lasted an hour and a half. He had a similar attack the day before admission. He was feverish, thirsty, and perspired freely.

State on Admission.—A rickety child, with slightly deformed chest. Pulse 156; respirations 68; temperature 100°. He is very cyanotic in appearance, with distended jugular veins; alæ nasi working, and sides of chest falling in during inspiration. The chest is resonant everywhere, and sibilant rhonchus is universally present. The child is drowsy.

In the evening the child became worse; respiration rapid, pulse 160. Very drowsy, at times crying out; rolling from side to side, and almost wriggling out of his cot. Died during the night, being convulsed before death.

On admission, the House-Surgeon ordered pulv. ipecac. grs. xxv. in divided doses, but, in spite of being repeated, no vomiting was produced. Hot fomentations with turpentine were applied externally.

Post-mortem Examination.—Chest : Veins of neck, superior and inferior venæ cavæ, and innominates distended with blood. Right side of heart distended; left side empty and contracted. Right lung—upper lobe: The surface shows numerous light-coloured (emphysematous) lobules raised above the level of the surface, and a few scattered lobules of a dark purple colour depressed below the surface (collapse). Middle lobe in a state of collapse, being of a dark prune colour, firm to pressure, and non-crepitant. Lower lobe resembling upper lobe, with alternately emphysematous and collapsed patches on the surface. Left lung partly emphysematous and partly collapsed, the anterior edge being especially emphysematous. Lower lobe : Upper and anterior border collapsed ; posteriorly, emphysematous state predominates. Bronchi, large and small, have mucous membrane swollen, injected, and contain tough viscid fluid. Other organs healthy.

Remarks.— Dyspnœa, cyanosis, and convulsions, coming on in the course of an attack of bronchitis, with only slight elevation of the temperature, are suggestive of collapse of the lung. The sequence of events in this case is tolerably plain. A mis-shaped rickety chest with pliable walls supplies the predisposing cause of collapse, namely, weakness of inspiratory power. Inflammation of the mucous membrane of the smaller bronchi, swelling, and secretion of viscid mucus, supply the exciting cause by completely stopping up their calibre. The experimental researches of Lichtheim and others have clearly demonstrated that complete stenosis or blocking up of the smaller bronchi is followed by collapse of the corresponding portion of lung. The imprisoned air, subject to compression by the elasticity of the alveoli walls, is quickly absorbed by the surrounding capillaries— the alveoli falling together and becoming emptied of air. Emphysema of the neighbouring lobules will take place, filling up the cavity of the chest. Thus two portions of lung are simultaneously damaged, the collapsed portions, and the emphysematous portions ; a state of things naturally giving rise to dyspnœa. Death in this case was clearly due to asphyxia. Scattered tracts of lung-tissue had been placed *hors de combat* by collapse, other portions damaged by over-distension of the air-cells, leading to imperfect aëration of blood and distension of the right side of the heart. The drowsiness, the restless tossing of the limbs, and the convulsions, betokened the venous condition of blood supplying the nerve-centres. The case illustrated the uselessness of emetics in such a condition. In bronchitis, when the mucous membrane is swollen, and there is but little secretion, as in the early stages of an acute attack, pulv. ipecac. in emetic doses constantly gives marked relief by producing vomiting and free secretion from the swollen mucous membrane. But when cyanosis, drowsiness, or collapse have set in, emetics are powerless for good and will never produce vomiting. In this case, moderate bleeding would probably have brought at least temporary relief.

TERMS OF SUBSCRIPTION.
(*Free by post.*)

British Islands	*Twelve Months*	.	£1 8	0
,, ,,	*Six* ,,	.	0 14	0
The Colonies and the United }	*Twelve* ,,	.	1 10	0
States of America . . . }				
,, ,, ,,	*Six* ,,	.	0 15	0
India	*Twelve* ,,	.	1 10	0
,, (*viâ Brindisi*)	,, ,,	.	1 15	0
,, ,,	*Six* ,,	.	0 15	0
,, (*viâ Brindisi*)	,, ,,	.	0 17	6

Foreign Subscribers are requested to inform the Publishers of any remittance made through the agency of the Post-office.

Single Copies of the Journal can be obtained of all Booksellers and Newsmen, price Sixpence.

Cheques or Post-office Orders should be made payable to Mr JAMES LUCAS, 11, *New Burlington-street, W.*

TERMS FOR ADVERTISEMENTS.

Seven lines (70 words)	.£0	4	6
Each additional line (10 words) .	. 0	0	6
Half-column, or quarter-page . .	. 1	5	0
Whole column, or half-page . .	. 2	10	0
Whole page	. 5	0	0

Births, Marriages, and Deaths are inserted Free of Charge.

THE MEDICAL TIMES AND GAZETTE *is published on Friday morning : Advertisements must therefore reach the Publishing Office not later than One o'clock on Thursday.*

Medical Times and Gazette.

SATURDAY, NOVEMBER 19, 1881.

OLD AND NEW LONDON.

THE sanitary condition and laws of mediæval and modern London was the subject of Dr. Tripe's inaugural address on his assuming the presidential chair of the Society of Medical Officers of Health. His description of the streets and houses of old London, and of the habits of our forefathers, though most graphic, was not new. Most of us, thanks to the attention of late directed to the early literature and the " history of the English people," are familiar with the mud-walls, the thatched roofs, and overhanging storeys, " the floors of clay strewed with rushes, under which lies unmolested an ancient collection of beer, grease, fragments of bones, spittle, excrements of dogs and cats, and everything that is nasty," as Erasmus wrote so late as the reign of Henry VIII.; the streets paved with round stones, down the middle of which ran an open channel, that received not only the surface waters, but into which were emptied " boles of urine and ordure ": but few, we think, have any idea of the antiquity of Sanitary, Nuisance Removal, and River Conservancy Acts; and Dr. Tripe has therefore done well to again set forth the accounts of them that have been exhumed from the records of the City. Rude as they may seem to modern notions, they ought to have sufficed for the prevention of the epidemics which from time to time decimated the population if they had not, like so many more recent enactments, been in advance of the age, and consequently remained for the most part dead letters. Such, for example, were the repeated prohibitions of slaughter-houses within the precincts of the city, and heavy penalties for casting blood, entrails, etc., into the river or streets, for selling putrid meat, and similar offences. There were laws regulating the removal of filth, the cleansing of ditches, the custody of conduits and water-courses, construction of cellars, penthouses, stalls, pavements, and gutters, precautions against fires, and others prescribing the distance of cesspools from adjacent houses. The conservancy of the city was committed to sworn "scavagers," who combined the duties of surveyors and inspectors of nuisances, the actual work being done by "rakers." The contents of cesspools and street refuse were taken in carts to laystalls in Whitechapel, Mile-end, or Dowgate, some of which were in existence as intolerable nuisances within the memory of the speaker himself.

The first Building Act, Fitz-Ellwynne's Assize of Building, was passed in the first year of Richard I., in consequence of a fire which spread from London-bridge to St. Clement's Danes. Party walls were to be of stone or brick three feet thick by sixteen high, to allow of ground and first floor or "solar," and the roofs of tiles. Penthouses to be raised above the roadways high enough for a man to ride beneath; while other regulations determined the rights and obligations of owners of adjacent property. From the frequent occurrence of fires it would appear that these rules were often evaded, and that many must have still have been of wood and plaster only. The laws against overcrowding were peculiar, consisting for the most part of prohibitions of the erection of new houses, which could only aggravate the evils against which they were aimed. The water-supply was originally drawn from the Thames and its tributaries (the Fleet, Langbourne, and Walbrook), as well as from numerous wells, public and private; but in the reign of Henry III. several conduits were opened, and water was brought in leaden pipes from Tyburn and other places. In the sixteenth century Peter Morris obtained a grant for 500 years empowering him to pump water from the Thames and to lay it on at high pressure to the houses in the city, and the New River was opened in 1613.

After the great fire in 1666 considerable improvement was made in the size and construction of the houses, but the new streets were mostly laid on the old lines. Had the grand scheme of Sir Christopher Wren been adopted, London would have been the finest city in the world; but the opportunity was lost for ever. The middle rows, however, were not rebuilt; and to the general improvement in the houses and habits of the people, rather than to the direct effects of the fire itself, we may attribute the gradual disappearance of the plague, which in preceding centuries had from time to time decimated the population.

In the absence of censuses, and with the imperfect registration of births and deaths, it is impossible to form any correct notion of the population in the middle ages. In 1631 we know that there were 75,000 within, and 55,000 without the city walls, or 130,000 in London proper, to which we may add, for Westminster, Islington, Stepney, Hackney, Lambeth, and Rotherhithe, perhaps half a million. The death-rate was little, if at all, under 50 per 1000. Indeed, all through the sixteenth and seventeenth centuries, it is probable that the deaths exceeded the births, the population being maintained by immigration. In the earlier part of the sixteenth century the causes of death, excluding the plague, were returned as fevers and ague 13·9 per cent., chest affections 24·1, dropsy 5·2, bloody flux 4·2, small-pox 5·7, deaths of infants (including teething and worms) 17·4, old age 8·6. Scarlatina is not mentioned, and can scarcely have been included under measles or sore-throat, since these are returned as only 0·4 and 0·3 respectively. The plague caused probably, on an average, 25 per cent. of the total deaths.

A hundred years later we find fevers 14·8, chest affections

19·6, small-pox 8, and old age 7·8. Classified according to age, 45 per cent. were under five years, 6·5 between five and twenty, 35 between twenty and sixty, and 13·5 above sixty, showing a high mortality in childhood, and, compared with these days, a still higher rate in adult life; the small number of deaths over sixty indicating the short mean duration of life.

Space forbids our following Dr. Tripe through the history of sanitary legislation in the last fifty years. Certainly, the condition of the metropolis has improved: the death-rate, which a hundred years ago was 50 per 1000, is now but 22 or 23, and the births exceed the deaths by 50 to 70 per cent.; but though the total mortality has slightly decreased since 1841, *the infantile death-rate has actually increased.* The proportion of deaths of infants under one year to the total deaths from 1841-50 was 19·97 per cent., from 1851-60 it was 21·91 per cent., from 1861-70 it was 23·56 per cent., and from 1871-80 it reached 24·89 per cent. Again, the mortality of infants under one year to 1000 births was in these four decades respectively 157, 155, 162, and 158.

These facts demand the serious attention of social reformers—indeed, of all who have the welfare of the masses of our fellow-men at heart. It is idle to sneer at sanitary measures or to insinuate that the vast expenditure on sewerage and other works has been productive of no result. People do live longer and are healthier than they were; more die at an advanced age, and fewer are cut off in the prime of life. It is to individual neglect and ignorance, not to general or unavoidable causes, that this fearful slaughter of the innocents is due. Among the professional and upper classes, 8 per cent. of infants die under one year; among the working classes, at least 20 per cent., in many quarters of our large town even double this number or more! Bad drainage, ventilation, and water-supply doubtless do their share, but the main causes are improper food, false notions of "hardening," exposure from sheer ignorance or thoughtlessness, maternal neglect, whether from the employment of married women in factories or as laundry and charwomen, or mere unacquaintance with the duties of mothers, and, last, but not least, the Demon Drink, the source of so much poverty, misery, and crime.

SYPHILIS AND LOCOMOTOR ATAXY.

ONE of the most interesting as well as best discussed subjects under review at the recent International Congress was that of locomotor ataxy (tabes dorsalis), and among the communications on the subject not the least important was that of Professor Erb, of Leipzig, on the *rôle* of syphilis as a cause of locomotor ataxy. As the result of his examination of 100 cases of typical tabes in male adults, he finds that 12 per cent. only had not been previously infected with that disease. Of the remaining 88 per cent., 59 had had secondary syphilis, and 29 had had chancre without secondary syphilis. This would be of little value in a community almost universally syphilised. But what is the proportion of syphilis among patients generally? Among 500 male adults over twenty-five years of age in his *clientèle*, neither suffering from tabes nor directly from syphilis, Professor Erb found there were 77 per cent. who had never been infected, 12 per cent. who had had secondary syphilis, and 11 per cent. who had had only a chancre. These facts, Professor Erb considers, show unquestionably an etiological connexion between syphilis and locomotor ataxy; and if we hold the unitarian view of syphilis, as Professor Erb is inclined to do, his statistics would show that in 90 per cent. of tabetic patients, syphilis is present as an etiological factor.

In the discussion, considerable doubt, of a more or less. à priori character, was thrown on Professor Erb's statistics, and of course it is manifest that their entire weight rests.

on the well-known clinical acumen and conscientiousness of the observer. In his original paper (*Centralblatt für die Medicinischen Wissenschaften*, Nos. 11 and 12, 1881), Professor Erb urges other observers to examine their cases in regard to this point, and Dr. Voigt has, in answer to this, recently (*Berliner Klinische Wochenschrift*, Nos. 39, 40, 1881) published statistics on the point, differing to a certain extent from Professor Erb's, but practically confirmatory of them.

Of 43 cases of typical tabes in adult males observed by Dr. Voigt, 29—i.e., 67 per cent.—had had primary syphilis, and had been specifically treated for it, 8 of them showing no secondary symptoms. Of the remaining 14 cases, only 9 gave definitely negative histories in the matter of syphilis. The percentage of syphilitic cases is lower than Professor Erb's, a fact which may partly depend on the smallness of the number on which it is calculated. Smaller though it is, however, it is much in excess of the proportion of syphilis among patients generally, which Professor Erb makes to be 23 per cent. As to causes of tabes other than syphilis, in 22 syphilitic cases, and 9 non-syphilitic, the patients were unable to state any cause whatever, while exposure and fatigue, the commonly alleged causes, were blamed by only two patients in each class. In no single case was sexual excess given as the cause of the disease, and it is to be noted that tabes occurs least often at that age when sexual excess is most common, and when the nervous system is least resistant. Comparison of the syphilitic and non-syphilitic cases naturally suggests itself, and this Dr. Voigt gives us, in respect to the following points:— 1. Age of occurrence. In both classes the maximum is from thirty to fifty years. 2. First symptom occurring. In both classes the large majority of patients complained first of the tabetic "lightning pains." 3. Other symptoms. These are in the main precisely parallel, any slight differences being evidently dependent on the small number observed. Seeing, then, that on these points a detailed and careful comparison fails to bring out any distinction between syphilitic and non-syphilitic cases, such, for example, analogically as exists between the syphilides and the cutaneous diseases they imitate, it is manifest that, so far as these statistics can prove it, syphilis does not in tabes act as a specific disease-producing influence, but as a general influence disturbing perhaps the nutrition of the organism generally, or of the nervous system specially.

Is tabes a manifestation of syphilis in the ordinary sense of the term? Then, as practical physicians, we should expect a strong corroboration in the effect on it of specific antisyphilitic treatment. Here, however, Dr. Voigt's results agree with those of other physicians. In four cases of recent tabes treated energetically with mercurial inunctions he saw no benefit whatever; in a few others there was a marked deterioration under the treatment; while in no single case was there the slightest improvement from the use either of mercury or iodide of potassium. Brine baths and galvanisation produced improvement of certain definite tabetic symptoms in twenty-one syphilitic and eleven non-syphilitic patients, and here again the general result, as well as the detailed improvements, were precisely parallel in the two classes.

While, therefore, the statistics given point to a causal connexion between syphilis and tabes dorsalis, it cannot be said that the question is more than *sub judice*.

MICROZOIC PATHOLOGY.

THE progress made during the past ten years in the study of what we may call microzoic pathology has been so vast, and scovery follows discovery with such bewildering rapidity,

that it is almost impossible for anyone not devoting special attention to the subject to keep abreast of the present state of our knowledge: the conjectures of last year or even of a few months ago being among the facts of to-day, while views long accepted as facts are as often found to be in need of modification or correction.

Not only in the fields of minute pathology, experimental inoculations, and the observation of epidemics has enormous progress been effected, but the collateral sciences, and above all the almost new study of mycetology, i.e., of microscopic fungi and organisms whose biological position is still undefined, have contributed much, and promise, while overturning many of our earlier notions, to shed a flood of light on the etiology and pathology—in short, the natural history—of infections, contagious, and infective disease. Such, for example, is the now well-ascertained fact that every phase and form from spore to mycelium of a large number, if not of all, of these organisms depend on and are determined by the surroundings of soil, pabulum, temperature, etc.; that though for mere convenience in communication we may speak of *Penicillium glaucum*, *Mucor mucedo*, *Aspergillus nigricans*, and *Oidium albicans* or *aurantiacum*, we must always do so with the mental reservation that they are not distinct genera and species, as are *Pisum* and *Faba*, *Brassica oleracea* and *Napa*, but that evolution and transmutation of species are actively and constantly at work, together perhaps with regular alternations of forms; that, consequently, what we recognise as an *Aspergillus* to-day may next week become a *Eurotium*, an *Oidium* turn into an *Erysiphe*, and so on with more than we know of at present. In the cultivation of pathophytes or bacilli the pathologist and mycetologist meet on common ground, and when we contemplate the transformation by Buchner of the harmless *Bacillus fœni* into the virulent *B. anthracis*, and vice versâ, and other similar developments effected by gradual changes in the pabulum, we are almost inclined to believe that measles and small-pox, enteric fever and scarlatina, cholera and dysentery, may be familiar to us under other conditions and in other forms as common moulds and fungi, though their relations are as yet unsuspected.

The Epidemiological Society, therefore, did well to inaugurate their new session by taking stock, as it were, of our knowledge on these questions. The President, Dr. Buchanan, opened with a thoughtful and suggestive address on "Aids to Epidemiological Knowledge," in which, after showing the necessity for an acquaintance with the general principles of mathematics, physics, chemistry, geology, and biology to success in epidemiological research, and illustrating by examples the aid rendered by adepts in each of these sciences, he traced the chief discoveries which during the past thirty or forty years have opened up fresh lines of thought in the investigation of these diseases. At the commencement of this period, when Farr proposed the name of zymotic, we were scarcely advanced beyond the notions of humours and influences of the ancients, and knew little more of fermentation. The idea of particulate matter, advanced by Beale, was confirmed by the diffusion experiments of Chauveau and Sanderson on the pus of small-pox and its allies. The guesses of Snow and Budd as to cholera and enteric have been partially established by Klein and others, though Hallier's alleged discoveries still lack confirmation. Schroeder and Pasteur as chemists showed the relations of cause and effect subsisting between specific vegetable forms and the several fermentive processes; while Pasteur, Lister, Roberts, Koch, and others have in like manner connected bacteria with putrefaction, septicæmia, gangrene, and erysipelas. Skin diseases have been largely traced to fungi, as have the diseases of the potato, vine, silkworm, fishes, and insects.

A host of workers, too numerous to recount, but among whom Obermeier, Koch, Buchner, Klebs, Kolbe, Chauveau, Pasteur, Toussaint, Davaine, Klein, and Sanderson stand in the foremost rank, have step by step exhibited the presence of bacilli, spirilla, or micrococci in nearly every one of the so-called zymotic class of diseases, have occasionally proved by artificial cultivation *extra corpus* the absolute identity of the disease and the pathophyte, and have produced modified forms of the latter capable of conferring, by a mild febrile disturbance, more or less complete protection against the graver form. Lastly, Tommasi-Crudeli, Klebs, and others have brought the malarial fevers under the class of bacterial diseases, and venereal and tubercular affections are awaiting admission to the same category.

Dr. G. C. Henderson followed with a paper, marked by his indefatigable erudition, in which he went over the same ground in detail, tracing every step and describing every discovery from those of Pollender in 1855 down to the present year. It was too long for him, even there, to read it *in extenso*, but we hope ere long to give an abstract of it. He concluded by pointing out several cautions to be observed by investigators in future; the identity of the disease and the pathophyte, he maintained, could not be positively and finally asserted unless three conditions were fulfilled:—1. The constant presence of an organism in the tissues in, and only in, the disease; 2. The communication of the disease by inoculation of blood or fluids containing such organisms, but not by blood or fluids from which they are absent or from which they have been mechanically separated; and 3. Its communication by inoculation of these organisms after cultivation in artificial fluids with no change in form or intensity. All these conditions have been realised in the case of anthrax, pneumo-enteritis of pigs, the so-called fowl cholera, and in septicæmia. The first and second only have been attained in variola and its allies, in malaria, in enteric fever according to Klebs, and in several others. He directed attention to the "pure cultivation" of Koch by employment of gelatinous instead of fluid media, by which the intrusion of foreign forms is averted as a procedure of the highest importance for securing trustworthy results, and suggested that the mitigation of intensity obtained through successive cultivations by Pasteur might be due to the antagonism of intrusive forms, just as on the setting-in of putrefactive changes the *Bacillus termo* exterminates the *B. anthracis*.

To the solution of the problem why certain diseases render the individual more susceptible to future attacks, while others confer a more or less complete immunity against its recurrence, we have, he said, at present no clue, and he expressed himself doubtful as to the permanence of the protection alleged by Pasteur, Toussaint, and Greenfield to have been obtained by their respective procedures.

THE WEEK.

TOPICS OF THE DAY.

THE position of the Metropolitan Asylums Board at the present time must be very unpleasant and unsatisfactory to the members. Not only are the Board hampered in the fulfilment of their duties by threatened actions and injunctions for spreading infectious disease, but they are also accused in many directions of a too lavish expenditure of the money of the ratepayers. At a recent meeting of the City of London Union the debate upon the following motion was continued:—"Considering that the Metropolitan Asylums District Board has called upon the ratepayers of the metropolis for £240,000 for this half-year, of which £23,700 falls upon the City of London, this Board is of opinion that the time has now arrived when a Parliamentary Commission should be appointed to inquire into the working of the Acts under which the said Board was formed; and further to inquire and report fully upon the management, expenditure, and results in respect to the establishments under control." It was urged that the Asylums Board had unduly strained their powers, and had burthened the ratepayers with liabilities amounting to four millions of money. Their expenditure was declared unnecessary, extravagant, and profligate; and they were accused of having failed in the trust committed to them, after having abused and betrayed the generous confidence of the guardians, whose representatives they were. One speaker proceeded to analyse and condemn certain payments of the Board, specially referring to the sums expended in fitting up the hospital-ships employed in the recent epidemic of small-pox. Dr. Fowler, a member of the Asylums Board, who was present, admitted that the facts and figures adduced were, from a ratepayer's point of view, exceptional. The Act under which the Board was created was a necessity, as, prior to its passing, the general treatment of the sick poor of the metropolis was most unsatisfactory. Many of the mistakes of the Board were due to the mistakes of medical science, but many more were due to the mistakes of the guardians themselves. The excessive expenditure was traceable to the neglect of the sanitary authorities in relation to non-pauper cases, and to the selfish opposition of the ratepayers. In short, according to him, everybody was in fault but the Asylums Board. Eventually the debate was adjourned.

The next census in France is to be taken before the end of the present year, and, for the first time, is to be got through in a single day. It is intended to show sex, age, birthplace, nationality, status (whether married, etc.), and occupation. The intention now expressed is to fix the next census for the year 1885, on the ground that most countries take the census in years ending with 5. Hitherto the forms have been filled in by municipal officers, who have been allowed a margin of several weeks, but forms are now to be delivered to the heads of families a few days before the date of the census.

The authorities of Cambridge University have decided that the examinations for medical and surgical degrees shall commence on the following days:—First M.B. Examination, Tuesday, December 13; Second M.B. Examination, Tuesday, December 13; Third M.B. Examination (part 1), Tuesday, December 13, and (part 2) Friday, December 16; for the degree of M.C., Thursday, December 15. The names of candidates for the various examinations for the degree of M.B., with the necessary certificates, are to be sent to Mr. G. B. Atkinson, Trinity Hall, on or before December 3; the names and certificates of candidates for the degree of M.C., to the Regius Professor of Physic (Dr. Paget), on or before December 3.

The distributors of Crane's Charity for the relief of sick scholars recently met at Peterhouse Lodge for the purpose of considering and determining the claims of applicants for the benefits of this charity, and grants were made on account of medicine, medical attendance, nursing, diet, and other necessaries in sickness.

At a recent meeting of the Vestry of the parish of Paddington, it was unanimously resolved—"That this Vestry regrets that, owing to the passing of the Valuation (Metropolis) Act of 1869, the charges made by the Grand Junction Waterworks Company for water are continually being raised, while no additional benefit whatever is conferred upon consumers; and that the various vestries and district boards in the metropolis be requested to urge upon Parliament the desirability of their introducing a Bill during the ensuing session, restraining the metropolitan water companies from taking advantage of the gross value as created by the above-mentioned Act, it never having been the intention of the Legislature that such gross value should be used for other than Imperial and local purposes."

The Committee for arranging the details of the forthcoming Smoke Abatement Exhibition recently held a meeting at 48, Berners-street. Amongst those present were Lord Harberton, Sir Frederick Pollock, Professor Chandler Roberts, F.R.S., Mr. Lowry Whittle, Sir Antonio Brady, and Mr. Ernest Hart. It was announced that the Society of Arts had resolved to add to the other prizes a special medal, to be given in the name of the Society, and Lord Alfred Churchill, President of the Society, was nominated to act with the Committee. Professor Chandler Roberts reported that he had arranged for chemically examining the products of combustion during the course of trials of grates and stoves. Several interesting exhibits have been received, and it was reported by the Honorary Secretary that the arrangements for completing the Exhibition were being pushed on as fast as practicable. It was agreed that arrangements should be made with the School of Cookery for illustrating, by lectures and practically, the use of some of the exhibits. Lectures by Professor Chandler Roberts and Captain Galton were arranged to be given during the Exhibition, and lectures by other distinguished men were in negotiation.

It is reported from Alexandria, under date 11th inst., that a telegram was received that morning by the Sanitary Commission, dated Djeddah, November 6, announcing that the outbreak of cholera at Mecca is increasing. The mortality from this cause on the 3rd inst. amounted to fifty-five, but on the two following days the number of fatal cases increased to 215 and 214. The pilgrims, the telegram adds, left Mecca on the 6th inst., and it was feared the Egyptian troops stationed at Elwedj (460 strong) would be either unable or unwilling to prevent them from entering that place. The pilgrims in the united caravans number upwards of 5000 men. The Sanitary Commission will probably decide upon establishing a rigorous quarantine at Elwedj. The public health at Djeddah is reported to be satisfactory; a local representative committee has been formed to improve the sanitary condition of the town, which is at all times dangerous, but no alarm exists in the locality.

At a recent meeting of the Indian Medical Service Defence Committee, it was determined, after conference with several members of the Service, to take steps to obtain compensation for those officers who entered the Department under the Honourable East India Company's rules, and whose prospects have been injuriously affected by changes introduced since the transfer to the Crown. The following resolution was accordingly submitted and unanimously carried: "That the report of a consulting actuary be obtained on the losses sustained by the members of the Indian Medical Service through changes made since 1858. That the actuary's fees be defrayed from the general fund, but, to provide for any possible deficiency, all officers who entered prior to 1860 be invited to guarantee the probable amount."

The St. Petersburg correspondent of the *Daily Telegraph* reports that the epidemics which have been devastating the centre and South of Russia have greatly increased in severity during the last two months, and their ravages are now in excess of anything that has hitherto been known, even in those sorely plagued provinces. Diphtheria, scarlet fever, small-pox, and other infectious diseases are carrying off the population by hundreds, and even thousands. It is supposed that the impoverished condition of the peasants, and their consequent insufficient nourishment, is the chief cause of the present mortality. Children, being more sensitive to the ills resulting from defective nourishment, form the greater number of the victims. The towns of Orel, Rostoff-on-the-Don, Voronesh, Tamboff, Charkoff, and Kiev are the special centres of the present pestilence.

Our contemporary the *Globe* says:—"Mr. P. A. Taylor, M.P., and his anti-vaccinationist friends should try Chicago. In the foreign quarter of that city the sacred right of every man to have the small-pox if he likes is upheld by force, all attempts to carry out the law having failed. Forty thousand persons are in the enjoyment of unvaccinated freedom within a small area, and eighty-one of them died of small-pox during the month of September last."

The following classes for the instruction of soldiers' wives in elementary nursing are now formed, and the interest and attention of the pupils are stated to be most encouraging. At Eastney Barracks there is a class of thirty-five pupils, which meets by permission of Colonel Mawbey; at Parkhurst, a class of fourteen, by permission of Colonel Hogge; at Taunton, a class of twelve, by permission of Colonel Montgomery; and at the Royal Military College, a class of fourteen wives of non-commissioned officers.

THE VIVISECTION PROSECUTION.

On Thursday, Dr. Ferrier appeared at Bow-street, charged with one or more infractions of the Vivisection Act. We indicated that there would probably be a good answer to those who had summoned Dr. Ferrier before a court of justice. That has so turned out, and the magistrate has so dealt with the summons that Dr. Ferrier goes scot-free. Persecution and prosecution are two different things: we do not like either, but of the two the former is the worse. We shall have something more to say on this subject.

FEVER AND SMALL-POX IN THE METROPOLIS.

At the last meeting of the Metropolitan Asylums Board, after allusion had been made to the lamented decease of the late chairman, Dr. Brewer, Mr. Hodges referred to the fever statistics. Should the same rate of increase in the number of cases which generally took place at this period of the year in the metropolis be sustained this year, he said, he did not see what was to be done, or how the patients were to be accommodated. The returns from the fever hospitals showed during the past fortnight a total increase of 60 upon the numbers admitted in the previous fortnight: 79 had been admitted to the Stockwell Hospital, 113 to the Homerton Hospital, and 14 to the Deptford Hospital. The totals showed that 205 had been admitted to the various hospitals, 30 had died, and 75 had been discharged, leaving 471 under treatment, and 38 beds available. The small-pox returns showed a decrease of 20 in the total number remaining under treatment, as compared with the figures of the previous fortnight, the total number of patients in the Asylums hospitals being 430.

SANITARY CHRONICLE OF THE PARISH OF ST. MARYLEBONE.

Mr. Alexander Wynter Blyth, the Medical Officer of Health for the parish of St. Marylebone, in his sanitary chronicle for the quarter ending September 30 last, shows that during the month of July four weeks of summer heat were recorded, the mean temperature ranging from 60° to 79°, while the maximum heat was as high as 98°. Both the remaining months (August and September) were of a very different character to July, and, in one sentence, they may be summed up as cool, dull, and showery. During the period under notice there were 1219 births and 716 deaths recorded in the parish. Of these 716 deaths, 51 were non-residents, and should properly be subtracted, leaving a total of 665 deaths, which gives the low death-rate of 17·1 per

1000. Similarly the birth-rate was 31·4 per 1000. Although the new infirmary at Notting-hill erected for St. Marylebone is not actually in the parish, it is in point of fact an outlying part of it, and Mr. Blyth rightly thinks it is very important that there should be some record of the diseases, etc., of the parishioners received in it. Altogether 991 cases were under treatment in this institution during the September quarter, and 45 deaths occurred; the mortality, therefore, appears at present to be a little under 5 per cent. of the admissions. The admissions for constitutional syphilis—2·2 per cent.—would appear, he thinks, to be somewhat high. An outbreak of typhus fever is recorded as having taken place in the immediate neighbourhood of Charles-street, Lisson-grove; the patients were removed as soon as possible to the fever hospitals, and the bedding, etc., destroyed. Some of this latter is described as having been most offensive; in one case in which Mr. Blyth accompanied the inspector of nuisances to a room in this locality, the clothing and persons of the wife and children were so exceptionally dirty, and had such an indescribable odour, that it was actually impossible to remain in the room five minutes.

A CURIOUS COINCIDENCE.

IN the *British Medical Journal* for November 5 is to be found a review of a book by Mr. Oakley Coles; in the number of the *London Medical Record* just issued the same book is reviewed, and almost in the same words. True, the latter review is shorter than the former, and the wording is not everywhere the same, but in some parts it is identical. The one has all the appearance of having been cut down from the other in such a way as literary work should not be done. Records of facts are one thing: opinions and reviews must rest in a different category. Hence to quote facts and to quote opinions is likewise different. Let anyone compare the two reviews, and they can frame their own judgment. We should scarcely have cared to say anything on this subject had it not been for a total want of any reference to the work of Mr. Ramsay, from whose papers, read before the Odontological Society many years ago, some of the best illustrations are drawn. That Mr. Coles' book is not the best of its kind we should be far from denying, but any notice of it must remain incomplete which contains no reference to the work of Mr. Ramsay.

ON THE USE OF PILOCARPIN IN DIPHTHERIA.

DR. ADOLFO FASANO, in a recent number of the *Giornale Internazionale delle Scienze Mediche*, offers some observations on the use of pilocarpin in diphtheria, a mode of treatment which has been said to be attended with the most favourable results. He quotes the reports of Dr. Guttman, who extols most highly the use of pilocarpin in this malady. Dr. Guttman administers it internally in solution in the form of hydrochlorate combined with pepsin, the dose varying according to the age of the patients. Dr. Fasano also quotes a case reported by Professor Cantani as having been treated successfully by pilocarpin alone. Professor Lepidi-Chioti, who has reported this case in all its particulars, describes two other cases of the same kind which were equally benefited. But it is stated that large doses may disturb the stomach and cause spasm and vomiting, and therefore it is necessary to be very careful in the mode of administering the drug. The anti-diphtheritic properties of pilocarpin are said to be due to the great salivation induced, by which means the detachment of the false membrane is much accelerated, and thus the course of the disease is shortened. Lepidi-Chioti also regards the sweating as a true depurative, eliminating a quantity of the virus circulating in the blood, in the same way as pyrogenic matters are expelled by the perspiration in fevers. The human skin is a true filter, and, as such, various products are eliminated by it from the system. The success of pilocarpin is therefore due, according to some authors, to the salivation detaching the false membrane, or, according to Lepidi-Chioti, to the copious perspiration. Dr. Fasano, in relating these views, adds his own testimony to the efficacy of pilocarpin in diphtheria, but proposes some questions as to the theoretical reasoning on which the treatment is founded; and he gives his opinion, in the first place, that the detachment of the false membrane, although an important element in the treatment, is by no means the only curative object to be attained. He asks, accordingly, to be informed as to the exact therapeutical value of the detachment of the false membrane, and whether it is certain that the diphtheritic virus, circulating in the blood and in many of the internal organs, is really eliminated with the sweat. Again, if it be admitted that it is eliminated, is it all eliminated? and has pilocarpin a local and general antiseptic action which enables it to destroy the products and the factors of the diphtheritic virus? If an explicit and experimental solution of these doubts should be afforded, then, Dr. Fasano thinks, it may be said that a great remedy has been discovered for diphtheria; and the easy administration of pilocarpin, its rapid action and its innocuous nature, are so many further recommendations for its use. In the meantime, he himself proposes to make further trials of the remedy, and recommends his colleagues to do the same, and if trustworthy results should confirm the observations of Lepidi-Chioti, Dr. Fasano, regarding the ultimate object, namely, the cure, will withdraw the doubts which he now entertains on the subject.

THE PARIS WEEKLY RETURN.

THE number of deaths for the forty-fourth week, terminating November 4, was 960 (528 males and 432 females), and among these there were from typhoid fever 42, smallpox 6, measles 3, scarlatina 5, pertussis 1, diphtheria and croup 39, erysipelas 2, and puerperal infections 3. There were also 36 deaths from tubercular and acute meningitis, 22 from acute bronchitis, 70 from pneumonia, 58 from infantile athrepsia (24 of the infants having been wholly or partially suckled), and 22 violent deaths. The number of deaths has diminished by 74 from that of the preceding week, and the amelioration is all the more significative, as it has been chiefly due to the fewer deaths from athrepsia and the epidemic diseases to which the young are most liable. The births for the week amounted to 1015, viz., 527 males (395 legitimate and 132 illegitimate) and 488 females (359 legitimate and 129 illegitimate); 89 infants (40 males and 49 females) were born dead or died within twenty-four hours.

WHOLESOME PUNISHMENT FOR SELLING UNWHOLESOME MEAT.

WE should be well pleased could we assume that two recent decisions in cases of exposure of unwholesome meat would be regarded as precedents by magistrates generally. In the first case, at the Guildhall Police-court, George Dunkley and Henry Bagley, butchers, of Holbeach, Lincolnshire, were summoned for sending four quarters of a cow to market in a diseased state and unfit for human food. The meat was seized on September 14 last, was brought to the court, and condemned, on evidence given by the Chief Inspector of Meat at the London Central Market, and by Dr. Sedgwick Saunders, that it was totally unfit for the food of man. Dr. Sedgwick Saunders said that it was pale, emaciated, and commencing to become putrid. It was evidently the carcase of some animal that had suffered from a wasting disease, and, in his opinion, was totally unfit for human food; it would, in fact, be dangerous for people to eat it. Alderman Hadley remarked that the case was not one that would be met by a fine, and, as a warning to men in the defendant's position, he should sentence them each to one month's imprisonment. In the second case, W. Bailey, a butcher, of Liverpool, was summoned at the police-court in that city for exposing for sale seven pieces of the carcase of a cow in a state unfit for human food. An inspector went to the defendant's place of business, and found the meat, which was in a state of "fermentation," cut up and openly exposed for sale. The meat was submitted to Dr. Vacher, Medical Officer of Health, and he pronounced it to be part of the carcase of a cow that had died from some complication consequent on parturition. The magistrate ordered the defendant to be imprisoned for a month, remarking that, had he the power, he would have added, "with hard labour."

SANITARY CONDITION OF THE BOROUGH OF GREAT GRIMSBY.

DR. FRANKLIN PARSONS has recently submitted to the Local Government Board a report upon the present sanitary condition of the borough of Great Grimsby. The last public inspection of the locality was made by Dr. Home (now Sir Anthony Home, V.C., K.C.B.), in 1871, when grave imperfections in the arrangements for the conservation of health were brought to notice. Dr. Parsons is able to bear testimony to the fact that in all the shortcomings enumerated by Dr. Home, improvements, more or less considerable, have been effected. A growing population, he remarks, such as that of Grimsby (which has increased from 1524 in 1801 to 26,182 at the present time), consists, in greater measure than a stationary population, of young adults, of persons in the prime of life, and of children. In such a locality the birth-rate should be high, and the death-rate (sanitary and social conditions otherwise being favourable) should be low, and this the present inquiry elicited to be, to a considerable extent, the case. The most unsatisfactory features in the death statistics of Grimsby were the high mortality among infants and the large number of deaths from diarrhœa, the latter twice as great in proportion to the population as in the United Kingdom at large. But, as Dr. Parsons observes, these may be almost looked upon as two phases of the same phenomenon, the large infant mortality being in considerable part due to the fatal prevalence of diarrhœa among children. Of 239 fatal cases of diarrhœa recorded for the six years 1875-80, 206 were children under five years old, and probably four-fifths of them were infants under one year. Apart from these, the deaths of infants in Grimsby would not be in any remarkable excess of the average of the kingdom. With a view of ascertaining the cause of the prevalence of diarrhœa, Dr. Parsons endeavoured, with the assistance of the Medical Officer of Health and Inspector of Nuisances, to obtain particulars respecting the children who had died from that disease in 1880; the lapse of time, however, and the difficulty of tracing the parents, prevented his arriving at any satisfactory conclusion on the subject. Judging by the recommendations which Dr. Parsons has appended to his report, the sanitary arrangements of Great Grimsby are certainly very much more satisfactory than those of the great majority of places dealt with in these Local Government Board inquiries. He suggests that ample means of ventilation should be provided in the trunk sewers for the relief of the air displaced by the accumulation of sewage when the outfalls are tide-locked; and that house-drains should be disconnected from the sewer by a trap, the drain on the house side of the trap being ventilated by a double set of openings for inlet and exit. The hospital for the isolation and treatment of persons suffering from infectious diseases, erected during the small-pox epidemic of 1870-71, is not sufficiently large to meet the probable wants of the locality, and, moreover, on the occasion of Dr. Parsons' visit, was in such a condition that some time must have elapsed before it could have been got ready to receive patients. This should be remedied, so that infectious cases might be removed thither immediately on their occurrence, and the disease be thus prevented from getting a footing amongst the inhabitants. These are not very difficult or costly details to carry out, to meet the requirements of the great central sanitary authority.

NERVE-STRETCHING.

MR. MACKELLAR, at St. Thomas's Hospital, on Wednesday last, stretched the whole brachial plexus of a man, whom some of our readers may remember to have seen at the late International Congress. The man had what has been styled a "mad" or "possessed" arm—that is to say, that the arm was the subject of violent, uncontrollable muscular movements, hitting out in all directions. It is needless to say that these movements greatly exhausted the man; and that every other means of treatment had been tried without success.

THE NORTH-WESTERN ASSOCIATION OF MEDICAL OFFICERS OF HEALTH.

AT an adjourned meeting of the members of the North-Western Association of Medical Officers of Health recently held at Manchester, Dr. Tatham, of Salford, read a paper on "Vital Statistics." He urged that, as we are entering on a new decade, and health officers will soon have to prepare their annual reports for 1881, the first year of the new decade, some endeavour should be made by those who had to administer the Public Health Act to secure something like uniformity in the statistical records which for the future each sanitary authority would contribute to the national stock. The present unsatisfactory condition of our national vital statistics was due, he said, to the fact that, with respect at least to the large urban districts, the health officers were working solely with regard to local requirements, and entirely without reference to a national statistical system; and their reports were well-nigh worthless, from the want of uniformity in the tabular forms employed. It was not probable that statistical forms issued by local associations or individuals would enjoy more than very local and partial adoption, and he therefore ventured to suggest that the Association should petition the President of the Local Government Board to instruct its medical department to prepare, and issue officially, a set of forms such as they would recommend for adoption by medical officers of health acting for urban authorities. He felt certain that such a set of forms would be gratefully received, and loyally acted upon by medical officers generally. At the conclusion of Dr. Tatham's address, the meeting resolved to adopt the principle of Dr. Tatham's communication, and a sub-committee was appointed to draw up a memorial in accordance therewith. A discussion on a paper on "Milk-Supply," read at a previous meeting by Dr. Vacher, of Birkenhead, was afterwards resumed, and resulted in a resolution to memorialise the Local Government Board to issue a memorandum urging upon local associations the necessity of efficiently enforcing the present regulations for the control of milk-sellers and the inspection of milk, and to grant to local associations additional powers to require all licensed milk-sellers to notify all cases of infectious disease appearing on their premises, with ability to close such premises until the removal of the infected animal or person, and the disinfection of the premises; and to enable a local association to veto the sale of milk by vendors coming from without the boundary, on evidence of infectious disease existing on their premises.

INDIAN MEDICAL SERVICE.

THE special correspondent of the *Times* in India states in a recent communication to that journal that the scheme for the re-organisation of the Indian Medical Department has lately been somewhat modified. It is now proposed to form an Indian Medical Staff Corps, to be recruited partly from the Army Medical Department and partly by competition among the students of British and Irish medical schools. The chief administrative officer of the new corps will be styled Director-General of the Medical Department in India. He will control the medical staffs of the *three* Presidencies, discharging the duties hitherto performed by *all* the surgeons-general of the Indian and Army Medical Departments. The estimated saving to the Government of India by uniting all these offices in one individual will be Rs. 22,000 annually. Should the proposal be sanctioned, it is expected that Dr. Cunningham, the present Surgeon-General of the Indian Medical Department, will be appointed the first Director-General on a salary of Rs. 3500 per mensem, which, we may add, will be an increase of Rs. 800 to his present monthly rate of pay, or Rs. 9600 per annum. While the pay of the *individual* is augmented to this very large extent, the total amount of pay to the *Department* will be diminished by something more than twice as much.

Considering that Dr. Cunningham has very recently, and to the great chagrin of a large number of men senior to him in his own branch of the Service, been promoted to the rank of surgeon-general from that of surgeon-major, without having passed through any of the intermediate portals through which ordinary men have to struggle in order to attain surgeon-general's rank; further, that this promotion was actually over the heads of other men of no mean standing; we can hardly believe that this further advancement of the one to the detriment of the many is likely to receive the sanction of the Secretary of State and the Council for India.

Everyone knows the high estimation in which Dr. Cunningham has been held by the Government of India in connexion with his duties as Sanitary Commissioner, which appointment he filled for many years. But few will deny that the reputation which he acquired while in that capacity was to a very great extent based upon the admirable system of statistics organised and developed by the late Surgeon-Major James Bryden, to whom, however, only scant credit was accorded by the Sanitary Commissioner, and it was only within a few months of his lamented death that Bryden received from the Government of India recognition at all commensurate with the value of his services.

The duties of the Sanitary Commissionership with the Government of India are so entirely different from those of the administrative medical charge of the large force of British troops serving in India, that it is difficult to believe that the Imperial Government will consent to hand over the latter to a medical officer whose experience has been entirely confined to the former.

ALL SAINTS' CONVALESCENT HOSPITAL, EASTBOURNE. —On the 10th of the present month two new wards and a new sitting-room, with attendant offices, for the reception of twenty-four male convalescents, were opened at the All Saints' Convalescent Hospital, Eastbourne. The opening ceremony consisted of a service, with sermon by the Rev. Geo. Body, M.A., conducted in the beautiful chapel attached to the Hospital. The sanitary and other arrangements of this liberally managed institution are admirably efficient; and the spacious and lofty wards and dining-halls are all that could be desired. More sitting-room accommodation is still wanted, and in this direction further extension will, when possible, be made. With the additional beds just added, the Hospital holds 324 patients, of whom the great majority are admitted free, by subscriber's letter. The children's wards and dining-rooms occupy a separate wing of the Hospital. We may remind our readers that private bedrooms, with a separate common sitting-room, are provided for a limited number of patients who can pay from 14s. to 18s. a week.

ON CONJUNCTIVAL TRANSPLANTATION FROM THE RABBIT.

THE new number of the *Annales d'Oculistique* contains the following letter from Dr. Wolfe on this subject:—

"At the recent Medical Congress in London, reported in the current number of the *Annales d'Oculistique*, M. Dufour, of Lausanne, reported cases of transplantation of conjunctiva from the rabbit. In that report I find the following sentence : 'The flap being provided with its ligatures, is placed upon a vapour bath until the place has been prepared to receive it.' I have lately been assisted in a similar operation by Dr. Eugene Smith, of Detroit, who, after watching the progress of the case for a week, and satisfying himself as to its success, informed me that he had some years ago assisted an eminent Paris surgeon in the same operation. From what he had then seen, he could only regard it as a complicated procedure, and had, therefore, never practised it himself; but now, after having seen how the operation ought to be performed, he is determined to take it up, and I have no doubt of his success.

"I have to thank M. Dufour for the description of his procedure, which comes quite opportunely. It explains why the operation has not been extensively practised, and why some surgeons have preferred cutting off mucous membrane from the mouth or vagina, while they could have bought a rabbit for a trifle, or two rabbits, if a large surface was to be supplied. If, for example, the conjunctival sac be kept upon steam for half an hour, the chance of success will be very remote. Perhaps I have not sufficiently accentuated the difficulties of the procedure, and the methods of overcoming these difficulties. I shall therefore mention some modifications which I have recently introduced for this purpose.

"1. To remove such a thin membrane as the conjunctiva, and transplant it in another place, is rather difficult. The moment it is dissected off it curls up, and it becomes impossible to say which is its epithelial surface. The ligatures do not help us to overcome entirely this curling and twisting tendency. Hence I am sure that many a membrane must have been transplanted inside-out or in a twisted condition. I therefore, immediately after removal, spread out the flap by means of a spatula upon the dorsum of my left hand, and leave it there while I am arranging the place for its reception, which has already been prepared. In the meantime the conjunctival flap dries up and sticks to the hand ; but when the place has been well arranged, a single drop of warm water makes the flap relinquish its hold without rendering it too soft. It is then gently raised upon a spatula and spread out in its new position.

"2. It is by no means easy to keep the lid everted for such a length of time as to enable one to fix the membrane as far as the *cul-de-sac*. The lid is apt to slip just at the moment when you wish to introduce the stitches and the membrane becomes twisted and displaced. I therefore commence the operation by introducing three silk threads through the whole thickness of the lid at its border. By means of these the eyelid can be everted and kept steady during the whole operation. No forceps can supply the efficiency of this contrivance.

"3. The practice of covering the new membrane with innumerable stitches rests on a pure misconception of the case. Four to six stitches of fine silk at the borders are the utmost that are required. If properly applied, the conjunctiva sticks like court-plaster, so that after a few days it cannot, even if we try, be removed by friction. Studding it with ligatures can only do harm.

"I am glad that an American *confrère* has witnessed this operation, for it is through an American surgeon, Dr. Wadsworth, of Boston, that my transplantation of skin-flap has obtained such popularity, and is now a recognised ophthalmic operation. After he had exhibited successful cases at the Congress in New York, the operation again came up for discussion at Amsterdam and Milan, and the adoption of it was thus extended.

"I may take this opportunity of expressing my conviction that transplantation of conjunctiva, skin, and even cornea, is yet destined to play an important part in plastic operations on the eye, and that at no distant date."

SOME ACCOUNT OF THE NEW DOCTRINE OF TISSUE-GROWING.

(From a Correspondent.)

BEFORE relating the experiments and views on the changes which grafted sponge may undergo, we may just remind our readers that the organisation of a blood-clot or of fibrinous lymph depends essentially on its vascularisation. Pathologists are agreed on this point; but as to how this vascularity is brought about, there are wide differences of opinion. The first change noticeable is dilatation and tortuosity of the existing bloodvessels of the part on which the lymph rests; next, the tissue becomes "infiltrated" with a vast number of cells. It is at this point that divergence of opinion commences. Whence come these cells? Virchow and his immediate followers regard them as the offspring of the fixed "connective-tissue corpuscles" of the part; while Cohnheim and his disciples regard them as "wandering cells" derived from the bloodvessels. The majority of pathologists at the present time would probably adhere, more or less, to this latter view, although a more correct view would perhaps be an amalgamation of the two. These infiltrated cells, however, cannot organise and form tissue (cicatrise) without becoming vascular, and this is another bone of contention among practical pathologists— How are the earliest vessels formed? Dr. Hamilton boldly rejects the outgrowth of shoots from the sides of the vessels, as taught by Arnold and others: he substitutes the doctrine that the tortuous and distended vessels are displaced and pushed outwards towards the clot or lymph lying on the surface of the wound. These bloodvessels carry with them great numbers of actively proliferating connective-tissue corpuscles. "The vascular loops, surrounded by their tissue-forming cells, continue to penetrate further and further into the clot; and as successive meshes of the fibrinous network are filled by them, so they appear to cause its destruction, until the whole clot becomes in this way removed, its place being taken by new vessels and the above-described cicatricial elements. The latter soon elongate into spindle cells, and these in from three weeks to a month become transformed into fibrous tissue.

"It was from observing the merely passive part played by the blood-clot when undergoing organisation in wounds, in bloodvessels, and in other parts, that I was led to suppose that a porous substance like sponge, if applied under the same circumstances, would serve a similar purpose." We may now attempt to follow Dr. Hamilton's experiments, five of which on the human subject are recorded. We may say that the sponge to be used is carefully selected; it must be soft and fine in texture. All siliceous and calcareous salts are dissolved out by steeping in weak nitro-hydrochloric acid. The sponge is then soaked in liquor potassæ, and finally steeped in carbolic solution 1-20 strong. We will quote experiment No. 3. This was carried out under Mr. Bell's direction in the Royal Infirmary. In one of his wards was "a patient suffering from an intractable ulcerating wound of old standing on the left leg. It had been previously healed, and had again broken out, and there was great cicatricial contraction of the surrounding parts. Several methods of treatment had been employed, but apparently with no benefit, the cicatricial contraction of the skin and deep tissues around preventing the wound from closing. . . . . Seeing that it was proposed to amputate the limb if it would not heal, Mr. Bell thought it right to make a trial of sponge grafting. The object in doing so was to grow sufficient young tissue to allow of the necessary contraction, and at the same time to afford a healthier—that is, a more embryonic—surface for the epithelium to spread over." The wound measured two inches and a half by two inches, and on January 3 of this year it was covered by a layer of fine sponge rising a little higher than the level of the skin. It was dressed with Listerian antiseptics, but, at the time of application, was in a septic condition, and remained so throughout. The patient's age was twenty-nine.

"In from a week to a fortnight after application it had taken a firm hold on the exposed surface, and Mr. Bell noticed in dressing it that it appeared to be slightly vascular, and bled when pricked. The daily record of the case it will be unnecessary to follow out; but suffice it to say that it shortly became filled with young vascular cicatricial tissue, which grew up from below, filling the cavities of the sponge as in the first case. The discharge from the wound was considerable, and remained of a septic nature throughout the course of the organisation.

"The patient in time was dismissed with the sponge completely organised and the wound healed. There did not appear, moreover, to be any injurious stretching of the parts, the newly formed tissue having allowed for this."

In order to study the changes which had taken place, or were taking place, pieces of the organising sponge were cut off for microscopical investigation. It was remarked that the patient did not feel any pain, and hence it was surmised that nerves had not at that period found their way into the organising sponge. The case from which the sponge was taken was a recurrent mammary tumour, in which a large gap of raw surface had been covered over with a layer of fine prepared sponge. It had become completely organised, and was healed, all except a small patch of the size of a shilling. Microscopic sections of little bits, which had been removed and hardened in Müller's fluid, showed that "the whole of the sponge interstices were filled with what would generally be called young connective-tissue cells," among which, and for the most part hugging the keratode framework of the sponge, were to be seen great numbers of unusually large giant-cells. Dr. Hamilton has illustrated his paper by some drawings of the microscopical appearances; and, without which it will be difficult to accurately reproduce his descriptions. In some of the giant-cells there were as many as thirty nuclei; around them lay spindles and round cells of a connective-tissue type. "In fact, the appearance was like that of a typical giant-cell sarcoma."

"The sponge framework appeared somewhat altered from its usual homogeneous aspect. It was marked by many little lines, and at its ends was thinner than usual—appearances which seemingly indicated that it was dissolving. That such will be the ultimate result I cannot fail to believe. Being an animal texture, it will, like catgut, in course of time undergo tissue digestion."

It is right to state that one experiment failed. This was in a case of old necrosis of the lower end of the tibia communicating with a wound of considerable size. The want of success appears to have been due to a want of granulating power in the wound.

With the view to further test and study this process, some experiments were tried in Vienna on animals by Dr. Woodhead (who had formerly assisted Dr. Hamilton), Dr. Stricker having placed his laboratory at disposal. One set of experiments consisted in placing pieces of sponge within the peritoneal cavity; another set comprised the introduction of sponge into muscular parts; a third series was made by inserting two thin glass plates, with a layer of sponge between them, into the subcutaneous tissue. The result in all cases which went on favourably was invariably the same, namely, that the sponge in a few days after insertion began to organise in the same manner as in the human subject.

Dr. Hamilton describes minutely the changes which a piece of sponge underwent after being ten days in the peritoneal cavity. He says, "There was considerable peritonitis, and this occurrence, either of a local or a general nature, is extremely liable to be set up in all such experiments on the peritoneum of the lower animals, chiefly from the difficulty of avoiding septic contamination. The sponge, as generally happens, was found to be adherent to a loop of the intestine. The union was so firm that it could with difficulty be detached. Throughout the abdominal cavity there was a considerable quantity of fibrinous lymph, but the part of the sponge not attached to the intestine was only partially covered by it. The greater part of the unattached surface was still porous, and did not present any evidence of organisation."

Sections were made through different parts: the first thing noticed is the infiltration of the interstices of the sponge with a certain amount of fibrinous lymph; subsequently, cicatricial or organising tissue invades this, displaces the fibrin and destroys it. The fibrinous lymph, when examined microscopically, is seen to consist of a delicate network of fibrin, containing within its meshes many blood leucocytes, all more or less in a state of disintegration. This disintegration, both of the leucocytes and of the fibrin, becomes more obvious as we approach the area of cicatrisation. This latter adjoins the area by which the sponge is adherent to the intestine. As regards the intestine itself, it may be said that it remains unchanged in all parts except its peritoneal covering, and it is in this that the earliest changes ensue, and from these that subsequent organisation proceeds. The earliest change noticed in the serous coat is distension of its bloodvessels; at the same time they become tortuous; the fibrous tissue around them then becomes œdematous.

As Dr. Hamilton holds views of his own on this point, we will transcribe what he says :—" On examining these distended vessels in other parts, long straight offshoots could be seen arising from them, and running directly upwards into the cicatrising layer. The large number of these was in some parts very remarkable, forming a dense bundle in certain places. For a considerable distance after they left the parent trunk in the peritoneal or sub-peritoneal tissue they gave off only a very few divisions.

" Nearer the fibrinous layer, however, they could be seen to give off branches enclosing wide meshes, and at the extreme internal limit of the cicatricial layer they ended in a network of wide loops. Now, the convex side of these loops was, without exception, always towards the distal extremity of the vessel, the concave towards the proximal, and in no instance could I find anything but loops in this situation." The bloodvessels are the primary cause of the vascularisation of the sponge, and they bear into its interior actively dividing connective-tissue corpuscles derived from neighbouring connective tissues, and it is not of the latter that the new cicatricial tissue is evolved. The bloodvessels are the primary, the connective-tissue elements the secondary, factors in the organising process.

Here our readers will observe that Hamilton is at variance with a widely accepted doctrine as to the growth of new bloodvessels by budding out, first advocated by Arnold. It is no intention of ours, in this place, to criticise the work now before us; our readers must study for themselves. Suffice it to say that the cicatricial layer is that in which the new bloodvessels are formed and forming, and that its vitality depends on this formation of vessels. It increases gradually in extent, and, by invading the fibrinous layer, as gradually destroys it until nothing is left but organised material.

The practical outcome of this interesting work appears to establish the principle that a porous body may become vascularised, and be used for the purpose of facilitating the cicatrisation of wounds. It would seem especially applicable to those cases where there is great loss of substance, but in which there is, however, healthy action.

Whether a wider experience will confirm Dr. Hamilton's views remains yet to be seen. The original article, from which we have taken the foregoing particulars, is worthy of careful study, for it contains many points of histological interest besides the clinical one to which we have chiefly alluded.

EXCISION OF THE PYLORUS.—We are informed that the condition of the patient upon whom Dr. Wölfler operated for carcinoma of the pylorus, exactly half a year since, is in every way satisfactory, no sign of relapse having appeared. It is the fourth case in Dr. Wölfler's book, " Ueber die Resektion des carcinomatösen Pylorus." This book, we may mention, has already been translated into Russian and Italian, and is about to appear in an English dress, so great is the interest everywhere taken in this important operative procedure inaugurated in Billroth's clinic.—*Wien. Med. Woch.*, October 15.

THE INDIAN MEDICAL SERVICE.—A rumour has got about that competition is no longer to constitute the portal to the Indian Medical Service, but that a certain number of nominations will be placed at the disposition of the principal medical schools. The native papers have it that the reason of this is that so many natives have obtained entrance into the Service, and that the authorities are afraid that the European candidates will not be able to hold their own against Indian competitors! We should be sorry to see competition abolished. If the Service is made and kept worth competing for, there will be no lack of good men to compete for it.—*Indian Med. Gaz.*, September.

FROM ABROAD.

TREATMENT OF PLEURISY.

PROF. DIEULAFOY, in a lecture upon this subject (*Gaz. des Hop.*, No. 83), observes that the medical treatment of pleurisy has for its object the relief of the initial phenomenon of the disease, the pain—pain which irradiates over the whole side of the chest, and which may be localised in a point that may be exactly indicated by the patient. One of the most simple and efficacious means of relieving it is to apply dry cupping-glasses or with scarification to the painful part. Or hypodermic injections of morphia may be employed; and a very simple formula for this consists of ten centigrammes of chlorhydrate of morphia and ten grammes of distilled water, furnishing the proportion of one centigramme of morphia to one gramme of the whole, from half a gramme to not more than a gramme being injected at first. If these means do not succeed we must have recourse to anodyne mixtures and to blisters applied *loco dolenti*. Blisters are of no other use than assuaging the pain, and should not be employed under the idea of effecting a derivation and diminishing effusion. They should not be made larger than a five-shilling piece. The first thing we are expected to do by the friends is to apply a blister, and the refusal to do this will incur blame; but the blister, without at all hastening the cure, impedes effectual auscultation and percussion, and therefore may prevent our ascertaining the amount of liquid effused. If, then, forced by the prejudices of the patient or his friends, we are compelled to apply the blister, this should be made as small as possible.

" When the fluid tends to increase, the family of the patient should at once be informed that an operation will probably be required. Its indications may be urgent or debatable. As to the first of these, if the patient has somewhat pronounced dyspnœa, complete dulness, and the tubular *soufle*, while from 2500 to 3000 grammes of liquid are supposed to be present, the operation should be performed at once, without waiting for to-morrow, when the patient may be dead. Hesitation here is entirely out of place. But under other circumstances, although the patient may have dulness, this is not absolute. There may even be a little sonority behind, above the spine of the scapula, and in front, opposite the clavicle. The heart is a little displaced if the effusion is on the left side; and the liver, if it is on the right side. The dyspnœa is not very considerable, and the liquid may be estimated at 2000 grammes. What are you to do here? Naturally enough, you are disposed to wait. The patient breathes pretty well, the cavity of the thorax is not filled, and you call to mind that thoracentesis has been accused of inducing purulency. Nothing seems very pressing, and you go away, saying you will decide to-morrow. Next day you receive a message that the patient, without apparent cause, had been seized with a fainting-fit and died. These cases are by no means so rare as you may suppose, death taking place when the liquid has not amounted to more than 1800 or 2000 grammes, as a consequence of syncope or of asphyxia due to pulmonary thrombosis formed *in situ*. Read Trousseau, and the examples which he gives of sudden death in his chapter on Thoracentesis. For my own part, I do not hesitate to lay down the rule, that whenever we estimate the quantity of liquid effused at about 2000 grammes, we must operate. If this is refused, give up the case, and do not accept the responsibility of what may happen. Remember that dyspnœa is a treacherous sign, and that the only true guide is the quantity of liquid effused, while complications do not contraindicate the operation.

" Thoracentesis is not always so clearly indicated, and there are cases in which it is debatable. You meet with cases in which there are effusions of 1200 or 1500 grammes that will not absorb. Are you to leave the patient with this fluid in his chest? This would not be prudent. Are you to apply blister after blister? I have punctured patients who have borne eight, ten, or twelve blisters without a drop of the effusion having been absorbed. In such cases, if there is any tendency to absorption, I merely wait. I order neither sudorifics, diuretics, nor blisters, and if at the end of thirty or thirty-five days the effusion has continued stationary, I propose thoracentesis, with which both the patient and myself have always been satisfied.

"For the operation, you puncture with the needle No. 2 in the eighth intercostal space on a line springing from the inferior angle of the scapula. I recommend you *never to remove more than a litre of the liquid at once*; for I do not hesitate to affirm that if any terrible accidents have succeeded the operation, this has been because two or three litres have been withdrawn at a time. It is much better to remove another litre next day, and the 300, 400, or 500 grammes that may still remain will be absorbed without any attention being required."

As to the transformation of a simple into a purulent pleurisy by thoracentesis, Prof. Dieulafoy entirely denies its possibility when the operation is properly performed with *quite clean instruments*. Those used at the hospitals are often very dirty. He maintains that thoracentesis is a very simple operation, which should be performed without hesitation.

OBSTETRIC APHORISMS.

Dr. Webster Jones, of Chicago (*New York Med. Record*, October 8), closed his report to the Obstetrical Committee of the Illinois State Medical Society with the following valuable and suggestive sayings. With these as his guide, the practice of the obstetrician of to-day would furnish less work for the gynæcologist :—1. An intelligent confidence once established between patient and physician does much to banish the terrors of the lying-in room. 2. It is possible to foresee and prevent the occurrence of the almost always fatal form of eclampsia gravidarum. 3. Cleanliness is especially next to godliness in the case of the accoucheur, its absence rendering one liable to professional homicide. 4. Modern midwifery must not be meddlesome, but must be mediatorial in the sense of palliating suffering, expediting nature's processes by well-proven means, and removing scientifically all inexplicable, accidental, or morbid states and conditions. Idleness is no longer an approved qualification for a degree in obstetrics. 5. The hand is the best uterine dilator. 6. The forceps should never be employed until the os uteri is dilated or dilatable, and then not unless the membranes have been ruptured and labour delayed unnaturally for at least an hour. Every practitioner should become skilful in their use, and they should never be left at home for fear of temptation. 7. Unnecessary and avoidable delays in labour are fruitful sources of gynæcological practice : they promote inflammation and sepsis. 8. The patient's hopeful confidence and the physician's industrious attention actually contribute to the physiological elements of labour. Anæsthetics here are, to say the least, superfluous. 9. Bi-manual aid in delivering the placenta is not only proper, but advisable. Skilfully rendered, the cry of "uterine inversion" is no longer a bugbear. 10. The continuous and intelligent counter-pressure over the fundus uteri during the child's exit, the delivery of the placenta, and the period of frequent oscillation (be that a shorter or longer time), form a safeguard never to be neglected. 11. Pursuant to the same end, the application of the bandage, and its continuance as long as the uterine globe can be felt and embraced by it above the pubes, contributes not only to comfort, but to speedy involution. After the seventh day, close pressure must be interdicted. 12. Puffiness of one ankle, with tenderness of the corresponding groin, and an abnormally quickened pulse, with or without copious sweating, noticed within the first ten days after labour, betoken the presence of phlebitis, and the possibility of embolism or thrombosis, and resultant sudden death. 13. The duties of an obstetrician are not concluded until a careful examination, from six to eight weeks after parturition, proves the integrity of the organs involved.

THE HUNTERIAN COLLECTION.—At a quarterly meeting of the trustees of the Museum of the Royal College of Surgeons, on the 11th inst., the Right Hon. the Earl of Aberdare was unanimously elected a trustee in the vacancy occasioned by the decease of Sir Philip de Malpas Grey Egerton, Bart., who was elected in 1840 with his Grace the Duke of Devonshire and the Earl of Enniskillen.

THE CHAIR OF SYPHILIS AT THE VIENNA MEDICAL FACULTY.—The *Allg. Wien. Med. Zeitung* of October 25 congratulates its readers that Prof. Neumann has been definitively appointed the successor of Hofrath Prof. Dr. von Sigmund, in the Chair of Syphilis (*syphilodologie*).

REVIEWS.

A Manual of Histology. Edited and prepared by THOMAS E. SATTERTHWAITE, M.D., of New York, in association with numerous contributors. Pp. 478, with 196 woodcuts. London : Sampson Low, Marston, and Co. 1881.

THIS manual of histology, issuing from the American press, is a well-printed volume of under five hundred pages and with about two hundred woodcuts. It is framed on the model of the well-known handbook edited by Stricker : the editor, Dr. Satterthwaite, writes the first nine articles, on general methods and on some of the simple tissues; the other articles, amounting to about three-fourths of the book, being contributed by sixteen writers, most of whom are teachers of histology in the medical schools of New York, Boston, and Philadelphia. The illustrations include a good many of the best woodcuts in Stricker's handbook, such as F. E. Schultze's drawings of the lung structure, Eberth's of the supra-renal and of bloodvessels, Waldeyer's of the teeth and of the ovary, Verson's of the intestinal canal, Klein's of the external organs of generation, Rollet's of blood and of bone, and others. Original woodcuts are most abundant in the chapters on the Connective Tissues, on the Central Nervous System, and on the Kidney. The important subjects of the testis, uterus, and placenta. are without illustrations, as indeed they are, for the most part, also in Stricker's handbook. We miss also woodcuts to make clear the development of long bones and of the membrane bones ; the admirable diagram of Rollet, showing the development of the tibia, ought certainly to have been taken from Stricker's handbook along with so many others. Also, it would not have been superfluous to have inserted woodcuts of fat-tissue and of its development, and of the cell-plates of tendon. Low-power drawings of the section of a lymphatic gland, and of the Malpighian corpuscles of the spleen, would have been useful to the student. Coming to the text, we note a certain inequality, which was perhaps inevitable, in the merit of the various chapters. The articles by the editor at the beginning of the book combine both systematic information and technical instruction in a judicious manner, and the same combination is found in several of those written by other contributors ; but this excellent plan has not been followed quite uniformly. Most of the writers appear to have worked through their respective subjects, and to have obtained the authority of their own observation for a large proportion of the statements that they make ; and throughout the book generally, there is not only much fairness in the statement of conflicting opinions, but there is sometimes also the valuable addition of a critical judgment on points at issue. We are bound to say, however, that the process of verification and of critical decision might have been carried a good deal farther. The example of Dr. Warren in re-writing the general anatomy of the cutis vera might have been followed by others, and doubtless the results would have been equally fresh and welcome. The article on the Supra-renal is too obviously a condensation made at the writing-desk, and the list of authors at the end of it, no less than the copious illustrations interspersed through it, might have been in great part omitted so far as any connexion with the text goes. Another rather meagre article, that on the Female Organs of Generation, might easily have been enriched by some account of the menstrual process as described by Dr. John Williams, and by an attempt at least to deal with the histology of the placenta.

The bibliography at the end of each chapter is too much restricted to the traditional string of German names, and is. frequently not quite appropriate to the text. The authorities named are of very unequal value, and while important monographs and memoirs are omitted, references are made to other pieces of work, which would have been found, if they had been examined at first hand, to be of too slight and casual a kind to occupy the valuable space of a text-book.

Having said or indicated thus much as to the defects of this work—defects which are to some extent inseparable from its plan, and to some extent due also to the unsifted condition of much that is published in the name of histological research,—we have pleasure in adding that Dr. Satterthwaite has produced a volume which fairly well comes up to the ideal that he set before himself of a manual of histology summarising "in concise and plain language" our present.

knowledge in that fundamental branch of medicine. Compared with the handbook edited by Stricker, it has not the same authority based upon strict verification of statements, and it is not so exhaustive; at the same time it is much more convenient to the student and practitioner, both in size and in cost. The recent admirable work of Klein and Noble Smith has furnished the writers in this volume with constant occasions of reference, and that fact is one indication, among others, of the entirely distinct and unique position occupied by the English atlas and text.

Fracture of the Patella. A Study of 127 Cases. By FRANK H. HAMILTON, A.M., M.D., LL.D., Visiting Surgeon to Bellevue Hospital; Consulting Surgeon to the Hospital for the Ruptured and Crippled, New York; Author of " A Practical Treatise on Fractures and Dislocations," "A Treatise on Military Surgery," "A Treatise on the Principles and Practice of Surgery," etc. New York: Charles L. Bermingham and Co. 1880. Pp. 106.

A TREATISE on an important subject such as fracture of the patella, from the pen of Dr. Hamilton, was sure to attract notice; for he is the author of the best modern work in his own or any other language on fractures and dislocations. Fracture of the patella is a frequent accident. The modes of treating it are numerous. The results of treatment are not as satisfactory as one would wish. In all cases of fracture of the patella there is for a time some anchylosis of the knee-joint, less or more marked according as passive movements have or have not been resorted to during the period of treatment; in perhaps the majority of cases this partial anchylosis continues for a period varying from one to two years after the accident; and in some few instances union never takes place, and permanent lameness is the result. But what, it will be asked, has Dr. Hamilton to say in a monograph which he could not have said in the recently issued sixth edition of his classical work? It is difficult to give an answer to this question, unless it be that the author desired to put his readers in possession of all the facts and materials from which he has drawn his conclusions. Thus we find this treatise consisting of four papers. The first gives the notes, more or less incomplete, of fifty-four cases which have come under his own observation. The second, the records, also more or less imperfect, of cases not seen by himself, but which have been admitted to Bellevue Hospital. The third paper is a summary of all these cases; and the fourth being the substance of two lectures on fracture of the patella, delivered by the author in 1879, contains his remarks on the etiology, anatomy and pathology, prognosis and treatment, of the injury. He points out that the large proportion of cases are simple transverse fractures, and that comminuted fractures are infrequent, and compound very rare. The predominance of muscular action as the cause of the fracture is proved from the greater frequency of the accident in males than in females, and during the active and most muscular periods of life. Thus ninety-nine happened in males to twenty-eight in females; and only three cases of any kind occurred to persons under twenty years, and only five to persons over sixty years.

Under the head of Anatomy and Pathology he draws attention to the frequency of early joint-effusion and of the presence of blood in the joint; the conditions which limit the degree of separation of the fragments; the effect and importance of tilting and lateral displacement of the fragments; the association of synovitis and bursitis as inevitable complications; and the hypertrophy of the fragments, which was noticed in nine cases out of 127.

Under Prognosis he refers to the uniformity of fibrous union with some separation; the frequency of anchylosis and its proportion to the time the limb is kept in splints; the great time which elapses before the functions of the limb are restored; the remarkable power of restoration of the functions of the limb after a time, when no union of the fragments has taken place, if only the patient continue to use the limb, and thus develope the muscles; the frequency of a re-fracture, i.e., of the rupture of a bond of union, and the much more serious results from it than from the primary accident, for the reason that a majority of re-fractures do not unite again, no matter what means may be employed to make them.

As regards Treatment, mention is made of the great variety of methods, and the frequent changes resorted to in the treatment of individual cases, either because of their inefficiency, or because of the pain and excoriations or other more serious injuries which they caused; and attention is drawn to the fact that equally good results have been attained where the attempts to get close union have been less assiduous.

The author's investigations led him to conclude that in a large majority of cases, under any plan of treatment, a fibrous union is all that can be expected, and that probably a fibrous union, with only a separation of half or three-quarters of an inch, is as useful as a bony union. The only methods which could encourage a reasonable hope of procuring a bony union are Malgaigne's hooks, and wiring the fragments together. Malgaigne's hooks have hitherto not been proven to have accomplished this result, and there seems no reason why, in ordinary cases of simple transverse fracture, where the separation does not exceed one inch and a half, this method should be employed; "but in cases in which the original separation exceeds this, and especially in cases of a re-fracture or rupture of the fibrous band, accompanied with great separation, it is my opinion that Malgaigne's hooks are entitled to a further trial." As to the method of wiring the fragments together under carbolic acid spray, Dr. Hamilton—as we think, rightly—remarks: "I feel in duty bound to say that it is offering a very grave and dangerous substitute for other perfectly safe and, so far as yet proven, equally efficient methods: it is hazarding the life of the patient without offering any equivalent." It is a piece of surgery in which the limb, if not the life, of the patient is staked, not against any great advantage which will accrue to the patient if successful, but against a possible triumph for an antiseptic proceeding. It is consequently to be condemned.

"Cutting the quadriceps . . . . demands a very extensive subcutaneous incision; . . . . and I venture to say that no surgeon has divided all of its fibres, or even the fibres of the rectus, in his subcutaneous incision." This treatment is not recommended. The method now employed and recommended by Dr. Hamilton is to elevate the foot of the extended limb six or eight inches, for the purpose of relaxing the quadriceps muscle, and then to apply a long splint to the back of the thigh and leg. This splint may be made of leather, or gum-shellac cloth, or any other substance having the necessary qualities of firmness, lightness, and plasticity, so that it can be properly moulded to the limb. The splint when moulded is covered with a firm cotton or woollen sac, and the sac is stitched along the back of the splint. The chief object of this covering is to supply a basis to which the bandage, which is to enclose the limb and splint, may be stitched. A roller of unglazed cotton is then applied from below upwards, and another from above downwards to about three inches of the knee. While the fragments are approximated, two or three turns with a third roller are made round the limb and splint close above the knee, after which the roller descends below the knee, and an equal number of circular turns are made close below the lower fragment of the patella; and finally a succession of oblique and circular turns are made above and below the fragments, until the whole of the patella is covered. The rollers are carefully stitched to the cover of the splint throughout its whole length on both sides. Thus Dr. Hamilton no longer uses the wooden inclined plane figured and recommended in his "Treatise on Fractures and Dislocations." The principle of its construction is, he maintains, correct, and the results have been satisfactory, but it is unnecessarily cumbrous. We cannot suppose that it was for the purpose of publishing this slight modification in treatment that the book was written. It was rather, as we have suggested above, to give the reader the chance of studying a large number of cases for himself, and of making his own inferences. Not many, however, do we think, will read through the first eighty pages of the work, which consists solely of the hospital notes of cases, not always too well taken. It is to be regretted that there is no index and no table of contents to assist the reader in extracting such information as he may desire. To us it seems that the great merit and chief value of the work is that the author brings into notice forcibly and with the whole weight of his undeniable authority the practical impossibility of obtaining bony union; and the further important fact that, after all, a short ligamentous bond is as good as a uniting osseous medium. It is a very well-timed address to the profession, as there has been a tendency to overlook what is the practical end to be obtained, and what the most desirable means of obtaining it.

GENERAL CORRESPONDENCE.

THE TESTIMONIAL TO PROFESSOR VIRCHOW.
LETTER FROM DR. J. S. BRISTOWE.

[To the Editor of the Medical Times and Gazette.]

SIR,—Permit me to acknowledge the receipt of the following additional contributions in respect of the above testimonial, and to say that, though I have already transmitted to Professor Küster, of Berlin, the sum of £88 16s., in order that it may reach him before the 19th inst., I shall still be happy to receive subscriptions.　　I am, &c.,　　J. S. BRISTOWE.

11, Old Burlington-street, W., November 17.

Sir Thos. Watson, Bart., £3 3s.; T. B. Curling, Esq., £1 1s.; Dr. Pye-Smith, £1 1s.; Dr. Wilson Fox, £2 2s.; Dr. Swanzy, £1 1s.; Dr. Vacher, £2 2s.; Dr. T. Edmonston Charles, £5 5s.; John Simon, Esq., £1 1s.; Dr. F. Chance, £2 2s.; Spencer Wells, Esq., £2 2s.; Dr. C. T. Williams, £1 1s.; Dr. W. M. Allchin, £1 1s.; Dr. Grigg, £1 1s.; Dr. E. B. Baxter, £1 1s.; Joseph Lister, Esq., £2 2s.; Dr. M. Watson, £2 2s.; Dr. A. R. Simpson, £5; from Manchester, per Dr. Dreschfeld, £17 17s.; Dr. A. B. Shepherd, £1 1s.; Dr. Cheadle, £1 1s.; Dr. Broadbent, £1 1s.; Dr. Hermann Weber, £3 3s.

THE FOULIS SCHOLARSHIP FUND.
LETTER FROM DR. M. CHARTERIS.

[To the Editor of the Medical Times and Gazette.]

SIR,—Dr. Foulis' death is exciting great sympathy here. Upwards of £200 has been already obtained from the profession in the West of Scotland, and it is proposed to institute a "Foulis Scholarship" when the subscriptions have reached a capital sum the interest of which will amount to £50 per annum.

This scholarship will be awarded to the most deserving student in pathology connected with the Glasgow Medical School.

Subscriptions from friends at a distance, or former pupils, will be gratefully received and acknowledged by the secretaries to the fund—Dr. J. G. Lyon, 276, Bath-crescent; or Dr. Eben. Duncan, 4, Royal-crescent, Glasgow.

I am, &c.,　　M. CHARTERIS.

8, Blythswood-square, Glasgow.

P.S.—Should the subscriptions not amount to such a sum as would give £50 annually, the scholarship will be awarded biennially or triennially.

DR. HARLEY ON ORTHOGRAPHY.
LETTER FROM DR. KESTEVEN.

[To the Editor of the Medical Times and Gazette.]

SIR,—I would ask permission to suggest, with much deference to Dr. George Harley, that the vowel letters of the English language deserve some consideration at his hands, as well as do the consonants. I admit that some reduction in their number might possibly be made with advantage, but I submit that he overlooks the relationship of the one set of letters to the other. Dr. Harley's own communication in your last impression affords an illustration of the confusion that would be introduced into our language by the adoption of the rules of orthography suggested by him. The reading of Dr. Harley's interesting pathological contribution is hampered and obscured by his arbitrary orthography.

I would not rashly engage in a war of words with so formidable and bold an innovator, but I would ask his leave respectfully to remind him that the sounds and value of the vowels in our language are largely controlled by the reduplication of the consonants. It is only necessary to consult the examples given in any "pronouncing" dictionary to see that vowels are short in the English language before double consonants, and long before single ones. I cite from the paper of Dr. Harley a few examples of the violation of established pronunciation, and no gain in the way of accuracy, exhibited in Dr. Harley's proposed orthography—e.g., spěling (spělling), compěled (compělled), áfect (éffect), láter

(lětter), crǎming (crǎmming), intěligent (intělligent), prěty (prětty), cǒmon (cǒmmon), bǐten (bǐtten). Scores more of examples might be quoted. I will merely add a few orthographical puzzles, referring for the key thereof to the Medical Times and Gazette of to-day's date :—Useles, reckles, al, ofer, cal, smal, caling, egs, stil, tel. Surely we need not further imitate the curtness of our American relatives, who have already thrown overboard letters, syllables, and words.

It is still as true as it was in the days of old, that "Life is short and art is long"; but surely life is long enough for us to take time to speak and write intelligibly ! I can see no advantage in augmenting the breathless rush, the wear and tear, of life. Art has already enabled us to distance our forefathers in the saving of time. Post-cards and telegrams have cut down our correspondence to symbols and ciphers; and now, forsooth, phonetic spelling is to crystallise our once flexible language into lifeless stenographic signs !

I am, &c.,

Enfield, November 13.　　W. B. KESTEVEN, M.D.

REPORTS OF SOCIETIES.

ROYAL MEDICAL AND CHIRURGICAL SOCIETY.
TUESDAY, NOVEMBER 8.

ANDREW WHITE BARCLAY, M.D., President, in the Chair.

TWO CASES OF CONGENITAL MACROSTOMA, ACCOMPANIED BY MALFORMATION OF THE AURICLES AND BY THE PRESENCE OF AURICULAR APPENDAGES.

MR. J. H. MORGAN read a paper on two cases of congenital macrostoma, accompanied by malformation of the auricles and by the presence of auricular appendages. The first case was that of a patient a year old, and very small. The deformity consisted of a fissure-like prolongation of the mouth downwards and backwards into the left cheek, and extending about three-quarters of an inch, and involving all the structures of the cheek. The lower maxilla was considerably smaller than normal, and the movements were not symmetrical; the external auditory meatus was larger outwardly and placed more anteriorly than usual, and ran backwards, where it became narrow in front of the membrana tympani, which, with the ossicula, was believed to be natural. Two so-called auricular appendages were placed in a line, one below the other, on the cheek between the tragus and the extremity of the fissure; one similar growth existed on the right cheek; and there was a similar but less morbid condition of the meatus on that side. The hearing was believed to be good. There was no history of hereditariness. The second case was that of a child aged five, delicate, and presenting an almost identical condition on the opposite side of the face. The mouth was prolonged into the cheek on the right side of the face, and there were two similar growths on the cheek, and the external meatus of both ears was expanded outwardly. The malformation of the lower jaw was not so evident, but it was smaller than usual. Hearing was fairly good in both ears, and the child talked naturally. There was no history of hereditariness. The two cases justify the observation that malformations of these parts are more frequent in females; but the only two cases hitherto described of macrostoma have not been accompanied by any deformity of the ears and their appendages. It is suggested that the deformity of the mouth is due to non-union of those parts of the first branchial arch which form the upper and lower jaw, and not to any error of formation of the oral opening ; whilst the auricular appendages are probably aberrant remnants of the opercular skin-fold of the first post-oral branchial cleft. They are much more common in all domestic animals than in man; but the author has found them in two cases lately, in neither of which was there any branchial fistula, whilst they were not present in a case of branchial fistula in front of the right sterno-mastoid in a boy. The patients were exhibited to the Society.

MR. FRANCIS MASON had seen two cases of enlarged mouth : one in the practice of Sir W. Fergusson, at King's College Hospital, in which there was also deformity of the ears; the other at St. Thomas's Hospital. In a work of which he was the author, he had quoted a case with the photograph.

Mr. HOLMES said that the theory of the connexion of the malformation with imperfect development of Meckel's cartilage was new to him, and had not been mentioned by other authors. It was, however, very interesting to hear two cases together, which bore out the explanation given by Sir James Paget and Mr. Morgan. There was no reason why the defect should not be remedied by sewing the parts together.

Mr. SAVORY had under his care, in St. Bartholomew's Hospital, four years ago, a young woman with a similar malformation of the mouth, but without deformity of the ear. A cure was effected by paring the edges of the cleft and bringing them together, a piece of the tissue being brought round at the angle of the mouth, so as to avoid the inconvenience which would be caused by a cicatrix.

Mr. BARWELL had shown the case at the International Medical Congress, and the foreign visitors who were present said that they had never seen such a case. He agreed with Mr. Morgan's explanation.

Mr. BERKELEY HILL said that Professor Virchow had described a case of the kind in his *Archiv*.

Mr. BARWELL said that Professor Virchow was unfortunately unable to be present when he showed the case.

Mr. THOMAS SMITH had had a case of cleft cheek at St. Bartholomew's Hospital, which was successfully treated by paring the edges of the cleft, and sewing them together. The orbicularis oris in this case was perfect. He had seen two or three cases of supernumerary cartilaginous auricles, without deformity of the mouth; but he had never seen such cases as these exhibited by Mr. Morgan.

Mr. CLEMENT LUCAS asked whether Mr. Morgan had examined into the condition of all the members of the families, so as to ascertain whether the deformity might not have been foreshadowed by some previous defect. He had, some time ago, a child under his care with a branchial fistula, whose mother had a similar malformation.

Mr. DALBY said that it was not very uncommon to find supernumerary ears, with perfect hearing; but, in cases of great deformity of the ears, the hearing was almost always greatly impaired.

Mr. MORGAN expressed regret that Sir James Paget, who had taken much interest in the subject under discussion, was unavoidably prevented from being present. Two questions were suggested by the cases. Why should the deformity be more frequent in females than in males? What was the influence of maternal impressions in the prevention of such deformities? If the influence of such impressions were admitted, why should small portions of the germinal membrane go wrong? No doubt, an imperfect development of the first branchial cleft was connected with the deformity of the ear and the defect of the mouth. As regarded operation, he did not anticipate much difficulty; but the younger child was in an unfavourable condition. He thanked Mr. Barwell for having placed the elder child under his care. He had endeavoured to ascertain through the parents, by means of correspondence, whether there was any similar malformation in other members of the family; but none could be discovered.

SUCCESSFUL CASE OF SIMULTANEOUS LIGATURE OF THE SUBCLAVIAN AND CAROTID ARTERIES FOR INNOMINATE ANEURISM.

Mr. H. W. LANGLEY BROWNE related a successful case of simultaneous ligature of the subclavian and carotid arteries for innominate aneurism. Suffering from this disease in an advanced form, J.A., aged thirty-two, was admitted into the West Bromwich Hospital on June 29, 1881. The sac-walls and coverings were thin and liable to rupture. There was a loud bruit over the swelling. The man was very weak and suffered intense pain in the chest. On July 11, the two arteries were tied with chromic catgut ligature, which Professor Lister had himself prepared. Antiseptic measures were used throughout. The highest temperature was 100·6°. Pulsation returned in the right temporal four days, and the right radial nine days after ligature, and is even yet very slight at the radial. There is much less pulsation in the tumour, which has strong thick walls. There is no bruit nor pain. The man feels so well that he has already tried to work. The condition of the tumour on October 28 was still one of improvement.

Mr. BARWELL congratulated Mr. Browne on the success of the case. He asked what was the condition of the aorta and heart before the operation. This had great influence on success. From an examination of statistics of the operation, he had arrived at the conclusion that, when there was extensive atheroma of the aorta, with dilatation, the ligature of the two great vessels was likely to be soon followed by death; if dilatation were not present, it would probably soon follow. It was important, before operation, to examine the state of the heart and aorta. The heart was hypertrophied in cases of aneurism of the divisions of the aorta; and there was, in many instances, aortic insufficiency.

Mr. HOLMES said it was a mistake to call the case successful at so early a period after operation. The author had rightly said that the danger of rupture of the aneurism had been reduced; but it was not correct to assume that there was no danger of a return of the aneurism. He was not aware that anyone operated in such cases without examining the heart and aorta.

Mr. C. HEATH referred to the difficulty of diagnosis between innominate and aortic aneurism; there was no positive diagnostic test during life.

Mr. BROWNE said that, as far as could be ascertained before the operation, the heart was sound. The case was one of successful ligature of the carotid and subclavian arteries; but he did not say that the aneurism was altogether cured—it was too early to say this. He concluded by referring to the advantage of the chromicised over the carbolised catgut—the latter, in his experience, having become too rapidly absorbed when used for ligature.

THE CLINICAL SOCIETY OF LONDON.
FRIDAY, NOVEMBER 11.

JOSEPH LISTER, D.C.L., F.R.C.S., F.R.S., President, in the Chair.

HONORARY MEMBERS.

SIR JAMES PAGET and several distinguished foreigners were unanimously elected Honorary Members of the Society.

FIVE CASES OF CANCER OF THE ŒSOPHAGUS, IN FOUR OF WHICH GASTROSTOMY WAS PERFORMED, CONSIDERED IN REGARD TO THE ADVISABILITY OF THIS OPERATION.

Mr. GOLDING-BIRD presented brief abstracts of these cases, together with one of a case in which the operation, though commenced, had to be abandoned, from the occurrence of œsophageal hæmorrhage that threatened immediate death. He pointed out that, being a palliative and not a radical operation, it could not be judged by bare statistics, for it dealt with the effect of the disease, not the disease itself; that his cases showed that the chances of giving relief were inversely as the length of time the patient had suffered (the man who lived five months after gastrostomy was sixty-six years of age, but had only had symptoms two months—all the others had much longer histories); that gastrostomy of itself was not a fatal and hardly a risky operation, the one case of peritonitis that occurred being due to an accident, the causes of which were not likely to be often met with; that, as with most other medical or palliative operations, the patient had the better chance the earlier he was operated upon, and this was especially so in gastrostomy, where the surgeon only fed, but the patient still required power to digest; yet he would not withhold gastrostomy even from cases presenting themselves late in the disease, where starvation was the only prospect, though he thought the anæsthetic added much to the existing share of depression in the patient. He would here, however, modify the usual plan, and open the stomach at the time of operating, and give nourishment at once. He believed that he lost two of his cases by not doing this, fearing vomiting, etc. He was distinctly opposed to œsophagotomy as a substitute. Four out of the five cases quoted had the growth in the chest, and therefore would not have been benefited by œsophagotomy; while, when the growth was at the cricoid level, it was operating dangerously close to a growth liable to fungate or increase on irritation. Dilatation of a cancerous stricture high up might be fairly tried, but when in the chest it was, in his opinion, more dangerous than gastrostomy itself.

Dr. COUPLAND related the case of a man aged sixty years, who had suffered from dysphagia for six months, and was almost moribund upon his admission to the Middlesex Hospital. The fluid which was given him was heard, upon auscultation, to trickle as far as the eighth dorsal spine. Stimulants were administered, and the patient rallied. As a bougie could not be passed through the stricture, Mr. Morris opened the stomach through a vertical incision in the abdominal wall, and fixed the stomach to the outer wound by quill sutures, the union being accomplished in three days. The patient was meanwhile fed with enemata, then by a little food introduced into the stomach; but he sank on the fifth day. The disease extended beneath the diaphragm, pushing forward the pericardium; and the gastric fistula was found to have been made within an inch and a half of the pylorus. As in most other cases coming to hospital, the time for operative interference which might benefit the patient had passed. The passage of food through the diseased œsophagus irritated the growth. The operation should be done at an earlier stage of the disease.

Dr. CAVAFY inquired if a canula had ever been fixed in the stomach, as was done by physiologists when performing the operation for the sake of obtaining gastric juice. The animals survived the operation. With some such precaution, the accident of pouring beef-tea into the peritoneum could not take place.

Mr. DURHAM thought cases of cancer of the œsophagus some of the most painful the physician or surgeon could have to treat. He had performed gastrostomy years ago, and thought Mr. Howse's suggestion of stitching the stomach-wall to the skin-wound some few days before the opening of the stomach was very good. The objection to the operation was, that patients would not permit it until the period of operation had almost come by. But the same objection applied to œsophagotomy. The dangers of gastrostomy had been overrated; the operation itself was not dangerous if the patient had sufficient recuperative power left in him to enable him to recover. The operation of œsophagotomy for a foreign body in the gullet was most excellent, and admitted of happy results; but when the operation was done for disease, the result was not equally good, and naturally a conspicuous wound in the neck was highly repellent to most patients. He would not have it done upon himself in such an unhappy contingency. He would suggest a third alternative. A female patient of his, now in Guy's Hospital, who had a growth involving the larynx and œsophagus, had after a time complete dysphagia, even for liquids. She was then fed through a No. 7 elastic catheter passed into the stomach from the mouth, and which found its way between the growth springing from the posterior wall of the larynx and the wall of the pharynx. Such catheter, changed every fourth day, had now been kept in for four months, and the size of it had been increased, so that she now wore a No. 12 instrument. Dr. Krishaber, at the recent International Medical Congress, had detailed four cases, and had reported that in most cases the œsophagus tolerated the presence of a bougie, but it would not do so in all cases. Before attempting the operation of gastrostomy, Mr. Durham advised that the plan of leaving a tube in the œsophagus should be first tried. The instruments should be passed carefully; they must be soft, and should find their own way without forcing, so as to avoid perforation of the diseased gullet. The tube should not be passed day by day at each time of feeding, but should be retained in position. Dr. Krishaber had advised the passing of the tube through the nostril; but a "nice little pipe in the mouth" was to most patients less disagreeable than one passed through the nose. If feeding through a tube could be accomplished, it should certainly be attempted before either œsophagotomy or gastrostomy was performed.

The PRESIDENT suggested that Dr. Coupland and Mr. Durham should furnish notes of their cases for insertion in the Transactions of the Society.

Dr. D. POWELL remarked that there was a danger of injecting the fluid food into the pleural cavity through a perforation in the œsophagus, however skilful the surgeon might be. He had seen the growth extend to the pleura. He had also recently seen, at the Eastbourne Convalescent Hospital, a young woman with traumatic stricture of the œsophagus, upon whom Mr. Bryant, at Guy's Hospital, had formerly performed gastrostomy, with the result that the patient was now rosy and well-fed, in a condition indeed of hypernutrition. She had been easily fed through the gastric open-

ing, and no regurgitation had occurred. He considered the operation should not be done in cases which were far advanced.

Dr. GOODHART said that, as regarded the extent of the disease, he thought the simple annular stricture was rare. The disease usually extended from the level of the cricoid cartilage nearly to the cardia. So that, from the pathological point of view, gastrostomy was the preferable operation.

Mr. RIVINGTON thought no surgeon would open the stomach if he could pass a bougie through the œsophagus. In one of Mr. Reeve's cases, no bougie could be passed, and the disease was evidently high up in the œsophagus. In such a case he would choose œsophagotomy, so as to pass a tube beyond the disease, and therewith feed the patient. When possible, a bougie should, of course, be passed.

Mr. DAVIES-COLLEY desired to remove some of the dislike of gastrostomy still entertained. Mr. Howse had, by modifying the operation, given to patients an extension of life of several months' duration, even when the disease was cancerous. When the malady of the œsophagus was not cancerous, the result was still more beneficial. He had performed gastrostomy upon two patients. In one, the disease was very extensive, and already sloughing at the time of operation; that patient soon died. The second patient was a woman, who, after the operation, and the consequent rest given to her œsophagus, from which it once more became patulous, was able to swallow; the wound in the stomach was consequently sewed up, and she had since done well, being able to swallow even solids. Mr. Howse's method of operation consisted in stitching the wall of the stomach, by two circles of sutures about an inch apart, to the abdominal wall around the abdominal opening. There was thus about an inch of the serous membrane enclosed between the two circles; and not until union of the apposed serous surfaces occurred, i.e., after about four or five days, was the stomach opened, and the patient fed through the fistula. Nutrient enemata were meanwhile administered.

Dr. ANDREW CLARK had a small addition to make to the discussion. Some months since, a little boy had come under his care, at the London Hospital, who had swallowed ammonia, which had caused ulceration of his mouth. After three months of treatment, he had gone out able to swallow liquids, but in two or three months subsequently was re-admitted, and could not then swallow even liquid food. Application being made to the surgeon to open the stomach —they were not like the Guy's surgeons!—they declined to perform gastrostomy. After a time, the house-surgeon, Mr. Oxley, with care managed to pass a bougie through the œsophagus, and now, after nine months, the little patient could swallow a meal of mutton-chop or other solid food. He wished to know if any and what care had been taken to make the food given to gastrostomised patients easy of digestion, as by peptonising it. He thought information on this subject desirable.

The PRESIDENT asked the question, where was cancer of the œsophagus most frequently situate. Mr. Reeves, in his paper, had seemed to think it was most often found at the upper part; but his own experience would place the most favourite site lower down. In the case of cancer, no operation could be expected to be over-successful; but in the case of traumatic stricture, life might by an operation be indefinitely prolonged. Of course, if the bougie could be, it should be, passed. Œsophagotomy had seemed to him to be a difficult operation, especially if the œsophagus were flaccid; and he asked if it was easy to feed the patient through the wound. The operation of gastrostomy was easier, but should not be deferred until the patient became too low to rally.

Mr. GOLDING-BIRD had hitherto been afraid to pass the œsophageal tube in cases of cancer for fear of perforation; but to-night's discussion had modified his opinion on this point. In his operations of gastrostomy, he had adopted Mr. Howse's precautions. In the case of accident, a stitch had been out at the time of the operation, the stomach had great tension upon it, and so the opening between that viscus and the abdominal wall into the peritoneal cavity had occurred.

Mr. REEVES said that in two of his cases the cancer of the œsophagus had not extended far down that tube, and the stricture was small. Such he had found to be the case in most specimens in museums; whilst it was generally easy to pass a finger or bougie through the stricture. In cases of gastrostomy, a Danish surgeon had distended the stomach through a tube passed into that viscus down the œsophagus. Verneuil, in 1876, made two rows of stitches in the manner which had been described to-night as Mr. Howse's modification of the operation. The mortality after gastrostomy was so high, that almost anything was justifiable before resorting to it. Therefore, he would say, first do œsophagotomy, which was not a difficult operation, and dilate the stricture. As in cancer of the rectum he had performed forcible dilatation with the finger without the occurrence of serious hæmorrhage, so he considered cancer of the œsophagus might be in a somewhat similar manner dilated without bad result.

Mr. LUCAS explained that Mr. Howse's operation consisted not only, like Verneuil's, in the stitching of the wall of the stomach to the abdominal wall by two circles of sutures, but, in addition thereto, in the deferring of the opening of the stomach for three or four days after that; whereas Verneuil opened the stomach directly after the external operation. This was a great distinction between these two methods of performing gastrostomy.

CASE IN WHICH A PEBBLE WAS REMOVED BY TRACHEOTOMY FROM THE RIGHT BRONCHUS.

Mr. R. CLEMENT LUCAS read notes of this case. A little boy, aged four, sixteen days before admission into Guy's Hospital, was playing with a pebble, and accidentally swallowed it. He was immediately seized with violent paroxysms of coughing and dyspnœa, which lasted for some time, and then passed away. From that time he was usually seized about twice daily with these paroxysms of coughing, which were always accompanied by distressing dyspnœa. During the attacks, the face became blue, and the veins prominent and turgid. It was especially on awaking from sleep that the coughing became violent. In the intervals between the paroxysms he suffered no distress, and was able to laugh, sing, and swallow without the slightest discomfort. When seen by Mr. Lucas, on July 14, 1881, the child was breathing with difficulty, and a physician who examined his chest had heard râles over the right bronchus. The cough was violent, rasping, and jerky, unaccompanied by whooping or wheezing. When the paroxysm came on, the child became blue, and almost suffocated. Mr. Lucas further noticed that during the effort of coughing, with his finger on the trachea, the foreign body could be felt to rise and strike that tube, and then fall back again. The trachea was opened, under Mr. Lucas's direction, by the House-Surgeon, Mr. Wood, and held open by retractors. At this time the child ceased breathing, but was restored by artificial respiration. The coughing which followed failed to dislodge the foreign body. A silk suture was next passed, by means of a semicircular needle and needle-holder, through the margin of the wound in the trachea on either side. The trachea could by means of these be drawn widely open. The child was then inverted and percussed on the back. The body did not become dislodged till the child was again placed on its back, when a fit of coughing brought it into sight. It was two or three times sucked back by the inspiration which follow after it had been driven up in the trachea, but was eventually dislodged, and prevented by forceps from re-entering. The foreign body proved to be a hard white pebble about the size of a cherry-stone. The after-treatment consisted in placing the child in a steam-tent, with moistened lint. For several days the child breathed chiefly through the wound. There were râles in the chest, and muco-purulent expectoration. The temperature rose on the third day as high as 102° Fahr., but gradually subsided to normal at the end of a week. The child left the hospital well on August 4, the wound being at this time soundly healed. Mr. Lucas remarked that tracheotomy was the only treatment in such cases, as it was highly improbable that the vocal cords, irritated by the presence of a foreign body in the trachea, would allow that body, when of considerable size, to repass the rima. Left alone, the case would almost certainly after a time have proved fatal. He strongly advocated the use of sutures to draw open the tracheal wound, as being infinitely superior to any form of retractor or dilator that could be invented. The weight of the pebble in this case caused delay in its expulsion. Had it been a cherry-stone, as the parents thought, it would probably have been more readily coughed up. Some foreign bodies, as tracheotomy-tubes, could not be expelled by coughing, owing to the air passing by or through them. He alluded to a case

of this kind that he brought before the Royal Medical and Chirurgical Society in 1877, and said that a narrow curved forceps was the best instrument to use in such cases.

The PRESIDENT exhibited a pair of forceps devised by himself, and intended for use in such a case as that of Mr. Lucas. The peculiarity in their construction consisted in the fact that when the blades were open they occupied less space than when closed. The blades were fenestrated; and, in cases of impaction in the urethra or larynx, they might be used with much advantage. The curve of the blades would vary with that of the canal in which they were to be employed.

OBITUARY.

PROFESSOR BOUILLAUD.

JEAN (or, according to some, Joseph) Bouillaud, who has occupied so prominent a place in French medical life during the last half-century, was born in September, 1796, so that when he died, almost suddenly, on October 29 last, he had entered his eighty-sixth year. And yet so vigorous were still both his mental and bodily powers, and so obedient did his remarkable memory continue, that only a very few weeks since, in one of the discussions on virulent and infectious diseases, which have of late so much engaged the attention of the Academy of Medicine, he delivered with clear and unfaltering voice a discourse of more than an hour's duration, giving a retrospective view from remote antiquity on the doctrines which had prevailed as to putridity in disease.

Although of very humble origin, he had an uncle who, being a military surgeon, enabled him to embrace the medical career. In 1818 he became an *interne* of the Paris hospitals, and especially devoted himself to physiological investigation, which Magendie was then making so attractive. As early as 1823, while still an *interne* at the Cochin, he published his first treatise on the influence of the Obliteration of the Veins in the formation of Passive Dropsies, which at once proved a work of mark, and has been regarded as one of the best of his productions. From this time, communication after communication continued to appear, among which some of the most interesting were those on the functions of the anterior lobes of the brain and of the cerebellum. His various memoirs on cerebral localisation constituted, indeed, important contributions to a branch of study which has since undergone so much expansion. This first bent of his studies induced him to contest the Chair of Physiology with Berard in 1831, and great was his disappointment in not obtaining it. The Chair of Clinical Medicine at La Charité, however, having become vacant in the same year, he succeeded in wresting it from such competitors as Louis, Rostan, Gendrin, and Piorry, and this success diverted his energies into the channel of practical teaching, which engaged his chief attention during the long period of thirty-five years. His clinic during this time acquired an immense popularity, for it was generally acknowledged that, as a clinical teacher, he was unsurpassed. His successive publications, "Traité Clinique des Maladies du Cœur," in which physical diagnosis was carried to its highest perfection, his works on Rheumatism and its Relation to Disease of the Heart, and his "Clinique de la Charité," offer ample evidence of the justice of the reputation he thus gained as one of the most successful teachers of the then celebrated Paris school. When his views on pathology and therapeutics come into question, however, a very different verdict has to be delivered. An ardent follower of Broussais, he devised and practised with great energy his *coup-sur-coup* mode of venesection, and aroused great hostility in consequence of his determined and arrogant advocacy of doctrines which the advance of medical science was fast leaving in the background.

Admitted early to the Académie de Médecine, Bouillaud became one of its most active members, memoir after memoir flowing from his pen; and, gifted with eloquence and a highly combative disposition, while possessed of no mean appreciation of the value of his own labours, there was scarcely a discussion of importance in which he did not take part, and many are the pages which he has contributed to the *Bulletin* in those prolonged discussions which Frenchmen seem never to weary in listening to. When admitted to the Académie des Sciences he was just as assiduous and laborious.

Bouilland had left directions that no addresses should be delivered at his grave, and no military honours should be rendered him as a Commander of the Legion of Honour. The concourse of practitioners, professors, and academicians at his funeral was, however, immense. It was felt that there had passed away one of the medical glories of the epoch, and one who, amidst a life of controversy, had yet endeared himself to all who knew him, and had cast great lustre on the famous school to which he belonged.

MEDICAL NEWS.

KING AND QUEEN'S COLLEGE OF PHYSICIANS IN IRELAND.—At the usual monthly examinations for the Licences of the College, held on Monday, Tuesday, Wednesday, and Thursday, November 7, 8, 9, and 10, the following candidates were successful:—

For the Licence to practise Medicine—

Callan, Richard.
Gelston, John Seymour.
Kisby, James Henry.
Ledwich, Edward L'Estrange.

McCabe, Alfred Alexander Donald.
McCormack, William Lane.
O'Carroll, Joseph Francis.
Skerrett, Patrick de Basterot.

For the Licence to practise Midwifery—

Gelston, John Seymour.
Kisby, James Henry.
Ledwich, Edward L'Estrange.
McCabe, Alfred Alexander Donald.

McCormack, William Lane.
O'Carroll, Joseph Francis.
Peyton, Henry Reynolds.
Skerrett, Patrick de Basterot
Sugrue, Jeremiah.

The following Licentiates of the College, having complied with the by-laws relating to membership, were admitted Members of the College—

MacDowel, Benjamin George, M.D. Dub. 1888, F.R.C.S.I. 1845, Licentiate of the College 1850.
Rae, William Masters, Surgeon R.N., Bermuda, Licentiate 1875.

ROYAL COLLEGE OF SURGEONS OF ENGLAND.—The following gentlemen passed their Primary Examinations in Anatomy and Physiology at a meeting of the Board of Examiners on the 10th inst., and, when eligible, will be admitted to the Pass Examination, viz.:—

Bailey, William E., of St. Bartholomew's Hospital.
Campbell, Ernest E., of St. Bartholomew's Hospital.
Edwards, Charles E., of St. Bartholomew's Hospital.
Goode, Ernest H., of University College Hospital.
Miller, Thomas H., of Guy's Hospital.
Molesworth, Robert E., of St. George's Hospital.
Push, Wilson, B.A. Cantab., of the London Hospital.
Penhall, Wm., B.A. Cantab., of St. Bartholomew's Hospital.
Scutt, Tom, of St. Thomas's Hospital.
Squire, Walter F., of St. George's Hospital.
Warner, Frederick A., of St. George's Hospital.
Webster, Ernest, of the Manchester School.

Seven candidates, having failed to acquit themselves to the satisfaction of the Board of Examiners, were referred to their anatomical and physiological studies for three months, making a total of thirty-one out of the ninety-one candidates examined, including three who were referred for an additional three months.

The following were admitted Members of the College at a meeting of the Court of Examiners on the 14th inst., viz.:—

Castañeda y Triana, T. P., M.D. Madrid, Habana.
Conway, John, M.B. Glasg., Glasgow.
Fligg, William, M.B. Edin., Edinburgh.
Fryer, John, L.S.A., Batley Carr, near Dewsbury.
Greaves, Thomas, M.D. New York, Charlotville, Virginia.
Hurtley, William M., L.S.A., Leeds.
Karanjia, Merwanji D., L.S.A., Bombay.
Lewers, Thomas R., M.B. Melb., Melbourne, Australia.
Line, William H., M.B. Dub., Daventry.
Ochiltree, Edward G., M.B. Glasg., Victoria, Australia.
Richmond, James, Preston, Lancashire.
Riordan, Daniel, M.D. Queen's Univ. Ire., Llandore, near Swansea.
Summerhill, Thomas H., Wolverhampton.
Sykes, Matthew C., L.R.C.P. Lond., Barnsley, Yorkshire.
Taylor, Benjamin R. A., L.S.A., Botesdale, Suffolk.
Viljoen, Anthony G., M.D. Edin., Caledon, Cape of Good Hope.

Eight candidates were rejected. At this meeting of the Court, Mr. John Croft, of St. Thomas's Hospital, the recently elected member of the Court, took his seat. The following gentlemen were admitted Members on the 15th inst., viz.:—

Adeney, Edwin L., Reigate.
Archer, Henry E., Anerley, S.E.
Chittenden, Thomas H., Maidstone.
Coles, William J., L.S.A., Croydon.
Dannt, Elliot, Leamcoston.
Evans, John D., L.R.C.P. Edin., Llandovery.
Gordon, Bryce, Bombay.

Hart, William H., L.S.A., Streatham.
Hingston, Richard, L.S.A., Liskeard.
Marshall, John G., L.S.A., Wallingford.
Martyn, Ernest, M.B. Aberd., Southall.
Rayner, Hugh, Liverpool.
Shaw, Lauriston E., Hastings.
Square, James E., Plymouth.
Williams, Robert, Liverpool.

Thirteen candidates were rejected. The following gentlemen passed on the 16th inst., viz.:—

Bertram, Benjamin, Cape Colony.
Birkett, Ernest, Ramsgate.
Cleaver, William F., M.D. Kingston, Stamford-street
Cowan, Richard H., L.S.A., Southsea.
Deane, Herbert E., L.S.A., St. Peter's-park, W.
Edwards, Thomas R. C., Gloucester-crescent, N.W.
Fox, George, Huddersfield.
Garrard, Charles B. O., Tickenhall, Derbyshire.
Gotch, Francis, Bristol.
Greenwood, George, Dalston.
Harrison, James, L.R.C.P. Edin., Manchester.
Harvey, Eldon, L.R.C.P. Edin., Bermuda.
Husband, John C. R., Ripon, Yorks.
Kershaw, U., Brighouse, Yorks.
Pitt, George N., M.A. Cantab., Sutton, Surrey.
Style, Robert G., Chichester.
Thomson, St. Clair, L.S.A., St. Mark's-crescent.
Williams, Herbert E., Abertillery, Mon.

Twelve candidates were rejected.

Pass Examinations.—The following were the questions on Surgical Anatomy and the Principles and Practice of Surgery submitted, on the 11th inst., to the candidates now undergoing their vivâ voce examination for the diploma of Membership of the Royal College of Surgeons; they were required to answer at least four, including one of the first two, out of the six questions:—1. Give the relations of the sartorius muscle throughout its entire length, and mention the chief points of surgical interest connected with it. 2. Mention, in order, the several structures necessarily divided in removal of the entire upper jaw-bone. 3. What circumstances would lead you to suspect the presence of a foreign body in the air-passages, at some point below the glottis? What are the risks which it entails, and what treatment would you adopt? 4. Describe the various conditions which are known popularly under the name of whitlow, and their complications. What treatment is appropriate to each? 5. Describe the probable course of syphilis during the first year from the date of infection, in the absence of treatment; giving carefully the probable dates and duration of the various symptoms. 6. What symptoms would lead you to suspect an abscess in the middle ear? What is the usual course of such abscesses, and what are the later risks they entail? The following were the questions on the Principles and Practice of Medicine, viz.:—1. State exactly the physical signs of the different recognised varieties of disease of the aortic and mitral valves; and enumerate and discuss the consequences of lesions of the mitral valve. 2. What are the causes of abdominal dropsy? How would you recognise its presence? And how would you discriminate its several varieties, having regard not only to the condition of the abdomen and its contents, but to associated phenomena? 3. What are the medicinal properties of opium, belladonna, aconite, Indian hemp, strychnia, elaterium, colchicum, arsenic, zinc, and iron? And give the ordinary dose for an adult of at least two preparations of each of them.

APOTHECARIES' HALL, LONDON.—The following gentlemen passed their examination in the Science and Practice of Medicine, and received certificates to practise, on Thursday, November 10:—

Cortis, Herbert Liddell, Guy's Hospital.
Cowan, Richard Hamilton, London Hospital.
Dunmore, Howard House, Victoria Dock-road, E.
Hingston, Richard, London Hospital.
Richardson, Adolphus Joseph, London Hospital.
Rowall, Robert Henry, Houghton-le-Spring.
Yeatman, John Walter, R. S. B. Infirmary, Margate.

The following gentleman also on the same day passed the Primary Professional Examination:—

Edwards, Charles Augustus, London Hospital.

APPOINTMENTS

** The Editor will thank gentlemen to forward to the Publishing-office, as early as possible, information as to all new Appointments that take place.

DASHWOOD, EDMUND S., M.R.C.S.E., L.S.A.—Assistant House-Surgeon to the Sussex County Hospital, Brighton.

BIRTHS.

BELLAMY.—On November 16, at 17, Wimpole-street, the wife of Edward Bellamy, F.R.C.S., of a daughter.

COX.—On November 11, at 3, Dean-street, Park-lane, W., the wife of Frederick Augustus Cox, M.R.C.S., of a son.

CUTHBERT.—On November 14, at Walsham-le-Willows, near Bury St. Edmunds, the wife of W. W. Cuthbert, M.R.C.S., of a daughter.

HARLEY.—On November 13, at Saffron Walden, Essex, the wife of Edward Harley, L.R.C.P., of a daughter.

HAWARD.—On November 13, at 16, Savile-row, Burlington-gardens, the w.fe of Warrington Haward, F.R.C.S., of a son.

KING.—On November 12, at Ambleside, Westmoreland, the wife of William Moore King, M.R.C.S., of twins, girls.

MALLAM.—On November 14, at Shepherd's Bush, the wife of W. P. Mallam, L.R.C.P., of a daughter.

POTTS.—On November 5, at Leatherhead, the wife of Laurence Potts, M.R.C.S., of a son, prematurely.

THOMAS.—On October 20, at Palamcottah, South India, the wife of Surgeon G. T. Thomas, L.R.C.P., Indian Medical Department, of a daughter.

MARRIAGES.

ATKEY—ANDERSON.—On November 8, at Chichester, William T. Atkey, L.R.C.P., of Chichester, to Mary Catherine, daughter of J. Anderson, Esq., of Stockbridge, Chichester, and late of Alresford, Hants.

AUSTIN—DAVEY.—On November 8, at Walmer, Corneby Austin, L.R.C.P. and S. Edin., of Gayton, King's Lynn, Norfolk, to Mary Elizabeth, daughter of Richard Staines Davey, M.D., J.P., of Hill House, Walmer, Kent.

BLYTH—FINDLATER.—On November 12, at Kingstown, John Blyth, M.D., of Fitzwilliam-square, Dublin, to Jane, widow of the late Adam B. Findlater, Esq., of The Slopes, Kingstown.

BOMFORD—ETESON.—On October 17, at Simla, Gerald Bomford, M.D., Bengal Medical Service, to Mary Florence, only daughter of Lieutenant-Colonel Eteson, Assistant Adjutant-General, Army Headquarters in India.

GRIFFITH—WRIGHT.—On November 9, at Sydenham, Arthur Gerald, elder son of Griffith Griffiths, M.D., of Taltreudyn, Monmouth, and of Hydras, Var, France, to Mary Camilla Braybrooke, daughter of W. Dumaresq Wright, Esq., of the Ceylon Civil Service.

KILNER—DAVIS-GOFF.—On November 9, at Horetown, Charles Scott Kilner, M.B., youngest son of John Kilner, F.R.C.S., of Bury St. Edmunds, to Lucy Ussher, youngest daughter of S. Davis-Goff, J.P., of Horetown House, County Wexford.

SNEYD—ELIN.—On November 10, at Hertford, James Alexander Parsons, Sneyd, Esq., of the Bengal Constabulary, to Florence Caroline, eldest daughter of George Elin, M.D., of Leahoe, Hertford.

DEATHS.

BUCKNILL, SAMUEL BIRCH, M.D., at Rugby, on November 12, aged 66.

GORE, RICHARD THOMAS, F.R.C.S., at Bath, on November 14, in his 83rd year.

McNICOLL, JAMES W., only son of Robert McNicoll, M.R.C.S., of St. Helen's, Lancashire, at Southport, on November 12, aged 30.

SCOUGAL, MARGARET THERESA, wife of Edward Fowler Scougal, M.B., M.A., at Lydgate, New Mill, Huddersfield, on November 12, aged 37.

TRENNEL, EDWARD ALFRED, M.D., Surgeon-Major, of Chingleput, at Madras, on October 23, in his 54th year.

WATKINS, WALTER, M.R.C.S., at Eccles House, Demerara, on October 6, aged 45.

UNION AND PAROCHIAL MEDICAL SERVICE.

. The area of each district is stated in acres. The population is computed according to the census of 1871.

RESIGNATIONS.

Beverley Union.—The First District and the Workhouse are vacant by the death of Mr. Thomas John Thompson: area 14,026; population 7494; salary £34 per annum. Salary for Workhouse £40 per annum.

Burton-upon-Trent Union.—The Repton District is vacant: area 14,313; population 3930; salary £49 per annum.

APPOINTMENTS.

Billingham Union.—Robert Jackson, M.D. St. And., M.R.C.S. Lond., to the Fourth District.

Machynlleth Union.—David Edwards, B.M. and M.C. Edin., to the Darowen District.

Malling Union.—Thomas Holyoake, M.R.C.S. Eng., L.S.A., to the Second District.

St. Columb Major Union.—Frederick Dunbar Sutherland McMahon, L.R.C.P., L.R.C.S., L.M. Edin., to the Third and Sixth Districts.

Solihull Union.—Mm. Huey, L.K. & Q.C.P. Ire., M.R.C.S., L.R.C.S., and L.M. Edin., to the Tamworth District.

South Molton Union.—Joseph Tucker, M.R.C.S. Eng., L.S.A., to the Eighth District.

Ticehurst Union.—Charles Hoar, B.M. and M.C. Aber., to the Hurstgreen District.

VACANCIES.

In the following list the nature of the office vacant, the qualifications required in the candidate, the person to whom application should be made and the day of election (as far as known) are stated in succession.

BELGRAVE HOSPITAL FOR CHILDREN, 79, GLOUCESTER-STREET, WARWICK-SQUARE, S.W.—House-Surgeon. Candidates must be qualified. Applications, with testimonials, to be sent to the Hon. Sec., at the Hospital, on or before November 23.

CHARING-CROSS HOSPITAL, WEST STRAND, W.C.—Assistant-Physician. *particulars see Advertisement.*)

EVELINA HOSPITAL FOR SICK CHILDREN, SOUTHWARK-BRIDGE-ROAD, S.E.—Physician. (*For particulars see Advertisement.*)

NORTH-EASTERN HOSPITAL FOR CHILDREN, HACKNEY-ROAD.—Assistant House-Surgeon. Candidates must be duly registered practitioners. Applications and copies of testimonials to be sent to Alfred Nixon, Secretary, 27, Clement's-lane, E.C., on or before November 21.

GENERAL INFIRMARY AT GLOUCESTER, AND THE GLOUCESTERSHIRE EYE INSTITUTION.—Ophthalmic Surgeon. Applications, enclosing qualifications and testimonials, to be forwarded to the Committee, under cover to the Secretary, on or before December 7.

LIVERPOOL DISPENSARIES.—Assistant House-Surgeon. Candidates must be duly qualified and unmarried. Applications, stating age, with testimonials and registration certificate, to be sent to the Secretary, Leith Offices, 34, Moorfields, Liverpool, not later than November 22.

GATESHEAD DISPENSARY.—Resident House-Surgeon. Candidates must be doubly qualified. Applications, with copies of testimonials, to be sent to Mr. Joseph Jordon, Hon. Sec., 2, Side, Newcastle, not later than November 23.

ST. PETER'S HOSPITAL FOR STONE AND URINARY DISORDERS, ETC., 54, BERNERS-STREET, W.—House-Surgeon. Applications, with copies of testimonials, to be sent to R. G. Salmond, Secretary, on or before November 22.

MEDICAL MAYOR.—On the 9th inst., Mr. Alfred Emson, J.P., was appointed Mayor, for the second time, for the borough of Dorchester.

THE KING OF SWEDEN AND NORWAY has just conferred upon Dr. Alfred Meadows the Commandership of the Second Class of the Order of the Wasa. The insignia of the Order were officially presented to Dr. Meadows by his Excellency Count Piper, the Swedish Minister Plenipotentiary at the Court of St. James.

STRETCHING THE LINGUAL NERVE IN FACIAL TIC DOULOUREUX.—Dr. Le Dentu presented a patient before the Société de Chirurgie, in whom he had successfully stretched the lingual nerve for facial tic douloureux, accompanied by epileptiform convulsions. The pain had its seat in the temporal region, the ear, the lower jaw, and the left side of the tongue. It dated back five years, but since last June the pain had become insupportable, especially at the side of the tongue. Dr. Le Dentu, determining to perform stretching of the lingual nerve, fixed the point of the tongue by means of a strong ligature, and by the aid of a small hook gently raised the nerve to a height of about twelve millimetres above the buccal mucous membrane, and retaining it there for some seconds, he let it descend again into the mouth, having ascertained that in consequence of the stretching it had become quite flaccid and of a kind of zig-zag form. Seeing the old date of the case no immediate result was expected, but after the second day the patient had already begun to enjoy sleep, and now—thirteen days after the operation—she was quite free of pain, not only in the tongue itself, but also in the temporal region—a little pain above the angle of the jaw alone remaining. She eats and sleeps well, and must be considered to be, at all events provisionally, cured. Dr. Polaillon observed that three months since he performed stretching of the inferior dental nerve for very violent neuralgia affecting it, and the patient has continued cured.—*Union Méd.*, November 8.

THE CINCHONA CULTIVATION IN BENGAL.—Dr. King's reports on cinchona cultivation and manufacture for the year 1880-81, together with an appreciative resolution on them by the Government of Bengal, furnish an interesting and altogether hopeful account of this important and beneficent enterprise. Both cultivation and production are progressively increasing, and effort is now being made to propagate the finer qualities of cinchona and those yielding a larger proportion of quinine. Thus 90,000 plants of a hybrid variety of the *Calisaya* species, the bark of which gives a large yield of quinine, were put out during the year, and 99,415 of the *Ledgeriana* variety, which is peculiarly rich in the same valuable alkaloid. There are now more than four million trees of the *Succirubra* species on the plantations. The amount of dry bark husbanded during the year was 377,525 lbs., which exceeds the production of any previous year. Most of this was red bark, some 81,000 lbs. being yellow (*Calisaya*). Dr. King points out that the object of Government in maintaining its cinchona plantation in Sikkim is not to grow bark for England or elsewhere, but to produce raw material for the manufacture of the febrifuge for the use of the people of the country. The amount of the alkaloid manufactured during the year was 9296 lbs. There were 8650 lbs. disposed of in the year, 5500 lbs. having been sent to the medical depôts and 3150 lbs. sold to the public, being 393 lbs. more than last year.—*Indian*

CASE OF ACUTE CHOREA.—Dr. Gary reports, in the *Transactions of the South Carolina Medical Association* for 1881, the following case:—F. B., while at college during the last winter, suffered from a very severe attack of acute rheumatism, and when he was supposed to be nearly well, the irregular movements so characteristic of chorea were observed. Confined at first to the left side, as the disease advanced they became general. The usual remedies were tried without benefit, and as the symptoms were becoming aggravated (such as difficult deglutition, drawing the mouth to one side, rolling of the eyes, flushed face, pain in the head, constant movements of the hands and feet, quick pulse, etc.), and threatened a fatal termination from congestion of the brain, it was determined to put him on veratrum viride, ten drops every two hours, increasing each dose by two drops until nausea or a considerable reduction of the pulse should be observed. Just after the administration of the fourth dose of eighteen drops there was free emesis and a reduction of the pulse to fifty beats, with great prostration. This, however, under a dose of stimulant soon passed off, when it was observed that there was great improvement in the choreic movements, which just before were so violent and so serious. This treatment was continued in smaller doses, adapting the quantity according to the amount of movement. The patient continued to improve, and at the end of two months was dismissed cured.—*New York Med. Record*, October 8.

APPOINTMENTS FOR THE WEEK.

November 19. *Saturday* (*this day*).

Operations at St. Bartholomew's, 1½ p.m.; King's College, 1½ p.m.; Royal Free, 2 p.m.; Royal London Ophthalmic, 11 a.m.; Royal Westminster Ophthalmic, 1½ p.m.; St. Thomas's, 1½ p.m.; London, 2 p.m.

21. *Monday*.

Operations at the Metropolitan Free, 2 p.m.; St. Mark's Hospital for Diseases of the Rectum, 2 p.m.; Royal London Ophthalmic, 11 a.m.; Royal Westminster Ophthalmic, 1½ p.m.

MEDICAL SOCIETY OF LONDON, 8½ p.m. Mr. Henry F. Baker, "On a Case of Congenital Displacement of the Head of the Tibia Backwards in both Legs, with Double Clubfoot." Dr. Stephen Mackenzie, "On Pityriasis Rubra (four cases) and its Allies" (a postponed paper). Dr. Routh, "On the Necessity of adopting a Different Mode of Burying Bodies the subjects of Infectious Disease."

22. *Tuesday*.

Operations at Guy's, 1½ p.m.; Westminster, 2 p.m.; Royal London Ophthalmic, 11 a.m.; Royal Westminster Ophthalmic, 1½ p.m.; West London, 3 p.m.

ANTHROPOLOGICAL INSTITUTE (Council Meeting, 4½ p.m.), 8 p.m. Dr. E. B. Tylor, "Notes on the Asiatic Relations of Polynesian Culture." Rev. R. H. Codrington, "Notes on the Affinity of the Melanesian, Malay, and Polynesian Languages." Rev. Lorimer Fison, "Fijian Riddles." Dr. J. Beddoe, "On the Stature of the Inhabitants of Hungary."

ROYAL MEDICAL AND CHIRURGICAL SOCIETY, 8½ p.m. Mr. Spencer Wells, "On a Case of Excision of a Gravid Uterus with Epithelioma of the Cervix; with Remarks on the Operations of Blundell, Freund, and Porro." Mr. T. M. Girdlestone (of Melbourne), "On the Surgical Uses of Kangaroo Tendons."

23. *Wednesday*.

Operations at University College, 2 p.m.; St. Mary's, 1¼ p.m.; Middlesex, 1 p.m.; London, 2 p.m.; St. Bartholomew's, 1½ p.m.; Great Northern, 2 p.m.; Samaritan, 2½ p.m.; Royal London Ophthalmic, 11 a.m.; Royal Westminster Ophthalmic, 1½ p.m.; St. Thomas's, 1½ p.m.; St. Peter's Hospital for Stone, 2 p.m.; National Orthopædic, Great Portland-street, 10 a.m.

24. *Thursday*.

Operations at St. George's, 1 p.m.; Central London Ophthalmic, 1 p.m.; Royal Orthopædic, 2 p.m.; University College, 2 p.m.; Royal London Ophthalmic, 11 a.m.; Royal Westminster Ophthalmic, 1½ p.m.; Hospital for Diseases of the Throat, 2 p.m.; Hospital for Women, 2 p.m. Charing-cross, 2 p.m.; London, 2 p.m.; North-West London, 2½ p.m.

25. *Friday*.

Operations at Central London Ophthalmic, 2 p.m.; Royal London Ophthalmic, 11 a.m.; South London Ophthalmic, 2 p.m.; Royal Westminster Ophthalmic, 1½ p.m.; St. George's (ophthalmic operations), 1¼ p.m.; Guy's, 1½ p.m.; St. Thomas's (ophthalmic operations), 2 p.m.; King's College (by Mr. Lister), 2 p.m.

QUEKETT MICROSCOPICAL CLUB (University College), 8 p.m. W. H. Gilburt, F.R.M.S., "On the Structure and Division of the Vegetable Cell."

CLINICAL SOCIETY, 8½ p.m. Dr. Mahomed and Mr. Cripps, "On Two Cases of Direct Transfusion of Blood for Hæmorrhage in Typhoid Fever." Dr. Whipham, "On Three Cases of Continued Fever with Affection of the Spleen and unusually High Temperature." Mr. W. H. Bennett, "On a Case of Talipes Equino-Varus treated by Resection of a Portion of the Tarsus" (patient will be shown). Mr. J. R. Lunn, "On Two Cases of Myxœdema, Male and Female" (patients will be shown).

VITAL STATISTICS OF LONDON.

Week ending Saturday, November 12, 1881.

BIRTHS.

Births of Boys, 1404; Girls, 1334; Total, 2738.
Corrected weekly average in the 10 years 1871-80, 2701·8.

DEATHS.

	Males.	Females.	Total.
Deaths during the week	860	776	1636
Weekly average of the ten years 1871-80, corrected to increased population ...	848·1	819·3	1667·4
Deaths of people aged 80 and upwards ...	...	...	57

DEATHS IN SUB-DISTRICTS FROM EPIDEMICS.

	Enumerated Population, 1881 (unrevised).	Small-pox.	Measles.	Scarlet Fever.	Diphtheria.	Whooping-cough.	Typhus.	Enteric (or Typhoid) Fever.	Simple continued Fever.	Diarrhœa.
West	668993	2	6	6	...	2	...	4	...	2
North ...	905677	4	7	17	11	10	1	12	1	1
Central ...	281793	...	...	1	1	6	...	4	...	...
East	692580	1	1	8	6	16	1	5	...	4
South	1265578	20	27	17	5	9	1	10	...	6
Total	3814571	27	41	49	23	43	3	35	1	13

METEOROLOGY.

From Observations at the Greenwich Observatory.

Mean height of barometer	29·992 in.
Mean temperature	51·6°
Highest point of thermometer	59·5°
Lowest point of thermometer	42·0°
Mean dew-point temperature	49·1°
General direction of wind	E. & S.W.
Whole amount of rain in the week	0·25 in.

BIRTHS and DEATHS Registered and METEOROLOGY during the Week ending Saturday, Nov. 12, in the following large Towns:—

Cities and boroughs (Municipal boundaries except for London.)	Estimated Population to middle of the year 1881.*	Persons to an Acre. (1881.)	Births Registered during the week ending Nov. 12.	Deaths Registered during the week ending Nov. 12.	Temperature of Air (Fahr.)			Temp. of Air (Cent.)	Rain Fall.	
					Highest during the Week.	Lowest during the Week.	Weekly Mean of Daily Mean Values	Weekly Mean of Daily Mean Values.	In Inches.	In Centimetres.
London	3829751	50·8	2738	1636	59·5	42·0	51·6	10·90	0·25	0·63
Brighton	107934	45·9	74	45	59·0	44·0	51·2	10·67	0·04	0·10
Portsmouth ...	128335	28·6	92	51	...	...	...	...	...	...
Norwich	88038	11·8	60	27	...	...	...	...	...	...
Plymouth	75262	54·0	38	23	62·6	47·8	54·4	12·44	0·34	0·86
Bristol	207140	46·5	138	93	58·0	42·5	51·4	10·78	0·41	1·04
Wolverhampton ...	75934	22·4	51	20	...	...	...	...	...	...
Birmingham ...	402296	47·9	322	169	...	...	...	...	...	...
Leicester	123120	38·5	87	28	61·2	40·8	49·8	9·89	0·06	0·15
Nottingham ...	188035	18·9	133	88	58·3	38·5	49·2	9·55	0·33	0·84
Liverpool	553988	106·3	415	303	58·0	43·5	51·7	10·95	0·16	0·41
Manchester ...	341269	79·5	254	161	...	...	...	...	...	...
Salford	177760	34·4	152	99	...	...	...	...	...	...
Oldham	112176	24·0	82	36	...	...	...	...	...	...
Bradford	184037	25·5	105	59	58·0	43·0	50·6	10·34	0·08	0·20
Leeds	310490	14·4	217	129	59·0	41·0	49·7	9·83	0·07	0·18
Sheffield	285621	14·5	261	115	59·0	42·0	51·3	10·73	0·18	0·46
Hull	155161	42·7	119	91	57·0	40·0	48·4	9·11	0·15	0·38
Sunderland ...	116753	42·2	99	37	63·0	43·0	52·5	11·39	0·01	0·03
Newcastle-on-Tyne	145675	27·1	91	57	...	...	...	...	...	...
Total of 20 large English Towns ...	7608775	38·0	5531	3264	63·0	38·5	51·0	10·56	0·17	0·43

* These figures are the numbers enumerated (but subject to revision) in April last, raised to the middle of 1881 by the addition of a quarter of a year's increase, calculated at the rate that prevailed between 1871 and 1881.

At the Royal Observatory, Greenwich, the mean reading of the barometer last week was 29·99 in. The lowest reading was 29·83 in. on Wednesday evening, and the highest 30·10 in. on both Friday morning and at the end of the week.

NOTES, QUERIES, AND REPLIES.

Be that questioneth much shall learn much.—Bacon.

India.—Consult the "Guide to European Universities," by Dr. J. H. Hardwicke, published by Messrs. Churchill, 11, New Burlington-street, W.

S. A. G. asks—" Would you kindly, through your paper, tell me if you know of anything that will remove Indian ink tattoo-marks from the flesh; and if I could do it myself, or get a surgeon to do it ?"

Colonial Items.—Yellow fever still prevails at St. Louis on the river Senegal, and the malady has also made its way to Dakar and Gorée, where deaths have taken place. The fever, which appeared in a severe epidemic form at St. Louis, is said to have caused terrible havoc amongst the population. So devastating has been the visitation that it is stated the island will be little fit for business during the ensuing season. New South Wales : The second reading of the Licensing Bill has been moved in the House of Assembly by Sir Henry Parkes. It will repeal all existing Acts relating to publicans, and insure, as far as possible, that intoxicating drinks shall not be supplied to aborigines, children, or inebriates. It also includes the trade of brewer, the members of which will, in future, have to pay for licences on a graduated scale. The leading principles of the Bill are—" That the power of granting licences will be taken from the magistrates, and given to licensing boards, and the people will have a voice in deciding whether a licence should be granted or not."

Generosity.—Mr. T. H. Woods (of Messrs. Christie, Manson, and Woods) has generously constructed and fitted up a new coffee-tavern in the largely populated hamlet of Croxley Green, Rickmansworth, where extensive paper-mills are situated. Mr. Woods is a resident in the locality.

A Misconception.—A somewhat unusual action has just been tried at the County Court, Exeter. Some time ago the members of several friendly societies formed themselves into a Medical Association, and appointed their own medical officer, who was to give his whole time to the appointment. He was sent for to attend the wife of a member, but on calling, he said there was nothing the matter with her. The woman still feeling ill, her husband called in another medical man, when it was discovered she was suffering from typhoid fever, which subsequently developed into a very bad attack. The present action was brought to recover £5, paid to the second medical man. The defendant urged that he called at the house and expressed surprise at the letter he had received, when the wife talked to him in such a manner that he concluded she was suffering more from bad temper than anything else. From her condition he did not consider the case one of emergency, and told her so, upon which she declined his attendance. The Judge remarked that a sick woman would naturally feel irritated on being told nothing was the matter with her. The jury found a verdict for the amount claimed, his Honour refusing permission to appeal.

Food-Supplies to the Metropolis.—Some American consignors of meat, unable to discover the mystery of the enormous difference between the prices they receive and those the public have to pay, have resolved, it is stated, to apply to the Corporation for shops in the new Leadenhall Market, in order to sell their meat direct to the public. One of the principal firms in the Leadenhall Market has just issued a circular "To the small farmers, cottiers, and farm labourers of England," calling attention to the fact that 200 tons of rabbits are sent over from Ostend to London every week during the season. These are not wild rabbits, as is generally supposed, but are reared, for the most part, by Belgian cottiers. The circular asks why the example of the Belgian cottiers is not followed by the same classes in this country.

Filthy Condition of a Registered Lodging-house.—The keeper of a registered house in Brooke-street, Holborn, has been fined 40s. by the Clerkenwell police magistrate for neglecting to thoroughly clean the floors, blankets, and sheets, and to keep the same in a wholesome condition. The defendant had been several times cautioned by the police, but with no effect.

Jerry Builders.—The Edmonton magistrates have fined a builder of St. George's-road, Seven Sisters-road, in the sums of £10 and £2 7s., for erecting two separate houses with improper materials. The Tottenham Local Board prosecuted. Samples of the mortar used were submitted to the Bench, which, on being rubbed between the fingers, crumbled to pieces, and it was totally unfit for the purposes of building. Many similar instances of infringing the sanitary by-laws of this district have come under our notice. A commendable vigilance is evidently exercised by the local officials over these speculative house-builders.

As St. Pancras Workhouse Difficulty.—An official notice and order have been issued by the Local Government Board, directing the removal of St. Pancras from the Asylums District from December 26 next ; at the same time ordering the transfer of the Highgate Infirmary to the Guardians of St. Pancras. Simultaneously, the Local Government Board has officially announced its assent to the reconstruction of the existing workhouse of St. Pancras on its present site.

Prosecution against a "Medical Man" at Didcot.—The county magistrates, after a protracted investigation of a series of charges preferred by the Glasgow College of Physicians and Surgeons against a medical man practising at Didcot, have committed the defendant for trial at the next Berkshire Assizes. He was admitted to bail, himself at £200, and two sureties of £150 each. There were four charges—the forgery of a document purporting to be a diploma of the Faculty of Physicians, Glasgow ; the forgery of and for uttering a certificate that he was a licentiate of the said College ; and for obtaining money in two instances by false pretences.

Antagonism.—The second refusal of the Local Government Board to sanction the Coventry City Council to borrow £889 for improving the river Sherbourne has produced considerable surprise and irritation. The Council have formulated a scheme to obviate the periodical floods, which are a great nuisance, and the cause of disease and death. It appears the Local Government Board considered it would be a work of river conservancy, and consequently refused to sanction the project. Subsequently, however, at the request of the City Council, they deputed an inspector to hold an inquiry into the matter and to view the river. He made his report, which, it was understood, would be favourable to the proposed improvements ; and this ultimate refusal from the central authority was not anticipated. There is an undivided opinion that something must be done, and the subject has been referred to the General Works Committee of the Council to consider and report.

COMMUNICATIONS have been received from—
The Registrar of the Apothecaries' Hall, London; Mr. J. Croft, London; Mr. H. H. Dickson, Atlanta, U.S.; Mr. Snell, Sheffield; Mr. C. R. Francis, London; Dr. Norman Kerr, London; Dr. W. Alexander, Liverpool; Dr. De Bartolomé, Sheffield; Dr. W. B. Kesteven, London; Messrs. J. Allen and Sons, London; Mr. Alfred Enson, Dorchester; Messrs. F. Edwards and Sons, London; The Secretary of the Indian Medical Service Defence Committee, London; Dr. Creighton, London; Dr. Garth Wilkinson, London; Surgeon-General Gordon; Messrs. F. Newbery and Sons, London; Mr. Sidney Jones, London; Dr. Russell, Birmingham; Mr. Parker, London; Dr. W. H. Day, London; Dr. Arthur Ransom, Altrincham; Dr. Aury Lawrence, Clifton; Dr. Douglas Powell, London; Mr. W. Bacot, London; Mr. J. Chatto, London; The Honorary Secretary of the Medical Society of London; Mr. C. Higgens, London; Dr. Crichton Browne, London; The Director of the Anthropological Institute, London; The Secretary of the Clinical Society of London; Dr. Ridge, London; Dr. Bryan Waller, Edinburgh; Dr. Shaw, Clifton; The House-Surgeon, King's College; Surgeon Gilligan, Bengal Medical Service; The Secretary of the Quekett Microscopical Club, London; Dr. Shingleton Smith, Bristol; Messrs. Street and Co., London; Messrs. Bates, Hendy, and Co., London; Mr. Doreitt Stone, London; Professor Chaveau, Glasgow; Dr. Langmore, London; Mr. Field, St. Mary's Hospital; Mr. Wickham Barnes, London; Dr. J. W. Moore, Dublin; Mr. Bacot, Seaton; Mr. G. S. Perkins, Exeter; The Honorary Secretary of the Royal Medical and Chirurgical Society of London; Mr. John Langton, London; Mr. T. M. Stone, London.

BOOKS, ETC., RECEIVED—
Étude du Processus Histologique des Néphritée, par le Dr. Ch. Hortolès—Excision of the Tongue, by Walter Whitehead, F.R.C.S.—Annual Report of the Taunton Sanitary Hospital, 1880-81—On Enteric Fever, by Christian Baümler, M.D., F.R.C.P.—The Latin Grammar of Pharmacy, by Joseph Ince, F.C.S., F.L.S.

PERIODICALS AND NEWSPAPERS RECEIVED—
Lancet—British Medical Journal—Medical Press and Circular—Berliner Klinische Wochenschrift—Centralblatt für Chirurgie—Gazette des Hopitaux—Gazette Médicale—Le Progrès Médical—Bulletin de l'Académie de Médecine—Pharmaceutical Journal—Wiener Medizinische Wochenschrift—Centralblatt für die Medizinischen Wissenschaften—Revue Médicale—Gazette Hebdomadaire—National Board of Health Bulletin, Washington—Nature—Deutsche Medicinal-Zeitung—Boston Medical and Surgical Journal—Louisville Medical News—Atlanta and Neurological—Boston Journal of Chemistry—Atlanta Medical Register—La Presse Médicale—L'Impartialité Médicale—El Observator—Manchester Examiner and Times, November 12—Christian Commonwealth—Daily Courier, November 12—Centralblatt für Gynäkologie—Revue Médicale—Science—Western Medical Reporter—The Colonies and India—New York Medical Journal—Canada Lancet—Chemist and Druggist—Scientific Roll—Canadian Journal of Medical Science—Birkenhead and Cheshire Advertiser, November 12—Daily Telegraph, November 11—Liverpool Daily Post, November 16—Irish Times, November 12—Journal of the British Dental Association—Gazzetta Medica Italiana.

IMPROVEMENTS IN HOSPITAL CONSTRUCTIONS IN FRANCE.—The *Gazette Hebdomadaire* (November 11), after describing two new *hopitaus-hospices* which have been recently opened in Paris, observes, " These new hospital constructions exhibit the attention which architects are beginning to pay to the teaching of hygiene, and are the more gratifying as they stand in contrast with some examples still recent. We are at last beginning to understand in France that patients should not be accumulated in magnificent edifices, the ostentatious product of ambitious conceptions, and that all we have to do is to insure the well-being of the sick and the salubrity of their abodes. Air, space, and the completest possible isolation are the indispensable requisites that have to be provided, after which questions of detail will no longer present difficulties."

ORIGINAL LECTURES.

ON

AIDS TO EPIDEMIOLOGICAL KNOWLEDGE.

By GEORGE BUCHANAN, M.D.,
President of the Epidemiological Society. (a)

Our Society enters to-day on the thirty-first year of its life. It has experienced its ordinary share of difficulties, and its full measure of success. In no small degree its difficulties have been the creation of its success. That greater concern is now felt about scarlatina, typhus, small-pox, etc., than at the time of the Society's creation, and that public bodies and their officers compete with us in their interest for the problems which we study, is a result to which our Society has contributed in a foremost degree, but we still continue to hold our place as pioneers. We have among us people who study the subject from different standpoints at the bedside, in the post-mortem room, or in the camp, the ship, etc., but we want for success to study the δῆμος under other aspects than the technically medical, to study other δῆμοι than our own, and to identify ourselves with statesmen, geographers, and with travellers, to obtain help from chemistry and physics, from meteorology, botany, and zoology; indeed, it would be difficult to name a department of human knowledge to which we do not hope some day to become indebted.

Our first thought is of the place we shall gratefully assign to mathematics. So identified is epidemiology with mathematics that there has occasionally been a confusion in the popular mind, and the study of epidemics has been regarded as essentially an affair of statistics. Epidemic disease claims the aid of numbers, but it would be a serious error to think of this relation ending with records of quantity of disease, of death-rate, sickness-rate, etc. It is by arithmetical analysis of coincident circumstances of one and another sort that a clue is often got about the relation of effect to cause, as to efficiency of cause to produce effect. The case of relation between cholera and elevation of soil is an example familiar to us of an experience noted by the arithmetician to have something in it for the physician to inquire about. Of another sort of arithmetical help an evidence was afforded to me in the investigation of a fever outbreak, when, of two competing sets of circumstances, either of which might contain the cause of the outbreak, I was told the probabilities in favour of the one set were as 375 to 1, while the probabilities in favour of the other set (putting aside any probabilities against it) were but as 6 to 1. As another illustration :—An investigation is being made as to the possible influence of an infectious centre upon its neighbourhood. Putting aside influences that may destroy it, there is necessarily more of it at a spot near the centre than there is at a spot further off—that is, so long as the distribution is effected after the fashion of a something radiating from centre to circumference. The question arises: How much more infection will there be at a given nearer point, than at a given more distant point? because an answer to this question is wanted before we can go on to consider the meaning of the facts we observe. In reply to this question we shall see that the distribution of our infection will be affected according as it is effected along a single plane or into space of three dimensions. In the former case the relative amounts of infection present in two given places will be inversely as the distance of each place from the centre; in the latter they will be inversely as the squares of the distances. Now, there is reason for thinking the contagious matter is subject to the laws of gravitation, wherefore it is to the plane of the earth's surface that the contagion will tend, and its distribution in that plane will come to be effected according to the law that governs radiation in one plane. In this way we can appreciate the rate at which the spread of infection should manifest itself, and we can understand the significance of the actually observed distribution. The best example of our indebtedness to physical science may be taken from the lessons that the physicist has taught

(a) Address delivered before the Epidemiological Society on November 2

us of the characters of infection itself. At the foundation of our Society there was but a half-formed recognition of the fact that every disease of the class with which we concern ourselves has a material of its own. The earlier addresses of our first President contain many exhortations to the use of the microscope as a means of understanding the nature of diseases which we had to study, and from the microscope in the hands of Dr. Beale we soon came to know of the existence of particulate matter in infective liquids, but it was not until the resources of the physicist had been applied to separate out the particle from the fluid that any conclusion could be formed about the inherence of the quality of contagiousness in the one or the other element of the infectious liquid. The method of diffusion was used by Chauveau to such liquids, and first to vaccine lymph : the soluble was separated from the particulate, and the potency of the lymph was found to be in the particulate only. It was soon found that other contagia, like small-pox, exhibit the same quality.

At this time the pathologist had been cautiously tracking other lines of research ; and so long ago as 1841 a happy inspiration had led Dr. Farr to insist upon the use of the word," zymotic " as best expressing the character common to epidemic, endemic, and contagious diseases ; and then in 1848-49 Dr. John Snow had satisfied himself that the best explanation of the phenomena of cholera and its spread was to be found in the existence of a specific cholera " cell " capable of passing into other bodies and producing cholera in them.

Further, Dr. Budd reached the judgment, alike for diseases propagated through air and for those communicated by water, that " the contagious agent which issues in the excreta is the fruit of its own prior reproduction within the already infected body."

In study of the nature of various fermentative and putrefactive processes, it has appeared to Professor Schroeder and M. Pasteur that certain microscopic bodies are essential to such changes. From the standpoint thus reached by the chemist, the chemist himself came to regard similar organisms as probably concerned in processes of disease also; and the researches of M. Pasteur in 1865 into the disease which was so fatal to silkworms, gave sufficient demonstration. This was a true view of the case in respect of that disease, and afforded a stronger presumption that the material of contagion was in nature a parasitic being having a life and life-history of its own. This strong presumption rapidly led to further inquiries ; one after another the characteristic staff-shaped bodies of splenic fever, the spirillum of relapsing fever, and the microzymes of vaccine, of small-pox, and of sheep-pox have been made out.

For years before this period, the suggestion that particulate contagium must, almost of necessity, be contagium vivum had been one that had its attractions for the botanist. What if it should be the reproductive matter of some vegetable thing? At one time it did seem that we should find the genesis of cholera in that direction. It is to be admitted that Dr. Sanderson's critical examination of Professor Hallier's experiments relegated to the domain of the unproved this promising vision, but we are coming more and more to expect that the materials of some contagia have another habitat, perhaps in a known, but not yet recognised, alternative form. As time has gone on, and one disease after another has been found to be accompanied by organisms that are apparently concerned in their pathological processes, as the several members of the epidemic and contagious groups have been brought, with more or less of probability, into the list of those which have parasitic vegetable organisms for their actual cause, we are invited further to observe in the natural history of the various organisms affinities of botanical classes broadly corresponding to the nature of the groups of diseases with which they are found associated.

Unquestionably the prospects held out to the epidemiologist are of the most fascinating kind. As there was a period when we were promised in the behaviour of metallic oxides in the presence of peroxide of hydrogen the line of explanation of what constituted contagiousness, so now we seem to have reached a point where the botanist offers us the most promising insight into the nature of what is epidemic.

I wish to spend the time that remains to me in pointing out some of the interesting and important consequences that follow from the doctrine which would regard the material of infectious disease as something in its essence having a place and mode of life beyond the infected body. One of these is the possibility that is appearing of being able to cultivate that material outside the body in ways that shall give it different degrees of potency. So long ago as 1867, Dr. Sanderson had distinguished two sets of consequences producible by local inflammations artificially set up in the lower animals—the one a chronic disease having the characters of tubercle, the other an acute disease presenting the features of pyæmia, and both infective and being producible at the will of the experimenter by the inoculation of the same material. In 1872 he demonstrated in a number of acute infective processes, microzymes abounding in the exudation liquids and in the blood; he showed how by successive transmissions of infective material an intensely virulent material could be obtained, the original product and the cultivated material having certain microscopical and physical characters distinguishing the one from the other. Dr. Koch, of Wolstein, made a notable advance, and found the bacilli of splenic fever grow and multiply in blood serum or aqueous humour, and even in artificially prepared cultivating liquids, and that this could be done through successive generations. More than this, he found that mice inoculated with matter that contained numerous spores died of splenic fever in twenty-four hours, whereas mice inoculated with liquid in which spores were scarce did not die until later. And shortly afterwards our own Dr. Klein found this same property of cultivability outside the body in the very similar bacilli of the disease of the pig known as pneumo-enteritis, and that liquid of the eighth generation inoculated in a pig produced a disease reduced in intensity.

In 1879, Dr. Sanderson found that the cultivation of anthrax in the body of rodents modified the poison so that the subsequent inoculation of a bovine animal did not destroy the life of the latter, but protected it from subsequent attacks of disease. At the same time M. Pasteur made out for the disease called "fowl-cholera" the same quality of cultivability by multiplication of its bacilli in inorganic, but not vitalised, liquids.

We cannot help having before us the dazzling prospect of being able to offer to men and animals the protection of a trivial disease against each more fatal disease, to achieve what M. Pasteur calls the "vaccination" of animals against the several dangerous contagia.

But perhaps as valuable are the indications we are gaining of possible means of preventing epidemic disease in other ways. Suggestions arise of material of contagion having, like tape-worm, an alternative mode of life outside the animal body, or in one animal body leading a different sort of existence from that in the other animal body. What if the material of cholera, or of yellow or of enteric fever, should have another habitat than as a contagium, and there exist, having no power of producing disease until its conditions were changed, but then altering its mode of life, and becoming the active material of disease in animals into whose bodies it was introduced? What if we could recognise it in its other fashion of life, and destroy it or prevent the conditions necessary for its development? In 1875, Dr. Klein recognised in a particle peculiar to enteric fever a microphyte which had been identified by Professor Cohn, of Breslan, as occurring in the water of a well at Breslan, and the district of the city supplied by that well had long been famous for the amount of enteric fever in it. The relation between milk and outbreaks of enteric or scarlet fever or diphtheria has been thought of as a mere affair of disease entering milk-cans by the aid of water used in washing or of hands used in milking cows. It may turn out that the disease-producing milk has received some organism that under other conditions of life would have been impotent, or such organism have been derived from the body of the cow itself.

Indeed, the hygienist is coming to suspect that he may often have to do with organised material not far developed from perfectly non-specific germs. It is impossible not to recollect the inquiries of Dr. Ballard at Welbeck and Nottingham, in which he heard of strange maladies occurring in groups of people, and having their cause in some common article of food.

Such are a few examples of the aid which pathology is rendering to an understanding of epidemics. It must be of concern to our Society in the future to have regard to the many new considerations that are presenting themselves to us, and to put the views of the pathologist to the test of our manifold experiences.

CLINICAL LECTURES
ON DISEASES OF THE ABDOMEN.

By FREDERICK T. ROBERTS, M.D., B.Sc., F.R.C.P.,
Professor of Materia Medica and Therapeutics at University College,
Physician to University Hospital, and Professor of
Clinical Medicine, etc.

LECTURE IV.
A CLINICAL CLASSIFICATION OF DISEASES OF THE ABDOMEN—Continued.

IN my last lecture I gave you a classification of cases belonging to the sudden or hyper-acute, and the acute or sub-acute groups. I now proceed to consider the third great division, namely—

III.—CHRONIC.

Cases which are of a more or less chronic nature, as regards their mode of onset, symptoms, and duration, are more difficult to arrange than those included under the other divisions; but I will endeavour to indicate approximately the classes to which the majority of them may be referred.

1. There is a class of cases in which there is no actual disease; but the patient complains of various symptoms in connexion with the abdomen, being either a hypochondriac, hysterical or nervous, or a malingerer. Or it may be that there is some abnormal objective condition of little or no moment, but which such patients make a great deal of, and imagine, or pretend to think, that they are very serious. Cases of this kind are by no means uncommon or unimportant, and they must be definitely recognised and borne in mind, else serious mistakes are liable to be made. Allusion may also be made here to cases of supposed neuralgia affecting abdominal organs. Whether they are really of this nature is a matter of considerable doubt.

2. Conditions of the Abdominal Walls.—These may be the seat of painful or other abnormal sensations without any objective changes, as in cases of neuralgia, myalgia, and certain forms of spinal disease. They are, however, also liable to evident morbid conditions, and these may cause more or less troublesome symptoms, or even more obvious effects. Those chiefly deserving of mention are:—(a) Excessive accumulation of fat; (b) Flabbiness and want of tone of the muscles, with consequent relaxation of the walls; (c) The presence of an abnormal opening in the muscles or aponeuroses in some part of the abdomen, especially about the umbilical region, through which a hernial protrusion of variable size is liable to take place; (d) Subcutaneous œdema, which is not uncommon as a chronic condition.

3. Chronic Peritoneal Affections, of a Local Nature.—In this group I include, mainly, two classes of cases, namely—(a) Those of ascites or dropsy of the peritoneum, which is almost always secondary to some other disease; (b) Those of so-called simple chronic peritonitis, in which adhesions or other conditions remain after acute peritonitis, or are produced gradually from certain causes. It may be also mentioned that the peritoneal folds, especially the great omentum, may be the seat of a large collection of fat.

4. Chronic Congestion and its Effects.—This is a much more frequent class of cases than those of acute congestion, and they demand due recognition, on account of the importance of the clinical phenomena which they often present. They belong to the following groups:—(a) Those due to general plethora; (b) Those resulting from embarrassment of the circulation on the right side of the heart, or in the lungs; (c) Those in which more or less continuous congestion of the alimentary canal and liver is set up by the habitual ingestion of irritating articles; (d) Those due to some obstruction affecting the portal system; (e) Those dependent upon some local disorder of the renal circulation; (f) Congestion from continued malarial influence, especially affecting the spleen; (g) Local interference with particular veins, such as the inferior vena cava, the mesenteric veins, or the veins of the abdominal walls. In these different forms of chronic congestion it will be seen that it is the venous circulation which is in most instances affected, and that the congestion is chiefly mechanical or passive. The nature and range of the symptoms

will depend upon the structures which are congested, as a little consideration will show ; while it must be remembered that the condition in course of time leads to permanent organic lesions.

5. *Disorders of the Digestive Organs.*—By this expression I mean affections of the alimentary canal, or of its related organs, the liver and pancreas, which are not due to any evident organic disease, at least of an important character, or such as can be positively recognised. Here would be included a large proportion of cases of so-called "dyspepsia," with its varied combinations of symptoms ; as well as many cases of constipation, some of diarrhœa, and certain functional derangements of the liver. It must be remembered that many cases of grave and even fatal organic disease appear in the early part of their course as if they belonged to this group ; and indeed there are not a few instances of a doubtful and obscure nature, which might almost be put into a separate class.

6. *Organic Disease of the Alimentary Canal, of Local Origin.*—There are numerous cases in which the digestive canal is the seat of some organic mischief, due to causes acting locally, and, with few exceptions, these have to be recognised by symptoms alone, there being no evident physical signs. They may be divided into :—(a) Those of chronic mucous inflammation or catarrh, gastric, intestinal, or general ; (b) Those of simple ulceration, almost always gastric ; (c) Those of chronic dysentery. Chronic poisoning by irritants must be borne in mind in connexion with this group.

7. *Cirrhosis of the Liver and Neighbouring Structures.*— The liver is particularly liable to become the seat of the condition termed cirrhosis (generally from chronic alcoholism), which usually leads to chronic diminution in size of the organ, but it is not uncommonly enlarged. It must be noted, however, that though, as a rule, the condition of the liver is the cause of the prominent symptoms, it is not always so ; and in some instances the gall-bladder, the biliary ducts, the duodenum, and the pancreas are similarly affected, and their implication makes matters more serious. This class of cases demands distinct and special recognition. It may be called to mind here that chronic venous congestion tends to set up a cirrhotic condition after a time.

8. *Chronic Bright's Disease.*—Although different morbid conditions of the kidneys characterise cases thus denominated, they may for clinical purposes be conveniently included under one group, and it is a very important one, on account of their frequency and serious nature.

9. *General or Constitutional Diseases.*—Cases belonging to this group constitute a large proportion of the chronic diseases of the abdomen. The nature of these maladies has already been pointed out ; but it will be well to mention them here again, and, in my opinion, it is far preferable to study them from a general point of view as regards the abdominal structures, than to consider them in relation to particular organs or tissues. Those general diseases which may manifest themselves as chronic affections of abdominal structures, and which I would include here, are :—(a) Carcinoma of all kinds ; (b) Albuminoid or waxy disease ; (c) Chronic tuberculosis or scrofulosis ; (d) Gout, and perhaps rheumatism ; (e) Syphilis ; (f) The fatty diathesis and degenerations ; (g) The malarial condition. The different diseases tend to affect different structures, as will be pointed out in future lectures.

10. *Chronic Suppuration and its Remains.*—A chronic abscess may be left behind after one which has commenced acutely, or it may be chronic from the outset. The collection of pus may occupy any of the sites indicated when speaking of acute suppuration. Subsequently sinuses or fistulæ may remain. A chronic discharge of muco-pus or pus with the urine is also to be recognised as the result of pyelitis or cystitis, and other conditions.

11. *Malformations and Malpositions of Organs.*—These are not uncommonly met with as chronic conditions in the abdomen, and ought always to be borne in mind.

12. *Hypertrophy and Atrophy.*—The only organs in the abdomen likely to come under clinical observation as the result of hypertrophy are the spleen and liver ; but other parts may be thus affected. Symptoms may also arise from atrophy of various structures, such as those of the alimentary canal, the liver, or the kidneys.

13. *Obstruction of Orifices, Tubes, or Canals ; Dilatation ; and Accumulations in connexion with Tubes or Hollow*

Organs.—I have grouped these conditions together, as they are often necessarily associated, and it is not easy to separate them. The cases that come under notice belong to one or other of the following subdivisions, according to the organ affected :—(a) Gastric ; (b) Intestinal ; (c) Hepatic, in which the bile-duct is obstructed ; (d) Renal, where the ureter is closed up in various ways, so that materials accumulate in the pelvis of the kidney ; (e) Vesical, where fluid collects in the bladder, this being due to obstruction of the urethra and other causes.

14. *Cystic Diseases, and Fluid Accumulations.*—These may be arranged under one division, although collections of fluid have already been alluded to in the previous class. Ovarian cysts must necessarily be mentioned here ; and also hydatid cysts, but these rightly belong to the next group.

15. *Animal Parasites.*—The most common class of cases belonging to this group are those of intestinal worms. Hydatid disease is the next common, and this is chiefly noticed in connexion with the liver. Rare and exceptional instances occur in which special parasites inhabit the liver or kidney.

16. *Calculi.*—These are chronic in their formation ; and they not uncommonly give rise to clinical phenomena of a chronic character.

17. *Morbid Conditions of Arteries.*—Aneurism is an important lesion to be recognised in connexion with the abdominal arteries, especially the aorta. Aortic pulsation is also a condition demanding special notice.

18. *Peculiar and Rare Diseases.*—Under this head it will suffice to mention the following affections :—(a) Leucocythæmia and lymphadenoma ; (b) Addison's disease ; (c) Pernicious anæmia ; (d) Non-malignant growths ; (e) Embolism, with infarctions in the spleen and kidney, which, as a chronic condition, however, is rarely indicated by any clinical signs.

Such, then, is the arrangement of abdominal diseases which I would submit for your consideration, and it is one according to which, in the main, I propose to study these diseases clinically. This classification, however, must not be taken too strictly, and it is only intended to bring within a somewhat more intelligible compass the very numerous affections to which the abdominal structures are liable, and to afford you a practical basis upon which they may be conveniently studied. You must remember that the three main divisions run into each other, and that a sudden or acute lesion may supervene on a chronic disease, or *vice versâ* ; also that more than one structure may be implicated at the same time ; and that the same organ may be the seat of two or more morbid conditions.

IDENTIFICATION ON THE FIELD OF BATTLE.—With the object of identifying soldiers killed or severely wounded on the field of battle, the Minister of War has decided that every man shall be provided in the time of war with a medal termed an identity-plate. It is to be oval in form, and measuring thirty-five millimetres in length, twenty-five in breadth, and one in thickness.

EXTIRPATION OF THE KIDNEY.—Dr. Le Dentu related to the Académie de Médecine (*Union Méd.*, November 17) the case of a gentleman aged thirty-two, who applied to him in March, 1875, with a fluctuating tumour in the left flank and iliac fossa, arising from hydronephrosis and perinephritic abscess. The severe suffering of the patient led to the incision of the tumour, giving issue to a clear liquid mixed with blood. In a few days urine flowed abundantly by the wound ; and as its issue caused frequent attacks of inflammation, which put the patient's life in danger, it was resolved to remove the kidney of that side. The operation was performed on April 14, the decortication of the organ being easily effected. The upper two-thirds of the kidney were converted into a sac with flaccid walls, the lower third remaining normal, and the hilus being voluminous. The kidney, being secured by means of two ligatures, was excised with the scissors. Lister's dressing was employed for some days, until the mortified parts had been eliminated by means of the ligatures and the thermo-cautery. The lumbar wound cicatrised in the course of two months. The fistulous track remained open, but now only yields a few drops of purulent serosity. The patient, who is a distinguished dramatic artist, made a brilliant reappearance on the stage in October. This is the first example of successful nephrectomy in France.

ORIGINAL COMMUNICATIONS.

—◆—

CHILDREN IN HOT CLIMATES.

By F. R. HOGG, M.D., Surgeon-Major.

It has been recorded that Alexander the Great could easily command enormous armies, yet failed to *force* the simple ivy of Greece to flourish near Babylon. In the beautiful garden encircling that peerless gem, the Taj at Agra, delicate plants and lovely flowers from all parts of the world can be cultivated *so long* as unremitting studious care in climatic adaptation *never relaxes*. To a certain extent the parallel applies to the human body. European girls landing in India, after suffering with amenorrhœa, prickly heat, mosquito bites, or thermal fevers, gradually become seasoned for awhile, and, unless enfeebled by rapid procreation, get on very well during the early years of married life. Heat often militates against cerebral or nervous affections, whilst organic diseases of heart or liver, dyspepsia, deafness, and rheumatism do not improve at several sanitaria. Morning sickness, neuralgia, cramp, insalivation, dysentery, diarrhœa, or leucorrhœa may be excessive; and in wet, relaxing locali-ties, phthisical symptoms neither abate, divert, nor amelio-rate. Typhus and enteric, and even cholera, as contrasted with relapsing fever, need not induce the premature birth of still-born children. Distressing instances of insomnia occur at Mount Aboo, and children elsewhere may inherit cerebral affections from unfortunate mothers struggling as school-teachers in hot stations. Calcutta formerly had a bad reputation for childbirth mortality, which diminished ex-ceedingly as sanitary measures and obstetric teaching improved.

By all accounts old traditions never change as regards profound belief in castor oil, butter and sugar, applications of burnt linen to funis, tight bandaging of infants, also in stimulating diet during pregnancy and after delivery. English nurses, the wives or widows of soldiers, travel long distances, and receiving from 100 to 120 rupees per month or broken period, are invaluable when sober, experienced, and strong. Eurasians may be weakly, dirty, and untrust-worthy. In some places small means, overcrowding, still, sultry, muggy air, and sanitary defects, may invite diph-theria, erysipelas, scarlet or puerperal fever. For the latter, early inunction with mercurial ointment, vaginal injections of warm carbolic acid solutions, and turpentine by mouth are valuable remedies. Turpentine next to ergot is extremely useful in menorrhagia, and the perchloride of iron injec-tions in post-partum hæmorrhage are increasing in esti-mation. Quinine prescribed during pregnancy may induce premature labour. At the commencement of menstruation, during suppression or excess, whilst quickening, or after abortion, tetanus during the rains has attacked European females. Cold, privations, chills caused by sleeping on the house-top, will thus tell on native girls. Chloral, cannabis indica (alone, or combined with bromides), have answered with many practitioners. A half-caste woman at the change of life in October, at Meerut, for fourteen days had her jaws so locked that with extreme difficulty beef juice, milk, beef-tea could be slowly trickled in. I gave her large doses of iodide of potassium by day, chloral at night; blistered her neck and temples; rubbed the spine with opium and belladonna; relieved the bowels by ene-mata, the bladder by catheter; kept her quiet in a warm, dark room; ordered stimulants somewhat liberally; and gradually good food, with quinine, facilitated recovery. In many months women cannot take exercise, nor will heat permit the wearing of supporting-belts. They injure themselves by jumping out of carriages, playing lawn tennis, dancing, or over-lifting; else are shaken on elephants, in camel-carts, on the line of rail, are jolted on stretchers or any form of conveyance from the plains up to 6000 feet elevation, during pregnancy. Some ladies remaining at Calcutta almost until the last moment, risk a long railway journey to Umballa, a drive to Kalka, and thence somehow an ascent to Simla. Labour may occur on board ship, in the train, the rest camp, or in carriage, cart, or dooly, perhaps in a desert, without any disaster; and in the furnace heat of Mooltan there may be equal safety as amongst the fragrant pines and cedars of the blue hills beneath the silver glistening snows. At Mooltan, careful people shut up doors at 9 a.m., and, trusting to punkahs and thermantidotes, can keep house temperature about 86° Fahr. The careless or im-pecunious contrive to exist for months in a temperature exceeding 100°. At night it is customary to court sleep out in the open, perhaps on the house-top, else amongst the palm trees in the garden, surrounded by wet matting, under a punkah, and the ground covered with wet sand. The mean temperature in June of 95° contrasts with 98° at Agra, Lahore, and Delhi, 91° at Lucknow and Benares, about 85° at Calcutta. At Lahore, where the hot winds of May and June cannot frequently be mitigated in their fury often by watered matting, the temperature of a closed house without cooling appliances may average from 90° to 98°, and that of the outer air at night may exceed 105°. During the hot season, careful women and well-managed children may escape sickness, but tight clothing, the weight of bed-clothes, cold feet, noise, excitement, glare, bad smells, oppres-sive air, cramp, colic, and teething troubles must be con-sidered, especially during night-chills after refreshing rain. Then do cases of fever, measles, whooping-cough, or dysentery require special care. At Meerut, in April or May, an infant almost immediately after birth can be taken out early in the morning or late in the afternoon in the garden, and the mother's bed placed in the verandah. Cramp, colic, and especially earache, may be traced to the splashing of the sweet-smelling kus-kus tatties. An enervating climate and an artificial life will partially explain inability or dis-inclination for nursing. On the other hand, scarcely a week passes at Netley, but some wonderful specimen of a soldier's wife comes under observation, in bright con-trast with the majority of sickly women with climate-stricken children. Frequently the favourable exceptions are thrifty, temperate women, with good husbands and comfortable homes, who, cooking and performing house-hold duties all the year round in the plains, are still able to suckle their infants for eighteen months and bring them to England. In many instances, firm flesh, ruddy cheeks, and lusty limbs are due to entire or prolonged residence in the hills, such as Darjeeling, Dalhousie, Ranikhet, Landour, or Murree. Very bad places for children are the plain stations of Mean Meer, Morar, and notably Peshawur; and yet the latter place is greatly liked by ladies, who contrive to be absent in sickly months.

The first child born in India may be sacrificed to ignorance and inexperience of climate. The next two or three do well, but the remainder often are weakly, and may die of dysentery, diarrhœa, convulsions, or some form of atrophy. About the age of fifteen are many soldiers' daughters married, soon to fall pregnant, and, with comparatively easy labours, to bear infants, who are looked upon as dolls by the girlish mothers. Mammary abscesses are uncommon. Now and then such children, entirely mismanaged, are carried off by trismus in crowded habitations during bleak and variable weather, especially if the mother be prone to malarial epilepsy. Eruptive fevers, notably measles, may swell the bills of mortality. Thanks to vaccination, variola is mild, and so far scarlatina does not do much mischief. In 1879 the mortality of children amounted to 87 per 1000 in Bengal, 78 in Bombay, and 44 in Madras. From measles 60 deaths occurred in Bengal, 5 at Rawul Pindee, the re-mainder widely distributed. In Bengal, 13 cases out of 15 of cholera died, mostly at Rawul Pindee and Murree. At Pindee, crowded with soldiers' wives, whilst husbands fought in Afghanistan, 4 of 17 cases of scarlatina proved fatal to children. At Mean Meer their death-rate was 218, at Neemuch 227, and at Gwalior 245. Under six months the mortality was 319, between this and twelve months 216, after three years declining, so that between the ages of three and four it only equalled 36 per mille. A dirty bottle, a careless nurse, sickly cows or goats, native adulteration tricks, sour, decomposed, maggotty patent foods, mixed with unreliable condensed milk, have much to answer for in hot climates. Not a few poor, blanched, bloodless women go on suckling, beside cramming their wasting children with cornflour, sago, rusks, biscuits, or boiled bread, only to encourage exhausting diarrhœa. All this time, too, the fretting, the broken rest, another pregnancy, else menstruation during early lactation, will be a terrible drain on maternal constitution. Dental convulsions in May or June are not infrequently connected with brandy or opium drugging. Improper food, night-chills, unsuitable clothing, may derange the liver even at certain hills—specially Simla, where diarrhœa occasionally resists all treatment until the patient is removed. In August and September, malarial fevers in the plains prostrate weakly mothers, and their infants, suddenly deprived of breast-milk, perhaps utterly collapse. During October and November, cold nights succeeding hot days partially account for dysentery. At Mean Meer and Peshawur, fevers, complicated with vomiting, diarrhœa, or rheumatism, run on to February; so, before broken constitutions can temporarily be repaired by bracing, cold weather, the hot sun again commences cruelly to torment.

In the battle with climate the physician of to-day often has the advantage of the rail, the telegraph, cooling appliances, besides the modern inventions of condensed milk and patent foods, to supplement his skill. The first point to be discussed is that of lactation.

AN ACCOUNT OF

ONE HUNDRED AND TEN CONSECUTIVE CASES OF ABDOMINAL SECTION

PERFORMED SINCE THE 1ST OF NOVEMBER, 1880.(a)

By LAWSON TAIT, F.R.C.S.

(Continued from page 546.)

FOUR of the cases of single cystoma were pregnant at the time of the operation, and all recovered. In two cases I operated in the course of acute peritonitis, with completely successful results.

There are, of course, many of the cases having features of special interest, such as suppurating and gangrenous tumours, and operations performed during pregnancy, but these have now been reduced by extended experience to the compass of ordinary treatment, so that I need not trouble you with their details.

One case, however (74), deserves some brief notice, for there I had to deal with a rotten, gangrenous, and adherent tumour, which gave me trouble of a most unusual and unexpected kind, which I had to meet as best I could, and I am glad to say I did successfully.

In turning out the stinking, rotten mass, I suddenly caused a most alarming hæmorrhage, which, of course, I controlled with Kœberle's forceps, and proceeded with the removal. I could find no pedicle, but the point from which the hæmorrhage came was undoubtedly the pedicle which I had torn across before I had recognised it. When Mr. Harmar tried to tie its bleeding points, the more he tied the more it bled. The cautery equally failed me, and I was at my wits' end. Nine pairs of forceps were fastened upon something in the pelvis—I knew not what,—and from it I dared not move them. I therefore closed the wound over them, went up to the hospital next morning, and reopened it. Then, in fear and trembling, I released the forceps, one pair after another. No bleeding came. I fastened in a drainage-tube, the patient recovered slowly, and went home on August 9.

I now come to a group of twenty-one cases of removal of the uterine appendages for various conditions, and these had best be divided into two groups, according to the nature of the two leading symptoms—hæmorrhage and pain. This division, however, like every other, is unsatisfactory, because it is quite impossible in some of the cases to say to which group they ought properly to belong, for pain and hæmorrhage were often so pronouncedly in combination as to afford a double justification for surgical interference. I must, however, enter here the protest which I have again and again advanced, so far in vain, against these operations being styled "oöphorectomies," or "cases of Battey's operation." I do so, in the first place, because I have completely established the fact that removal of the Fallopian tubes is quite as necessary as removal of the ovaries; in fact, I think it is far more necessary in all cases, for upon the tubes, it seems to me, the periodic function of menstruation exists, and ovulation and menstruation are wholly independent the one of the other. As Dr. Battey limited his definition of the operation he performed to the removal of the ovaries, I would plead for this that I advocate, if we are to indulge in clumsy pedantry, the name of *salpingo-oöphorectomy*, or

(a) Read before the Midland Medical Society, November 2, 1881.

prosthekotomy. If the names of the advocates of the various proceedings are to be employed—a practice I object to—then it should be called "Tait's operation," but not "Battey's." Dr. Battey practically purposed his operation for the "production of the menopause or the arrest of ovulation." I am wholly indifferent on the question of ovulation in most of my cases, and I care not about the menopause in a large number. Therefore, in the whole of my large experience I have only three cases of "Battey's operation." One has been a complete success ; the second I am not sure about, as I have lost sight of her ; and the third I am afraid will turn out a failure, though it is too soon yet to pronounce judgment.

For my own part, I speak always of the operation as one "for the removal of the uterine appendages," and for the treatment of uterine myoma it is one of the most brilliant additions to modern surgery. It is perfectly absurd for any one to start the discussion of this subject with the assumption that uterine myoma is not a fatal disease. If this is so, why do we hear on all hands of the employment of surgical proceedings for its treatment, which have had, up to the present, a perfectly murderous mortality? I have condemned them utterly ; and though, in the present list, four such cases are given, I will not willingly perform another. It will be seen, in explanation of this, that every now and then hysterotomy will be performed, and till the operation is finished, or almost so, the surgeon will be ignorant of what he is doing. Removal of a uterine polypus, already completely extruded, or nearly so, is the only operation for uterine myoma which is safer than removal of the uterine appendages. Enucleation I shall never again attempt ; and hysterotomy I shall equally avoid, if I can.

To tell us, as was practically done in a recent discussion, that hæmorrhage due to uterine myoma is only exceptionally fatal, is wholly opposed to my own experience since the first death I saw from it, nearly twenty years ago, in which case I made a post-mortem examination. But even if this were true, our operative practice, like our therapeutics, is surely not to be limited to the saving of life, but is to be extended to the restoration of health and the relief of physical distress. I ask anyone who has had such a case under his care, what ill-health is more distressing to the patient or her friends, or what suffering greater than that endured by a woman who bleeds profusely for ten or fourteen days every month, and who spends the rest of her time vainly endeavouring to replace what she has lost? Even if it were true that the deaths from removal of the uterine appendages in such cases were more numerous than the deaths from the disease, I urge that it is in the interests of the majority we have to consider, and that it is far better to cure ten women out of eleven, and that the eleventh should die, than that the whole eleven should spend year after year in a state of misery to themselves and their surroundings. But this will not be the proportion in the hands of extended experience. I have now a larger experience of this operation than any yet published by any other operator, and I know that every failure points out the road for future success, and will ultimately yield me a mortality as low as that of any other operation in my province. The only death in my present series would, I think now, have been obviated by the use of a drainage-tube. Of the ten cases in the present list which recovered, I have to report complete arrest of the hæmorrhage up to the present date, and in one of them (47) a large tumour, which I estimated to weigh at least five pounds, has completely disappeared (*Lancet*, October 22, 1881) within six months of the operation.

The diseases which I have classed as hydro- and pyosalpinx arise from a glueing of the fimbriated extremity of the tube to the ovary, and an occlusion of the uterine extremity. These alterations are due, of course, to inflammatory action, arising from gonorrhœa or exanthematic peri-oöphoritis ; and the method in which it occurs is probably something like this. The ovary is in a condition of subacute or even acute inflammation when the trumpet-shaped extremity of the tube approaches it and grasps it in the ordinary method. What would have been a mere cellular adhesion, lasting only a few hours, becomes intimate and permanent by the inflammatory action. The uterine end of the tube becomes occluded probably by exfoliation of epithelium—a process common enough in ducts.

The contents of the tube may consist of simple serum, the most common variety ; of pus, much less common ; or of menstrual blood, of which I have seen only two examples. The patients suffer terrible pain during menstruation, and are rarely free from distress at any time. They wander about from hospital to hospital, or from doctor to doctor, seeking relief and finding none. Menorrhagia is a very frequent symptom. Drugs do no good whatever; and of the opinions concerning the nature of the disease, given by the various men consulted, we may fairly say, "Quot homines, tot sententiæ." On careful bimanual examination, it is quite possible to diagnose exactly many of these cases; and in all cases where the history of the patient indicates the presence of this condition I open the abdomen. In all of those in the present list my diagnosis has been correct: I have removed the appendages, the patients have recovered, and many doubtless will be permanently cured; so far, they are all relieved. In one of my recent cases I operated on the patient in order that she might be married. She was a helpless cripple by reason of a pint of curdy pus in the right Fallopian tube, and about half as much in the left; and, as she was, marriage was altogether out of the question. She consulted a lady from whom I had removed both tubes and ovaries in order that she should be married, and who has been married for quite a long time now, and the result of the conference was so satisfactory that the operation was promptly accepted.

I may be asked, Why do I remove the ovaries when the tubes only are at fault? For the reason that without the tubes the ovaries are useless, and nothing will be gained by having an ovum dropped into the peritoneum every now and again; and removing the ovaries complicates the operation very little. The results of these cases, so far, are all that could be desired; and only let me say further about this class of operations, that anyone who imagines that their performance is an easy matter—no more difficult than sow-gelding—will speedily find out his mistake after he has seen one or two.

In the present list I have removed the appendages for chronic oöphoritis in two cases only. They occurred in servant-girls, who had been rendered wholly unable to make their living on account of their sufferings. Such cases will rarely be operated on in the better ranks of life; but in such a case as that sent to me by Dr. McFie Campbell of Liverpool (17), the operation affords the only prospect of relief. Dr. Campbell (and others) had in this case completely exhausted the whole range of other plans of treatment, and only after that did he send me his patient as one in whom he thought the operation ought to be tried. The operation was as difficult as can well be imagined, and in my earlier practice it would have been left incomplete. The patient was not so steady as she might have been, and the result was that she got a big hæmatocele, and menstruated regularly after. This effusion ultimately suppurated, and I had to readmit her, open the abdomen, and drain the abscess (95). She is now perfectly free from pain, and, I trust, is permanently cured. The second case was very like this, but she unfortunately died from septic infection caught from a patient who had preceded her in the ward. It happened that this operation was performed with complete Listerian details, and it was one of the experiences which convinced me of the uselessness of this practice. I wish now that I had re-opened her abdomen and cleansed her out as soon as the symptoms were marked, though, as the disease was more systemic than local in its manifestation, this might have failed.

I have performed eleven operations in this series for the treatment of pelvic abscess, upon the principles which I advocated for the first time in a paper read before the Royal Medical and Chirurgical Society on May 11, 1880. Every case which I have treated in this way has yielded, so far, brilliantly successful results, and I have no doubt that it will become the established practice.

After having opened the abdomen, I open and empty the abscess, and stitch the margins of the opening into it to the margins of the parietal opening, and then insert a drainage-tube. In a few cases I have made a circular drainage, that is, I make a counter-opening in the vagina and tie the two ends of the tube together. Two of these cases (75 and 96) have been collections of pus in the Fallopian tubes, where removal of the tubes was impossible.

Of my four cases of hepatotomy, two have been already published (Birmingham Medical Review, October, 1881), and the others will form the subject of a special paper. The operation consists in opening the abdomen, then opening the liver,

stitching the edges of the two apertures in accurate adaptation, and draining the cavity. This is a departure of surgery which is altogether novel, which we owe to the brilliant example of Dr. Marion Sims in performing cholecystotomy, and the success of which is as yet limited to Birmingham. I can now count seven cases without a death, and these are all that have been performed up to the present date.

The performance of abdominal section for intestinal obstruction is a subject which has received much attention, and many efforts have been made, as a dernier ressort, for the avoidance of impending death.

The usual practice has been to open the abdomen in the middle line, and search for the obstruction—a search which has been very exceptionally successful. I have only once found the obstruction in seven cases in which I have made an exploratory incision for the purpose, and then it was due to malignant adhesions in the pelvis. I have therefore given up the search, and my rule now is to open the intestine and make an artificial anus as low down in the canal as I can, and trust to nature for the rest. In the two cases in which I have carried out this practice the results have been perfectly successful. One of these instances (50) I show here to-night in the person of one of my few male patients, who was placed under my care by Mr. Hall Wright. Obstruction had existed for eighteen days, and the abdomen was distended to a size relative to the patient's body such as I never saw before, and could not have believed possible had I not seen it. After the establishment of the fistula, some gallons of liquid fæces were passed. On the twelfth day fæces passed by the rectum, and the boy rapidly recovered, the fistula having now closed completely. Here the obstruction must have been due to volvulus or to mere paralysis, which was overcome by the relief of the distension.

The second case was operated upon on October 9, and had a history which pointed to suppuration of the gall-bladder, and the probable rupture of that organ into the intestine. Such was the combined opinion of Dr. Foster and Mr. Langley Brown. The result was intestinal obstruction, and they asked me to make an exploratory incision. This I did, and opened into a cavity close to the umbilicus, from which came a large quantity of pus and liquid fæces. What that cavity was I do not know; it was either the cæcum or the gall-bladder—more probably the latter. On the third day the fæces came by the rectum, and, as the patient is rapidly recovering, we shall probably never know the exact conditions which were dealt with. A detailed account of the case will form the subject of a special publication.

Hysterotomy is one operation I would gladly get rid of, and the last time I wittingly performed it was in a case (2) from Liverpool, of malignant sarcoma, and I had resolved that it would be the last. In March last, however, Dr. Leacroft, of Feckenham, sent me a case (38) which I had seen five years before, and had diagnosed as a parovarian cyst; which he had tapped many times without discovering anything to modify this view; yet in which we were entirely mistaken. The patient had resolutely refused to have any operation performed till she was very much exhausted. When I came to operate I found the tumour unusually adherent, and the process of removal was most difficult and protracted. The tumour had no pedicle, but consisted of one huge sessile cyst arising from the pelvis. It was only when I cut across its base that its true nature—that of a huge fibrocyst of the uterus—became apparent. The patient died on the sixth day of suppuration of the pelvis, and I regret that I did not drain the cavity. The third case occurred in a patient from Durham (78), with two large sessile cystic tumours, which I could remove only by cutting off the uterus close to the vaginal insertion, along with a large myoma. She made a perfect recovery. The fourth seemed to me to be a solid tumour of the broad ligament, but on examination it turned out that it was a uterine myoma, and that I had cut through the right uterine cornu.

It thus seems that it is quite impossible to avoid an occasional ablation of the uterus, and this proceeding is always very risky. The chief trouble is hæmorrhage, for the uterine tissue seems little inclined to yield security with ligatures. Those cases which have been successful have had both the ligature and the cautery applied to the stumps—a proceeding which I advocated for the first time a few months ago. But so had one of my fatal cases (38), where the absence of drainage seemed to me to account for the failure. Therefore I shall always in future add the precaution of a drainage-tube where I am at all in doubt as to the security of the pedicle. Where we can use the clamp we shall get a security on this point which the ligature cannot give, but then we shall have all the risks of the extra-peritoneal treatment, and I doubt if this would be any improvement. I have had one case of Cæsarian section, in a rickety dwarf, thirty-eight inches high, with a pelvic area like the crest of the Isle of Man. She died, apparently of embolism, on the fourth day; but the child is alive and flourishing. I shall publish this case separately.

The last group of my series consists of two most remarkable cases of huge cysts altogether outside the peritoneum, in the removal of which the peritoneum was never opened, and in both of which the operation was, unfortunately, fatal. I could not obtain in either case a post-mortem examination, so that the exact nature of the cysts remains quite uncertain, though I have reason to believe they grew from the remains of the urachus. I can offer no other explanation of their relations.

The first (26) was under the care of Dr. Lamb, of Albrighton, and had been seen by Dr. Saundby and Dr. Heslop. For twelve months she had complained of pain in the abdomen, apparently depending on flatulence, and also of pain at the scapula. In October, 1880, she began to suffer from occasional vomiting, and up to the time of my seeing her in February had taken no solid food. Some swelling of the lower part of the abdomen was noticed, and was regarded as ascitic. The liver dulness was much diminished. The urine was free from albumen, and continued so.

On February 11 she was tapped by her attendants, and ten pints of fluid were removed. It was of a dark brown colour, and gave an abundant flaky yellow deposit on settling, and this was composed almost entirely of pus and disintegrating blood-corpuscles. When shown to me, I unhesitatingly expressed the opinion that it had been obtained from a cyst, and could not have been the result of peritoneal effusion. When I saw her on February 13, the abdomen was largely distended with fluid, and the signs were all those of a unilocular cyst, and therefore I thought it was a parovarian cyst in a condition of suppuration. Under the circumstances, the clear course was to attempt its removal. This was agreed to, and was at once proceeded with. I made an incision five inches in length, and exposed a cyst which was outside the peritoneum. I opened it, and emptied out at least thirty pints of the same fluid, in which floated masses of disintegrating clot. I then tore off the cyst from the transversalis fascia for about five inches on either side, and came upon a reflection of the peritoneum on to the posterior wall of the cyst. I separated onwards till I came round to the corresponding point on the opposite side. Then upwards I found the same relation almost as far as the margin of the ribs, and down to the brim of the pelvis in front. When I got the cyst all out, the peritoneum was quite unopened, and the viscera could be felt through the posterior covering of the cyst, which really was, of course, the parietal layer of the peritoneum. The uterus and ovaries could be made out quite easily. I closed the abdominal wound, leaving in a small drainage-tube. She rallied very well, and gave us no reason for anxiety till the third day, when diarrhœa came on, and on the morning of the fourth she vomited. She sank, and died late that night.

No post-mortem examination could be obtained, so that we are entirely without exact information as to the relations of this extraordinary extra-peritoneal cyst, or as to the cause of death. I can see no other explanation than that it was a cyst of the urachus, and I fear that the cause of death was the gangrene of the denuded peritoneum. I believe it would have been better had I removed a great portion or the whole of the great peritoneal sac, which I left bereft of the source from which it derived its blood-supply.

The second case was operated upon on May 19. During my absence from home she had been sent to me, and was found in my waiting-room by my wife, in an apparently moribund condition. They were glad to get her out of the house alive and placed in lodgings. On my return I found evidence of a large tumour suppurating, and I at once proceeded to remove it. I found it extra-peritoneal, just like the other, quite rotten, and full of pus. The condition of the patient was entirely due to her obstinate refusal to have anything done for three years during which her attendant had recognised it. When she at last consented it was too late. The removal of the tumour was a matter of the utmost difficulty. She lingered till June 7—nearly three weeks—and died of exhaustion.

As far as these cases go they speak for themselves, and I do not think I need say that the series marks in many respects a distinct advance in abdominal surgery; and it is a matter of no small pride to me to have taken a part in a line of practice in which I venture to think that results have been obtained in this, the town of my adoption, which are second to none on record.

I cannot conclude without paying a tribute, well deserved, to one whose modesty will not permit that he should speak for himself. Much of my success I must attribute to the loyalty and skill of my assistant, Mr. Raffles Harmar.

REPORTS OF HOSPITAL PRACTICE
IN
MEDICINE AND SURGERY.

EAST LONDON HOSPITAL FOR CHILDREN.

TWO CASES OF TETANUS NEONATORUM.

Case 1.—Tetanus—Treatment by Chloral—Death.

(Under the care of Dr. EUSTACE SMITH.)

[For these notes we are indebted to Mr. J. Scott Battams, Resident Medical Officer.]

George R., aged four days, was admitted October 18, 1881. Died November 20.

Family and Previous History.—It is an Irish child. Parents appear healthy; there are three other children. No history of miscarriages or marks or signs of syphilis. The patient is the fourth child; labour was natural in all respects. The umbilical cord was tied with thread, and the remnant covered with clean rag; it had fallen off on the day of admission. There is no unhealthy action about the umbilicus. The whole family occupy one and the same room, which, however, is said to be clean and large. The child has been in bed with the mother constantly; the bed is so situated as to be in a direct draught, of which the mother has constantly complained. When born, the child appeared very healthy; took the breast well up till the day before admission to hospital, when for the first time it was noticed that it was unable to suck. Early on the morning of admission it cried out with a strong voice, but constantly screwed up its legs, and had no rest all night.

Condition on Admission.—When first seen (about noon), the child appeared to be well nourished; was dirty, but otherwise there was nothing abnormal about its exterior; umbilicus appeared healthy. The child was having spasms about every five minutes, not very severe, and not interfering with respiration: during the spasm, the legs were drawn up rigidly, the forearms flexed, the fingers outstretched and widely separated one from the other. The lips pouted a little; there was risus sardonicus. The jaw was slightly fixed, and the head was only slightly retracted. Any kind of irritation aggravated the spasms (such as attempting to open the eyes or mouth). The person in charge of the child refused to leave it without first getting the mother's consent; at 6.30 p.m. it was brought back again to the hospital, and admitted. The spasms had continued all the afternoon, and were somewhat more severe. The child had not swallowed any food since 11 p.m. of the previous day. Its general condition appeared less favourable even since noon (18th).

Shortly after admission (no bath was given) an enema was ordered, which brought away a rather large and constipated stool. After being put to bed, an ice-bag was ordered to the back for three hours. Between 7 p.m. and midnight three enemata of milk with, respectively, four grains, six grains, and six grains of chloral, were administered. At midnight, the child not being at all relieved, and still being unable to swallow, was chloroformed; and three ounces of its mother's milk, with four grains of chloral, were administered through a catheter passed into the stomach. This was repeated at 4.30 a.m., after which the catheter was passed without difficulty and without chloroform; and between two and three ounces of its mother's milk, with ten drops of brandy, were given every two or three hours. The convulsions had varied in intensi as well as in number during this time. They were manifestly influenced by the chloral, so that from 5 a.m. (19th) until 10 a.m. it slept quietly.

October 19.—10 a.m.: The limbs are now quite relaxed; the child's face is somewat dusky; very little air is entering the lungs. On passing the catheter into the stomach, no spasm was excited. 2 p.m.: Mr. Battams was sent for, as the child was thought to be dead. On making artificial respiratory movements, the child gave a gasp. From this time until 5 p.m. it continued to breath *eight times per minute*. The conjunctivæ were insensible; the surface was cold; but there was less cyanosis. Some brandy was administered. 10.30 p.m.: Condition unaltered, except that the respirations are now reduced to four per minute.

20th.—2.30 a.m.: The child was again thought to be dead, but artificial respiration again revived it for a while. It, however, finally sank about 3 a.m.

The temperature was 96° on admission (October 18); 99° at 9 p.m.

On the 19th it was 100·6° at 12 p.m., 99·8° at 2.15 p.m., 94·8° at 5.30 p.m., 95·8° at 7.30 p.m., and 96° at 10.30 p.m.

Remarks (by Mr. Battams).—It is to be regretted that a post-mortem examination in this case could not be obtained. The child's body was removed almost immediately by its parents (Irish) to be "waked." The diagnosis in this case was easy, the prominent condition being a permanent rigidity of the voluntary muscles, varying in intensity, with temporary exacerbations excited by trivial causes, during which time rigidity of the jaws and suspended respiration occurred. Not having the advantage of Dr. Smith's advice at the time, and guided to some extent by observations made in Mr. Parker's case, three indications for treatment presented themselves—viz., removal of all external and internal sources of irritation, keeping up the child's nutrition, and dominating the spasms. An enema relieved the constipated bowels. A spinal ice-bag seemed too theoretical in its probable results to be continued; and warm baths rather aggravate than relieve the spasm, so were not given. Quietness, subdued light, and avoidance of too frequent examination, are obvious indications. The rapid emaciation —always a striking feature of the disease—was met by feeding the child with its mother's milk through a catheter introduced into the stomach by the mouth, chloroform being given for the purpose. Unfortunately, emotional causes limited the supply of milk from this source, but we obtained some from a nursing mother. I venture to think this means of supplying nourishment and potent remedies is too little used in diseases of this class. Since the introduction of chloral several successful cases have been recorded. Dr. Widerhofen (*Lancet*, March 18, 1871) states that he has saved six out of twelve cases. In this child the violence of the spasms was markedly diminished after a few doses, and for twelve hours before death they occurred only at long intervals. An interesting feature was the slow breathing: for five hours before death only four inspirations occurred per minute, each accomplished apparently by a slight jerk of the diaphragm. For some hours before death the face was dusky; the heart could neither be heard nor felt. The body was cold, in spite of hot bottles and cotton-wool; the temperature, too, was very low. I am inclined to think the chloral had a large share in producing this condition.

(*To be continued.*)

DEVON AND EXETER HOSPITAL.

EXOSTOSIS OF FEMUR, INVOLVING KNEE-JOINT —REMOVAL ANTISEPTICALLY—PERFECT RECOVERY OF MOVEMENT IN THE JOINT.
(Under the care of Mr. BANKART.)
[Reported by Mr. A. G. BLOMFIELD, M.B., House-Surgeon.]

HENRY D., aged sixteen, was admitted into the Devon and Exeter Hospital in September, 1881, with an exostosis of the femur, of which he gave the following account:—Two months ago he first noticed a swelling on the outer side of the thigh, just above the knee-joint. He complains of it paining him at times, and inconveniencing him in his work as a farm-labourer.

On September 17, Mr. Bankart removed the exostosis under antiseptic precautions. An incision was made over the swelling, which was then exposed, together with the capsule

of the knee-joint. A small opening into the joint was therefore necessary to get at its base; it was then detached with bone-clippers and a gouge. The growth was found to be partly soft bone and partly cartilaginous, with a soft cartilaginous surface attached by two pedicles to the junction of the anterior and outer surface of the femur within the joint. A medium-sized long drainage-tube was then passed into the knee-joint, and the antiseptic dressings applied before Esmarch's bandage-tourniquet was removed, and the joint confined in a long back splint. The temperature on the evening of the operation was 98·6°.

18th.—First dressing. Temperature 100·2°. Slight sanious oozing. Evening temperature 101°. No pain. Throughout the case he never complained of pain, swelling, or any inconvenience about the joint.

20th.—Morning temperature 98·6°, evening 99°.

21st.—Temperature normal, and after this it never varied. Eight days after the operation, at the second dressing, the drainage-tube was removed, and the wound was found to be completely healed, except at the opening for the tube. There was no heat or swelling about the joint. The splint was still kept on for a time.

A week afterwards the opening left by the drainage-tube was found healed. Dry lint was applied, and over this a bandage, and the splint done away with. The boy was, however, kept in bed for a time. On October 15 he was discharged perfectly cured, the movements of the knee-joint being perfect.

Remarks.—The case is of interest as showing, along with other recorded cases, how large joints can now be opened with perfect immunity under antiseptic precautions. The time too (eight days) during which the drainage-tube was kept in the joint without causing any synovitis or pain is also worthy of note. The rise of temperature to 101° on the evening of the second and third day after the operation is probably accounted for by the fact that the dressings were applied while Esmarch's bandage-tourniquet was still on above the site of operation, and consequently a slight oozing of blood subsequently took place between the edges of the wound. The absence of all pain in or about the joint, and no constitutional disturbance all along, are worthy of note, and the subsequent restoration of perfect movement in the knee-joint allowed the boy to resume his accustomed occupation without the pain and inconvenience which the exostosis had caused. From its partly bony and partly cartilaginous nature it is highly probable that if it had been left it would have increased in size, and necessitated eventually a more formidable operation.

THERAPEUTICAL EMPLOYMENT OF RESORCINE.—Drs. Dujardin-Beaumetz and Callias terminate an elaborate paper upon this subject with the following conclusions :— 1. Resorcine possesses the same properties as carbolic acid, salicylic acid, and other substances of the aromatic series. It is anti-fermentescible at 1 per cent., and anti-putrescent at 1½ per cent. 2. Its poisonous power is inferior to that of carbolic acid. 3. It is a stimulant of the central nervous system. 4. It exerts no influence on the morphological condition of the blood, except when it is brought in direct and prolonged contact with that liquid. 5. It is a medicinal substance that may be employed internally and externally in all diseases due to contagious germs, or in diseases which favour their development, and for which other benzols are employed. The anti-rheumatismal, febrifuge, and antithermic power of resorcine is not as yet well defined, and calls for repeated investigations. 6. We feel very desirous that resorcine, in consequence of its extreme solubility, its scarcely perceptible smell, its slight toxicity and causticity, should be tried in surgical cases under the same conditions as carbolic acid, in the serious inconveniences of which it does not participate.—*Bull. de Thérap.*, July 30.

PRINTER'S ERRORS WITH A VENGEANCE.—Dr. Aahhurst of Philadelphia, referring to some typographical errors in a recent report of a clinical lecture in the *New York Med. Record*, writes :—" I wish to protest that I do *not* use *in* gonorrhœa injections of *six ounces* of acetate of lead to *two ounces* of water, nor do I attempt to cure *chancre* with camphor-and-opium suppositories. I think *two scruples* to *six ounces* of *water* quite strong enough for the injection; and it is *chordee*, not chancre, the pains of which I attempt to relieve by the rectal administration of anodynes."

TERMS OF SUBSCRIPTION.
(Free by post.)

British Islands	. . . . .	Twelve Months	.	£1 8 0
,, ,,	. . . . .	Six ,,	.	0 14 0
The Colonies and the United States of America	. . . }	Twelve ,,	.	1 10 0
,, ,, ,,	. . . . .	Six ,,	.	0 15 0
India	. . . . .	Twelve ,,	.	1 10 0
,, (via Brindisi)	. . .	,, ,,	.	1 15 0
,, ,,	. . . . .	Six ,,	.	0 15 0
,, (via Brindisi)	. . .	,, ,,	.	0 17 6

Foreign Subscribers are requested to inform the Publishers of any remittance made through the agency of the Post-office.

Single Copies of the Journal can be obtained of all Booksellers and Newsmen, price Sixpence.

Cheques or Post-office Orders should be made payable to Mr JAMES LUCAS, 11, New Burlington-street, W.

TERMS FOR ADVERTISEMENTS.

Seven lines (70 words)	.	.	.	.	£0 4 6
Each additional line (10 words)	.	.	0 0 6
Half-column, or quarter-page	.	.	1 5 0
Whole column, or half-page	.	.	2 10 0
Whole page	.	.	.	.	5 0 0

Births, Marriages, and Deaths are inserted Free of Charge.

THE MEDICAL TIMES AND GAZETTE *is published on Friday morning: Advertisements must therefore reach the Publishing Office not later than One o'clock on Thursday.*

Medical Times and Gazette.

SATURDAY, NOVEMBER 26, 1881.

THE ROYAL COMMISSION ON HOSPITALS FOR INFECTIOUS DISEASES.

OUR readers are well acquainted with the woes and troubles of the Managers of the Metropolitan Asylums Board; with their almost utter failure to provide adequate hospital accommodation for small-pox patients in London during the present year, and the fear now felt lest they should be unable to provide efficiently for fever cases. They are acquainted also with the helplessness of the Local Government Board, either to aid the Asylums Board or to make or carry out arrangements for the control of small-pox. The Asylums Board brought all their troubles upon their own heads, it will be remembered, by their persistence in establishing the Small-pox Hospital at Hampstead; and, very naturally, the success that attended the action brought against them in that case encouraged the inhabitants of other parts of the metropolis to resist the establishment of small-pox hospitals, or to seek to restrict the employment of existing Asylums Board hospitals. An interlocutory injunction was obtained in the Queen's Bench Division of the High Court of Justice to restrain the Managers from bringing patients to the Fulham Hospital from any district lying beyond the radius of one mile from the Hospital; injunctions were applied for, and with some success, against the establishment of temporary small-pox hospitals in Fulham and at Wormwood Scrubs; and, in short, nearly every attempt to provide new hospital accommodation for small-pox patients met with determined and vigorous opposition. The Managers appealed to the Local Government Board over and over again for help, but obtained nothing more than official courtesy. In May they urged upon the Local Government Board the necessity of immediate legislation "to enable them to deal with epidemic disease in a successful and satisfactory manner, without molestation, and to discharge the duties which the Act of

1867 imposed upon them," but without any effect; and again, in the present month, they repeated their appeal in almost piteous terms. At last, however, Her Majesty's Government has come to the rescue; and the *Gazette* of Friday last week contained the appointment of a Royal Commission to consider the hospital accommodation in the metropolis in relation to infectious diseases. The *personnel* of the Commission and the specified subjects of inquiry are given at length elsewhere in our columns, and it must be acknowledged that the Commissioners have plenty of work before them—if they can obtain reliable evidence upon the subjects they have to deal with. These subjects are arranged under six heads. The Commissioners are to examine into, and report upon, the nature, extent, and sufficiency of the hospital accommodation for small-pox and fever patients provided by the Asylums Board and the various vestries and district boards in the metropolis; upon the relative advantages and disadvantages, to patients and the public, of providing for these patients by a limited number of hospitals for the whole metropolis under one authority, such as the Metropolitan Asylums Board, or by parochial and district hospitals under vestries and district boards; on the expediency of continuing the existing small-pox and fever hospitals of the Asylums Board, and, should it be considered desirable to close any of them, on the substitutes to be provided; and on the expediency of the establishment of additional hospitals by the Asylums Board, and of making special provision for convalescent cases. It will take not a little time and labour to obtain and sift evidence upon these several points, but it will be still more difficult to deal to any purpose with the subjects further set out for inquiry. Under heads 5 and 6 are included, first, the conditions and limitations under which the present Asylums Board hospitals should be continued, and the general conditions and limitations to be applied to any new hospitals established by the Managers, or by any other authority, so as to insure in all practicable degree the recovery of patients and the protection of the public against contagion; and, secondly, the Commissioners are to report on the operation of the Acts authorising the establishment of small-pox and fever hospitals in the metropolis, on the provisions (if any) required for obtaining sites for such hospitals, and for the protection of the authorities providing and managing these hospitals from liability to legal proceedings so long as the hospitals are conducted with reasonable care and according to prescribed regulations. The Local Government Board and the Asylums Board ought to be able by this time to produce clear and decided evidence—not opinions only—upon these subjects; but though the Hampstead Hospital trial ought to have taught them to consider and be able to provide remedies for every weak point in the establishment and management of these hospitals, we have no proof that they are one whit better prepared to justify the establishment of large hospitals rather than small ones, and *vice versâ*, to formulate and support by clear evidence well reasoned-out systems and conditions of management, or to discuss with knowledge and intelligence the question of the protection of the public against contagion from the hospitals, than they were three years ago. But we do know that it was not until the beginning of the present year that any effort was, apparently, made by the Local Government Board to obtain, through its medical department, evidence as to whether hospitals for infectious disease are instrumental, and, if so, by what means, in causing the spread of infection in their neighbourhood; and that a few months ago the President of the Local Government Board professed, in one of his public utterances, that he did not know whether the risk of the propagation of small-pox would be less by a small hospital than by a large one. It does not seem probable that the Commission will obtain much assistance from the President of the Local Government Board, or from the Managers of the Asylums Board. The Commissioners must obtain the evidence they will need whencesoever they can, and sift and judge it with intelligence and without prejudice. And for their purposes the Commissioners seem well selected. Lord Blachford is a man of great and approved ability; he took a double first-class at Oxford in 1832, and many other marked university distinctions, has filled many important Government appointments, and was Permanent Under-Secretary of State for the Colonies for ten years. Mr. Peel has considerable Parliamentary experience, and is Parliamentary Under-Secretary of the Home Office. Both he and Mr. Leigh Pemberton are men of known ability. Sir Rutherford Alcock has had very wide experience, has filled important posts with great distinction, and had the advantage of being educated and trained for the medical profession. Of the merits of the professional members of the Commission we need not speak. Their qualifications, merits, and talents are well known to all our readers. Clearness of intellect, power of judging and appreciating evidence, breadth of view, and freedom from narrow prejudices, are the qualities specially needed for the task before the Commission; and surely these qualities are possessed in full sufficiency by the gentlemen who have accepted the task; and who, it may be added, have already begun their work.

MEDICAL EDUCATION IN FRANCE.

WE recently drew attention to the state of medical education in the United States of America. We may now contrast with that the way in which the French manage the same matter.

As everyone knows, the French people have a strong tendency to, or instinct of, order, classification, and precision. Wagner defines a Frenchman as a being who is endowed with a special faculty of dressing, moving, and expressing himself; and whose mission it is to teach the world the arts of dress, deportment, and expression. In French scientific literature, we can nearly always admire the orderly way in which the different branches of the subject are arranged and defined, and the neatness and clearness with which the author's thoughts are expressed. And in their arrangements for the education of the medical practitioner, French statesmen would never tolerate the existence of a cloud of varying qualifications, a scale exhibiting every gradation in kind and degree of fitness for practice, all of them being alike in the eye of the law. On the contrary, in France the conditions under which a youth is to be brought up to practise medicine are as definite as most other things in that country.

There are six great faculties; but the conditions under which they are allowed to fulfil their functions are minutely laid down by the central Government. The faculties are, Paris, Montpellier, Nancy, Bordeaux, Lille, and Lyons. There are two other schools (écoles de plein exercice) which are allowed (also under conditions laid down by the State) to educate students, but do not confer degrees. They are at Nantes and Marseilles. There are also preparatory schools at Algiers, Amiens, Angers, Arras, Besançon, Caen, Clermont-Ferrand, Dijon, Grenoble, Limoges, Poitiers, Reims, Rennes, Rouen, Toulouse, and Tours. At these the medical student may pass the first three years of his course of study, but the fourth year must be spent either in a faculty or in an école de plein exercice.

The course of study is mapped out for the student with careful precision. It extends over four years, and there are five examinations which have to be passed. Three of these examinations are divided into two parts, so that the exa-

minations may even be described as eight in number. The time at which each of these is to be passed is laid down for the aspirant by the central authority. A failure to pass any examination at the proper time causes the candidate to be put back for a certain time; that is, not merely is his passing the examination deferred in date, but his whole period of study becomes so much the longer for his failure. The first examination comprises Physics, Chemistry, and Medical Natural History. The second consists of two parts: the first being in Anatomy and Histology, the second in Physiology. The third is also divided: External Pathology (i.e., Surgery), Midwifery, and Operative Surgery coming first; Internal Pathology (Medicine) and General Pathology following. The fourth examination is in the subjects of Hygiene, Legal Medicine, Therapeutics, Materia Medica, and Pharmacology. The fifth, and last, is again divided: the first part being in Clinical Surgery and Obstetrics, and the second part including Clinical Medicine, practical demonstrations in Pathological Anatomy, and a thesis on a subject chosen by the candidate. The State requires that the student's work shall be practical, in the laboratory and in the dissecting-room. Its paternal care over him goes to the length of insisting that for two years he must live near the hospital. And the French student cannot avoid the disgrace of being plucked by simply not going up; for at the proper time his name is called, and if he does not present himself, and cannot show a good reason for his absence, he is sent back as if he had been plucked, and forfeits the fees which he has paid.

The fees for the degree of Doctor of Medicine amount in all, including "inscriptions" (somewhat analogous to our lecture fees) as well as examinations, come to 1360 fr., about £55. These fees do not go, as in England, either to the lecturers or examiners, but to the public treasury. Professors and examiners are remunerated by the State. The medical schools, therefore, are not, as in England, private adventures, the expenses of which have to be borne by private individuals, and the prosperity of which is profitable to those who manage them. The professors, though they have not such stimulus to exertion as may be given by the hope of a larger class, and therefore increased fees, if their teaching is made attractive, yet are not beset by any temptation to court popularity by lax discipline, or by lowering the quality of their teaching to suit the tastes of the majority. The examiners, too, having in no way to consider how the funds of the institution with which they are connected will be affected by the number of candidates whom they pass or reject, may also be considered as free from a temptation to let down their standard which besets nearly all (and, it is thought, with effect in some cases) of our own examining boards.

It is exceedingly difficult, when we have compared the systems of medical education in different countries, and the status and capacity of the average medical practitioner in each, to say how much is due to the rules and regulations, and how much to national peculiarities, the general average of education, taste, and moral and religious principle, and the other social forces which cannot be measured and can scarcely be defined, but which are much more powerful in modifying the individual type than written law. But, comparing France and America, we think few will dispute that in the average French doctor we are pretty certain of a man who knows something of his business; that among the laity the sick Frenchman probably is more sure of getting competent medical skill applied to his case than the American invalid; that the medical profession occupies a higher place in public esteem in France than it does in America; and that the average of French medical literature exhibits greater knowledge and a more general application of scientific method than the average of

American medical literature. (Of course, we are not comparing the leaders of medical science in the two countries). It is obvious that such a result might be expected from the different systems in vogue in each. The one government takes care that the medical advisers of its people shall be well educated, that no one shall practise whose training has not been thorough and his knowledge tested, and that no one shall profess to have qualifications which he does not possess. The other takes no precautions to insure this.

When we compare France with England, the points of difference which we have to note are more of detail than of principle. The Government in France prescribes in much more detail the course of the student, and leaves much less to the discretion either of teachers or students than is compatible with our insular ideas of liberty. Whether, if we ourselves were to follow in some points the French example, the result would be advantageous or not, is a question we have not space here to discuss. Possibly we may do so on a future occasion.

THE "OSTOMIES."

THE recent meeting of the Clinical Society, the proceedings of which were recorded last week, was enlivened by a discussion on two papers, by Mr. Reeves and Mr. Golding-Bird. The questions dealt with seemed from the first hopelessly obscured. One would seem to contend for opening the œsophagus when there was stricture; another would point out the danger of opening the stomach under similar circumstances. But various facts were obviously overlooked: strictures of the œsophagus are not always in the same place; and some are malignant, while some are cicatricial. Often we have seen malignant disease of the œsophagus spreading from disease of the larynx. But it may be situated much lower down. A simple stricture is one thing; an obviously malignant growth is another: for the one, an opening may give the power of waiting until the stricture be permanently overcome; in the other, any kind of operation must evidently be palliative merely. So, too, there must be a great difference between operating on a healthy (though emaciated) patient, and one the subject of fatal disease. Opening the stomach—as has been done, we were going to say, from time immemorial on dogs and other animals for physiological purposes—is, comparatively speaking, an easy operation, whatever may be said as regards the intense importance of one or more rows of quilled sutures. Opening the œsophagus cannot be such a light matter, as anyone accustomed to post-mortems (to say nothing of earlier dissections) must know. The tube itself is never patent in a state of rest, like the trachea; consequently its seizure, its opening, its connexion with the external integuments, are more or less matters of difficulty: and certainly the movements of the neck must at all times interfere with any permanent apparatus which may be thought of as desirable in these cases. There is no good record as yet of a successful case where the stomach had been opened, except that of the famous Alexis St. Martin, where assuredly the operation was performed in the rudest possible way by means of a gunshot, but who, nevertheless, survived the injury perfectly well. But why compare things which are totally different? St. Martin was in perfectly good health when his little accident occurred. Or, why talk of the fatal results of opening the stomach when a patient is sure to die in a short time of malignant disease? If cases are to be compared they should be similar in some kind of degree. Opening the œsophagus and opening the stomach are clearly two different things, even though the operations may be associated by the same bastard Greek terms which some nowadays, when Greek is proscribed as a part of medical education, seem so fond of using—not, we may say, altogether

with advantage. Such tender and delicate words as œsophagostomy (that is, if it means anything in plain English, "mouthing the food-pipe") are a little beyond us. Nevertheless, they seem in favour with some gentlemen, just as some fearful compounds of a like type find favour in the eyes of various kinds of tradesmen. At all events, and words notwithstanding, operations of a much more serious character are readily undertaken by skilled surgeons: witness that narrated this week by Mr. Spencer Wells at the Royal Medical and Chirurgical Society.

THE WEEK.
TOPICS OF THE DAY.

A SHORT time since we were obliged to remark upon the difficulties which had been placed in the way of post-mortem inquiries through the parsimonious conduct of the Middlesex magistrates in unduly cutting down the expenses of coroners. Another complaint has now been publicly made on the subject, and it is to be hoped that some steps will be taken to remove a state of things which must, if not modified to a reasonable extent, become exceedingly detrimental to the interests of justice. Dr. Diplock, the Coroner for West Middlesex, recently held an inquiry in Chelsea touching the death of a lady aged twenty-seven, the wife of a gentleman residing there. The circumstances of the case were very peculiar, many of the symptoms being apparently identical with those produced by the administration of an irritant poison. Dr. Edwards Crisp, of Beaufort-street, Chelsea, who attended the deceased during her illness, deposed that he had made a post-mortem examination, but he wished to state that four days and seven or eight hours had elapsed before he received the necessary warrant, and the consequence was that the body was by that time in such an advanced stage of decomposition that the results obtained could not be of a positive and satisfactory character. The spinal cord ought to have been examined in this case; but it would have been quite useless, owing to the advanced stage of decomposition. The Coroner very much regretted the circumstance; but said there had been no delay on his part, for directly he received information he sent off the warrant. He had spoken of the inconvenience of the present state of affairs over and over again, without avail. Some time ago it used to be the practice of medical men to make post-mortem examinations on their own responsibility if they thought the cases justified them; but one of these cases having been brought under the notice of the Middlesex magistrates, they refused to allow the costs of an examination made before the receipt of the warrant. Further delay was occasioned by the travelling expenses of his officers being disallowed. The inquiry was ultimately adjourned to admit of an analysis of the stomach and intestines being made.

A deputation, which amongst others comprised the names of Lord Harberton, Sir Antonio Brady, Captain Galton, C.B., Colonel Festing, R.E., Professor Chandler Roberts, F.R.S., and Mr. Ernest Hart, recently waited upon the Lord Mayor and requested him to consent to open the exhibition and trials of smoke-preventing appliances now about to be held at South Kensington. The earnest effort, they said, of the committee had been to encourage general improvement in the methods and appliances by which heat is obtained, and thus to secure the advantages of greater economy of fuel and diminished production of smoke. That effort had been so far successful that a very considerable number of economical and effective grates, stoves, and furnaces had been brought forward, and many improved methods of firing and other smoke-preventing means had been introduced. The Lord Mayor acceded to the request of the deputation, and the committee promised to communicate with him at the earliest possible date as to the day of opening the exhibition.

It having been reported by the Engineer and Chemist to the Metropolitan Board of Works that the nuisance arising from the chemical works at Hackney Wick has been abated, and that the fluid flowing from those works into the sewer is now of an innoxious character, Mr. Reginald Ward, solicitor to the Board, intimated that the adjourned summons against the proprietors of the works would be withdrawn. In a letter to Mr. Portwell, the Chief Inspector of Nuisances for the Hackney district, Mr. Ward has further stated that samples of the fluid flowing from the chemical works in question will be taken from time to time, in order to make certain that the nuisance is not revived.

Mr. Langham, Deputy Coroner for Westminster, recently held an inquest at St. Martin's Vestry Hall on the body of a child, aged eleven months, who, it was alleged, had died from blood-poisoning through sanitary defects at its parent's residence, Hanover-court, Long-acre. The mother deposed that they lived in a room on the first floor back; that the child had been taken ill, and expired before a doctor, who had been sent for, arrived; and, in answer to the coroner, she said that she considered that the stench arising from the water-closet and the dust-bin had hastened the death. They had occupied the room eighteen months, and the stench had been very bad the whole of the time. The husband also said that he had frequently complained of the smell, which arose immediately beneath their window. Dr. Dunn stated that upon going to the house he found it in such a condition that he felt it his duty to communicate immediately with the medical officer of health for the district. He had ascertained that the child died from convulsions due to natural causes. But he is reported to have said, in answer to the jury, that the house ought to be inspected by the sanitary authorities; unless precautions were at once taken, typhoid fever or some other contagious disease would arise. He could not, however, interfere with the duties of the medical officer of health. The jury, after some discussion, returned a verdict in accordance with the medical evidence, and requested the coroner to communicate with the medical officer of health, with a view to having the house in question thoroughly inspected.

A somewhat important decision was recently given in an appeal case brought by the Secretary of the Chemists' and Druggists' Association of Great Britain, in order to have the law declared as to whether a trader can sell by retail poisons supplied to him by a duly qualified chemist and druggist, under cover of a label bearing the name and address of the chemist, and not of the actual vendor. In this case, a grocer at Oxford had received packets of drugs from a chemist to sell for him on commission, and it was proved that a small quantity of red oxide of mercury was procured from him to test the question. The magistrates would not convict, but stated a case in which they found that defendant was a servant, and referred it to the Court whether the sale was legal, and whether the packet was duly labelled. The defendant was not represented by counsel—a circumstance regretted by Mr. Justice Grove in giving judgment; it was, however, decided that the magistrates had not drawn the proper inference from the facts as to the sale, and that the packet was not duly labelled within the Act. In the present case it was clear that the chemist who first sent the poison to the defendant could not be deemed the seller of the packet of poison as he was not on the premises, and was not, therefore, in a position to comply with the Act. The person who sold poisons was to enter the names of purchasers in his books, and a person living at a distance could not do so; it was

impossible that the chemist who carried on business at a different place could, as the magistrates had supposed, have been the "seller" of the poison in the present case. Mr. Justice Lopes concurred, and the case was ordered to be sent back to the magistrates to be decided in accordance with that judgment.

The Council of University College, Liverpool, have recently appointed Dr. W. A. Herdman to the Professorship of Natural History, founded by Lord Derby. Dr. Herdman is a graduate of the University of Edinburgh, and took the degree of Bachelor of Sciences in the department of Natural Science in 1879. The Council have also appointed Dr. J. Campbell Brown to the Professorship of Chemistry in the University College. Dr. Campbell Brown has for several years held the offices of Borough and County Analyst, and of Lecturer upon Chemistry at the Royal Infirmary School of Medicine.

The agitation in favour of a public park for Paddington still continues. A meeting has just been held at the Presbyterian Church, St. John's-wood, to further this object; the Rev. J. M. Gibson, D.D., who took the chair, enforced the necessity of a vigorous and liberal effort, whilst the chance still existed, of rescuing from the builders this remnant of the Paddington Estate for the benefit of all classes. The Rev. Canon Duckworth, D.D., proposed— "That it is of high importance for the physical and moral welfare of the population of London that every effort should be made to preserve for public use any open spaces still available for the purposes of parks or recreation grounds within metropolitan limits." The object, he said, was one which concerned not only London, but the whole country. Thickly built districts fostered disease and crime, and statistics proved that the death-rate increased in proportion to the lesser space allotted to each individual. The resolution, having been duly seconded, was unanimously carried, and it was agreed that it would be highly beneficial to secure the land in question as a people's park; also that a public subscription be raised, and offered to the Metropolitan Board of Works as a voluntary contribution towards the expenses.

A public meeting was held at Willis's Rooms, King-street, St. James's, on Monday last, ostensibly "to discuss the moral right and true philosophy of painfully experimenting upon animals for scientific purposes." The President of the Society for the Abolition of Vivisection, Rev. C. W. Grove, occupied the chair, and, in opening the proceedings, stated that the object of the meeting was to invite physiologists, biologists, and members of the medical profession to expound their views on the subject of vivisection. It was desirable to hear both sides of the question, and to know the results of the vivisection experiments which had already been made. The honorary secretary availed himself of the opportunity to give some particulars of the Society for the Abolition of Vivisection, and openly stated that the Government were now in opposition to the Colleges of Physicians and Surgeons, and refused to grant licences to physiologists of widespread repute. He did not know whether that was the beginning of the end; but (presumably in the opinion of the Society) the time had arrived for a public meeting to discuss a question so momentous, not only to animals, but to the human race, and to hear the statements of those gentlemen who advocated vivisection, and whether they had any claim upon the support of the Society. The chairman then invited medical gentlemen to express their views, and as a result several speakers addressed themselves to a wholesale condemnation of vivisection. In conclusion, the Chairman expressed his gratification that the Government had refused licences to eminent physiologists to carry on vivisection experiments.

Mr. Firth Groves, the Medical Officer of Health to the Lambeth Vestry, recently reported that a man who had been informed by his doctor that he was suffering from small-pox, rode to the Stockwell Small-pox Hospital in a tramcar, at a time when these vehicles were most crowded. On his recommendation of Dr. Groves, it was unanimously resolved to prosecute the man when he left the Hospital.

ROYAL COLLEGE OF SURGEONS OF ENGLAND.

At the last meeting of the Council of the Royal College of Surgeons, held on the 10th inst, Mr. John Croft, F.R.C.S., Surgeon to St. Thomas's Hospital, was admitted a member of the Court of Examiners. Mr. Edward Hadduck, L.S.A., of Biddulph, Congleton, was elected a Fellow of the College, his diploma bearing date October 21, 1842. The sitting of the Council was mainly occupied by the discussion of the report of the Committee appointed to consider and report on the questions sent to the Council by the Medical Acts Commission. The report was fully discussed, amended, and adopted. We shall publish it, more or less at length, soon; but, meanwhile, we may state that, in replying to the question whether any, and what, alterations of the present licensing are, in the opinion of the College, required, the Council in effect recommend the establishment of conjoint schemes; and, further, we understand that they recommend that twenty-two years shall be the earliest age at which any person shall be legally admissible to a qualifying examination. This recommendation, of course, implies an expectation of fresh legislation.

THE FERRIER PROSECUTION.

As we indicated last week, the violent attack of the anti-vivisectionists on Dr. Ferrier failed. It was a pity the case fell through simply on account of the summoning of the wrong person. It would have been better had the question been dealt with on its own merits. Were the experiments of such a thing as firing a capped pistol, containing no gun-powder (as was, we believe, the case here), of a painful kind? If a monkey was deaf, surely it could not be so. Was the exhibition of a monkey recovering from artificially induced hemiplegia a painful thing either to the monkey or the spectators? Such absurd prosecutions seem much as if they were got up on the principle of O'Donovan Rossa's brags—to raise the wind. At all events, they will probably fail in that respect. We are as greatly opposed as men can be to needless experimentation and cruelty to animals. We favour no experiments made only to acquire dexterity or to demonstrate the operator's skill. All, we hold, should be done with a clear and distinct purpose and by no bungler, but by men well skilled as to what they seek to attain and how to attain it. We should be the last in the world to back up such experiments, or rather tortures, as those which used to be common at the Veterinary School of Alfort. We take it that if such a question as having a slight wound inflicted, or that of sudden death, were proposed to a congress of animals—international or otherwise—they would prefer the former. But when we find men and women practically advocating that all experiments intended to aid the art of healing are to be performed on human beings, there is little good to be got from argument.

"A CURIOUS COINCIDENCE."

With regard to the paragraph that appeared under the above heading in our pages last week, we are assured on the highest authority that any idea that one of the reviews referred to had been cut down from the other would be absolutely contrary to the fact. Of course, we accept the assurance as frankly as it has been given; and the "curious coincidence" remains one of the "curiosities of literature."

THE ROYAL MEDICAL AND CHIRURGICAL SOCIETY.

At the meeting of this Society on the 22nd inst., a paper by Mr. Spencer Wells, describing his case of successful removal of the cancerous gravid uterus, was read. This unique case attracted a large meeting. The operation, although Mr. Wells was not aware of it at the time (former cases not having been published), had been performed before, but never successfully. Drs. Graily Hewitt, Playfair, Matthews Duncan, Mr. Knowsley Thornton, Mr. Doran, and Dr. Harris of Madras, were among the speakers. We shall deal more fully with the subject next week.

THE PARIS WEEKLY RETURN.

The number of deaths for the forty-fifth week, terminating November 11, was 1037 (550 males and 487 females), and among these there were from typhoid fever 28, small-pox 9, measles 8, scarlatina 3, pertussis 5, diphtheria and croup 53, dysentery 1, erysipelas 3, and puerperal infections 6. There were also 37 deaths from tubercular and acute meningitis, 32 from acute bronchitis, 92 from pneumonia, 87 from infantile athrepsia (23 of the infants having been wholly or partially suckled), and 29 violent deaths. For the last three months the mortality of Paris has been about stationary, oscillating between 851 and 1037 deaths per week. The present week's contingent, which is the largest of the three months, is perhaps the commencement of the increase which must be necessarily expected as autumn passes into winter. Diphtheria exhibits one of its highest figures for the present year. The births for the week amounted to 1164, viz., 586 males (436 legitimate and 150 illegitimate) and 578 females (435 legitimate and 143 illegitimate); 88 infants (51 males and 37 females) were born dead or died within twenty-four hours.

RESIGNATION OF PROF. VULPIAN.

Prof. Vulpian, in consequence of changes of which he disapproves being about to take place in the Faculty of Medicine, has resigned the post of Dean of that body, which he has filled now for some years to the general satisfaction. The loss of his services will be greatly felt by his colleagues. Prof. Béclard has been appointed his successor.

AN INQUEST IN JAMAICA.

There come to us from various quarters some curious details of an inquest in Jamaica, held, apparently, with unusual solemnity. Briefly, it would appear that a medical man was accused of poisoning his wife with morphia or prussic acid, or both. This lady had recently aborted, or been prematurely confined, and had, as a consequence, "white leg," that is, plugging of the veins on one side. The pain was, as is usual in such cases, intense, and undoubtedly large doses of morphia had been given. On one occasion, after, or just as she was being raised in bed, she suddenly screamed out, and in a few minutes was dead. Somehow or other, strange stories got abroad, and a post-mortem was made with a view to giving evidence at an inquest. In the right heart was found a mass of partially white clot, extending into both cavities. The stomach was removed, and in it was found, according to the analyst, no morphia, but plenty of prussic acid. Now, as it was well known that the morphia had been given, this is somewhat surprising. Alkalies of the free kind are not so frequently found as to be already present in the stomach for the purpose of fixing the hydrocyanic acid, and if they are not, the poison has a tendency to disappear (so we believe), especially after the opening of the stomach in a hot climate. But be this as it may, and making allowance for Jamaica climate and Jamaica analysis, the facts are well known to all in this part of the world that, given a plugged vein, a portion of the plug is apt to break off and to be carried to the right side of the heart. Here, in this case, some slow coagulation had taken place, probably extending to the pulmonary. Raising a patient up often breaks off a portion of this, and then there is no need for prussic acid—pulmonary embolism soon does its work.

VITAL STATISTICS OF SCOTLAND.

THE monthly return of the Registrar-General for Scotland for September last shows that during that month there were registered in the eight principal towns the births of 3365 children and the deaths of 1780 persons. This latter number is 389 under the average for the month of September during the last ten years, allowance being made for increase of population. A comparison of the deaths registered in the eight principal towns shows that the mortality during this month was at the annual rate of 14 deaths per thousand persons in Aberdeen, 15 in Perth, 16 in Dundee, 17 in Edinburgh and in Leith, 19 in Glasgow and in Paisley, and 20 in Greenock. The zymotic class of diseases proved fatal to 306 persons, and constituted 17·3 per cent. of the whole mortality. Diarrhœa was the most prevalent epidemic, and caused 70 deaths; fever was responsible for 45, of which 14 were tabulated as typhus, 20 as enteric, and 2 as simple continued fever. The deaths from inflammatory affections of the respiratory organs (not including consumption, whooping-cough, or croup) amounted to 321, or 18·0 per cent. Those from consumption alone numbered 215, or 12·1 per cent. Three females were aged ninety years and upwards, the eldest of whom was the widow of a shoemaker, and was ninety-five years of age.

THE HOWARD MEDAL OF 1881.

THE Howard Medal, offered by the Statistical Society for the best essay on "Gaol Fever," has been awarded to Dr. Frederick Pollard, of Liverpool, M.D. of London. Dr. Pollard was Cheselden Medallist and Senior Prizeman of St. Thomas's Hospital in 1868, and is a contributor to current medical literature.

THE SANITARY CONDITION OF PORTSMOUTH FOR THE YEAR 1880.

DR. WALTER J. SYKES, the Medical Officer of Health for the Borough of Portsmouth, in his annual report on the sanitary condition of the district for the year 1880, calls attention to the fact that as he only came into office on December 17 of that year, he can scarcely do more than give the statistics of it, with a few comments thereon. He points out that, although Portsmouth has the lowest death-rate of any large town in the kingdom, yet there are each year, on the average, nearly 500 deaths from preventable diseases—a fact which ought to stimulate every endeavour to get rid of those sanitary defects upon which, in a great measure, the prevalence of these diseases depends. In a carefully prepared table, Dr. Sykes shows the mortality of the principal large towns of England, with the deaths from the seven principal zymotic diseases reduced to the population of Portsmouth, also the mean age at death calculated at the same birth-rate as that of Portsmouth. By this table it can be seen at a glance the number of deaths from each disease there would have been in this borough had persons died at the same disease-rates as obtained in other towns. In mean duration of life Portsmouth heads the list, the average lease of life of its inhabitants being two years more than that of any town on the list. In the absence of scarlet fever it stands second; in measles, diphtheria, and whooping-cough it occupies a medium position; in diarrhœa it ranks amongst the lowest. But in fever

it occupies a most unenviable position, being the worst or the last, with the exception of Sheffield and Salford. Portsmouth, Dr. Sykes remarks, ought certainly not to have a higher death-rate from fever than such places as London, Birmingham, Leeds, and Liverpool. Attention is called to the large amount of the trashy kind of building, known as "jerry building," which is going on all over the borough, and the report suggests that if the authorities are not possessed of sufficient powers under the Public Health Act to alter this, from a sanitary point of view, very unsatisfactory state of affairs, it would be well to acquire further powers under a Private Improvement Act.

THE ARMY MEDICAL DEPARTMENT.

IN October last the Army Medical Department issued or published a newly drawn " Schedule of Qualifications necessary for Candidates desirous of obtaining Commissions in the Army Medical Department, with the Conditions of Service"; and this new Schedule presents some variations of arrangement and expression, as compared with the Schedule which was published immediately after the issue of the Army Medical Warrant of November 27, 1876. Our readers need not be told that these "Schedules" are not Royal Warrants; but they are supposed to embody, for the information of candidates, some of the most important provisions of the Royal Warrant, which is the authoritative exponent of the relations between Army Medical Officers and the Government; and they are official documents. But in the new Schedule the regulations as to rank and pay, although also component parts of the Army Medical Warrant of November, 1879, are quoted as "Extracts from the Royal Warrant of June 25, 1881," which is otherwise known as the "Pay, Promotion, and Non-effective Pay Warrant" of that date, and is the sole official authority on these points as concerns the whole Army.

This change has given rise to the idea that a new Army Medical Warrant has been published; and, in connexion with some other alterations in the Schedule, has created a good deal of very undesirable and unnecessary confusion and alarm. It is desirable, therefore, to assure our readers, on the best authority, that the new Schedule means exactly the same as the Schedule of December, 1879, and that the differences between the two have no significance whatever. We will, however, note some of these differences; and as it appears, from questions addressed to us from time to time, that many of those most interested in the matter are greatly at a loss to understand certain parts of the Army Medical Warrant, it may be not amiss to take this opportunity to elucidate some of the less explicit or more involved sections of that Warrant.

We shall notice the several points just as they strike us, or appear likely to strike persons of ordinary intelligence, on reading the Warrant; we do not, therefore, propose to notice each section of it seriatim.

Section 12 indicates the relative " precedence among each other as surgeons," of surgeons on probation who pass out of the Army Medical School at the same qualifying examination, being divided into two classes:—"(a) Those appointed on nomination according to their date of joining on probation." " (b) Those appointed on competition according to the last day of the competitive examination, and in the order of merit at such examination, with priority over any joining under sub-section (a) on the last day of the competitive examination." Now, the fact is that, as yet, in consequence of the steadily advancing degree of competition, no surgeons on probation have been appointed by nomination. We further take it that so long as candidates present themselves in sufficient numbers to confer a really competitive character upon each half-yearly examination, it is not the intention of the authorities to appoint any surgeons by nomination. Should it, however, become necessary to do so, in consequence of dearth of competitive candidates, it is provided in Section 9 that such nomination, up to half the number of vacancies, shall be made by the Secretary of State from among "such qualified candidates as may be proposed by the governing bodies of public schools of medicine in our United Kingdom, or in our colonies, as we may think proper." It may be presumed that the recommendation of the governing bodies of public schools of medicine in such cases would be likely to insure a degree of eligibility to which the precedence accorded to such candidates in sub-section (a) of Section 12 may be considered to be a suitable expression. To competitors, however, the inducement is still held out by the concluding sentence of sub-section (b), Section 12, that candidates who succeed in entering by competition shall have " priority over any joining under sub-section (a) on the last day of the competitive examination."

The publication of the Warrant of November, 1879, rendered necessary the division of the officers of the Army Medical Department into the classes A and B, the former (A) containing three sub-classes, viz., those who entered before April 28, 1876, those who entered after November 29, 1879 (the date of the present Warrant), and those who, having entered between the two dates above given, have been (under Article 2) permitted to exchange their terms of service for those of class A ; the latter (B) containing those who entered on or after April 28, 1876, and before November 29, 1879, generally known as the ten years' men, being liable, with a small proportion of exceptions, to discharge from the service, with a gratuity, on the expiration of that period of service. All medical officers of class B having, within the two years laid down in Section 2 of the Warrant now in force, been transferred at their own request to class A, all sections of the late Warrant referring to them may now be pronounced obsolete. For these reasons the rates of pay and half-pay to Class B are omitted from the new Schedule.

The regulations as to promotion to the grade of surgeon-major (Sections 15 and 17) appear sufficiently explicit, and are to the effect that medical officers on completing twelve years' service, of which at least three years shall have been abroad, shall, on the recommendation of the director-general, and, we may add, without further examination, be promoted to the rank of surgeon-major, and in case of distinguished service may be promoted to that rank without reference to seniority, the services for which the promotion may be given being published in the Gazette in which such promotion may appear.

The omission in the new Schedule of these regulations is to us entirely unaccountable, except on the grounds of the fact being now so generally known as no longer to require special statement. We may, however, state that the rule as to promotion is actually applied and acted on in the case of every medical officer on the completion of the prescribed term of service, provided, of course, no special objections exist.

In the section of the new Schedule detailing the relative rank of medical officers, is inserted a paragraph to the effect that deputy surgeons-general shall " rank among themselves according to their commissions as such," their relative rank in the Army being that of colonel. It certainly appears to us that this intimation is redundant as referring to the rank of deputy surgeons-general among themselves, which appears to be sufficiently defined by the dates of their respective commissions in the Army List. But as regards the rank of brigade surgeons among themselves there seems to be some necessity for such a definite ruling, as opposite to the name of each of the medical officers of that rank in the official Army List there are two dates, the first being that of appointment as brigade surgeon, and the second being "that from which they have the relative rank of lieutenant-colonel." Among the brigade surgeons now serving, instances exist of medical officers who, notwithstanding their having attained the relative rank of lieutenant-colonel on the completion of twenty years' full-pay service, hold a lower position in the official Army List, and we take it that to them more correctly than to deputy surgeons-general should be applied the ruling above referred to. In this opinion we are confirmed by the fact that among the Army Circulars of March, 1831, appears clause 48, publishing a Royal Warrant dated February 5, 1881, on the " Precedence of surgeons-major on promotion to the rank of brigade surgeon," which, referring to brigade surgeons and surgeons-major after twenty years' service having the relative rank of lieutenant-colonel, directs that "a surgeon-major of the Army Medical Department who, on promotion to the rank of brigade surgeon, is granted, under the provisions of our said Warrant, the relative rank

of lieutenant-colonel, shall take precedence of all surgeons-major who may be holding such relative rank." The full bearing, however, of this Warrant will affect the case of surgeons-major of less than twenty years' service promoted by selection to the rank of brigade surgeon, and will be thoroughly appreciated as soon as the system of promotion by selection becomes an actual fact, instead of being, as it now still is, a vision of the future among the many other "things hoped for."

In the matter of half-pay the rules are now much more to the advantage of the medical officer than they have ever been before. In all previous Warrants the allowances on retirement were graduated according to the number of years' service in each rank, the consequence being that senior medical officers naturally held on in the hope of attaining the largest possible amount of pension. Under the present Warrant the retired pay of surgeons-general and de_uty surgeons-general is fixed according to the rank attained, so that immediately even on promotion a medical officer of either of those ranks may retire on the pension of his rank. In the lower grades, the advantage of higher attainable pension may be found at some future time to induce medical officers of the ranks of brigade-surgeon and surgeon-major to hold on to the completion of thirty years on full-pay service ; but none have as yet achieved such a length of service without having been promoted into the administrative rank.

Under the terms of the Warrant of November, 1879, medical officers of all ranks who may voluntarily retire before having attained the full period of age—sixty years for the administrative and fifty-five years for the executive ranks—are liable, in case of national emergency, to be called on to serve again, but not beyond the limit of age ; and their half-pay at the various rates is granted as to officers on the active list. So also is the half-pay of officers who from ill-health may be temporarily unfit to serve. In the cases, however, of officers who, while still under full pay, may have been pronounced by a Medical Board to be permanently unfit for further service, half-pay, although issued without any alteration in the several rates, is designated retired pay. It may probably be inferred that surgeons and surgeons-major retiring before the expiration of twenty years' service on the specified rates of gratuity are considered to have permanently retired and not to be liable again to serve, inasmuch as their gratuities are classified with the retired pay. No case, however, has yet arisen in which this question has been submitted for definite official decision.

METROPOLITAN HOSPITALS FOR INFECTIOUS DISEASES.

THE urgent appeals of the Metropolitan Asylums Board would seem at last to have secured attention, since a recent Gazette announces the appointment of a Royal Commission to inquire into metropolitan hospital accommodation for infectious diseases. The Commissioners are to be Baron Blachford, Sir James Paget, Sir Rutherford Alcock, Arthur Wellesley Peel, Esq., Edward Leigh Pemberton, Esq., M.P., John Burdon Sanderson, M.D., Alfred Carpenter, M.D., William Henry Broadbent, M.D., and Jonathan Hutchinson, Esq. The inquiry, it is stated, will include—

1. The nature, extent, and sufficiency of the hospital accommodation for small-pox and fever patients, provided by the Managers of the Metropolitan Asylums Board, and the several vestries and district boards in the metropolis, including the Commissioners of Sewers for the City of London.

2. The relative advantages and disadvantages to patients and the public of providing for small-pox and fever patients, whether amongst persons of the pauper class, or persons of the non-pauper class without proper means of isolation, or both, by a limited number of hospitals for the whole metropolis under one authority, such as the Managers of the Metropolitan Asylum District, or by parochial and district hospitals, under vestries and district boards.

3. The expediency of continuing the several existing small-pox and fever hospitals now under the Managers of the Metropolitan Asylum District ; or, if it be considered desirable that any should be closed, the accommodation for small-pox and fever cases which should be substituted.

4. The expediency of the Managers of the Metropolitan Asylum District establishing additional hospitals and of making special provision for convalescent cases.

5. The conditions and limitations under which the hospitals provided by the Managers should be continued, and the general conditions and limitations which should be observed in the case of the establishment of new hospitals, whether by the Managers or any other authority, so as to insure, as far as practicable, the recovery of the patients and the protection of the public against contagion.

6. The operation of the Acts relating to the establishment of hospitals for small-pox and fever patients in the metropolis, and the provisions, if any, required for the acquisition of sites for such hospitals, whether by agreement or otherwise ; and for the protection of the authorities providing small-pox and fever hospitals, subject to the same being conducted with reasonable care, and according to prescribed regulations, from liability to legal proceedings, so as to secure the public against the loss of the benefits arising from such institutions ; and to make such suggestions as may be deemed expedient in connexion with all or any of the matters aforesaid.

FROM ABROAD.

CASE OF GENERALISED HYPEROSTOSIS.

M. LELOIR (Revue Médicale, September 3) brought before the Paris Biological Society the highly interesting case of a man about fifty years of age, in whom for the last ten years all the bones of the body have been undergoing a slow but progressive and perfectly regular development. No cause can be assigned for it, as the patient has no morbid history either as regards himself or relatives. Formerly he had some symptoms of lead-poisoning from working with preparations of lead, but he abandoned this occupation long ago, and became a bill-sticker. He exhibits no trace of scrofula, rheumatism, syphilis, or other diathesis. It was shortly after the siege of Paris that his attention was called to his present affection, first feeling pains in the back and loins, with some œdema of the latter. He then found his cap became by degrees much too small for his head, and afterwards his limbs increased in size. At present he can hardly walk, breathes with difficulty, suffers from constant headache, and is almost always in a half-comatose state. The whole skeleton is symmetrically hypertrophied, without the general configuration of the body having undergone much change. The ribs, increased in size, almost touch each other, and impede the play of respiration. The bones of the cranium, by compressing the brain, produce that intellectual torpidity which the patient now continues in ; and the strangulation of the cerebral nerves at the apertures by which they leave the base of the cranium gives rise to disorders of smell, vision, and hearing. Finally, darting pains, which radiate from the spinal cord towards the lower limbs, and are comparable to the fulgurant pains of locomotor ataxy, are probably due to the obliteration of the intravertebral foramina by the recent bony production. There has doubtless taken place here what Prof. Charcot terms pseudo-neuralgia in the spinal disease of cancerous subjects, when the softened vertebræ, sinking in, compress the nerves on their exit from the spinal canal. But in the patient in question, nowhere is there any vestige of bony ramollissement. Moreover, analysis of the urine has always shown it to be of normal composition.

M. Joffrey observed that it is of primary importance that this patient should be exactly weighed. In this manner we should derive the valuable information whether there is a true osteoplasia present, or whether there is an increase in the volume of the bones without any new production of bone—a kind of osteo-porosis. M. Hanot believed that, curious as the case of this man is, it is not an exceptional one. It is simply an example of osteomalacia. This disease may present itself in two stages—the one of induration, and the other of ramollissement ; and Sir James Paget has well described this succession. In this case the disease is only at its first stage, but it is to be expected that its evolution will go on, and before long it will resemble the ordinary cases of osteomalacia. M. Hanot has published a case in which the individual passed through these two phases.

FERRIER'S RESEARCHES IN THE BRAIN :
THEIR CHARACTER AND RESULTS.

(From a Correspondent.)

AT a time when public attention has been strongly directed towards Dr. Ferrier's experimental investigations into the functions of the brain, it may be well to indicate, in a form intelligible even to the non-professional reader, the nature of these investigations, the practical results which have already flowed from them, and the influence which they are likely to exercise on the future progress of medicine.

Had Dr. Ferrier's discoveries been mere barren knowledge, yielding no benefit to man nor beast, and promising none as far as the scientific foresight of the day can penetrate into " the wonder that shall be," they would still have deserved the grateful recognition of all educated and reflecting men. For knowledge is good for its own sake, and, strictly speaking, no true knowledge is barren, absolutely and finally. It may lie long dormant and apparently dead, like wheat in the immemorial cerements of the mummy, but sooner or later it is brought into the conditions of growth, and buds and burgeons, and bears fruit in due season. The most isolated and ineffectual-looking observations are to be welcomed into the storehouse of scientific truth, and treasured there until the hour and the man arrive for their practical utilisation. And indeed some of those observations that have revolutionised the history of the world have been isolated and ineffectual-looking enough when first made and recorded. Galvani's discovery in 1780, that the limbs of a recently killed frog, when hung by the nerves from a metal support, contracted convulsively at the recurrence of each spark from an adjacent electric machine, seemed doubtless, at the time it was made, a mere curiosity of physiological research. His friends probably dinned in the philosopher's ears that miserable Cui bono ? that has blighted so much fair scientific promise, and he himself cannot have thought much of the value of the fact which he had noted, as he allowed ten years to elapse before he published it. And yet this insignificant and disregarded observation was the germ from which have sprung all the marvellous developments of dynamical electricity, and to which we owe the innumerable and ever multiplying applications of it in art, science, and manufacture, which add so immensely to the comfort, convenience, and refinement of our daily lives. And so it has been with many other scientific discoveries, which have stood for a time detached and useless, with no promise of fertility, but which have ultimately become the parents of progress and material advantages. And this desirability of knowledge for its own sake, or with a view to remote and contingent, rather than immediate and direct, advantages, has surely been fully recognised in this country, which has gained world-wide renown by its polar expeditions, which have involved a sacrifice of life and treasure, and no little suffering, in hitherto futile attempts to obtain knowledge, which, if gained, would not be at once available for any purpose of practical utility.

With Dr. Ferrier's discoveries, however, the case has been different: they have had no period of waiting and inutility. For science has been long waiting for them, and from the first statement of them their importance and direct bearing on the healing art were recognised by all who were able to understand them. Aristotle was the first who attempted localisation of function in the brain, his view being that three faculties, which he named common sense, phantasy, and memory, were seated in the fore, middle, and hinder regions of the cerebrum respectively. And since his time frequent attempts have been made to obtain proof of the ever-strengthening conviction that the brain does not act as a whole, and to distinguish the plurality of organs of which it was assumed to be composed. Gall and Spurzheim for a time succeeded in convincing many that they had solved the great problem ; but although their method was sound, and their contributions to cerebral physiology of some value, they failed alike in their analysis of mind and topography of brain, and their system, yielding to opposition and ridicule, fell gradually into disrepute. Since their day the need of trustworthy information about the brain, and of some insight into its obvious but baffling complexities, has been constantly and urgently felt. But until Fritsch, Hitzig, and Ferrier set to work, all efforts to read the great riddle had proved unavailing. Notwithstanding untold labour and ingenuity expended in the study of it, the brain proper was still a mystery when they commenced their luminous work. It was then —about ten years ago—a great dark continent, and their explorations have done for it what the travels of Livingstone, Stanley, Grant, and other intrepid geographers have done for Africa. They have dissipated many foolish speculations which hovered over it ; they have marked out its natural highways ; they have revealed the distinctive characters of its different regions, and disclosed its resources. The brain is no longer an inexplicable mass of convolutions —of curved ridges and rounded valleys between,—with no individuality of function, but a series of centres, distinct and yet in intimate relations, in definite sequence, presiding over all the movements of the body, and receiving and elaborating all the communications of the senses.

Ascertaining that, contrary to current belief, the tissue of the brain may be stimulated into activity by electricity, they have, by the use of the constant current and of faradisation, compelled that organ to deliver up its well-kept secret and declare its own constitution. Exposing the living brain in animals, and travelling over its surface with the electrodes, Ferrier (for his researches have far transcended those of Fritsch and Hitzig) has been able to demonstrate that each convolution or gyrus of the brain has its own work to do, and is a separate and independent centre. He touches one gyrus, and the paw is raised as if to strike ; he touches another, and the ear is pricked as if to listen ; another, and the mouth is opened as if to emit a cry. And not only has he been able by his divining-rod to fix on the hidden springs of all simple and combined movements, but by a combination of the method of electrical irritation with that of experimental destruction of a part he has succeeded in tracing the senses to their cerebral homes. Stimulating electrically one gyrus, he has produced movements of the eye and its pupil, and then, removing this centre from both hemispheres by cauterisation, he has caused permanent blindness, thus proving that this particular gyrus is the centre where visual impressions are received and harboured. As in the various animals experimented on the several motor and sense centres are invariably arranged in the same order, and as there is no difficulty in making out the convolutions in the human subject homologous with these, the functions of which have been determined in the lower animals, it was an easy step to proceed to make out on the human brain the areas of diverse functional endowments. And the correctness of the localisation of function thus arrived at has been incontestably proved by that ruthless vivisector, disease, which is always performing such cruel experiments upon our kind. In many cases now in which convulsions, or paralysis of certain groups of muscles, has been observed during life, it has been shown after death that there was some pathological change—a tumour, a clot of blood, or a patch of inflammation—in the precise spot indicated as the centre presiding over the movements which were troubled or abolished by disease.

It has been imagined that Ferrier's experiments were of a peculiarly painful nature, and involved protracted torture of the animals submitted to them. Excruciating images are conjured up in the lay mind by a description of the removal of the skull, the exposure of the palpitating brain—the holy of holies, the very quick of the whole organism,—and of the application to it of electrodes or white-hot platinum wires. But pictures are fanciful, and arise out of ignorance of the conditions necessary for the success of such experiments, and of the nature and endowments of the crown of the nervous system. The brain, although the home of feeling, is itself insensitive. When laid bare, as it has often been by accident in the human subject, it may be sliced away, as portions of it have been repeatedly for surgical reasons, without any suffering being occasioned ; and in animals, when uncovered, it may be probed or cauterised without the faintest sign of inconvenience being manifested. The membranes covering the brain are intensely sensitive, but the wonderful organ they enclose is as destitute of feeling as the tips of our finger-nails or hair. The removal of the brain-coverings, as pre-

paratory to Professor Ferrier's explorations, must have entailed brief and exquisite pain but for the merciful administration of anæsthetics, which has never been neglected. Even a vivisector may, we presume, be credited with a desire to obviate unnecessary suffering ; but should this safeguard to humanity be denied, we have still a guarantee that anæsthetics were not neglected in the fact that without them the designed experiments could not have been properly carried out. An animal exhausted by pain and struggling would not, when electrically stimulated, yield satisfactory results ; and more than that, an animal retaining the power of voluntary movement could not exhibit in an intelligible way the effects of artificially-induced activity in certain regions of the brain. Professor Ferrier's aim was to ascertain the definite movements induced when certain portions of the brain were stimulated, and that would obviously have been frustrated had the subject of his experiment remained capable of spontaneous movements. In order that he might recognise the effects of his experimental procedure it was necessary that the animal should be absolutely quiescent ; and absolute quiescence in an animal is only to be obtained through deep anæsthesia : we say " deep anæsthesia," for it is well known that ether, chloroform, and other anæsthetics in common use extinguish feeling long before they paralyse motion, and that a patient may writhe and struggle through an operation which has involved no pang of pain. To insure muscular stillness, anæsthesia must be carried far beyond the point at which the sense of pain is abolished ; and this is what was necessarily and invariably done in Dr. Ferrier's investigations. But his non-professional critics have hitherto failed to realise this truth. Because, in playing with his electrodes on the brain of the prostrate and insensible animal before him he has evoked movements and cries which are ordinarily expressive of pain or distress, the conclusion has been jumped at, that these were to be taken as betokening subjective states such as usually correspond with them, and that the anæsthesia was incomplete. But the truth is that these movements and cries no more betokened suffering than other movements and cries induced in like manner— those of laughter, barking, and wagging of the tail—betokened comfort and gratification. All movements and cries elicited by the process were mechanical, and no more betokened sensibility than do the movements, snortings, and shrieks of a locomotive. A man, whose neck has been broken, looks with no feeling but curiosity at the contortions of his legs when his feet are pricked, pinched, or burned ; and an animal deeply anæsthetised may exhibit all the signs of suffering or of joy in the most purely automatic manner.

But had Dr. Ferrier's experiments involved all the suffering that has been ascribed to them, and ten times as much, they would still have been not only justifiable, but commendable. Even then they would not have been responsible for one tithe of the torture that the crimping of cod entails daily, while, instead of merely refining the flavour of an already palatable article of food, and so tickling the palate of the gourmet, they have conferred a heritage of untold alleviation upon all future generations of mankind. " Localisation," says Virchow, " is the principle of modern medicine." Whatever benefit has accrued to the sick in modern times in any branch of practical medicine is attributable directly or indirectly to localisation, for before we can rationally treat disease we must know its " where " and its " what," we must have an anatomical and a pathological diagnosis. But in diseases of the brain, until Ferrier buckled to his work, no anatomical diagnosis was possible. Guesses might be made, but scientific precision was unattainable. Now, however, as has been already hinted, we can in many cases definitely fix on the foci of cerebral disease, and, in no metaphorical sense, put our finger on the spot beneath which the morbid change lies concealed. And day by day our power of accurate diagnosis in brain-disease becomes enlarged by the observation of cases in the light of Ferrier's discoveries. It is no exaggeration to say that our knowledge of the functions of the brain has been extended more during the last ten years than in the ten centuries preceding them, and that this remarkable extension of knowledge is due entirely to experimental interrogation of the living tissue of the brain.

And surely this extension of our knowledge of brain-function comes opportunely at a time when diseases of the brain are, if we may believe those most competent to speak on such a subject, increasing rapidly amongst us, and are cutting off not the waifs and strays of civilisation, the brutish and the ignorant, but the noblest and best amongst us, scholars and men of genius. Diseases of the nervous system, the Registrar-General tells us, destroyed 70,345 persons in England and Wales during 1879, of whom 14,205 died of apoplexy, and 12,593 of paralysis. But these figures, startling though they are, give but a faint idea of the number of lives sacrificed to morbid changes in the brain and its appendages, for an immense number of persons who are brought to the brink of the grave by nervous diseases are actually toppled into it by some intercurrent complaint, such as congestion of the lungs or diarrhœa, and these intercurrent complaints are, of course, set forth in the certificates of death, which do not go into pathological history, and so swell the columns of the Registrar-General's Report representing other than nervous diseases. It is characteristic of nervous diseases that, being mostly of a chronic nature, they may run on for years, causing disability and great distress, and sometimes ruin, not only to those immediately afflicted by them, but to whole families. Could a just estimate be presented of the wretchedness and suffering caused by diseases of the nervous system, a very urgent demand would arise for the discovery of more effectual means of amelioration than we now possess, and the practical benevolence of Dr. Ferrier's enterprise would perhaps be recognised.

But here, doubtless, the objection will be intruded, that, admitting that Ferrier's researches have thrown light on the physiology of the brain, they have not afforded any assistance in the treatment of the diseases of that organ. Granted it may be said that he has afforded guides to diagnosis, which aid doctors in forming a neat theory of a case; but what has he done for patients, how has he helped them in their forlorn condition? Now, it is undeniable that Ferrier's discoveries in cerebral localisation have not and cannot of themselves insure any advance in the treatment of disease. But the same cannot be said of them if they are viewed in relation to discoveries in other directions. It is from the colliding of truths that light to lighten the nations is evolved, from the congress of discoveries that practical results are begotten. And an illustration of this has been already afforded in connexion with Ferrier's discoveries. Standing alone, as we have said, they gave no help in treatment; but united with Lister's discoveries in antiseptic surgery, they have at once yielded valuable results, and promise to bear fruit an hundred-fold. Suppose a case of tumour or local growth in the brain. Formerly, it might have been possible to say that there was a tumour in the cranial cavity, but beyond this no one would have dared to go. Now it is possible, thanks to Ferrier's inquiries, to define in many cases the exact situation of the growth. And in future it will sometimes be possible, thanks to Mr. Gerald Yeo's application of Lister's method, to cut down upon the tumour and remove it with safety. What was formerly a necessarily fatal complaint, is thus converted into a curable one. Without Ferrier's discoveries, the position of the tumour could not have been defined; without Lister's discoveries, which were also achieved by experiments on animals, the tumour could not have been removed, because of the dangers attending operative interference with the skull, which had, indeed, brought the use of the trephine into discredit. But now Mr. Gerald Yeo's ingenious investigations have made it certain that the inflammation which follows exposure of the cranial contents is caused by septic agencies, and may be prevented by the exclusion of these, and that strong carbolic solutions have no dangerous effect when applied to the meninges of the brain. Of twenty-six monkeys that had performed on their brains operations of a more formidable character than would usually be required for the removal of a tumour, and involving extensive loss of cerebral substance, nineteen recovered completely; while of the seven that died, at least four were lost from causes which were independent of the operation, such as an overdose of chloroform, and the intense cold of the weather bringing on catarrh. Reducing his numbers to a percentage, Mr. Yeo states that 100 per cent. of the animals treated with antiseptic dressings were cured without any inflammation of the meninges, and that 100 per cent. of those treated without antiseptic dressing died of acute encephalitis. And those teachings of Mr. Yeo, bringing together the discoveries of Lister and Ferrier, have already been adopted in the domain of practical surgery. Mr. MacEwan, of Glasgow, has recently described in

the Lancet a brilliant example of their application—the case of a patient from whose brain he removed antiseptically a tumour, the position of which he determined by Ferrier's method. The patient recovered, and owes his life to Ferrier and Lister, as interpreted by Yeo and MacEwen. At the same time, Mr. MacEwen narrates another case in which, also by means of Ferrier's discoveries, he felt justified in marking out on the skull the position of an abscess beneath, and in which, so great was his confidence in his method, he was anxious to trephine and evacuate the pus. The patient and his friends, however, could not believe in such scientific divination, and so declined the proposed operation. Death took place, and Mr. MacEwen was then allowed to demonstrate the accuracy of his diagnosis. He trephined, and found the abscess at the very spot which he had indicated.

Similar cases have been reported in France, and no one with any acquaintance with the subject can for a moment doubt that henceforth tumours, clots of blood, and abscesses on the surface of the brain will cease to be the utterly hopeless maladies which they have hitherto been. Many lives will be saved and prolonged, that must have ended speedily and miserably had not Ferrier braved the rancorous attacks of the old enemies of science in alliance with humanitarian jingoes and those well-disposed imbeciles who do so much social mischief with the best intentions.

It is satisfactory to note that the benefits of the practical applications of Ferrier's discoveries will not be confined to the human species, but that the lower animals that have been sacrificed to secure them will also have some share in them. Dr. Beaston, of Glasgow, has successfully removed from the brain of a sheep, affected by sturdy, a cyst which Ferrier's observations enabled him to localise. The animal, which was dull and lethargic, and had lost vision in both eyes, in a few days after the operation recovered its sight, and was soon in its usual health. Sturdy is a common disease amongst sheep that are tended by dogs, and consists in the presence in the brain of a cyst of an hydatid, the Cœnurus cerebralis, which is the larval stage of the Tænia cœnurus, one of the six varieties of tape-worm infesting the dog. It is marked by symptoms of congestion of the brain, such as redness of the eyes and contraction of the pupils, and subsequently by rotatory movements, emaciation, exhaustion, and death. The animals affected by it suffer much, and it will be an incalculable boon to many sturdy-stricken sheep, as well as a great saving to farmers, when, by means of Ferrier's discoveries, the site of the cyst can be at once defined, and its removal safely effected.

But it is not probably in the domains of surgery that the grandest results of Ferrier's discoveries will be achieved. They have facilitated the study of pharmacology, and it is the offspring of that study that will, in all likelihood, bring them their proudest rewards. It has long been known that certain drugs act principally and specially upon certain nerve-centres, and specifically modify certain nerve-functions. Digitalis slows the heart, belladonna dilates the pupil, jaborandi stimulates the salivary secretion, and strychnia operates on the motor centres in the cord. Is it too much to hope, then, that the progress of pharmacology will yet furnish us with the means of operating on each centre, or group of centres, which Ferrier has marked out for us, so that we may exalt or depress their action at pleasure, and so effectually control those functional derangements in which cerebral diseases begin? Crichton Browne has endeavoured to show that, in many cases of mania, the starting-point of the pathological process may be detected by watching the disordered movements that are exhibited. Could we then apply the appropriate "drowsy syrup of the world" to that centre at the moment of its initial fretfulness, should we not "medicine it again to that sweet sleep" which it previously enjoyed, and so cut short the maniacal paroxysm? The same physician has pointed out—and in this he is confirmed by Dufour, and to some extent by Mickle—that in general paralysis of the insane, that grievous malady, one of the infirmities of "noble minds," which carries off year by year in the flower of their days a large contingent of intelligent and energetic men and women, there is localisation of the lesions after death, pointing to a definite line of march over the brain, and holding out the hope that it may yet be arrested in the centres which it first invades.

That Ferrier's discoveries will yet prove serviceable in the treatment of epilepsy, of chorea, and of many other cerebral diseases, few who have looked into the matter will deny. The difficulty, indeed, is not to multiply, but to limit, the possibilities of usefulness that lie before them, for what department of human activity is there that may not be influenced by the revelation of the structure of the organ of the mind. We have sketched only some of the more immediate results of these discoveries. Among their remote consequences it can scarcely be necessary to refer to the sway which they may exert over psychology and education. They may revolutionise the one, and remodel the other. As regards education, it is plain that if the brain is composed of a series of centres, evolved, not simultaneously, but in definite sequence, and if training can be best applied to each centre when it is undergoing development and before it becomes permanently organised, then Ferrier's work must afford the key to the natural order in which the different branches of education should be arranged, so as to attain the highest results. Speculation has ample scope in shadowing forth the future of Ferrier's discoveries, but the most prosaic nature cannot fail to perceive that they are charged with vast potentialities, and that they have already accomplished practical results of no mean importance.

REVIEWS.

Minor Surgical Gynæcology. A Manual of Uterine Diagnosis and the Lesser Technicalities of Gynæcological Practice, for the use of the advanced student and general practitioner. By PAUL F. MUNDÉ, M.D., Professor of Gynæcology in Dartmouth Medical College, Obstetric Surgeon to the Maternity Hospital, New York, etc. With 300 illustrations. New York : William Wood and Co. London : Sampson Low and Co. 1880. Pp. 381.

THIS work is undeniably a very laborious, full, and clearly written account of the subject of which it treats, and if certain premises which it takes for granted be admitted, it will follow that the book is one of great value; if, on the contrary, these premises are erroneous, then the volume is a great heap of misdirected industry.

It contains very minute and detailed descriptions of many methods of treatment of uterine diseases : as to some of these methods there is great doubt whether they ever do any good; as to others, it is questionable whether the possible benefit is worth the trouble or risk of the treatment; others, again, are only called for in rare and exceptional cases. If it be granted that each manœuvre described here is sometimes necessary or desirable, then the book is most valuable; if, on the contrary, it should be thought that many of them are useless and objectionable, then the merits of the book will only make us regret that the ability and toil displayed in it should not have been directed to a better purpose.

The first 115 pages are devoted to a description of the different methods of examining the female pelvic organs. Most elaborate accounts are given of every possible way of investigating by finger, sound, speculum, etc., the condition of the parts. However useful this may be to one who intends to make gynæcology a speciality, it is possible, we think, that its effect upon an ill-informed student or general practitioner might sometimes be one which we think the author would not wish, viz., to induce him to think physical examination all-important, to think too much of alterations in the configuration or aspect of the genital parts, and to forget the part played by disease elsewhere in producing or modifying functional disorders of the pelvic organs. The author seems as if he occasionally forgot that these methods of gynæcological examination are painful, and, if resorted to without good reason, objectionable. We think, for instance, that the practitioner who should make it his rule to act on this permissive precept, "When a patient complains of painful, too frequent or too scanty micturition, or when the finger in the vagina detects an unusual sensitiveness of the urethral body or vesical base, it may be desirable to explore the urethra or bladder by means of instruments or the finger" (page 58), would do himself and his patients a good deal of harm. The author shows by the use of the word "may" that he is aware that some other reason than the presence of these symptoms should be

present; but he does not give the general practitioner any further guidance.

The rest of the book is devoted to the minor gynæcological operations. Here again we have the same fault to find—that the book recommends what seem to us unnecessary, or needlessly prolonged and multiplied, local interferences. Thus, the author tells us (page 163), "I rarely treat a case of areolar hyperplasia or subacute or 'chronic' pelvic peritonitis or cellulitis, otherwise than by the application with a swab once or twice a week through the speculum of pure tincture of iodine. . . . By the persistent use of these remedies (by persistent I mean for from three to six months, and we should expressly caution the patients not to expect even the sign of an improvement sooner) we may confidently hope to relieve our patients, at least, if we cannot actually cure them." Has it never occurred to Dr. Mundé that it is the characteristic of all inflammatory changes, that, when the cause is removed, and the patient put under favourable conditions, they tend to recovery; and that consequently his patients might have got well as quickly (perhaps more quickly) without this bi-weekly swabbing ? Dr. Mundé seems to have observed facts in accordance with this law, although the explanation does not seem present to his mind. He says (page 162), "It is a good rule, after using any local remedy for a reasonable length of time without appreciable benefit, either to interrupt it for a short time to give the *vis medicatrix naturæ* time to assert itself, or to change the remedy." Might it not be inferred that the remedy in these cases had retarded recovery ? We may give a few other instances. In describing the treatment of dysmenorrhœa and sterility by dilatation of the uterine canal, we are told, "If a systematic gradual dilatation of the uterine canal is intended (as in stenosis, sterility, dysmenorrhœa, flexion), the sitting should be repeated *every day or two*, according to the necessity and endurance of the patient. . . . In the latter cases (of sterility), the treatment, in order to achieve permanent results, generally requires to be continued for some months"—the italics are ours—(page 236). Again (at page 240), with reference to the same subject, "I have repeated it three times a week for several months in dysmenorrhœa and sterility, with decided benefit as regards the former difficulty, and occasional relief of the latter." Further (at page 258), "In dysmenorrhœa from constriction of the canal or flexion, a few sittings, say two a week for a couple of months, . . . will generally result in decided improvement or cure." Surely this is *nimia diligentia!* We know that there are cases in which one dilatation will completely cure, and it has yet to be proved that in those in which one sufficient dilatation fails, a repetition of the operation every alternate day is more successful. Again, with regard to pessaries, we are told (page 301) that "the frequent replacement of a dislocated uterus is in itself a valuable method of gradual cure by restoring tone to the ligaments, and giving the vagina a proper shape for a supporter." At page 318 we read, "The rule is to remove, as far as possible, all counter-indications before applying a pessary, and this preparatory treatment may occupy months." At page 330, "Every patient wearing a pessary . . . . should be examined from time to time. This interval with soft pessaries should not exceed two weeks, with hard instruments one to two months." The importance which the author attaches to mechanical treatment may be judged of from the fact that there are no less than seventy pictures relating to pessaries. But if pessaries can give no better results than this—if they are only useful after months of preparatory treatment, and, to be safe, require a fortnightly or monthly examination all the time they are worn,—then the mechanical treatment of uterine displacements would not be a thing to be very proud of. With regard to this and the other instances we have quoted, we cannot think that Dr. Mundé's book is likely to improve the art of gynæcology. These local manipulations repeated so frequently for such long periods may perhaps be necessary in complicated or exceptional cases : we do not for a moment question Dr. Mundé's judgment as to those which have come under his own care ; but such cases are quite exceptional, and we cannot but think that the commencing practitioner will be ill advised if he follows, in the instances we have quoted, the advice of this work. The book tells him *how* to do all these things, but does not tell him *when*, and the latter question is much more difficult than the former, and quite as important.

If we had to choose between two men, one of whom went into practice utterly ignorant of the diseases of women, and treating them all with some simple tonic mixture, and the other blindly followed out the teachings of a book like this, resorting to these surgical measures, and multiplied and persistent local treatment for the cure of every disease, real or supposed, of the pelvic organs, we believe that patients would be better off under the care of the first. This book is one only safe in the hands of an experienced gynæcologist, who knows what is to be expected from the treatment and when to apply it. It is by no means a book for students or general practitioners.

The Venereal Diseases, including Stricture of the Male Urethra. By E. L. KEYES, M.A., M.D. London: Sampson Low, Marston, Searle, and Rivington. 1881.

THIS work is one of a series of volumes published by Messrs. Low and Co. for the use of the general practitioner. Dr. Keyes' writings on venereal diseases, and more especially on the treatment of syphilis, are well known, and advocate what he terms the tonic treatment of syphilis. He has reduced the tonic dose from a half to a third of that required to produce slight salivation, and this is continued for a long period of time. When severe outbreaks occur this dose may be increased; and afterwards, when the attack has subsided, be reduced to the former quantity. The dual theory of syphilis, and the new views on gleet and stricture of the urethra, are discussed at great length and very ably. The volume is a most interesting one and will repay careful perusal; it is well suited for the purpose for which it is intended.

We do not admire the style of the book. It is bound in a semi-æsthetic style, the type is very close, and the paper thin, thus being difficult and disagreeable to read.

How to use the Forceps; with an Introductory Account of the Female Pelvis and of the Mechanism of Delivery. By HENRY G. LANDIS, A.M., M.D., Professor of Obstetrics and Diseases of Women and Children in Starling Medical College. Illustrated. New York: E. B. Treat. 1880. Pp. 168.

THIS little work is a very thoughtful, original, and valuable contribution to the literature of the subject. It consists, as will be seen from the title, of two parts: the first dealing with the mechanism of labour, the second with the forceps. Of these, the former is the more interesting, from the freshness and clearness of the author's view. The special point of his description is that he regards the right and left oblique diameters of the pelvic brim as two distinct canals, overlapping one another in front, and merging into one at the pelvic outlet. We cannot quote or condense the manner in which the author applies this principle to explain the pelvic mechanism; it will be enough to say that it deserves the careful study of obstetricians, and will be found highly interesting as well as instructive.

The second part of the work displays the same power of vigorous and independent thought, but contains less that is novel. One of the chief points is that the author defends, in opposition to the views of Barnes and his followers, the application of forceps to the sides of the head, instead of on each side of the pelvis. In treating of the indications for their use, he rightly keeps in view, and puts prominently before the reader, the large part which personal knowledge and skill play in determining the good or ill result of the frequent use of forceps. He says—"The mere application of the forceps contains not a single element which is detrimental, and is not even painful" (page 151). This statement applies to the mother only. The harm which sometimes follows the use of forceps is usually the result of their being applied in improper cases or in an improper manner. In short, this work is a practical, thoughtful, and scientific contribution to our knowledge.

CHOLERA IN CALCUTTA IN 1880.—There was less cholera in 1880 than in any year since 1871, the registered mortality being 805. The hospitals show a marked decrease of cases treated, the mortality also being more favourable than usual. The number treated was 356, of which 183 died, or 514 per 1000.—*Indian Med. Gas.,* August.

GENERAL CORRESPONDENCE.

THE PROSECUTION OF DR. FERRIER.
LETTER FROM DR. S. WILKS.

[To the Editor of the Medical Times and Gazette.]

SIR,—The prosecution of Dr. Ferrier has become so serious a matter to the cause of medicine and science that it is to be hoped there will be a universal rallying of the whole of the profession to support him and any others who may be placed in a like position. As a very general desire has been expressed to show our sympathy with Dr. Ferrier, I think we cannot do better, when his expenses have been paid, than apply our subscriptions towards the formation of a " Defence Association," which will not only assist persecuted individuals, but show to the world that there is a great principle at stake.　I am, &c.,

Grosvenor-street.　SAMUEL WILKS.

[We have much pleasure in publishing Dr. Wilks' letter. Seeing that the expenses of Dr. Ferrier's defence have, we understand, been undertaken, fully and entirely, by the British Medical Association, Dr. Wilks' proposal commends itself to us much more than does the proposition which we have seen made and approved of elsewhere, for a direct testimonial to Dr. Ferrier. We venture, moreover, to think that Dr. Ferrier himself would much prefer the matter not being made in any public sense a personal one.—ED. Med. Times and Gas.]

THE TESTIMONIAL TO PROFESSOR VIRCHOW.
LETTER FROM DR. J. S. BRISTOWE.

[To the Editor of the Medical Times and Gazette.]

SIR,—I beg leave to acknowledge the receipt of the undermentioned sums since my letter to you of last week. The total amount of the subscriptions I have received is £99 6s., of which all but three guineas has been forwarded to Prof. Küster.　I am, &c.,　J. S. BRISTOWE.

11, Old Burlington-street, W., November 24.

Dr. Southey, £1 1s.; Dr. Barratt, £1 1s.; Dr. Beddoe, £1 1s.; J. Croft, Esq., £1 1s.

A VOLUNTEER HOSPITAL CORPS AT DURHAM.
LETTER FROM MR. W. P. MEARS.

[To the Editor of the Medical Times and Gazette.]

SIR,—For some time the idea of the formation of a Volunteer Hospital Corps has been mooted among the students of this College, and in furtherance of the project a meeting was held on October 28, Dr. Mears presiding. A large number of the students attended, and resolutions were passed appointing a Committee, consisting of Dr. Mears and Messrs. C. H. C. Milburn, F. W. Gibbon, and D. J. P. McNabb, to carry the project into effect, and engaging the students to support the movement. As the Committee were at first unable to see in what way the full strength of a bearer company on the model of the Army Hospital Corps might be made up (although nearly sixty students had given in their names), they waited on Lieut.-Col. Potter, C.B., of the 1st Northumberland Artillery, who evinced great interest in the matter. He pointed out that there were two plans open, viz., for the corps to be attached to a regiment, such as his own, detachments being lent to other regiments; or for the corps to be independent, having for its cadre the students of the College, the strength being made up by drafts from the regiments in the district. The former plan at the time appeared the more feasible, as Colonel Potter kindly undertook all negotiations with the War Office, and at the same time offered the use of the Drill Hall and other advantages to the corps. No reply has as yet been received from the War Office; but whatever it may be, there can be little doubt, from the interest taken in the matter in the district, that the movement will be ultimately successful.

I am, &c.,　W. P. MEARS, M.B.

University of Durham College of Medicine, Newcastle-upon-Tyne, November 22.

REPORTS OF SOCIETIES.

THE OBSTETRICAL SOCIETY OF LONDON
WEDNESDAY, NOVEMBER 2.

Dr. MATTHEWS DUNCAN, President, in the Chair.

THE LATE DR. McCLINTOCK.

THE PRESIDENT having referred to the loss sustained by the Society in the death of Dr. McClintock, Dr. BARNES proposed, and Dr. PRIESTLEY seconded, the following resolution:— "That the Obstetrical Society of London, having learned with deep sorrow of the death of Dr. Alfred H. McClintock, one of its Honorary Fellows, hereby records its sense of the heavy loss which this Society, his profession, and science sustain by that event, hereby expresses its heart-felt sympathy with his widow and family in the still greater loss which falls upon them."

Dr. BEVERLEY COLE (of San Francisco) supported the resolution, which was carried unanimously.

LARGE FIBROID UTERINE POLYPUS.

Dr. HEYWOOD SMITH showed a large fibroid polypus removed in pieces from a single woman aged thirty-five. The tumour distended the vagina, and it was impossible to touch the os uteri, or to reach more than half-way up the tumour. About one-fourth of the mass was first removed by steel wire écraseur. The perineum was then incised up to the sphincter, as it seemed likely to give way, and the neck of the polypus divided by the wire loop. The detached tumour was then divided into three parts by the écraseur, and so removed. The tumour weighed one pound ten ounces. The perineum was united by three sutures, and was found completely healed on the eighth day.

Dr. MURRAY mentioned a case in which he had seen the perineum ruptured in removal of a fibroid tumour. He would advise previous slicing of the mass.

Dr. BARNES thought Dr. Smith had done right in incising the perineum. He had seen a similar case in which a ruptured perineum seemed to be a main factor in producing fatal septicæmia.

Dr. ROUTH mentioned a case in which he had removed a large fibroid in slices. The patient did well at first, but eventually died from tetanus. If the perineum were not sewn up, or antiseptic injections were not used, in the case mentioned by Dr. Barnes, the fatal result might be accounted for.

Dr. AVELING thought it was undoubtedly proper to incise the perineum when there was fear of laceration. He would suggest, however, that it might be better to make the incisions laterally.

Dr. WYNN WILLIAMS said that implicit confidence could not be placed in Dr. Heywood Smith's écraseur, as he had had a case in which the rivet on which the square button worked broke, when he was many miles in the country, and he had to get an ingenious local watchmaker to rivet it as a fixture.

Dr. WILTSHIRE thought that the perineum should very rarely be torn or incised during the removal of large uterine fibroids. The growths might be so diminished by cutting portions away, either in wedge-shaped masses or otherwise, as to render injury to the perineum, as a rule, unnecessary.

The PRESIDENT had known great laceration of the perineum, even through the sphincter, to occur in removing fibroids. If only a little laceration, as was usual, was expected, he would prefer that the perineum should take its chance. He did not think incision would afford any appreciable degree of security against septicæmia as compared with laceration. Lacerations of considerable extent might be avoided, as a rule, by cutting up the tumour, especially by the spiral cut, whereby the tumour was by cutting made into a long strip.

Dr. HEYWOOD SMITH said that, in his case, it would have been impossible to remove the tumour without injury to the perineum, as the tumour had already distended the vagina, and the vulval outlet was small.

INSTRUMENTS.

Dr. BEVERLEY COLE showed the following instruments:—
1. A pessary for retroflexion or version. The instrument

had a short and flat Hodge's pessary as basis, with an upper bar of vulcanite or celluloid connected with the lateral arms by segments of watch-spring. 2. A spring anteversion pessary. This had an anterior bar attached to the lateral arms by springs running forwards. 3. A gas-cautery, furnished with a series of platinum points. It could be attached to any ordinary gas-burner, and never failed to work perfectly.

ON SHORTNESS OF THE CORD AS A CAUSE OF OBSTRUCTION TO THE NATURAL PROGRESS OF LABOUR.

Dr. MATTHEWS DUNCAN read this paper. He said the obstruction arose from the morbidly early establishment of a solidarity of, or union between, the fœtus and the genital passages, in which it should be easily moved. The cord was taut, then stretched, and advance of the fœtus was difficult or impossible without injury. The cord might be absolutely short, or it might be made relatively short by encircling the neck or other parts of the fœtus. Its length when stretched had to be considered, as well as that when not stretched. Twelve inches of cord would stretch about two inches before breaking. Most cords would break with gradually applied tension by a weight of about eight pounds. Labour power, if it breaks the cord, must, of course, be greater than its tensile strength. When the cord was shortened by encircling the neck, its fœtal attachment was, so far as delivery is concerned, the neck, not the navel, and the measurement from the placental attachment to the neck was about two inches longer than to the navel; hence a greater length was required in this relative shortening than in absolute shortening when the measure is to the navel. Disturbance of mechanism rarely occurred till the child was partly born. The cord might then be torn across, or the placental end freed by separation of the placenta, or inversion of the uterus might occur, or the fœtus might be born by a kind of spontaneous evolution. In this evolution, taking place after partial birth, the anterior surface of the body was by rotation made to look forwards, so as to make the most of the length of the cord. The cord-insertion was the fixed point. The cord was tight, and passed below the lower border of the symphysis between its two insertions. A cord of twelve inches measured to umbilicus, or one of fourteen inches measured to neck, in both cases inclusive of gain by stretching, would permit birth by spontaneous evolution, if it was strong enough. A cord measuring under ten inches when stretched would necessitate rupture or cutting of cord, or inversion of uterus, or separation of placenta.

Dr. BARNES was surprised to hear Dr. Duncan describe the cord as sometimes springing from the upper edge of the placenta. Levret had pointed out long ago that the cord, if it sprang from an edge, always sprang from that nearest the os, and he had himself constantly verified this conclusion. He would submit, as a means of lessening the tension of a cord artificially shortened, the method of compressing the uterus downwards during the second stage. Instead of losing time in trying to slip the loop over the head or shoulders, he had found it better to cut the cord at once.

Dr. HICKINBOTHAM mentioned a case in which obstruction from short funis was diagnosed by the fact that with roomy pelvis, sufficient pains, and movable fœtal head, yet no progress was made. He advocated immediate forceps delivery, and prompt division of the cord.

Dr. GERVIS had met with cases of forceps delivery in which the cord around the neck proved both an obstacle to delivery and a cause of danger to the child. He called attention to the advisability of ascertaining as soon as possible in forceps cases whether the cord encircled the neck.

Dr. WYNN WILLIAMS had known of two cases. One in his own practice, in which, with shortened cord, the child was forcibly expelled, breaking the cord at its insertion into the child's abdomen, the vessels being drawn almost within the abdomen. Fortunately he had a tenaculum with him, and succeeded in hooking out the vessels and tying them.

Dr. W. B. ROBERTSON mentioned a case in which a child had been born five minutes before his arrival. He found the cord of average length and thickness, but severed five or six inches from the umbilicus. Hæmorrhage had ceased, and the child did well.

Dr. BRAXTON HICKS mentioned a case of twins, the cord of the first of which was very short, so that it could hardly be tied and divided. The second presented by the feet, and became arrested when the breech reached the vulva. Chloroform being given, he passed up his hand, and found the funis very tense, the umbilicus being stretched up. He divided the funis with Sir J. Simpson's osteotome, and the child was then expelled. The funis was about four inches long. He thought it was the general plan, in case of a shortened funis, to divide it without attempting to tie. The fœtal portion could be easily seized.

Dr. MURRAY, in reference to Dr. Barnes' suggestion to press down the fundus uteri from above, mentioned a case in which partial inversion of the uterus had thus been produced.

Dr. BRUNTON said that it had been stated, as a sign of shortness of the cord, that if the placental attachment were at the usual place, with every pain there was a depression of the fundus uteri to be seen and felt.

Dr. HAYES inquired whether in Dr. Duncan's experiments to test the strength of the cord any note had been taken of the thickness, number, and condition of vessels. He had never met with inversion of the uterus from pulling on the cord, or from its undue shortness. He thought that where inversion had occurred with an abnormally short cord there must have been some other factor in its causation.

Dr. EDIS thought in some instances where the cord was twisted several times round the neck, and forceps were employed, as soon as traction was exerted the undue strain upon the cord interfered with the fœtal circulation, giving rise to convulsive movements on the part of the fœtus. He had witnessed such cases, the child being apparently still-born, and resuscitated with difficulty if the delivery were delayed.

The PRESIDENT found the valued criticisms on his paper had reference chiefly to practice, and to this he had no positive objection; but the paper was written with a view mainly to the description of mechanism. He thought Dr. Hayes would find that the variations of thickness of the cord made little variation in its tensile strength; the matter was one that could easily be settled by experiment, and in no other way. He hoped that the rare case of Dr. Murray and the unique and most valuable case of Dr. Braxton Hicks would be well recorded in the reports of their speeches. With Dr. Barnes he concurred in supposing that the cord was, in battledore placenta, at least generally, inserted in the lower border; but it was only supposition, and he knew no physiological reason why it should not be inserted in the upper border.

THE PATHOLOGICAL SOCIETY OF LONDON.
TUESDAY, NOVEMBER 15.

SAMUEL WILKS, M.D., F.R.S., President, in the Chair.

PULSATILE LIVER.

Dr. SAMUEL WEST showed a patient with this condition. He was a bootmaker, and aged twenty-two. He was the subject of heart-disease following on acute rheumatism, from which he suffered when seven years of age. Two years previously he had suffered from ascites, and had been tapped repeatedly for it. Two months after leaving hospital, he returned with the abdomen full of fluid; this was removed, and then the pulsation of the liver was remarked. The area of pulsation was confined (or nearly so) to the right of the median line, just below the margin of the ribs. The liver was enlarged. At present there was no ascites or anasarca, and no venous congestion. The heart was enlarged, especially on its right side. Dr. West asked whether this was pulsation in the liver, or communicated to it.

Dr. MAHOMED thought it might be conveyed from the heart through a wasted and atrophied diaphragm.

Dr. D. POWELL thought the pulsation was due to aortic regurgitation. If the man had a diaphragm so flaccid as to allow the heart to communicate its pulsation to the liver, he ought to be more cyanosed than was the case.

Dr. WEST replied that the pulsation was systolic in time. He could not accept Dr. Mahomed's explanation.

EXTRA-UTERINE (TUBAL) FŒTATION.

Dr. S. WEST showed this specimen. It was removed from the body of a woman who had died in collapse a few hours after her admission to hospital. The woman had suffered

from abdominal pain for some days, and had had discharge of blood per vaginam. She had suffered also from diarrhœa. At the autopsy, the abdominal cavity was found filled with blood (partly fluid, partly in clots), and connected with the right side of the pelvis there was a tumour which, on examination, proved to be an extra-uterine fœtation. The uterus was enlarged, and lined with a deciduous membrane. The right ovary was attached to the tumour, but distinct from it. The placenta was adherent to the rectum; the hæmorrhage was due to partial detachment of the placenta. The tumour contained a three-months' fœtus. The right Fallopian tube was closed; the left ovary contained a corpus luteum; the left tube was open and normal. The woman had two living children. The special points of the case were—1. The condition of the uterus and its lining membrane; 2. The presence of the corpus luteum on the opposite side to the tubal gestation; 3. The attachment of the placenta, and its detachment as the cause of death.

The PRESIDENT asked how Dr. West explained the presence of the corpus luteum in the opposite ovary, and how the ovule had travelled across.

Dr. WILTSHIRE related an analogous case.

Dr. WEST replied that he presumed the ovule had crossed the fundus of the uterus and got into the opposite tube.

RICKETY THORAX, WITH SPONTANEOUS FRACTURE OF RIBS.

Mr. R. W. PARKER showed this specimen, which he had removed from a child aged twelve months, who had died of bronchitis and collapse of lung in the East London Children's Hospital. The chest presented a twofold deformity—(1) an anterior one, the usual incurving of the ribs, just external to their junction with the cartilages; and (2) a more posterior bending, amounting to actual fracture in many of the ribs, which seemed to occur at the mid-point of the ribs proper. The former deformity was well known and familiar to all; but the latter, Mr. Parker thought, was much less common. Many writers (Virchow among others) had referred to the tendency which rickety bones showed to spontaneous fracture. The child had been many times, and carefully, examined during life, but the fractures were not detected. He would suggest that they had been brought about at the moment of death.

The PRESIDENT remarked that the specimen was a typically rickety chest.

Dr. BARLOW had often seen nodosities on the ribs posterior to their chondral junctions, and questioned whether they were not of the same nature as the fractures in this case. He could not accept Mr. Parker's view, that they occurred after death.

Mr. HAWARD thought the anterior incurvation in this case had occurred at the point where it is usually found, which is in the rib proper, and not at the chondral junction.

Dr. PAYNE could not think that atmospheric pressure was greater after death than before. He thought it possible that these fractures might have been produced after death by force.

Dr. SHARKEY had recently made an autopsy on the body of a child in whom several ribs were found broken. There was no history of injury, or mark of violence on the body. He would ask, Could fractures occur spontaneously in healthy children. Mr. Sharkey, in answer to Mr. Parker, said there was no sub-pleural extravasation of blood about the fractures. In his case there was also peritonitis, but nothing to show from what cause it originated.

Mr. PARKER replied. He was struck by the acuteness of the bend in the bone about half an inch from its extremity; the junction with the cartilage appeared quite normal. He thought in the majority of cases the curve was not so strictly limited to the bone itself as in the present case. In suggesting that the fractures had occurred at the last moment of life, he thought that changes in the bone had been going on for some time; and that at the moment of death, when atmospheric pressure was entirely unopposed by any inspiratory (muscular) effort, the ribs, bent before, finally fractured. There were no signs of extravasation of blood, as in Dr. Sharkey's case. (The specimen will be sent to the Museum of the College of Surgeons.)

ANEURISM OF AORTA, WITH SECONDARY POUCH.

Dr. DOUGLAS POWELL showed this specimen. It had been removed from a woman aged fifty-five years. She had suffered from dyspnœa. On admission to hospital she was suffering from aphonia and cough of a laryngeal quality. Her tongue was scarred with old syphilitic ulcerations. A slight impulse with a bruit and some dulness were found over the aortic cartilage. There was no inequality of the pulses. She died in about ten days. At the autopsy the aorta was found somewhat dilated. Just below the origin of the large vessels there was the orifice of a sac as large as a walnut, growing directly backward towards the trachea (on which it doubtless pressed). There was a smaller sac connected with the left subclavian, filled with laminated clot. The left recurrent laryngeal nerve was blended with the sac of the larger aneurism.

The PRESIDENT asked whether all the muscles of the larynx were affected, or only the abductors of the larynx.

Dr. FELIX SEMON said, if all the muscles were affected, the cords would be in the cadaveric position, in which case there ought not to have been any dyspnœa. Dr. Ferrier and others had pointed out the greater liability to disease of the fibres of the abductors, or their less power of resistance.

GREAT HYPERTROPHY OF TOE-NAIL.

Dr. I. OWEN showed this specimen, which was seven inches long, and which had not been out for upwards of forty years.

The PRESIDENT remarked that the finger-nail grew its own length in six months, but that the toe-nails required a much longer time.

Mr. GOULD stated that his finger-nails grew one-thirty-second of an inch per week.

Mr. MORRIS mentioned that his thumb-nail had required five days less than five months to regrow.

AORTIC STENOSIS.

Dr. I. OWEN also showed this specimen, which he had removed from a man aged seventy, recently under the care of Dr. Dickinson. The orifice now hardly admitted a probe. He had suffered lately from dyspnœa and dropsy. The pulses were almost inappreciable at the wrists. The temperature was subnormal. The other arteries were all exceedingly atheromatous.

ENLARGED THYROID GLAND, PRESSING ON THE TRACHEA.

Mr. BERNARD PITTS showed the trachea from which the thyroid gland had been removed on account of urgent dyspnœa. The patient was a young man aged fifteen or sixteen years, who had suffered from the enlargement for about five years. He was brought to St. Thomas's Hospital during the night, suffering from intense dyspnœa. Tracheotomy was performed, but it was a most difficult operation on account of the enlarged condition of the gland. As relief was not afforded, and as the case was extremely urgent, Mr. Pitts removed the entire gland. The lad was temporarily relieved by this, but died of lung-troubles thirty-six hours later. The enlargement was due to simple hypertrophy of all the elements of the gland. Mr. Pitts stated that within the last twelve months they had had two other deaths in St. Thomas's Hospital from pressure caused by bronchoceles. The dyspnœa in all three cases was worse at night. In one case, incision of the enlarged gland had brought temporary relief.

Dr. OWEN asked as to the condition of the tracheal rings, whether they were of the usual size and thickness.

Mr. PITTS replied in the affirmative.

VACCINATION GRANT.—The Local Government Board have awarded to Mr. William Ernest Good, Public Vaccinator of the Dorchester Union, a first-class grant for efficient vaccination in his district.

PROF. BENEKE'S NORTH SEA SANATORIUM.—Writing from Norderney, October 23, Prof. Beneke speaks in the warmest terms of his new establishment. His little colony of sixteen patients is doing admirably, and the results already obtained in the cases of phthisis are quite surprising. The hurricane of October 14.15, which committed such devastation, did not do the least harm to any of the patients, who yet were out of doors daily. He believes that with time this place will become an important therapeutical resort for a variety of patients. If the unusually stormy character of this month has been attended with no mischief, how much may be expected during the usually tranquil and softer atmospheric conditions!—*Berlin. Klin. Woch.*, October 30.

MEDICAL NEWS.

UNIVERSITY OF LONDON.—The following is a list of the candidates who passed the recent M.B. examination:—

First Division.—Anundrao Atmaram, B.Sc., University College; Charles Alfred Ballance, St. Thomas's Hospital; Alexander Barron, Liverpool Royal Infirmary; Henry Thurstan Bassett, Guy's Hospital; Richard Bredin, Liverpool Royal Infirmary and Guy's Hospital; Wm. Chisholm, B.A., Sydney, University College; Charles Alfred Dagnall Clark, B.A., Bartholomew's Hospital; Ernest Clarke, St. Bartholomew's Hospital; Mark Purcell Mayo Collier, St. Thomas's Hospital; William Job Collins, B.Sc., St. Bartholomew's Hospital; David Samuel Davies, St. Thomas's Hospital; Thomas Vincent Dickinson, St. George's Hospital; Philip Rhys Griffiths, University College; James Harper, St. Bartholomew's Hospital; William Lenton Heath, St. Bartholomew's Hospital; John Hodgson, Manchester Royal Infirmary; Victor Alexander Haden Horsley, University College; William Arbuthnot Lane, Guy's Hospital; Robert Maguire, Manchester Royal Infirmary; Henry Maudsley, University College; Frederick Walter Mott, University College; Beaven Neave Rake, Guy's Hospital; Bernard Rice, St. Bartholomew's Hospital; Amand Jules McConnel Routh, University College; John Reynolds Salter, University College; Thomas Dixon Savill, St. Thomas's Hospital; Tom Henry Sawtell, St. Bartholomew's Hospital; John Edward Squire, University College; Thomas George Stonham, London Hospital; Fredk. Rufenacht Walters, St. Thomas's Hospital.

Second Division.—John Mitford Atkinson, London Hospital; Wayland Charles Chaffey, St. Bartholomew's Hospital; Thomas Crisp, St. Thomas's Hospital; John Davidson, King's College; Alfred Edgar Drysdale, University College; Ben Hall, St. Bartholomew's Hospital; Henry Hoole, Charing-cross Hospital; Eugène Arthur Laurent, University College; Greville Matheson MacDonald, King's College; George Ryding Marsh, Guy's Hospital; Charles Sanders, St. Bartholomew's Hospital; John Frederick William Silk, King's College; Henry Smith, St. Bartholomew's Hospital; John Smith, Guy's Hospital; Samuel Walter Sutton, St. Thomas's Hospital; Harold Swale, St. Thomas's Hospital; William Ainley Sykes, St. Bartholomew's Hospital; Edward Sabine Tait, St. Bartholomew's Hospital; Walter Duncan Thomas, St. Bartholomew's Hospital.

ROYAL COLLEGE OF SURGEONS OF ENGLAND.—The following gentlemen, having undergone the necessary examinations for the diploma, were admitted Members of the College at a meeting of the Court of Examiners on the 17th inst., viz.:—

Booth, George, Chesterfield.
Foxwell, William A., B.A. Cantab., Weston-super-Mare.
Gardner, Percy H., Ilfracombe.
Green, Edwin C., Clapham.
Grimsdale, Thomas B., Liverpool.
Johnston, Thomas, Barnstaple.
Knight, Alfred O., L.S.A., Tewkesbury.
Lofthouse, Arthur, L.S.A., Bishopsthorpe, Yorks.
Morton, Charles A., Canonbury.
Pook, William J., L.S.A., New Cross, S.E.
Stonham, Charles, Maidstone.
Streeton, John L., Kidderminster.
Walker, Francis J., Spilsby, Lincolnshire.

Fourteen candidates were rejected. The following gentlemen passed on the 18th inst., viz.:—

Bissill, Austin C., Sleaford, Lincolnshire.
Campbell, Harry, Belsize-park, N.W.
Colville, Ernest G., Eastbourne.
Cooper, George F., Reading.
Giles, Oswald, Oswestry.
Hayes, James, Leigh.
Humphrey, Francis W., Albion-street, Hyde-park.
Kempster, William H., M.B. Durh., Battersea.
Longman, George P., Southampton.
Pollock, William E., Hanworth, Middlesex.
Rackham, Arthur R., Norwich.
Stevsking, Herbert E., Manchester-square.
Stuart, Sidney O., Woolwich.
Williams, John F., L.S.A., Cotham, Hants.
Wray, Charles, Marston, Yorks.

Seven candidates were rejected. The following gentlemen passed on the 19th inst., viz.:—

Adams, William C., Regent's-park-road.
Andrews, Archibald G., Wolverhampton.
Benham, Robert F., King's Bench-walk, Temple.
Benson, Ernest W., M.A. Cantab. and L.S.A., Gloucester-street.
Bevan, Henry C., Talsarn, Cardiganshire.
Carter, Thomas E., Uxbridge.
Dendy, Walter C., Forest Hill.
Elliott, Edgar, Wimborne, Dorsetshire.
Harris, David P., Watling-street, E.C.
Ingoldby, Frederick J., Shepherd's Bush.
Jones, Henry L., B.A. Cantab., Hendre, Carmarthenshire.
Marston, Francis E., Ludlow, Shropshire.
Sanders, Francis C. S., B.A. Cantab., Lower Belgrave-street.
Sanderson, Robert, B.A. Oxon., Lancing, Sussex.
Strachan, William H. W., Penge.
Stroyan, Frederick, Norwich.
Treadwell, Oliver F. N., Brixton.
Wood, Henry S., M.B. Melb., Palace-road, S.E.

Seven candidates were rejected. The following gentlemen passed on the 21st inst., viz.:—

Coombe, Albert T., Gloucester-road, N.W
Davies, Sidney, Anerley, S.E.

Dodd, Henry W., Hilldrop-crescent, N.W.
Hewkley, Frank, Dalston.
Nicholson, Gerald, Wimbledon Park.
Pike, Charles J., L.S.A., Hobart, Tasmania.
Pocock, Alfred G. C., Streatham.
Pollard, Joseph, M.A. Cantab. and L.S.A., Hitchin, Herts.
Pope, Percy, Woodridings, Pinner.
Walker, Ernest G. A., Retford, Notts.
Waller, Theodore H., Bedford.
Warlters, W. Scott, Warwick-street, S.W.
Webster, George L., L.S.A., Portsdown-road, S.W.
Unsworth, Francis H., L.S.A., Derby.

Eight candidates were rejected, making a total of sixty-nine out of the 173, who, having failed to acquit themselves to the satisfaction of the Court of Examiners, were referred to their professional studies for six months.

Fellowship of the College of Surgeons.—At the half-yearly Primary or Anatomical and Physiological Examination for the above distinction there were thirty-one candidates, whose dates of Membership ranged from April, 1868, to January, 1881. The following were the questions submitted to them on the 18th inst. in Anatomy and Physiology, when they were required to answer at least three out of the four questions on each subject (from 9 a.m. to 12 o'clock noon), viz.:—Physiology : 1. Describe the development of the alimentary canal. 2. State approximately the relative proportions of albuminous and starchy food-stuffs in beef, egg, wheaten bread, peas, potatoes, and rice. Write dietaries for an adult male prisoner with and without hard labour. 3. Explain the mechanism of voice and speech. 4. What are the functions of the pneumogastric nerve? Give the evidence on which your statements are founded. Anatomy: 1. Describe the surfaces and borders of the several bones which form the walls and boundaries of the spheno-maxillary fossa. 2. Describe the dissection necessary to expose the two ganglia of the pneumogastric nerve. Enumerate their branches of connexion and of distribution. 3. The neck having been properly dissected, and the clavicles and anterior wall of the chest removed, describe the course and relations of the several cardiac nerves as thus brought into view; and state how you would further proceed in order to display completely the nervous supply to the heart. 4. The whole of the skin and fascia and the first layer of muscles having been removed from the under surface of the foot, describe the parts brought into view, and their relative positions.

The following gentlemen (the last two of whom were not Members of the College),[out of the sixteen who presented themselves at the oral examination on the 22nd inst., were successful, viz. :—

Gunn, Robert Marcus, of the Edinburgh, Vienna, and London Hospitals, diploma of membership dated July 21, 1878.
Suckling, Cornelius William, of the Birmingham School, April 22, 1879.
Albert, Henry Louis, of St. George's Hospital.
Knaggs, Robert Lawford, B.A. Cantab., of Guy's Hospital.

The following gentlemen passed on the 23rd inst. :—

Kempe, John A., of University College Hospital, diploma of Membership dated January 29, 1875.
Hull, Walter, of St. Thomas's Hospital.
Pruen, Septimus T., of St. Bartholomew's Hospital.
Berry, James, of St. Bartholomew's Hospital.
Targett, James H., of Guy's Hospital.
Brown, John M., of the Edinburgh School.
Shearer, Thomas L., of the Edinburgh School.
Dyson, Herbert J., of St. Mary's Hospital.

Nineteen candidates having failed to acquit themselves to the satisfaction of the Board of Examiners, were referred to their anatomical and physiological studies for six months.

Clinical Examinations.—At the pass examinations for the diploma of Membership of the Royal College of Surgeons, which were brought to a close on Monday last, the following well marked typical cases selected by the Court of Examiners from the metropolitan hospitals were submitted to the candidates, viz. :—Hydrocele of the tunica vaginalis; ulceration of one leg; enlarged lymphatic glands; hæmatocele after hydrocele; chronic periostitis; secondary eruption; tertiary syphilis; inflammation of the knee-joint; gummata; granular eyelid, trichiasis entropion, vascular opaque cornea, ulcers, synechia anterior (all in the same subject); chronic abscess; lipoma, enlarged cervical glands; eczema; old fracture of the clavicle; epithelioma labii; old compound dislocation of the ankle-joint; syphilitic inflammation of the cornea; disease of the hip-joint, excision; ecchymosis, ruptured biceps; syphilitic nodes; hydrocele and undescended testicle; periostitis and necrosis; orchitis, lumbar abscess; curvature of the spine with rib (a very interesting case); popliteal bursa

epithelioma linguæ and enlarged glands; enlarged saphena vein, tortuous; loose cartilages (a very puzzling case to some of the candidates); injury to the musculo-spiral nerve; rodent ulcer; syphilitic ulceration of the tongue; blood tumour (hæmatoma); fatty tumour (lipoma); malignant disease of the floor of the mouth; enlarged femoral gland, etc.; psoas abscess; gangrene of the middle finger; epithelioma of the lower lip, right commissure; large mammary glands and eruption; disease of the elbow-joint; cleft palate; ulcer of the scrotum; cancer of inguinal glands; hydrocele and inflamed testicle; monorchis and enlarged inguinal gland; chronic enlargement of cervical glands and lymphadenitis; hydro-sarcocele; periostitis, etc.

APOTHECARIES' HALL, LONDON.—The following gentlemen passed their examination in the Science and Practice of Medicine, and received certificates to practise, on Thursday November 17 :—

Lofthouse, Arthur, Bishopthorpe, York.
Mitra, Jogendra Nath, 29, Keppel-street, S.W.
Roy, Shira Prasad, 99, Camden-street, N.W.

The following gentleman also on the same day passed the Primary Professional Examination :—

Maye, John, London Hospital.

APPOINTMENTS.

*** The Editor will thank gentlemen to forward to the Publishing-office, as early as possible, information as to all new Appointments that take place.

Good, William Ernest, M.R.C.S., L.R.C.P., etc.—Medical Officer to Her Majesty's Prison, Dorchester, Dorset, vice John Good, superannuated.
Hadden, W. B., M.D., M.R.C.P.—Demonstrator of Morbid Anatomy to St. Thomas's Hospital, vice R. W. Reid, M.D., resigned.

BIRTHS.

Armstrong.—On November 19, at 136, Parrock-street, Gravesend, the wife of John C. Armstrong, M.R.C.S., of a son.
Gayton.—On November 21, at the Homerton Hospital, the wife of W. Gayton, M.D., M.R.C.P., of a son.
Turtle.—On November 20, at Kirkmead, Woodford, Essex, the wife of Frederick Turtle, M.D., of a son.
Wood.—On November 17, at 2, Peel-terrace, Gosport, the wife of Staff-Surgeon J. Wood, M.D., R.N., H.M.S. Duke of Wellington, of a daughter.

MARRIAGES.

Brodie—Sutherland.—On October 31, at Dalkey, Dublin, Arthur James Brodie, L.R.C.P.& S. Edin., of Ambleside, to Mary Emilia, daughter of George Sutherland, Esq., of Forse, Caithness, J.P. and D.L.
Chadwick—Musgrove.—On September 29, at Toorak, Melbourne, John William Chadwick, eldest son of Charles Chadwick, M.D., J.P., of Tunbridge Wells, to Rebecca H., eldest daughter of A. W. Musgrove, Esq., of South Yarra, Melbourne.
Corbett—Lefroy.—On November 19, at St. Marylebone, Daniel Corbett, jun., Esq., B.A., T.C.D., L.R.C.S.I., son of Daniel Corbett, Esq., M.R.C.S.E., of 12, Clare-street, Dublin, to Louisa Florence, widow of Edward T. Lefroy, Esq., daughter of Maurice Brooks, Esq., M.P., of York-terrace, Regent's-park, London, and Sackville-place, Dublin.
Dunn—Blundell.—On November 23, at Westbourne-park, Holt Dunn, L.S.C.P., of Bayswater, to Marie, only daughter of the late William Blundell, Esq., of Trinidad.
Moore—Fitch.—On November 16, at Chaddesley Corbett, Worcestershire, Edward Moore, Esq., Executive Engineer, State Railways, India, to Frances, youngest daughter of F. Fitch, M.D., of Chaddesley Corbett.
Payne—Whitmore.—On November 21, at Calcutta, India, Arthur J. L. Payne, eldest son of Surgeon-General A. J. Payne, M.D., of Bengal, to Grace Emily, youngest daughter of the late William Lechmere Whitmore, K.C.H., R.E., of Lower Slaughter, Gloucestershire.
Raye—Fox.—On November 21, at Marylebone-road, D. O'C. Raye, Surgeon-Major Indian Medical Department, to Kate Mary, second daughter of Anthony Fox, Esq., late of Runnymede, co. Dublin.
Watson—Ransome.—On November 15, at Mount Risco, New York, Barclay Seebohm Watson, M.D., of Iowa, to Adah, daughter of the late Sheppard Ransome, Esq., of St. Anne's House, Wandsworth Common.

DEATHS.

Bucknill, Samuel Birch, M.D., at Rugby, on November 12, aged 66.
Camden, Sarah, wife of G. J. S. Camden, M.R.C.S., at 18, West-parade, Rhyl, on November 15, aged 81.
Cleghorn, Harriett Louisa, wife of George Cleghorn, M.R.C.S., at Blenheim, New Zealand, on September 21, aged 23 years.
Coote, Michael, M.D., M.R.C.S., at Ashby-de-la-Zouch, on November 17, aged 59.
Denny, John, L.R.C.P., at Stoke Newington Dispensary, on November 18, aged 62.
Erskine, Archibald, M.D., at Sandys-place, Newry, on November 7.
Hayne, Frederick Greaves, M.R.C.S., at 1, The Hill, Northfleet, on November 19, in his 30th year.
Head, Edward A. H., M.B., M.R.C.P., at Fishwick, Newton Abbot, Devon, on November 11, aged 59.
Oldfield, Edmund, M.D., of Paris, at Leasowes Coronie, Surinam, West Indies, on October 17, in his 49th year.

ROBERTSON, ANDREW, M.D., of Hopewell, late Commissioner for Her Majesty the Queen and His Royal Highness the Prince of Wales, at 15, Bonaccord-square, Aberdeen, on November 18, aged 82.

SCOTT, WILLIAM EDWARD, M.R.C.P., at Lancaster House, Lincoln, on November 17, aged 80.

TAYLOR, ADAM, Surgeon-Major Bengal Army, at Delhi, India, on October 21, aged 47.

TRIMMELL, Surgeon-Major E. A., at Madras, on October 20, aged 36.

WILSON, ROBERT, M.D., M.R.C.S., L.S.A., Surgeon-Major of the 3rd Battalion Northumberland Fusiliers, at Bondgate-street Without, Alnwick, Northumberland, on November 19, in his 53rd year.

WRIGHT, ALEXANDER, Surgeon-General (retired) Bombay Army, at Hollyoot, Leeswade, on November 22, aged 71.

VACANCIES.

In the following list the nature of the office vacant, the qualifications required in the candidate, the person to whom application should be made and the day of election (as far as known) are stated in succession.

CENTRAL LONDON OPHTHALMIC HOSPITAL GRAY'S-INN-ROAD.—Assistant-Surgeon. Candidates must be members of the Royal College of Surgeons of England, and must produce certificates of having attended the practice of some ophthalmic institution for at least six months. Testimonials to be addressed to the Secretary, on or before December 6.

DENTAL HOSPITAL OF LONDON, LEICESTER-SQUARE.—Dental House-Surgeon. (For particulars see Advertisement.)

GENERAL INFIRMARY AT GLOUCESTER, AND THE GLOUCESTERSHIRE EYE INSTITUTION.—Ophthalmic Surgeon. Applications, enclosing qualifications and testimonials, to be forwarded to the Committee, under cover to the Secretary, on or before December 7.

KENT COUNTY ASYLUM, BARMING HEATH, NEAR MAIDSTONE.—Assistant Medical Officer. Applications, together with testimonials of recent date, to be sent to F. Pritchard Davies, M.D., Superintendent, on or before November 30.

LOWESTOFT FRIENDLY SOCIETIES' MEDICAL INSTITUTE.—Surgeon. Candidates must be duly qualified. Applications, with testimonials, to be sent to Mr. John Hammond, 86, Bevan-street, Lowestoft, on or before December 1.

MIDDLESEX COUNTY LUNATIC ASYLUM, COLNEY HATCH.—Assistant Medical Officer. (For particulars see Advertisement.)

READING AMALGAMATED FRIENDLY SOCIETIES' MEDICAL ASSOCIATION.—Resident Medical Officer. Candidates must be duly qualified, and from thirty to forty-five years of age. Applications, stating qualifications, with testimonials of recent date, to be sent to Samuel Griffin, Secretary, 9, Alfred-street, Reading (of whom further information can be had), not later than November 30.

STAMFORD-HILL, STOKE NEWINGTON, CLAPTON, ETC., DISPENSARY.—Resident Medical Officer. (For particulars see Advertisement.)

UNION AND PAROCHIAL MEDICAL SERVICE.

** The area of each district is stated in acres. The population is computed according to the census of 1871.

RESIGNATIONS.

Ashby-de-la-Zouch Union.—The Second and Third Districts are vacant by the death of Mr. Michael Coote. Second District: area 5691; population 2713; salary £30. Third District: area 7098; population 2969; salary £26. Wilton Union.—Mr. Frederick J. Flower has resigned the Bishopstone District: area 19,580; population 3840; salary £122 per annum.

APPOINTMENTS.

Burton-upon-Trent Union.—Daniel H. Bastable, L.K. & Q.C.P. Ire., L.R.C.S. Ire., to the Lullington District.

DURHAM UNIVERSITY.

At a Convocation held on November 15 the following gentlemen were appointed Examiners for degrees in Medicine and Surgery:—Professor G. H. Philipson, M.A., M.D. Durh., F.R.C.P. Lond.; W. C. Arnison, M.D. Durh.; C. J. Gibb, M.D. Durh.; C. Gibson, M.D.; Mr. Frederick Page; Mr. H. E. Armstrong; Mr. H. G. Howse, M.S. Lond., F.R.C.S. Eng., Surgeon to Guy's Hospital.

MEDICAL PRACTITIONERS' FEES FOR EVIDENCE.—At the Metropolitan County Court of Bloomsbury, this week, the case of Whiteford v. Fitzgerald was heard, before Mr. Judge Bacon, in which the plaintiff, a medical man, of 117, Albany-street, W., sued the defendant to recover the sum of two guineas for professional services rendered as a witness, in January and February last, in the case of Fitzgerald v. Butler, in which the plaintiff recovered £18 for having one of his ribs fractured, and in which case the present plaintiff gave medical evidence. After the plaintiff had stated his case, the learned Judge said the claim could not be allowed, whether the plaintiff attended on subpoena or at the simple request of the defendant. His Honour was then informed that after action brought the defendant's solicitor had sent the plaintiff a postal order for one guinea. In the case of Whiteford v. Smith, heard in this Court in December, 1878, his Honour had allowed the same plaintiff two guineas for his attendance at the Marylebone Police-court for similar evidence given there. His Honour, however, ruled that the plaintiff in the present instance was not entitled to recover, and gave judgment in favour of the defendant, but without costs.

VITAL STATISTICS OF LONDON.

Week ending Saturday, November 19, 1881.

BIRTHS.

Births of Boys, 1330; Girls, 1293; Total, 2623.
Corrected weekly average in the 10 years 1871-80, 2643·9.

DEATHS.

	Males.	Females.	Total.
Deaths during the week	683	751	1434
Weekly average of the ten years 1871-80, corrected to increased population ...	871·9	864·4	1736·3
Deaths of people aged 90 and upwards ...	...	...	44

DEATHS IN SUB-DISTRICTS FROM EPIDEMICS.

	Enumerated Population, 1881 (unrevised).	Small-pox.	Measles.	Scarlet Fever.	Diphtheria.	Whooping-cough.	Typhus.	Enteric (or Typhoid) Fever.	Simple continued Fever.	Diarrhœa.
West ...	668993	...	3	6	1	8	...	4	...	...
North ...	905677	3	9	10	4	7	6	10	1	2
Central ...	281793	...	...	3	2	1	...	5	...	...
East ...	692530	1	2	6	...	10	...	8	1	3
South ...	1265578	9	21	15	8	11	3	8	...	1
Total ...	3814571	13	35	40	15	43	9	33	2	6

METEOROLOGY.

From Observations at the Greenwich Observatory.

Mean height of barometer ...	...	29·977 in.
Mean temperature ...	...	49·0°
Highest point of thermometer ...	...	60·9°
Lowest point of thermometer ...	...	34·0°
Mean dew-point temperature ...	...	45·3°
General direction of wind ...	...	S.W.
Whole amount of rain in the week ...	...	0·18 in.

BIRTHS and DEATHS Registered and METEOROLOGY during the Week ending Saturday, Nov. 19, in the following large Towns:—

Cities and boroughs (Municipal boundaries except for London).	Estimated Population to middle of the year 1881.*	Persons to an Acre, 1881.	Births Registered during the week ending Nov. 19.	Deaths Registered during the week ending Nov. 19.	Temperature of Air (Fahr.). Highest during the Week.	Lowest during the Week.	Weekly Mean of Daily Mean Values.	Temp. of Air (Cent.). Weekly Mean of Daily Mean Values.	Rain Fall. In Inches.	In Centimetres.
London	3829751	50·8	2623	1434	60·9	34·0	49·0	9·44	0·18	0·45
Brighton	107934	45·9	69	53	57·3	38·0	48·7	9·28	0·28	0·71
Portsmouth	128335	23·6	77	58	...	...	...	...	...	...
Norwich	88036	11·8	53	29	...	...	...	...	...	...
Plymouth	75292	54·0	43	26	59·5	39·0	51·9	11·06	0·42	1·07
Bristol	207140	46·2	151	71	59·9	31·6	49·9	9·94	0·59	1·50
Wolverhampton	75934	22·4	45	31	...	...	...	...	...	...
Birmingham	402296	47·9	256	147	...	...	...	...	...	...
Leicester	123120	38·5	89	45	61·8	31·0	47·5	8·61	0·27	0·71
Nottingham	188335	19·9	107	72	61·8	29·5	47·7	8·72	0·51	1·30
Liverpool	553988	106·3	419	284	...	...	...	...	...	...
Manchester	341289	79·5	203	153	...	...	...	...	...	...
Salford	177780	34·4	119	80	...	...	...	...	...	...
Oldham	112176	24·0	73	42	...	...	...	...	...	...
Bradford	184037	25·5	92	87	58·4	34·7	49·4	9·66	1·14	2·90
Leeds	310490	14·4	217	106	64·0	33·0	49·5	9·72	0·43	1·9
Sheffield	285691	14·5	219	102	63·8	34·0	48·9	9·39	0·85	2·16
Hull	155161	42·7	115	82	60·0	30·0	46·9	8·28	0·25	0·63
Sunderland	116753	42·2	74	55	63·0	35·0	49·7	9·83	0·18	0·46
Newcastle-on-Tyne	145875	27·1	94	58	...	...	...	...	...	...
Total of 20 large English Towns...	7605775	38·0	5201	3000	64·0	29·5	49·0	9·44	0·40	1·17

* These figures are the numbers enumerated (but subject to revision) in April last, raised to the middle of 1881 by the addition of a quarter of a year's increase, calculated at the rate that prevailed between 1871 and 1881.

At the Royal Observatory, Greenwich, the mean reading of the barometer last week was 29·98 in. The highest reading was 30·26 in. on Sunday evening, and the lowest 29·46 in. on Thursday morning.

NOTES, QUERIES, AND REPLIES.

He that questioneth much shall learn much.—Bacon.

Algernon.—1. The Apothecaries rank as the fifty-eighth in the list of City Companies. 2. Of the charitable institutions of the metropolis, one-quarter consist of general hospitals, medical charities for special purposes, dispensaries, and societies for the preservation of life and public morals, which are chiefly supported by voluntary contributions and annual subscriptions.

A Curiosity.—At the Food Exhibition at the Agricultural Hall was a brownish-coloured object about the size of a skin of lard, and labelled "Zulu cheese, made by the youngest wife of Cetewayo."

Insuring Children's Lives.—At an inquiry before the Sheffield Coroner touching the death of a poor girl, twelve years of age, whose life was insured for £5, and who had been cruelly beaten by her father when almost dying of "typhoid fever and consumption," the jury found that death had been accelerated by the brutal treatment, and the Coroner said he would try to vitiate the insurance.

Workmen's Views on Workmen's Dwellings.—Respecting the workmen's dwellings of the metropolis, the Trade Councils of London are providing themselves with evidence, and answers to the following questions (formulated by Mr. Broadhurst, M.P.) are solicited from the trade committees in every district, viz.:—Are the present block buildings suitable? Are they built in convenient places? Are they better or cheaper than the present house accommodation? Should dwellings be provided in the suburbs? and if so, what alterations in railway arrangements will be necessary? The object of this information is to supply the Artisans' Dwellings Committee of the House of Commons, next session, with the views of the workmen themselves on the question, preparatory to framing the proposed new Bill.

Statistician.—The superintendent of the census reports that the population of the United States by the last census, as finally determined, was 50,155,783.

Exposing an Infected Child.—A resident of Blackwall Cross, Poplar, has been charged at the Rochford Petty Sessions by, respectively, the Southend Board of Health for exposing his child suffering from scarlet fever without taking proper precautions, and by the London, Tilbury, and Southend Railway Company for unlawfully travelling with the child in one of the Company's carriages without having obtained the special permission of the Company. The defendant was fined on each charge in the sums of £3 10s. and £2 9s. 6d. and costs.

Unregistered Dairies.—Two persons were convicted last week, at Glasgow, for keeping dairies not registered in terms of the statute, and fines of £2 and £4 respectively were inflicted.

A Prize for a Vivisection Essay.—The Danish Society for the Protection of Animals has issued an offer of a prize of £80 or 2000 frs. for the best scientific essay, and an "accessit" of £40 or 1000 frs. for the second best, on a particular aspect of the vivisection question. The competitors are to treat the subject of the employment of freshly killed animals in the place of living animals in physiological experiments. The writers must illustrate their argument from cases in which the substitution has actually been made. The essays are to be sent to the President of the Society, Oberst Stattmeister A. von Haxthausen, Copenhagen, on or before September 30, 1882.

Women Doctors, France.—From the Faculty of Paris, Madame Perrée, aged thirty-two, has recently obtained a doctor's decree. It is stated that she is only the second lady-doctor authorised to practise in France. After being successfully treated by an American "doctoress" in a severe illness, she was induced to undertake the study of medicine with a view of entering the profession.

Apparently a Hardship.—On the hearing of a summons at the Highgate Police-court against a builder, of Hamilton-road, Finchley, for infringing the by-laws of the Finchley Local Board, by using inferior materials in the construction of several houses at Finchley, Mr. Bodkin, a magistrate, remarked that it seemed hardly fair to builders that they should be allowed to almost complete the houses before they were summoned for not complying with the Local Board by-laws. The solicitor to the Local Authority said it would want a dozen surveyors to watch the progress of all builders' houses in the parish. He assured the Bench they took immediate action in all cases brought under their notice. The magistrate rejoined, if there were not sufficient persons to do the work, others ought to be appointed. It was a great pity the Local Board had not the power to stop the work of builders when they found it was not being carried on in accordance with the by-laws. However, the defendant had clearly infringed them, and was fined altogether in the sum of fourteen guineas.

Erudite.—In itself, demography is somewhat a new term, and probably its exact significance is not yet clearly established. But in Littré's great work it is defined as "a didactic expression: descriptive of peoples as regards the population, considered in relation to ages, professions, dwellings, etc."; also as the "natural history of society."

The Temperance Movement in City Warehouses.—Under the patronage of the City of London Total Abstainers' Union, a series of weekly temperance meetings and lectures have been commenced in City warehouses. The first meeting augured well for those which will follow in various warehouses up to the 16th proximo.

COMMUNICATIONS have been received from—

Mr. W. B. Kesteven, London; The Secretaries of the Harveian Society, London; Mr. Jacobson, London; The Secretary of the Statistical Society, London; The Registrar of the Apothecaries' Hall, London; Mr. Kenneth Millican, Kineton; Dr. Crichton Browne, London; Messrs. Goodall, Backhouse, and Co., Leeds; Dr. Whipham, London; Mr. John Dougall, Glasgow; Mr. G. B. Jenn, London; The Town Clerk of Hastings; Mr. A. G. Blomfield, Exeter; The Honorary Secretary of the Medical Society of London; Mr. Teale, Scarborough; The Secretary of the Obstetrical Society of London; Mr. R. J. Godlee, London; The Honorary Secretary of the Royal Medical and Chirurgical Society of London; Messrs. J. Smith and Co., London; Dr. Mears, Durham; The Secretary of the Medical Department of the Durham University; Mr. Watson Cheyne, London; Mr. R. C. Lucas, London; Mr. Hulke, London; Mr. W. E. Good, Dorchester; Mr. Boyle, London; Dr. A. W. Edis, London; Dr. Graily Hewitt, London; The Sanitary Commissioner, Punjaub; Dr. Sedgwick Saunders, London; Dr. Stephen Mackenzie, London; Dr. Cockle, London; Dr. Semple, London; The Secretary of the University of London; The Editor of the "Christian World"; Dr. Little, Dublin; Dr. John Williams, London; The Honorary Secretary of the Midland Medical Society, Birmingham.

BOOKS, ETC., RECEIVED—

Ophthalmic and Otic Memoranda, by D. B. St. John Roosa, M.D., and Edward T. Ely, M.D.—Cutaneous and Venereal Memoranda, by Henry G. Piffard, A.M., M.D., and George Henry Fox, A.M., M.D.—The Prevention of Stricture and of Prostatic Obstruction, by R. Harrison, F.R.C.S.—Monaco, by Dr. T. H. Pickering—The Middlesex Hospital Reports for 1879—The Communicability to Man of Diseases from Animals used as Food, by Dr. Henry Behrend—On the Action of Water upon Lead Pipes, by W. Sedgwick Saunders, M.D., F.S.A.—Die Parasitären Krankheiten des Menschen, von Sigmund Theodor Stein—Thoughts on the Source of Life, by An Octogenarian.

PERIODICALS AND NEWSPAPERS RECEIVED—

Lancet—British Medical Journal—Medical Press and Circular—Berliner Klinische Wochenschrift—Centralblatt für Chirurgie—Gazette des Hopitaux—Gazette Médicale—Le Progrès Médical—Bulletin de l'Académie de Médecine—Pharmaceutical Journal—Wiener Medizinische Wochenschrift—Centralblatt für die Medizinischen Wissenschaften—Revue Médicale—Gazette Hebdomadaire—National Board of Health Bulletin, Washington—Nature—Deutsche Medicinal-Zeitung—Boston Medical and Surgical Journal—Louisville Medical News—Students' Journal and Hospital Gazette—Martin's Chemists' and Druggists' Bulletin—Church of England Pulpit and Ecclesiastical Review—The American—Chicago Medical Review—Philadelphia Medical Times—Keene's Bath Journal, November 19—Leeds Mercury, November 18—Monthly Military Budget—Science—Weekblad—Physician and Surgeon—Boston Medical and Surgical Journal.

APPOINTMENTS FOR THE WEEK.

November 26. *Saturday (this day).*

Operations at St. Bartholomew's, 1½ p.m.; King's College, 1½ p.m.; Royal Free, 2 p.m.; Royal London Ophthalmic, 11 a.m.; Royal Westminster Ophthalmic, 1½ p.m.; St. Thomas's, 1½ p.m.; London, 2 p.m.

28. *Monday.*

Operations at the Metropolitan Free, 2 p.m.; St. Mark's Hospital for Diseases of the Rectum, 2 p.m.; Royal London Ophthalmic, 11 a.m.; Royal Westminster Ophthalmic, 1½ p.m.

Medical Society of London, 8½ p.m. Dr. Routh, "On the Necessity of adopting a Different Mode of Burying Bodies the Subjects of Infectious Disease." Dr. Gilbert Smith will give the details of a Case of Hæmorrhage into the Mesentery."

29. *Tuesday.*

Operations at Guy's, 1½ p.m.; Westminster, 2 p.m.; Royal London Ophthalmic, 11 a.m.; Royal Westminster Ophthalmic, 1½ p.m.; West London, 3 p.m.

30. *Wednesday.*

Operations at University College, 2 p.m.; St. Mary's, 1¼ p.m.; Middlesex, 1 p.m.; London, 2 p.m.; St. Bartholomew's, 1½ p.m.; Great Northern, 2 p.m.; Samaritan, 2½ p.m.; Royal London Ophthalmic, 11 a.m.; Royal Westminster Ophthalmic, 1½ p.m.; St. Thomas's, 1½ p.m.; St. Peter's Hospital for Stone, 2 p.m.; National Orthopædic, Great Portland-street, 10 a.m.

December 1. *Thursday.*

Operations at St. George's, 1 p.m.; Central London Ophthalmic, 1 p.m.; Royal Orthopædic, 2 p.m.; University College, 2 p.m.; Royal London Ophthalmic, 11 a.m.; Royal Westminster Ophthalmic, 1½ p.m.; Hospital for Diseases of the Throat, 2 p.m.; Hospital for Women, 2 p.m. Charing-cross, 2 p.m.; London, 2 p.m.; North-West London, 2½ p.m.

Harveian Society, 8½ p.m. Dr. Alfred Meadows, "On Menstruation and its Derangements." (First Harveian Lecture.)

2. *Friday.*

Operations at Central London Ophthalmic, 2 p.m.; Royal London Ophthalmic, 11 a.m.; South London Ophthalmic, 2 p.m.; Royal Westminster Ophthalmic, 1½ p.m.; St. George's (ophthalmic operations), 1¼ p.m.; Guy's, 1½ p.m.; St. Thomas's (ophthalmic operations), 2 p.m.; King's College (by Mr. Lister), 2 p.m.

ORIGINAL LECTURES.

CLINICAL LECTURES
ON DISEASES OF THE ABDOMEN.

By FREDERICK T. ROBERTS, M.D., B.Sc., F.R.C.P.,

Professor of Materia Medica and Therapeutics at University College,
Physician to University Hospital, and Professor of
Clinical Medicine, etc.

LECTURE V.

ON THE CLINICAL INVESTIGATION OF ABDOMINAL CASES.

GENTLEMEN,—My subject to-day is the general clinical investigation of abdominal cases, and in dealing with this subject the opportunity will be afforded me of indicating in outline the plan of investigation applicable to all kinds of cases, the details being varied in particular instances, and in different groups of diseases. Probably I shall be going over ground that is familiar to many of you, but possibly some points may be brought out which may give you all hints of practical value.

From what has been said in preceding lectures, it is clearly my duty in discussing this subject to urge at the very outset, and to lay particular stress upon this point, namely, that your investigation of every abdominal case should be *satisfactory*. It should, at any rate, always be sufficiently careful to guard you against making inexcusable and obvious blunders in diagnosis. I have known a doctor explain certain grave symptoms on the assumption that a man was slowly poisoning his wife, when all the while there was evident cancer of the stomach, and a cancerous liver filling the abdomen, which he had never examined! Such instances of extreme and flagrant carelessness are, of course, rare, but there is a rather prevalent tendency to think lightly of many abdominal symptoms, and to take it for granted that they do not indicate anything of much importance. This may be illustrated by the way in which cases of supposed "dyspepsia" or "indigestion" are but too commonly investigated. Such terms are often very misleading, and have led to many serious mistakes in diagnosis. They really have no definite meaning, and to be satisfied with applying them to a particular case without due inquiry, so as to ascertain what is actually wrong, cannot but lead to untoward consequences from time to time. On the whole, I think it may be affirmed that the investigation of abdominal cases needs to be more cautious and complete than that of any other class; and this not only from a diagnostic point of view, but because it often brings out facts which are of considerable practical importance with reference to treatment. Of course, different cases demand more or less minute and elaborate inquiry, according to circumstances. Some are obvious in every respect after a very superficial examination; others require close and thorough investigation. And it must be borne in mind that not only cases presenting difficulties in their diagnosis may need such investigation, but also those of a simple, and perhaps even trivial, nature, especially with reference to points bearing upon treatment. Your safest and best plan will be to make it a rule to aim at thoroughness and completeness in your investigation of abdominal as of other cases, and you will then generally be right, or, at any rate, will have the consciousness that you have done your duty.

The points bearing upon the investigation and clinical observation of any individual case of disease may be gathered under the following heads:—

I.—The ÆTIOLOGICAL HISTORY, or the facts relating to its causation.

II.—The CLINICAL HISTORY: that is, the history of the case with reference to the present illness.

III.—The CLINICAL CONDITION when the patient is first seen.

IV.—The CLINICAL PROGRESS of the case, while the patient continues under observation.

In briefly discussing these points in succession, I will endeavour to indicate the more important practical facts relating to abdominal affections, and to illustrate their application in particular instances.

I.—ÆTIOLOGICAL HISTORY.

I have already in a former lecture pointed out the principal causes which are concerned in the production of abdominal affections, and it is to determine which of these have been at work in any individual case, whether as predisposing or exciting causes, that we investigate as to its ætiological history. The facts elicited in this direction are conveniently arranged under the following separate heads :—

1. *General History.*—Here we have to deal with certain matters relating to the patient himself, and bearing upon his ordinary life and mode of existence, and his surroundings. These are often of much consequence in all classes of cases, and they have particular significance in many abdominal affections. We may notice briefly some points deserving of special notice.

a. *Climate, Season, and Residence.*—These ætiological factors are not, on the whole, of such direct importance in abdominal cases as in connexion with chest affections, but there are certain conditions which have a more or less powerful influence in originating some diseases in this part of the body. The following may be mentioned as the most striking illustrations of this point, indicating the directions in which inquiry may be demanded. A tropical climate is peculiarly favourable for the development of such affections as dysentery, acute and severe disorders of the alimentary canal, and hepatic abscess. Choleraic attacks are prevalent in hot seasons. Prolonged residence in a tropical climate may originate important morbid changes in the liver. The influence of malarial districts in causing temporary or permanent lesions in the spleen and liver is well known. A cold and damp climate or season, and exposure to cold and wet, are certainly important factors in producing some forms of renal disease. Similar conditions are supposed to affect the alimentary canal and other abdominal structures in some cases. Unfavourable hygienic conditions connected with a patient's residence may certainly account for many cases of gastric or intestinal disorder, as well as partly for other more serious affections.

b. *Occupation.*—The patient's employment has an important bearing in relation to many cases of abdominal disease, and may need to be carefully inquired into with regard to several points. For example, it may explain the introduction of definite and obvious exciting causes of disease into the system, such as lead, or certain animal parasites, which give rise to well-known abdominal complaints or lesions. Again, a person's occupation may involve exposure to cold and wet, or allied causes; or it may lead to habits of intemperance, which seriously affect abdominal organs. Sedentary habits, want of exercise, long hours, unsatisfactory hygienic surroundings, and irregularities in feeding, associated with various employments, are prolific sources of abdominal disorders, and often need full and close investigation in individual cases. It is believed, and probably on good grounds, that occupations involving much pressure upon the epigastrium may originate serious organic diseases within the abdomen—even malignant disease. Those which necessitate prolonged standing may act injuriously on certain abdominal structures, especially in females.

c. *Food and Drink.*—The ætiological relations of diet to abdominal diseases are so evident that they are universally recognised. At the same time they are often not studied sufficiently in all their bearings, and the subject is so important that it will demand special consideration on a future occasion. In the meantime it will suffice to mention a few facts in illustration of the influence exercised by food and drink in originating various complaints, and of the principal points to which attention has to be directed in the ætiological history. Errors in diet are prolific sources of acute affections of the alimentary canal, as well as of chronic disorders and organic diseases in the digestive organs. The mischief depends not only on the quantity or quality of the food or drink, but also on the cooking of food, the frequency with which it is taken, imperfect mastication, and other conditions. Again, certain direct causes of disease are often introduced into the body in this way, such as poisons or animal parasites. The habit of taking strong condiments with meals may be injurious, and needs to be remembered in investigating certain cases. Questions relating to drink frequently demand special inquiry; and this refers particularly to the quantity and quality of water consumed, tea-drinking, and alcohol. The improper use of various alcoholic drinks not only causes disorders of, and organic changes in, the alimentary canal, but also often seriously damages the liver, kidneys, and other structures. Moreover, it must be borne in mind that food and drink have an important influence in originating the gouty condition, which tends to affect several of the abdominal structures.

d. Clothing.—This is not of much consequence in relation to abdominal affections, as a rule. Deficient clothing may have a certain influence in originating some cases of renal disease. Pressure caused by tight articles of clothing, such as stays or belts, is an important factor in producing displacement of certain organs, especially the liver, or even some degree of malformation.

e. General Habits.—Apart from the questions already considered, a patient's habits may need more or less investigation in different cases, in such circumstances as circumstances seem to indicate. For instance, quite independent of occupation, a person may lead a sedentary, indolent, and perhaps luxurious life, which may have an important bearing on the ætiology of several abdominal affections. Such habits as excessive smoking or snuff-taking unquestionably tend to cause disorders of the digestive organs. Habitual indulgence in narcotics must also not be forgotten. Want of cleanliness of the skin may be a factor in the causation of renal disease. Sexual habits must not be overlooked, and in some instances need to be closely inquired into.

f. Mental Condition.—A person's natural mental state may be worth attention in relation to disorders of the digestive organs, as to whether he is morbidly low-spirited and desponding. What is most important in this connexion, however, and what may need very careful and sometimes delicate investigation, is to ascertain if the patient has any reason for much anxiety, or has some great worry weighing him down. This not only causes disorders connected with the digestive organs, but there is every reason to believe that it may lay the foundation for malignant disease; and I have met with cases strongly suggestive of this relationship. Besides, worry and anxiety often lead to secret intemperance, a most prolific cause of abdominal affections.

Such are the most important points in a patient's general history to which your attention needs to be directed in cases of abdominal disease. You must remember that many of the causes which have been indicated not only tend to affect the abdominal structures immediately, but also to produce certain general conditions or diseases which are liable to implicate these structures. Allusion has already been made to gout; and general debility affords another illustration.

2. *Family History.*—The main object of inquiring into the family history of a patient is, as you are probably aware, to ascertain whether there is any hereditary morbid tendency or family disease. The investigation may need some tact and discrimination, and its results must be taken with due caution, as patients sometimes give a positive history of a hereditary condition which never existed; while, on the other hand, they conceal or are ignorant of some family taint. In illustration of the danger of error with regard to this matter, I may mention a case which recently came within my knowledge. The patient died from what was believed, without any doubt, by several physicians to be malignant disease of the stomach and liver. A post-mortem examination was made, and revealed that the morbid changes were not in the slightest degree malignant, but of a cirrhotic character, and involved several structures of importance. Had this examination not been made, the history of cancer in the family would have been handed down; and my impression is that I have met with other cases of a similar kind, in which no autopsy was made, and so the cancerous taint is attached to the family, perhaps without reason.

The chief diatheses which have to be remembered in the family history, in relation to abdominal diseases, are the cancerous, the gouty, and the tuberculous or scrofulous. Congenital syphilis must be thought of in exceptional cases; for instance, a form of enlarged spleen in infants may be due to this cause. There may be a hereditary history of predisposition to certain particular symptoms or diseases, such as dyspeptic symptoms, habitual constipation, biliary disorders, or calculus.

3. *Previous Health and Past Illnesses.*—Investigation with regard to these points is often of essential value in cases of abdominal disease; and the subject will require a little detailed consideration.

a. In the first place, there may be a history of some permanent morbid condition, of longer or shorter duration, congenital or acquired, which it may be important to recognise, not only in itself, but in relation to other abdominal affections. An intestinal hernia will serve to illustrate this point.

b. Any previous illness of the patient is always worthy of note, although it may have no special bearing upon the case. So far as the abdomen is concerned, particular attention needs to be directed in different instances to a past history of typhoid or scarlet fever; of attacks of gout or gouty symptoms; of syphilis; of chronic suppuration from any part; or of malignant disease in other regions of the body. A little consideration of what was stated in a former lecture will indicate where these affections may be of ætiological importance, and this matter will be further elucidated hereafter.

c. A history of any local abdominal disease likely to leave permanent morbid conditions behind, or to originate others of a secondary kind, is of the greatest consequence, and often deserves particular attention. For example, there may be well-authenticated evidence of a previous attack of acute peritonitis, intestinal accumulation or obstruction, ulceration of the stomach or bowel, local injury, an abscess in some abdominal structure or organ, and various other conditions. These may explain not only subsequent symptoms and functional disorders, but even more or less serious organic lesions; and it must be remembered that the knowledge of the existence of certain diseases may account for the occurrence of others.

d. It is not uncommon of decided service to inquire definitely as to the manner in which the digestive functions are habitually performed, and as to certain particular symptoms connected with the digestive organs. A history of frequent dyspeptic disorders, so-called "bilious attacks," habitual constipation, or liability to diarrhœa, may be of no little moment in some instances. In this connexion it may also be stated that it is often well to ascertain whether patients have been addicted to taking much aperient medicine, especially strong purgatives, or such as are liable to accumulate in the alimentary canal.

e. In dealing with females, a knowledge of the way in which the menstrual functions are performed habitually is always essential. Not unfrequently it may be necessary to inquire as to the number and frequency of pregnancies; any symptoms or conditions noted during their progress; the ease or difficulty of parturition, and other points connected therewith; and any untoward events happening subsequently. These points may have a bearing on morbid conditions quite apart from those associated with the genital organs themselves.

f. Lastly, a history of previous attacks or paroxysms of a certain kind may be of great help in the diagnosis of some abdominal cases, often of a severe or urgent character—such as gastric spasm, intestinal colic, or the passage of hepatic or renal calculi.

4. *History of Direct Exciting Cause or Causes.*—Of course, it is essential to trace an illness to its immediate and actual cause or causes, if this can be done. In many instances this is perfectly easy, and only the most superficial questioning is needed; or patients will tell you of their own accord. In other cases more or less elaborate investigation is required; and this must be left to individual judgment and skill, founded upon the probable nature of the complaint, and the known relations between particular causes and particular diseases. It may be impossible to discover any immediately antecedent cause, and then the whole ætiological history may have to be taken into account, and the causation is more or less complex and intricate; or the ætiology may even be quite indefinite or unknown.

II.—CLINICAL HISTORY.

The ætiology of the illness from which the patient is suffering when he comes under observation having been considered under the preceding heading, it only remains to notice the following points to which attention has to be directed with reference to its clinical history.

1. *Duration.*—Of course, one of the first points to be ascertained with regard to any illness is whether it is recent and acute, or more or less chronic in its duration. But beyond this, it is often of great service in chronic cases to take into account the time during which symptoms have

been noticed, in relation to the conditions actually found to exist when a patient comes under treatment. For instance, this may afford valuable assistance in the diagnosis of cancer from other forms of disease.

2. *Mode of Onset, Rapidity of Progress, Nature, and Course of Symptoms.*—Each one of these elements in the clinical history has to be borne in mind, and may have to be more or less carefully investigated in different cases. Some discrimination is needed in taking the statements of patients or their friends on these points, but, with due care in estimating their value, they frequently afford most useful information bearing upon diagnosis.

3. *History of Abnormal Physical Conditions.*—When any unusual physical condition is discovered by examination of the abdomen, it is often of essential importance to inquire into the history of this particular condition. For example, if there should be a solid enlargement or tumour, it might be of the greatest service in diagnosis to ascertain the part in which it was first noticed, and the direction in which it grew; its rate of progress; whether it was constant or variable; and other points which individual cases might suggest. General enlargements of the abdomen might also need similar investigation.

III.—CLINICAL CONDITION.

The actual clinical examination of the patient is necessarily in most cases the principal part of the investigation, and, as regards abdominal cases, little or nothing can be known about them unless this is performed properly and efficiently. The process often requires not only considerable knowledge, but also no small amount of skill on the part of the practitioner, and needs to be conducted intelligently and systematically, with due recognition of the meaning of the facts ascertained from the examination. Of course, cases present very different degrees of difficulty, both in determining the symptoms and signs present, and in interpreting their significance. At present I shall only direct your attention to the groups of phenomena which you may have to investigate in individual cases of abdominal disease.

1. It is always well at the outset to take a note of the *sex, age,* and apparent *general condition* of the patient. These points may have more or less significance in diagnosis.

2. The local *symptoms* referred to the abdomen, or associated with either of its contained organs and structures, should then be ascertained and investigated, whether of a subjective or objective character. This may have to be done very thoroughly, and with close attention to details.

3. It must be remembered that symptoms directly connected with particular abdominal organs may be observed in some *remote* part, or may even affect the *entire system;* and these have to be recognised and duly considered. Jaundice and renal dropsy will serve to illustrate this point.

4. In the next place it is frequently of great consequence to determine whether any *general symptoms* are present; and to study carefully their nature when present. The absence of such symptoms may be of essential aid in diagnosis. Special attention should be paid to the signs of any particular diathesis. Be also on the watch for hysteria and allied conditions.

5. It may be confidently affirmed, that in a considerable proportion of cases of abdominal disease a correct diagnosis is absolutely impossible without satisfactory *physical examination,* and sometimes very elaborate examination is needed, directed to particular points. Therefore, let me emphatically impress upon you not to neglect this part of the clinical examination, if you see the slightest need for it. I have already given you an illustration of the grave errors into which a practitioner may fall by such neglect, and I could give many more from personal knowledge. We are, of course, all liable to mistakes, but let us at any rate so act that such mistakes are not due to any fault of neglect on our part. I shall, on a future occasion, consider the subject of physical examination of the abdomen at some length; in the meantime, I will merely observe that it may have to be directed to the investigation of the abdomen generally; of particular organs; or of special diseases.

6. In cases of abdominal disease it is not uncommonly of practical importance that attention should be specially paid to symptoms and physical signs connected with the *chest.* These may be mere effects of the abdominal conditions, and may help to throw light upon them; or some

thoracic disease may be recognised as the cause of the abdominal symptoms or morbid changes.

7. Sometimes it is requisite to look for other *remote* conditions besides those in the chest, as having an important relation to those found in the abdomen. Thus, the existence of chronic suppuration in any part of the body might account for certain morbid states of some of the abdominal organs, such as albuminoid disease. The discovery of cancer in some other structure might throw much light upon the diagnosis of a similar disease in the abdomen.

IV.—CLINICAL PROGRESS.

The importance of watching the clinical progress of many abdominal cases cannot be over-estimated. The chief points to be noted in any particular instance are its duration and rate of progress; the development of new or additional symptoms or physical signs, or the disappearance of those already present; and the effects of treatment. This waiting and watching may be absolutely necessary before a positive diagnosis can be made; but, moreover, it must be remembered that in many abdominal cases fresh complications and morbid conditions are very apt to supervene from time to time, and these demand due recognition. The repetition of physical examination under various conditions is often of the greatest service in making out obscure cases, and also in discovering new complications.

VACCINATION IN COCHIN CHINA.—Small-pox having committed great ravages in Cochin China, the French Local Government itself compelled to insist upon effectual vaccination being put into force, and entrusted its execution to naval medical officers. The country was mapped out into districts, and two inspectors were appointed to superintend the operations. One of these, Dr. Vantalon, has published an interesting report upon his proceedings during 1880. According to this, at the beginning of that year, in a population of 2,000,000 there were about 50,000 already vaccinated, and during the year he inspected the nineteen districts into which the colony was divided, and in which 50,798 children had been vaccinated. Upon an average 190 vaccinations from arm to arm were performed at each sitting. The successful results amounted to 83 per cent.; and it was found that while five-day lymph produced 96·36 per cent. successful results, the eight-day lymph only produced 47·70 per cent. As the lymph furnished by the five-day pustules is, however, very sparing, Dr. Vantalon advises that that of the sixth or seventh day should be employed. The cost of vaccination was estimated at about a franc and a half per child.—*St. Petersb. Med. Woch.,* November 12.

ANTISEPTIC TREATMENT OF CYSTS OF THE WRIST.—Alluding to a discussion which recently took place upon this subject at the Paris Société de Chirurgie, Dr. Daniel Mollière observes (*Lyon Méd.,* October 23) that synovial cysts of the wrist have been successfully treated in this way at Lyons since Dr. Létiévant introduced the Listerian method at the Hotel-Dieu in 1875. Prior to that time, operations upon these cysts had over and over again given rise to pyæmia, and it was only with trembling that iodine injections were ventured upon; so that the prudent surgeon wherever possible declined meddling with these bodies. Dr. Létiévant opened the cyst widely under the spray, scraped away the vegetations which covered its surface (removing sometimes a portion of the walls of the cyst when these were very large or very thick), and on closing the wound left a small piece of drainage-tube at its upper and lower angles. Union took place in a few days, and the cure was definitive. This practice was so successful as soon to become generalised at the Lyons hospitals. For this method Dr. Mollière substituted three years since what he terms "antiseptic capillary drainage," which, however, is only applicable to cases in which the hordeiform or riziform bodies are free—i.e., when there are few or no vegetations on the surface of the cyst. The operation is very simple, consisting in making only an incision a centimetre in length at the palm of the hand, and another above the wrist, and passing through them, under the annular ligament of the carpus, a large tent of hair carefully disinfected and well soaked in carbolised oil. The wound is dressed antiseptically, and the limb immobilised. The success that has attended this procedure shows that a large operation is not always required for the cure of these cysts.

ORIGINAL COMMUNICATIONS.

———◆———

ON A CASE OF EXCESSIVELY HIGH AND VARIABLE TEMPERATURE.

By JAMES LITTLE, M.D. Edin., F.K.&Q.C.I.,

Physician to the Adelaide Hospital ; and Professor of the Practice of Medicine in the Royal College of Surgeons, Ireland.

———

THE following case, carefully reported almost day by day, and carefully observed by Dr. Little himself, affords one of the most important contributions to the literature of exaggerated temperatures which has yet appeared. The records given are, in point of fact, the highest we yet have had, and the character of the girl helps us to a clue as to their causation.

K. M., aged twenty-three ; admitted April 15, 1880.

April 15, 1880.—Morning, pulse 108, temperature 102° ; evening, pulse 112, temperature 102·2°. Has considerable supra-orbital headache, with noises in her ears, and feeling of depression and lassitude. Her arms tremble on being raised. Respirations hurried and shallow ; spat up some blood this morning, which she thinks came from her nose. Complains of considerable pain in right iliac fossa ; the abdomen is here painful on pressure ; descending colon dull to percussion. Tongue brilliant red, moist, and not furred. Says her bowels were very loose the last three days. Urine : Has considerable difficulty in making water. No mottling or spots. Skin very hot, and covered with perspiration.

16th.—Morning, pulse 96, temperature 103·5°, respirations 48 ; evening, pulse 104, temperature 105·2°. Headache still very severe. Was moaning all the evening, and did not sleep until 1 a.m., when she had three hours' restless sleep. In the early part of the night complained of feeling very cold. Respirations shallow, hurried, and jerky. Bowels not moved since admission. No spots or mottling. Treatment : A purgative enema at once ; a leech to each mastoid. ℞. Sodæ salicyl., sodæ bicarb., āā ʒj., aquæ ad ʒvj., m. ; and ℞. Acid. salicyl., acid. citrici., āā ʒj., aquæ ad ʒvj., m. ; one ounce of each to be mixed together and taken every three hours ; potassii bromidi gr. xxx. at bedtime. Leeching did not seem to relieve her headache, which is still very painful. Was restless during the evening, moaning repeatedly, but quite rational until about 11 p.m. 11 p.m. : Got the bromide. She then began to wander, and was more restless, wanting to get out of bed. She was very hot, and perspiring very freely. She was then sponged over with vinegar and tepid water, which quieted her, and she was comparatively quiet until about half-past twelve, when she became very delirious. Her hair was closely cut behind, and her head was douched with tepid water. 1 a.m. : Got ten grains more of bromide, and an ice-bag was applied to the nape of her neck. 2 a.m. : Got her medicine, and remained quiet until 3 a.m., when she fell asleep, and slept quietly, without moaning, until 6 a.m. Bowels moved twice after enema ; stools dark-coloured scybala, very offensive.

17th.—Morning, pulse 108, temperature 103·7°, respirations 52 ; evening, pulse 120, temperature 110°, respirations 60. 9 a.m. : Headache as before. Complains of considerable pain in her back ; is quite sensible now ; still complains of pain in right iliac fossa. Tongue coated behind with creamy fur, clean and bright red at tip and edges. No spots. Treatment : To get a castor-oil draught at once. Two leeches to be applied to each mastoid. To continue her other medicine. 10 a.m. : Took a cup of tea. Leeches seemed to have relieved her head, for she remained quieter until 1 p.m., when she fell asleep, and slept until 3 p.m. 3 p.m. : Bowels were moved ; the stool consisted of a few light-brown softer masses, in a thick and very offensive fluid. She now got very delirious, and complained of great pain in the precordial region. An additional leech was applied to each mastoid, and she was given ten grains of potassii bromidi, and her head was douched with tepid water. 5.30 p.m. : As she still complained of great pain in her head a blister 4 × 3 in. was applied to the nape of her neck. 6 30 p.m. : Says she is intolerably hot. Her temperature was now taken, and, although she was perspiring freely, was found to be 105·8°. Ordered sixty grains of potassii bromidi

to be taken at 9 p.m. ; to discontinue her other medicine after 8 p.m. 9 p.m. : Gave her the bromide. Is complaining of being intensely hot, and of a "bursting" sensation in her head, and is very restless. Her temperature was now taken by two thermometers (Mr. Beeston's and Mr. Scott's), their indications being as follows :—By No. 1, which registers 0·2° too low, 109·8° ; by No. 2, which registers about 1° too high, 111°, thus agreeing in making the temperature 110°. Tepid water was now poured over her head, and as she was very restless she was allowed to sit up with a shawl around her shoulders. 10.30 p.m. : Says she feels much cooler. The temperature is now only 104° by Dr. Little's thermometer. Her head was thoroughly douched with two jugs of tepid water, and the remainder of her hair cut off. 10.45 p.m. : Got twenty grains quiniæ sulphatis. Is quieter now. At 11.15, as some of the quinine was ejected, she was given ten grains more, suspended in milk. Did not taste last dose so much as former. 12.30 p.m. : Fell asleep, and slept till 3.15 a.m. 3.15 a.m. : Complains of pain in her stomach. 3.45 a.m. : Slept from this time until 4.45. 4.45 a.m. : As her head is rather worse, tepid water was poured on it, and again at 6 a.m., which seemed to relieve her head. Passed water twice during night ; no vomiting. From 5 a.m. was rather delirious, but not so when sleeping. Towards morning complained of great pain in her chest.

18th.—Morning, pulse 124, temperature 105·4°, respirations 60. The morning temperature was taken by Mr. Brooke's thermometer (which is 0·3° lower than Dr. Little's) twenty minutes after she had been sponged over with vinegar and water. 10.15 a.m. : Temperature has fallen to 99° by Dr. Little's thermometer. She is shivering slightly. Pulse very compressible ; heart-sounds feeble. Respirations much as before. Tongue coated with thick yellow fur. Bowels not moved since yesterday. Urine very pale-coloured, faintly opaque, acid, specific gravity 1007, no albumen, chlorides abundant. Is now perspiring freely. Treatment : To get twenty grains of quiniæ sulph. at once. Diet as before. Her head is not so painful. She has no pain in her back, but is still intolerant of light. Complains of feeling of coldness, and has some pain in her stomach. Up till twelve o'clock was very restless, her head being very painful. She has had a troublesome hiccup for the last hour. 1 p.m. : As she was complaining of great pain in her head it was douched with tepid water, which relieved it for some time. She is still very thirsty, and has a sour taste in her mouth. 2 p.m. : Has great pain in her right iliac fossa. A poultice was applied, which has relieved her a little. At 2.5 p.m., temperature 102·4°, pulse 132. 3.10 p.m. : As she was complaining of her head being much worse, her temperature was taken, and found to be 104·6°. 3.30 p.m. : Has been douched with two jugfuls of tepid water, and is at present quieter. Remained in much the same condition until 5.15 p.m., when she got into a very excited state, and her temperature was found to be 106°. The bath was brought to the side of the bed, and a jugful of tepid water poured on her head. She then suddenly become quite collapsed, with stertorous breathing, very feeble pulse, pains in legs, with tonic half-flexion of her fingers, and violent rigor. All available clothes were put on the bed, and her arms and legs were rubbed with eau-de-cologne. She began to get warmer, and the cramp left her hands. 6.15 p.m. : The nurse called me to see her in a most excited condition, her head "bursting," and her body in a state of great heat. Her temperature was now taken, and found to be 109·2° by Mr. Beeston's thermometer. As her pulse was only 100, very thin and compressible, it was thought inadvisable to give her another douche. Two leeches were applied to the right mastoid, one of which took very well. 7.15 p.m. : Is in much the same condition as regards her head, and is now perspiring freely. Temperature 103° by Dr. Little's thermometer. Got twenty grains of quinine sulphatis in milk, and one-sixth of a grain of morphia hypodermically. She now states that about a fortnight ago she got a fall from a sofa, by which her head was knocked against a wall. It was sore for a few days. From this time (7.45) until 9.30 she was quieter, and did not complain of any pain in her head, but was rambling until 10 p.m. At 9.30 p.m. her temperature was taken, and found to be 103·4° by Dr. Little's thermometer ; pulse 136. 9.55 p.m. : As she got more restless her temperature was again taken, and found to be 105·5° by Dr. Little's thermometer ; pulse 140. She now got twenty-five minims of hypodermic solution of ergotine injected into the cellular tissue of her chest, and one-sixth of a grain of morphia into her arm. She became somewhat quieter, although still rambling, until twelve o'clock, when she fell asleep, and slept till 1.30 a.m., when she awoke complaining of pain in right breast; had poultice, which did not relieve her. At 2.30 a.m. gave her an additional injection (twenty minims) of ergotine and one-sixth of a grain of morphia. Temperature 106·8° by Mr. Brooke's thermometer, pulse 104. She now got into a very collapsed condition; her pulse was very feeble, and, although very hot, she had a violent rigor, her teeth chattering, with pains in her arms. 2.45 a.m.: Patient suddenly vomited three spitting-cupfuls of fluid—the tea, milk, and soda-water, of which she had taken a quantity during the evening. 3 a.m.: Her pulse has improved in tone very much since the hypodermic. She is quieter, and seems likely to sleep. Slept from 3 a.m. until 4 a.m., then awoke and had some tea; fell asleep, and slept for half an hour; then vomited, and soon after got quieter, and slept until 6 a.m.

19th.—Morning, pulse 132, temperature 112·4°; evening, pulse 128, temperature 115°. When the thermometer was put into her axilla at 8.45 a.m., she appeared to be quite quiet and did not seem to be very hot, but when it had been under her arm about six minutes she began to complain of intense pain in her head, as is always the case when her temperature is very high. 9 a.m.: Temperature 112·4° by Dr. Little's thermometer. Urine, specific gravity 1025, acid, no albumen. Treatment: To get one-sixth of a grain of morphia if not asleep in two hours; the quinine to be discontinued. 11 a.m.: Got the hypodermic, and in a short time became quieter and did not complain so much of pain in her head. Slept quietly from 12.5 to 12.40 p.m. She then awoke, had a drink, and fell asleep again. Awoke soon after 1 p.m., and was then perspiring freely. Fell asleep again, and slept until 2 p.m. She then awoke, and slept immediately fell asleep, and slept till 2.40 p.m. She then had a drink of soda-water and a small cup of tea. 2.45 p.m.: Dr. Little's and Mr. Brooke's thermometers were placed one under each axilla. When put in they were both at 96·2°, and on being taken out at 3 p.m., Dr. Little's (left) registered 105·6°, Mr. Brooke's (right) 105·3°. 3 p.m.: As she was complaining of pain in her chest, a poultice was applied, which relieved her a little. She also has some pain in the left side of her abdomen (about the left iliac fossa). Was quite quiet until 9 p.m., and, as she was complaining of pain in her head, the thermometer was placed under her left axilla at 9.10 p.m., and on being taken out at 9.20 p.m., was found to have risen to 115° by Dr. Little's thermometer. 9.30 p.m.: Got six minims of hypodermic solution of morphia (five grains of solution equal one-sixth of a grain of morphia), which, as has always been the case, converted her delirium from a wildly excited condition to one of comparative quietness, although still very loquacious. 10.10 p.m.: Is much cooler now, and does not complain so much of her head. Temperature 106·2° by Dr. Little's thermometer. 11.30 p.m.: Fell asleep, and slept until 12 p.m.; she then awoke complaining of her head, but went to sleep again soon after.

20th.—Morning, pulse 88, temperature 106·5°, respirations 72. 1 a.m.: Awoke complaining of a bursting sensation in her head, and her temperature was found to be 111·1° by Dr. Little's thermometer. She now got eight minims of hypodermic solution of morphia, which, however, did not quiet her, and she was restless until 4 a.m. From 4.30 till 5 a.m. she slept. 5 a.m.: Awoke complaining of great heat, and the usual "bursting" sensation in her head. Her face was dusky, and her temperature was over 115°. Her head was sponged with tepid water and ice was applied to it, and at 5.35 a.m. her temperature was again taken, and found to be 103·8° (by Mr. Brooke's thermometer, as Dr. Little's was kept that the indication might be seen), pulse 108. As she still complained of her head she got two minims of hypodermic solution of morphia, and in a short time became quieter. Had short sleeps between 6 a.m. and 7 a.m. On awaking was always found to be freely perspiring. Passed water twice during the night; no vomiting. 7.30 a.m.: Patient was sponged all over with vinegar and water, which made her much cooler and more comfortable. Passed water at 8 a.m. Complains of considerable pain of a burning character during and after micturition. Urine acid, specific gravity 1015, no albumen. 9 a.m.: Pulse 88; temperature 106·5° by Mr. Brooke's thermometer; respirations 72. 10.30 a.m.:

As she was complaining of her head being worse, her temperature was taken, and found to be 108·6° by Dr. Little's thermometer. Her head was sponged with tepid water, and she is now somewhat better. 11.15 a.m.: Had turpentine enema, after which her bowels were twice moved. Motions confined. Feels better since her bowels were moved. Up to 1.30 p.m. has taken half a pint of whey, one cup of tea, half a pint of milk, one cup of beef-tea, and two oranges. 12.45 p.m.: At 12.45 a water-cap consisting of a number of coils of india-rubber piping in connexion with an elevated can of iced water was placed on her head. Is perspiring freely. 2 p.m.: Her temperature was now taken by Dr. Moore, of the Meath Hospital, and found to be 108° by a new (Casella's registered) thermometer from Fannin's. 3 p.m.: Feels much better; has no unpleasant sensation in her head. 3.45 p.m.: As she seemed hot and was rather restless, her temperature was taken by the new thermometer, and found to be 107·4°. Remained quite quiet until 7 p.m., when she had a purgative enema which did not move her bowels. 8.30 p.m.: Has been sponged over, and feels cooler. Has some pain from the right anterior superior iliac crest to the spine and along lower lumbar and sacral vertebræ. 9.14 p.m.: Temperature 107·4° by new thermometer, pulse 108, respirations 68. 9.50 p.m.: Her temperature was taken, and found to be 103·4° by new thermometer. She now got eight minims of Dr. Little's hypodermic solution.

(To be continued.)

SOME NEW FACTS CONECTED WITH THE ACTION OF GERMS IN THE PRODUCTION OF HUMAN DISEASES.

By Dr. GEORGE HARLEY, F.R.S.

Reformed Speling—No Duplicated Consonants except in Personal Names.

CHAPTER II.

THE ETIOLOGY OF THE PERIODICITY OF INFECTIOUS, CONTAGIOUS, AND INOCULABLE DISEASES—GROUNDED ON THE GERM THEORY.

To the reflecting philosophicaly trained mind there apears scarcely anything more surprising than the fact that, in this the last half of the suposed to be enlightened nineteenth century, there should stil exist a disposition among medical writers to atempt to explain al non-self-evident clinical facts, where and whenever legitimate theory is wanting, through the instrumentality of hazy hypotheses. Rather than to seek for their solution among the understood analogous facts abundantly provided for their use in the realms of the sister natural siences. Just as if they imagined it were more desirable to find explanations of obscure natural phenomena in the aërial regions of fancy than to humbly cul them from among already recognised data. This remark has been drawn forth from my having frequently had hazy hypothetical explanations given to me regarding what their authors have almost invariably characterised as the " obscure causes of the periodicity of disease."

To my way of thinking there is nothing realy obscure about the mater. If one only takes the trouble to cast his mental eyes, not only over the whole range of animated nature, but over the Universe at large. For then he sees that one great law of periodicity governs everything. Not alone everything that liveth, but everything that moveth. For the night suxeeds the day. Light folows upon darkness. Sunshine upon shower. The tides eb and flow. Winter comes, and sumer goeth. Just as the leaves bud and the leaves fal. Sleep suxeeds waking. The heart's cavities dilate and contract. The lungs inhale and exhale air. Hunger foloweth upon satiety. The blader fils after having emptied itself, and menstruation obeys periodic law. In fact, every action in nature, as wel as every animal function, is more or les periodic. Why, then, should we wonder at diseases asuming a periodic character, when we, as physiologists, know that every diseased, like every healthy function, is subservient to the same chemico-physical laws? I shal cast al the hypotheses of periodicity entirely on one side as if they never had existed, and at once atempt an explanation of its phenomena on a natural rational basis.

The maner in which I explain the apearance of paroxysmal signs and symptoms, their retrocesion, disapearance, and subsequent recurence after longer or shorter, regular or iregular, intervals of quiesence in Infectious, Contagious, and Inoculable diseases, such as Hooping-cough, Ague, Malarial Jaundice, Hydrophobia, and al kinds of Hectic fevers, is on the grounds that there is, in the patient's body continualy at work, an alternating process of destruction and reproduction of the miasmatic and epizootic germs which produce them. This is not a hypothesis, but a legitimate theory, as wil be presently seen. It is founded upon the suposition that each suxeeding paroxysm is acompanied by a destruction of germs, and that it is not until the germs have again reproduced spawn, rehatched, re-multiplied, and reacumulated in the patient's system to a suficient extent to upset the nervous functions that the paroxysm recurs. This may be said to be the case in Ague, Hooping-cough, Hydrophobia, and Malarial Jaundice. So likewise the rigor which is almost the invariable premonitory sign of germ disease, and precedes the apearance of constitutional disturbance. Such, for example, as ocurs in Smal-pox, Scarlatina, Measles, and the other forms of Exanthematæ. Also in cases of Blood-poisoning, Puerperal fever, and Erysipelas. And in al metastatic and other forms of secondary supurations which are ushered in by rigors. In fact the rigors ocuring in the course of any disease in which supuration is likely to ocur, and which is usualy regarded as a pathognomonic sign of its advent, are al more or les periodic.

Again, atacks of Hectic, which, although usualy ocuring only once, frequently ocur twice, in the twenty-four hours in Tuberculosis, Pyæmia, and Typhoid, are other forms of periodicity, and are closely allied, especialy in having a sweating stage, to the periodic aguish paroxysms of true malarial disease. Now, although it is easy enough to give an explanation of the cause of the quiesent stage after the paroxysm, on the grounds of the destruction of the germs which produced the atack, it is not so easy to tel by what means their destruction was acomplished. Though the mere fact of a quiesent stage suxeeding the paroxysm favors the belief that during the actual paroxysm itself must have been destroyed the agents that excited it.

But whether this is acomplished directly by the paroxysm-exciting germs themselves being destroyed, or it is merely the pabulum necesary for their existence which is got rid of, we know not. In both cases, however, the imediate result would be the same—the germs' anihilation. For, of course, if the germs' food be destroyed, they would, as a natural consequence, perish by starvation. For, be they animal or vegetable, or a mixture of both, it would not be logical to supose that they, any more than four-foot beasts, or forest trees, can exist for beyond a limited period of time without a suply of materials suited to their requirements.

The period, or interval, as it is caled, of quiesence, in my opinion represents the period of the absence of a suficiency of germs from the circulation to cause visible functional disturbance in the host.

As Periodic disease does not usualy abruptly end with the first paroxysm, or even after the first dozen of paroxysms; but only remains for a time in abeyance, and again reapears, we are forced to imagine that it hapens with germs as it hapens with al other animals placed under like circumstances. Namely, that the weakest, as the food gets scarce, sucumb first, and they being swept away before al the food has uterly vanished, the few of the strongest individuals, that chance to be left behind, manage to drag on a miserable half-starved sort of existence until once again "the gras has grown," and they not only find a suficiency for their wants, but enough upon which to increase and multiply. Til at length, as things go on improving, they once again flourish apace, and in course of time become a suficient multitude to re-upset their host's functions, and reinduce another paroxysm. This theory of periodicity is, as seen, an ofshoot of Darwin's grand principle of the "Survivorship of the Fitest." Coupled with the idea of an alternately repeated proces of germ destruction and reproduction. The intervals between the paroxysms must in this way be regarded in the light of merely fresh periods of Incubation. The germs, or germ-egs, which escaped destruction requiring time to propagate their species in suficient numbers to be able once again to throw their host's working gear out of order.

The sweating stages of germ diseases—in Ague, Hectic, and al kinds of fevers—I regard as being due to an efort of nature to eliminate the destroyed germs through the skin along with the sweat. For the sweating stage invariably, we know, precedes amelioration of the symptoms or complete convalesence. Which is in itself a good reason for my suposing that it has something or other to do with the elimination of the agents that produced the atack.

Next, as regards the cause of the longer and shorter intervals of quiesence which exist in the diferent cases of the same periodic disease.

The duration of the intervals between the paroxysms in any given case, I look upon as being directly proportionate, not only to the inherent fecundity of the germs themselves; but also to the rapidity with which the host has the power of reproducing the pabulum requisite for their sustenance. For just as some hapily constituted persons never produce any pabulum at al, and consequently remain inocuous to germ influence, so others again, unfortunately for themselves, poses the power of regenerating it with abnormal facility, and the paroxysmal atacks recur in them with proportionate rapidity. The total cesation of the periodic atacks of germ disease may be said to be due to the total extinction of the germs' pabulum from the system. No food—no germs.

Although I believe that the periodicity of al kinds of epizootic and miasmatic diseases may thus be philosophicaly acounted for, there yet apears to me to be a large clas of nervous periodic diseases lying entirely outside its pale. And as I am not writing for mere writing's sake, but with the view of aiding my litle mite to the great heap of facts which must be colected, analysed, and generalised ere the fabric of Rational Medicine can be firmly fixed on its pedestal. I wil here digres for a minute and say a few words regarding those artificialy producible convulsive periodic diseases which according to the present state of our knowledge canot be explained on the suposition that they are due to the alternate reproduction and destruction of living germs. To wit, the periodic tetanus of strychnia poisoning, and such like.

Strychnia being suposed to be a dead vegetable alkaloid, the convulsions it induces can no more than the periodic convulsive atacks of epilepsy folowing upon injury to the skul be imagined to be due to germs.

I shal cite an example of artificialy induced periodic convulsive disease which presents the question to us in a most unusual and—to me at least—totaly inexplicable light; but which nevertheles, when iluminated by the colateral data, which wil no doubt soon be discovered, may not itself alone be found to be capable of a philosophic interpretation, but be the means of throwing considerable aditional light on the whole theory of the periodicity of disease.

Strange to say, notwithstanding my having performed, and re-performed, the same kind of experiment on precisely the same species of animal, aparently under the identical same circumstances, dozens of times over, I have never on one single ocasion been able to obtain the same result, and consequently there is at present but one way left for me to acount for it. Namely, that it was chiefly due to the posession by the individual experimented upon of a special and rare form of constitutional idiosyncrasy. A suposition which in no wise, however, detracts from the importance of its bearing upon the etiology of the cause of periodicity in certain forms of nervous afections. For, as everyone knows, one positive is worth more than one thousand negative results in the interpretation of a sientific problem. It is, therefore, with feelings of unfeigned pleasure that I submit the facts of the case to the consideration of the learned among my readers. Some of whom perhaps wil be able to find a clue to the physiological as wel as pathological mystery which hangs around the case. Which is as folows:—

On November 5, 1856, at a time when I was, in consequence of Palmer's Rugby murder, specialy engaged in experimentaly studying the physiological and pathological action of strychnia on animal life,[a] I injected under the skin of the back of two perfectly healthy-looking, similarly sized and sexed frogs $\frac{1}{10}$ of a grain of the acetate of strychnia, disolved in distilled water. In four minutes both animals became tetanic. After waiting ten minutes more I injected under the skin of the back of one of them $\frac{1}{10}$ of a grain of

(a) George Harley, "De la Strychnine et de son Mode d'Action," Archiv. Gén. de Méd., 1856, pages 564,79. "Recherches sur Strychnine," Comptes Rendus, xliii., 670.72. "Physiological Action of Strychnia," Lancet, 1856, June 7, 14, and July 12.

wourali poison; and for the sake of distinction I shal cal one frog K, and the other L, and subjoin the results obtained in a tabular form, with the view of making the comparison of the efects produced in the two cases more easy to the reader.

K.—*Frog with Strychnia alone.*	L.—*Frog with Strychnia and Wourali.*
Nov. 5.—In two hours. Frog stil tetanic.	Quite flacid, and seemed dead.
6th.—In twenty hours. Becomes violently tetanic on slightest touch.	Siting up, aparently quite well, and does not become tetanic on being touched.
7th.—Violently tetanic.	Violently tetanic. As the efects of the wourali apeared to have pased of, injected an aditional ⅛ gr. wourali. Became in fifteen minutes flacid and totaly insensible to stimulus.
8th.—Seems quite wel.	Stil flacid and insensible.
9th.—Being Sunday, no observations made.	
10th.—Violently tetanic; cries ocasionaly as if in pain.	so. Injected ¹⁄₁₀ gr. wourali.
11th.—Tetanic.	Flacid; but legs ocasionaly twitch spontaneously, and yet do not twitch when touched.
12th.—Tetanic, as yesterday.	Same state as yesterday; but legs twitch when touched with galvanic forceps.
22nd.—Seems quite wel. Not tetanic when touched.	Seems quite wel. Not tetanic when touched with galvanic forceps.
24th.—Stil apears quite wel.	Again violently tetanic.
28th. Do. do.	Do. do.
Dec. 3. Do. do.	Is stil violently tetanic, and is always found lying on his back, though he is every day turned by me on to his bely.
6th. Do. do.	Apears to be quite wel; not even tetanised when touched, though starts when the dish containing him is taped.
Feb. 14, 1857. Do. do.	Now violently tetanic without any asignable cause to excite the spasm.
16th. Do. do.	Siting up aparently quite wel, but the mere taping the glas jar in which he sits not only makes him start, but throws him into violent tetanic spasms.
18th. Do. do.	At 10 a.m. was found violently tetanic, whereas at one o'clock, three hours later, he apeared perfectly wel, and did not even so much as start when his dish was taped, or himself touched.
25th. Do. do.	Quite wel—aparently—and remained so until— .
Mar. 18. Do. do.	Found violently tetanic from no known cause whatever.
19th. Do. do.	Stil tetanic.
20th. Do. do.	This morning found the frog dead, and what was very extraordinary, stretched out and quite stif as if rigor mortis had set in, while he was yet in a state of tetanic spasm. I never before or since saw an animal whatever remain in the tetanic position after death, beyond a minute or two. A flacid interval always preceding rigor mortis.

Strychnia is, of course, a poison, the very esence of whose nature is to produce periodic disease. For the atacks of tetanic convulsions it produces are never continuous. No mater how severe they may be, there are always quiescent intervals between each recuring spasm. The strange thing in this case, therefore, consists not in the mere fact of

the periodicity; but in the very unusual length of the periods of quiesence, and yet stil more in that of the long duration of the atack of artificial disease induced by one single and smal dose of the toxic agent. The efect of which almost infinitesimal quantity extended over a period of no les than four and a half months, and ultimately only terminated with the death of the animal—which might, or might not, be due to the mere efects of confinement, at the spring season of the year(b)—furnishes the scientifically medical trained mind with ample materials for reflection. As an aid to any ingenious-minded reader who may feel inclined to try and solve the mater, I wil tabulate a few facts which I think ought not to be lost sight of in endeavouring to do so.

1st. Strychnia is a dead alkaloid poison, and the diference in the mode of action between a dead and a living poison is that, while the former can only produce artificial disease and extinguish the life of the individual into whose body it enters, without, however, posesing the power of reproducing itself. The later can not only produce artificial disease and death; but reproduce its species within the precincts of its host.

2nd. Strychnia is suposed to poses a direct deleterious chemical or physical action on the Nervous System through the instrumentality of the blood.

3rd. We have it within our power to make this dead alkaloid (strychnia) cause almost instantaneous death by the very first manifestation of its toxic power—as when it is introduced into the jugular vein; and we have it equaly in our power to defer its action for half an hour or more—by introducing the same quantity into the stomach.

With living germs we have no such controling power.

4th. By introducing strychnia into a healthy animal body in moderate doses, that is to say, those suficient to convulse though not to kil, its power of producing a true periodic form of disease is seen in the greatest perfection. For then it is that each convulsive paroxysm is folowed by a shorter or longer interval of complete quiesence. Making it apear as if the preceding violent tetanic explosion exhausted or destroyed—as in the case of the germs—the materials which produced it, and here, in the case of strychnia too, is required the same element of time to enable the strychnia to regenerate the materials by which it would be re-enabled once more to work up the nervous system into a suficiently oxidisable state as to compel it again to relieve itself by another explosion. Precisely in the same way as the urinary blader, after having expeled its contents, has to wait until it refils before its nerves are again suficiently excited to demand once more the expulsion of its contents.

5th. Strychnia, although a violent and deadly poison to animals, is not only inocuous, but even highly advantageous, to certain low forms of vegetable life. Certain kinds of fungi are, for example, not only not kiled when put into aqueous solutions of strychnia or its salts, but grow and flourish apace in them. Strychnia may therefore be regarded—in certain cases—as a favorer of germ growth. So that its introduction into the animal body may perhaps be the means of favoring, in it, the rapid development of convulsive disease producing germs.

(*To be continued.*)

THE ST. PETERSBURG LYING-IN HOSPITAL.—During the years 1873-76, 8800 women were admitted. There took place 8742 deliveries, 7706 of these being at full time, 807 premature, and 229 abortions. Twins occurred in 203 instances, and triplets in 4. The births were normal in 5651 and pathological in 3091, interference being required in 1660. The forceps were applied 148 times, or 1 in 28·8 primipara, and 1 in 120·8 multipara. Expression of the fœtus was efected 42 times, turning 106 times, and manual removal of the placenta 144 times—the reporter allowing that the interference in this last item was sometimes unnecessary. Perforation and cranioclasis were executed 34 times, narrow pelvis being the cause in 24 cases. The number of deliveries has constantly increased from 1907 in 1873 to 2675 in 1879, while the puerperal mortality has constantly diminished from 6 per hundred in 1873 to 1·3 per hundred in 1879. This favourable result has been brought about by the enforcement of prophylactic rules.—*St. Petersb. Med. Woch.,* October 15.

(b) Almost al the frogs that have been kept in confinement during the winter months die in the spring of the year.

A CASE OF
REMOVAL OF THE UTERINE APPENDAGES FOR THE ARREST OF HÆMORRHAGE
DUE TO A MYOMA.
By LAWSON TAIT, F.R.C.S.

MRS. B., aged thirty-five, was brought to me on October 18, 1880, in a condition of extreme anæmia. She had been married thirteen years, but had never been pregnant, and had been perfectly regular till three months previously. At that time hæmorrhage began to occur every ten or twelve days, and became very profuse. Dr. Somerville, of Bloxwich, recognised the presence of a pelvic tumour, and, finding all his efforts to arrest the loss were in vain, he brought her to me. I found a multinodular myoma as large as the head of a full-time fœtus, and I advised the removal of the uterine appendages. This was at once agreed to, and, with the assistance of Mr. Raffles Harmar and Dr. Somerville, I performed the operation on October 26, 1880. Both ovaries were cystic, and were removed without much difficulty. The tubes were cut off close to the uterus. Owing to the extreme condition of anæmia to which the hæmorrhage had reduced her, the recovery was very slow, and she did not return home till November 20, and even after that for some weeks her permanent recovery seemed doubtful. She had the appearance of menstruation usual after the operation, but has never menstruated since. In January, 1881, she began to gain strength, and improved so rapidly that she was soon able to conduct the laborious work of her business as the keeper of a butcher's shop. I saw her on October 11, the first time since her recovery, and I completely failed to recognise her when she presented herself. She is in perfect and robust health, and her sexual functions are wholly uninterfered with. The tumour seems to be about one-third of the size which it was at the time of the operation.
Birmingham.

HYPODERMIC INJECTION IN SCIATICA.—M. Lereboullet employs the following injection:—Chlorhydrate of morphia thirty centigrammes, neutral sulphate of atropia two centigrammes, distilled water ten grammes. Half a Pravaz's syringe full is to be injected every six hours (until relief is obtained) into the cellular tissues of the posterior surface of the thigh, from opposite the sciatic notch to the popliteal space. Relief is in this way rapidly obtained, without any of the accidents so often produced by intolerance of morphia.—Union Méd., November 22.

CASE OF APHASIA.—M. Chauffard relates in the France Médicale a curious case. A man sixty-five years of age was admitted with decided aphasia, coming on after an attack of apoplexy. He was able to give his name and address correctly, but was unable to indicate his profession, or to pronounce a connected sentence, a word, a substantive continually failing him, notwithstanding great efforts to recover it. His writing was as hesitating as his speech, and his cerebral energy soon came to a stop. When interrogated urgently, which led to his making great efforts, he was seized with another cerebral attack, whence he emerged still more weak and with the aphasia aggravated, complaining also of a continuous and severe pain at the left fronto-parietal region. Under the influence of absolute rest and some purgatives, with bromide and iodide of potassium in small doses, his general condition somewhat improved, but the cerebral activity remained defective, the patient speaking as if the language was not familiar to him; although his expressions were just and correct, and there being scarcely any lacunæ in his vocabulary. On the other hand, all intellectual effort was impossible, and led to cerebral fatigue and failure. M. Chauffard observes that two points are deducible from this case: first, that the subjects of aphasia should not be fatigued by too minute or too prolonged examination, under the penalty of producing a new cerebral attack, especially in those in whom the aphasia seems connected with a localised thrombosis or a faulty "cortical irrigation"; and next, never to forget in our Prognosis that the patient may well-nigh recover the use of his speech, but that he is still always under the imminence of new accidents which may prove promptly fatal.—Rev. Méd., November 12.

REPORTS OF HOSPITAL PRACTICE
IN
MEDICINE AND SURGERY.

EAST LONDON HOSPITAL FOR CHILDREN.

TWO CASES OF TETANUS NEONATORUM.
Case 2.—Tetanus—Treatment by Calabar Bean—Death—Autopsy.
(Under the care of Mr. PARKER.)

JOHN F., aged one week, was admitted into the hospital on October 11 of this year, and died on the following day.
Family History.—The mother had had five children; the two eldest children are alive and well, the others died in early infancy. There had been four miscarriages. There did not appear to have been any very active or obvious signs of syphilis.
Previous History of Patient.—When born, the arms were noticed to be stiff; they could not be flexed. For a day it had sucked without much difficulty; then the milk was seen to run out of its mouth, as if it could not swallow it. It began also at this time to have slight spasms (it was two-days old). The spasms were immediately set up on putting the nipple to the mouth. The navel-string fell off on the fifth day early; a few hours later, the first series of spasms began, and it was quite unable to swallow any milk. At this period it was brought to the hospital.
Present Condition.—The cranial bones present no abnormality. The child lies with the eyelids screwed up. Its mouth is not quite closed; any attempt to open it wider brings on a tetanic spasm. There is no risus sardonicus. When stripped, the child's body is seen covered over with hæmorrhagic flea-bites. The umbilicus is slightly red and inflamed; there is no discharge from it. There are no marks of violence or sores of any kind about the body. The limbs are rigid and outstretched, the legs rather less so than the arms; the hands are clenched. The abdominal and thoracic walls are also rigid during the spasm, but they partially relax after the spasm has passed. The limbs never quite relax during the intervals of the spasms. The spasms are of short duration (quarter to half a minute), and affect the whole body at once; they recur very rapidly, and the slightest touch suffices to set them up. Respiration is quite arrested during the spasm. There is no opisthotonus.
Treatment.—A hot bath was ordered at once; several spasms occurred during the bath. Afterwards the spasms occurred less often for a while. One-sixth of a grain of Calabar-bean extract was ordered to be given every half-hour until some physiological effect was produced. At 3 p.m. (four hours after admission) it was noted that the spasms were occurring at longer intervals, but that they seemed quite as severe. When milk was put into the mouth it was not swallowed, but came out again at the angles of the mouth. 6 p.m. to 10 p.m.: The Calabar bean is now to be given every hour. The improvement has become more marked; the eyes are opened, and food can be swallowed. 11 p.m.: A warm bath was again given. Some spasms occurred during the bath, and a few others followed, but at midnight they had ceased entirely.
October 12.—½ to 3 a.m.: The child seemed to be doing well, taking its nourishment rather greedily, when the spasms again recurred. 4.30 a.m.: The child died of asphyxia during a spasm.
From 10 p.m. until 4 a.m., the Calabar bean was given every two hours. So that, altogether, about three grains of the extract (B.P.) were administered in the fifteen or sixteen hours during which the child was under observation. As regards the physiological effect of Calabar bean, there were two or three periods of comparative quietness: but it would be difficult to say that the spasms, when they occurred, were less strong; perspiration was increased slightly. The eyelids being closed, it was not possible to record the state of the pupils. The child never once cried while it was in the hospital.
Temperatures.—The temperature on admission (about noon, October 11) was 103·8° Fahr., 102·8° at 4 p.m., 99° at 6 p.m., 100° at 8 p.m., 100·8° at 10 p.m., 100·4° at midnight.

October 12: 101·6° at 2 a.m., 102·4° at 4 a.m., 101·4° at 4.30 a.m., when death occurred.

Post-mortem Examination (twelve hours after death).— There was no rigor mortis. Lungs were healthy, but collapsed in part. Heart: Left side empty and contracted; right side full of blood. Liver was healthy, and weighed four ounces and a half. The umbilical vein was partially closed between the umbilicus and the liver; it contained loose, healthy-looking clot, not yet wholly decolourised. The two hypogastric arteries presented similar appearances. Spleen, healthy. Kidneys: The lobules still quite distinct. When cut into, the cortex appeared very thin; at the bases of the cones, which were conspicuously marked out by congestion, the cortex was hardly a quarter of an inch thick. Skull: Nothing remarkable about the bones. The pia mater was not even congested. There were no meningeal hæmorrhages anywhere. The ventricles did not contain any excess of fluid; the brain substance was soft, but otherwise appeared normal. Pons and medulla normal. Spinal cord: On opening the spinal canal, the loose connective tissue around the cord was found to be ecchymosed in patches from the middle to the lower end of the dorsal portion of the cord. On opening the spinal dura mater, the pia mater did not present any unusual appearance; it did not appear abnormally congested. The cord itself was firm to the touch. On cutting into it, its grey matter was clearly mapped out by its pinkish colour, when compared with the white substance. There were no extravasations into its substance at any point. (The nerve-centres were preserved for microscopic examination, and will be more fully reported on elsewhere.)

Remarks (by Mr. Parker).—The result of the autopsy does not throw much light on the *pathology* of this fatal malady. Meigs and Pepper state that the brain and meninges are frequently "intensely congested," and that "even an actual effusion of blood, either between the skull and dura mater, into the arachnoid cavity, or into the ventricles," may occur. "In some cases, instead of hæmorrhage, there has been found serous effusion, with a diminution of consistence of the cerebral substance." In my case I was struck by the total absence of all congestion; even the choroid plexuses were empty. The brain substance was certainly soft, but whether because of "serous effusion" into its substance or not, I cannot say. Even if meningeal apoplexies were constantly found after death, it would be difficult to prove that they were the cause of death, and not due to the circulatory disturbance which the tetanus brings about. (*A propos* of meningeal congestion, I may just mention that the head was examined last, after the other organs had been removed. I have constantly noticed that this influences the amount of "congestion" in the head.) There was nothing to support Dr. Marion Sims's view that the tetanus "is a disease of centric origin . . . . the result of displacement of the occipital bone."

Rarity of the Disease.—To judge from recorded cases, infantile tetanus is exceedingly rare in this country. I believe that only one other case, besides the two now recorded, have been observed (and that was by Dr. Eustace Smith) in this hospital since its foundation, thirteen years ago. Dr. West only records one case observed in London during his long experience. When we bear in mind, however, how many infants die of "convulsions" who are not seen by skilled observers, it would seem just possible that some cases die unrecorded and unrecognised. And yet most of the conditions which are supposed to favour its onset prevail *par excellence* in London. Thus draughts and variations of temperature, impure air and surroundings, among general causes, while cases of unskilful and rough treatment of the navel-string by incompetent midwives, and various kinds of bodily injury, as possible local causes, are matters of constant occurrence among the patients of a children's hospital.

As regards *the period of onset*, in this case the mother stated distinctly that the arms were rigid from the birth, and that "something was wrong with the sucking." Authors vary a little on this point—from the third to the tenth day. The average age appears to be about three or four days. Dr. West speaks of a case which commenced fifteen hours after birth, while in two others it commenced on the fifth and sixth days respectively. I find no mention made of congenital tetanus, though if the history of this case can be relied on, rigidity commenced at a very early period of life, while the general attack was marked on the second day.

Causation.—The house and the room in which this patient was born were squalid in the extreme, as were its immediate surroundings. The mother only had the assistance of a midwife during her confinement, but it was an easy one in all respects, and I could not gather that the infant had received any fall or been subject to cold or in any way neglected. When first seen there was some redness about its umbilicus, but it was quite superficial and did not appear to affect either the umbilical vein or the hypogastric arteries, for the clot in these vessels was healthy. The child was very dirty, as were its clothes. Dr. Joseph Clarke, while Master of the Dublin Lying-in Hospital, where "sixty years ago every sixth child born in that institution died within a fortnight after birth, and trismus was the cause of the death of nineteen-twentieths of these children" (quoted from Dr. West's book), became impressed with the view that dirt and defects of ventilation were the prime causes of the disease. On adopting means to secure efficient ventilation, the mortality from this cause very considerably decreased. Similar experience has been made in other lying-in hospitals. I now very much regret that I did not examine the blood of this patient both during life and after death. For the above facts, together with the epidemic character of this disease, as well as of the traumatic form, suggest a micro-zootic origin. Tetanus often occurs during war-time epidemically, especially in hot climates; zymotic disease is usually present in an aggravated form at the same time. It is not a little remarkable that infantile tetanus is also most common in the same regions, and that it too occurs in epidemics. I have no means of knowing whether zymotic fevers prevail at the same time as epidemic tetanus in civil practice, but think it extremely probable that they do.

THE CROCODILES AT THE JARDIN DES PLANTES.—It will be recollected that, some time since, ten crocodiles which were presented to Prof. Paul Bert were placed in the Jardin des Plantes until he had leisure to make an examination of them. Five of these animals have now been dissected, and Prof. Bert has found that the encephalic mass is insignificant in the crocodile, whence it may be inferred that they are devoid of intelligence. The assistants of the Professor had an unexpected treat in dining off crocodile, which proved excellent meat, a little musky, and having some flavour of salmon. It seems that the tail is the most delicate part of the animal. Five of the crocodiles are still living in the Jardin in a state of repletion, not having as yet partaken of any food. In the intestinal canal of their dissected companions some fish, belonging to the species found in the marshes of the Nile, were discovered absolutely intact.—*Union Méd.*, November 17.

HYPODERMIC INJECTIONS OF HYDROCHLORATE OF MORPHIA IN INSANITY.—Dr. Voisin, of the Salpêtrière, has published twenty-seven cases of insanity so treated, in addition to those which he published in 1874, and repeats the statement then made, that these injections have furnished the most satisfactory results. In this second memoir he calls attention to the importance of combating the neuralgic pains met with in the insane, experience having shown that a good number of these patients called hypochondriacs become, after a period of more or less years, the subjects of organic cerebral or spinal affections, the evolution of which would have been prevented had the pains been effectually treated. The new cases are almost all examples of lypemaniac insanity. They are the depressive forms of insanity, and especially those which have been preceded by anæmia and asthenia, that are most amenable to the morphia treatment, which is also very efficacious in hysterical insanity. It is not suitable for acute cases unless no secondary changes have occurred in the vessels and cells, and when the cerebral substance and the membranes are not hyperæmic. The doses required are very variable, for while in some patients very large doses may be given without any physiological or therapeutical effect being produced, in others very feeble doses are not tolerated. Thus, one patient received daily in two injections two grammes without any ill effect; another could not receive the tenth of a milligramme without vomiting during the whole day. It is of importance to know that any patient improving under this form of treatment becomes less and less tolerant of the remedy, the intolerance thus becoming a favourable symptom.—*Gaz. des Hop.*, Sept. 24.

TERMS OF SUBSCRIPTION.
(Free by post.)

British Islands	. . . .	*Twelve Months*	.	£1 8	0
"	"	*Six*	"	. 0 14	0
The Colonies and the United }	*Twelve*	"	. 1 10	0
States of America . . . }					
"	"	*Six*	"	. 0 15	0
India	*Twelve*	"	. 1 10	0
" *(viâ Brindisi)* . . .	"	"	. 1 15	0
" *Six*	"	"	. 0 15	0
" *(viâ Brindisi)*	"	"	. 0 17	6

*Foreign Subscribers are requested to inform the Publishers of
any remittance made through the agency of the Post-office.*

*Single Copies of the Journal can be obtained of all Booksellers
and Newsmen, price Sixpence.*

*Cheques or Post-office Orders should be made payable to Mr.
James Lucas, 11, New Burlington-street, W.*

TERMS FOR ADVERTISEMENTS.

Seven lines (70 words)	. . .	.£0 4	6
Each additional line (10 words)	.	. 0 0	6
Half-column, or quarter-page	.	. 1 5	0
Whole column, or half-page	.	. 2 10	0
Whole page	. . . . .	. 5 0	0

Births, Marriages, and Deaths are inserted Free of Charge.

*The Medical Times and Gazette is published on Friday
morning: Advertisements must therefore reach the Publishing Office not later than One o'clock on Thursday.*

Medical Times and Gazette.

SATURDAY, DECEMBER 3, 1881.

THE GENERAL MEDICAL COUNCIL.

The Executive Committee of the General Medical Council
met on November 11. The official notifications of the
appointments of the following members of the General
Council were received:—Dr. Pitman, as Representative of
the Royal College of Physicians of London, for five years
from May 16; Thomas Collins, Esq., as Representative of
the Apothecaries' Hall of Ireland, for one year from
August 1, in place of Dr. Leet; Dr. Aquilla Smith, as Representative of the King and Queen's College of Physicians
in Ireland, for one year from October 18; and Dr. Storrar, as
Representative of the University of London, for one year
from October 27. Dr. Pitman and Dr. Aquilla Smith were
elected members of the Executive Committee; and then
the names of sixty-eight persons were restored to the
Medical Register, from which they had been erased
in conformity with the provisions of Section 14 of the
Medical Act. Such a list shows how negligent the members
of the profession are in observing the legal requirements
for continuance on the Register. We have called attention
to the importance of their notifying any change of address to
the Registrar by whom they were registered. This is absolutely necessary to secure the accuracy of the Register, and
neglect of it may, and, as is seen, often does, lead to names
being struck off. Then, men who have brought the punishment
upon themselves are—unjustifiably, though perhaps not unnaturally—surprised and indignant. The Committee were
next occupied in considering the applications of eighteen
persons for permission, in various exceptional circumstances, to be registered as medical students. Sixteen
of the applications were acceded to. Some of them were
rather remarkable. One gentleman had passed a preliminary examination at Oxford in all the subjects required
by the Council in 1857, and now desires to enter the profession; and another, more than fifty years of age, had passed

an examination in Latin, English, and Mathematics prior to
his receiving a commission as ensign in the late East India
Company's Service. In reply to a communication on the
subject, the Committee resolved—"That a University student
desiring not to pass in Natural Philosophy as an optional
subject at his preliminary examination, must, at that examination, pass in some other one of the optional subjects
named in the Regulations."

As regards dental business, applications were received
from dental apprentices, whose articles commenced at
various dates from July 10, 1876, to June 28, 1878, requesting to be allowed to be registered pursuant to the provisions of Section 37 of the Dentists Act (1878); and
the Committee resolved that those students who had completed their apprenticeship before January, 1880, be admitted to the Register, and that the rest be recommended
to apply to one or other of the licensing bodies for examination. The Committee further directed the Registrar to
suggest to the licensing authorities in dentistry whether it
may not be desirable to admit to examination, under conditions more or less exceptional, those students whose apprenticeship began before the passing of the Dentists Act, and
did not terminate before January 1, 1880. The tenderness
of the Committee towards their dental subjects and friends
must strike everyone. It shows itself in all ways. Several
applications were before the Committee from persons who
alleged that they had been deterred from making or proceeding with applications for dental registration, when such
registration was open, owing to erroneous advice as to who
were entitled to be registered under the Act; and requesting
permission to be now placed on the Register. The general
fitness of these applicants may be guessed from the fact
that one of them stated that he was, and we suppose is still,
"engaged in business as a jeweller." But the Committee
are ready to consider even the openly-avowed jeweller's
application, only asking for a little more information
as to the nature of his dental practice; and the other
cases were "deferred for further consideration." Probably
this hesitation to at once admit the applicants to the
congenial society to be found in the Dentists' Register
may have been due only to want of time; but it may, perhaps, have been accentuated—to employ a pet phrase of
medical writers at present—by a letter received from that
troublesome body the Representative Board of the British
Dental Association; which letter led the Committee to place
"the several documents and legal opinions in the possession
of the Council, having reference to registration under the
Dentists Act," in the hands of Mr. William James Farrer,
the newly appointed Solicitor to the General Council, in
order that he may further advise the Committee thereon.

THE EXCISION OF THE CANCEROUS UTERUS.

The Royal Medical and Chirurgical Society discussed at
their last meeting the most recent triumph of British
surgery, viz., the successful removal of the cancerous gravid
uterus. The operation had been performed before, but each
time with a fatal result; although, as former operators had
not published their cases, the fact was not known to the bold
surgeon who undertook the responsibility of the case we
speak of. To him, therefore, belongs the credit of originality,
if not of priority; and his operation is, without doubt, the
first that has proved successful.

Cases such as the one operated upon are so rare, that with
regard to them alone we should have little more to say than
to congratulate the profession upon possessing a surgeon
with the courage to undertake, and the skill to successfully
carry out, an operation of such magnitude, difficulty, and
risk. Whatever doubts might have been entertained befor

the operation as to its justifiability are now set at rest. Mr. Wells has shown that the cancerous gravid uterus can be excised with success; and given another case similar in all respects to the one on which he operated, anyone with competent skill in abdominal surgery will now be fully justified in performing the same operation.

Pregnancy, however, with cancer of the cervix uteri is rare, and with cancer of the body of the uterus impossible. When pregnancy occurs with cancer of the cervix, it is seldom that the surgeon is consulted at the precise period at which this operation is suitable: the time, viz., when the disease has advanced so far that it cannot be got rid of by merely amputating the vaginal portion, and yet has not advanced into the tissues which adjoin the uterus. Even Mr. Wells, with his wide-reaching reputation, may never see another case.

Cancer of the uterus, without pregnancy, is so common, so fatal, and so little amenable to treatment, that anything which promises a cure demands most careful consideration. The extirpation of the cancerous uterus has been performed largely abroad, and taking the cases all together, the results have not been encouraging. When we find that 90 per cent. have either died immediately from the operation, or from a speedy return of the disease for which it was done; and that the 10 per cent. who recovered have not as yet been watched more than two or three years at the outside, so that it is possible that in them relapse may yet take place; we should, unless we can find circumstances which give reason to hope for improved results, be driven to condemn the operation.

There are, however, important differences in the kind of cancer affecting the uterus, and in the seat of such cancer. Secondary infection of internal organs is known to be less frequent in cancer of the uterus than with most other kinds of cancer; and we know that with some kinds of uterine cancer such infection is more common than with others. But the criteria which we at present possess for clinically predicting the probability of constitutional infection are very insufficient. This is one direction in which we think advance is needed. We want to distinguish cases in which the disease is so far constitutional that relapse may be expected, from those in which we may fairly hope that it is entirely local.

Cancer of the uterus is not only met with in different forms, but affecting different parts of the uterus. It may affect the body of the womb, in which case it can be effectively treated in no other way than by excision of the whole organ. It may grow as a warty papillary growth from the vaginal portion of the cervix, so that by amputation of this part we may reasonably hope to free the patient from her disease, and consequently that operation becomes here the proper one to perform. But the most frequent cases are those in which the malady, beginning either in the cervical canal or near the external os, forms a tumour apparently in the substance of the cervix, spreads up to the os internum, downward along the vaginal wall, and around into the cellular tissue. It is these cases which form the debateable ground for Freund's operation. The difficulty is mainly a diagnostic one. Where we have simply more or less irregular swelling of the cervix, without fixation, the diagnosis of cancer is so open to doubt, that the physician hesitates to advise an operation so dangerous as extirpation of the uterus until he is certain. The sign which makes him sure of the correctness of his opinion— viz., the advance of the disease to the surrounding parts, and consequent loss of mobility of the uterus—is, as Dr. Playfair pointed out in the discussion, the condition which contra-indicates operation. And in these cases the disease sometimes advances with terrible rapidity. Dr. Playfair and Mr. Knowsley Thornton both narrated cases in which

the physician first consulted had felt doubtful, either as to the nature of the disease, or as to the propriety of undertaking so grave an operation for disease so limited in extent; and when, after only such an interval as was necessary for arranging a consultation, the advice of some one else was obtained, the disease had so quickly spread that any attempt at operation was inadmissible.

In cancer of the cervix, therefore, it is only when the disease is in an early stage that the operation of Freund is admissible. In such cases it comes into competition with the different methods of removing the new growth per vaginam. It has long been recognised that it was sound practice to remove cancerous disease of the cervix uteri either by écraseur, scissors, scoop, or caustic, whenever it could be certainly diagnosed and the removal safely done; and operations of this kind have been familiar to gynæcologists for years. Dr. Marion Sims has described the way in which he does this, but his method has nothing in it novel except that he—using the knife first, and then caustic —removes more tissue than most people formerly thought safe. The result of Dr. Sims's operations at Vienna goes to show that the older opinions were fairly correct. Mr. Spencer Wells showed at the meeting a slough which had come away from a uterus on which Dr. Sims had operated, and which comprised nearly the whole uterus, including a bit of its peritoneal covering. After this severe and radical treatment the disease recurred.

At present we think the cases in which Freund's operation is justified are very few. In the future it may be otherwise; but what we want before it can be generally adopted, is knowledge which will help us to the following desiderata: more certainty in the diagnosis of uterine cancer in its early stages; a sharper distinction between the form of that disease which is local in kind and limited in extent, and the variety which tends to spread deeply and soon infect the system; and a lower death-rate from the operation itself. The latter, no doubt, will come with increased experience, but without knowledge as to the other points we have named, the operator's hopes will continually be frustrated by the occurrence of relapse.

"GASTRO-ENTEROSTOMY."

UNDER the above title we hear of a new operation from Germany, performed for the first time by Dr. Anton Wölfler, who is Professor Billroth's assistant, and afterwards by that distinguished surgeon himself. The operation (an account of which will be found in the Centralblatt für Chirurgie for November 12) appears to have been devised on the spur of the moment, after an exploratory incision had been made into the abdomen of a man who was suffering from cancer of the pylorus, and in whom the operation for removal of the tumour proved to be impossible. It consisted in making an incision into the stomach near the middle of the great curvature, and a similar cut into a coil of small intestine, we presume as near as possible to the commencement of the jejunum, and carefully sewing to one another the margins of the two openings thus formed. The object of the operation is thus twofold—in the first place, to allow the materials swallowed to pass into the intestine; and in the second place, to prevent any obstruction to the escape of the biliary and pancreatic secretions. Strict antiseptic precautions, "with the exception of the use of the spray," were observed during the operation, and not only did healing take place without any fever and by first intention, but the patient experienced very marked relief, and at the time of the report had survived the operation nearly four weeks. Not only had he survived, but a marked improvement had taken place in his symptoms:

the vomiting had stopped, and he had been able to take increasing quantities, first of liquid, and afterwards of solid food. He had also had daily evacuations of the bowels, the stools being firm and brown.

Billroth's case was also one of a cancer of the pylorus too far advanced for removal. The operation was apparently carried out in the same way; it was easy of performance, and lasted only an hour. The patient, however, was seized with biliary vomiting, which continued till he died on the tenth day. An explanation of the vomiting was found post-mortem: there was not peritonitis; but the result of drawing the intestine towards the stomach had been to form a spur which divided the opening between the two viscera into two unequal parts, the larger of which communicated with the proximal portion of the intestine. The result of this was that the bile and pancreatic secretion, instead of passing into the intestine, were poured into the stomach, and the consequence was that which has been described. The author points out the necessity of making sure, to begin with, which is the proximal and which the distal portion of the coil of intestine selected, and then taking care that a thoroughly free communication shall exist between the latter and the stomach, while the former shall be, in a way, valved by making the stomach-wall overlap it. He also suggests that this method of procedure may possibly prove of value in cases of malignant growths in connexion with the intestine.

THE WEEK.
TOPICS OF THE DAY.

FEW forms of food find more favour among the lower orders than sausages; and, unfortunately, in no other article of diet can sophistication be more successfully resorted to. The Poplar District Board of Works have recently instituted a searching investigation into the circumstances under which the manufacture of " German " sausages is carried on, this industry forming one of the principal features of the locality over which the Board presides. A report has accordingly been issued, in which it is stated that, from inquiries made in the Metropolitan Meat Market and other places, horse-flesh is largely used in the manufacture of these German sausages, and there can be no doubt, even if the flesh is sound, as far as regards its freshness, that as the horse is commonly slaughtered on account of either age or disease, it cannot be considered fit for human food. The Poplar Board have therefore determined to employ an extra staff of officials for the purpose of inspecting the sausage manufactories, and all other places in their district where food is sold or manufactured for human consumption, with a view of suppressing the issue of unwholesome compositions, if possible to detect the use of horseflesh in the making of German sausages, and to bring the offenders to justice. It would appear that the regulations enforced at horse-slaughtering establishments in London make it impossible that they are the sources of supply to the sausage-makers; but suspicion is directed to certain persons who are known and described as horse-dealers and cattle-dealers. It is from them that the flesh is supposed to be obtained, as they slaughter clandestinely, but do not themselves boil down the flesh or prepare the other parts of the animal for their respective uses. The Metropolitan Board of Works, as the "local authority" in the metropolis, the Commissioners of the City, and the various local boards around London, have been urgently invited to use increased energy, with a view to discover, if possible, any persons who may be supplying the flesh of horses or other animals unfit for food to sausage manufactories; and a representation has also been made to the Local Government Board, to the effect that such manufactories should by law be placed under strict supervision, in order to secure the examination of all material intended for conversion into sausages.

At the last meeting of the Metropolitan Board of Works a report was brought up from the Works Committee, recommending that the reservoirs at the Crossness Pumping Station and Barking Outfall Works be enlarged, at an estimated cost of £160,000, and that it be referred to the Finance Committee to see that proper provision be made in the Board's Money Bill of next session for meeting the contemplated expenditure. Mr. Dalton moved the adoption of the report, and explained that the enlargement of the reservoirs was most desirable, because, owing to the main sewers being charged with an increased amount of sewage, it was found impossible at times to discharge all the sewage at the ebb-tide. As a consequence, some of it flowed back into the sewers again. By making the extension proposed, the reservoirs could be made to hold the largest quantity of sewage that could be received. The report was ultimately agreed to. Somewhat singularly, it is authoritatively stated that the Port of London Sanitary Committee intend to represent to the Government the urgency of the sewer outfalls being removed further down the river. The Government will, therefore, have to decide the question raise by the two public bodies.

An increase in the efficiency of the Birmingham Lunatic Asylum is likely to result from an inquiry which has been recently held as to the death of one of the inmates. From the evidence adduced, it appears that deceased was admitted into the Asylum, and on the following day his wife visited him, and found him unconscious, and disfigured with bruises on the face and body. It was also stated that he had been kicked about the body by an attendant named Hughes. Mr. Gamgee, who had made a post-mortem examination, said that the immediate cause of death was inflammation of the bowels, and a shock caused by rupture of the bladder, which might have been due to a kick or fall; there was a bruise on the back which he described as about the size of the toe of an average boot. Under certain conditions, such a blow, if inflicted by a kick, would probably cause rupture. Two witnesses, formerly inmates of the Asylum, stated that they had seen Hughes strike the deceased. The official report made by Hughes was simply " David Pullman : nose bruised, caused by a fall in a struggle with the attendant." The Coroner having summed up, the jury returned a verdict of manslaughter against the attendant Hughes, coupled with a censure of the medical staff for their negligence; which was, however, to some extent excusable, owing to the inadequacy of the present medical staff for so large an institution, there being only two officers for 683 patients. The jury expressed a strong feeling as to the necessity for an increase, both in the medical staff and in the number of attendants, and recommended that there should be a further inquiry into the case by the Lunacy Commissioners.

The Sanitary Inspector to the Whitechapel Board of Works recently reported a somewhat novel nuisance in his district. He stated that he had received a complaint from the Surveyor of Her Majesty's Customs, stationed at the St. Katharine Docks, as to enormous consignments of tortoises, which gave rise to an unbearable stench. There was a large number of barrels containing dead, as well as dying and live tortoises, which had been allowed by the consignees to remain on the quays for some weeks, without being fetched away. The heads and legs of the tortoises projected from the holes left in the barrels for the purpose of ventilation, and the creatures were so tightly wedged together that great numbers of them died. A similar nuisance had also been found to exist in a cellar in Old-street, beneath a milk-shop, and in another underground apartment in Wentworth-street, Mile-end New Town, where small land tortoises were stored in thousands. Major Munro said this nuisance arose from commercial transactions in the Port of London, and the only thing the Board could do was to put in force, as far as possible, the powers of the Act for the Prevention of Cruelty to Animals.

The Peabody Trustees were recently summoned, at the instance of the parish authorities of St. Giles's and St. George's, Bloomsbury, for allowing certain premises owned by them in Chapel-place, and Marchmont-place, Brunswick-square, to be a nuisance and unfit for habitation. The District Surveyor deposed that the buildings in question were ruinous, filthy, badly ventilated, and had defective drainage; there was no water-supply, and all the sanitary arrangements were very defective. The premises were extremely unhealthy, unfit for human habitation, and quite incapable of being made so. Dr. Lovell, Medical Officer of Health, entirely agreed with the evidence given by the previous witness. There had been twenty cases of typhus and typhoid fever in these houses during the past few months, and four deaths had resulted. The houses, he thought, ought to be shut up at once. Mr. Lea, who appeared for the Trustees, said they were not really responsible for the state of things described. They acquired the freehold of the buildings some time since, and finding it quite impossible to alter their condition, an arrangement was made with the Metropolitan Board of Works to enforce the provisions of the Artisans' Dwellings Act, but the Home Secretary would not grant an order for the demolition of the houses until there was a batch of fifteen. It would not be long before this number was reached, and the whole of the buildings would then be demolished, and the ordinary blocks of Peabody Buildings would be erected in their place. Eventually the magistrate made an order that the houses should not be used for habitation until further notice.

A very sad and startling case of poisoning by misadventure, by which no less than three children met their deaths, was investigated by Sir John Humphreys, Coroner of East Middlesex, on Saturday last. The mothers of the children, two of which belonged to one family, had gone to the surgery of Dr. Harvey, of Poplar, for medicine for their children, and in each case received powders to be administered; these were duly given, the result being that serious symptoms shortly supervened, and although a Dr. Cross promptly attended at both of the houses, and the stomach-pump was promptly used, all three of the sufferers succumbed. Edward Cavan stated that he acted as assistant to Dr. Harvey. He sold the powders in question, which he believed must have consisted of morphia. In the surgery was a cupboard in which only poisons were kept, and the morphia was supposed to be kept in that cupboard. The bottle containing the morphia was of the same size and colour as the one in which the cooling powder was kept; he had previously been using the morphia, and pushed that bottle along the counter for the shop-boy to replace in the cupboard, but he must have neglected to do this, and have placed it on the shelf with the ordinary bottles. Some of the labels on the bottles were illegible, and this was the case with the label on the bottle containing the cooling powder. Dr. Cross deposed to having been summoned to all three patients; in each case he used the stomach-pump, and everything was done that was possible, but the children died shortly afterwards from the effects of poisoning by morphia. The jury, after a short deliberation, returned in all the cases a verdict of "Death by misadventure"; and added that they considered Mr. Cavan deserved grave censure for not exercising greater carefulness. They also recommended Dr. Harvey to have his poisons put up in bottles clearly distinguishable from all others, and Dr. Harvey promised to comply with their suggestion.

The reports of the Medical Officer of Health for Sandown show that that portion of the Isle of Wight has enjoyed an exceptionally low death-rate during the present year. The report for the quarter ended June 30 last gave a rate of mortality of only 5 in the 1000 on the year; and he further states that during the September quarter it was still but 6·4 per 1000. The Registrar-General has also made special reference to Sandown as having the lowest death-rate of any town reported since 1832. This is considered in Sandown to be an answer to the reports of a contrary character made by Dr. Ballard, Inspector to the Local Government Board, at the beginning of the summer.

The Medical Acts Commission met at Victoria-street, Westminster, on the 18th, 19th, and 22nd ult. Evidence was given by Dr. Quain and by Mr. F. W. Crick (Medical Herbalists' Association). There were present the Earl of Camperdown (Chairman), the Bishop of Peterborough, the Right Hon. W. H. F. Cogan (the Master of the Rolls), the Right Hon. G. Sclater-Booth, M.P., Sir William Jenner, Mr. Simon, C.B., Professor Huxley, Dr. McDonnell, Professor Turner, and the Secretary.

THE ROYAL COMMISSION ON THE MEDICAL ACTS.

WE understand that the Royal Commission on the Medical Acts will meet once more before the end of the year, but that it is not at present intended to call further witnesses. The Commission will probably arrange to assemble again about Easter, and not earlier; so that we need not look for their report until some time after the meeting of Parliament.

THE ST. BARTHOLOMEW'S INQUEST.

AFTER repeated adjournments, the coroner's jury which sat with regard to the death of a medical man who was carried to St. Bartholomew's Hospital in a dying condition, but was not instantaneously admitted, has come to an end. The Hospital authorities, as is usual in such cases, did not get off clear from blame; but, as far as we know, no blame was reflected on two—estimable, doubtless, but excited—men who imagined that it was the usual course of things to have house-physician, nurse, and porter all waiting for their arrival with their patient. Perhaps it might not have been mal à propos to suggest that these gentlemen erred in insisting on the removal of a patient already in the jaws of death, but with regard to whose maladies they seemed to know little. We cannot commend the mode of receiving in-patients at St. Bartholomew's; but two and two do not make five.

THE YELLOW FEVER AT BARBADOS.

ACCORDING to latest accounts, the yellow fever has become localised at Gun Hill, the station at which the troops had been placed in camp in order to avoid it, nine deaths having occurred among them within a few days previous to their embarkation on H.M.S. Orontes, on 26th ult., for their complete withdrawal from the island, and transfer to England. It is stated by the civil practitioners that the disease is disappearing from Bridgetown, and is now confined to the country districts. Surgeon-Major Bennett suffered from a severe attack of the disease, but happily is now reported as being convalescent. Lieut. Pemberton, 2nd West India Regiment, died on October 9. One death has occurred among the men of departmental corps remaining at Gun Hill after the withdrawal of the troops, and three men are still under treatment. The camp is about to be broken up, and the men transferred to quarters in Bridgetown. During the voyage of H.M.S. Orontes five fatal cases of yellow fever occurred among the troops. Since the disembarkation o the 1st Royal Lancaster Regiment at Devonport several me have been transferred to hospital in a very low condition from the results of remittent fever, and two men suffering from recent attacks of the same disease of very severe form. The men of the Royal Artillery who disembarked at Dover from the same ship are reported as being in good health. Deputy Surgeon-General H. T. Reade, V.C., has arrived in England, suffering, we regret to state, from general debility, the result of overwork during the epidemic. On his departure from the island a highly complimentary General Order was published by Major-General Gamble, C.B., recording his appreciation of the services rendered by Deputy Surgeon-General Reade, the medical officers under him, and by the men of the Army Hospital Corps. The mortality among the Medical Department amounted to 33 per cent. of their strength.

THE PARIS WEEKLY RETURN.

THE number of deaths for the forty-sixth week, terminating November 18,' was 1036 (555 males and 481 females), and among these there were from typhoid fever 40, small-pox 5, measles 17, scarlatina 2, pertussis 3, diphtheria and croup 54, erysipelas 8, and puerperal infections 8. There were also 40 deaths from tubercular and acute meningitis, 27 from acute bronchitis, 95 from pneumonia, 65 from infantile athrepsia (31 of the infants having been wholly or partially suckled), and 34 violent deaths. There is nothing to note particularly for the present week, the *statu quo* being complete, inasmuch as the number of deaths was the same as in the preceding week. The same stationary condition is observable in the entries and discharges of the hospitals. The births for the week amounted to 1220, viz., 617 males (429 legitimate and 188 illegitimate) and 603 females (444 legitimate and 159 illegitimate); 87 infants (51 males and 36 females) were born dead or died within twenty-four hours.

EXTRAORDINARY CASE OF DISPUTED MEDICAL CHARGES.

A REMARKABLE case of disputed charge for medical services was heard in the Edmonton County Court, before Judge Abdy and a jury, on November 16. Mr. John Lloyd Whitmarsh, of New Southgate, brought an action to recover £26 14s., for medical attendance upon Mr. Wingrove, of New Southgate; his wife, Lady Travers; his brother-in-law, the Earl of Traquair (said to be the last of the Stuarts of Scotland); and Mrs. Morrell, nurse in the establishment, who had represented herself as the foster-mother of the Earl. The medical services sued for were rendered between January and March of this year. The Earl, who was suffering from rheumatic fever, was attended day and night from February 18 to March 5, when he died; and other members of the family were attended. The defence contended that the charges made (5s. for a day visit, and 7s. 6d. for a night visit) were exorbitant; but it seems impossible, in the circumstances, that this contention could be maintained, though we regret to observe that one member of the profession was found to swear that he thought the charges too high. The defendant swore that he had not retained the plaintiff to attend his brother-in-law, nor requested that he should have every attention, as the plaintiff had stated; but the Judge decided, as to this, that the probabilities were in favour of the plaintiff, as he had called Dr. Garrod in consultation, and the defendant paid the physician's fee. But, not content with this ordinary kind of defence, the defendant stated that Mr. Whitmarsh had said to him, "I have a nice quiet place at Southgate for young fellows to come to if they don't wish their friends to know. I am thinking of having some circulars printed, and if you know of any young fellows who wish to be treated privately, I hope you will recommend them to me." The plaintiff wholly denied this conversation; and the Judge commented on this part of the defence with great

and just severity. If true, he remarked the defendant ought to have kicked the plaintiff out of the house; while, if the proposal had not been made, a more disgraceful scandal could not have been invented against the profession. The jury were ready, with one dissentient, to give the full amount claimed: and in the end, as the defendant declined to accept the verdict of the majority, plaintiff's counsel accepted an offer of £20 1s. as carrying costs upon the higher scale. Mr. Whitmarsh, if he is correctly reported, made one mistake in his statement in court—a very curious mistake, and one that in a less strong and plain case might have mischievously affected the jury. He stated that "medical men are entitled to charge according to the rental of their houses; and not according to the rental of the houses inhabited by patients." The Judge very rightly remarked that this must be a mistake; it must mean that a medical man would gauge the position of the people he attends by the character of the houses they occupy, and make his charge accordingly. When entering a verdict for the amount accepted, the Judge addressed the defendant as follows: "By your offer you practically admit that plaintiff's claim is a proper one; and let me tell you, sir, in open court, that a more mean and harsh attack than that which you made against a professional man was never uttered in a witness-box. For you to have imputed such a foul charge against an innocent man is a disgrace to the name of a gentleman. I say with the greatest confidence that the plaintiff leaves this court without a stain upon his character." We congratulate Mr. Whitmarsh on having had the courage to fight his case, and stand upon the reasonableness of his charges; and we congratulate him on the result.

OBSTETRICAL SOCIETY OF DUBLIN.

THE opening meeting of the forty-fourth annual session of this Society took place on the evening of Saturday, November 26, in the College of Physicians, Kildare-street, Dublin. The chair was taken by the President, Dr. John A. Byrne, who delivered an address, in which he alluded to the death of Dr. McClintock and of others who had passed away during the year. He alluded also to the proposal for the amalgamation of the medical societies of Dublin, of which he expressed his disapproval. In conclusion, he hoped that the vacancy on the General Medical Council caused by the death of Dr. McClintock would be filled by the appointment of another representative of the obstetric branch of medicine. It was moved by Dr. Kidd and Dr. Denham—"That we desire to record our deep sense of the loss sustained by this Society and the profession at large in the death of Dr. Alfred McClintock, one of the most distinguished, energetic, and active of our members, whose many contributions to our *Proceedings* and whose writings have, by their high scientific and literary merit, added much to the reputation of the obstetrical school of Dublin; and we beg also to express our deep and heartfelt sympathy with his family in their bereavement." Professor Beverley Cole, of California, in supporting the resolution, said the people from whom he came in America all spoke the same language, and it was well known there what Dr. McClintock had done in his profession. The motion was unanimously adopted. The Hon. Secretary, Dr. Roe, read the report of the Council, which, on the motion of Dr. Pollock, seconded by Dr. Henry, was adopted. The following members of the Society were elected officers for the ensuing year:—*President:* John A. Byrne, M.B. *Vice-Presidents:* Arthur Vernon Macan, M.D., and R. J. Kinkead, M.D. *Committee:* Fleetwood Churchill, F.K.Q.C.P.; John Denham, M.D.; George H. Kidd, M.D.; John Rutherfoord Kirkpatrick, M.B.; Richard D. Purefoy, M.B. *Honorary Treasurer:* John J. Cranny, M.B. *Honorary Secretary:* William Roe, M.D.

THE NORWOOD HOUSE CASE.

AFTER a three days' trial the jury have disagreed on a question which is undoubtedly of the first importance to all householders. Briefly, the case was this. Was a house taken and assured to be healthy, but which really turned out to be in a most insanitary condition, to be returned on the hands of the lessor with damages, or no? Perhaps the most interesting part of the evidence—worthless for the most part—was that one gentleman swore that a cesspool, close by the conservatory, and only a short distance from the house, was a perfectly healthy appendage. It contained four feet of solid sewage (mostly, we presume, fæcal), but this was nothing—there was a foot of water over it!

LINACRE CHAIR OF PHYSIOLOGY, OXFORD.

THE Linacre Professorship of Physiology at Oxford, made vacant, it will be remembered, by the death of Dr. George Rolleston, F.R.S., was filled up on Saturday last by the election of Mr. H. N. Moseley, M.A., F.R.S., Assistant-Registrar of the University of London. Mr. Moseley had already distinguished himself by his researches in comparative anatomy when he was selected as one of the naturalists to make the great exploring voyage round the world in the *Challenger*; and he has been chiefly occupied, we believe, since his return to England, in work on the records of the *Challenger* exploration.

ON THE PHYSIOLOGICAL ACTION OF THE ASCLEPIAS CURASSAVICA.

WE read in a recent number of the *União Medico*, of Rio Janeiro, that Dr. Guimarães has made a series of experimental investigations on the physiological action of the *Asclepias curassavica*—a common plant in Brazil, and known to European botanists under that name, and also in England under the name of *bastard ipecacuan*. Dr. Guimarães made twenty-five experiments on various animals, such as dogs, rats, guinea-pigs, etc., and he obtained some well-marked results, among which were the following:—The active principle is a cardiac poison, resembling digitalis in its action; and, like almost all such poisons, the asclepias affects all the striated muscles, and causes them to lose their contractility. It does not exercise any injurious action on the nervous centres presiding over the life of relation, nor on the sensitive or motor nerves. An alcoholic solution of the roots, injected into the veins, immediately causes a great constriction of the small vessels, resulting in a considerable increase of blood-tension in the large ones, and a more or less rapid reduction of the normal temperature. It is an excitant of the vaso-motor centres. Besides these primary effects, the asclepias produces others which are secondary, among the most notable of which are disturbances of respiration, from a state of slight dyspnœa to great orthopnœa; and disorder of the digestive system, marked principally by vomiting and diarrhœa. The solution obtained by maceration from the stems and the roots acts on the heart and the vessels, but with unequal intensity—that from the stalks exercising a more marked and rapid action on the heart than the solution from the roots; but the reverse takes place when the action is exerted on the vaso-motor centres.

MICROSCOPICAL SECTION OF THE MANCHESTER MEDICAL SOCIETY.

AT the meeting of this Society in October, Mr. E. H. Howlett showed some granular elements which are present in normal blood, stained with methyl-aniline after the manner of Koch. In addition to the red and white corpuscles, groups of smaller elements could be seen in various parts of the field. These groups were made up of from five to twelve separate corpuscles, varying in size from 2·5 to 5 micro-millimetres in diameter. Spherical in shape, they were readily seen, from the fact that they stained with aniline similar to, but in a less degree than, the nuclei of the white corpuscles. Isolated specimens were also seen. It is probable that these small "racemose bodies" exist in normal blood, as they can be seen on the warm stage; they could also be seen on the cold stage. By irrigating the specimen with corrosive sublimate solution, the red and white corpuscles are washed away, whilst the "racemose body" is left sticking to the slide or cover-glass; but it is seen to have become somewhat flattened, and to have assumed a faint greenish-yellow colour. The works of various observers in the same field were alluded to, more especially that of Hayem. Attention was drawn to the great similarity between the "hæmatoblast" described by Hayem and the "racemose corpuscle," whilst doubt was expressed as to the accuracy of Hayem's description of their shape, which he found to be discoidal. In conclusion, it was suggested that, owing to their manner of staining, these little elements were either broken-up leucocytes or detached portions of the same bodies during life. Mr. Stocks showed sections of kidney of a young woman who died from the effects of taking chlorate of potash, some one ounce and a half in about thirty-six hours. The symptoms observed were cyanosis with prostration. The cyanosis was followed on the fourth day by decided anæmia. During this time she had almost complete ischuria, secreting only about two ounces of urine, which was obtained by catheterism; on the day preceding her death only half an ounce was passed. The urine was highly albuminous, and of a dark colour resembling porter, evidently from the admixture of blood. No blood corpuscles could be seen. The sections of the kidney showed the glomeruli free from change, but the convoluted tubes in the majority of instances were packed with solid granular blood-casts, and others seemed denuded of their epithelium; the straight tubes were normal.

THE ENTRIES IN THE MEDICAL SCHOOLS OF DUBLIN.

THE last day for medical students to enter their names for the present session in the various schools was November 25. The following returns of entries have since that day been made to the Anatomical Committee by the authorities of the Dublin schools. We append the corresponding figures of 1880 for comparison:—

	1881.	1880.
School of Physic, University of Dublin	216	192
School of Surgery, Royal College of Surgeons	140	183
Ledwich School of Medicine	221	230
Carmichael College of Medicine	159	149
Catholic University School of Medicine	100	94
Total number of entries	836	848

It will be seen that there is a substantial increase in the number of entries in three of the five schools, whereas there is a falling off in the Ledwich School, and a very considerable falling off in the School of the Royal College of Surgeons. The total number of entries is 12 below that of 1880.

LAPLAND AS A HEALTH-RESORT.

IF what M. Paul du Chaillu tells us of the land of the Lapps be correct, it is possible that health-resorts rivalling Davos Platz may spring up in the northern regions of Scandinavia. Consumption, he says, cancer, chills, and fever, are unknown in Lapland. The water is as pure as in granitic countries, and the drinking of sour milk seems to prevent many complaints elsewhere common. But acute diseases are prevalent, often brought on by the perspiration which comes on when ascending steep mountains being suddenly checked by the piercing winds of the summits. The Lapps are subject to measles, and sometimes get small-pox from the seashore people. Hernia is not infrequent, owing to their driving with their legs reversed and acting as a drag on their sleighs. Ophthalmia is quite common, owing to the cold winds and glare of the snow. In the spring, great care has to be taken with the eyes, as the reflection of the sun is very bright in April, May, and the beginning of June, and without blue or green goggles one easily becomes snow-blind. The men and women are active to a great age. Their life in the open air and constant wanderings on foot pre-serve the elasticity of the muscles; their simple habits, the keen, invigorating, dry air, and the pure water, all con-tribute to secure longevity to those who have been able to pass through the severe ordeal of childhood. Many attain a very great age—some more than a hundred years. Although the Lapps live chiefly on animal food, barley-flour is almost always found in the *kata*, to be used for *mush*, unleavened bread, or blood-pudding. They often mix their milk with sorrel grass. They are great drinkers of coffee, inveterate smokers and snuff-takers. The vice of drunken-ness, once so prevalent, has now almost entirely disappeared at home, but whenever they go to a town, and can procure spirituous liquors, they generally have a frolic for a day or two.

A COMMISSION OF INQUIRY INTO CHOLERA IN THE PUNJAUB.

OUR contemporary the *Indian Medical Gazette* states that a Commission has been appointed to investigate the recent prevalence of cholera in the Punjab. The Commission is instructed to visit the localities where the disease prevailed during the past "rains," to investigate the circumstances, sanitary and otherwise, which existed during its prevalence, and to specify, if possible, the conditions which determined or favoured the development and spread of the disease. The Commission is composed as follows:—Colonel Hall (Com-missioner of Lahore), President; Major Stephen (Rifle Bri-gade) and Major King-Harman (Assistant Quartermaster-General), members; and Surgeon-Major Bellew, C.S.I., Secretary. We shall be agreeably surprised if the result should be any real addition to our knowledge of the causa-tion or the spread of cholera. A report has also been called for by the Punjaub Government on the value of dilute sul-phuric acid in cholera. It is stated that the drug has been tried on a large scale in Lahore, and that Dr. Bellew holds a high opinion of its value.

A RARE FORM OF PREGNANCY.

IN a recent number of the *Archiv für Gynäkologie* a case is recorded which, on account of its exceeding rarity, deserves notice. It occurred in the clinique of Professor Litzmann of Kiel, and is reported by Dr. Werth. It was one of preg-nancy in the imperfectly developed horn of a bicorned uterus, the fœtus, fully developed, being retained beyond the full term. The patient was thirty-nine years old, and had had two children. She last menstruated in December, 1878. Fœtal movements were felt about the end of May, 1879. In the latter end of October the fœtal movements were un-usually vigorous, and then ceased. Then came pain; and, at the end of November, feverishness, serious vaginal dis-charge, and wasting. She was taken into the hospital, and as, on examination, the os uteri was found large enough to admit the finger, and the fœtal head could be felt within it, the diagnosis was made that it was a case of retention of a dead child in the uterus. On February 14, laparotomy was performed: a decomposing, but fully developed, child was removed; and then the sac, at first supposed to be the uterus, which had contained the fœtus was extirpated. On exami-nation this sac, was found to have only one set of uterine appendages. The patient died on the 16th from peritonitis. It was then found that the uterus was bicorned, the fœtus having developed in the right horn. The right kidney was absent. A corpus luteum was present in the right ovary. The author has only been able to find one case on record which at all resembled this, viz., one published by Turner.[a] We may add that Dr. Barnes (in his work on *Diseases of Women*) has, hazarded the speculation that many cases reported as extra-uterine gestation, in which fœtal bones, etc., were discharged per vaginam, were really cases like this one.

VITAL STATISTICS OF IRELAND FOR THE SECOND QUARTER OF 1881.

THE Registrar-General for Ireland has recently published his report for the second quarter of the year 1881. During this period, ended June 30 last, there were registered in the 800 Registrar's districts in that country 34,202 births—a number equal to an annual birth-rate of 26·7 in every 1000 of the estimated population—and 23,614 deaths, representing an annual rate of 18·4 per 1000. The birth-rate during the quarter under notice is under the average of the rate for the corresponding quarter of the previous five years, to the extent of 0·7 per 1000 of the population, but it is 0·5 per 1000 over the rate for the second quarter of the year 1880. The death-rate is also below the average of the corresponding quarter of the five years 1876-80, to the extent of 1·6 per 1000, and is likewise 3·2 below the rate for the second quarter of 1880. In the present report, various modifications have been introduced, consequent upon the information obtained at the recent census. The populations for all the urban sanitary districts have been extracted from the original returns, or from the enumerators' abstracts, and thus the birth and death rates have been calculated for the principal Irish towns, which may be considered correct for all practical purposes. Another important modification is a revision of the estimated population of Ireland, which, as estimated to the middle of the present year, is 5,129,950. The highest county birth-rate was 33·8 per 1000 in Antrim, and the lowest 21·7 for Mayo. Of the intermediate rates, the highest five were—Dublin, 29·7; Kerry, 29·7; Waterford, 29·2; Armagh, 28·9; and Down, 28·5: whilst the lowest five were —Fermanagh, 21·9; Meath, 21·9; Tyrone, 22·5; Sligo, 22·5; and Clare, 22·9. The death-rate in the province of Leinster was 20·5 per 1000; in Munster, 18·0; in Ulster, 18·8; and in Connaught, 14·3. Of the 23,614 deaths registered during this quarter, 2929, or 12·4 per cent., were of children under one year old, and 9448, or 40·0 per cent., were of persons aged sixty years and upwards. The deaths of infants under one year old were equal to 85·6 per 1000 of the births registered. In commenting on the general health of the people, the report observes that the various registrars' returns for the second quarter of the present year are of a favourable character. The death-rate is below the average, and below that for the corresponding period of last year, although at that time the population was estimated at too high a number, and consequently the death-rate was then calculated to be lower than the correct rate. The death-rate was, in fact, lower than in any of the corre-sponding quarters since the year 1874. The notes furnished by the registrars contain accounts of local outbreaks of disease, and many interesting particulars regarding sanitary improvements, sanitary defects, and the ages of those who were remarkable for longevity. The mortality from zymotic diseases during the quarter is given as 1306, or 7·6 per cent. of the total deaths, equal to a rate of 35 in every 100,000 of the population. This number is 1354, or 41·0 per cent., under the number for the corresponding quarter of last

(a) "On Malformations of the Organs of Generation." Edinburgh, 1865.

year, and is the lowest number of deaths from these diseases ever returned for the second quarter of the year since registration commenced in 1864. The decrease in the general and zymotic death-rates during the first half of the present year is, the report considers, no doubt owing to the unusually plentiful harvest of 1880, and the consequently abundant supply of wholesome food at a reasonable rate.

THE TREATMENT OF SNAKE-BITES.

IT is reported from India that Dr. Vincent Richards, of Bengal, who was a member of the committee for the investigation of snake-poisoning, and is joint author of "Reports on Indian and Australian Snake-Poisoning," has commenced a series of experiments to test the efficacy in cobra-poisoning of Dr. Lacerda's plan of injecting permanganate of potash; and that he states that the experiments, although not absolutely conclusive, have yet, so far as they have gone, led to much more hopeful results than any previously instituted, and believes that the ground for hoping for a practical remedy has at last been found. Unquestionably the progress of Dr. Richards's experiments will be watched with much interest.

PATHOLOGICAL SOCIETY OF DUBLIN.

THE first ordinary meeting of this Society for the session 1881-82 was held in the Anatomical Theatre, Trinity College, on Saturday, November 12; Mr. William Stokes, President, in the chair. The President showed two examples of necrosis of the tibia. The first occurred in a lad aged fifteen, who was suddenly attacked with pain and swelling about the middle of the left leg. An abscess formed, and numerous sinuses gave exit to a sanious watery discharge. The limb was at last amputated by a modified supra-condyloid operation, and the lesion was found to be acute necrosis of the tibia, with immunity of the fibula. The epiphyses at both extremities of the bone shared in the disease. Firm anchylosis had occurred at the knee-joint and at the ankle, welding the tibia to the astragalus. The second case was that of a boy aged nine years, who had been kicked on the shin. The entire diaphysis of the tibia was stripped of its periosteum, and was carious. Dr. E. H. Bennett exhibited a series of united fractures of the metacarpal bones. They were examples of fracture of the shaft of the third and fifth, from the same hand; one of the shaft and one of the base of the fifth, both from right hands; and five of the first metacarpal, all of the right side. It would thus appear that fracture of the first metacarpal was that most commonly observed. Also in each of the five metacarpal bones of the thumb the fracture was the same, and placed in a position not hitherto described: the plane of the fracture passed obliquely through the proximal extremity of the bone, detaching the palmar projection with the greater part of the articular surface. In all the cases union had occurred with but little displacement of the fragment. In a case observed in the living, Dr. Bennett had verified the existence of the lesion as the result of a fall upon the ball of the thumb.

THE BLANE GOLD MEDAL.

ON the recommendation of the Director-General of the Medical Department of the Royal Navy and the Presidents of the Royal Colleges of Physicians and Surgeons, the following medical officers of the Royal Navy have just had the fine gold medal founded by Sir Gilbert Blane, Bart., awarded to them—viz., Fleet-Surgeon Belgrave Ninnis, M.D. St. And. and M.R.C.S. Eng., of H.M.S. Garnet; and Staff-Surgeon Alexander McDonald, M.D. and L.R.C.S. Edin., of H.M.S. London.

SCIENCE DEFENCE FUND.

THE letter from Dr. Wilks, which appeared in our columns, has already called forth strong influential support. Preliminary meetings are being held for the establishment of an association for the defence of those engaged in physiological, pathological, and pharmacological experiments, against unjust attacks, and for the diffusion of information calculated to combat popular prejudices on the subject. Several of the most influential members of the profession have taken an active part in the matter, and a considerable sum has already been subscribed. Communications may be addressed to Dr. Lauder Brunton, F.R.S., 50, Welbeck-street, who is acting as interim secretary.

THE MAN WITH AN ELASTIC SKIN.

THE Wiener Med. Wochenschrift states that a man is now exhibiting in that city a peculiarity highly interesting to medical men. This consists in an enormous and astonishing elasticity of his skin. He is able to raise this in folds from his trunk or limbs to the extent of more than a foot; and as soon as the traction ceases the skin resumes its normal position, neither folds nor depressions being visible. The procedure is entirely painless. When the skin is touched it imparts a sensation as if one had hold of a fine sponge, and as if it were much too large for what it covers. Even the hairy scalp and the skin of the nose and palm of the hand exhibit the peculiarity, but to a less extent than that of the trunk or arm. So delicate is the skin, and especially of the upper extremities, that when it is raised in a fold and held before a light, it is found to be transparent, exhibiting the course of the vessels. The "india-rubber" man is thirty-two years of age, and the peculiarity in question was first observed in his twenty-first year.

ON THE WATER-TREATMENT (IDROTERAPIA) IN ORGANIC DISEASES OF THE HEART.

IN a recent number of the Giornale Internazionale delle Scienze Mediche there is an article by Dr. Raffaele Maturi, Director of the Hydrotherapeutical Institution of Naples, on the application of baths in organic diseases of the heart. The author sets out by noting the cases of heart-disease in which the use of baths is contra-indicated—as, for instance, where there is insufficiency of the aortic valves, with diffused atheroma and recurrent hyperæmia in the head; and also where there is cardiac wasting, with irregularity of the pulse and threatened fainting; and the same rule, of course, holds good where there is aneurism or violent palpitation. But all lesions of the heart are not of this kind; and a neoplastic pericarditis, which has left some proliferation of the connective tissue in the form of excrescence, adhesion, or thickening, without any notable derangement of the cardiac functions, without œdema or suffering, cannot receive any injury from the use of baths, but may even be benefited. Again, there are cases of endocarditis which may be similarly benefited—as when the valves, though normal in texture, volume, and form, yet, from deficient energy of the papillary muscles, want the tension necessary for the uniformity and the number of the vibrations taking part in producing tonicity. To all these considerations it may be added that medicine has no power to remove valvular alterations, and the only hope in such cases rests upon the compensatory hypertrophy of the heart and the power of accommodation of the valves. Mineral baths do not interfere with this salutary proceeding, and they may assist in improving the general nutrition, for which tonics are usually prescribed. Quinine, iron, good living, ergotine, and even the preparations of iodine, are given to promote the healthy change of materials in the body; and Dr. Maturi asks whether mineral baths are inconsistent with such treatment. It appears to him, on the contrary, that the moderate excitement caused by the baths improves the nutrition of the myocardium, and regulates and sustains the ventricular contractions. He quotes from the opinions of various authors on the treatment of heart-disease, and, making due allowance for cases in which the water-treatment is inapplicable, he shows that in certain instances it may not only be harmless, but beneficial.

DR. PARSONS' REPORT ON FEVER IN THE CHORLEY URBAN DISTRICT.

In April last Dr. Franklin Parsons was deputed by the Local Government Board to make an inquiry on the prevalence of fever in the Chorley Urban District, and also to report on the general sanitary condition of the locality. Chorley, it should be premised, lies on the high road between Wigan and Preston, and has a population of over 19,000 inhabitants. The prevalence of scarlet fever in Chorley in 1879, Dr. Parsons found to be a part of the general epidemic of that disease which overspread Lancashire in 1878-79, and in which the adjoining registration districts of Preston, Blackburn, and Wigan suffered very severely, the disease having reached its greatest height in the two former before, and in Wigan later than in Chorley. Of the mode in which scarlet fever was propagated little can be said, Dr. Parsons observes, except that it appeared to be through the usual channels of personal intercommunication. Of enteric fever about fifty cases, twelve of which were fatal, were ascertained to have occurred since the beginning of 1880 up to the date of the inspection. Twenty households had been attacked, there being in some instances four, five, six, and even eight cases in succession in one household. The cases were distributed through various parts of the district, though groups occurred in particular streets, and they commenced also at various periods throughout the year, though most numerous in the latter half of 1880. As regards the mode of origin and propagation of the disease, inquiries in many instances failed to elicit satisfactory evidence. The report adds, that there was no reason for suspecting the public water-supply, which is in universal use, to have been at fault, and milk was obtained from various sources by the families attacked. The scattered distribution of the cases in point of time further negatives the idea of any common simultaneous cause; while the fact of a number of cases having followed each other in the same house, or the same street, points rather to local circumstances being concerned in their production. After explaining his reasons for arriving at such a conclusion, Dr. Parsons observes that it seems most probable that the morbid poison has been conveyed by the medium of sewer-air. Hospital isolation was not largely resorted to, the only hospital for infectious diseases in the district being the fever wards at the Chorley Union Workhouse, into which the working-classes as usual, strongly object to be taken. The Medical Officer of Health also complained much of the difficulty experienced in dealing with infectious diseases in the locality, through want of early information as to its existence, and he has advised the Sanitary Authority to apply for powers to render the notification of cases of such diseases compulsory. The result of Dr. Parsons' inquiries into the sanitary condition of the district may be gathered from the recommendations which he has appended to his report. In these he advocates the more frequent flushing of the sewers, when necessary, with disinfectants such as solution of sulphate of iron, while the discharge of heated liquids into the sewers should, if possible, be prevented. This practice is followed by certain manufacturers in the locality, and is highly objectionable, since it promotes decomposition, and by expanding the air in the sewers, increases its pressure. The house-drains, he recommends, should be disconnected from the sewer by a trap, and ventilated by inlet and exit openings on the house side of the latter. Proceedings should also be taken against persons exposing themselves, and others, or infected articles, in contravention of the Public Health Act; whilst it would be well if hospital accommodation for infectious cases could be secured, free from the objections attaching to the use of workhouse wards for the purpose.

THE MEDICAL PROFESSION IN LIVERPOOL AND THE "SANITARY ACTS."

THE third ordinary meeting of the Liverpool Medical Institute, which was held on November 3, was entirely devoted to the consideration of the proposed amendments by the City Council of the Building and Sanitary Acts. The meeting was an exceptionally large and representative one, and it soon became evident that the proposed amendments would meet with a determined and unanimous opposition. By these amendments the Corporation would have power to close schools, dairies, and shops, where the presence of contagious disease may render such closure necessary. Every occupier, head of a family, or person in charge of a house where contagious disease appears, would require to give notice to the medical officer of health immediately he becomes aware of the existence of such disease amongst those in any way under his charge. Every medical practitioner called in to see a patient suffering from contagious disease would be required to give a certificate to that effect to the person in charge of the patient, and the latter to forward it to the "health office." Certain fees are given to the medical practitioner for the certificate, and penalties are inflicted on medical men and householders if they infringe these regulations. The following letter was sent to the Town Clerk as the result of the discussion:—

"To the Town Clerk, Liverpool.

"After a prolonged and careful consideration by the members of the Medical Institution, at a meeting especially convened for the purpose, of the clauses proposed to be inserted in an amended Building and Sanitary Act for the city, they regret that they feel themselves unable to recommend their adoption for the following reasons, viz.:—

"1. They are of opinion that the risk of propagation of disease by means of dairies or milkhouses is greatly lessened by the Dairies, Cowsheds, and Milkshops Orders of 1879, and that a much longer trial should be given to these orders before new powers are asked for.

"2. They are of opinion that the danger of introducing infectious diseases into schools would be effectually met by requiring each child to bring medical certificates of freedom from such diseases after holidays or other absence from school, and would suggest a trial of this course instead of adopting the more stringent plan of compulsory closure.

"3. They are of opinion that the householders, fearing the effects of publicity under a compulsory system of registration, may be tempted to conceal the existence of infectious disease, and that during each period of concealment the danger of multiplication will be greater than at present, when, under the skilled guidance of medical men, more or less effectual means are taken to effect isolation.

"4. They are of opinion that the experience collected from other towns (so far as members have been able to obtain it up to date) tends to prove that the anticipated advantages to the public health have not followed the adoption of similar clauses, and that serious inconveniences to the community have resulted therefrom.

(Signed)   "REGINALD HARRISON,
             "President Liverpool Medical Institution.

"November 7, 1881."

The matter came before the Health Committee of the City Council on November 10, when Dr. Hamilton moved that the obnoxious clauses be removed from the Bill on the grounds mentioned in the letter. Dr. Taylor (Medical Officer of Health) did not think he received sufficiently early notice of infectious disease at present. The proposed amendments did not confer any greater powers of compulsory removal than were now possessed, and in *Liverpool*, where there was such a large floating population, early notification seemed to him especially necessary.

The consideration of the matter was postponed for further information.

The medical profession do not seem to have any objection to notify the presence of infectious disease to the medical officer of health. What they especially object to is the unnecessary interference of "inspectors" between them and their patients. If the health officers only interfered where the medical attendant of the patient considered interference necessary, very little difficulty would be experienced in getting early notification of every case of contagious disease.

FROM ABROAD.

THE OPIUM HABIT.

DR. MANN, in an article published in the October number of the *New York Journal of Medicine*, observes that, although so much less known than the effects of the excess of alcohol, inebriation by opium affects thousands of persons. Generally commencing with small doses, the victim of this habit succeeds in keeping it a secret until the irresistible craving that becomes established renders him insensible to the shame of the indulgence. The amount that can be taken at last seems incredible, for Dr. Mann states that several of his patients were taking from two to seven or eight grains of morphia daily; while one lady suffering from cancer was able to take 150 grains of morphia, equivalent to 480 grains of opium! According to Dr. Mann's experience, most of the victims of this habit have originally commenced the use of opium for the relief of pain, but in other cases it has been resorted to in order to counteract domestic unhappiness or to mitigate mental suffering. Its habitual use seems to induce a peculiar type of moral insanity, leaving the intellectual powers untouched. The patient's views of right and wrong are perverted, and while he still goes on with his routine duties, he often manifests an utter disregard for truthfulness, honesty, and sincerity, and after a time shows a seeming inability to exert his will in any other direction or for any other purpose than the gratification of his morbid appetite. "Hearing and vision are not infrequently affected, and insomnia is very common. Tremors and an unsteady, ill-balanced gait are generally observed in well-developed cases. Opium rather suspends the operation of the mind than causes disease, for it does not seem to act directly on the cerebral structure. If it did, insanity would be the result; and I have never met with a case of mental disease that I could trace to indulgence in opium, and I have had many cases of this nature under my care."

After a graphic description of the effects produced by the habit (for which we regret we have not space), Dr. Mann proceeds to the consideration of its treatment. One of the saddest things connected with it, he observes, is the fact that voluntary renunciation of opium by one who has become addicted to its use is unknown to the profession. Opium-takers make many well-intentioned resolves towards reform, but they are invariably frustrated by the revival of the appetite, and a relapse follows. And yet—

"The opium or morphia habit is a curable disease, as other diseases are, and I only desire to know that an opium sufferer honestly desires a cure to assure him that this result can be accomplished. If the opium habit is not eradicated when the physician has the moral support of the patient in desiring a cure, it is because the treatment is at fault in some respect. I know of no disease that yields a better percentage of cures to the proper treatment. Primarily, the patient must put himself under the necessary control, and must, as I have said, desire a cure himself. The nervous system of most of our modern Americans is too delicate to bear the shock of a total deprivation of the opium at once. Grave nervous disorders follow such a course. In my own plan of treatment I employ a reductionary course of treatment, keeping the patient's nervous system quiet with a combination of the bromides, gradually *increasing* the bromides as I decrease the *morphia*, until, on the tenth day after admission [Dr. Mann is physician to a private hospital at Sunnyside, for diseases of the nervous system, the opium habit, and inebriety], my patient is taking no opium and has avoided all suffering and nervous prostration. I generally combine the bromides of sodium and ammonium, and eliminate them from the system, after I stop the opium, by warm baths, sweet spirits of nitre, and digitalis. The reflex action of the spinal cord, which has been purposely kept depressed by the bromides during the reductionary treatment, is now excited by strychnia, and the central nervous system is stimulated and invigorated by the daily use of the induced or faradic current of electricity employed as general faradisation. Nerve-tonics are also employed, and an emaciated patient generally gains in a month's time from twenty-five to thirty pounds of flesh; his shattered constitution is built up; and in from four to six weeks he is generally well enough to be discharged, and to resume his position in society, entirely free from all craving for opium or morphia. Nothing but a thorough, systematic course of treatment can restore such patients to health, and there is no greater delusion than the belief in any specific to counteract the effect of opium on the human system and to eradicate the craving for the narcotic; but with such thorough, systematic treatment success is certain and invariable."

Dr. Mann has some interesting remarks on the relation of this opium habit to nervous exhaustion. "The wear and tear of our hurried life, and the nervous prostration so common among fashionable women, are temporarily relieved by this habit. There is also a great deal of brain-fatigue among professional and business men, resulting from the preponderance of waste over repair, which induces grave nervous prostration. This state of neurasthenia, or nervous exhaustion, is one of the most important predisposing causes of severe neuralgia, and these sufferers generally resort to opium to assuage the pain; and as these attacks are not only severe, but frequent, the opium habit is thus often insensibly acquired by repeated recourse to it to allay pain. In neurasthenia the brain is irritable, and the patient is apt to become sleepless; and if a professional man not unfrequently resorts to morphia to obtain sleep, before he is aware of it he has acquired an irresistible craving for the drug, which, even against his will and in defiance of it, has enslaved him. I have found, as the results of excessive mental labour, anxiety, depressing mental emotions, hæmorrhages, and sleeplessness—a state of things which in women is associated with uterine displacements and spinal irritation, and in men with irritability, mental depression, and impending mental disorders. I have seen many cases of opium-eating developed amongst this class, as they are very prone to resort to opium for temporary relief. Modern nervous diseases are rapidly increasing and multiplying, and our morbid nervousness, which is developing itself in modern society, is making itself manifest by a great increase in neuralgia, sick-headache, dyspepsia, and nervous exhaustion. Opium or morphia is too often the principal medicine or sedative resorted to in these cases to relieve pain or procure sleep, and, before long, those who resort to it habitually find that they cannot live without it. As one lady expressed herself to me, the opium is taken, not because these persons want it, but to relieve the terrible sensations which attack them when they are without it, and they are thus forced deeper and deeper into a habit which they may honestly detest, because they can see no way out of the dilemma into which they have plunged themselves by their habitual use of opium to relieve nervousness. The opium *habitué* is thus an opium sufferer. When he wakes to a consciousness of his real position it is pitiable in the extreme to know that this state can only be mitigated by new, and perhaps increased, indulgence. There is probably no more terrible suffering than the complete exhaustion, the prostration of mind and body, which these patients suffer. The control over the muscles is lost, and epilepsy, paralysis, and an unsteady, ill-balanced gait are all frequent symptoms of this terrible disease. Such patients have a full consciousness of their position, but are powerless to emancipate themselves from the opium habit. Their miseries and anguish are extreme; but, in spite of all efforts, they find themselves forced back again into the habit. It is just such cases that need medical aid and systematic treatment. There are no patients with any disease who more require to be lifted out from the depths of their suffering, and are in greater necessity of careful nursing, consideration, and attention."

VITAL STATISTICS OF PARIS AND VIENNA.

THE report on the movement of population in Vienna for the five years 1875-79 having just been published, M. Loua takes the opportunity (*Journal de la Société de Statistique*, October) of instituting a comparison between Vienna and Paris—the two capitals, he says, resembling each other in the magnificence of their palaces, the beauty of their boulevards, the elegance of their houses, the charm of their promenades, and also, it is said, by the easiness of their manners. It will be interesting to inquire, therefore, how far the resemblance holds good with regard to the movement of their populations.

The population of Paris is 1,988,306, including a garrison of 18,360 men; and that of Vienna is 726,015, including a garrison of 20,703 men. 1. *Marriages.*—The mean annual number of these for the five years 1875-79 was 18,436 for Paris, and 5515 for Vienna; and in relation to the population there were 9·3 marriages per 1000 inhabitants in Paris, and 7·6 per 1000 in Vienna: so that marriage was more frequent in Paris than in Vienna. 2. *Births.*—Of living children for the five years there was an annual mean of 55,119 in Paris, and 27,658 in Vienna, which gives 27·7 births per 1000 inhabitants to Paris, and 38·1 per 1000 to Vienna: the fertility of the population being thus incomparably higher in Vienna than in Paris. With respect to *sex*, there were 104 male births to 100 female in Paris, and 106 male to 100 female in Vienna. Of the 55,119 mean annual births in Paris, 40,611 were legitimate and 14,509 natural; and of the 27,658 in Vienna, 16,032 were legitimate and 11,626 natural. In Paris there were, therefore, 26·3 *natural infants* in 100 births, and in Vienna 42 per 100! In Paris there were 2·2 legitimate births per marriage, and in Vienna 5. Of infants *born dead* there were 6·82 per 100 of the entire number of deaths in Paris, and 4·25 in Vienna; but the numbers were much higher in relation to illegitimate infants born dead, these being 7·86 per 100 in Paris, and 4·46 in Vienna. The number of infants born dead (and probably of infanticides) is much less, therefore, in Vienna than in Paris. As seen above, the male births of living children preponderate, but this is much more so the case in regard to children born dead. Of these there were 131 males to 100 females in Paris, and 125 males to 100 females in Vienna. 3. *Deaths.*—The annual mean number of deaths for the five years was in Paris 48,115, viz., 24,827 males and 23,288 females; and in Vienna 21,123, viz., 11,403 males and 9270 females. Relatively to the population, there were 24·2 deaths per 1000 in Paris, and 29·1 in Vienna. The mortality was thus far greater in Vienna than in Paris, which is easily explained by the fact that many more children are born in Vienna. Although the mortality was relatively greater at Vienna than at Paris, it was not sufficiently so to sensibly attenuate the fertility of that capital —a fertility so considerable that it sufficed to procure the annual increase of its inhabitants at the rate of 9 inhabitants per 1000, while that of Paris increased only at the rate of 3·5 per 1000. At Paris, as at Vienna, the female deaths were less than the male in the same number of births; but that is a law which is observed everywhere. Of the mean annual number of deaths (48,115) that occurred in Paris, 36,399 took place à domicile, and 11,716 in hospitals (charitable institutions); and in Vienna 7429 out of a total of 21,123 also took place in hospital. So that a fourth of the deaths in Paris took place in hospital, which, although a large number, is exceeded at Vienna, where a third of the deaths occurred in hospital. At Vienna, one-third of the deaths which took place in hospital occurred among a floating population, strangers to the city; and at Paris in 1879 (when the distinction was first made) one-half the deaths were those of persons who were strangers to the capital. It is thus seen that it is a floating population which furnishes the most habitual inmates of hospitals; and at Paris, as well as Vienna, it is the foreign element that is the most dangerous.

SANITARY INSTITUTE OF GREAT BRITAIN.—The announcement of the award of the prize of £200, offered by the Rev. E. Wyatt Edgell, for an essay on the "Range of Hereditary Tendencies in Health and Disease," will be made by the adjudicators at the first ordinary meeting of the Institute for the session 1881-82, which will be held on Wednesday, December 7, at 7.45 p.m. The inaugural address will be delivered by Dr. Alfred Carpenter.

REVIEWS.

União Medica : Publicação Mensal. (*Medical Union :* A Monthly Journal.) Edited by DRS. CYPRIANO DE FREITAS, MONCORVO, JULIO DE MOURA, MOURA BRAZIL, and SILVA ARAUJO. Nos. II. to VIII. Rio de Janeiro. 1881.

WE have received seven numbers of the above Journal, which is a new serial, and is written in the Portuguese language. It is arranged on the same plan as that of some of the European medical journals, each monthly number containing forty-eight pages. The contents are varied and interesting, and consist of editorial articles, original communications, scientific reviews, memoirs of distinguished Brazilian physicians, miscellaneous news relating to medicine, and notices of medical appointments, bibliography, obituary, etc. The editorial articles relate chiefly to the necessity for sanitary measures in the city of Rio de Janeiro, which seems very deficient in this respect; and to the organisation of the new Faculty of Medicine, which appears to have occupied the attention of the profession in Brazil for a long time, and is now in a high state of efficiency, both in its appliances for the treatment of disease and in its arrangements for medical teaching. The original communications treat of a variety of subjects, both surgical and medical, but perhaps the most interesting are those which illustrate the pathology and treatment of diseases peculiar to tropical countries in general, and to the Brazilian Empire in particular; such as marsh fevers, elephantiasis, and beri-beri, on all of which subjects much important information is given. The botany of Brazil, in particular relation to the medicinal plants growing wild, receives special attention; and it need scarcely be mentioned that in a country so fertile in vegetable productions of all kinds there is a wide field for medico-botanical exploration. There is in the journal some lack of information regarding the progress of medicine in Europe, but still there are some miscellaneous notices of French, German, and English medical literature.

La Contrattilità dei Vasi Capillari in relazione ai due Gas dello Scambio Materiale. Nuove Ricerche di LUIGI SEVERINI, Prof. Ord. di Fisiologia nella Università di Perugia.

The Contractility of the Capillary Vessels in relation to the Two Gases concerned in the Change of Material. New Researches by LUIGI SEVERINI, Professor of Physiology in the University of Perugia. Perugia. 1881. Pp. 201.

IN this monograph Professor Severini contributes some new researches on the influence of oxygen gas and carbonic anhydride respectively upon the capillary vessels. He has already published in 1878 some observations in which he showed that oxygen has the property of constricting the lumen of the capillaries directly and in great part by the swelling it produces in the parietal nuclei; and, on the other hand, that carbonic anhydride enlarges their lumen by causing a shrinking of the same nuclei. Since then Dr. Charles Roy, of Cambridge, Dr. Mering, and others, have repeated the experiments described by Professor Severini, and have been unable to perceive the least change in the dimensions of the vessels in question, either by oxygen or carbonic anhydride. Their experiments were made on the *membrana nictitans* and the mesentery of the water-frog, and others were repeated on the same tissues of the *Hyla arborea*; and these writers maintained that all due precautions were taken to insure accuracy in the results. Professor Severini therefore determined to institute a fresh series of microscopical and other researches which he communicates in his present publication, and he expresses himself as being unconvinced of having fallen into any error, and, on the contrary, he asserts that renewed investigations have only confirmed his former conclusions. Professor Severini's experiments and arguments are very elaborate, and are well deserving of careful study by physiologists.

THE VICTORIA HOSPITAL FOR CHILDREN.—His Royal Highness the Prince of Wales has been graciously pleased to signify his intention of presiding at the anniversary festival to be held in aid of this Hospital in the coming year.

GENERAL CORRESPONDENCE.

DR. HARLEY'S ORTHOGRAPHY.
LETTER FROM MR. KENNETH W. MILLICAN.

[To the Editor of the Medical Times and Gazette.]

SIR,—May I add a rider to the remarks of Dr. Kesteven in the current number of the *Medical Times and Gazette?* It is to this effect:—

Dr. Harley defends his innovations on the orthography of the English language against the attacks of those who argue that his method obscures the etymology of the words employed, by calling attention to the fact that the larger number of the reduplicated letters are in themselves destructive of etymological considerations, being the product of the pompous pedantry of the Elizabethan age. That this is largely true will be evident to readers of Chaucer and other older English writers, to whom "wel" for "well" and "al" for "all" will be tolerably familiar. But Dr. Harley's remark, though applying to useless reduplications, can scarcely be said to hold good in the substitution of "vaxinated" for "vaccinated" and "axidentaly" for "accidentally." Surely the verbal descendants of "vacca" and "accido" (*ad cado*) have a right to complain.

Nov. 23. I am, &c., KENNETH W. MILLICAN.

ONE RESULT OF THE CONGRESS.

[To the Editor of the Medical Times and Gazette.]

SIR,—I imagined that the result of the late International Congress of doctors would have been the unquestioned acceptance by foreigners of British habits and customs, but I regret to say I am disappointed. When I was at Krankenbad the other day, I was astounded by the outrageous ignorance still displayed by German medical men of some eminence. I was discussing with Herr Krauts, the celebrated physician, the difficult subject of hospital management, and happened to ask him if there were any paying wards for private patients in any of the great Krankenbad hospitals. You never saw a man become so furious as Krauts when I put the question. "No, a thousand times no!" he shrieked. "But why not?" I exclaimed. "Hospitals are for the poor!" he shouted. "Yes," said I, "but the rich need charity sometimes. In a large city like Krankenbad there are many wealthy people who have no homes, no friends; what are they to do when they are ill?" "Go to bed, and send for me," replied Krauts. "Nothing could be better," I answered; "but how about the nursing? It is not likely that the doctor's orders would be carried out by mercenary and careless attendants." "That is true," said Krauts; "I found a bottle of brandy under the pillow of a noble lord who is suffering from delirium tremens, and also another bottle in his riding boots. But for all that I will admit no noble lords into a public hospital. Better that the nobility should perish than that the medical profession should be disgraced!" "Who dares speak of disgrace," I exclaimed hotly, "in the presence of an M.R.C.S. London, and L.S.A. of Blackfriars?" "Silentium!" roared Krauts, "I know your English love of gold! Ich seh' wahrhaftig schon die Zeit. I mean, I know the time of the clock." "What time?" I asked. "The time," said Krauts, "when competition will ruin the great hospitals of London. I shall live to see your omnibuses and your railway-stations stuck all over with flaring advertisements. Yes, thus it shall be: 'Here you are! Try St. George's Hospital! Bones skilfully set and a first-rate diet for 7s. 6d. a day!' 'Now is your time! Great reduction at St. Bartholomew's! Entirely new set of pulleys for dislocations, four meals a day, and smoking permitted. Charge 6s. 3d., and no extras!' And there is worse than this," continued Krauts. "Doctor will be pitted against doctor. We shall read—'Dr. Jones for hernia, always ready at the Middlesex; come quickly!' 'Dr. Smith for tumours at St. Thomas's! Size no object! Omnibuses pass the door every ten minutes!' And women, too, will be made to play their parts upon the stage of the operating theatre. We shall see placards—'Where's Maria? Head nurse at Guy's, of course!' 'Who is Jemima? Why, the champion poulticer at Bartholomew's!'" "How dare you insinuate the possibility of such a state of things in England!" I

exclaimed. "Because," said Krauts, "since I was in London I have carefully read your journals. Is this your English *Standard?*" he continued, as he handed me the following:—

"Sir,—In these days of hospital mismanagement, it may be refreshing to chronicle my recent experiences as an invalid in the 'Home' ward of the St. Thomas's Hospital, Westminster.

"Having succumbed to severe accidental illness, which baffled my regular medical attendants, I followed a friend's advice, and took up my quarters in this establishment, where, for the small charge of 8s. per day, I have had medical attendance, skilled nursing, eating and drinking, all of the very best.

"I cannot avoid writing this letter, if only as a sincere thanks-offering to Dr. Edmonds and the management generally. I can only again repeat my gratitude to the attendants, especially to the particular nurse under whose care I was placed. Throughout, everything has been done that could tend to alleviate my sufferings, and I can only strongly urge anyone, whether male or female (there are female wards), to at once follow my example should illness occur.

"I may add that a male dresser (formerly a member of the Army Hospital Corps) is always in attendance, and that a sitting-room, with books, etc., is provided. Smoking on the pleasant gallery overlooking the Thames is permitted.

"I am, Sir, your obedient servant,

"London, November 17." "A LATE PATIENT."

"Krauts," I said, "this is only the letter of a patient still weak from an operation—probably trephining." "That is so," replied Krauts; "I can make allowances for patients, but why did the Editor of the *Standard* put it in?"

I could not answer him, so I have written to you, sir, for an explanation. I am, &c., ROBERT SAWYER.

ON THE TRAMP.

[To the Editor of the Medical Times and Gazette.]

SIR,—In April last, the Master of the Axminster Workhouse said the short-service system had flooded the country with idle and dissolute scamps, too proud or too lazy to work as civilians.

I ventured to suggest that injured constitutions might be added to the list of causes which made discharged soldiers prefer tramping the country to steady work at their former trades.

Besides, it was the happy spring time then, and who could tell but that these military vagabonds might find employment? But I am sorry to say that in November the Relieving Officer at Honiton makes the same complaint as that made at Axminster by his brother official in April. He says that a large number of tramps, who had visited the town lately, were soldiers and short-service men, and that many had entered barefooted.

These men must either be unsuccessful candidates for work, or idle objectors.

But the question I want to have answered is this—What proportion of these tramps is due to sickness *from disease acquired in the service?* How many can get no work because they can do no work?

There may be better times in store for those who are willing and able to labour, but what prospect is there for men with injured constitutions? Is there no resource for them but to join the great army of the predatory classes?

I believe that occupation could be found by the State for men of good character who have been injured by short service, and find themselves unfit to compete with civilians. But, before discussing remedies, I should like to be sure that the disease of "military vagabondism" is pretty general. It may be that Devonshire is particularly unfortunate. I confess that I am anxious to know if the experience of relieving officers *along the great vagabond tramp roads of England* points to the same conclusion, that the number of military paupers is steadily increasing?

I think that if you, sir, were to express a wish for information on this point, numbers of medical men would be able to obtain statistics from relieving officers which would enable the public to form an opinion of their own on short service *as it is at present.* Surely it is a professional subject affecting the general health of an ever increasing class. I am, &c., A WANDERER.

EXHIBITION JUDGES.

[To the Editor of the Medical Times and Gazette.]

SIR,—It must, I think, be admitted that for the permanent success of exhibitions, the judges appointed should be men of position, possessing the full confidence of the medical profession, pre-eminently qualified for the duties they are expected to perform, and against whose impartiality there is not a scintilla of evidence—*i.e.*, if any value is to be attached to the awards by the public or the exhibitors themselves. The awards are given rise to very great discontent. The same dissatisfaction was expressed last year at the first—grandiloquently, but erroneously, termed "International"—Food Exhibition, and, as a consequence, several of our leading firms, it is stated, declined to put in an appearance this year. It is furthermore asserted that for the same reason upwards of one hundred (or more than half) of the exhibitors at the first show were conspicuous by their absence at the Agricultural Hall this year. From what I myself saw and heard, the complaints made appear to be fully justified. It would be a very easy matter to adduce facts in support of my statement; regard for your space, however, deters me from doing more than simply pointing out the bane and the antidote. Of course, judges are not immaculate, and it is not to be expected that their decisions would meet with general favour.

"'Tis with our judgments as our watches—none
Go just alike, yet each believes his own."

But when we find the complaints loud and numerous, and the decisions opposed to the expressed opinions of men whose notices and awards are never questioned, I submit that *attention*, at least, should be drawn to the matter. Surely it is "worse than a crime, it is a blunder," for a man to adjudicate on articles the virtues (?) of which he has extolled only a few weeks previous to the opening of an exhibition! I am, &c., SCRUTATOR.

OBITUARY.

THOMAS MICHAEL GREENHOW, M.D. DURH., F.R.C.S.

ON October 25, Thomas Michael Greenhow, M.D. Durh., F.R.C.S. Eng., Consulting Surgeon to the Newcastle-upon-Tyne Infirmary, died at Newton Hall, Patternewton, near Leeds, in his ninetieth year. After becoming M.R.C.S. in 1814, and serving as Assistant-Surgeon in the Army for about two years, he settled at Newcastle in 1817. He soon became Surgeon to the Lying-in Hospital, and obtained great experience in obstetric practice; but his taste lay in the direction of surgery, and in 1832 he was elected Surgeon to the Newcastle-upon-Tyne Infirmary, an office which he held for twenty-three years, during many of which he was Senior Surgeon. In conjunction with the late Sir John Fife, he established the Newcastle Eye Infirmary; and his reputation and skill in ophthalmic practice were considerable. His surgical success was great, his boldness as an operator being only equalled by the skill and resource with which he conducted the most serious undertakings in surgery.

On August 15, 1848, Dr. Greenhow performed the successful excision of the os calcis, being himself the author of the operation. Dr. Greenhow had been a Lecturer in the University of Durham College of Medicine, Newcastle-upon-Tyne, and in 1855 had the degree of M.D. conferred on him by the University. In 1843 he was appointed one of the original Fellows of the College of Surgeons of England, and at his death was the Senior Fellow but one on the list. Dr. Greenhow's vast experience of all matters connected with the healing art are but imperfectly represented by his writings. He was too fully occupied to be able to work much with his pen; but he published, in 1824, "The Remuneration of General Practitioners," an "Estimate of the True Value of Vaccination" in 1825, an "Essay on Cholera as it appeared in Newcastle and Gateshead" in 1832, and "A Description of a Sling Fracture Bed" in 1833. He also contributed to various medical journals, papers on "Stricture of Intestines," "Ovariotomy," and other subjects.

REPORTS OF SOCIETIES.

ROYAL MEDICAL AND CHIRURGICAL SOCIETY.

TUESDAY, NOVEMBER 22.

ANDREW WHYTE BARCLAY, M.D., President, in the chair.

CASE OF EXCISION OF A GRAVID UTERUS, WITH EPITHELIOMA OF THE CERVIX; WITH REMARKS ON THE OPERATIONS OF BLUNDELL, FREUND, AND PORRO.

MR. T. SPENCER WELLS read a paper descriptive of a case of excision of a gravid uterus with epithelioma of the cervix; with remarks on the operations of Blundell, Freund, and Porro. In this case a uterus with malignant disease of the cervix, and containing a fœtus at the sixth month, was removed through the divided abdominal wall, and the patient recovered. She was thirty-seven years old, mother of five children, six months pregnant, and her cervix uteri surrounded by a mass of epithelioma. The uterus was extirpated entirely on October 21 : the incision in the abdominal wall was eight inches long ; the uterus was brought out through the incision, separated from the bladder after tying the main arteries on each side ; the liquor amnii and fœtus removed through the anterior uterine wall ; the vaginal attachments separated all round ; the uterus removed ; all bleeding vessels tied ; and the communication between the vagina and peritoneal cavity closed by sutures. The abdominal wound was closed in the usual way. Phenol spray and all the usual antiseptic precautions were adopted. The various steps of the operation were described, and several modifications suggested as improvements in future operations. The uterus, preserved in the Museum of the College of Surgeons, was shown to the meeting. Total extirpation of the uterus both by the hypogastric and vaginal methods, and by a combination of the two methods, was briefly discussed. It is believed that this is the first case on record where excision of a gravid cancerous uterus has been followed by the recovery of the patient. Similar cases must be rare, but total extirpation of a cancerous uterus where pregnancy does not complicate the case will hereafter, much more frequently, become the subject of anxious consultation.

Dr. GRAILY HEWITT said that, having shared with Mr. Spencer Wells the responsibility of advising the operation which was performed in this case, he thought it well that the grounds on which this decision was arrived at should be mentioned. He saw the patient first in consultation with Dr. Tucker, her medical attendant. She had previously seen Mr. Wells. In accordance with the speaker's suggestion a consultation was subsequently held with Mr. Wells. The patient was unmistakably affected with epithelioma of the cervix uteri, the vaginal portion being hypertrophied and presenting a very distinct warty projection, running round it like an irregularly shaped cord just outside the orifice of the os uteri. The patient was, it was thought, a little over four months advanced in pregnancy, but it proved to be somewhat further advanced. She was in a very depressed and prostrate condition, having had little sleep, and having suffered from almost continuous pain in the pelvic region for several weeks past. There was a brownish irritating vaginal discharge. It was evident that the disease was rapidly progressing, but it appeared that, as yet, it was limited to the cervix uteri. One course of action which suggested itself was the speedy induction of abortion, followed as quickly as possible by amputation of the cervix uteri. Another was to remove the whole uterus at once. A third course of procedure would have been to allow the pregnancy to proceed to the viable period, then to effect delivery, and afterwards deal with the cervical disease. The objections to this latter course were, that the disease being in rapid progress it was probable that delivery *per vias naturales* of a viable child could not be counted on ; the cervical infiltration and thickening were fast increasing, and the operation of vaginal delivery would imply laceration of the cervix ; while in order to secure a live child the Cæsarian section might even be rendered necessary. Moreover, the delay in procedure would allow the patient to be subjected for some time longer to the deadly influence of the disease. The first and second procedures were discussed. On the one hand was the extreme danger of the immediate excision of the whole uterus, giving, however, a better chance, in the event of the patient's surviving the operation, of a considerable prolongation of her life. On the other, the possible bad effect of a premature induction of labour, followed by necessity for the further operation of excision of the cervix. Mr. Spencer Wells expressed himself very hopefully as to the result of the immediate excision plan, and, after duly discussing the matter, it was resolved that he should undertake the operation, and this was accordingly done. Dr. Hewitt stated that this is the first occasion in which the pregnant uterus has been removed entire in this country, and the profession must all congratulate Mr. Wells on his having so skilfully and successfully surmounted the difficulties attendant upon it. The operation differs from Porro's operation in some important particulars. In this operation performed by Mr. Wells the peculiarity is that the whole of the uterus was removed, whereas in the ordinary Porro operation the cervix uteri is not removed, or at all events not entirely removed, as in this case. The operation performed in this case is probably the more dangerous for the reason that the risk of injuring the ureters would seem to be greater. In this case Mr. Spencer Wells separated the uterine cervix from the adjacent tissues by a process of tearing rather than cutting. It may not be possible to adopt this plan in all cases, but it seems likely that it may conduce to the safety of the ureters.

Dr. PLAYFAIR said that the patient first came to him complaining of a vaginal discharge. There was then, he thought, epithelioma of the os, and he advised that labour should be brought on at once, after which the disease might be dealt with. This advice was not taken, and the disease spread rapidly. In such cases, no doubt, complete extirpation was the best thing to be done. Pregnancy and epithelioma were seldom found together; but when we had to deal with epithelioma alone, the question was, what was the best thing to be done. Under certain circumstances, no doubt, it was better to extirpate the whole uterus, but when the neck alone was affected, then the disease might be removed by cutting, scraping, and applying chloride of zinc, till the whole diseased mass sloughed off. In five or six cases this had done well in his hands. Even after this, abdominal section still remained. But when medullary cancer affected the body of the uterus, then abdominal section might be of the greatest importance; but the diagnosis was most difficult, and the mere fact of fixation of the uterus rendered the operation almost inadmissible. He had seen a case where, at the time, Freund's operation might have been successful, but it was not done, and in a fortnight fixation had taken place. In another case, seen with Dr. Matthews Duncan, there was much bleeding in a pregnant woman, suspected to be caused by malignant disease. Labour came on spontaneously, and the disease was found to be too far advanced for operation.

Dr. MATTHEWS DUNCAN said that, though it had been demonstrated by Mr. Spencer Wells that it was possible to remove a gravid uterus with success, its possibility and advisability were totally different things. In operations for uterine cancer, where even the disease had penetrated some distance from the cervix into the body of the organ, there had been considerable success. The cases of supra-vaginal cancer had generally done well, but in ordinary cancer of the cervix the reverse had been the case. In Mr. Wells's case the operation had the additional advantage of obviating the risks of labour.

Mr. KNOWSLEY THORNTON believed that Mr. S. Wells had tied both the spermatic and uterine arteries. Were it possible to tie off the ovaries and the spermatic arteries, the uterus might be easily and safely removed. Few ligatures would be required: Freund used too many. The extension of the disease into the uterus showed that a partial operation would have been of no use. Sometimes disease spread so fast that in a single week operation became out of the question. He thought drainage should be used in these cases. His experience of Marion Sims's operation was not so good as that of Dr. Playfair.

Mr. DORAN observed that hardening round the lower portion of the uterus was of the greatest importance. When Dr. Playfair saw this case there was none, but it soon made its appearance. This hard tissue contained many leucocytes, and, though not cancerous itself, was generally to be found round cancerous organs. After an operation, this hard tissue frequently disappeared in other organs, but it was very apt to become cancerous; hence the necessity for early operation when it was present.

Dr. HARRIS (of Madras) mentioned a case where he had removed portions of the cervix and then of the uterus, finally extirpating the uterus per vaginam. The patient died three days after; still, he preferred the vaginal operation.

Dr. BANTOCK had operated on a cancerous uterus in a very stout woman. The uterus was easily removed. He had been obliged to leave an opening in the vagina whereby the effused blood might escape. There formed, however, a considerable collection of blood in Douglas's pouch, where, perhaps, it would have been better to have placed a drainage-tube.

Dr. HEYWOOD SMITH said it was important to distinguish between the extension of cancer by contiguity and continuity.

Mr. SPENCER WELLS, in reply, said he had seen Dr. Marion Sims perform his operation, and never certainly was anything more complete, for the whole uterus came away, including a portion of the peritoneum. The patient died some time afterwards from extension of the disease. The question of the existence of leucocytes would be important if the surgeon could always tell what was inflammatory and what cancerous. No doubt a kind of induration might exist which would be no bar to operation. The spermatic and uterine arteries were too far apart to be conveniently tied together, and in tying the uterine there was always a risk of including the ureter.

THE CLINICAL SOCIETY OF LONDON.

FRIDAY, NOVEMBER 25.

JOSEPH LISTER, D.C.L., F.R.C.S., F.R.S.,
President, in the Chair.

TWO CASES OF DIRECT TRANSFUSION OF BLOOD FOR HÆMORRHAGE IN TYPHOID FEVER.

DR. F. A. MAHOMED read a paper on two cases of direct transfusion of blood for hæmorrhage in typhoid fever. The first case was that of an unmarried man, twenty-six years of age, who was stout, rather bloated-looking, and thoroughly out of condition. He passed through an anxious attack of enteric fever, complicated during the latter part of it by wakeful, excited delirium, resembling that of "delirium tremens," a complication not unfrequent during the defervescence of the specific fevers, and perhaps more especially liable to occur in persons addicted to the excessive use of alcohol. He relapsed on the twenty-fifth day of his illness; on the tenth day of his relapse, and the thirty-fifth of his fever, he had a severe hæmorrhage, which recurred twice on the following day. Exhausted, anæmic, restless, with cold extremities, and a very small, thready, and often irregular pulse, about 160 per minute, he was evidently fast sinking, when transfusion was performed, with the immediate result of bringing down his pulse rate from 160 to 144. After this he rallied for a few days, and even gained ground so much as to give great hopes of his ultimate recovery. Six days after the operation, hæmorrhage recurred to a small amount, which caused a sudden change for the worse, one or two more slight discharges of blood soon reduced him to a state of exhaustion, from which he could not recover. He died nine days after the operation, on the nineteenth day of his relapse, and the forty-fourth of his fever. The second case was that of a married man, who had a young family dependent upon him. He was twenty-five years of age—a powerful, well-made man, who during his attack of fever suffered a probably irrecoverable injury by collapse of a large part of his right lung, while in addition to this he had severe general bronchitis. On the twenty-sixth day of his illness he too had a relapse. On the fifth day of his relapse, and the thirty-first of his illness, he also had a severe hæmorrhage; four days later he had three more severe hæmorrhages, and relapsed into a state of complete exhaustion and impending dissolution. On the following day, when he appeared to be in extremis, transfusion was performed with the best possible effects; for two days he rallied greatly, when, during the exceptionally cold weather, his bronchitis increased, and he died from the lung complication on the fifth day after the operation, on the fifteenth of the relapse, and the fortieth of his fever. Dr. Mahomed gave some statistics showing that the average frequency of hæmorrhage in enteric fever was about 7 per cent. of all cases, and that about 50 per cent. of these were fatal; more than half of the fatal cases of hæmorrhage lost their lives as a direct result of the bleeding, and that it was in these cases more especially that the operation might be called for. He estimated that it might prove of service in about twenty cases out of 1400 cases of enteric fever. Each case must be judged on its own merits, and he would advise its performance whenever the patient was sinking into a dangerous condition, as a direct result of the loss of blood. He claimed that by means of it fatal exhaustion and syncope might be warded off, and time given for the action of remedies; a ready stimulant and food supplied to the heart and tissues; and the danger of destructive ulceration of the intestines during exhaustion and anæmia diminished. He advocated only direct transfusion of human blood by means of Aveling's transfusor, with a small expansion and no valves. He referred to Professor Schäfer's report to the Obstetrical Society in 1879, as proving the uselessness of the blood of the lower animals or saline solutions for this purpose.

Mr. HARRISON CRIPPS, in describing this operation, said that it was difficult to get good statistics with regard to the results of transfusion, the operation having been done for so many causes and with so many fluids. He would speak of blood in its natural state only, for defibrinated blood was of no use. Moreover, too many instruments had been employed to enable us to get a good knowledge of any one of them. The three chiefly in vogue were Roussel's, the simple tube, and Aveling's apparatus. As regards the first of these, the operation was clumsy—it meant machinery instead of anatomy. The simple tube could act only by gravitation, and was liable to cease to act altogether. Aveling's apparatus, on the other hand, was simple and good, but, as ordinarily sold, the tubes were too large. He found, moreover, that clips were better than stop-cocks. It was best first to expose the vein of the recipient, as it was usually much easier to open the vein of the giver, but it was best only to expose the vein, not to open it. After this the vein of the giver should be opened, and next that of the receiver, when the two should be immediately connected. The quantity used by him in the case under discussion he estimated at from twelve to fourteen ounces.

Mr. BARKER spoke of a case of pernicious anæmia where the patient's brother freely supplied the blood. The apparatus leaked somewhere, so that the blood coagulated, and the operation broke down. He then tried defibrinated blood, but that did not do much good.

Dr. COUPLAND asked whether it was better to take the blood from an artery or a vein. In certain respects arterial blood would seem to be the better, but was a wound in an artery as serious a thing as a wound in a vein. It would not be easy to measure the exact quantity transmitted from an artery.

Mr. PARKER was present at one of Roussel's operations when Mr. Adams gave from his arm a quantity of blood to a patient in risk of dying on the operation-table. The instrument acted perfectly.

Mr. WARRINGTON HAWARD said that it was plain that in such cases the simpler the apparatus the better. He had seen Roussel, and that gentleman had said that with his apparatus the blood was least likely to coagulate, but that was not so. He had tried it in a case of pernicious anæmia under Dr. Cavafy. He encountered no difficulty to begin with, but after about four ounces had been injected no more would pass; a coagulum had formed in the apparatus. There was no material gain, but no harm. Further experiments on the dead body showed it to be unsatisfactory; the valves could not be used. He had seen defibrinated blood used, certainly with good effect for the time being.

Mr. PARKER remarked that Roussel had insisted on the necessity of employing pure rubber tubes, as the others tended to favour coagulation.

Mr. W. HAWARD said that the apparatus he used was one of Roussel's own.

The PRESIDENT likewise thought that the simpler the apparatus the better; and he recommended the ordinary glass syringe, as it could be washed out if any coagula formed. India-rubber, if kept for a time, almost always goes out of order. There was little danger to the patient in these cases if antiseptics were used. Many years ago he had found that coagulation was really due to contact with foreign solid matter. Even the veins might act in this way, yet the blood does not coagulate in the veins.

In reply, Dr. MAHOMED said that he did not think that more than about four ounces of blood had been transfused in his last case; certainly less than ten would do good. In these cases he did not think it fair that the resident officers, living in a more or less vitiated atmosphere, should be asked to give the blood, and he saw no reasonable objection to having a strong, healthy person for this purpose. Opening a vein and introducing a tube was not the same thing as making a longitudinal slit with a lancet. In his case all antiseptic precautions broke down. A transverse incision was the best. It really did not matter greatly whether the blood taken was venous or arterial; in either case it had to pass through the lungs before reaching the left heart.

The PRESIDENT said that Dr. Fox had present an interesting case of chromidrosis, and he would appoint a committee to examine into it. This was accordingly done.

THREE CASES OF CONTINUED FEVER, WITH AFFECTION OF THE SPLEEN, IN TWO OF WHICH AN EXTREMELY HIGH TEMPERATURE OCCURRED BEFORE DEATH, AND ONE OF WHICH CLINICALLY RESEMBLED ENTERIC FEVER.

Dr. T. WHIPHAM related three cases of continued fever, with affection of the spleen, in two of which an extremely high temperature occurred before death, and one of which clinically resembled enteric fever. The cases had come under the author's observation during the past three years. Case 1 was a domestic servant, aged twenty; had enjoyed excellent health, and save that she was an inordinate meat-eater, was guilty of no excesses. Five weeks before admission into hospital she was attacked by headache; vomiting and profuse sweats set in about nine days before she came under observation. At this time she complained of abdominal tenderness. While under treatment the symptoms were but little altered, and on the thirty-eighth day she was suddenly attacked with severe pain in the left iliac region. So severe was this pain, that she never ceased screaming until her death in the evening. At the autopsy a few yellowish-white masses of irregular shape were found in the spleen, giving the general impression of infarcts; no other organ showed any appreciable change from the normal condition. Case 2.—A domestic servant, aged twenty-one, had been remarkably free from illness, and had never been seriously ill, save when she had chicken-pox as a child. She was in perfect health four days before admission, when she took a warm bath, after which the catamenia appeared, but ceased in about three hours, and she was then attacked by abdominal pain, chiefly in the hypogastrium, and also in the legs and back. She had lost two brothers and a sister from phthisis. After four days' rest in hospital she was so much better that she was allowed to get up, but eleven days later she was unable to stand, and had fits of alternate laughing and crying; was constipated, and complained of pains at the top of her head. On July 1, 1878 (eighteen days after admission), her pulse was 104, and the temperature still normal, but she was delirious and so noisy that she was removed to the separation ward. She became gradually worse, and died on July 11. The temperature had risen to 109° F. shortly before her death. At the autopsy a few circumscribed dark red patches were found in the spleen, which contrasted strongly with the general brick-red colour of the organ. Beyond some congestion of the lungs, no other morbid change was found. Case 3.—A domestic servant, aged twenty-six, was attacked about November 10, 1880, with many of the symptoms of enteric fever, and was admitted on November 24. Next day several rose-coloured spots were found on the abdomen, indistinguishable from typhoid spots. Diarrhœa persisted; the patient became very weak, and then delirious. The abdomen tympanitic. On December 1 the diarrhœa was profuse, pulse 168, and she died in the afternoon. About ten minutes before death her temperature rose to 108·6° F. At the autopsy the spleen weighed sixteen ounces; in its substance was a large infarct, partially broken down; the tissue of the organ was diffluent. The solitary glands of the intestines were unusually conspicuous, but no other abnormality was found. The cause of the disease was in each case obscure. Two explanations suggested themselves—viz., blood-poisoning or local inflammation of, or in the neighbourhood of, the spleen, the weight of evidence pointing rather to the latter. The absence of any history pointing to splenic affection is remarkable, as also is the fact that these three patients were all female domestic servants, and of about the same age. The high temperature which was observed in Cases 2 and 3 is noteworthy.

Dr. C. T. WILLIAMS asked if the spinal cord and brain had been examined in these cases.

The PRESIDENT said that many different diseases were produced in animals by organisms, and this was probably the case in man too. He thought that in such cases the blood ought to be examined after having been duly prepared.

Dr. WHIPHAM said that the brain in all, and the spinal cord in one, had been examined, but not the blood.

NEW INVENTIONS AND IMPROVEMENTS.

MURRAY AND LANMAN'S FLORIDA WATER.

WE have no hesitation in recommending this preparation, for which Messrs. Burroughs, Wellcome, and Co., Snow-hill, E.C., are the European agents. It is a simple floral extract, and has a very delicate, refreshing fragrance and perfume. In America it has been well known for many years; and in tropical climates it is largely used in the bath, and to freshen the atmosphere by sprinkling or spraying through the room. A like employment of it in the sick-room would, we have no doubt, be found especially grateful and useful. It deserves to gain the favour of the public.

SCHIEFFELIN AND CO.'S SOLUBLE PILLS.

WE have already spoken of the excellence of manufacture of these pills. They are admirably made in all points, and the coating is easily and quickly soluble. And we now only add to our former notice of them the additional testimony to their merits afforded by the fact that Messrs. Allen and Hanburys, of Plough-court, are the sole agents for them for Great Britain and Ireland.

KANDOLT'S TAMARIND LOZENGES.

THESE lozenges, which are manufactured by C. Kandolt, of Gotha, may be recommended as a convenient and trustworthy laxative for children and delicate women. They are made from the fruit of the tamarind tree; are got up so as to look like sweetmeats rather than medicine; are not at all unpleasant to take; and act well and quickly, without causing griping. The dose required will of course vary much in different individuals, but, as a rule, a quarter or a half of a lozenge will be sufficient for a child, while an adult may take a whole one, or rather less, daily. They may be obtained from Mr. P. Metz, 10, Jewin-street, E.C.

ALLEN AND SON'S PORTABLE BATH.

FROM Messrs. James Allen and Son, the well-known manufacturers, of Marylebone-lane, we have received the following:— "Will you allow us to call the attention of your readers to a hospital-bath we are about to introduce to the profession. This bath is 5 ft. 6 in. long, and made of strong tinned iron,

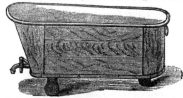

japanned in and out, fitted with a large draw-off tap, and drainer-plate over same; is mounted on a wood bottom, with iron wheels with india-rubber tyres, to be noiseless for ward use. We believe the bath is being much used for scarlet fever, and as this is very prevalent just now, and the fever hospitals are re-opening, we think this would meet a want."

THE ROYAL COMMISSION ON SMALL-POX AND FEVER HOSPITALS.—The Royal Commission on Small-pox and Fever Hospitals in the Metropolis has already held several meetings in No. 10 Committee-room of the House of Commons.

MEDICAL NEWS.

APOTHECARIES' HALL, LONDON.—The following gentlemen passed their examination in the Science and Practice of Medicine, and received certificates to practise, on Thursday, November 24 :—

Clarke, Albert Blockly, Chatteris, Cambridgeshire.
De Woolfson, Louis Eslevan Green, Holles-street, Cavendish-square.
Gordon, Edward, Hazel Grove, Stockport.

The following gentleman also on the same day passed the Primary Professional Examination :—

Power, Charles Frederick, Manchester School of Medicine.

APPOINTMENTS.

** The Editor will thank gentlemen to forward to the Publishing-office, as early as possible, information as to all new Appointments that take place.

CORSOULD, HENRY FRANCIS, L.R.C.P. Lond., M.R.C.S. Eng.—Resident Obstetrical Officer to the Charing-cross Hospital, vice F. J. Grindon.
CRANE, CHARLES R., M.R.C.S. Eng., L.S.A.—Resident Surgical Officer to the Charing-cross Hospital, vice F. E. Taylor.
DUNCAN, W. A., M.D., L.R.C.P., M.R.C.S., L.S.A.—Resident Accoucheur at St. Thomas's Hospital.
GULLIVER, G., M.B., M.R.C.P.—Assistant-Physician to St. Thomas's Hospital, vice W. S. Greenfield, appointed Professor of Pathology to the University of Edinburgh.
LYSTER, C. R. C, M.R.C.S. Eng.—Resident Medical Officer to the Charing-cross Hospital, vice J. S. Baker.
PITTARD, M., M.R.C.S. Eng.—Assistant Surgical Officer to the Charing-cross Hospital, vice H. R. Mosse.
SUTTON, S. W., M.B. Lond., L.R.C.P., M.R.C.S.—Senior Assistant House-Physician to St. Thomas's Hospital.
WELLS, A. E., L.R.C.P., M.R.C.S.—Junior Assistant House-Physician to St. Thomas's Hospital.
WHITE, E. F., M.R.C.S., L.S.A.—Assistant House-Surgeon to St. Thomas's Hospital.
WIGAN, C. A., L.S.A.—Assistant Medical Officer to the Charing-cross Hospital, vice C. R. C. Lyster.

NAVAL, MILITARY, ETC., APPOINTMENTS.

ADMIRALTY.—Staff-Surgeon Henry Ashlin Close to be Fleet-Surgeon in Her Majesty's Fleet, with seniority of the 19th inst.—Staff-Surgeon William Denson Isaac has been placed on the retired list of his rank from the 7th inst.—Surgeon William Henry Boland has been placed on the retired list of his rank from the 4th inst.

BIRTHS.

CLARK.—On November 24, at 19, Cavendish-place, W., the wife of Andrew Clark, F.R.C.S., of a daughter.
DEBENHAM.—On November 23, at Heath House, Stepney, the wife of Robert Debenham, M.R.C.S., of a daughter.
DRUMMOND.—On November 18, at 3, Piazza di Spagna, Rome, the wife of Edward Drummond, M.D., of a daughter.
FRY.—On November 26, at 24, Cornwallis-gardens, Hastings, the wife of Surgeon-Major Walter Fry, Her Majesty's Indian Army, of a daughter.
HILLIARD.—On November 26, at Fairmead House, Upper Holloway-road, N., the wife of R. Harvey Hilliard, M.D., of a daughter.
HOAR.—On November 23, at Robertsbridge, Sussex, the wife of Charles Hoar, M.B., of a daughter.
HOLLIS.—On November 29, at Park Gate, Brighton, the wife of W. A. Hollis, M.D., of a son.
MACSWINNEY.—On November 23, at Westall House, Brook Green, W., the wife of G. H. MacSwinney, M.D., of a daughter.
PERIGAL.—On November 20, at New Barnet, Herts, the wife of Arthur Perigal, M.D., of a son.
SAWTELL.—On November 7, at 102, Florence-road, Stroud Green, N,, the wife of Tom Henry Sawtell, M.B., L.R.C.P., of a son.

MARRIAGES.

DE DENNE—WEIGHELL.—On November 24, at Hove, Sussex, Thomas Vincent de Denne, M.R.C.S., of Cradley Heath, Staffordshire, youngest son of William Denne, F.R.C.S., of Eastbourne, to Margaret Anne, third daughter of the late Rev. John Weighell, B.A., rector of Cheddington, Bucks.
BEFITT—LIEPMANN.—On November 22, at Berlin, Paul Eberty, M.D., to Katie, only daughter of Julius Liepmann, Esq., formerly of Victoria park, Manchester.
MITCHELL—MILLS.—On November 17, at Galway, Robert Mitchell, M.D., of Nelson, Lancashire, to Agnes Halleburton, eldest daughter of John Miller, J.P., of Weir House, Galway.
PENSON—SPACKMAN.—On November 23, at Faringdon, Richard, youngest son of the late Rev. J. P. Penson, vicar of Clanfield, Oxon, to Clara, only daughter of F. C. Spackman, M.R.C.S., of Faringdon.
ROBERTSON—MORRALL.—On November 24, at Dudleston, Shropshire, W. H. Robertson, M.D., F.R.C.P., J.P., of Buxton, Derbyshire, to Margaret, second surviving daughter of the Rev. Cyrus Morrall, of Plas Yolyn, Shropshire.

DEATHS.

BEAN, WILLOUGHBY JOHN, Esq., C.E., son of Surgeon-Major John Bean, late of the Bombay Medical Service, on a voyage to Australia, on September 7, aged 23.

BLAKE, VALENTINE WALSHMAN, F.R.C.S., late of 6, Old-square, Birmingham, at Bishopstone, Moseley, on November 24, in his 64th year.
CHEESBROUGH, HENRY A., M.D., Consulting Physician to the East Lancashire Infirmary, at Blackburn, on November 20, aged 44.
DAVIS, EDWARD WILLIAM STEPHEN, M.R.C.S., at Duffryn Efrwd Mountain Ash, on November 22, aged 63.
JOHNSTON, JOHN, M.B.C.S., at 27, Huskisson-street, Liverpool, on November 29, aged 30.
MILLER, DAVID GRAHAM, M.R.C.P., Fleet-Surgeon R.N., at 113, Camberwell New-road, on November 26, in his 51st year.
POLLOCK, TIMOTHY, M.D., late of 26, Hatton-garden, at Rose Hill, Hornsey, on November 26, aged 53.
PRESCOTT, ELIZABETH LYDIA MONRO KNIGHT, wife of Surgeon-Major A. K. Prescott, at Grays, on November 25.
TURTLE, NEWTON, infant son of Frederick Turtle, M.D., at Kirkmead, Woodford, Essex, on November 24.
YELD, HENRY JOHN, M.D., at Sunderland, on November 18, aged 47.

VACANCIES.

In the following list the nature of the office vacant, the qualifications required in the candidate, the person to whom application should be made and the day of election (as far as known) are stated in succession.

BECKETT HOSPITAL AND DISPENSARY, BARNSLEY.—House-Surgeon. Candidates must hold a diploma from one of the recognised Universities of the United Kingdom, or from one of the Royal Colleges of Surgeons, and must be a Licentiate of the Apothecaries' Company, London, and be unmarried, and, if elected, must agree not to engage in private for a period of three years. Applications, with testimonials, to be sent to the Honorary Secretary, on or before December 10.
CENTRAL LONDON OPHTHALMIC HOSPITAL GRAY'S-INN-ROAD.—Assistant-Surgeon. Candidates must be members of the Royal College of Surgeons of England, and must produce certificate of having attended the practice of some ophthalmic institution for at least six months. Testimonials to be addressed to the Secretary, on or before December 6.
GENERAL INFIRMARY AT GLOUCESTER, AND THE GLOUCESTERSHIRE EYE INSTITUTION.—Ophthalmic Surgeon. Applications, enclosing qualifications and testimonials, to be forwarded to the Committee, under cover to the Secretary, on or before December 7.
HUNTINGDON COUNTY HOSPITAL.—House-Surgeon. (For particulars see Advertisement.)
ISLE OF MAN GENERAL HOSPITAL AND DISPENSARY, DOUGLAS.—Resident Medical Officer. Candidates must be members of some of the Royal Colleges of Surgeons of London, Edinburgh, or Dublin, and have a thorough knowledge of the compounding of medicines, and be unmarried. Applications and testimonials to be sent to the Secretary, not later than December 5.
MIDDLESEX COUNTY LUNATIC ASYLUM, COLNEY HATCH.—Assistant Medical Officer. (For particulars see Advertisement.)
VICTORIA HOSPITAL FOR CHILDREN, QUEEN'S-ROAD, CHELSEA, S.W.—Assistant-Physician. Candidates must be graduates in medicine of a University recognised by the Medical Council, and not practising pharmacy. Applications, with copies of testimonials, to be sent to the Secretary, at the Hospital, on or before December 12.

UNION AND PAROCHIAL MEDICAL SERVICE.

. The area of each district is stated in acres. The population is computed according to the census of 1871.

RESIGNATIONS.

Lincoln Union.—Mr. William Edward Scott has resigned the Second and Eleventh Districts. Second District : area 15,560 ; population 2184 ; salary £30 per annum. Eleventh District : area 9535 ; population 2296 ; salary £30 per annum.
Scarborough Union.—Mr. W. C. Everley Taylor has resigned the Workhouse. Salary £70 per annum.
Wareham and Purbeck Union.—Mr. William Todman Boreham has resigned the Morden and Wareham First Districts. Morden District : area 11,467 ; population 1562 ; salary £32 per annum. Wareham First District : area 7579 ; population 2965 ; salary £40 per annum.

APPOINTMENTS.

Dunmow Union.—William Sunderland, M.R.C.S. Eng., L.R.C.P. Edin., to the Thaxted District.
Leeds Union.—Jas. Allan, C.M., M.D. Aber., as Medical Superintendent to the Infirmary.
Maldon.—Thomas A. Poole*, F.C.S., as Analyst for the Borough, *vice* Dr. Whitmore, deceased.
Pontesbury Union.—David McConbrey, M.D., M.C. Queen's Univ. Ire., to the Silkstone District.
Thame Union.—L. Williams, M.R.C.S. Eng., L.S.A., to the Waterperry District.

DR. EDGAR SHEPPARD has resigned his Medical Superintendentship at Colney Hatch Asylum, after a service of twenty years ; and one of the Assistant Medical Officers, W. J. Seward, M.B. Lond., has been elected to succeed him. The Middlesex magistrates have granted Dr. Sheppard a pension of £450 a year.

VACCINATION IN BENGAL.—It is stated, in the *Indian Medical Gazette*, that the number of persons vaccinated in Bengal in 1880-81 was 1,394,312 ; of which total 1,339,012 were contributed by vaccine circles, and 55,300 by dispensaries and municipalities. The percentage of success in primary operations was 98·60. There are ten vaccine circles in Bengal. The Government states that the reports of the year indicate that the attitude of the people towards vaccination is improving.

ENGINEER VOLUNTEERS.—Surgeon M. Baines, M.D., 1st Middlesex Engineer Volunteers, has been granted the rank of Honorary Surgeon-Major—dated July 1, 1881.

COLLEGE OF PRECEPTORS.—The half-yearly certificate examination of the College of Preceptors, which opens on Tuesday next, will be carried on for the rest of the week, simultaneously in London and at about forty local centres in various parts of England and Wales, will be attended by the large number of 7500 candidates. At Midsummer 3890 candidates were examined by the College, so that the total for the year falls little short of 11,500. This is the largest examination which has ever been held in this country by any examining body ; and, taken in connexion with the various University local examinations, which attract about 10,000 candidates annually, furnishes a striking evidence of the great extension which the system of middle-class examinations has now attained. The higher certificates of the College having been recognised by Her Majesty's judges and by the General Medical Council as guarantees of a good education, exempting the holders of them from the "preliminary literary examinations" required by the Incorporated Law Society, and by the various medical corporations of the United Kingdom, the College has arranged for holding two supplementary examinations, in March and September each year, for these higher certificates, which will be open to legal and medical students, as well as to candidates desirous of qualifying for the Royal Veterinary College, the Pharmaceutical Society, and other bodies by whom the certificates of the College are recognised.

DEAFNESS OF RAILWAY EMPLOYÉS.—In a communication to the *Bulletin de Thérapeutique*, August 30, Prof. Terrillon observes that the absence of sufficient acuteness of hearing of railway *employés* is no less deserving attention than the anomalies of vision that have of late attracted notice. This dulness of hearing, which is of so much importance in all those who have to attend to the whistle as a signal, sometimes comes on very slowly and almost imperceptibly to the subject of it. Prof. Terrillon refers to two important papers on the subject, one by Prof. Moos of Heidelberg, and the other by Dr. Burckner of Göttingen.

ROYAL COLLEGE OF SURGEONS.—At the half-yearly examinations for the Fellowship of the College, which were brought to a close on the 28th ult., eight candidates out of the twenty-five examined were reported to have acquitted themselves to the satisfaction of the Court of Examiners. The following were the questions on Pathology, Therapeutics, and Surgery submitted to them at the written examination on the 24th ult., viz. :—1. Explain, with precision, what is understood by the term reduction of a hernia "*en masse.*" Describe the clinical history of such a case, and the treatment you would adopt. Mention other conditions which have been included under this term. 2. Describe in detail the symptoms and course of traumatic tetanus, and state what is known of its pathological anatomy. What principles would guide you in its treatment, and by what circumstances would your prognosis be influenced ? 3. Discuss the symptoms, supervening at an interval of several days after a blow on the head, which would lead you to infer the occurrence of inflammation within the skull. Mention the forms such inflammation may assume ; state the circumstances which might aid you in distinguishing between them, and detail the treatment you would adopt in each. 4. What are the chief causes of paralysis of the muscles of the eyeball ? Give examples of some of the principal forms, and state the appropriate treatment. The candidates were required to answer all four questions. At the clinical examination on cases selected from the metropolitan hospitals, the following were the Medical, viz. :—Syphilitic ostitis and choroiditis ; chronic abscess in neck, strumous disease of testis ; herpes frontalis ; chronic disease of hip ; varicose aneurism ; cancer of œsophagus ; subcutaneous nævus ; syphilitic ostitis ; rodent ulcer ; paralysis of fifth pair (sensory only) ; paralysis of left arm (motion only) ; curvature of the spine, with necrosis of rib ; hydrocele and disease of testis ; syphilitic disease of finger ; cheloid, and scars of acne ; lupus ; curvature of spine and abscesses, disease of epididymis ; fluctuating tumour, chronic abscess ; disease of testis and hydrocele ; tertiary syphilitic disease ; syphilitic disease of testis ; chancre in the palm ; gangrene from pressure ; eruption—lupus lymphaticus (Hutchinson) ; abscess in tibia.

APPOINTMENTS FOR THE WEEK.

December 3. *Saturday (this day).*

Operations at St. Bartholomew's, 1½ p.m.; King's College, 1½ p.m.; Royal Free, 2 p.m.; Royal London Ophthalmic, 11 a.m.; Royal Westminster Ophthalmic, 1½ p.m.; St. Thomas's, 1½ p.m.; London, 2 p.m.

5. *Monday.*

Operations at the Metropolitan Free, 2 p.m.; St. Mark's Hospital for Diseases of the Rectum, 2 p.m.; Royal London Ophthalmic, 11 a.m.; Royal Westminster Ophthalmic, 1½ p.m.

Royal Institution, 5 p.m. General Monthly Meeting.

Odontological Society, 8 p.m. Mr. Coleman, "On the Economical Methods of Preparing and Administering Nitrous Oxide." Casual communications by Messrs. Varier and Pedley, etc.

Medical Society of London, 8½ p.m. Dr. Gilbart Smith, "Notes of a Case of Hæmorrhage into the Mesentery." Dr. Isambard Owen will read notes of two similar Cases. Dr. Habershon, "On Cold Shock in its Action on the Branches of the Pneumogastric Nerve." Dr. Dowse, "On some Points in the Differential Diagnosis of Intracranial Disease, General Paralysis of the Insane, and Tabes Dorsalis."

6. *Tuesday.*

Operations at Guy's, 1½ p.m.; Westminster, 2 p.m.; Royal London Ophthalmic, 11 a.m.; Royal Westminster Ophthalmic, 1½ p.m.; West London, 3 p.m.

Pathological Society, 8½ p.m. Specimens: Dr. Norman Moore—Joints from a Case of Gout. Dr. Wickham Legg—Tissues of a Patient with Hæmophilia. Mr. Lawson Tait—Specimens of Hydro- and Pyo-Salpinx. Mr. Eve—Calcified Adenoma of Scalp. Dr. Pye-Smith—Cirrhosis of Liver in a Child. Dr. Bedford Fenwick—Diseased Supra-Renal Capsules. Mr. A. P. Gould—1. Bones from Genu Valgum; 2. Case of Lateral Asymmetry. Mr. A. Barker—1. Fracture of Femur; 2. Congenital Dislocation of Hip; 3. Spinal Caries. Dr. Goodhart—Specimens of Ulcerative Endocarditis. Mr. Shattock—Adenoma of Scalp.

7. *Wednesday.*

Operations at University College, 2 p.m.; St. Mary's, 1¼ p.m.; Middlesex, 1 p.m.; London, 2 p.m.; St. Bartholomew's, 1½ p.m.; Great Northern, 2 p.m.; Samaritan, 2½ p.m.; Royal London Ophthalmic, 11 a.m.; Royal Westminster Ophthalmic, 1½ p.m.; St. Thomas's, 1½ p.m.; St. Peter's Hospital for Stone, 2 p.m.; National Orthopædic, Great Portland-street, 10 a.m.

Epidemiological Society, 8 p.m. Dr. Cobbold, "On Filaria Sanguinis Hominis" (sent by Dr. Wykeham Myers, stationed at Formosa); followed by a short paper of his own on the same subject.

Hunterian Society (London Institution) (Council Meeting, 7½), 8 p.m. Dr. Francis Warner, "On a Case of Empyema treated by Antiseptic Drainage." Dr. F. C. Turner, "On a Case of Cerebral Hæmorrhage."

Obstetrical Society, 8 p.m. Specimens will be shown by the President, Mr. Thornton, Dr. Percy Boulton, Mr. Outhwaite, and Dr. Herman. The following papers will be read:—Dr. Godson, "On Five Cases of Spasmodic Dysmenorrhœa associated with Sterility successfully treated by Dilatation with Graduated Metallic Bougies." Dr. Herman, "On a Case in which Dilatation of the Cervical Canal was followed by Removal of Sterility." Mr. N. W. Jastreban, "On the Normal and Pathological Anatomy of the Ganglion Cervicale Uteri." Dr. W. S. Playfair, "On Trachelorraphé, or Emmet's Operation."

8. *Thursday.*

Operations at St. George's, 1 p.m.; Central London Ophthalmic, 1 p.m.; Royal Orthopædic, 2 p.m.; University College, 2 p.m.; Royal London Ophthalmic, 11 a.m.; Royal Westminster Ophthalmic, 1½ p.m.; Hospital for Diseases of the Throat, 2 p.m.; Hospital for Women, 2 p.m. Charing-cross, 2 p.m.; London, 2 p.m.; North-West London, 2½ p.m.

Harveian Society, 8½ p.m. Dr. Alfred Meadows, "On Menstruation and its Derangements." (Second Harveian Lecture.)

Ophthalmological Society, 8½ p.m. Mr. R. J. Pye-Smith, "On a Case of Glaucoma cured by Eserine." Dr. Gowers—1. "Sequel to a Case of Cerebral Tumour"; 2. "On Two Cases of Optic Neuritis in Chorea"; 3. "On a Case of Axial Neuritis in Spinal Disease"; 4. "On a Case of Hemiopia in Locomotor Ataxy." Mr. G. E. Wherry, "On a Case of Paralysis of Fifth and Facial Nerves in a Young Child." Dr. Stephen Mackenzie, "On a Case of Acute Vascular Disease with Retinal Hæmorrhages." Mr. Nettleship, "Note on a Case of Diabetic Cataract" Mr. C. E. Fitzgerald, "On Unilateral Exophthalmos." Living specimens at 8 p.m.: Mr. Mules—General Retinal Periarteritis. Mr. Nettleship—1. Cystic Tumour of Eyebrow; 2. Diabetic Retinitis. Mr. Cowell—Case of Retinitis Pigmentosa."

9. *Friday.*

Operations at Central London Ophthalmic, 2 p.m.; Royal London Ophthalmic, 11 a.m.; South London Ophthalmic, 2 p.m.; Royal Westminster Ophthalmic, 1½ p.m.; St. George's (ophthalmic operations), 1¼ p.m.; Guy's, 1½ p.m.; St Thomas's (ophthalmic operations), 2 p.m.; King's College (by Mr. Lister), 2 p.m.

Clinical Society, 8½ p.m. Mr. W. H. Bennett, "On a Case of Talipes Equino-varus treated by Resection of a Portion of the Tarsus." Mr. J. R. Lunn, "On Two Cases of Myxœdema (Male and Female)." Dr. Cavafy, "On Two Cases of Myxœdema." Mr. W. H. Kesteven, "On a Case of Unilateral Xanthopsia" (patient will be exhibited).

VITAL STATISTICS OF LONDON.

Week ending Saturday, November 26, 1881.

BIRTHS.

Births of Boys, 1221; Girls, 1180; Total, 2401.
Corrected weekly average in the 10 years 1871-80, 2566·8.

DEATHS.

	Males.	Females.	Total.
Deaths during the week	791	810	1601
Weekly average of the ten years 1871-80, corrected to increased population ...	892·4	867·8	1760·2
Deaths of people aged 80 and upwards ...	...	...	51

DEATHS IN SUB-DISTRICTS FROM EPIDEMICS.

	Enumerated Population, 1881 (unrevised).	Small-pox.	Measles.	Scarlet Fever.	Diphtheria.	Whooping-cough.	Typhus.	Enteric (or Typhoid) Fever.	Simple continued Fever.	Diarrhœa.
West	668993	2	12	2	1	3	...	5	...	1
North ...	905677	1	8	17	7	6	2	12	1	2
Central ...	281793	...	1	2	3	10	...	7	1	...
East	692530	1	4	7	4	8	...	6	2	1
South	1265578	16	25	24	11	23	3	11	...	6
Total	3814571	20	50	52	26	50	5	41	4	10

METEOROLOGY.

From Observations at the Greenwich Observatory.

Mean height of barometer ...	29·619 in.
Mean temperature ...	49·5°
Highest point of thermometer ...	58·3°
Lowest point of thermometer ...	41·0°
Mean dew-point temperature ...	45·6°
General direction of wind ...	S.W.
Whole amount of rain in the week ...	1·07 in.

BIRTHS and DEATHS Registered and METEOROLOGY during the Week ending Saturday, Nov. 26, in the following large Towns:—

Cities and boroughs (Municipal boundaries except for London.)	Estimated Population to middle of the year 1881.*	Persons to an Acre. (1881.)	Births Registered during the week ending Nov. 26.	Deaths Registered during the week ending Nov. 26.	Temperature of Air (Fahr.): Highest during the Week.	Temperature of Air (Fahr.): Lowest during the Week.	Temperature of Air (Fahr.): Weekly Mean of Daily Mean Values	Temp. of Air (Cent.): Weekly Mean of Daily Mean Values.	Rain Fall: In Inches.	Rain Fall: In Centimetres.
London	3829751	50·8	2401	1601	58·3	41·0	49·5	9·72	1·07	2·72
Brighton	107934	45·9	55	44	55·7	41·5	49·1	9·50	2·04	5·18
Portsmouth ...	128335	28·6	89	48	...	...	...	...	...	...
Norwich	88038	11·8	49	37	...	...	...	...	...	...
Plymouth	75262	54·0	43	27	58·0	43·0	52·0	11·11	1·19	3·02
Bristol	207140	46·5	133	76	58·0	38·5	49·3	9·61	1·54	3·91
Wolverhampton ...	75934	22·4	41	19	55·4	32·3	45·0	7·22	1·07	2·72
Birmingham ...	402296	47·9	264	165	...	...	...	...	...	...
Leicester	123120	38·5	69	47	58·5	34·0	47·5	8·61	1·23	3·12
Nottingham ...	188035	18·9	125	78	57·3	36·0	46·7	8·17	0·72	1·83
Liverpool	553988	106·3	378	299	56·9	35·5	46·7	8·17	0·75	1·90
Manchester ...	341269	79·5	230	147	...	...	...	...	...	...
Salford	177760	34·4	130	92	...	...	...	...	...	...
Oldham	112176	24·0	59	46	...	...	...	...	...	...
Bradford	184037	25·5	111	58	54·2	38·6	47·4	8·55	1·32	3·35
Leeds	310490	14·4	191	94	...	...	...	...	...	...
Sheffield	285621	14·5	186	102	56·0	36·0	45·8	7·67	1·57	3·99
Hull	155161	42·7	95	91	56·0	35·0	45·5	7·50	1·10	2·79
Sunderland ...	116753	42·2	88	43	59·0	36·0	47·1	8·39	0·21	0·53
Newcastle-on-Tyne	145675	27·1	92	47	...	...	...	...	...	...
Total of 20 large English Towns ...	7608775	38·0	4828	3161	59·0	32·3	47·6	8·67	1·15	2·92

* These figures are the numbers enumerated (but subject to revision) in April last, raised to the middle of 1881 by the addition of a quarter of a year's increase, calculated at the rate that prevailed between 1871 and 1881.

At the Royal Observatory, Greenwich, the mean reading of the barometer last week was 29·62 in. The highest reading was 29·91 in. on Wednesday evening, and the lowest 28·75 in. at the end of the week.

NOTES, QUERIES, AND REPLIES.

Be that questionest much shall learn much.—Bacon.

BORED EARS—IN REGARD TO WEAK EYES.
TO THE EDITOR OF THE MEDICAL TIMES AND GAZETTE.

SIR,—Can you kindly inform me whether there is any medical or anatomical foundation for the widely-spread idea throughout the globe, that having the ears bored and wearing gold rings in the holes strengthens eyesight. Several ladies, whose veracity I cannot doubt, have assured me of this "fact, derived from their own experience." They state that before this operation of having their ears bored, styes were frequent on the eyes, and caused much pain, but this inconvenience entirely disappeared immediately after boring, when the ear-rings were inserted. They give as reason that the hole in the ear and the weight of the ear-ring draw any humours or affections from the eyes to those parts. My friends recommend highly this custom, and never, even in bed, remove from their ears the small gold wires which are commonly called "sleepers," for fear the holes would close and require to be re-bored. The *British Medical Journal*, August 10, London, 1867, page 120, has an "almost painless mode of boring ears with a needle heated to a red heat." The ear rings are adjusted and occasionally rotated. Neither suppuration, inflammation, nor inconvenience of any kind is the consequence. In Germany, boys have their ears bored for rings when very young. Gold metal is considered better to use than copper: the former is purer, hence ear-wires are made of gold. Cardinal Manzoliant always wore broad gold rings in his ears for weak eyesight. In Germany, sore eyes are a rarity, resulting from this simple precaution in boring at an early age the ears of both sexes, and wearing ear rings always. Islington, N. I am, &c., JOHN BEAUMONT.

"Better Late than Never."—It appears from the monthly report of Colonel Frank Bolton, the Metropolitan Water Examiner, that all the companies are at present, in some portion of their districts, voluntarily giving a constant supply under the Act of Parliament of 1871.

Healthy Lodging-houses, Oxford.—Congregation has passed the revised statute for the sanitary control of lodging-houses. An annual fee of half a guinea is to be paid by all undergraduates residing in licensed lodgings, and the fund thus collected is to provide for an annual inspection by a competent medical sanitary officer.

The Gravesend and Milton Dispensary and Infirmary.—The governors have resolved to raise a fund to establish a children's ward in connexion with this institution. The President, the Earl of Darnley, has given a site on which to erect the proposed building.

Lennox, Bayswater.—At Brussels the medical inspection of schools is under the direction of Dr. Janssens, the Chief of the Bureau d'Hygiène, with the assistance of five physicians connected with the Hygienic Service.

In Memoriam.—We learn from New York that the Garfield Memorial Hospital Committee have received upwards of $50,000 subscriptions, and they have promises of large additional sums.

Iago.—At the close of last year the estimated population of New South Wales was 784,288 persons—an increase during the twelve months of 40,559, which exceeds any that has been recorded for many years. The number of males exceeded that of females by rather more than 11½ per cent.

Urban and Rural Sanitary Works.—The Stoke Town Council have resolved to purchase twenty-one acres of land, in front of the infirmary, for a cemetery, at an estimated cost of about £5000.——The districts of Sirhowy and Dukestown have just been supplied with water from the Ebbw Vale Water Company's mains.——Works for extending the water mains of the Merthyr Local Board of Health to the village of Vorchrtw are in progress.——The Hendon Board of Guardians have adopted plans for additions to the workhouse at an estimated cost of £18,000.——Part of the works in connexion with the additions and improvements of the Armagh Lunatic Asylum is finished and in occupation. The remainder is drawing towards completion. The principal object of the work is to provide accommodation for upwards of one hundred patients. The estimated cost is £90,000.——The Kidderminster Board of Guardians are considering plans for rebuilding the workhouse at an expenditure, if entirely rebuilt, of £30,000.——The Newberry Town Council have authorised the Town Clerk to procure a provisional order for carrying out a sewerage plan, and to schedule Greenhorn Mills and Bone Mill as alternative sites for a pumping-station.——The governors of the Cardiff Infirmary have authorised the trustees to receive from the Marquis of Bute the conveyance of a site in Newport-road for a new infirmary. The speedy erection of the building may now be looked for.——The main sewerage of Market Harborough and the adjoining parishes of Great Bowden and Little Bowden (these parishes forming a united district under one local board) is now being carried out. The cost will be £11,260.——A new cemetery is about to be formed at Stoke-next-Guildford, upon a site of eight acres of land adjoining the South-Western Railway.——At Cardiff, new workhouse buildings have been erected at a cost of £32,000.——A new building is to be erected in Woodthurch-road, Birkenhead, for the Wirral Hospital for Sick Children.——The three boring operations at Birdlip, Gloucester, at the respective depths of 195, 186, and 54 feet from the surface, have been successful, yielding in each case a supply of good water, which up to the present time has been abundant.——New sewerage works have just been completed at Newmarket.

An Experiment.—Large quantities of tea have been supplied, as an experiment, by the French military authorities, to be served out in rations to the troops engaged in North Africa. The men had complained of the disagreeable flavour of the Tunisian water when drunk in its natural state. The step is stated to be popular with them.

The Imperial Reformer.—It is stated that a Bill will be brought before Parliament next session in respect to the City of London parochial charities. It will provide for the appointment of Royal Commissioners, to inquire into them, their revenues and administration, and the appointment of trustees under the Charitable Trustees Act, to administer the property belonging to them.

Disused Burial Grounds: Marylebone.—The Vestry of St. Marylebone has just appointed a committee to confer with the vicar and churchwardens on the subject of utilising the disused burial-grounds in Paddington-street, Marylebone, by adapting them for a public garden and recreation ground.

Juvenile Smoking.—It is said that there is a police regulation in Germany that no persons shall smoke in the streets or public places till they have attained the age of sixteen.

Army Coffee Taverns.—"The Guardsman" coffee tavern is a success financially. A surplus remains for the Central Council to appropriate to the establishment of similar taverns in other garrisons. The new Army coffee tavern at Sandgate is just completed. The Secretary of State for War has granted a site for a coffee tavern on the Lynchford-road, Aldershot, which will be forthwith erected.

Philanthropist.—The Peabody Buildings comprise, we understand, 3355 dwellings of 5170 rooms, and are occupied by nearly 10,000 persons, at weekly rents averaging 4s.

COMMUNICATIONS have been received from—
Dr. HERMAN, London; Mr. TEEVAN, London; THE SECRETARY OF THE CAMBRIDGE MEDICAL SOCIETY; Dr. EDGAR SHEPPARD, Colney Hatch; Dr. D. W. FINLAY, London; THE ACTUARY OF THE CLERICAL, MEDICAL, AND GENERAL ASSURANCE SOCIETY; THE REGISTRAR OF THE APOTHECARIES' HALL, London; Dr. F. T. ROBERTS, London; Dr. R. H. SEMPLE, London; Mr. J. W. BACOT, Seaton; Dr. MERCIER, London; THE HONORARY SECRETARY OF THE MEDICAL SOCIETY OF LONDON; Dr. J. W. MOORE, Dublin; Dr. F. CHURCHILL, London; Mr. MARK H. JUDGE, London; Mr. CLEMENT LUCAS, London; THE SECRETARY OF THE ROYAL INSTITUTION, London; THE HONORARY SECRETARIES OF THE ODONTOLOGICAL SOCIETY OF LONDON; THE DIRECTOR OF THE EPIDEMIOLOGICAL SOCIETY OF LONDON; THE DIRECTOR OF THE OPHTHALMOLOGICAL SOCIETY OF LONDON; THE REGISTRAR-GENERAL, Scotland; THE HONORARY SECRETARIES OF THE HARVEIAN SOCIETY OF LONDON; THE SECRETARY OF THE CLINICAL SOCIETY OF LONDON; Mr. W. H. D. BAINES, London; THE SECRETARY OF THE VICTORIA HOSPITAL FOR CHILDREN, Chelsea; Mr. JOHN BEAUMONT, Islington; THE SECRETARY OF THE SANITARY INSTITUTE OF GREAT BRITAIN, London; Mr. J. D. CAMPBELL, London; Mr. J. CHATTO, London; THE HONORARY SECRETARY OF THE PATHOLOGICAL SOCIETY OF LONDON.

BOOKS, ETC., RECEIVED—
Eczema, by L. Duncan Bulkley, A.M., M.D.—The Right Hon. James Stansfeld, M.P., on the Failure of the Contagious Diseases Acts, etc.—The Sanitary Chronicle of the Parish of St. Marylebone, October, 1881 etc.—Guide for Inspectors of Nuisances, by F. R. Wilson.—Transactions of the Medical and Chirurgical Faculty of the State of Maryland.

PERIODICALS AND NEWSPAPERS RECEIVED—
Lancet—British Medical Journal—Medical Press and Circular—Berliner Klinische Wochenschrift—Centralblatt für Chirurgie—Gazette des Hopitaux—Gazette Médicale—Le Progrès Médical—Bulletin de l'Académie de Médecine—Pharmaceutical Journal—Wiener Medizinische Wochenschrift—Centralblatt für die Medizinischen Wissenschaften—Revue Médicale—Gazette Hebdomadaire—National Board of Health Bulletin, Washington—Nature—Deutsche Medicinal-Zeitung—Boston Medical and Surgical Journal—Louisville Medical News—Medical News and Collegiate Herald—Dublin Journal of Medical Science—Maryland Medical Journal—Detroit Lancet—Nordisk Medicinskt Arkiv—Centralblatt für Gynäkologie—Gazzetta Medica Italiana—Indian Medical Gazette—The American—La Independencia Médica—Boy's Own Paper—Girl's Own Paper—Leisure Hour—Friendly Greetings—Sunday at Home.

EDINBURGH UNIVERSITY AWARDS.—The awards of the following "Van Dunlop Scholarships," of £100 each per annum, tenable for three years, were reported and confirmed at the meeting of the Senate on the 26th ult. :—Faculty of Medicine: One scholarship to Eustace B. Pilgrim, as the student who obtained the highest total number of marks in the subjects of the preliminary examination in Arts for medical students. One to B. E. Jastrzebski, as the student who, having attended for the first time a systematic course of lectures on Botany, Zoology, Chemistry, and Anatomy, obtained the highest total number of marks in the class examinations in those subjects. One to George Fisher, as the student who, having attended for the first time a course of lectures on Physiology and Surgery, obtained the highest total number of marks in the class examinations in those subjects. One to Frederick Ashwell, being the student who, after having attended the classes of Anatomy, Physiology, Materia Medica, and Pathology, obtained the highest number of marks in an examination specially conducted for the purpose in those subjects.

ORIGINAL LECTURES.

ON RETINITIS HÆMORRHAGICA, MORE ESPECIALLY IN ITS RELATIONS WITH GOUT.

By JONATHAN HUTCHINSON, F.R.C.S.,

Senior Surgeon to the London Hospital ;
Consulting Surgeon to Moorfields Hospital ; and Professor of Surgery
and Pathology in the Royal College of Surgeons.

GENTLEMEN,—The term Retinitis Hæmorrhagica is not one which is beyond criticism as regards its appropriateness, because hæmorrhages occur in various forms of inflammation of the retina and optic nerve. It has, however, come into employment as fairly descriptive of a group of cases in which very numerous hæmorrhages, streaking the whole fundus of the eye, are the most prominent condition. In other cases the hæmorrhages may be few and inconspicuous, or very large and almost solitary ; here they are at once of considerable size and countless in number. They present usually another peculiarity, often absent in other cases, that they are all linear in shape, or, more correctly, flame-like, their points being directed away from the optic disc. Well-marked examples of the condition are not very common, and when once seen will be easily recognised. As a rule, there are none of the white streaks, dots, or patches which imply renal disease; but there is no reason why these should be absent in all cases, since albuminuria is not very infrequently present. The conditions are, however, very distinct both generally and locally, from those which we meet with in renal retinitis. In the best-marked cases there is always swelling of the optic disc and of the retina in its neighbourhood, but in others there may be comparatively little, and the multiplicity and form of the hæmorrhages may be the chief feature of distinction.

You will find an excellent illustration of this disease in Jaeger's Atlas, a copy from which I now show you ; and I produce also a good portrait from one of my own cases, which was done for me by Mr. Burgess. It is not my intention on the present occasion to trouble you with the details of single cases, but rather to invite your attention to some general facts suggested by a table which has recently been compiled for me, and which comprises all the cases that I can find in my note-books. To my own list I have added the case given by Jaeger, since an excellent narrative of the patient's history accompanies that portrait. The table which I now produce contains twenty-four cases. It reveals to us at a glance the fact that hæmorrhagic retinitis is a disease of the middle or senile periods of life. Nine of the patients were above sixty, and not one was younger than forty-five. It shows a nearly equal proportion of the two sexes—thirteen men and eleven women. Most of them were at the time of the attack in apparently good health, but I know respecting several that death has since occurred from cerebral apoplexy or other causes. In not many had there been any previous evidence of tendency to rupture of bloodvessels (epistaxis, conjunctival hæmorrhages, etc.), but it may be that I did not inquire in detail on this point in all cases. In connexion with this absence of general tendency to hæmorrhage we may note that in only seven cases out of the twenty-four (less than one-third) were both eyes affected. In all the others the conditions were strictly limited to one eye. Respecting not a few of the cases, I can speak to the fact that the other eye remained free during the whole period that the patient was under my observation. This tendency to occur in but one eye suggests the probability that there must be some accidental locating or exciting causes in addition to those which predispose. We will return to that point presently.

I desire in the first place to say a few words as to the predisposing causes, and especially as to the association of the disease with the state of health which causes gout. It was indeed chiefly in reference to this latter point that I had the cases put together. My impression was that I had encountered a history of gout in nearly every instance

of hæmorrhagic retinitis which had come under my notice. I find, however, on counting the cases, that in seven out of twenty-four, or nearly one-third, such history was absent. Its absence, we must remember, by no means proves that the patients were not gouty, but merely that they had never experienced a gout paroxysm, nor known of such in any near relative. In counting seventeen as gouty, I do not exactly mean that all these had had acute attacks of gout, but rather that in all there was good reason to suspect a gouty constitution. In only twelve, or exactly one-half, had the patient actually experienced an attack of unmistakable gout. I count Jaeger's case as probably one of gout, though nothing definite is said on the point The man was an innkeeper, and is said to have had a bloated face, and to have suffered from piles ; and with three such facts we can scarcely doubt that gout was, at any rate potentially, present. Let me say that the recognition of gout as a cause of hæmorrhagic retinitis, or at least as frequently met with in association with it, is not novel. Most writers on ophthalmic diseases mention it, though I am not aware that anyone has devoted much attention to the subject.

If we ask in what way gout acts in predisposing to this affection, several possibilities may be discussed. We know well that in gout there is a general tendency to disease of bloodvessels, thickening of arterial walls, and increase of pulse-tension. With this increase of tension there goes strain upon the capillaries and risk of rupture. This proneness to hæmorrhage in the gouty has been noticed by several observers, and especially by Sir James Paget. Epistaxis and recurring blood-patches in the conjunctiva are both of them of frequent occurrence in the gouty. But it is not only the arterial system which suffers in gout : the veins also become dilated, and are liable to thrombosis ; piles and other forms of varicose veins are well known to be common; and the patchy congestion of nose and cheeks not rarely seen is another piece of evidence in the same direction. Now, extreme turgescence of the veins is a conspicuous feature in most examples of this form of retinitis, and, although I do not know that I have ever been able to prove absolute arrest of circulation, yet in several I have believed that there was evidence of partial stoppage. An incomplete thrombosis of the vena centralis is, I think, no improbable hypothesis as to the immediate cause of the attack. It is especially probable in those cases in which the attack is sudden and only one eye affected. In many cases the attack is very sudden indeed, and, as I have already stated, in not a few the affection confines itself to one eye. Another suggestion to be made is that the heart itself is the cause of the attack, and that cardiac hypertrophy may be suspected whenever this form of retinal hæmorrhage is observed. The suddenness of onset and the limitation to one eye are facts which strongly militate against this view.

I have said that hæmorrhagic retinitis is never met with in the young; nor does it occur, so far as I know, in cases of hypertrophy of the heart in middle life. There is, however, in youth another form of intra-ocular hæmorrhage, which, although rare, is well recognised. In it there is little or no inflammation of retina or optic nerve, but simply a liability to rupture of vessels. The bleedings are usually free and almost always escape from the retina into the vitreous humour. In this affection we never see the retina spotted over with flame-shaped streaks as in the cases we have been considering. A liability to sudden repetitions of hæmorrhage is almost always a marked feature. My own experience had led me to believe that this affection, like the hæmorrhagic retinitis of the aged, was usually seen in connexion with gout; but the cases collected by others, and especially by Mr. Eales, of Birmingham, have not borne out this supposition. It is found to be almost always attended by constipation and increased arterial tension. The fact that its subjects are always young lads, and never females, suggests the explanation that its attacks are in some way connected with that state of recurring vascular disturbance, which in the female sex finds its relief in menstruation.

In connexion both with these cases of intra-ocular bleeding in young lads, and with those of true hæmorrhagic retinitis, we have the fact that the subjects of hæmophilia (the hæmorrhagic diathesis in a definite sense) are usually liable to joint-pains, and of gouty families. So strongly are the facts on this subject that one writer has even contended that all hæmophilia is due to gout. It may be that the gouty state developes, as above suggested, a modification in the arterial coats, with increase of the risk of rupture, and that this structural peculiarity becomes specialised in hereditary transmission, and finally survives as a family peculiarity after all tendency to gout has, under altered circumstances of life, died out. A careful examination of the facts as to hæmophilia, with its most remarkable tendency to prevail in families, leads me to think that what I have suggested is by no means an improbable hypothesis. It begins in gout; it survives as a transmissible peculiarity of vascular structure. I fear you will think I am wandering from our subject. My object has been to impress upon your minds the fact that in gout there is a remarkable liability to hæmorrhage from small vessels, and to disease not only of the central organ, but of both arteries and veins. The sum of our clinical knowledge respecting retinitis hæmorrhagica appears to be this—that it never occurs till past middle life, that it is usually in association with gout, that it is often confined to one eye, and, I may add, that it is irremediable. For purposes of prognosis we must regard it much as we do attacks of epistaxis or of conjunctival hæmorrhage under similar circumstances. It is a proof of degeneration of tissue, and may be the precursor of some form of apoplexy.

Table of Twenty-four Cases of Retinitis Hæmorrhagica, chiefly in reference to its Connexion with Gout.

No.	Name.	Age.	History of gout.	Nature of attack.	One eye or both	Characters of Hæmorrhages, Retinitis, etc.
1	Mr. L.	50	Gout; albumen		Both	Not flame-shaped.
2	Richard S. ...	67	No gout; diabetes		„	
3	James S. ...	67	No gout	Sudden ...	„	Not flame-shaped.
4	Edmund L. ...	62	Gout probable; no albumen ...	Not sudden	Left	Hæmorrhage; confined to yellow spots.
5	Miss B.	56	Gout; some albumen...		Both	Small and flame-shaped.
6	Miss B.	49	Gout in sister; no albumen ...	Sudden after premonitory symptoms	One	Some flame-shaped; others small blots.
7	Mrs. A.	53?	Gout in family; albumen... ...		Right	Neuro-retinitis, with numerous flame-shaped hæmorrhages.
8	Mrs. W.	56	Gout in family and in patient ...	Gradual ...	„	One large clot, and many very small lines.
9	Mrs. P.	45	Probably gouty. (No note.) ...	Sudden ...	Left	Hæmorrhage, without neuritis.
10	Henry S. ...	63	Stout man; albumen, a trace ...		„	Well marked.
11	George G. ...	50	Good health...	Sudden ...	Right	Large extravasations.
12	Mrs. A.	...	No gout; no albumen		„	But little neuritis.
13	Joseph D. ...	70	Gout; no albumen	Sudden ...	Left	Well marked.
14	William P. ...	44	Gout from lead; much albumen	Sudden ...	„	Hæmorrhage, without neuritis.
15	James D. ...	50	Gout severely; albumen		„	Liable to conjunctival hæmorrhages.
16	Jaeger's case ..	53	Innkeeper; stout and bloated ...		Both	Flame-shaped hæmorrhages.
17	Mrs. J.	72	Gout; no albumen	Not sudden	Left	Numerous, and in all parts.
18	Mrs. M.	73	Gout in her family	Sudden ...	Right	Very numerous small hæmorrhages.
19	Mrs. J.	69	Gout in family and in patient ...	...	Both	Numerous flame-shaped hæmorrhages; some retinitis.
20	Mr. J.	46	Slight diabetes and chronic rheumatism	...	Left	Had had iritis; large white patch, and numerous hæmorrhages.
21	Mrs. A.	48	No gout known	...	Right	Retinitis, and many hæmorrhages.
22	Joseph T. ...	58	No proof of gout; albumen ...	...	Left	Numerous hæmorrhages with white dots.
23	Mrs. P.	62	Gout in patient	...	Right	Numerous flame-shaped hæmorrhages.
24	David Y. ...	51	Gout in patient and inherited ...	...	Both	Slight neuritis; some white dots.

COMMUNICATION OF SYPHILIS BY SKIN-GRAFTING.— Dr. Deubel communicated the following case to the Paris Hospital Society :—A man, aged forty-nine, who had never contracted venereal disease, became the subject of gangrenous erysipelas of the thigh, which was attended with a large ulceration, that, except at some isolated points, refused to cicatrise. On March 7, 45 dermo-epidermic grafts, furnished by five persons, were inserted, and 33 of these contracted adhesions; and 20 other grafts taken from seven persons were placed on another part of the wound on the 23rd, 30 of the number retaining their vitality. Cicatrisation went on satisfactorily until April 5, when ulceration commenced in the now almost cicatrised wound where the first grafts had been planted, and soon destroyed the cicatrisation. The grafts applied on the second occasion did not ulcerate, but became pale and fell off. The new ulceration had a syphilitic aspect; but the man's wife, who had nursed him, having also been seized with erysipelas which proved fatal, and a lodger suffering from lymphangitis, it was concluded that the whole had arisen from infectious causes due to the very unsanitary condition of the abode in which they all resided. The ulcerations improved on being touched with nitrate of silver, but new ones kept appearing during the next three months, and ten weeks after the first application of the grafts the skin and scalp became the seat of syphilitic eruption, and some weeks later the mucous membrane of the mouth was affected. A mercurial and iodide treatment was put into force, and eight months after the first appearance of the erysipelas the breach of surface became entirely cicatrised. It turned out that a son, who had furnished some of the grafts, was the subject of syphilis.—*Gas. Méd.*, November 5.

FACULTIES OF MEDICINE OF LYONS AND BORDEAUX. —During the scholastic year 1880-81, the Lyons Faculty conferred 44 diplomas of doctor, none of *officiers de santé*, 18 diplomas of *pharmaciens*, 32 of midwives, and 12 of *herboristes*. During the same year the Faculty of Bordeaux conferred 21 diplomas of doctor, 2 of *officiers de santé*, 34 of *pharmaciens*, and 26 of midwives.—*Lyon Méd.*, December 4.

CASE OF RECOVERY FROM POISONING BY MORPHIA AND CHLORAL.—Dr. Chipman relates (in the *Canada Medical Journal*, October) the case of a middle-aged lady who, while having charge of sick relatives, had become addicted to alcohol, and who had just taken a dose of medicine containing about two grains of morphia, sixty of chloral, and forty of bromide of potassium. She became unconscious, her countenance being deeply livid, the pupils contracted to the size of pin-heads, and the breathing very slow and stertorous. The stomach was well washed out with a stomach-pump extemporised from an enema-syringe with a gum-elastic catheter tied to its end. A powerful electric battery was kept constantly going, and twenty minims of a solution of one-third of a grain of atropia to a drachm of water were injected hypodermically. This soon affected the pupils, and after a time the breathing increased from four to twelve per minute. The pulse was small and frequent, and could be counted only with difficulty. The rest of the atropia was given in two doses some hours after. Strong tea and coffee were injected into the bowels, and frequent shaking and slapping of the body with wetted cloths were resorted to. Her case seemed desperate, the respirations again sinking to four, when, about twenty-nine hours after taking the poison, consciousness began to return, and from that time she gradually recovered.

ON THE TREATMENT OF THE DIFFERENT FORMS OF NERVOUS AND NEURALGIC HEADACHE.

By WILLIAM HENRY DAY, M.D.,
Physician to the Samaritan Hospital for Women and Children.

It is important to recognise the fact that nervous headache, or migraine, is purely neurosal, and not dyspeptic in its origin. The violent vomiting which often follows prolonged nausea is attended, it is true, with the vomiting of bile, but this is no indication in these nervous headaches that the liver is congested or even disordered. It merely points to the violence of the retching which causes the contents of the duodenum to regurgitate into the stomach, as in violent sea-sickness. There must be other accompaniments of hepatic disorder, as sallowness of skin, foul tongue, or clay-coloured stools, with altered bile, to prove that the hepatic functions are primarily disordered. The more the brain is attacked as the source of the evil, and the less the stomach is worried with mercurials and aperients, the better, for by irritating the alimentary canal the general health is lowered, and the patient's increasing debility renders him or her the more liable to frequent recurring attacks. Put aside, then, the liver, and the stomach, and the intestines, as the origin of the evil, and seek its explantion in some excitement or other alteration in the cerebral ganglia, for it is essentially cerebral. All successful treatment must be based on this understanding. The intimacy between nervous and neuralgic headache is so close that we have, however, to remember that nervous headache which may be entirely frontal for years does frequently become, with the lapse of time, trigeminal, or one-sided.

The treatment must be considered from two points of view. 1. *That during the paroxysm.* 2. *That during the interval of freedom from acute suffering.*

1. *Treatment during the Paroxysm.*—This will in some measure depend on the severity and situation of the pain. If frontal and moderately severe, the patient wanders about the house in misery, and is unable to do anything. All the functions of the brain are disturbed, and life is almost unendurable. It is difficult to know how best to approach the enemy; for the remedy that will do good at one time will fail at another, and no amount of experience in the same individual even appears to help us. In some cases relief comes from the constant application of cold to the head when the pain is frontal, and the vessels are full and throbbing. Cold seems to contract the dimensions of the cerebral vessels by its action on the nervous ganglia. The head should be elevated on a hard pillow, and a bottle of hot water applied to the feet, so as to draw the blood towards the lower extremities. A nervous headache may be now and then cut short by a drachm of the syrup of chloral, and this may be safely given if the head be hot and the pulse good—if, in short, there be vascular excitement, and the vessels of the brain are too full of blood. I have known this remedy bring relief over and over again to the same sufferer, either within a very short space of time, or on awaking after sleep. If the pulse be small and contracted, and the vessels of the head are full and throbbing—if, in fact, the capillaries are in a state of tension, whilst the hands and feet are cold, it is a good plan to put the patient into a warm bath at 97° for ten minutes, and then to bed. It is astonishing the relief this simple remedy sometimes brings: the skin becoming moist, the pulse softer and fuller, and the "opening and shutting" feeling in the head is diminished as the force of the circulation is lessened.

I may briefly direct attention to *guarana*. Now, I cannot say a great deal in its favour, because I have not been very successful with it, and I seldom employ it. In many cases I have found that it has aggravated the nausea and vomiting, and rather increased than lessened the headache, whilst in a few cases it has proved serviceable, and cut short the headache when other remedies had failed. Perhaps it is that I have employed it in rather severe cases, which do not readily yield to any remedy, whereas in some mild cases it might prove beneficial. A few persons tell me they are never without the powders, taking some occasionally in a little water or tea when they are going out, and that it always averts a severe seizure.

But if the pain continues in spite of all drugs taken by the mouth, if it defies emetics, stimulants, counter-irritants, absolute rest, cold to the head, and warmth to the extremities, then the patient at any risk, and at any cost, must have relief from suffering. Acute pain, depriving the patient for several nights of sleep, cannot go on without inducing great nervous exhaustion, especially to women of anxious temperament, whose nervous power is not strong.

Chloroform inhalation will occasionally relieve a severe nervous and neuralgic headache when one drug after another has been tried in vain. It does this by inducing sleep. The patient has perhaps endured the most miserable discomfort in the head for a day or two, and the usual remedies afford no relief. Then towards night the pain is aggravated, and the patient cannot obtain rest. A few drops of chloroform should be sprinkled on a piece of spongio-piline, and then cautiously inhaled. It ought only to be administered by a competent person, and the sufferer should not be allowed to do it of his own accord. Such a practice is about as bad as dram-drinking. I should consider myself very culpable if I allowed patients to do it themselves. It should only be attempted by a medical man, who would be as careful in its administration as if he were sending a person to sleep for a surgical operation. A person may be kept slightly under its influence for an indefinite period, and safely so, if the ordinary precautions are observed.

The utility of *hypodermic injection of morphia* in the acute forms of nervous and neuralgic headache is, in my opinion, under-estimated by the profession. It deserves to be placed in the first rank of all remedies for the relief of this agonising affection when it has reached a certain crisis. It is impossible to over-estimate its value when there is nothing in prospect but an increase of pain, and a degree of restlessness and irritability over which the patient can exert no control whatever. Then the wakefulness adds to the exhaustion and increases the pain. If the injection only brings temporary relief, it enables the patient to recover strength a little, and to bear the return of suffering with some degree of fortitude. If not much exhausted, it never makes her really worse, but it repeatedly diminishes or even cuts short the paroxysm altogether. Experience fully justifies me in saying that the hypodermic injection is most safely employed when the circulation and pulse are good, before the pain has caused much exhaustion. Given under these circumstances, the patient, who just before has been twisting and rolling about in agony for hours, will turn round in bed and fall off to sleep till morning, dozing perhaps the entire day following, being happy and composed, and scarcely caring to be disturbed to take a morsel of food. Still, there are cases that yield to the subcutaneous action of the drug when there is great sickness and prostration, and the extremities are cold and the pulse is weak. If the patient has reached this terrible stage, I believe we ought to employ it in very small quantity, watching the patient meanwhile to guard against a comatose condition. The gr. $\frac{1}{8}$ to gr. $\frac{1}{4}$ of morphia and gr. $\frac{1}{80}$ to $\frac{1}{40}$ of sulphate of atropia will often send off a patient speedily into blissful rest. I usually employ double this quantity to a patient who has been a miserable victim to these nervous and neuralgic headaches.(a) It has a most magical and instantaneous effect. The morphia, when it acts in this way, appears to lull and tranquillise the nervous system, to induce sleep at once, and that sleep is both restorative and refreshing. The atropia obviates the tendency to sickness, and is a most valuable addition.

The primary effect of the hypodermic injection is sedative—a condition in some degree retarded, if not in a few cases prevented, when the pain has so prostrated the system as to induce nausea and vomiting, or even collapse. Then the patient rests for a few minutes, or obtains a little sleep, but is soon disturbed by an increase of vomiting and return of the pain. Vomiting interferes with the action of the morphia by its partial ejection. A large portion, however, is absorbed into the blood, and by that means it exerts its action on the nervous centres.

In carefully considering the subject, it is clear that there

(a) ℞. Morph. acet. gr. v., atropia sulph. gr. $\frac{1}{4}$. aquam ʒi.—m.; twelve minims contain one grain of morphia and one-twentieth of a grain of sulphate of atropia.

can be no valid objection to the employment of the drug, for acute pain must not be allowed to persist; this is the first symptom that demands relief, and it is of supreme importance to check it.

The substantial point is, Does the remedy cut short the paroxysm? It does unquestionably. Is there any condition that contra-indicates its employment? No! There are certain drawbacks to the use of the drug which ought to be kept in mind. If the patient has suffered for many days, and there is much depression and exhaustion; if the pulse be slow and weak, as it often is, and a very limited supply of food has been taken, then it must be used with caution. But I maintain that we cannot stand by and see the patient hour after hour in pitiable agony, and do nothing.

2. *Treatment during the Interval of Freedom from Acute Suffering.*—This consists in endeavouring to correct any disorder of the general health, for until this has been attended to, no special drug for the relief of the head will be of any service. If there be menorrhagia, or bleeding piles, leucorrhœa, uterine or ovarian disease, these conditions must be first attended to, and until they are relieved the headache is certain to continue. I cannot now enter into details, but they will be apparent to every intelligent practitioner. The avoidance of fatigue, excitement, and all other common causes of headache, with a rigid dietary, is sometimes efficacious in warding off these attacks. If the brain be overtaxed in any way, and certain articles of diet and fermented liquors are indulged in, they disorder the stomach, and forthwith throw the nervous system off its balance.

Now, change of place and scene has a most important bearing on the treatment of nervous headache. Some persons suffer mostly at home where they cannot escape the daily anxieties and duties of life; others suffer when on a damp soil, and during the prevalence of cold winds.

Having made our diagnosis of the particular form of headache, and selected our remedy, we ought to give it a fair trial. A remedy should not be lightly abandoned in chronic disease, for over and over again it will be found to cure when persevered with, and the system is slowly brought under its influence. The tendency is to hastily exchange it for some other if it fails to do good at once, but this is an error to be avoided.

(*To be continued.*)

HONOURS FOR DOCTORS IN CHINA.—The *Pekin Gazette* publishes a decree of the Emperor Ouang-su, announcing that the second reigning empress, who had been ill for some weeks, has recovered her health and resumed the direction of the affairs of the State. The same decree confers a whole crowd of honorary distinctions, such as peacock feathers, red and blue buttons, etc., on the members of the college of physicians of the court, twenty-four in number, who daily visited the august patient and felt her pulse one after the other.—*Lyon Méd.*, November 27.

DEVELOPMENT OF A SINGLE BREAST IN GIRLS.—M. Desprès took occasion of the presence of a girl at his clinic to draw the attention of his class to a circumstance that causes alarm to mothers, and is sometimes judged wrongly of even by practitioners. This was an example of the development of only one breast at the age of puberty, when the belief is often entertained that this arises from the presence of a tumour. This girl was thirteen years of age, and was brought to the hospital under the idea that she had a tumour of the right breast, the left one not yet having undergone any change. Her attendant had prescribed iodide of potassium. M. Desprès at once assured the mother that it was only the natural development of the organ, and would be soon followed by the appearance of the menses and the development of the other breast. He observed to his class that while it is natural for mothers to be deceived in these cases, it should be impossible for the surgeon to be so. In fact, there exists beneath the breast a regular prominence in the form of a movable disc on the chest, without the slightest adherence to the skin, and accompanied by no pain whatever. The nipple is exactly in the centre of the tumefaction, and although the developing gland is resistant, it is never irregular, and never presents lumps. A tumour of new formation, such as a sarcoma, is always harder, and is never found exactly in the centre of the mammary region.—*Gaz. des Hop.*, November 24.

ORIGINAL COMMUNICATIONS.

ON A CASE OF EXCESSIVELY HIGH AND VARIABLE TEMPERATURE.

By JAMES LITTLE, M.D. Edin., F.K.&Q.C.I.,
Physician to the Adelaide Hospital; and Professor of the Practice of Medicine in the Royal College of Surgeons, Ireland.

(*Concluded from page 651.*)

APRIL 21, 1880.—From the time of last note until 12.30 a.m., remained quiet and had some short sleeps. She then awoke and began to get very restless and talkative. 12.50 a.m.: Her temperature was taken by new thermometer, and found to be 106·8°. 1.50 a.m.: Got three minims of hypodermic solution, after which she got quieter, but did not sleep until 3.30 a.m., when she slept until 4.45 a.m. 5 a.m.: Her temperature was now taken by new thermometer, and found to be 106·1°. Passed water. Slept from 5.30 a.m. with water-cap on until 7 a.m., when she awoke, perspiring freely, and complaining of a burning pain in lower part of back. Took during night one pint of whey, two cups of tea, two oranges and a half, five ounces of milk, and soda-water. 7.30 a.m.: Upper part of back was sponged over with vinegar and water, before which her temperature was taken, and found to be 104·6°. 10.5 a.m.: Her temperature was now taken, and found to be 107·8°; pulse 88; respirations 80, very shallow. 10.30 a.m.: Head much better, although still very hot. Still complains of pain in her back at the same part. Tongue thickly coated behind with a creamy yellow fur which extends almost to the tip. Pulse feeble and compressible. No pain in stomach. Urine acid, specific gravity 1011, very limpid; no albumen. Remained comparatively quiet, singing and talking, until 1 p.m., when she had a turpentine enema, by which her bowels were well moved once; motion rather confined. 1.30 p.m.: Had a cup of beef-tea, and slept from 1.30 till 2.35 p.m., when she awoke, feeling very hot, and covered with perspiration. At 2.45 p.m. her temperature was taken, and found to be 111·5° by a new thermometer sent by Dr. Little this morning. After being dry-rubbed, the thermometer was again placed under her left axilla at 2.55 p.m. She now complained of intense heat and the usual bursting sensation in her head, which when the hand was placed on it, was found to be throbbing violently. At 3.5 p.m. the thermometer was taken out, and found to register 125·5°. On being taken out the indication was witnessed by Mr. Brooke (Medical Resident) and Mr. Scott (Surgical Resident), and the thermometer was then looked up, to be afterwards seen by Dr. Little, Dr. Franks, and Mr. Beeston. 3.15 p.m.: She was now placed in a hip-bath at 85°, and her body was well sponged over, her head being douched with an artificial shower-can. She remained in the bath five minutes. 3.25 p.m.: Is now cooler, and has not shown any signs of faintness. She was given a cup of beef-tea, and at 3.30 p.m. had eight minims of hypodermic solution of morphia. After the hypodermic injection she became less excited, and although she says her head is throbbing unpleasantly, she is, on the whole, freer from pain. 5 p.m.: Her temperature is now 108° by Mr. Brooke's thermometer. 6.30 p.m.: Her temperature was now taken by Dr. Franks, and found to be 111·4°. The thermometer used on this occasion was one which was sent up from Fannin's this evening, as the thermometer at 125·5° was kept for Dr. Little to see. Up till 8 p.m. she was rather restless. She then fell asleep, and awoke at 8.30 p.m., complaining of feeling hot. Up to this time she has taken—milk, one pint and a half; beef-tea, one pint; tea, four cups; three oranges, and ice. Slept from 8.45 until 9.35 p.m., and then awoke, complaining of feeling very weak and of her stomach being sick. She seemed very heavy; her eyes were turning up, and she felt much colder. Her temperature at 10.45 p.m. was 101·4°; pulse 84; respirations 64. Her pulse was very feeble and scarcely to be felt. She now got a cup of coffee, and from this period until 11.24 p.m. she got gradually better. Her temperature was then found to be 107° by the new thermometer. 12 midnight: Patient got weak again, and said she thought she was dying. She, however, got gradually better.

22nd.—12.35 a.m.: Her temperature was now taken, and found to be 103·5°. Slept from 1 till 1.30, and from 2.45 till

3.45 a.m., with the water-cap on. She awoke at 3.45, and got very excited, and complained of pain in her head. 4 a.m.: She got eight minims of the hypodermic solution of morphia, and seemed much easier after it. After 5 a.m. she got restless again, and remained so until 6.50 a.m., when she fell asleep and slept till 7.25 a.m. Passed water twice. Took during night—milk, sixteen ounces; tea, one cup; beef-tea, one cup; oranges, two. 7.30 a.m.: Patient awoke complaining of being very hot. Her face was very flushed. She was very excited, and was perspiring freely, her night-dress being quite saturated. She was sponged over with tepid vinegar-and-water, and at 8 a.m. her temperature was taken, and found to be 105·6°. Remained quiet till 12.30 p.m., then fell asleep, and slept till 1.10 p.m. 1.30 p.m.: Had a cup of beef-tea, and went to sleep again, and slept till 4.50 p.m. As she awoke complaining of feeling very cold, her temperature was taken at 5.5 p.m., and found to be 107·6°. 5.30 p.m.: Passed water. Is not complaining of head. Until 9 p.m. was comparatively quiet; she then fell asleep. During day has taken—beef-tea, two cups; milk, two cups; tea, five cups; oranges, two. 10 p.m.: Her temperature was now taken, and found to be 109·5°.

23rd.—Was restless until 11.25 last night. She then went to sleep, and slept until 12.30 a.m. She then awoke, complaining of her head. The water-cap was put on, and she slept from 1.15 till 5.15 a.m. Her temperature was taken at 5.30 a.m., and found to be 108·2°. Complains of slight pain in her back. During the night had—tea, two cups; milk, two cups; oranges and grapes. 7.30 a.m.: Is quite quiet now, and does not complain of pain in her head. Was now sponged over with vinegar-and-water, and had a cup of tea. 9 a.m.: Temperature 104·5°. After the class went away she began to get very excited, and complained of great pain in her head. Her temperature at 10.3 a.m. was 110·8°; and as she got much worse, it was taken again at 10.25, and found to be 119°. Her pulse was 112. She got somewhat quieter, and at 10.53 a.m. her temperature was found to be 112·6° (taken by Dr. Little). 11 a.m.: Head much as before. Has a crop of herpes on the right side of upper lip. Her pupils are very much dilated. Complains of pain in upper cervical and sacral vertebræ. Tongue thickly coated with a creamy yellow fur; cleaner at the tip. Bowels not moved since day before yesterday. Treatment—To get a turpentine enema at once, and to have her head shaved. Urine acid, specific gravity 1010, no albumen, very limpid. 11.30: Had a turpentine enema, by which her bowels were well moved; motion natural. Passed water; has still pain in doing so. 1 p.m.: Had a cup of tea. Complaining very much of her back. Temperature taken at 2.10 p.m., and found to be 109·8°. 2.30 p.m.: Passed water. Pain in back less severe. Temperature 109·4°. Remained awake until 5 p.m., when she fell asleep, and slept till 5.25 p.m. She then awoke, perspiring freely. 7 p.m.: Her temperature was now taken, and found to be 116°. 7.20 p.m.: Passed water. Had during the day—tea, five cups; beef-tea, one cup; oranges, three; milk, one pint. Slept from 8.30 until 10.25 p.m., when she awoke, complaining of sickness of stomach and of feeling cold. Pulse 80, very feeble. Temperature at 10.40, 101·3°. Treatment—℞. Spirit. chlorof. ℨij., tinct. lavand. co. ℨiij., aquæ ad ℨvj.—m.; ℨss. every two or three hours, if stomach inclined to be sick. 11.15 p.m.: Had a dose of medicine, and went to sleep.

24th.—Slept till 2 a.m., and awoke complaining of sickness, great pain in her back and head. Had a dose of medicine, which did not seem to relieve her. Water-cap was put on her head, and she slept from 3.30 to 4.30 a.m., her sleep being very restless. Remained awake for some time; had another dose of medicine, and slept till 6 a.m. 6.30 a.m.: Temperature 113°. Looks dull and weak, but is not complaining of pain. Passed water twice during the night, and had—tea, three cups; milk, one pint; oranges, one; grapes. 7.30 a.m.: Patient is now quiet. Has had a cup of tea, and was sponged over with vinegar and water. 8 a.m.: Her bowels were moved without medicine. She is now complaining of her head. At 11.15 a.m. her temperature was 110·2°, pulse 96. She is complaining of her tongue being sore; it is very red, covered with enlarged papillæ, and marked by three transverse fissures. She has a red rash on her cheeks and on the back of her left wrist. It is observed that the rash is most vivid when she gets excited. Her pupils vary—are at times immensely dilated (as at present), and later on are quite a natural size. Urine acid, specific

gravity 1010, no albumen. 11.20 a.m.: Had a cup of tea. Says her head is easier. Fell asleep, and slept for twenty minutes; and awoke complaining of severe pain in her back, running up to her shoulder. It is observed that the pain in her back is chiefly in the upper cervical and lower lumbar and sacral regions; it also shoots along the left shoulder behind. She is now, for the first time, complaining of not being able to see properly. 12.30 p.m.: Is now very much excited, and complaining of great pain in her head and back. 12.50 p.m.: The (new) thermometer put into her left axilla at 12.40 p.m., at 12.50 registered 125·5°. 1 p.m.: She was now put into a hip-bath at 85°, and left in for five minutes. She enjoyed the bath very much, and although shivering for a few minutes after, did not show any signs of faintness. 1.40 p.m.: Temperature 122·6°; pulse 140. 2 p.m.: Fell asleep, and awoke at 2.20 p.m. At 2.30 fell asleep again, and slept till 3 p.m. Remained quiet, but did not sleep until 8 p.m., when she slept for half an hour. Passed water thrice during the day; and had tea, six cups; oranges, three; milk, one cup; beef-tea, one pint; lemonade, one pint. Patient complained of her head and throat in the early part of the night. 11.20 p.m.: As she was complaining of her head, she now got eight minims of hypodermic solution. Slept from 11.30 till 12 p.m., from 12.15 till 6 a.m., and from 6.40 to 7 a.m.

25th.—6.20 a.m.: Temperature 117·4°. Passed water once during night, and had milk, a pint and a half; tea, two cups; oranges, two; ice. 7 a.m.: Awoke complaining of sickness, and seeming dull and heavy. Had a cup of tea, which revived her considerably. Remained quiet until 12 noon, when she complained of her head being very bad, of sore throat, of dimness of vision, and also of great heat. At 12.15 p.m.: Temperature 122·6°; pulse 88. She was now given a bath at 85°, and had ten minims of hypodermic solution. The rash on her face is very vivid, and she has an elevated pustular eruption between the shoulders, and a few spots scattered over the front of chest. Was very restless all day, and during the day did not sleep more than one hour. 7 p.m.: Complaining of dimness of vision in left eye, of soreness of throat, which is a little inflamed. 7.10 p.m.: Temperature 122·4°. Given a bath, after which she complained of pain across the abdomen. 7.30 p.m.: Soon after the bath, temperature 122·2°. Says she is fainting with heat. 8.10 p.m.: As she was complaining of her head being very bad, she was given ten minims of hypodermic solution, and poultice applied to abdomen. Had during day—tea, three cups; coffee, one cup; milk, one pint; beef-tea, two cups; oranges, four. Was wakeful in early part of night. 10.45 p.m.: Pulse 104. As she was complaining of her back, got a hypodermic injection of water, and, as she was very hot, a bath at 85°. Slept, shortly after bath, for twenty minutes, and awoke at 11.55, complaining of faintness, with inclination to vomit. She then got ℨj. of medicine, and slept very restlessly from 12.15 till 2 a.m.

26th.—From a little after 2 a.m. she slept quietly until 5.15 a.m. On awaking, said she felt a cold sort of sensation in her back, and was perspiring slightly. Temperature 113·4°. 5.30 a.m.: Had a cup of tea. Water-cap put on, and slept soon after for half an hour. Passed water once. Had tea, two cups; milk, one pint. Slept from 6.50 until 8 a.m. Had a cup of tea, and was sponged with tepid water and soap. Still complains of pain in back and sore throat. Was quiet up till 10 a.m. Temperature 114·2°; pulse 120. Urine acid, specific gravity 1010, no albumen. Pupils normal. Rash on forehead and cheeks and on upper part of back. Tongue very red, slightly furred at the back and the sides. 11.30 a.m.: Passed water. Bowels moved; motion natural. 11.48 a.m.: Slept from 11.48 a.m. till 12.30 p.m. Temperature 109°. 2.20 p.m.: Slept from 2.20 p.m. till 4.20 p.m. Passed water. 6.35 p.m.: Complaining of pain in back. Head not paining much. Temperature, after shaking index to 85°, was 125°; pulse 100. To get bath at 85°. 7 p.m.: Crying with pain in head and back. Seven minims of hypodermic solution administered. Temperature 122·2°. 8.35 p.m.: Pain still very bad in back, not so bad in head. Temperature 125·5°. Had during day—tea, four cups; beef-tea, two cups; milk, one pint; oranges, four. Remained restless and crying with pain in back until 11 p.m., when she slept for an hour. 12 p.m.: Awoke complaining of throbbing in head. Had some tea, and had short disturbed sleep until 1.20 a.m.

27th.—1.20 a.m.: Awoke complaining of sickness and pain in back of head and back. Got sedative medicine, and remained restless until 2.30 a.m., when she fell into a quiet sleep, and slept till 6.20 a.m. At 6.40 a.m., temperature 120·2°. Did not perspire during the night. Passed water once. Had beef-tea, half a pint; tea, two cups; oranges, milk, grapes, ice. 7.30 a.m.: Patient had half a cup of tea, and was washed. Remained quiet until 11.15 a.m., when she fell asleep. 8.30 a.m.: Passed water. 11 a.m.: Bowels moved; motion natural. Remained quiet until 3.5 p.m. 3 p.m.: Bowels moved again. 5 p.m.: Complaining of her head being very bad. 7.30 p.m.: As she was still complaining, got hypodermic injection, and remained quiet until 9 p.m. Had tea, four cups; milk, one pint; beef-tea, one cup; oranges, four; grapes. No night report.

28th.—8 a.m.: Patient quiet. Had breakfast of tea and bread-and-butter. Remained quiet until 11 a.m., when she began to complain of pain in her back and head. 12 noon: Had a bath at 85°, after which she said she was much better, fell asleep at 12.20 p.m., and slept till 1.20 p.m. 3 p.m.: Bowels moved; motion natural. 3.30 p.m.: Complained of feeling weak. She soon, however, revived after a cup of beef-tea. 5 p.m.: Complaining still of pain in head. 7.30 p.m.: Got five minims of hypodermic solution, and fell asleep at 8 p.m. Had oranges, four; tea, four cups; milk, one cup; beef-tea, one cup.

29th.—Slept quietly until 1 a.m.; awoke complaining of pain in head and of cramps in stomach. A poultice on stomach. Lay awake until 3.15 a.m., and then slept till 6 a.m. Passed water twice. 8 a.m.: Patient quiet, but complaining of feeling weak; is hiccuping. Hiccup continued during day. At about 11 a.m. got eight minims of hypodermic solution, and afterwards ice, and mustard-and-water, but nothing seemed to relieve the hiccup. She refused to take any tea during the day except tea and soda-water. Complained of pain in the abdomen at the left iliac fossa. Linseed-and-mustard poultice relieved her. She vomited several times during day. Tea, four cups; milk, one cup; soda-water, etc. Had some lemonade and milk-and-egg.

May 12.—6 p.m.: Temperature 129·2° between labia and thigh. Eight minims of hypodermic solution were given. 6.20 p.m.: Temperature 121·5°, taken by Dr. Little in the rectum.

13th.—10.45 a.m.: Says she did not sleep; complains of pain in her ear. Pulse 86; temperature 130 8° between thighs.

14th.—11.30 a.m.: Temperature 101·2°, taken by Dr. Smith in vagina.

15th.—Temperature 97·2°.

16th.—11 a.m.: Temperature 114°. Says she feels very weak.

18th.—11.15 a.m.: Temperature 106°. Complains of pain in chest.

19th.—10.45 a.m.: Temperature 129·2°. Right conjunctiva is very red; complains of pain in side of head.

22nd.—11 a.m.: Temperature 107·8°.

June 5.—9.20 p.m.: Temperature 110°.

10th.—Temperature 119·8°.

12th.—Morning temperature 122·4°.

14th.—Morning temperature 126·5°.

15th.—Morning temperature 127·5°.

16th.—Morning temperature 129·6°. Tongue very sore; head very hot.

17th.—Morning temperature 129·6°.

18th.—Morning temperature 130·3°. Was very hot all last night.

19th.—9.15 a.m.: Morning temperature 130·3°. 11 a.m.: Morning temperature 130·3°; feels very hot. Got up to-day, though told to stay in bed.

20th.—Got up out of bed, went to far end of ward, took thermometer out of box, and carried it over to her bed, where she broke it accidentally.

22nd.—Gets up every day.

24th.—Her appetite is increasing; able to go out to garden, and seems very well.

30th.—Not complaining of much wrong with her. 7 p.m.: Says her catamenia have come on badly since June 26, for third time within the month.

July 1.—Menorrhagia. Ordered inf. ergotæ ad ℥ss, spt. chloroformi ℳv., liq. ferri perch. ℳv.

2nd.—Discharge as bad as before. Complains of great pain in bowels; pain in cardiac region. Pulse 86.

3rd.—Discharge much the same. Head very hot. Pulse 84. 1 p.m.: Temperature in axilla with new thermometer of Casella, 133·6°, witnessed by two gentlemen. 2 30 p.m.: Temperature again taken in axilla. Head not so hot, 127·6°; left in arm—a few minutes after felt head getting hotter; thermometer taken out—registered 133·6° Fahr. 6.15 p.m. Taken by Dr. Little in rectum, 99 6°. 8·15 p.m.: Sudden rush of blood to head; feels brain "turning round," and a commotion inside of skull. Pulse 148; temperature in rectum 99·8°. A few minutes afterwards, in axilla, temperature 123·7°. Face looks very flushed, and great burning pain at back of neck. Chest and neck feel very hot; legs and feet very cold—says they feel like ice. Head and neck burning.

4th.—Feels hot this morning. 11 a.m.: Temperature 114·6°.

5th.—Discharge better; does not feel very hot. Temperature taken by Dr. Little in rectum, 108·1°. Thermo-cautery used at back of neck.

7th.—Says she feels pretty hot. 11 a.m.: Temperature 98·5°.

8th.—Has been up last two days. Temperature in axilla, 10 p.m., 97°. Discharge from uterus began again to-day.

9th.—Temperature normal. Walking about the ward, apparently much better. Allowed to go to Convalescent Hospital to-morrow. Went out for a walk.

10th.—Got up at 8.30 a.m., feeling a great deal better. Went to Convalescent Hospital, Stillorgan, at 9 a.m.

OBSERVATIONS BY DR. LITTLE.

I saw K. M. a few hours after her admission to hospital, and she then had the appearance of a patient who had been severely attacked by one of the essential fevers, and in whom the brain was specially affected. I thought the case was one of the epidemic cerebro-spinal meningitis. When very high temperatures were first observed, they were accompanied by symptoms of great distress, the complaint of a bursting feeling in the head, and restlessness, and the whole body conveyed to the hand of the observer the impression of pungent heat. Subsequently such was not the case; the thermometer often rose to 115° to 120° in the axilla, when the patient showed no special oppression, and when to the hands of the attendants the body did not seem preter-naturally warm. There was nothing truly hysterical about the girl, but she appeared to have led a wild life, and to be thoroughly bad and unreliable. She was caught several times tampering with the thermometers, and I have no doubt would not have hesitated to use any means to render herself an object of interest and attention. At the same time, I cannot conceive any artificial way in which she could have raised the mercury in the thermometers, as she was often surrounded by observers at the time when the instrument was in the axilla. My own conviction is that the girl really had cerebral mischief, probably in consequence of the injury of the head, and of the dissipated life which she appeared to have been leading; but the highest temperatures were found after all symptoms of this condition had passed off, and certainly did not affect any large portion of the body, and, as it appears to me, they must either have been produced in some artificial way, or have been the result of a special state of the nervous system, which enabled her to determine active change of tissue in a part by an effort of the will.

INCREASE OF NEGROES IN THE UNITED STATES.—

M. Chervin, in a communication to the Paris Société de Médecine, draws attention to the fact that while up to the census of 1860 the negroes in the Northern States numbered 4,880,000, in that of 1880 they had increased to 6,577,151, i.e., an augmentation of 35 per cent. This is a result well worthy of attention, for it has always been hitherto admitted that when an inferior race is placed in contact with a superior one, with which it has to maintain the struggle for existence, it is always, in a future more or less near, condemned to disappear in consequence of the excess of deaths over births. M. Chervin attributes this great fertility of the negro race in the United States to the liberty which they now enjoy there, and believes that a very different result would have been observed had it continued in a state of slavery.—Union Méd., November 27.

TREATMENT OF TETANUS BY CHLORAL.
By JOHN T. FAULKNER, M.B. Lond.

THE following case well illustrates the use of chloral in the treatment of tetanus:—

. B. S., a robust, healthy girl, aged ten years, fell on a tile in the garden on Wednesday, July 13, 1881, causing a superficial abrasion of left knee. This was carefully washed and plastered up according to domestic custom, and the plaster was not disturbed for many days. She appeared quite well until the evening of Thursday, 21st, when she was out playing on the damp grass, and, on going to bed, complained to her mother of slight sore-throat. When seen the following morning the tonsils were a little inflamed, and the neck was rather stiff. Temperature in axilla 98·4°. On 23rd her sister said she had passed a restless night and had been "twitching" very much. The mouth was so nearly closed that a quill could scarcely be got between the teeth; there was opisthotonus, the abdominal muscles rigid; and spasmodic contractions of trunk and limbs recurred from four to six times per minute. For a few minutes they would be very severe, and then abate in violence for a time. The child kept asking for milk every few minutes; this she preferred to take from a spoon. The spoon was placed between her lips, and she sucked the milk through her teeth with much force, only being interrupted by the more violent spasms. This state continued without any sleep until about 4 a.m. on the 24th, when the spasms had become so violent that an attempt was made to administer chloroform. With the first inhalation there was produced a violent spasm of larynx, which lasted until the whole body was relaxed in a state of asphyxia. Artificial respiration was immediately resorted to, and after a little while the breathing was re-established; but as soon as she had recovered, the spasms commenced again. Chloral was then given by the mouth in small and frequently repeated doses, and the effect watched. In a few minutes the spasms were less violent, and patient quieter in every way. Twenty grains sufficed to keep her quiet for two hours, and there was a quarter of an hour's unbroken sleep. Then followed an interval of about an hour without any more chloral—none being at hand. During this time the paroxysms became worse, and culminated in another severe spasm of larynx and respiratory muscles, producing asphyxia, and the patient was again resuscitated by artificial respiration. This process was repeated many times during the subsequent course of the case. At 6.45 a.m. chloral occurred; twenty grains given in small repeated doses by 7.20 a.m., from which time the patient slept, with only three slight spasms, till 8.30. She then took fifteen grains in ten minutes, and afterwards slept for two hours, having only slight spasms occasionally. At 10.30 took ten grains more; quiet for an hour. She now refused to take any medicine by the mouth, though she constantly asked for and took milk. The intellect was remarkably bright and clear, and the voice quite natural. Pulse 120; temperature in axilla 99°. 11.50: Had thirty grains of chloral and two drachms of brandy per rectum. The introduction of the syringe caused violent opisthotonus and tetanic spasms of the whole body, which lasted five minutes. She became extremely cyanotic, but this condition passed away gradually, and sleep followed. At 1.35 p.m. another enema of half a drachm of chloral and two drachms of brandy was administered; and at 3.15 a further one. As the injections per rectum always caused such violent contractions, and as the difficulty in giving the injections while there was opisthotonus was great, this method was abandoned, and at 4.30 five minims of a solution of one grain of chloral to one minim of water was injected subcutaneously. This rapidly produced a profound sleep, which lasted nearly an hour. An enema of brandy and milk or brandy and beef-tea was given a few minutes after this and every subsequent injection of chloral, while the patient was quiet. The wound on the knee, which had an "angry" look, was dressed with a lotion of No. 40 carbolic and tinct. opii in equal parts. This was applied for its local antiseptic and sedative action, keeping in view the reflex theory of tetanus. Temperature in axilla 101°, pulse 125. At 5.20, three grains of chloral were injected; at 5.40, four grains (temperature in axilla 101°, pulse 120); at 6.50, four grains; at 8 5, four grains (temperature in axilla 101·6°, pulse 120); at 9.5, four grains; at 10.5, four grains (temperature in axilla 101·8°, pulse 120). There then followed

a sleep a little longer than usual, and about 11.20 she was becoming cyanotic even during sleep. In this paroxysm the muscles of face and larynx and the respiratory muscles seemed to be chiefly affected; there was scarcely any opisthotonus. Shortly respiration was completely arrested. Artificial respiration was carried on and the breathing re-established. On recovery four grains of chloral were injected; temperature in axilla 102·4°, and pulse 130. 25th: At 12.30 a.m., four grains more injected; at 1.35, four grains chloral (pulse 130, respirations 52 per minute, temperature 102·4°); at 2.30, artificial respiration; at 2.30, five grains chloral (temperature 101·2°—this was probably taken soon after resuscitation); at 3, artificial respiration. On recovery, sleep came on without any more chloral. At 3.20, artificial respiration; at 3.30, four grains chloral injected (temperature 102·8°); at 4, three grains chloral (temperature 103·2°, pulse 120, respirations 51); at 4.30, four grains chloral (temperature 101·8°). About twenty minutes after this injection she wakened up more than previously—she recognised her sister, called her by name, and asked for milk; she took a little, but the attempts to swallow threatened to cause another paroxysm, so no more was given. She quietened, and seemed to be half asleep, but at 4.55, while lying flat on her back and very quiet, the lips and face became blue, the chest-walls moved, but no air entered. With a view of preventing further asphyxia, chloral (five grains) was immediately injected, but the spasm continued, and after it artificial respiration had to be kept up for some minutes before breathing was re-established. About 5.30 another paroxysm occurred; face getting blue. The child struggled with her arms, and muttered with closed teeth, "Oh, lift me up!" Artificial respiration was begun this time before the paroxysm had completely passed away, and was kept up for a prolonged period, but the patient did not recover.

Dr. Dreschfeld and Mr. Lund saw the case in consultation on the 24th.

Remarks.—Whatever be the true pathology of the disease —whether it be that a poison is generated in the wound and thence absorbed into the circulation, or that the symptoms are purely reflex, or that there are actual changes in the nerve-centres as Dr. Ross ("Diseases of Nervous System") adduces some slight evidence to show—it is admitted that chloral has no direct influence on the morbid process. A feature worthy of notice is the change in character of the paroxysms. At first chiefly spinal (opisthotonus, etc.), later on they became more and more respiratory (obstruction of larynx, pharyngeal spasm, and especially an accumulation of fluid in the bronchial tubes). This gradual accession of medullary symptoms upon the spinal, together with the fact of the higher centres being unaffected—the pupils responded to light, and the intellect was clear so far as could be made out through the effects of the chloral—points, I think, to an affection of the nerve-centres. but the present condition of our knowledge we can only treat symptoms, and that chloral has a decided effect on the most prominent of these will be admitted by everyone; and if, as Dr. Boon of the West Indies says, and many others believe, the disease has a tendency to right itself, it is an eminently rational plan of treatment to tide the patient over the spasms, and so gain time. I believe this patient would have died many hours earlier if chloral had not been given. Dr. Boon says he has never seen any die except from spasm of respiratory muscles. The best way of giving chloral is by the mouth, as long as the patient can swallow without any very great distress; it should be given in small quantities, and frequently repeated. Liquid food can be given alternately with the medicine; the administration should be guided entirely by the effects produced, and not by the total quantity taken, as patients in this condition will take enormous quantities. This patient took sixty-five grains by mouth, ninety grains by rectum, and sixty-one grains subcutaneously, in twenty-six hours. If swallowing becomes very distressing, it is better to resort at once to the subcutaneous injection, as the injection per rectum, in my experience, causes greater distress than swallowing, and is a matter of difficulty if there be opisthotonus.

Stretford.

THE COLLECTIVE INVESTIGATION COMMITTEE.—-Dr. William Robert Smith, of Cheltenham, has been appointed Secretary to the Collective Investigation Committee of the British Medical Association.

REPORTS OF HOSPITAL PRACTICE
IN
MEDICINE AND SURGERY.

ST. PETER'S HOSPITAL.

STONE IN BLADDER—BIGELOW'S OPERATION—GOOD RESULT.

(Under the care of Mr. TEEVAN.)

JAMES S——, a hairdresser, aged sixty-six years, was admitted into the hospital on February 1, 1881, suffering from a stone in the bladder, which had been detected by Mr. Teevan when the man had visited the hospital as an out-patient. From notes taken by Mr. W. Neale, the House-Surgeon, it appeared that about four years ago the patient noticed that he suffered pain at the tip of the penis when making water, which was the colour of coffee-grounds. Since then he had been troubled with frequency of micturition. For the past three months the pain in the penis had been very severe when riding or walking, so that he was often obliged to stop. The patient was a tall thin man, in good health, and of very cheerful spirits. He was born at Sittingbourne, Kent. His mother was a native of Suffolk. He did not know where his mother was born. His urine was clear, faintly acid, its specific gravity being 1020 ; there was no deposit or albumen in it.

On February 2, at 3 p.m., the patient was put under the influence of ether by Mr. Knott. Mr. Teevan introduced a strong but slender lithotrite, and caught hold of a stone about the size of a hazel-nut, which was exceedingly hard to crush. Having completely pulverised the calculus, the *débris* were evacuated with a No. 27 tube. The stone was composed of oxalate of lime, and weighed forty-five grains.

3rd.—9 a.m.: Patient is very well. Has not had any sickness or rigor. Urine slightly tinged with blood. Temperature 98°. 9 p.m.: Temperature 100·4°.

4th.—9 a.m.: Has passed a bad night; has been sick several times, and for some hours voided very little urine. Temperature 100°. 10 p.m.: Temperature 97·8°.

6th.—Slept well; better. Temperature 97°. Urine clear.

7th.—Feels quite well. No pain in making water, which is quite clear. Mr. Teevan sounded the patient, but could not find anything.

11th.—The man left the hospital, quite well in all respects.

May 23.—The patient called at the hospital to say that he had been uninterruptedly at work ever since he left the institution, and was in all respects quite well.

STONE IN BLADDER—LITHOTOMY—RECOVERY.

(Under the care of Mr. TEEVAN.)

John F. W——, twelve years old, was admitted into the hospital, March 21, 1881, suffering from a stone in the bladder, which had been detected by Mr. Teevan when the child had been brought to the out-patients' department by his mother. From notes taken by Mr. W. Neale, the House-Surgeon, it appeared that about one year ago the mother noticed the boy commenced to suffer pain in making water. At times the stream of urine would stop, and on one occasion he passed blood. For the past month he has complained of pain in the lower part of the abdomen, and has walked with his body bent forwards. The boy and his father were natives of London, but the mother was born in Yorkshire. The child seemed in fair health, but when only two years old had been an out-patient for some time at the Children's Hospital, Great Ormond-street, for chronic diarrhoea.

On March 30, at 3 p.m., the boy was put under the influence of chloroform by Mr. Knott, and a rectangular staff having been passed by Mr. Teevan, was taken charge of by Mr. Heycock. Mr. Teevan then introduced the point of a broad-bladed knife into the angle of the staff, and having opened the bladder, extracted a phosphatic calculus, like a cocked hat in shape, measuring one inch and one-eighth by one inch in diameter.

31st.—9 a.m.: Patient has had a good night, but is rather weak this morning. Skin cool and moist. Tongue clean. Temperature 99°. 10 p.m.: Has been sick several times. Ordered sp. ammon. aromat. with sp. æther. nit., and to take lime-water and milk.

April 1.—Has had a good night (temperature 99°), but during it the urine passed several times " per penem." 10 p.m.: Temperature 97·8°.

2nd.—Patient seems very well, is bright and cheerful. All urine flows through the wound, which looks very healthy.

18th.—No urine has to-day come through the wound, which is nearly healed.

19th.—Water very cloudy to-day, and contains much mucus. Ordered buchu and dilute hydrochloric acid.

May 1.—The boy left the hospital to-day, quite well and water-tight, and not suffering from incontinence.

WEST NORFOLK AND LYNN HOSPITAL.

CASE OF SUPPURATION OF THE KNEE-JOINT, FOLLOWING INJURY — FREE INCISIONS AND DRAINAGE.

(Under the care of Mr. S. M. W. WILSON, Senior Surgeon.)

[Reported by Mr. S. H. LINDEMAN, House-Surgeon.]

J. P., aged five, in good health, but of the dark type of strumous diathesis, was admitted into the hospital on May 31, with the following history :—He was crawling through an attic window, when his foot slipped, causing his knee to come in contact with the edge of a broken window-pane. The wound resulting therefrom was on the outer and lower part of the right knee, about one inch and a half long, and, as far as could be seen, quite superficial ; it was clean, and free from fragments of glass. After carefully cleansing the surrounding skin, the edges were drawn together by a silver-wire suture and dry dressing applied. The limb was then accurately bandaged to a back splint, some pressure being applied over the wound.

June 1.—Leg quite comfortable ; no pain ; not dressed.

2nd.—Dressings removed. Wound quite healthy, and apparently healed by first intention.

3rd.—Has great pain in knee. Temperature at noon 104° Fahr. Skin hot ; has vomited. Wound angry-looking ; knee-joint hot and very tender to the touch. The suture was removed and an ice-bag applied. Temperature at night 101° Fahr.

4th.—Passed fair night. Knee still hot, but fever less.

5th.—Slightly delirious at night. Wound looks sloughy and unhealthy. Knee hot. Poultices were now applied, and the ice-bag removed. The joint became much swollen, and the child's condition remained bad till the 11th, when the wound was dressed with carbolic oil and tenax. Temperature at nights ranges from 100° to 105° Fahr.

16th.—The knee looks rather better. Wound freely discharging.

July 1.—The diseased knee was half as big again as the other. On pressure over the patella, pus freely oozed from the original wound. As the child's condition was now precarious, it was determined to incise the joint freely. Under strict antiseptic precautions a grooved director was passed into the joint, and through the primary wound (the outer side). Along this a bistoury was passed upwards and downwards. The length of the incision was three inches and a half, and the interior of the joint was freely exposed. It was found to be full of pus. It was syringed out with a (one in forty) solution of carbolic acid, and a drainage-tube passed through.

3rd.—Patient better. Copious discharge of pus. Dressed twice daily. In spite of this the discharge came through the dressings. The gauze was on this account abandoned, and tenax, well teazed out, applied all round the joint.

8th.—One week since operation. Patient decidedly better. Wound granulating up. But as the inner side of the knee was puffy, another incision was made into it, and a drainage-tube inserted. The two wounds from this time steadily healed. First one and then the other drainage-tube was removed. A month after the last was removed a collection of pus formed behind the joint, but quite superficial to it. This was evacuated. With this exception the case has done extremely well. It is now five months and a half since the accident. The sites of the two incisions are now only marked by firm cicatrices. There is no pain, and the child walks with no other inconvenience than that of a stiff knee-joint. As would be expected, there is little or no movement in any direction.

Remarks.—It is probable that had the antiseptic mode of treatment been adopted at the commencement, the knee would not have suppurated, as in that case the dressings would not have been disturbed for a week or more. For this reason, if for no other, it would have done good. Till the first dressing took place all was well. Although there was, so far as could be made out, no opening into the joint at first, yet the inflammation extending thereto from the wound would soon break down the slight barrier; and when once suppuration had taken place, nothing availed except free incisions combined with perfect drainage. It is an example of the reparative power in children, and shows how chary one should be to resort to extreme measures in cases of the sort. At one time the condition of the patient was as bad as it could be, and amputation of the limb above the joint was seriously considered. Happily this was not carried out.

TERMS OF SUBSCRIPTION.
(*Free by post.*)

British Islands	. . . . .	*Twelve Months*	.	£1 8 0
,,	,, ...	*Six*	,,	. 0 14 0
The Colonies and the United States of America	. . . }	*Twelve*	,,	. 1 10 0
,,	,, ...	*Six*	,,	. 0 15 0
India	,, ...	*Twelve*	,,	. 1 10 0
,, (*viâ Brindisi*)	. . .	,,	,,	. 1 15 0
,,	,, ...	*Six*	,,	. 0 15 0
,, (*viâ Brindisi*)	. . .	,,	,,	. 0 17 6

Foreign Subscribers are requested to inform the Publishers of any remittance made through the agency of the Post-office.

Single Copies of the Journal can be obtained of all Booksellers and Newsmen, price Sixpence.

Cheques or Post-office Orders should be made payable to Mr. JAMES LUCAS, 11, New Burlington-street, W.

TERMS FOR ADVERTISEMENTS.

Seven lines (70 words)	. . .	. £0 4 6
Each additional line (10 words)	.	. 0 0 6
Half-column, or quarter-page	. .	. 1 5 0
Whole column, or half-page	. .	. 2 10 0
Whole page	. . .	. 5 0 0

Births, Marriages, and Deaths are inserted Free of Charge.

THE MEDICAL TIMES AND GAZETTE *is published on Friday morning. Advertisements must therefore reach the Publishing Office not later than One o'clock on Thursday.*

Medical Times and Gazette.

SATURDAY, DECEMBER 10, 1881.

THE FULHAM HOSPITAL CASE.

ONE more stage in the action which will be generally known as "The Fulham Hospital Case" was completed last week in the Court of Appeal. The matter is worthy of notice in full for several reasons, but chiefly as showing the growing dissatisfaction in the mind of the public, and in the judicial mind, with the system of hospitals for infectious diseases in the metropolis, as managed by the Metropolitan Asylums Board. The action, that of "Chambers and others against the Managers of the Metropolitan Asylums District," is a consequence or product of the Hampstead Hospital Case; and, as in that case, so in this, the defendants fight every inch of the ground. The plaintiffs are owners of property in the neighbourhood in which the Asylums Board Hospital at Fulham has been erected. Mr. Chambers is lessee, under Colonel Gunter, of the well-known Lillie-bridge Grounds, which are used not only for athletic and other sports, but for lawn tennis, for garden parties, and as a playground for the children of schools in the neighbourhood; and he also holds, on the north side of the Hos-

pital, some land which he took as a building speculation. Colonel Gunter, another of the plaintiffs, owns valuable estates, known now as the "Beaufort House Estate," the "Redcliffe Estate," the "Boltons" and "Earl's Court" estates, and other property near, and some of it adjacent to, the land of the defendants. And a third plaintiff, Mr. Richard Pickersgill, is now, and was before the opening of the Hospital, lessee of several houses in Walham-grove, Fulham, one of which he has occupied as a dwelling-house. The defendants, the managers of the Metropolitan Asylums Board, are owners of a piece of land in Fulham, and built upon it, and in March, 1877, opened, a hospital for the reception and treatment of small-pox and other infectious diseases, and it has been used in that way till lately; but during the epidemic of small-pox this year cases of small-pox have been brought into it from other parts of London besides Fulham, and the defendants had proposed to enlarge it. The plaintiffs, consequently, early in May this year, issued a writ against the defendants on the ground that the Hospital is injurious to the neighbourhood. On July 21 a summons for an injunction was issued, and came before Mr. Justice Bowen, who referred it to a Divisional Court; but no such court was available, and he therefore, on August 5, heard it, and refused to grant an injunction. The plaintiffs then appealed to a Divisional Court, consisting of Mr. Justice Cave and Mr. Justice Kay, who granted an interim injunction restraining the defendants from receiving into the Hospital patients from any district beyond a radius of one mile, until the trial of the action; and from this decision the defendants appealed to the Court of Appeal of the Supreme Court of Judicature The case was heard before Lords Justices Brett, Cotton, and Lindley, on the 1st and 2nd of the present month. The plaintiffs complained that by reason of the danger and inconvenience caused by the presence of the Hospital the safety and the enjoyment of themselves and their tenants had been seriously interfered with, and the value of the property diminished, so much that houses remained for a long time unlet, and that persons no longer frequented the Lilliebridge Grounds as in former days before the Hospital was erected. And the plaintiffs claimed damages as well as an injunction.

On the part of the defendants, counsel complained that Mr. Justice Cave had referred to the Hampstead Hospital case, while in that case the only question that had been decided was whether the defendants were protected by statute, the question of nuisance having been ordered for a new trial. And against the affidavits of the other side they read affidavits by medical men, officers of the Hospital, and others, to the effect that the Hospital was well constructed, properly ventilated, and admirably managed; and they contended that it had not been made out that small-pox had increased in the neighbourhood by reason of the introduction of an increased number of patients into the Hospital; that the defendants had, by standing by and delay, precluded themselves from a right to an interim injunction; and, further, that the benefits to the public from the Hospital preponderated over the inconvenience caused to the neighbourhood. For the plaintiffs it was argued that there had been no delay, because they had not until lately known facts which, if proved, would entitle them to succeed in their action; and that there was still pending the Hampstead Hospital Case, in which the same defendants raised points which, could they have maintained them, would have decided the present case. The plaintiffs altogether denied that the balance of convenience preponderated in favour of the defendants.

Lord Justice Brett held that the decision of the Divisional Court ought to be affirmed. The question was, he said, whether the plaintiffs had not made out a preponderating case of great probability; whether, if the case stood, as at present, without further evidence, there would not be a great probability of an action by the plaintiffs being maintained on the ground that where a large number of small-pox patients were brought together from remote districts into a hospital, so that it became filled to the extent to which the hospital in question had been filled, infection would be spread roundabout. If the evidence showed that, it showed a probability that it would be found that a hospital so conducted would be a nuisance to the neighbourhood; and if the plaintiffs could show that they were injured by a public nuisance, they would be entitled to damages and an injunction. The Court had not to deal with the question whether a jury would give damages, but ought an injunction to be declared? He was of opinion that the plaintiffs had made out a preponderating case of probability. As to delay, he was of opinion that the plaintiffs' delay, if any, in instituting an action was explained by the litigation then going on between other persons and the same defendants in the Hampstead Hospital Case, which was a similar suit. And as to the balance of convenience, that was a difficult question to decide. The impression on his mind was in favour of the defendants. It must be a great benefit to poor people afflicted with small-pox in small dwelling-houses that the sick should be removed from their neighbourhood and placed in an excellent hospital. On the other hand, there was the injury to the poor, and to those not poor, from the bringing in a large number of patients into the district in which the Hospital stood. In a question of convenience or inconvenience, a consideration of the justice or injustice of a proceeding should be taken into account; and it appeared to him that such consideration was strongly in favour of prevention of the probability of a great infliction like small-pox being brought by the hands of men to persons who would not otherwise have suffered from it. Lords Justices Cotton and Lindley delivered judgments to the same effect as Lord Justice Brett, and the appeal was dismissed, and the injunction granted by the Divisional Court supported.

We will add only one observation, suggested by the perusal of the above case. At the commencement of the present year the Local Government Board instituted an investigation, by its medical officers, for the purpose of ascertaining whether hospitals for infectious diseases, and notably small-pox hospitals, are instrumental in causing the spread of infection in the localities in which they are situated. But it does not appear from the reports of the trial in the Court of Appeal that the Managers of the Asylums Hospital brought forward any new evidence on that vital question. If this was so, may it not be considered that there is "a preponderating case of probability" that no new evidence in favour of the Asylums Board Hospitals has been discovered?

SCHÜLLER'S EXPERIMENTAL RESEARCHES ON SCROFULOSIS AND TUBERCULOSIS OF THE JOINTS.(a)

Although a whole year has passed since the publication of Dr. Schüller's work, it may still be useful to readers to receive a somewhat detailed account of it, more particularly as the author's opinions on the essential cause of tuberculosis appear to be receiving a rather easy—we do not say an undeserved—currency in extra-professional circles.

(a) "Experimentelle und histologische Untersuchungen über die Entstehung und Ursachen der skrophulösen und tuberculösen Gelenk leiden." Von Prof. Dr. Max Schüller in Greifswald. Pages 256, with 80 woodcuts. Stuttgart, 1880.

We must pass over briefly the first, and not the least valuable, part of the work (pages 17 to 48), in which the author ingeniously argues that tuberculosis, artificially produced in rabbits by means of tuberculous and allied substances introduced through the trachea, is a close analogy for the assumed scrofulous or tuberculous diathesis in man which predisposes an injured joint to scrofulous or tuberculous changes. He injured (by blows with a mallet, or by twists and dislocations) the right knee-joint in two sets of rabbits, one set that had been on the same day infected with tubercle, and another set that had remained uninfected, and had been, for the most part, carefully isolated from those infected. The changes in the injured joints were, as regards the first set, either true scrofulous changes or "pannus-like" inflammation; but for the second set (with the exception of a certain number of rabbits which had been allowed to remain beside the infected), they were simple inflammatory and transient effects, and in most cases merely extravasations of blood. Not content with finding, by tuberculous infection of the rabbit, an analogy for the scrofulous taint which so often causes injured (not to mention uninjured) joints in man to take on the characteristic structural changes, Dr. Schüller went on to discover the essential cause of tuberculosis in the joints (and in general) by a series of experiments, the narrative of which occupies the greater part of the volume. Grains of colouring matter and other finely divided substances, when introduced into the trachea along with tuberculous matter, were discoverable in the injured joint in close association with those structural changes that were due to the co-existing tubercular infection. That apparently irrelevant circumstance somehow led him to think that the tuberculous virus might also exist in the form of minute particles which behaved like the pigment particles, and, in particular, circulated in the blood and got deposited in the joint through the extravasations of blood caused by the injury. The particles of pigment behaved so, and it was reasonable to suppose that the tuberculous virus which had borne them company from the windpipe onwards might exist also in the form of particles, and not as a soluble virus. If that reasoning should appear a little queer, it is right that the reader should further know that pigment particles introduced into the trachea by themselves (and unmixed with tuberculous substance) do not show a decided tendency to get deposited in the injured joint. Leaving, as it were to its fate, that ingenious analogy of the pigment particles, the author very soon lets us know that all this is merely by way of leading up to the well-known micrococcus question; and it is into that question that we have now to follow him.

Dr. Schüller took pieces of tuberculous human lung, pieces of freshly extirpated scrofulous lymphatic glands, the detritus of caseous glands (avoiding pus, if possible), and pieces of lupus of the nose, carefully cleansed by water from all crusts and adhering purulent matter, which, as experience showed, were apt to encourage the growth of all kinds of fungi. These things formed what he calls his raw material. Portions of each kind of raw material were ground in a mortar to the consistence of a fluid, and then, filtered; the filtered fluid was put aside in a test-tube stopped with cotton-wool. A series of test-tubes were then carefully cleansed and filled with a fluid called Bergmann's solution, or simply with white of egg; and after being subjected to heat, they were stopped with cotton-wool. After a short time the plug of cotton-wool was half withdrawn (sometimes this was done under the spray), and one, two, or three drops of the tuberculous substance which had been ground in a mortar were introduced into each. In the course of twenty-four hours the white of egg (or the Bergmann's solution) began to get cloudy, owing to the rapid multiplication of organisms of various kinds, and it attained a uniform milky appearance in the course of a few days. From that milky fluid, one, two, or three drops were taken, and introduced into other test-tubes filled with white of egg or with Bergmann's solution. These test-tubes became turbid in their turn from the presence of organisms that were less varied in kind than in the first set of test-tubes. From No. 2 a drop or two were taken and put into white of egg No. 3, which became cloudy with organisms that were now practically of one kind, viz., spherical bacteria of various sizes mixed with more or less numerous rod-shaped bacteria having flask-shaped swellings at one end (pages 76, 77). The author leaves it to professed botanists to determine their life-history. The test-tube No. 3 proved to be the one best adapted for the subsequent experiments; the earlier mixtures of white of egg and bacteria were too virulent, and the latter were too mild. As a variation on the above procedure, the piece of tuberculous lung (or other raw material) was not ground in a mortar so as to be mixed with the white of egg only to the extent of two or three drops, but it was taken just as it came from the body, and deposited in the albumen. The results of that procedure were not only as good as those of the pounded and filtered tuberculous substance, but even better, inasmuch as the cloudiness in the first set of test-tubes was much more intense (page 58). Test-tubes of the third generation being accordingly prepared in either way, and allowed to stand till the white of egg had reached its point of greatest turbidity, a Pravaz syringe was filled from them, and discharged into an aperture made in the trachea. The syringeful of bacteria-containing fluid was in some cases injected, not down the windpipe, but into the pleura, peritoneum, jugular vein, or subcutaneous tissue; but that proved to be too vigorous a manner of proceeding, and usually led to the death of the animal in a few days from pleurisy, pneumonia, or peritonitis. The organs in these rapidly fatal cases contained numerous micrococcus-deposits, and that circumstance made it probable that the animals had died of an acute mycosis which was, perhaps, tubercular (page 60). It was only when the virulent fluid was introduced by the gentler way of the windpipe that the due effects followed. The wound in the neck was left to itself, and in the majority of cases it healed under a scab "after the tracheal opening had remained patent for a longer or shorter time"; but, in a few cases, fistulæ remained. On the same day as the injection was made into the lungs, the right knee was injured.

At this stage of the narrative, the interest of the reader reaches its highest point. What effects followed the introduction of the virulent fluid in each case? Unfortunately, the author gives no synoptical tables of the experiments, and the exact information that we would gladly get at has to be sought for in sections of the book widely apart. Notes were kept of forty-two animals used in this experiment with the bacterium-containing albumen: many more animals were used, and we regret to find that no notes were kept of these. However, as we gather from various parts of the book, the results for the forty-two were sufficiently various. So many exceptions, reservations, and deductions have to be allowed for in one place or another, that the reader begins to wonder how many of the original forty-two were left to support the author in his conclusions. What with those that were too young, those that died in the first few days from pleurisy or peritonitis, those that survived for many months and were not killed after all, and those that had benzoate of soda administered to them and recovered,—what with those exceptions which confront one in various parts of the work—we can form hardly an approximate estimate of the degree of success of the experiments.

Again, most of the animals that die or are killed after a sufficient interval belong to that group (more than half the original forty-two) which had the bacterial solution introduced direct into the bronchi and air-vesicles, the tuberculosis that followed being in some cases desquamative pneumonia, and in other cases interstitial tubercles, which were not, however, always visible to the naked eye. The macroscopic appearances of the lesions following the experiments are (with the exception of a swollen joint) entirely omitted from the illustrations. Taking, however, the result of the experiments at the author's own valuation, we find that there was always tubercle produced in the lungs, and sometimes in the liver, and that certain changes occurred in the injured joint very like those that occurred when the raw material itself was used. That much, he says, was common to all the cases, whether it was tuberculous lung that had been added to the white of egg, or scrofulous gland, or lupus-tissue, or synovial granulations. But for the rest "there were manifold differences in the general as well as in the local phenomena." Tuberculous and scrofulous micrococci produced the greatest local changes; synovial granulation and lupus-micrococci produced changes much less marked. Curiously enough, that was the order of intensity also when the raw material was used; and it is in that parallelism that the author finds strong support to his conclusion that the micrococci are the determining or potent element in the infectiveness of the raw material. With the unaided reason (not to mention the method of concomitant variations) one would be disposed to conclude that anything rather than the micrococci present in the raw material, or in the fluid, was accountable for the effects following tuberculous, scrofulous, and lupous infections respectively. The organisms, at least, were the same in all (barring certain differences among themselves); they were cultivated with equal ease from all of the various tissues used. In another set of experiments the various cultivations were injected direct into the knee-joint, and, curiously enough, it was the cultivation from lupus-tissue that produced the best-marked tuberculous changes both in the joint and throughout the body. But in most of those direct injections the changes in the joint were very much the same as followed the injection of the common bacteria of putrefaction.

The limits of an article do not permit of our dwelling longer on this rather celebrated work, and in particular the therapeutical part of it must be passed over. The author writes learnedly, in the first section, on the history of the names given to, and of the views held about scrofulous joints, and he writes intelligently on the ordinary pathological histology of tubercle. One cannot but commend his candid inability to discover any rational connexion between the clinical and morphological features of tuberculosis and the bacteria by which the disease is caused; he willingly admits that the mechanical presence of micrococci in the tissues and in the blood will not account for the phenomena. His account of micrococci in the tissues shows them as occurring in singularly casual groups, considering the important part that they play: some few cells are occupied by them, and their nearest neighbours are spared; and, on the whole, the pathological histology of tubercle stands very much where it did. Dr. Schüller's work, we fear, will have to be placed in that class which his countrymen call motivirt. Those who have a leaning towards the germ theory of tuberculosis will find much in the author's manner of statement to encourage them; but those of us who are sceptical, and yet willing to be instructed, will find that the observations in this work are too much lacking in precision, numerical and other, for an independent critical judgment to be formed upon them.

THE DISINFECTION OF CLOTHING AND BEDDING.

It is recognised as important for the safety of the public that all clothing, bedding, etc., which has been used by patients suffering from infectious disease should, with the least possible delay, be disinfected; and as people cannot be depended on to do this themselves, it becomes one of the most important duties of the sanitary authorities to see to it on behalf of the public. In an able and interesting report on the health of Bethnal Green, the Medical Officer of Health for that parish, Dr. G. Paddock Bate, has enabled us to see at a glance the methods of sanitation in this respect which are adopted in the different London parishes, and to form some idea of their relative efficiency. Dr. Bate has made careful inquiries as to each parish, brought together in a tabular form the information gained, and added to it an account of the different kinds of apparatus used. The labour he has expended in investigating this subject makes the report one of much value, and, on account of the interest and importance of the subject, we think we shall do well to summarise the facts to which he has thus drawn public attention.

The sanitary authority of London is vested in fifty-one different vestries, each of which can in this matter choose its own way of fulfilling its public duties. In regard to the disinfection of clothing and bedding, the things to be disinfected have to be divided at once into two classes—those worth disinfecting, and those not worth it. We may dispose of the latter first. Things not worth disinfecting are destroyed by fire, except in six parishes, where no distinction is made, but everything alike disinfected, nothing destroyed. These six parishes are Mile End, Clerkenwell, Wimbledon, Strand, Paddington, and St. Martin's-in-the-Fields—parishes so different as to the social classes which inhabit them, that there seems no especial reason for this conservative tendency. In twenty of the parishes which destroy infected rubbish the owners receive compensation; in five they are never compensated; and in the rest compensated if too poor to replace the articles burnt. The five districts which never compensate are mostly rich ones—the Port of London, Fulham, Kensington, Hampstead, and St. Giles's, Bloomsbury. In the latter parish, however, they only burn at the owner's request.

Articles too valuable to be destroyed are disinfected in thirty-five parishes by a special apparatus, while the remaining sixteen have no such provision. Out of these sixteen, in ten disinfection is accomplished by fumigation with sulphur, in two with bisulphide of carbon, in one (Wanstead) with carbolic acid and steam, and in one (Hornsey) with chlorine. One parish (Wandsworth) burns everything; and Bethnal Green everything except feather beds, which are sent to a private firm to be disinfected. Among those which have a special apparatus, Fraser's is the favourite, thirteen parishes using it. Five parishes contract for the work with private firms. Five employ a hot-air chamber. Three use sulphurous acid at a high temperature. Three parishes possess Leoni's apparatus, and three Nelson's. One uses a gas-oven, another May and Sons', and one Lyon's.

Fraser's apparatus, the oldest and most generally in use, consists of a brick or iron chamber, into which a truck containing the things to be disinfected is run. The doors are then closed, a furnace by the side of the chamber is lighted, and by an ingenious arrangement of flues, air, the heat of which is about 250° Fahr., is kept circulating through the chamber. This apparatus is perfectly efficient, safe, and is no nuisance. The objection to it is, that the efficacy of the whole process depends upon the care of the attendant in charge. Unless he is constantly on the watch while the disinfection is going on, the temperature rises too high, and the articles put in the chamber are scorched. If the attendant be careless and untrustworthy, he soon finds that the easiest way of not getting into trouble for this mishap is to keep the temperature low, and then, of course, there is no disinfection. This is not an imaginary fault, for Dr. Bate says he has been told that articles have been returned to their owners after being through this apparatus and pronounced thoroughly disinfected, in which lice still remained alive.

As to Nelson's apparatus, the medical officers of health for two out of the three parishes which use it are not perfectly satisfied with it. Leoni's and May's are essentially gas-ovens, and have been improved upon by Dr. Ransome, of Nottingham. With an ordinary furnace it is difficult to attain that nice regulation of the degree of heat which is required; for a few degrees of heat make all the difference between inefficiency on the one hand, and scorching on the other. It is, on the contrary, easily managed by means of gas. The special feature of Ransome's apparatus is that, by an automatic arrangement, the gas is turned off when the mercury registers a certain temperature. It also has an ingenious arrangement for the prevention of fire. It has sometimes happened that matches have been left in the pockets of clothing put in the disinfector, and these, when the temperature reaches a certain point, become ignited. Should this happen, of course the heat rapidly rises. To guard against this, dampers suspended by chains are placed over both inlet and outlet, and one link of each chain is made of fusible metal which melts at 300°. Therefore, when this temperature is reached, the chain breaks, the dampers fall, and the gas is turned off. Of course, combustion cannot go on in a close chamber, and so the fire soon dies out, without extending beyond the articles first ignited.

The apparatus which Dr. Bate gives good reasons for considering the best is Washington Lyon's, in which superheated steam is used. It consists of a close chamber, into which steam is admitted at a pressure of 28 lbs. on the square inch, the temperature being about 264° Fahr. This chamber is surrounded by an outer jacket, the object of which is to prevent loss of heat, and therefore condensation of the steam and wetting of the articles disinfected. This apparatus has several advantages. The fabrics (bedding, etc.) which require disinfection are bad conductors of heat. In the case, for instance, of a mattress put inside a hot-air chamber, it is a long time before the heat reaches the centre of the mattress. The hot air outside the article has to part with its heat to the cold air occupying the interstices of the horsehair stuffing, and be in its turn again heated or replaced by currents of hot air; and in the same way the heated air at the periphery of the mattress has to impart its caloric to the air in the centre. As circulation of air in the interior of such a thing as a mattress is very slow, the transference of heat is proportionately tardy. But in Lyon's apparatus other forces are made of service—first, the hot vapour is forced in by pressure; second, when the steam comes into contact with the cool air in the mattress it is immediately condensed; this condensation brings about a great diminution in volume, and fresh steam immediately rushes into the area of low pressure thus produced. The consequence of these two forces is that the penetration of the heat to the interior of the mattress is extremely rapid. This has been proved by experiment. A mattress with a registering thermometer sewn in the middle of it was put in the apparatus. In a few minutes the thermometer showing the interior temperature was at 260° Fahr. The mattress was left in half an hour, and on removal the thermometer in its centre was found to register 259° Fahr. Experiments made by the inventor, with the assistance of Dr. Sedgwick Saunders, the Medical Officer of Health for the City of

London, show that insect life is destroyed by the apparatus. The articles submitted to it are not injured, because when the pressure is removed the water in them quickly evaporates, and they remain almost dry. The disadvantages of the apparatus are that it is rather more expensive than the others, and requires a skilled stoker to manage it. In Dr. Bate's opinion, however, its rapidity and certainty of action counterbalance these drawbacks.

THE WEEK.

TOPICS OF THE DAY.

IT was hardly a happy decision on the part of the Managers of the Metropolitan Asylums Board to try once more an appeal in the higher courts of law against the interim injunction obtained relating to the Fulham Hospital, while evidence is now being received by a Royal Commission on the risk caused to the public by the Asylums Board Hospitals. They, however, appealed in the Supreme Court of Judicature from the decision of a Divisional Court, granting an interim injunction by which they were restrained until the trial of the action from receiving into their Hospital at Fulham patients beyond a radius of one mile. The summons for an injunction was issued on July 21 last, and originally came before Mr. Justice Bowen, who refused it; this judgment was reversed by the Divisional Court, and the defendants, in consequence, appealed. Sir H. Giffard, Q.C., argued the case for the defendants; and read affidavits by medical men, officers of the Hospital, and others, to show that the building and the arrangements were all that could be desired; and he contended that the allegation of the plaintiffs, that small-pox had increased in the neighbourhood by reason of the introduction of an increased number of patients into the Hospital, had not been made out. Lord Justice Brett, however, in delivering judgment, held that it was right that the injunction granted by the court below should be continued, counsel for the plaintiffs having left it clear that the Divisional Court was right in confirming the limits within which patients should be received, rather than the number of patients to be received. Lords Justices Cotton and Lindley concurring, Lord Justice Brett said it would be a condition of this judgment that the plaintiffs should make no opposition to any application which the defendants might make to the High Court of Justice to expedite the trial of this cause as much as possible. The appeal was then dismissed with costs, and the interim injunction stands.

A meeting of the Council of the Hospital Sunday Fund was recently held at the Mansion House to receive the report for the past year. The chair was taken by Bishop Claughton, and the report was read; it stated that the ninth year of the operation of the Fund has resulted in the largest collection since its institution in 1873. The total collection on the last occasion was £31,856, as compared with £30,423 in 1880, and £26,501 in 1879. There had been also a considerable increase in the number of contributing congregations. The surgical appliance branch of the Fund was allowed 2 per cent. of the gross annual receipts; this year the proportion was about £640. Of the sum collected, £27,402 went to ninety-four hospitals, and £2513 to fifty dispensaries. The working expenses had amounted to £1054, or a trifle over 3 per cent. of the gross receipts. The Council desired to express their thanks to the clergy and ministers of all religious denominations for their valuable co-operation in pleading the cause of Hospital Sunday. The adoption of the report was carried unanimously.

After some unavoidable delay, the Smoke Abatement Exhibition was last week opened by the Lord Mayor. A distinguished company assembled in the Albert Hall to meet Her Royal Highness the Princess Louise and the Marquis of Lorne, including Lord Aberdare, Lord Mount-Temple, Earl De la Warr, Mr. Childers, M.P., Mr. Shaw Lefevre, M.P., Captain Douglas Galton, Sir H. Thompson, Sir F. Pollock, Dr. Siemens, F.R.S., etc. The necessary preliminaries having been got through, the distinguished visitors proceeded to inspect the Exhibition, which is arranged in the galleries to the east of the Albert Hall. It includes a great number of improved fire-grates, furnaces, kitcheners, cooking, warming, and other apparatus devised to prevent smoke or to consume smokeless fuel, together with varieties of bituminous and anthracite or smokeless coal, and special fuel for household fires. These are to be practically tested during the period that the Exhibition remains open. The exhibits are roughly divided into six sections—the first contains open coal fire-grates, stoves of all kinds, kitcheners and kitchen ranges; the second, gas-heating apparatus of all kinds; the third, hot air, hot water, and steam appliances; the fourth, gas-engines, boiler-furnaces, and appliances for steam-engine and general industrial purposes; the fifth, anthracite, bituminous, and semi-bituminous coals; and the sixth, all the foreign exhibits, improvements in chimney-flues, and ventilating apparatus. It is proposed to award certain prizes and medals to the best exhibitors, and the arrangements under which these will be awarded will be made known as soon as practicable. Among the donors for this purpose is Dr. Siemens, who has offered a prize of one hundred guineas. A ladies' prize of one hundred guineas, divided into two sums, for the best domestic open grate and best kitchener, will be given. The Society of Arts have offered a medal; the Manchester Association for Controlling the Escape of Noxious Vapours have added a prize of £50; and other prizes will also be offered. So far, the National Health and Kyrle Societies have succeeded in carrying out the programme laid down by them some time ago. It remains to be seen whether their efforts will result in securing in any appreciable degree a purer atmosphere for the denizens of overgrown London.

Amongst other business transacted by the Metropolitan Board of Works at their last meeting, a recommendation from the Works Committee was brought up and agreed to, submitting a schedule of the lands proposed to be taken compulsorily for the purpose of the Metropolis (Little Coram-street, St. Giles' District, and St. Pancras) Improvement Scheme, 1879, under the Artisans' and Labourers' Dwellings Improvement Acts, 1875 and 1879, and recommending that it be forwarded to the Secretary of State for the Home Department; and that an application be made to the Home Secretary, as the confirming authority under the Acts, to appoint an arbitrator between the Board and the persons interested in the land and hereditaments comprised in the said schedule, or in the lands injuriously affected by the execution of such scheme.

Recently, at the Wandsworth Police-court, a butcher was summoned, at the instance of the Wandsworth Board of Works, for having twenty-four joints of unwholesome meat deposited on his premises, intended to be used for the manufacture of sausages, and being unfit for human food. The sanitary inspector deposed that he called on the defendant, and went down to the basement, where a sausage-machine was kept; he found there three tubs of pickle, one containing the joints of beef complained of. In answer to defendant's counsel, the inspector said the defendant told him that the meat was sent by a man to be cut into German sausages for himself. The magistrate said the Act referred to meat in preparation for sale; the case would therefore come within its scope. In answer to another question, the inspector said the defendant told him that it was the practice of the trade to lend the machines. Mr. Joseph Oakman, the Medical Officer of Health for the Western Division of Battersea, proved that the meat was putrid, and unfit for the food of man. Mr. Haynes called witnesses to prove that the meat did not belong to the defendant, who only allowed it to be sent to his place to be cut up by the machine; but the magistrate ruled that the Act was intended to meet such a case. It was to him a wonder, he said, that people continued to eat sausages after all the revelations concerning their manufacture. He imposed a penalty of £15 with 2s. costs. While on this subject it will not be out of place to remark that, at a recent meeting of the City Commissioners of Sewers, Dr. Sedgwick Saunders, their medical officer, reported that from January 1 last to that date there had been seized in the City of London no less than 479½ tons of meat unfit for human food, representing, approximately, one-sixth per cent. of the whole quantity received by the toll-clerks of the Central Meat Market during the same period. He called the early attention of the Commissioners to the significance of the fact, as bearing immediately on the question of the disposal of a "disease-carrying factor," which, despite the statistics of irresponsible persons, was ever on the increase. The proper treatment of the difficulty involved many considerations seriously affecting the reputation of the Commission as the sanitary authority; and it appeared that some modification would be required of the present system of selling the condemned material by contract, at prices absurdly below its commercial value, and without adequate security respecting its ultimate use. Dr. Saunders added to his report a letter from the chief inspector of meat and slaughter-houses, who complained that great difficulties had been experienced by inspectors of meat through the want of co-operation on the part of salesmen at the Central Meat Market. They had fallen, as it was delicately phrased, into the practice of concealing putrid meat by placing it in any corner of their premises, or by covering it over with cloths; sometimes even the ice-safes—recently fitted in the shops—were used as receptacles for stinking meat. The matter was referred to a committee for investigation.

The contention of the metropolitan water companies, that they have a right to base their charges on the gross value of property, has been challenged by Mr. Archibald E. Dobbs, barrister, of 34, Westbourne-park, who has summoned the Grand Junction Waterworks Company for making a claim for £4 10s., the amount alleged to be due to them for two quarters' supply of water to his house, to Michaelmas, 1881, the claim being based upon the annual value of £140 of the said premises. The complainant disputed the amount, and contended that the annual value should be taken at £118; and he urged that by the Act of the 10th Victoria, the magistrate had power to determine disputes of this character. Up to Lady-day last his water-rate had been £5 per annum, but the Company had since raised it to £9. The Grand Junction Waterworks Act of 1852 provided that the Company was to give a proper supply, the rate was to be 4 per cent. when the annual value did not exceed £200, and 3 per cent. if the value was over that amount. That Act did not repeal the Act of 7th George IV., section 27, which provided that the rate should be payable on the amount of rent if it could be ascertained, and if not, the annual value should be the amount at which it was rated to the poor-rates. The complainant paid no rent, the house being his own, and he submitted that the water-rate should be reckoned on the rateable value assessed for the poor-rate, and not on the gross value. Mr. Cooke, the Marylebone magistrate, said it was a very important matter. It wanted some consideration, and he would adjourn the hearing that he might look into the authorities. Mr. Dobbs deserves the gratitude of all house-occupiers in London for contesting the tyranny of the water companies.

At the Clerkenwell Police-court, a duly qualified medical man, practising in the West Central district, was summoned by Frederick Bunyan, of Judd-street, to answer his complaint of having wilfully made a false certificate or declaration concerning the death of Lilian Bunyan. It was stated that an unqualified assistant to the defendant had attended the complainant's child, who afterwards died, and the defendant drew up a certificate to the effect that the child died from diarrhœa, brought on by an overdose of chlorodyne administered by some one else five weeks before. The defendant pleaded guilty, and the magistrate ordered him to pay a fine of £10 and £2 2s. costs, but allowed him a few days in which to pay.

An epidemic of typhoid fever has broken out at Oldham, and many cases have been taken into the Corporation Hospital there. The epidemic is attributed either to impure milk or water, and the medical officer of health is inquiring into the cause of the outbreak.

THE METROPOLITAN WATER-SUPPLY DURING OCTOBER LAST.

THE report of Colonel Bolton, the Metropolitan Water Examiner, for the month of October last, shows that the state of the water in the Thames at Hampton, Molesey, and Sunbury, where the intakes of several of the London companies are situated, was good in quality during the greater part of the month; on the 24th, however, it became indifferent, and remained in that condition until the end of the month. The water in the river Lea was good during the whole of the month. The foregoing remarks, of course, refer to the condition of the water previous to filtration. Regarding its quality when issued for consumption, Dr. Frankland reports that, taking the average amount of organic impurity contained in a given volume of the Kent Company's water during the nine years ending December, 1876, as unity, the proportional amount contained in an equal volume of water supplied by each of the metropolitan water companies and by the Tottenham Local Board of Health was—Colne Valley 1·2, Kent 1·5, Tottenham 1·5, New River 1·9, Chelsea 3·2, West Middlesex 3·4, East London 3·4, Southwark 3·6, Grand Junction 3·7, and Lambeth 4·4. The Thames water sent out by the Chelsea, West Middlesex, Southwark, Grand Junction, and Lambeth Companies maintained the superior average quality which has characterised the supply since March last. Notwithstanding, the filtration was less efficient than usual, for the water of the West Middlesex and Grand Junction Companies was slightly turbid, the former containing fragments of decayed leaves, and the latter moving organisms and fungoid growths, whilst the Lambeth Company's water was turbid and exhibited moving organisms and fragments of leaves. The water drawn from the Lea by the New River and East London Companies also preserved the improved quality of the last and preceding months, and both waters were efficiently filtered before delivery.

THE SANITARY CHRONICLES OF ST. MARYLEBONE FOR OCTOBER, 1881.

IN his remarks on the sanitary condition of the parish of St. Marylebone for the month of October last, the Medical Officer of Health, Mr. A. W. Blyth, refers to the recent outbreak of typhus fever in Charles-street, Lisson-grove, and points out the difficulties under which the sanitary authorities labour in such matters. Much that has been written, he says, has been based upon a misapprehension of the powers possessed by the sanitary staff, and of the real history of the locality. They can only proceed under Torrens's Act;

but, though a medical officer may condemn houses as unfit for human habitation, his report must be sent to the surveyor, and if that official reports the buildings capable of repair, the Vestry are powerless to touch a single brick. The houses in Charles-street were condemned by Dr. Whitmore five years ago, but the surveyor, on being consulted, could not say they were incapable of being repaired, and repairs were accordingly ordered. It was only through the accident of the houses becoming still more dilapidated that Mr. Blyth was enabled to make a second report, which obtained the order for their destruction. This has now been done; but Mr. Blyth thinks it will be a great mistake to suppose that this will have an appreciable effect in staying future epidemics. The only way the outbreak could have been successfully grappled with at the onset would have been by conveying the inhabitants of the affected houses to a bathing and disinfecting establishment, and cleansing them thoroughly, as well as their clothes, while applying a similar process to their rooms. But this cannot be done under the law as it now stands; yet it is mainly infected clothes and infected persons that spread the disease. People may, it is true, be prosecuted for exposing infected clothing; but to do this they must be brought into a crowded court, with the risk of repeating the results of the "black" assizes of old times, and with the chance of spreading the epidemic much more certainly and more widely than if they had been left alone. The house-to-house sanitary inspection, begun in September, is still actively progressing. Local sanitary defects have been discovered in many instances, but hitherto little illegal over-crowding has been found. It must, however, be remembered, Mr. Blyth adds, that the inspectors may be often grossly deceived with regard to overcrowding, no power of entry existing after six o'clock p.m.

GENERAL MEDICAL COUNCIL.

THE London *Gazette* of December 2 gives the information that Her Majesty has been pleased to nominate Robert Dyer Lyons, Esq., M.P., Doctor of Medicine, of Merrion-square, Dublin, to be, for five years, a Member of the General Council of Medical Education and Registration of the United Kingdom, for Ireland, in place of the late Dr. Alfred Henry McClintock. Dr. Lyons is Physician to the Richmond, Whitworth, and Hardwicke Hospitals, and M.P. for the city of Dublin.

THE USE OF THE AMBULANCE IN CIVIL PRACTICE.

MR. REGINALD HARRISON, President of the Liverpool Medical Institution, has published, in the form of a pamphlet, the portion of his inaugural address to that Institution which referred to the necessity at present existing for organising some less imperfect method of removing patients to hospital. Mr. Harrison approaches the subject fresh from a visit to the United States, where he was especially struck with the provision he found in some of the most important hospitals for the conveyance of the sick and injured. He contends, with much reason, that for want of proper appliances to convey to hospital those suffering from accidents, a simple fracture not unfrequently is converted into a compound one, while extra and avoidable pain is entailed on the patient, and extra expense and trouble on the institution. The remedy proposed by Mr. Harrison for this would certainly prove effectual if it could be carried out in our large cities, as it is in the recently constructed City of New York Hospital. New York is divided into police precincts, and these latter are assigned to the different hospitals having an ambulance service. On the occurrence of an accident, information is given to the nearest police-station, and the hospital is directed by tele-

graph where to despatch its ambulance. In the hospital there are electric bells, in the room and within hearing of the surgeon who is told off for ambulance duty, as well as in the driver's room and stables; these are all simultaneously acted upon by a switch in the hospital office where the telephone is placed and the messages received. All these details, including a brief record of the message, notifying the porter to open the gates, harnessing the horses, and starting the ambulance, can be, and are, effected in less than a minute from the time the call reaches the hospital. The ambulance—a neat, solidly-built, easy-running vehicle —is provided with a sliding bed, which is pulled out to receive the patient, and also with a certain quantity of emergency medicines, splints, dressings, etc. If expense is to be urged against the adoption of some such plan on this side of the Atlantic, Mr. Harrison is of opinion that the saving it would effect by reducing the number of compound fractures (always expensive to treat) would go a long way towards providing the necessary funds. At any rate, it would afford an excellent opportunity to the benevolent to endow the larger hospitals with one of these ambulances complete. Mr. Harrison's views on the subject have excited, we are glad to see, some amount of interest, as a second issue of his pamphlet has already been called for; and we trust that something practical will result from this extended publicity.

THE PARIS WEEKLY RETURN.

THE number of deaths for the forty-seventh week, terminating November 25, was 1022 (548 males and 474 females), and among these there were from typhoid fever 43, small-pox 13, measles 12, scarlatina 4, pertussis 6, diphtheria and croup 48, dysentery 2, erysipelas 5, and puerperal infections 5. There were also 36 deaths from tubercular and acute meningitis, 35 from acute bronchitis, 69 from pneumonia, 68 from infantile athrepsia (23 of the infants having been wholly or partially suckled), and 35 violent deaths. The condition of the public health remains with-nigh stationary, and with the exception of variola, which shows a considerable increase, the other epidemic diseases exhibit nearly the same figures as for some time past. The proportion of civil burials for this month has increased from 20·5 to 21·4 per cent. The births for the week amounted to 1189, viz., 617 males (429 legitimate and 188 illegitimate) and 572 females (414 legitimate and 158 illegitimate); 97 infants (54 males and 43 females) were born dead or died within twenty-four hours.

COMPULSORY REPORTS OF INFECTIOUS DISEASE IN LIVERPOOL.

AT the Health Committee of the Liverpool City Council, held on December 1, the subject of the proposed amendments to the Sanitary Acts again came up for discussion. These amendments include compulsory closure by the medical officer of health of premises supposed to be infected, and compulsory notification by the medical profession of all cases of infectious disease that may come under their notice. A letter was read from Dr. Jacobs, of Dublin, in contradiction of Dr. Ransome's statement in the *British Medical Journal* that medical men are generally in favour of the Acts; and another letter from Dr. Littlejohn, of Edinburgh, showing the utility and practicability of the proposed amendments. Dr. Hamilton, in an able speech, opposed the amendments on the grounds that they had failed elsewhere; that it would be impossible in Liverpool for the sanitary staff to carry them out; and that compulsory removal to hospital would increase the mortality. Dr. A. M. Bligh said that at a meeting of medical men held in the Stanley Hospital, lately, twenty out of twenty-three voted against the proposed amendments, and the three abstained from voting because they did not understand the matter. Dr. Bligh objected to the interference of inspectors, and mentioned a case where the father of a patient of his had to bribe an "inspector" by a "drink" to cease insisting on the removal of his child to hospital, although the child was not suffering from infectious disease! The Committee generally expressed the feeling that it would be desirable to obtain the co-operation of the medical profession, and, at the suggestion of Dr. Hamilton, the following amendment was carried—"That it is not expedient to proceed further with the clauses referring to the prevention of infectious diseases and the closing of premises."

THE YELLOW FEVER.

THE French Minister of Marine has addressed a letter to the Academy of Medicine, calling their attention to the recent prevalence of yellow fever in the colonies, and asking that learned body to undertake an inquiry into the various important questions relating to the disease similar to that which it conducted concerning the plague in 1879. The letter was referred to a committee consisting of MM. Pasteur, Davaine, Fauvel, Rochard, Le Roy de Méricourt, and Léon Colin.

PATHOLOGICAL SOCIETY OF DUBLIN.

AT the meeting of this Society held on Saturday, December 3 (Dr. Stokes, President, in the chair), Dr. J. W. Moore showed an immense aneurism of the ascending aorta in a discharged soldier, aged forty-three years, who had served eight years and a half in India, and who presented a clinical history of syphilis and rheumatism. The aneurism contained a mass of solid fibrin which weighed twenty ounces. The whole ascending aorta was atheromatous, dilated, and sacculated, rendering the aortic valves incompetent. The left cardiac ventricle was hypertrophied, dilated, and soft from fatty degeneration. The mitral orifice was dilated. The liver was rather large; it was a nutmeg liver. There was some cirrhotic change in the kidneys and spleen. Dr. Stokes (the President) showed a large tumour of the thigh, which was of traumatic origin. A blow had been followed by hæmorrhagic effusion, and the resulting hæmatoma had been incised freely two years previously. Amputation was ultimately performed at the hip-joint. The centre of the tumour was occupied by a large cyst filled with blood. Otherwise the new growth was partly soft and brainlike, partly firm. The microscopical characters were those of round-celled sarcoma. Mr. W. Thornley Stoker exhibited two specimens of fracture of both bones of the leg—of the tibia in its lowest third, of the fibula in its uppermost third in the vicinity of its head. He thought the latter injury was consecutive to the oblique fracture of the tibia, and was caused by the weight of the leg and foot, and the efforts of the patient after the injury. Professor Bennett said the specimens illustrated oblique fracture of both bones, and that, as pointed out by Malgaigne, the obliquity of the fibular fracture was in the opposite direction to that of the tibial. One of Mr. Stoker's specimens was an example of Gosselin's "fracture en-V" of the tibia. Dr. G. F. Duffey presented the bladder and kidneys of a discharged soldier, aged fifty-four, who had suffered from a very tight stricture. The urine was intermittently albuminous. Severe attacks of hæmaturia occurred at intervals, and ultimately proved fatal. The lungs, heart, and liver were healthy; the spleen was enlarged and diffluent; the bladder was hypertrophied, and its mucous membrane was ecchymosed. The right kidney, with its surroundings, weighed seventeen ounces and a half. Both kidneys were the seat of a new growth, which was probably a carcinoma. Mr. W. Thomson laid on

the table an interesting series of five fractures of bones of the skull; for an opportunity of showing which he was indebted to Dr. Jacob, of Maryborough. The first specimen was a depressed fracture of parietal and occipital bones, caused by the blow of a spade. In the second case, a pistol-bullet lodged in the occipital bone, having passed through both plates and almost escaped from the outer one. The third specimen was a fracture of the frontal bone in a female who died of an abscess of the brain three weeks after the receipt of the injury. In the fourth a fracture of the right parietal bone was caused by the kick of a horse. The outer table was crushed in, and the inner table pushed up into three plates. Violent maniacal symptoms set in half an hour after the injury, but at once ceased on the trephining of the bone. The fifth case was also a fracture of the right parietal from the kick of a horse. In this instance, too, trephining was performed.

THE FRENCH DECREE AGAINST AMERICAN PORK.

THE decree issued by the French Government, February 18, prohibiting absolutely the admission of American pork on account of the danger from the trichina said to infest it, has given rise to great dissatisfaction and many complaints. It has interfered greatly with large commercial interests, and has pressed hardly upon the poorer classes, who in France make great use of pork. All this might have been borne had the danger been as great as it was at first represented to be, but it is now believed that it was in a great measure imaginary, seeing how little mischief has resulted in those countries which took no similar precautions. The decree was passed very precipitately, without the consultation with the Académie de Médecine which is usual on such occasions. The proposed organisation of laboratories for the microscopical examination of pork has never been carried out, and it is expected that the decree will be in a short time withdrawn.

THE REPORT OF THE COMMISSIONERS IN LUNACY FOR 1880.

THE thirty-fifth Report of the Commissioners in Lunacy to the Lord High Chancellor, dated March 31 last, shows that, from returns furnished to that body, the total number of registered lunatics, idiots, and persons of unsound mind in England and Wales on January 1 last was 73,113, being an increase of 1922 upon the cases recorded on January 1, 1880. This number does not, however, include 234 lunatics so found by inquisition, and residing in charge of their committees in unlicensed houses, nor 189 male prisoners who, having become insane whilst undergoing sentences of penal servitude, were on January 1 last detained under care and treatment in the wards of convict prisons. The 73,113 cases remaining on January 1 last were made up of 774½ classed as private patients, and of 65,372 paupers, and the increase already mentioned was divided between 121 private patients and 1801 paupers. During the previous ten years the average annual increase was 184 of the private class and 1518 among the paupers, and the report explains that the excess in the average annual increase of numbers shown by the figures of January 1 last, as compared with those of January 1, 1880, is fully accounted for by the diminished death-rate in asylums, hospitals, and licensed houses of the year 1880, as compared with 1879. Among the private patients the deaths were 119 less in number, and amongst the paupers they were less by 449 in 1880 than in the previous year. It is further pointed out that the annual increase in the number under care, as compared with population, continues to be among the paupers, and not in the private class. A table of a novel character has been compiled to accompany the present report, showing the yearly ratio of fresh admissions to population. For this purpose the transfers and the admissions into idiot asylums have been excluded. It is, the Commissioners think, an established fact that the legislation of 1874 has tended to encourage the removal of pauper lunatics from workhouses into asylums, and has thus helped annually to swell the total admissions. It is, however, shown that, notwithstanding this fact, the ratio of the yearly increase of the admissions to population has been but slight, and not constant, suggesting that the large increase in the total number of the insane under care in asylums, hospitals, and licensed houses during the twelve years to which this table refers, is mainly due to accumulation, and not to a greater annual production of insanity. The statistics of the different counties show that the increase of cases during 1880 was above the average in Middlesex, Surrey, Nottingham, Warwick, Devon, Essex, Norfolk, Stafford, and Bedford. On the other hand, in Lancashire and Yorkshire the increase was below the average annual increase of the past ten years. The total number of deaths during the year 1880 was 4498. Post-mortem examinations were made in only 1656 of the deaths, which, the Report observes, shows a falling off much to be regretted in the practice of making these very necessary examinations, as compared with previous years; and the attention of medical superintendents is particularly directed to the omission. Of the deaths, twenty were by suicide, besides one case where the act was committed before admission into the asylum, and in five instances the patients destroyed themselves whilst absent on leave. In estimating the recoveries, the idiot asylums have been excluded as not receiving curable cases, and all transfers have been eliminated. Thus calculated, the total recoveries, as compared with the admissions of the year 1880, were 37·06 per cent. for the males and 43·28 per cent. for the females, or 40·29 per cent. for both sexes. These ratios are nearly the same as for 1879, and are somewhat above the average rate for the last ten years. The general result, the Report remarks, must be considered satisfactory, bearing in mind that a large proportion of the admissions of every year are chronic and incurable cases. Still excluding the idiot asylums, the death-rate in the other establishments, calculated on the average daily number resident during the year, has been 11·10 per cent. for males, and 7·61 per cent. for females, or 9·22 per cent. for both sexes. This ratio is more than 1 per cent. lower than that for 1879, and nearly 1 per cent. below the average of the last ten years. The average weekly cost per head of maintenance, medicine, clothing, etc., during 1880 was in county asylums 9s. 6½d., and in borough asylums 11s. 4½d.

BATTEY'S OPERATION FOR INTERMENSTRUAL PAIN.

AN interesting and instructive case is recorded by Fehling in a recent number of the Archiv für Gynäkologie. The patient was aged thirty-one, married for eight years, but sterile. Menstruation was painless, but the patient said that she suffered from severe attacks of pain, which came on from fourteen to sixteen days after one menstrual period, and lasted till three days before the beginning of the next. The cervix uteri had been incised and dilated; the uterus had been depleted; the patient had tried one of the bath cures,—but without benefit. She had had an attack of scarlet fever, during which the pain was quite absent. It was thought that the pain was connected with the maturation of Graafian follicles, and therefore spaying was advised; Professor Hegar concurring with Dr. Fehling in this recommendation. The operation was performed in June, 1880, both ovaries being completely removed; and the patient recovered. The ovaries were thought to possess an unusually tough and hard tunica albuginea, and the number of follicles was considered unusually small; but examination, both

with the naked eye and the microscope, failed to detect anything else abnormal about them. The patient left the hospital four weeks after the operation, and remained well for six or eight weeks later. Then the pains began to return, and soon became as bad as ever. Hæmorrhage, similar to that of menstruation, also recurred. The patient, therefore, was not benefited by losing her ovaries. We have had occasion to speak strongly on the wrong done to medical science by authors who rush to announce their cases as cures before there has been time to ascertain whether the ultimate result has been beneficial or not. This case shows the necessity for caution before assuming that benefit immediately following extirpation of the ovaries will be permanent. Only in cases which have been watched for a long time can anything be safely said as to whether they have been cured or not.

THE BRIGHTON HEALTH CONGRESS AND DOMESTIC AND SCIENTIFIC EXHIBITION.

THE arrangements for this Congress and Exhibition are being pushed forward with great energy and success. The Exhibition, over which Lord Chichester presides, will be opened in the afternoon of Monday, December 12. The Congress, over which Dr. Richardson, F.R.S., presides, will be opened on Tuesday evening, the 13th, by the delivery of his inaugural address. The sittings of the Congress will be continued every day until Friday. The Congress will be composed of three sections. The first, presided over by Mr. Edwin Chadwick, C.B., relates to the Health of Towns; the second, presided over by Mr. J. R. Holland, M.A., M.P., relates to Food; and the third, presided over by Dr. Alfred Carpenter, C.S.S., relates to Domestic Health. There will be introductory presidential addresses in each section. On Wednesday, the Mayor and Mayoress will hold a reception in the Pavilion. On Thursday, Dr. Taaffe, Medical Officer of Health for Brighton, will deliver a public lecture. On Saturday, excursions will be made to various places of interest in and about Brighton; and in the evening of Saturday the proceedings of the Congress will be brought to a close by a lecture to the working-classes from Mr. Brudenell Carter, F.R.C.S.

UCKFIELD URBAN SANITARY DISTRICT.

A SHORT notice of Mr. W. H. Power's report on an outbreak of enteric fever in this district appeared in our pages two months ago; but as it is in some points one of unusual interest, it seems well to refer to it with more minuteness. Uckfield Parish—a Local Board district—contains about 2400 inhabitants, of whom some 2000 reside in the village or "town" of Uckfield. In September, last year, an outbreak of enteric fever began, in Uckfield town, in the almost simultaneous attack of three persons belonging to two separate households in Church-street, and of a fourth person living in another street nearly a quarter of a mile off. In October four other cases occurred, in November two, and in December three. Towards the end of January of the present year a rapid increase of the fever occurred, continuing into February; the attacks during the two months numbering twenty. In March there were only five cases; and in April, when Mr. W. H. Power inspected the town, no more cases had been reported. The town stands upon the Hastings sands of the Wealden, on "hills" or slopes formed north and south of a tributary of the Ouse; and as to its dwelling-houses, its water-supply, drainage, sewerage, etc., it is like numberless other old high-road villages that have gradually developed or are developing into towns. That is to say, the houses vary much in class and character, and the degree of crowding also varies; the water-supply is from wells commonly situated close to and even under dwellings which in their turn occupy sites that have for generations been fouled by soakage from privies, cesspools, ashpits, defective drains, and the like. The wells are sunk in the sand rock of the lower Tunbridge Wells sand, which is mostly within a few feet of the surface, and some of them are from forty to sixty feet deep, but it appears that most of them are, from characters of construction, from the lie of the ground and its geological character, liable to pollution. The sewers are almost quite unventilated, and flushing is so entirely neglected that even the exact whereabouts of the flushing boxes once provided is no longer known; traps shutting off house-drains from the public sewers are almost unknown, and ventilation of house-drainage can hardly be said to exist; excrement is disposed of by a form of water-carriage, but instead of the closets being properly supplied with water, they are, as a rule, dependent for flushing on an occasional pail of water cast into them by the tenants of the dwellings to which they belong. Considering the existence of these, and of some other similar, grave defects in the sanitary arrangements of the place, there is no room for surprise at the outburst of enteric fever in January last. The origin of the four cases that occurred in the previous September is not clear. There is some probability that in the case in High-street the disease was acquired in Worthing; but the source of infection in the other cases is much more doubtful. Afterwards, the wonder is, not that fresh cases occurred, but that the cases were not more numerous and more widely spread. But still more interesting and noteworthy is the fact that for some years cases of enteric fever had from time to time occurred in Uckfield, and the disease had not spread. In 1877, and in January and in the autumn of 1878, small groups of cases occurred, in single families, without any extension of the disease; and in 1879, again in the autumn, two occurred, almost simultaneously, in separate houses in one street, and in September and October and November eight cases in the grammar-school in the same street. Then no more were observed till the autumn of last year. Mr. Power remarks on this—"There is here a history of enteric fever, whether imported or of home production, repeatedly failing to propagate itself under conditions apparently singularly favourable for its reproduction, but in the end tending to become seasonal in its occurrence. Also there is a history of autumnal enteric fever, infertile at first in circumstances apparently conducive to its fertility, but suddenly in a particular season developing reproductive powers, to be in a subsequent season fully maintained with widely increased range. Suggestions of this sort concerning the natural history of enteric fever are of no little interest."

DEATH OF DR. BRIQUET.

WITHIN a month of the death of Professor Bouillaud, the Nestor of the Academy of Medicine, the other Nestor, Dr. Pierre Briquet, has passed away at the same age—eighty-six. They resembled each other in their constant attendance at the meetings of that learned body. Indeed, of Dr. Briquet it has been declared that he never missed a meeting since his nomination in 1860. Like Bouillaud, too, shortly before his death he read a memoir, being a kind of supplementary chapter ("Prédisposition à l'Hystérie") to his well-known work on hysteria. He was for a long period Physician to La Charité, and was as regular and as punctual there as at the Academy. He attained a very large private practice among a good circle of patients, so that he has left a large fortune; but this has been in part due to his economical habits, owing to which he never kept a carriage, even when at the height of his practice, always walking to see even his most distinguished patients. Besides various reports and minor publications, his three principal works were

—"Traité du Choléra," "Traité Thérapeutique de Quinquina, et de ses Préparations"—a work to which the Académie des Sciences adjudged a prize, and which may still be consulted with advantage,—and "Traité Clinique et Pratique de l'Hystérie."

ROYAL COLLEGE OF SURGEONS OF ENGLAND.

WHEN we noticed, some time ago, the business transacted at the meeting of the Council of the Royal College of Surgeons on November 10, we stated very briefly the purport of the report of the Committee appointed to consider the questions sent by the Medical Acts Commission, which, after considerable discussion, and some amendment, had been adopted by the Council. But the report is one of considerable importance, and we therefore now give more fully what, so far as we have been able to learn, the document really contained. In reply to the questions, whether, in the opinion of the College, any alteration of the present licensing system is required; and what, if any, changes would be most likely to prove beneficial to the public and the profession? the Council state briefly that it has for many years been engaged, from time to time, in attempts to arrange some plan by which complete examinations in medicine, surgery, and midwifery might be held under the combined authority of all the licensing bodies in England. Then, believing that some amendment of the Medical Act of 1858 will follow the report of the Royal Commission on the Medical Acts, the Council place before the Commission the following resolutions:—That no person should be registered as a legally qualified practitioner unless, after a duly recognised general and professional education, he shall have passed complete examinations in Medicine, Surgery, and Midwifery. That such complete examinations would be most likely to prove beneficial to the public and the profession if, in each division of the United Kingdom, there were a combination of licensing bodies, under the sanction of the General Medical Council, to conduct the examinations. That persons who have passed such examinations should be entitled, under conditions agreed to by the corporations, and sanctioned by the General Medical Council, to the diplomas of the combining corporations; and that a medical and a surgical diploma should be necessary for registration. That it should be enacted by legislation that no person be admitted to a qualifying examination under the age of twenty-two years, in order that another year may be added to the time assigned to professional education. And that no university should be permitted to grant a licence in medicine or in surgery independently of its degrees. These resolutions in general practically recommend, it will be observed, the establishment of conjoint schemes; but the last resolution but one—that recommending an enforced extension of the period devoted to professional study—is of great importance. As respects the present constitution, powers, and functions of the General Medical Council, the Council of the College replies that it is not agreed in opinion in regard to the question of any alteration in the constitution of the General Medical Council; but, in reference to the powers and functions of that body, the Council holds that these should not be increased or extended. The rest of the report gives, in answer to a request from the Commission, in a concise and convenient form for reference, the number of candidates who have in each of the last five years obtained from the College each of the registrable titles granted by it: the amount of emolument derived from this source, and the annual income derived from any other sources. And in this part the Council explains the College expenditure, and shows, among other things, that since the beginning of the present century it has expended not less than £40,000 on its library; and that while it has received, at different dates, Parliamentary grants amounting to £43,500 for the enlargement of the buildings devoted to the reception of the Hunterian Collection, it has contributed £42,000 for the same purpose, and about £200,000 for the preservation and improvement of the Anatomical Collection, the guardianship of which it has undertaken for the use of the scientific world, and therefore for the benefit of the public.

OPIUM IN CHINA.(a)

It seems at first sight somewhat remarkable that, because two-thirds of 1 per cent. of the 300,000,000 of the people of China choose to consume opium—some only of these to an immoderate extent,—the well-wishers of the country should so earnestly desire to do away with the consumption of the drug altogether. They admit that, whilst it adds considerably to the revenue of India, it does not diminish the wealth of the people nor affect the growth of the population of China; and that its injurious effects are infinitesimal. Still, they advocate the discountenance of its use. Our surprise is lessened when we remember that the percentage above mentioned means 2,000,000 of human beings, a number equal to half the population of the metropolis of London. Opium-smoking, to this limited extent even, is regarded as a canker that is annually increasing its proportions. Chinese philanthropists would therefore prevent its further development. Chinese merchants and agriculturists, especially in the far West, would exclude foreign products for their own. It appears from this valuable paper that 100,000 chests (each chest containing 100 Chinese pounds of opium) are annually imported from India into China; 30 per cent. being lost in the boiling down and conversion into prepared opium, and a Chinese pound equalling one pound and one-third of an English pound avoirdupois, the actual amount of foreign opium when ready for use is over 900,000 pounds avoirdupois. A similar quantity is produced in China itself; and for the possession of the luxury from these two sources £25,000,000 are paid annually. The foreign opium is much preferred to that of indigenous origin, it being less astringent, and devoid of the grassy taste which the latter is apt to have. It is calculated that each of the 2,000,000 smokers daily consumes from one to five drachms of the drug; and it is added that, if this amount be exceeded, the result is detrimental. But the tolerance of opium is so much a matter of idiosyncrasy and habit, that with many the single drachm must be more than enough. The money value of the quantity consumed by each individual varies from 5d. to 11d. per day. Taken in the first instance to allay pain or for sickness, the craving for opium after a while is developed. The regular smoker becomes a slave to the habit, whilst those who smoke irregularly can more readily give it up. As a rule, opium at first disagrees; the habit is quite an acquired one. Immoderate smokers die early, and, having got rid of pretty well all they possess to gratify their morbid appetite, usually in misery. Those who smoke temperately rarely suffer. Partly owing to the aversion of the Chinese to give information, and partly owing to the difficulty of ascertaining the extent of any social evil, it is impossible to say exactly how far the practice of opium-smoking is carried, especially amongst the upper classes; but it is doubtless very considerable. Opium has a dietetic as well as a medicinal value. It is customary for the reformers of society, with reference to this drug and alcohol, to bracket them together in one sweeping condemnation; but, while the latter is simply a temporary stimulant, for which there are substitutes equally powerful, though not so pleasant to swallow, the former tranquillises, arrests waste of tissue—being in this respect to the poor Chinaman what tea is to the same class in the United Kingdom,—and in time of famine takes the place even of food; to say nothing of its incommutable value as a medicine. Its reception into the heart of society is too universal and deep for Acts of Parliament or Imperial decrees to be efficacious in preventing its consumption. If the cultivation of opium was interdicted, except for medicinal purposes, the country of its growth, as Sir C. E. Trevelyan has pointed out, would be overrun with smugglers; leading to social convulsions that would seriously strain the resources of Government, diminished as they would be by loss of revenue from opium. If Government gave up the monopoly, adds Sir Charles, and levied only an excise, its responsibility would still remain, whilst the control of the growth and manufacture would be rendered more difficult.

"China: Imperial Maritime Customs." II. Special Series, No. 4. Published by order of the Inspector-General of Customs.

THE A B C PROCESS.

In a former article on Sewage Farming, we pointed out that, while on economic grounds downward intermittent filtration seemed to be superior to other methods of disposal or utilisation of sewage, there were, or might be, circumstances which would render its adoption impracticable. Such, for example, would be the case of a town surrounded on all sides by lofty hills, or where the land for several miles round is required for building, or is too costly, as in the neighbourhood of rapidly growing or manufacturing centres. We maintained that sewage farming, judiciously conducted, might be a source of considerable profit, as the Craigentinny meadows and Breton Farm amply prove, but that, since sewage may no longer be allowed to pollute our rivers, any method of rendering it innocuous, at an expense not absolutely prohibitive, may be accepted as at least a provisional expedient. Utilisation of sewage must not be approached from a merely commercial point of view, and if a method be found a sanitary success, although it may not yield a profit, the cost must be considered as the price paid for pure watercourses and uncontaminated soil. Unfortunately, the chemical processes for the most part do not fulfil even these requirements, their effluents being often only slightly mitigated sewage, quite unfit for discharge into rivers whose waters may later on be drunk. From this general condemnation we must, however, except the A B C process, Sillar's patent, as carried on at the Company's works at Aylesbury, which we recently had an opportunity of inspecting.

The sewage as it issues from the culvert is passed through a grating, which breaks up fæcal masses, and intercepts rags, sticks, and occasionally babies. At the same time the deodorant—a mixture of finely divided clay, crude animal charcoal, and a small proportion of blood—enters the stream of sewage by a pipe just above a weir; a few feet lower down, a solution of alum, which is precipitated by the ammonia and organic matter as a hydrate, is added in like manner; and the mixture of sewage and chemicals passes into a subsiding tank, the overflow from which is carried much clarified into a second, and in the same manner still further cleared into a third, whence the effluent passes finally into the river. The first tank is cleared out every third day, the others at longer intervals, two only being used while one is being emptied. The freedom of the effluent from suspended or colouring matters is conspicuously seen where it meets and drives back the turbid water of the river. We have several analyses by Professor Wanklyn of this effluent, one of the most recent showing chlorine 3·2 grains per gallon, free ammonia 0·05 parts per million, and albuminoid 0·30, or one-tenth of the standard fixed by the Rivers Pollution Commissioners. Though it varies .with the rainfall, etc., it never transgresses or even approaches the limits prescribed by the Commissioners.

Before the sludge is put into the driers a little sulphuric acid is added to fix the ammonia, but no lime is used, since it is found to detract from the value of the manure. Throughout the whole process there is no effluvium or nuisance whatever; the space required for the works is surprisingly small; the effluent is fit to pass into any river (though not immediately above the pumping station of a water company); and, in short, as a sanitary measure the success of the A B C seems complete. As to the financial questions—whether the process, as a mere mode of disposal, can be carried on at a reasonable cost, and whether the product is really capable of utilisation as a valuable and saleable manure—there may be more difference of opinion.

The Town Council of Leeds, after careful observations, extending over three years, estimate the cost of purifying one million gallons of sewage at from £1 7s. to £1 17s., or for the whole sewage of the borough, say £7000 per annum—no intolerable burden on a rateable value of over £1,000,000.

Secondly, what is the real value of the manure as an application to crops? It has been asserted that its value is due chiefly to the ingredients added. It is a fact that in the early days of the Company a pretty well-known analyst was convicted of fortifying the manure without the knowledge of the directors; but, seeing that the chemicals are only clay, charcoal, and alum, the proportion of blood being insignificant (although aiding in some ill understood way the deposition of suspended and precipitated matters), and that, after drying, the manure weighs nearly twice as much as the materials employed, as well as taking into account the evidence of analyses of the effluent, we may dismiss this objection. To exhibit its results in a practical way, the Company hold an annual show of farm and garden produce grown solely with the help of the Native guano. So far as we could judge, the results were very satisfactory, though much more so in the case of some crops than others—*e.g.*, mangels 56 tons, and swedes 24 tons per acre; the potatoes also were remarkably fine. And we have the testimony of eminent agriculturists and practical farmers in different parts of the country, who unanimously report favourably of it, especially for grass, gardens, and certain root crops. Compared with Peruvian guano (now nearly exhausted) at £15 per acre, general consent fixes the Native at from £3 10s., the selling price, to £3 by some who recommend its more lavish employment.

In short, the A B C process gives us no nuisance, an effluent as pure as we can demand, and a manure not only of intrinsic value, but capable of transport to distant places; the process can be carried on anywhere, and at a cost which, if not remunerative, is at least within the resources of every urban authority.

FROM ABROAD.

Professor Verneuil on Phimosis.

In a clinical lecture delivered at La Pitié, Prof. Verneuil observed (*Gaz. des Hop.*, November 15) that phimosis is a tolerably frequent affection, which is sometimes attended with rather serious accidents, as might be seen in a case now in the hospital, in which amputation of the penis became necessary. It was a case of phimosis complicated with balano-posthitis, predisposing to papilloma, and that to epithelioma.

The object of the lecture is not a general account of phimosis, but an account of its treatment. When it is characterised by mere narrowness of the orifice of the prepuce, a *débridement* carried parallel to the axis of the prepuce, either by means of scissors, bistoury, or elastic cord, will suffice. It is a good operation when the narrowing is especially due to the formation of cicatricial tissue, as is observed, for example, after chancre. It is sufficient then to make the *débridement*, and leave the parts to themselves. There is also circumcision—an operation, in fact, far more difficult than is usually supposed. Sometimes it succeeds very well, but most frequently union does not take place by first intention, and the results of the operation are very prolonged. In some cases, too, it gives rise to more or less hemorrhage, and in others to more or less dangerous consequences. It is for these reasons that M. Verneuil often opposes its performance. A considerable time since, dilatation of the prepuce had been proposed, but was abandoned in favour of circumcision, which was regarded then, quite erroneously, as a very simple operation. Dilatation, thus, if it had not become quite disused, was of very little account until Nélaton took it up, employing for this purpose a small special forceps which he had devised. It was on the faith of the results which he obtained that Prof. Verneuil resorted to dilatation, which he has now performed for a long time, reserving circumcision for some special cases. Even in phimosis produced by cicatricial contraction the prepuce yields to dilatation, except in the very rare cases in which the tissue is very hard. Special forceps have been invented, which are all very well in Paris, where every variety of instrument is obtainable; but in country practice such facilities do not exist, and it is therefore well to know that the common dressing-forceps is just as convenient.

"As to the operative procedure, it is a very simple one. I put my patient to sleep because I wish to proceed as slowly as necessary, and to obviate the pain inherent to the operation. I draw out the prepuce, and commence by introducing a grooved director between the prepuce and the glans, and then I pass a second grooved director along the groove of the first. In this way a commencement of dilatation takes place, and then I introduce a common dressing-forceps, open it, and withdraw gradually, distending the prepuce, just as the anus is dilated by a speculum. Since I have had recourse to this procedure I have never yet met with a failure. All that can happen is a slight rupture of the preputial mucous membrane, giving rise to a few drops of blood. When the prepuce thus dilated is everted, you wash the glans with some carbolised water. If the dilatation has been very considerable, you then close the prepuce over the glans. If not, you will have a paraphimosis, which you should dress with lead lotion, without any fear that gangrene of the glans or the penis will be produced by strangulation. Still, gangrene of the glans does occasionally take place, of which we have had an interesting example during this year, without being able very well to explain how it came to occur."

Vulcanised Indiarubber Bandages.

In a communication to the Société de Chirurgie (*Union Méd.*, No. 97), Dr. Marc Sée gave an account of the various advantages derivable from these. 1. In œdematous infiltration of the limbs, whatever may be its cause—affections of the heart or liver, various forms of cachexia, compression produced by tumours of the abdomen, etc. Under all these circumstances, the elastic bandage, properly applied, prevents the too great distension of the skin, as well as the development of the erysipelatous redness to which so frequently succeed partial mortifications of the integument. It is especially efficacious in those distressing infiltrations of the upper extremities in the subjects of cancer of the breast, with extension to the axillary glands. The same may be said of the œdema which persists after the cure of phlebitis, lymphangitis, etc. 2. Sero-plastic infiltrations consecutive to diffuse phlegmons, which leave behind them articular stiffness and an impediment to motion proceeding from rigidity of the skin and subcutaneous cellular tissue. The frictions and kneading which are so useful in these cases are powerfully aided by the application of the elastic bandage in the intervals of their performance. The rigidity due to the dwelling of the fingers left after phlegmon of the hand and forearm are successfully treated by the same means. 3. Infiltrations and effusions of blood consecutive to contusions, subcutaneous lacerations, and ecchymoses of all kinds. The bandage here hastens the absorption of the extravasated blood by acting on it as does the thumb of the surgeon which crushes a sanguineous tumour of the hairy scalp—differing, however, by acting gently, without violence, and in a continuous manner. 4. Serous effusions into the joints, and especially in hydrarthrosis of the knee, elbow, and ankle, which so often resist other means of treatment, or recur whenever the patient attempts to use his limb—as is often seen in certain cases of blennorrhagic arthritis. In several cases of this kind Dr. Sée has procured, by means of the bandage, permanent cures in some days, after the failure of immobility and superficial cauterisation. 5. Circumscribed or diffused phlegmon at any period of its evolution. Whenever the bandage can be applied, it advantageously replaces the emollient cataplasm, over which it has the advantage of moderating the afflux of blood by its compression of the tissues. 6. Ecthyma of the limbs, and ulcers which remain after the fall of crusts, atonic ulcers of the leg, callous ulcers, and varicose ulcers. In all these cases the bandage causes the rapid disappearance of complications, and favours cicatrisation. 7. In recent wounds, whether accidental or surgical, united by means of sutures. The bandage applied over Lister's dressing greatly promotes union by first intention, and allows of the intervals of dressing being much longer than usual. Dr. Sée has left a first dressing on for three weeks, and then found the wound almost completely healed. This is, however, a very important point, which is now only indicated, M. Sée intending to enter into details about it on a future occasion.

Certain precautions are necessary in the application of the bandage. The compression which it exerts on the soft parts ought to be extremely moderate and in nowise impede the circulation. While putting it on, the gentlest traction should be employed, only sufficient to insure the exact application of the various turns of the bandage throughout their whole extent. These should cover over each other to the extent of a third or a fourth of their breadth, leaving no intervals between their edges, for the parts freed from pressure would soon swell from infiltration of serosity. Except under special circumstances when it has to remain applied as long as possible, the bandage should be removed every two or three days, and only reapplied after having been washed in carbolised water. The effects produced by the bandage are due to two properties which it possesses in the highest degree—its elasticity and its impermeability. By its elasticity it exerts upon the parts which it covers a pressure which, while it is always very gentle, is none the less efficacious, in consequence of its continuousness and the slight extent to which it is influenced by the small changes in volume that the parts undergo. It is needless to insist upon the influence which such pressure may exert on the local circulations and on effusions. By its impermeability the bandage establishes an impassable barrier between the parts it covers and the external air. On the one hand, it amasses under itself the products of transpiration and the secretions of the skin, which, as well as the wounds, it maintains in a constant condition of warmth and humidity, similar to that produced by cataplasms. On the other hand, it prevents the wounds becoming contaminated by the germs permeating the air, and the putrefaction of effused liquids, thus proving a very useful adjuvant to antiseptic dressing.

In the discussion which followed, M. Nicaise stated that he had several times found the bandage irritate the tissues. He always employs the red or black caoutchouc, which are less irritating than the grey. M. Lucas-Championnière has found the grey rapidly effect changes in the liquids with which it comes in contact, while, with the red or black, organic liquids may be kept in contact for any length of time. Prof. Verneuil suggested that compression produced by the bandage on the œdematous tissues of persons suffering from cardiac or renal affections may prove injurious by repelling into the general circulation a mass of extravasated liquids, and thus cause the re-entrance into the blood of principles which should be eliminated by these liquids. Is it not to be feared, for example, that urea, deprived of this kind of excretory, may accumulate in the blood and give rise to the accidents of uræmia? Injudicious applications, made with the object of suppressing this kind of "serous dew," have, in fact, been followed by the most serious consequences. M. le Dentu, while succeeding in diminishing the œdema of the arm in cancer of the breast by means of the bandage, has found such an amount of dyspnœa produced as to oblige him to abandon its use. Dr. Sée observed that the irritation from the bandage may occur both with the red and the grey caoutchouc; and the latter undergoes change very rapidly on exposure to air, becoming very friable. This is prevented by keeping it in a bottle, closed by emery, and containing a little water. He stated that he had never met with the ill consequence of the use of the bandage referred to by Prof. Verneuil; but he always accompanies its application by the administration of diuretics.

ROYAL INSTITUTION.—At the general monthly meeting of the Royal Institution of Great Britain, held on Monday last, the managers reported that they had that day appointed Professor John Gray McKendrick, M.D., F.R.S.E., of the University of Glasgow, Fullerian Professor of Physiology for three years.

PARSLEY AS AN ANTILACTIC.—Dr. Stanislas Martin, after observing that the use of mineral waters interrupted the secretion of milk, states that, as an external application, parsley-leaves act most efficaciously in dispersing it, and that they were used for this purpose by the Roman matrons of old. The breasts should be covered with freshly plucked leaves, and these should be renewed several times a day as fast as they begin to fade. The dispersion of the milk soon takes place.—Bull. de Thérap., July 30.

COD-LIVER OIL.—Dr. Fonssagrives recommends the following formula:—Cod-liver oil 96 grammes, iodoform 20 centigrammes, essence of anise 4 drops. The addition of the last two articles completely masks the taste and smell of the oil. Patients to whom the preparation is still repugnant may add to each spoonful of oil a very small quantity of salt, which modifies its taste and facilitates its digestion.— Gaz. des Hop., November 15.

REVIEWS.

Lectures on Diseases of the Nervous System, especially in Women. By S. WEIR MITCHELL, etc. With five plates. London : J. and A. Churchill. 1881. Pp. 238.

THIS work is—as, indeed, from the name of the author, most will have expected—a very original, valuable, and interesting contribution to scientific medicine. It deals with that important, but little, if at all, understood, class of symptoms which stand on the doubtful territory between recognisable and definite organic disease on the one hand, and malingering on the other. It tries to introduce order and precision into the vague and various phenomena which are called hysterical. Dr. Weir Mitchell truthfully says (page 191), "The natural history of many of the forms of hysteria is still an open study. One reason for that is, I presume, the disgust with which the general practitioner encounters this malady. It is hysteria, and with that seems to end all need for observation of details and varieties of symptoms, such as more manageable disorders obtain." Another, and rather longer quotation, will give a better idea of the scope of these lectures, and the importance of their subject, than any words of ours :—" Perhaps no cases are more common in general practice, none more annoying, and none more dreaded, than those of hysteria in its infinite number of forms and its infinite variety of masquerade. The lighter troubles, the spasms, rigors, nervousness, and curious mental states, which haunt the times of sexual changes in a woman's life, and especially her passage into womanhood, are more or less easily dealt with. . . .. But, beside these every-day manifestations of hysteria, we meet in practice with a growing class of disorders in which change of social circumstances, love affairs, disappointments, and what the French call vies manquées, combine with physical accidents to create invalids, who unite neurasthenic states with a bewildering list of hysterical phenomena. These are the 'bed cases,' the broken-down and exhausted women, the pests of many households, who constitute the despair of physicians, and who furnish those annoying examples of despotic selfishness which wreck the constitution of nurses and devoted relatives, and, in unconscious or half-conscious self-indulgence, destroy the comfort of everyone about them. These are the cases of chronic hysterical invalidism which are so difficult to deal with. There must be in every country thousands of these unhappy people. They weary doctor after doctor, go hopelessly through the various cures, and at last end in therapeutic inactivity, or find a refuge in homœopathy, which promises a pill for every symptom, and leaves them at last where it found them."

This book is devoted to a careful analysis and classification of the different nervous symptoms which are met with in these people, and to a description of the mode of treatment—by rest, seclusion, massage, and electricity—which the author has found remarkably successful as a means of cure. The first two chapters deal with hysterical paralysis. We have heard a good deal lately in the daily papers about American nervousness. Judging from Dr. Weir Mitchell's experience, we should think the strange hysterical developments which are to be seen at the Salpêtrière must be commoner in America than in England. Doubtless differences of race and of habits affect the frequency of these phenomena in different countries. Although Dr. Mitchell seems to have seen plenty of hysterical anæsthesia and hysterical ischæmia, we notice that he has not observed the phenomena of transference by magnets. Then we have two chapters on mimicry of disease—occurrences not so unfamiliar to English medical men. Next, Dr. Mitchell narrates some cases of unusual forms of spasmodic affections in women, and then takes up the subject of tremor and chronic spasms. Two lectures on chorea follow. A curious fact which he brings out is that lines showing the greater or less prevalence of chorea, and the greater or less frequency of storms (rain, snow, or thunder), seem to rise and fall together. Dr. Mitchell is cautious in his inferences, and suggests possible explanations of this fact which prevent him from asserting that chorea is produced by atmospheric variations. There is one which, as he does not mention it, we may—viz., that fright is known to produce chorea, and that thunderstorms are often very alarming to children. In the remaining lectures, the author treats of nervous symptoms more commonly observed—

disorders of sleep, vaso-motor and respiratory disorders, hysterical aphonia, hysterical gastro-intestinal disorders, and, lastly, describes his new treatment.

So little is this class of cases understood, common though they are, that it is hardly going too far to describe Dr. Weir Mitchell's book as an attempt to introduce order into chaos. There has been too great a disposition, among those who try, by precision of statement and rigid verification of hypothesis, to raise medicine to the position of an exact science, to take trouble only with such conditions as, by the simplicity of their symptoms, and the presence of demonstrable ana- tomical lesions, give good prospect that patient labour may be rewarded with the discovery of some new fact. The vagaries of hysteria have been looked on by such as an in- soluble problem, a kind of maze, in which the pathologist might wander for any length of time, and only increase his bewilderment by trying to find the way out. Consequently, symptoms of this kind have too often made their patient the prey of quacks. Specialists of the bad kind which Dr. Russell Reynolds denounced the other day, have seen in hys- terical phenomena only reflex results of irritation of the par- ticular organ it was their business to treat. The only way to rescue the subjects of these diseases from such a fate is to get the symptoms, causes, and effects of hysteria put on a scientific basis. Dr. Weir Mitchell has here made a step towards doing this, for which we heartily thank him. His book should be studied by all who have to treat women, either from the point of view of the neurologist or that of any other specialist.

Notes on Midwifery. Specially designed to assist the Stu- dent in preparing for Examination. By J. J. REYNOLDS, M.R.C.S. Eng. London: J. and A. Churchill. 1881. Pp. 134.

IT has been our disagreeable duty to notice other books of this kind—works designed not to make men understand the subject, but to enable them to conceal from examiners their ignorance of it.

This one is avowedly a compilation from the works of Playfair, Leishman, and Braxton Hicks; and it is not a good one. We hope, for the credit of the examiners, that anyone who goes up to a midwifery examination only pre- pared by reading this book may be given the occasion of studying a better one. It cannot teach anyone to practise midwifery; and therefore we cannot recommend anyone to read it.

THE MOSCOW AND ST. PETERSBURG FOUNDLING HOS- PITAL.—According to the report recently published, there were admitted into the Moscow Hospital 12,719 infants in 1877, 13,612 in 1878, and 13,812 in 1879, with an increasing mortality of 22, 24, and 30 per cent. This increase is ex- plained by the augmented numbers of admissions having led to overcrowding, and by the impossibility of procuring a sufficient number of nurses, so that some of the infants have to be brought up by hand. As to the relative frequency of the causes of death, 22 per cent. died of broncho-pneu- monia, 1 per cent. of congenital atelectasis of the lung, 24 per cent. of acute intestinal catarrh and colitis, 10 per cent. of chronic intestinal catarrh, 6 9 per cent. of congenital syphilis, 15 per cent. of septicæmia and "dissolution" of the blood, and 4 per cent. of eclampsia. In the St. Peters- burg Hospital there were admitted 8860 infants during 1879, with a mortality of 14 per cent. Since 1874, when the mor- tality was 36 per cent., this has been constantly decreasing, the explanation of which is that of late years the infants have been sent into the country at a much earlier age than formerly. Most of them (80 per cent.) were sent away during the first month of their residence in the hospital. Here, as at Moscow, the majority of the infants (70 per cent.) had not reached their tenth day when they were ad- mitted. The relative proportion of causes of death is very similar to that of the Moscow Hospital. During the first week atelectasis of the lung is the predominant cause of death; while during the two following weeks catarrhal pneumonia, and especially acute intestinal catarrh, are the predominant diseases; from the fourth week pneumonia and intestinal catarrh form the chief contingent; but from the fifth month the latter becomes less frequent, pneumonia constituting the predominant disease during the rest of the first year.—*St. Petersb. Med. Woch.,* October 15.

ECONOMICS OF THE CALCUTTA HOSPITALS.
LETTER FROM SURGEON-GENERAL IRVING.

[To the Editor of the Medical Times and Gazette.]

SIR,—In your issue of February 14 you were good enough to insert a letter of mine on the Hospitals of Calcutta, in which I told you that the dietary had recently been considerably lowered, on the recommendation of a committee appointed by the present Lieutenant-Governor of Bengal, and com- posed entirely of officers, medical and civil, serving under his orders. I mentioned that in my annual report for the year 1878, alluding to the Campbell Native Hospital, I showed that for years past the general mortality had been at the rate of 25 per cent. on the admissions, and that I had expressed to Government a doubt whether the diet-rate recently fixed would be sufficient, considering the nature of many of the cases that come to this hospital—viz., cases greatly reduced by long-continued disease. I also stated to you that I had ventured to suggest whether a mortality so dreadful might not be reduced by the employment of a more liberal diet-rate than had yet been tried. Being at this time Surgeon-General to the Government of Bengal, I considered it my duty to make these observations, which were surely mild enough; but they made the Lieutenant-Governor very angry, and in a resolution which he wrote on the subject he pro- fessed to construe what I had said into a proposal for feed- ing the poor in the streets of Calcutta at the public expense! Sir A. Eden's words of wisdom are worth repeating :—" It is no doubt the case that there are many hundreds of persons in the streets of Calcutta whose health might be improved, and, indeed, from whom disease might be averted, by a 'liberal use of generous soups, milk stimulants, and other kinds of food,' and the Lieutenant-Governor knows of no town in the world of which the same might not be said; and he is not aware that any Government in the world has recognised it as a part of its business to raise taxes for the purpose of averting disease by a system of general public diets."

Since I addressed you the annual reports of the medical institutions of Calcutta for 1879 and 1880 have been printed, and during these years the most rigid economy as to diets and the expenditure on medicines has been the rule; and I was therefore anxious to compare the death-rate during those years with that of other years before the introduction of the new system, among the cases for which I had advocated " a liberal use of generous soups, milk," etc. Now, I am unable to separate all the cases admitted in states of great exhaustion, but I know that dysentery and diarrhœa fur- nish many such, and I have selected these two diseases, and compared the results of 1879 and 1880 with those of 1875, 1876, and 1877. The figures refer to native patients only, and in the Medical Native, Campbell, and Howrah Hospitals. During the three years there were 3640 admissions from dysentery, and 1425 deaths, or at the rate of 336·5 per 1000. During 1879-80 the admissions amounted to 2222, the deaths to 1076, and the rate was 485·5 per mille. The admissions on account of diarrhœa from 1875 to 1877 were 2505, the deaths 973, or 388·4 per thousand. In 1879-80 the admis- sions were 1968, the deaths 1087, or at the rate of 552·3 per mille.

Now, without making too much of the result of so short a period as two years, I submit that the experiment, so far as it has gone, and as affecting the two diseases, dysentery and diarrhœa, is not favourable; and, notwithstanding the sneers of the Lieutenant-Governor, I reiterate that it might be well to try the effect of a liberal diet, such as I suggested, in reducing the frightful mortality above indicated. Such a state of matters should not long be allowed to exist in this country, anywhere, or under any circumstances—or cost what it might to remedy it. I am fully aware that the report for 1880 alleges that the dietary is more than suffi- cient for all requirements; but against this I put the fact, of which I have reliable information, received from a non-medical friend, that patients in the Calcutta hospitals still get food sent to them from outside—which is certainly unusual in well-regulated establishments where ample provision is made for the sick. I am, &c.,

JAMES IRVING, Surgeon-General.

Edinburgh, November 30.

REFORMED SPELING!—REPLY TO CRITICISMS ON OMISION OF DUPLICATED CONSONANTS.

LETTER FROM DR. GEORGE HARLEY.

[To the Editor of the Medical Times and Gazette.]

SIR,—As there is a Silence of Contempt as wel as a Silence of Consent, if I do not reply to Mears. Kesteven and Millican's leters, some of your readers may perhaps be in doubt as to which category my Silence belongs. I send you a few words in answer to their courteously worded and no doubt kindly meant strictures on my proposed method of improving English Speling.

It is, however, with great reluctance that I take up my pen to do so, from being conscious that it is at best but a thankles task to criticise the criticism of self-constituted critics who have ventured to give opinions on a subject with which they are evidently so litle acquainted as the history of the orthography of their own language. For as I shal presently have to show, had they only posesed a trifling knowledge of Modern Comparative Philology they would not only have held other opinions, but also would have restrained themselves from exposing their limited acquaintance with the subject in print.

I wil refrain from expresing opinions on their individual remarks, and only bring forward some data in conection with the orthographical construction of the English language which wil enable them to see for themselves the false position they have unconsciously asumed.

I thought that I had said enough in my Prologue regarding the comon, though mistaken, idea that English words are spelt in obedience to etymological principles, to restrain persons with no more than a school-acquired knowledge of the subject from ventilating old and now utterly exploded opinions; but, as such apears not to have been the case, I reply to my critics' strictures by furnishing them with the folowing incontrovertible data, with which they apear to be wholy unacquainted.

Even in the palmiest days of old English (before the speling of its words became corrupted by ignorant and pedantic writers), the words taken, almost in their entirety, from other languages were not alowed to retain their original spelings. From the simple fact that the majority of the leters in the alphabet are transmutable, and were transmuted. "P's" became "d's," "v's" became "f's," "b's" became "t's," "t's" became "d's," "a" was replaced by "o," "o" was changed into "u," "k" transformed into "c," etc. So that, by this mere transmutation of leters, even the comonest words were not alowed to retain their original speling. Thus, "vater" is writen "father," "mutter" as "mother," "bruder" as "brother," "une" as "one," "deux" as "two," and so on. Even holy names that were adopted in their entirety had their speling completely changed. Thus, "Heilige Geist" became "Holy Ghost," and "Gott" had its two "t's" changed into one "d." In fact, neither rhyme nor reason had anything to do with the employment or disemployment of either single or duplicated consonants in any word whatever. Thus, while "bal" was changed into "ball," and "glas" into "glass," "mann" was transmuted into "man," "omelette" into "omelet," "pouding" into "pudding," "carotte" into "carrot," and so on. Where, then, are the philosophic grounds for objecting to my replacing the actualy unpronounceable duplicated "cc" by the phonetic pronounceable leter "x"?

Duplica*ted* "c's," mouth them as you will, never did, nor ever can, yield the sound they are intended to represent in words such as "accident" and "vaccination," which is that of the leter "x," and the leter "x" alone. And the first Roman who pened the duplicated "cc," with the intent of symbolising the sound of "x," did so, not out of the superabundance of his etymological knowledge, but, alas! poor felow, out of the profundity of his orthographical phonetic ignorance. And is to be pitied, rather than copied. Is it, then, realy incumbent upon us to go on to al time perpetuating the mistake out of a morbid sentimentality not to wound the susceptibilities of the poor dead Roman? I think, as we are told not to copy the vices but only the virtues of the dead, it would be equaly wisdom not to copy their eroneous, but only their corect orthographical symbolism.

Again, one of the critics naïvely informs me that by omiting duplicated consonants I destroy the clue to pronunciation. Surely this remark must be meant as a kind of joke. For the writer can scarcely be suposed to be ignorant that this is not a fact. I should think he has already lived long enough to have discovered—even by personal observation—that pronunciation is not alone a fluctuating quantity, but is never alike in two separate districts at the same time. Nay, more, he surely knows how to read aloud the folowing sentence:—"As he made a bow, he shot an arrow from his bow, which killed the sow, that was eating the corn he intended to sow!" If he fails to see the pith of this bit of pronunciation-speling dogrel, let him try for himself to discover in which of the leters in the folowing words lie the symbols of their pronunciation:—

Cough, pronounced, if I mistake not, as				Kof.
Plough	„	„	„	Plow.
Enough	„	„	„	Enuf.
Through	„	„	„	Threw.
Dough	„	„	„	Doe.

Moreover, can it be posible that he is unaware that every yokel knows that when he says that he is going to Sitcoster, Copersmith, and Kassalton, he is actually going to Cirencester, Cockburnspath, and Carshalton? If, then, even a yokel has no dificulty in understanding the name of a place spelt diferently from what it is pronounced, is it likely that an educated man wil be unable to pronounce words corectly when merely spelt without a duplicated leter, which it is imposible even for him to articulate with more than the sound of a single one? Let my critic tel me in what way the pronunciation of the folowing words is obscured by the omision of what I cal their redundant, and consequently totaly uncaled-for, duplicated consonants:—

Is wel-come more dificult to understand than welcome?				
„ wag-on	„	„	„	waggon?(a)
„ ful-fil	„	„	„	fulfill?
„ op-res	„	„	„	oppress?
„ sup-res	„	„	„	suppress?
„ co-mand	„	„	„	command?
„ co-ment	„	„	„	comment?
	etc. etc. etc.			

I think it is further necessary to cal my critics' atention to the fact that, in discusing the question of reforming our speling, they must not lose sight of the salient fact that orthography has but one great, primary object in view. Namely, to convey an idea through the instrumentality of the eye, which canot be conveyed through the instrumentality of the ear. The greatest number of ideas, then, that can be conveyed in the fewest number of words, and the shorter each individual word is (so long as it is inteligible), the beter it is for both the writer and the reader. Further, let me remind them that, even at its very best, English orthography is nothing beyond a general index to pronunciation, and, as seen in the few cited cases, frequently not even so much as that. Were our speling required to be a corect index to pronunciation it would be imperatively necessary to alter the present speling of nearly Every Word in the Language, and reconstruct it on a phonetic basis. Nay, more; as the pronunciation is diferent, and not only in some districts, but in many towns, from what it is in others, in order to be logical, we would require a modified system of orthography for each.

A litle reflection on these remarks wil, I think, show my critics the uter inaplicability of their objections to my proposed plan of omiting redundant duplicated consonants. And in conclusion, as I think it is a wise maxim for a man who presumes to teach, to condescend to learn, in case my knowledge of the orthographical construction of our own language is much more deficient than I imagine, and I have underated the knowledge of my oponents, I shal feel extremely obliged if my two critics wil turn to their Bibles (which I presume

(a) The orthographical history of this word is a capital comentary on the logic of my scheme of reforming our speling. For originaly it was spelt " wagon." Exactly according to its derivation. Then some ignorant pedant thrust an aditional " g " into it, and his equaly ignorant suxesors blindly perpetuated his eror at the expense of both time, trouble, and money. At length some one, either by axident or design, in obedience to the great law of linguistic evolution—which is simplification—restored the speling of the word to its original purity. By omiting from it the redundant and consequently totaly useles, duplicated consonant. Which had no right ever to have been thrust into it. And now we equaly blindly folow his example. But, fortunately, in this instance to our own convenience and advantage. In this lies the gist of my schema. For it is nothing more nor les than an ofshoot of natural linguistic evolution. The simplification of orthography.

they wil admit are writen and spelt in typical English), and furnish in your next number a list of the words spelt etymologicaly in the first chapter of Genesis. It may also be as wel for them, at the same time, to give their derivations, in case I and some other of your readers may be unable to discover them for ourselves.　I am, &c.,
25, Harley-street, W., December 3.　GEORGE HARLEY.

"AUDIPHONE."
LETTER FROM MR. J. DIXON.

[To the Editor of the Medical Times and Gazette.]

SIR,—Before it is too late, I would enter a protest against the admission of this barbarous word into our medical vocabulary. I see it already figures in the surgical instrument makers' advertisements. A Latin word (audio) and a Greek one are pieced together in a manner repugnant to all sound etymology; and yet the change of one letter would make the word legitimate.

The instrument is intended to increase the voice—not as regards the speaker, but as regards the hearer; and to the latter anything which makes a voice more audible becomes an *increaser* of that voice. Now, there is a real Greek adjective (αὐξίφωνος) which means *increasing the voice*, and *Auxiphone*, therefore, would be a perfectly well-formed and expressive word for the instrument.

December 1.　I am, &c.,　JAMES DIXON.

THE TESTIMONIAL TO PROFESSOR VIRCHOW.
LETTER FROM DR. J. S. BRISTOWE.

[To the Editor of the Medical Times and Gazette.]

SIR,—Permit me to acknowledge the receipt during the past week of the following contributions to the above fund :—Dr. Grainger Stewart, Edinburgh, £5; Dr. Philip Frank, Cannes, £2; Dr. Saundby, Birmingham, 10s. 6d. ; W. Bowman, Esq., London, £5 5s.　I am, &c.,　J. S. BRISTOWE.
11, Old Burlington-street, W., December 1.

THE LINACRE CHAIR OF HUMAN AND COMPARATIVE ANATOMY IN THE UNIVERSITY OF OXFORD.

[To the Editor of the Medical Times and Gazette.]

SIR,—In the printed Regulations of the University of Oxford we read, that "The subjects of the first examination are Human Anatomy and Physiology, Comparative Anatomy and Physiology to a certain extent." Other branches are included, but with these this chair has nothing to do. Allow me to ask, through your correspondence column, if it is true, first, that the recent vacancy in the Chair of Anatomy and Physiology in the University of Oxford has been filled up by the appointment of a gentleman who is not a medical man, and who knows little or nothing of human anatomy ? Second, whether the appointment has been hurried on so as to get a gentleman introduced who could not, even by his friends, be considered eligible for a chair in which the teaching of human anatomy held a prominent place?

It is believed, rightly or wrongly, by most Scotchmen that the claims of Dr. D. Y. Cunningham, the unsuccessful candidate, have been set aside because he is only a Scottish graduate, and we are naturally anxious to know whether professorships in science are practically shut against men who, whatever their claims, have no direct connexion with that ancient seat of learning. That Dr. Cunningham could have been passed by, and Mr. Moseley appointed to a chair of human and comparative anatomy, with such men as Sir William Jenner and Sir Erasmus Wilson on the list of patrons, appears perfectly inexplicable on any other supposition than that no outsider can be allowed to enter as a teacher the sacred precincts of an Oxford lecture-room. Is it possible that Church influence could have been brought to bear against a Presbyterian, seeing that the Archbishop of Canterbury is one of the patrons ? Mr. Moseley can teach well—perhaps none better—a class of students in some of the branches of zoology, but how he is to teach human anatomy and physiology puzzles some of us in Scotland. We are sorry for Mr. Moseley; his reputation is wide and deserved, and his friends have placed him in a very false position—one

in which that reputation must suffer, unless it be that the patrons intend that Oxford shall cease to be a medical school, and Mr. Moseley's class become one of zoology only.

If such be their intention it ought to have been made public, and intending candidates informed of the proposed change. But how can this be, when under the new statutes the Chair is more than ever one of Human Anatomy? The patrons may not trouble themselves to solve our difficulties ; but some of them occupy a position in scientific circles, which, if they value that position, demands that their conduct be explained. If ever an appointment to a university chair required explanation this does, and unless some satisfactory explanation is forthcoming, there is not a graduate of any Scottish university, perhaps not a medical man or student of medicine in Great Britain, who knows anything of the merits of the respective candidates, who will not believe that motives other than the good of the University have influenced the choice of the patrons.

Such an appointment could not have been made in Germany or France, and the sooner our mode of election to high scientific positions is changed the better. If not, our teaching power must soon fall low enough, seeing that good men are sent to teach what they cannot, and placed in a position where they have no opportunity of teaching what they really know.　I am, &c.,　M.D. EDIN.

[WE sympathise not a little with our correspondent, but he appears not to have known either that Oxford long since ceased to be a medical school ; or that the late Linacre Professor did not teach either human anatomy or human physiology. Hence "M.D.'s" surprise and disappointment at the way in which the Linacre Chair has been filled are keener much than ours. He believed in a living medical school, and fears that it is now doomed to cease to be ; we knew that the school was dead or sleeping, but we hoped that a new Linacre Professor might revive it. "M.D.," moreover, appears to regard the matter too entirely from a Scotch point of view.—ED. *Med. Times and Gas.*]

REPORTS OF SOCIETIES.

EPIDEMIOLOGICAL SOCIETY OF LONDON.
WEDNESDAY, NOVEMBER 2.

GEORGE BUCHANAN, M.D., President, in the Chair.

THE first meeting of the session was held at University College, Gower-street, on November 2, when the newly elected President, Dr. BUCHANAN, delivered the inaugural address on "Aids to Epidemiological Knowledge," of which an abstract has already appeared.

THE PROGRESS OF ZYMOTIC MICRO-PATHOLOGY.

Dr. G. C. HENDERSON then read a paper on the progress of zymotic micro-pathology. After alluding to the great importance which the question of the relation of micro-organisms to disease had recently assumed, the speaker enumerated the various affections in which their occurrence had been noticed. He then gave a brief summary of the researches of Pollender, Bravel, Davaine, Klebs, Sanderson, Cohn, Koch, Greenfield, Pasteur, and Toussaint, in anthrax or splenic fever, showing how gradually our knowledge of the life-history of the *Bacillus anthracis* was obtained. Special reference was made to the "protective inoculation" of modified virus as recommended by Pasteur and Toussaint in France, and by Sanderson and Greenfield in this country, as well as the criticisms on the method recently published by Koch. The process adopted by the latter for "pure cultivation," to prevent the unchecked mixture of the original bacillus, micrococcus, etc., stock with accidentally introduced aërial germs, was to grow them on media rendered semi-solid by gelatine instead of in liquids. Gaffky's experiments on the cultivation of aspergillus and other "moulds" by this method were referred to as tending to show that Grawitz's results on the development of "moulds" ordinarily harmless into toxic products were due to contamination of the fluids used. In septicæmia the researches of Billroth, Klebs, Rindfleisch, Cohn and Feltz, Davaine, Sanderson, Lister, and many others were enumerated, and the recent observations of Semmer and Krajewski on the protective inoculation of a modified virus in that group of affections were noticed. Bacilli, bacteria, and micrococci were also mentioned as the supposed causes of erysipelas, diphtheria, variola, vaccinia, enteric fever, malarial fevers, leprosy, scarlatina, and several other complaints; whilst the researches of Obermeier, Cartar, Heydenreich, and others on the occurrence and the connexion between relapsing fever and the spirillum in the blood were alluded to. In infectious pneumo-enteritis of pigs, fowl-cholera, and glanders, as well as other infectious diseases of animals, the presence of microphytes was referred to. In conclusion, the author of the paper expressed his opinion that the reasons for admitting the micro-organisms to be the causes of the diseases in anthrax, pneumo-enteritis, fowl-cholera, and some forms of septicæmia were as strong as those for holding the *Trichina spiralis* to be the cause of trichinosis. In the other affections, when the malady was communicable by inoculation from one person or animal to another, and the same organism was present in the blood or tissues of both, he was, while inclined to admit the organisms as causes of disease, obliged to look upon the case as not absolutely settled till cultivation and inoculation experiments had been made. The doubts raised by Koch, Œmler, and Loeffler as to the real conferring of immunity against the original malady by protective inoculation were next discussed, and the writer of the paper felt obliged to refrain from a full acceptance of Pasteur's results till the question of the non-recurrence of anthrax after one attack was definitely proved.

In the discussion which followed Dr. Henderson's paper, Sir Joseph Fayrer, Sir William Smart, Dr. Cobbold, Dr. Vandyke Carter, Mr. John Spear, and others took part.

ODONTOLOGICAL SOCIETY OF GREAT BRITAIN.

Monday, November 7.

Mr. THOMAS ARNOLD ROGERS, President, in the Chair.

Specimens were exhibited, and casual communications read, by Messrs. S. J. Hutchinson, J. R. Mummery, Charles Tomes, and Lawrence Read.

ON THE ORIGIN OF DENTAL CARIES, CONSTITUTIONAL AND LOCAL.

Dr. B. W. RICHARDSON, F.R.S., read the paper of the evening, on the Origin of Dental Caries, constitutional and local. The present widespread prevalence of caries was, he said, a matter of more than mere professional—it was of national importance. For some years past he had noted on his clinical records the condition of the teeth of the patients who came before him, and the result of these inquiries had astonished him not a little. He found that of over 4000 persons of both sexes, and of all ages, over 80 per cent. were affected more or less severely with dental caries, whilst it was rare to meet with a person in whom both sets of teeth were altogether free from the disease. He believed also that it was now more prevalent among the young than it was twenty-two years ago, when he first commenced medical practice. For such a general development of disease general causes must be looked for, and there were two such which he believed to be of chief importance, viz., hereditary syphilis and dyspepsia. With regard to the first, he quoted the statements of Professor Gross and Dr. Holland respecting the proportion of the adult population in the United States and in Great Britain respectively who acquired the primary disease, estimated in each case at about one in eight. Contracted in adult life, syphilis did not materially affect the teeth, but the hereditary constitution left by it was undoubtedly indicated in the next generation by disease of the teeth and by a constitutional condition in which caries was readily developed. It was hard to say whether dyspepsia should be placed before or after syphilis in point of importance. The form of the disease which produced the greatest amount of evil was that which was induced in the first months of life by improper feeding. In children who were deprived of their natural food, the tissues generally were imperfectly constructed; and although, in the case of tissues which were constantly undergoing reconstruction, some of this harm might be redeemed, in the case of such structures as the teeth, made for the whole of life in a few short months, perfection was impossible if the start was bad. Dr. Richardson did not think that the strumous or tuberculous diatheses caused of themselves any marked tendency to caries; nor did he find that the epidemic diseases of children had any such effect. Passing on to speak of local causes, he mentioned four—viz., the action of heated fluids taken into the mouth, the action of acids upon the teeth, deficient cleanliness of the teeth, and exposure of the teeth to the action of certain chemical substances during work at some special occupations. He believed, however, that these causes were comparatively of slight importance; that caries was rarely of purely local origin, though when there was a low state of nutrition within the tooth, very slight external causes, acting physically or chemically, would produce rapid results. In conclusion, he urged upon the dental profession the importance of impressing upon all with whom they came in contact the necessity of leading a more natural life if they wished to exorcise the terrible disease which was demoralising civilised humanity, and of assisting to promulgate the natural law that it was the duty of every mother, of whatever rank, to nurse her child, and gradually to lead its vital steps into healthy independent existence.

A prolonged discussion followed.

NEW INVENTIONS AND IMPROVEMENTS.

A VACCINATION SHIELD.

THE Vaccination Shield, of which the annexed is an illustration, was devised by Dr. John C. Hogan some months ago (when the small-pox epidemic in London was causing considerable uneasiness,) to obviate the pain and inconvenience attended on the rubbing or adhesion of the sleeve to the vaccinated part. This it satisfactorily accomplishes; and moreover, as, from its construction, no pressure is made either above or below the part operated on, no hindrance to the free circulation of the blood occurs, an advantage which he thinks will recommend it for use in cases of vaccination or adult revaccination. It is made in various sizes by Messrs. Arnold and Sons, West Smithfield, E.C.

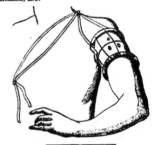

ŒTTLI'S SWISS MILK FOOD.

WE have received from Messrs. Lehmann and Co., 106, Fenchurch-street, E.C., samples of Œttli's Swiss Milk Food, one of the latest additions to our foods for infants and children. We have taken opportunities of having its value tested in the best possible way—i.e., practically,—and find that it is taken very readily, and to good purpose, by both infants and children. The food is prepared from condensed pure milk from cows pastured on the Swiss mountains, and from, we imagine, malted wheat; or, at any rate, wheat that has been so treated that the starchy matter is converted into a substance easily digestible in the infant's stomach; and the food is made sufficiently sweet to render any further addition of sugar unnecessary. The directions for use are simple, and the food can be prepared quickly and with very little trouble. For an infant three months old a tablespoonful is carefully mixed with twelve or fourteen tablespoonfuls of water, and then boiled for eight or ten minutes. For a child of six months or more the same quantity is mixed with rather less water, and boiled for five or six minutes. It is very palatable, and is likely to come largely into use.

MEDICAL NEWS.

ROYAL COLLEGE OF SURGEONS OF ENGLAND.—The following Members of the College, having undergone the necessary examinations for the Fellowship at the half-yearly meetings of the Court of Examiners, terminating on the 28th ult., were reported to have acquitted themselves to the satisfaction of the Court, and at a meeting of the Council yesterday, the 8th inst., were admitted Fellows of the College, viz. :—

Barling, Harry Gilbert, M.B. Lond., Newnham, Gloucestershire, diploma of Membership dated July 25, 1879, student of St. Bartholomew's Hospital.
Gill, Richard, M.B. Lond., Prince-street, Hanover-square (not a member of the College), of St. Bartholomew's Hospital.
Griffith, Walter Spencer Anderson, Guilford-street, W.C., April 16, 1878, of St. Bartholomew's Hospital.
Leahy, William Denis, L.S.A., Warwick-street, S.W., November 11, 1878, of the Charing-cross Hospital.
Lockwood, Charles Barrett, L.S.A., Serjeant's-inn, April 17, 1878, of St. St. Bartholomew's Hospital.
Shattock, Samuel George, L.S.A., Downshire-hill, Hampstead, January 25, 1878, of University College Hospital.
Uhthoff, John Caldwell, M.D. Lond., Hove, Brighton, July 25, 1877, of Guy's Hospital.

And one candidate who had not attained the legal age, but to whom the diploma will be presented on reaching the age of twenty-five. Seventeen candidates out of the twenty-five examined having failed to acquit themselves to the satisfaction of the Court of Examiners, were referred to their professional studies for twelve months.

At the same meeting of the Council, Mr. Richard Cross, M.D. St. And., of Scarborough, was elected a Fellow of the College, his diploma of membership bearing date November 13, 1840; and Mr. Edward Haddock, L.S.A., of Biddulph, Congleton, elected a Fellow at a previous meeting of the Council, was admitted as such, his diploma of membership bearing date October 21, 1842.

Mr. Henry Power, M.B. Lond., F.R.C.S., was elected a member of the Board of Examiners in Anatomy and Physiology; and the following gentlemen were re-elected members of the Board :—Messrs. W. M. Baker, E. Bellamy, J. Langton, B. T. Lowne, J. McCarthy, T. Pickering Pick, W. Rivington, and G. F. Yeo.

APOTHECARIES' HALL, LONDON.—The following gentlemen passed their examination in the Science and Practice of Medicine, and received certificates to practise, on Thursday, December 1 :—

Day, John Roberson, 121, Camden-road, N.W.
Phillips, Frank Leslie, National Hospital, Ventnor.
Stuart, Ernest Offord, Nightingale Vale, Woolwich.

The following gentleman also on the same day passed the Primary Professional Examination :—

Parakh, Nasarwanji N., Grant Medical College, Bombay.

NAVAL, MILITARY, ETC., APPOINTMENTS.

BENGAL MEDICAL ESTABLISHMENT.—To be Surgeons-Major : Olliver Thos. Duke, Francis Cobham Nicholson, Thos. Holbein Hendley, William Henry Gregg, Albert Baird Seaman, Frederick Augustus Smyth, Herbert Boyd, John Lloyd, M.D., William Michael Courtney, Edward Butler Ruttledge, Thomas Robinson, Daniel Nicholas Martin, M.D., Alexander Bannerman Strahan, William Alexander Crauford Roe, Charles John Walford Meadows, William Napier Keefer, Andrew Deane, William Flood Murray.
MADRAS MEDICAL ESTABLISHMENT.—To be Deputy Surgeons-General : Brigade-Surgeon Michael Cudmore Furnell, M.D., Brigade-Surgeon William Henry Bean, M.D., Brigade-Surgeon William Pearl. Surgeons to be Surgeons-Major : David Sinclair, John North, Edward Fawcett, William Joseph Hastings, M.D., Thomas Charles Howell Spencer, Henry George Hall.

BOMBAY MEDICAL ESTABLISHMENT.—Surgeons to be Surgeons-Major : William Coleridge Kiernander, Selim Myer Salaman, M.D., Frederick Charles Barker, M.D., Randolph Caldecott, George Waters, Patrick Murphy, M.D., William McConaghy, M.D., Arthur Hy. Hughes, M.D.
MILITIA MEDICAL DEPARTMENT.—Surgeon-Major David Simpson Penrice, 3rd Battalion the Norfolk Regiment, resigns his commission, also is permitted to retain his rank, and to wear the prescribed uniform on his retirement.

BIRTHS.

BUCKLE.—On November 29, the wife of John Buckle, M.R.C.S., of Great Bardfield, of a son.
DENNISTON.—On November 1, at Dunoon, Argyllshire, the wife of J. Denniston, M.D., of a son.
GEOGHEGAN.—On October 20, at Pietermaritzburg, Natal, the wife of Surgeon-Major Geoghegan, of a daughter, who survived her birth only a few hours.
LOWE.—On November 27, at Stapenhill, Burton-on-Trent, the wife of Henry Charles Lowe, M.R.C.S., of a daughter.
PRESTON.—On November 4, at 148, Union-street, Plymouth, the wife of Theodore J. Preston, L.R.C.P., M.R.C.S., Royal Naval Hospital, Plymouth, of a daughter.
REYNOLDS.—On December 5, at Stamford-hill, N., the wife of W. Percy Reynolds, L.R.C.P., M.R.C.S., of a daughter.
WALSH.—On November 25, at Jersey, the wife of Thomas Walsh, Surgeon-Major A.M.D., of a daughter.

MARRIAGES.

BURCHELL—BUTT.—On December 1, at Stoke Newington, James Lodwick, eldest son of P. L. Burchell, M.B., F.R.C.S., of Kingsland-road, E., to Annie Eliza, only daughter of Charles Butt, Esq., of Amhurst-road, Stoke Newington, N.
HARMER—EDEN.—On December 6, at Wandsworth, Robert Harmer, M.D., of Court Lodge, Richmond, Surrey, to Jane Ann, eldest daughter of James Eden, Esq.
KANE—CARDEW.—On December 1, at Bath, John Seymour Kane, B.A., M.D., of Almondsbury, Gloucestershire, to Emma, eldest daughter of G. S. Cardew, M.D., of Marlborough-buildings, Bath, Inspector-General of Hospitals, H.M. Indian Army, retired.
MARGETSON—SPARKS.—On December 3, at Notting-hill, Parker Margetson, M.R.C.S., L.S.A., of Barnes, Surrey, to Agnes Helen, third daughter of the late Lieut.-Col. T. P. Sparks, Madras Staff Corps.
YOUNG—PROCKTER.—On November 15, at Penzance, Charles, son of Edward Young, M.D., Hounslow (late Salisbury), to Laura, third daughter of the late John Prockter, Esq., of Penzance.

DEATHS.

FINCH, ROBERT, M.D., at Stainton Lodge, Blackheath, on November 28, aged 58.
GREEN, THOMAS, M.R.C.S., L.S.A., Medical Superintendent of the Borough Asylum, Winson Green, of Birmingham, on November 29, aged 81.
JUNOD, VICTOR THEODORE, M.D., of Bonvillar, Switzerland, at 46, Omaburgh-street, Regent's-park, on November 26, in his 77th year.
MARTIN, ALFRED HENRY, M.B.T.C.D., of the Colonial Medical Service, at Port of Spain, Trinidad, on October 29, aged 33.
STRIDE, EDWARD, M.R.C.S., L.S.A., at 72, High-street, Sheerness-on-Sea, on December 3, aged 58.
STEELE, ELMES YELVERTON, M.R.C.S., L.S.A., at Abergavenny, on November 27, aged 69.

VACANCIES.

BECKETT HOSPITAL AND DISPENSARY, BARNSLEY.—House-Surgeon. Candidates must hold a diploma from one of the recognised Universities of the United Kingdom, or from one of the Royal Colleges of Surgeons, and must be a Licentiate of the Apothecaries' Company, London, and be unmarried, and, if elected, must agree not to engage in private for a period of three years. Applications, with testimonials, to be sent to the Honorary Secretary, on or before December 10.
CHORLTON-UPON-MEDLOCK DISPENSARY, MANCHESTER.—Honorary Surgeon. (For particulars see Advertisement.)
LINCOLN GENERAL DISPENSARY.—Resident Medical Officer. Candidates must be M.R.C.S. England, and either licentiates of the Society of Apothecaries, London, or licentiates of the Royal College of Physicians, London, duly registered, and unmarried. Applications, with testimonials, to be sent to William Dean, Secretary, on or before December 14.
METROPOLITAN FREE HOSPITAL, 81, COMMERCIAL-STREET, SPITALFIELDS, E.—Assistant House-Surgeon. Candidates must be qualified. Further information may be obtained on application to George Croxton, Secretary.
MONMOUTH UNION.—Medical Officer. (For particulars see Advertisement.)
NORWICH FRIENDLY SOCIETIES' MEDICAL INSTITUTE.—Assistant-Surgeon. Candidates must be duly qualified, and not above thirty years of age. Recent testimonials to be sent to W. C. Brundell, Messrs. Dawson Bros., Pitt-street, Norwich.
SHEFFIELD GENERAL INFIRMARY.—House-Surgeon. (For particulars see Advertisement.)
VICTORIA HOSPITAL FOR CHILDREN, QUEEN'S-ROAD, CHELSEA, S.W.—Assistant-Physician. Candidates must be graduates in medicine of a University recognised by the Medical Council, and not practising pharmacy. Applications, with copies of testimonials, to be sent to the Secretary, at the Hospital, on or before December 12.
VICTORIA HOSPITAL FOR CHILDREN, QUEEN'S-ROAD, CHELSEA, S.W.—House-Surgeon. Candidates must be Fellows or members of the Royal College of Surgeons of England, and licentiates of the Apothecaries, or of the Royal College of Physicians, or graduates in Medicine of any University recognised by the Medical Council. Applications, with copies of testimonials, to be sent to the Secretary, at the Hospital, on or before December 12.

UNION AND PAROCHIAL MEDICAL SERVICE.

*** The area of each district is stated in acres. The population is computed according to the census of 1871.

RESIGNATIONS.

Petersfield Union.—Mr. Edward Noott has resigned the First District: area 18,857; population 2559; salary £67 10s. per annum.

Risbridge Union.—Mr. John Francis Vincent Bent has resigned the Second District: area 11,130; population 3868; salary £56 per annum.

Uxbridge Union.—Dr. C. J. Carr has resigned the West Drayton District: area 810; population 2626; salary £20 per annum.

APPOINTMENTS.

Blything Union.—Charles E. Lay, L.R.C.P. Edin., L.R.C.S. Edin., to the Third District.

Cannock Union.—John C. Blackford, M.R.C.S. Eng., L.S.A. Lond., to the Cannock District. John A. Masters, L.R.C.P. Lond., M.R.C.S. Eng., to the Hednesford District.

Easthampstead Union.—Charles J. Denny, M.R.C.S. Eng., L.K.&Q.C.P. Ire., to the Sandhurst District.

Nottingham Union.—John W. Inger, L.R.C.P., M.R.C.S., L.S.A., to the Fourth District.

Warminster Union.—Frederick J. Flower, M.R.C.S. Eng., L.S.A., to the Workhouse.

Professor Flower, LL.D., F.R.S., F.R.C.S., has just been appointed by the President and Council of the Royal Society a Trustee of Sir John Soane's Museum, in the vacancy occasioned by the decease of Sir Philip de Malpas Grey Egerton, Bart., M.P.

Smith's "Visiting List" for 1882.—We have received this long-known and well-tried medical practitioners' friend and help for the coming year. As it has now reached the thirty-sixth year of publication, we need not say more of it than that it will be found the same trustworthy, complete, convenient, and useful companion as in former years.

APPOINTMENTS FOR THE WEEK.

December 10. *Saturday (this day).*

Operations at St. Bartholomew's, 1½ p.m.; King's College, 1½ p.m.; Royal Free, 2 p.m.; Royal London Ophthalmic, 11 a.m.; Royal Westminster Ophthalmic, 1½ p.m.; St. Thomas's, 1½ p.m.; London, 2 p.m.

12. *Monday.*

Operations at the Metropolitan Free, 2 p.m.; St. Mark's Hospital for Diseases of the Rectum, 2 p.m.; Royal London Ophthalmic, 11 a.m.; Royal Westminster Ophthalmic, 1½ p.m.

Medical Society of London, 8½ p.m. Dr. Hilton Fagge will open a discussion on the Salicylate Treatment of Acute Rheumatism, when numerous Hospital Statistics will be laid before the Society by the President (Dr. Broadbent), Dr. Coupland, Dr. De Havilland Hall, Dr. Charles Hood, Dr. Isambard Owen, Dr. Warner, and Dr. Gilbert Smith.

13. *Tuesday.*

Operations at Guy's, 1½ p.m.; Westminster, 2 p.m.; Royal London Ophthalmic, 11 a.m.; Royal Westminster Ophthalmic, 1½ p.m.; West London, 3 p.m.

Anthropological Institute, 8 p.m. The Discussion on the Rev. R. H. Codrington's paper "On the Melanesian, Malay, and Polynesian Languages" will be resumed. Mr. M. J. Walhouse, "On some Vestiges of Girl-Sacrifices, Jar-Burial, and Contracted Interments in India and the East." Mr. G. Bertin, "On the Origin and Primitive Home of the Semites."

Royal Medical and Chirurgical Society (Ballot, 8 p.m.), 8½ p.m. Mr. Reginald Harrison (of Liverpool), "On a Case of Lithotomy where a Tumour of the Prostate was successfully Enucleated; with Remarks on the Removal of such Growths." Mr. Berkeley Hill, "On a Case of Fibrous Polypus of the Bladder successfully Removed."

14. *Wednesday.*

Operations at University College, 2 p.m.; St. Mary's, 1¼ p.m.; Middlesex, 1 p.m.; London, 2 p.m.; St. Bartholomew's, 1½ p.m.; Great Northern, 2 p.m.; Samaritan, 2½ p.m.; Royal London Ophthalmic, 11 a.m.; Royal Westminster Ophthalmic, 1½ p.m.; St. Thomas's, 1½ p.m.; St. Peter's Hospital for Stone, 2 p.m.; National Orthopædic, Great Portland-street, 10 a.m.

Royal Microscopical Society, 8 p.m. Mr. A. D. Michael, "Further Observations on British Oribatidæ." Mr. W. H. Symons, "On a Hot and Cold Stage for the Microscope."

15. *Thursday.*

Operations at St. George's, 1 p.m.; Central London Ophthalmic, 1 p.m.; Royal Orthopædic, 2 p.m.; University College, 2 p.m.; Royal London Ophthalmic, 11 a.m.; Royal Westminster Ophthalmic, 1½ p.m.; Hospital for Diseases of the Throat, 2 p.m.; Hospital for Women, 2 p.m. Charing-cross, 2 p.m.; London, 2 p.m.; North-West London, 2½ p.m.

Harveian Society, 8½ p.m. Dr. Alfred Meadows, "On Menstruation and its Derangements." (Third Harveian Lecture.)

16. *Friday.*

Operations at Central London Ophthalmic, 2 p.m.; Royal London Ophthalmic, 11 a.m.; South London Ophthalmic, 2 p.m.; Royal Westminster Ophthalmic, 1½ p.m.; St. George's (ophthalmic operations), 1¼ p.m.; Guy's, 1½ p.m.; St. Thomas's (ophthalmic operations), 2 p.m.; King's College (by Mr. Lister), 2 p.m.

VITAL STATISTICS OF LONDON.

Week ending Saturday, December 3, 1881.

BIRTHS.

Births of Boys, 1280; Girls, 1228; Total, 2508.
Corrected weekly average in the 10 years 1871-80, 2578·8.

DEATHS.

	Males.	Females.	Total.
Deaths during the week	734	726	1460
Weekly average of the ten years 1871-80, corrected to increased population ...	891·5	905·4	1796·9
Deaths of people aged 80 and upwards ...	...	...	47

DEATHS IN SUB-DISTRICTS FROM EPIDEMICS.

	Enumerated Population, 1881 (unrevised).	Small-pox.	Measles.	Scarlet Fever.	Diphtheria.	Whooping-cough.	Typhus.	Enteric (or Typhoid) Fever.	Simple continued Fever.	Diarrhœa.
West	668993	...	8	6	1	8	1	3	...	3
North ...	905677	3	5	16	10	7	...	12	...	3
Central ...	281793	...	4	5	2	7	...	2	...	...
East	692530	5	4	9	5	24	...	5	1	1
South	1265578	20	24	14	3	16	...	10	1	8
Total	3814571	28	45	50	21	62	1	32	2	15

METEOROLOGY.

From Observations at the Greenwich Observatory.

Mean height of barometer	29·696 in.
Mean temperature	44·6°
Highest point of thermometer	58·5°
Lowest point of thermometer	35·5°
Mean dew-point temperature	40·5°
General direction of wind	S.W. & S.S.E.
Whole amount of rain in the week	0·80 in.

BIRTHS and DEATHS Registered and METEOROLOGY during the Week ending Saturday, Dec. 3, in the following large Towns:—

Cities and boroughs (Municipal boundaries except for London.)	Estimated Population to middle of the year 1881.*	Persons to an Acre. (1881.)	Births Registered during the week ending Dec. 3.	Deaths Registered during the week ending Dec. 3.	Temperature of Air (Fahr.) Highest during the Week.	Temperature of Air (Fahr.) Lowest during the Week.	Temperature of Air (Fahr.) Weekly Mean of Daily Mean Values	Temp. of Air (Cent.) Weekly Mean of Daily Mean Values.	Rain Fall. In Inches.	Rain Fall. In Centimetres.
London	3829751	50·8	2508	1460	55·0	35·5	44·6	7·01	0·80	2·03
Brighton	107934	45·9	64	45	55·7	36·4	44·7	7·06	0·84	2·13
Portsmouth ...	128335	28·6	83	41	...	...	...	...	...	...
Norwich	88038	11·8	57	34	...	...	...	...	...	...
Plymouth	75262	54·0	46	28	56·7	34·0	47·3	8·50	1·44	3·66
Bristol	207140	46·5	144	74	55·0	38·2	45·8	7·67	1·32	3·35
Wolverhampton ...	75934	22·4	42	22	53·7	33·3	42·5	5·84	0·60	1·52
Birmingham ...	402296	47·9	260	135	...	...	...	...	...	...
Leicester	123120	38·5	88	46	54·5	33·8	44·4	6·89	0·55	1·40
Nottingham ...	188035	18·9	127	82	56·2	32·4	44·2	6·78	0·73	1·85
Liverpool	553988	106·3	431	262	52·8	37·7	45·8	7·67	0·71	1·80
Manchester ...	341269	79·5	229	176	...	...	...	...	...	...
Salford	177760	34·4	120	72	...	...	...	...	...	...
Oldham	112176	24·0	80	40	...	...	...	...	...	...
Bradford	184037	25·5	118	64	55·0	38·0	45·1	7·28	1·41	3·58
Leeds	310490	14·4	231	129	57·0	38·0	45·2	7·33	1·93	4·90
Sheffield	285621	14·5	173	106	51·0	34·5	43·9	6·61	0·89	2·26
Hull	155161	42·7	112	79	51·0	34·0	42·2	5·67	0·33	0·84
Sunderland ...	116753	42·2	78	55	56·0	36·0	45·7	7·61	0·78	1·98
Newcastle-on-Tyne	145675	27·1	115	55	...	...	...	...	...	...
Total of 20 large English Towns ...	7608775	38·0	5106	3005	57·0	32·3	44·7	7·06	0·95	2·41

* These figures are the numbers enumerated (but subject to revision) in April last, raised to the middle of 1881 by the addition of a quarter of a year's increase, calculated at the rate that prevailed between 1871 and 1881.

At the Royal Observatory, Greenwich, the mean reading of the barometer last week was 29·70 in. The lowest reading was 28·71 in. on Sunday morning, and the highest 30·10 in. on Friday morning.

NOTES, QUERIES, AND REPLIES:

Ye that questioneth much shall learn much.—Bacon.

Enquirer, Bolton.—You will find information as to "Surgeoncies in Emigration Agencies" in Dr. E. Diver's little work entitled, "The Young Doctor's Future; or, What shall be my Practice ?" lately published by Smith, Elder, and Co., Waterloo-place, London.

A Member.—The number of rejections at the recent pass examination for the Fellowship of the College of Surgeons was unusually high. On referring to the Calendar we find that at the corresponding period last year the number of candidates was exactly the same, viz., twenty-five, and the rejections only twelve, against seventeen this year.

Dairy Husbandry.—The Royal Agricultural Society has appointed a standing Dairy Committee to watch dairy husbandry.

A Graceful Recognition.—Dr. W. A. Guy, F.R.S., one of the earliest friends of the Hospital for Consumption, Brompton, has presented to that institution a portrait of the Honorary Secretary, Sir Philip Rose, Bart., to whose benevolence and energy the foundation of the charity, in 1841, is due.

A Competitor.—Essays for the Jacksonian Prize of the Royal College of Surgeons must be delivered at the College on or before Saturday, the 31st inst. The subject for this prize for the ensuing year has already been announced as "Wounds and other Injuries of Nerves: their Symptoms, Pathology, and Treatment."

Staff Surgeon.—Sir Gilbert Blane, the founder of the medal bearing his name, was the first baronet. The title has descended to Major Sir Seymour John Blane.

J. A. J., Wandsworth.—The duty of providing hospitals for infectious diseases is divided at present between the Metropolitan Asylums Board and the vestries as the sanitary authorities—the former for paupers; the latter for persons other than paupers, who must be removed from their homes for treatment on public protective grounds.

Felix.—1. First in 1876. 2. The Melbourne University admits ladies as students, excepting the classes for medicine.

A Metropolitan Teacher.—A special notice will be sent by the Secretary of the College of Surgeons in a day or two to the Deans or Secretaries of all medical schools in the provinces as well as in the metropolis, that in future candidates for the professional examinations of the College will be required to give not less than a fortnight's instead of ten days' notice, as heretofore, of their intention to present themselves for examination; and in future all candidates will be required to undergo an examination in midwifery and medicine unless holding a recognised medical degree or licence which includes midwifery.

Poor-Law Guardian.—We believe there is no absolute rule requiring the medical officers of Her Majesty's prisons to vaccinate all children born in the prisons before they are allowed to go out.. As a general rule, a child is vaccinated in prison when it is old enough, and the mother makes no objection. It has been stated that there could be no regulation on the subject, because it is uncertain at what age a child may be at the time its mother is discharged.

The Anti-Vaccination Association.—It is somewhat of a scandal if no steps can be taken to check the action of this body towards encouraging defiance of the law.

Veræ.—The water sources of the valley of the Thames are drawn upon by the water companies for upwards of 130,000,000 gallons per diem. The original sources—the wells and springs over the City area, and the brooks that fed the Thames within the limits of the suburbs—have been for the most part abandoned on account of contamination by the percolation of sewage.

Sloley.—Read "The Ocean as a Health Resort: a Handbook for the use of Tourists and Invalids," by W. J. Wilson, L.R.C.P., published by Messrs. Churchill. The author describes the climate and weather usually experienced during a passage to and from Australia, and gives some useful hints as to the management of the health.

A Farmer fined for Adulteration.—A farmer residing near Whitchurch, Manchester, has been fined £30 and costs, or two months' imprisonment, for selling milk impoverished by the addition of 30 per cent. of water. The milk had been supplied to the Royal Infirmary, Manchester.

Barbarism Superseded.—The story runs, that the United States Government applied to the German Government for information as to the extent to which patent medicines were sold in Germany, and the number of them; and the reply was, that patent medicines had now no existence in that country, as it was civilised!

"Official Pressure."—In consequence of pressure put on the Town Council by the Local Government Board, an influential and numerously attended meeting has been held at Margate on the drainage question. The Mayor presided. The Medical Officer of Health and the Registrar of Deaths stated that the town had been exceptionally healthy for many years, the death-rate being only a fraction over 14 per thousand. It was, however, admitted that in the low-lying districts the drainage should be improved. Ultimately the meeting was adjourned.

Bad Eyesight: Germany.—"J. B." writes :—*A propos* of the letter in your last week's journal as to wearing gold rings in the ears with a view of the habit being beneficial to eyesight, and to the alleged prevalence of the practice in Germany, where "boys have their ears bored for rings when very young." I send you the results of a long series of careful experiments carried out by a Saxon oculist with some six hundred scholars of the Royal School at Chemnitz, for the purpose of determining the proportion of normal eyesight to near-sightedness, which show that in the sixth or lowest class 90 per cent. of the scholars possessed normal sight; in the fifth, 88 per cent.; in the fourth, 80 per cent.; in the lower third, 75 per cent.; in the upper third, 85 per cent.; in the lower second, 56 per cent.; in the upper second and upper first also, 56 per cent.; and in the lower first, actually only 36 per cent. of the scholars were not near-sighted. The continuous and rapid increase of short-sightedness from the lower to the upper classes is highly suggestive. Of all the scholars in this school, over 28 per cent. were near-sighted and 1 per cent. far-sighted."

Economist.—The income of |Bethlem and Bridewell Hospitals amounts to about £83,000 per annum, mostly the accumulations of private benevolence.

Cholera in India.—An official return of the deaths from Cholera in the Bombay Presidency since of January 1 last, shows that the total number of fatal seizures was 14,922 out of 30,986 cases. According to the *Bombay Gazette*, the disease had early in the past month entirely disappeared throughout the Presidency.

The Antiquity of Food Adulteration.—Upwards of two hundred years ago a cynical poet, Cornelius May, wrote thus on the "The Knavery of the World" :—

> "Thy baker and thy brewer
> Do wrong thee night and morn,
> And thy miller he doth grind thee
> In the grinding of thy corn.
> Thy goldsmith and thy jeweller
> dire leagued in knavish sort,
> And the ell-board of thy tailor
> It is an inch too short."

Laws against adulteration date back to the time of Edward the Confessor, if not earlier, and it is remarkable that in many cases the same ingredients of adulteration appear to have been in use for centuries.

Successful Sewage Farming.—In his official report, Mr. Campbell, inspecting officer, calls the attention of local authorities in general to the sewage farm at Forfar as " a great sanitary benefit, combined with a commercial success." The system known as "intermittent downward filtration" appears to have been adopted.

COMMUNICATIONS have been received from—

Mr. S. H. Sayersan, Lynn; The Registrar of the Apothecaries' Hall, London; Dr. Ward Cousins, Southsea; Dr. Bristown, London; Dr. Stirling, Edinburgh; Dr. James Dixon, Dorking; Dr. Hehran, London; Mr. R. Whyte Wallis, London; Dr. MacCormack, Belfast; Dr. John R. Wolfe, Glasgow; Dr. W. R. Smith, Cheltenham; The Secretaries of the Harveian Society of London; Dr. James Irvine, Edinburgh; Dr. Sutherland, Whitehall; Dr. Norman Chevers, London; Dr. J. W. Moore, Dublin; Messrs. E. Chapman and Co., London; Dr. E. J. Moses, Bordeaux; The Honorary Secretary of the Royal Microscopical Society of London; Dr. Alexander, Liverpool; Mr. J. Chatto, London; The Honorary Secretary of the Medical Society of London; The Registrar-General, Scotland; Dr. Charles Glacier, Bolton; The Secretary of the Royal Institution of Great Britain, London; The Secretary of the Anthropological Institute of Great Britain and Ireland, London; The President of the Brighton Health Congress; Dr. R. H. Semple, London; The Honorary Secretary of the Royal Medical and Chirurgical Society of London.

BOOKS, ETC., RECEIVED:—

The Use of the Ambulance in Civil Practice, by Reginald Harrison, F.R.C.S.—Über den Werth der Infusion Alcoholischer Kochsalzlösung, etc.—Visible Muscular Conditions as Expressive of States of the Brain and Nerve Centres, by Francis Warner, M.D., M.R.C.P.—Report on the Sanitary Condition of the Whitechapel District for the Quarter ended October 1, 1881.—Reports on the Royal Lunatic Asylum of Montrose for 1881—Medical Reports of the China Imperial Maritime Customs—How to Use the Bromides, by G. M. Beard, A.M., M.D.—Naval Hygiene, by John D. Macdonald, M.D., F.R.S.—Transactions of the Clinical Society of London—Caso di Tumore Tubercolare della Midolla Allungata, pel Prof. Francesco Orsi—Handbuch der Allgemeinen Therapie, von Prof. H. Von Ziemssen—Health Lectures for the People : The Human Body, by D. J. Cunningham, M.D., F.R.S.E.—Health Lectures for the People : Some Lessons from Modern Medicine, by Dr. James A. Russell—Sessional Proceedings of the National Association for the Promotion of Social Science—Notes on Books, by Messrs. Longmans and Co.

PERIODICALS AND NEWSPAPERS RECEIVED:—

Lancet—British Medical Journal—Medical Press and Circular—Berliner Klinische Wochenschrift—Centralblatt für Chirurgie—Gazette des Hopitaux—Gazette Médicale—Le Progrès Médical—Bulletin de l'Académie de Médecine—Pharmaceutical Journal—Wiener Medizinische Wochenschrift—Centralblatt für die Medizinischen Wissenschaften—Revue Médicale—Gazette Hebdomadaire—National Board of Health Bulletin, Washington—Nature—Boston Medical and Surgical Journal—Louisville Medical News—Gazzetta Medica Italiana—Journal of Science—Archives Générales de Médecine—Ophthalmic Review—The Veterinarian—La Independencia Medica—Medical News and Collegiate Herald—Medical Inquirer—Monthly Homœopathic Review—Maryland Medical Journal—Medical Education—Glasgow Medical Journal—Monthly Index—Ilkeston Pioneer, December 1—Analyst—Students' Journal and Hospital Gazette—Philadelphia Medical Times—Australian Medical Journal—Chicago Medical Review—Unità Medica—Edinburgh Medical Journal, December—Night and Day—Practitioner, December—Ceylon Observer.

ORIGINAL LECTURES.

ON THE TREATMENT OF
THE DIFFERENT FORMS OF NERVOUS AND NEURALGIC HEADACHE.

By WILLIAM HENRY DAY, M.D.,
Physician to the Samaritan Hospital for Women and Children.

(Concluded from page 676.)

I SHALL consider the action of the chief remedies in the order in which I have elsewhere enumerated them.(a)

Bromide of potassium is a valuable remedy, and many a headache is kept in check, and the seizure cut short, if a full dose be taken as soon as discomfort is felt, particularly if the patient can go to bed and obtain sleep. Again, if compelled to keep about, twenty grains taken in a little sal volatile and water will lull the nervous centres, and so calm the cerebral circulation; or ten-grain doses with carbonate of ammonia in effervescence with citric acid will sometimes have an equally good effect. I know many persons who never undertake a journey without being provided with this remedy, and yet with it they can travel the whole day and awake next morning perfectly free from headache or nervous disturbance. When the remedy exerts such a speedy and good effect, the headache is not of a severe type. The physiological action of bromide of potassium is to diminish the functions of the brain, and to allay reflex irritability of the whole system of spinal nerves. By its sedative action on the stomach, the sympathetic nerve is quieted, and this has a corresponding effect upon the cerebral nerves. Then it may do good by its tendency to lower cardiac excitement and to contract the smaller vessels by which a diminished quantity of blood circulates through the brain. I have never known any ill-effects to ensue from the administration of the bromide, and I have given it in considerable doses for a long time together.

Bromide of ammonium is a drug which sometimes exerts an excellent effect upon nervous headache, relieving it, in fact, when the potassium salt fails. I generally give it with a few drops of sal volatile in a wineglassful of water on first awaking in the morning, before the patient gets up, and in this way a mild form of headache is kept at bay. The remedy would be altogether useless in a severe form.

Hydrate of chloral is a popular and excellent drug. When an attack is threatening, and the patient knows from former experience that unless sleep can be procured at once he is doomed to many hours, if not to days, of misery, a full dose will rest the brain, and so act upon its vessels as to control the hyperæmic condition upon which, in a great measure, the pain depends. Excitement of the cerebral circulation, flushing of the face, and fulness of the pulse, are the chief indications which justify its exhibition; but there is no danger of giving it now and then, even if the pain seems chiefly to depend upon some peculiar excitability of the nerve-centres. There is no fear of depression in such cases, but the habitual resort to it will lull the senses into a state of drowsiness and lethargy, just as habitual indulgence in alcohol will damage the nerve-tissue, and lower the activity of both respiration and circulation. The brain is certain to become weakened and the mental functions impaired if a person acquires the habit of taking the drug for any lengthened period. Occasionally taken at the onset of a headache, or when the patient is nearly worn out with suffering, it is most valuable; but indiscriminately resorted to, the patient is certain to pave the way to mischief in the brain and nervous centres. The best chance of its doing good is to give it when the patient feels an approaching seizure, for, if the pain has reached an acute stage, it will repeatedly cause nausea and vomiting, and then several doses may be taken with an increase of suffering rather than any abatement of it.

Croton-chloral is formed by the action of chlorine gas upon aldehyde, and, like hydrate of chloral, was introduced by Dr. Liebreich. In some forms of nervous and neuralgic

headache it is a most useful remedy. In doses of from five to ten grains it will relieve pain and procure sleep, but if there be any nausea present the tendency is to increase it. The dose must be varied, according to the circumstances of each case, delicate, nervous women being affected by a small dose, whilst strong people require a larger quantity. I begin with five grains in a little syrup and water at night, and if this has no effect in an hour, then I repeat the dose. As a rule, I have given ten grains for a dose at bed-time, but this has not in all cases procured sleep. The symptoms occasioned by an overdose of croton-chloral are said to be precisely similar to those of chloral hydrate.

Arsenic is a remedy of the greatest utility in neuralgic and periodic headache. Alone I have seldom employed it, generally combining it with iron or quinine, according to circumstances. It is one of the remedies that ought to be continued a sufficiently long time. I remember a little girl who had severe frontal headache and chorea, for which various remedies were prescribed in vain, all judiciously selected, but abandoned too soon. Under the prolonged use of Fowler's solution the choreic movements eventually ceased, and the headache vanished at the same time. In order, therefore, to bring about a successful issue, this remedy must be taken long enough to produce its specific effects.

I find, on looking over my notes, that some cases of neuralgic headache have yielded to a combination of bromide of potassium, quinine, and arsenic, when none of them alone brought any relief. The attacks diminished in severity, and in the case of one patient where headache occurred periodically, instead of being confined to the couch during each menstrual period, she could get about at this time in comparative comfort. This headache was of seventeen years' duration, and the relief derivable from the plan of treatment, carefully carried out, in the intervals of the attack was very remarkable. Arsenic is especially serviceable in depressed states of the nervous system; neuralgic headache, like neuralgia generally, indicates lowered vitality, and for this arsenic is a valuable remedy, by giving a stimulus to the vital forces. Again, in all cases of neuralgic headache associated with eczema or psoriasis, or the absorption of miasmata, arsenic is very serviceable, and should be given till its specific effects are produced. Granules of arsenious acid (gr. 1-66th) is a very good form of administration. One may be given twice a day after food.

Quinine is a remedy so well known and so generally administered in headache that it will require only a short notice. Frontal headache is rarely relieved by it, unless it is paroxysmal, and resembles the neuralgic form in other respects. If the pain originates from disorder of the digestive apparatus, or if it be due to sympathetic disturbance in some other organ of the body, then quinine will aggravate the suffering; but if the attack is purely neuralgic, if one-sided, or even if it seize the occiput, the remedy will be found of service. Five grains dropped on a little plain water, and instantly swallowed, may be given for a dose when the pain affects one side of the head and face. This dose may be repeated every hour till the suffering subsides. Sometimes a single dose will take away the pain in a few minutes. After this, drachm doses of the tincture of quinine with ten minims of spirit of chloroform will be found very serviceable, and may be continued for some days.

Iron, from its direct action on the blood, and its power to remove anæmia, is of great value in nervous and neuralgic headache. When the pathological change in the brain is one of anæmia, and the ganglionic cells are disturbed there, some soluble preparation of iron will be needed. Those that are the least astringent and stimulating are to be preferred; but where the conjunctiva is very pale, and the tongue is large, flabby, and indented by the teeth, then the tincture of the perchloride may be given with a few drops of spirit of chloroform twice a day after food. When the anæmic condition is removed, and the digestive functions are stronger, the headache is often relieved. The preparation I have most frequently used is the ammonio-citrate of iron, in five-grain doses, given three times a day, combining it with bromide of ammonium, or with arsenic where the headache is one-sided. Dialysed iron is an excellent preparation, and I have often employed it successfully in the case of children. The syrup of the hypophosphite, occasionally combined with ten-grain doses of bromide of potassium, is well borne in many cases of nervous headache.

(a) *British Medical Journal,* November 16, 1878.

Phosphorus may be often given with advantage in some forms of nervous and neuralgic headache. It acts as a general tonic to the nerve-centres, and is undoubtedly of value when the nervous system is exhausted from any cause. The phosphorus *perles* are the best form of administration. The drug should be commenced in small doses (gr. 1-60th) directly after food, and be gradually increased to gr. 1-30th daily, or even twice a day. I never exceed this dose. I have known uncomfortable symptoms follow very small doses in the shape of sickness, abdominal irritation, and weak pulse. In large doses its action is that of an irritant poison. It should only be given in the intervals of the headache due to nerve exhaustion, and it is useless if there is nausea, or a seizure is coming on. The most striking instance I have seen of its utility was in a case of neuralgic headache arising from malarial poisoning.

Gelseminum will occasionally relieve a neuralgic headache when the bromides and quinine fail. In one case of occipital and neuralgic headache, ten minims administered in an ounce of water quickly gave relief. In another case, a grain of the powder given in a pill at bed-time warded off a threatening paroxysm and induced sleep. It is important to begin with a small dose, say five minims of the tincture, as a case is recorded where ten minims, followed in half an hour by a repetition of the same dose, produced drowsiness, shivering, frontal headache, dizziness, and symptoms of collapse.(b)

Tea, as a rule, should be prohibited to the victims of nervous headache. If it is ever consumed in the place of food, it is a still more baneful excitant. Notwithstanding that long-established habit has made it an indispensable article of daily consumption, and some persons are peculiarly adapted to tolerate it, it is certain to be productive of evil when the nervous system is reduced in strength. In one person a severe nervous headache will vanish quickly on taking a strong cup of tea, and in another it will increase the headache by causing severe nausea or vomiting.

Coffee will ward off an attack in some persons by acting as a powerful stimulant or as a brisk aperient. So much for idiosyncrasy and habit of constitution, which ought to be considered when we are prescribing for a patient. If in persons of delicate constitution we can encourage the consumption of the purest and the lightest cocoa or chocolate well prepared, and give it when the stomach is at its strongest, in the absence of headache, we shall strike at the origin of the evil by conveying into the system a large amount of nourishment which exercises a most salutary effect on the nervous system.

The therapeutic action of *caffein* is like that of strong coffee. It is a stimulant to the brain and nervous system, augmenting reflex action, increasing the frequency of the pulse, and removing the sensation of fatigue. A moderate nervous headache arising from exhaustion will often yield to it at once. From one to four grains of citrate of caffein is the proper dose. Bishop's granular effervescent citrate of caffein is a convenient form of administration. A teaspoon-ful may be taken in a little water, twice or three times a day. Each drachm contains one grain of caffein.

As with medicinal remedies employed for the relief of an irritable and sensitive brain, the danger is that the stomach may be over-burdened or excited, and so transmit evil messages through the complex arrangement of nerves that are scattered over its surface.

With reference to the use of *alcoholic stimulants* by persons suffering from headache it is impossible to lay down any precise rules of guidance, for it cannot be gainsaid that all persons are not alike affected by them. In considering any advantages derivable from their moderate employment in the disorder under consideration, I pass by the important question of their action on the mind and body in health, and of the prejudice which is now being raised against them by such a large section of the community.

I think it is very questionable whether there is any headache benefited by alcohol, except that which attacks one side of the cranium. When the headache is not of this character I rarely prescribe a stimulant. It is wiser and safer to assume that the cause is rather within the reach of good food, rest, tonics, and change of air, than alcohol in any form. Alcohol increases the energy of the heart, and dilates the capillaries, whilst a small portion only of it is

exhaled by the lungs, or thrown out by the other excretory organs. Dr. Richardson, speaking of the physiological action of alcohol, which he believes is no longer speculative, as it was at one time, says, "That the ultimate action of alcohol on the animal temperature is to reduce the temperature; that alcohol relaxes organic muscular fibre; that alcohol produces four destructive physiological states of the body; that alcohol reduces oxidation; that alcohol interferes with natural dialysis; that alcohol induces, even when it is taken in small quantities, a series of morbid changes and diseases which were not formerly attributed to it."(c) I am in possession of sufficient data to justify the opinion that these nervous headaches have been kept at bay by relinquishing stimulants altogether, and following a strictly careful and temperate diet. So many sufferers from headache have feeble digestive power, through their anæmic or debilitated condition, that they falsely imagine stimulants compensate for the scanty food which they consume, taking wine or brandy habitually, from which they derive passing relief. If alcohol occasions a degree of excitement in the system, so as to induce heat of surface, a quickened pulse, and flushing of the face, then it has been carried too far, and there is every chance that the patient will pass a night of discomfort, and the next morning will find him a sufferer. Many persons unfortunately believe that alcohol supplies the place of food; and among poor women I have found in hospital practice this error so deeply rooted, that they go on with the indulgence under the notion that, as they have lost their appetite for food, they must "take something to keep them up." So surely as they fall into this pernicious practice they will injure their nervous system, and favour a condition which demoralises their feelings and destroys every remnant of energy.

There is a condition of the vascular system arising from the excitement of alcohol, not unlike that produced by anger and violent excitement, into which, in fact, the mind, when fatigued and disordered by pain, sometimes passes, warping the judgment, and letting passion take the place of reason. A man afflicted with headache at an early stage will, if thwarted in his plans, sometimes pass into this excited state, and the fury and passion will produce just these effects, the face becoming flushed, and the veins turgid with blood.

> "Ora tument irâ, nigrescunt sanguine venæ,
> Lumina Gorgoneo sævius igne micant."(d)

In bringing this lecture to a conclusion, let me urge that it is of primary importance to ascertain the causes of these headaches, so that we may be prepared to guard against them if possible; to search into the family history of the patient for the interpretation of whatever is obscure and unproven, and to formulate, from the inquiry, definite rules of management in accordance with the facts as they have been ascertained, and further to establish some proposition or general truth which is both irresistible and convincing.

What we want is careful observation, made without bias or intention (conscious or unconscious) to establish a theory; and then, when the observations have been recorded, we may venture to construct an hypothesis, and not till then. A handful of fact is worth a waggon-load of theory—at least it is so at present, and must be so until our assured facts have grown to a far bigger heap than they have yet attained.

PET ANIMALS AND CONTAGIOUS DISEASES.—The fact that pet animals can carry contagion, and thus be the means of spreading fatal diseases, is not widely enough known or duly appreciated. We have heard of authentic cases in which scarlet fever was communicated from one person to another by means of a cat. Dr. Hewit, of Lake Superior, relates a somewhat similar instance in which diphtheria was communicated by the same animal, two or three of his children dying in consequence thereof. We refer to the subject in the hope that more facts bearing upon it may be communicated. These are at present scarce, but a little attention paid to the matter would, no doubt, secure much that would be of importance to comparative and preventive medicine.—*Journal of Comparative Medicine* (in *New York Med. Record*, November 5).

(b) *British Medical Journal*, 1881, vol. i., page 199.

(c) Inaugural Address, delivered before the British Medical Temperance Association, May 30, 1879.
(d) Ovid, De Art., iii., page 502.

ORIGINAL COMMUNICATIONS.

SOME NEW FACTS CONECTED WITH THE ACTION OF GERMS IN THE PRODUCTION OF HUMAN DISEASES.

By Dr. GEORGE HARLEY, F.R.S.

Reformed Speling—No Duplicated Consonants escept in Personal Names.

CHAPTER III.

CAN THE SUDEN REAPEARANCE OF INFECTIOUS DISEASES IN A LOCALITY WHICH HAS LONG BEEN FREE FROM THEM BE PHILOSOPHICALY ACOUNTED FOR BY THE GERM THEORY? *Answer*—YES.

IF germs are exterminated when disease ends, how is it posible, it has been asked, to philosophicaly acount for the recurence of Epidemic diseases—due to germs—in a neighbourhood, into which they have not been imported. After a long lapse of years of perfect imunity from the scourge, without axepting of the Spontaneous Generation theory? It has further been asked—How it is posible even to acount for the ocasionaly equaly suden apearance of eratic sporadic cases of virulently Infectious diseases in districts which, both at the time and long before their ocurence, have been not only perfectly free from an Epidemic of that special kind of disease, and from any other examples of a similarly Sporadic kind of that species of germ disease? Except by admiting the posibility of germs being generated *de novo*. My answer is—Wait, and you shal see.

No doubt there was a time—and that time in many people's minds has not yet gone by—when, owing to our imperfect knowledge of the existence of Latent-life, it was utterly imposible to reconcile the suden apearance, after long periods of quiescence, of Epidemic Contagious and Infectious Diseases. Suposed to be due to germs, without at the same time giving credence to the theory of the Spontaneous generation of animal or vegetable life. That day, however, pased, or ought to have pased away, when Mr. Worthington Smith discovered in the spawn of the *Botrytis basiana*—the germ which produces one of the forms of vine and potato blight—what he was pleased to name a "Resting-spore." A spore which might lie dormant, though not dead, in the soil, or in the tisues of the vine and potato plant during nine months of the year—throughout the whole autumn, winter, and spring—and then under the influence of the sumer's heat vivify and burst into active developmental life.

Upon the Resting-spore discovery, the folowing very judicious remarks fel from the lips of Sir James Paget during the adres he delivered at Cambridge in 1880. While speaking of the causes of Epidemics in the human body, and comparing them with parasitic vegetable Epidemics—which they in many respects closely resemble—he said that the dificulty hitherto experienced in explaining the aparent long periods of latency which are ocasionaly noticed to ocur between the production of one virulent epidemic of a particular form of disease, and the subsequent suden outburst of another, of precisely the same nature, in the same district, vanishes when we regard them from the same point of view as vegetable Epidemics, and imagine that they poses Resting-spores—Germ-spores. Like that of the fungus which produces one of the forms of the potato-blight and vinedisease. As Sir James said, it has already been, in fact, demonstrated with great probability that, in the case of the anthracoid disease of catle, such a Resting-spore does exist, and is preserved in the soil. Beside the germs which inhabit the blood, and which are transmited from one animal to another.

Having a particular bearing on this Resting-spore theory, I may here alude to the researches (1880) of Drs. Klebs and Tommasi-Crudeli, who examined the air of the Pontine Marshes, and found in it a microphyte of the genus *Bacilus*, to which the name *Bacilus malariæ* has been given. They injected water taken from malarious localities under the skin of animals, with the result of producing intermitent fever, with enlargement of the spleen. The lymph and spleen were found to contain oval shining bodies exhibiting active movements—probably Brownian granules. On the other hand, the injecta of *Bacilus*-obtained from a liquid

soil produced only very slight intermitent fever. Showing that cultivation of the soil diminished the number as wel as, perhaps, the strength of the malarial germs—Restingspores. The bacilus was also found in the spleen and bones of three individuals who died of pernicious malarial fever.

From the above it is seen that neither the theory of Spontaneous generation nor even that of the posibility of Regeneration of germs *de novo* is by some any longer considered necesary to acount for the existence of either individual Sporadic cases or Epidemics of Contagious and Infectious diseases. Moreover, what is of equal importance to the mere discovery of the existence of a Resting-spore can have its quiescent habitat somewhere else than in the tisues of the human body. For a knowledge of this fact greatly facilitates the understanding of how it is a single Sporadic, as wel as the first case of an Epidemic of disease, is al at once sudenly brought into existence. Which would most asuredly not be the case if we were bound to believe that the natural and only quiescent *habitat* of the Resting-spore was the human body itself. For how, then, it would be asked, could children or other persons born long after the disapearance of an epidemic disease get into posesion of a Resting-spore and become the victims of the first Sporadic or Epidemic case of the same kind of disease? When, however, it is known that the soil itself may even be the quiescent *habitat* of a human disease germ, the mater is at once simplified.

An anonymous writer in the *British Medical Journal* of October 23, 1880, under the heading, "The Etiology of Typhoid Fever," judiciously remarks that although in many epidemics there is oftentimes no history of any previous local case before the outbreak begins; and, unles the later is to be acounted for on the pythogenic theory, the most natural explanation seems to be that which rests upon the presence of old disease germs lying latent in the soil. A prolonged drought, by drying the subsoil, and sinking considerably the level of the water in the wels. On a heavy rainfal coming and rapidly refiling the wels the water would percolate quickly through the dry subsoil, and cary with it the unaltered germs, which would then be taken into people's stomachs along with the water, and give origin to the disease. So much for the Resting-spore Theory. The *rationale* of which I most cordialy endorse. BUT the idea in which it originates I most heartily condemn. For, as I shal now proceed to show, there is in reality no such thing in nature as a Special Resting-spore. Therefore the term is misleading, and consequently objectionable, and ought at once to be abandoned. For every germ spore, when regarded in the same sense, is a resting-spore. That is to say, every germ spore posese Latent-life, and when placed under favorable circumstances for remaining dormant, and yet not dying, wil retain its vitality, and in the end vivify, just as the seed of a plant, or the chrysalis of a silkworm bursts forth into active life when placed under the conditions necesary to and favorable for its vivification. Any single germspore, without exception, does this. But just as al individual wheat-seeds are not alike strongly constituted—some being capable of retaining their vitality longer than others—yet from al of them posesing the comon property of Latent-life, no one ever speaks of "Resting-wheat-seeds." So, though al individual germ-spores are not alike strongly constituted—some being capable of retaining their vitality longer than others—yet al posesing the comon property of Latent-life, philosophicaly speaking, there is no such thing as a specific form of Resting-spore. Consequently from hence forth I shal cease to employ the misleading term of "Resting-spore" in my exposition of the Why and the Wherefore of the suden reapearance of epidemic diseases in localities which have remained long free from their presence.

I shal now try and substantiate the view I take of the quiescent intervals ocuring between the outbreaks of similar kinds of Epidemic and Sporadic diseases being the direct result of germs posesing, like many other species of animated nature, peculiarly persistent powers of Latent-life.

To begin with, I must first point out what I regard as Latentlife, and give my reasons for believing that germs, no mater whether they belong to the animal or the vegetable kingdom, may, presumably, naturaly and normaly poses it to such an extent as to be capable of lying torpid, but not dead. Not alone for many months, but for many years, and afterwards wake up into active life with al their relative state ———

Not only germs, but EVERY THING that liveth, I believe, posesse Latent-life in one form or another. Without the posesion of Latent-life nothing could live. For alternating periods of repose and activity are the indispensable concomitants of animated existence. To be active when awake, even man himself, the boasting lord of creation, must be torpid while asleep. The being capable of lying dormant for eighty minutes, eighty hours, eighty months, or eighty years, which distinguishes some of the diferent durations of Latent-life posessed by diferent species of animals and plants, are merely diferences in degree. Not in kind. For Latent-life, acording to my way of regarding it, is a specific physiological atribute of al animated nature. Depending on no special and peculiar form of organisation, and on no solitary exciting cause, but being equaly the posesion of animal and plant, and the concomitant of cold and of heat, of fatigue ,and of poison. In fact, merely a condition of animated creation, where, for a longer or shorter time, al the functions of organic life, though incompatible with an active, are nevertheles compatible with a lethargic, state of animated existence. The lethargy may be periodic, and diurnal, as in the sleep of animals and plants. Or anual, and due to the influence of atmospheric temperature. As in winter hibernation, and sumer æstivation. Or it may be non-periodic, and due to exceptional abnormal bodily conditions. Such as prolonged fatigue of body. Or mind (so-called mesmerism), catalepsy, and the imbibition of certain foreign materials.

I shal now endeavour to substantiate these opinions, by aducing demonstrable data in their suport, and to begin with I shal point out how normal physiological Latent-life, both in animals and plants, manifests itself to us in three welmarked ways.

Firstly.—In the form of ordinary diurnal sleep.

Secondly.—In the form of hibernation. The name aplied by naturalists to denote the peculiar state of torpor in which many kinds of animals pas the cold winter months.

Thirdly.—As æstivation. The name given to the torpid state in which certain animals in the tropics pas the hotest months of the year.

Al three are, I believe, perfectly analogous examples of Latent-life. But the first—ordinary sleep—difers very materialy from the other two, from being so imperfect a form of Latent-life that the function of consciousness alone is in complete abeyance. Al the animal functions are stil in moderated activity. Respiration, circulation, digestion, secretion, and excretion stil go on, and even the senses of hearing and feeling are so slightly in abeyance that a loud noise or a rough touch imediately recals the ordinary sleaper to consciousness. This state, however, may merge in disease, or by taking toxic substances, or from mere fatigue, into as profound a torpor as exists in hibernation and æstivation. In cataleptic trance, for example, the pulse is not only imperceptible, and the heart's action insaudible, but respiration is invisible. While, again, the death-like sleep of fatigue or poison may be so profound that neither the pulse may be detectable nor the respiration visible, and the senses of hearing and feeling exageratedly in abeyance, but the processes of digestion and secretion corespondingly diminished.

The conditions of hibernation and æstivation difer stil further from ordinary sleep in being not only more profound, but much more prolonged. In them, as in trance, or any other kind of death-like sleep, every function of the body, besides consciousness, is in marked abeyance. Even not so much as a feeble action of the heart being visible until it is exposed. And that may be the only sign of life. In some animals the heart seems, even on exposure, to be motionles while they are hibernating. Such is at least said to be the case with the heart of the comon large brown-sheled snail of our gardens. Which, although it powerfuly pulsates at the rate of from sixty to one hundred while in active life during the sumer months, lies aparently quite stil while the animal is in its profound winter's sleep. Usualy, however, so tenacious is the heart's power of action found to be, that animals in a hibernating and æstivating state have been decapitated, and yet the feeble pulsations of the heart gone on for a considerable time, aparently uninfluenced by the mutilation. That respiration is likewise in marked abeyance during hibernation is proved by the fact that frogs and lizards can be kept from breathing by placing them under water for at least eight times longer than it would take to drown them when in their usual state of active life.

The best example I can give of the respiration being in complete abeyance in profound hibernation is that of the comon bat, whose sleep more closely resembles the sleep of death than does that of most other hibernating animals, for it is said not only not to eat, but not even to breathe. This fact has, it is suposed, been proven by suspending it in a vesel filed with a poisonous gas. In which it remains for hours unscathed. Whereas when woke up it imediately inspires, and with the first inspiratory efort closes its earthly career. Although this fact seems almost imposible, a litle reflection wil, I think, show that there is nothing improbable about it. As it is easy enough for a physiologist to imagine that a bat while in a hibernating state need not respire for exactly the same reason as it does not require to eat. Namely, from its vital as wel as its animal functions being reduced to a minimum—it can proportionately require as litle oxygen as it does food to suply the modicum of tisue waste. And consequently its respiration, like its digestion, may easily be in an almost complete state of abeyance. Suficient oxygen, like suficient nutritive materials, for its smal requirements existing in the blood slowly and almost imperceptibly circulating through its torpid tisues.

It is not, however, alone animals whose vital functions may be suposed to be specialy constituted for the purposes of hibernation, upon whom the influence of cold is such as to enable them to live in a state of torpor for an exceptionaly long period without being suplied with food. For it is an established fact that not only mountain hares, but ordinary Highland sheep, have been known to lie asleep buried in snow-drifts in Scotland for several weeks without, aparently, sustaining any injury to their constitutions.

I have next to point out that it is not cold alone, as is comonly suposed, which leads to hibernation. On the contrary, any other clas of physical conditions not destructive to, but merely incompatible with, active life, causes hibernation. Or its analogous æstivation, both in plants and animals. For example, certain reptiles and fish entirely disapear from the dried-up water-tanks in India during the hot season, and imediately reapear with the return of the cold wet season. Certain eel-like fish—the Lepidosiren—indigenous to the river Gambia lie torpid in the hard sun-baked mud during the hot season. When the water has disapeared from the river's bed. And reawaken into active life with the return of the water after the rainy season has set in.

Even warm-blooded animals æstivate. The Tanrec of Madagascar, an animal of the hedgehog species, is said to sleep in its burow during the whole of the hotest three months of the year.

Æstivation is not an atribute posessed by the animal kingdom alone. Many plants in tropical climates poses it. Whenever the amount of atmospheric humidity is insuficient for the maintenance of their leaves, they shed them as ours do in autumn, and go into an equal state of torpidity. This may be designated as a state of vegetable æstivation. The winter torpor of plants in temperate zones may equaly apropriately be denominated vegetable hibernation.

There exists a far more intimate similarity, not only in the structure and chemical constitution, but even as regards the vital functions, of plants and animals, than is usualy dreamed of. This is, perhaps, no where more manifest than in their mutual posesion of the atribute of Latent-life. Plants sleep, as wel as animals; some even close their petals, as animals close their eyes. Moreover, just as al kinds of animals in temperate zones do not hibernate, neither do al kinds of plants. For example, we have what are caled evergreens in abundance. Evergreen shrubs, and Evergreen forest trees. The diference between the two kingdoms, then, is only limited by the fact that while the majority of animals don't, the majority of vegetables do, annualy hibernate.

Neither an elevated nor a diminished temperature is, however, necesary to produce Latent-life. Either of the hibernating or æstivatory kinds. In proof of the truth of this asertion that neither heat nor cold are elements absolutely necesary to produce profound states of torpor, I may here refer to what is known of the life-history of the chrysalis of the comon smal Eggar moth of our hedge-sides (E. Lanestris)-Which, as is wel known, often remains for two whole years in the pupa state, and from its being, while in this condition, encased in a wel-closed hard shel, can receive no food whatever. Beyond the limited amount of atmospheric air and moisture which permeates to it through its self-made prison-wals.

(To be continued.)

DISEASE OF THE BRONCHIAL GLANDS.

By JAMES C. DE CASTRO, M.B., M.R.C.P.

DR. R. QUAIN has recently drawn the attention of the profession to the fact that "diseases of the bronchial glands," occurring in adult and advanced periods of life, are frequently overlooked or mistaken for other maladies of the lungs. My own experience goes to substantiate this statement by Dr. Quain, and, out of many cases of which I have notes, I select a few which seem illustrative of the main propositions referred to.

Case 1.—A gentleman about thirty years of age consulted me for a chest affection which had existed more or less from early childhood. The symptoms were—habitually imperfect respiratory power, shown by a certain amount of embarrassment in breathing, especially under stress of exertion; liability to asthmatic attacks; slight cough and expectoration; some pain in the chest; slight attacks of hæmoptysis; a strangely altered state of the voice, which was weak and "squeaky" to a ludicrous degree—an altered condition which varied somewhat in degree, but which was always remarkable; generally feeble health, and extreme thinness, without progressive emaciation. Aspect strumous; severe and intractable eczema. Physical Signs: Slight dulness anteriorly, a hand's breadth below the left clavicle, under rather strong percussion. Breath-sounds somewhat weak; occasional râles. Posteriorly, decided dulness below and between the margins of the scapula, most pronounced on left side, at points slightly tubular in character. Breath-sounds generally weak, at points harsh. The form of the thorax was rather narrow, approximating to "pigeon-breasted," without any marked contraction on one side more than the other. The dulness anteriorly, feeble health, want of flesh, and attacks of slight hæmoptysis, had led to an opinion that this patient was phthisical; but, finding that the anterior dulness was manifestly elicited through the overlying lung, from the posterior condensed tissues, and looking to the facts that the delicacy had dated from childhood, that there was no progressive emaciation, that the strangely abnormal condition of the voice, and the tendency to paroxysmal attacks of difficulty of breathing, indicated some intrathoracic centripetal pressure, the diagnosis of disease of the bronchial glands was given. This patient was under my observation for many years, and enjoyed intervals (especially whilst residing at Nice) of very tolerable health, and I gave a favourable prognosis as regarded the prolongation of life; but in this prognosis I was unfortunately mistaken, since, without any very manifest retrogression in health, or warning of the coming event, profuse hæmoptysis came on, proving fatal in a few hours—hæmoptysis caused, as was proved on inspection, by the suppuration of a bronchial gland involving the coats of a rather large pulmonary bloodvessel; an accident not of frequent occurrence, but one the possibility of which must be borne in mind.

Case 2.—A lady about twenty years of age consulted me for rather severe chest symptoms, for which she had been sent to Pau by an eminent Dublin physician. No definite diagnosis had been given, as far as I could learn, nor at first could I get a clear history of the case as to the length of time the symptoms of chest-delicacy had existed. Ultimately I found that these had dated from an attack of measles in childhood, complicated with pulmonary symptoms. The aspect of this patient was unhealthy, with a tendency to swelling of the lymphatic glands of the neck; there was some turgescence of the face, and a look of distress; no emaciation. The general symptoms were—considerable embarrassment of breathing, increased to a painful degree by much exertion, such as quick walking or going up stairs, and this embarrassment assumed at times a spasmodic character; slight cough, little expectoration; some pain complained of in chest, passing back to between the shoulders; voice weak and very husky; no hæmoptysis. Physical Signs: Some dulness in front on right side below the clavicle (this anterior dulness, as in the first case, required strong percussion for its development). On the left side there was some extension of the cardiac dulness. Decided dulness posteriorly, below the margins of the scapula, extending to the spine. Breath-sounds irregularly weak and harsh at points over the front of the chest, with occasional rhonchi; posteriorly, over the seat of dulness, deficient and at points bronchial in character. Cardiac sounds rather prolonged with the systole

without distinct murmur. From the aspect of this patient and the character of the respiration I was rather prepared to find bronchitis, with emphysema and cardiac hypertrophy; but the chief seat of the dulness being over the region of the bronchial glands, the indications afforded by the state of the voice, paroxysmal difficulty of breathing, of intrathoracic pressure decided the diagnosis in favour of bronchial gland disease. This patient was under observation, "off and on," for twelve years with varying conditions of amendment and the reverse, and ultimately succumbed to some pulmonary attack (the precise nature of which I did not learn) when on a visit to Ireland; but the diagnosis of diseased and enlarged bronchial glands was confirmed.

Case 3.—A little girl aged five years had a severe attack of typhoid fever, complicated with pulmonary mischief. She rallied from the fever, but remained very feeble, with persistent emaciation, cough and purulent expectoration, with the physical signs of consolidation of the lung, and a cavity pronounced to be tubercular; and a hopeless prognosis was given. I did not see the child during the attack of typhoid fever, but, finding that the dulness was very pronounced over the region of the bronchial glands, looking to the fact that the condition existing was a sequela to typhoid fever, and bearing in mind how fallacious physical signs of cavities are in young children, as regards the extent of the mischief, I gave a more hopeful prognosis, upon the ground that the stress of the disease was in the bronchial glands, and such destruction of tissue as existed the result of the laying down and softening of typhoid matter. The little patient was taken to a warm, dry climate for two successive winters; recovered flesh and strength, and all the prominent chest-symptoms subsiding; the physical signs of dulness over the region of the bronchial glands, with strong tubular breath-sounds over the same region, remaining, and some slight contraction of the left side. Of course the correctness of diagnosis is not proved by this result, but is made infinitely probable.

Some of the most desperate cases, both in adults and children (judged of solely by the physical signs), have occurred to me in my practice, as a consequence of the laying down of tubercular deposit in the bronchial glands, and substance of the lung undergoing softening destruction of tissue and formation of vomicæ, yet resulting in recovery, barring a certain amount of persistent, but unprogressive, structural damage, manifestly because there is not the tendency to constantly renewed deposit and destructive softening that there is in true tuberculosis.

A very, very important difference of opinion exists as to the age at which "bronchial gland disease" most frequently commences. Whilst Dr. Walshe notes that in regard to clinical importance it is essentially a disease of childhood, Dr. Quain holds a precisely contrary opinion. My own experience, as far as it goes, leads me to the conclusion that though it occurs as a substantive disease in adult and even advanced life, and may originate at any age, it can, in the majority of instances, be traced by careful inquiry to childhood or infancy. There seems no antecedent reason why it should not commence at an adult or advanced period of life, but there are very cogent reasons why the disease should more frequently originate in childhood, inasmuch as it is a frequent sequela to the exanthemata complicated with pulmonary mischief, and to whooping-cough, and that the lymphatic glands (including the bronchial) are more prone to become the seat of deposits, more or less aplastic, in childhood and early life than at later periods. When the disease can be clearly traced to early life, it of course facilitates the "diagnosis" by excluding most other forms of tumour, with which, supposing it to have commenced in adult or advanced life, it might possibly be confounded.

The history of "bronchial gland disease," when occurring in early life, is almost identical with that of "acquired collapse of the lung" or "apneumatosis"—both originating in some pulmonary attack, simple or complicated, and in whooping-cough, leaving various chest-symptoms as a consequence. But the developed diseases have certain differences as to general symptoms and physical signs. To defective respiratory power and embarrassment of breathing, characteristic of "apneumatosis," there are in bronchial gland disease generally superadded indications of intrathoracic centripetal pressure, viz., alterations in the character of the voice, paroxysmal attacks of difficulty of breathing, hæmoptysis, pain; and the same differences exist as between the malady under consideration and pneumonic and fibroid consolidations of the lung, excepting always hæmoptysis, which is not unfrequent in fibroid disease of the lung (cirrhosis).

The chief seat of dulness in "apneumatosis" is the mammary region and the base of the lung. In "bronchial gland disease" the dulness is most marked posteriorly about the margins of the scapula; what dulness exists anteriorly generally requires rather strong percussion for its development, and is manifestly derived from the posterior condensed tissues.

Little can be added to Dr. Quain's remarks on the treatment of disease of the bronchial glands. I have found a moderately warm, dry, and tonic climate suit these cases best; avoiding the decidedly warm, relaxing climates—Madeira, for instance,—and the rainy, cloudy, and often cold climates of the South-west of France, such as Pau, Biarritz, etc.

11, Hinde-street, Manchester-square, W.

COMPARISON OF THE WEIGHT OF THE HEART AND OTHER VISCERA IN THE SANE AND THE INSANE.
By R. BOYD, F.R.C.P.

ON this subject so little appears in the current treatises of physiology and pathology, and still less in the general medical mind, that it may be well to give a few of the results in a brief summary of my researches, so as to ventilate some of the leading points more distinctly than they are shown in my extended memoir in the *Philosophical Transactions*, or in any other publication. Whatever theory or further inquiries a consideration of the weights may give rise to, at present the bare facts only are recorded, quite independently of any opinion or speculation.

In my Tables recently published by Messrs. Churchill, as regards the weight of the body and brain and several of the internal organs in the sane and insane, when compared at decennial periods of life, it is very remarkable that although the weight of the body was on the average heavier in the insane, the heart was as much as one ounce lighter in males, and one and a quarter ounces in females. This difference was greatest in the two earliest decennial periods, when it amounted to two ounces in each sex. The average weight of the liver at the four earliest decennial periods was also considerably less in males, varying from nearly thirteen to two ounces; in insane females the average weight was also less at the three earliest decennial periods, varying from nine to four ounces. After sixty years the average weight of the liver gradually diminished in both sane and insane, and the difference became less in the two classes. On the average of the whole, the liver was four ounces less in insane than in sane males, and three and one-third ounces less in insane than in sane females.

The spleen, likewise, was less in the insane of both sexes. At the first four decennial periods of life the average weight being—in sane males 6·6, and in females 5·5 ounces; in insane males it was 5·5, and in females 4·7 ounces. After sixty years the weight of the spleen gradually declined in both classes. On the average of the whole the spleen was about half an ounce less in the insane than in the sane, both in males and females, the average being 5·5 in sane males and 4·5 ounces in sane females, and 5 ounces in insane males and 4·1 ounces in insane females.

The kidneys, too, were less on the average of the whole, in the insane being in the males 9·2 and in the females 7·7 ounces, whilst in the sane the average was in the males 10 and in the females 8·6 ounces.

The average weight of the cerebellum in males, sane and insane, was 5 ounces, and in females 4·64 in the sane and 4·75 ounces in the insane.

Whether or not the apparent difference in the weights of the metropolitan (sane) paupers and the paupers of the agricultural class in Somersetshire is owing to local circumstances, or to circumstances attributable to other causes, might be worthy of further inquiry. The records of Hanwell or Colney Hatch might settle the point so far as regards metropolitan pauper lunatics. The visiting justices have not, like the Poor-law Guardians of St. Marylebone, pro-

hibited such investigations, although, like them, they are blundering in proposing to make an addition for 500 patients at Colney Hatch, instead of providing a separate asylum for that number, large enough for the proper management of acute cases. Alas for Sydney Smith! Although dead, he yet speaketh respecting boards of guardians.

REPORTS OF HOSPITAL PRACTICE
IN
MEDICINE AND SURGERY.

GENERAL HOSPITAL FOR SICK CHILDREN, PENDLEBURY, MANCHESTER.

TWO CASES OF ACUTE ENDOCARDITIS—PYREXIA—EMBOLISM—DEATH.
(Under the care of Dr. H. ASHBY.)
[Reports by H. B. WALKER and C. R. GRAHAM, Resident Medical Officers.

Case 1.—W. W., aged thirteen years, admitted to hospital on July 11, 1881. Father died of heart-disease and dropsy. Patient had acute rheumatism six years ago, being laid up for some time. Latterly has been languid and poorly. A fortnight ago he fainted, and since then has felt very weak and ill.

Present State.—Spare boy, with flabby tissues; looks languid; no œdema. He has a loud systolic mitral bruit, heard all over the chest in front and at the angle of the scapula behind. Apex-beat in sixth space near junction with cartilage; deep cardiac dulness extends to nipple line, and shades away gradually to left. No enlargement of liver or spleen. No albumen.

August 1.—Since admission, boy has continually had a somewhat furred tongue, has become paler and thinner; frequently complained of pain over the præcordial region, extending to shoulder and down left arm. His temperature constantly goes up in the evening to 101° to 103°, falling to normal in the morning.

September 1.—Boy's condition much the same, only worse. He is languid, listless, does not care to leave his bed. Temperature rises regularly to 101° to 103° every night, and is again normal in the morning. Still has pain over region of heart, mostly every night, which is relieved by fomentations. Bruit has somewhat a musical character, and occasionally there is a small quantity of albumen in the urine. No optic neuritis.

October 5.—Condition the same. Temperature still intermits. Two days ago complained of pain in left foot. It was noticed that there was a tender swelling, tense and red, on the inner side of the dorsum of the foot. Pulsation normal in both tibial arteries. To-day the swelling is increased. Urine albuminous.

7th.—Swelling on dorsum of foot much less. Unfortunately the boy was removed home by his friends. He was, however, visited at his home till his death on November 28. Whilst at home he gradually wasted, lost strength, was hectic at night, and apparently died of exhaustion.

Post-mortem.—Chest: Lungs normal, except some hypostatic congestion at the bases. Heart: Right side normal. Left ventricular wall hypertrophied; edges of mitral valve rough, thickened, studded with fibrinous concretions; no ulceration; no endocarditis elsewhere in ventricle. In the left auricle, extending up the left wall, the endocarditis is rough, with numerous fibrinous tags attached, one or two a quarter of an inch long; granulations on corpus Arantii of aortic valves. Liver large and pale. Spleen enlarged, soft, with numerous infarcts, for the most part of soft, cheesy consistence; some lymph on surface. Kidneys pale, not fatty; supra-renals and other organs healthy. Head not opened.

Case 2.—Julia H., aged nine years, was admitted to hospital June 27, 1881. Has had a cough for three years. Three weeks ago cough became troublesome. Frequently cried with pain over the region of the heart, and feet began to swell a week ago.

Present State.—A pale girl, with some œdema of legs and puffiness about face. Some rhonchus in chest. A loud systolic apex-murmur traced into axilla. Spleen enlarged;

lower end nearly on level with umbilicus. Liver enlarged; edge felt three inches below ribs. Urine contains a quantity of albumen.

July 13.—Since admission, heart, liver, and spleen much in same condition. Urine still contains albumen, and the temperature has regularly risen to 101°-102° every evening, becoming normal, or nearly so, in the morning. No œdema.

August 25.—Still intermittent temperature. Albumen and casts in urine. Pain over præcordial region. For the last three days she has had severe frontal headache, crying out with pain; is very cross and irritable; no sign of paralysis. Left optic disc swollen, and is partly surrounded by a recent hæmorrhage; in one place the blood-clot is as large as the disc; veins full, arteries distinct, but small. Right optic disc swollen, pink; veins full and tortuous, arteries small. No loss of vision.

August 28.—Still complains of pain in head; is drowsy and irritable; no paralysis, paresis (?) of both arms. Exaggerated tendon-reflex on right side.

October 7.—Somewhat improved up to-day, but still drowsy and irritable; no sign of paralysis. Optic discs less swollen, and blood-clots mostly disappeared. This morning, whilst at breakfast, she fell back on her pillow; became unconscious, with stertorous breathing. Later on, she could be roused with some difficulty, and face was drawn to left side. Right arm seems weak, and falls when lifted up, but she moves it at times. Vomited several times. Knee reflex on right side exaggerated. On touching the soles of the feet both legs are almost violently drawn up. Examination of discs impossible on account of the irritability of patient.

17th.—Remained since the 7th in a drowsy state, crying out sometimes with pain in head. Evident weakness of right side of face and right arm, but no decided paralysis. Passes urine and fæces into the bed. Died early this morning, convulsions preceding death. No ophthalmoscopic examination possible for the last ten days.

Post-mortem.—Brain : Subarachnoid hæmorrhage on left side of parietal region extending from Sylvian fissure. Embedded in Sylvian fissure is an aneurism of middle cerebral artery of the size of a small walnut, situated beyond arteries to anterior perforated space, and surrounded by softened brain-substance. Aneurism nearly filled with laminated clot. White substance of nearly the whole of parietal region in a state of softening, and containing much blood-clot. Basal ganglia and internal capsule normal. Heart : Left ventricular walls much hypertrophied. Edges of mitral valve and chordæ tendineæ swollen and rough; numerous fibrinous concretions of irregular shape, some one-third of an inch in length, attached to valves and chordæ; several are cretaceous. Extending from the valve up the left wall of auricle there is recent endocarditis, and numerous fibrinous tags are attached. Aortic and other valves normal. Spleen large and soft; no infarcts. Liver large and pale. Kidneys pale; early stage of nephritis (verified by microscopical examination); no infarcts.

Remarks (by Dr. Ashby).—These two cases of acute or subacute endocarditis are of great interest. Endocarditis, as a rule, save for the murmur it produces, gives rise to no definite symptoms, or none apart from the disease which it accompanies. We meet occasionally with cases of "ulcerative endocarditis" or "endocarditis maligna" running a short course of a few days or weeks, and resembling pyæmia more than any other disease. In the two cases of which a short summary is given above, we have a condition apparently occupying a position midway between the ordinary run of endocarditis cases and the malignant form. Acute heart-disease terminating fatally in a few months, and producing symptoms not unlike tuberculosis, is not infrequent in young people. Clinically, this condition is illustrated by the cases above narrated, and is accompanied by a systolic mitral murmur, angina-like pain in the præcordial region, pyrexia of an intermittent type, wasting, increasing weakness, the phenomena of inflammatory emboli, and more or less enlargement of the liver and spleen. The first case ran its course in about five months, having what was probably embolism of dorsal artery of foot, and later splenic embolism. The career of the second case was cut short by embolism of the left middle cerebral, softening of the arterial wall, aneurism, and finally hæmorrhage and softening of brain. In this case the enlarged liver and spleen were noteworthy, and there was an early condition of nephritis, which in all probability was secondary to the cardiac

trouble. The condition of both hearts was almost exactly similar : the roughened edges of the mitral valve, the numerous fibrinous tag-like concretions attached, were alike present in both; also a similar condition of endocarditis extending into the left auricle, creeping up the left wall for some inch and a half. Possibly this latter condition was due to a current of blood impinging on the surface of the auricle, produced by regurgitation through the mitral valve. It is interesting to note that the effects produced by embolism in these cases were not mechanical alone, but the inflammatory processes set up were due to the nature of the emboli. The red, painful swelling on the dorsum of the foot, the lymph on the surface of the spleen, the aneurismal swelling of the middle cerebral, were silent witnesses to the inflammatory processes affecting the valves of the heart.

TERMS OF SUBSCRIPTION.
(Free by post.)

British Islands	. . . .	Twelve Months	.	£1 8	0
,,	,,	Six	,,	. 0 14	0
The Colonies and the United }	Twelve	,,	. 1 10	0
States of America . . }				
,,	,,	Six	,,	. 0 15	0
India	,,	Twelve	,,	. 1 10	0
,, (viâ Brindisi)	. . .	,,	,,	. 1 15	0
,,	,,	Six	,,	. 0 15	0
,, (viâ Brindisi)	. . .	,,	,,	. 0 17	6

Foreign Subscribers are requested to inform the Publishers of any remittance made through the agency of the Post-office.

Single Copies of the Journal can be obtained of all Booksellers and Newsmen, price Sixpence.

Cheques or Post-office Orders should be made payable to Mr. JAMES LUCAS, 11, New Burlington-street, W.

TERMS FOR ADVERTISEMENTS.

Seven lines (70 words)	. . .	. £0 4	6
Each additional line (10 words)	. .	. 0 0	6
Half-column, or quarter-page .	.	. 1 5	0
Whole column, or half-page	.	. 2 10	0
Whole page	. . . .	. 5 0	0

Births, Marriages, and Deaths are inserted Free of Charge.

THE MEDICAL TIMES AND GAZETTE is published on Friday morning. Advertisements must therefore reach the Publishing Office not later than One o'clock on Thursday.

Medical Times and Gazette.

SATURDAY, DECEMBER 17, 1881.

"UNFIT FOR HUMAN FOOD."

A WEEK or two ago, before Alderman Sir Thomas Owden, a man in a small way of business as a butcher in Derbyshire was prosecuted and fined £10 for sending to the Smithfield Market the dressed carcase of a cow which he had bought for the moderate sum of 20s. The farmer who sold the animal for 20s. gave evidence in court. Not being a scientific pathologist, nor even a veterinary surgeon, he did not admit that the animal was diseased; it was only an old and wasted cow, of no more use to him as a milker. All that he got for his cow was 20s., and it was probably all that he asked; that sum is, in fact, the conventional price in all such cases throughout the whole of Great Britain and Ireland. The purchaser recouped himself to the extent of 9s. by selling the hide, and he had still the hoofs and tallow (if, indeed, the wretched animal had any fat left), as well as the flesh, to balance the account with. A certain acuteness of conscience led him to offer the flesh, in the first instance, for the use of a kennel of foxhounds in the neighbourhood, but his offer was not accepted. He then dressed and packed the four quarters in the usual way, and consigned them to a salesman at Smithfield Market. The Market Inspector was dissatisfied with the appearance of the meat, and condemned it, and he even went so far as to have the consignor summoned to the Guildhall Court, with the result that we have mentioned. The case is one that recurs at the Guildhall Court about once a month with a monotonous sameness in the details. There is always a butcher in a small way of business in a country district who buys an animal for 20s., and consigns it to a salesman at the Central London Meat Market, with instructions to do the best with it that he can. There is also the farmer who sold the animal, protesting that it was sold for the value of the hide and hoofs, and that he had no idea of the flesh being used as human food. These cases come into court and are reported in the newspapers from time to time. The Aldermen at the Guildhall Court must have come to think that there are a good many diseased cows about, and the Inspector at the Central Meat Market has begun to suspect that there may be cases which escape his vigilance. He has within the last week or two reported that the salesmen throw obstacles in the way of the detection of meat unfit for human food, and the salesmen have drawn up a counter-statement full of generous indignation.

But we say, with the confidence derived from accurate information, that neither the Aldermen, nor the Inspector nor the salesman, nor the public, have even an approximate idea of the extent to which meat unfit for human food is sold as human food. The Inspector judges only by the appearance of the quarters of beef which enter the market; the meat has a dull, sodden, pale, or abnormally dark appearance, it is sticky or glutinous to the touch, and it wants the due admixture of fat. The Inspector at the Central London Meat Market is in the same position for detecting disease in slaughtered animals as a hospital pathologist would be for the diseased states of the human body if he had only the muscles to look at. It is not in the meat market that the inspector should be stationed, but in the slaughter-house; and as there are a good many thousands of slaughter-houses all over the country, the efficient control of the meat-supply would require a good many thousand inspectors. Slaughter-houses may be licensed, but they are not inspected; there is hardly any limit to the number of them, and many of them are situated in sufficiently obscure corners. They are among the dark places of the earth, and—we say it advisedly, and with no rhetorical intention—they are full of abominations. Let the Inspector of the Central London Meat Market betake himself to one of the great slaughter-houses (or rather, groups of small slaughter-houses) in London; let him especially direct his attention to the old cows, or to other animals of the skin-and-bone kind; let him observe especially the lungs, the lymphatic glands, and the serous membranes,—and he will find occasion to condemn, not one animal in a month, but half a dozen animals a day. If he looks merely at the dressed carcase, he will be surprised that the "rickle of bones" which he saw alive should look so presentable when skinned, eviscerated, and hung up by the heels. But the chances are that the carcase, however presentable, would never have come under his notice if he had remained at Smithfield. No one pretends to say that the meat from a cow whose lungs are riddled with purulent cavities is prime meat; on the contrary, it is fit only for sausage-meat, and it is sold at the moderate rate of about fourpence per pound. The butcher who sends the quarters of an old tuberculous cow to a great public meat market is either too ambitious or he does not know his business. Those of them who are caught and are fined at the Guildhall Court are weaker brethren. The unscrupulous members of a class of tradesmen which is for the most part a respectable class, are also knowing

enough to have the joints and parts of a suspected carcase reduced as soon as possible to the small and safe condition in which it is introduced into sausages, and sometimes even into tins.

The present state of the law regarding the meat-supply of the kingdom is barely befitting the intelligence, the wealth, and the business capacity of the nation. Those of us who stand nearest to the law-making and administrative class have perhaps little to complain of; we buy prime joints, and, generally speaking, we avoid beef-sausages, sausage-rolls, meat pies, and all other manufactured forms of bovine flesh. But the multitude, which has little money to spend, and much appetite, requires to be protected from the ignorance, if not the conscious villany, of those who supply it with meat. It is a disgrace to the municipal government of London that there are no public *abattoirs* open to the light of day and to official inspection. It is a not less discreditable circumstance—one that carries us back to the time when there were witches and wise women—that there should be in almost every agricultural centre, be it large village or small town, a butcher or dealer of shady reputation, who is known to the farmers round about to have always a market for a wasting or diseased animal. The farmer asks a price which is calculated independently of the flesh, and he makes no further inquiries. The business of the shady butcher is known in its further details only within a small closed circle. There is, in the minds of all parties concerned, a vague consciousness of something not quite right; but there is naturally a want of pathological knowledge such as would be a law unto itself, and there is equally a want of restraint imposed by a paternal legislature. It is the duty of our profession and of the veterinary profession to announce that there may be injurious properties in meat which neither the eye of the Inspector at Smithfield nor the palate of the consumer are likely to detect. It is our duty to point out that the juices of the flesh are largely the same as the fluid of the blood; that all the blood of the body is constantly being sent through the lungs; and that the lungs of many old cows, and of not a few young bulls, steers, and heifers, present a spectacle of tuberculous disease which is no less revolting to the eye of an uninstructed person than it is alarming to the comprehensive intelligence of a pathologist.

THE NATURAL HISTORY OF UTERINE FIBROIDS.
I.

IN deciding as to whether a method of treatment is worth trying or not, the first thing we want to know is, what will be the course of the disease if it be let alone? There are only too many morbid conditions in which this elementary and fundamental question cannot be answered with any degree of precision. Among these stands the one mentioned in our title. Although we know in a general way what changes *may* take place in a uterine fibroid, yet we are still unable, in any particular case, to predict its course; to say how big it will grow, what symptoms it will cause, whether such symptoms will spontaneously cease or not, or even whether life will be endangered. Not only is this the case, but opinions differ much as to the frequency with which the different terminations which are possible actually occur.

Any record of experience which bears on these points is therefore worthy of study. Dr. Roehrig, a physician practising at Kreuznach—a place which, as everyone knows, is much frequented by those who suffer from uterine fibroids,—has analysed the cases which have come under his care, and published in the *Zeitschrift für Geburtshülfe und Gynäkologie* an account of what he has seen.

Dr. Roehrig has had under his charge 570 cases of these-tumours. Of these, 108 he has had under observation for five or more years, some as long as ten years; 165 he has watched for periods between three and five years; and the remaining 297 cases have been under his notice for less than three years.

The first point Dr. Roehrig speaks of is the *rate of growth* of these neoplasms. Here he can find no law. Not only do tumours of apparently the same kind grow, some slowly, some quickly, but even the same tumour will for a time grow, and for a time remain stationary or appear to diminish. Five times he has seen tumours grow to the size of a child's head within a year; in forty-two other cases the growth in the space of ten years did not get larger than a hen's egg; and in one case a tumour of the bigness of an apple remained stationary for twelve years, and then suddenly within two years grew till it equalled a man's head in volume. There are conditions which favour and hinder rapid growth : soft vascular tumours having a large attachment to the uterus grow faster than hard, slightly vascular, or pedunculated tumours ; and tumours having a thick pedicle are more likely to grow fast than those that have a thin one. Their growth is also stimulated by the determination of blood to the pelvic organs which attends menstruation and pregnancy. But it does not follow that amenorrhœa has any effect in retarding their growth; our author has seen nineteen cases, all of them subperitoneal tumours, in which during periods of amenorrhœa varying from six to fourteen months the new growths steadily increased in size; in one case, a fibroid the size of an apple grew, during fourteen months' absence of menstruation, to be as large as a man's head, and naturally led to the supposition that pregnancy existed—an idea negatived by the return of menstruation. Any cause leading to congestion of the pelvic organs, active or passive, tends, in Dr. Roehrig's opinion, to favour the growth of neoplasms; thus diseases leading to increased menstrual congestion, valvular disease of the heart, portal congestion, injuries to the generative organs, constipation, too active local treatment of uterine disease, anæmia, etc. —all have more or less effect in stimulating the production and growth of uterine fibroids. Out of his 570 cases, 46 suffered from valvular disease of the heart. The effect of pregnancy upon such tumours is well known. Our author has seen a tumour quadruple its bulk during pregnancy. He has never known a patient who had a submucous tumour become pregnant, and only two in whom interstitial tumours were present; in both of these, at the termination of the lying-in, the tumour had become submucous.

The most important part of the subject relates to the methods by which nature sometimes effects a cure, and the frequency with which such spontaneous cures occur. First, it is the rule, especially with subperitoneal tumours, that at the climacteric they cease to grow, and undergo retrograde changes. They generally retard the occurrence of the menopause ; thus in more than 60 of our author's cases menstruation persisted to the fifty-sixth year, and in 4 as late as the age of sixty. The rule was, that in from one to three years after the climacteric, it became evident that the tumour had ceased to grow. Only in 19 cases has Dr. Roehrig known it otherwise ; in these the interval between the menopause and the quiescence of the tumour was from four to ten years.

Spontaneous *cure* takes place either by the absorption or expulsion of the tumour. Out of our author's 570 cases, there were 10 in which the tumour disappeared by *absorption*. Of these, in 7 it took place during the involution of the uterus after labour, and in 1 after abortion; in 2 it occurred independently of pregnancy. The author very correctly says, that many of the so-called cases of spontaneous absorption of uterine fibroids are simply instances of diagnostic errors; the exudations due to pelvic peritonitis and hæmatocele being

especially likely to lead to this mistake. Spontaneous absorption is so rare as to be a kind of clinical curiosity, not at all to be counted on in framing a prognosis for a particular case.

Spontaneous *expulsion* takes place indubitably, and much more frequently. Four times Dr. Roehrig has seen this take place by suppuration of the capsule of interstitial tumours, which were thus spontaneously enucleated and expelled. This process, in his experience, seems to be almost free from risk. Far more commonly, the suppurative process is not confined to the capsule, but affects the tumour itself. Our author has seen this 57 times. In 3 only of these were the growths subperitoneal, and in them the inflammation appeared to have been started by a contusion. In 28 there was more or less calcareous degeneration of the expelled tumour, leading to the supposition that diminished blood-supply had led first to degeneration, then to necrosis. In 5 the process took origin in an abortion; in 4 it was thought due to the irritation of pessaries; and in the same number to strangulation of a partly expelled tumour by the contracting uterus. In the remainder the cause could not be made out. Of the 57 only 5 ended in complete cure. Seventeen times a considerable part of the tumour was expelled, and then the eliminative process and the growth of the tumour alike came to a standstill. Twenty-six of the patients died. The termination in the remaining 9 the author was not able to ascertain. Thus, putting together all the cases in which nature attempted to effect a cure, we have 22 in which her efforts were successful, against 26 in which the patient succumbed during the process.

Dr. Roehrig holds that fibroids become the subject of *cancerous* change oftener than is supposed. In 24 out of his 570 cases he believes this has happened. In 7 of these the primary disease was seated in some other part; in 14 no such primary disease was discovered; and in 3 it was demonstrated by autopsy that all the other organs were healthy.

The next point upon which the author has analysed his experience is the effect of fibroids upon the uterus. It is known that they distort the shape and alter the position of this organ. In 120 of Dr. Roehrig's cases such was their effect. As the precise kind of deviation produced is subject to almost infinite variation, we need not quote the author's classification of the deformities so produced.

IS MARSH POISON A MYTH?

THE transitional progress of the medical agnostic from the point at which, having emerged from the darkness of plausible theory, he struggles honestly, cautiously, and laboriously forward, through the twilight of speculation and experiment, into the full dawn of perfected discovery, is deeply interesting to all true men of science. Nevertheless, sympathy with the doubter is liable to be suspended whenever we observe that, in a blind struggle for change, he blunders into some new darkness, imagining it to be light, and is satisfied to prefer a shallow new theory to a well-grounded old one. None can be more willing than we are to admit that those physicians who, in the present day, refuse to adhere to the old belief in the existence of a marsh poison as a true entity, are doing good, if it be only in promoting discussion upon an unsettled question of vast practical importance; but we consider it to be undeniable that, when they endeavour to convince us that the paludal influence is simply the combined effect of climatic causes, such as cold, heat, damp, and extreme vicissitudes of temperature (which used to be recognised, not as the true causes, but merely as the *exciting* causes of marsh fever), they do no more than conduct us into new obscurity, offering us doctrines which are quite as theoretical as those held by

Lancisi and Maculloch, and very far less probable. The profession are indebted to Deputy Surgeon-General W. J. Moore for a monograph(a) in which he sets forth the steps by which he has succeeded in persuading himself that such a thing as marsh poison has no existence. The compilation of opinions which Dr. Moore adduces, as leading him up to this conclusion, is long and careful. We regret that we cannot accept it as a perfectly full and fair exposition of all the facts at issue. Anyone who may desire to enter into a thorough investigation of this question will find it useful, but its practical value would be enhanced ten-fold if it could be re-edited by two other scientists, one an advocate of the old views, the other a practical investigator of the germ-doctrine; or perhaps we should rather say, by one who, having in mind the observations of the Maculloch school, follows diligently in the path of microscopical research thrown open by Klebs, Tommasi-Crudeli, and Sternberg. We think it especially to be regretted that men who, like the propounders of the climatic theory of paludal influence in America and India, dwell in the very hotbeds of that influence, whatever it may be, with every facility for practical observation in their hospitals and at their very doors, should, at this very critical stage of inquiry, prefer theory to physical research, employing the pen instead of the microscope and test-tube in their attempts to elicit new truth. Dr. Moore is by no means the only clever advocate of the Climatic theory who, without, as it would appear, having attempted to follow practically the researches of the *savants* of Austria, Rome, and New Orleans, puts aside the whole doctrine of paludal microphytes with easy incredulity. It is by no means impossible that future research may dismiss the at present much-vexed *Bacillus malariæ*, as a detected pretender to the status of a specific virus, "to the base mud from which it sprung—unwept, unhonoured, and unsung." Still it is, just now, a very substantial little entity, which will not allow itself to be reasoned into space, any more than the hind leg of a sagacious domestic quadruped admits of being resolved by argument into its elements. We should occupy unnecessary time and space in attempting to combat the reasonings upon which Dr. Moore has succeeded in convincing himself that marshes are not the source of a specific poison, but that arid sandy wastes and dry mountain ravines are the natural *habitats* of ague and remittent fevers. We have merely to remark (1) that a sandy desert, destitute of trees and hill-ranges, capable of arresting the course of malaria, is no defence against winds laden with the emanations of very distant terais, jheels, and jungles; and (2) that, although Dr. Moore has been rather cautious in citing the authority of William Fergusson (who, true man of science as he was, was not strong upon the doctrine of microphytes), those who deny that there is a marsh-poison attach the greatest weight to Fergusson's narrative of a remittent fever which arose among troops encamped in "the half-dried ravine," "which had lately been a water-course," "from the stony bed of which (as soil never could lie for the torrents) the very existence even of vegetation was impossible."(b) Upon this we have to suggest that botany has made some progress since the year 1809, and that "the half-dried ravine" and "the stagnant pools of water that were still left among the rocks" are, we apprehend, precisely the localities in which our microscopists would expect to discover the *Bacillus malariæ* in its highest perfection.

Dr. Moore further argues, "It is stated that the *Bacillus* prevails in the greatest quantity during the heat of the summer, while we, in India, know that malarial fevers are most common in the autumnal season, and for some time after the commencement of the cold weather. It is therefore believed that *Bacillus malariæ* will not account for the universal prevalence of malarious disease." Upon this we have to remark that the autumnal and cold seasons of India are what may be termed the *drying up* time, at which the leaves of deciduous plants die and rot, and the water of tanks, jheels, and mountain torrents either disappears or becomes "thick and slab" with the products of organic decomposition. This autumnal and cold weather follows immediately, with little or no break, upon that terrible hot season which immediately succeeds the rains, and which leaves everyone more or less debilitated and prone to suffer from the diseases of that climate. Again, would it not be better to search for the *Bacillus* in the marshes which lie only too close to the Bombay Club, to inoculate monkeys (which are not subject to ague and remittent fever), as Dr. Vandyke Carter did with the *Spirillum*, and then to discuss this question further? We thank Dr. Moore for his thoughtful memoir, which is a very well-assorted piece of medical mosaic work; but its subject is one upon which, in our present state of mind, we should prefer one observation by, say, Burdon-Sanderson to any number of arguments, however elaborate. An Indian anecdote will fairly illustrate our opinion of this narrative. A high official, having received a report which contained a great deal of showy argument, handed it to his Hindoo clerk, saying, "Read that, Baboo, and give me your opinion upon it." The reply was, "Very fine report, O protector of the poor, *but vouchers not got!*" The sensible Indian practice being not to look at a bill unless the voucher be attached to it.

<hr>

THE WEEK.

TOPICS OF THE DAY.

THE inaugural address at the Sanitary Institute for the session 1881-82 was recently delivered, by Dr. Alfred Carpenter, at the rooms in Conduit-street. In the outset of his address Dr. Carpenter congratulated his hearers on the position attained by the Institute, and asserted that the list of surveyors and inspectors of nuisances who had come forward to obtain its diploma testified to the work which was being done, while the ignorance evinced by some of the rejected candidates, already holding office under local boards and town councils, proved the necessity for that work. The Institute, by its diplomas, sought to remove one of the many evils exposed by the Social Science Association, viz., that there were no means of knowing the duties of sanitary inspectorship except learning them after appointment. The existence of fever in our midst was, Dr. Carpenter said, one of the subjects interesting to the members as students of the science of health. Unfortunately, in grappling with this, we were hindered by a conflict of authority; the police had the care of lodging-houses, but had nothing to do with the houses unregistered, and the sanitary authority had no right of entry at night. Germs of typhus and relapsing fever were sometimes spread broadcast before the disease was suspected. The right of entering any house let out in tenements and suspected of being overcrowded, should be given, he considered, to the sanitary authority, who should also look after lodging-houses with the assistance of the police. Dr. Carpenter next referred to the quality of the London water-supply, and predicted a fearful epidemic some day for every part of the metropolis but that supplied by the Kent Water Company. The only remedy was the exclusion of crude sewage from the Thames above the intake of the water companies, and making the sewers self-cleansing, instead of being, as they now are, simply sewers of deposit. In conclusion, he said the Institute proposed to educate the community by imbuing

(a) "Malaria v. Recognizable Climatic Influences" (*Indian Medical Gazette* for November 1, 1881).
(b) "Notes and Recollections of a Professional Life," page 187.

sanitary authorities with the conviction that the best way to do a thing was to know how to do it, and that the diploma of the Institute afforded the best guarantee that a surveyor or inspector was thoroughly competent. He hoped before long they would obtain a charter of incorporation from the Government.

A conference of the friends and supporters of the Association for Promoting Trained Nursing in Workhouse Infirmaries was recently held in the board-room of the Marylebone Infirmary. Mr. Boulnois, chairman of the Marylebone Board of Guardians, was called to the chair, and amongst those present were Sir Francis Burdett, Bart., Drs. Dallas, Rogers, Lloyd, Sieveking, and Baker, etc., with several ladies, including Miss L. Twining, the Honorary Secretary of the Association. Several papers were read, including a letter from Miss Florence Nightingale, recording her deep sympathy with the objects of the Association. An animated discussion followed, in which several members of boards of guardians and others took part, all recognising the urgent necessity for trained superintendents and nurses in all workhouse and other infirmaries.

The West Ham Local Board is to be commended for taking action under the following circumstances. Charles Hiscock, of Plaistow, was summoned for wilfully disobeying an order, made on September 30 last, for his removal to a small-pox hospital whilst suffering from small-pox. Mr. Layard, on behalf of the Local Board, said that these proceedings had been taken under Section 124 of the Public Health Act, which provided for the isolation of diseases of an infectious nature. The Local Board in this case did not wish a heavy penalty to be imposed, but only desired that their powers in the matter of infectious diseases might be made known to the public. The Chief Sanitary Inspector to the Local Board deposed that he received from the magistrate, under his signature and seal, an order to remove the defendant, his wife, and child, to the small-pox hospital of the West Ham Union, but that order the defendant refused to obey, although he, his wife, and the child were at that time each suffering from the disease. The child has since died. The dimensions of the room in which they were living was 1000 cubic feet, while the poor-law regulations required 1200 cubic feet for each person. The magistrate, after pointing out the importance of isolation in diseases of an infectious nature, said that as the Local Board did not wish to press the charge vindictively, he would only impose a fine of 10s., and the costs 8s.

At the last meeting of the Whitechapel District Board of Works the sanitary inspector reported that, upon visiting some houses in Pelham-street, Spitalfields, he found a serious case of overcrowding in the ground-floor back room of No. 11 in that street. The room is used by a foreigner for a school in which young children are taught the Hebrew language, and at the time of the visit there were twenty-five children in the place, besides the master and his wife. The room was nine feet long, eight feet wide, and eight feet high, thus giving only twenty-one cubic feet of space for each child. The inspector ascertained that at times a much larger number of children attended the school. Independently of the size of the room, the place was totally unfit for a school in consequence of its confined situation. The atmosphere of the room was overpowering, and the children looked pale and sickly. The authorities had to deal with the same offender for a similar nuisance in Spitalfields a few years ago. An order was issued to enable the inspector to take legal proceedings for the suppression of the nuisance.

The Board of Trade has obtained from America one of the instruments devised by Dr. William Thomson, Professor of Ophthalmology in the Jefferson Medical College, for detecting colour-blindness. The instrument is arranged on the system of Professor Holmgren of Sweden, and has been used in examining the employés of the Pennsylvania Railway, its great utility consisting in the fact that any intelligent non-medical person may, by its means, make what may be called the coarse examination needed to decide whether anyone should be passed on to the ophthalmic surgeon for further and closer examination. The instrument consists of two flat narrow sticks, each about two feet long, hinged together at one end. To one of these sticks forty worsted skeins are attached to little buttons hung upon hooks, so arranged that the buttons can be readily unhooked. The buttons are numbered from 1 to 40, and the other stick is shut down over the buttons so as to conceal the numbers and keep them in their places. When presented to the person to be examined, the instrument appears simply as forty skeins of different coloured worsted yarns hanging from a stick. The forty skeins are arranged upon a theory (which has been proved by experience) that it is only necessary to use the genuine tints of the three test-colours—green, rose, and red —and the "confusion" colours. This reduces Holmgren's 150 skeins to 40, and helps to shorten the examination. Beginning at the left hand, the first twenty numbers are devoted to the green test; the ten odd numbers are shades of green; the ten even numbers are "confusion" colours, such as greys, tans, light browns, etc. The skeins from 21 to 30 have rose or purple tints on the odd numbers, and blue tints on the even numbers. The remaining skeins—from 31 to 40 —have red tints on the odd numbers, and the "confusion" colours for red on the even numbers, such as browns, sages, and dark olives. A man placed before the instrument is first told to select ten skeins to match the green test skein which is shown him. If his sight is normal he quickly throws the ten green skeins over the stick, and a clerk recording the result will examine the buttons and put down the series of odd numbers from 1 to 19 as the entry upon a blank report arranged for the purpose. The normal eye will select only the odd-numbered green tints from the first half of the stick, while the colour-blind will hesitatingly select at random odd and even numbers all along the stick. The blank reports, properly filled up and sent to headquarters, tell the result in the case of each employé by the odd or even numbers recorded, and determine those men, if any, who should be further examined by a medical officer. On the Pennsylvania Railway 4·2 per cent. of the employés were detected to be colour-blind by this simple instrument, and it is stated that its adoption on both railways and vessels all over the United States will only be a question of time.

The Board of Delegates appointed to administer the Hospital Saturday Fund held last week their annual meeting at Charing-cross Hospital, Mr. S. Morley, M.P., presiding. The report of the Council showed that the total amount collected for the year was £8174, or £1540 more than the sum realised in 1880—an advance which is rightly not considered to adequately represent the artisans of the metropolis. It is satisfactory to learn that the expenditure has fallen from 14·66 to 13·15 per cent. on the total collected. The annual street collection of this year resulted in a gain of £2050, or 50 per cent. on the collection of 1880. Besides gold and silver, nearly two tons of bronze money were received from the 750 street stations. The next item of the report was the question of the direct representation of the Fund on the governing bodies of participating hospitals, and the results of an experiment made upon St. George's Hospital to obtain the concession of a life-governorship of that Hospital for the Fund. We are glad to observe that Mr. Morley said he regretted the step that had been taken in this direction by the Board, and warned them against attempting any principle of seeking a quid pro quo for their awards. The report was certainly more satisfactory when it recorded the labours of a special committee appointed to consider the question of establishing seaside convalescent homes for the benefit of London workmen. The need of more institutions of this kind being generally admitted, an appeal is suggested for a separate and special annual collection for this purpose. The report wound up by stating that since its institution, in the year 1874, the Fund had distributed £40,351 to the metropolitan hospitals and dispensaries. Before the adjournment of the meeting it was arranged, at the suggestion of the Chairman, that a general meeting should be held on January 21 next, to consider the important question of the proposed establishment of seaside convalescent homes in connexion with the Fund.

The annual general meeting of the friends and supporters of the Hospital Sunday Fund movement is announced to be held at the Mansion House on the 20th inst. In reference to previous discussion which has taken place on the subject, the Rev. Canon Spence, Vicar of St. Pancras, has given notice of motion to alter the constitution of the Fund, so as to allow a grant of 4 per cent. of the collection each year to be expended in the purchase of surgical appliances, instead of 2 per cent. as heretofore. To our view this would seem to be questionable policy, unless Canon Spence can adduce very special arguments to justify the alteration.

At a recent meeting of the Oldham Town Council, the Medical Officer of Health reported, in reference to the prevailing epidemic of typhoid fever in that town, that 72 cases had been notified to him. Of these 38 had been treated at their own homes, and 34 in the Corporation Hospital; 5 deaths had occurred amongst the former, and 3 amongst the latter; 9 patients had been discharged cured, and 55 were still under treatment. He believed that it might be said that the worst of the epidemic was now over.

THE ROYAL COLLEGE OF PHYSICIANS OF LONDON.

THE Gulstonian Lectures of the Royal College of Physicians for next year will be delivered at the College on March 3, 8, and 10 by Dr. W. Ewart, who has taken for his subject "Pulmonary Cavities: their Origin, Growth, and Repair." On March 15, 17, and 22 the Croonian Lectures will be given by Sir J. Fayrer, "On the Climate and Fevers of India." And on March 24, 29, and 31, Dr. Burdon Sanderson will give the Lumleian Lectures, taking for his subject "The Pathology of Inflammation." Dr. Long Fox, of Bristol, has been appointed Bradshaw Lecturer for 1882, and will deliver his lecture in August, "On the Position of the Sympathetic in the Causation of Disease."

SMALL-POX AND FEVER IN THE METROPOLIS.

AT the last meeting of the Metropolitan Asylums Board for the present year the returns from the various small-pox hospitals were presented, and showed an increase of 6 in the total number of patients remaining under treatment. At the Stockwell Asylum, 21 had been admitted, 3 had died, and 23 had been discharged, leaving 64 under treatment; at Deptford, 96 had been admitted, 21 had died, 67 had been discharged, leaving 152 under treatment; at Fulham, 9 had been discharged, and 24 remained under treatment; on the Atlas and Endymion, 31 had been admitted, 5 had died, and 25 had been discharged, leaving 151 under treatment. The fever returns showed an increase of 2 in the total number remaining under treatment. At Stockwell, 31 had been admitted, 4 had died, and 45 had been discharged, leaving 173 under treatment; at Deptford, 46 had been admitted, 4 had died, and 72 remained under treatment. After the transaction of other business, the Board adjourned until January 7, 1882.

UNIVERSITY HONOURS TO MEDICAL MEN.

AT a meeting held on the 10th inst., the Trustees of the University of Aberdeen unanimously resolved to confer the Honorary Degree of LL.D. of the University upon Dr. Andrew Clark, Physician to, and Lecturer on Medicine at, the London Hospital; and upon Sir Erasmus Wilson, President of the Royal College of Surgeons of England.

ON A NEW AID TO THE DIAGNOSIS OF UNILATERAL DISEASE OF THE KIDNEY.

DR. M. GLUCK sends a communication to the Centralblatt für Chirurgie for December 10, in which he refers to a new method of discovering in a case in which removal of one kidney seems advisable, whether or not the kidney of the opposite side retains any secreting substance. He proposes that as small an incision as possible shall be made over the kidney to be removed, and that then the ureter shall be sought, and compressed either by a temporary ligature or the application of a pair of forceps. When this is done, some material which is certain to make its appearance rapidly in the urine, such as ferrocyanide of potassium or iodide of soda, is to be injected subcutaneously, and successive drops of urine are to be tested for the presence of the drug by means of a catheter introduced into the bladder. It seems to be suggested that the appearance of the material injected in the secretion of the opposite kidney will be a justification to proceed with the operation, though we must confess to certain misgivings on this head. We can conceive a very imperfect kidney—that is to say, one that would be far from sufficiently healthy to fulfil the whole requirements of the body—which might still secrete enough of the injected material to allow of its being rapidly discovered in the urine; and thus it appears to us that the test might give undue confidence to the operator. If, after a sufficient time has been allowed to elapse, the urine from the presumably unaffected side gives no reaction, it is advised to release the ureter of the diseased side, and test the urine coming from it. The writer adds that the experiment could not be made in cases where, owing to anatomical complications, the ureter of the affected kidney could not be reached; and that it would prove delusive if there happened to be a horse-shoe kidney, the existence of which would, of course, seriously interfere with the diagnosis under any circumstances.

INFECTIOUS HOSPITALS IN LIVERPOOL.

Now that a Royal Commission has been appointed to inquire into the subject of hospitals for the treatment of infectious diseases in the metropolis, it will not be uninteresting to consider what provision is made in the second city of the kingdom for isolating patients suffering from zymotic disorders. The required information is afforded in the last annual report of Dr. J. Stopford Taylor, Medical Officer of Health, on the health of Liverpool during the year 1880. From this report it is to be gathered that for the accommodation and treatment of infectious disease the Select Vestry have a hospital at Brownlow-hill, the West Derby Guardians one in Mill-road, Everton, and the Toxteth Guardians another in Smithdown-road. Patients are admitted into these institutions free of charge. There is also another hospital for infectious disease, situated in Netherfield-road, supported by voluntary contributions and payment by patients, the charges being from 10s. 6d. to £2 2s. per week, according to accommodation. The Corporation contributed £5000 towards its erection; and owing to the diminishing number of fever cases the funds were so reduced that further application was made for assistance. In order to extend its usefulness, and offer an inducement to the public to avail themselves of its advantages, the Corporation have since undertaken to pay an annual sum of £250, provided that twenty-five beds be placed at the disposal of the Medical Officer of Health at the reduced charge of 7s. a week payable by each patient. The importance of early isolation of cases of infectious disease, Dr. Taylor adds, cannot be too strongly urged upon the attention of the public, as affording the most effectual measure for limiting the spread of contagion ; and the small charge thus made will enable many persons to avail themselves of private hospital treatment who had hitherto objected to entering parish hospitals. Dr. Taylor makes no complaint on the score of sufficiency, but relatively this would appear to be a much smaller provision than what is required to meet the wants of London.

THE PARIS WEEKLY RETURN.

THE number of deaths for the forty-eighth week, terminating December 1, was 948 (547 males and 401 females), and among these there were from typhoid fever 31, small-pox 10, measles 11, scarlatina 3, pertussis 5, diphtheria and croup 64, erysipelas 11, and puerperal infections 7. There were also 41 deaths from tubercular and acute meningitis, 38 from acute bronchitis, 52 from pneumonia, 80 from infantile athrepsia (29 of the infants having been wholly or partially suckled), and 30 violent deaths (27 males and 3 females). The mortality is very low for the time of year—a circumstance due to the fineness of the weather,—and diphtheria and erysipelas are the only diseases that have exhibited any increase. It is observable that all ages have participated in this attenuation of mortality except infants under a twelvemonth, 180 of these having died in place of 159—doubtless due to the fact that the mild temperature which has proved so favourable to the higher economies does so also to minute organisms, and consequently to the fermentations which so easily induce alterations in the food given to young infants. The births for the week amounted to 1136, viz., 561 males (415 legitimate and 146 illegitimate) and 575 females (414 legitimate and 161 illegitimate) ; 92 infants (43 males and 49 females) were born dead or died within twenty-four hours.

THE ELASTIC LIGATURE IN THE ABDOMINAL EXTIRPATION OF UTERINE FIBROIDS.

ONE of the chief difficulties in the extirpation by laparotomy of uterine fibroids has been to find some trustworthy method of securing the stump. The pedicle, being formed of muscular tissue, contracts, so that the clamp or ligature, a few hours after it has been applied, will have become loose. In a recent number of the *Archiv für Gynäkologie* a case is recorded in which the elastic ligature was successfully employed. It occurred in the clinique of Professor Olshausen, and is reported by Dr. E. Schwarz. The tumour, before operation, was supposed to be ovarian ; its smoothness, the sense of pseudo-fluctuation which was felt over it, and the facts that it pressed down the uterus (which could thus be palpated per vaginam apparently throughout its whole length) and that a rounded elastic segment of the tumour could be felt below the uterus, being the features which led to this error. An incision having been made, and the tumour exposed, a trocar was thrust into it, but nothing escaped. The opening was then enlarged with the knife, and a quantity of opaque, reddish-brown, thin fluid, and a mass of decolourised blood-clot as big as two fists (in all, weighing about thirty pounds), was removed. The incision having been prolonged upwards, and thus the bulk of the tumour (which was found to grow from the upper and posterior part of the uterus) got outside the abdomen, a piece of india-rubber drainage-tubing was made fast round its pedicle to control hæmorrhage. Then the tumour, the solid, part of which weighed twelve pounds and a half,

was excised the pedicle, being left of a funnel shape; the arteries visible were separately taken up and tied, and the sides of the hollowed-out pedicle were brought together by superficial and deep sutures. The india-rubber tubing was then taken off ; but blood welled up from the pedicle in such quantity as to call for some mode of stopping it which would not involve delay. A piece of india-rubber tubing about the thickness of a goose-quill was therefore put twice round the pedicle and tied. Between the two bands of tubing the stump was transfixed with a long needle, and it was then made fast to the abdominal walls, drainage-tubes were inserted, and antiseptic dressings applied. The part outside the ligature was nearly as big as the fist. The operation lasted one hour and three-quarters. In the evening the dressings were found soaked through, and on removing them, it was discovered that the needle had broken, and the stump dropped into the abdominal cavity. The ends of the elastic ligature were still outside. As there were no bad symptoms, it was not thought necessary to interfere further. The drainage-tubes were removed on the fourth day. The elastic ligature and the detached part of the pedicle came away on the seventeenth day. The patient did well. Dr. Schwarz suggests some ingenious modifications in the mode of applying the elastic ligature ; and Professor Olshausen (who adds some comments) expresses himself as without doubt that the elastic ligature is destined to play a large part in the treatment of cases similar to the one described. We may add that a volume of *Beiträge* recently published to commemorate the jubilee of Professor Credé's occupation of his chair, contains a communication by Dr. Leopold, of Leipzig, bearing on the same subject.

OBSTETRICAL SOCIETY OF LONDON.

THE following gentlemen have been nominated by the Council as officers of this Society for 1882 (those marked with an asterisk did not hold the same office, or were not on the Council, during 1881) :—*Honorary President :* Arthur Farre, M.D., F.R.S. *President :* J. Matthews Duncan, M.D. *Vice-Presidents :* John Bassett, M.D. ; Jonathan Hutchinson, F.R.C.S. ; *John Brunton, M.D. ; *Clement Godson, M.D. ; John Thorburn, M.D. ; John Williams, M.D. *Treasurer :* *J. Baptiste Potter, M.D. *Secretaries :* A. L. Galabin, M.D. ; *G. Ernest Herman, M.B. *Honorary Librarian :* F. H. Champneys, M.D. *Council :* Henry Oldham, M.D. ; Robert Barnes, M.D. ; J. Hall Davis, M.D. ; Graily Hewitt, M.D. ; J. Braxton Hicks, M.D., F.R.S. ; E. Till, M.D. ; W. O. Priestley, M.D. ; T. Spencer Wells, F.R.C.S. ; W. S. Playfair, M.D. ; *H. C. Andrews, M.D. ; *J. Ford Anderson, M.D. ; *G. P. Bate, M.D. ; J. Henry Bennett, M.D. ; *P. L. Burchell, M.B. ; C. H. Carter, M.D. ; *E. Charles, M.D. ; Edward Malins, M.D. ; G. E. Ord, Esq. ; D. Lloyd Roberts, M.D. ; F. W. Salsmann, Esq. ; C. Brodie Sewell, M.D. ; *J. Knowsley Thornton, Esq. ; *W. H. Strange, M.D. ; F. Wallace, Esq. ; G. E. Yarrow, M.D.

PATHOLOGICAL SOCIETY OF DUBLIN.

AT the meeting of this Society held on Saturday, December 10 (the President, Dr. W. Stokes, in the chair), Dr. J. M. Finny showed a specimen of pericarditis in a man aged forty-two, a discharged soldier of ten years' service, who had suffered severely from scarlet fever six or seven years ago. Chest symptoms set in a year back. The patient was intemperate. There were great dyspnœa, cyanosis, and ultimately evidences of pleuro-pneumonia and capillary suffo-cative bronchitis. The feet were œdematous, and a triple murmur was heard at the base of the heart. After death both pleuræ were found adherent. There was œdema and hepatisation of the right lung; in the left lung there was a hæmorrhagic infarction. Four ounces of reddish fluid escaped from the pericardium, which was the seat of a recent dry pericarditis. The heart, with the pericardium and vessels, weighed thirty-two ounces and a half; the left ventricle was excentrically hypertrophied; the mitral orifice was dilated; one of the aortic valves was incompetent. Cretaceous matter was deposited in the aorta. There was a small aneurism of the descending aorta. The liver showed the nutmeg appearance and commencing cirrhosis. The kidneys were enlarged and firm; the left kidney weighed nine ounces and a half, the right ten ounces. The spleen was hard and firm. Mr. W. T. Stoker showed the right upper extremity, portion of the thorax and of the spinal column and spinal cord of a cabman, aged sixty years, who presented a five years' history of progressive muscular atrophy. The patient had been obese, but of temperate habits. Nearly all the muscles supplied by the branches of the brachial plexus below the clavicle were much wasted, and in a condition of advanced fatty degeneration. The latissimus dorsi, deltoid, triceps, and the two teres, were all fatty; there were fatty streaks in the biceps. The muscles of the front of the forearm were much altered, with the exception of the pronator quadratus, which was spared. The muscles on the back of the forearm had suffered to a less degree. The interossei and lumbricales with the muscles of the thumb and little finger were much atrophied. An exostosis engaged the fourth, fifth, sixth, and seventh cervical vertebræ, causing anchylosis of the last three. The anterior nerve-roots on the right side were atrophied, and Mr. P. S. Abraham, who examined the cord microscopically, reported that two portions near the anterior horns of grey matter stained more deeply with picrocarmine than elsewhere. Mr. Stoker pointed out that probably all the assigned causes of Cruveilhier's paralysis—viz., overwork, exposure, and injury—were present in this case. An interesting discussion followed, in which Dr. R. McDonnell, Dr. H. Kennedy, and Professor Bennett took part. Mr. H. G. Croly exhibited a specimen of the rodent ulcer described by the late Dr. Arthur Jacob in the *Dublin Hospital Reports*, vol. iv., in 1827. The subject of the disease was a man aged fifty-eight. The new growth had been of thirteen years' standing, and, as is usual in these cases, it had commenced as a little pimple near the inner canthus. A discussion ensued, in which most of the speakers maintained the epitheliomatous nature of the neoplasm. Mr. Abraham, who had examined the present specimen, described it as a cylindroma.

THE REGISTRAR-GENERAL OF SCOTLAND'S REPORT FOR THE THIRD QUARTER OF THE YEAR 1881.

THE births registered in Scotland during the third quarter of the present year amounted to 31,158; they were consequently at the rate of 333 to every 10,000 of the estimated population, and represent an annual birth-rate of 3·33 per cent. Of the eight principal towns, Leith had the highest and Perth the lowest birth-rate. The illegitimate births were most frequent in the North-Eastern, and least frequent in the North-Western Division; thus, in Wigtownshire the rated exceeded 17 per cent., while in Ross and Cromarty it was only 3·3 per cent. The number of deaths registered in Scotland during the period was 15,602, being in the proportion of 167 deaths to every 10,000 of estimated population. The average death-rate of the corresponding quarter of the ten preceding years having been 192 per 10,000 of population, the death-rate of this third quarter of the year 1881 must be regarded as unusually favourable. Of the principal towns, Paisley had the highest and Aberdeen the lowest death-rate. Zymotic diseases caused 293 deaths

in July, 374 in August, and 354 in September; these deaths constituted 17·9 per cent. of all deaths registered during the quarter and referred to specified causes. There were 3 deaths from small-pox, 1 occurring in Leith, 1 in Perth, and 1 in Edinburgh; all the patients had attained the age of at least twenty years. To violent deaths 57 cases were referred in July, 79 in August, and 60 in September; of these only 8 were returned as from suicide, but it must be remembered that, as there are no coroners' inquests in Scotland, the registrars there cannot present an accurate or complete list of the cases of suicide that occur from time to time. The remaining features of the quarter's mortality call for no special comment. During July the weather was characterised by great prevalence of west wind, accompanied by a barometric pressure slightly below the average; the mean temperature was lower than the average. The main characteristic of August was its low mean temperature, accompanied by a low barometer, small range of temperature, greater depth of rainfall, but rather less humidity in the air, and more north wind than usual for the month. September was of a-dull, cloudy, rather cold and humid character, with preponderance of east over west winds. The barometric pressure did not vary much, and the strength of the wind was less than usual.

ELECTION OF PROFESSOR PASTEUR.

PROFESSOR PASTEUR was elected, December 7, a member of the Académie Française, in place of the late M. Littré, by the votes of twenty of the thirty-three members who were present.

SURGICAL INTERFERENCE IN PULMONARY AFFECTIONS.

IN a recent number of the *Nordiskt Medicinskt Arkiv*, Dr. Edouard Bull, of Christiania, discusses the question of treating certain serious kinds of pulmonary disease by surgical means. He thinks that when a sufficient supply of materials is obtained to show in what cases such treatment is applicable, it will be seen that internal diseases offer a new field for successful surgical operations, and he contributes two cases from the practice of the Christiania Hospital in support of his views. One of these was treated successfully by operative means; the other was not so treated, and terminated fatally. But Dr. Bull conceives that in this also a successful result might have been obtained by the aid of surgery. The first case was one of circumscribed pulmonary gangrene in a female of twenty-three years old. It was found that there existed a gangrenous cavity in the superior lobe of the left lung, pretty clearly limited in extent and very near the thoracic wall. The general condition of the patient was bad, and the chances of cure by purely medical treatment were unpromising, but as the local position of the disease seemed favourable for operative proceedings, Dr. Bull determined to open the gangrenous cavity from without. The operation was accordingly performed, and a quantity of fœtid pus was discharged. The cavity in which this pus had been contained was circumscribed, and, on feeling within it, the pulsations of the heart could be perceived. It was slightly washed with a weak solution of carbolic acid, and drainage was established. Soon afterwards the local and general symptoms rapidly improved, and although at first the wound discharged some dirty and fœtid pus, yet at the end of three days the expectoration became scanty and without fœtor; and, after some fluctuations, convalescence was set up in about six weeks from the admission of the patient; and the cure, although slow, was at last complete. In the second case, which was that of a female of fifty-four years old, there was pleuro-pneumonia resulting in an abscess in the superior lobe of the left lung. The patient was awoke in the night with coughing and choking, and she died in about a quarter of an hour after expectorating a large quantity of fœtid pus. On the autopsy a circumscribed cavity was found in the left lung, from which the pus had passed into the pharynx, the larynx, the trachea, and the large bronchi, thus producing suffocation. The author conceives that the fatal result might have been prevented by an operation, which could have been performed without the least danger, and, at the worst, might have led only to a permanent pulmonary fistula. In commenting upon the cases, Dr. Bull observes that the pathological alterations of the lung which may become the subjects of surgical operation are cavities of all kinds—namely, limited gangrenous excavations, pulmonary abscesses, and phthisical and bronchiectatic cavernous spaces. The first two are perfectly curable if the loss of substance be not too great, and the lungs are in all other respects sufficiently healthy; but in all cases the pulmonary cavity should be near the surface of the lung, for unless it be so it is impossible to determine its position with accuracy or to reach it without danger. In cases of cavities due to phthisis or bronchiectasis, Dr. Bull expresses himself more doubtfully, but he still thinks that operative interference might be justifiable where there are large isolated cavities with stagnant contents, or where their evacuation by coughing is exceedingly distressing to the patient. In the case of phthisical cavities there would remain undoubtedly a permanent fistula; but in those due to bronchiectasis, obliteration might be possible, and consequently a radical and perfect cure.

DEATH OF PROFESSOR BUSCH.

THE University of Bonn has sustained a great and unexpected loss of its celebrated Professor of Surgery, who died recently, after a short illness, of typhlitis, in the fifty-fifth year of his age. A short time since the jubilee of the twenty-fifth year of his professorship was celebrated with great enthusiasm; and a few months since he had the opportunity of exhibiting the precision of his diagnosis and his great operative skill in the severe affection of which the Empress of Germany was the subject. He belonged to that group of the pupils of John Müller—as Billroth, Wilms, and others (Deutsche Med. Woch.)—who, first inspired by their great master with the love of anatomico-physiological studies, afterwards became celebrated surgeons. After officiating for two years and a half as assistant to Müller, Busch took part in the Schleswig-Holstein War in 1848, and when this had terminated he devoted himself, under the direction of Langenbeck, exclusively to surgery. Having qualified himself as Privat-docent in Berlin in 1851, he received the appointment of Professor of Surgery at Bonn in 1855. He went through the wars of 1866 and 1870-71, the latter as consulting-surgeon. His earliest works related to comparative anatomy, and the later to surgery, in which the subjects of the influence of the mechanism of the joints in inflammation and dislocation, the mechanism of strangulated hernia, and gunshot wounds, became, among many others, objects of predilection.

SLOW PULSE.—Dr. Rice, of Bridgeport, Connecticut, gives the following account of personal observations on the rate of his heart-beat:—"Lying-down, 36; sitting, 36; standing, 41; after walking one mile, 48; after walking two miles, 46; after violent exercise, 52 per minute. Beats counted at the apex-beat to avoid error. The other members of my family have natural pulses. I first noted my peculiarity eight years ago, since which time it has not changed. I have no valvular lesion or other trouble of the organ, though it is at times a little irregular. My health is at all times excellent; my age is under thirty. I know of no cause for the slow rate."—New York Med. Record, Oct. 29.

THE BRIGHTON HEALTH CONGRESS AND SANITARY EXHIBITION.

(From our Special Correspondent.)

THE present is an age of "big" advertisements, and the caterers for popular entertainments in our big cities seem evidently imbued with the notion that the public are, moreover, omnivorous. As Brighton is the English home of the octopus, so a Sanitary Exhibition, to be a success, must include in the arms of its octopean embrace every collateral subject that is "likely to take" the popular fancy. The Executive at Brighton have shown great enterprise in the general get-up of this "nine-days' wonder," and considerable success is attending their efforts to interest and instruct their fellow-townsmen.

So varied is the nature of the several exhibits as displayed in the Corn Exchange and in the iron building specially erected in the Pavilion grounds, that it would be easy for a busy person not an epicure to make a fair meal en passant from the comestibles which delicate fingers offer for his reception. Here are dainty chops being grilled by gas-heat, the products of the gas being carefully drawn away from contact with the articles in the grill-chamber. In another department of the same furnace are potatoes being steamed and apples roasted. A few yards off is a slicing machine which will cut up a loaf of bread in a few seconds. The rambling excursionist is further admonished that if he wishes to avoid the half-cleansed forks and spoons of a café or restaurant, he can get a dozen such articles thoroughly cleaned by a few turns of the machine called "The Butler's Friend."

As he passes from the cooking stalls to the section for Food Products, the visitor is requested to take a savoury meat lozenge about the size of a sixpence, and supposed to contain the concentrated essence of a cup of strong beef-tea, and to give substantial support in a simple and convenient form. The Swiss Alpine Milk Company next attract attention. They are offering pure Swiss cow's milk preserved in its natural fluid state, maintaining the relative proportion of its constituents, without the addition of sugar or any other substance, and preserving all the properties of unskimmed milk. It is alleged in its support that "condensed milk" products are manufactured by a process which necessitates the removal of all the cream and most of the water of the milk, and the substitution thereof by cane sugar, so that the nutritious part of the milk is wanting, and a large quantity of sugar, which is injurious and liable to turn acid, is given to the infant; whereas, in the preparation under consideration, "nothing is taken from or added to the milk." Of course the taste is somewhat different to that of "new milk," and there are flocculi looking like curds floating in the milk. These solid particles are said to be condensed cream, and therefore easily dissolved.

As a finish-off to the varied repast I should recommend a "white wash" at the stall of one of the aërated water companies. The several manufacturers of hedozone, khushi, ferroxodone, sparkling vinita, ferroine, phosphodone, etc., are most anxious, each in his own way, to impress the thirsty traveller through the mazes of the Exhibition with the superlative excellence of their sparkling beverages. Certainly little is wanting to give satisfaction to the most critical palate of our worthy total abstainers, Dr. Richardson as President of the Congress notwithstanding. They can now offer at their dinner-tables, without stint or measure, a really drinkable champagne without "the fire" (as they call it).

In case the diner in transitu should be overcome or feel surfeited by the varied ingredients of his hasty meal, a final visit to the stall of Messrs. Savory and Moore, Wyeth and Co., Corbyn and Co., etc., will set all right. A pearl-coated pill, or a dose of tasteless castor oil, or an encapsuled hydragogue cathartic, will rectify all disturbing influences, and smooth the way for a second and more critical visit. I hope next week to give some account of the exhibits in the section for House Sanitation, etc.

As regards the Health Congress, which is being held in the Dome, the attendance of Brightonians was not up to the mark. Sanitation is still an unsavoury subject with most of the idler and gentler sex, though the Ladies' Sanitary Association are fairly represented at the Congress.

Dr. Richardson, the President, opened the Congress on the evening of Tuesday, the 13th; and in the shape of an introductory address, entitled, "The Seed-time of Health," treated his hearers to one of the eloquent and graphic discourses which he has accustomed his audiences to expect from him on occasions of this sort.

On Wednesday, Section A—the Health of Towns, including Sanitary Legislation—commenced its sittings, under the presidency of Mr. Chadwick.

Papers were read by the President and also by the following gentlemen:—H. S. Mitchell, M.A.: Comparison of English and Foreign Watering Places. Dr. Mackey: Geology and Climate of Brighton, from a Health point of view. Edward Easton, M.Inst.C.E., F.G.S.: Water Supply. Dr. Edward F. Fussell (Medical Officer of Health for East Sussex): Recreation Spaces in Large Towns. E. B. Ellice-Clark (Town Surveyor of Hove): The Administration of the Sanitary Laws. Edward F. Griffith, C.E.; Escape of Gases from Ventilating Covers in Towns. Mr. Fred. Walsh: Sanitation in Japan—a Comparative Study. Dr. Benj. Browning (Medical Officer of Health for Rotherhithe). C. E. Parker-Rhodes, on Water Reform. W. Hempson Denham: Improved Disposal of Sewage.

FROM ABROAD.

The Eyesight in Public Schools.

The number of the *Philadelphia Medical Times* for July 30 contains an important paper in the shape of a report by Dr. Risley, Lecturer on Ophthalmology in the University of Pennsylvania, as chairman of a committee appointed by the Philadelphia Medical Society to examine into the state of the eyesight of the children in the public schools in Philadelphia. The report is a very elaborate one—too elaborate for insertion in our columns,—and at present we must content ourselves by transcribing the editorial comments upon it in the number of the journal for August 15 :—

"The report of the Committee of the County Medical Society on the examination of the eyes of children in the public schools of Philadelphia contains facts and conclusions so interesting and important as to merit the careful attention, not only of physicians, but also of the intelligent public generally. Too little importance has heretofore been attached to the conditions of study in relation to the preservation of eyesight; and although the attention of parents and instructors has in recent years been drawn more and more to the subject, yet, from the necessity of the case, this interest has been that of inquiring ignorance asking for that guidance which it is clearly the duty of the medical profession to furnish to the community at large. The desired information has now been at last to some extent obtained, and although the investigations of Dr. Risley's Committee were not extended over as great a number of cases as might have been desired, yet, from the results of examination of some 2400 eyes in children attending all grades of the public schools, a fair estimate may be made of the conditions of eyesight among the school children of Philadelphia.

The conclusions drawn are in some degree unexpected. Thus, for example, it has generally been thought that improperly lighted schoolrooms were perhaps the chief factors, and more and more attention is being paid to this subject by school authorities. But, as Dr. Risley points out, other causes are also at work, among which are the habit of reading and study carried on at work, among which are the habit of reading and study carried on at home to an excessive degree, and under more or less unfavourable and injurious conditions; the custom of sending children to school at too early an age (which the investigations of the Committee show to directly favour the occurrence of defective vision); and chiefly, the pre-existence of more or less abnormal eyesight. To these, perhaps, may be added the use of books improperly printed on poor paper and with defective type. While we believe the books in use in our schools are usually of the proper kind in this respect, yet the prevalence and popularity of those cheap but abominably printed editions of standard authors must unquestionably exert a pernicious influence on the eyesight.

"The conclusions of the committee—to the careful perusal

of whose report we urge all medical men who may be personally or officially connected with the mental training of our citizens of the future—point directly to the following measures, which should be carried out if the subject of eyesight in the public schools is to receive the attention it demands :—1. The proper lighting and seating of our schools should receive the earliest attention, with the view of remedying well-known existing defects and preventing for the future those errors in architectural construction which exist in the present school-buildings. 2. Children should not be permitted to enter schools at too early an age. 3. *A careful examination should be made of the eyes* of all children on entering upon school life, and such precautions should be taken as to correct or prevent injury to the eyes from study. 4. Parents should be warned of the harm and injury which may result from over-study, and especially from excessive reading at home, and they should be told to take heed to the conditions of light and position occupied by children during their hours of reading and study. It is the duty of the medical profession to urge these views on the community at large as occasion offers, with the hope of influencing public opinion."

Naphthalin as a New Antiseptic.

Dr. Fischer, Privat-docent of Strasburg, strongly recommends (*Berliner Klinische Woch.*, November 28) naphthalin ($C_{10}H_8$) as a most energetic and cheap antiseptic and "antibacteriticum." Urine exposed to a local naphthalin atmosphere will remain clear for a week, no minute organisms developing in it; while a fluid, on the surface of which fungus formations have occurred, ceases to produce these in a similar atmosphere. Offensive wounds and ulcers, on powdered naphthalin being sprinkled over them, in a very short time cease manifesting any bad odour. This produces no pain in the wound, is not absorbed by it, favours granulation, and does not excite eczema of the surrounding skin. Deep wounds, abscesses, etc., may be filled with it, just as is the case with iodoform, without any ill effect being produced. The naphthalin is insoluble in water and by the secretions at the surface of wounds; but it is easily soluble in ether (one part to four), and this mixed with alcohol forms a suitable means of impregnating the materials for dressings, such as gauze, etc. In order to impregnate gauze at the rate of 10 per cent. of naphthalin, 100 parts of naphthalin, 400 of ether, and 1200 of alcohol may be employed. The rapid evaporation of the ether and alcohol allows of gauze which has only been prepared a short time before the visit to be at once applied; and the only objection to applying it while still wet is the unpleasantness of the cold produced by the evaporation. By means of the above mixture, from thirty to forty metres of gauze may be impregnated at a cost of 1s. 9d., the cost of naphthalin being 1s. 3d. per kilogramme, contrasting with the prices of some recently recommended antiseptics, such as iodoform at 30s. or 40s., salicylic acid at 15s., thymol at 50s., resorcin at 50s., chinolin at 60s., etc. The easy miscibility of naphthalin with fatty matters, vaseline, etc., should render it, in the form of ointment, serviceable in diseases produced by vegetable or animal parasites.

A Fat Girl.

Dr. Hillairet brought before the Académie de Médecine recently (*Bulletin*, November 29), and the Hospital Medical Society (*Gaz. Médicale*, December 10), a case of corpulence, which is remarkable as occurring in a child aged five years and some months. The daughter of peasants who neither themselves nor their other children exhibited any abnormality, she was brought up exclusively at the breast until she was fifteen months old. When born, she was of an average size, but by the fifth or sixth month her weight had much increased, and at her third year she had attained an amount of corpulence that attracted attention. Having a good appetite, all the functions of the body were performed regularly, and she never has had occasion to take any physic. Her intellectual condition is much the same as that of children of her position, and she is lively and playful with her sisters. Her food is that of her parents, but she has a preference for bread-and-cheese, drinks but little, and sleeps soundly. Her external aspect is deformed. Tumefied by the fat, her features are still those of a child of her age, and her cheeks are fresh-coloured. Her ears, except the lobules, are but slightly developed; her hair is abundant, fair, and curled, and resembles a true fleece. She is one metre fifteen centimetres in height, and weighs about 124 (French) pounds. Her head sinks into her shoulders; and the trunk, and especially the abdomen, are extraordinarily developed. The skin is delicate and supple, and does not retain the impression of the finger. The subcutaneous venous network is very distinct, especially over the abdomen, which is very hard. The integuments are of a violaceous colour, especially at the legs and forearms. At the lower part of the abdomen and on the breasts (which are as large as those of an adult, contain hardly any glandular structure, and hang down over the chest) there are some suggillations. Her limbs are something colossal, and the bony projections disappear amidst the fatty tissue. The child moves about easily, but cannot walk far without being out of breath and stopping. She is strong enough to be able to carry her sister, who is three years old, with ease. The heart beats regularly without any abnormal sound, and the pulse is 100, the respirations being 24. The circumference of the child's body opposite the navel is one metre seven centimetres; that of the chest on a level with the armpits is 1·2 metres; and of the neck, which is very short, thirty-seven centimetres. The back measures from one shoulder to the other thirty-nine centimetres, and the thighs at their highest part are fifty-seven centimetres, and at the knee thirty-eight centimetres in circumference. The calf of the leg measures thirty-four centimetres, and the ankle twenty-five centimetres.

THE PRODUCTION OF DIPHTHERIA.

The *Boston Med. Jour.* (November 3) states that Prof. H. Wood of Philadelphia and Dr. Formad are engaged, under the auspices of the National Board of Health, in researches on the nature of the diphtheritic contagium, and that the results of their labours will soon be published in full. Among these is the demonstration, in cases occurring during an epidemic, that the blood is more or less full of micrococci, some free, others in zooglœa masses, and others in the white corpuscles. The viscera, and especially the kidneys, also contain them. Prof. Wood's theory of diphtheria (as stated in an address by him reported in the *Philadelphia Med. Times*, October 22) is as follows:—"A child gets a catarrhal angina or tracheitis. Under the stimulation of the inflammation-products the inert micrococci in the mouth begin to grow; and if the conditions be favourable, the sluggish plant may be finally transformed into an active organism, and a self-generated diphtheria result. It is plain that if this be correct there must be every grade of case between one which is fatal and one which is checked before it fairly passes the bounds of an ordinary sore-throat. Every practitioner knows that such diversity does exist. Again, conditions outside of the body favouring the passage of inert into active micrococci may exist, and the air become at last well loaded with organisms, which, alighting on the tender throats of children, may begin to grow, and themselves produce violent angina, tracheitis, and finally fatal diphtheria. In the first instance we have endemic diphtheria as we see it in Philadelphia; in the second, the malignant epidemic form of the disease. It is also apparent that in the endemic cases the plant whose activity has been developed within the patient may escape with the breath, and a second case of diphtheria be produced by contagion. It is also plain that as the plant gradually, in such a case, passes from the inert to the active state, there must be degrees of activity in the contagium, one case being more apt to give the disease than is another; also that the malignant diphtheria must be more contagious than the mild endemic cases. We think that there is scarcely a practitioner who will not agree that clinical experience is in accord with these logical deductions from our experimentally determined premises. It yet remains for us to investigate as to what are the conditions outside of the body which will especially favour the production of active micrococci, and also to study the effect of agents in killing these organisms, for it is very apparent that local treatment of the throat must often be of the utmost importance, and that it will be far more effective if it be of such character as to kill the micrococci, and not simply be antiphlogistic in its action." The influence of this theory, if it shall be confirmed and accepted, will be felt particularly in two directions: in the first place, more attention will be paid to the favouring and predisposing conditions, with a view to prophylaxis;

and secondly, local applications to the throat will assume, relatively, a highly important place in the treatment, and be placed on a sound scientific and clinical basis. What these conditions are, and what the best agents to be used to kill the micrococci, are questions still under consideration.

REVIEWS, NOTICES OF BOOKS, &c.

Ueber den Werth der Infusion alkalischer Kochsalzlösung in das Gefässystem bei Acuter Anämie. Von Dr. E. SCHWARZ, Assistant an der gynäcologischen Klinik der Universität Halle-Wittenberg.
On the Use of the Injection of an Alkalised Solution of Common Salt into the Vascular System in Acute Anæmia. By Dr. E. SCHWARZ, Assistant Obstetric Clinical Teacher in the University of Halle-Wittenberg. Halle. 1881. Pp. 41.

IN this essay, presented to the Medical Faculty of the combined Friedrichs University of Halle-Wittenberg, the author proposes a new method for restoring animation in threatened death from extensive losses of blood—as, for instance, in uterine puerperal hæmorrhage. Dr. Schwarz in the first place examines the question as to the cause of the failure of the vital powers in sudden losses of blood, and, although the result has been usually attributed to the diminution of the blood corpuscles and the withdrawal of oxygen, he is inclined to doubt this explanation and to offer the following. He asks whether the imperfect filling of the vascular system, and consequently the diminished blood-pressure, are not the real causes which induce the striking disturbance of the circulation, and eventually death; and whether the organism in the first place does not fall a sacrifice, not so much to chemical changes as to the mere mechanical disproportion between the quantity of the blood and the capacity of the vessels. This hypothesis has appeared to him to be most consistent with the principal symptoms of acute anæmia and with recovery from that condition, and he therefore determined to submit it to experimental investigation.

He quotes in support of his view a striking experiment recorded by Kronecker and Sander in a recent number of the *Klinische Wochenschrift* of Berlin, showing that those physicians withdrew from two dogs a large quantity of blood, and when the pulsation of the heart had become very feeble they injected into each of them as large a quantity of a weak alkalised solution of common salt as corresponded to the amount of blood withdrawn. Both the dogs recovered and were quite well in a few days. Dr. Schwarz was further encouraged in his views by the perusal of the work of Goltz in *Virchow's Archiv*, "Ueber den Tonus der Gefässe und seine Bedeutung für die Blutbewegung" (On the Tone of the Bloodvessels, and its Importance in the Movement of the Blood). According to Goltz's opinion, in which Dr. Schwarz coincides, death from excessive bleeding is caused principally by the disturbance of the circulation, and this again results from the insufficient movement of the blood caused by the purely mechanical disproportion between the capacity of the vessels and their contents. The nutritive material still present in the remaining blood would in most cases of excessive bleeding have sufficed some time for the support of the organism if the blood had only continued in due motion, and had reached the organs which require a continuous supply of that fluid for the maintenance of life. Dr. Schwarz does not deny that there are cases of acute anæmia in which the remaining proportion of the red corpuscles is no longer sufficient to support life, but he is persuaded that in such cases the disproportion between the capacity of the vessels and their contents is fatal before the excessive impoverishment of the red corpuscles can exercise an injurious influence.

Such being the opinion of Dr. Schwarz, his experiments (which were numerous) on rabbits and dogs were carried out to test its accuracy. The general plan of operation was first to withdraw about half the normal quantity of blood from the living animal, and, when death was threatening, to inject into the vessels a quantity of the alkalised solution of salt equal to the amount of blood withdrawn; and the results proved, not only that the proceeding was quite harmless in itself, but that it was followed by restoration of the animal to its former health and vigour. All the experiments showed that the injection of this fluid, even when it exceeded in quantity the amount of blood in the body, was absolutely innocuous. Not in a single case, either during or after the operation, did any bad symptoms supervene—such as excessive dyspnœa, irregularity and weakness of the heart's action, shivering, spasms, or other ill effects which have occasionally been observed in transfusion of blood,—and no impairment of important functions was ever noticed which could indicate any injury to the system from the injection of the saline solution.

The general conclusions at which Dr. Schwarz arrives are chiefly the following, viz., that as death is caused in excessive bleeding by the mechanical disproportion between the capacity and the contents of the vessels, the rational treatment of acute anæmia must keep in view, in the first place, the rapid adjustment of this disproportion; that when the usual methods, such as laying the head down, medicinal appliances, etc., are unsuccessful, then the direct injection of a weak alkalised solution of salt is not only a harmless, but a safe and rapid means of saving life; that the influence of this injection (as shown in rabbits and dogs) on the action of the heart, the increase of the blood-pressure, the respiration, and the other functions of life, when the animals were on the point of death from the loss of half or two-thirds of their normal blood, was quite surprising; and that the injection is indicated not only in threatened death from bleeding, but also in cases of extreme collapse in which there is reason to suspect a paresis of a large system of vessels, as, for instance, after operations in the abdominal cavity. The minimum quantity of fluid to be injected into the human body should amount, according to Dr. Schwarz, to 500 cubic centimetres (about 125 fluid drachms).

Boy's Own Paper. Published at the *Leisure Hour* Office. Vol. III.
Girl's Own Paper. Published at the *Leisure Hour* Office. Vol. II.

THESE two papers fully keep up to the high standard of merit that so early gained them the warm approval of the public. They are admirable in every way, and contain, besides stirring and well-written stories, a remarkable amount of sound, practical, and clearly-conveyed information on various subjects—domestic, scientific, literary, artistic, etc. The volumes now before us are well and handsomely bound in cloth, and marvellously cheap considering their contents. The binding of the volume of the *Girl's Own Paper* is especially praiseworthy; it is charming for elegant simplicity and taste. Any of our readers seeking a Christmas present for boy or girl may rest on these volumes; and be thankful, as would be the happy recipient.

THE prize of £200 offered by the Rev. E. Wyatt-Edgell, late Treasurer of the Sanitary Institute, for the best essay on "The Range of Hereditary Tendencies in Health and Disease," has been awarded by the adjudicators—Drs. W. Farr and B. W. Richardson—to Mr. George Gaskoin, of 7, Westbourne-park, W. There were twelve competitors, several of whose essays possessed considerable merit.

DR. SIMS ON WOUNDS OF THE ABDOMEN.—Dr. Marion Sims terminates a paper read at the New York Academy of Medicine (*New York Med. Record,* October 22), bearing the title "The Recent Progress of Peritoneal Surgery: Does it lead to a Better Treatment of Gunshot and other Wounds of the Abdominal Cavity?" with the following conclusions:—1. Wounds of the peritoneal cavity, however produced, have to run a common course. 2. They have a common termination in death, and that death is by septicæmia. 3. This is the general law in deaths from ovariotomy. 4. This is the general law after gunshot and other wounds of the abdomen. 5. The septicæmia is the result of the absorption of bloody serum remaining in the abdominal cavity after wounds or operations. 6. In gunshot wounds of the pelvic cavity the tendency is to recovery, on account of the natural drainage in this situation. 7. Gunshot wounds of the abdominal cavity prove fatal from septicæmia, because there is no natural drainage, and the bloody serum poured out becomes absorbed. 8. In order to prevent this it is necessary to open the abdomen, clear out the peritoneal cavity, tie the bleeding vessels, suture the intestines or other tissues requiring it, and possibly insert a drainage-tube. 9. If the operation be properly performed it is rarely necessary to make use of a drainage-tube.

GENERAL CORRESPONDENCE.

DR. HARLEY'S ORTHOGRAPHY.
LETTER FROM MR. KENNETH W. MILLICAN.

[To the Editor of the Medical Times and Gazette.]

SIR,—In replying to Dr. Harley's letter in your last issue, I feel bound to enter a protest as to its tone. I trust to avoid being personal, however, and shall merely content myself with stating that had I, as Dr. Harley regretfully wishes, "only possesed a trifling knowledge of modern comparative philology," I might possibly have been more inclined to agree with him.

Dr. Harley appears to me to have completely "run off the lines" in his reply. He seems to argue thus—"My modification of English spelling may be recommended, not only on utilitarian, but also on etymological grounds, as tending, in fact, to render English etymology less obscure." And when I ask him how he reconciles the abortion of "vaxination" from "vacca," and "axidentaly" from "accido" with this statement, he practically replies—"Hang etymology! The poor deluded Roman who first endeavoured to represent the sound of 'x' by a double 'c' made an ass of himself!"

Now, suppose this point be conceded, nevertheless, as he did write "accido," and as we do derive "accidentally" therefrom, the substitution of "x" for double "c" would, I still maintain, obscure the etymology.

But the fact is, "modern comparative philology," to which Dr. Harley refers in words at once majestic and consoling (as the old lady said of the word "Mesopotamia"), presents an explanation of the double "c" quite different from that so feelingly advanced by him.

In point of fact, the written double "c" is prior to the sound. The process was as follows:—The misguided Roman found himself in the presence of a word compounded of the two parts, "ad" and "cado." In trying to pronounce them he found the change of position by the tongue required for the pronunciation of a hard guttural after a soft dental somewhat trying, so by the process of "assimilation" he said "ac-cádo" instead. Then, still finding a difficulty with the hard vowel, "a," he quietly substituted a short "i," thus producing "ak-kído." If Dr. Harley will pronounce (1) ad-cído, (2) ac-cído, (3) ac-cído, he will find the steps very easy, and the result fairly satisfactory.

The softened "c," making "ak-sído," is a further and later transmutation on the score of easiness; and only occurred long after the orthography of the word was well established; as I should have thought would have been known to anyone with even "no more than a school-acquired knowledge of the subject." It thus follows that the laboured and utterly ineffectual attempt on the part of the poor defunct Roman grammarian to pen a duplicated "cc" with the intent of symbolising the sound of "x," though touchingly pathetic in Dr. Harley's hands, is purely mythical and legendary.

Moreover, with all due deference to Dr. Harley, whose knowledge, I presume, he would have me to understand is not "school-acquired," I desire to point out that modern English, so far as it comes from a German stock, comes from the Low, and not from the High German, and the transmutations which occur are so thoroughly in accordance with "Grimm's law" as to clearly indicate that fact.

I take the first word to which Dr. Harley refers—viz. "father." Cf. *pater*—Indo-European represented by Latin. Change the hard labial and hard dental into their corresponding aspirates, and you get *father*; but this is the rule for transmutations from Indo-European to Low German.

Moreover, Dr. Harley's scheme itself, so far as utilitarian reasons go (and my "limited acquaintance with the subject" will not yet allow me, in the "profundity of my orthographical phonetic ignorance," to perceive the etymological ones), to be consistent should omit also double and mute vowels. Why write "blod" when "blod" would do, or "school" when "schol" would suffice?

Why not write "croneus" and "virtus"? And above all, when such bitter exception is taken to "vaccination" and "accidentally," why should "susceptibilities" and "acquaintance" each remain in triumphant possession of an unnecessary consonant? The same etymological reasons which would retain the one would retain the other; and the utilitarian grounds which are cogent enough to dispense with a duplicated " c " can surely dismiss a useless " c " behind an " s " in " susceptibilities," and an equally lazy " c " in "acquaintance."

I think I have now said enough—too much, perhaps, Dr. Harley will think, save for the purpose of clearly demonstrating my very " limited acquaintance with the subject " ! Moreover, as it is doubtless your intention to retain the medical sciences as your chief *raison d'être*, you will probably not care to have your pages converted into a dialectical debating society, nor yet assimilated to a comic journal.

In conclusion, Dr. Harley sneers at Dr. Kesteven and myself as " self-constituted critics." May I suggest that sneers, like most other double-edged tools, are dangerous, for they cut in two directions. A " self-constituted critic " does not appear to me to be a greater anomaly in the economy of literature than a self-constituted reformer.

I am, &c., KENNETH W. MILLICAN.

EXHIBITION JUDGES.

[To the Editor of the Medical Times and Gazette.]

SIR,—Exception has been taken, by the two chemists employed by Mr. Black to adjudicate at the recent Food Exhibition, to the statements contained in my letter of the 28th ult., published in your columns on December 3. I now beg to reiterate my avowal as substantially correct, in proof of which I adduce the following facts. A few weeks prior to the opening of the Exhibition, Mr. H. C. Bartlett, in his private capacity, gave a testimonial in favour of Zoedone, and in his public capacity as one of the judges at the show in question (of course in conjunction with his coadjutors) awarded the proprietors of the said non-alcoholic beverage a silver medal —the highest award! For the donor of a testimonial to adjudicate under such circumstances is, I still contend, a mistake. Last year, Mr. H. C. Bartlett, in his private capacity, pronounced a certain whiskey "the purest he ever examined." The proprietors, no doubt thinking, very naturally, that if they exhibited it at the forthcoming Exhibition they would obtain an award—seeing that Mr. H. C. Bartlett was one of the judges—were not a little chagrined, I am told, on finding that it had not even received honourable mention ! Thirdly, Brand's specialties, which are universally admitted to be extremely good articles, obtained a bronze medal only—which was, I am informed, " declined with thanks." Fourthly, shortly before the opening of the first Food Exhibition, Mr. H. C. Bartlett gave a testimonial in favour of a certain " corn-flour," advertised as a " most famous article for infants' diet." He spoke of it as " this unique preparation of Indian corn." " Its peculiarities," he further states, " are very striking." He finds it differs from all the " corn-flours " he has examined, and " in its texture, colour, and delicate characteristic odour of ripe maize, it alone maintains the agreeable flavour and appearance of the pure flour of that cereal"; and he is " happy to testify that the recipes and directions on the wrapper may be implicitly followed." The " corn-flour " in question was exhibited and received an award ! This is the more curious from the fact that Mr. H. C. Bartlett some years since spoke and wrote very strongly against so-called " corn-flour," and, still more extraordinary, the very preparation Mr. H. C. Bartlett spoke of in such glowing terms, no less an authority than the late Dr. Alfred Swaine Taylor, F.R.S., for upwards of forty years Professor of Chemistry at Guy's Hospital, certified to contain " no flesh-forming principles ; it is pure starch, and therefore unfit to supply the necessary nutriment to young children. I find in it no gluten and no albumen ; its nutritious properties—to use a Hibernicism —depend on the *milk* and other nitrogenous matters associated with it. People are deceived by its forming a good jelly, but this is simply starch-jelly. To pass it off, to the public as highly nutritious food is either a delusion or something worse."

The next subject to which I would draw attention is that of foods for children and invalids. Several were exhibited, but not one received an award, though, strange to relate, two, viz., Savory and Moore's, and Lloyd's Universal Food, have both been commended by the medical press—the latter not only by the *Medical Times and Gazette*, but by the *British Medical Journal*, the *Lancet*, the *Medical Record*, and the *Medical Press and Circular*—as being "skilfully devised, highly

nutritious, easily digestible, suitable for the use of adults as well as of infants and young children."

I will now append, without comment, the names of a few of the more conspicuous firms who expressed dissatisfaction, nearly all of whose wares have been spoken of in high terms by the medical press; also by English and continental physicians—men certainly not inferior to Mr. Black's judges at the late grandiloquently-termed International Food Exhibition :—Nestlé's Infants' Food ; Gittli's Infants' Food ; Professor Redwood's Cocoa ; Möller's Cod-liver Oil ; Liebig's Cocoa ; Kopf's soups ; Harzer Water ; Glacialine ; Sulis Water ; Dolby's Beef-tea Extractor ; Blatchley's Diabetic Foods ; the Consolidated Soup and Food Company ; Anglo-Swiss Milk Food ; Hedosone, Vinita, Rubine, and several other non-alcoholic beverages ; the Alpine Milk Exporting Company ; preserved meats, too numerous to mention.

In conclusion, I may observe that I can quite understand many of the unsuccessful competitors complaining, and I can also understand many of the exhibitors who had prizes awarded them feeling anything but elated on being told that nearly half of the firms represented in the Hall had received awards !

I have now finished. That I was fully justified in drawing attention to the above matter, the facts I have adduced conclusively prove. Whether Messrs. Bartlett and Wigner will confess to having committed errors of judgment remains to be seen. In the language of Rochefoucault, " Few are so wise as to prefer the censure which may be useful to them to the flattery which betrays them."

December 12. I am, &c., SCRUTATOR.

RARE FORM OF PREGNANCY.

[To the Editor of the Medical Times and Gazette.]

SIR,—At page 662 is a report of a case under this heading. Will you allow me to refer Dr. Werth to the many similar cases he will find recorded in Yours truly,

SECTION 1110 : 5 MEDICAL DIGEST.

Since I saw the light there have appeared cases in the *Lancet*, vol. ii. 1877, page 87 ; and in the *British Medical Journal*, vol. ii. 1878, page 372, and vol. ii. 1879, page 695.

[We have examined the references which our esteemed correspondent gives in his postscript, and find that the cases referred to are not "similar." They only resemble the one we mentioned in that a malformation of the uterus was present.—ED. Med. Times and Gaz.]

BATTEY'S OPERATION.

LETTER FROM MR. W. E. PORTER.

[To the Editor of the Medical Times and Gazette.]

SIR,—The interesting part of the case of spaying you chronicle at page 691 in your last week's journal I am unable to see. The instruction to be gleaned from it is, that the operation should not be done except for incurable disease threatening life. Fashionable it may be, and profitable I have no doubt it is, to the surgeons who perform it ; but even the powerful incentives of fashion and greed, though clothed in their softest and most apt sophistry, will not convince plain honest men that it is right to cut away a healthy organ or a simply disordered one.

Excising the clitoris, or a part of it, was a fashion some years ago, and, though nothing when compared with the mutilation in question, yet it raised such a storm of indignation that its career was very short ; and the sooner this operation is abandoned, the better for the credit of the profession, and perhaps the morality of society. I am, &c., Lindfield, Dec. 14. WILLIAM ELLIOTT PORTER.

ROYAL MEDICAL BENEVOLENT COLLEGE.—Sir Erasmus Wilson, President of the Royal College of Surgeons, will preside at the [ensuing biennial festival of supporters and friends of the Royal Medical Benevolent College, Epsom.

DE LA RUE'S OINTMENT IN ERYSIPELAS.—Creosote four parts, and lard thirty parts. The erysipelatous parts to be anointed every two hours.—*Union Méd.*, No. 162.

REPORTS OF SOCIETIES.

THE CLINICAL SOCIETY OF LONDON.
FRIDAY, DECEMBER 9.

JOSEPH LISTER, D.C.L., F.R.C.S., F.R.S.,
President, in the Chair.

TALIPES EQUINO-VARUS TREATED BY RESECTION OF A
PORTION OF THE TARSAL BONES.

MR. WILLIAM H. BENNETT exhibited a man, aged forty-seven, who had been the subject of the above description of talipes in a severe form. The patient had been born lame, and when an infant had been under surgical treatment: tenotomy had been performed, with temporary relief only. For thirty-five years the patient had been walking much on the deformed limb, wearing an ordinary boot padded and adapted by himself. At times there had been most severe pains from the bursæ which had developed, and the deformity had gradually increased. When admitted to St. George's Hospital under Mr. Bennett's care in June 25, 1881, the patient hobbled about in an unsightly manner. The left lower limb was wasted and shortened; the foot was much drawn up at the heel, and the sole was so twisted inwards that it was directed towards the median line of the body. The patient in walking or standing bore his weight entirely on the outer edge of the foot, over which the skin was greatly thickened, and beneath this thickening bursæ had formed. No alteration in the shape of the foot could be made by any force applied. On June 30 a portion of the central part of the tarsus was resected. A flap was turned back from the dorsal aspect of the mid-tarsal region, and with a chisel sufficient of the tarsus was chipped away, piece by piece, to allow the anterior part of the sole to be placed in a perfectly flat position. The tendo Achillis was divided, and the heel brought down as much as possible. The parts were accurately adapted, a drainage-tube introduced, and the limb placed on a splint with a foot-piece. The operation was performed antiseptically, and the wound dressed in the same way. The portions of bone removed included the cuboid and the scaphoid. No constitutional disturbance of any kind followed the operation. The dressings were changed for the first time eight days later; the wound had then healed excepting at its extremities where the drainage-tube was lying. By July 8 the whole wound had soundly healed excepting a small sinus at the lower part. At this date antiseptic dressing was discontinued in consequence of irritation produced by the carbolic acid. A few days later, erysipelas attacked the foot; cellulitis followed; the wound had to be opened up; all union between the bones, which before had been remarkably firm, broke down by degrees this attack passed off, and after much trouble the foot was brought again into a good condition. By September 8 the wound had again healed, and the bones were again consolidating. The progress from that time was uninterrupted. On November 3 he was provided with a boot with iron supports, and was allowed to walk. The condition of the foot when the patient was exhibited was described as follows :—The foot is somewhat shortened; the anterior part of the sole is as nearly as possible flat, and is planted firmly on the ground in standing and walking ; the heel is still somewhat inverted, but can be made to touch the ground. The union at the point where the bones were resected is firm but not bony. The gait is altogether better than on the patient's admission into the hospital, and is gradually improving. Mr. Bennett thought the case might fairly be considered successful, and also that it demonstrated the desirability of performing this operation in certain examples of talipes. The case itself was peculiarly suitable for the form of treatment adopted, inasmuch as the long continuance of the deformity and the age of the patient rendered relief impossible by any milder procedure. It was suggested that fibrous union would be preferable to bony anchylosis, as it would allow a certain amount of movement in a position where a joint is naturally provided. It was then submitted that the operation was one of extreme severity, and although performed with a successful result in a considerable number of cases recorded by other surgeons, should be resorted to only in those instances in which no other milder form of treatment could be adopted with success.

Mr. DAVEY expressed the satisfaction that he felt at the general sanction which was being accorded to this class of operations. His own experience of them was limited to seventeen cases, and the success obtained justified him in anticipating that by-and-by resection would be regarded as the only reliable treatment in all cases of the kind. He exhibited a foot taken from a post-mortem subject, and from which he had removed a wedge-shaped mass of bone, as would be effected in his mode of operating for excision of the transverse tarsal joint as a remedial measure for the malformation under discussion. This operation had been performed on a boy, aged ten, who had been suffering from talipes equinus, and after remaining two months in hospital he could walk easily on the foot, which thus had been transformed from a useless to a useful member. The operation had been simplified as compared with its original form. A quadrilateral fold of skin should be removed from the outer side of the foot, and a special wedge-shaped director employed as a guide to the knife in making the subsequent incisions prior to removal of the bony mass, the form of which followed that of the director. All the seventeen operations had been performed with no other antiseptic precautions than a scrupulous cleanliness, and but one death had occurred out of the number. Mr. Bennett's case was undoubtedly the oldest patient yet operated on, but it should be recollected that children who are submitted to surgical interference for remedying the defect of club-feet, had been for years subject to interference of one kind or another; and in their case a radical procedure of even so serious a description might be expected to produce good results. In fact, the operation was pre-eminently beneficial, substituting a strong useful limb for a weak, useless, and malformed one, and the risk attending it might be estimated by the fact that no relapse had occurred in any of his cases, and only one death. He thought fibrous union between the bones might produce a valuable extremity.

Mr. HOWARD MARSH, admitting that talipes was a difficult subject to understand thoroughly, thought it would conduce to a better comprehension of the claims of the operation if an opportunity were afforded for examining the cases described by Mr. Davey, and watching their future progress. Mr. Bennett's case was certainly so far successful, but it ought to be noted in the future. The operation was undoubtedly a dangerous one, and it ought to be had recourse to only as a final measure of affording relief. It seemed to him that Mr. Bennett's proceeding almost necessitated the formation of what might be termed a "wooden" foot, a consequence of the treatment pursued, since this involved the severance of the anterior and hinder portion of the foot so far as articular connexion was concerned. A committee might, perhaps, he thought, be appointed to watch and examine the progress of the cases described.

Mr. HAWARD said no one who had seen Mr. Bennett's patient when exhibited at the preceding meeting of the Society could doubt the successful issue of the operation. This, however, by reason of its severity, should be adopted with the utmost caution. He believed that the usefulness of such recovered limbs might even increase with time, and concurred in the opinion that their progress should be observed. In the case of children, it would rarely happen that a simpler and less dangerous operation could not be more wisely undertaken for the cure of these deformities, and it should be remembered that the previous treatment they had endured might favour relapse—this treatment, as a rule, being only half carried out, from the ignorance, or impatience, or misplaced kindness of persons in charge of the patients. For instance, it not rarely occurred that the tendons were divided, the foot put into position, and directions given for maintaining it so; and there all treatment ended, the limb returning to its malformed state, owing to unwillingness of the parents to continue painful applications of apparatus, etc. If rightly and persistently followed, such treatment would rarely prove ineffectual. The few cases of talipes found in persons of advanced years might be proper subjects for the proposed operation, but it would be a matter for regret if, on this account, enthusiastic surgeons should be led away to its adoption with children.

The PRESIDENT thought there could be no doubt that, in this particular instance, Mr. Bennett had performed an operation which was indicated by the circumstances, and which resulted very satisfactorily. For children, however, it was inappropriate and uncalled for. Patient treatment of such cases would effect wonderful improvement, and by simple, unheroic measures. He was interested to learn the good results obtained by Mr. Davey in the employment of antiseptic precautions; but he considered that, had he adopted them, instead of experiencing any surprise at the favourable consequences, he would rather have been astonished had they not ensued as a matter of course. Mr. Bennett would have done well to substitute eucalyptus oil gauze for the carbolic dressing when he discovered the injury done to his patient by the antiseptic, thereby avoiding any necessity for remitting the precautions against the introduction of septic influences. Erysipelas had been of very rare occurrence in cases treated antiseptically; only one instance had come under his notice in King's College Hospital. He had seen four cases where septic conditions existed which could not be removed, notwithstanding this treatment. They were, however, of a nature to indicate the difficulty of meeting the conditions surrounding them. One was a case of epithelioma of the vulva, and was necessarily out of the sphere of cases in which antiseptics could hopefully be employed. He would, however, perform such an operation as Mr. Bennett described without any feeling of risk being incurred, pursuing it, of course, antiseptically. In the case of children, however, he should look upon such a proceeding as unnecessary mutilation.

Mr. Bennett, in reply, said he had never met a single case of a child in which it would, in his estimation, have been justifiable to perform the operation; but in adults the conditions were different. When, in his case, carbolic irritation set in, strict antiseptic treatment was for a time discontinued, and this doubtless accounted for the attack of erysipelas. He expressed a doubt whether Mr. Davey would have had to chronicle the single death he mentioned in his series of cases if these had been treated antiseptically. That gentleman's mode of operating was, in every respect, admirable. He thought the progress of all cases of this kind, after operation, should be carefully watched.

Two Cases of Myxœdema, Male and Female.

Mr. Lunn read a paper on two cases of myxœdema, male and female. Case 1: G. M., aged forty-seven, male. Family history good. A stout man, well nourished; movements of locomotion slow; skin dry, harsh, and translucent, does not pit on pressure. Whole of face puffy, especially under lips, suggesting renal disease; several moles on face; nose flattened; lips thickened; teeth fairly good; breath offensive; articulation slow, with a nasal intonation; hair on head thin, especially on vertex, thin on pubes, none in axillæ. No apparent disease of fundus with the ophthalmoscope; fulness about supra-clavicular regions. Thyroid gland not to be felt; drowsy at times; does not perspire; temperature 90° to 97·2°, both sides alike; pulse small and weak, 80; respirations 18; no anæsthesia or hyperæsthesia; taste good; no apparent chest symptoms; appetite good; has had delusions lately. Urine, specific gravity 1015, contains a trace of albumen at times, no sugar, no apparent increase of urea with nitric acid; only passing thirty-four to thirty-eight ounces daily, averaging 5·72 grains of urea per ounce, equal to 194·48 per cent. grains in the twenty-four hours. Case 2: Mrs. J., aged forty-five, mother of eight children, four of whom are dead, cause unknown. She had had five miscarriages. No history of syphilis, gout, intemperance, or fright. The woman has the appearance of a cretin, being drowsy, movements slow; hands look puffy; skin harsh and dry, never perspires; also nasal thickened; always feels cold, temperature 97·4° to 95°; pulse 76, slow; respirations 18; taste good; hair dark and thin; no thyroid gland to be felt; hearing not good; appetite fairly good; slight hyperæsthesia of whole body when pricked with a pin; slight bronchitic signs in chest, latter otherwise normal. Uterus soft, axis normal; no disease. Catamenia stopped 1880. Urine amber-coloured, specific gravity 1020, vesical epithelium; distinct trace of albumen at times; no sugar; urea diminished in the twenty-four hours 6·78 grains in each ounce. Often has horrid dreams, but no distinct delusions.

Two Cases of Myxœdema.

Dr. John Cavafy related two cases of myxœdema. The first case was that of a woman, aged fifty-nine, married, who had had six healthy children and four miscarriages. The catamenia ceased at the age of forty-five. She had good

health until eight years ago, when she suffered from dyspeptic attacks, which have come on at intervals ever since. Five years ago she was subjected to a severe mental shock; after which she gradually became very weak and low-spirited, walking with difficulty, and the characteristic swelling of the disease slowly supervened, but was not sufficiently marked to attract attention until two years ago. On admission there was moderate tense swelling of the cheeks, nose, and lips, with a bright patch of dilated capillaries on the cheeks, the skin of the face being waxy. The hair was scanty, the eyebrows raised and scanty, and the eyelashes largely wanting. The hands were rather broad and swollen, covered with dull reddish, dry, and rough skin. The rest of the skin was dry and harsh. Her expression was dull and listless, and speech slow and nasal; the gait awkward and slow; common sensation blunted; special sense unaffected, and intelligence good. The thoracic and abdominal viscera were normal, and the urine free from albumen. She was very chilly, and her temperature was always subnormal, averaging 96·5°. The pulse was very slow, about 48, and urine scanty. She had two sudden attacks of dyspepsia and diarrhœa during her stay in the hospital, lasting a week and three days respectively, and was discharged feeling rather stronger, but with no appreciable change in her condition. Case 2: A married woman, aged thirty-three; she had had five children in eleven years, of whom two survive and are healthy, the remaining three having died in infancy during teething. Five years ago, after the birth of one of her children, she began to feel very weak, and at the same time her eyelids were swollen. In the course of a year the swelling became general, and her speech slow, with great awkwardness in all movements, so that she fell occasionally. On admission the face was much swollen, the upper eyelids especially pearly and semi-transparent, the nose very broad, and the lips much thickened. The hands were large, clumsy, red, and rough; the feet and ankles swollen, and the whole skin very dry and rough. She had a placid expression and slow speech, but intelligence and special sense were unaffected. Her movements were slow and awkward; common sensation rather dull; she felt constantly chilly. Heart, lungs, and abdominal organs were normal, and there was no albumen in the urine. The pulse was constantly slow, varying from 45 to 65, and the temperature averaged 97·6°. She remained in the hospital nearly a month without alteration, and has since been an out-patient. She has lately felt worse owing to grief from the death of one of her children from bronchitis, and the eyelids are more swollen, but there is no other change. It seems probable that the œdema and other nervous symptoms are both due to a common cause in the central nervous system, as the former predominated in the second case and the latter in the first case. This view is supported by the slow pulse and subnormal temperature, which was highest in the second case, in which there was most œdema. The acute dyspeptic attacks in the first case somewhat resembled the gastric crises of locomotor ataxia.

Dr. Ord read notes of another case of the same kind.

Dr. Mahomed wished to draw attention to certain points in these cases which assimilated them in character to those of renal dropsy. He had collected together for the Guy's Hospital Reports a number of examples of this kind, and dwelt on the concurrence of evidence pointing to the existence of similar conditions in the two classes of disease, and especially the non-albuminous nature of the urine. He had regarded these cases (one having been recorded as an example of myxœdema by Dr. Goodhart) as instances of chronic Bright's disease without albuminuria, under which term he would also include Gull and Sutton's cases of arterio-capillary fibrosis. The result of his own experience and comparison of published cases had been to compel him to regard myxœdema as having much in common with such forms of Bright's disease; and even the changes in the spinal cord favoured this view, the nervous changes not being, moreover, an invariable accompaniment of myxœdema. On all grounds, therefore, and particularly on these afforded by the variability of albuminuria in both myxœdema and in the forms of Bright's disease he referred to, he thought that the explanations afforded of the myxœdematous state should be carefully reconsidered.

Dr. Stephen Mackenzie moved the adjournment of the debate, and the motion was carried.

ASSOCIATION OF MEDICAL OFFICERS OF HEALTH.

Friday, November 18.

Dr. J. W. Tripe, President, in the Chair.

The following gentlemen were elected Members of the Society:—Mr. H. J. F. Groves, of Lambeth; Mr. G. H. Fosbroke, of Stratford-on-Avon; Dr. A. Downes, of Chelmsford and Maldon; Dr. Simpson, of Aberdeen; and Dr. Hime, of Sheffield.

A letter was read from the Société Française d'Hygiène de Paris, with a diploma conferring the honorary membership of the Société on the Society of Medical Officers of Health.

A letter was read, asking the opinion of the Society how near to small-pox hospitals dwelling-houses might be built with safety.

Dr. Jacobs moved—"That the Council be requested to consider and report the steps which should be taken so as to obtain for members of this Society the valuable reports on infectious diseases made by the medical inspectors of the Local Government Board."

Dr. Corner introduced to the Society Mr. Robert Parker, Surveyor to the Board of Works for the Poplar district, who exhibited a model of a ventilating shaft for sewers.

Mr. Parker first dwelt upon the necessity which existed for sewer-ventilation, and claimed for his own method that it could be easily adapted to existing sewers. His method was to utilise the force of the wind for the purpose of causing a current of air to pass through the sewers. With this object it would be necessary to have a number of cast-iron shafts erected, twelve feet high and ten inches in diameter, in convenient and open places; and also pipes, of various sizes according to circumstances, from the sewers and existing drains at the rear of houses to the housetop, as high as the chimney-stack; and these ventilating shafts should be surmounted by a cowl, guided by a vane attached to it, so that its opening or aperture should always be facing the wind. The wind impinging on it will pass down the sewer and travel along it, entering all drains to find an outlet so that it may escape. Mr. Parker had carried out experiments showing that there was always a downward current in the shaft, and an upward rush of pure air in all the gulleys. Mr. Parker exhibited a model of his cowl, and gave the results of various experiments showing the velocity of the wind at different temperatures. In reply to Mr. Blyth, he stated that if the air had a velocity of even less than two miles an hour, this was found sufficient to produce a current through the sewer.

Dr. Tripe said some points in Mr. Parker's method commended themselves to him, but that, to be successful, the shaft should be placed at the lower level of the sewer so as to permit air to escape at the upper level. He objected to Mr. Rogers Field's method of disconnecting the house-drain from the sewer, except in cases where the latter was badly constructed. He thought the air of sewers less injurious than that of drains.

Dr. Dudfield, on the other hand, looked upon sewer-air as very prejudicial.

Dr. Carpenter thought the best method was that which took advantage of the natural circulation of the air. If every soil-pipe were ventilated, and no sewer caused deposit, no other apparatus would be needed.

Dr. Corfield said that, with regard to house-drainage, an opening at the lower and upper levels presented a perfect system.

In reply to Dr. Dixon, Mr. Parker stated his apparatus would remain a long time in good working order.

Mr. Shirley Murphy exhibited a diagram, showing the behaviour of enteric fever during each week of the present and ten preceding years. The mean temperature, barometric pressure, and the rainfall for each of these weeks was also shown.

Dr. Tripe, in moving that the diagram be published, noted the fact that during the first three quarters of the present year the number of deaths from this disease was much below the average, and that it was only in the fourth quarter that they were so much more numerous than usual. He also gave the distribution of cases admitted into the —ton Fever Hospital.

Mr. Wynter Blyth gave a brief account of the recent outbreak of typhus in Marylebone, and spoke of the inadequacy of existing laws to deal with such outbreaks. It is first necessary to remove the sick person to hospital, and then to disinfect his room; for this purpose his family must be turned out, often into the street. The bodies of these people should be disinfected, but this of course could not be done. More power was needed to deal with infected clothing and infected persons, for burning old clothes, and replacing them with new ones.

Mr. Lovett gave his experience of the help that could be obtained in dealing with such outbreaks. Each outbreak with which he had had to do had begun in a condemned area, but as soon as the sick were removed to hospital, and the houses closed under a magistrate's order, the extension of the disease was checked.

Dr. Buchanan raised the question whether the present prevalence of enteric fever might in any part be due to cases of typhus which had not been recognised.

Dr. Dudfield was of opinion that the existing laws would be found to be of much avail in limiting an outbreak of typhus.

Dr. Carpenter discussed the present prevalence of enteric fever in association with water-supply.

Mr. Shirley Murphy said that cases in St. Pancras did not appear to be due to contaminated milk or water, but occurred at distinct intervals between successive cases. If one case were introduced into a house there was a great tendency for subsequent cases to occur.

Dr. Carpenter, in reply to Dr. Dudfield, made a few remarks on the Royal Commission appointed to consider metropolitan hospital provision for infectious diseases.

ODONTOLOGICAL SOCIETY OF GREAT BRITAIN.

Monday, December 5.

Mr. Thomas Arnold Rogers, President, in the Chair.

POISONING BY ARSENICAL PASTE.

Amongst other "casual communications," Mr. W. E. Harding, of Shrewsbury, related a remarkable case of poisoning by arsenical paste. A lady came to him, complaining of acute pain in a lower molar. Finding the pulp exposed, Mr. Harding applied a small quantity of a preparation known as Baldock's nerve-killing paste, closing the cavity with cotton-wool and sandarach. Within a few hours the patient was seized with symptoms of poisoning by arsenic —burning pain at the epigastrium, vomiting, etc.,—and a rash appeared resembling measles, but slightly raised, and which was followed by desquamation. The stopping was at once removed, but the patient was very ill for several days, and did not altogether regain her health for a fortnight. A remarkable feature in the case was that this lady had suffered in the same way three times previously: once from arsenic used by another dentist, and twice from prescriptions containing it ordered by medical practitioners.

The President remarked that it was very important that patients who were the subject of such idiosyncrasies should mention them when they came to a stranger for treatment; and any practitioner discovering such peculiarities should impress upon the patient the necessity of doing this.

ON ECONOMICAL PROCESSES OF PREPARING AND ADMINISTERING NITROUS OXIDE.

The paper of the evening was by Mr. Alfred Coleman, F.R.C.S., on "Economical Processes of Preparing and Administering Nitrous Oxide." In proof of the importance of the subject to hospitals and large consumers, Mr. Coleman mentioned that the one item of nitrous oxide cost the Dental Hospital of London over £70 a year. After describing the various ways in which the gas could be obtained, he said that he believed it could be manufactured on a large scale most cheaply by the action of dilute nitric acid on zinc. As a plan for making nitrous oxide alone this method would be extravagant, since only about one-third as much gas could be obtained by this means as could be obtained for the same money by the decomposition of nitrate of ammonia. But by treating the residual nitrate of zinc with sulphuric acid the nitric acid could be recovered and sulphate of zinc obtained, which was a well-known article of commerce. By making this the main object of the manufacture he believed that the gas could be obtained as a bye-product at an almost nominal cost. Mr. Coleman then passed on to describe various devices for securing economy in administration. He hoped, however, that these might be superseded in large institutions by a plan for saving all the products of respiration during the administration of the gas, and then separating the latter for use over again. This might be effected by conducting the respired air and gas into a closed vessel containing a certain quantity of water in which a little caustic potash had been dissolved; this would fix the carbonic acid, the nitrous oxide would be absorbed by the water, and the remaining air might then be allowed to escape. Heat being applied, the gas would be driven off again from the water, and re-collected in another gasometer. The process was much facilitated by agitating the vessel containing the mixture of air, gas, and water, and by reducing the temperature of the latter as low as possible in the first instance. It would be attended with some trouble and expense, but might probably be found to pay in the case of large institutions, and where circumstances were favourable for its application.

OBITUARY.

PHILIP BEVAN, M.A., M.D. Univ. Dub., F.R.C.S. Irl.
After a prolonged period of ill-health, Dr. Philip Bevan died at his residence, Pembroke-road, Dublin, on Tuesday, December 6. He is much regretted among his professional brethren in Dublin, where he spent a long and useful life. Educated in Trinity College, Dublin, and at the Royal College of Surgeons in Ireland, Dr. Bevan took the degree of Bachelor of Medicine in the University of Dublin in 1833, and about the same time joined the Royal College of Surgeons, of which he became a Fellow in 1837. He proceeded to the degrees of Master of Arts and Doctor of Medicine in his Alma Mater in 1845. Among his earliest professional appointments was that of Surgeon to St. Peter's Dispensary. He was next appointed Lecturer on Anatomy and on Physiology in the Dublin School of Medicine, and became Surgeon to Mercer's Hospital.
Ultimately, Dr. Bevan, who had previously enjoyed a seat on the Council of the Royal College of Surgeons, was elected Professor of Surgical Anatomy in the School of Surgery of the College. This post he filled up to the time of his death. Dr. Bevan resigned the Surgeoncy to Mercer's Hospital some ten or twelve years ago, when his health first became impaired. He was a member of the Royal Irish Academy, of the Royal Dublin Society, and of the Council of the Surgical Society. He was not a prolific writer, but he contributed occasionally to the medical journals. Among other contributions he mentioned papers on "Fracture of the Femur," and on "An Apparatus for Fracture of the Femur" (Dublin Quarterly Journal of Medical Science, 1850), on "Fracture of the Odontoid Process of the Axis" (Medical Press), and on "Scalds of the Larynx" (Dublin Quarterly Journal of Medical Science, 1860).

CARRIER PIGEONS AS DOCTORS' ASSISTANTS.—We learn from reports in the papers that carrier-pigeons are being made very useful by country doctors in this State and Pennsylvania. One doctor in Hamilton County, N.Y., uses them constantly in his practice, and considers them an almost invaluable aid. After visiting a patient he sends the necessary prescription to his dispensary by a pigeon, or any other instruction the case or situation may demand. He frequently, also, leaves pigeons at places from which he wishes reports of progress to be despatched at specified times or at certain crises. He says that he is enabled to attend to at least a third more business through the time saved him by the use of pigeons. In critical cases he is able to keep posted up by hourly bulletins from the bedside between daylight and nightfall, and he can recall case after case where lives have been saved that must have been lost if he had been obliged to depend upon ordinary means of conveying information.—New York Med. Record, October 29.

MEDICAL NEWS.

UNIVERSITY OF DUBLIN.—SCHOOL OF PHYSIC IN IRELAND.—At the Michaelmas Term Examination for the degree of M.B. (Medicinæ Baccalaureus), held on Monday and Tuesday, November 28 and 29, the following candidates were successful, their names being arranged in order of merit:—

Windle, Bertram C. A.	Scott, William S. J.
Henry, William.	Nolan, Chaworth L.
Turpin, Sidney G. (Clk.).	Gillespie, Thomas R.
Kingsbury, George C.	Nevell, Frank T. P.
Archer, Arthur M.	Craig, James.
Marshall, George.	Wilson, Edmund F. B.

At the examination for the degree of B.Ch. (Chirurgiæ Baccalaureus), held on Monday and Tuesday, December 5 and 6, the successful candidates passed in the following order of merit:—

Turpin, Sidney G. (Clk.).	Archer, Arthur M.
Kingsbury, George C.	Henry, Dawson.
Windle, Bertram C. A.	Pope, Henry R.
Wilson, Edmund F. B.	Johnstone, Alexander R.

KING AND QUEEN'S COLLEGE OF PHYSICIANS IN IRELAND.—At the usual monthly examinations for the Licences of the College, held on Monday, Tuesday, Wednesday, and Thursday, December 5, 6, 7, and 8, the following candidates were successful:—
For the Licence to practise Medicine—

Browne, Danby.	Jacob, William Gardiner.
Cahill, Thomas Esmonde.	Magner, Thomas.
Coolican, John Patrick Joseph.	Murphy, Patrick Joseph.
Elderton, Frederick Dundas.	Treston, Maurice Joseph.
	Wilkin, Loftus Ralph.

For the Licence to practise Midwifery—

Browne, Danby.	Jacob, William Gardiner.
Cahill, Thomas Esmonde.	Magner, Thomas.
Coolican, John Patrick Joseph.	Murphy, Patrick Joseph.
Elderton, Frederick Dundas.	Treston, Maurice Joseph.
	Wilkin, Loftus Ralph.

The following Licentiates in Medicine of the College, having complied with the by-laws relating to membership, have been duly enrolled Members of the College—

Gunn, Christopher, 1877, Dublin.
McLaren, Agnes, 1878, Edinburgh.
Horne, Andrew John, 1878, Dublin.

The dates after the names indicate the year in which the Members respectively became Licentiates in Medicine of the College.

APOTHECARIES' HALL, LONDON.—The following gentlemen passed their examination in the Science and Practice of Medicine, and received certificates to practise, on Thursday, December 8:—

Case, William, Cockthorpe Wells, Norfolk.
Cole, George Milner, Cambridge-gardens, Notting-hill.
Ghandy, Rastanji Dinshaji, Bombay.
Lane, James Oswald, Bridge-street, Hereford.
MacCulloch, Charles, Abbey Town, Cumberland.
Marras, Ernest Adrian, Halsey-street, S.W.
Puddicombe, Francis Morgan, Dartmouth.
Tyrrell, Charles Robert, Hornsey-lane, Highgate.

The following gentlemen also on the same day passed their Primary Professional Examination:—

Openshaw, Thomas H., London Hospital.
Honan, Lynton M., St. George's Hospital.
Webster, John Arthur, St. Mary's Hospital.

APPOINTMENTS.

. The Editor will thank gentlemen to forward to the Publishing-office, as early as possible, information as to all new Appointments that take place.

SELLERS, W. H. IRVIN, M.B., C.M. Edin., M.R.C.S.E.—Junior House-Surgeon to the Royal Southern Hospital, Liverpool.

BIRTHS.

CÆSAR.—On December 10, at Tottenham, N., the wife of Charles Augustus Cæsar, L.F.P.S., of a son.
GODSON.—On December 11, at 9, Grosvenor-street, W., the wife of Clement Godson, M.D., M.R.C.P., of a son.
GRIEVE.—On November 1, at Fort Canje, Berbice, the wife of Robert Grieve, M.D., of a daughter.
HAWARD.—On December 9, at St. Leonards on-Sea, the wife of F. Robertson Haward, M.R.C.S., of a daughter.

LEE-STRATHY.—On December 6, at Woodleigh House, Harborne, Birmingham, the wife of Frederick R. Lee-Strathy, M.D., of a daughter.
WOOD.—On December 9, at Bethlem Royal Hospital, S.E., the wife of W. E. Ramsden Wood, M.A., M.D., of a daughter.

MARRIAGES.

HO KAI—WALKDEN.—On December 13, at Upper Norwood, Ho Kai, M.B., and Member of Lincoln's-inn, to Alice, eldest daughter of the late John Walkden, Esq., of Blackheath, and Lawrence-lane, E.C.
KEYS—HEYNES.—On November 17, at Cape Town, Eliza Keys, M.R.C.S., to Lorne, daughter of John Heynes, Esq., of Cape Town.
LITTLE—MOUNSTEPHEN.—On December 10, at Compton-terrace, E. S. Little, M.D., of Wimbledon, to Clara Jane, only daughter of the late Robert Mounstephen, Esq., of Milnar-square, Islington.
SMITH—KOHLHOFF.—On November 14, at Tranquebar, F. Clarence Smith, L.R.C.P., Madras Medical Service, to Ada, daughter of the Rev. C. S. Kohlhoff, of Erungalore.

DEATHS.

COX, HENRY LAWRENCE, M.B., Surgeon A.M.D., at Dilkusha, Province of Oudh, India, on November 14, aged 28.
HEMMING, WILLIAM DOUGLAS, F.R.C.S., youngest son of William B. Hemming, M.R.C.S., of 25, Notting-hill-terrace, W., at Glenalmond, Bournemouth, on December 9, aged 33.
HENRY, EMERSON WILSON, M.D., M.Ch., at 10, Lowther-street, Whitehaven, on December 4, aged 37.
HOPGOOD, JOSEPH, M.R.C.S., at Slough, Bucks, on December 6, in his 80th year.
MACMILLAN, MARY ELIZABETH, wife of Angus Macmillan, M.D., at Hull, on December 11.

VACANCIES.

In the following list the nature of the office vacant, the qualifications required in the candidate, the person to whom application should be made and the day of election (as far as known) are stated in succession.
BROMPTON HOSPITAL FOR CONSUMPTION AND DISEASES OF THE CHEST.—Physician. (For particulars see Advertisement.)
GENERAL HOSPITAL, BIRMINGHAM.—Honorary-Surgeon. Candidates must be Fellows of one of the Royal Colleges of Surgeons of the United Kingdom. Diplomas to be sent to the Medical Committee at the Hospital on or before December 24.
LONDON LOCK HOSPITAL.—Female Department. Assistant House-Surgeon. Applications, with testimonials, to be sent to the Secretary, Lock Hospital, Westbourne-green, Harrow-road, W., on or before December 20.
LOUGHBOROUGH DISPENSARY AND INFIRMARY.—Resident House-Surgeon. Candidates must possess medical and surgical registered qualifications. Applications, stating age, etc., with testimonials, to be sent to William Berridge, Secretary, not later than December 17.
MONMOUTH UNION.—Medical Officer. (For particulars see Advertisement.)

UNION AND PAROCHIAL MEDICAL SERVICE.

*** The area of each district is stated in acres. The population is computed according to the census of 1871.

RESIGNATIONS.

Brackley Union.—Mr. Robert Barry Hooter has resigned the First District: area 16,250; population 3681; salary £60 per annum.
Castle Ward Union.—Mr. James Marr has resigned the Ponteland District and the Workhouse: area 19,520; population 2083; salary £20 per annum. Salary for the Workhouse £20 per annum.
Hailsham Union.—Mr. James Herring Eogle has resigned the First District: area 10,581; population 3040; salary £68 per annum.
West Derby Union.—Dr. H. Wilson has resigned the Wavertree District: area 1390; population 7880; salary £35 per annum.

APPOINTMENTS.

Beverley Union.—John F. Park, M.D., M.Ch. Queen's Univ. Ire., to the First District. Francis Calvert, M.R.C.S. Eng., L.S.A., to the Workhouse.
Scarborough Union.—Michael Collins, M.D. and M.C. Queen's Univ. Ire. and L.M., to the Workhouse.
Ulverstone Union.—Francis C. McNalty, M.D., M.Ch., L.A.H. Dub., to the Colton District.
West Ward Union.—William Bain, M.D. Glasg., to the Patterdale District.

PENETRATING WOUND OF THE AORTA.—Dr. Zillner exhibited at the Vienna Medical Society a specimen of a penetrating wound of the aorta, the man living for sixteen days after (a very unusual duration of life after such an injury), and then dying from pericarditis. The course of the wound ran from underneath the right clavicle, through the pectoralis major and the second intercostal space into the aorta, in which an aperture four millimetres in length, and situated three fingers' breadth above the valves, was visible. The small size of the wound, a considerable atheromatous degeneration of the aorta, the slight retraction of its inner coat, and a possible plugging by the pericardial covering, may perhaps account for the prolongation of life in this case. Prof. Chiari observed that even a spontaneous rupture of the aorta may heal. Last year, while dissecting the body of a man who had died of phthisis, he met with a false aneurism of the ascending aorta, with a transverse rupture of the vessel by the side of it, which had healed.—Wien. Med. Zeitung, November 29.

PARSLEY AS AN ANTILACTIC.—In allusion to M. Stanislas Martin's strong recommendation of this plant for the purpose of arresting over-secretion of milk in puerperal women, Dr. Dujardin-Beaumetz (Bulletin de Thérapeutique, August 30) confirms the statement of the great utility of this plant, always so conveniently at hand. His attention was drawn to the matter while travelling in Asia Minor, where it is one of the ordinary domestic remedies; but in place of applying the leaves in their fresh out state, as recommended by M. Martin, the women there make them into cataplasms large enough to cover the entire breast, which are renewed three times in the twenty-four hours. Dr. Dujardin has since that often employed the parsley for this purpose, and always with success.

UNIVERSITY COLLEGE, LIVERPOOL.—Dr. Wallace's lectures on Midwifery and Diseases of Women at this College have been recognised by the University Court of Edinburgh University; and as extra-academical lectures which shall qualify for graduation in medicine in the University.

MEDICAL STATISTICS OF THE GERMAN EMPIRE.—According to an extract from "Börner's Calendar" for 1882, which appeared in the Deutsche Med. Woch., December 3, there were, in the middle of 1881, in the German Empire, 17,591 medical practitioners, and 4457 apothecaries. There were also 2576 hospital establishments, having 127,063 beds. In the entire German Empire there were 3.56 practitioners to the 100 square kilometres; in Prussia, 3.47 (varying from 0.60 in the Government of Gumbinnen to 9.25 in that of Düsseldorf); in Bavaria there are 5.05 to the 100 square kilometres (varying from 3.98 in Lower Bavaria to 7.32 in the Palatinate); in Saxony, 6.61 (varying from 3.72 in the Government of Bautzen to 9.02 in that of Leipzig); in Würtemberg, 5.39; in Baden, 3.79; in Hesse, 4.98; in Mecklenburg-Schwerin, 1.67; in Saxe-Meiningen, 2.58; in Lubeck, 11.25; in Bremen, 34.51; and in Hamburg, 74.4. There are per 10,000 inhabitants of all Germany 3.89 practitioners; in Prussia, 3.15 (9.55 in Berlin); in Bavaria, 7.27; in Saxony, 3.40; in Würtemberg, 5.34; in Baden, 3.64; in Hesse, 4.06; in Mecklenburg-Schwerin, 3.84; in Saxe-Meiningen, 3.09; in Lubeck, 5.18; in Bremen, 5.63; and in Hamburg, 6.72. Similar differences of distribution are observed among apothecaries. In the twenty medical faculties of the German Empire there are 195 professors, 136 extraordinary professors, and 186 privat-docenten.

PREVENTION OF DIPHTHERIA.—At the Paris Hospital Medical Society, M. Descroizilles read the report of the committee appointed to consider the prophylactic measures which should be adopted in relation to diphtheria, which prevails in such excess in the hospitals. Although there exists no certain prophylactic, the committee expresses its opinion.—1. That the hospital administration should establish in the wards in which diphtheria exists pulverisation of carbolic acid—these wards being kept isolated, especially in children's hospitals; 2. The minutest precautions should be taken as regards the cleanliness of these wards, their ventilation, and the rapid destruction of old dressings; 3. They should be abundantly provided, as well as the post-mortem amphitheatres, with every means for effecting the ablution of the hands and face of the operators and their assistants; 4. The material condition of the internes and externes employed in the diphtheria wards should be ameliorated as completely as possible; 5. Special prophylactic measures, such as the wadding respirator, and any others of probable utility, should have an effectual trial.—Gas. Hebd., December 9.

A CINCINNATI HEALTH PROBLEM.—There are half a dozen distilleries in the western part of Cincinnati where cattle and hogs are fattened by the thousand on the warm meal-slops from which the alcohol has been obtained. These establishments give rise to very offensive odours, and it is proposed by the Board of Health to remove them, on the ground that the odours are injurious to health. The vital statistics of the city, however, show that there have been fewer deaths in the district in question since the pens were built than there were before, and fewer than there are in the cleaner portions of the city, which are sought for their supposed healthfulness. This is an anomaly that is hard to explain, but it seems to be well established. In consequence, it is something of a problem that the Board of Health has a right to do.—New York Med. Record, November 5.

VITAL STATISTICS OF LONDON.

Week ending Saturday, December 10, 1881.

BIRTHS.

Births of Boys, 1200; Girls, 1180 ; Total, 2380.
Corrected weekly average in the 10 years 1871-80, 2385·0.

DEATHS.

	Males.	Females.	Total.
Deaths during the week	784	737	1521
Weekly average of the ten years 1871-80, corrected to increased population ...	996·1	903·0	1839·1
Deaths of people aged 80 and upwards	...	...	48

DEATHS IN SUB-DISTRICTS FROM EPIDEMICS.

	Enumerated Population, 1881 (unrevised).	Small-pox.	Measles.	Scarlet Fever.	Diphtheria.	Whooping-cough.	Typhus.	Enteric (or Typhoid) Fever.	Simple continued Fever.	Diarrhœa.
West ...	668900	...	4	4	9	11	...	2	...	...
North ...	905677	...	16	16	9	9	...	13	1	3
Central ...	281798	...	...	3	3	4	...	2	...	...
East ...	692580	1	8	11	3	17	...	7	1	5
South ...	1265878	21	25	16	8	28	...	7	...	5
Total ...	3814571	22	53	49	25	68	...	31	2	13

METEOROLOGY.

From Observations at the Greenwich Observatory.

Mean height of barometer ...	... ...	29·751 in.
Mean temperature	... ...	40·4°
Highest point of thermometer	... ...	50·4°
Lowest point of thermometer	... ...	31·2°
Mean dew-point temperature	... ...	38·2°
General direction of wind ...	... ...	S.W.
Whole amount of rain in the week	... ...	0·91 in.

BIRTHS and DEATHS Registered and METEOROLOGY during the Week ending Saturday, Dec. 10, in the following large Towns :—

Cities and boroughs (Municipal boundaries except for London.)	Estimated Population to middle of the year 1881.*	Persons to an Acre, (1881.)	Births Registered during the week ending Dec. 10.	Deaths Registered during the week ending Dec. 10.	Highest during the Week.	Lowest during the Week.	Weekly Mean of Daily Mean Values.	Temp. of Air (Cent.) Weekly Mean of Daily Mean Values.	In Inches.	In Centimetres.
London ...	3829751	50·8	2380	1521	50·4	31·2	40·4	4·66	0·91	2·31
Brighton ...	107934	45·9	55	32	56·4	32·4	41·1	5·06	1·32	3·35
Portsmouth ...	128236	25·6	70	44	...	...	...	...	...	...
Norwich ...	88038	11·8	51	29	...	...	...	...	...	...
Plymouth ...	75362	54·0	36	22	55·0	32·2	45·3	7·39	1·07	2·72
Bristol ...	207140	46·5	140	73	54·0	27·4	46·7	4·83	0·73	1·85
Wolverhampton ...	75934	22·4	43	19	50·3	22·0	37·9	3·23	0·37	0·94
Birmingham ...	402296	47·9	234	143	...	...	...	...	...	...
Leicester ...	123120	38·5	65	58	50·0	26·0	37·8	3·23	0·35	0·89
Nottingham ...	189235	13·9	108	89	50·3	23·7	38·2	3·44	0·28	0·71
Liverpool ...	553268	106·3	375	274	49·9	28·3	40·4	4·63	0·17	0·43
Manchester ...	341260	79·5	248	141	...	...	...	...	...	...
Salford ...	177790	34·4	136	72	...	...	...	...	...	...
Oldham ...	112176	24·0	73	55	...	...	...	...	...	...
Bradford ...	184037	25·5	118	71	52·0	26·0	41·6	5·34	0·61	1·55
Leeds ...	310490	14·4	237	135	51·0	28·0	40·8	4·89	0·31	0·79
Sheffield ...	285621	14·5	209	115	50·0	25·0	39·4	4·11	0·48	1·22
Hull ...	155161	42·7	124	100	50·0	24·0	36·8	2·67	0·26	0·66
Sunderland ...	116758	42·2	92	41	50·0	31·0	41·3	5·45	0·28	0·71
Newcastle-on-Tyne	145675	27·1	97	63	...	...	...	...	...	...
Total of 20 large English Towns ...	7608575	38·0	4891	3090	56·0	22·0	40·2	4·55	0·59	1·50

* These figures are the numbers enumerated (but subject to revision) in April last, raised to the middle of 1881 by the addition of a quarter of a year's increase, calculated at the rate that prevailed between 1871 and 1881.

At the Royal Observatory, Greenwich, the mean reading of the barometer last week was 29·75 in. The highest reading was 30·09 in. on Sunday morning, and the lowest 29·39 in. on Friday afternoon.

NOTES, QUERIES, AND REPLIES:

Ye that questioneth much shall learn much—Bacon.

Universal Schools of Cookery.—The Liverpool Training School of Cookery—representing, however, the United Kingdom—has had an interview with Earl Spencer at the Privy Council Office, to ask the Government to give a grant in aid of cookery being taught throughout the country, and to allow cookery to supersede less useful "class" subjects for which grants are now given. It was urged that a knowledge of cookery would vastly conduce to the comforts of men's homes, save much drunkenness, and confer other advantages. Earl Spencer said it would create quite a consternation amongst both school teachers and the ratepayers if the suggestion made were adopted, but he would give consideration to the views of the deputation.

London Smoke.—"Make all chimneys chew the cud.
　　Like hungry cows, as chimneys should !
　　And since 'tis only smoke we draw
　　Within our lungs at common law,
　　Into their thirsty tubes be sent
　　Fresh air, by Act of Parliament."

A Fellow, Manchester.—The following are the metropolitan hospitals represented by the gentlemen elected at the last meeting of the Council of the College of Surgeons as members of the Board of Examiners in Anatomy and Physiology, viz. :—St. Bartholomew's—Messrs. J. Langton, H. Power, and W. M. Baker ; the London—Messrs. W. Rivington and J. McCarthy; St. George's—Mr. T. P. Pick ; Charing-cross—Mr. E. Bellamy ; Middlesex—Mr. B. T. Lowne; and King's College—Mr. G. F. Yeo. Mr. Power has since been elected Chairman of the Board.

Dingley P., Mile End.—What the Local Government Board did in reference to the scare last year of the alleged frequency of trichinosis in American and other hams and pork, was to issue a circular to the several sanitary authorities in the country, calling their attention to precautions in cooking, and urging them to require of their medical officers especial vigilance in carrying out the regulations of the Public Health Act in regard to the examination of ham and pork exposed for sale.

Good Templar.—The Middlesex District Lodge of the Independent Order of Good Templars has resolved to complete the contribution of £1000 for the establishment of a Good Templars' Ward in the London Temperance Hospital, Hampstead-road. About £850 has already been collected.

M., St. Bartholomew's.—The Common Crier of the City of London is Capt. W. H. R. Skey, a son of the late surgeon to your Hospital. His salary is £295 per annum. The Medical Officer, Dr. W. S. Saunders, receives £600 per annum. Mr. G. B. Childs, Chief Surgeon to the City Police, receives £700 per annum. The salary of Mr. Timothy Holmes as Chief Surgeon of the Metropolitan Police is £500 per annum.

Water Supply, South-west of London.—Application is to be made to Parliament next session to sanction a scheme of water-supply from springs at Epsom and Carshalton, for Wimbledon, Putney, Kew, Richmond, Petersham, Ham, and Roehampton.

Female Guardians.—An influential meeting has been held at Leeds, under the presidency of the Mayor, to consider the advisability of promoting the election of a certain number of ladies to serve on the Leeds Board of Guardians, which body has just adopted the triennial system of election. A resolution in favour of female guardians was unanimously carried, and two or more lady candidates will be selected for the election in April next.

A Benefactor.—The Duke of Buccleuch has intimated his intention of presenting to the town of Thornhill the large field near the parish church, where the cattle show is annually held, for a public recreation ground, subject only to a reservation in favour of the Agricultural Society.

Colonial Items.—Victoria : Corrected census returns have been issued, showing the population of the colony on April 3 last ; the total population is 862,346, being 8764 more than shown by the approximate tables published in May. New South Wales : Small-pox still continues to give cause for anxiety in Sydney ; several deaths have occurred, and fresh cases are reported. South Australia : On account of the threatened epidemic of small-pox, 12,000 persons have been vaccinated during the past two months. Queensland : The Government has decided to expand a certain sum in the search for water on the artesian plan.

Balsall Heath.—During the past month the death-rate in this district—a favourite suburb of Birmingham—has been only 13·8 per 1000, as compared with 17·1 in the corresponding period last year.

A Volunteer Hospital Corps.—The students of the University of Durham College of Medicine have appointed a Committee to carry out a project for forming a Volunteer Hospital Corps, subject to the approval of the War Office.

Gregson P., Essex.—The Local Government Board issued, under the Public Health Act, 1875, model by-laws, but the actual making of these laws rests with the local authorities, and not with the Board.

Pro Bono Publico.—Wormwood Scrubs is vested in the Metropolitan Board of Works by the Wormwood Scrubs Act, 1879, upon trust, for the perpetual use of the grounds by the inhabitants of the metropolis for recreation purposes, subject to their use by the military authorities.

Septimus.—The census to be taken in France to-morrow, the 18th, differs from those of all its predecessors. Instead of its occupying a month, as hitherto, the enumeration of the people will be completed in a single day. For the first time in France, papers are left to be filled up, as with ourselves. The enumerator has on former occasions interrogated the inhabitants.

E. M. S., Hove.—The Lord Chancellor was not aware, when he submitted the name of the gentleman in question to the Town Council of the borough as a fit and proper person to be appointed a borough magistrate, that he had been twice convicted and fined by the magistrates for offences against the Vaccination Act. These offences were subsequently brought to his lordship's notice, who naturally came to the conclusion that a gentleman who had not himself recognised the duty of obeying the law was hardly a suitable person to add to the roll of magistrates, and consequently withdrew the nomination.

Eye Hospital, Birmingham.—The governors of this institution have resolved to erect a new building in New Edmund-street, at an estimated cost of £17,000. The present building was originally an hotel; the dispensary was a bar, and it is on record that the house-surgeon's room was once occupied by the Queen, when she passed through the town as Princess Victoria.

A Sanitary Exhibition, Berlin.—During the coming spring a hygienic exhibition will be opened in this city, under the patronage of the Empress and Crown Prince. Foreign inventions appertaining to the subject will be exhibited.

The London Hospital.—Among the railway schemes to be brought before Parliament in the next session is one of the East London Railway Company. It proposes to run a line under the eastern part of the London Hospital, and to take certain portions of the Hospital property. An organised opposition is in course of formation, for the purpose of holding public meetings throughout the East of London to protest against the scheme.

G.O.O., Bayswater.—The drugs for the Army in England are supplied by either the Apothecaries' Company or Messrs. Savory and Moore, according to the price tendered. In Ireland they are supplied by the Apothecaries' Company of Dublin.

L. Donald N., Marylebone.—Much praise has been bestowed on the public health institutions of France, and the plan of a council of experts for each district would appear, *primâ facie*, to be good, and likely to be satisfactory in its working; but practically the councils of health of the smaller areas, it is stated, do nothing, and the advice of the others is often not attended to.

The Welsh Sunday-Closing Act.—The decision was given in the Queen's Bench Division last week as to when this Act comes into force. It appears, in the appellant's case, the annual licensing meeting for one of the divisions of Flintshire had been appointed before, and not after, the Act came into operation, and the Court held the Act would not take effect, therefore, until next year, after "the next appointed day" for the licensing meeting. The appellant was, consequently, wrongly convicted.

Water Supply, United States.—Artesian wells are beginning to command attention in Boston and New York. They have been tried in the latter city with doubtful results. Most of the brewers have sunk them, but in many cases without success. It is stated, however, that if the well which is being sunk in Providence-street, Boston, at a great expense, should prove successful, the water problem will then be speedily solved.

Hygienist.—1. Baths and washhouses for the working classes originated in 1844, with an "Association for Promoting Cleanliness among the Poor," who fitted up a bathhouse and a laundry in Glasshouse-yard, East Smithfield. It was a successful experiment, and led to the passing of the Act 9 and 10 Vic., c. 74, "To encourage the establishment of baths and washhouses." 2. Public burial-grounds, planted and laid out as gardens, around the metropolis were suggested just after the Great Fire of 1666, when Evelyn regretted that advantage had not been taken of the calamity to rid the city of its burial-places and establish a necropolis without the walls.

PERIODICALS AND NEWSPAPERS RECEIVED—

Lancet—British Medical Journal—Medical Press and Circular—Berliner Klinische Wochenschrift—Centralblatt für Chirurgie—Gazette des Hopitaux—Gazette Médicale—Le Progrès Médical—Bulletin de l'Académie de Médecine—Pharmaceutical Journal—Wiener Medizinische Wochenschrift—Centralblatt für die Medizinischen Wissenschaften—Revue Médicale—Gazette Hebdomadaire—National Board of Health Bulletin, Washington—Nature—Boston Medical and Surgical Journal—Louisville Medical News—Deutsche Medicinal-Zeitung—Evening Chronicle, December 7—Medical News and Collegiate Herald—North American Journal—Centralblatt für Gynäkologie—Therapeutic Gazette—Scienze Mediche—Australasian Medical Gazette—Sanitarian—Western Medical Reporter—Church of England Pulpit, etc.—Argosy, Demerara, November 19—Western Daily Mercury, December 10—Boston Journal of Chemistry, etc.—North Carolina Medical Journal—Archives of Medicine.

BOOKS, ETC., RECEIVED—

The Surgeons of Baltimore and their Achievements, by B. Bernard Brown M.D.—Aural Surgery, by Macnaughton Jones, M.D.—Rudolf Virchow, by A. Jacobi, M.D.—Leprosy in British Guiana, by J. D. Hillis, F.R.C.S., M.R.I.A.—The Smoke Difficulty Conquered, by Frederick Edwards, jun.—The Garden of Hyères, by Adolphe Smith—The Seed-Time of Health, by B. W. Richardson, LL.D., F.R.S.—Descriptive Catalogue of Surgical Pathology, by Marcus Beck, M.S., M.B., F.R.C.S., and S. G. Shattock, M.R.C.S.—Report of the Port of London Sanitary Committee—National Temperance League's Annual, 1882.

COMMUNICATIONS have been received from—

Mr. J. B. Barnes, London; Messrs. Kilner Bros., London; Dr. Dowett Stone, London; Mr. A. G. Blomfield, Exeter; Dr. Neale, London; Dr. Buzzard, London; The Registrar of the Apothecaries' Hall, London; Mr. S. S. Forster, Worcester; Mr. Kenneth W. Millican, Kineton, Warwick; Mr. Lawson Tait, Birmingham; Dr. Herman, London; Messrs. Allen and Hanburys, London; The Secretary of the Smoke Abatement Exhibition, London; Dr. C. Creighton, London; The Honorary Secretary of the Medical Society of London; Dr. J. W. Moore, Dublin; The Registrar-General, Scotland; Dr. R. H. Semple, London; The Secretary of the East London Mission; Dr. Ballota Taylor, Santillana; The Secretary of the Odontological Society of Great Britain; Mr. J. Chatto, London; Mr. T. M. Stone, London; Dr. W. H. Barlow, Manchester; Mr. Rickman J. Godlee, London; The Secretary of the Richmond Hospital, Surrey; Mr. Storrs Turner, London; The Sanitary Commissioner, Punjab; Dr. Wallace, Liverpool; Dr. D. Colquhoun, London; Mr. W. W. Yates, Dewsbury; Dr. R. Boyd, London; Dr. Yarrow, London; Brigade-Surgeon Kidd, London; Dr. Benjamin Ward Richardson, Brighton; The Honorary Secretary of the Pathological Society of London; Mr. William Elliott Porter, Lindfield.

APPOINTMENTS FOR THE WEEK.

December 17. *Saturday* (*this day*).

Operations at St. Bartholomew's, 1½ p.m.; King's College, 1½ p.m.; Royal Free, 2 p.m.; Royal London Ophthalmic, 11 a.m.; Royal Westminster Ophthalmic, 1½ p.m.; St. Thomas's, 1½ p.m.; London, 2 p.m.

19. *Monday.*

Operations at the Metropolitan Free, 2 p.m.; St. Mark's Hospital for Diseases of the Rectum, 2 p.m.; Royal London Ophthalmic, 11 a.m.; Royal Westminster Ophthalmic, 1½ p.m.

Medical Society of London, 8½ p.m. The discussion on the Salicylic Treatment of Acute Rheumatism will be resumed, when further Statistics will be furnished by the President, Dr. De Havilland Hall, Dr. Warner, Dr. Charles Hood, Dr. Coupland, Dr. Fowler, and Dr. Gilbert Smith.

20. *Tuesday.*

Operations at Guy's, 1½ p.m.; Westminster, 2 p.m.; Royal London Ophthalmic, 11 a.m.; Royal Westminster Ophthalmic, 1½ p.m.; West London, 3 p.m.

Statistical Society, 7¾ p.m. Monthly Meeting.

Pathological Society, 8½ p.m. Specimens: Dr. Pye-Smith—Cirrhosis of the Liver in a Child. Dr. B. Fenwick—Disease of Supra-Renal Capsules. Dr. Goodhart—Ulcerative Endocarditis. Mr. A. Barker—1. Dislocation of Hip; 2. Spinal Caries. Dr. Sharkey—1. Cyst of Liver; 2. Cyst of Cerebellum; 3. Gummata in Spleen. Dr. Stephen Mackenzie—Stricture of Intestine. Dr. Fowler—Intestinal Obstruction. Card Specimens: Attached Fœtus; Fracture of Femur; Absence of Radius; Filaria Medinensis.

21. *Wednesday.*

Operations at University College, 2 p.m.; St. Mary's, 1¼ p.m.; Middlesex, 1 p.m.; London, 2 p.m.; St. Bartholomew's, 1½ p.m.; Great Northern, 2 p.m.; Samaritan, 2½ p.m.; Royal London Ophthalmic, 11 a.m.; Royal Westminster Ophthalmic, 1½ p.m.; St. Thomas's, 1½ p.m.; St. Peter's Hospital for Stone, 2 p.m.; National Orthopædic, Great Portland-street, 10 a.m.

Association of Surgeons Practising Dental Surgery (Council Meeting, 8 p.m.), 8½ p.m. Monthly Meeting.

22. *Thursday.*

Operations at St. George's, 1 p.m.; Central London Ophthalmic, 1 p.m.; Royal Orthopædic, 2 p.m.; University College, 2 p.m.; Royal London Ophthalmic, 11 a.m.; Royal Westminster Ophthalmic, 1½ p.m.; Hospital for Diseases of the Throat, 2 p.m.; Hospital for Women, 2 p.m. Charing-cross, 2 p.m.; London, 2 p.m.; North-West London, 2½ p.m.

23. *Friday.*

Operations at Central London Ophthalmic, 2 p.m.; Royal London Ophthalmic, 11 a.m.; South London Ophthalmic, 2 p.m.; Royal Westminster Ophthalmic, 1½ p.m.; St. George's (ophthalmic operations), 1¼ p.m.; Guy's, 1½ p.m.; St Thomas's (ophthalmic operations), 2 p.m.; King's College (by Mr. Lister), 2 p.m.

Quekett Microscopical Club (University College), 8 p.m. Ordinary Meeting.

The Examination in Subjects relating to Public Health of the University of London.—The following gentlemen have passed this examination:—Hutton Castle, M.B.; Edward F. Willoughby, M.B.

ORIGINAL LECTURES.

CLINICAL LECTURES
ON DISEASES OF THE ABDOMEN.

By FREDERICK T. ROBERTS, M.D., B.Sc., F.R.C.P.,
Professor of Materia Medica and Therapeutics at University College,
Physician to University Hospital, and Professor of
Clinical Medicine, etc.

LECTURE VI.
THE SYMPTOMATOLOGY OF ABDOMINAL DISEASES.

THE symptoms connected with the abdomen are not only numerous, but in individual cases they are not uncommonly more or less complicated. It will, therefore, perhaps help you in your study of these symptoms, and will enable you to understand them better, both in themselves and in particular instances, if we consider them as a whole at some length, before discussing them in relation to individual organs or diseases. From the preceding lecture you will have gathered that we may have, in any abdominal case, to deal with four groups of symptoms having a direct bearing upon it, namely:—1. Local abdominal symptoms. 2. Remote symptoms, but known to be associated with one of the abdominal structures. 3. General symptoms. 4. Thoracic symptoms. Each of these groups will need to be discussed, but before doing so there are certain important practical facts which I desire to impress upon you at the outset.

1. Remember that there are some abdominal diseases which have no obvious symptoms, and which cannot possibly be recognised during life. As a rule these affections are of little or no consequence, but they may be important. It will suffice to mention, as illustrations, atrophy of the spleen and some other structures; fatty and other forms of degeneration of certain organs; chronic infarctions; and new growths in viscera, not large enough to affect their functions or to produce any other obvious disorder, such as syphilitic deposits, small hydatids, or fibrous and other benign growths. You must be prepared to meet with these and other morbid conditions at post-mortem examinations, when there has been no sign whatever of their existence during life.

2. The seriousness and gravity of an abdominal case can by no means always be judged of by the symptoms present. This statement demands a few words of explanation and illustration.

Abdominal symptoms may be very marked and prominent, and yet be merely indicative of some temporary disorder of no particular importance, and not dependent upon any actual disease, or, at least, any disease of much consequence. This is observed commonly enough as regards pain and other subjective feelings; but it may also apply to objective phenomena, such as vomiting, diarrhœa, or jaundice. On the other hand, it not infrequently happens that a complaint of the most grave character is unattended with any definite symptoms, or they are quite out of proportion to the seriousness of the case. For example, in some instances of dangerous or fatal acute inflammatory disease connected with the abdomen, the symptoms may be absolutely latent from first to last. This is particularly noticed in certain forms of acute peritonitis, and in connexion with septic or pyæmic inflammations or abscesses. Even in typhoid fever there may be none of its ordinary abdominal symptoms. Again, many cases of certain chronic grave diseases start and progress in such an insidious manner, that it may be a long time before any symptoms at all, or merely those of a very indefinite character, are noticed. Sometimes their existence is only revealed by the onset of sudden or acute symptoms. Such diseases may be exemplified by cancer of various organs, tubercular affections, cirrhosis of the liver, some forms of Bright's disease, and renal or hepatic calculus. Indeed, certain organs may be gradually changed, and their structures ultimately destroyed, without the occurrence of any evident symptoms connected with them—at any rate such as indicate disturbance of their functions. But what is still more remarkable is this—

namely, that there may be some obvious and prominent abdominal morbid condition—so obvious that only the most superficial physical examination is needed to discover it—and yet no symptoms arise to draw either the patient's or the practitioner's attention to such condition. Patients, however, are sometimes quite aware of its existence, but, because there are no symptoms, think it of no consequence; or, even if they are conscious of symptoms, they conceal them from the practitioner, or will not tell him of what they have every reason to know or suspect is their cause. I remember a case in which a patient consulted me for neuralgic pains in the left leg, from which she had suffered severely, and for which she had been treated for some time. For certain reasons I suspected that the pains depended upon some pressure on the nerves within the abdomen or pelvis, and, on inquiry, ascertained that there was a swelling in the lower part of the abdomen, on the left side, of the existence of which the patient had not informed her medical attendant, because she thought it was of no consequence, and did not like to be examined. I insisted upon an examination, and found a large accumulation of fæces, which afterwards led to serious local inflammation and suppuration. But, further, it is very curious what abnormal physical conditions may be present in the abdomen, of which the patient is quite unconscious. This applies to some very large livers and spleens, tumours of considerable size, fæcal accumulations, and other conditions. We have at present in the wards a youth who has an enormous spleen. He came to me as an out-patient at the Brompton Hospital, complaining of chest-symptoms, and it was only as the result of my examination that the enlarged spleen was discovered. Even now, however, he will not acknowledge to any abdominal symptoms whatever, although he has this large mass within the abdomen.

3. It must be remembered that there may be prominent symptoms connected with abdominal organs, and yet without the existence of any evident disease in this part of the body. I need scarcely again remind you of the frequency with which symptoms connected with the alimentary canal are met with in many general and remote morbid conditions. Vomiting is an important symptom of certain cases of cerebral disease. One of the complaints most strikingly illustrative of the point now under consideration, however, is diabetes. Some of the most prominent clinical phenomena observed in this affection are connected with certain abdominal viscera; and whatever its pathology may be, it certainly does not depend on any lesion of the organs with which these symptoms are associated.

4. Most of the organs and structures within the abdomen have a definite set of symptoms belonging to each, of which it is your obvious duty to acquire an adequate knowledge at the outset, before you proceed to study their several diseases. In the first place you should learn merely what these symptoms are, but this is far from being sufficient. A mere repetition of the clinical phenomena connected with a certain organ may be of no value in any particular case, for these may equally belong to several of its diseases, and give no hint as to their differential diagnosis. What you have further to do, then, is to try to understand the symptoms, founded on a knowledge of the general and histological anatomy of the various structures, and of their functions, as determined by the most recent observations and physiological researches. Having done this, you are then in a position to study any special morbid condition, such as cancer, as well as the several diseases of each structure; and, recognising their nature and the pathological effects which they are liable to produce, you will comprehend what clinical phenomena each several condition or disease is likely to originate, and so will be prepared for their occurrence in actual practice.

5. I now come to a point for which I claim your special attention and consideration, and which I would impress upon you never to forget in dealing with abdominal cases. Symptoms obviously connected with a particular organ may be due, not to any disease in itself, but to disease affecting some other organ or structure within the abdomen, which may be of a very grave nature. I have already hinted at this in a former lecture, when explaining to you that a morbid condition in one organ or structure often sets up pathological changes in others; and you will readily understand how mere symptoms may be similarly produced. Indeed, it may be stated that organic disease of certain

organs, as of the pancreas, is commonly recognised, not by any clinical signs directly referable to such organ, but by those associated with neighbouring structures. Jaundice may be said, as a rule, not to be due to anything wrong with the liver itself; gastric and intestinal symptoms are very often dependent upon diseases in other organs; and the same remark applies, to a less degree, to urinary symptoms. The obvious lesson from these facts is, that you must not carelessly refer symptoms connected with an organ to disease of that organ, or jump at the conclusion that such disease exists. From a want of due consideration of this matter, I have known several most serious errors in diagnosis committed.

Now, it is worth a little study on your part to try to comprehend how abdominal symptoms may arise outside the seat of actual disease, and it appears to me that they may originate in the following ways:—

a. By mere *contiguity.* Structures which are in contact with each other are liable to cause mutual irritation, and thus may excite symptoms. We have recently had a case in the hospital, in which a mass of glands so irritated the stomach as to cause very troublesome vomiting. I recollect an interesting case in which there were such severe gastric symptoms, that ulcer of the stomach was diagnosed; but at the post-mortem examination it was found that the transverse colon was ulcerated, and had become adherent to the stomach, the interior of this viscus being quite healthy. The contiguity of the pelvic organs often accounts for symptoms in this region external to the seat of disease.

b. By *mechanical pressure and obstruction.* While these conditions are liable to cause actual organic lesions, they also frequently produce mere symptoms, at any rate for a time. Thus, the pancreas may cause jaundice by obstructing the bile-duct; or gastric symptoms by pressing upon the stomach or its pyloric orifice, or upon the duodenum. An enlarged organ or tumour tends to interfere with any structure in its vicinity. It must also be borne in mind that organs are sometimes displaced, and may thus mechanically originate symptoms at a point more or less distant from their normal seat.

c. By the anatomical arrangement of *blood-vessels.* This is best illustrated by diseases of the liver, the symptoms of which, when present, are most frequently due to obstruction of the portal circulation. Not only is ascites thus caused, but prominent symptoms often occur in connexion with the stomach and intestines, on account of the congestion of these structures which is induced. Indeed, I have known a case where these symptoms were so severe and grave, with urgent vomiting and hæmorrhage, but without ascites, that the liver was entirely overlooked, and the diagnosis of malignant disease of the alimentary canal was arrived at; yet the post-mortem revealed that the case was one of extreme cirrhosis.

d. By *disordered secretions* and *functions.* When certain secretions or excretions are abnormal in quantity or quality, they are often the cause of symptoms beyond their source. For instance, deficiency of bile, and perhaps of pancreatic juice, frequently accounts for constipation and other intestinal symptoms. Excessive quantity or irritable quality of the bile may probably excite bilious vomiting or diarrhœa; and the pancreatic juice has been made answerable for some cases of pyrosis and diarrhœa. Disorders affecting the functions of the stomach, secretory and motor, certainly have an important influence in originating intestinal symptoms, for if the food is rapidly propelled out of the stomach, or if the products of imperfect digestion reach the intestines, disturbances are very likely to be produced here. Abnormal conditions of the urine, as regards quantity or quality, often set up symptoms connected with the bladder or urethra as it passes over the surface of the mucous membrane, quite independent of any disease in these parts.

e. By the *physiological relations of organs,* or *nervous influence.* Undoubtedly, thus is explained, in some instances, the occurrence of abdominal symptoms away from the seat of actual disease. The different parts of the digestive organs may be mutually affected in this way. Uterine and ovarian diseases or disorders are frequently credited with originating symptoms by their physiological relations to organs, or through some reflex nervous influence; at any rate, symptoms are often associated with these conditions, which seem to have no other explanation. We speak of organs being affected by sympathy, and this is through the agency of the nervous system.

f. By altering the *blood.* This may be illustrated by the occurrence of vomiting or diarrhœa as phenomena of uræmia due to renal disease.

These are the principal ways in which it appears to me that symptoms may be set up in abdominal organs away from the seat of actual mischief, and I would again urge upon you the importance of recognising and remembering them.

6. From what has been already stated, it will be at once evident that abdominal symptoms may be very numerous and complicated. But they become still more so from the fact that some symptoms are liable to give rise to other secondary symptoms; or that more than one—it may be several organs—are implicated at the same time. Under these circumstances it frequently becomes very difficult, and sometimes impossible, to unravel all the symptoms, and to refer them to their several causes.

7. You must not forget that symptoms directly due to some definite morbid condition in the abdomen may be localised in other parts of the body. This is generally the result of irritation or pressure, and the phenomena are principally noticed in the lower extremities, such as neuralgic pains, or œdema from pressure on veins.

8. It may be worth while to notice, that you might possibly meet with a case in which the symptoms present seem to be readily explained by some morbid condition you discover, and yet they are actually due to a totally different cause. This was much impressed upon my mind by a case in which certain urinary symptoms appeared to be attributable to a movable kidney, combined with uterine disease and displacement, and yet they were really caused by diabetes, which was immediately revealed by examination of the urine.

(To be continued.)

RECURRENT SYMMETRICAL HERPES ZOSTER.—Dr. Zinsser related a case of this to the New York Society of German Physicians, occurring in a man aged nineteen. He had suffered occasional attacks of zoster for many years, each attack being ushered in by constitutional disturbance, with a feeling like sea-sickness. In the intervals of the attacks he seemed in apparent health, barring slight anæmia. The bilateral symmetry, with the recurrence of the eruption, constituted the case one of great rarity, and Kaposi has observed but a single one of the kind, and refers only to two others. Neuralgic pains were never experienced by this patient, nor was his constitution of a nervous type, and the local pains incident to the eruption have never been severe. Dr. Zinsser believed that the disease in this case is of central origin. Dr. Jacobi said that there could hardly be any doubt of the situation of the disturbance in such cases, and he located it in the vaso-motor centre of the medulla oblongata.—*New York Med. Record,* November 12.

VITAL STATISTICS OF MASSACHUSETTS IN 1880.—Some interesting facts connected with the death-rate and its causes in Massachusetts have appeared in the *Boston Med. Journal* for October 6. They relate to the year 1880. With a population of 1,783,085, the rates for the year per 1000 were—births 24·80, deaths 19·79, and marriages 8·71. The number of deaths (35,292) was considerably in excess of that of any year in the previous quarter of a century. The very fatal epidemic of diphtheria and croup has caused 18,714 deaths in the ten years ending with 1880, the number in that year being 2394. The order of fatality of the twelve causes producing the greatest number of deaths places consumption easily at the head of the list, as usual; pneumonia is second, and is always a leading source of mortality in Massachusetts; cholera infantum, from having steadily fallen from the second place in 1872 and 1873, the third in 1874 and 1875, the fourth in 1876 and 1877, the fifth in 1878, and the sixth in 1879, has again risen in 1880 to the third; heart-disease is fourth; diphtheria stands fifth (but if croup were included with it the deaths would be 2394 instead of 1769, and its place would be third); old age is sixth; paralysis is now, for the fourth year, seventh; cancer has risen from the tenth, eleventh, and twelfth places to the eighth; "cephalitis" is ninth; typhoid fever has shown an extraordinary decline from the fourth place in 1872, sixth in 1873, seventh in 1874, eighth in 1875 and 1876, ninth in 1877 and 1878, and thirteenth in 1879, but has risen again in 1880 to tenth.—*New York Med. Record,* November 12.

ORIGINAL COMMUNICATIONS.

ASCITES IN THE FŒTUS, OBSTRUCTING DELIVERY.

By G. ERNEST HERMAN, M.B. Lond.,
Assistant Obstetric Physician to the London Hospital; Physician to the
Royal Maternity Charity; Examiner in Midwifery to the
Royal College of Surgeons of England.

THE following case deserves record on account of its unusual character. It occurred in the practice of the London Hospital Maternity Charity, and the account which I give is taken from notes by Mr. W. F. Dale, who was in attendance on the case.

Eighth Pregnancy—Small Conjugate Diameter—Face Presentation—Podalic Version—Delay in Extraction, owing to Ascites of Fœtus—Perforation of Fœtal Abdomen— Delivery.

E. M., aged thirty-nine, pregnant for the eighth time. None of her former labours had been attended with any great difficulty, so far as she knew. During pregnancy she said she had often felt very unwell, suffering from faintness, and dimness of sight, and difficulty in moving herself in bed; but there was no history of any more definite symptoms than these. Mr. Dale was sent for on June 29, at 10.30 a.m. The os uteri was then about the size of a crown-piece, soft and dilatable. The membranes were protruding through it, and the presenting part was high up. The pains were occurring regularly, about every five minutes. The face was presenting, with the chin posterior. Soon after Mr. Dale's arrival, the membranes ruptured, and a large quantity of liquor amnii escaped, and the pains became more feeble and less frequent. Mr. Fenton Jones, the resident accoucheur, and subsequently Dr. Herman, were then sent for. With the combined manipulation of one hand in the vagina and the other externally, an attempt was made about 2 p.m. to turn the chin forwards and then deliver with forceps. The chin could be turned forwards and the forceps applied, but when traction was made the chin rotated back again. The forceps was therefore removed, and podalic version performed by Mr. Fenton Jones without much difficulty. During the turning a good deal of liquor amnii escaped. A foot was brought down, and the breech was thus got to enter the pelvic brim, but in spite of vigorous traction, continued for about an hour, no further progress was made. About 3.15 p.m., therefore, the fœtal abdomen was perforated with Smellie's scissors. When the abdominal walls were penetrated, a good deal of serous fluid escaped. Upon traction by the foot, the breech now descended, and as it did so more fluid flowed from the abdomen. Delivery was completed without further difficulty. Some of the fluid which escaped after perforation of the abdomen was collected in a vessel, and was estimated to be more than a pint in quantity, and it was thought that at least as much more ran into the bed. It was judged that altogether probably about three pints of fluid must have been let out from the abdomen. The vessel used to receive it was the first that came to hand, and unfortunately happened not to be quite empty; therefore the fluid could neither be measured nor examined.

The mother made a good recovery. After delivery the internal conjugate diameter was found to measure three inches and a half.

The body of the child was examined by Mr. Fenton Jones. The bladder and kidneys were healthy. The liver was healthy. The portal vein was dissected up, but not found occluded. There was no evidence of peritonitis, old or recent. The only abnormality noticed was a cyst in the right supra-renal capsule, which contained blood. Together with the capsule it was about equal to the kidney in size, and it extended upwards so far that it pressed on the portal vein at its entrance into the liver.

I have thought this case worth publication on account of the rarity of the morbid condition present, and the paucity of recorded cases of it. Dr. Madge (a)says he has seen a few cases, but does not give particulars of any. Spiegelberg(b)

says he has once seen delivery hindered by this condition. Dr. Galabin(c) showed, at a meeting of the Obstetrical Society of London, a fœtus in which ascites, of inflammatory origin, coexisted with distension of the bladder. Another ascitic fœtus was exhibited to the same Society by Mr. Ashburton Thompson.(d) In this case the head presented and was born without much trouble, but the body offered so much resistance that the head was pulled off by the traction used. After this had been done, the body was expelled by the natural efforts. Mr. Thompson offered the ingenious explanation that by pulling on the trunk the fluid was driven up into that part of it which was above the pelvic brim; but when this pressure was left off, the fluid gravitated, expanding that part of the fœtal trunk which was below the pelvic inlet; and then, the part above the brim being no longer so voluminous, it was able to pass the strait. The specimen was referred to a committee, who verified the fact that ascites was present, but were unable, owing to the advanced decomposition of the body, to ascertain the cause of the dropsy. Dr. Keiller(e) has put on record a case in which ascites was the result of peritonitis. Delivery was effected without mutilation of the child. Another such has been described by Virchow.(f) The mother was aged thirty; it was her seventh pregnancy, and her last three children had been still-born, and were said to have had dropsical bellies. She had complained of pain in her right side during her pregnancy, but had been otherwise well. The child was born at seven months: the labour was easy, the liquor amnii abundant, and the placenta is described as "enormous." Examination of the fœtus showed ascites, with traces of past peritonitis, and the liver and spleen were large. In speaking of the pathology of this case, Virchow remarks that although it is abundantly evident that fœtal disease may arise independently of maternal influence, yet a disturbance in the organism of the mother during gestation may affect the fœtus. Küstner(g) has published a case in which the ascitic fœtus was one of twins, and hydramnios was also present—with which fœtus was not ascertained. With the ascites there was commencing induration of the liver, and hypertrophy of the heart. There is also a case recorded by Steinberg,(h) in which, in the last mentioned, the child was one of twins. It was born prematurely and dead, there being no difficulty in its delivery. Ascites is said to have been the only morbid condition present, the different organs all being apparently healthy. Another has been published by Schlesinger,(i) in which we are told there was ascites, and the liver and kidneys were of unusual size; but no further information is given as to the pathological conditions present. Porak(k) has put on record a remarkable case, in which the head, both arms, and both legs were successively pulled off in vain attempts at delivery. The abdomen of the fœtus was afterwards found to measure forty-five centimetres (about seventeen inches and a half) in circumference. The peritoneum was thickened; the liver was hypertrophied, and contained a cyst. There is also one mentioned by Herpin,(l) in which the head was detached by traction made in vain to effect delivery. The belly had then to be opened. The fœtus had been long dead; it is said that there was ascites, but there is no detailed account of the examination of the fœtus.

These are all the authenticated cases of ascites in the fœtus which I have been able to find. There are many others scattered through the older authors under this name, but they are simply instances of distension of the fœtal abdomen with fluid, the exact situation of which was not ascertained by anatomical examination. Depaul(m) has shown reasons for thinking that these were mostly cases of distension of the urinary passages—a condition which in the fœtus is commoner than ascites.

These few cases are not enough, even if they were all well reported, to justify any generalisations as to the natural history of the morbid condition present. It may,

(a) "On Diseases of the Fœtus."　(b) *Lehrbuch der Geburtshülfe*, S. 598.

(c) *Obstetrical Transactions*, vol. xix., page 119.
(d) *Ibid.*, vol. xvii., pages 4 and 65.
(e) *Edinburgh Medical Journal*, 1855, page 135.
(f) *Schmidt's Jahrbuch*, Bd. 102, S. 308. (The original paper, which I. have not been able to see, is in the *Monatsschrift für Geburtskunde*, Bd. xi. S. 181.)　(g) *Archiv für Gynäkologie*, Bd. x., S. 134.
(h) *Schmidt's Jahrbuch*, Bd. 8, S. 29?.　(i) *Ibid.*, Bd. xiv., S. 46.
(k) *Bulletin de la Société Anatomique de Paris*, 1875, page 534.
(l) *Gazette des Hopitaux*, 1822, page 351.
(m) *Gazette Hebdomadaire*, 1860.

nevertheless, be instructive to concisely put together the facts, such as they are, which appear. Out of ten cases, in three either there was no other morbid condition, or, if present, it was not recognised. Of the remaining seven, in four the dropsy was of inflammatory origin. In three the liver was enlarged (in one containing a cyst), and in one it was indurated. In two the spleen was large. In one there was general dropsy and distension of the bladder. In one there was hypertrophy of the heart. In one there was a cyst in the supra-renal capsule, which appeared to have pressed on the portal vein. In one there was some slight reason for thinking that former children of the same parents had been the subjects of similar disease. In one the placenta was unusually large, and in two the liquor amnii was in excess. In two cases the child affected was one of twins. Three were born prematurely. In three the abdomen had to be opened and the fluid let out before delivery could be accomplished, the obstruction to delivery from the size of the belly being so considerable that traction sufficient to detach the head or limbs was ineffectual. In the remainder the effusion was not enough to prevent natural delivery.

SOME NEW FACTS CONECTED WITH THE ACTION OF GERMS IN THE PRODUCTION OF HUMAN DISEASES.
By Dr. GEORGE HARLEY, F.R.S.

Reformed Speling—No Duplicated Consonants except in Personal Names.

CHAPTER III.

CAN THE SUDEN REAPEARANCE OF INFECTIOUS DISEASES IN A LOCALITY WHICH HAS LONG BEEN FREE FROM THEM BE PHILOSOPHICALY ACOUNTED FOR BY THE GERM THEORY? *Answer*—YES.

(*Concluded from page* 700.)

I WIL further show that the mere element of bodily and mental exhaustion (without the intervention of mesmerism) is suficient to induce for a time in the human being a sleep almost equivalent to hibernation.

This I know for a fact, by what was during the Crimean War rather an unpleasant personal experience. When I was in danger of being caught trespassing on territory where I had no right to be. It is briefly as folows :—

After having been exposed for eight consecutive days and nights to great bodily fatigue and personal danger, I was at length able to throw in safety my exhausted frame, dressed and dirty as I was, on to a bed in a smal out-of-the-way roadside *Wirthshaus*. I slept,. while lying flat on my back, without either moving or waking, for no les a period than twenty-six consecutive hours. This I can vouch for, as at the end of that time I found myself in the identical (what at another time would have been an uncomfortable) atitude I asumed when I threw my exhausted body down to rest. Now comes the strangest part of the story. Not only did I not empty my blader during' these twenty-six hours, but I felt no particular inclination to do so on waking up, and I could not, from my bodily sensations, for a time bring myself to believe that I had had more than a few minutes' refreshing sleep. The French have a saying, that he who sleeps dines, and certainly that saying was most extra-ordinarily verified in my case. For, notwithstanding that not a particle of food had pased my lips for over thirty hours, I neither felt particularly hungry nor thirsty on waking out of my twenty-six hours' profound sleep. They who have experienced the exhausting efects of prolonged fatigue, danger, and excitement, will apreciate these remarks.

I have another example to give of a different form of, what may be equaly apropriately designated, artificialy induced Latent-life. Namely, that which is the result of the intro-duction into the animal economy of toxic agents. During my career as a Teacher of Practical Physiology at University Colege, I made it a rule to experiment, when posible, on al subjects which excited my thirst for knowledge ; and after saying this it wil not surprise the reader to hear that I tried my hand upon the artificial production of Latent-life in animals by means of drugs. After having made several more or les satisfactory trials with diferent toxic agents, I at length discovered a poison which acts in this way far

more efectualy than any species of ordinary narcotic—bang, opium, or such like. The substance I alude to is the Indian's arow poison—Woorara,—and the most striking example I can give of its efects in this way is to quote the result of an experiment which I published in the *Field* in 1861, at the special request of Frank Buckland, under the title of " A Dead Animal's Heart Pulsating."

The history of the experiment is briefly this :—In a few minutes after a ful-grown and vigorous frog was pricked with the sharp point of a smal poisoned arow he became completely paralysed. Ceased to give visible signs of breath-ing, and looked and felt to the touch like a dead animal. Dead, however, he was not, for the circulation of the blood could be seen going on in the web of the foot when it was microscopically examined. On the fourth day—that is to say, ninety-six hours after the animal was poisoned—not only did the frog look dead, but its lower limbs were already shrunk and withered. A portion only of the heart, when ex-posed, seemed to be stil alive. At least, only the left auricle continued to pulsate. Exactly 100 hours after the animal ceased to show signs of active life, I began to atempt its resuscitation by placing it in the chamber of a water-bath in a warm moist atmosphere, and there retaining it until the temperature of its body was slightly raised. This had the desired efect. Within a quarter of an hour I had the satisfaction of seeing organic life return. First both auricles, and afterwards the single ventricle, of the frog's heart began to pulsate rhythmicaly. Then the large vessels atached to it folowed suit. In a few hours the animal could move its fore limbs. On the folowing day it jumped when pricked with the point of my steel pen. Here, then, is a case of resuscitation after 100 hours of artificialy produced complete Latent-life.

Dead poisons, even of an organic nature, if kept dry, re-tain their toxic properties for an almost indefinite period. I have now in my posession woorara arow poison, which was brought home from Guiana by the celebrated Charles Waterton in 1812—which he gave to me twenty-five years ago—and it stil retains, though it must now be seventy years old, its virulency. It was with some of this very poison that the foregoing experiment was made in 1861. That is to say, when it was half a century old. And what is stil more surprising—and I have no doubt it stil astonish the reflecting reader as much as it astonished me—is that on one ocasion the efects of two minute hypodermic doses of this same specimen of woorara, asociated with a minute dose of strychnia, actualy lasted for four and a half months. Fact is said to be often stranger than fiction, and this fact proves the truth of the adage. I recorded the experiment with al its details, in the previous chapter, when treating of the causes of the periodicity of certain forms of germ diseases.

Having thus paved the way to the establishment of my theory that the recurence of Epidemic diseases after long periods of quiesence is not due to the existence of any specific form of Resting-spores. But to the general posesion by germs' of marvelously prolonged powers of Latent-life. I shal now proceed to aduce data, both from the animal and vegetable kingdoms, in suport of the logical tenability of this view. In order to do this satisfactorily I shal bring forward the best examples of prolonged Latent-life with which I am acquainted. And these I think wil be found suficient to confirm my theory.

To begin with, I may refer to the results of Richter and Verloren's experiments made in 1853-4, by which we became aware that the egs of certain of the parasites afecting the human system—the Trichina, for example—lie perfectly dormant during the winter season, and only burst into developmental activity in the warm months of spring and sumer. It has been equaly conclusively shown that the em-bryos of some nematoid worms—like those of the Ascarides,. which lie dormant in tanks and other such like damp localities during the winter time—imediately resume active vitality on being transfered to the warm human ali-mentary canal. This canot surprise us when we recolect the astounding powers of certain members of the Molusca species, which have a special contrivance for protecting themselves from hurtful external agents during their winter's sleep. For example, the edible snails of the French and Italian markets close the mouths of their shels with a calcareous plate, caled the epiphragm, at the begining of winter, and in that state lie dormant until spring. Indeed, epicures do not consider them worth eating until they have been some time in this torpid condition—certainly not, at least, until after the first sharp frost.

I now come to the best, as it is the most startling, of all examples of latent animal life with which I am acquainted. And to it my attention was first kindly directed by Sir John Lubbock. It is the case of a snail—the *Helix maculosa*—an inhabitant of the arid Egyptian and Syrian deserts, which was on March 25, 1846, when thought to be only a dead and dry empty shel, fastened by gum to a tablet, and placed away among the other similar specimens in the British Museum. Where it remained, sumer and winter, until the month of March, 1850—that is to say, four entire years,—without its guardian having the remotest idea of the shel's containing a living ocupant, when Mr. Baird axidentaly noticed an epiphragm on its mouth. Which speared to him to have been newly formed. So he detached the shel and placed it in tepid water. When, to his intense surprise, a living head soon projected from the shel, and in a few minutes more the animal began crawling about in the basin. Next day it was suplied with a piece of cabage-leaf. Of which it imediately partook. On June 24, when Mr. Baird published his observations upon it in vol. vi. second series of Taylor's "Anals of Natural History," from which I have extracted the above, the animal was stil alive and wel.

In my corespondence with Dr. Günther about the above recorded case, he kindly related to me the folowing examples of natural dormant life artificialy complicated, which I think are worthy of record, as they prove the falacy of the comon belief that al animals, while hibernating from cold, poses the power of resisting the efects of frost-bite. He says:—

"I have never made methodical experiments as to the latent life of animals or their own, with the exception of spawn of frogs, which in the earliest stage of development may be frozen into ice without life being destroyed." But to this he sols:—

"In the winter 1853-54 during a strong frost with snow on the ground, a servant in my house at Bonn, where I was staying at the time, found three dormice (*Myoxus nitela*) in a lumber-room in a state of perfect torpidity; they are a hibernating species. She threw them into the garden; and from four to six hours had elapsed before I heard of the ocurence. I found one lying on the ice of a tank, frozen to the ice; the second with the body in the snow, and with the tail on the ice; the third in the snow.

"About an hour after their removal into the house the last had fuly revived; the second also recovered, but lost its tail; whilst the third had been frozen to death."

In case of my being misinterpreted, I have a word or two to say regarding the fabulous tales of Latent-life in reptiles, insects, and men. Such, for example, as that a living frog has jumped from a cavity in a solid piece of sandstone rock when it was axidentaly laid open by the hewer's pickaxe. That a whole swarm of bees has flown busing out from the holow centre of a solid tree, the entrance into which had been closed up for years. And that the Fakirs of India can at pleasure go into a state of vital torpidity, and remain in it, with impunity, for months. The two former tales are, I believe, founded upon erors in observation. The existing chanels into the hole in the sandstone, and the holow of the tree, simply having escaped the narators' notice. This is, I believe very likely to ocur. For I myself discovered a domestic bee-hive in the top-stone of the celebrated Druidical cromlech in Kent, caled Kits-Coty-House.

While one day, in 1872, taking shelter from a shower of rain under the enormous mas of solid unhewn stone which forms its covering, I noticed a number of domestic bees; and wondering what they were doing in such an out-of-the-way locality, I watched their movements, and found that they one by one disapeared through an almost undetectable opening, just big enough realy to admit them, in the under surface of the midle of the great mas of solid stone, directly above my head. Which hole would never have been detected by my eye had I not seen the bees enter and come out of it. They were in such numbers that I had not the slightest doubt that there existed in the interior of the block a regular hive, and for aught I know it may be there stil. As I stood gazing at the strange sight I said to myself: "As this opening is not only so smal, but so placed that it would have escaped my notice had I not seen the bees apearing and disapearing

through it; it is not improbable that, suposing this stone had been axidentaly or intentionaly fractured at this point during the winter time, when the bees were in a state of torpidity; from the hole escaping the observer's notice, the discovery of the hive within this stone would undoubtedly be reported as an undeniable and indisputable example of Latent-life of a most extraordinary character. We would be sure to be told that as there was no opening into the stone from without, the hive of bees must have formed there ages ago, when the stone, in fact, was in course of geological formation. And who could gainsay it if no opening into it was found?"

No wonder, then, that I put down the presence of living reptiles in stones, and insects in solid trees, as mere instances of imperfectly observed facts!

The tales of Fakir's torpidity for months, on the other hand, I regard as real and nothing extraordinary, up to a certain time. For he begins by taking a good dose of powerfuly stupefying Bang, and therefrom becomes for a time a narcotised, inert mass of humanity. In which state he is lowered into a quiet and cool tomb. Which stil further favors the prolongation of the artificialy induced vital lethargy. Again, as human life can be prolonged even in activity for forty days without food or drink, there is nothing whatever surprising at the Fakir's being found alive after a six or even eight weeks' entombment. Braid, in his treatise on Human Hibernation, published in 1850, states, on the authority of Sir Claude Wade, that a Fakir was buried in an unconscious state at Lahore, in 1837, and when dug up six weeks afterwards (though every precaution had been taken by guarding his grave night and day with soldiers to prevent anyone from disturbing it in the interval), restored to consciousness. Notwithstanding that when he was exhumed, he had al the apearances of a corpse. The legs and arms were shrunken, and stif. The face, however, was ful. The head reclined on the shoulder like that of a dead person. No pulsation of the heart, or in the arteries of the arm, or temples, could be felt.

It is quite posible that some of my readers, though perceiving the direct and interesting bearing al these facts conected with Latent-life have upon the Germ theory of disease, may stil consider that the examples of prolonged Latent-life as yet cited are al of them of too brief a duration to acount for the very prolonged lapses of time which ocasionaly exist between the cessation of one epidemic and the outburst of another of precisely the same sort, in the same district—five, ten, twenty, aye, even sixty, or more years, ocasionaly intervening between them. However, that dificulty is not insurmountable.

Let us now, then, briefly see what the vegetable world tels us regarding the marvels of Latent-life. Mushroom spawn has been suxesfuly planted after having been kept stored up dry for fourteen years. And who amongst my readers has not heard of the Raspbery seeds, the produce of Pharaoh's daughter's last meal, having been taken from her mumified stomach by the late Mr. London, and planted in his garden? From which raspbery bushes grew, which flowered, and in due course fruited, notwithstanding that the seeds from which they sprung had lain dormant, though not dead, in an Egyptian tomb for over 2000 years!

If such, then, be the exceptional vitality of the highly organised and complex constituted seed of a raspbery, why should we hesitate to believe that ocasionaly an equal amount of latent vitality may exist in a simply constituted germ spore? Even, however, if we hesitate to acord to the germ spore the posibility of the posesion of a 2000 years' Latent-life, can we not acord to it a twentieth, or even a fortieth part of that vital power? In which case a fifty years' quiesence between the end of one and the begining of another Epidemic of the same disease would be readily acounted for. I am not, however, satisfied with that computation, for I believe that germ spores may poses a much more prolonged vitality than this; and my reason for thinking so is, that if we aply the same mode of reasoning to the germ spore as we may philosophicaly do to the raspbery seed, then we arive at a 333 years' Latent-life duration for them. Thus, a raspbery seed is thought, as a rule, to retain its vitality for only six years, and yet we know that it may actualy retain it 333 times longer. This being the case, and we knowing for a fact that the germs of vacine lymph under ordinary circumstances retain their vitality for at least twelve months, what prevents us imagining that they, like the raspbery seeds, might, under exceptional circumstances, retain it 333 times longer? Namely, for 333 years. Koch found that the blood of animals, containing Bacili germs, may be kept dry for four years, and then, when pulverised, mixed with water, and injected into healthy animals, readily infect them with disease. Such being the case, and if a snail has a Latent-life of four, mushroom spawn of fourteen, and raspbery seeds of 2000 years, I see no reason to doubt for a moment, without having recourse to a special Resting-spore theory, that the recurence of Epidemic contagious diseases in localities which have long been free from them may be due to the Latent-life in the posession of the germs giving rise to them. They, like the mushroom spawn and the raspbery seeds, sudenly vivify and fructify when their surroundings become favorable for their germination, after having lain dormant for years under circumstances and in situations unsuited for their vivification and development.

REPORTS OF HOSPITAL PRACTICE
IN
MEDICINE AND SURGERY.

MANCHESTER ROYAL INFIRMARY.

CASES OF CEREBELLAR DISEASE.
(Under the care of Dr. DRESCHFELD.)

Case 1.—Persistent Vomiting for Three Months—Gradually Increasing Vertigo—Death—Hæmorrhages into the Left Cerebellar Lobe, implicating the Vermiform Process.

G. F., aged sixty-one, married, salt-miner, was admitted into the Infirmary on June 8, 1880, and died on July 19, 1880. The following is a brief outline of the case from the notes taken by Mr. H. W. Pomfret, then Clinical Clerk.

Family History of patient is good. Patient has four children; all healthy.

Previous History.—Patient has been a salt-miner for nearly forty years. Was a heavy drinker when young, but for the last thirty years has been a total abstainer from alcoholic drinks. Has never had syphilis. Enjoyed excellent health up to January, 1880, when he commenced to feel giddy and to vomit, and to feel some weakness in his legs. He was still able to follow his work up to April, when he had to give it up, owing to the giddiness, persistent vomiting, and increasing weakness. His appetite has been very bad for the last few months. The vomiting came on only after taking food, sometimes immediately, at other times some hours after a meal. He has lost a great deal of flesh.

Condition on Admission.—Patient is a very tall and well-built man. He has all the appearance of having been a strong, muscular man. He looks thin; his muscles are flabby, but he has no cachectic appearance. The physical examination of the thoracic and abdominal organs reveals normal relations. Pulse 70, firm and strong; the abdomen is not tympanitic and not painful on palpation or pressure, and no tumour of any kind can be detected; the tongue is clean; bowels regular. Urine of light straw-colour, specific gravity 1009; contains neither sugar nor albumen. The temperature of body is normal. The patient complains of slight frontal headache, and giddiness, which becomes worse on walking. The examination of the special-sense organs shows nothing abnormal: his vision is good; the fundus of the eye normal; the pupils react well; no arcus senilis; his hearing is good. There is no affection of any of the other cerebral nerves. The patient is able to walk, but does so with some difficulty, owing to the vertigo; when walking he staggers slightly—sometimes to the right, sometimes to the left; he walks much worse with his eyes shut; can, however, stand for some time with his eyes shut without falling. There is no loss of power in either the upper or lower extremities. The sensibilities are normal; "tendon reflexes" are present, but not exaggerated.

Progress.—During the first few days of his stay in the hospital the patient vomited but little; the vomiting was, however, always preceded by nausea; the vertigo slowly increased. His general condition also became worse, and he continued to lose flesh. From June 8 to June 24 he lost six pounds in weight. The vomited matter consisted of undigested food, and bile. Some gastric juice removed by

stomach-pump showed the presence of hydrochloric acid on testing with tropeolin and methylaniline violet.

On July 5 his condition became much worse. The vertigo increased to such an extent that it was impossible for him to walk or even to stand. The temperature rose that day from normal to 102°; the vomiting continued; and a very marked pulsation of the abdominal aorta became visible. During the next few days the patient's temperature showed a marked evening elevation, while in the morning it was nearly normal. On July 16 the patient was found semi-conscious, refused to take any food; his breathing became laboured and stertorous. The temperature rose to 103·2°, and remained high both evening and morning. The coma deepened on the next day. The patient sank gradually, and died on July 19 without any convulsions supervening.

Post-mortem Examination.—The chest was not opened. The abdominal viscera were found perfectly normal. The bones of the skull, the membranes of the brain, and the brain itself, showed nothing abnormal on external inspection. On making sections of the brain after its removal it was found that the cerebellum was the only seat of any lesion. Externally the cerebellum showed no changes, except that the upper surface on the left side felt softer than on the right. Sections through the cerebellum showed the presence in its interior of a small hæmorrhagic cyst, filled with serum tinged red; this cyst had a longitudinal diameter of one inch, and a transverse diameter of three-quarters of an inch; it occupied chiefly the white substance in the left lobe of the cerebellum, close to the inner border, and it extended right into the superior vermiform process, the anterior portion of which was found tunnelled out and filled with red serum. The outline of the cyst was irregular, and no cyst-wall could be detected. External to this cyst, and closely connected with it, was found a small, but fresh, hæmorrhagic focus, filled with a fresh coagulum. This second hæmorrhage, evidently of very recent date, implicated and replaced a portion of the corpus dentatum. The cerebral and meningeal vessels were found healthy, and the origin of the hæmorrhages could not be traced to any large vessel. No miliary aneurisms were found in any portion of the brain.

Remarks.—The case is interesting from several points of view. Cerebellar hæmorrhage in itself is very rare, and when it does occur is either so insignificant as not to give rise to any very definite symptoms, or else so extensive as often to produce speedy death. Few cases have, therefore, been observed where such hæmorrhages could be made use of for the purpose of localising the lesions. On the other hand, hæmorrhages, more than any other lesions, especially if they are not too extensive, form the best test cases for localising purposes. Viewed from this point, the above case is an important one, for we had here to do with two separate hæmorrhages—the one of old date, to which all the symptoms observed on admission and during the further progress of the case were due; and the other of very recent date, and most probably taking place during the last few days of life, when the temperature suddenly showed an evening rise and marked daily oscillations, and when the patient's condition became rapidly worse. The chief symptoms observed were the persistent vomiting, the vertigo, and, later on, the staggering; and to account for these we found, after death, a hæmorrhagic cyst, situated on the inner side of the left cerebellar hemisphere, and extending into the superior vermiform process. The case, then, forms an important support to the well-known theory of Nothnagel, according to which the incoördination of movement seen in cerebellar disease is due to the affection of the vermiform process. The vomiting in this case was so persistent, and was observed from the very commencement of the illness, and that I am inclined to believe it to be due to the cerebellar lesion rather than to an implication of the medulla, which was neither pressed upon nor found in any way affected.

Case 2.—Headache, Vomiting, Staggering, Convulsions, Blindness from Optic Neuritis—Gradually Increasing Paresis of the Lower Extremities—Gradual, but very Marked, Increase in the Size of the Head—Death—Excessive Internal Hydrocephalus, causing Distension of all the Ventricles, and also of Left Lobe of Cerebellum—Sarcomatous Tumour in Cerebellum.

E. S., a boy aged thirteen, came under treatment in the out-patient room of the Manchester Infirmary on April 11, 1878, and died on July 21, 1880.

The following is a brief history of the case previous to his admission:—When six years old had scarlet fever, which left a slight otorrhœa from the right ear for some months, but which quite subsided; he had also, afterwards, measles and chicken-pox, but quite recovered, and remained well till the autumn of 1877, when, whilst playing with some schoolfellows in a public park, he fell from a swing. He did not seem much hurt by the fall, continued to go to school, and complained only of occasional headache. The headache increased in intensity, and was also associated with pain in left side of face and arm; he also commenced to stagger and complained of his eyesight. Owing to these troubles, he took to his bed about January, 1878. Since then he had become much worse; he had several general convulsions, was often troubled with vomiting, and became so weak in his legs as not to be able to walk. A month ago he became quite blind.

On admission the following notes were taken:—Patient is a healthy-looking, well-nourished boy. His intelligence is perfect, and his memory is good. There is no affection of any of the cerebral nerves or special-sense organs, except the eyes; he is quite blind, the pupils are dilated and do not react to light, and there is marked atrophy of both discs. The hearing on the right side is slightly diminished. The patient is not able to walk, except with assistance, owing to the excessive staggering; when staggering, he has the tendency to fall to the left side. There is slight left hemiparesis of the arm and of the leg, but the power in them is still considerable. There is no anæsthesia and no trophic disturbance. The tendon reflex is normal on the right side, slightly exaggerated on the left side. The appetite is good; bowels regular; the urine normal. The examination of the chest and of the abdominal organs shows nothing abnormal.

The case was diagnosed then as that of a cerebellar tumour situated in the left cerebellar hemisphere. The further progress of the case is briefly the following:—For a time the patient remained in the same state as on admission; then the incoördination became so great that it was quite impossible for him to stand or to walk; the weakness of the left arm and leg slightly increased; the patient suffered from intense headache occasionally, and from convulsions, which were sometimes unilateral and confined to the left side, at other times general. The intelligence of the patient remained perfect. There was occasional vomiting; the appetite remained good, and the patient's body weight increased and he grew fat; but it was noticed, during the summer of 1879, that the head grew quite out of proportion to the rest of the body, and assumed a distinct hydrocephalic appearance. Measurements taken on September 28, 1879, showed the head to have a circumference of twenty-five inches; to measure transversely from ear to ear fourteen inches, and longitudinally from the root of nose to occiput thirteen inches and three-quarters. During the winter of 1879 the condition remained unaltered; there were, however, no more convulsions, and the headache diminished in intensity. On July 19, 1880, the patient had a very severe attack of general convulsions. After the convulsions had passed off he remained unconscious, and died on July 21, 1880.

With the assistance of Dr. Lindemann, I made a post-mortem examination on July 22. The patient having been a home-patient for the last eighteen months of his life, and the autopsy having to be made in the patient's residence, the head only was allowed to be examined. The bones of the skull were found to be very thin; the sutures, especially the parietal ones, stretched considerably, and thickened by fibrous tissue. The convolutions of the brain were very much flattened. On cutting through the brain the lateral ventricles were found enormously distended by fluid; the cortical part of the brain forming a mere envelope of only about half an inch in thickness to this large accumulation of fluid. The basal ganglia were equally compressed and anæmic. The third and fourth ventricles were likewise very much distended; the opening into the fourth ventricle posteriorly was found sufficiently large to admit a crow-quill. The right cerebellar hemisphere showed no change, except being very much compressed. The left hemisphere was found larger, softer, and fluctuating, and on section it was seen distended with clear yellow serum (about three ounces), which had replaced nearly the whole of the white substance, under-mining the superior vermiform process, and compressing it.

On evacuating the fluid the large cavity thus formed in the left cerebellar hemisphere was found to have no proper lining membrane; anteriorly it communicated with the dilated fourth ventricle, while on its outer and posterior border there was found a tumour, about one inch long and half an inch broad, of soft gelatinous consistence, reddish in appearance, irregular in its outline. The greater portion of this tumour-mass lay free in the cavity; its base, attached to the cerebellum, passed gradually into the surrounding cerebellar tissue. The right cerebellar hemisphere was found on section anæmic, but otherwise not altered. The tumour, on microscopic examination, proved to be a glio-sarcoma, with excessive preponderance of bloodvessels.

Remarks.—The presence of hydrocephalus in cerebellar tumours is not of uncommon occurrence, and its production is due to pressure on the venæ Galeni. This was specially marked in one case reported by Hughlings-Jackson (Medical Times and Gazette, 1871), and some other cases published since (Guéneau de Mussy, etc.). It is difficult, however, to understand how in our case such a pressure could be exerted by the tumour. A case very similar to the above, both as regards the situation of the tumour and the distension of all the ventricles of the brain, is reported by Mosler (Virchow's Archiv, 1868, page 220). Another noteworthy feature of the case is the expansion of the cranial cavity, considering the age of the patient. Cases of acquired chronic hydrocephalus with expansion of the cavity are very rare after the ninth or tenth year; in our case the enlargement of the head commenced some time after the boy had been under observation, that is, after his thirteenth year.

(To be continued.)

CENTENARIANS.—There are at this time 3108 centenarians in Europe, in a population of 243,000,000 inhabitants; of these 1864 are women, and only 1244 men. In France there are most sexagenarians, octogenarians, and nonagenarians; but France possesses fewer centenarians than any other European state, with the exception of Belgium, Denmark, and Switzerland. Longevity is decreasing in France, but mean old age is on the increase, so that there are fewer centenarians but more septuagenarians, octogenarians, and nonagenarians than formerly. Centenarians attribute their longevity to temperance, sobriety, regular habits, heredity, the absence of powerful emotions, healthy occupations, and a country life.—Lyon Méd., December 11.

PROF. PETTENKOFER AND THE CHOLERA BACTERIA. —A novel prediction (Louisville Med. News, November 26) has recently been made by Prof. Pettenkofer before the Society of German Naturalists and Physicians. The influence exerted by the soil as a hygienic factor has been with him a favourite study. In his address he reiterated the theory of cholera with which his name has long been identified. He still holds that an epidemic of this disease is the result of certain relations of the ground, its water, and its organic matter. By this theory he accounted for the remarkable immunity enjoyed by Lyons during the cholera. This is so uniform an experience that dwellers in neighbouring cities in times of danger resort to Lyons as a place of refuge. He thinks that theories of production in or transmission by air direct, or by water, fail to account for the security of Lyons. It is not considered to be better off in water-supply or non-exposure to contagion than other cities. He holds the view that in infected places the porous soil, open to the reception of diarrhœal filth, allows of easy diffusion by underground currents in water of the specific organisms, which breed there, and engender cholera in man. He thinks it not unlikely that some soils are already occupied by benign bacteria to such a degree as to render them sterile to noxious bacteria when introduced from without. These lowest representatives of organic life, he says, can therefore be made useful to us, and we must not be surprised if in future times the useful bacteria will be actually cultivated, and those only which are noxious thwarted in their struggle for existence. By domesticating the innocent forms in the soil under our houses, the supply of organic matter may be so exhausted that the diseased bacteria will not have the common necessaries of life, and will therefore be literally starved out. It is rather a happy thought to fight these terrible mites with good fellows of their own size.

TERMS OF SUBSCRIPTION.
(*Free by post.*)

British Islands	*Twelve Months*	.	£1	8	0
,, ,, ...	*Six*	,,	.	0	14	0
The Colonies and the United }	*Twelve*	,,	.	1	10	0
States of America . . . }					
,, ,, ,, . .	*Six*	,,	.	0	15	0
India ,, ...	*Twelve*	,,	.	1	10	0
,, (*viâ Brindisi*) . . .	,,	,,	.	1	15	0
,, ,, ...	*Six*	,,	.	0	15	0
,, (*viâ Brindisi*) . . .	,,	,,	.	0	17	6

Foreign Subscribers are requested to inform the Publishers of any remittance made through the agency of the Post-office.

Single Copies of the Journal can be obtained of all Booksellers and Newsmen, price Sixpence.

Cheques or Post-office Orders should be made payable to Mr. JAMES LUCAS, 11, New Burlington-street, W.

TERMS FOR ADVERTISEMENTS.

Seven lines (70 words) . . .	.	£0	4	6
Each additional line (10 words)	. .	0	0	6
Half-column, or quarter-page .	. .	1	5	0
Whole column, or half-page .	. .	2	10	0
Whole page	.	5	0	0

Births, Marriages, and Deaths are inserted Free of Charge.

THE MEDICAL TIMES AND GAZETTE *is published on Friday morning; Advertisements must therefore reach the Publishing Office not later than One o'clock on Thursday.*

Medical Times and Gazette.

SATURDAY, DECEMBER 24, 1881.

HOSPITALS FOR INFECTIOUS DISEASES.

THE Royal Commission on Hospitals for Infectious Diseases having intimated to the Society of Medical Officers that they would be glad to receive a communication from them on the subjects submitted to the Commission, the Society, on Friday last week, considered a draft report prepared by the Council. Some parts of the report excited, we understand, considerable discussion; but the document was finally adopted with some amount of amendment. The Society consider that the available accommodation in the metropolis is insufficient to meet the demands which might at any moment be made upon it by a recrudescence of fever or existing epidemic; and there certainly could not, we imagine, have been any difference of opinion on that point. As to fever cases, the Society consider that the beds available are, perhaps, sufficient for present wants; but as the hospitals are few in number, and necessarily remote from many parts of the metropolis, probably double the number would be required under improved sanitary legislation—a somewhat infelicitously expressed opinion, as it might be taken to mean that improved sanitary legislation will cause an increase of fever; but the ambiguity may be due to the reporter. The advantages of a limited number of hospitals for the whole metropolis, and under one central authority. preponderate, the Society think, over any other system. And they express the opinion that the hospital authority should provide for all classes of persons, and that admission to such hospitals should not entail pauperisation. In connexion with this, the Society might, we venture to think, have insisted that the management and administration of the hospitals should be entirely separate from the Poor-law administration. One part of the draft report referred to particular existing hospitals, and the evils possibly arising from them; and this excited much criti-

cism. It was proposed to say that, as regarded Stockwell, the Society had no evidence; but the Medical Officer of Health of Stockwell parish pointed out that the published report showed that in one year 174 small-pox cases out of 219, and in the next year 210 cases out of 221, occurred within a very short distance of the hospital; and, finally, the Society evaded the point by agreeing that no opinion should be expressed respecting particular hospitals, as they are the subject of inquiry or of litigation. Proceeding with the matters before the Commission in the order of the reference, the Society agreed that provision ought to be made for mild cases of small-pox and for convalescents outside the metropolis; and that were this done, probably eight well-placed hospitals, containing 150 beds each, would suffice for such cases as must be treated in the metropolis—that is, for cases too severe or too ill to be removed any great distance. A like provision should be made for fever cases. To each hospital for fever and small-pox cases a district should be allocated, and only overflow cases (no small-pox hospital is ever to contain more than 150 cases at any one time) in emergencies should be removed to any other hospital than that of the district properly assigned to it. This would, the Committee consider, meet many of the objections to the existing system of hospital accommodation. Perhaps so, but other objections would arise, and whatever site might be chosen for any district hospital, obstinate opposition to that site would most assuredly be made. The Society, therefore, next expressed the opinion that the hospital authority should possess power to acquire sites compulsorily; and that, subject to the hospitals being conducted with reasonable care and according to prescribed regulations, the authority should be protected from legal proceedings, "so as to secure the public against the loss of the benefits arising from such institutions." We do not understand that the Society offered any suggestion as to what authority is to be the judge of whether a hospital has, or has not, been "conducted with reasonable care"; and that will be a very important point for the Commission to consider. Lastly, the Committee agreed that legislation is required to secure compulsory notification of infectious diseases, and compulsory powers to enable the sanitary authority to enforce the removal to hospital of the infectious sick not possessed of lodging or accommodation where they could be properly treated and isolated. We are not aware that the subjects into which the Royal Commission are directed to inquire include the advisability or otherwise of compulsory notification of infectious diseases; and we do not know whether the Commission addressed any question to the Society upon that subject; but, however all that may be, we hope that the Society expressed a clear and definite opinion on the much-vexed question of who is to be responsible for the notification of the existence of infectious disease, and state how any plan for it is to be worked. And we think that if the Society chose to go outside the terms of the Royal Commission, they had better have represented the paramount importance of *preventing* small-pox. If we do really believe in vaccination, we must believe that no great permanent hospital accommodation for small-pox patients ought to be necessary. In such a kingdom of houses as the metropolis we can never look to be absolutely free from small-pox; but that amount of the disease always present in London is a standing reproach to the vaccination department of the Local Government Board, and the occurrence of anything like an epidemic is a flagrant scandal. With a thoroughly efficient and thoroughly well administered Compulsory Vaccination Act, the permanent provision of the tenth part of the number of small-pox beds mentioned by the Society of Medical Officers of Health would amply suffice for the needs of the four millions of inhabitants of the metropolis.

THE NATURAL HISTORY OF UTERINE FIBROIDS.
II.

In a former article we noticed some of the conclusions which a physician—Dr. Roehrig—practising at Kreuznach had drawn from his experience as to the natural history of uterine fibroids. We would ask yet a little more of our readers' attention to the subject.

It is generally known that fibroids attract blood to the uterus, which, in consequence of its being more vascular, becomes more liable to congestive and inflammatory changes than in health. Of more or less acute *metritis* complicating fibroids, Dr. Roehrig has seen 32 cases, 5 of which ended fatally. We have already quoted his experience of suppuration of fibroids. In 8 cases he has known inflammation and ulceration of the endometrium lead to adhesion of the tumour to the surface to which it was opposite. Once he has seen suppuration in Douglas's pouch.

Dysmenorrhœa is a recognised and frequent result of fibroid tumours of the uterus. Out of Dr. Roehrig's 570 cases, in 112 this symptom was present.

Hæmorrhage from the uterus is at once the most common and most important symptom which fibroids occasion. As to its frequency, our author tells us that in 318 of his patients menstruation was either increased in quantity or returned with undue frequency. It was present in all the cases of submucous tumours, 212 in number; out of 79 interstitial fibroids, excessive losses of blood were complained of in 69; while of the remaining 279 subserous growths, in only 73 was hæmorrhage a factor worth consideration. With regard to its importance, death directly from hæmorrhage is a rare occurrence; in all his experience Dr. Roehrig has only seen it once, and in that case there was suppuration of the tumour. But much oftener hæmorrhage undermines the health, and so renders the patient an easy victim to other diseases.

Sterility is an effect which depends greatly upon the situation and size of the tumour, but seems not so common as is generally supposed. In no less than 147 out of the 570 cases, conception occurred. All of these, except 2, in which the growths were interstitial, were cases of submucous tumours. Dr. Roehrig has never known pregnancy occur where a submucous tumour was present. Eliminating those of his patients who were unmarried, he finds that in two-thirds of those who were married, their fertility was put a stop to by the growth. Considering the risk attending labour or abortion under such circumstances, he regards this as fortunate.

When pregnancy has taken place, *abortion* is exceedingly common. In 129 of Dr. Roehrig's 147 cases, the pregnancy thus ended; and the perils which attend labour at term make this termination a very desirable one. If delivery take place at or near the full period of pregnancy, it brings with it especial risk of rupture of uterus, of dangerous hæmorrhage, of subsequent metritis and peritonitis. Of the possibility of spontaneous cure during puerperal involution we have already spoken.

Of other ill-understood accompanying phenomena, such as the so-called "reflex" symptoms, we need not quote our author. And those exceptional phenomena which result from dragging on or compression of other parts by bands of adhesions attached to the fibroids, it is not necessary to particularise; nor need we specify those which may arise mechanically from the weight and bulk of the tumours themselves.

The last branch of the subject upon which the author enters is the prognosis. Out of 570 cases, in 66 death resulted in some way from the tumour, being a mortality of 11·4 per cent. These 66 deaths were thus occasioned:

26 from suppuration, sloughing, and disintegration of the tumour (*Verjauchung*); 24 from cancerous degeneration; acute metritis and peritonitis as a result of injury, 5; in delivery or childbed, 3; from premature labour and its results, 5; 2 from obstruction of the bowels caused by the tumour; and 1 from hæmorrhage.

Dr. Roehrig mentions a fact of pathological interest—viz., that out of these 570 cases, in 35 fibrous tumours existed in the mamma, and in 3 in the vagina.

The figures we have quoted seem to show that uterine fibroids bring with them a degree of injury to health and danger to life much greater than is generally attributed to them. We must, however, bear in mind that Dr. Roehrig's cases are in a measure selected. He practises in a place the waters of which have a popular reputation as being efficacious in curing fibroids. It is unlikely that patients would go to the trouble and expense of a residence there unless their symptoms were really such as to make them think their illness serious. One eminent pathologist has expressed his opinion that 20 per cent. of women between the ages of forty and fifty suffer from uterine fibroids. If this estimate even approach the truth, it will be manifest that Dr. Roehrig's mortality of 11·4 per cent. must be far too high. It represents, in fact, the death-rate among those already bad enough to go to Kreuznach, not that among fibroids generally.

A point which has an important bearing upon a question of present interest is the remarkably small number of deaths from hæmorrhage, only one such occurring out of 570 cases selected for their gravity. We think the experience of gynæcologists generally, concurs with that of Dr. Roehrig, that for a uterine fibroid to cause death directly from hæmorrhage is a rare event. It will be in the recollection of our readers, that during the past year papers have been read at our leading medical society, and elsewhere, advocating the removal of the ovaries to arrest hæmorrhage from uterine fibroids. In one communication more than thirty cases were recounted which had occurred in the practice of one operator in a provincial town in the space of about two years, and in nearly all it was stated that the hæmorrhage was so profuse as to endanger life. We cannot call in question the correctness of the prognosis given in the individual cases, for two reasons: first, because it is unfortunately at present impossible to formulate in any precise terms either the amount of hæmorrhage of this kind, or its effects on the system, and, consequently, when the reporter has expressed his opinion as to the gravity of the danger from bleeding, he has said all that he can say; and, secondly, because it is impossible for anyone who has not seen the cases to controvert the opinion formed by one who has. But it is a very surprising thing that in a provincial town such a number of these rare cases should be met with in so short a time—so astonishing that it must occur to the mind as a possibility that the enterprising surgeon by whom the prognosis was made may have taken in some cases too unfavourable a view; that in some of the cases the hæmorrhage might have diminished, and the patient lived in comfortable health, even without the removal of the ovaries. We should be sorry to say anything to throw cold water on the zeal of those who advance by untrodden paths, or to show a want of appreciation of the boldness and dexterity of the surgeon by whom these cases were brought forward; the more so as this operation has been already freely criticised from other quarters, in a manner with which we cannot altogether agree. But before this operation can take its proper place, the profession must be satisfied that the cases in which it has been performed have been such as to exclude the possibility that the benefit following the operation might have only been part of the natural course of the disease, instead of a result of the surgical interference.

PROVIDENT DISPENSARIES.

AT a district meeting of the British Medical Association, held in Hackney last week, the subject of Provident Dispensaries was brought under consideration by Mr. Timothy Holmes. As most are aware, there is a Metropolitan Association for promoting the establishment of these institutions; and of this Mr. Holmes is a leading, or the leading, member. That the motives of those who are moving in it are purely disinterested, need not be said; the association of Mr. Holmes with the movement is a guarantee that it is untainted with corrupt or selfish intrigue. The scheme is a complex one: so complicated that, as Mr. Holmes said, no one is so devoid of ingenuity as to be unable to pick holes in it. We shall not weary our readers by again going into the details of the project, but we wish to state certain broad general objections which make us feel very doubtful whether the working of the system will be as satisfactory as its promoters hope.

The objects of the scheme are these. It is said, with some truth and not a little exaggeration, that the out-patient departments of hospitals are greatly abused. There are so many out-patients that it is impossible for each to get proper attention, and the patients therefore suffer. Many go to hospitals who otherwise would pay medical men, and therefore medical men suffer. Many hospital out-patients are suffering from trivial maladies, and the time of consulting physicians and surgeons is wasted in prescribing for such; therefore the hospital staff suffers. It is proposed, in order to remedy all this, to establish dispensaries where, by a small weekly payment, the class which is above taking parish relief, but unable to pay long doctors' bills, shall be entitled to whatever medical attendance they require.

First, as to the hospitals. It is said that the hospital out-patient departments should be purely consultative. They should be fed from these dispensaries—the simple cases being treated there, the difficult ones sent to the hospital for the consultant's advice. If this change should take place, we believe it would greatly injure the staff, retard the progress of medical science, and hamper medical education. Among the most important steps in medical science are the discovery of new means of diagnosis; the isolation, as separate forms of disease, of different cases hitherto massed together as alike; and, above all, the recognition of diseases in earlier and earlier stages. Now, if the experience of hospital consultants is to be confined to seeing, once only, those cases that the general practitioner has failed to cure and considers of gravity, how is he to get at those slight beginnings of disease, marked by symptoms which both patient and practitioner think little of, and which only tell their tale to the investigator who is on the alert for them? Again, it is well known that some of our most successful physicians and surgeons say that they taught themselves how to *treat* disease in the out-patient room. How are the rising consultants to do this if their hospital practice is to be consultative only? We must consider also the student. The *slight* cases are those which form the bulk of a general medical practitioner's work. The student who goes into practice not knowing how to treat porrigo or flatulent dyspepsia, will suffer from his ignorance more than if he were uncertain as to acute atrophy of liver or ligature of the external iliac. The slight, common, everyday diseases and the opportunity for treating them are wanted at hospitals for the sake of students and staff alike.

Next, as to medical men. In poor neighbourhoods, the incomes of medical men are of course derived from the class ··· if this scheme should be extensively put in practice,

would be asked to join the provident dispensaries. The more cheaply they got their medical attendance, so much the less would be the doctor's earnings, or so much the more the work he would have to do. If the effect stopped here, we should say little about it, for we could not expect much public sympathy simply because we feared our own pockets might be touched. But the effect of diminished income would be this: that educated and capable men would go where they could get remunerated properly, the low scale of payment would only attract men of inferior quality, and the poor would consequently be the sufferers. We think, however, that this effect will correct itself, although it might press hardly on medical men for a time. A medical man who is known and trusted, if he find the dispensary payments insufficient, can withdraw from it without loss; it would be those commencing practice who would have to work for scanty emolument.

But let us admit, whether it be likely or not, that the provident dispensaries will fairly and adequately remunerate the medical men, and that the arrangement will work well on both sides. Then we would ask, What is the need for a dispensary, and a committee, and the rest of the machinery? Why not leave the medical men and their poorer patients to make a bargain between themselves, without the intervention of any organisation? Roughly speaking, the expenditure of the provident dispensary is distributed somewhat as follows:—About half goes to the doctors, about a quarter in drugs, and about a quarter in expenses of management. Why should not the doctors manage it themselves, and have thus the whole of the proceeds? The amount spent in drugs is probably more than would be so disbursed in a private surgery, for this reason: that in a dispensary where drugs have to be kept for the use of several different prescribers, there is more waste. An individual medical man knows what drugs he is in the habit of using, and about how much he is likely to require, and orders in supplies from his chemist accordingly. The dispenser who has to guess at the needs of several different practitioners is pretty sure to order a good deal that will never be used.

Let us now go a little farther, and assume, not merely that the dispensaries work well, but that they are a great success, and have become as popular as the hospital out-patient rooms. What reason is there for supposing that the dispensary doctors will do their work better than those who at present see hospital out-patients? If the rooms are crowded, the work will be hurried. The amount of crowding will depend on the popularity of the dispensary. The truth is, that it costs, in travelling expenses and loss of time, as much, on an average, for a working man or woman to attend for several weeks at a hospital, as would cover a year's subscription to a provident dispensary. The attraction of a hospital is not the cheapness of the advice, but the reputation of the staff. When the medical man proposes a consultation, and names the physician or surgeon whose opinion he would like to have, he probably, if the patient does not happen to have heard of the gentleman in question before, backs his recommendation by the name of the hospital to which the consultant belongs. "Mr. X, of —— Hospital." He thinks that is a sufficient guarantee of skill, and so does the patient. When the latter gets well, he thinks and says that it is worth while to submit to some inconvenience for the sake of getting the advice of so eminent a man. The collective reputation of the medical men who in the past and the present have been and are on its staff, makes the renown of the hospital; and the fame of the hospital surrounds and strengthens its out-patient staff. This is why the out-patient rooms are crowded; and we do not think competition on a pecuniary basis will divert patients elsewhere. The provident dispensaries will not be "in it" in the race for public favour with the hospitals; they will only compete with the medical men in general practice who do not join the dispensaries.

If general practice is to be worked on an amended plan, we think that plan is best settled by medical men for themselves. We happen to know that the "provident" system (viz., that of a regular payment in health as well as in sickness, to cover attendance during the latter) is already a good deal acted on without the intervention of any committee; and we are at present inclined to think this mode of adopting it the preferable one.

THE WEEK.

TOPICS OF THE DAY.

THAT the International Smoke Abatement Exhibition has created a certain amount of interest cannot for one moment be denied, but whether that interest will be sufficient to bring about any amelioration of the present unsatisfactory state of affairs yet remains to be proved. With every wish to see carried out many of the reforms which the present Exhibition advocates, it is useless to shut one's eyes to the fact that in this country we are notorious for the persistency with which we adhere to the manners and customs of our ancestors. Nothing short of legal enactment will ever induce the general bulk of the public to fit up stoves for consuming the smoke, instead of sending it up the chimney to the detriment of the community at large. Many of the inventions exhibited at South Kensington are unquestionably excellently adapted to the wants of the largest coal-burning city in the world. But it is impossible to forget that all this array of ingenious contrivances has not been called into existence by the present Exhibition; and as all their advantages have been allowed to lie dormant in the past, so far as any general adoption has taken place, such, it is to be feared, will be their fate in the future, unless the societies who have been instrumental in bringing together the collection can induce the Government to take up the question. From the number of firms competing for custom, it is evident that the London householder may exercise a considerable choice in the method adopted for getting rid of our great enemy—Smoke. Messrs. Barnard, Bishop, and Barnards, of Norwich; the British Sanitary Company, of Glasgow; Messrs. Brown and Green, of Luton; Messrs. Boyd and Sons, of New Bond-street; and Messrs. Edwards and Son, of Great Marlborough-street, are prominent amongst the exhibitors; and Captain Galton has also sent his well-known open grate for reducing the smoke, and effecting the ventilation of rooms and buildings. This is an ordinary open fireplace so arranged as to insure complete combustion with economy of fuel, proper ventilation, and uniformity of temperature, which is maintained in a room for a long time after the fire has gone out.

A great difficulty which threatened the successful taking of the present census in France was only just averted in time by the authorities there. Instead of the enumerators waiting on heads of families, and themselves filling up the forms as hitherto, the Government had proposed that the forms should be filled up by the parties themselves, and deposited with the concierges, who were to deliver them to the enumerators when called for. But a concierge is regarded in France as a natural enemy, and such an outcry arose at the prospect of his being thus enabled to possess himself of information regarding the ages, family relationships, means of livelihood, etc., of the occupants, that the Prefect of the Seine considered it expedient to obtain from the municipality a vote of 40,000 francs for envelopes to accompany each form sent out, so that every

family might hand over its return under seal, either to the enumerator direct, or to the concierge. Paris alone is estimated to contain about 76,000 houses, each having, on the average, five sets of apartments. Even after this concession it is rumoured that there is a probability of some families refusing information as to the ages of children, from the fear of its being used under the impending compulsory education system; and as the Government is possessed of no power of enforcing returns, it is extremely probable that for the future a Census Law will have to be passed by the Chambers, similar to the Census Act in this country.

The Greenwich magistrate seems to have dealt somewhat lightly with an offender summoned before him by the Local Board for exposing himself in the public streets while suffering from small-pox. A witness deposed that on November 2 last he saw the defendant, whom he knew to have been recently suffering from small-pox, walking along London-street, Greenwich, his face being covered with the eruption. Mr. H. W. Roberts, surgeon, said on November 5 he called at the defendant's house to see a patient, when defendant opened the door for him. Knowing he was just recovering from small-pox, he told him it was very wrong of him to open the door. He was then "scabbing," and, in reply to the magistrate, Mr. Roberts stated that this was as infectious a stage as any period of the disease. The defendant had been seen in the street as early as October 29, and it was stated that he only took the disease on the 17th of that month. Defendant said that on the last occasion, for which he was summoned, he went for a doctor, his wife being in a critical state from heart-disease; and on the first date he only went across the road to the butcher's. The magistrate said he saw no possible excuse for defendant's being in the public street as proved, and it was a very improper thing to do; and he inflicted a fine of £3 for the first case. No evidence was published as to the position in life of the offender, but the unenviable notoriety of London for its small-pox mortality is not likely to be removed unless a strong example is made in cases of such selfish and reckless exposure.

A report has been issued in connexion with the recent census in the United States of America, indicating the distribution of rainfall in the States, and that of population relatively to rainfall. It appears that the highest annual rainfall has been 150 inches. This was reached one year in Paget Sound. The average annual fall in the United States, exclusive of Alaska, was, in 1880, 29 inches. This average implies a large area of land unfit for the purposes of vegetation, which, with the rapid evaporation that occurs, requires much more moisture. Hence population is found to centre chiefly on such parts as have 08·13 per cent. of rain. From a table compiled by Mr. Gannet, it appears that that portion of the country has 68·13 per cent. of the total population, while the classes between 30 and 60 inches comprise 92·3 per cent. The densest settlement is in the class 45 to 50 (the population per square mile being for that area 57·7). That portion of the country also contains the greatest absolute population. It is calculated that the total rainfall in the United States, exclusive of Alaska, in 1880, is an amount about double the water contents of Lake Erie and Lake Ontario combined. It is 1,796,532,642,000,000 gallons, while the surface of evaporation is about 3,000,000 square miles.

The evil of employing unqualified assistants to represent medical practitioners was further illustrated by the proceedings recorded at a recent inquest held by Dr. Danford Thomas, at the St. Pancras Coroner's Court, on the death of a child aged twenty-one months, the son of a working jeweller, of Brill-street, Somers Town. The father deposed that the child was taken ill with measles, and at four o'clock in the morning he ran off to a dispensary kept by a Dr. Dyte in Judd-street, Euston-road, and after some difficulty obtained the services of a young man, who administered a powder to the child. As the infant became worse he went to the dispensary again, when the same young man told him if he would pay 3s. 6d. for his attendance and 3s. 6d. for a week's dispensary subscription Dr. Dyte would make his case the first one. Dr. Dyte, however, never appeared till after ten o'clock in the morning, just two hours after the child was dead. He did not decline to give a certificate of death, but it was not on the regular form, and was moreover worded in such a manner that the Registrar of the Somers Town district very properly refused to accept it. The Coroner regretted to have to remark that this class of cases was becoming more common every day; these dispensaries were supposed by the ignorant to be public dispensaries, whereas they were only the private speculation of a medical man, who, although he might himself be qualified, frequently left persons in charge who were not. The poor who went to them thought they were receiving proper medical advice, but were greatly deceived. After some very strong animadversions on the part of the coroner and jury on this practice, a verdict of ." Death from convulsions supervening upon measles " was returned, with the following rider :—"In returning this verdict the jury desire to strongly condemn the system of medical practice which the evidence in this case has revealed, as they consider the employment of unqualified assistants to take charge of dispensaries, where the principal is non-resident, most pernicious in its practice, and in many cases a fraud upon the public and the sick poor. The jurors further regret that in the present case the deceased did not receive skilled medical attendance, more especially as an extra fee had been paid for the same." We commend the most grave scandal of this employment of unqualified assistants to the very serious consideration of the Medical Acts Commission.

A complaint was made at a recent meeting of the Greenwich District Board of Works, as to the condition of about one hundred gipsies encamped in about thirty vans and tents in Greenwich Marshes, and amongst whom there had been a case of small-pox. The children were described to be in a wretched condition; and not even a School Board officer had visited these squatters! It was suggested that some steps should be taken with regard to these people, who were entirely without sanitary arrangements, and stole all the water they used, it was believed, from the Kent Water Company. A member of the Board corroborated the statements, and remarked that it was surprising to find men, women, and children in their deplorable condition within a few miles of the metropolis. Mr. Richardson, the Metropolitan Board member, said all they could do was to drive them away. Eventually the matter was referred to the Greenwich Parish Committee to report upon. "Alas for the rarity of Christian charity!"

On Saturday evening last, at Exeter Hall, Dr. B. W. Richardson delivered the last of a second series of discourses on Domestic Sanitation, under the auspices of the Ladies' Sanitary Association. The subject chosen was the question of Sleep. In the course of his remarks the lecturer referred especially to the importance of warmth during sleep, particularly in the case of the aged, who should always, during sleeping hours, be protected from the influence of cold. The bedroom, he said, should have a temperature of 60° Fahr., and care should be taken to keep up the temperature of the air of the bedroom in winter-time late into the spring. In conclusion, Dr. Richardson referred to the nervous function in reference to mental and physical education, the effect of work and overwork, the influence of physical training, and

the great importance of maintaining a healthy nervous activity in order to insure the longest duration of useful life.

It is announced that the Corporation of London will contribute £5000 out of the City grain duty in aid of the sum necessary for acquiring a park and recreation-ground for Paddington and North-west London, provided the Metropolitan Board of Works eventually take the requisite steps for forming it, and subject to the necessary funds being raised amongst the inhabitants and the public generally. The Grocers' Company has also promised a grant of £500 towards the furtherance of the same scheme.

THE RECENT DAY CENSUS OF THE CITY OF LONDON.

THE result of the recent day census instituted by the Corporation of the City of London has lately been made public. This is the second occasion upon which an inquiry of this nature has been undertaken, the first dating back so far as the year 1866. It would appear that 261,061 persons were actually resident or employed within the City on the day of investigation, being an increase since 1866 of 90,928, or 53·4 per cent. The adult males were 195,577, the adult females 44,179, and the children of both sexes under fifteen years of age 21,305. This total is more than five times the number given by the Registrar-General as the "sleeping population" on April 4 last. The report further gives an exhaustive analytical classification of trades, professions, and employments made with great care by the City Chamberlain. From this it is to be gathered that there are 57,503 individual employers, estimated to have in their employ 162,253 persons, and, adding to these the 21,305 children, and 20,000 of the adult females being caretakers and others, the total of 261,061 is accounted for.

THE PARIS WEEKLY RETURN.

THE number of deaths for the forty-ninth week, terminating December 8, was 1089 (589 males and 500 females), and among these there were from typhoid fever 33, small-pox 8, measles 12, scarlatina 4, pertussis 3, diphtheria and croup 53, dysentery 3, erysipelas 9, and puerperal infections 6. There were also 56 deaths from tubercular and acute meningitis, 48 from acute bronchitis, 78 from pneumonia, 65 from infantile athrepsia (22 of the infants having been wholly or partially suckled), and 25 violent deaths (18 males and 7 females). The number of deaths for the preceding week (948) was so small that an increase of 91 in the present one is not surprising. The increase chiefly arises from the greater number of deaths due to diseases of the respiratory organs (191 from bronchitis and pneumonia, instead of 145) and from cerebro-spinal diseases (110 instead of 86), the exacerbations of which usually correspond to declensions of temperature. This decline of temperature, on the other hand, seems, as noticed last week, to act favourably in regard to deaths from infantile athrepsia, which are only moderate in number. The births for the week amounted to 1146, viz., 559 males (403 legitimate and 156 illegitimate) and 587 females (434 legitimate and 153 illegitimate); 100 infants (59 males and 41 females) were born dead or died within twenty-four hours.

THE CHARGES OF THE LONDON WATER COMPANIES.

WE recently noticed the action taken by Mr. Archibald Dobbs against the Grand Junction Waterworks Company; he contending that the water-rate must be charged on the rateable value to the poor-rate, and not on the gross value or rent. As the former is in amount about one-sixth less than the latter, the question is one of great importance to all ratepayers and water companies throughout the country, and when the summons was first heard, Mr. Cooke, the magistrate at the Marylebone Police-court, decided to take time to consider the question. Last week he gave his decision, and explained, at length, his view of the different Acts of Parliament quoted by both parties, concluding by observing that the gross value, as laid down in Section 45 of the Valuation (Metropolis) Act, 33 and 34 Vic., chap. 67, seemed to be exactly the definition he had given of "annual value" applicable in the case before him, and he thought as the Company had assessed on that basis there was no reason for altering the amount they claimed of the complainant. Mr. Cooke was, however, willing to grant a case if it was desired. Mr. Dobbs said he would take a case. Mr. Clerk, who appeared for the Company, asked for costs, and remarked that the complainant was backed by other persons. Mr. Dobbs observed that he had acted entirely by himself, but he had received many assurances of sympathy. Mr. Cooke then dismissed the summons, and allowed the defendants 5l. 5s. costs. The case excited a great deal of interest, and several large owners of property, and persons connected with water companies, were present. We trust that Mr. Dobbs will have the courage, and meet with sufficient practical sympathy, to enable him to fight the question through. It appears to be contrary to common sense and to public morality that the water companies should be legally able to largely raise their rates without giving the consumer even the shadow of a quid pro quo.

DEATH THROUGH ANÆSTHESIA.

A CASE of death under sulphuric ether is reported from the Radcliffe Infirmary, Oxford. At the inquest it appeared that the patient was a labouring man, sixty-seven years of age, who had received a lacerated wound on his face, and fracture of his jaw, from being knocked down by the shaft of a cart. It was intended to unite the ends of the fractured bone with wire, but the patient died from blood passing into the trachea during inhalation of ether before the operation was commenced.

THE ENGLISH REGISTRAR-GENERAL'S RETURN FOR THE THIRD QUARTER OF 1881.

THE Quarterly Return for the third quarter of 1881, published by the authority of the Registrar-General for England, gives the total number of births registered during the period as 215,586, being 3437 fewer than in the corresponding quarter of last year. The annual birth-rate, therefore, did not exceed 32·8 per 1000 of the estimated population, which was 1·8 below the average rate in the corresponding periods of the ten years 1871-80, and was lower than in the third quarter of any year since 1860. It is satisfactory to learn from the Return, that although 109,956 deaths were registered during the September quarter, these figures showed a decline of no less than 21,285 from the number recorded in the corresponding period of 1880. The annual death-rate during these three months did not exceed 16·7 per 1000 of the estimated population in the middle of this year, and was no less than 2·9 below the average rate in the ten preceding corresponding quarters. In the third quarter of 1879 (the year so celebrated for its continuous downpour of rain) the English death-rate was as low as 16·3; with this single exception, the rate of the quarter under notice was lower than in any summer quarter since civil registration was commenced in 1837. The average rate in the third quarters of the forty-three years 1838-80 was equal to 20·4 per 1000, and as the recorded rate last quarter was 3·7 below this rate, it is tantamount to saying that 24,000 persons survived the three months who would have died had the death-rate corresponded with the average rate in the forty-three preceding

corresponding quarters. In twenty of the largest English towns, including London, and having an estimated population of seven millions and a half, the death-rate averaged 20·5 per 1000, although this was 2·7 below the rate that prevailed in the third quarter of last year. The lowest rates were 16·0 both in Plymouth and Bradford, and they ranged upwards to 25·8 in Liverpool, 26·2 in Hull, and 26·5 in Leicester. The high death-rates in the three last-mentioned towns were in a great measure due to excessive zymotic fatality—a fatality which, it must also be remarked, considerably influenced the rates of Stoke-upon-Trent, St. Helen's, and Gateshead. It must not, however, be imagined from this that the zymotic mortality was generally in excess, since in only one of the ten preceding summer quarters was the death-rate from these diseases lower than in the quarter under notice. The most prevalent, as is the rule in the summer quarter, was diarrhœa, which caused 8307 deaths; these figures are lower than any recorded for the previous ten summer quarters, always excepting 1879. This low rate is attributed to the cold weather which prevailed through August and September last, and which more than counterbalanced, so far as the production of diarrhœa was concerned, the burst of excessive heat and high diarrhœa mortality of last July. The only other zymotic disease which need be noticed is small-pox: the deaths from this cause, which had been 750 and 1213 in the two immediately preceding quarters, fell (as is the rule in the summer quarter), and were only 674, which, however, is a higher number than in any summer quarter since the great outbreak in 1871 and 1872. It is most unsatisfactory to be compelled to record that of these 674 deaths no less than 461 occurred in London, and 61 more in the Outer Ring; while of the remainder a considerable proportion occurred in the immediately adjoining counties. In addition, there were 84 deaths in Lancashire, and 15 in Yorkshire, while a localised outbreak causing 9 deaths occurred in the sub-district of Wokingham.

PRIZE FOR THE RADICAL CURE OF CANCER.

IN an advertisement in the Boston Med. Journal (November 10), Dr. Collins Warren offers a prize of $300, and another of $100, for the best and second best essays on the following subject:—"The Probability of the Discovery of a Radical Cure of Malignant Disease, and the line of Study on Experimentations most likely to bring such cure to light." The essays must be sent in to Dr. Warren (58, Beacon-street, Boston, Mass.) by February 15 next, legibly written, and neatly bound, and they will all become the property of the donor of the prize, who also constitutes himself (together with any assistance he may select) the judge of their merits. [What with this clause and the short time allowed for the preparation of the essays, we doubt if any satisfactory result will be obtained. A hopeful passage as to the curability of cancer, expressed by Sir James Paget during the discussion on the subject at the Pathological Society, is appended to the advertisement.]

PATHOLOGICAL SOCIETY OF DUBLIN.

AT the meeting of this Society on Saturday, December 17 (Dr. W. Moore, Vice-President, in the chair), Dr. Lombe Atthill showed two large uterine fibroids which were removed from the body of an unmarried woman aged forty, who had suffered from profuse uterine hæmorrhage for several years. A solution of ferric chloride in the proportion of one part to four was injected into the uterus; the patient did well for some days, but sank and died suddenly in less than a fortnight. On the removal of the sternum, the right lung did not collapse, being the seat of a septicæmic or metastatic pneumonia; it was firmly adherent to the pleura. The heart was large; it contained a firm decolourised clot of considerable size in the right auricle; this clot extended into the right ventricle. The liver was probably fatty; the gall-bladder contained 150 small-sized gall-stones. The kidneys were fatty. A small submucous tumour lay between the vagina and the bladder. The cervix uteri was elongated; the cavity of the uterus was encroached upon by a large intramural myoma, situated at the fundus. This tumour measured four and a half inches in its vertical diameter, and three and a half inches in its transverse. There was also a sub-peritoneal tumour, the size of a small pear, attached to the lower portion of the uterus posteriorly by a broad pedicle. On the left anterior surface of the uterus there was a dark soft place, from which, on section, a dark green (purulent) fluid exuded. This was probably an abscess, the contents of which were coloured by the solution of ferric chloride, and which perhaps gave rise to a fatal embolic pneumonia. The ovaries were healthy. Mr. W. T. Stoker presented two specimens of intracapsular fracture of the neck of the femur. The first had occurred not very long before the patient's decease, for no ligamentous union had taken place. In the second case—one of fracture of the right femur—partial ligamentous union had occurred; there was considerable absorption of the head and neck, and erosion of the head on its articular surface. Large exostoses had grown from the anterior intertrochanteric line, and developed so as to articulate with and give support to the anterior edge of the acetabulum, thus giving colour to the theory of Vidal that such bony outgrowths were designed to support the weight of the body carried through the acetabulum. Commenting on this case, Professor Bennett suggested that the cause of the exostoses was the fact that the fracture passed through the capsular ligament and became partly extracapsular. Mr. W. T. Stoker exhibited a rare specimen—a skeleton of the index finger illustrating union of fracture of the second phalanx. The first phalanx was entire and healthy. The articulation between the first and second phalanges had disappeared, and there was firm osseous union between these bones. Strong ligamentous union existed between the second and third phalanges.

VITAL STATISTICS OF IRELAND FOR THE THIRD QUARTER OF 1881.

THE quarterly return of the Registrar-General for Ireland, for the period ended September 30 last, shows that 31,431 births were registered during the three months, a number equal to an annual birth-rate of 24·5 in every 1000 of the estimated population. The total number of deaths registered was 17,958, representing an annual rate of 14·0 per 1000. These returns may be considered of a favourable character, since the births are in excess of those for the corresponding period of 1880 by 1170, and the birth-rate is above the average of the third quarter of the past five years to the extent of 0·3 per 1000. On the other hand, the deaths are below those registered in the corresponding quarter of the previous year to the extent of 3402, and the death-rate 2·0 per 1000 lower. The death-rate has not been so low at this period of the year since 1876, when it also stood at 14·0 per 1000 for the third quarter. The return also shows that the birth-rate was very level all over the country, the figures given being—24·0 per 1000 for Leinster, 24·3 for Munster, 24·6 for Ulster, and 24·4 for Connaught. The death-rate was not quite so even, having been in Leinster 15·2 per 1000, in Munster 14·1, in Ulster 14·1, and in Connaught only 11·4. The return further points out that the notes of the different registrars, both in urban and rural districts, are of a generally favourable character, and the outbreaks of infectious diseases have

been few in number and not of a very grave character. The improved condition of the public health is to be attributed, we are told, to the continuance of a plentiful supply of provisions at moderate prices, and the cool weather of the late summer and autumn. Many of the registrars refer to considerable sanitary improvements having taken place in their districts, but these have not been so long executed, or of such a very general character, as to have yet borne fruit in the shape of diminished disease- and death-rates. The tables for registration provinces and counties show that the number of deaths was below the average of the past three years in each of the four provinces, and in each of the counties except Tipperary. The number of deaths during the quarter referred to the principal zymotic diseases was 1580, or 8·8 per cent. of the total deaths. This number is no less than 1477 (or 48·0 per cent.) under that for the corresponding quarter of last year, and shows that the low death-rate from infectious diseases, commented upon in the return for the second quarter of the present year, still continues. It is certainly a subject for congratulation that small-pox caused only 11 deaths, against 76 in the corresponding quarter of 1880, and compared with 13 in the preceding quarter; but it is not so satisfactory to learn that in the north-eastern division this disease shows a tendency to become epidemic, several cases having occurred, although no fatality is recorded. The mortality from all the other zymotic diseases exhibits a decrease, in some very marked, but fever is reported to be still very prevalent in many parts of Ireland, the continued spread of typhus in Munster forming, probably, the most unfavourable feature in the returns for the quarter under notice.

PROFESSOR VIRCHOW'S REPLY TO CONGRATULATORY ADDRESSES.

AT the end of the newly issued number of his Archiv, Professor Virchow publishes the following, under date Berlin, November 26 :—" In the course of the last few weeks, the occasion being partly the twenty-fifth anniversary of the Pathological Institute of our University, and partly my sixtieth birthday, congratulations and honorary distinctions have reached me in so rich abundance, even from the remotest parts, that it is impossible for me, who already find my load of daily duties heavy to bear, to reply to them all in person. I am obliged to express my thanks to many friends in the present form. Let them believe me that I am most reluctant to forego a personal answer. I am deeply sensible that they have joined in these congratulations from their heart, and I could have wished to assure each individual that I also replied with my whole heart. The very circumstance that the intimate nature of the relations which unite me to my friends has everywhere found full expression, readily suggests to me that the external distinctions which have been bestowed on me at this time far exceed the measure of that which the most strained self-esteem could lay claim to. My friends know that I am accustomed to do my work without thought of reward, and I will say that I still know no higher satisfaction than that which comes of knowledge gained by work. But it was always my endeavour to win independent comrades in work, and therefore it is that I find the highest gratification and a true encouragement in receiving the addresses of so many men who so recognise themselves as comrades. Not a few among them, who formerly worked with me in the Pathological Institute, including those with whom I have from time to time had differences in opinion, came to assure me that in our endeavours we are still at one. Many others, with whom only the common bond of science unites me, assured me of their sympathy in the heartiest way, and even more than that—of their active participation in the common work. Let them all be assured that I have entirely and fully appreciated this demonstration, and the memory of it will be dear to me all my life. What I may still be able to achieve, time will decide. I can only give the assurance that I have not lost the taste for work, and that I shall give all my strength to complete that which I have begun. Age has the advantage that it can make use of many experiences that are wanting to youth, and can preserve the recollection of many things which have disappeared from the literature of the day. But it has also the drawback that it makes us somewhat reluctant to enter into controversies which have been fought out already once or several times, but which are ever anew taken up by the succeeding generation. I do not blame this repetition, for I have myself gone through it. I too have had my time of polemics, and I cannot imagine that I always attained to the full height of that wisdom which would have been necessary to decide the question outright. Everyone has my excuses who seeks in controversy to strive after truth, and for whom controversy is only the means of securing the victory of truth. If I have now little disposition to throw myself into the fight, that will certainly be forgiven by everyone who knows that there is still fighting enough notwithstanding. My silence may not always be taken for assent. Where great matters are in question, there, I think, shall I always be to the fore. This *Archiv*, which contains so many memories of the scientific development of our research, bears witness to the fact that I willingly give free course to every movement, even when it goes against myself, so soon as I recognise that it is an earnest endeavour to find out the truth. And so may I this day carry my hearty greeting and thanks to all those who recognise themselves to be at one with me in endeavour; may it bring them my wish in return, that, in the prosecution of our common work, we may find still further the means of giving to Science the certain pledge of progress in knowledge."

HARVEIAN SOCIETY OF LONDON.

THE following is a list of the names of gentlemen proposed by the Council as officers of the Society for the year 1882 :—
President : *W. Hickman, M.D. *Vice-Presidents :* *J. Milner Fothergill, M.D.; H. Sewill, Esq.; *W. B. Cheadle, M.D.; *H. Cripps Lawrence, Esq. *Treasurer :* James E. Pollock, M.D. *Honorary Secretaries :* Malcolm Morris, Esq.; W. H. Lamb, M.B. *Council :* *Henry Power, Esq.; *George P. Field, Esq.; T. T. Whipham, M.D.; Alfred Cooper, Esq.; F. A. Mahomed, M.D.; Osman Vincent, Esq.; Robert Argles, Esq.; W. Rayner, Esq.; *D. Ferrier, M.D.; *J. Knowsley Thornton, Esq.; *H. W. Kiallmark, Esq.; *J. H. P. Staples, M.D. An asterisk is prefixed to the names of those gentlemen who did not hold the same office the preceding year. Mr. Wheelhouse, of Leeds, has been elected a Corresponding Member of the Society, in place of the late Professor Rolleston.

INSANITY IN NEW SOUTH WALES.

THE Report of Dr. Manning (the official Inspector-General of the Insane in the colony of New South Wales) for the year 1880 is interesting in so far as it records the statistics of lunacy in a comparatively new country. It is first shown that on December 31, 1880, the number of patients on the registers of the hospitals was 1964, giving an increase for the year of 88, which is only very slightly above the average for the last ten years. The proportion of insane persons to population was one in 367, a trifle less than at the close of the preceding year, and exactly the same as at the close of the year 1872. The proportion to population in England at the close of the year 1879 was one in 357. The number of patients admitted for the first time during the

year was 412, while the readmissions numbered 58; these numbers are in excess of those for any previous year. The readmissions formed 12·39 per cent. of the total admissions; in English asylums during the year 1879 the readmissions constituted 13·62 per cent. of the whole number. In 146 cases, or 31·06 per cent., the cause of the malady was unknown. Among the physical causes, to which, as a whole, 57·44 per cent. are attributed, hereditary influence was the cause in 42 cases, or 8·93 per cent.; intemperance in 35 cases, or 7·44 per cent.; and epilepsy in 23 cases, or 4·89 per cent.; congenital defect was ascertained in 20 cases, or 4·25 per cent.; whilst sunstroke, parturition and the puerperal state, diseases of the skull and brain, bodily diseases, and chronic ill-health, all show a high percentage. Amongst moral causes, to which, as a whole, 11·48 per cent. are attributed, domestic trouble, mental anxiety and "worry," and religious excitement, proved the most potent. Spring and autumn, or rather the advent of summer and winter, are distinctly marked, the former by an increase, the latter by a decrease, in the number of cases admitted into hospital. The Report also calls attention to the number of patients admitted, either directly from the ships in which they arrived in the colony, or very soon after landing. A certain number of insane patients are to be expected amongst emigrants, but owing to the closure of the Victorian and Queensland ports to these cases, the number admitted to New South Wales is certainly larger than it would otherwise be, and the hospitals for the insane in this colony are made the receptacle for the homeless insane from the whole of the South Pacific, several cases having occurred in which patients have been sent from New Caledonia and the South Sea Islands. The proportion of recoveries, as in former years, compares favourably with that in asylums in England; whilst the death-rate, 7·10 per cent., is somewhat above that of the colony for the preceding year. In the English asylums the average mortality for the ten years from 1870 to 1879, inclusive, was 10·14; the average for the past five years in New South Wales has been 6·92. Dr. Manning thinks that it is desirable to consider, at once, the extent and character of the existing accommodation for patients, both with regard to the steps which have already been taken to increase it, and to those which may be necessary in the future, since increased accommodation will soon become a necessity.

ST. GILES'S DISTRICT AND INFECTIOUS HOSPITALS.

IN the course of some remarks on hospital accommodation for small-pox and other infectious diseases, Mr. S. R. Lovett, Medical Officer of Health for the St. Giles's District, in his annual report for the year 1880, points out that that parish, in common with the whole of London, suffers when the power of the law is brought in to prevent sanitary authorities from properly isolating those who may be suffering from infectious fevers, and speaks of the difficulty of making new arrangements. It has, he says, been suggested that in the event of the closing of the several hospitals of the Asylums Board, the different parishes should establish hospitals of their own for the isolation and treatment of infectious disorders; but if such a suggestion could be carried out by suburban parishes having an open country at their disposal for choice of a locality, it is quite clear that parishes like St. Giles's, without open country on any side, could not possibly act on such a suggestion. As the nuisance authority, the local board could not allow the erection of hospitals for an infectious disease in the midst of its crowded streets, for any such hospital would no doubt be a nuisance *per se*, and render the board liable to legal proceedings. As an instance of the necessity for a contagious hospital, Mr. Lovett's report remarks that his district, in common with the rest of the metropolis, suffered severely from an epidemic of scarlet fever which continued throughout the year 1880, reaching its intensity in August during the hot weather, at which time more than fifty children (chiefly belonging to the poor) were reported to be suffering from it, and of the total number of cases reported during the year, twenty were removed to hospital—a number which should have been considerably more but for the difficulty of persuading parents to allow their children to be isolated by removal to a fever hospital.

BRIGHTON HEALTH CONGRESS AND SANITARY EXHIBITION.

(From our Special Correspondent.)

HAVING given some account of the food products, specially the novelties, at this Exhibition, I promised to report upon the exhibits in Class 1, viz., House Sanitation. Before doing so, however, I may remark that it is currently reported in the town that at the breakfast given by certain leading practitioners of Brighton to their medical *confrères* from a distance, a ham which was partaken of by many of the visitors (your correspondent among the number) was actually trichinised! The fact of the carver selecting the knuckle of the ham aroused the suspicions of your correspondent. Dr. Richardson, who also partook, is said to have verified the suspicion by microscopic examination. We all believe that the ham was, happily, thoroughly well cooked, but we shall look with anxiety and expectation for a protest from the Anti-vivisection Society against this attempt of the refreshment contractors to experiment upon the distinguished *savants* at the breakfast, however innocent they may have been of any *malice prepense.*

But to resume my peregrinations through the corridors of the Exhibition. I note that the building specially erected by Mr. Humphreys is well adapted for such a temporary purpose. It is lofty, well ventilated, and so constructed (partly of iron and partly of wood) that the materials can be easily taken down and reconstructed elsewhere. I allude to this because an offshoot of this building is a model cottage hospital, fitted up with every appliance for the accommodation of two or three patients. At a place like Brighton, with so many schools—and combating, as the authorities are just now, with an epidemic of small-pox and typhoid fever—it would be well for the Town Council to keep a few of these model hospitals in stock, and to fit them up when required in the playgrounds and gardens of schools, so as to effectually isolate the first cases, which are so likely to infect the whole school unless placed at once under proper quarantine regulations.

Among the novelties in Class 1 is a fountain urinal exhibited by Underhay. The whole of the china basin is continually flushed by a spray of water, which, filling up to a certain height, instantly empties itself automatically, and refills. In this way urine is carried away without being left to make the urinal offensive. The inventors also registered, in November last, a new valve resembling that used for valve closets, to be applied to sinks and hand-basins, and thus to shut off all smell from the trap below.

Mr. Banner exhibits a closet, of which the basin and container may be removed and cleansed by merely lifting them from their sockets. It is not likely, however, that servants would care to undertake this duty; and the mechanism of the closet seems clumsy, and certainly exposes an unusually large surface for fouling. The basin is constructed on the bell-trap principle, and this is generally considered unscientific.

Messrs. Doulton, Jennings, and others show modifications of the wash-out closet, but the objection to this is that the soil and hard lumps of excrement often fail to be flushed out of these closets. The outlet is at the back or side; consequently the centre of the basin is where the deposit collects, requiring a very powerful flush of water to raise it up to the outlet.

Mr. Botting, of Brighton, shows the self-ventilating "Disjuncta" closet, entirely cut off from all drain connexion. The mechanical arrangements for flushing and emptying are the same as in most other valve closets, but the valve-box is separated from the trap by an air-space of two inches, so that the contents of the closet fall through a current of pure air (introduced through the external wall) before passing through the trap.

Mr. Waller shows a model hospital arranged for heating and ventilating without draught. By placing the hot-water pipes in separate casings, and connecting the casings with outlets to the open air, and those outlets guarded by valves, the air introduced to the building passes over the hot pipes, and thus becomes duly warmed in transit.

In this class Prof. Flower has sent some drawings showing "fashions in deformity." Placed side by side with the latest edition of Paris fashions are face deformities, etc., of Caffres, Hottentots, etc.—the head flattened into a sugarloaf form by the gradual pressure of a board worn on the forehead of the infant; lips pouted and elongated by a tablet fixed to the mucous membrane; teeth chiselled and tatooed. It is greatly to the discredit of our more highly civilised race that some of the drawings show physical deformities artificially induced by habits of tight-lacing, etc. A drawing of the Venus of Milo is also shown with the well-known spinal deformity. The deformed foot of the Chinese lady and the high arching foot of the English lady of fashion contrast with the bunioned foot of the mechanic.

Mr. Hansell shows a combination cot, the supports of which are taken from the legs of a reversed table, which may be also used as a table in the daytime. This secures the infant at a convenient height by the mother's bedside at night, and is easily adjustable.

Several inventors of cowls and exhaust-pipes show their inventions in action. All claim to be free from downdraught, though unfortunately this is not our experience with many that we have tested.

A tubular water-bed is shown for localising heat or for protection from bedsores. It is especially serviceable for lunatic asylums and bedridden patients. Any of the tubes may be removed, cleansed, and refilled without disturbing the patient.

Mr. Hamilton, of Brighton, showed several invalid couches, among them a novelty called the "Siesta," with movable arms and head supports, adjustable to any desired position without the patient being required to move.

Messrs. Wright and Stephens show a new water regulator to take the place of the ball lever for cisterns and tanks. The advantages claimed for it are—"silent delivery, regularity of supply, no waste-pipe required, non-disturbance of sediment, durability, and small expense for repair, etc."

Mr. Stott exhibits a self-acting gas-valve. The gas being passed through a bath of mercury after leaving the meter, the pressure is regulated, and thus the waste and noise of gas forcing through the burner when the pressure is great are prevented.

Messrs. Gilmore and Clark show a self-acting ventilator, which opens by the expansion of metal when the heat of the room is sufficiently raised.

In addition to the list which we gave last week of the papers read at the Congress, we would add that Dr. Taaffe read a paper on the Propagation of Disease through Food and Drink—a fortuitous commentary by one of the hosts after the practical illustration already mentioned of the trichinised ham on the breakfast-table at the Pavilion.

Messrs. Savory and Moore show many elegant preparations, some of them introduced this year—especially some Indian febrifuge novelties. Also a fumigator, consisting of a lamp and two trays, with a reservoir for the disinfectant overhanging the top tray. When in use, the fluid falls *guttatim* upon the heated tray, and is thus vaporised.

THE HEALTH CONGRESS.

We subjoin a summary of some papers that were read at the Congress.

Dr. CARPENTER read a paper on "Domestic Health," being a consideration of the means by which individual health is raised or lowered, and the period of life lengthened or shortened by domestic agencies. There are, or were, some streets in Liverpool in which 90 out of every 100 of the children who were born into the world died within the first five years of their existence, whilst the children belonging to the same class of people taken from their wretched homes and sent to such schools as those of Anerley, or to the Beddington Female Orphan Asylum, have a mortality of about 8 in the 1000 per annum. In one case 900 die out of 1000 in five years; in the other only 15! When does health cease, and disease begin? There is a border line in which the conditions necessary for the establishment of disease must have time to produce their results before the disease actually arises. A knowledge of, and obedience to, the laws which regulate health and prevent disease is of the greatest importance, for unhealthy home influences prevent the throwing off of disease, which works its way in many directions, and by a thousand and one means. The presence of zymotic disease in our midst is evidence that some kind of excreta is retained somewhere in too close proximity to particular individuals for it to be safe for those persons to continue in contact with it. The first principles of sanitary work are embodied in the immediate and direct removal of all excreta from our midst, and its conveyance to, and utilisation or destruction in, those districts which Providence has designed for its reception. Six to twelve or twenty-four hours are required, according to temperature and seasons, before mischief can arise, but this margin of time is ample for its removal. There is scarcely a house in the kingdom in which excreta are not to some extent retained. Pure air, pure water, pure food, and temperate habits will diminish the amount of pabulum in which disease factors can develope, and with those benefits we shall have a diminishing amount of impurity in the blood of individuals. If the products of the act of life are removed from the body as soon as formed, or as soon as nature requires them to be removed, the germs of disease may be admitted. Dr. Carpenter holds, without material risk; but being admitted, the result of their action will be manifest according to the quantity of débris which is present for them to feed upon. Time would fail to deal with all the diseases which arise from a want of proper knowledge among the people of the first principles of domestic hygiene, and of the evils which follow from a non-removal of the products of excretion, and the retention within ourselves and our houses of those deadly poisons which are manufactured by the human frame in the act of living. Every region of the body is liable to tubercular deposit, and it is most certain that its greatest factor is the want of ventilation in our dwelling-houses, our workrooms, and our places of public resort; and nowhere is it more deadly than in the counting-house of the city merchant, and the offices which are inhabited by the clerks who have made his fortune. (Your readers will remember that all these assertions are Dr. Carpenter's,—not your correspondent's.) The first proof of this is afforded by the fact that death-rates increase in an alarming ratio among populations according to the density of the people upon the soil, and the number in individual houses. This increase of mortality among children under five is progressive so far that the number of persons living upon each acre of land being known, the number of children per thousand dying under five years of age will certainly mount up in a very rapid manner with each addition of persons per acre. Dr. Farr has proved that mortality is progressive according to the extent of overcrowding. The influence of overcrowding is shown most fatally in its effects upon children under five, for whilst the death-rate at all ages in the most crowded populations is 38·6 per 1000, it is 139·5 for children under five years of age. Compare this with Brighton mortality, and the advantages of situation and pure air are manifest, although it is probable that the mortality among children in the Brighton houses is very much higher than it ought to be. This increase in the death-rate is mainly caused by impure air, and it ought not to be. Poverty assists, but it is impure air which allows tubercular disease to be so prevalent. We may take it that tubercular diseases are as certainly preventable as typhoid fever or cholera, and that a dense population may exist if architects provide adequate ventilation, so that individuals do not poison each other. Alter the proportion of air by a very small degree, and the excretion of carbonic acid from the lungs is interfered with; oxygen is not absorbed in its usual rapid way; and as a consequence the débris (the result of the act of living) is no longer thoroughly oxidised, but is retained in some of the blood-cells, or some parts of the tissues of the body, and the blood is not purified as it ought to be. The cells are unequal to

the work which they have to perform, some used-up matter is kept back, and the foundations for tubercular and other disease are laid. If it were not for other circumstances connected with poverty, the poor would be rapidly swept from the face of the earth by tubercular disease, but it happens, fortunately for them, that their houses cannot be kept entirely draught-proof; wind and storm find their way into their lodgings, and diminish the evil by diluting it; and that which they consider a misfortune is a real blessing, for dilution of the poison is an impediment to its effects. This good fortune does not apply, to the same extent, to the houses of the rich. The old-fashioned open fireplace and imperfectly fitting windows kept the enemy at bay for a time; but the chimney-corner is gone, window-frames are made so tight that not a breath of fresh air can get in by their means, and carpets, curtains, and other so-called comforts remove from the air all its freshness.

Mr. Griffith read a paper on the "Escape of Foul Gases from Ventilating Gratings on the Main Sewers of Towns: the Cause of the Evil and its Remedy." The defective house drainage throughout the whole country, he said, is the great cause of emanations of foul gases from street ventilators on the main sewers. The house drains generally being drains of deposit, or elongated cesspools, the main sewers, instead of receiving fresh sewage, receive putrid sewage, it having been lying in the house drains for months, and sometimes even years. The house drains gradually discharge putrid matter into the sewer; this is immediately put into motion, being churned up by the velocity of the flow into the sewer, and gives off the foul air, which passes at once out of the ventilators into the street. An evil, with regard to house drainage, which is rapidly increasing in the neighbourhood of London, is one caused by the fact that large tracts of land are bought up by speculating companies, roads are laid out, sewers constructed, under their supervision, and only when the district has obtained sufficient importance are the authorities of the parish in which it is situated asked to take it over—and generally do so without giving a thought to the state of the drainage! The real mode of prevention is that in every house the soil-pipe should be carried up above the roof as a ventilator, so that it not only ventilates the house drains, but also the main sewers in the street. If so adopted, the ventilators in the street would act as inlets for air, and the soil-pipes as outlets for foul air. Supposing surveyors have the power of insisting on everything being carried out on the soundest principles, the staff at their disposal is invariably too small to really insure good workmanship.

Mr. Chadwick, on the "Prevention of Epidemics," made some general observations upon the prevention of the occurrence and spread of epidemics. His paper may be summarised as follows:—That cases of small-pox, of typhus, and of others of the ordinary epidemics, occur in the greatest proportion, in common conditions of foul air, from stagnant putrefaction, from bad house drainage, from sewers of deposit, from excrement-sodden sites, from filthy street surfaces, from impure water, and from overcrowding in foul houses. That the entire removal of such conditions by complete sanitation and by improved dwellings is the effectual preventive of diseases due to these causes; and of ordinary as well as of extraordinary epidemic visitations. That where such diseases continue to occur, their spread is best prevented by the separation of the unaffected from the affected, by home treatment if possible; if not, by providing temporary accommodation; in either case obviating the necessity of removing the sick to a distance, and the danger of aggregating epidemic cases in large hospitals—a proceeding liable to augment the death-rates during epidemics. The skilful and complete work of sanitation, and the removal of conditions of stagnation and putrefactive decomposition, are the most efficient means of reducing the expenses of excessive sickness and death-rates.

Mr. Ellice-Clark read a paper on "Some Anomalies in the Administration of the Sanitary Laws." Thirty years' experience of what were practically novel laws for England has demonstrated the fact that the public in the aggregate take but slight interest in the administration of the sanitary laws—an apathy in itself so remarkable as to call for inquiry and discussion. Any demonstration which attracts the attention of the public to sanitary matters is therefore of great value. The division of all sanitary areas into wards is so practical that it should form the subject of a clause in the next Public Health Bill. Of all the learned professions whose members would be of the highest value to a sanitary board, the medical is frequently conspicuous by its absence. The assimilation of the Sanitary Laws is much needed. While the Public Health Act contemplated uniform laws for all towns, its provision for making by-laws and its permissive character have produced quite the contrary result. Not only are the laws of adjoining districts different, but in the same area two separate sanitary authorities administer the law. In local board districts the Poor-law authorities are armed with sanitary powers, distinct, yet clashing with the powers of the sanitary authority. Two sets of officers go over the same ground; two legally constituted bodies exercise their powers in dealing with epidemics in the same area; both have power to isolate disease. Such a conflict of authority can have but one result—that of impairing the Acts they administer. Is not the relief of the poor a question itself of sufficient importance to demand a separate authority? County or watershed boards appear to offer the most practicable machinery for giving effect to rural sanitary legislation. A grave defect of the Sanitary Acts is the non-interference with existing buildings: remembering that the very nature of old streets and buildings was the primary cause of sanitary legislation, it would seem temporising with the case not to deal with streets and buildings where sanitary evils exist. Any house erected previous to the adoption of the Act by the local authority may be enlarged, or dealt with in such a way as its owner wishes—it may be rebuilt with every sanitary defect (except drainage) perpetuated; there may be rooms of any height, without any ventilation, walls of any thickness, every inch of area within the curtilage may be covered, in short, all those evils for which by-laws are made, may remain, and worse still, may be exaggerated and intensified, for there is no difficulty in so rebuilding a house as to place it outside the pale of the Act of 1875. Is it not practicable to deal with the cardinal points of sanitation—rooms to be of a minimum height, walls of a standard thickness, air space of a minimum area when not previously built on, water-closets or privies to be erected next to an external wall, and to have external ventilation? A most important omission is the inability to control the direction of streets. A property owner may so lay out new streets as to render inconvenient for all time streets which in a few years pass into highways, unable and repairable by the public purse, entailing great sacrifice in the carriage of burdens on succeeding generations. These might have been arranged with immediate advantage to landowners, and perpetual positive convenience to the public, at little or no cost. They can now be only attained by sacrificing property, at great cost to the public rates. If the public are to bear the burden of maintaining in perpetuity any road, they have a right to determine its direction. If an owner of property proposes to construct houses without stables he must give a large area for street purposes; if he makes provision for both man and beast, then his own will is law, and he may crowd double the number of human habitations on a given area. A great disadvantage possessed by by-laws is the difference existing between them in the same neighbourhood. This is the result of the permissive nature of the Act and the elastic wording of the section. No sanitary requirements that the necessities of the case demand should be omitted because of the value of land, building materials, or the social position of the inhabitants. The Tottenham Board passed plans for 5000 houses in one year. To imagine that all these houses are built in accordance with sanitary requirements, even if the strictest by-laws are in force, is a delusion that the public should have exposed as soon as possible. Sanitary authorities may not confess it in public, but those who see what is daily going on know that the most insanitary evils are being perpetuated, and modern speculative builders are forging a rod for the backs of our immediate descendants, which must kill its thousands and tens of thousands. The Local Government Board have recently issued a set of by-laws to be observed in the construction of buildings. There are fifty-two pages of closely printed matter, contained in ninety-nine by-laws to be observed—enough and to spare for any surveyor to have at his finger-ends,—and yet under these a house may be built without doors, floors, or windows, or restrictions as to the height of rooms, nor is there one word about plumbing! To properly supervise a district having houses completed at the rate of 200 a month, at least six inspectors are required.

TYPHUS FEVER IN SWEDEN.

Dr. Warfvinge, of Stockholm, published last year a treatise on Typhus Fever, based on his own experience, which has lately come into our hands, and we think the medical profession in England will be much interested to learn how closely the opinions of so useful an observer with regard to typhus agree with those taught here at home.

We are indebted for the following notes to a summary in French which is appended to Dr. Warfvinge's work:—

Typhus exanthematicus, which had not appeared in Stockholm for twenty-five years, prevailed epidemically in that city during the years 1870, 1872, 1874, and 1875; and the author's work is based on the study of 2239 cases of this disease observed during the epidemics in question in a hospital for "typhoid" affections.

Commencing with the etiology of typhus, Dr. Warfvinge insists on the specific difference which exists between this form of continued fever and typhoid fever; he quotes all the arguments in favour of this distinction, and refutes the objections which have been put forward against it. Typhus has raged epidemically from time to time in Stockholm, while typhoid was endemic there at the same time, the number of cases of this latter malady varying from year to year only in an insignificant manner. From this the complete mutual independence of these diseases in their perfectly accidental coincidence is a necessary sequence.

Typhus continues to increase in prevalence from the commencement of winter until spring—a period during which the poor remain crowded together in rooms badly, or not at all, ventilated—and it disappears when summer comes. But exactly the opposite is observed in regard to typhoid fever, and this is well shown in a table given by Dr. Warfvinge.

Typhus occurred most frequently in foci (often of as many as from twenty to fifty cases) which developed in the city and in houses tenanted by a too numerous and indigent population, whereas not a single case of typhoid had taken its origin from these foci. A person who had recovered from typhoid most usually remained henceforth inaccessible to that disease, while he was not so as regards typhus, and vice versâ. In support of this view the author cites a good many cases—at the hospital twelve convalescents from typhoid contracted typhus, and in the same way the author observed four cases in which individuals recovered from typhus subsequently took typhoid. The specific distinction between the two diseases also declared itself under the other etiological factors.

Typhus is transmitted directly from one individual to another; it presupposes a "contagium," and Dr. Warfvinge gives, in illustration of the eminently contagious nature of the disease, a number of examples, such as:—At the hospital, four physicians, twenty-two attendants on the sick, and nurses, besides fifty-five patients under treatment for other diseases, contracted typhus from contact with persons affected with it, and several took it in other hospitals. It was quite a common occurrence for all the members of the same family to come into hospital simultaneously or at short intervals stricken with typhus, and for them to be frequently followed by all or almost all the other inhabitants of the infected house. The author calls attention to this tendency of the disease to form foci of infection, as well as to the fact that the danger of contagion increases directly as the frequency of contact between the healthy and the sick, but that it diminishes in the presence of ventilation, which dilutes the contagious matter, and that the separation of those infected puts a stop to the further spread of the disease. He also cites examples of typhus transmitted, by infected individuals, into places which had been previously free from the disease. Just the reverse was noted in the cases of typhoid fever observed by the author.

Dr. Warfvinge shows that typhus generally began to prevail epidemically in the month of December, and its frequency thence increased very rapidly, to attain its maximum between January and May. Afterwards, it diminished so quickly during June and July, that August presented only

(a) "Om Typhus Exanthematicus; Afhandling grundad på egen Erfarenhet jemförd med andras." (" A Treatise on Exanthematic Typhus, based on individual experience compared with that of others.") By Dr. F. W. Warfvinge. Stockholm: P. A. Nyman. 1880. 8vo. Pp. 199.

a few cases, and the epidemics almost entirely ceased during the months of September, October, and November. The proof that this fact is not accidental is that it repeated itself with slight differences during four epidemics.

The author connects these facts with the circumstance that in Stockholm the indigent class, within the limits of which the disease almost exclusively confined itself, was obliged—principally of late years—in consequence of the want of lodgings, to live crowded together in close and non-ventilated dwellings. When winter, with the want of ventilation which accompanies it, had lasted a certain time, typhus epidemics broke out, to decline rapidly and to cease with the warm season, during which the indigent class live much more in the open air.

The author had not met with a single example to prove that a spontaneous origin should be attributed to typhus, and he attempts to show that all the cases cited, especially by Murchison, in support of an autochthonous origin of the disease can be explained in quite another way, remembering how easily the disease is communicated, and how protracted is the retention of the virus by walls, clothing, etc.

Sex.—Of the patients, 1359 were males, and only 880 females. From this, however, it does not follow, Dr. Warfvinge maintains, that typhus has a predilection for the former. The preponderance of male patients held only in the year 1874 and 1875 (in the proportion of two to one), when a large number of labourers out of work were crowded together in Stockholm; and for this reason it was confined exclusively to the ages between fifteen and forty-five years; in the other two epidemics, the two sexes were equally represented.

As regards *age*, the youngest patient was only eleven months old; the most aged was seventy-seven years. And the author shows that age predisposes in a different way to typhus and typhoid. Up to ten years the frequency of both diseases remains the same; but, whereas the number of typhus cases undergoes only slight variations from ten to fifty years, the frequency of typhoid fever rapidly increases from ten to twenty years, to fall subsequently quite as quickly.

Having described the course of the disease, illustrating his remarks with a clinical history of some cases, Dr. Warfvinge passes on to an account of the different symptoms of typhus.

He first gives a detailed sketch of the conditions of the axillary *temperature*. With a rise sufficiently abrupt, it may sometimes go as high as 40·5° Cent. (105° Fahr.) on the evening of the second day, and ordinarily attains its acme on that of the fourth or fifth day. From this date and with morning remissions of half a degree Centigrade (0·9, Fahr.), or a little more, the same temperature is generally maintained for six or seven days—sometimes (in the most benign cases) for a shorter time, only two or three days; sometimes for a longer time, up to twelve days. During this period of acme of temperature, the maximum fell on the fourth to the sixth day, sometimes a little later; it was rarely below 40° C. (104° F.), and never above 41·6° C. (107·3° F.), with the exception of elevations to 42·3° C. (108·3° F.) in the death-agony. With more decided morning remissions, the temperature then decreased during two or three days (the period of decline or defervescence), to present towards the end a fall which was generally very rapid. Rarely, however, was this defervescence rapid enough for the fall of temperature to normal or below it—that is, to 35° C. (95° F.) and less—to be brought about in the space of twelve hours; and there was never a lysis, properly so-called. In typhoid fever the increase of pyrexia goes on more slowly; but, on the other hand, the temperature remains longer at a typical height, whence it descends only by degrees and by morning remissions, which are more and more pronounced.

Dr. Warfvinge shows that it is not, as has been contended, the degree of temperature which renders an attack of typhus more or less grave. It can only be said (as in the case of typhoid fever) that the graver the type of typhus, the better marked is the elevation of temperature simultaneously with the other symptoms; but this rule presents numerous exceptions.

The rapidity of the *pulse* corresponded tolerably closely to the temperature. *Epistaxis* occurred in 5·09 per cent. of the cases, with a mortality of 8 per cent. In the *blood* the red corpuscles showed a continued but slight reduction in number (from 5,000,000 to 4,200,000 per cubic millimetre).

The Cutaneous Exanthem.—This very important symptom of typhus showed itself tolerably soon, most frequently on the fifth day. The maculæ appear all at once in the course of a day or two, and not by degrees; they are at first of a pale red colour, and disappear on pressure. Then they become darker, taking on a brownish tint, when they can no longer be made to disappear altogether on pressure; later on their colour becomes livid, and some are in the serious cases transformed into true petechiæ. The fully developed eruption, as a rule, commenced to disappear with the subsidence of the temperature; the petechiæ persisted after death. In 16·4 per cent. of the patients the exanthem was wanting or was very slightly marked, and this most commonly in children.

A *bronchial catarrh*, most frequently very benign in character, was present in 78 per cent. of the patients.

As to the *digestive system*, the *tongue* was in the majority of cases (63·8 per cent.) moist and more or less furred, dry in only 36·2 per cent.; this usually at the end of the first or the beginning of the second week, and with a greater frequency according as the patients were aged and the cases severe (mortality 24·2 per cent. in the cases in which the tongue was dry). The *bowels* were generally regular (in 55·5 per cent.) or costive (24·5 per cent.); in the remaining 15·1 per cent., in which they were relaxed, this occurred—with some exceptions, 4·9 per cent.—only to a very trifling extent, and the symptom was essentially transitory (mortality in these cases with diarrhœa 23·3 per cent., against 15·1 per cent. in the others). *Vomiting* was not a very common symptom (7·9 per cent.), and appeared more frequently at the beginning of the illness than in the course of it or during convalescence. *Enlargement of the spleen* was observed in the majority of the cases, but usually in a moderate degree.

As regards the *urine*, Dr. Warfvinge made quantitative analyses of the urea and of the chlorides in three cases—the results of which was that the urea was increased to such a degree that it was from 1·7 to 2·6 times more abundant than in healthy men on the same diet. The excretion of urea, which did not, however, correspond with the degree of temperature of the body, was greatest during the stage of crisis. As to the chlorides, they were considerably diminished during the fever, so that often only traces of them remained. The urine was albuminous in 67·7 per cent. of the 1660 cases which were examined, and the frequency of albuminuria increased, with the age, from 20 per cent. in children under five years to 82 per cent. in patients above fifty-five years. The mortality rose successively from 4·3 per cent. to 32·0 per cent. with the degree of albuminuria—a symptom which was observed at the earliest on the fourth day, and generally lasted about eight days—sometimes longer, sometimes shorter.

The symptoms referable to the *nervous system* most usually assumed the form of a certain degree of stupor and of somnolence. The loss of muscular power was very common and well-marked, so that as a rule the patients took to their bed after one or two days. Delirium was present in 31·1 per cent. of the cases (mortality 24·1 per cent.), impairment of hearing in 9 per cent. (mortality only 5·5 per cent.), subsultus tendinum in 3·7 per cent., involuntary dejections with profound prostration in 6·8 per cent. The author disputes the alleged dependence of the nervous symptoms on the rise of the temperature, the intensity of these symptoms not being in direct ratio to the amount of the rise of temperature, and their character presenting a manifest resemblance to certain narcotic poisons.

Grave *complications* and *sequelæ* were not frequent. There occurred, amongst others, thirty-five cases of erysipelas, fifty-two of parotitis, twenty-nine of suppurative adenitis and of subcutaneous or intermuscular abscess (amongst these were three cases of abscess in the borders of the larynx, of which two proved fatal and one was cured by tracheotomy), thirty-five of bedsore, five of spontaneous or embolic gangrene (of a toe, the prepuce, the nymphæ, the cheek, a circumscribed piece of lung with consecutive pneumothorax), sixty-three of pneumonia, forty of pleurisy, seven of icterus, one of peritonitis, two of intestinal hæmorrhage.

As to the *periods* of the disease, that of incubation was generally about two weeks. There was no prodromal period, properly so called, and the period of invasion, during which the temperature underwent a rapid rise, lasted from four to five days. Almost simultaneously with the eruption of the exanthem came the period of some of temperature, which most often lasted from six to seven days—the extreme limits being from two to twelve days. We may then estimate the period of defervescence at about three days. The *duration* of the fever varied, therefore, from eight to twenty days—most frequently, in 35·7 per cent. of the cases, from fourteen to fifteen days,—the mean being 14·39 days. It was in general shorter in children than in adults. Convalescence was usually rapid.

The *mortality* varied during the four epidemics between 10·78 and 19·49 per cent., the mean being 15·94 per cent. It seems to depend little or not at all upon the seasons. Higher amongst males (17·8) than amongst females (13·06 per cent.), it presented this peculiarity—that it always rose more with the age of the patients—namely, from 1·1 per cent. in children to 80 per cent. in subjects above sixty-five years. During these epidemics it was proved that the mortality is in direct proportion to the crowding together of the patients. Of fifteen pregnant women, none died, two only aborted. The mean duration of the fatal cases was 14·49 days.

As regards the *pathological anatomy* of the disease, the author, in more than 300 autopsies of persons dead of typhus, never observed those alterations in the lymphatic system of the intestinal canal which are so characteristic of typhoid fever; at most the spleen was, as a rule, found slightly enlarged and rather soft, but by no means to the same extent as in typhoid.

In *treatment*, prophylaxis occupies the first place. Therapeutical treatment, properly speaking, was expectant ; fresh air, refrigerant beverages, ablutions with cold water, and sometimes baths between 30° and 25° C. (67·5° and 56·3° F.), acids, quinine, wine.

It will be seen from the foregoing analytical abstract of Dr. Warfringe's treatise that he adds little to our knowledge of typhus and its epiphenomena. His book is, however, useful as a brief compendium on the subject of which it treats, and is interesting as showing how closely the type of typhus observed in Sweden corresponds to that of this form of continued fever with which we are unfortunately so familiar in some parts of the United Kingdom. With pardonable pride we note that Dr. Murchison is constantly quoted by the author, who fully recognises the inestimable service rendered to medicine by our illustrious countryman in his splendid monograph on the "Continued Fevers of Great Britain."

Dr. Goodell's Formulæ in Amenorrhœa.—When this is due to torpid action of the uterus, Dr. Goodell orders Ext. aloes, ferri sulph. exsic., āā ʒ ij., assafœtida ʒ iv. ; divide into 100 pills, one pill to be taken after each meal, increasing to two, and then to three pills. If the bowels become too much affected, the patient is to stop, and begin again with one pill. When the amenorrhœa is due to arrested development, he has derived the best results from the constant use of Blaud's pills.—Pulv. ferri sulph., potass carb. pure, āā ʒ ij., mucil. tragacanth q.s., in pil. xlviij. To be taken daily until three pills are taken after each meal. If these pills cause constipation, Dr. Goodell prescribes—Pulv. glycyrrhizæ, pulv. sennæ, āā ʒ iv., sulph. sublim., pulv. fœniculi, āā ʒ ij., sacchar. ʒ xij. ; a teaspoonful in half a cup of water at bedtime. When the suppression is due to change of habits and loss of health, tonics are employed ; and when the suppression comes on suddenly from cold or exposure while in the midst of the menses, and is accompanied by severe lumbar pains, the patient is placed in a mustard hip-bath, a Dover's powder is administered, she is put to bed, and hot drinks are given to provoke copious diuresis and diaphoresis.—*Louisville Med. News*, November 26 (from *New York Med. Record*).

Bromide of Potassium in Orchitis and Inflamed Breast. Dr. Gramner states that he always has found, both in orchitis and in inflamed breast (from milk), that five grains of the bromide given three times a day, or in smaller doses more frequently repeated, are all that is required to effect a speedy cure. In some cases he has seen the disease kept in abeyance for weeks, although the patients committed the grossest imprudence in riding or walking; yet even these cases recover without atrophy or suppuration.—*Louisville Med. News*, December 7.

FROM ABROAD.

The Paris Hospital Mortality Returns.

Dr. E. Besnier, in his report for the third quarter of 1881 (*Union Médicale*, November 17 and 27, and December 3 and 11), states that the mean temperature of the quarter was 17·4° C., and scarcely differed from the thermometrical mean of the corresponding quarter calculated for the period 1803-70. The fall of rain, without being excessive, exceeded the mean of the period, being 175 millimetres in place of 147. The prevailing winds blew from the north and west in July and August, and were very variable in September.

The *general mortality* only exhibited its normal declension at a late period, and after having undergone an intense exacerbation in July. In consequence of this, the mortality for the quarter in the hospitals and hospices (3650) exceeded the mean mortality of the quarter for the nine previous years (3011) by 640 deaths—an excess much beyond that explicable by increase of population.

1. *Affections of the Organs of Respiration.*—Of all the diseases of these organs, it is pneumonia that is most manifestly subject to the action of the seasons. From the month of May its monthly declension is constant and regular, both as regards numbers and gravity. This is the normal course of the disease, which is each year exhibited in an invariable manner. In pleurisy there is observed a similar diminution of cases, but its mortality varies little with the seasons. As to the various affections designated as bronchites, their statistical collation is so absolutely defective that their enumeration, under such conditions, is without any interest whatever. Of phthisis there were admitted 1676 cases, with 815 deaths; of pneumonia, 568 cases, with 158 deaths (27 per cent.); bronchitis, 1411 cases, with 103 deaths (7 per cent.) ; and pleurisy, 366 cases, with 88 deaths (10 per cent.).

2. *Diphtheria.*—The epidemic of diphtheria, continuing to exhibit its gravity and intensity, has, nevertheless, undergone a slight attenuation, as usual at the season; but the annual progression of the disease continues, and augurs ill for the approaching winter. This ever-increasing peril to the population must before long compel the institution of a special inquiry as to the appropriate measures to be employed. During this quarter in all Paris 596 deaths occurred from diphtheria. In the hospitals there were admitted during the quarter 157 cases of diphtheria, with 76 deaths (48 per cent.), and 126 cases of croup, with 97 deaths (75 per cent.). Distributed according to age and sex, there were 9 adults (2 males and 7 females) admitted with diphtheria, and of these 3 died. Of the 81 boys admitted for diphtheria, 37 (45 per cent.) died, and of 59 admitted for croup, 46 (77 per cent.) died. Of the 67 girls admitted for diphtheria, 36 (53 per cent.) died, and of 69 admitted for croup, 51 (73 per cent.) died.

3. *The Eruptive Fevers.*—These have in general, from the month of August, undergone a positive attenuation both in regard to number and mortality. Scarlatina, the annual evolution of which is on the increase, alone forms an exception. During the quarter there were admitted 505 cases of *small-pox*, with 87 (17 per cent.) deaths ; 158 cases of *measles*, with 25 (15 per cent.) deaths ; 216 cases of *scarlatina*, with 17 (7 per cent.) deaths ; and 121 cases of *erysipelas*, with 13 (11 per cent.) deaths.

4. *Small-pox.*—As predicted in former reports, small-pox pursued during the summer its regular and normal course of diminution; so that while there were (in all Paris) 35 deaths during the first quarter of 1881, these diminished to 296 during the second quarter, and now, in the third quarter are only 211. The general annual diminution also continues: for instead of 211 deaths there were, in the corresponding third quarter of 1880, 449 deaths. The same decrease is observable in the hospitals ; for while during the first quarter of 1881 there were 723 admissions, with 173 (23 per cent.) deaths ; and in the second quarter 694 admissions, with 164 (23 per cent.) deaths ; there were in this third quarter but 504 admissions, with 87 (17 per cent.) deaths. So that both the number of the cases and their mortality alike obey the seasonary law, the operation of which may always be predicted.

5. *Scarlatina.*—Dr. Besnier reminds his readers that it is now several years since he called their attention to the

extraordinary difference which separates Paris from other capitals as regards "the fecundity of the scarlatina ferment." Thus, while London registers 1500 or 2000 deaths from scarlatina, Paris can scarcely count 100. In 1879, London had 2706, Berlin 461, and Paris only 105; and this has been the case from a remote period, in spite of the incessant mixture of men and things induced by modern manners and the rapidity of intercommunication. Here is an affection of the most contagious character, which during a long series of years has propagated itself to a great excess in London, and yet during the same period is limited to a most narrow range in Paris. During the nine years 1871-79 there were but 951 deaths in Paris, three times less than London furnishes in a single year, and only equal to that which Berlin registers sometimes in a year. And even this annual mean of 105 deaths for the nine years is only attained because in the anomalous year 1871 alone there were registered 205 deaths from scarlatina. For the other eight years the mean is but 80 deaths per annum, with a diminution to 60 in 1878; while in that same year (1878) there occurred in Berlin 871 deaths, or fourteen times as many.

"The cause of these extraordinary differences in the diffusion of a contagious disease at the same epoch, in different countries, between capitals so near and so united by relations of all kinds as London and Paris, escapes us absolutely; but we may affirm it is upon conditions appertaining to the localities, and not to individuals, that these great oscillations of fermentative diseases depend. But this long immunity of the Parisian soil would seem to be exhausted, and the benign years of scarlatina are passing away. A continuous progressive movement in this direction has unexpectedly appeared, and is becoming more marked even at the present time. We must be made aware of this, and practitioners must not ignore it. The disease is becoming more frequent and more fatal, and complications which formerly were unusual and exceptional have become, if not common, at least relatively frequent. The prognosis in a case of scarlatina should, then, be delivered with more reserve, the surveillance of the patient should be more close, and isolation and private and public prophylactic measures should be more rigorous."

The following is a list of the mortality from scarlatina year by year in Paris since 1871, when it was 205 :—1872, 124; 1873, 86; 1874, 68; 1875, 88; 1876, 183; 1877, 92; 1878, 60; 1879, 95; 1880, 356; 1881 (nine months), 406.

6. *Typhoid Fever.*—The epidemic of typhoid fever takes its place in severity after the epidemic of 1876; but, in spite of its extreme intensity, it has none the less been subjected to the rule of a seasonary diminution in the spring. With the summer it has resumed as regularly its ascensional course, giving for the three months, July, August, and September, 435 deaths—that is, 25 per cent. higher than the mean of the corresponding quarter calculated for the nine preceding years, which is 322 deaths. The different parts of Paris have been affected very unequally, without any *fixed conditions*—whether absolute or specific, population, altitude, riches or indigence, etc.—being discoverable capable of explaining the disparities. A table is given, comparing the distribution of deaths from the epidemic in the third quarter of 1876 (655) with that of 1881, which confirms the above statement. There were admitted into the hospitals during this quarter 942 cases, with 201 (21 per cent.) deaths. These were distributed as to sex as follows: 536 men, with 110 deaths; 59 boys, with 12 deaths; 296 women, with 70 deaths; and 51 girls, with 9 deaths.

INFANTILE DIARRHŒA.—Dr. Lewis Smith recommends the following as a very efficacious formula for diarrhœa due to indigestion and acidity :—Pulv. ipecac. gr. ss., p. rhei gr. ij., sod. bicarb. gr. xij.; in pulv. xij. One from every four to six hours for infants a year old.—*Louisville Med. News*, December 3.

BLOOD OF CROCODILES.—Detailing to the Société de Biologie the analyses of the gases of the blood which he has performed on the crocodiles lately sent to M. Paul Bert, M. Blanchard states that, owing to the large quantity of fibrin contained in the blood of these animals (seven grammes and a quarter per kilogramme), if an arterial trunk be opened, hæmorrhage is immediately arrested. The lymph also contains much fibrin, so that if a lymphangitis be induced it is also at once arrested.—*Gaz. des Hôp.*, December 6.

REVIEWS.

A Treatise on Orthopædic Surgery. By J. WARRINGTON HAWARD, F.R.C.S. London: Longmans, Green, and Co. 1881. Pp. 167.

THIS book will doubtless receive considerable attention, because it proceeds from the hands of a general surgeon, while it nevertheless treats of a special subject. It is divided into eight chapters, which deal respectively with Talipes; Torticollis, or Wry Neck; Distortions of Upper Extremity; Distortions of Lower Extremity; Contracted Cicatrices; Anchylosis; Rickets; and Lateral Curvature of Spine. We notice that in defining talipes, or club-foot, the author makes no mention of a primary bone lesion as a possible factor in its production; and yet authors have shown that the tarsal bones are deformed at so early a stage of uterine life that it becomes difficult not to associate the deformity as a cause rather than as a consequence of the talipes. It seems difficult for us to account for "muscular contraction" in the fœtus. The rest of this chapter is excellent. The importance of careful and long-continued manipulation is more than once alluded to: "The result will certainly fall far short of complete success unless these measures are followed by a long course of systematic exercise of the weak muscles." It will not be an exaggeration to say that herein lies the gist of the whole treatment. We should not have looked for a notice of "ingrowing toe-nail" in a special work on orthopædic surgery, but here it is nevertheless, and is well worth reading. Dupuytren's treatment of finger-contraction seems somewhat less out of place. The information, however, on these two subjects is none the less accurate or worthy of account.

We find Mr. Haward regards flat-foot as a result of genu valgum (when the two deformities co-exist), and not the cause, as advocated by one well-known orthopædic surgeon. It is our own view also. We must differ from him somewhat when he says that genu extrorsum is not usually associated with any corresponding overgrowth of the external condyle. In cases of true extrorsum the external condyle is, we believe, more often overgrown than not.

In the chapter on Lateral Curvature, our author, after discussing causes and treatment, says :—"I am quite sure that far more harm than good is done by spinal supports in the slighter cases of lateral curvature. . . . . Such treatment is as unscientific as it would be to apply irons to support the legs of a person recovering from fever because he is unable to walk steadily." With this we entirely agree. The muscles require strengthening. If they are too weak to perform their functions, it is hardly rational to overweight them further by the application of so-called iron supports.

Mr. Haward has quite ignored the subject of angular curvature (Pott's disease). It is, nevertheless, one of very frequent occurrence in practice, and one which presents many difficulties. It may be argued, perhaps, that it is only part of a very much larger subject. True; but why exclude it on that account from a "treatise" which discusses rickets, for instance, and the means by which bodily deformities generally may either be alleviated or remedied?

Mr. Haward thinks, and very justly, that the average student, as a rule, knows very little about this subject; and, while he deprecates the separate practice of orthopædic surgery, he advocates its separate teaching, on the ground that "such separation permits the more elaborate consideration and explanation of minutiæ, without which it cannot be understood." His argument does not appear quite as clear as it might be, and there seems at first sight a little inconsistency about it. But we take it that his meaning is, let a man who is a good general surgeon devote special attention to orthopædics if he has a taste that way; but let him not give up the study and practice of general surgery. With this we are quite ready to agree. We have always felt that the exclusive practice of any one speciality is a mistake; but we must carefully abstain from ascribing all the evils of specialism simply to this fact. It is the practitioner who goes wrong rather than the speciality he practises; and it is as often owing to a deficient education as to any other cause that an "exclusive devotion to one part of surgery is apt to interfere with a just appreciation of the relation which that part bears to the whole."

Mr. Haward's book is short, and eminently readable; it may be safely recommended both to the practitioner and the student. They will both obtain from it a clear and just insight into a class of disease which is at present but little understood, because it has not yet become a matter either of general study or of general teaching.

The Bible and Science. By T. LAUDER BRUNTON, M.D., D.Sc., F.R.S. London: Macmillan and Co. 1881.

IT is but seldom that members of our profession venture on the debatable ground of the relations between science and religion—too seldom, we think, for the many-sided studies of the really educated physician render him far more competent to speak on such subjects than is the divine who has not had the advantage of a scientific training, or the man who has concentrated his whole attention on a single department of science, as chemistry or physics. Such men cannot but be more or less one-sided, whereas the accomplished physician must be a man *in seipso totus, teres atque rotundus*. Dr. Brunton is eminently qualified for the task he has undertaken—familiar with every branch of science, an avowed believer in revelation, and well acquainted with the Bible and Bible lands. His work is essentially popular, and consequently he has devoted twelve out of the eighteen lectures to an outline of botany, zoology, geology, and anthropology, in order that his readers may be enabled to appreciate the arguments to which he introduces them in the concluding three or four. The three opening lectures contain a picturesque description of Egyptian and Arab life in the time of Joseph and Moses, with the purpose of better illustrating the sacred narrative. With no wish to eliminate the supernatural element, he ventures to explain the mechanism of certain miracles on physical grounds: as, for instance, the darkness that might be felt, during which the Egyptians could not stir from their houses, as a sandstorm of unusual denseness; the passage of Jordan by an upheaval of the land—an idea which occurred to him on viewing the spot, and which he sees confirmed in Psalm cxiv.; and he gives plausible reasons for regarding the phenomenon commonly supposed to have been a prolongation of daylight, at the battle of Gibeon, as rather an eclipse, preferring the translation given in the margin of the A.V., "Be dumb," in the sense of darkened, to the received one of "Stand still."

But the gist of the whole book is contained in the concluding chapters, in which he ably maintains that the doctrine of evolution is in entire harmony with revelation, and the very opposite of atheistic in its tendencies. He courageously contends that the popular notions on creation, the state of our first parents, and so on, are drawn from the Miltonic mythology, rather than from the Bible as read in the light of modern science. By a few well-chosen illustrations he puts in the clearest light the evidence of evolution as against the doctrine of permanent and independent species. And in fearlessly facing its logical conclusion as applied to man himself he employs two arguments which we do not remember to have seen used before—first, that though we were not individually made out of lumps of clay, we have no hesitation in telling our children that God made us, or as to the scientific accuracy of the statement that "dust we are, and unto dust we shall return"; and secondly, that as we watch the development of the embryo, for a long time absolutely indistinguishable from that of lower animals, and devoid of consciousness or independent life, we must admit that the making of man a "living soul" need not necessarily imply the putting of a rational and fully developed soul into a full-grown body ready made to receive it.

Many, we know, will be staggered at the plain speaking of the author, but all must allow that the mature opinions of a man of Dr. Brunton's scientific and religious character are deserving of thoughtful and respectful consideration.

A New Analogy. By CELLARIUS. London: Macmillan and Co. 1881.

WE have received this work from the same publishers, but its more strictly theological character precludes our noticing it as fully. The pseudonym of its author, who is, as he informs us, a layman, is a play on that of the immortal author of the "Analogy" between religion and nature, and his work is based on that of Bishop Butler; but the order of the argument is, to a certain extent, reversed, in consequence of the changed aspect and method of science.

Butler argued, to a large extent, from our *ignorance* of the laws of nature; modern scepticism appeals to the completeness of our *knowledge*, and the author accepts the challenge. Again, when Butler wrote, men believed that the world was created as it is, and the laws impressed on it afterwards. Geology and evolution have reversed this view of things, and shown that the present order is the result of the working of laws: so, while Butler speaks of the constitution and course of nature, "Cellarius" reasons from its course to its constitution. The work may be regarded as a not unworthy sequel to the "Analogy" of Butler.

The Classics for the Million: Being an Epitome in English of the Works of the Principal Greek and Latin Authors. By HENRY GREY. Second Edition, revised and enlarged. London: Griffith and Farren, St. Paul's-churchyard. 8vo. 1881.

THIS well-brought-out volume contains a fairly good summary of the chief works of some four-and-thirty of the best known Greek and Latin writers, illustrated by quotations from good and approved English translations. The Greek authors selected are—Homer, Hesiod, Æschylus, Pindar, Herodotus, Euripides, Sophocles, Thucydides, Aristophanes, Xenophon, Aristotle, Demosthenes, and one or two others; the Latin—Plautus, Terence, Catullus, Lucretius, Cæsar, Cicero, Sallust, Virgil, Tibullus, Propertius, Horace, Livy, Ovid, Martial, Pliny, Juvenal, Tacitus, and Quintillian. A brief history or sketch of each author is given, and an appendix contains the names of the principal English translators of the classics. The book contains a wonderful amount of information for its size—only 350 pages; but the work of analysis and condensation has been well and clearly done, and the result is a pleasantly written handbook to an acquaintance with the classics. The intelligent student who has little Latin and no Greek will find it well worth reading carefully; and the classical scholar may find it useful and interesting as a book of reference and a spur to his recollection of past studies.

GENERAL CORRESPONDENCE.

"REFORMED SPELING."
LETTER FROM MR. J. DIXON.

[To the Editor of the Medical Times and Gazette.]

SIR,—I have read with astonishment Dr. Harley's last letter on spelling reform. If he thinks that our present spelling should be changed, why does he merely nibble at a few details? Why not take in at once the whole phonetic system? A great deal is to be said in favour of it, as regards the learning and skill with which it has been constructed by the labours of Mr. Ellis, Mr. Pitman, and others. Ingenious characters have been invented for more clearly expressing the sounds of our speech, and many small changes have also been suggested, which might, at once, be easily adopted, such as the enclosing of an interrogative sentence between two notes of interrogation, etc. The only objection to the phonetic system is, that it is impracticable. Before it could be generally adopted, we must either learn two languages, or utterly ignore all English written before the Phonetic Era. And what would become of the poor children who are now being taught in our schools? No doubt they learn there a great deal that is useful and necessary; but in many cases they are crammed with much that is perfectly useless to them, seeing that they are hereafter (to gain their living as artisans, servants, and labourers. Are they also to learn two written forms of language—current English, and phonetic or reformed? The thing is too absurd to be entertained.

English is no doubt a very difficult language; its vowel sounds being so various, and its spelling so arbitrary. But then it only requires study and application to master all this; and surely the effort to overcome difficulties constitutes the most valuable part of a child's education.

To write "vaxination" (why not vaxinashun?) will not make the word easier to a poor child; while to an educated adult, who knows that the origin is vacca, the word is hideous and revolting.

Dr. Harley seems to think that modern English was derived from High-German. Does he not know that Anglo-

Saxon, the basis of our present language, was a Low-German dialect? And why does he derive our numerals "one" and "two" from French "une" and "deux," instead of from the Anglo-Saxon án and twa? Surely the Saxons could count before Norman-French came over to them!

Reformed spelling is to represent our pronunciation. But whose pronunciation? I go to Paddington Station: the porter says, "Bath, sir?" sounding the word like lath. In less than two hours another porter appears, and he cries "Bath, Bath!" sounding it like hath; and throughout the city I hear the word so pronounced. Who is right?

Professor Earle sums up his remarks on the phonetic system thus:—"When we enter on the path of spelling reform, we pass from that on which we are tolerably agreed, namely, conventional orthography, to raise a new structure on a foundation of unascertained stability. The moment you resolve to spell the sound, you bring into the foreground what before lay almost unobserved—the great diversity of opinion which exists as to the correct sound of many words."

I am, &c.,
Dorking, December 15.   JAMES DIXON.

THE NEW ORTHOGRAPHY.

[To the Editor of the Medical Times and Gazette.]

SIR,—The new orthography not only has its advantages in allowing us to curtail the length of words, but it moreover renders them so much more comprehensive. On the other hand, however, I confess that this comprehensiveness is sometimes rather confusing. An old friend of mine is an enthusiast for this reformed spelling; and the consequence is, that I am obliged to study his letters before I dare read any portions of them to my wife. I send you a few extracts from some of them, italicising some of the words in which the wicked reduplicated consonants have been omitted. Thus, one day he wrote:—"On meeting this morning in the street a man who much dislikes me, he exclaimed, 'Who's your hater?' and as I made as if to poke him in the abdomen with my umbrela, he yeled out, 'Don't boly me.' Whereupon a man on the top of the house—he seemed rather 'cut'—caled out, 'What's that below there?' and had for an answer, 'You're a toper.' Returning home, I picked branches of the holy, with its bright red beries. You know I always do this in remembrance of the plant which gave the name to our holydays. Then I took my Turkish bath, and rasped myself wel; and next, being very hungry, gave my stomach a good filing, having joined the early diners, and realy eaten a diner. Then my wife gave me my smoking-cap (she would make, I can tel you, an exelent caper)." Another time he wrote:—"Little Nelly looked pale this morning, and I thought she pined for fresh air, so I invaded the schoolroom, caried her of, pined a shawl over her chest, and bade her run and get her hat. She did my biding, and, after biding our oportunity for escaping strict mama's remonstrances, we got out, I taking my favorite malaca walking-stick. Mama saw us, however, and caled out that I was not cosy, that I was as mad as a hater to spoil the child, and that I had no right or title to change a jot or title of the school rules. The litle one was soon hoping along merily by my side, hoping for some fun. We were pasing the cathedral when a batery of artilery came along, and the eclesiastical dignitaries coming out at the same time, we stoped to see the canons pas." And this morning my friend says, "The pug is as noisy as ever. I punished him, but the efect was not satisfactory. The dog was not cured, and I incured his mistres's displeasure for my 'cruelty.' Our old servant Joe, as you predicted, did not get better of his chronic dysentery, and I was obliged to 'get rid of him, but I gave him a fair sum per anum."

Yours faithfully and grammatically,   M.D.

SOUTH LONDON SCHOOL OF PHARMACY.—The prizes were presented to the following successful competitors in the lecture-room of the institution on December 17:— Senior Chemistry — Medal, E. John Bull; Certificate, Herbert Shaw. Junior Chemistry—Medal, W. T. Mignot-Tucker; Certificate, Walter Lloyd. Botany — Medal, Clement Caldecott; Certificate, F. E. Tozer. Materia Medica—Medal, H. Hardy White; Certificate, W. J. M. Tucker. Practical Pharmacy and Dispensing — Medal, Frederick E. Tozer; Certificate, C. Caldecott.

REPORTS OF SOCIETIES.

THE PATHOLOGICAL SOCIETY OF LONDON.

TUESDAY, DECEMBER 6.

SAMUEL WILKS, M.D., F.R.S., President, in the Chair.

THE PRESIDENT announced the approaching completion of the volume of Transactions for last session; and, in explaining its late appearance, referred to the large number and excellence of the woodcuts with which the volume would be illustrated.

SPECIMENS FROM A CASE OF GOUT.

Dr. NORMAN MOORE showed the knee-joint, the kidneys, the larynx, and some pia mater which he had removed from a man (a painter by trade) who had recently been in St. Bartholomew's Hospital under the care of Dr. Southey. The man died a few hours after his admission. He had suffered from profuse diarrhœa for some five weeks previously, and was greatly exhausted. His knees were much swollen, and so painful that he could not walk. At the autopsy, deposits of urate of soda in very considerable quantities were found in both knees, in the great-toe joints, in the index metacarpophalangeal joints, the elbows, and hips. There were no deposits in the lower-jaw articulation, nor in the shoulders, nor in the vertebral joints. In the knee-joints the urate of soda was very abundantly deposited, while in the right knee there was also a considerable collection of pus. This pus, when analysed, gave no uric reaction. Larynx: There was a small deposit in one of the vocal cords. Kidneys were small and contracted. There was extensive interstitial nephritis, the epithelium of the tubules was gone, and the Malpighian bodies were atrophied and degenerated. Brain : On the pia mater of the left lobe of the cerebellum there was a small hæmorrhage, in which a minute deposit was found; to which he drew special attention, as Dr. Garrod doubts, even when it occurs, whether it has any direct connexion with the gout. The Bones : On examining them, they did not give any uric acid reaction. The man had been a plumber; he had never suffered from colic, but frequently from gout. He had a faint blue line on the gums. On testing the liver no trace of lead could be found. Dr. Moore thought that the lead checked the excretions generally; and as these men were often intemperate, the excretion of uric acid was interfered with, and the condition above described was thus brought about.

Dr. DYCE DUCKWORTH had seen the autopsy, and thought that this case filled up one or two gaps. The occurrence of urate of soda in the pia mater and in the larynx was interesting ; but more so the pus in the knee-joint. This occurrence was doubtless rare in gout; and only a few cases were recorded. Sir Benjamin Brodie and Dr. Todd had each related a case, but as the patients had suffered from erysipelas, it was thought that this, rather than the gout, explained the presence of pus. In another case it was thought to be due to typhoid fever; whereas the present case was really a true case of gout, in which the lesion could hardly be attributed to any other or outside cause.

Dr. CURNOW had made two autopsies at King's College Hospital on extensively diseased gouty joints. In none of the affected joints had he found any signs of inflammation or suppuration. He doubted whether from this single case any precise conclusions as to the occurrence of suppuration could be drawn; and, for his own part, he regarded it rather as accidental.

Dr. MAHOMED inquired whether there had been any convulsions in this case. He had himself described similar cases of hæmorrhage, but with convulsions. He would now ask whether it was probable that insufficient excretory organs did or did not render patients liable to be affected by slighter causes than others.

Mr. MORRIS asked whether the phalanges were affected. Very slight causes occasionally lead to pus in the joints; he related a case in point.

The PRESIDENT asked for more information regarding the presence of urate of soda in the bones.

Dr. MOORE replied: he had not analysed the metacarpal

bones, though sections through them showed no naked-eye traces. There had been no convulsions in his case.

The PRESIDENT believed that he had not infrequently seen urate of soda in the bones after section.

Dr. SOUTHEY said that there had been no convulsions while the man was in the hospital. He had, however, only seen him once; and the history of his previous health was not very clear.

Dr. FELIX SEMON said that two other cases of urate of soda deposits were recorded in *Virchow's Archiv*—one by Professor Virchow himself, and one by Dr. Litten.

TISSUES FROM A PATIENT WITH HÆMOPHILIA.

Dr. WICKHAM LEGG showed specimens of tissues which he had removed from the body of a young lad who had died of hæmorrhage consequent on an insignificant injury. While sitting on a doorstep, the lad had been knocked over by some old woman; in the fall he had sustained a slight wound on the lip. Spite of the surgeon's art, the hæmorrhage had persisted, and he died fourteen days after his accident, of syncope. Portions of different tissues were put into Müller's fluid nine hours after death. After due preparation, they were carefully examined, but no changes whatever were found in them. Up to the present time only five cases of examination of the tissues were recorded. In three of these no changes were found, while, in the other two, slight changes had been found. In one of the latter, Dr. Percy Kidd recorded that the nuclei in the veins were increased, while the middle coat of the arteries was thickened and transparent. The tissues all presented traces of fatty degeneration and infiltration, but this was common to all forms of loss of blood (as in purpura). As regards the joints, the knees were found to contain some brown blood-stained fluid. The cartilage was white and appeared healthy. It is interesting to note that the hereditary tendency is transmitted by girls, but only manifests itself in the males of a family. A family tree going back over two hundred years was shown, in which this remarkable peculiarity was well illustrated. This peculiarity seemed, however, not to be confined to hæmophilia, but was observed in the case of colour-blindness and in some other diseases.

The PRESIDENT thought that the occurrence of small hæmorrhages in the acute fevers pointed to an altered relation between the blood and the bloodvessels.

FOURTEEN SPECIMENS OF HYDRO- AND PYO-SALPINX.

Mr. LAWSON TAIT, who exhibited the above specimens, said that thirteen of them had been removed by abdominal section on account of pain and hæmorrhage, in every case the patients recovering from the operation, and up to the date of the paper complete relief had been obtained. On account of adhesions the operations were all difficult, in some cases extremely difficult, but the removal of the uterine appendages was complete in every instance. The features common to such cases are—(1) a history of some pelvic inflammation, though sometimes this cannot be obtained with precision. Its origin is variously ascribed, as from gonorrhœa, a chill or sudden stoppage of menstruation, and, most frequently, an attack of inflammation occurring after labour or a miscarriage. There is always (2) pain, which comes on after exertion, and especially after intercourse, and becomes greatly intensified when menstruation appears. At this time the pain is often described as excruciating, and it lasts throughout the period. In the majority of instances there is (3) irregular and profuse menstruation, often amounting to hæmorrhage. The physical signs are, swellings at the seats of the ovaries, which are always tender, and generally quite fixed. Distinct fluctuation can often be felt, and their peculiar sausage-like shape has frequently enabled a correct diagnosis to be made of the condition previous to the operation. No treatment short of removal of the uterine appendages has been found to relieve such cases, though most of the cases under notice had been, previous to coming under the author's care, under the care of eminent specialists who had treated them with infinite variety of therapeutical means, by pessaries and even by division of the cervix, etc. At the operations the organs were nearly always found to be matted to the pelvic wall and to the viscera, and the hæmorrhage was often severe during the separation of the adhesions. All the operations of this character which had been performed by Mr. Tait (nineteen in number) had recovered completely. Menstruation was in

the great majority immediately arrested, but in a few it lingered for a month or two. In those cases where the marital function had been destroyed, it was restored, and had been injuriously affected in none of them. The pathological condition of most importance is practically the same in all of these cases, and arises, it seemed to the author, from an attack of acute or sub-acute oöphoritis or peri-oöphoritis. During this process the trumpet-shaped extremity of the tube approaches the ovary for its normal temporary attachment; and this, by the inflammatory action, becomes permanent. Certain it is that, in nearly all the cases, permanent attachment of the tube to the ovary is to be seen. Probably after this attachment has occurred the inflammatory process extends to the tube, there is a desquamation of the ciliated epithelium, and occlusion of the tube at its uterine extremity occurs. The nature of the contents of the tube is determined by causes which he did not understand. The most common of the varieties is hydrosalpinx, and the rarest is hæmatosalpinx. Sometimes these tubal cysts ruptured into the peritoneal case, and a post-mortem specimen of this was exhibited, in which several ruptures, followed by peritonitis, had been watched. Mr. Tait had no doubt that many mysterious cases of peritonitis were due to this cause.

Mr. ALBAN DORAN demonstrated the true relation of the Fallopian tube and its fimbriæ to the ovary. He could not agree with the descriptions contained in the text-books, which stated that the ovary lies transversely in the pelvis below the tube, which ran directly outwards from the uterus. On the contrary, the ovary would be found to lie almost vertically close below the brim of the pelvis, and resting on the fimbriæ. Hence it was that in all these cases the dilated tube, was found closely attached to the outer side of the ovary, and to its lower part. He believed that one common cause of pyosalpinx was the constant passage of unclean sounds. Most of Mr. Tait's cases had been repeatedly examined by different practitioners.

Mr. KNOWSLEY THORNTON bore out the general correctness of Mr. Doran's views on the position of the Fallopian tubes. It would be interesting to know how often the condition of pyosalpinx would prove fatal if not operated on. As regards hydrosalpinx, he knew of cases of spontaneous cure, where the women had since borne children—a fact to be borne in mind before subjecting them to such an operation as this.

CALCIFIED ADENOMA OF SCALP.

Mr. EVE showed a specimen of this condition. It was a small, firm tumour, lobulated and encapsuled. At first it was thought to be fat. Before microscopic preparations could be made it had to be softened in an acid solution. It was then found to consist of columns of epithelial cells in a fibroid stroma. These columns varied in size; some were branched, some were tortuous. The epithelial cells were small, about the size of those found in the sudoriparous glands, having nuclei. The family history of the young man from whom the tumour was removed was interesting. His father and his father's sister had both suffered from similar tumours. These tumours resembled some which were shown at the International Medical Congress by M. Malherbe, who described them as calcified epitheliomata of the sebaceous glands. He could not agree to regard them as epithelioma, as there was no infiltration of the surrounding tissues, no leucocytes, and the size of the cells also differed. He thought that they most resembled what English pathologists agreed to call adenoma. He also showed sections of a second tumour of the same nature.

SEBACEOUS ADENOMA.

Mr. SHATTOCK showed this specimen, which, he stated, resembled an ordinary adenoma of the breast.

Dr. PYE-SMITH drew attention to the difference in the signification of the word epithelioma in this country and on the Continent.

The following were exhibited as

CARD SPECIMENS.

Dr. HADDEN—Stomach and Œsophagus, showing Dilated Œsophageal Veins, which had given rise to Fatal Hæmorrhage in a Case of Cirrhosis of the Liver. A second Stomach and Œsophagus, also showing Dilated Œsophageal Veins and Enlarged Follicles.

Mr. TREVES—An Attached Fœtus, from the Sacrum.

ROYAL MEDICAL AND CHIRURGICAL SOCIETY.

TUESDAY, DECEMBER 13.

ALEXANDER WHITE BARCLAY, M.D., President, in the Chair.

CASE OF LITHOTOMY, WITH ENUCLEATION OF TUMOUR OF PROSTATE.

MR. REGINALD HARRISON read a paper on a case of lithotomy where a tumour of the prostate was successfully enucleated, with remarks on the removal of such growths. The case is recorded as bearing upon the remedying of prostatic enlargement by means other than those commonly recognised. It was considered that a study of what, for the most part, have been regarded as accidents occurring during lithotomies might contribute to our resources in the treatment of this affection. The patient was admitted into the Liverpool Royal Infirmary with a stone in the bladder and enlarged prostate, for which lithotomy was performed on September 5, 1881. The stone was so large that bilateral section of the prostate became necessary. Though this extension of the incision gave additional room for extraction, a tumour of the prostate proved to be an additional obstacle. This was enucleated with the finger, when the stone was easily removed with the forceps. One patient made a good recovery. The tumour was about the size of a walnut, and proved to be an adenoma. The calculus (oxalate of lime) weighed two ounces and five drachms. An analogous case occurring in the practice of Mr. Bickersteth, where a prostatic adenoma, and a stone weighing two ounces and a half, were successfully removed in a somewhat similar manner, was also recorded. From these instances, together with others of the same kind, published by the late Sir William Fergusson, Mr. Cadge, and Dr. C. Williams, Mr. Harrison considered the following conclusions might be drawn:—1. That lateral cystotomy may be practised in certain cases of enlarged prostate which are attended with symptoms producing great distress, with the view of exploring and, if possible, of removing the growth. 2. That in all cases of cystotomy for calculus where the prostate is found to be enlarged, a careful search should be made with the finger with the view of effecting the removal of the growth, should such be found practicable. 3. That, in determining the selection of lithotomy or lithotrity in a case where stone in the bladder is complicated with enlargement of the prostate, regard should be had to the possibility of removing both of these causes of annoyance by the one operation—namely, by lithotomy. Further, these cases seem to indicate the best mode of removing these tumours when met with during the performance of cystotomy. It was suggested that where the third lobe was found to be enlarged and pendulous a simple form of écraseur might be advantageously substituted for avulsion with the finger.

Sir HENRY THOMPSON considered the suggestion practical, and well worthy of consideration. Tumours of the prostate complicating stone in the bladder were not uncommon, and they had sometimes been removed during lithotomy. In 1862 he presented Mr. Cadge's cases to the Pathological Society, and at that meeting the late Dr. Keith, of Aberdeen, said he had removed an outlying portion of the prostate seven or eight times, without any bad effect; whilst Sir William Fergusson had removed a prostatic growth four or five times. There were two distinct kinds of these—namely, outgrowths from the prostate itself, and tumours encapsuled in the interior of the gland. He preferred the general term " prostatic tumour" to that of " adenoma," even though, as in tumours of the breast, the new growth approached the gland in structure. Encapsuled tumours existed in almost every specimen of hypertrophied prostate. Median or lateral lithotomy had been performed for the relief of enlarged prostate even where there was no stone, but he had been disappointed in his results. It was not very large prostates which were so troublesome, but those with small nipple-like projections which blocked the orifice of the urethra. He would be glad to see his way to any reasonable chances of success by operation in these cases, but in old persons between sixty and seventy the mortality was about one in four.

Mr. SAVORY said that it would greatly aid in surgical treatment were it possible to diagnose between simply enlarged prostate and tumour of the prostate. Some tumours could be enucleated, but nothing could be done for hypertrophied prostate. He would scarcely propose an operation except there were some means of diagnosing the two.

Mr. C. HEATH mentioned a case where Sir William Fergusson tore off a portion of the prostate during lithotomy. The patient died.

Mr. R. HARRISON said he wanted to see if the so-called accident might not be utilised. He did not propose the operation for simple enlarged prostate, and though a diagnosis could not always be made between the two forms, he thought that an exploratory incision could do no great harm.

CASE OF REMOVAL OF FIBROUS POLYPOUS TUMOUR OF BLADDER.

Mr. BERKELEY HILL read a paper on a case of fibrous polypous tumour of the bladder, successfully removed. The patient, aged forty, had suffered from January to October with irritable bladder. The earliest symptoms were fever with rigor, hæmaturia, and strangury. Then followed abortion at three months, diminished gravity of symptoms, and marked improvement for some months after voiding a mass of clot and phosphates. Return of the suffering; digital exploration of the bladder; removal of polypus with rapid recovery—structure of polypus being mainly fibrous, but in part villous and in part resembling alveolar sarcoma. Statistics of the number of recorded successful removals of vesical tumours are twenty-eight, with nineteen recoveries.

Dr. CHARLES CARTER had seen a patient at the Hospital for Women with a reddish mass projecting from the urethra. Next day it had disappeared, and she left. Some time afterwards she returned, as a reddish mass always projected from the urethra when she passed water. By digital examination a polypus was found adhering to the posterior part of the bladder. A portion of it was torn away during examination, and the patient had since remained well.

Mr. HARRISON CRIPPS believed that the polypi both of bladder and rectum were villous outgrowths, the deeper epithelial cells being transformed into elongated fibre-like bodies.

Mr. MORRIS advised early examination, and removal if necessary. In one case he had seen a papilla hanging over and obstructing either ureter. Both ureters were dilated, and on one side the kidney destroyed.

Mr. B. HILL asked if there was not a chance of the tumour returning in Dr. Carter's case. He quite agreed as to the importance of early detection, but dilatation of the ureters might precede any active symptoms.

MEDICAL NEWS.

For the degree of M.D. (for Practitioners)—

Carter, Frederick, M.R.C.S., L.R.C.P.
Cullingworth, Charles James, M.R.C.P., M.R.C.S., etc.
Deane, Andrew, M.R.C.S., etc.
Walford, Walter G., L.R.C.P., M.R.C.S.

Three failed to satisfy the Examiners.

For the degree of M.B.—

Breet, James, M.R.C.S.
Doudney, George Herbert.
Hudson, Theodore James, L.R.C.P., M.R.C.S.
Paley, William Edmund, F.R.C.S. Eng.

One failed to satisfy the Examiners.

For the degree of M.S., two candidates presented themselves, and both failed to satisfy the Examiners.

Examiners: Charles Gibson, M.D.; Charles John Gibb, M.D.; G. H. Philipson, M.A., M.D.; W. C. Arnison, M.D., M.R.C.S.; H. E. Armstrong, M.R.C.S.; Frederick Page; T. W. Barron, M.A., M.B.; Octavius Sturges, M.D.; and H. G. Howse, M.S., F.R.C.S.

UNIVERSITY OF DUBLIN.—At the Winter Commencements in Michaelmas Term, held on Thursday, December 15, in the Examination Hall of Trinity College, the following degrees in Medicine and Surgery were conferred, in the presence of the Senate of the University, by the Right Hon. John Thomas Ball, Vice-Chancellor of the University; the Rev. John H. Jellett, D.D., Provost of Trinity College; and the Rev. James W. Barlow, Senior Master Non-Regent:—

Baccalaurei in Chirurgiâ.—Arturus Montfort Archer, Alex. Richmond Johnston, Henricus Brougham Pope, Edmundus FitzGerald Bannatyne Wilson.

Baccalaurei in Medicinâ.—Arturus Montfort Archer, Thomas Ricardus Gillespie, Gulielmus Henry, Alexander Richmond Johnston, Franciscus Thorpe Porter Newell, Gulielmus Sidney Jebb Scott, Edmundus Fitz-Gerald Bannatyne Wilson.

Doctores in Medicinâ.—Gulielmus Henricus Line, Henricus Singer Gabbett, Ricardus Dormer White, Ricardus Carolus Studdert.

APOTHECARIES' HALL, LONDON.—The following gentlemen passed their examination in the Science and Practice of Medicine, and received certificates to practise, on Thursday, December 15:—

Barnes, Walter Stanley, 82, Caversham-road, N.W.
Edensor, Arthur, Heath Mount, Hampstead.
Fletcher, John, Park-street, Southport.
Hoolis, Robert, Carshalton.
Hudson, Theodore Joseph, Kedley Vicarage, Hull.
Murch, Wilfred, Gilbert-terrace, Kilburn.
Rodwell, John Lyndsay, Loddon, Norwich.
Rogers, Thomas Edward, 184, Aldersgate-street, E.C.
Shannon, Robert Alexander, Llanidloes, Montgomeryshire.
Webster, James Arthur, R.A.E. Infirmary, Wigan.

The following gentlemen also on the same day passed their Primary Professional Examination:—

Barry, Donald Moore, St. Bartholomew's Hospital.
Bush, James Paul, Bristol School of Medicine.
Clarke, Charles Frederick, Charing-cross Hospital.
Erulkar, Solomon A., Grant Medical College, Bombay.
German, Harway, King's College.
Leach, Arthur Herbert, Charing-cross Hospital.
Schön, Charles Henry, University College.
South, George, Charing-cross Hospital.
Verity, Herbert W. S., King's College.
Wilson, Thomas, Westminster Hospital.

BIRTHS.

WASKALLY.—On December 14, at Sidmouth, South Devon, the wife of C. B. Faskally, F.R.C.S., of a son.
HUTCHESON.—On December 19, at Brighton, the wife of Surgeon-Major G. Hutcheson, M.D., H.M.'s Bengal Army, of a daughter.
NEWMAN.—On December 17, at St. Martin's, Bowness, Windermere, the wife of A. J. Newman, L.R.C.P., M.R.C.S., of a son.
PARAMORE.—On December 19, at 13, Hunter-street, Brunswick-square, W.C., the wife of Richard Paramore, M.R.C.S., of a daughter.
SMITH.—On December 12, at 18, Harley-street, the wife of Heywood Smith, M.D., of a daughter.
SUTCLIFF.—On December 17, at Great Torrington, North Devon, the wife of Edward Sutcliff, M.D., of a son.
TEEVAN.—On December 14, at 116, Netherwood-road, West Kensington-park, the wife of Alfred Teevan, L.R.C.P., M.R.C.S., L.S.A., of a daughter.

MARRIAGES.

CALEEN—BERRYMAN.—On December 13, at Bath, William Bruce Clarke, F.R.C.S., of St. Bartholomew's Hospital, to Annie Euphemia, daughter of the late Rev. J. W. Berryman, Rector of Tyd St. Giles, Cambridgeshire.

HUNT—LANGLEY.—On December 15, at Bristol, Joseph William Hunt, M.D., B.S. Lond., of 101, Queen's-road, Dalston, to Maria Beatrice, only daughter of J. N. Langley, LL.D., of Redland, Bristol.
KENNY—LISTON.—On December 19, at Kensington, Edward Sebastian Kenny, son of Dr. Kenny, L.R.C.P., to Effie Marguerite Lauder Liston, daughter of the late W. H. Liston, Esq.
KIDD—BENN.—On December 17, at Blackheath, Walter Kidd, M.D., second son of Joseph Kidd, M.D., to Alice, daughter of the late Rev. J. W. Benn, M.A., rector of Carrigaline and Douglas, co. Cork.
KIDD—HARRISON.—On December 15, at Blackheath-park, Percy Kidd, M.B., eldest son of Joseph Kidd, M.D., to Gertrude Eleanor, daughter of Colonel T. B. Harrison.
PETHEBRIDGE—WELLS.—On December 15, at Penang, Walter S. Pethebridge, Esq., to Mary Dalzell, eldest daughter of S. S. D. Wells, Deputy Inspector-General of Hospitals and Fleets, Haslar.
SIMONS—SIMPSON.—On December 14, at Finsbury, Charles N. Simons, Esq., of 1, Somerfield-road, Finsbury-park, N., son of P. A. Simons, M.D., of Luton, Beds, to Emily, only daughter of Frederick Simpson, Esq., also of Luton.
WARBURTON—COMBER.—On October 8, at Shillong, G. A. Warburton, Surgeon Bengal Army, to Augusta Maud, second daughter of Colonel Comber, Bengal Staff Corps.

DEATHS.

CLAPHAM, MARY FREDERICA, wife of Lawrence Clapham, M.R.C.S., at Thorney, near Peterborough, on December 17, aged 36.
ELLIS, ROBERT WILLIAM, M.R.C.S., at 9, Redcliff-parade, Bristol, on December 19, aged 56.
MANLEY, MARY ANDERSON, wife of John Manley, M.D., at Knowle, Fareham, Hants, on December 20, aged 51.
NEALE, ELLEN MARIE, wife of John Edward Neale, M.R.C.S., Cape Copper Mining Company, Port Nolloth, at Klipfontein, Namaqualand, South Africa, on November 18, aged 26.
OMOND, ROBERT, M.D., F.R.C.S., at 48, Charlotte-street, Edinburgh, on December 18, in his 75th year.
RAMSBOTHAM, JOSEPH MEREDITH, M.D., at 15, Amwell-street, Myddleton-square, London, on December 19, in his 81st year.
ROBERTS, R. PRICE, M.D., at Shamrock House, Rhyl, North Wales, on December 17, aged 65.

VACANCIES.

In the following list the nature of the office vacant, the qualifications required in the candidate, the person to whom application should be made and the day of election (as far as known) are stated in succession.

BOROUGH OF SHEFFIELD.—Resident Medical Officer. (*For particulars see Advertisement.*)
GENERAL HOSPITAL, BIRMINGHAM.—Honorary-Surgeon. Candidates must be Fellows of one of the Royal Colleges of Surgeons of the United Kingdom. Diplomas to be sent to the Medical Committee at the Hospital on or before December 24.
GRAVESEND INFIRMARY AND DISPENSARY.—House-Surgeon and Dispenser. (*For particulars see Advertisement.*)
MONMOUTH UNION.—Medical Officer. (*For particulars see Advertisement.*)
NATIONAL DENTAL HOSPITAL, 149, GREAT PORTLAND-STREET, W.—Dental Surgeon. Candidates must be Licentiates of Dental Surgery. Applications and testimonials to be sent to Arthur G. Klugh, Secretary, on or before January 10, 1882.
QUEEN'S HOSPITAL, BIRMINGHAM.—Non-Resident Physician for Out-patients. Candidates must be graduates in medicine of a British or Irish University. Copies of the regulations, etc., can be obtained from the General Superintendent, to whom applications, with testimonials, must be sent on or before January 3, 1882.
ROYAL COLLEGE OF SURGEONS IN IRELAND.—Professor of Practical and Descriptive Anatomy. (*For particulars see Advertisement.*)
WARNFORD HOSPITAL, LEAMINGTON.—House-Surgeon. Candidates must be Members of the Royal College of Surgeons of London, Edinburgh, or Dublin, and Licentiates of the Apothecaries' Company of London, or of the College of Physicians, London, or possess a medical degree from some of the British Universities, and appear on the Medical Register. Applications, with testimonials, to be sent to William Maycock, Secretary, on or before December 27.
WORKSOP DISPENSARY.—Resident Surgeon. Candidates must be unmarried, and will be required to act as Secretary to the Committee. Applications to be sent to J. Easterfield, Hon. Secretary, Gateford-road, Worksop.

UNION AND PAROCHIAL MEDICAL SERVICE.

*** The area of each district is stated in acres. The population is computed according to the census of 1871.

RESIGNATIONS.

Chapel-en-le-Frith Union.—Mr. John Bennett has resigned the Chapel-en-le-Frith District and the Workhouse: area 24,390; population 7000; salary £40 per annum. Salary for Workhouse £40 per annum.

APPOINTMENTS.

Chipping Norton Union.—Arthur H. Orpen, L.R.C.S. Edin., L.K. & Q.C.P. Ire., to the Second District.
Fordes Union.—James John Robertson, M.B. and C.M. Glasg., to the Montgomery District.
Newtown and Llanidloes Union.—Daniel Ferguson, L.R.C.P. Edin., L.R.C.S. Edin., to the Workhouse.
Settle Union.—Richard Ernest Williamson, L.R.C.P., L.R.C.S., M.B. and C.M. Edin., to the Kirkby Malham District.
Thetford Union.—Alfred J. G. Waters, L.R.C.P. Edin., M.R.C.S. Eng., to the Brandon District.

Bromide of Sodium in Epilepsy.—Dr. Hammond's experience has proved the following to be one of the best methods of treating epilepsy:—Dissolve eight ounces of the bromide in a quart of water, and give a teaspoonful three times a day. After three months add another teaspoonful to the night dose, and after another three or four months add another spoonful to the afternoon dose also. At the expiration of a year do the same with the morning dose, and continue thus for a year or more. If no symptoms of the disease have meanwhile appeared, then gradually reduce the doses, and at the end of the third year stop. The attacks do not usually return after this course of treatment. Ordinarily, however, patients stop the medicine after a week or two, and in such cases the attacks almost invariably return. It is then almost impossible to bring these patients under the influence of the bromides again. The doses will have to be at least doubled, and this may so derange the system as to make it impossible to take the medicine longer.—*Louisville Med. News*, December 3.

Royal College of Surgeons of England.—Mr. William Frederic Haslam, L.S.A., of St. Thomas's Hospital, whose diploma of membership of the College is dated May 22, 1878, having passed the necessary examinations, was admitted a Fellow at the last meeting of the Council.

Iodide of Potassium in Frontal Headache.—Dr. Haley states in the *Australian Med. Journal* for August that for some years past he has found minimum doses of iodide of potassium of great service in frontal headache. A heavy dull headache, situated over the brow, and accompanied by languor, chilliness, and a feeling of general discomfort, with distaste for food, which sometimes approaches to nausea, can be completely removed by a two-grain dose dissolved in half a wine-glass of water, and this quietly sipped, the whole quantity being taken in about ten minutes. In many cases the effect of these small doses has been simply wonderful. A person who, a quarter of an hour before, was feeling most miserable and refused all food, wishing only for quietness, would now take a good meal and resume his wonted cheerfulness. The rapidity with which the iodide acts in these cases constitutes its great advantage.

APPOINTMENTS FOR THE WEEK.

December 24. Saturday (this day).

Operations at St. Bartholomew's, 1½ p.m.; King's College, 1½ p.m.; Royal Free, 2 p.m.; Royal London Ophthalmic, 11 a.m.; Royal Westminster Ophthalmic, 1½ p.m.; St. Thomas's, 1½ p.m.; London, 2 p.m.

26. Monday.

Operations at the Metropolitan Free, 2 p.m.; St. Mark's Hospital for Diseases of the Rectum, 2 p.m.; Royal London Ophthalmic, 11 a.m.; Royal Westminster Ophthalmic, 1½ p.m.

27. Tuesday.

Operations at Guy's, 1½ p.m.; Westminster, 2 p.m.; Royal London Ophthalmic, 11 a.m.; Royal Westminster Ophthalmic, 1½ p.m.; West London, 3 p.m.

Royal Institution, 3 p.m. Professor R. S. Ball, "The Sun."

28. Wednesday.

Operations at University College, 2 p.m.; St. Mary's, 1¼ p.m.; Middlesex, 1 p.m.; London, 2 p.m.; St. Bartholomew's, 1½ p.m.; Great Northern, 2 p.m.; Samaritan, 2½ p.m.; Royal London Ophthalmic, 11 a.m.; Royal Westminster Ophthalmic, 1½ p.m.; St. Thomas's, 1½ p.m.; St. Peter's Hospital for Stone, 2 p.m.; National Orthopædic, Great Portland-street, 10 a.m.

29. Thursday.

Operations at St. George's, 1 p.m.; Central London Ophthalmic, 1 p.m.; Royal Orthopædic, 2 p.m.; University College, 2 p.m.; Royal London Ophthalmic, 11 a.m.; Royal Westminster Ophthalmic, 1½ p.m.; Hospital for Diseases of the Throat, 2 p.m.; Hospital for Women, 2 p.m.; Charing-cross, 2 p.m.; London, 2 p.m.; North-West London, 2½ p.m.

Royal Institution, 3 p.m. Professor R. S. Ball, "The Moon."

30. Friday.

Operations at Central London Ophthalmic, 2 p.m.; Royal London Ophthalmic, 11 a.m.; South London Ophthalmic, 2 p.m.; Royal Westminster Ophthalmic, 1½ p.m.; St. George's (ophthalmic operations), 1½ p.m.; Guy's, 1½ p.m.; St. Thomas's (ophthalmic operations), 2 p.m.; King's College (by Mr. Lister), 2 p.m.

VITAL STATISTICS OF LONDON.

Week ending Saturday, December 17, 1881.

BIRTHS.

Births of Boys, 1283; Girls, 1197; Total, 2480.
Corrected weekly average in the 10 years 1871-80, 2611·2.

DEATHS.

	Males.	Females.	Total.
Deaths during the week ...	819	817	1636
Weekly average of the ten years 1871-80, corrected to increased population ...	951·4	915·3	1866·7
Deaths of people aged 80 and upwards ...	...	...	61

DEATHS IN SUB-DISTRICTS FROM EPIDEMICS.

	Enumerated Population, 1881 (unrevised).	Small-pox.	Measles.	Scarlet Fever.	Diphtheria.	Whooping-cough.	Typhus.	Enteric (or Typhoid) Fever.	Simple continued Fever.	Diarrhœa.
West ...	668998	...	15	2	1	13	1	4	1	2
North ...	905677	1	13	9	6	9	1	11	1	2
Central ...	281793	...	2	2	2	11	...	2	1	1
East ...	692530	2	11	8	...	22	1	6	...	1
South ...	1265578	22	31	21	3	23	2	10	1	5
Total ...	3814571	25	72	42	12	78	5	33	4	9

METEOROLOGY.

From Observations at the Greenwich Observatory.

Mean height of barometer ...	29·694 in.
Mean temperature ...	38·8°
Highest point of thermometer ...	52·1°
Lowest point of thermometer ...	30·3°
Mean dew-point temperature ...	35·6°
General direction of wind ...	Variable.
Whole amount of rain in the week ...	0·71 in.

BIRTHS and DEATHS Registered and METEOROLOGY during the Week ending Saturday, Dec. 17, in the following large Towns:—

Cities and boroughs (Municipal boundaries except for London.)	Estimated Population to middle of the year 1881.*	Persons to an Acre. (1881.)	Births Registered during the week ending Dec. 17.	Deaths Registered during the week ending Dec. 17.	Temperature of Air (Fahr.): Highest during the Week.	Temperature of Air (Fahr.): Lowest during the Week.	Temperature of Air (Fahr.): Weekly Mean of Daily Mean Values.	Temp. of Air (Cent.): Weekly Mean of Daily Mean Values.	Rain Fall: In Inches.	Rain Fall: In Centimetres.
London ...	3829751	50·8	2480	1636	52·1	30·3	38·8	3·78	0·71	1·80
Brighton ...	107934	45·9	66	51	45·0	31·0	39·3	4·03	0·76	1·93
Portsmouth ...	128335	28·6	83	48	...	...	...	...	...	...
Norwich ...	88038	11·8	56	32	...	...	...	...	...	...
Plymouth ...	75262	54·0	36	23	50·0	28·7	38·8	3·78	1·04	2·64
Bristol ...	207140	46·5	152	62	50·1	27·0	37·0	2·78	0·68	1·73
Wolverhampton ...	75934	22·4	48	36	41·2	23·0	32·2	0·11	1·40	3·56
Birmingham ...	402296	47·9	200	212	...	...	...	...	...	...
Leicester ...	123120	38·5	78	55	46·0	23·5	34·5	1·39	1·08	2·74
Nottingham ...	188035	18·9	138	85	42·9	21·4	33·7	0·95	0·50	1·27
Liverpool ...	553988	106·3	338	341	44·0	28·2	36·2	2·33	1·28	3·25
Manchester ...	341269	79·5	208	226	...	...	...	...	...	...
Salford ...	177760	34·4	121	99	...	...	...	...	...	...
Oldham ...	112176	24·0	65	53	...	...	...	...	...	...
Bradford ...	184037	25·5	108	71	42·3	27·5	36·1	2·28	1·45	3·68
Leeds ...	310490	14·4	182	125	42·0	28·0	36·5	2·50	0·95	2·41
Sheffield ...	285621	14·5	214	128	41·0	27·0	35·4	1·89	1·61	4·09
Hull ...	166161	42·7	125	92	42·0	27·0	35·9	2·17	1·00	2·54
Sunderland ...	116753	42·2	76	46	46·0	30·0	38·6	3·67	1·16	2·95
Newcastle-on-Tyne	145675	27·1	96	55	...	...	...	...	...	...
Total of 20 large English Towns ...	7608775	38·0	4960	3476	52·1	21·4	36·4	2·44	1·05	2·68

* These figures are the numbers enumerated (but subject to revision) in April last, raised to the middle of 1881 by the addition of a quarter of a year's increase, calculated at the rate that prevailed between 1871 and 1881.

At the Royal Observatory, Greenwich, the mean reading of the barometer last week was 29·69 in. The highest reading was 30·17 in. on Tuesday evening, and the lowest 28·84 in. on Saturday afternoon.

NOTES, QUERIES, AND REPLIES:

Be that questioneth much shall learn much.—Bacon.

S. C., Boulogne.—The time for sending in essays for the Jacksonian Prize will expire on Saturday, the 31st inst. We understand that up to the present time only one essay has been received; and this one, from "B. I. M.," was nearly being rejected by the housekeeper on account of the non-prepayment of the carriage.

"The Blane Medal."—The notice which appeared in the *Medical Times and Gazette* was quite correct, and given in the order indicated by the Director-General of the Medical Department of the Royal Navy, in his official letter to the College of Surgeons. Dr. Belgrave Ninnis was placed *first* in order of seniority. This officer narrowly escaped in the severe attack on a slaver, just recorded, where the captain fell a victim.

A Local Authorities' Association.—A meeting has been held at Manchester of the representatives of the local boards throughout the country, for the purpose of completing the promotion of an association of local authorities for protecting the various interests entrusted to their charge. Among the objects set forth are—opposition to centralisation, and the obtaining of Acts of Parliament to facilitate the absorption of local board districts by town councils.

Juvenile Factory Labour, Russia.—By the proposed new law, relative to the employment of children in manufactories in Russia, the minimum age is fixed at twelve years; but children already employed in such establishments are excepted from the benefits of this regulation. Up to eighteen years of age the day's labour is not to exceed twelve hours, inclusive of two hours for rest and meals. Night-work is absolutely prohibited.

Reorganisation of the Local Government Board.—It is said that steps are being taken by the officials of this department, and a committee has been appointed, to promote this object. It is probable that the office will be reorganised on the basis of the report of the Commission presided over by Dr. Lyon Playfair.

The Excise and Proprietary Clubs.—The first case under the new rule of the Inland Revenue with regard to clubs has taken place at Aberdeen. The proprietor and nominal manager of a club was summoned before a Justice of the Peace Court, at the instance of the Excise authorities, charged with having on five different occasions sold drink without a licence. The offence was proved, and the mitigated penalty of £40 imposed.

Confirmed Drunkards.—The official returns of persons of each sex apprehended by the police in England and Wales show that, during the official year 1879-80, 10,063 women were classed as habitual drunkards, while of men in the same category there were only 27,873.

An Unsuccessful Protest.—The Local Government Board has replied to the protest of the ratepayers of the parishes comprised in the St. Saviour's Union, Southwark, against the erection of a workhouse at Champion Hill, that the Board still retains the opinion that the existing establishments are insufficient to meet the present and increasing requirements of the Union, and fails to see any sufficient objection to the employment by the Guardians of the site at Champion Hill selected by them and approved of by the Board. Further, that the sum of £300,000, the alleged cost of the proposed new buildings, appears to be far in excess of the amount which will actually have to be expended. The ratepayers have resolved to continue pressure upon the central authority to induce it to accede to their wishes, and a deputation is appointed to confer with the Board of Guardians on the subject.

Damp Dwellings.—The Medical Officer of Health, Galashiels, having certified that a newly erected house, which was inhabited by a family, was injurious to health, as the water was running down the walls, the Health Committee procured the opinion of counsel, which was, that under the Public Health Act they could not close the house simply because it was damp. They have, in consequence, taken no action in the matter.

Fire Burial, France.—The last report of the French Cremation Society shows the present number of members to be 408. The receipts for the first year had been 7000 fr. Efforts are to be made by the Society to induce the Minister of the Interior to withdraw his prohibition of cremation experiments. It is stated that the average cost of incinerating a body will be three francs.

Sick-Leave, India.—The Secretary of State for India, it is announced, has placed a restriction on the period of all sick-leaves out of India granted by the Indian Governments. Heretofore the period has been two years in almost all cases; in future, only one year will be granted under any of the furlough rules now in force on medical certificate, and the question of its extension will be left to the decision of the standing Medical Board at the India Office.

Goat's Milk.—The British Goat Society have resolved, in consequence of the large demand for goats, together with the increasing popularity of goat's milk as a food for infants, to form a Goat Supply Company for the importation, breeding, and supply of goats. The matter has been referred to the Committee of the Society to carry out.

Young Seamen and Spirit Rations.—An Admiralty Order has been issued, discontinuing the spirit ration to seamen under twenty years of age, and giving all seamen the option of receiving, in lieu of spirits, cocoa, chocolate, or sugar.

Edgar N. W.—Mr. Murray, the British Consul at Portland, reported on the Prohibitory Liquor Law (Maine), as the result of his own observation and inquiries, that, however well the law had succeeded in country villages and places easy of supervision, in Maine it was impossible to prevent the sale of liquors and drunkenness in the larger towns. If, he says, this be the real state of the case, and as two distinct laws (one for the country, and another for the towns) could not be thought of, it appeared to follow that a stringent Licence Law, efficiently enforced, would further temperance more than the Prohibitory Law, which was rendered inefficient and obnoxious by its severity.

Unqualified Doctors.—At an inquest held by Mr. Hooper, the Coroner at West Bromwich, it was shown in evidence that an unqualified practitioner had not only given a certificate of death of a child which he had not seen, but charged 5s. for it. A caution from the Coroner to the Registrar with respect to such certificates was the consequence of the inquest.

Extraordinary Overcrowding, Hawarden.—Several cases of overcrowding in cottages at Pentrehaden were brought before the Petty Sessions last week. In one small room a man, his wife, and eight children slept. There was no ventilation, and the house had been condemned by the Medical Officer of Health. In another case a man, his wife, three sons (the eldest being twenty-four), and three daughters (the eldest twenty-one), all slept together in one room. In the third case a man and six other persons slept in a very small room. These families had been reared up in the cottages, and there was a difficulty in ejecting them. An order was made that the cottages be vacated in a month.

The Dangers of the Electric Light.—The fatal accident to a young man at Hatfield, by touching the wires when charged and conveying electricity, to Hatfield House, should be a warning to others. In the ensuing session of Parliament several applications are to be made for legal powers for electric lighting, and provision will, we should hope, be made for the protection of the public against dangers which at present are little understood, from the general inexperience of the risks connected with this new system of illumination. The fatality at Hatfield will, no doubt, draw public attention to the necessity of the wires being enclosed or cut of harm's way, that the recurrence of a similar disaster may be averted.

COMMUNICATIONS have been received from—
The Registrar of the Apothecaries' Hall, London; The Secretary of the Royal National Hospital for Consumption, Ventnor; Mr. A. Knight, Hackney; The Secretary of the Royal Victoria Hospital for Children, Chelsea; Dr. Wynter Blyth, Marylebone; Mr. J. Dickson, Harrow; The Sanitary Commissioner, Punjab, India; Dr. A. Wiltshire, Manchester; The Secretary of the International Smoke Abatement Exhibition, London; The Secretary of the Harveian Society, London; The Secretary of the Midland Medical Society, Birmingham; Messrs. Budall, Carte, and Co., London; Dr. Herman, London; Mr. E. W. Parker, London; The Secretary of the Shop Assistants' Twelve Hours' Labour League, London; Dr. E. F. Willoughby, London; Dr. C. Creighton, London; The British and Foreign Blind Association, London; Dr. E. T. Armitage, London; Mr. E. L. Hussey, Oxford; Messrs. T. J. and J. Smith, London; Messrs. Whitworth and Co., London; The Registrar-General for Scotland; Messrs. Allen and Hanburys, London; Dr. J. W. Moore, Dublin; The Registrar of the University of Durham; The Secretary of the Royal Institution, London; Mr. W. Watson Cheyne, London; The Secretary of the South London School of Pharmacy; The Secretary of the Cambridge Medical Society; Messrs. E. and C. Coler, London; The Secretary of the Poor-Law Medical Officers' Association; Dr. J. Ward-Cousins, Southsea; Mr. T. M. Stone, London; Mr. J. Chatto, London; The Secretary of the Hospital for Women, London.

BOOKS, ETC., RECEIVED—
Diseases and Injuries of the Eye, by J. R. Wolfe, M.D., F.R.C.S.—Chronic Clubfoot, by James S. Green, M.D.—Report of the Manchester Medico-Ethical Association—The Water-Supply of England and Wales, by Chas. E. De Rance—On Cross-Legged Progression, by E. Clement Lucas, B.S., M.B.—On Artificial Respiration in Stillborn Children, by Francis Henry Champneys, M.A., M.B., etc.—On the Pain in Pelvic Cancer, by Francis Henry Champneys, M.A., M.B., etc.—Notes on Uterine Polarity, by Francis Henry Champneys, M.A., M.B., etc.—Comparison between the Scoliotic and Obliquely Contracted (Naegele) Pelves, by Francis Henry Champneys, M.A., M.B., etc.—Case of Delivery through a Scoliotic Pelvis, by Francis Henry Champneys, M.A., M.B., etc.—Report on the Health, etc., of Kensington to December 3, 1881.

PERIODICALS AND NEWSPAPERS RECEIVED—
Lancet—British Medical Journal—Medical Press and Circular—Berliner Klinische Wochenschrift—Centralblatt für Chirurgie—Gazette des Hôpitaux—Gazette Médicale—Le Progrès Médical—Bulletin de l'Académie de Médecine—Pharmaceutical Journal—Wiener Medizinische Wochenschrift—Centralblatt für die Medicinischen Wissenschaften—Revue Médicale—Gazette Hebdomadaire—National Board of Health Bulletin, Washington—Nature—Boston Medical and Surgical Journal—Louisville Medical News—Deutsche Medizinal-Zeitung—Journal of the British Dental Association—Medical News and Collegiate Herald—Sanitary Chronicles of the Parish of St. Marylebone—Students' Journal and Hospital Gazette—L'Imparzialité Médicale—Canada Lancet—New England Medical Monthly—Anales del Circulo Medico Argentino—Gazzetta Medica Italiana—Canadian Journal of Medical Science—New York Medical Journal—Gazzetta degli Ospitali—Swansea Debating Society's Magazine—Sussex Daily News, December 13, 14, 15, 17, 19, 20, 21—Nordiskt Medicinskt Arkiv—Daily Free Press, December 21.

ORIGINAL LECTURES.

ON CERTAIN RARE CASES OF CHRONIC RHEUMATISM,

IN WHICH PARTS SUFFERED THAT ARE USUALLY ATTACKED ONLY IN GOUT.

Part of a Clinical Lecture.

By JONATHAN HUTCHINSON, F.R.C.S.,

Senior Surgeon to the London Hospital ; Professor of Surgery and Pathology in the Royal College of Surgeons.

GENTLEMEN,—I have in to-day's lecture to ask attention to a class of facts which have hitherto, I think, been much overlooked. I refer to certain rare cases in which, in the course of what, in all other respects, appears to be chronic rheumatism, parts are affected which are usually regarded as the especial domain of true gout. It is true that in these the result is not lithate of soda—or, at any rate, not always ; but still, the fact is a very remarkable one, that precisely the same regions and tissues suffer in the two. Of course, we have known all along that the joints suffer both in rheumatism and gout, but it is a new and somewhat startling observation to find rheumatism attacking the cartilages of the ears, the cellular tissue near to joints, and the bursa at the tip of the elbow. These, I repeat, have been hitherto deemed to be positions in which gout alone shows its power. I may at once say that I attach more importance to these facts than to any other as proving that the two maladies are closely connected. To state the proposition in another form, it might be said that we seem to have proof that gout may occasionally end in causing local deposits which are not chalky. This I have long believed and taught. In cases of inherited gout a form of iritis or ophthalmitis occurs, which runs a very peculiar and special course, and in which there is never any evidence of lithate of soda deposit. Further, in a few of these cases joints are disorganised by chronic inflammation and thickening occurs near to them again wholly without deposit of chalk. I have cut out such deposits for examination, and found only a gelatinous granulation substance. If to such facts we add those I am about to cite, which show rheumatism attacking the ears, etc., and producing swellings in all respects exactly like those of gout, excepting in the absence of lithate of soda, the line of distinction between the two maladies appears to be very gravely endangered.

The patient whose case has suggested these remarks is a married woman named Mrs. C., aged thirty-eight. She first began to suffer from "rheumatism in her wrists" thirteen years ago. It began first in the right wrist, and soon afterwards in the other. Then she had general pain in joints, "a sort of rheumatism." The knees were "bad and she could scarcely bend them." There was no great swelling of the larger joints, but all the smaller joints were puffy and stiff. This beginning of the rheumatism was just after her marriage. But previous to this she had been threatened occasionally with rheumatic pains. A paternal great-aunt was quite crippled with rheumatism. "She lived to be old, and could not help herself in the least."

Nothing is known as to "chalk gout" in any member of the family. Her father lived to be sixty-two, and had no definite rheumatism or gout. He suffered much from piles, and had also "tender feet." He was a pewterer. His brothers all died young, and some were known to have suffered from rheumatism.

Mrs. C. herself had, as she and her sister both assured me, enjoyed excellent health up to the date of the advent of rheumatism, and had been florid and robust. Her only ailment had been too profuse menstruation. She had never had rheumatic fever.

I saw Mrs. C. for the first time in March, 1877, and her condition was then much as follows :—Her fingers were, several of them, considerably distorted, and nearly all their

joints were swollen. The wrists were slightly swollen, but moved freely. The shoulders were somewhat stiff, so that she could not lift her arms except by giving a peculiar swing round. Her knees and elbows were almost wholly free from symptoms, though she complained of their being somewhat stiff. She could open her mouth wide, but the jaw-joints grated somewhat in the movement. Her spine was somewhat stiff, and she moved slowly and with care. The pisiform-bone joints grated most decidedly. The small joints of her feet suffered almost in the same manner as those of her hands. Thus you will see that we had the usual conditions of chronic rheumatism (with absorption of cartilage), falling with especial severity on the smaller joints, and attended by thickening and comparatively little synovial effusion. None of her joints were much swollen, and none had effusion enough to fluctuate. None were anchylosed. The deformity was but moderate. She was able to walk about well, and did not lose much rest at nights, but the state of her hands disabled her from most household occupations. She was tall, thin, and somewhat wan-looking.

Next I have to mention certain curious features in which the disease differed from chronic rheumatism in that we had proof of other than the joint structures being affected. With the exception of iritis I am not aware that as yet any structure not a joint has been proved to be inflamed in rheumatism. We have of course affections of fascia and of muscles, lumbago and sciatica, but of these as yet we cannot assert that they are attended by structural change. It is at any rate improbable that they are attended by changes which are permanent. Now, in gout we have very frequently deposits of urate of soda with inflammatory thickening around them in many parts not joints. We may have tophi in the cellular tissue, in the lymphatics, in or near to bursae, and above all in connexion with the cartilages of the ears. Now, it was precisely those structures which were affected in Mrs. C. On the anti-helix of each ear, exactly where gout concretions are so often met with, and with the most exact symmetry, were little inflamed nodules. These nodules were red at their bases and paler in their middles. They showed no tendency to suppurate, and they had been present for some months. At first we did not feel certain that they were not deposits of chalk, with somewhat more than the usual amount of inflammation about them, but I obtained her consent to cut into one of them, and the result proved that no chalk, only a little pale gelatinous substance, was present. Had there been but one we might have been inclined to consider it as the result of some accidental irritation, but as there was one in each ear, such a suggestion was out of the question. Nor did the similarity to gout in respect to the parts affected end with the ears, for on the tip of the left elbow was a lump, probably a much thickened bursa, with deposit in its interior which occasionally discharged, and which exactly resembled those so frequently seen in this position in gout. It had no fellow on the opposite side, but there was often tenderness in the position, as if one were threatened. On various parts of the fingers, too, near to joints, but not in them, nor adherent to them, were lumps of thickening, not of stony hardness, nor, I think, containing chalk, but again exactly those of gout in all other qualities. I had a sketch made of one hand and one ear, which I now show you. The conditions in the two hands were almost exactly symmetrical, and in each there were four or five of the lumps which I refer to. In the sketch they are difficult to distinguish from the nodosities due to joint-changes, but in the living hand it was easy, by moving them, to become certain that they were connected with the skin and cellular tissue, and not with bones, tendons, or ligaments.

Nor is this the only case of the kind which I have seen. A man named T., whose leg I amputated here ten years ago, and in whose joints no urate deposits were found, has now deposits or growths on his fingers and ears exactly like those I have been describing to you. They are so like gout that several good observers have suggested that they are gouty, but most certainly they contain no urate of soda. He is crippled by chronic rheumatism.

"LA RUE LITTRÉ."—A street in Paris, situated in the arrondissement in which Littré died, is to be called after him. It is a new street, which will be opened into the end of the Rue de Rennes, and will be 600 metres in length.—*Gas. Hebd.*, December 23.

ORIGINAL COMMUNICATIONS.

ON AMYGDALOTOMY AND SUICIDE.

By R. B. TAYLOR, L.R.C.P.

In the course of an interesting and instructive clinical lecture on Amygdalotomy, delivered a short time since by the well-known operator Dr. Rubio, at the Madrid Institution for Medical Practitioners, attention was drawn by the lecturer to the frequency of suicide in young persons subsequent to excision of tonsils. Four cases of the kind, which have come under the personal notice of Dr. Ambrose Rodrigues, one of the able Professors of the Institution, formed the subject-matter of Dr. Rubio's theme ; and I hardly need say that this novel subject has aroused a considerable degree of interest in medical circles and societies.

On broaching the question of relationship between amygdalotomy and [suicidal mania—a relationship which will in all probability elicit a variety of conflicting opinions and hypotheses,—Professor Rubio calls attention to the immature age of the four individuals whose cases are recorded, one of whom had just completed his fourteenth year. This tender age precluding, as it does, all idea of thwarted passions, financial losses, blemished honour, *tedium vitæ*, or other etiological factors which in more advanced years commonly play so important a part in the production of suicidal mania, Dr. Rubio offers another view of the cause of this peculiar mental aberration.

The Professor's point of departure is the remarkable property which every portion of the pharyngeal isthmus, and especially the uvula, possesses, of causing reflex action in many and distant organs. The slightest touch of the uvula excites contraction of the whole digestive apparatus, from the jaws and their muscles, to the pylorus, diaphragm, and sphincters, creating gastric spasm and sickness. The most insignificant inflammation of the pillars or of the soft palate interferes with deglutition to a degree out of all proportion to the swelling of the affected part, just as a trivial pharyngeal angina causes violent efforts at swallowing, and simultaneous over-action of all the facial muscles, not excluding even those of the eyes and eyelids.

The supposed naso-pharyngeal-obstructing and voice-modulating functions of the uvula having been disproved by modern research, and no other special physiological uses having as yet been assigned to this organ, Dr. Rubio, taking into consideration the sympathetic responses of the digestive and respiratory organs to the balls of the palatal appendage, regards it as a *centre of gastric and respiratory reflex actions.* Bearing in mind the fact that *the symptoms of disease in an organ of special reflex action are transmitted to every other organ with which they are physiologically connected,* it is easy to account for those most diverse and apparently anomalous morbid phenomena which, due to a simple elongation of the uvula, betray their presence in larynx, lungs, stomach, heart, and head. We can on the same grounds explain, as Dr. Rubio has so forcibly pointed out, why certain apparently insignificant pharyngeal irritations give rise to those strange pseudo-hypochondriacal and pseudo-hysterical groups of symptoms which, as occurring in both sexes, he has denominated pharyngeal hypochondriasis and pharyngeal hysteria.

According to Dr. Rubio, these pharyngeal reflex diseases possess features to some extent similar to those present in persons suffering from fissure of the anus. Just on the same principle as the sufferings of these latter patients induce a state of terror and mental depression bordering upon hypochondriasis, so also a fissure of the pillars of the pharynx, caused by the nipping of a portion of the same during excision of the tonsils, inducing thereby a state of incessant irritation of the unhealed pharyngeal fissure, kept up by the act of deglutition and the contact of solid and liquid food, may influence the reflex action on the brain sufficiently to lead to perversion of the affective faculties, despondence, or anger, and ultimately to self-destruction.

Whatever may be the fate allotted to Dr. Rubio's ingenious theory, the relationship between amygdalotomy and suicide is, beyond doubt, a topic well worthy of careful and attentive consideration.

Santillana.

REPORTS OF HOSPITAL PRACTICE
IN
MEDICINE AND SURGERY.

DEVON AND EXETER HOSPITAL.

EPITHELIOMA OF LEG IN A YOUNG MAN—AMPUTATION BELOW KNEE—PRIMARY, AND TWO ATTACKS OF SECONDARY HÆMORRHAGE—SUBSEQUENT RECOVERY.

(Under the care of Mr. CAIRD.)

[Reported by A. G. BLOMFIELD, M.B., House-Surgeon.]

NICHOLAS S., aged thirty-six years, was admitted into the hospital in May, 1881, with an excavated and apparently spreading ulceration, commencing over the internal malleolus, and running five inches up the right leg. He is a florid and healthy-looking man.

History.—He broke the right leg in its lower third when fourteen years of age ; since then he says it has been somewhat crooked and smaller than the opposite limb.

History of Present Attack.—He had always enjoyed good health, and been able to get about in his work as a farm-labourer, until twelve months ago, when he first noticed a small sore breaking out without any apparent cause (there is no history of any recent injury), about two inches above the internal malleolus. The ulcer spread somewhat rapidly, getting deeper, and was attended with a good deal of pain, but his general health had not suffered. His father died at the age of forty-five, six months after having an epithelial cancer removed from the lower lip.

Present Condition.—Lately this ulcer has increased rapidly in size, and he feels weaker. There is an irregularly excavated ulceration, the lower edge of which corresponds to the right internal malleolus, extending up the limb five inches. Over the internal malleolus is an elevated, bright-red-coloured mass, with edges slightly hardened, and on pressure discharging little masses of a yellow colour, apparently epithelial *débris.* There has been occasional hæmorrhage. The edges are not raised above the surrounding skin, except over the malleolus, in which direction the disease appears to tend to spread. The deepest part of the ulcer has, as its floor, the lower third of the shaft of the tibia, which is soft and necrosed, and evidently involved in the disease. It discharges a thin puriform fluid. The femoral glands are enlarged, but he cannot say how long he has noticed this. Small portions of the growth were cut off, hardened in spirit, and examined microscopically by Mr. Blomfield. The examination showed the growth to be well-marked epithelioma, nests being very numerous and prominent in the sections examined. He was kept in bed, put on ordinary diet, and the wound dressed with carbolic oil. He appeared to be the better for the rest in bed ; his appetite was good, and he complained very little of pain in the leg. The temperature before the operation was taken on several occasions, but was never above 99°.

On June 15, Mr. Caird amputated the leg in its upper third. The bone appeared to be quite healthy at this point. No blood was lost during the operation, and, after being left open for some hours, the flaps were brought together with wire sutures, and the stump exposed to the air with a small piece of gauze over it. The evening temperature was 98·8°. At 10 p.m., hæmorrhage (primary) came on ; pressure failed to control it, and it was necessary to remove the sutures. Several muscular branches were tied, and the bleeding ceased ; the stump, however, was left open for ten hours, and then the flaps were brought together with silk sutures tied in a bow.

June 16.—Temperature : morning 98·4°, evening 98·8°. Doing fairly well.

18th.—Free discharge of pus. Sleeps well, and does not complain of much pain.

20th.—Slight, but sharp, attack of secondary hemorrhage from the top flap at 8.15 a.m. Evening temperature 99·2°.

21st.—Violent secondary hæmorrhage at 8.30 a.m. It was necessary to apply a tourniquet above, and again take out the sutures. The bleeding did not appear to come from any large vessel in particular, but depended on a general hæmorrhage from the numerous vessels in the flaps and in the bone itself. Tinct. ferri perchlorid. was applied. The flaps appeared congested and dark-coloured. A consultation of the surgical staff was held to-day as to the advisability or otherwise of secondary amputation. As it appeared, however, that amputation higher up would not probably do away with his tendency to hæmorrhage, and seeing that, though there had been three attacks on the first, sixth, and seventh days after the amputation, the hæmorrhage had been brought rapidly under control, so that the actual amount of blood lost in the three attacks had not been so great as to reduce him to a desperate state, it was thought best for the patient to leave the flaps open and allow the wound to heal by granulation.

The subsequent history of the case may be briefly stated as follows :—The sloughs formed on the surface of the flaps by the tincture of iron gradually separated, on one occasion being attended with some considerable hæmorrhage, which was checked by applying a little more of the iron. The surfaces became gradually covered over by healthy granulations, from which there was an abundant discharge of healthy pus. His general health kept up remarkably well during the trying time through which he passed. In July a special splint was applied, and the limb kept suspended. During the next two months the flaps gradually contracted by granulations, and it was possible by pressure and strapping to bring the lower flap over the face of the amputation. Towards the end of September it had completely healed over; his general health was excellent; the glandular enlargement in the groin had disappeared; and he was discharged cured on September 29.

Remarks.—The patient was of middle height, with dark hair and blue eyes; of florid complexion, there being two bright red patches on both cheeks. Medically, after the amputation, he was treated with large doses of steel and liquid extract of ergot. From the repeated hæmorrhage, it is probable that there exists a hæmorrhagic diathesis. The large glandular swelling in the groin, though it eventually disappeared, suggests the probability of some secondary deposit, and this led Mr. Caird to elect to amputate below the knee, because amputation above would have been attended by greater shock to the system, which might have so reduced his strength as to hasten return of the disease in the glands. The original disease no doubt began as an epitheliomatous ulceration of the skin, and by extension involved the shaft of the tibia, which was superficially softened and ulcerated. The glandular enlargement may possibly be accounted for partly by the irritation caused by the large extent of suppurating surface; at any rate, the removal of the limb has had a beneficial effect in causing the enlargement to disappear.

MICROCOCCI IN MUMPS.—MM. Cabitan and Charrin, at a recent meeting of the Biological Society of Paris, gave an account of the investigations which they have for some time been engaged in on the presence of minute organisms in the blood of persons suffering from mumps. These are multipliable by cultivation in Liebig's broth, and are found to consist of minute *batonnets*, but chiefly of micrococci all in a state of motion. These minute organisms, they consider, corroborate the clinical observations which tend to place mumps among the infectious diseases. The absolute proof that this disease is due to these minute existences, by reproducing it by inoculation of the "cultures," has not been attained by the experiments made to that end.—*Gazette Méd.*, December 17.

DEAF AND DUMB ASYLUM, MARGATE.—At the recent distribution of prizes to the children of this institution, the treasurer stated that sixty new pupils will be trained in lip-reading.

THE DUKE DOCTOR CARL THEODORE OF BAVARIA.—The King of Bavaria has requested Duke Dr. Carl Theodore to make himself thoroughly acquainted with the military hospitals of Munich and the military medical service of all Bavaria, preparatory, as it is understood, to the Duke being put at the head of the Military Medical Department of Bavaria. We shall welcome such an appointment with great satisfaction; for then for the first time will the highest post in military medicine of a country be in the hands of so influential a person as a member of the Royal family must be. In such a post the Duke may render inestimable service, and the action of his beneficial influence may be felt far beyond the boundaries of his own country.— *Wiener Med. Woch.*, November 26.

TERMS OF SUBSCRIPTION.
(Free by post.)

British Islands	*Twelve Months*	.	£1	8	0
	Six	"	. 0	14	0
The Colonies and the United } *States of America* . . . }	*Twelve*	"	. 1	10	0
" " "	*Six*	"	. 0	15	0
India " "	*Twelve*	"	. 1	10	0
" (*viâ Brindisi*)	"	"	. 1	15	0
" "	*Six*	"	. 0	15	0
" (*viâ Brindisi*)	"	"	. 0	17	6

Foreign Subscribers are requested to inform the Publishers of any remittance made through the agency of the Post-Office.

Single Copies of the Journal can be obtained of all Booksellers and Newsmen, price Sixpence.

Cheques or Post-office Orders should be made payable to Mr. JAMES LUCAS, 11, New Burlington-street, W.

TERMS FOR ADVERTISEMENTS.

Seven lines (70 words)	.£0	4	6
Each additional line (10 words) .	. 0	0	6
Half-column, or quarter-page . .	. 1	5	0
Whole column, or half-page . .	. 2	10	0
Whole page	. 5	0	0

Births, Marriages, and Deaths are inserted Free of Charge.

THE MEDICAL TIMES AND GAZETTE *is published on Friday morning: Advertisements must therefore reach the Publishing Office not later than One o'clock on Thursday.*

Medical Times and Gazette.

SATURDAY, DECEMBER 31, 1881.

ANNUS MEDICUS 1881.

THROUGHOUT nearly the whole of the first three months of the year 1881 the weather was unusually cold, and, according to general ideas, "trying" to health. The barometer ruled rather low; each monthly mean was below the average, and the mean of the whole quarter was below the average reading in the corresponding periods for forty years. Very cold weather set in early in January, and lasted till almost the very end of the month, more or less snow falling every day (with but one exception) from the 9th to the 27th. February was cold, wet, and gloomy, with excess of east wind and frequent falls of snow; and it was cold in March also, except during a week or so in the middle of the month. Taking the three months together, the mean temperature was 37·3°, being about 1·5° below the average for—the Registrar-General tells us—a hundred and ten years. The rainfall (which includes melted snow) measured at Greenwich was considerably in excess of the average quantity for these months for sixty-six years; but the number of hours of bright sunshine recorded at Greenwich was greater than of late years—it was 175·7, against 141·0, 137·5, and 235·9 in the three preceding quarters. We may suppose, therefore, that throughout England generally there was some increase of clear sunshine; and this may perhaps account, in part, for the unusual healthiness of the quarter. For, notwithstanding the severe cold, and that there were forty frosty days, and we are told the amount of cold weather exceeded that recorded in the corresponding period of any year since 1855, the annual death-rate did not exceed 21·8 per 1000 of the estimated population, and was 2·1 below the average rate in the ten preceding corresponding quarters. So low a death-rate in the first quarter of the year has, in fact, not been recorded since that of 1856. The rate of infant mortality, measured by the proportion of deaths under one year to births, was equal to 134 per 1000; while in the ten preceding corresponding quarters this proportion averaged 149 per 1000, and ranged from 167 in 1875 to 138 in 1877. And, in short, comparing it with the average rates in the ten preceding corresponding quarters, the death-rate in the first quarter of 1881 was considerably below the average among infants, children, and adults; while, though it showed a slight excess among elderly persons—i.e., among those above sixty years of age—this excess was not nearly so marked as might have been expected to occur from the exceptionally severe weather in January.

In the second quarter, taken as a whole, the mean reading of the barometer, at Greenwich, was 29·84 inches, and was slightly above the average for the corresponding period in forty years. The mean was slightly in excess in April and May, and in June corresponded with the average. The mean temperature of the quarter was 52·9°, being a little more than half a degree above the average of the same quarter in 110 years. April showed a slight deficiency, while in May and June the mean of the temperature was above the average. The measured rainfall, at Greenwich, was 4·1 inches for the quarter, which amounts to 1·6 inches above the average for sixty-six years. Rain was measured on only eight days in April, on thirteen days in May, and on nine in June. There were 514·0 hours of bright sunshine recorded at Greenwich, against 352·1 and 457·8 in the two preceding corresponding periods. The annual death-rate of the quarter did not exceed 18·6 per 1000 of the population, and was 2·3 below the average in the ten preceding quarters ; and this is the lowest rate recorded in the second quarter of any year since civil registration was established in 1837. The nearest approach to it was made last year, when the rate of the same quarter was 19·5; and if the rate of the quarter in this year be compared with the average rate of the second quarters of the forty-three years 1838-80, viz., 21·8 per 1000, it shows a decline of 3·2. The rate of infant mortality was lower in the quarter than in the second quarter of any year on record. It was equal to 121 per 1000; in the ten preceding quarters the proportion averaged 181 per 1000, and ranged from 139 in 1875 to 123 in 1880. Among persons aged between one and sixty years the rate was equal to 10·6 per 1000, against an average rate of 12·3 in the ten preceding corresponding quarters. Among persons aged upwards of sixty years the annual death-rate averaged 66·3 per 1000, being about the same as that of the same quarter last year, but considerably below the rates in previous corresponding quarters since 1872.

Again, in the third quarter of the year, the public health of England and Wales, judged according to the rate of mortality, was as satisfactory as in the first and second quarters. The death-rate did not exceed 16·7 per 1000, being no less than 2·9 below the average rate in the ten preceding corresponding quarters. It was lower than in the third or summer quarter of any year since civil registration commenced, with the single exception of 1879, when the rate was only 16·3; the average death-rate in the summer quarters of the forty-three years 1838-80 was 3·7 (nearly one-fifth) higher. The low death-rate of the quarter was no doubt due in large measure to the unusually small fatality of infantile diarrhoea, owing to the low temperature in August and September. But the decline in the death-rate was not confined to infancy. The mortality at all ages was 15 per cent. below the average rate in the ten preceding corresponding quarters ; and this decline, which was equal to 18 per cent. among infants under one year of age, was 18 per cent. among children and adults under sixty years of age, and 5 per cent. among persons aged upwards of sixty years. The mean reading of the barometer was slightly below the average for the same period in forty years; the mean showing a slight excess in July, but being below the

average in August and September. Part of July was very warm ; with the exception of four days (from the 6th to the 9th), the temperature of the first nineteen days was much above the average, and the 4th, 5th, 15th, 18th, and 19th were exceptionally hot days. During the remainder of the month the weather was very variable ; and it was generally wet, cold, and cloudy throughout August, excepting during a few days at the beginning of the month. September also was cold during the first half, but moderately fine afterwards. The mean temperature showed an excess of 3·8° in July ; but was 1·8° deficient in August, and 1·2° in September. The rainfall, measured at Greenwich, 8·19 inches, was nearly an inch below the average of the same period in sixty-six years. In was below the average in July and September, but considerably in excess in August. The number of hours of bright sunshine recorded was 430·4, against 410·6, the average amount in the corresponding quarters of the four years 1877-80.

As regards the ZYMOTIC FATALITY, the total number of deaths referred to scarlet fever, whooping-cough, fever, diarrhoea, measles, small-pox, and diphtheria in England and Wales was, in the first quarter of the year, 12,158, corresponding to an annual rate of only 1·91 per 1000, against an average of 2·96 in the ten preceding corresponding quarters. The rate from those diseases was, without any exception, considerably lower than that recorded in any quarter since the beginning of 1870, when this information was first given in the Quarterly Return. The deaths from small-pox, which had been 69 and 208 in the last two quarters of 1880, rose to 730 in the first quarter of 1881 ; and of these 650 occurred in London and its Outer Ring of suburban districts. The deaths from "fever" (including typhus, enteric, and simple continued) were fewer than in any previous corresponding quarter on record; they equalled an annual rate not exceeding 0·26 per 1000, while in the ten preceding corresponding quarter the death-rate from "fever" averaged 0·48.

In the second quarter also the zymotic fatality was low. The total number of deaths from zymotic diseases was 12,167, and the death-rate from them was 1·87, "the lowest yet recorded in the Quarterly Return." And the death-rate from each of the diseases was below the average. The deaths from small-pox rose still further to 1213, the highest record since the second quarter of 1877. The deaths were equal to an annual rate of 0·19, against an average of 0·32 for the ten preceding corresponding quarters. Of the 1213 deaths from this disease, 1010 occurred in London. The deaths from fever were 1443, a number considerably below the lowest previously recorded in any single quarter. The rate was 0·22 against an average of 0·41 for the ten preceding corresponding quarters; but it must be remembered that it is in the second quarters that enteric fever—to which, without doubt, most of the deaths from fever were due—is, as a rule, at its minimum.

Again, in the third or summer quarter the mortality from zymotic diseases was below the average. The total number of deaths from these causes amounted indeed to 18,222, but, large as that number is, it means a death-rate of only 2·77, against an average rate of 4·21 for the ten preceding corresponding quarters. It was lower in one of those ten quarters —namely, in that of 1879—when the cold season, and consequent absence of summer diarrhoea, reduced the rate to 2·25. This year the cold, low temperature of August and September more than counterbalanced the excessive heat and consequent high diarrhoea mortality of July; and the death-rate from diarrhoea for the summer quarter was 1·26 per 1000, against an average of 2·27 for the ten preceding summer quarters. The deaths from small-pox fell, as is the rule in the summer quarter, and were 674. But that is a higher number than in any summer quarter since the great epidemic of 1871 and 1872. Of the 674 deaths, 461 occurred in London, and 61 more in the Outer Ring; and a considerable proportion of the remainder occurred in the immediately adjoining counties. The deaths attributed to *fever* were 1705, corresponding to an annual rate of 0·26, against an average of 0·44 for the ten preceding corresponding quarters.

The month of October was, as a whole, colder than in either 1879 or 1880. The maximum readings of the thermometer fell very short of those recorded in 1880, and the minimum readings were lower than those of either 1880 or 1879; but England in general, especially the southern parts, escaped the heavy storms of snow and rain that marked the month of October in 1880. The recorded hours of bright sunshine during the month did not exceed more than a quarter or a third of the time during which the sun was above the horizon. During November the weather was exceptionally mild—so much so that the temperature of the month was actually higher than that of October. Along the coasts of England the increase was about 2° in Cornwall, 3° in the neighbourhood of the Isle of Wight, and about 1° along the east coast. Inland the rise ranged from 2·5° to 3·5°. In all parts the maximum, the minimum, and mean readings of the thermometer were several degrees higher than in either 1880 or 1879; and indeed there has not been so warm a November for many years. The first week of the month was cold, and over part of England wet, and there was very little sunshine. In the second week the temperature was *much* higher, and the sky was almost continuously overcast, but there was very little rain. The third week was still mild, though less so than the second, but an excess of rain fell over all but the eastern parts of England, and we had frequent southerly and south-westerly gales. The fourth week was mild, but very wet and rough. On the whole, however, the air was soft and humid through the month; and the Registrar-General tells us that strawberries and some other fruits ripened in the open air at our southern watering-places. The public health was good. The deaths from small-pox in London were continuously above the average. Scarlet fever was rather prevalent, and in the last week the deaths attributed to diphtheria increased to more than double the average. In October, typhoid fever carried off many more than the average. But it seems very probable that the Registrar-General will report that the general death-rate in England, and the zymotic fatality, were markedly below the average.

Parliament met on January 7; and the session did not close till August 27; but it was practically devoted to one measure, carried by one man, for one division only of the United Kingdom—namely, Ireland. Looked at from the medical point of view, the session was indeed a very barren one. An Alkali Works Bill was passed, but it cannot be considered in any sense a great measure; nor can the Coroners (Ireland) Bill be regarded with any admiration. Hardly any other Bill, Government or private, that had any medical bearing became law during the prolonged session; though the Sunday Closing (Wales) Act may, from our point of view, be counted as a sanitary Act. One measure was, however, passed, which affects to some extent medical graduates in one division of the kingdom. Personal experience of any particular grievance and wrong will, no doubt, have a marked effect in quickening a legislator's sense of the necessity of reform. The costliness of a contest for the honour of representing the Universities of Scotland in Parliament had become so great as to amount to a scandal; and Mr. Lyon Playfair, the member for the Universities of Edinburgh and St. Andrews, and a member of the present Government, had had cause to vividly appreciate this. But out of this evil came good. He introduced a Bill, almost as soon as Parliament met, into the House of

Commons, to reform "the manner of voting in the election of members of Parliament for the Universities of Scotland," and it was so drawn that it was backed by Scottish members on both sides of the House. Thus fathered, and the attention and the mental powers of our legislators being absorbed to exhaustion by the Irish difficulty, the measure slipped through the two Houses without receiving, we think, very close or critical attention, though some useful amendments were made in it, and it became law. The great object of the Act is to lessen the expense of contesting the University seats; and, looking at this only, we welcome the Act. But some of the provisions for obtaining that desirable end are entirely new in character, and it seems hardly possible that the significance of them was fully or generally recognised. It is enacted by Section 16 of the Act that on and after the passing of it, "No person shall be allowed, after examination, to graduate at any of the Universities of Scotland until he shall have paid, as a registration fee, a sum not exceeding twenty shillings to the general University Fund of the University at which he wishes to graduate." His name, designation, qualification, and ordinary place of residence will then be entered in the registration book, and he, having become a member of the General Council of his University, will be entitled to all the privileges of a member of Council during his life, provided, of course, that he does not incur any legal incapacity. Before the passing of the Act a graduate might register when he liked, or not at all, if he preferred that course. But now he must be registered, or suffer the penalty of not being permitted to graduate; while if he registers he is fined for doing so. It is a wonderful clause to find in a new Act of Parliament, and an Act affecting Scotland. Section 17 enacts that "Any person either directly or indirectly corruptly paying any fee for the purpose of enabling any person to be registered as a member of the General Council, and thereby to influence his vote at any future election, and any candidate or other person either directly or indirectly paying such fee on behalf of any person for the purpose of inducing him to vote or to refrain from voting, shall be guilty of bribery, and shall be punishable accordingly; and any person on whose behalf and with whose privity any such payment as in this section mentioned is made shall also be guilty of bribery, and punishable accordingly." What, it may be asked, is " corrupt payment "? and may a parent, any next-of-kin, a guardian, or a trustee of a youth, safely pay his registration fee for him? It seems more than possible that legal ingenuity may often use the clause as an instrument of vexatious litigation. It is true that a most objectionable practice had obtained with regard to the registers of the Universities. Political agents of all parties used to search out unregistered graduates, and on some sort of understanding or intimation of how they should vote, would undertake that they should, by some ill-defined means, be put on the register without trouble or expense. It is manifest that some less drastic means of remedying this scandal might have been found than the clauses above quoted. It is enacted that in case of a poll at an election, the votes shall be given by voting-papers *only*; that the voting-papers shall be issued by, and returned to, the Registrars of the Universities; and that each voter, who desires to vote, shall duly fill up and subscribe his voting-paper in the presence of one witness who personally knows him, and who shall attest, by his own signature, the fact that the voting-paper has been duly signed in his presence. These provisions of the Act will unquestionably save the voters much trouble, and largely lessen the expenses of the candidates.

It may be noted that a Veterinary Surgeons Act was passed, as it may be expected that any measure to protect educated and qualified veterinary surgeons will encourage and promote the study of comparative pathology, and so be of service to medical science. The Veterinary Surgeons Act does not forbid veterinary practice, but it establishes a Veterinary Surgeons' Registry, and enacts that after 1883 it shall be illegal for any unregistered person to assume the title of Veterinary Surgeon, or in any description to state that he is one. The Royal College of Veterinary Surgeons is created the examining body; and all British practitioners must, to entitle them to be registered, be members of that College.

The subjects of the water-supply and the fish-supply of the metropolis were frequently mentioned in Parliament, but without any real effect in advancing either of them. Some words let fall by the Home Secretary, indeed, moved the Corporation of the City of London and the Metropolitan Board of Works to institute inquiries with a view to promote and cheapen the fish-supply; but the inquiry by the Board of Works came to an end without any useful result; and that instituted by the Corporation has not as yet been more fruitful.

Two or three Bills for the amendment of the Medical Acts were again introduced into the House; but no effort was made to procure their consideration this year. The Government felt that the subject was not yet ripe for legislation, and that further inquiry, or inquiry of a different kind than that carried out by the Select Committee of 1879, was necessary. The reappointment of a Select Committee was asked for, but Government decided to empower a Royal Commission to carry out the desired investigation. The *London Gazette* of May 3 published the terms of the Commission, and the names of the Commissioners, viz.:—The Earl of Camperdown, the Bishop of Peterborough, the Right Hon. W. H. F. Cogan, the Master of the Rolls (Sir George Jessel), the Right Hon. G. Sclater-Booth, M.P., Sir William Jenner, Bart., K.C.B., John Simon, Esq., C.B., Professor Huxley, Dr. Robert McDonnell (Dublin), Professor Turner (Edinburgh), and James Bryce, Esq., M.P., with John White, Esq., barrister-at-law, as Secretary. The well-known and thoroughly proved ability and character of the Commissioners gave assurance that their work would be well and fully performed in a broad and liberal spirit; and the subjects of the inquiry were so well chosen and set forth, that the appointment of the Royal Commission was received with general satisfaction by the profession. The terms of the Commission are given at some length at page 547 of our first volume for the year; but we may note here that it states, by way of preamble,—"Whereas it is of importance to all classes of our subjects that the conditions under which persons are permitted to represent themselves as qualified practitioners should be such as to afford the best attainable security for their skill and knowledge in medicine and surgery"; and "Whereas powers in relation to the education and examination for a grant of medical degrees, diplomas, or licences to medical practitioners are by various statutes and charters vested in certain universities, medical colleges, and other bodies in the United Kingdom," and representations had been made in relation to the unsatisfactory position of the above matters," Her Majesty has thought it expedient that, with a view to legislation, further inquiries should be made into the grant of medical degrees, memberships, fellowships, licences, and other diplomas, by universities, colleges, and other bodies in the United Kingdom; into the courses of education and examination, payments, and other conditions required as a preliminary to such grant; and into the skill and knowledge which such degrees, fellowships, licences, or diplomas represent; into the conditions and manner under, or in which medical practitioners are entered in, or struck

off the Medical Register; the privileges of registered and the disabilities of unregistered practitioners, the position of registered practitioners in British possessions abroad, and the position in the United Kingdom of medical practitioners educated in those possessions, or in a foreign State; and further to inquire into the constitution, functions, powers, and procedure of the General Medical Council, and their relation to the various universities, colleges, and other bodies, and to the medical profession; and into the result of "the Medical Act, 1858," and the Acts amending the same, and into all matters dealt with by those Acts. It would have been difficult to make the terms of the inquiry larger and more comprehensive. The Commission set promptly and steadily to work, and by the end of November had examined some forty witnesses. That these witnesses were selected in a most catholic spirit will be apparent from the following list of their names:—Dr. Acland, Sir James Paget, Mr. Erichsen, Professors Paget and Humphry (of Cambridge), Dr. A. H. Jacob (of Dublin), Dr. Glover, Dr. Scott Orr, Professor Marshall, Dr. Haldane, Dr. D. R. Haldane, Dr. T. S. Byass, Dr. Edward Waters (Chester), Mr. J. Sampson Gamgee (Birmingham), Professor Spence (Edinburgh), Dr. R. H. Semple, Dr. Pitman, Mr. Christopher Heath, Mr. C. Macnamara, Dr. F. E. Pocock, Dr. G. Y. Heath (Newcastle), Mr. Henry Morris, Professor Gairdner (Glasgow), Dr. Billings (United States of America), Mr. Thomas Cooke, Dr. J. K. Barton (Ireland), Mr. W. Stoker (Dublin), Dr. J. Magee Finny (King and Queen's College of Physicians, Ireland), Dr. J. W. Moore (for the Irish Medical Association), Dr. B. W. Richardson (for the Medical Defence Association), Mr. Thomas Collins (Apothecaries' Hall, Ireland), Professor Struthers (Aberdeen University), Professor P. Redfern (Queen's University), Professor T. R. Fraser (Edinburgh University), Mr. J. Tomes (British Dental Association), Mr. Thomas Edgelow (Association of Surgeons Practising Dental Surgery) Rev. Samuel Haughton, M.B. (Dublin University), Professor Young (Glasgow University), Dr. J. G. Greenwood (Victoria University), Dr. Quain; and Mr. F. W. Crick, as representing a medical herbalists' association.

With the beginning of the year the prevalence and the mortality of small-pox in London increased, and rapidly attained epidemic proportions; and as quickly the unwelcome fact of the incapacity of the Local Government Board and the Metropolitan Asylums Board to deal with the epidemic was forced upon the public. The Asylums Board failed altogether to provide adequate hospital accommodation for small-pox patients, and the Local Government Board did not even attempt to limit or prevent the spread of the disease, by any extraordinary arrangements for widespread, prompt, and efficient vaccination and revaccination. The President of the Local Government Board was night after night questioned in the House of Commons upon all these subjects. With regard to hospital accommodation, he was obliged to admit that the authorities had been paralysed by the successful legislation against the Managers of the Asylums Board in the Hampstead Hospital Case, and the hostility roused against them by that success; and when asked how such a deplorable state of things was to be remedied, showed himself as unready to advise the House of Commons in the matter as he had been to help the Asylums Board. While, as regarded the supply of vaccine lymph by the Vaccine Department, he was content with the dry official statement that the duty of that Department is only to supply lymph to those medical practitioners whose stock of it had failed. The Department had met with fresh difficulties in making the arrangements, promised last year, for the supply of calf-lymph, and the public have had to depend for such supply on private enterprise.

The difficulties of the Managers of the Metropolitan

District Asylums at last induced Government to come to their aid, and in November a Royal Commission was appointed "to consider the hospital accommodation in the metropolis in relation to infectious diseases." The Commissioners are—Lord Blachford, Sir James Paget, Sir Rutherford Alcock, Mr. Arthur Wellesley Peel, M.P., Mr. E. Leigh Pemberton, M.P., Dr. John Burdon Sanderson, Dr. Alfred Carpenter, Dr. W. H. Broadbent, and Mr. Jonathan Hutchinson; with Mr. N. Baker, barrister-at-law, as Secretary. The duty imposed upon them is complicated and large. They are to inquire into and report upon the nature, extent, and sufficiency of the hospital accommodation for small-pox and fever patients provided by the Asylums Board and the various vestries and district boards in the metropolis; upon the relative advantages and disadvantages, to patients and the public, of providing for these patients by a limited number of hospitals for the whole metropolis under one authority, or by parochial and district hospitals under vestries and district boards; on the expediency of continuing the existing small-pox and fever hospitals of the Asylums Board, and should it be considered desirable to close any of them, on the substitutes to be provided; and on the expediency of the establishment of additional hospitals by the Asylums Board, and of making special provision for convalescent cases. Then, further, the Commissioners are to inquire into the conditions and limitations under which the existing Asylums Board hospitals should be continued, and the general conditions and limitations to be applied to any new hospitals established by the Managers, or by any other authority, so as to insure as far as practicable the recovery of patients, and the protection of the public against contagion. And, finally, inquiry is to be made into the operation of the Acts authorising the establishment of small-pox and fever hospitals in the metropolis; and into the provisions (if any) required for obtaining sites for such hospitals, and for the protection of the authorities from liability to legal proceedings so long as the hospitals are conducted with reasonable care and according to prescribed regulations. The Commission is empowered, therefore, to re-open questions which it was supposed had been settled by the Sanitary Act (1866) and the Public Health Act (1872), as well as to settle, or to endeavour to settle, the many questions raised by the Hampstead Hospital Case; and their report will necessarily be a very important paper, and will be looked for with great interest and anxiety. The Commission sit, like the Medical Acts Commission, with closed doors, so that the tenor of the evidence given will not be known with any degree of certainty before the report comes out, for the profession, even should they learn the names of all who may be called upon to give evidence, will not have in this instance the foreknowledge of their opinions that they possessed so largely as regards the witnesses called before the Medical Acts Commission. The probability, possibility, or certainty of these hospitals being a source of danger to the neighbourhoods in which they are placed seems to lie at the very foundation of all the complaints made against them. The Local Government Board directed an inquiry to be made, by their medical officers, on this subject at the beginning of this year; and it seems somewhat remarkable that none of the evidence that must have been obtained by them was made known when the Fulham Hospital Case was before the court of appeal in November.

The General Council of Medical Education and Registration met twice during the year. They were summoned very unexpectedly, and at but short notice, to hold a special session, commencing on February 3, for the purpose of considering questions arising under the Dentists Act. The time of meeting was as inconvenient as could well be, as all the medical schools were in full work; and further, the Council met under the disadvantage of having just lost one of their oldest, most active, and clear-headed members, Dr. Andrew Wood, the Chairman of the Business Committee. He was probably by much the most practical business man among them, and there had not been time either to fill up his place in the Council as representative of the Royal College of Surgeons of Edinburgh, or to select from among the Council a new Chairman of the Business Committee. The President, in his brief address at the opening of the session, stated that a question had been raised as to the accuracy of the Dentists' Register in over 500 cases, and that it seemed improper to delay the publication of a corrected Dentists' Register till a later period of the year, when the Council might meet for ordinary business. The urgency of the business did not become clearly apparent to the ordinary observer; but neither did it appear that any member of the Council at all questioned the necessity of the session. Anyhow it cannot be denied that the Council worked with a will at the business before them, for though it concerned the purity of the Dentists' Register, and, as the President stated, involved the right of some 500 persons to remain on that Register, the whole matter was settled in a session of one day's duration. It may be remembered that in July, 1880, the Council received communications from the Association of Surgeons Practising Dental Surgery, and from the British Dental Association, setting forth the grounds upon which they considered that the names of a great number of persons ought to be erased from the Dentists' Register. These documents were referred to the Dental Committee, in order that the facts of the several cases named might be ascertained; and the reports of the Dental Committee came before the Council for consideration at the special session of which we now speak. In no case had the Committee found that a name had been entered on the Register on a declaration "fraudulently" made; but then came the question, Had any of the names been entered on declarations "incorrectly" made? Section (C) of Clause 6 of the Dentists Act (1878) entitled to registration "any person who is at the passing of this Act bona fide engaged in the practice of dentistry or dental surgery, either separately or in conjunction with the practice of medicine, surgery, or pharmacy." A great number of the persons, whose right to be on the Register was questioned, had declared that they had been bona fide engaged in the practice of dentistry in conjunction with the practice of medicine, surgery, or pharmacy, while their names were not to be found on the Medical Register, the Pharmaceutical Register, or the Register of Chemists and Druggists. Very many of them justified their declarations on the ground that they had been managers, assistants, or apprentices to chemists. Some eighty others, to whom the Solicitor to the Council had written, stating that it had been represented that their names had been entered on the Register on declarations "incorrectly or fraudulently" made that they were bona fide in the practice of dentistry with pharmacy, and inviting explanations, had not returned any answer; while others contended that their declarations were correct, though their names were not in either the Pharmaceutical or the Chemists' and Druggists' Registers. Again, the report of the Committee gave a list of some seventy persons who had replied to the Solicitor that they had desired their names to be removed from the Register. Some stated they had done so "in consequence of threatening letters from the Secretary of the British Dental Association," and it may well be taken that the rest had been alarmed by all that had been written and said about the abuse of the term "in conjunction with pharmacy." The Dental Committee, recognising that it would undoubtedly much perplex and trouble the Council to have to give any clear and positive decision as to the interpretation of that term, or of almost t any term of real importance in the Dentists Act, had the forethought to obtain counsel's opinion as to the interpretation of Clause (C) of Section 6 of the Act. A "case" was stated for the joint opinion of the Solicitor-General (Sir Farrer Herschell) and a junior barrister (Mr. M. Muir Mackenzie), and the result was almost magical. The joint opinion made a royal road through the Act, along which the Medical Council drove in triumph, making a clean sweep of all objections and difficulties. The form of declaration required to be made by persons claiming to be registered under the Act, as contained in the schedule, differs from Clause (C) of Section 6, in that it omits the words, "either separately or in conjunction with the practice of medicine, surgery, or pharmacy"; but the Council, in accordance with what they believed to be the intention of the Act, included the omitted words in the form of declaration which they issued. The joint opinion declared that this was wrong, and that the Council had no right to demand anything more than was required by the schedule of the Act, or to insert anything more in the Register; that the "Dentists' Register" is a *Dentists'* Register, and nothing more; and that it "should contain the names of the practitioners, with any dental diplomas or qualifications to which they may be entitled, but should not contain any reference to their qualifications or practice either in medicine, surgery, or pharmacy." The learned counsel made Clause (C) of Section 6 simply a mockery, a delusion, and a snare, and left it without a shadow of excuse, not to speak of justification, for its appearance in the Act. They declared that "the words '*bona fide* engaged in the practice of dentistry or dental surgery, either separately or in conjunction with medicine, surgery, or pharmacy,' have no reference to any legal qualifications to practise medicine, surgery, or pharmacy," except to show that such qualification to practise does not disqualify an applicant if he is *bona fide* in practice as a dentist; that "the question whether the name of a dentist seeking to be registered in conjunction with medicine, surgery, or pharmacy, is or is not on the Medical Register or the Pharmaceutical Register is quite immaterial"; that it is also immaterial whether or not he be an assistant only; and immaterial what kind of pharmacy he may practise, "provided he satisfies the dental qualifications necessary for registration"; the only dental qualification necessary for registration up to August 1, 1879, having been, for 90 per cent. of the applicants, an affirmation or a statutory declaration that they had been "*bona fide* engaged in the practice of dentistry" when the Act passed. The Council "bowed unreservedly," as Mr. Simon put it, "to the legal opinion"; and without any more ado resolved that "all statements with reference to the practice of medicine, surgery, and pharmacy now appearing in the Dentists' Register be erased therefrom"; they resolved also that they had not been put in possession of evidence to show that any of the registered dentists to whom objection had been made "were not at the time of their registration *bona fide* engaged in the practice of dentistry"; and therefore the Council were not prepared to order the removal of any of them from the Register; and they decreed that facilities should be afforded for letting the gentlemen who had been frightened into taking their names off the Register, get on again without paying any fee. Having thus put the assailants of the Dentists' Register to rout, and made the Dentists Act ridiculous, the Council "lightly went back" to their homes.

The great question of the purity and the proper formation of the Dentists' Register were, however, not yet settled. When the Council met in April, applications were laid before them from some registered dentists, claiming to have certain medical or surgical qualifications held by them added o their descriptions in the Dentists' Register. They rested their claims on that part of the famous joint opinion which says that the only additional qualifications which should appear in the Register are those which express or imply fitness to practise dentistry, and argued that a registrable medical or surgical diploma will by itself admit the holder to the Dentists' Register, and that, at any rate, the possession of a registrable *surgical* diploma must imply a higher degree of fitness to practise dental surgery than does a dental licence only. On this it was moved that—"Every registered dentist holding any of the surgical qualifications recited in Schedule (A) of the Medical Act shall be entitled to have such qualification or qualifications recorded in the Dentists' Register as evidence of the possession of a higher degree of knowledge": and the resolution was agreed to, in spite of the fact that the Solicitor to the Council stated that, in his opinion, the Council could not put in the existing column of the Register any additional titles—they could only put the qualifications which entitled persons to be registered under the Act; and though the Council had, in March, 1879, passed a resolution—"That the column for additional diplomas, memberships, degrees, licences, or letters, be omitted from the Dentists' Register." The Council further resolved that the additional surgical qualifications be entered in the fourth column of the Dentists' Register, and after the original qualification. Two days later, on the last day of the session, the President informed the Council that the Registrar had requested some guidance as to whether registrable surgical diplomas that are not registered in the Medical Register are to be entered in the Dentists' Register; and as to which are to be considered as *surgical* qualifications; was the licence of the Royal College of Physicians of London, for instance, such a surgical qualification, registrable in the Dentists' Register? These queries gave rise to a discussion on the meaning of the expression "a *surgical* qualification"; and in the end the Council, who had two days before rejected their Solicitor's advice on a point of law, resolved: "That the President be authorised to answer these questions, and any other questions that may arise in respect of the registration of additional titles in the Dentists' Register, after consultation with the Solicitor to the Council."

It may be stated here that the British Dental Association are not at all inclined to join the Council in bowing unreservedly to the joint opinions of the Solicitor-General and Mr. Muir Mackenzie as to the interpretation of the Dentists Act. Before they sent in to the Medical Council their black list of names, they had been advised by counsel that a person who could not practise pharmacy without contravening the Pharmacy Act was not entitled to be admitted to the Dentists' Register on the ground of having practised "dentistry in conjunction with pharmacy" before the passing of the Dentists Act; and a copy of this opinion had been sent to the Medical Council, but the Council regarded it not. After the emasculation of the famous Clause (C) of Section 6 of the Act in February, the Association submitted the section, together with the opinions of Sir F. Herschell and Mr. Muir Mackenzie, to Sir John Holker and two junior counsel, and received from them a joint opinion directly opposed to that upon which the Medical Council had acted. The Association had also, in reply to a question put to their counsel, received the opinion that practically the only means of obtaining a judicial decision on the section, supposing Sir F. Herschell to have been wrong, would be "for the Council to expunge from the Register the name of some person who, according to the view we have taken, was not entitled to be registered. The question can then be tried on a mandamus to restore the name." This opinion the Association sent in July to the Executive Committee, inviting the Medical Council to be so obliging as to take the necessary steps to try the correctness of the course taken by them. The Executive, acting for the Council, replied, on July 28, that in their opinion it rested with the Dental Association to take the requisite measures, and not, as suggested, " by the removal of a name which, in the judgment of the Council, is registered in conformity with law "—a polite way of saying that if the Association wanted the chesnuts they must themselves pluck them out of the fire. The Representative Board of the Association replied that they were advised that the point in question could not be settled by action taken under Section 35 of the Dentists Act (the section respecting penalties for obtaining registration by false representations) ; and requested, inasmuch as the Council had, in February last, declared that sufficient evidence of error in registration had not been adduced to justify the erasure of the names under consideration, that " the memorial, with the appended legal opinions (constituting strong additional evidence), addressed to the Council, and in part considered by the Executive Committee on July 28, be laid before the Council at its next session." In fact, the Association appealed from the Executive Committee to Cæsar. The Committee considered the communication on November 11, and appear to have been puzzled what to do, for they resolved—" That the several documents and legal decisions in possession of the Council having reference to registration under the Dentists Act be placed in the hands of Mr. Farrar, the Solicitor to the General Council, for the purpose of his further advising the Committee thereon." There the matter rests at present.

The Medical Council met again, for their thirty-second session, on April 26. In his opening address the President stated that the business for which it had been thought desirable to call the Council together need not detain them long. It had seemed to himself and members of the Council of urgency " to consider, without delay, certain questions affecting the education and examination of schools and colleges throughout the country "; which meant that the resolutions respecting general education and preliminary examinations passed, after six days' discussion, in July, 1880, would not work, and required reconsideration. The Council had made alterations in their requirements regarding preliminary examinations, without considering the effect of these alterations in connexion with their resolution, repeatedly insisted on, that " the superintendence of the general education of the medical profession should be left to the great national educational bodies, meaning thereby the Universities of the United Kingdom "; and the result had been that none of the examinations conducted by the University of Oxford, by the University of Cambridge, or by the College of Preceptors, would fulfil the required conditions, were these strictly enforced. Communications upon the subject had been received from all those bodies ; and were considered and reported upon by the Executive Committee. In accordance with that report, the Council, with commendable promptness, agreed that—" The Executive Committee be requested to communicate with the Universities of the United Kingdom, and with the College of Preceptors, with a view to promote that such of their examinations as most nearly correspond to the minimum requirements of the Medical Council in respect to preliminary education, and are open to all classes of candidates, should be held, or in part held, at times which may be generally convenient to medical students intending to enter on their professional curriculum in the winter or the summer session "; and also, that the examination in general education conducted by the Universities be accepted as heretofore ; but that, if any of them did not include the elementary mechanics of solids and fluids, a knowledge of those subjects should be required at a subsequent examination.

A report was received from the Executive Committee on cases of students from India who had passed the Matricula-

tion Examination of Indian Universities. That examination classes Latin among the optional subjects, and as a rule the students take up Sanscrit, or some other language, in place of Latin, which the regulations of the Council make obligatory. Certain students had applied to be admitted to professional examination with or without now passing in Latin, and the Executive Committee had in all cases granted the requests made, considering that Sanscrit might very well be accepted in place of Latin. And further, the Committee suggested that they should be empowered to make exception to the recommendations of the Council on Education and Examination, when such exception should seem reasonable. The report gave rise to not a little discussion and consideration. Some members of the Council considered the Executive Committee had usurped the functions of the Branch Councils, and wanted to override the recommendations of the General Council. Dr. Quain pointed out the importance, and at times the urgency, of the matter, as the students affected by the decree that an examination in Latin is obligatory come not only from India, but from Syria, Constantinople, and the East generally, " where a knowledge of Latin is not in the least useful." In the end, power was given to the Branch Councils for Scotland and Ireland respectively, and the Branch Council for England, or the Executive Committee, to make exception in the case of a student from any Indian, colonial, or foreign university or college who has passed the matriculation or other equivalent examination, " provided such examination fairly represents a standard of general education equivalent to that required in this country." Answers were received from a very large proportion, but not from all, of the medical licensing bodies to the Council's resolutions respecting the institution of a preliminary scientific examination, and a report of the Committee which had been appointed to consider them ; and these documents gave rise to a lengthy discussion. The result was that the Council decided to recommend to the licensing bodies to consider whether a preliminary scientific examination can be carried out, and how ; and the answers were referred, when received, to the same Committee as before for consideration and report. Some dental business, which is noted elsewhere, was transacted ; a name was ordered to be erased from the Medical Register ; and the financial report was received, which showed that for the last year or two the income of the General Medical Council has considerably exceeded its expenditure. The dental financial account was, however, as unsatisfactory as are most things connected with the dental administration of the Council ; the estimated annual expenditure of dental registration will be £1407, but the estimated income only £524. Some additions were made to, and some alterations in, the standing orders ; and the Council adjourned, after a sitting of five days.

The President and Censors of the Royal College of Physicians delivered in January their judgment on the complaint laid before them last year by Dr. Pavy as to the evidence given by Sir William Gull in the case of Regina v. Ingle. It is not necessary to recall to our readers the particulars of that case. The Guy's Hospital nursing dispute will be well remembered ; as will the case in question, which arose out of it. It will suffice to record as a matter of history the judgment delivered to the College. It was as follows :—" The President and Censors of the Royal College of Physicians having carefully considered Dr. Pavy's complaint, and Sir William Gull's reply to that complaint, do not deem the character of the evidence which a Fellow or Member of the College has given an oath in a court of justice a proper subject to investigate, when the court has expressed itself satisfied in regard of the truth and sincerity of the witness. They consider Sir William Gull, holding the opinions he

expressed on oath, justified in going into court. They are further of opinion that Dr. Pavy's diagnosis and treatment of the woman afford no grounds for any remarks calculated to disparage his well-deserved reputation as an eminent and skilful physician." The judgment was signed by Dr. (now Sir) Risdon Bennett (President), Sir William Jenner, and Drs. J. C. Bucknill, Hermann Weber, and E. Headlam Greenhow. The logic of the judgment—if it contains any logic—may be questioned; but the meaning of it is plain enough. The annual meeting for the election of a Fellow of the College to the high office of President was held this year on April 7, when, in an unprecedentedly large Comitia, Sir William Jenner was elected to the chair by a very large majority of votes. The retiring President, in a brief address on the affairs and condition of the College, stated that 2260 names were on the roll of the College, viz., 304 Fellows, 462 Members, and the rest Licentiates of various grades. In April, nine members of the College were elected to the honourable distinction of the fellowship. At the same meeting the College accepted fully the conditions of a legacy of £1000 from Mrs. Bradshawe for the purpose of establishing and endowing a lecture on Physic, to be called the Bradshawe Lecture, in memory of the late Dr. Bradshawe, and to be delivered at the College every year on August 18. The President afterwards appointed Dr. Vivian Poore to be the first Bradshawe Lecturer; and in that capacity he delivered on the appointed day at the College a lecture on "Nervous Affections of the Hand." The Harveian Oration of the year, a scholarly, thoughtful, and very eloquent address, was delivered by Dr. Andrew Whyte Barclay. The Gulstonian Lectures were given by Dr. Sidney Coupland, who took "Anæmia" for the subject of them; the Croonian Lectures, by Dr. Moxon, were on "The Influence of the Circulation upon the Nervous System"; and the Lumleian Lectures were delivered by Dr. Reginald Southey, on "Bright's Disease." These lectures, for all of which we gladly found room in our pages, were of, at the least, the usual interest and excellence, and well worthy of the College and the lecturers. The Baly Medal of the College was awarded to Dr. Burdon-Sanderson, and was presented to him on June 18, immediately after the Harveian Oration, by Sir William Jenner, who seized the opportunity of expressing his admiration of the high character and value of Dr. Sanderson's physiological work. In the last week of the year, the College, for the guidance and help of its Fellows, Members, and Licentiates, and for the information and benefit of the public, passed the following resolution:—
"That while the College has no desire to fetter the opinions of its members in reference to any theories they may see fit to adopt in connexion with the practice of medicine, it nevertheless considers it desirable to express its opinion that the assumption or acceptance by members of the profession of designations implying the adoption of special modes of treatment is opposed to those principles of the freedom and dignity of the profession which should govern the relations of its members to each other and to the public. The College therefore expects that all its Fellows, Members, and Licentiates will uphold these principles by discountenancing those who trade upon such designations."

The Council of the Royal College of Surgeons of England, at their quarterly meeting held on January 13, received, approved, and adopted a report from the Committee on Preliminary Examination. The report recommended that the preliminary examinations for the diplomas of Member and Fellow of the College, conducted by the College of Preceptors under the authority of the College, should cease from and after December 31, 1881, in accordance with the resolution of the Council of November 11 of last year. The resolution thus finally adopted was conveyed to the General Medical Council, with the intimation that the giving up of the College preliminary examinations rendered it in the highest degree desirable that the General Medical Council should, as far as possible, require that examinations recognised in lieu of the College examinations should be held at such times and places as may best suit the convenience of the candidates who desire to enter the medical profession. The Council reserved to themselves the right of determining the conditions of admission to examination for the diploma of the College in the case of any colonial, Indian, or foreign student not registered by the Medical Council; and resolved that, in future, candidates for the diploma of Fellow should not be required to undergo any preliminary examination beyond that required for the diploma of Member of the College. The Council continued the work of making arrangements to render their professional examinations complete. The Committee appointed to consider and report on the necessary arrangements for the institution of additional examinations for the diplomas of Member and Fellow of the College, reported, at the above-mentioned meeting of the Council, that, in pursuance of the resolution of the Council adopted in May last year, the President had addressed a letter to the President of the Royal College of Physicians of London, inviting a conference on the practicability of making arrangements for a joint examination for qualification to practise medicine, surgery, and midwifery. The invitation was declined on the ground that the Royal College of Physicians was bound by the terms of the Conjoint Scheme, dated May 1, 1877, and therefore could not take part in the formation of any other examining board till after the expiration of five years from October 1, 1877, the shortest time fixed by the Scheme for its duration; and though the President of the Royal College of Surgeons pointed out that this interpretation of Section 12 of the Scheme was not tenable, as it seemed quite clear that that section is binding on the several medical authorities only on the condition that the Conjoint Scheme has come into actual force, his argument did not avail. Consequently the Council of the College of Surgeons proceeded with arrangements for the reform of their own examinations. They resolved: That there be four instead of two examiners in medicine; that the examinations [on the Principles and Practice of Medicine, both written and vivâ voce, be extended, and do include the examination of patients; that from and after January 1, 1882, every candidate for the final examination, whether for the diploma of Member or of Fellow, be required to pass an examination in midwifery, unless he shall possess a recognised qualification in midwifery, or before obtaining the diploma shall produce a certificate of having passed the necessary examination entitling him to a recognised qualification in midwifery; and that there be two examiners in midwifery, and that the examination be partly written and partly vivâ voce. And regulations were made as to the conditions entitling to exemption from the College examination in medicine or in midwifery. In March the Council adopted a reply, formulated by their Committee on Preliminary Examinations, to certain inquiries contained in a communication from Dr. Haldane, chairman of a Committee of the Medical Council, as to the desirability of candidates for the profession being required, before entering on the purely medical curriculum, to have been instructed and examined in the rudiments of Natural Science—physical, chemical, and biological. The Council replied that, in their opinion, it is desirable that intending medical students should be encouraged to study in one or more of the branches of natural science not included in the compulsory subjects of the preliminary examination; and that the having passed an examination in one or more of such subjects should exempt a student from attendance on lectures on those subjects, and from similar examinations in them during his professional education, but not from the practical instruction and examinations now required by any of the medical authorities; and further, that proficiency in the subjects, as ascertained by examination, should suffice, without any other evidence of special instruction. The Council have since appointed the additional Examiners in Medicine, and the Examiners in Midwifery, and have otherwise completed the arrangements for the extended examinations in those subjects; but have deferred instituting examinations in Chemistry, Materia Medica, Medical Botany, and Pharmacy. Some further changes have been made in the Erasmus Wilson Trust; and in future (till some fresh change be made) the proceeds of the Fund are to be employed in part towards the payment of the salary of a Pathological Curator of the Museum, and in part for the payment of lectures or demonstrations on the pathological contents of the Museum, to be given either by the Pathological Curator or some other person appointed for the purpose. Three vacancies in the Council of the College had to be filled up, for which six candidates presented themselves: of whom the Fellows elected Sir James Paget, Mr. J. Whitaker Hulke (of Middlesex Hospital), and Mr. Christopher Heath (of University Hospital). Mr. Frederick S. Eve, F.R.C.S., has been appointed Pathological Curator of the Museum of the College, and Erasmus Wilson Lecturer. We do not learn that the Council have decided yet how to give effect to the conditions of Mrs. Bradshawe's bequest of £1000 to the College. The Council promptly accepted the legacy, and the conditions are similar to those of the like bequest made to the College of Physicians; but the first Bradshawe lecture at the College of Physicians has already been delivered. Two lectures were given at the College by Professor Henry Trentham Butlin, "On the Relations of Sarcoma to Carcinoma," and one lecture by Professor Frederick Treves, "On the Pathology of Scrofulous Affections of the Lymphatic Glands," being lectures delivered under the (then) conditions of the Erasmus Wilson Trust. The Jacksonian Prize was awarded to Mr. Watson Cheyne, M.B. Edin., F.R.C.S., for his essay on "Antiseptic Surgery."

Of all the various Congresses that met in the present year of the Congress Age, the most important, and the greatest event of the medical year 1881, was the seventh meeting of the International Medical Congress, which was held in London on August 3 and the six following days. The Congress had met six times previously—in Paris, in 1867; in Florence, in 1869; in Vienna, in 1873; in Brussels, in 1875; in Geneva, in 1877; and in Amsterdam, in 1879. On those occasions the numbers of the members had ranged from 400 to 700; while at the meeting held in London the members numbered some 3000, and of these about 1000 were foreigners, the list of whom included very many men of the highest eminence and distinction in the profession. Delegates were sent by the Governments of France, Germany, Austria, Italy, Russia, Belgium, Spain, Hungary, Sweden and Norway, the Netherlands, Switzerland, Roumania, Brazil, the Argentine Republic, the United States, and from Canada, besides the well-known physicians and surgeons who travelled from far and wide to attend the meeting as private members; so that the Congress was most fully and truly representative of the science and art of medicine. Sir James Paget was President of the Congress, and the work of it was distributed among sixteen sections—Anatomy, President Professor W. Flower; Physiology, Dr. Michael Foster; Pathology and Morbid Anatomy, Dr. Samuel Wilks; Medicine, Sir William Gull; Surgery, Mr. Erichsen; Obstetrics, Dr. McClintock; Diseases of Children, Dr. Charles West; Mental Diseases, Dr. Lockhart Robinson; Ophthalmology, Mr. Bowman; Diseases of the Throat, Dr. George Johnson; Diseases of the Ear, Mr. W. B. Dalby; Diseases of the Skin, Mr. (now Sir) Erasmus Wilson; Diseases of the Teeth, Mr. Edwin Saunders;

State Medicine, Mr. John Simon, C.B.; Military Surgery and Medicine, Surgeon-General T. Longmore, C.B.; and Materia Medica, Professor T. R. Fraser, M.D. Each section was complete in itself for the carrying out of its work, being provided with a vice-president, a council, and a secretary; and, besides the morning and afternoon meetings of the sections, there were six general meetings of the Congress.

To carry out such a scheme with any prospect of success, extensive and well-organised machinery was necessary. There was a large and very influential general committee, presided over by the President of the Royal College of Physicians, who till April this year was Sir Risdon Bennett, and thereafter Sir William Jenner. The Honorary Treasurer was Mr. Bowman, and the Honorary Secretary-General Mr. William Mac Cormac, with Mr. G. H. Makins as Under-Secretary. There was an Executive Committee, with Sir Risdon Bennett as chairman; and a Reception Committee, of which Mr. Prescott Hewett was chairman, and Professor John Marshall vice-chairman. Everybody worked well, but the chief labour of organisation and administration fell, of course, upon Sir James Paget, the Executive Committee, and the Secretaries; and their unflinching and incessant industry, administrative talents, patience, and tact, shown in attention to the minutest details of the whole scheme, insured a brilliant and unparalleled success. The Royal College of Physicians placed their rooms at the service of the Congress from the end of July till August 10; and the sections were provided with rooms by the University of London, the Royal Academy of Arts, the Royal Institution, the Royal, the Linnean, the Chemical, the Astronomical, the Antiquaries', the Asiatic, and the Geological Societies, and the Royal School of Mines; the Geological Society also housed the temporary Museum; and the general meetings were held in St. James's Great Hall. A reception of the members of the Congress was held at the Royal College of Physicians, on Tuesday, August 2, which was crowded for some hours. The first general meeting, for the election of officers and the constitution of the Congress, and the inaugural address by the President, was held on Wednesday, the 3rd, in the morning. The Great Hall was crowded, and the meeting was attended by H.R.H. the Prince of Wales, and H.R.I.H. the Crown Prince of Germany; and by Cardinal Manning, the Archbishop of York, and some lay dignitaries.

The proceedings were commenced by the President of the Royal College of Physicians, Sir William Jenner, in an admirable and most effective address; the necessary formal business followed; and then the President, Sir James Paget, having taken the chair, the Prince of Wales delivered one of his telling speeches, and declared the Congress opened. The inaugural address of Sir James Paget, which followed, was worthy alike of the occasion—extraordinary and great as that was—and of the man: higher praise could not well be given to it. On the same day, in the afternoon, the second general meeting was held, and Virchow delivered to a large and appreciative audience an address on "The Value of Pathological Experiment." Five other addresses-in-chief were delivered during the Congress: by Dr. Billings, of the United States Army, on Our Medical Literature; by Professor Pasteur, on the Germ Theory; on Scepticism in Medicine, by the late Dr. Maurice Raynaud; by Professor Volkmann, on the Changes in Surgery during the last Ten Years; and by Mr. Huxley, on the Connexion of the Biological Sciences with Medicine.

They all were masterly addresses, but perhaps that from Dr. Billings was the most remarkable for its practical value, its originality, the wit and humour that illumined it through out, and the skill with which it was delivered; while a special and tender interest attached to the address written by Dr. Maurice Raynaud (who died a week or two before the Congress met), and ably read by his intimate friend, Dr. Féréol. All the addresses in-chief, except that by Volkmann, are published in our second volume for this year, and they will long be read with profit and pleasure.

The work in the several sections was carried on very actively and steadily, and the attendances were, as a rule, large, and sometimes very large. Many valuable communications were made, and some extremely interesting discussions excited, and we do not doubt that the results have been real and solid gain to both the science and the art of medicine. But for the addresses given by the Presidents of Sections, and reports of the work day by day, we must again refer our readers to the full record of the Congress given in our pages throughout August. It is due to the Secretaries of the Congress and the Secretaries of Sections to record here, that a large volume, of over 700 pages, was prepared for the members before the Congress met, giving abstracts, in English, French, and German, of every paper sent in to be read in the sections; programmes of the day's work, and amusements were published every morning, also in these languages; and many other most useful and efficient aids were provided. And since the termination of the Congress the Secretaries have been engaged in preparing the volumes of the *Transactions*, which are to contain a very complete record of the whole of the proceedings, including the discussions in the sections, revised by the several speakers. The Museum connected with the Congress was altogether very successful. It constituted a valuable companion to the work done in Congress, and an interesting illustration of great workers of the past as well as of contemporary research. In a room adjoining it living examples of rare or very interesting diseases were shown every morning; and these demonstrations formed one of the most popular and successful features of the Congress.

A few lines must be given to a note of the social side of the Congress. Only one entertainment, a *conversazione* at the South Kensington Museum, was given by the Congress—that is, of course, by the English members. It was held on August 3, and, though it was attended by some 5000 persons, the courts, galleries, rooms, and garden of the Museum gave ample space for that large assemblage. The admirably skilful arrangements of the whole made it a perfect success. There was no overcrowding or other discomfort anywhere, and we know that the brilliancy and entire management of the *soirée* excited the admiration and astonishment of our foreign guests. The Prince of Wales, the Crown Prince of Prussia, and his son Prince Henry, attended it, and stayed a considerable time. On Thursday, the 4th, the Lord Mayor entertained nearly three hundred members of the Congress at dinner at the Mansion House; and in the evening of August 5 the Lord Mayor and the Corporation of London gave a brilliant *conversazione* at the Guildhall, which was attended by more than 3000 persons, including all the foreign members. On the afternoon of the 5th, garden parties were given by Sir J. D. Hooker at Kew Gardens, Dr. and Mrs. Langdon Down at Normansfield, Mr. and Mrs. Spencer Wells at Hampstead, and Mr. and Mrs. Saunders at Wimbledon; and in the evening the Countess Granville gave a reception to which many members of the Congress were invited. On that day also a considerable number of members visited Folkestone, to be present at the unveiling of Mr. Bruce Joy's statue of Harvey; and were entertained at luncheon by the Corporation of the town. On Monday, the 8th, the Baroness Burdett-Coutts (Mrs. Ashmead Bartlett) gave a garden party to a large number of members; and in the evening the Master and Wardens of the Society of Apothecaries entertained about 120 in their hall at Blackfriars; and the Royal College of Surgeons invited all the members of Congress to a very brilliant *conversazione*,

which was very largely attended, in their museums and library. Other semi-public entertainments were given, which we have not space to mention, as that by Sir Erasmus Wilson to a large party to view the Infirmary at Margate, for which he is doing so much; and the private hospitalities of the London members of the Congress were unbounded. It must be added also that the weather throughout the time of the Congress was simply perfect, rain having fallen on one day only—on Monday afternoon.

The several medical societies held very active sessions, and many of the meetings were more than usually interesting. No special subject was appointed for debate this year, except at the Medical Society of London, where a discussion on the Salicylate Treatment of Acute Rheumatism was opened by Dr. Hilton Fagge, on December 12. It proved highly attractive and instructive, was continued on the evening of the 19th, and then adjourned to January. Many hospital physicians have taken part in it, and a large number of hospital statistics have been brought forward, so that it seems not improbable that some definite conclusions may be formulated as to the employment and value of the salicylates in rheumatic fever. At the Pathological Society, the debate on Rickets, which was continued into the present year from 1880, elicited a great difference of opinion as to the heredity of the disease, as to the etiology, and indeed as to most points regarding it. But it added no new fact to our knowledge of its pathology or its clinical history. As the President of the Society observed, there "had been an interchange of ideas," rather than "a citation of new facts." The debate may, however, have served the very good purpose of inciting to a new and thorough study of rickets. The report of the Clinical Society's Special Committee on Hip-joint Diseases was presented in May. It is the result of much very careful consideration, is ably drawn up, and constitutes a valuable contribution to surgical literature. At both the Clinical and the Royal Medical and Chirurgical Societies, surgery loomed very large; and not only there, but everywhere, and throughout the year. Indeed, nothing has been more remarkable than the audacity with which surgeons have extended the domain of operative interference except the wonderful degree of success that has in many instances made the audacity a happy one. In January, on the 29th, Billroth removed the pyloric portion of the stomach on account of cancerous disease in a woman, who recovered, and lived an active life for some time, but died on May 23, from a recurrence of cancer. In four other cases, however, the operation was speedily fatal. Lately, Billroth and his able assistant, Dr. Wölfler, modified the operation, changing it to one called gastro-enterostomy, the name signifying that the stomach is not surgically interfered with, but that a mouth is made into the intestine: this operation has been reported unsuccessful. Dr. MacEwen reported to the Royal Society a remarkable case of successful transplantation of bone in a child three years old; by which, after necrosis of the right humerus, a useless arm was made a thoroughly useful one. Portions of the intestinal tract have been removed in many instances (*Medical Times and Gazette*, vol. i., pages 431, 541, 622), but without encouraging results. Extirpation of the kidney has been performed with success, for the first time in England by Mr. A. E. Barker, and on the Continent (vol. ii., pages 496 and 623); Dr. Wolfe's operation of the transplantation of the conjunctiva of rabbits to the eye has been reported (vol. ii., page 608); and Mr. Spencer Wells has completed, for the first time in this country, the removal of the gravid uterus with cancerous cervix, on October 21, and with success. The surgeons have supplied us with several new, and rather uncouth, names for operative procedures, such as oesophagostomy, gastrostomy, duodenostomy, and enterostomy, enterectomy, and enterorraphy. There has been, at home and abroad, continued discussion and hostile criticism of some of the details and materials of *Listerism*, and the results have been that the spray has been less generally used, and that Mr. Lister himself now employs eucalyptic spray and dressings instead of carbolic. Surgeons are even taking destructive disease of the lung into the domain of operative surgery.

An International Medical and Sanitary Exhibition, organised by the Committee of the Parkes Museum of Hygiene, was held at South Kensington from July 16 to August 13. It was the greatest and most important exhibition of the kind that has ever been held, and was the outcome of an infinite amount of patient labour and care bestowed on its collection and arrangement by the Executive Committee. The Exhibition embraced all materials and appliances for the prevention, investigation, and treatment of disease and injury. The exhibits included in this wide range were classed in sections: Surgical Instruments and Apparatus; Appliances of the Ward and Sick Room; Electrical Instruments and Appliances; Microscopes and Optical Apparatus; other Apparatus used in the Investigation of Disease; Domestic and Hospital Architecture, Planning, Construction, Decorative Materials, Ventilation, Lighting and Warming, Water - closets, Sinks, etc., Sewerage and Drainage, Water Supply and Filtration; Appliances used for the Treatment of the Sick and Wounded during War, Street Ambulances, etc.; Drugs, Disinfectants, Dietetic Articles, and Mineral Waters; Applications of Hygienic Principles to Food and Dietaries, Clothing, etc.; School Furniture, etc. The intention and scope were ambitious, but on the whole the Committee were more than justified. The Exhibition was a very large and very important school for both the profession and the public, and it proved a very popular school. The recollection of it, however, is not, we regret to say, unclouded. Some trade jealousy or prejudice, or some other malign influence, appears to have affected the adjudication of awards of merit in the Drug Section. Very grievous and serious complaints, which seem only too well founded, have been made in the matter, but entirely without effect. The idea of the Exhibition was a grand one, and it was well carried out. The Exhibition was opened by its President, Earl Spencer, supported by Lord Granville and the President of the International Medical Congress; and it was a great success. Prizes and other awards of merit, which were offered by the Committee and eagerly competed for, were to have been publicly bestowed upon the competitors fortunate enough to gain any of these distinctions. But this last part of the programme appears to have been wiped out since the complaints to which we have alluded became widely known. Such an occurrence is a grievous pity, and cannot but be mischievous; but it is happily so rare as to be almost unprecedented.

Amongst the subjects of our annual retrospect, there is none that will excite more interest, or even a certain degree of anxiety, than the subject of Therapeutics, or treatment in the widest sense of the term, which, after all, is the end and aim of our profession. With respect to medicinal therapeutics, less brilliant results must necessarily be chronicled from time to time than those which reward the scientific surgeon; and again, the time of probation of any new method of treatment by drugs is necessarily much more than twelve short months. For these reasons we cannot expect to be able to congratulate our readers upon many additions to the armamentarium of medicine. What there chiefly are in the way of novelties have indeed been reviewed by us at a comparatively recent date, during the International Congress, and in our reports of the International Medical and Sanitary Exhibition. We would, therefore, refer those of our readers who may desire to have a more complete record of recent advances in pharmacology and pharmacy to the numbers of our journal for July 30, August 6, and August 27.

When we regard the character of the work that has recently been done in pharmacology, we are struck with the parallelism between the lines which advance has followed and is following in this subject, and the direction of progress in the allied subjects of pathology, hygiene, and practical surgery. Just as the germ-theory of disease is dominant in these three departments of our profession, so is the endeavour amongst therapeutists to put to the test every possible kind of antiseptic, apyretic, and disinfectant substance, and to search in the boundless field of the higher organic chemical compounds for new drugs. Our review naturally, therefore, begins with this class. Whilst some surgeons of eminence declare that they have abandoned the Listerian system of antiseptic operation and dressing, either in whole or in part, various modifications of the old method have been introduced in England and abroad (see page 304, vol. i.; and page 77, vol. ii.). Evidence, both of a theoretical and of a clinical kind, has been adduced against the necessity of the spray during operation (see pages 276, and 302, vol. i.). The number of new antiseptics that have been suggested is large. Professor Lister himself, as well as others, has drawn attention to certain advantages which the oil of the eucalyptus possesses over carbolic acid. Salicylated camphor has been used in France as a powerful antiseptic and stimulant to foul syphilitic and cancerous sores. Iodoform appears to be steadily gaining in reputation as a surgical dressing; and the quantities of the substance which are sometimes dusted on the surface of wounds, or applied otherwise to diseased parts, are little short of alarming. In the hands of dermatologists, iodoform also continues to give favourable results; and as its unpleasant and very persistent odour can, in a measure, be covered by the tonquin-bean (vol. ii, page 27), by tar (*ibid.*), or by musk (page 425, vol. i.), we may expect to find it come into still more extensive use. Thymol continues to be highly praised by some authorities; and boracic acid by others. Resorcin has probably received more attention during the year, both from the chemist and the practical physician and surgeon, than any of the other substances just mentioned. Its chemical relations appear to be now thoroughly understood, and it would seem to be a valuable but expensive antiseptic. Quite recently, naphthalin has been recommended in Germany both as an efficient and as a remarkably cheap antiseptic substance (see vol. ii., page 718).

The treatment of phthisis by constant inhalation of antiseptics from a "respirator," as noticed in our columns in former volumes, has been extensively employed during the year; and various refinements in the method of application and in the antiseptic material have been introduced. The combination in most favour at present appears to be that of Dr. Sinclair Coghill, consisting of ethereal tincture of iodine, carbolic acid, creasote or thymol, and rectified spirits; ether or chloroform being added if cough be severe.

Various recommendations have been offered of acids or salts which may acidify the urine in chronic cystitis with ammoniacal decomposition and bacterial development. Amongst these we may quote lactic acid in doses of fifteen to thirty grains in water three times a day, benzoic acid, and biborate of soda. The salicylates and other antiseptics continue to be used as vesical injections for the same purpose.

As usual, the name is legion of the new cures for whooping-cough, trial being made especially of the various antiseptics, including salicylic acid and carbolic acid, which might be supposed to arrest the activity of the hypothetical organism on which pertussis is believed by some authorities to depend. On the whole it cannot be said that trustworthy evidence signalises any of these substances as specially valuable in the disorder.

The intimate pathology of infectious diseases introduces us to another and very different kind of treatment. Probably the most remarkable, and certainly the most important, step that has been made by general therapeutics during the year is the *vaccination charbonneuse* of Professor Pasteur (see page 707, vol. i.; and page 133, vol. ii.). As applied to the lower animals, the method of inoculation with the artificially attenuated virus of anthrax promises to be worthy of comparison with vaccination in man; and both directly as preventing the spread of this deadly disease to the human subject, and indirectly as suggesting further investigations in the same direction, this discovery must be regarded as a great boon to the human race. Vaccination from the calf has been most extensively employed in London during the recent epidemic of small-pox. This system, which we have persistently recommended to the profession for years, has given such satisfactory results that it promises in a great measure to take the place of arm-to-arm vaccination, to which there are certain reasonable objections. The hope that was once raised, that the germ of the hydrophobic poison had been isolated, and that so far an advance had been made towards a possible prophylaxis of rabies, as of anthrax, in animals—that is, the diminution or disappearance of the risk of hydrophobia in man—has been unfortunately, but, we trust, temporarily only, disappointed (vol. i., page 387).

Diphtheria has been treated, with various results, by salicylic acid in strong solution applied locally, and benzoate of soda internally; by chlorate of potash; and by lactic acid. Various other "solvents" have been tried locally, such as pepsine and papayotin; the latter, prepared from the juice of the *Carica papaya*, being constantly kept in contact with the diseased surface by irrigation or by brush. But of all remedies for diphtheria most has been written during the year upon pilocarpin, which was greatly extolled by Guttmann (see page 101, vol. i.) as having *cured all his cases*. Very unfortunately, the latest accounts on the same subject from Germany are to the effect that of a series of cases of the disease treated by pilocarpin *all died!* The simple solution of the false membrane in diphtheria is surely but a small part of the proper treatment of the disease. American physicians appear to have arrived at the same conclusion (see vol. ii., page 82).

Amongst the newer drugs which have been investigated during the year are the Jamaica dogwood (*Piscidia erythrina*); the *Thalictrum macrocarpum*, which appears to closely resemble its congener, aconite, in action; maize (*Zea mais*), which seems to be a renal and vesical sedative, and possibly litholytic in its effects; and oolachan oil, which is derived from the candle-fish of North America, and appears to resemble cod-liver oil in its valuable properties, whilst its flavour is agreeable rather than the reverse.

An attempt has even been made to press the fluorides into the service of medicine, but apparently with little success, unless as a means of producing anorexia and vomiting, which may occasionally be desirable. The action of ergot upon the circulation has been taken advantage of in the local treatment of erysipelas, eczema, acne rosacea, and some other forms of disease on cutaneous and mucous surfaces.

The black walnut of America (*Juglans nigra*) is another new remedy, which is said to have proved of great value in the form of a gargle or spray in diphtheria, although no account is given of its physiological action.

Thapsia garginica is a plant which promises to furnish a useful rubefacient for general use in painful and inflammatory diseases. A species of cactus, the *Cereus Bonplandii*, has given remarkably favourable results in the hands of some American physicians in cardiac cases which resist digitalis.

Viscum album has also rewarded investigation by relieving cardiac distress under somewhat similar conditions. Dr. Wolfenden has recorded forty cases of sweating in phthisis in which remarkable benefit followed the administration of twenty to thirty grains of *agaricus* (see vol. ii., page 442).

Hamamelis virginica, or witch-hazel, has been favourably spoken of as an application to inflamed parts, such as the fauces, superficial contusions and ulcers, and inflamed piles. Attempts have been made to secure the advantages of the physiological effects of the nitrites in the treatment of disease without the disadvantages that attend the sudden and evanescent action of the amyl compound. With this end in view, the nitrites of potassium and sodium have been investigated and employed in America and Germany, apparently with promising results (see vol. i., page 71). The repeated and methodical inhalation of the amyl-nitrite six times a day, in doses amounting even to forty minims, has meanwhile been tried in epilepsy—not during, but between the attacks—and apparently with some success. The same drug seems to relieve chordee and priapism (vol ii., page 489).

Bromide of ethyl and iodide of ethyl have been fairly tried during the year, and variously reported on. The bromide has, on the whole, not gained in favour with anæsthetists, who generally regard it as a dangerous compound (see page 166, vol. ii.). The iodide, on the contrary, probably maintains its character as a useful antispasmodic in some cases of asthma. Citrate of caffeine has been commended not only as a diuretic, but as a nervous stimulant (see page 659, vol. i.). Dr. Shapter has shown in our pages (vol. ii., page 33) the extensive application which may be made of this drug, both generally and in some of the more special forms of nervous and visceral exhaustion. Naphthol has been extensively tried by Kaposi, of Vienna, in the treatment of skin diseases, and has yielded good results in cases of scabies, psoriasis, seborrhœa, prurigo, ichthyosis, and lupus erythematosus, as well as in particular stages of eczema.

The salts of ammonia have not fulfilled the expectations that were raised of their value in the treatment of diabetes by the previous reports of Adamkiewics. On the contrary, benefit has attended the employment of chloral hydrate in the same disease, for which its use had been suggested by experiments on animals. Picrate of ammonia has been used with possible success in malarial fevers (see vol. i., page 257).

Dr. Colley March, of Rochdale, has shown how the use of certain "old" and almost forgotten remedies may be revived with success (vol i., pages 237 and 319).

Defibrinated blood has been brought forward as a valuable form of substance for rectal alimentation, and means have been suggested for preparing and drying it, and for preventing its decomposition, as well as the odour that may cling to the patients using it (see vol. i., page 284).

Amongst the newer surgical operations which the practitioner has come to perform for the relief of what are ordinarily regarded as "medical" diseases must be mentioned nerve-stretching. Our columns have recently contained records of cases in which this method of treatment has been employed in locomotor ataxy (vol. i., page 107); in painful tic of the face (vol. i., page 688); in sciatica; and in neuralgia of the face and tongue (vol. ii., page 618).

Another kind of operation belonging to the same category—namely, trephining for the relief of traumatic epilepsy (if the expression may be used)—has been followed by various results (see vol. ii., page 85). Possibly the intravenous injection of a weak and alkalinised solution of common salt (as described on page 719 of vol. ii.) may prove of great service in syncope from anæmia. The method of treating lupus by scraping has been successfully employed in cases reported during the year (vol. i., page 317).

There is not much to record with regard to the Medical Services of the Army and Navy. A new Order in Council for reforming and improving the regulations governing the position of medical officers in the Royal Navy was published on April 5 (vol. i., pages 488 and 702); but it was not altogether satisfactory, and has not, so far, made the Service much more attractive. At the entrance examination for candidates, on February 14, 12 candidates presented themselves, of whom 3 were found physically unfit, 2 were rejected, and 7 were successful. At the examination on August 15, 18 candidates appeared, of whom 4 were physically unfit, 1 was rejected, and 13 were successful. The number of vacancies in the Service was not published, but it is believed to have been very large.

For the Army Medical Department 63 candidates appeared in February, 18 of whom were rejected, and 45 passed. In August 63 candidates sent in their names, of whom 3 failed to appear or retired from the examination, 1 was rejected, 59 qualified, and 25 obtained appointments.

The Indian Medical Service has become more attractive again since the appearance, in December last year, of the Royal Warrant on the Service. In February 22 candidates passed the entrance examination for the Service, and the list contained the names of only 3 who were apparently natives of India. In August 29 candidates competed for 10 vacancies; 27 qualified, and no Indian-like name appeared in the list of the 10 who obtained appointments. There are, unfortunately, rumours of further changes in the Service, which are hardly likely to be popular.

The forty-ninth annual meeting of the British Medical Association was held in Ryde on August 9, and the three following days. Thus it followed immediately on the Congress, and men having had a surfeit of addresses, and professional discussions and work, it was wisely held in a charming seaside health-resort, within easy distance of London, and had more than usual the character of a pleasant social holiday, with enough of business to add a zest to play. But it was a very pleasant meeting, with good addresses, and the profession and the inhabitants of Ryde did their utmost to entertain and please their visitors. Mr. Benjamin Barrow, of Ryde, the Consulting Surgeon to the Royal Isle of Wight Infirmary, was President, and in that capacity delivered an interesting address on the habits of medical men, and on the manner in which, both in ancient and modern times, they have carried on their manifold duties. Three addresses-in-chief were given: the Address in Medicine by Dr. Syer Bristowe, the Address in Surgery by Mr. Jonathan Hutchinson, and the Address in Obstetric Medicine by Dr. Sinclair Coghill, of Ventnor, Interim Lecturer on Midwifery in the University of Edinburgh. Dr. Coghill's address was a scholarly and thoughtful discourse on "the claims, intrinsic and relative, of obstetric medicine to increased recognition and cultivation, and the directions in which its development should be encouraged"; and it was the only one of the three addresses that dealt exclusively and directly with the special work of the speakers. Dr. Bristowe took for his theme Hahnemann and the system founded and taught by him. He showed that homœopathy is still, in its most modern form, "a protest against the best traditions of orthodox medical science," and that all science is on the side of the regular medical practitioner; and then proceeded to argue in favour of our meeting homœopaths in consultation. And Mr. Hutchinson, who discoursed on surgical ethics, on medical education, and on the best means of advancing the clinical study of disease, also spoke in favour of meeting homœopaths. This character of two of the addresses formed the most remarkable feature of the meeting, and caused not a little excitement and discontent. No discussion or criticism of the addresses is allowed, but it was made clear that the feeling of the meeting was not with Dr. Bristowe and Mr. Hutchinson as regards their opinions about meeting homœopaths at the bedside; and their opinions have since been widely and freely discussed, and generally condemned. At the third general meeting of the Association the report of the Parliamentary Bills Committee gave rise to a very lively debate. The Committee recommended that in the next session of Parliament a Bill should be introduced on the part of the Association with the object of making the registration of infectious diseases compulsory, but not imposing the duty of notification upon the medical attendant directly. An amendment was proposed, that it should be an instruction to the Committee to support a Bill, introduced last session by Mr. George Hastings at the instance of the Social Science Association, which would impose the duty of notification directly upon the medical man; and this amendment gave rise to a warm discussion, ending in the defeat of the amendment by a very large majority. Professor Humphry, of Cambridge, proposed a resolution expressing the deep sense of the Association of the importance of vivisection to the advancement of medical science, and its belief that any further prohibition of it would be attended with serious injury to the community. In a very effective speech he met ably and skilfully all the arguments used against vivisection—so called—and fully justified the practice of it; and his resolution was carried with only a single dissentient voice. The meetings of the sections were fairly well attended, and some valuable papers were read. The fiftieth anniversary of the Association will very appropriately be held next year at Worcester, the birthplace and place of residence of Sir Charles Hastings, the founder of the Association; and Dr. Strange, of Worcester, is the President-elect.

The Social Science Congress met at Dublin, on October 3 under the presidency of Lord O'Hagan, and sat for eight days. We must refer our readers to the record of its proceedings contained in the second volume for the year. It was a successful and busy meeting, and many important papers were read and discussed.

The British Association for the Advancement of Science held its jubilee meeting at York, in September. The meeting was attended by 2500 members, and was universally considered a great success. Sir John Lubbock was the president, and had a congenial and by no means difficult task in painting the marvellous progress made by science in the last fifty years. The presidents of sections were all, we believe, selected from among the past presidents of the Association, there were many valuable and important papers and discussions, and great activity and earnestness in scientific work was apparent in every section. Dr. Burdon-Sanderson, President of the Section of Anatomy and Physiology, ably reviewed the discoveries of the past half-century in relation to Animal Motion. His address will be found at page 354 of our second volume. Mr. Huxley discussed the rise and progress of Palæontology, and pleaded for the scientific soundness and the great biological value of the outcome of the work of palæontologists. Dr. J. C. Ewart gave an account of a recent epidemic of fever in Aberdeen; showed that the milk with which the sufferers had been supplied, from one dairy, contained abundant micrococci, fungi spores, and spores similar to those of the bacillus anthracis; and gave an account of the cultivation of the bacillus and of the results of inoculation experiments with it. Professor Tyndall also discoursed upon the cultivation and development of bacteria. These minute organisms at present dominate the theories of a great part of the scientific and the quasi-scientific world.

Among the honours conferred on medical men during the year we can record only a few here. Her Majesty was graciously pleased to confer the honour of knighthood upon —Dr. Risdon Bennett, F.R.S., then President of the Royal College of Physicians of London, for his eminent services to the profession and the public; on Mr. William Mac Cormac, " in recognition of his long-continued, laborious, and eminently successful work in arranging and managing in all ways the International Medical Congress of 1881 "; on Mr. Erasmus Wilson, " in consideration of his munificent gifts for the support of hospitals and the encouragement of medical study"; and on Dr. George Birdwood, C.S.I., who was for very many years an especially active and valuable member of the Medical Service in the Indian Army, and for two years has been Special Assistant in the Revenue, Statistics, and Commerce Department of the India Office; and Dr. John Kirk, C.M.G., Her Majesty's Agent and Consul-General at Zanzibar, was promoted to the grade of a Knight Commander of the distinguished Order of which he was already a Companion.

The decoration of the Victoria Cross was bestowed upon Surgeon John Frederick M'Crea, 1st Regiment Cape Mounted Rifles, for conspicuous bravery in South Africa during a fight with the Basutos at Tweefontein (vol. ii., page 42); and on Surgeon-Major Edmund Baron Hartley, Cape Mounted Rifles, for conspicuous gallantry in attending the wounded under fire on June 5, 1879, in Basutoland (vol. ii., page 469).

Her Majesty also conferred the Albert Medal upon two medical men—Surgeon Henry Grier, of the Army Medical Department, and Dr. David Lawson, of Huddersfield—for gallantry in attempting to save life. In each instance the practitioner, at the risk of his own life, cleared by suction with his own lips the choked trachea of his patient, after the operation of tracheotomy for diphtheria. This act of unhesitating devotion has often—too often—been performed by members of the profession; and it is well that Her Majesty should recognise such acts of " conspicuous gallantry" when they are brought to her knowledge. For notice of the honours and other rewards bestowed—all too sparsely and grudgingly—upon military medical men during the year, we must refer the reader to our volumes.

This imperfect record of the medical year would be glaringly imperfect without some mention, however brief, of the deaths of two men, eminent rulers and statesmen, at the doors of whose sick-chambers the civilised world waited and listened, with absorbing interest and anxiety, for tidings of the struggle between life and death. The illness and death of each has had a very special interest for the medical profession. President Garfield was shot by an American named Guiteau on July 2, and, notwithstanding the extreme gravity of his wound, lived until September 20. The whole record of his illness, the treatment adopted by the able and well-known surgeons who attended him, and of the post-mortem examination, will be one of extreme interest, but that record has not yet been made known. Meanwhile, the surgical conduct of the case, while the outside knowledge of it is very imperfect, has been made the subject of hostile comment in the medical as well as the lay press of America—an example which happily has not been, and we trust never will be, followed in this country. The Earl of Beaconsfield died, after an illness of many weeks, on April 19. At the end of March the anxiety of the public began to be excited about Lord Beaconsfield's condition, and in a day or two later it was known that Her Majesty had expressed a wish he should have further medical advice than that of his usual attendant, Dr. Joseph Kidd. We need not remind our readers of all that happened before Her Majesty's desire could be complied with. All the matter is detailed in our pages for the month of April; but they will remember that it was commonly believed that Dr. Kidd

practised homœopathically; in fact, he had been well known as one of the legally qualified medical men who practised homœopathy; and hence the difficulty that arose when a scientific physician was asked to meet him. Dr. Quain, however, wrote to Dr. Kidd on this point, and received his assurance that he was not treating and never had treated his patient homœopathically, and his written promise that every wish and direction of Dr. Quain's should be carried out most faithfully. In brief, Dr. Kidd was ready to hand over the treatment and management of his patient to Dr. Quain. Under these circumstances, and supported by the advice of some of the best known and most trusted heads of the profession, Dr. Quain took charge of the patient. We held then, and hold still, that he was more than justified in so doing under the circumstances. It was not a case of consulting with a homœopath. But, not unnaturally, very different opinions were held on the matter. The whole question of the right conduct of the profession towards homœopaths was again brought up; and public and professional feeling and opinions on the subject were stirred further by an episode during the meeting of the British Medical Association. Nor is the question settled yet. An important and dignified contribution towards the settlement has, however, just lately been made by the London College of Physicians, and is recorded elsewhere in our columns.

We have had again, during the past year, to record the losses the profession has suffered, and again they have been heavy. The list contains the names of some who were known far and wide as teachers and leaders, and of men who worked well and worthily in narrower fields; of not a few who lived to a ripe old age, but of some who had hardly time to well begin their work. We do not pretend to give here anything like a full death-roll, but will only enumerate some representative names. Dr. H. H. Cruicknell died at the age of 50; Dr. Ed. Ferdinand Jencken, of Dublin, at 58; Mr. Nathaniel H. Clifton, at 62; Dr. Andrew Wood was 60 when he died; Dr. Peter David Handyside, of Edinburgh, was 72; Professor Rutherford Sanders, only 58; Mr. T. Wemyss Bogg, M.B., was 44; Dr. Robert Cryan, of Dublin, 54; Dr. Edmund Peele, of the same city, 48; Dr. John Day, of Geelong, died at the age of 64; Mr. C. Harriott Roper, of Exeter; Mr. William Hardwicke, the Coroner for Central Middlesex, at 64; Dr. Wilbraham Falconer, at 65; Mr. Heckstall Smith, of St. Mary Cray, at 74; Dr. Humphrey Sandwith, at 58; Dr. James Sherlock, of Worcester, at 53; Dr. Day, of Stafford; Mr. Donald Napier, at 50; Dr. Milner Barry, of Tunbridge Wells, at 66; Professor Rolleston, at 51; Mr. Stephen Alford, at 60; Mr. James Luke, at 83; Mr. H. Holman, of Hurstpierpoint, at 60; Dr. Archibald Billing, at 90; Dr. William Addison, adopted at 79; Mr. F. Symonds, of Oxford, at 68; Dr. Robert Smith, at 32; Dr. Joseph Brown, at 32; Dr. Alfred H. McClintock, at 60; Dr. Thomas Hayden; Dr. David Foulis, at 35; Dr. William Brewer; Dr. Denham, of South Shields, at 61; and Dr. E. A. H. Head, formerly of the London Hospital staff, at 53.

Not a few among those of our professional brethren of all grades who went over to the majority during the year attained to an age that may still be called remarkable, though, happily, not nearly so unusual now as thirty years ago. To give a few instances:—Dr. C. Fleming, of Dublin, Mr. Richard Freer, of Rugeley, Mr. John Merriman, and Mr. G. R. Hilliard, died at the age of 80; Mr. J. E. Stacey, at 81; Mr. Richard T. Gore, of Bath, at 82; Mr. Thornley Bond, of Stoke Newington, at 83; Dr. Abraham Toulmin, of Kensington, and Inspector-General of Army Hospitals Charles Whyte, at 85; Mr. Wm. Gwillim, of Burton-on-Trent, at 86; Dr. William Scott, of Edinburgh, and Dr. E. Shettle, of Reading, at 87; Mr. W. Knott, retired Army

Surgeon, Dr. J. J. Bigsby, F.R.S., of Jersey, and Dr. Thomas Radford, of Manchester, at 88; Dr. T. Michael Greenhow, of Leeds, at 89; Dr. R. C. Griffiths, of London, within three days of 90; and Dr. John Metge Bartley, formerly of the Army Medical Department, at 93. On the other hand, many, besides the few already mentioned, have died young—some of disease caught in the discharge of their duties at home; and not a few have died at their post abroad, with the sound of battle in their ears, as Surgeon-Major Cornish and Surgeon A. J. Landon; or in battle with pestilence, like young Mr. Rawdon Macnamara, of the Colonial Medical Service; or calmly facing danger and disaster on the ocean, as Dr. James Rose-Innes, who at the age of 26 was lost in the *Teuton*.

Among the eminent medical men on the Continent and in America who died during the year may be mentioned Max Perls, Professor of Pathology and Director of the Pathological Institute, Giessen, who died in the prime of life; M. Littré, who died' at the age of 80; Skoda; Professor Heschl, who succeeded Rokitansky as Professor of Pathological Anatomy at Vienna; Dr. Maurice Raynaud, Dr. Gustave Chantreuil, and Bouillaud, of Paris; Surgeon A. Otis, United States; Professor Spiegelberg, of Breslau; Professor Schutzenberger, who was for thirty-five years Professor of Clinical Medicine at Strasburg; Dr. Giovanni Cabiadis, of Constantinople; Wilhelm Busch, of Bonn; and Nicholas Pirogoff, of St. Petersburg.

As regards the contents of our volumes during the year, we note first the lectures contained in them. We were enabled to place before the profession, at full length, Sir Joseph Fayrer's valuable and learned "Lettsomian Lectures on Tropical Dysentery and Diarrhœa"; Dr. F. T. Roberts's "Clinical Lectures on Diseases of the Abdomen" were continued, five of them having been published in our pages this year, on the "General Etiology and Pathology" of Abdominal Diseases, a "Clinical Classification" of them, "The Clinical Investigation of Abdominal Cases," and "The Symptomatology" of these diseases; from Mr. Hutchinson we have published a clinical lecture "Introductory to the Study of the Arthritic Diathesis," a valuable and suggestive paper "On the Local Origin of Cancer" read many years ago at one of our medical societies, but never published, and a lecture on "Retinitis Hæmorrhagica, more especially in its Relations with Gout"; two clinical lectures by Mr. J. W. Hulke, "On a Punctured Wound of the Skull, Recovery," and "On a Case of Trephining for Anomalous Convulsive Attacks supervening Several Months after Injury to the Head"; a clinical lecture by Mr. Christopher Heath, on "The Treatment of Whitlow"; one by Dr. Handfield Jones, on "Four Cases of Pneumonia"; and lectures by Dr. J. R. Wolfe, of Glasgow, on "Formation of Artificial Pupil," and on "Glaucoma." We have also given a lecture by Dr. E. A. Sansom, "On the Causes and Significance of Reduplications of Sound of the Heart"; one by Dr. T. Stretch Dowse, "On Ataxia and the Pre-ataxic Stage of Locomotor Ataxy"; by Dr. W. H. Day, on the "Treatment of the Different Forms of Nervous and Neuralgic Headache"; and a lecture by Dr. W. Osler, of Montreal, on "Some of the Effects of the Chronic Impaction of Gall-stones in the Bile-passages, and on "The Fièvre Intermittente Hépatique of Professor Charcot." We have also had the pleasure of giving at length the Gulstonian, Croonian, and Lumleian lectures of the Royal College of Physicians, and the "Bradshawe Lecture" delivered by Dr. Vivian Poore; and some very able addresses delivered before various societies—as Mr. Lister's Presidential Address to the Clinical Society; Dr. Matthews Duncan's Presidential Address to the Obstetrical Society; Dr. J. Russell Reynolds' address on

"Specialism in Medicine"; Dr. J. W. S. Greenfield's inaugural address on "Pathology, Past and Present," delivered in the University of Edinburgh; Mr. Spence's inaugural address delivered in the Department of Surgery in the new buildings of the University of Edinburgh; Dr Tripe's presidential address on "The Sanitary Condition and Laws of Mediæval and Modern London," delivered before the Society of Medical Officers of Health; and Dr. George Buchanan's address on "Aids to Epidemiological Knowledge," delivered before the Epidemiological Society.

Many of the articles published as "Original Communications," and other papers, have treated of diseases or disorders of the nervous system: as—Dr. Hughlings-Jackson's remarkable communication, "On a Case of Temporary Left Hemiplegia, with Foot-Clonus and Exaggerated Knee-Phenomenon, after an Epileptiform Seizure beginning in the Left Foot"; an abstract of Professor Westphal's Address to the Medical Society of Berlin, stating the results of his enlarged experience and research as to the significance and the diagnostic value of the Knee-Phenomenon; Dr. P. McBride's paper on "The Etiology of Vertigo"; Dr. Saundby's communication on "Hysteria in the Male Sex"; an abstract of Professor von Stoffella's Address to the Medical Society of Vienna, on "Epilepsy and its Differential Diagnosis from Hystero-Epilepsy"; Dr. Octavius Sturges' article on "The Place in Nature of Functional Nervous Disease," and his "Note on Chorea of the Hand"; Dr. Hughlings-Jackson's address to the Ophthalmological Society on "Optic Neuritis in Intracranial Disease"; Dr. James Russell's "Cases of Acute Spinal Disease, in which Muscular Atrophy and Paresis were Prominent Symptoms," and his "Clinical Illustrations of Emotional Excitement as a Cause of Chorea." Dr. Dickson, the Physician to the British Embassy, Constantinople, enabled us to publish a summary of the report made on the "Outbreak of the Plague in Russia" by the late Dr. G. Cabiadis to the Constantinople Board of Health. Among other valuable and practical papers, we published a series of "Cases of Hydatid Disease of the Lungs," by Dr. J. Davies Thomas, of Adelaide; a case of "Ilio-cæcal Intussusception in an Infant, with Rapid Strangulation, and Death in Thirty-six Hours," by Dr. Judson Bury; an interesting paper on "Some New Uses of Old Remedies," by Dr. Colley March, of Rochdale; a paper from Mr. J. C. Cullingworth, of Manchester, on "A Case of Acute Atrophy of the Liver," and a very interesting "Account of the Successful Removal, thirty-eight years ago, of a Persistently Recurring Tumour of the Breast"; from Mr. Rickman Godlee, "A Case of Lupus treated by Scraping with Volkmann's Sharp Spoon"; Mr. E. L. Hussey's "Cases of Retention of Urine"; Mr. R. W. Parker's "Remarks on the Curvature of the Long Bones in Rickets"; Mr. Spencer Watson's papers on "A Case of Primary Chancre in the Nostril," and on "The Advantage of Opening the Capsule before making the Corneal Section in the Operation for Cataract"; Dr. J. Brassey Brierley's "On the Diagnosis and Treatment of Pleuritic Effusions"; one by Dr. R. H. Smith, of Cheltenham, "On the Pathology of Pneumokonioses"; by Dr. Joseph Ewart, "On Scrofula, Tuberculosis, and Phthisis in India"; papers by Surgeon-Major F. R. Hogg, M.D., on "Hooping Cough," and on the management of "Children in Hot Climates"; Mr. Henry Morris's paper on "Naso-Pharyngeal Polypi, and the Operations for their Removal"; and Dr. Morell Mackenzie's, "On the Use of the Œsophagoscope in Diseases of the Gullet." We also published a paper by Dr. Thomas Oliver, of Newcastle-on-Tyne, on "A Case of Aneurism of the Aorta, simulating Aneurism of Pulmonary Artery"; Dr. G. Ernest Herman's papers, "On Prolapse of the Ovaries," and on "A Case of Ascites of the Fœtus obstructing|Delivery"; Dr. Alexander's, of Liverpool, "Ovariotomies at Liverpool Workhouse," and "An Attempt to Cure Epilepsy by Ligature of the Carotid Arteries"; Surgeon-General C. R. Francis's "Note of a Case of Conception with Imperforate Hymen"; and Mr. Lawson Tait's "One Hundred and Ten Consecutive Cases of Abdominal Section" performed since November 1, 1880, and a "Case of Removal of the Uterine Appendages for the Arrest of Hæmorrhage due to a Myoma."; an article by Dr. W. H. Pearse, of Plymouth, on "Instances of the Evolution of Epidemics and the Alliances of some Diseases"; and remarks by Surgeon-General C. A. Gordon, C.B., "On certain Assigned Causes of Fever "; articles by Dr. Patrick Manson, of Amoy, on "Distoma Ringeri, a Human Parasite infecting the Lungs, discovered by Dr. Ringer, of Formosa," and on "Filaria Sanguinis Hominis"; one by Mr. Reginald Harrison, on "Acute Prostatitis"; and one by Mr. Henry Hoole, on "Acute Laryngitis in the Adult, Tracheotomy, Recovery"; Dr. Lewis Shapter's paper on "The Medicinal and Dietetic Uses of Citrate of Caffeine"; Dr. R. Norris Wolfenden's, "On Agaricus in the Treatment of Night-Sweats"; and Dr. William Murrell's, on "A Case of Poisoning by Resorcin." Papers by Dr. Stephen Mackenzie, Mr. Walter Rivington, and Dr. James Little, of Dublin, on cases of "Excessively High and Variable Temperature"; and by Mr. Chauncy Puzey's, of Liverpool, "Remarks on a Case of High Temperature, with Scarlatinoid Rash (Roseola), occurring after Excision of the Knee-joint"; a "Case of Treatment of Tetanus by Chloral," by Mr. John T. Faulkner, M.B., of Stratford, a paper by Mr. James C. de Castro, M.B., on "Disease of the Bronchial Glands"; Dr. R. Boyd's note on the "Comparison of the Weight of the Heart and other Viscera in the Sane and the Insane"; and Dr. George Harley's long, interesting, and original article concerning "Some New Facts conected with the Action of Germs in the Production of Human Diseases." And communications from Dr. J. W. Hunt, of Wolverhampton; Dr. C. V. Guisan, of Vevey; Dr. J. B. Hellier, of Leeds; Dr. E. Symes Thompson, Mr. Tom Bird, Dr. C. J. Thorowgood, Dr. Charles Bryce, Dr. Brinsley Nicholson, Mr. E. Thurston; and many other friends and contributors.

In another department of the journal, many papers, in full or in abstract, by distinguished medical men in America or on the Continent, have been placed before our readers; such as—by Professor Verneuil, on "The Inutility and Danger of Pharmaceutical and Topical Treatment of Surgical Epithelioma," and on "Steatosis of the Liver"; by Professor Billroth, "On Lithotripsy and Poisoning by Chlorate of Potash"; by Dr. Brown-Séquard, on "The Effects of the Local Application of Chloroform and Chloral"; by Professor Pasteur, on "Anthracoid Vaccination"; a Note of MM. Krishaber and Dieulafoy's communication to the Académie de Médecine, on Experiments on the Inoculation of Tubercle; and the conclusions arrived at after a careful and exhaustive review of recent investigations on that subject, by Dr. Whitney, Curator of the Warren Anatomical Museum, Boston; by Professor Benjamin Ball, of Paris, on "The Pathological Anatomy of General Paralysis"; Dr. Emil Noeggerath's "New Method of performing Ovariotomy," communicated to the Medical Society of New York; a paper by Dr. Pepper, of Philadelphia, on "The Treatment of Typhoid"; and lately (vol. ii., page 746), a resumé of Dr. Warfringe's work on "Typhus Fever in Stockholm "; papers by Dr. Lewis Smith, of New York, on "The Treatment of Pleurisy in Children "; and by Dr. W. S. Brown, of Boston, on "The Obstetrical and Gynæcological Employment of Chloral Hydrate." Also, we may mention, as of much interest, a note of the elaborate report made by Surgeon Sternberg, U.S.A., on the results of the investiga

tion made by him, at the request of the National Board of Health, on the "Bacillus Malariæ." Dr. Sternberg's inquiries tend to show that the observations of Tommasi-Crudeli and Klebs do not justify their conclusion that the bacillus malariæ is the special organism that gives rise to malarial fever; but Dr. Sternberg has not discovered anything to indicate that the bacillus malariæ, or some other of the minute organisms associated with it, is not the active agent in the causation of malarial fever in man.

Editorially, also, we have put before the profession Drs. Krause and Felsenreich's investigation on "The Atrophic Lines of the Abdomen in Pregnancy "; Professor König's article on "The Treatment of Empyema"; one by Dr. Max Runge on "Pregnancy and the Acute Infectious Fevers "; Drasche's, of Vienna, paper on "Temporary Aortic Insufficiency and Triple Aortic Sound"; one by Rosenstein, of Leiden, on "A Case of Purulent Pericarditis in a Boy of Ten Years, treated successfully by Incision and Drainage "; Török and Wittelshöfer's Statistics of Mammary Cancer, being the result of the analysis of 72,000 post-mortem examinations; the experience as to "Tracheotomy for Diphtheria in Children" from a report of the Bethany Hospital for Children; M. Parrot's article on "Desquamative Syphilis of the Tongue "; Heitler's paper on "Acute Miliary Tuberculosis "; Dr. Balding on the value of the aspirator in "The Diagnosis and Treatment of Hydatid Disease of the Liver "; Dr. Finlayson's very interesting account of "Diphtheria in Glasgow at the Beginning of the Nineteenth Century "; Dr. Seller's address to the Dresden Medical Society on "Ascites during Childhood "; an article by M. Vincent, of Lyons, on "Intra-peritoneal Wounds of the Bladder "; Professor Stoffella's article on "Fatty Heart, its Diagnosis, Pathology, and Treatment "; and Dr. Voigt on "Syphilis and Locomotor Ataxy."

Among the subjects of general public interest dealt with we may mention "Nervous Strain on Railway Pointsmen," "Preservation of Health in India," "The Economics of the Calcutta Hospitals," "Lunatic Asylum Casualties," "Small-pox Hospitals in London," "Vaccination and Small-pox," "The Sanitary Condition of the Roman Hotels," "Modern Sanitary Science," "The Contagious Diseases Acts," "The Sanitary Condition of the Isle of Wight," and "Sanitary Gains." We have spoken on "Colour-Blindness," on "Criminal Lunatics," on the "Monomania of Suspicion," on "Waiting for Trial," on "Work in the Treatment of Insanity," on "Medical Education" in America and in France, and on other like public matters.

Finally, we most cordially thank all our contributors for the assistance they have so kindly given us; and wish them, and all our friends and brethren, at home and abroad, a happy, peaceful, and prosperous New Year.

1882.

In addition to our record of the principal events of the year, the course of which has been so nearly run, we have a few words to say as to the provision made, as regards Lectures, for the pages of the Medical Times and Gazette in the coming year. We shall continue, with such regularity as we can command, Dr. F. T. Roberts' clinical lectures on Diseases of the Abdomen; and we shall begin with the new year a course of lectures on Diseases of the Skin, by Dr. McCall Anderson, Professor of Clinical Medicine in the University of Glasgow, and Physician to the Glasgow Western Infirmary, and Cutaneous Wards. We shall be enabled also to publish clinical or other lectures by Mr. Timothy Holmes, of St. George's Hospital; Dr. George Johnson, of King's College Hospital; Dr. O. Sturges, of the Westminster Hospital; Dr. J. F. Goodhart, of Guy's Hospital; Mr. Francis Mason, of St. Thomas's; Dr. John Williams, of University College Hospital; Dr. George Buchanan, Professor of Clinical Surgery in the University of Glasgow, and Surgeon to the Western Infirmary; Dr. Bryan Waller, Lecturer on Pathology in the Edinburgh School of Medicine; Dr. J. R. Wolfe, of Glasgow; Dr. T. Grainger Stewart, Professor of the Practice of Physic in the University of Edinburgh; Dr. James Russell, Senior Physician to the Birmingham General Hospital; Mr. J. Whitaker Hulke, of the Middlesex Hospital; Mr. Jonathan Hutchinson, of the London Hospital; and from some other well-known metropolitan and provincial teachers of medicine and surgery: while from several of these physicians and surgeons, and from many others, we have promises of Original Communications, and other practical and scientific papers. We shall publish contributions from Mr. Arthur Durham, Mr. John Croft, Dr. F. Warner, Dr. Stephen Mackenzie, Dr. Hughlings-Jackson, Mr. G. P. Field, Mr. W. Whitehead, of Manchester; Dr. K. Duncanson, of Edinburgh; Dr. Nunneley and Mr. H. C. Allbutt, of Leeds; Dr. T. Whipham, Dr. Edis, Dr. Norman Chevers, Dr. James Ross, and other known workers in the science and art of medicine. We have neither space nor need to give the names of all who have kindly undertaken to help us. Our readers will not require any further assurance that our pages will be richly and fruitfully supplied throughout the coming year.

IODOFORM.

WE were lately tempted to take down the volumes of Virchow's *Jahresbericht* for the last few years, in order to see for how long the medical papers had contained any account of the properties and virtues of iodoform. The drug is one that seems so comparatively lately to have occupied a prominent position in surgical practice, that we were prepared to find that, except quite recently, no notice had been taken of it by practical men. It is well known that it had for many years been looked upon rather as a chemical curiosity—" one of the innumerable compounds," to quote from " Miller's Chemistry," 1867, " which may be formed from the simple and compound ethers by the substitution of chlorine, bromine, and iodine for hydrogen," and which, " with one exception, which occurs in the case of chloroform, present but little to arrest the attention of the chemist." He adds that they have been minutely studied by Malaguti, Cahours, and Cloez, and refers the reader to the various papers by these authors in the *Annales de Chimie*. It was not altogether without surprise, therefore, that we found that as long ago as 1857 there appeared a paper by A. Maître in the *Annuaire de Thérap., par Bouchardat*, 1857, describing its therapeutic properties, the proportionally large amount of iodine that it contains as compared with the other iodine compounds commonly in use, its absence of irritating qualities, and its slow absorbability. It was administered by this authority in doses of five, fifty, and sixty centigrammes, and was given in cases of scrofula, rickets, endemic goitre, syphilis, etc., apparently in some cases with good result. Possibly, there may be still earlier accounts of its employment, but the *Jahresbericht* before this date has so unintelligible an index, that we felt indisposed to pursue our investigations further. The next then that we happened upon was a paper by E. Franchino, in the *Gazzetta Sarda*, 28, 1858, describing the anæsthetic effect of the drug when inhaled by small animals, such as fowls, pigeons, and rabbits, and hinting at the possibility of iodoform equalling, if not excelling, chloroform in this direction. This is a property which seems in later times to have been altogether lost sight of. In 1865 appeared a monograph by Eighini, in the *Ann. Univ. di Med.*, Milan, April, 1865,

which carries us still further back. This gentleman appears to have been experimenting, since the year 1846, on the therapeutical effect of the administration of iodoform, its appearance in the various secretions, and its physiological action. He gave as much as three grammes daily, apparently without any evil result, but acknowledged that from three to four grammes proved fatal to small animals. He seems to have employed it with a considerable amount of success in a variety of affections. He used it, as well, as an external application by means of ointment, baths, and plasters, and arrived at the happy conclusion, which later observers have unfortunately not confirmed, that from such applications no absorption of the drug need be feared. Between 1871 and 1876 numerous papers appeared by American authors, who seem to have adopted the use of iodoform as an application to venereal sores, for which, it is needless to say, it was found it of the greatest possible service; but it was also employed by them internally in a great variety of diseases, such as rheumatic and neuralgic affections, and other painful conditions, including painful menstruation; and externally for ulcers of the nose, pruritus, prurigo, etc. In 1875 McKendrick published a series of experiments on the manner in which it produces poisoning, in the *Edinburgh Medical Journal*, July, page 1, comparing its action with that of chloral and bromal. In 1878 appeared a notice of cases in which iodism, including acne, was produced by its administration; and in 1879 we find for the first time that medical literature begins to be flooded with communications upon the subject. Now also cases commenced to be reported, in which results were produced by its external application in large quantities. We have not space, and indeed it would be inexpedient, to enumerate all the articles which the volume for this year contains; suffice it to say that a number of affections of the eye and eyelids seem to have been benefited by its internal and external administration, both in Italy and America; but to two of them a special reference must be made. The first is by Binz (*Arch. f. exp. Path. u. Pharm.*, viii., 4.—5, s. 308, referring to one by Mœller, 8 Diss., Bonn, 1877); it describes the narcotic action of the drug upon cats and dogs, and the post-mortem appearances after they have succumbed to its administration. It seems that the animals all suffered from coma, as indeed has been the case with human beings who have absorbed too large a quantity. The principal post-mortem change was fatty degeneration of the viscera, which is attributed by these authors to the fact of free iodine being produced by the decomposition of the iodoform within the system, though they point out that it does not all become so decomposed, as the breath retains to a certain extent the characteristic smell. They refer to a case in which Busch gave a child ·02 grammes, and produced serious toxic effects. The other paper of importance is by Oberlander (*Deutsche Zeitschr. f. prakt. Med.*, 37, s. 433), describing two cases of iodoform poisoning. The first was a syphilitic patient, who in eighty days took 42·0 grammes, and was suddenly seized with giddiness, weakness of the legs, double vision, and two and a half days after the appearance of these symptoms, with vomiting, delirium, twitching of facial muscles, irregularity of breathing, and occasional apnœa. This patient, after recovering from these symptoms, was submitted to a second very cautious exhibition of the drug, when the same course of events began to make itself apparent. Another patient, after taking for seven days 6·0 grammes, had difficulty in walking, and drowsiness, and two days later complete coma; the dizziness and weakness remaining for some time after the coma had passed away. 1880 does not furnish very much that is new. There are further records of the poisonous effects upon the lower animals, with attempts at the theoretical explanation of the phenomena, which are not of much interest to the practical surgeon. The reader will gather from the foregoing observations how long it has taken to discover the wide practical application of this agent, although we have been, in degree, familiar with its virtues. We propose on another occasion to point out what these practical applications are, and to give a short account of the manner in which the drug is at present being very widely employed both here and on the Continent.

THE WEEK.

TOPICS OF THE DAY.

MR. T. HOLMES continues his earnest endeavours to bring about hospital reform. At a recent meeting of the Social Science Association he read a paper " On the Necessity of a Public Inquiry into our Hospital System," in the course of which he strongly advocated the advisability of applying to Government for a Royal Commission. He admitted that up to the present time such applications had been unsuccessful, but he felt convinced that Government will entertain the subject if once convinced that it is generally wished for. A Government inquiry, he said, would afford the public accurate information as to what the real functions of hospitals are, as to which undoubtedly much ignorance prevailed. In his opinion the teaching of medicine had become the most important function of voluntary hospitals. In the course of the discussion which followed, some opposition to Mr. Holmes's proposition was expressed, but that gentleman submitted that the objections raised to a Royal Commission were, after all, only imaginary. Finally a motion was carried, " recommending the Council to present a memorial to Government, praying that Her Majesty will issue a Commission to inquire into the administration of all hospitals; and further, that the Home Secretary be asked to receive a deputation."

At the annual general meeting of the constituents of the Metropolitan Hospital Sunday Fund, recently held at the Mansion House under the presidency of the Lord Mayor, the Committee were authorised to take out of the balance of the General Fund whatever sums might be necessary to cover the expenses which had been incurred over and above the sum for surgical appliances already voted. The Rev. Canon Spence moved an alteration in the laws constituting the Fund, of which he had previously given notice, so as to enable 4 per cent., instead of 2 per cent., to be paid out of next year's collection for the purchase of surgical appliances. He bore testimony from personal experience to the immense good effected by the regulation which enabled poor people requiring surgical aid to obtain immediate help, instead of begging from door to door for letters from subscribers, and expressed his belief that the proposed increase would have a large recoupment at the next Hospital Sunday. Cardinal Manning seconded the resolution, which was unanimously agreed to. Special donations were afterwards announced to provide surgical appliances until the Hospital Sunday collections in next year. June 11 was fixed for the Hospital Sunday collection of 1882, and the cordial co-operation of all ministers of religion in the metropolitan area was again invited. After the transaction of some purely formal business the meeting separated.

We recently published a short account of the ambulance accommodation provided in the large cities of the United States, which we suggested might be introduced into some of our leading towns. It is now announced that an ambulance waggon, built on very ingenious principles, has been presented to the London Hospital by Mr. J. H. Crossman. The vehicle has been constructed by Mr. J. Burt, of Swinton-

street, Gray's-inn-road, on the plans of Dr. Benjamin Howard, New York. It stands about 5 ft. 10 in. in height by 6 ft. 6 in. in width from the outside, and weighs about 6 cwt. The floor of the waggon is about fifteen inches from the ground, and a falling leaf is provided, which serves as a step; the patient, once laid on the stretcher, may be put in and taken out with the greatest ease, and without the infliction of any pain. This stretcher rests on a tramway with springs, independent of those of the waggon itself, and may, with its burden, be pulled forward and drawn back again with one hand. Jolting is guarded against by very easy springs on which the vehicle is hung, and by india-rubber tires with which the wheels are covered. Besides the stretcher already mentioned, there is room within the car for another, which can be suspended, and a seat within is provided for a surgeon or other person in charge of the patients. A box under the driver's seat is intended for the reception of medicines and surgical instruments. At a meeting of the Committee of the London Hospital to receive the ambulance, a resolution was carried for holding a conference at the rooms of the Society of Arts, with a view to the establishment of a general ambulance system for the metropolis.

A shocking instance of ignorance and incompetence was brought to light by the proceedings at an inquest recently held at Sheffield on a child aged eleven months. Her parents, when she became ill, procured the services of Thomas Garbutt, " medical botanist," under whose instructions they gave it five hot baths in one day, several doses of physic, bathed its head repeatedly with lotions, and finding it get worse, finally wrapped the child in blankets, and took it to Garbutt's premises at Attercliffe, two miles away. There the child was put into a Turkish bath, at a temperature of 120°; and it died whilst in the bath. Garbutt, who said he had no religious belief, declined to take the oath, and the Coroner refused to receive his evidence. In addressing the jury, the Coroner expressed his surprise that the medical profession did not prosecute these quacks. A verdict of congestion of the brain was recorded, but the jury added that the parents had acted very wrongly in taking the child out of the house, and that Garbutt's conduct in treating it was very reprehensible. The Coroner should know that anybody may practise medicine so long as he does not assume any title which implies that he is a legally qualified medical man. The medical profession have no power against the open quack.

A recent Government *Gazette*, published in Calcutta, contains a further minute of thanks to the officers connected with the Afghan war. After mentioning the services of certain civil officers in Scinde, and of Dr. Bellew and other political officers, it goes on to apologise for the previous omission of any allusion to the Medical Department. This, it says, arose from the fact that the late head of that department was included in the list of officers recommended by the Commander-in-Chief; but as the services rendered by both the Army and Indian Medical Departments, under Drs. Innes, Beatson, Crawford, and Cuningham, were valuable and conspicuous, they are now specially brought to the notice of Her Majesty's Government. A few words of thanks are also bestowed on the Survey, Clothing, Commissariat, and Transport Departments. It would be satisfactory to know who really is responsible for the omissions and "faint praise" invariably accorded to the non-combatant branches of the Army after any active operations. A General fitted for a high command should be above such petty jealousies as are indicated by endeavouring to reward only one branch of the service, when all have equally done their duty.

The Local Government Board have written to the Hackney Guardians on the case of a vagrant named Thomas Jones, who complained to the casual-ward-keeper that he was ill, and desired to see the workhouse doctor,—which was refused, the ward-keeper imagining that he was simulating illness; whereupon the man took his discharge, went to a neighbouring union, and was there found to be suffering from small-pox. The Local Government Board, in their letter, express their satisfaction that the Hackney Guardians have given implicit instructions that the attention of the medical officer of the workhouse should be drawn without delay to any vagrant who may desire to be seen by him.

THE ROYAL COLLEGE OF PHYSICIANS OF LONDON.

At a meeting of the Royal College of Physicians held on Tuesday this week, the following resolution was proposed by Dr. Wilks:—"The College considers it desirable to express its opinion that the assumption or acceptance by members of the profession of designations implying the adoption of special modes of treatment, is opposed to those principles of the freedom and dignity of the profession which should govern the relations of its members to each other and to the public. The College therefore expects that all its Fellows, Members, and Licentiates will uphold those principles by discountenancing those who trade upon such designations." Considering all the discussion that has been excited by the opinions expressed by two eminent members of the profession, at the meeting of the British Association at Ryde, in favour of the profession meeting homœopathic practitioners in consultation, and the utterances of the lay press on this subject during the year, we think the College amply justified in passing Dr. Wilks's admirably framed resolution. And if any justification was needed, it was amply supplied by the proposer and the speaker who supported him. There was, we believe, a rather lengthy discussion on the resolution. Dr. Wilks argued, we understand, that the question was not one of therapeutics, but of morals. That there is no doctrine of therapeutics, every man being at liberty to prescribe what drugs he likes, and in what doses he thinks best, or to prescribe no drugs at all. That the profession of any special doctrine of therapeutics, and the assumption of a special designation expressive of such a profession, is quackery; and this is what the homœopath has done and still does. He appeals to the public—advertises himself, as it were —as having other, special and superior, knowledge and skill in the treatment of disease than that possessed by the medical man pure and simple. This was contrary to good professional manner and morals; besides being without foundation in fact. Such, we believe, was his main argument. The resolution was supported with great force and ability by Dr. Wilson Fox. We should do grievous wrong to the science and art of medicine, and therefore wrong to the public, by meeting in consultation men who professed doctrine and practice that we entirely dissent from; such a consultation could not be productive of good to the patient, and must, in fact, be a farce—or rather, a false consultation —and therefore immoral. Sir William Gull, and several others of the Fellows, spoke, and there was a general agreement that the College ought to deliver some opinion on the subject in question, for the guidance of its Fellows, Members, and Licentiates, and of the profession at large, and for the instruction of the public. The opinions of the President are well known, but he stated them to the College strongly and clearly. He said the public have nothing to ask from us but that we shall do good to the patient; that is our object and aim, and that is the reason for consultations; but no good can possibly accrue to the patient from consultation with a true homœopath. And of course no man would knowingly meet a pretended homœopath. In short, Sir William Jenner, as others of the speakers, hold what was so well expressed by Sir Benjamin Brodie, whom we will once more quote:—"The object of a medical consultation is the good of the patient, and we cannot suppose that any such result can arise from the interchange of opinions, where the views entertained, or professed to be entertained, by one of the parties as to the nature and treatment of disease are wholly unintelligible to the other." In the end Dr. Wilks's resolution, with the addition, as a kind of preamble, of the following words at the commencement of it—"That while the College has no desire to fetter the opinions of its members in reference to any theories they may see fit to adopt in connexion with the practice of medicine, it nevertheless"—was agreed to without a single dissentient voice.

THE PARIS WEEKLY RETURN.

The number of deaths for the fiftieth week, terminating December 15, was 1040 (560 males and 480 females), and among these there were from typhoid fever 39, small-pox 9, measles 10, scarlatina 1, pertussis 9, diphtheria and croup 60, erysipelas 10, and puerperal infections 5. There were also 48 deaths from tubercular and acute meningitis, 42 from acute bronchitis, 74 from pneumonia, 77 from infantile athrepsia (38 of the infants having been wholly or partially suckled), and 33 violent deaths (24 males and 9 females). The numbers for the week are so nearly the same as those of the preceding week that there is little remark to be made beyond that there is some diminution in cases of typhoid, measles, scarlatina, and puerperal infections, and an increase in small-pox, pertussis, and diphtheria, this last numbering as many as 60 deaths. During the week there have been admitted into the hospitals 50 cases of typhoid, in place of 74 the week before; 26 cases of small-pox, instead of 30; and 37 cases of diphtheria, instead of 30. The births for the week amounted to 1150—viz., 583 males (428 legitimate and 155 illegitimate) and 567 females (389 legitimate and 178 illegitimate): 91 infants (45 males and 46 females) were born dead or died within twenty-four hours.

WOOL-SORTERS' DISEASE IN BRADFORD.

In his annual Report on the Health of the Borough of Bradford for the year 1880, Mr. Harris Butterfield, the Medical Officer of Health for the district, remarks that during that period several cases of disease, known in that locality as "wool-sorters' disease," have occurred, six of which proved fatal. Although, Mr. Butterfield observes, in Bradford and its neighbourhood the malady is peculiar to wool-sorters, yet the disease is not confined solely to them, but may affect all persons whose avocations bring them in contact with the tissues of animals infected with the complaint known as splenic fever or anthrax. Butchers, farm labourers, and workers in horsehair have contracted the disease, and it is probable that many hitherto unsuspected sources of infection exist. What is yet known of the disease as it occurs in the Bradford district is due, Mr. Butterfield continues, to the research and investigation of Dr. Bell. The Sanitary Committee of the town, assisted by delegates from the wool-sorters themselves, have drawn up a code of regulations to be observed in all factories where foreign wool is dealt with, and since the adoption of these rules no case of wool-sorters' disease has occurred in any of the establishments where they are in force. In addition to the precautions agreed to, some firms require the man who steeps the bales to wear a respirator and long gloves. It is still doubtful, Mr. Butterfield thinks, whether the hairs and wools admitted to be noxious are the only dangerous materials. Anthrax as an epizootic is not confined to the animals from which the admittedly dangerous hair is obtained, but is known occasionally to infect all animals. It is not because home and colonial sheep's wool is never infected that sorters engaged solely on this material do not contract wool-sorters' disease, but because the greasy nature of this description of wool prevents the germ-bearing particles from floating in the atmosphere.

THE "TRANSACTIONS" OF CONGRESS.

WE hear that the *Transactions* of the Congress are in an advanced state, and that they will be ready for distribution in a week or ten days' time. It is no secret that considerable pressure has been put on the secretaries of the various sections. Doubtless also the Executive Committee—as represented by the Hon. Secretary-General—have spared no efforts to get the work finished; it is highly creditable, but only in keeping with the excellent organisation of the whole Congress, that such a gigantic labour should have been carried out in such a short time. The *Transactions* of previous Congresses, though on a much smaller scale, have not been published under a year, at least, after the termination of the Congress. There will be four volumes. The first will contain the List of Members, Reports of the various Meetings, the Addresses-in-Chief, and the Proceedings of the Sections for Anatomy, Physiology, Pathology, and Materia Medica; and the Museum Report. Vol. II. will contain the Medicine, Military Medicine, and the Surgical Sections. Vol. III. will contain the Ophthalmology, Mental Diseases, Skin, Throat, Ear, and Teeth Sections. While in Vol. IV. will be included the Children's, Obstetrical, and State Medicine Sections. The papers will be published in their original language, while the discussions on them will all appear in English. Members of the Congress will each receive a copy of the *Transactions* free of all expense; to non-members the price will be 10s. 6d. per volume.

EPIDEMIOLOGICAL SOCIETY OF LONDON.

A MEETING of the Society will be held in the Council-room of University College, Gower-street, W.C., on Wednesday, January 4, at 8 p.m., when a paper will be read by Surgeon-General Joseph Ewart, M.D., entitled "Is the Climate of the Indian Hill Sanitaria beneficial in Scrofula, Tuberculosis, and Phthisis?"

"THE INDEX MEDICUS."

MR. LEYPOLDT, of New York, the enterprising publisher of this valuable work, who has made many sacrifices to keep it afloat while awaiting that adequate appreciation of the profession, both at home and abroad, which it should long since have received, has recently issued a circular to its subscribers. In this he declares his inability to carry it on longer unless insured from additional pecuniary loss by a guarantee fund of not less than $1000, applicable to the expenses of the volume for 1882. All those who are aware of the great service this "Index Medicus" is doing as the continuation of Dr. Billings' comprehensive, and almost exhaustive, "Catalogue-Index," must feel anxious that this appeal should be generously responded to; and we learn, with great pleasure, that the authorities of the Royal College of Surgeons of England have announced their intention of contributing $25 to this guarantee fund—a resolution which has given the greatest satisfaction in the quarter concerned, not only on account of the liberality of the procedure, but still more because of the effect which the example of so important a body is likely to produce.

FROM ABROAD.

TENDINOUS SYNOVITIS.

M. NICAISE, in a lecture delivered at the Hopital Laennec (*Gaz. des Hop.*, No. 115), relates the case of a postillion, fifty-seven years of age, who was admitted with a tendinous synovitis occupying the dorsal and palmar surfaces of the forearm—an affection which formerly, in the event of surgical interference, terminated fatally in the majority of cases; but the operation for which is now, thanks to the antiseptic method, one of the simplest. The man, who was strong and robust, had suffered from the affection for six years, this having commenced at the anterior surface of the thumb of the left hand. After increasing gradually in size, the tumour about eighteen months since disappeared, to gain the palm of the hand and forearm, and from there two bilobed swellings, the one in front and the other behind. Neither the skin nor the subcutaneous tissue had undergone any alteration. Very distinct fluctuation could be felt, and pressure gave rise to a crepitation which was very plain, and was continuous as long as the pressure was kept up. This was a case, then, of chronic tendinous synovitis with riziform granules, accompanied only with some difficulty in the movements of the fingers and wrist, and unattended by very severe pain. An interesting point to notice, as demonstrating the peculiar change in the tendons in this affection (and which has not hitherto been insisted on), is the loss of the movements of the thumb in consequence of the destruction of the flexor tendon. It was at the thumb the disease commenced six years ago. As to the nature of the affection, it cannot be confounded with a lipoma, which never is accompanied by crepitation, but which is absolutely characteristic of tendinous synovitis with riziform granules.

Prior to the antiseptic method, if in this kind of affection no surgical intervention took place, the disease made progress, the motions became more and more obstructed, the tendons underwent atrophy in their sheaths until they were completely destroyed, leading to the entire loss of all movements. If intervention were resorted to, several terminations might occur: the operation succeeded, but there was liability to relapse; or suppuration might follow the operation, and when it had ceased, and the synovitis was cured, then adhesion of the tendons to their sheaths had taken place, and there was more or less retraction and impotence of the fingers; or the suppuration might extend to the sheaths of all the tendons, to the palm, the forearm, arm, etc., developing diffuse phlegmons which rendered amputation of the arm necessary; or, finally, the suppuration might extend further still, giving rise to purulent infection, and ending fatally. This termination ensued in more than half of the cases, and that to such a point that some surgeons at last renounced all intervention in such cases, regarding this synovitis as a *noli me tangere*. So that, in fear of such a termination, they were reduced to the employment of treatment which was rather palliative than curative, such as obtaining the absorption of the liquid and granules by means of blisters and painting with iodine. Simple punctures were also tried, but they furnished very poor results, the contents of the sac being almost exclusively composed of a large quantity of small granules which would not pass through the canula. As to the curative treatment, it consisted in punctures and iodine injections, to which may be objected their inutility or their danger. Drainage has also been resorted to, after an incision at each extremity of the tumour, so as to obliterate the sac by suppuration. Simple incision itself was just as dangerous, and when total or partial extirpation was employed no better results were obtained.

" But having executed, thanks to Lister's dressing, several arthrotomies for various affections with success, I determined to act in the same manner in the present case, and I opened the tumour largely at the dorsal aspect of the forearm. On March 26, after having procured local anæsthesia by means of pulverised ether, I divided the skin, the slightly infiltrated cellular tissue, and the sheath of the tendons, hard and thickened to two millimetres, and gave issue to a flood of riziform granules, more or less agglutinated by a sparse, viscid, yellowish, and transparent liquid. After completely emptying the sac, I perceived on its smooth, regular, and highly vascular internal surface some small cysts appended by a little pedicle. I removed the whole with the forceps and scissors. One of the tendons had its fibres separated from each other by the riziform bodies. I washed out the interior of the tumour three successive times with a 20 per cent. carbolic solution. The operation was repeated on the palmar side, and exactly the same appearances were found. This double operation was rapidly performed under the carbolic spray, and was terminated by placing a very short and broad drain in each of the open cavities, and by Lister's dressing covered by a layer of wadding, applied so as to produce good elastic compression, and to maintain an equable temperature."

We need not pursue the details of the progress of the case, which ended by a cure on April 12. M. Nicaise goes on to observe that tendinous synovitis is an inflammation of the synovial sheath, and not, as has been erroneously stated, a cystic tumour. The sheath is always thickened, more or less regular, sometimes with small vegetations like polypi, at others with a smooth surface, and at others, again, having a granulated surface covered with fibrinous exudations, without vegetations. The state of the tendons has been but little investigated, but in the two cases that have come under M. Nicaise's care they seemed to have been wasted or destroyed. The small grains forming the contents in tendinous synovitis were considered by Velpeau as resulting from a fibrinous exudation from the synovial surface of the tendons becoming developed like foreign bodies in the joints ; and Virchow regards them as only small vegetations from the synovial sheath. In the first of the two cases which M. Nicaise has met with, the cavity was lined with a fibrinous, concrete, adherent exudation, removable in strata, and containing granules of various form, without any vegetation or excrescence. It was possible to observe the formation of these granules from the simple layer of exudation to the period when this became detached and rolled on itself by the movements of the tendons themselves, while others assumed the forms of more or less voluminous grains of rice. This case, therefore, would seem to confirm the opinion of Velpeau. But, in the present case, no fibrinous exudation was present, but vegetations or excrescences, in company with the riziform grains, and seeming to support the theory of Virchow. Histological and chemical investigation demonstrated the absence of conjunctive tissue in both cases. The present case is of especial interest, as it is the first time that a tendinous synovitis with riziform grains has been operated upon in France by largely opening the tumour and employing Lister's procedure.

GENERAL CORRESPONDENCE.

"A CURIOUS COINCIDENCE."

Letter from Mr. Oakley Coles.

[To the Editor of the Medical Times and Gazette.]

Sir,—The Medical Times and Gazette for November 19, page 606, contains the following statement, in a paragraph headed "A Curious Coincidence":—

"We should scarcely have cared to say anything on this subject had it not been for a total want of any reference to the work of Mr. Ramsay, from whose papers—read before the Odontological Society many years ago—some of the best illustrations are drawn."

Will you permit me to say that this statement as to the illustrations is not correct. There is not a single illustration in either the second edition of "Deformities of the Mouth" (published in 1870) or the third edition, published this year, drawn from any paper of Mr. Ramsay's, read before the Odontological Society.

In both these editions I have been careful to preserve the earlier prefaces, and to give full recognition to Mr. Ramsay's claims in the department of dental science of which the work treats.

I only saw the paragraph on Tuesday last, or I would have written sooner to correct the error in your issue of November 19.　　　I am, &c.,　　　Oakley Coles.
18, Wimpole-street, W., December 28.

A CORRECTION.

Letter from Mr. R. Harrison.

[To the Editor of the Medical Times and Gazette.]

Sir,—In your report of my paper on the enucleation of a prostatic tumour, at the Medical and Chirugical Society, in your issue of December 24, you state "one patient made a good recovery"—"one" should read "the." In both the instances recorded by me, where large tumours were removed from the prostate, the patients made complete recoveries. You will oblige me by inserting this correction.
　　　I am, &c.,　　　Reginald Harrison.

REPORTS OF SOCIETIES.

SOCIETY OF MEDICAL OFFICERS OF HEALTH.

Friday, December 16.

Dr. J. W. Tripe, President, in the Chair.

The minutes of the last meeting having been read and confirmed, the Council presented the following report, which was received and adopted :—" That the Society petition the Local Government Board to cause the reports of their medical inspectors on local outbreaks of disease to be printed in future as Parliamentary papers, or to be otherwise made available for those who may desire to purchase them."

A letter was read from Bury St. Edmunds, asking how near to a hospital for contagious diseases a dwelling-house might be built with safety to its occupants. It was resolved to reply that this question had been made the subject of investigation by two officers of the Local Government Board, who would be in a better position than the Society to answer such an inquiry.

The Royal Commission on Hospital Accommodation having made a verbal communication to the President that they would be glad to receive a report from the Society respecting the subjects of the better management of epidemics and the drafting of cases of small-pox and fever to neighbouring hospitals, the Council had drawn up a report, which, on being submitted to the Society for consideration, was somewhat modified, and then adopted.

The several questions which were submitted to the Royal Commission were considered and reported on seriatim.

Dr. Seaton proceeded to make some observations on "The constitution of a sanitary staff in large towns." His remarks were founded upon an unusual advertisement which had appeared in the papers for a medical officer of health in succession to the late Dr. Yeld, of Sunderland. The candidates were required by the terms of the advertisement to discharge the same duties as were undertaken by Dr. Yeld. Dr. Seaton pointed out the anomalous position occupied by this officer of health, seeing that in addition to his ordinary duties he had consented to act the part of "chief scavenger" (as Dr. Seaton called it) to the borough. This gentleman had placed under his immediate supervision eighty scavengers; he had further to make contracts for the supply of horse provender, and for the sale of manure. All such duties were, of course, totally foreign to those of a medical officer of health as they are generally understood. To make it more clear, Dr. Seaton enumerated the chief duties to which a medical officer of health in a large town is required to attend :—1. The general superintendence of hospitals for infectious diseases. In most provincial towns such hospitals are placed under his supervising care, and the patients are also, in some cases, under his treatment. 2. In some towns the officer of health has to attend at police-courts to prosecute defaulters against the Public Health Acts ; and this is often done creditably, but it is altogether foreign to his official duties. It might occur sometimes that he would be placed in the anomalous position of prosecutor, and then as a witness in the same case. In some towns the inspectors of nuisances are placed under the supervision of the medical officer of health. In towns having, say, 180,000 inhabitants or more, it is very important to have a man salaried at about £200 a year for superr intending the work of scavenging, and to have othe- officials under him. Besides this there should be a chief inspector of nuisances directly responsible to the local authority, and to undertake the legal prosecutions. It is hardly fair to expect a medical officer of health to undertake this. As regards the reporting upon dwelling-houses as fit for occupation and sanitarily perfect, every town has its competent surveyors, who should be employed for this purpose. Inspectors of meat and food are also distinct offices, which a medical officer of health has no right to interfere with except to supervise. The management of disinfecting stations, and certain clerking work, and the inspection of lodging-houses, should be undertaken by the respective officers reporting themselves to the local authority. There are certain duties under the Artisans' Dwellings Act, and the general management of epidemics, which devolve upon the medical officer of health. He has also important duties as an educator of public opinion. These, though not prescribed, are very important. Duties that do not require professional knowledge are not such as ought to be undertaken by a medical officer of health. From a public health point of view it is unwise for the medical officer of health to undertake work that he ought to be always criticising.

It was resolved to refer this question to the Council for consideration and report.

MEDICAL NEWS.

APPOINTMENTS.

Dickinson, T. Vincent, M.B. Lond., L.R.C.P.—Resident Obstetric Assistant to St. George's Hospital.

BIRTHS.

Barlow.—On December 25, at 10, Montagu-street, Russell-square, the wife of Thomas Barlow, M.D., F.R.C.P., of a son.

Brend.—On December 19, at 6, Argyll-road, Kensington, the wife of William Brend, M.R.C.S., of a daughter.

Blakiston.—On December 25, at Glastonbury, the wife of A. Alexander Blakiston, M.R.C.S., of a daughter.

Greathead.—On November 21, at Grahamstown, Cape of Good Hope, the wife of John Baldwin Greathead, M.B., of a son.

Wegg.—On December 23, at 15, Hertford-street, Mayfair, the wife of W. Wegg, M.D., of a son.

Walker.—On December 23, at 56, Ladbroke-grove-road, the wife of A. Dunbar Walker, M.D., of a son.

MARRIAGES.

Bruce—Connell.—On December 22, at Aberdeen, Alexander Bruce, M.A., M.B., to Annie Louisa, daughter of the late William Alexander Connell, H.E.I.C.S.

West—Frankland.—On December 22, at Reigate, Samuel West, M.B., of 15, Wimpole-street, Cavendish-square, to Margaret Nannie, daughter of Professor Frankland, D.C.L., F.R.S., of The Yews, Reigate.

DEATHS.

Bird, Henry, M.D., at Chelmsford, on December 17, in his 83rd year.

Cooper, Thomas Henry, M.R.C.P., Physician to the Great Western Railway, at The Limes, Slough, on December 25, aged 68.

Flower, Thomas, M.R.C.S., youngest son of Isaac Flower, M.R.C.S., of Codford St. Peter, Wilts, on December 19, aged 36.

Griffin, R. W. Waudby, M.D., at 11, East Park-terrace, Southampton, on December 24, aged 45.

Oldham, James, F.R.C.S., at Lucastes, Hayward's Heath, on December 26, aged 64.

Wotton, Charles, M.D., at King's Langley, Herts, on December 20, aged 44.

VACANCIES.

In the following list the nature of the office vacant, the qualifications required in the candidate, the person to whom application should be made and the day of election (as far as known) are stated in succession.

Huddersfield Infirmary.—Senior House-Surgeon and a Junior House Surgeon. Candidates for the former must be doubly qualified, and for the latter they must possess, at least, one registered qualification. Applications and testimonials to be sent to Fredk. Eastwood, Hon. Secretary, not later than January 21, 1882.

Leeds Amalgamated Friendly Societies' Medical Aid Association.—Two Medical Officers. Candidates must be duly qualified and registered. Applications, stating age, whether single or married, with not more than four testimonials of recent date, to be sent to G. Hackett, 3, Artillery-terrace, Roundhay-road, Leeds, on or before January 3, 1882.

Lincoln County Hospital.—House-Surgeon. Candidates must be members of the Royal College of Surgeons of England, Edinburgh, or Dublin, and Licentiates of the Apothecaries' Company, or of one of the Royal Colleges of Physicians; graduates in medicine of one of the Universities of Great Britain or Ireland; duly registered under the Medical Act; under forty years of age, and unmarried. Testimonials as to qualifications and character to be sent to J. W. Danby, Secretary (from whom further particulars may be obtained), on or before January 16, 1882.

National Dental Hospital, 149, Great Portland-street, W.—Dental Surgeon. Candidates must be Licentiates of Dental Surgery. Applications and testimonials to be sent to Arthur G. Klugh, Secretary, on or before January 10, 1882.

North Ormesby Cottage Hospital, Middlesborough.—House-Surgeon. (*For particulars see Advertisement.*)

Nottingham County Lunatic Asylum, Sneinton.—Assistant Medical Officer. Candidates must be registered under the Medical Act, unmarried, and able to produce testimonials of good moral character. Applications, stating age, with testimonials, to be addressed to the Chairman of the Committee of Visitors, under cover to Samuel Bunting, Clerk, on or before January 5, 1882.

Owens College, Manchester.—Demonstrator and Assistant-Lecturer in Physiology. Particulars may be obtained of J. Holme Nicholson, Registrar, to whom applications and testimonials are to be sent up to January 7, 1882.

Queen's Hospital, Birmingham.—Non-Resident Physician for Out-patients. Candidates must be graduates in medicine of a British or Irish University. Copies of the regulations, etc., can be obtained from the General Superintendent, to whom applications, with testimonials, must be sent on or before January 3, 1882.

Royal College of Surgeons in Ireland.—Professor of Practical and Descriptive Anatomy. (*For particulars see Advertisement.*)

UNION AND PAROCHIAL MEDICAL SERVICE.

⁂ The area of each district is stated in acres. The population is computed according to the census of 1871.

RESIGNATIONS.

Frome Union.—Mr. Joseph Henry Benson has resigned the Road District: area 11,199; population 3392; salary £90 5s. per annum.

APPOINTMENTS.

Ashby-de-la-Zouch Union.—Charles Robert Williams, M.B. and M.C. Edin., to the Second District.

Chester Union.—George Harrison, L.R.C.P. Edin., L.R.C.S. Edin., to the Workhouse and the City District.

Lincoln Union.—Charles G. Dalton, M.R.C.S. Eng., L.S.A., to the Second and Eleventh Districts.

APPOINTMENTS FOR THE WEEK.

December 31. *Saturday (this day).*

Operations at St. Bartholomew's, 1½ p.m.; King's College, 1½ p.m.; Royal Free, 2 p.m.; Royal London Ophthalmic, 11 a.m.; Royal Westminster Ophthalmic, 1½ p.m.; St. Thomas's, 1½ p.m.; London, 2 p.m.

Royal Institution, 3 p.m. Professor R. S. Ball, "Mercury, Venus, and Mars."

January 2, 1882. *Monday.*

Operations at the Metropolitan Free, 2 p.m.; St. Mark's Hospital for Diseases of the Rectum, 2 p.m.; Royal London Ophthalmic, 11 a.m.; Royal Westminster Ophthalmic, 1½ p.m.

3. *Tuesday.*

Operations at Guy's, 1½ p.m.; Westminster, 2 p.m.; Royal London Ophthalmic, 11 a.m.; Royal Westminster Ophthalmic, 1½ p.m.; West London, 3 p.m.

Royal Institution, 3 p.m. Professor R. S. Ball, "Jupiter, Saturn, Uranus, Neptune."

Pathological Society, 8½ p.m. Annual General Meeting. Specimens: Dr. Stephen Mackenzie—Annular Stricture of Intestine. Dr. Fowler—Intestinal Obstruction. Mr. Butlin—(1) Squamous Epithelioma of Upper Jaw; (2) Mixed-celled Sarcoma of Phalanx of Thumb. Mr. James Startin—(1) Xanthelasma; 2. Morphoea Alba. Dr. Carrington—Hour-Glass Contraction of the Stomach. Mr. W. H. Kesteven—Disease of the Stomach. Dr. Zamarol (of Alexandria)—Bilharzia Hæmatobia *in situ*. Election of Officers and Annual Report of the Council.

4. *Wednesday.*

Operations at University College, 2 p.m.; St. Mary's, 1¼ p.m.; Middlesex, 1 p.m.; London, 2 p.m.; St. Bartholomew's, 1½ p.m.; Great Northern, 2 p.m.; Samaritan, 2½ p.m.; Royal London Ophthalmic, 11 a.m.; Royal Westminster Ophthalmic, 1½ p.m.; St. Thomas's, 1½ p.m.; St. Peter's Hospital for Stone, 2 p.m.; National Orthopædic, Great Portland-street, 10 a.m.

Epidemiological Society (Council Meeting, 7½ p.m.), 8 p.m. Surgeon-General Joseph Ewart, M.D., "Is the Climate of the Indian Hill Sanitaria Beneficial in Scrofula, Tuberculosis, and Phthisis?"

5. *Thursday.*

Operations at St. George's, 1 p.m.; Central London Ophthalmic, 1 p.m.; Royal Orthopædic, 2 p.m.; University College, 2 p.m.; Royal London Ophthalmic, 11 a.m.; Royal Westminster Ophthalmic, 1½ p.m.; Hospital for Diseases of the Throat, 2 p.m.; Hospital for Women, 2 p.m.; Charing-cross, 2 p.m.; London, 2 p.m.; North-West London, 2½ p.m.

Royal Institution, 3 p.m. Professor R. S. Ball, "The Solar System further considered."

Harveian Society, 8½ p.m. Mr. Field, "On Cases of Removal of Osseous Tumours from the Auditory Canal." Mr. Knowsley Thornton, "On Encysted Purulent Peritonitis, with Cases."

6. *Friday.*

Operations at Central London Ophthalmic, 2 p.m.; Royal London Ophthalmic, 11 a.m.; South London Ophthalmic, 2 p.m.; Royal Westminster Ophthalmic, 1½ p.m.; St. George's (ophthalmic operations), 1¼ p.m.; Guy's, 1½ p.m.; St. Thomas's (ophthalmic operations), 2 p.m.; King's College (by Mr. Lister), 2 p.m.

NOTES, QUERIES, AND REPLIES:

Ye that questioneth much shall learn much.—Bacon.

Jacksonian Prize.—This day (Saturday) is the last day for sending in the essays, only two of which have as yet been received.

A. Hearn B.—The clerical part of the registrar's duty is checked by the inspectors, the superintendents, and by the Central Record Department. The Bank of England refuses to accept the death-certificate as a proof of death.

Forewarned.—The Local Government Board has just inquired what steps the Town Council of Stamford had taken to provide a small-pox hospital. It appeared, at a meeting of the Council, that nothing had been done, and notwithstanding the letter of the Central Authority, the consideration of the question was deferred, the ex-Mayor observing, however, that if the Corporation did not build a hospital, which it had been estimated would cost £800, the Local Government Board would compel them to do so, and at, probably, a much heavier expenditure.

G. G., Paddington.—A new edition of the Handbook of the Soane Museum, Lincoln's-inn-fields, is in preparation by Mr. Wild, the curator.

Guy's Hospital Jury Accommodation.—A few days since, on Mr. Payne, the Coroner, taking his seat in the inquest-room at this Hospital, the jury complained that there was neither fire nor fireplace, and that the room, in consequence, was so cold that they were all fearing serious results from having to sit in it for some length of time, and they appealed to him to do something to remedy the discomforts under which they assembled in that room. The Coroner, in reply, stated that the room was used for out-patients as well as for coroners' inquiries, and he thought the attention of the Hospital authorities ought to be drawn to it. After some discussion, Mr. Payne undertook to see the medical superintendent on the matter.

Public Hygiene.—Sir James Fitzjames Stephens' maxim was, " If the object aimed at is good, if the compulsion employed is such as to attain it, and if the good obtained overbalances the inconvenience of the compulsion itself, then the compulsion is good."

Alleged Death from Vaccination.—At Manchester, the city Coroner, Mr. Herford, has held an inquest on the body of a child, ten weeks old, which was vaccinated about a month ago at Birmingham, and appeared to go on well until the 7th inst., when a redness about the arm and shoulders became apparent. It was then taken to Dr. Sutherland, of Manchester, and died on the 18th inst. The father deposed that, at Birmingham, he objected to the child being vaccinated at all, but was told that it must be done. Four years ago another child of his, three months old, was vaccinated at Birmingham, and died within five weeks afterwards. The foreman of the jury stated that, sixteen years ago, he lost a child through vaccination, and the operation, in his case, was performed against his will. Dr. James Sutherland stated that the child was brought to him on the 7th inst. There were five distinct vaccination-marks on its arm. Erysipelas had then begun, and was extending. The jury returned a verdict to the effect that death had resulted from erysipelas caused by vaccination—an illogical verdict, but that was probably not the fault of the jury.

COMMUNICATIONS have been received from—

The Registrar of the Apothecaries' Hall, London; Dr. J. W. Moore, Dublin; The Editor of the "British Medical Journal," London; The Secretary of the Hunterian Society of London; The Secretary of the Epidemiological Society of London; The Secretary of the Harveian Society of London; Dr. Radcliffe Crocker, London; The Sanitary Commissioner, Punjab, India; Dr. Robert C. Smith, Ardwick, Manchester; Dr. Frederick Churchill, London; Mr. E. W. Parker, London; The Secretary of the Royal Institution, London; Mr. Reginald Harrison, Liverpool; The Secretary of the Obstetrical Society of London; The Secretary of the University of London; Dr. E. F. Willcoughby, London; The Registrar of the Royal College of Physicians of London; Mr. J. Chatto, London; The Honorary Secretary of the Pathological Society of London.

BOOKS, ETC., RECEIVED—

Treatment of Varicocele, by M. H. Henry, M.A., M.D.—The Propagation of Disease, etc., by R. F. B. Taaffe, M.D.—Malaria, by Deputy Surgeon-General W. J. Moore—The Opium Question, by Deputy Surgeon-General W. J. Moore.

PERIODICALS AND NEWSPAPERS RECEIVED.—

Lancet—British Medical Journal—Medical Press and Circular—Berliner Klinische Wochenschrift—Centralblatt für Chirurgie—Gazette des Hôpitaux—Gazette Médicale—Le Progrès Médical—Bulletin de l'Académie de Médecine—Pharmaceutical Journal—Wiener Medizinische Wochenschrift—Centralblatt für die Medizinischen Wissenschaften—Revue Médicale—Gazette Hebdomadaire—National Board of Health Bulletin, Washington—Nature—Boston Medical and Surgical Journal—Louisville Medical News—Deutsche Medicinal-Zeitung—Revue de Médecine—Gazetta degli Ospitali—Detroit Lancet—Sussex Daily News, December 22—Revue de Chirurgie—Night and Day—Chicago Medical Review—Martin's Chemists and Druggist's Bulletin—Musik-Welt—Antiquarian Magazine, etc.—Centralblatt für Gynäkologie—Philadelphia Medical Times—Deutsche Medicinische Wochenschrift—Leisure Hour—Colonist, December 3—Friendly Greetings—Girl's Own Paper—Boy's Own Paper—Sunday at Home—Unão Medica—Dublin Journal of Medical Science—Brighton Guardian, December 23.

VITAL STATISTICS OF LONDON.

Week ending Saturday, December 24, 1881.

BIRTHS.

Births of Boys, 1273; Girls, 1244; Total, 3457.
Corrected weekly average in the 10 years 1871-80, 2502·7.

DEATHS.

	Males.	Females.	Total.
Deaths during the week	793	862	1655
Weekly average of the ten years 1871-80, corrected to increased population	963·5	963·1	1926·6
Deaths of people aged 80 and upwards	...	...	53

DEATHS IN SUB-DISTRICTS FROM EPIDEMICS.

	Population, 1881 (unverified).	Small-pox.	Measles.	Scarlet Fever.	Diphtheria.	Whooping-cough.	Typhus.	Enteric (or Typhoid) Fever.	Simple continued Fever.	Diarrhœa.
West ...	669988	...	14	1	15	1	6	...	2
North ...	905877	...	15	11	5	13	...	9	...	3
Central ...	282178	...	8	1	7	3	11	...	2	...
East ...	692530	3	4	7	7	32	...	4	...	2
South ...	1265578	20	32	15	4	26	...	12	...	4
Total ...	3814571	23	73	35	19	96	3	33	...	11

METEOROLOGY.

From Observations at the Greenwich Observatory.

Mean height of barometer	29·636 in.
Mean temperature	36·6°
Highest point of thermometer	53·4°
Lowest point of thermometer	21·6°
Mean dew-point temperature	31·9°
General direction of wind	W.S.W.
Whole amount of rain in the week	0·69 in.

BIRTHS and DEATHS Registered and METEOROLOGY during the Week ending Saturday, Dec. 24, in the following large Towns:—

Cities and boroughs (Municipal boundaries except for London.)	Estimated Population to middle of the year 1881.[*]	Persons to an Acre. (1881.)	Births Registered during the week ending Dec. 24.	Deaths Registered during the week ending Dec. 24.	Temperature of Air (Fahr.) Highest during the Week.	Temperature of Air (Fahr.) Lowest during the Week.	Temperature of Air (Fahr.) Weekly Mean of Daily Values.	Temp. of Air (Cent.) Weekly Mean of Daily Mean Values.	Rain Fall. In Inches.	Rain Fall. In Centimetres.
London ...	3829751	50·8	2467	1655	53·4	21·6	36·6	2·67	0·69	1·75
Brighton ...	107934	45·9	77	44	51·6	30·0	38·8	3·78	0·38	0·97
Portsmouth ...	128335	28·6	85	52	...	...	...	...	...	...
Norwich ...	88038	11·8	56	32	...	...	...	...	...	...
Plymouth ...	75292	54·0	31	41	54·2	30·0	41·1	5·08	1·02	2·59
Bristol ...	207140	46·5	114	91	45·6	21·5	36·9	2·72	1·92	4·88
Wolverhampton ...	75934	22·4	48	31	44·3	20·4	34·0	1·11	0·53	1·35
Birmingham ...	402296	47·9	282	188	...	...	...	...	...	...
Leicester ...	123120	38·5	93	69	43·2	22·0	34·2	1·92	0·97	2·46
Nottingham ...	188235	18·9	137	84	43·6	21·9	35·1	1·73	1·17	2·97
Liverpool ...	553988	106·3	359	324	38·9	24·3	35·1	3·12	1·11	2·82
Manchester ...	341266	79·5	205	188	...	...	...	...	...	...
Salford ...	177760	34·4	109	57	...	...	...	...	...	...
Oldham ...	112176	24·0	67	55	...	...	...	...	...	...
Bradford ...	184057	25·8	97	87	42·0	26·4	35·6	2·01	0·70	1·78
Leeds ...	310490	14·4	216	184	44·0	25·0	36·4	2·44	1·06	2·69
Sheffield ...	285621	14·5	186	116	43·0	21·0	35·7	2·06	1·21	3·07
Hull ...	155161	43·7	98	91	41·0	24·0	33·6	0·90	0·44	1·12
Sunderland ...	116758	42·2	99	42	...	...	...	...	...	...
Newcastle-on-Tyne	145675	27·1	103	44	...	...	...	...	...	...
Total of 20 large English Towns ...	7636675	38·0	4936	3512	54·2	20·4	36·3	2·39	0·93	2·36

* These figures are the numbers enumerated (but subject to revision) in April last, raised to the middle of 1881 by the addition of a quarter of a year's increase, calculated at the rate that prevailed between 1871 and 1881.

At the Royal Observatory, Greenwich, the mean reading of the barometer last week was 29·63 in. The lowest reading was 28·57 in. on Sunday morning, and the highest 30·37 in. on Friday evening.

INDEX.

END OF VOLUME II. 1881.

Lightning Source UK Ltd.
Milton Keynes UK
UKHW021304221118
332685UK00010B/1895/P